Use these tabs to mark secti important pages in your *CPT* *Edition* codebook for quick ref

MW00843875

E/M	RAD
ANES	APP A-B
PA/LAB	APP C-F
SURG	URIN
INTEG	M/GEN
MUSC	F/GEN
RESP	NERV
CARD	OC/AUD
DIGES	MED

CAT II	CAT III
APP G-J	INDEX
APP K-P	APP Q-T
VACC	ALLERG
PSYCH	NEURO
DIALY	HEALTH BEHAV
OPHTH	ENDO
ENDO	
PULM	GASTRO

Customize your *CPT® 2025 Professional* codebook and make it work for you.

These removable and reusable tabs can be used to flag the code sections and codes that you refer to regularly.

- Use the printed tabs to flag the section openers of each section.
- Use the **red** tabs to flag key pages in Evaluation and Management, Radiology, Category II and Category III.
- Use the **blue** tabs to flag key pages in Anesthesia, Pathology and Laboratory, Appendixes, and Index.
- Use the **green** tabs to flag key pages in the Surgery and Medicine.
- Use the **yellow** tabs to flag codes that you commonly use in your practice, codes that you need to research further, or personal notes that you've written into your codebook.

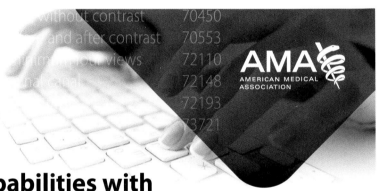

Elevate your coding capabilities with the CPT® Advanced Coding Pack from the authority on the CPT code set.

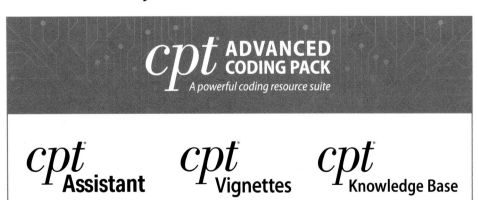

Learn more

Place-of-Service Codes for Professional Claims

Listed below are place-of-service codes and descriptions. These codes should be used on professional claims to specify the entity where service(s) were rendered. Check with individual payers (eg, Medicare, Medicaid, other private insurance) for reimbursement policies regarding these codes. If you would like to comment on a code(s) or description(s), please send your request to posrequest@cms.hhs.gov.

Place of Service Code(s)	Place of Service Name	Place of Service Description
01	Pharmacy	A facility or location where drugs and other medically related items and services are sold, dispensed, or otherwise provided directly to patients. (Effective 10/1/03)
02	Telehealth Provided Other than in Patient's Home	The location where health services and health related services are provided or received, through telecommunication technology. Patient is not located in their home when receiving health services or health-related services through telecommunication technology. (Effective 1/1/17)
03	School	A facility whose primary purpose is education. (Effective 1/1/03)
04	Homeless Shelter	A facility or location whose primary purpose is to provide temporary housing to homeless individuals (eg, emergency shelters, individual or family shelters). (Effective 1/1/03)
05	Indian Health Service Free-Standing Facility	A facility or location, owned and operated by the Indian Health Service, which provides diagnostic, therapeutic (surgical and non-surgical), and rehabilitation services to American Indians and Alaska Natives who do not require hospitalization. (Effective 1/1/03)
06	Indian Health Service Provider-Based Facility	A facility or location, owned and operated by the Indian Health Service, which provides diagnostic, therapeutic (surgical and non-surgical), and rehabilitation services rendered by, or under the supervision of, physicians to American Indians and Alaska Natives admitted as inpatients or outpatients. (Effective 1/1/03)
07	Tribal 638 Free-Standing Facility	A facility or location owned and operated by a federally recognized American Indian or Alaska Native tribe or tribal organization under a 638 agreement, which provides diagnostic, therapeutic (surgical and non-surgical), and rehabilitation services to tribal members who do not require hospitalization. (Effective 1/1/03)
08	Tribal 638 Provider-Based Facility	A facility or location owned and operated by a federally recognized American Indian or Alaska Native tribe or tribal organization under a 638 agreement, which provides diagnostic, therapeutic (surgical and non-surgical), and rehabilitation services to tribal members admitted as inpatients or outpatients. (Effective 1/1/03)
09	Prison/Correctional Facility	A prison, jail, reformatory, work farm, detention center, or any other similar facility maintained by either Federal, State, or local authorities for the purpose of confinement or rehabilitation of adult or juvenile criminal offenders. (Effective 7/1/06)
10	Telehealth Provided in Patient's Home	The location where health services and health related services are provided or received, through telecommunication technology. Patient is located in their home (which is a location other than a hospital or other facility where the patient receives care in a private residence) when receiving health services or health related services through telecommunication technology. (Effective 1/1/22)
11	Office	Location, other than a hospital, skilled nursing facility (SNF), military treatment facility, community health center, State or local public health clinic, or intermediate care facility (ICF), where the health professional routinely provides health examinations, diagnosis, and treatment of illness or injury on an ambulatory basis.
12	Home	Location, other than a hospital or other facility, where the patient receives care in a private residence.
13	Assisted Living Facility	Congregate residential facility with self-contained living units providing assessment of each resident's needs and on-site support 24 hours a day, 7 days a week, with the capacity to deliver or arrange for services including some health care and other services. (Effective 10/1/03)
14	Group Home	A residence, with shared living areas, where clients receive supervision and other services such as social and/or behavioral services, custodial service, and minimal services (eg, medication administration). (Effective 10/1/03)
15	Mobile Unit	A facility/unit that moves from place-to-place equipped to provide preventive, screening, diagnostic, and/or treatment services. (Effective 1/1/03)
16	Temporary Lodging	A short term accommodation such as a hotel, camp ground, hostel, cruise ship or resort where the patient receives care, and which is not identified by any other POS code. (Effective 1/1/08)
17	Walk-in Retail Health Clinic	A walk-in health clinic, other than an office, urgent care facility, pharmacy, or independent clinic, and not described by any other Place of Service code, that is located within a retail operation and provides, on an ambulatory basis, preventive and primary care services. (Effective 5/1/10)
18	Place of Employment/Worksite	A location, not described by any other POS code, owned or operated by a public or private entity where the patient is employed, and where a health professional provides on-going or episodic occupational medical, therapeutic or rehabilitative services to the individual. (This code is available for use effective January 1, 2013 but no later than May 1, 2013.)
19	Off Campus—Outpatient Hospital	A portion of an off-campus hospital provider based department which provides diagnostic, therapeutic (both surgical and nonsurgical), and rehabilitation services to sick or injured persons who do not require hospitalization or institutionalization. (Effective January 1, 2016)
20	Urgent Care Facility	Location, distinct from a hospital emergency room, an office, or a clinic, whose purpose is to diagnose and treat illness or injury for unscheduled, ambulatory patients seeking immediate medical attention. (Effective 1/1/03)
21	Inpatient Hospital	A facility, other than psychiatric, which primarily provides diagnostic, therapeutic (both surgical and non-surgical), and rehabilitation services by, or under, the supervision of physicians to patients admitted for a variety of medical conditions.
22	On Campus—Outpatient Hospital	A portion of a hospital's main campus which provides diagnostic, therapeutic (both surgical and non-surgical), and rehabilitation services to sick or injured persons who do not require hospitalization or institutionalization. (Description change effective January 1, 2016)
23	Emergency Room—Hospital	A portion of a hospital where emergency diagnosis and treatment of illness or injury is provided.
24	Ambulatory Surgical Center	A free-standing facility, other than a physician's office, where surgical and diagnostic services are provided on an ambulatory basis.
25	Birthing Center	A facility, other than a hospital's maternity facilities or a physician's office, which provides a setting for labor, delivery, and immediate postpartum care as well as immediate care of newborn infants.
26	Military Treatment Facility	A medical facility operated by one or more of the Uniformed Services. Military Treatment Facility (MTF) also refers to certain former U.S. Public Health Service (USPHS) facilities now designated as Uniformed Service Treatment Facilities (USTF).

27	Outreach Site/Street	A non-permanent location on the street or found environment, not described by any other POS code, where health professionals provide preventive, screening, diagnostic, and/or treatment services to unsheltered homeless individuals. (Effective October 1, 2023)
28-30	Unassigned	N/A
31	Skilled Nursing Facility	A facility which primarily provides inpatient skilled nursing care and related services to patients who require medical, nursing, or rehabilitative services but does not provide the level of care or treatment available in a hospital.
32	Nursing Facility	A facility which primarily provides to residents skilled nursing care and related services for the rehabilitation of injured, disabled, or sick persons, or, on a regular basis, health-related care services above the level of custodial care to other than individuals with intellectual disabilities.
33	Custodial Care Facility	A facility that provides room, board, and other personal assistance services, generally on a long-term basis, and which does not include a medical component.
34	Hospice	A facility, other than a patient's home, in which palliative and supportive care for terminally ill patients and their families are provided.
35-40	Unassigned	N/A
41	Ambulance—Land	A land vehicle specifically designed, equipped and staffed for lifesaving and transporting the sick or injured.
42	Ambulance—Air or Water	An air or water vehicle specifically designed, equipped, and staffed for lifesaving and transporting the sick or injured.
43-48	Unassigned	N/A
49	Independent Clinic	A location, not part of a hospital and not described by any other Place of Service code, that is organized and operated to provide preventive, diagnostic, therapeutic, rehabilitative, or palliative services to outpatients only. (Effective 10/1/03)
50	Federally Qualified Health Center	A facility located in a medically underserved area that provides Medicare beneficiaries preventive primary medical care under the general direction of a physician.
51	Inpatient Psychiatric Facility	A facility that provides inpatient psychiatric services for the diagnosis and treatment of mental illness on a 24-hour basis, by or under the supervision of a physician.
52	Psychiatric Facility—Partial Hospitalization	A facility for the diagnosis and treatment of mental illness that provides a planned therapeutic program for patients who do not require full time hospitalization, but who need broader programs than are possible from outpatient visits to a hospital-based or hospital-affiliated facility.
53	Community Mental Health Center	A facility that provides the following services: outpatient services, including specialized outpatient services for children, the elderly, individuals who are chronically ill, and residents of the CMHC's mental health services area who have been discharged from inpatient treatment at a mental health facility; 24 hour a day emergency care services; day treatment, other partial hospitalization services, or psychosocial rehabilitation services; screening for patients being considered for admission to State mental health facilities to determine the appropriateness of such admission; and consultation and education services.
54	Intermediate Care Facility/Individuals with Intellectual Disabilities	A facility which primarily provides health-related care and services above the level of custodial care to individuals with intellectual disabilities but does not provide the level of care or treatment available in a hospital or SNF.
55	Residential Substance Abuse Treatment Facility	A facility which provides treatment for substance (alcohol and drug) abuse to live-in residents who do not require acute medical care. Services include individual and group therapy and counseling, family counseling, laboratory tests, drugs and supplies, psychological testing, and room and board.
56	Psychiatric Residential Treatment Center	A facility or distinct part of a facility for psychiatric care which provides a total 24-hour therapeutically planned and professionally staffed group living and learning environment.
57	Non-residential Substance Abuse Treatment Facility	A location which provides treatment for substance (alcohol and drug) abuse on an ambulatory basis. Services include individual and group therapy and counseling, family counseling, laboratory tests, drugs and supplies, and psychological testing. (Effective 10/1/03)
58	Non-residential Opioid Treatment Facility	A location that provides treatment for opioid use disorder on an ambulatory basis. Services include methadone and other forms of Medication Assisted Treatment (MAT). (Effective January 1, 2020)
59	Unassigned	N/A
60	Mass Immunization Center	A location where providers administer pneumococcal pneumonia and influenza virus vaccinations and submit these services as electronic media claims, paper claims, or using the roster billing method. This generally takes place in a mass immunization setting, such as, a public health center, pharmacy, or mall but may include a physician office setting.
61	Comprehensive Inpatient Rehabilitation Facility	A facility that provides comprehensive rehabilitation services under the supervision of a physician to inpatients with physical disabilities. Services include physical therapy, occupational therapy, speech pathology, social or psychological services, and orthotics and prosthetics services.
62	Comprehensive Outpatient Rehabilitation Facility	A facility that provides comprehensive rehabilitation services under the supervision of a physician to outpatients with physical disabilities. Services include physical therapy, occupational therapy, and speech pathology services.
63-64	Unassigned	N/A
65	End-Stage Renal Disease Treatment Facility	A facility other than a hospital, which provides dialysis treatment, maintenance, and/or training to patients or caregivers on an ambulatory or home-care basis.
66	Programs of All-Inclusive Care for the Elderly (PACE) Center	A facility or location providing comprehensive medical and social services as part of the Programs of All-Inclusive Care for the Elderly (PACE). This includes, but is not limited to, primary care; social work services; restorative therapies, including physical and occupational therapy; personal care and supportive services; nutritional counseling; recreational therapy; and meals when the individual is enrolled in PACE. (Effective August 1, 2024)
67-70	Unassigned	N/A
71	Public Health Clinic	A facility maintained by either State or local health departments that provides ambulatory primary medical care under the general direction of a physician.
72	Rural Health Clinic	A certified facility which is located in a rural medically underserved area that provides ambulatory primary medical care under the general direction of a physician.
73-80	Unassigned	N/A
81	Independent Laboratory	A laboratory certified to perform diagnostic and/or clinical tests independent of an institution or a physician's office.
82-98	Unassigned	N/A
99	Other Place of Service	Other place of service not identified above.

current procedural terminology

cpt® 2025

Professional Edition

Current CPT Editorial Panel

Christopher L. Jagmin, MD, FAAFP*, *Chair*
Barbara S. Levy, MD, FACOG*, *Vice Chair*
Samantha Ashley, MS, *Secretary*
Sarah M. Abshier, DPM
J. Mark Bailey, DO, PhD, FACN
Linda M. Barney, MD, FACS†
Aaron D. Bossler, MD, PhD
Leo J. Bronston, DC, MAppSc
Daniel E. Buffington, PharmD, MBA†
Joseph S. Cheng, MD
Samuel L. Church, MD, MPH, CPC-I, FAAFP
Richard A. Frank, MD, PhD
Padma Gulur, MD
Daniel A. Halevy, MD, FASN, CPC
Steven C. Hao, MD, FACC, FHRS

Michael O. Idowu, MD, MPH
Kathy Y. Jones, MD
David M. Kanter, MD, MBA, CPC, FAAP
Craig H. Kliger, MD†
Janet L. McCauley, MD, MHA, CPC, FACOG
JoEllyn C. Moore, MD, FACC, FHRS†
Douglas C. Morrow, OD†
Daniel J. Nagle, MD, FACS, FAAOS
Judith A. O'Connell, DO, MHA, FAAO†
Robert N. Piana, MD, FACC*†
Daniel Picus, MD, FACR, RCC*
Gregory J. Przybylski, MD, MBA†
Lawrence M. Simon, MD, MBA, FACS*
Timothy L. Swan, MD, FACR, FSIR*

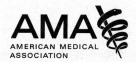

AMA
AMERICAN MEDICAL
ASSOCIATION

*Member of the CPT Executive Committee
†Former CPT Editorial Panel Member, who was active during 2025 content creation

Executive Vice President, Chief Executive Officer: James L. Madara, MD
Senior Vice President, Health Solutions: Lori Prestesater
Vice President, Coding and Reimbursement Policy and Strategy: Zach Hochstetler
Director, CPT Coding and Regulatory Services: Samantha Ashley
Director, CPT Content Management and Development: Leslie W. Prellwitz
Manager, CPT Editorial Panel Processes: Desiree Rozell
Senior Manager, CPT Content Management and Development: Karen E. O'Hara
Vice President, Operations Health Solutions: Denise C. Foy
Senior Manager, Publishing and Fulfillment: Elizabeth Goodman Duke
Manager, Developmental Editing: Lisa Chin-Johnson
Editorial Assistants: Laura Moreno; Samantha Bath
Vice President, Sales and Marketing: Sue Wilson
Director, Print, Digital and Guides: Erin Kalitowski
Director, CPT Operations and Infrastructure: Barbara Benstead
Marketing Manager II: Vanessa Prieto

Printed in the United States of America.   24 25 26/ BD-LBC / 9 8 7 6 5 4 3 2 1

Professional ISBN: 978-1-64016-304-1
ISSN: 0276-8283

1st Edition printed 1966
2nd Edition printed 1970
3rd Edition printed 1973
4th Edition printed 1977
Revised: 1978, 1979, 1980, 1981, 1982, 1984, 1985, 1986, 1987, 1988, 1989, 1990, 1991, 1992,
1993, 1994, 1995, 1996, 1997, 1998, 1999, 2000, 2001, 2002, 2003, 2004, 2005, 2006, 2007, 2008,
2009, 2010, 2011, 2012, 2013, 2014, 2015, 2016, 2017, 2018, 2019, 2020, 2021, 2022, 2023, 2024

To purchase additional CPT products, contact (800) 621-8335 or visit the AMA Store at amastore.com.

Refer to product number EP054125.

To request a license for distribution of products containing or reprinting CPT codes and/or guidelines,
please see our website at www.ama-assn.org/go/cpt, or contact the American Medical Association
CPT/DBP Intellectual Property Services, 330 North Wabash Avenue, Suite 39300, Chicago, IL 60611,
312 464-5022.

AC50:EP054125:9/2024

Disclaimers and Notices

Use of Copyright Protection Technology in *CPT*® *Professional 2025* Codebook

The American Medical Association (AMA) takes the copyright protection of its content very seriously and is committed to providing the most effective anti-piracy efforts for its authors and readers. To help combat print piracy, protect our intellectual properties, and ensure our customers' right to authentic AMA-certified content, the AMA has adopted copyright protection technology in the *CPT*® *Professional 2025* codebook.

To protect the copyrighted content and prevent counterfeiting of the *CPT*® *Professional 2025* codebook using scanners and photocopiers, this book is equipped with state-of-the-art anti-piracy technology within its pages. Therefore, you will notice light-yellow dots in a small rectangle at the bottom of most pages in this book. We have verified that these dots will not impede your ability to read or view the content of the book. As a result of the implementation of this anti-piracy technology, you will notice the pages in this codebook cannot be reproduced by photocopy or scan in accordance with current copyright rules and laws.

In addition to stopping counterfeit book production and protecting the copyrighted content of this manual, the use of anti-piracy technology is designed specifically to protect you, the end-user, by ensuring that you are using an accurate, high-quality, and authentic AMA-certified version of the reference manual. We appreciate your efforts and cooperation in reducing content piracy and improving copyright protections.

About CPT

Current Procedural Terminology (CPT®), Fourth Edition, is a listing of descriptive terms and identifying codes for reporting medical services and procedures performed by physicians and other qualified health care professionals. The purpose of the terminology is to provide a uniform language that will accurately describe medical, surgical, and diagnostic services, and will thereby provide an effective means for reliable nationwide communication among physicians and other qualified health care professionals, patients, and third parties. CPT 2025 is the most recent revision of a work that first appeared in 1966.

CPT descriptive terms and identifying codes currently serve a wide variety of important functions in the field of medical nomenclature. The CPT code set is useful for administrative management purposes such as claims processing and for the development of guidelines for medical care review. The uniform language is also applicable to medical education and outcomes, health services, and quality research by providing a useful basis for local, regional, and national utilization comparisons. The CPT code set is the most widely accepted nomenclature for the reporting of physician and other qualified health care professional procedures and services under government and private health insurance programs. In 2000, the CPT code set was designated by the Department of Health and Human Services as the national coding standard for physician and other health care professional services and procedures under the Health Insurance Portability and Accountability Act (HIPAA). This means that for all financial and administrative health care transactions sent electronically, the CPT code set will need to be used.

The changes that appear in this revision have been prepared by the CPT Editorial Panel with the assistance of physicians and representatives of other health care professions representing all specialties of medicine, and with important contributions from many third-party payers and governmental agencies.

The American Medical Association trusts that this revision will continue the usefulness of its predecessors in identifying, describing, and coding medical, surgical, and diagnostic services.

Maintenance and Authorship of the CPT Code Set

The CPT Editorial Panel (Panel) is tasked with ensuring that CPT codes remain up to date and reflect the latest medical care provided to patients. In order to do this, the Panel maintains an open process and convenes meetings at a minimum three times per year.

The Panel wishes to sincerely thank the many national medical specialty societies, health insurance organizations and agencies, and individual physicians and other health professionals who have made contributions. In particular, the Panel acknowledges the efforts of the following Panel Organizational and Coding Liaison Participants:

Sue Bowman, RHIA, *American Health Information Management Association*

Edith Hambrick, MD, JD, MPH, *Centers for Medicare & Medicaid Services*

Raemarie Jimenez, CPC, *American Academy of Professional Coders*

Douglas Kelly, MD, *Food and Drug Administration*

Mary E. Little, RN, CPC, *Blue Cross and Blue Shield Association*

Tammy R. Love, RHIA, CCS, CDIP, CMA, *American Hospital Association*

Lori Moore, PharmD, *Centers for Disease Control and Prevention*

Also key to authorship of the code set and resulting *CPT Professional Edition* codebook is AMA CPT staff. This experienced team prepares agenda materials for each panel meeting, facilitates the application process, compiles and reviews advisor comments, reconciles differences in opinions, and ultimately compiles all resulting information into a codebook filled with informative guidelines, practical tips, and procedural illustrations.

AMA CPT Staff

Shawn Agyeman
Jay T. Ahlman
Samantha L. Ashley, MS
Thilani Attale, MS
Jennifer Bell, BS, RHIT, CPC, CPMA, CPC-I, CEMC, CPEDC
Barbara Benstead
Andrei Besleaga, BS, RHIT
Meryl Bloomrosen, MBI, MBA, FAMIA, FAHIMA
Kemi Borokini, MSHI, RHIA, CCS
Kyle Dahl
Becky Dolan, MPH
Martha Espronceda
Desiree D. Evans, BS
Kerri Fei, MSN, RN
DeHandro Hayden, BS
Zach Hochstetler, MPP, MBA, CPC
Natasha Lafayette-Jones, MBA, RHIA
Mark Levine
Charniece J. Martin, MBA, RHIA, CCS, CCS-P
Caitlin Mora
Sara F. Nakira, BS
Karen E. O'Hara, BS
Leslie W. Prellwitz, MBA, CCS, CCS-P
Diane J. Regets, BS, RHIA
Desiree Rozell, MPA
Miroslava Rudneva, MS, RHIT, CCS, CRC, COBGC
Nancy Spector, BSN, MSC
Lianne Stancik, BA, RHIT
Keisha A. Sutton-Asaya, MHA, CPC
Okwara Uzoh
Ada Walker, CCA
Arletrice Watkins, MHA, RHIA
Chad Whitney
Rejina L. Young

AMA CPT Advisory Committee

American Academy of Child & Adolescent Psychiatry
Benjamin N. Shain, MD, PhD
Morgan Fallor, MD

American Academy of Dermatology
Alexander Miller, MD
Ann F. Haas, MD

American Academy of Family Physicians
Mary Krebs, MD
Michael Hanak, MD

American Academy of Neurology
Neil A. Busis, MD
Raissa Villanueva, MD

American Academy of Ophthalmology
Michael X. Repka, MD, MBA
John M. Haley, MD

American Academy of Orthopaedic Surgeons
Frank R. Voss, MD
Julie Y. Bishop, MD

American Academy of Otolaryngology Head and Neck Surgery
James Lin, MD, FACS
Jay R. Shah, MD

American Academy of Pain Medicine
Joseph Maxwell Hendrix, MD‡
Eduardo M. Fraifeld, MD

American Academy of Pediatrics
Renee F. Slade, MD
Kathryn Lalor, MD‡

American Academy of Physical Medicine and Rehabilitation
Joseph P. Shivers, MD
Antigone Argyiou, MD

American Academy of Sleep Medicine
Lawrence J. Epstein, MD
Vikas Jain, MD, FAASM

American Association for Thoracic Surgery
Scott C. Silvestry, MD
Charles C. Canver, MD

American Association of Clinical Endocrinologists
William C. Biggs, MD, FACE, ECNU
Pavan Chava, DO, FACE

American Association of Clinical Urologists
Jeffery Glaser, MD, FACS

American Association of Neurological Surgeons
Cheerag Upadhyaya, MD‡
Joshua M. Rosenow, MD, FAANS, FACS

American Association of Neuromuscular and Electrodiagnostic Medicine
Earl J. Craig, MD
John C. Kincaid, MD

American Clinical Neurophysiology Society
Marc R. Nuwer, MD, PhD, FAAN, FACP
Eva Ritzl, MD

American College of Allergy, Asthma and Immunology
James L. Sublett, MD
Gary N. Gross, MD

American College of Cardiology
Randall C. Thompson, MD
Barbara Pisani, DO, FAHA, FACC

American College of Chest Physicians
Steve G. Peters, MD
Michael E. Nelson, MD, FCCP

American College of Emergency Physicians
J. Mark Meredith, III, MD, MMM, FACEP
Michael J. Lemanski, MD, FACEP, FAAFP

American College of Gastroenterology
Christopher Y. Kim, MD, MBA, FACG, FASGE, AGAF, FACP

American College of Medical Genetics and Genomics
David B. Flannery, MD

American College of Mohs Surgery
David B. Pharis, MD, PC
Kishwer S. Nehal, MD

American College of Nuclear Medicine
Gary L. Dillehay, MD, FACNP, FACR
Alan K. Klitzke, MD, FACNM

American College of Obstetricians and Gynecologists
Judith Volkar, MD, MBA
Lisa Hofler, MD‡

American College of Physicians
Jeannine Z. Engel, MD, FACP

American College of Radiation Oncology
Sheila Rege, MD, FACRO
Salah Dajani, MD‡

American College of Radiology
Mark D. Alson, MD, FACR, RCC
Timothy A. Crummy, MD, RCC

American College of Rheumatology
Joseph E. Huffstutter, MD

American College of Surgeons
Megan E. McNally, MD, FACS
Jayme Lieberman, MD, FACS

American Dental Association
Joshua E. Everts, DDS, MD
Adam S. Pitts, DDS, MD

American Gastroenterological Association
Braden Kuo, MD
Joseph Losurdo, MD

American Geriatrics Society
Robert A. Zorowitz, MD, MBA, FACP, AGSF, CMD

American Institute of Ultrasound in Medicine
Fadi Bsat, MD

American Orthopaedic Association
M. Bradford Henley, MD
Adam Levin, MD

American Orthopaedic Foot and Ankle Society
John A. DiPreta, MD
Andrew Hsu, MD‡

---

‡New Advisors

American Osteopathic Association
Boyd Buser, DO, FACOFP

American Psychiatric Association
Sarah E. Parsons, MD

American Rhinologic Society
Bradford Woodworth, MD
Stacey T. Gray, MD

American Roentgen Ray Society
Eric M. Rubin, MD
Dana H. Smetherman, MD, MPH, FACR

American Society for Clinical Pathology
Lee H. Hilborne, MD, MPH, FASCP

American Society for Dermatologic Surgery
Murad Alam, MD, MBA
Ian A. Maher, MD‡

American Society for Gastrointestinal Endoscopy
Glenn D. Littenberg, MD, MACP
Edward Sun, MD

American Society for Metabolic and Bariatric Surgery
Joseph Northup, MD

American Society for Radiation Oncology
Catheryn M. Yashar, MD
Anita Mahajan, MD

American Society for Surgery of the Hand
Steven H Goldberg, MD
Thomas D. Kaplan, MD

American Society of Addiction Medicine
Joel V. Brill, MD, FACP, AGAF

American Society of Anesthesiologists
Edward R. Mariano, MD
Rene Przkora, MD‡

American Society of Breast Surgeons
Richard E. Fine, MD, FACS
Walton Taylor, MD

American Society of Clinical Oncology
Joseph J. Merchant, MD
Rahul Seth, DO‡

American Society of Colon and Rectal Surgeons
Eric Weiss, MD‡
Joshua M. Eberhardt, MD, MBA, FACS, FASCRS

American Society of Cytopathology
Carol A. Filomena, MD

American Society of Dermatopathology
Jonathan S. Ralston, MD
Aleodor A. Andea, MD, MBA

American Society of Echocardiography
Michael L. Main, MD
Susan A. Mayer, MD

American Society of General Surgeons
George K. Gillian, MD, FACS

American Society of Hematology
Samuel M. Silver, MD, PhD, MACP, FAHA, FASCO
Chancellor E. Donald, MD

American Society of Interventional Pain Physicians
Mahendra Sanapati, MD
Sheri Albers, DO‡

American Society of Neuroimaging
Ryan Hakimi, DO, MS

American Society of Neuroradiology
Colin M. Segovis, MD, PhD
Gaurang V. Shah, MD

American Society of Nuclear Cardiology
Friederike Keating, MD

American Society of Ophthalmic Plastic and Reconstructive Surgery
L. Neal Freeman, MD, MBA, CCS-P, FACS

American Society of Plastic Surgeons
Jeffrey H. Kozlow, MD, MS
David Schnur, MD

American Society of Regional Anesthesia and Pain Medicine
Houman Danesh, MD
David N. Flynn, MD

American Society of Retina Specialists
Gayatri S. Reilly, MD
Christopher R. Henry, MD

American Thoracic Society
Stephen P. Hoffmann, MD
Michael E. Nelson, MD, FCCP

American Urological Association
Jonathan N. Rubenstein, MD
Jay A. Motola, MD, FACS

American Vein & Lymphatic Society
Satish Vayuvegula, MD, MS
Michael S. Graves, MD

Association for Molecular Pathology
Samuel K. Caughron, MD, FCAP‡

Association of University Radiologists
Shiva Gupta, MD
Christina Marks, MD

College of American Pathologists
Ronald W. McLawhon, MD, PhD
Mark Synovec, MD‡

Congress of Neurological Surgeons
Henry H. Woo, MD, FACS, FAANS

Heart Rhythm Society
Christopher F. Liu, MD, FACC, FHRS
Sumeet Mainigi, MD

Infectious Diseases Society of America
Ronald E. Devine, MD

International Pain and Spine Intervention Society
Scott I. Horn, DO

International Society for the Advancement of Spine Surgery
James J. Yue, MD
Morgan L. Lorio, MD, FACS

National Association of Medical Examiners
Allecia M. Wilson, MD

North American Neuromodulation Society
Corey W. Hunter, MD
Dawood Sayed, MD

North American Spine Society
David Cohen, MD
David R. O'Brien, Jr, MD

Outpatient Endovascular and Interventional Society
Eric J. Dippel, MD

Radiological Society of North America
Timothy A. Crummy, MD
Cindy Yuan, MD

Renal Physicians Association
Timothy A. Pflederer, MD
Jeffrey Perlmutter, MD

Society for Cardiovascular Angiography and Interventions
Arthur C. Lee, MD, FSCAI
Andrew M. Goldsweig, MD

Society for Investigative Dermatology
Stephen P. Stone, MD

Society for Vascular Surgery
Sean P. Roddy, MD, FACS
Sunita D. Srivastava, MD

Society of American Gastrointestinal Endoscopic Surgeons
John S. Roth, MD, FACS
Kevin E. Wasco, MD, FACS

Society of Cardiovascular Computed Tomography
Ahmad M. Slim, MD

Society of Critical Care Medicine
Piyush Mathur, MD

Society of Interventional Radiology
Ammar Sarwar, MD
Ashok Bhanushali, MD

Society of Nuclear Medicine and Molecular Imaging
Scott C. Bartley, MD
Gary L. Dillehay, MD, FACNP, FACR

Society of Thoracic Surgeons
Francis C. Nichols, III, MD
Jeffrey P. Jacobs, MD, FACS, FACC, FCCP

The Endocrine Society
Ricardo Correa Marquez, MD
Sandhya Chhabra, MD

The Triological Society
Brian J. McKinnon, MD, MBA

United States and Canadian Academy of Pathology
Dennis P. O'Malley. MD
Ericka Olgaard, DO

AMA Health Care Professionals Advisory Committee (HCPAC)

Christopher L. Jagmin, MD, FAAFP*, Co-Chair
AMA CPT Editorial Panel

Leo J. Bronston, DC, MAppSc, Co-Chair
AMA CPT Editorial Panel

Academy of Nutrition and Dietetics
Keith-Thomas Ayoob, EdD, RD, FADA, CSP
Jessie M. Pavlinac, MS, RD, CSR, LD

American Academy of Audiology
Brad A. Stach, PhD
Annette A. Burton, AuD

American Academy of Physician Assistants
Patrick J. Cafferty, MPAS, PA-C

American Association of Naturopathic Physicians
Eva Miller, ND
Amy E. Hobson, ND

American Association for Respiratory Care
Susan Rinaldo-Gallo, Med, RRT, FAARC, CTTS

American Chiropractic Association
Kris Anderson, DC, MS

American Massage Therapy Association
Nancy M. Porambo, BA, MS, LMT, NCTMB

American Nurses Association
Jill Olmstead, MSN, NP-C, ANP-BC, FAANP
Julia Rogers, DNP, RN, CNS, FNP-BC

American Occupational Therapy Association
Leslie F. Davidson, PhD, OTR/L, FAOTA
Tippi S. Geron, MS, OTD, OTR/L, FAOTA

American Optometric Association
Rebecca H. Wartman, OD
Harvey B. Richman, OD, FAAO, FCOVD

American Physical Therapy Association
Kathleen M. Picard, PT, DPT
Jonathan Morren, PT, DPT

American Podiatric Medical Association
Ira H. Kraus, DPM

American Psychological Association
Neil H. Pliskin, PhD, ABPP-CN
Stephen Gillaspy, PhD

American Society of Acupuncturists
Chanta Sloma, DACM
Jessica Gregory, MSAOM

American Speech-Language-Hearing Association
Renee Kinder, MS, CCC-SLP

National Association of Social Workers
Mirean F. Coleman, LICSW
Nelda Spyres[‡]

National Athletic Trainers' Association
Karen D. Fennell, MS, ATC, LAT
Joseph J. Greene, MS, ATC

National Society of Genetic Counselors
Brian Reys, MS, CGC

Pharmacy Health Information Technology Collaborative
Brian J. Isetts, PhD, BCPS, FAPhA
Laura J. Hanson, PharmD, MBA, BCPS

*Member of the CPT Executive Committee
‡New Advisors

Contents

Contents

Introduction

Current Procedural Terminology (CPT®), Fourth Edition, is a set of codes, descriptions, and guidelines intended to describe procedures and services performed by physicians and other qualified health care professionals, or entities. Each procedure or service is identified with a five-digit code. The use of CPT codes simplifies the reporting of procedures and services. In the CPT code set, the term "procedure" is used to describe services, including diagnostic tests.

Inclusion of a descriptor and its associated five-digit code number in the CPT Category I code set is based on whether the procedure or service is consistent with contemporary medical practice and is performed by many practitioners in clinical practice in multiple locations. Inclusion in the CPT code set of a procedure or service, or proprietary name, does not represent endorsement by the American Medical Association (AMA) of any particular diagnostic or therapeutic procedure or service or proprietary test or manufacturer. Inclusion or exclusion of a procedure or service, or proprietary name, does not imply any health insurance coverage or reimbursement policy.

▶The main body of the Category I section is listed in six sections. Each section is divided into subsections with anatomic, procedural, condition, or descriptor subheadings. The procedures and services with their identifying codes are presented in numeric order with the exception of the resequenced codes and the entire **Evaluation and Management** section (98000-98016, 99202-99499), which appears at the beginning of the listed procedures. The evaluation and management codes are used by most physicians in reporting a significant portion of their services.◀

Release of CPT Codes

The CPT code set is published annually in late summer or early fall as both electronic data files and books. The release of CPT data files occurs annually between August 31 and early September. The release of the CPT Professional publication comes several weeks later. However, to meet the needs of a rapidly changing health care environment, the CPT code set is periodically updated throughout the year on a set schedule. Each update has both a release date and an effective date. The interval between the release of the update and the effective date is considered an implementation period and is intended to allow physicians and other providers, payers, and vendors to incorporate CPT changes into their systems. Changes to the CPT code set are meant to be applied prospectively from the effective date. The following table outlines the complete CPT code set update calendar.

New CPT codes have been created to streamline services related to the novel coronavirus. It is imperative to check the AMA CPT public website at https://www.ama-assn.org/practice-management/cpt/covid-19-coding-and-guidance throughout the year to obtain the necessary frequent updates to the CPT code set.

CPT Code Set Update Calendar

CPT Category/Section	Release Timeline	Effective Timeline
Category I Category II	August 31	January 1
Category III	January 1	July 1
	July 1	January 1
▶Immune Globulins, Serum, or Recombinant Products Vaccines, Toxoids	April 1	July 1
	July 1	October 1
	October 1*	January 1◀
Molecular Pathology Tier 2 Administrative MAAA	April 1	July 1
	July 1	October 1
	October 1*	January 1
PLA	January 1	April 1
	April 1	July 1
	July 1	October 1
	October 1	January 1

*Note that the release date may be delayed by several days due to the timing of the CPT Panel fall meeting.

It is imperative to check the AMA CPT public website throughout the year to obtain the necessary updates to the CPT code set. The following are several links on the AMA CPT website where these updates can be found:

- Category III codes: ama-assn.org/cpt-cat-iii-codes

- Immune globulins, serum, or recombinant products and vaccines, toxoids: ama-assn.org/cpt-cat-i-immunization-codes

- Proprietary Laboratory Analyses (PLA) codes: ama-assn.org/cpt-pla-codes

- Administrative MAAA codes: ama-assn.org/practice-management/cpt/multianalyte-assays-algorithmic-analyses-codes

- Molecular pathology tier 2 codes: ama-assn.org/mo-path-tier-2-codes

- General errata and technical correction updates: ama-assn.org/practice-management/cpt/errata-technical-corrections

Section Numbers and Their Sequences

Evaluation and Management. .98000-98016, 99202-99499

Anesthesiology. 00100-01999, 99100-99140

Surgery. 10004-69990

Radiology (Including Nuclear Medicine
    and Diagnostic Ultrasound) 70010-79999

Pathology and
    Laboratory. 80047-89398, 0001U-0520U

Medicine (except Anesthesiology). 90281-99199,
                                   99500-99607

The first and last code numbers and the subsection name of the items appear at the top margin of most pages (eg, "10004-11005 Surgery/Integumentary System"). The continuous pagination of the CPT codebook is found on the lower margin of each page along with explanation of any code symbols that are found on that page.

Instructions for Use of the CPT Codebook

►Select the CPT code of the procedure or service that accurately identifies the procedure or service performed. Do not select a CPT code that merely approximates the procedure or service provided. If no such specific code exists, then report the procedure or service using the appropriate unlisted procedure or service code. When using an unlisted code, any modifying or extenuating circumstances should be adequately and accurately documented in the medical record. Furthermore, all the language within a code descriptor should be assessed when selecting the appropriate procedure or service. This includes information directly in the descriptor that may be enclosed in parentheses.◄

It is equally important to recognize that as techniques in medicine and surgery have evolved, new types of services, including minimally invasive surgery, as well as endovascular, percutaneous, and endoscopic interventions have challenged the traditional distinction of Surgery vs Medicine. Thus, the listing of a service or procedure in a specific section of this book should not be interpreted as strictly classifying the service or procedure as "surgery" or "not surgery" for insurance or other purposes. The placement of a given service in a specific section of the book may reflect historical or other considerations (eg, placement of the percutaneous peripheral vascular endovascular interventions in the Surgery/Cardiovascular System section, while the percutaneous coronary interventions appear in the Medicine/Cardiovascular section).

When advanced practice nurses and physician assistants are working with physicians, they are considered as working in the exact same specialty and subspecialty as the physician. A "physician or other qualified health care professional" is an individual who is qualified by education, training, licensure/regulation (when applicable), and facility privileging (when applicable) who performs a professional service within his/her scope of practice and independently reports that profes-

sional service. These professionals are distinct from "clinical staff." A clinical staff member is a person who works under the supervision of a physician or other qualified health care professional and who is allowed by law, regulation, and facility policy to perform or assist in the performance of a specified professional service but who does not individually report that professional service. Other policies may also affect who may report specific services.

Throughout the CPT code set the use of terms such as "physician," "qualified health care professional," or "individual" is not intended to indicate that other entities may not report the service. In selected instances, specific instructions may define a service as limited to professionals or limited to other entities (eg, hospital or home health agency).

Instructions, typically included as parenthetical notes with selected codes, indicate that a code should not be reported with another code or codes. These instructions are intended to prevent errors of significant probability and are not all inclusive. For example, the code with such instructions may be a component of another code and therefore it would be incorrect to report both codes even when the component service is performed. These instructions are not intended as a listing of all possible code combinations that should not be reported, nor do they indicate all possible code combinations that are appropriately reported. When reporting codes for services provided, it is important to assure the accuracy and quality of coding through verification of the intent of the code by use of the related guidelines, parenthetical instructions, and coding resources, including *CPT Assistant* and other publications resulting from collaborative efforts of the American Medical Association with the medical specialty societies (ie, *Clinical Examples in Radiology*).

Because Category I or Category III codes may incorporate multiple components (bundled) that could be reported separately with other existing codes, "unbundling" of codes into their component parts for reporting purposes or combining those components with an unlisted code is inappropriate. For example, it would be inappropriate to separately report both codes 42825, *Tonsillectomy, primary or secondary; younger than age 12*, and 42830, *Adenoidectomy, primary; younger than age 12*, for removal of the tonsils and adenoids, because these two procedures are reported together using code 42820, *Tonsillectomy and adenoidectomy; younger than age 12*. Multiple Category I or Category III codes may be reported together to describe the totality of service rendered for a given patient encounter if they represent separately reportable services. Individual components of a procedure or service specified as part of a Category I or Category III code descriptor are reported neither separately with an existing CPT code nor with an unlisted code. Procedural steps necessary to reach the operative site and to close the operative site are also not reported separately, unless otherwise instructed by CPT guidelines or parenthetical notes. For example, a laparoscopic cholecystectomy should not be reported together with a code for the incision or a code for the repair of the surgical wound because these are inherent procedural steps needed to accomplish the cholecystectomy. However, if an excision of a benign lesion requires a complex repair for closure, both the lesion excision and the complex repair code are reported separately because the Repair (Closure) Guidelines indicate that "complex repair does not include excision of benign (11400-11446) or malignant (11600-11646) lesions."

Format of the Terminology

The CPT code set has been developed as stand-alone descriptions of medical procedures. However, some of the procedures in the CPT codebook are not printed in their entirety but refer back to a common portion of the procedure listed in a preceding entry. This is evident when an entry is followed by one or more indentations. This is done in an effort to conserve space.

Example

25100   Arthrotomy, wrist joint; with biopsy

25105   with synovectomy

Note that the common part of code 25100 (the part before the semicolon) should also be considered part of code 25105. Therefore, the full procedure represented by code 25105 should read:

25105   Arthrotomy, wrist joint; with synovectomy

Requests to Update the CPT Nomenclature

The effectiveness of the CPT nomenclature depends on constant updating to reflect changes in medical practice. This can only be accomplished through the interest and timely suggestions of practicing physicians and other qualified health care professionals, specialty/professional societies, state medical associations, organizations, agencies, individual users of the CPT code set, and other stakeholders. Accordingly, the AMA welcomes correspondence, inquiries, and suggestions concerning CPT coding and nomenclature for old and new procedures and services, as well as any matters relating to the CPT code set.

For information on submission of an application to add, delete, or revise codes contained in the CPT code set, please see www.ama-assn.org/go/cpt-processfaq or contact:

CPT Editorial Research & Development
American Medical Association
330 North Wabash Avenue
Suite 39300
Chicago IL 60611-5885

Code change applications are available at the AMA's CPT website at https://www.ama-assn.org/practice-management/cpt/cpt-code-change-applications.

All proposed changes to the CPT code set will be considered by the CPT Editorial Panel in consultation with medical specialty societies as represented by the CPT Advisory Committee, other health care professional societies as represented by the Health Care Professionals Advisory Committee (HCPAC), and other interested parties.

Application Submission Requirements

All complete CPT code change applications are reviewed and evaluated by the CPT staff, the CPT/HCPAC Advisory Committee, and the CPT Editorial Panel. Strict conformance with the following is required for review of a code change application:

- Submission of a complete application, including all necessary supporting documents;

- Adherence to all posted deadlines;

- Cooperation with requests from the CPT staff and/or Editorial Panel members for clarification and information; *and*

- Compliance with CPT Lobbying Policy.

General Criteria for Category I, II, and III Codes

All Category I, II, and III code change applications must satisfy each of the following criteria:

- The proposed descriptor is unique, well-defined, and describes a procedure or service that is clearly identified and distinguished from existing procedures and services already in the CPT code set;

- The descriptor structure, guidelines, and instructions are consistent with the current CPT Editorial Panel standards for maintenance of the code set;

- The proposed descriptor for the procedure or service is neither a fragmentation of an existing procedure or service nor currently reportable as a complete service by one or more existing codes (with the exclusion of unlisted codes). However, procedures and services frequently performed together may require new or revised codes;

- The structure and content of the proposed code descriptor accurately reflects the procedure or service as typically performed. If always or frequently performed with one or more other procedures or services, the descriptor structure and content will reflect the typical combination or complete procedure or service;

- The descriptor for the procedure or service is not proposed as a means to report extraordinary circumstances related to the performance of a procedure or service already described in the CPT code set; *and*

- The procedure or service satisfies the category-specific criteria set forth below.

Category-Specific Requirements
Category I Criteria

A proposal for a new or revised Category I code must satisfy all of the following criteria:

- All devices and drugs necessary for performance of the procedure or service have received FDA clearance or approval when such is required for performance of the procedure or service;

- The procedure or service is performed by many physicians or other qualified health care professionals across the United States;

- The procedure or service is performed with frequency consistent with the intended clinical use (ie, a service for a common condition should have high volume, whereas a service commonly performed for a rare condition may have low volume);

- The procedure or service is consistent with current medical practice; *and*

- The clinical efficacy of the procedure or service is documented in literature that meets the requirements set forth in the CPT code change application.

Category II Criteria

The following criteria are used by the CPT/HCPAC and the CPT Editorial Panel for evaluating Category II code applications:

- Measurements that were developed and tested by a national organization;

- Evidence-based measurements with established ties to health outcomes;

- Measurements that address clinical conditions of high prevalence, high risk, or high cost; *and*

- Well-established measurements that are currently being used by large segments of the health care industry across the country.

In addition, all of the following are required:

- Definition or purpose of the measure is consistent with its intended use (quality improvement and accountability, or solely quality improvement)

- Aspect of care measured is substantially influenced by the physician (or other qualified health care professional or entity for which the code may be relevant)

- Reduces data collection burden on physicians (or other qualified health care professionals or entities)

- Significant

  o Affects a large segment of health care community

  o Tied to health outcomes

  o Addresses clinical conditions of high prevalence, high costs, high risks

- Evidence-based

  o Agreed upon

  o Definable

  o Measurable

- Risk-adjustment specifications and instructions for all outcome measures submitted or compelling evidence as to why risk adjustment is not relevant

- Sufficiently detailed to make it useful for multiple purposes

- Facilitates reporting of performance measure(s)

- Inclusion of select patient history, testing (eg, glycohemoglobin), other process measures, cognitive or procedure services within CPT, or physiologic measures (eg, blood pressure) to support performance measurements

- Performance measure–development process that includes

  o Nationally recognized expert panel

  o Multidisciplinary

  o Vetting process

Category III Criteria

The following **criteria** are used by the CPT/HCPAC Advisory Committee and the CPT Editorial Panel for evaluating Category III code **applications**:

- The procedure or service is currently or recently performed in humans; *and*

At least one of the following additional criteria has been met:

- The application is supported by at least one CPT or HCPAC advisor representing practitioners who would use this procedure or service; *or*

- The actual or potential clinical efficacy of the specific procedure or service is supported by peer reviewed literature, which is available in English for examination by the CPT Editorial Panel; *or*

- There is (a) at least one Institutional Review Board–approved protocol of a study of the procedure or service being performed; (b) a description of a current and ongoing United States trial outlining the efficacy of the procedure or service; or (c) other evidence of evolving clinical utilization.

Audio-Video (Appendix P) and Audio-Only (Appendix T) Telemedicine Services Criteria

The following criteria are used by the Current Procedural Terminology/Health Care Professional Advisory Committee (CPT/HCPAC) and the CPT Editorial Panel for evaluating inclusion of services in Appendix P (synchronous audio-video) and Appendix T (synchronous audio-only) telemedicine services. Any request for inclusion in Appendix P and Appendix T must satisfy the following criteria:

- The totality and quality of the communication of information exchanged between the physician or other qualified health care professional (QHP) and the patient during the synchronous telemedicine service must be of an amount and a nature that would be sufficient to meet the requirements for the same service if services were to be rendered during an in-person face-to-face interaction; *and*

- The evidence supports the benefits of performing the service through telecommunications technology. These benefits may include, but are not limited to, the following:

  o Facilitate a diagnosis or treatment plan that may reduce complications

  o Decrease diagnostic or therapeutic interventions

  o Decrease hospitalizations

  o Decrease in-person visits to the emergency department

  o Decrease in-person visits to physician or other QHP offices, including urgent care centers

  o Increase rapidity of resolution

  o Decrease quantifiable symptoms

  o Reduce recovery time

  o Enhance access to care, such as for rural and vulnerable patients; *and*

- A service is ineligible for inclusion in Appendix T without also being requested for inclusion, or has current inclusion, in Appendix P.

(For a listing of CPT codes that may be used for synchronous real-time interactive audio-video telemedicine services when appended with modifier 95, see Appendix P)

(For a listing of CPT codes that may be used for synchronous real-time interactive audio-only telemedicine services when appended with modifier 93, see Appendix T)

Guidelines

Specific guidelines are presented at the beginning of each of the sections. These guidelines define items that are necessary to appropriately interpret and report the procedures and services contained in that section. For example, in the **Medicine** section, specific instructions are provided for handling unlisted services or procedures, special reports, and supplies and materials provided. Guidelines also provide explanations regarding terms that apply only to a particular section. For instance, **Radiology Guidelines** provide a definition of the unique term, "radiological supervision and interpretation." While in **Anesthesia**, a discussion of reporting time is included.

A written report (eg, handwritten or electronic) signed by the interpreting individual should be considered an integral part of a radiologic procedure or interpretation. Please see the guidelines regarding Imaging Guidance in each individual section.

Add-on Codes

Some of the listed procedures are commonly carried out in addition to the primary procedure performed. These additional or supplemental procedures are designated as add-on codes with the **+** symbol and they are listed in **Appendix D** of the CPT codebook. Add-on codes in CPT 2025 can be readily identified by specific descriptor nomenclature that includes phrases such as "each additional" or "(List separately in addition to primary procedure)."

The add-on code concept in CPT 2025 applies only to add-on procedures or services performed by the same physician. Add-on codes describe additional intra-service work associated with the primary procedure, eg, additional digit(s), lesion(s), neurorrhaphy(s), vertebral segment(s), tendon(s), joint(s).

Add-on codes are always performed in addition to the primary service or procedure and must never be reported as a stand-alone code. The inclusionary parenthetical notes following the add-on codes are designed to include the typical base code(s) and not every possible reportable code combination. When the add-on procedure can be reported bilaterally and is performed bilaterally, the appropriate add-on code is reported twice, unless the code descriptor, guidelines, or parenthetical instructions for that particular add-on code instructs otherwise. Do not report modifier 50, *Bilateral Procedures,* in conjunction with add-on codes. All add-on codes in the CPT code set are exempt from the multiple procedure concept. See the definitions of modifier 50 and 51 in **Appendix A.**

Modifiers

A modifier provides the means to report or indicate that a service or procedure that has been performed has been altered by some specific circumstance but not changed in its definition or code. Modifiers also enable health care professionals to effectively respond to payment policy requirements established by other entities. The judicious application of modifiers obviates the necessity for separate procedure listings that may describe the modifying circumstance. Modifiers may be used to indicate to the recipient of a report that:

- A service or procedure had both a professional and technical component.

- A service or procedure was performed by more than one physician or other health care professional and/or in more than one location.

- A service or procedure was increased or reduced.

- Only part of a service was performed.

- An adjunctive service was performed.

- A bilateral procedure was performed.

- A service or procedure was provided more than once.

- Unusual events occurred.

Example

A physician providing diagnostic or therapeutic radiology services, ultrasound, or nuclear medicine services in a hospital would add modifier 26 to report the professional component.

73090 with modifier 26 = Professional component only for an X ray of the forearm

Example

Two surgeons may be required to manage a specific surgical problem. When two surgeons work together as primary surgeons performing distinct part(s) of a procedure, each surgeon should report his/her distinct operative work by adding modifier 62 to the procedure code and any associated code(s) for that procedure as long as both surgeons continue to work together as primary surgeons. Each surgeon should report the co-surgery once using the same procedure code. Modifier 62 would be applicable. For instance, a neurological surgeon and an otolaryngologist are working as co-surgeons in performing transphenoidal excision of a pituitary neoplasm.

The first surgeon would report:

61548 62 = Hypophysectomy or excision of pituitary tumor, transnasal or transseptal approach, nonstereotactic + two surgeons modifier

and the second surgeon would report:

61548 62 = Hypophysectomy or excision of pituitary tumor, transnasal or transseptal approach, nonstereotactic + two surgeons modifier

If additional procedure(s) (including add-on procedure[s]) are performed during the same surgical session, separate code(s) may also be reported with modifier 62 added. It should be noted that if a co-surgeon acts as an assistant in the performance of additional procedure(s) during the same surgical session, those services may be reported using separate procedure code(s) with modifier 80 or modifier 82 added, as appropriate. A complete listing of modifiers is found in **Appendix A.**

Place of Service and Facility Reporting

Some codes have specified places of service (eg, evaluation and management codes are specific to a setting). Other services and procedures may have instructions specific to the place of service (eg, therapeutic, prophylactic, and diagnostic injections and infusions). The CPT code set is designated for reporting physician and other qualified health care professional services. It is also the designated code set for reporting services provided by organizations or facilities (eg, hospitals) in specific circumstances. Throughout the CPT code set, the use of terms such as "physician," "qualified health care professional," or "individual" is not intended to indicate that other entities may not report the service. In selected instances, specific instructions may define a service as limited to professionals or limited to other entities (eg, hospital or home health agency). The CPT code set uses the term "facility" to describe such providers and the term "nonfacility" to describe services settings or circumstances in which no facility reporting may occur. Services provided in the home by an agency are facility services. Services provided in the home by a physician or other qualified health care professional who is not a representative of the agency are nonfacility services.

Unlisted Procedure or Service

Category I and Category III codes describe the vast majority of procedures and services currently performed in the United States and should be used to report these procedures and services that are accurately described in existing CPT codes. It is recognized that there may be services or procedures performed by physicians or other qualified health care professionals (QHPs) that are not found in the CPT code set. Therefore, a number of specific code numbers have been designated for reporting unlisted procedures. When an unlisted procedure code is used, the service or procedure should be described (see specific section guidelines). Each of these unlisted codes (with the appropriate accompanying topical entry) relates to a specific section of the code set and is presented in the guidelines of that section.

The CPT code set's instructions to use an unlisted procedure code do not preclude the reporting of an appropriate code that may be found elsewhere in the CPT code set. It may be appropriate to report multiple Category I or Category III codes together to describe the totality of a service rendered for a given patient encounter, provided each code represents a separately reportable service. Similarly, it is appropriate to report an unlisted code together with a Category I or Category III code(s) for the same patient encounter on the same date of service when a separately reportable portion of a provided procedure or service is not described by an existing CPT code(s).

Example

Reporting unlisted code(s) with Category I code(s): When both radiofrequency ablation of the greater saphenous vein and stab phlebectomy using less than 10 incisions are performed in the same operative session, both codes 36475, *Endovenous ablation therapy of incompetent vein, extremity, inclusive of all imaging guidance and monitoring, percutaneous, radiofrequency; first vein treated,* and 37799, *Unlisted procedure, vascular surgery,* may be reported because there is no code for stab phlebectomy with less than 10 incisions.

While uncommon, if multiple separately reportable unlisted services are performed on the same patient on the same date of service by the same physician or other QHP, then multiple unlisted codes may be reported. If the two procedures are performed in the same anatomic region, then multiple units of the same unlisted code may be reported with modifier 59 appended to the additional unit(s). If two unlisted services are performed in two different anatomic regions, then two different unlisted codes may be reported.

Example

Reporting multiple separately reportable unlisted services: If two unlisted arthroscopic procedures are performed on two separate joints by the same surgeon on the same date of service, then two units of 29999, *Unlisted procedure, arthroscopy,* may be reported with modifier 59 appended to the second unit.

Note that unlisted codes are not used to separately report component(s) of an existing Category I or Category III service.

Example

It would not be appropriate to use 39599, *Unlisted procedure, diaphragm,* to separately report suturing of the diaphragm performed as a component of a paraesophageal hernia repair, which is reported with code 43281, *Laparoscopy, surgical, repair of paraesophageal hernia, includes fundoplasty, when performed; without implantation of mesh.*

Because unlisted codes do not include descriptor language that specifies the components of a particular service, modifiers that describe alteration of a service or procedure may not be used. For example, it would not be appropriate to append modifier 52, *Reduced Services,* to an unlisted code. However, modifiers to indicate laterality (ie, modifier 50, *Bilateral Procedure*); distinction (ie, modifier 59, *Distinct Procedural Service*); assistant-at-surgery (modifier 80, *Assistant Surgeon*); and place of service (eg, modifier 95, *Synchronous Telemedicine Service Rendered Via a Real-Time Interactive Audio and Video Telecommunications System*; modifier 93, *Synchronous Telemedicine Service Rendered Via Telephone or Other Real-Time Interactive Audio-Only Telecommunications System*) may be used, when indicated.

Results, Testing, Interpretation, and Report

Results are the technical component of a service. Testing leads to results; results lead to interpretation. Reports are the work product of the interpretation of test results. Certain procedures or services described in CPT involve a technical component (eg, tests), which produces "results" (eg, data, images, slides). For clinical use, some of these results require interpretation. Some CPT descriptors specifically require interpretation and reporting in order to report that code.

Special Report

A service that is rarely provided, unusual, variable, or new may require a special report. Pertinent information should include an adequate definition or description of the nature, extent, and need for the procedure and the time, effort, and equipment necessary to provide the service.

Time

The CPT code set contains many codes with a time basis for code selection. The following standards shall apply to time measurement, unless there are code or code-range–specific instructions in guidelines, parenthetical instructions, or code descriptors to the contrary. Time is the face-to-face time with the patient. Phrases such as "interpretation and report" in the code descriptor are not intended to indicate in all cases that report writing is part of the reported time. A unit of time is attained when the mid-point is passed. For example, an hour is attained when 31 minutes have elapsed (more than midway between zero and 60 minutes). A second hour is attained when a total of 91 minutes has elapsed. The evaluation and management (E/M) codes that use total time on the date of the encounter have a required time threshold for time-based reporting; therefore, the mid-point concept does not apply. See also the **Evaluation and Management (E/M) Services Guidelines**. When another service is performed concurrently with a time-based service, the time associated with the concurrent service should not be included in the time used for reporting the time-based service. Some services measured in units other than days extend across calendar dates. When this occurs, a continuous service does not reset and create a first hour. However, any disruption in the service does create a new initial service. For example, if intravenous hydration (96360, 96361) is given from 11 PM to 2 AM, 96360 would be reported once and 96361 twice. For facility reporting on a single date of service or for continuous services that last beyond midnight (ie, over a range of dates), report the total units of time provided continuously.

Code Symbols

A summary listing of additions, deletions, and revisions applicable to the CPT codebook is found in **Appendix B**. New procedure numbers added to the CPT codebook are identified throughout the text with the ● symbol placed before the code number. In instances where a code revision has resulted in a substantially altered procedure descriptor, the ▲ symbol is placed before the code number. The ▶ ◀ symbols are used to indicate new and revised text other than the procedure descriptors. These symbols indicate CPT Editorial Panel actions. The AMA reserves the right to correct typographical errors and make stylistic improvements.

CPT add-on codes are annotated by the ✚ symbol and are listed in **Appendix D**. The ⊘ symbol is used to identify codes that are exempt from the use of modifier 51 but have not been designated as CPT add-on procedures or services. A list of codes exempt from modifier 51 usage is included in **Appendix E**. The ⭠ symbol is used to identify codes for vaccines that are pending FDA approval (see **Appendix K**). The # symbol is used to identify codes that are listed out of numerical sequence (see **Appendix N**). The ★ symbol is used to identify codes that may be used to report audio-video telemedicine services when appended by modifier 95 (see **Appendix P**). The ◀ symbol is used to identify codes that may be used to report audio-only telemedicine services when appended by modifier 93 (see **Appendix T**).

Resequenced codes that are not placed numerically are identified with the # symbol, and a reference placed numerically (ie, Code is out of numerical sequence. See…) as a navigational alert to direct the user to the location of the out-of-sequence code (see **Appendix N**). Resequencing is utilized to allow placement of related concepts in appropriate locations within the families of codes regardless of the availability of numbers for sequential numerical placement.

Duplicate proprietary laboratory analyses (PLA) tests are annotated by the ⌘ symbol. PLA codes describe proprietary clinical laboratory analyses and can be either provided by a single ("sole-source") laboratory or licensed or marketed to multiple providing laboratories (eg, cleared or approved by the Food and Drug Administration [FDA]). All codes that are included in the PLA section are also included in **Appendix O**, with the procedure's proprietary name. In some instances, the descriptor language of PLA codes may be identical and the code may only be differentiated by the listed proprietary name in Appendix O. When more than one PLA test has an identical descriptor, the codes will be denoted by the ⌘ symbol.

Unless specifically noted, even though the Proprietary Laboratory Analyses section of the code set is located at the end of the Pathology and Laboratory section of the code set, a PLA code does not fulfill Category I code criteria. A PLA code(s) that has Category I status is annotated by the ⇅ symbol.

Alphabetical Reference Index

This codebook features an expanded alphabetical index that includes listings by procedure and anatomic site. Procedures and services commonly known by their eponyms or other designations are also included.

Use of Anti-Piracy Technology in *CPT Professional 2025* Codebook

The AMA takes the act of and/or the prospect of piracy of its books and copyrighted content very seriously, and is committed to providing the most effective anti-piracy service to its authors and readers. To help combat print piracy and protect our intellectual properties and customers' right to AMA-certified content, the AMA has adopted anti-piracy technology in the *CPT Professional 2025* codebook.

To protect the copyrighted content and prevent counterfeiting of the *CPT Professional 2025* codebook using color copiers, this book is protected and equipped with state-of-the-art anti-piracy technology within its pages. Therefore, you will notice light-yellow dots at the bottom of most pages in this book. As a result of the implementation of this anti-piracy technology, you will notice that the pages in this codebook cannot be reproduced by photocopy or scan in accordance with current copyright rules and laws.

In addition to stopping counterfeit book production and protecting the copyrighted content of this manual, the use of anti-piracy technology is designed specifically to protect you, the end-user, by ensuring that you are using an accurate, high-quality, and authentic AMA-certified version of the reference manual. We appreciate your efforts and cooperation in reducing content piracy and improving copyright protections.

CPT 2025 in Electronic Formats

CPT 2025 procedure codes and descriptions are available as downloadable data files. The CPT data files are available in ASCII and EBCDIC formats and provide a convenient way to import the CPT 2025 codes and descriptions into existing documentation or into any billing and claims reporting software that accepts a text (.TXT) file format. The data files contain the complete official AMA CPT guidelines, descriptor package, and new descriptors for consumers and clinicians.

The *CPT Professional* codebook is also available as an e-book. For more information about CPT electronic formats, call 800 621-8335 or visit **amastore.com**.

References to AMA Resources

The symbols ➋ ➋ and ➋ appear after many codes throughout this codebook, which indicate that the AMA has published reference material regarding that particular code.

The symbol ➋ refers to the *CPT Changes: An Insider's View*, an annual book with all of the coding changes for the current year, the ➋ refers to the *CPT Assistant* monthly newsletter. The symbol ➋ refers to the quarterly newsletter *Clinical Examples in Radiology*.

Example

36598	Contrast injection(s) for radiologic evaluation of existing central venous access device, including fluoroscopy, image documentation and report

➋ *CPT Changes: An Insider's View* 2006

➋ *Clinical Examples in Radiology* Winter 06:15

In this example, the blue reference symbol indicates that in the 2006 edition of *CPT Changes: An Insider's View* information is available that may assist in understanding the application of the code. The red reference symbol indicates that the 2006 Winter issue of *Clinical Examples in Radiology* (page 15) should be consulted.

CPT Assistant and *Clinical Examples in Radiology* are available online. Benefits exclusive to the online versions include:

• Monthly (*CPT Assistant*) and quarterly (*Clinical Examples in Radiology*) updates! The home screen notifies you when a new issue is available, and you can review the latest issue in its entirety.

• Unlimited access to every archived issue and article dating back to when the newsletters first published.

• A historical CPT code list that references when a code was added, deleted, and/or revised since 1990.

• Simple search capabilities, including intuitive menus and a cumulative index of article titles.

• A full archive of *CPT Assistant* articles (1990-2024) is also available in the *CPT Professional* print and digital app bundle (see the following information about the *CPT QuickRef* app).

The *CPT QuickRef* app is available for iOS (Apple) and Android devices (smart phones and tablets). The *QuickRef* app contains important coding and billing tools, including:

• The entire CPT 2025 code set (full codes, descriptions, icons, illustrations, and parenthetical notes), plus the entire 2024 code set to facilitate the year-end code set transition.

• Facility and non-facility RVUs and Global Days.

• Medicare Physician Fee Schedule calculator that can be set to a specific geographic region (GPCI).

• *CPT Assistant* Archive: all content and every issue of *CPT Assistant* from 1990 through 2024, linked to the pertinent CPT codes and available for browsing.

• Official AMA CPT coding guidelines linked to each CPT code.

• More than 200 AMA-created colorized procedural and anatomical illustrations

• Modifiers

• Keyword and code number search

• Favorites capability, to store most-frequently used codes or modifiers for easy access.

For more information, call 800 621-8335.

Illustrated Anatomical and Procedural Review

It is essential that coders have a thorough understanding of medical terminology and anatomy to code accurately. The following section reviewing the basics of vocabulary and anatomy can be used as a quick reference to help you with your coding. It is not intended as a replacement for up-to-date medical dictionaries and anatomy texts, which are essential tools for accurate coding.

Prefixes, Suffixes, and Roots

Although medical terminology may seem complex, many medical terms can be broken into component parts, which makes them easier to understand. Many of these terms are derived from Latin or Greek words, but some include the names of physicians.

Prefixes are word parts that appear at the beginning of a word and modify its meaning; suffixes are found at the end of words. By learning what various prefixes and suffixes mean, it is possible to decipher the meaning of a word quickly. The following lists are a quick reference for some common prefixes and suffixes.

Numbers

Prefix	Meaning	Example
mono-, uni-	one	monocyte, unilateral
bi-	two	bilateral
tri-	three	triad
quadr-	four	quadriplegia
hex-, sex-	six	hexose
diplo-	double	diplopia

Surgical Procedures

Suffix	Meaning	Example
-centesis	puncture a cavity to remove fluid	amniocentesis
-ectomy	surgical removal (excision)	appendectomy
-ostomy	a new permanent opening	colostomy
-otomy	cutting into (incision)	tracheotomy
-orrhaphy	surgical repair/suture	herniorrhaphy
-opexy	surgical fixation	nephropexy
-oplasty	surgical repair	rhinoplasty
-otripsy	crushing, destroying	lithotripsy

Conditions

Prefix	Meaning	Example
ambi-	both	ambidextrous
aniso-	unequal	anisocoria
dys-	bad, painful, difficult	dysphoria
eu-	good, normal	euthanasia
hetero-	different	heterogeneous
homo-	same	homogeneous
hyper-	excessive, above	hypergastric
hypo-	deficient, below	hypogastric
iso-	equal, same	isotonic
mal-	bad, poor	malaise
megalo-	large	megalocardia

Suffix	Meaning	Example
-algia	pain	neuralgia
-asthenia	weakness	myasthenia
-emia	blood	anemia
-iasis	condition of	amebiasis
-itis	inflammation	appendicitis
-lysis	destruction, break down	hemolysis
-lytic	destroy, break down	hemolytic
-oid	like	lipoid
-oma	tumor	carcinoma
-opathy	disease of	arthropathy
-orrhagia	hemorrhage	menorrhagia
-orrhea	flow or discharge	amenorrhea
-osis	abnormal condition of	tuberculosis
-paresis	weakness	hemiparesis
-plasia	growth	hyperplasia
-plegia	paralysis	paraplegia
-pnea	breathing	apnea

Directions and Positions

Prefix	Meaning	Example
ab-	away from	abduction
ad-	toward	adduction
ecto, exo-	outside	ectopic, exocrine
endo-	within	endoscope
epi-	upon	epigastric
infra-	below, under	infrastructure
ipsi-	same	ipsilateral
meso-	middle	mesopexy
meta-	after, beyond, transformation	metastasis
peri-	surrounding	pericardium
retro-	behind, back	retroversion
trans-	across, through	transvaginal

Word	Meaning
anterior or ventral	at or near the front surface of the body
posterior or dorsal	at or near the back surface of the body
superior	above
inferior	below
lateral	side
distal	farthest from center
proximal	nearest to center
medial	middle
supine	face up or palm up
prone	face down or palm down
sagittal	vertical body plane, divides the body into equal right and left sides
transverse	horizontal body plane, divides the body into top and bottom sections
coronal	vertical body plane, divides the body into front and back sections

Additional References

For best coding results, you will need to use other reference materials in addition to your CPT® coding books. These references include medical dictionaries and anatomy books.

Medical Dictionaries

Dorland's Illustrated Medical Dictionary, 33rd ed.
Philadelphia, PA: Elsevier; 2020.

Stedman's CPT® Dictionary, 2nd ed.
Chicago, IL: American Medical Association; 2009.
OP:300609

Stedman's Medical Dictionary. 28th ed.
Philadelphia, PA: Lippincott; 2005.

Anatomy References

Bernard, SP. *Netter's Atlas of Human Anatomy for CPT® Surgery.*
Chicago, IL: American Medical Association; 2015.
OP495015

Kirschner, CG. *Netter's Atlas of Human Anatomy for CPT® Coding*, 3rd ed.
Chicago, IL: American Medical Association; 2019.
OP490619

Netter, FH. *Atlas of Human Anatomy*, 6th ed.
Philadelphia, PA; Elsevier; 2014.
OP936714

Lists of Illustrations

To further aid coders in properly assigning CPT codes, the codebook contains a number of anatomical and procedural illustrations.

Anatomical Illustrations

Thirty-five anatomical illustrations are located on the following pages:

Procedural Illustrations

Procedural illustrations are placed throughout the codebook and are associated with the following specific CPT codes.

Figure 1A

Body Planes — 3/4 View

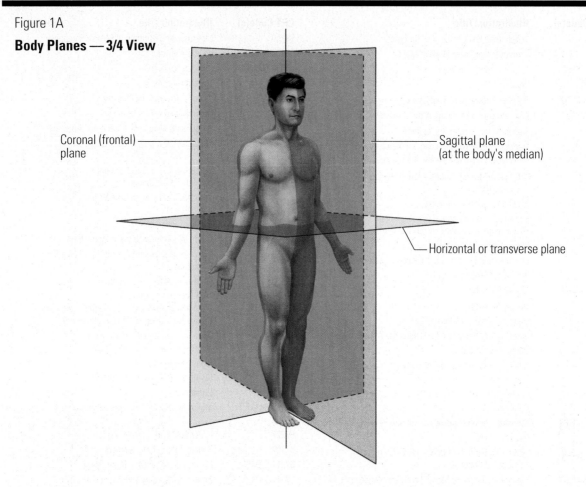

Coronal (frontal) plane

Sagittal plane (at the body's median)

Horizontal or transverse plane

Figure 1B

Body Aspects — Side View

Superior (cranial) aspect

Posterior aspect

Anterior aspect

Dorsal surface of hand

Palmar surface of hand

Dorsal surface of foot

Plantar surface of foot

Inferior aspect

Figure 1C

Body Planes — Front View

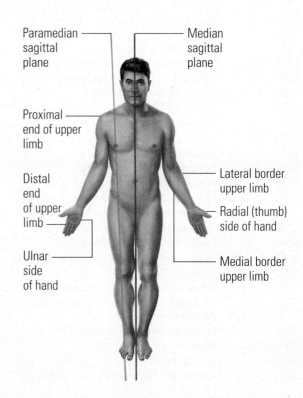

Paramedian sagittal plane

Median sagittal plane

Proximal end of upper limb

Distal end of upper limb

Ulnar side of hand

Lateral border upper limb

Radial (thumb) side of hand

Medial border upper limb

Office or Other Outpatient Services

Patient: New

Code	99202	99203	99204	99205
REQUIRED ELEMENTS				
Medically Appropriate History and/or Examination	X	X	X	X
Medical Decision Making (MDM) Level				
Straightforward	X			
Low		X		
Moderate			X	
High				X
Or				
Total Time (On Date of the Encounter)				
Minutes	15	30	45	60

Office or Other Outpatient Services

Patient: Established

Code	99211	99212	99213	99214	99215
REQUIRED ELEMENTS					
Medically Appropriate History and/or Examination	N/A	X	X	X	X
Medical Decision Making (MDM) Level					
Straightforward	N/A		X		
Low				X	
Moderate					X
High					X
Or					
Total Time (On Date of the Encounter)					
Minutes	N/A	10	20	30	40

Telemedicine: Synchronous Audio-Video E/M Services

Patient: New

Code	98000	98001	98002	98003
REQUIRED ELEMENTS				
Medically Appropriate History and/or Examination	X	X	X	X
Medical Decision Making (MDM) Level				
Straightforward	X			
Low		X		
Moderate			X	
High				X
Or				
Total Time (On Date of the Encounter)				
Minutes	15	30	45	60

Telemedicine: Synchronous Audio-Video E/M Services

Patient: Established

Code	98004	98005	98006	98007
REQUIRED ELEMENTS				
Medically Appropriate History and/or Examination	X	X	X	X
Medical Decision Making (MDM) Level				
Straightforward	X			
Low		X		
Moderate			X	
High				X
Or				
Total Time (On Date of the Encounter)				
Minutes	10	20	30	40

Telemedicine: Synchronous Audio-Only E/M Services

Patient: New

Code	98008	98009	98010	98011
REQUIRED ELEMENTS				
More than 10 Minutes of Medical Discussion	X	X	X	X
Medically Appropriate History and/or Examination	X	X	X	X
Medical Decision Making (MDM) Level				
Straightforward	X			
Low		X		
Moderate			X	
High				X
Or				
Total Time (On Date of the Encounter)				
Minutes	15	30	45	60

Telemedicine: Brief Synchronous Communication Technology Service

Patient: Established

Code	98016
Medical Discussion	5-10 Minutes

Telemedicine: Synchronous Audio-Only E/M Services

Patient: Established

Code	98012	98013	98014	98015
REQUIRED ELEMENTS				
More than 10 Minutes of Medical Discussion	X	X	X	X
Medically Appropriate History and/or Examination	X	X	X	X
Medical Decision Making (MDM) Level				
Straightforward	X			
Low		X		
Moderate			X	
High				X
Or				
Total Time (On Date of the Encounter)				
Minutes	10	20	30	40

Initial Hospital Inpatient Or Observation Care

Patient: New or Established

Code	99221	99222	99223
REQUIRED ELEMENTS			
Medically Appropriate History and/or Examination	X	X	X
Medical Decision Making (MDM) Level			
Straightforward or Low	X		
Moderate		X	
High			X
Or			
Total Time (On Date of the Encounter)			
Minutes	40	55	75

Subsequent Hospital Inpatient Or Observation Care

Patient: New or Established

Code	99231	99232	99233
REQUIRED ELEMENTS			
Medically Appropriate History and/or Examination	X	X	X
Medical Decision Making (MDM) Level			
Straightforward or Low	X		
Moderate		X	
High			X
Or			
Total Time (On Date of the Encounter)			
Minutes	25	35	50

Hospital Inpatient or Observation Care Services (Including Admission and Discharge Services)

Patient: New or Established

Code	99234	99235	99236
REQUIRED ELEMENTS			
Medically Appropriate History and/or Examination	X	X	X
Medical Decision Making (MDM) Level			
Straightforward or Low	X		
Moderate		X	
High			X
Or			
Total Time (On Date of the Encounter)			
Minutes	45	70	85

Office or Other Outpatient Consultations

Patient: New or Established

Code	99242	99243	99244	99245
REQUIRED ELEMENTS				
Medically Appropriate History and/or Examination	X	X	X	X
Medical Decision Making (MDM) Level				
Straightforward	X			
Low		X		
Moderate			X	
High				X
Or				
Total Time (On Date of the Encounter)				
Minutes	20	30	40	55

Inpatient or Observation Consultations

Patient: New or Established

Code	99252	99253	99254	99255
REQUIRED ELEMENTS				
Medically Appropriate History and/or Examination	X	X	X	X
Medical Decision Making (MDM) Level				
Straightforward	X			
Low		X		
Moderate			X	
High				X
Or				
Total Time (On Date of the Encounter)				
Minutes	35	45	60	80

Emergency Department Services

Patient: New or Established

Code	99281	99282	99283	99284	99285
REQUIRED ELEMENTS					
Medically Appropriate History and/or Examination	N/A	X	X	X	X
Medical Decision Making (MDM) Level					
Straightforward	N/A	X			
Low			X		
Moderate				X	
High					X
Total Time (On Date of the Encounter)					
N/A					

Subsequent Nursing Facility Care

Patient: New or Established

Code	99307	99308	99309	99310
REQUIRED ELEMENTS				
Medically Appropriate History and/or Examination	X	X	X	X
Medical Decision Making (MDM) Level				
Straightforward	X			
Low		X		
Moderate			X	
High				X
Or				
Total Time (On Date of the Encounter)				
Minutes	10	20	30	45

Initial Nursing Facility Care

Patient: New or Established

Code	99304	99305	99306
REQUIRED ELEMENTS			
Medically Appropriate History and/or Examination	X	X	X
Medical Decision Making (MDM) Level			
Straightforward or Low	X		
Moderate		X	
High			X
Or			
Total Time (On Date of the Encounter)			
Minutes	25	35	50

Home or Residence Services

Patient: New

Code	99341	99342	99344	99345
REQUIRED ELEMENTS				
Medically Appropriate History and/or Examination	X	X	X	X
Medical Decision Making (MDM) Level				
Straightforward	X			
Low		X		
Moderate			X	
High				X
Or				
Total Time (On Date of the Encounter)				
Minutes	15	30	60	75

Home or Residence Services

Patient: Established

Code	99347	99348	99349	99350
REQUIRED ELEMENTS				
Medically Appropriate History and/or Examination	X	X	X	X
Medical Decision Making (MDM) Level				
Straightforward	X			
Low		X		
Moderate			X	
High				X
Or				
Total Time (On Date of the Encounter)				
Minutes	20	30	40	60

Neonatal and Pediatric Critical/Intensive Care

Initial Inpatient Neonatal and Pediatric Critical Care

Code	99468	99471	99475	99291–99292
Age	28 days or younger	29 days–24 mos	2–5 yrs	6 yrs +

Subsequent Inpatient Neonatal and Pediatric Critical Care

Code	99469	99472	99476	99291–99292
Age	28 days or younger	29 days–24 mos	2–5 yrs	6 yrs +

Initial Neonatal Intensive Care

Code	99477
Age	28 days of age or younger
	Requires intensive observation, frequent interventions, and other intensive care services

Continuing Neonatal and Infant Inpatient Low Birth-Weight Intensive Care

Code	99478	99479	99480	99231–99233
Weight	less than 1500 g	1500–2500 g	2501–5000 g	+5000 g

Reporting Critical Care Time

Total Duration of Critical Care	CPT Codes
Less than 30 minutes	Appropriate E/M codes
30–74 minutes (30 minutes–1 hour 14 minutes)	**99291 x1**
75–104 minutes (1 hour 15 minutes–1 hour 44 minutes)	**99291 x1** and **99292 x1**
105–134 minutes (1 hour 45 minutes–2 hours 14 minutes)	**99291 x1** and **99292 x2**
135–164 minutes (2 hours 15 minutes–2 hours 44 minutes)	**99291 x1** and **99292 x3**
165–194 minutes (2 hours 45 minutes–3 hours 14 minutes)	**99291 x1** and **99292 x4**
195 minutes or longer (3 hours 15 minutes–etc)	**99291** and **99292** as appropriate

Evaluation and Management (E/M) Services Guidelines

The following is a listing of headings and subheadings that appear within the Evaluation and Management section of the CPT codebook. The subheadings or subsections denoted with asterisks (*) below have special instructions unique to that subsection. Where these are indicated, special notes or guidelines will be presented preceding those procedural terminology listings, referring to that subsection specifically. Note that all code ranges in each subsection are listed as they appear in the subsection, even if the code numbers are out of numerical sequence and/or repeated in the next subsection.

Evaluation and Management

Evaluation and Management (E/M) Services Guidelines

In addition to the information presented in the Introduction, several other items unique to this section are defined or identified here.

E/M Guidelines Overview

The E/M guidelines have sections that are common to all E/M categories and sections that are category specific. Most of the categories and many of the subcategories of service have special guidelines or instructions unique to that category or subcategory. Where these are indicated, eg, "Hospital Inpatient and Observation Care," special instructions are presented before the listing of the specific E/M services codes. It is important to review the instructions for each category or subcategory. These guidelines are to be used by the reporting physician or other qualified health care professional to select the appropriate level of service. These guidelines do not establish documentation requirements or standards of care. The main purpose of documentation is to support care of the patient by current and future health care team(s). These guidelines are for services that require a face-to-face encounter with the patient and/or family/caregiver. (For 99211 and 99281, the face-to-face services may be performed by clinical staff.)

▶In the **Evaluation and Management** section (98000-98016, 99202-99499), there are many code categories. Each category may have specific guidelines, or the codes may include specific details. These E/M guidelines are written for the following categories:

- Office or Other Outpatient Services
- Telemedicine Services
- Hospital Inpatient and Observation Care Services
- Consultations
- Emergency Department Services
- Nursing Facility Services
- Home or Residence Services
- Prolonged Service With or Without Direct Patient Contact on the Date of an Evaluation and Management Service◀

Classification of Evaluation and Management (E/M) Services

The E/M section is divided into broad categories, such as office visits, hospital inpatient or observation care visits, and consultations. Most of the categories are further divided into two or more subcategories of E/M services. For example, there are two subcategories of office visits (new patient and established patient) and there are two subcategories of hospital inpatient and observation care visits (initial and subsequent). The subcategories of E/M services are further classified into levels of E/M services that are identified by specific codes.

The basic format of codes with levels of E/M services based on medical decision making (MDM) or time is the same. First, a unique code number is listed. Second, the place and/or type of service is specified (eg, office or other outpatient visit). Third, the content of the service is defined. Fourth, time is specified. (A detailed discussion of time is provided in the Guidelines for Selecting Level of Service Based on Time.)

The place of service and service type are defined by the location where the face-to-face encounter with the patient and/or family/caregiver occurs. For example, service provided to a nursing facility resident brought to the office is reported with an office or other outpatient code.

New and Established Patients

Solely for the purposes of distinguishing between new and established patients, **professional services** are those face-to-face services rendered by physicians and other qualified health care professionals who may report evaluation and management services. A new patient is one who has not received any professional services from the physician or other qualified health care professional or another physician or other qualified health care professional of the **exact** same specialty **and subspecialty** who belongs to the same group practice, within the past three years.

An established patient is one who has received professional services from the physician or other qualified health care professional or another physician or other qualified health care professional of the **exact** same specialty **and subspecialty** who belongs to the same group practice, within the past three years. See Decision Tree for New vs Established Patients.

In the instance where a physician or other qualified health care professional is on call for or covering for another physician or other qualified health care professional, the patient's encounter will be classified as it would have been by the physician or other qualified health care professional who is not available. When advanced practice nurses and physician assistants are working with physicians, they are considered as working in the **exact** same specialty **and subspecialty** as the physician.

No distinction is made between new and established patients in the emergency department. E/M services in the emergency department category may be reported for any new or established patient who presents for treatment in the emergency department.

The Decision Tree for New vs Established Patients is provided to aid in determining whether to report the E/M service provided as a new or an established patient encounter.

── *Coding Tip* ──

Instructions for Use of the CPT Codebook

When advanced practice nurses and physician assistants are working with physicians, they are considered as working in the exact same specialty and subspecialty as the physician. A "physician or other qualified health care professional" is an individual who is qualified by education, training, licensure/regulation (when applicable), and facility privileging (when applicable) who performs a professional service within his or her scope of practice and independently reports that professional service. These professionals are distinct from "clinical staff." A clinical staff member is a person who works under the supervision of a physician or other qualified health care professional, and who is allowed by law, regulation and facility policy to perform or assist in the performance of a specific professional service but does not individually report that professional service. Other policies may also affect who may report specific services.

CPT Coding Guidelines, Introduction, Instructions for Use of the CPT Codebook

Initial and Subsequent Services

Some categories apply to both new and established patients (eg, hospital inpatient or observation care). These categories differentiate services by whether the service is the initial service or a subsequent service. For the purpose of distinguishing between initial or subsequent visits, professional services are those face-to-face services rendered by physicians and other qualified health care professionals who may report evaluation and management services. An initial service is when the patient has not received any professional services from the physician or other qualified health care professional or another physician or other qualified health care

professional of the exact same specialty and subspecialty who belongs to the same group practice, during the inpatient, observation, or nursing facility admission and stay.

A subsequent service is when the patient has received professional service(s) from the physician or other qualified health care professional or another physician or other qualified health care professional of the exact same specialty and subspecialty who belongs to the same group practice, during the admission and stay.

In the instance when a physician or other qualified health care professional is on call for or covering for another physician or other qualified health care professional, the patient's encounter will be classified as it would have been by the physician or other qualified health care professional who is not available. When advanced practice nurses and physician assistants are working with physicians, they are considered as working in the exact same specialty and subspecialty as the physician.

For reporting hospital inpatient or observation care services, a stay that includes a transition from observation to inpatient is a single stay. For reporting nursing facility services, a stay that includes transition(s) between skilled nursing facility and nursing facility level of care is the same stay.

Split or Shared Visits

Physician(s) and other qualified health care professional(s) (QHP[s]) may act as a team in providing care for the patient, working together during a single E/M service. The split or shared visits guidelines are applied to determine which professional may report the service. If the physician or other QHP performs a substantive portion of the encounter, the physician or other QHP may report the service. If code selection is based on total time on the date of the encounter, the service is reported by the professional who spent the majority of the face-to-face or non-face-to-face time performing the service. For the purpose of reporting E/M services within the context of team-based care, performance of a substantive part of the MDM requires that the physician(s) or other QHP(s) made or approved the management plan for the *number and complexity of problems addressed at the encounter* and takes responsibility for that plan with its inherent *risk of complications and/or morbidity or mortality of patient management*. By doing so, a physician or other QHP has performed two of the three elements used in the selection of the code level based on MDM. If *the amount and/or complexity of data to be reviewed and analyzed* is used by the physician or other QHP to determine the reported code level, assessing an independent historian's narrative and the ordering or review of tests or documents do not have to be personally performed by the physician or other QHP, because the relevant items would be considered in formulating the management plan. Independent interpretation of tests

Decision Tree for New vs Established Patients

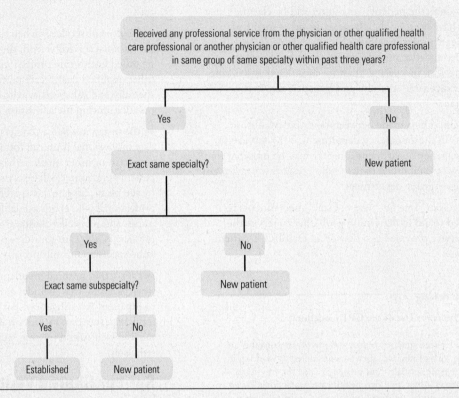

and discussion of management plan or test interpretation must be personally performed by the physician or other QHP if these are used to determine the reported code level by the physician or other QHP.

Multiple Evaluation and Management Services on the Same Date

The following guidelines apply to services that a patient may receive for hospital inpatient care, observation care, or nursing facility care. For instructions regarding transitions to these settings from the office or outpatient, home or residence, or emergency department setting, see guidelines for **Hospital Inpatient and Observation Care Services** or **Nursing Facility Services**.

A patient may receive E/M services in more than one setting on a calendar date. A patient may also have more than one visit in the same setting on a calendar date. The guidelines for multiple E/M services on the same date address circumstances in which the patient has received multiple visits or services from the same physician or other QHP or another physician or other QHP of the exact same specialty and subspecialty who belongs to the same group practice.

Per day: The hospital inpatient and observation care services and the nursing facility services are "per day" services. When multiple visits occur over the course of a single calendar date in the same setting, a single service is reported. When using MDM for code level selection, use the aggregated MDM over the course of the calendar date. When using time for code level selection, sum the time over the course of the day using the guidelines for reporting time.

Multiple encounters in different settings or facilities: A patient may be seen and treated in different facilities (eg, a hospital-to-hospital transfer). When more than one primary E/M service is reported and time is used to select the code level for either service, only the time spent providing that individual service may be allocated to the code level selected for reporting that service. No time may be counted twice when reporting more than one E/M service. Prolonged services are also based on the same allocation and their relationship to the primary service. The designation of the facility may be defined by licensure or regulation. Transfer from a hospital bed to a nursing facility bed in a hospital with nursing facility beds is considered as two services in two facilities because there is a discharge from one type of designation to another. An intra-facility transfer for a different level of care (eg, from a routine unit to a critical care unit) does not constitute a new stay, nor does it constitute a transfer to a different facility.

Emergency department (ED) and services in other settings (same or different facilities): Time spent in an ED by a physician or other QHP who provides subsequent E/M services may be included in calculating total time on the date of the encounter when ED services are not reported and another E/M service is reported (eg, hospital inpatient and observation care services).

Discharge services and services in other facilities: Each service may be reported separately as long as any time spent on the discharge service is not counted towards the total time of a subsequent service in which code level selection for the subsequent service is based on time. This includes any hospital inpatient or observation care services (including admission and discharge services) time (99234, 99235, 99236) because these services may be selected based on MDM or time. When these services are reported with another E/M service on the same calendar date, time related to the hospital inpatient or observation care service (including admission and discharge services) may not be used for code selection of the subsequent service.

Discharge services and services in the same facility: If the patient is discharged and readmitted to the same facility on the same calendar date, report a subsequent care service instead of a discharge or initial service. For the purpose of E/M reporting, this is a single stay.

Discharge services and services in a different facility: If the patient is admitted to another facility, for the purpose of E/M reporting this is considered a different stay. Discharge and initial services may be reported as long as time spent on the discharge service is not counted towards the total time of the subsequent service reported when code level selection is based on time.

Critical care services (including neonatal intensive care services and pediatric and neonatal critical care): Reporting guidelines for intensive and critical care services that are performed on the same calendar date as another E/M service are described in the service specific section guidelines.

Transitions between office or other outpatient, home or residence, or emergency department and hospital inpatient or observation or nursing facility: See the guidelines for **Hospital Inpatient and Observation Care Services** or **Nursing Facility Services.** If the patient is seen in two settings and only one service is reported, the total time on the date of the encounter or the aggregated MDM is used for determining the level of the single reported service. If prolonged services are reported, use the prolonged services code that is appropriate for the primary service reported, regardless of where the patient was located when the prolonged services time threshold was met. The choice of the primary service is at the discretion of the reporting physician or other QHP.

Services Reported Separately

Any specifically identifiable procedure or service (ie, identified with a specific CPT code) performed on the date of E/M services may be reported separately.

The ordering and actual performance and/or interpretation of diagnostic tests/studies during a patient encounter are not included in determining the levels of E/M services when the professional interpretation of those tests/studies is reported separately by the physician or other qualified health care professional reporting the E/M service. Tests that do not require separate interpretation (eg, tests that are results only) and are analyzed as part of MDM do not count as an independent interpretation, but may be counted as ordered or reviewed for selecting an MDM level. The performance of diagnostic tests/studies for which specific CPT codes are available may be reported separately, in addition to the appropriate E/M code. The interpretation of the results of diagnostic tests/studies (ie, professional component) with preparation of a separate distinctly identifiable signed written report may also be reported separately, using the appropriate CPT code and, if required, with modifier 26 appended.

The physician or other qualified health care professional may need to indicate that on the day a procedure or service identified by a CPT code was performed, the patient's condition required a significant separately identifiable E/M service. The E/M service may be caused or prompted by the symptoms or condition for which the procedure and/or service was provided. This circumstance may be reported by adding modifier 25 to the appropriate level of E/M service. As such, different diagnoses are not required for reporting of the procedure and the E/M services on the same date.

History and/or Examination

E/M codes that have levels of services include a medically appropriate history and/or physical examination, when performed. The nature and extent of the history and/or physical examination are determined by the treating physician or other qualified health care professional reporting the service. The care team may collect information, and the patient or caregiver may supply information directly (eg, by electronic health record [EHR] portal or questionnaire) that is reviewed by the reporting physician or other qualified health care professional. The extent of history and physical examination is not an element in selection of the level of these E/M service codes.

Levels of E/M Services

Select the appropriate level of E/M services based on the following:

1. The level of the MDM as defined for each service, **or**
2. The total time for E/M services performed on the date of the encounter.

Within each category or subcategory of E/M service based on MDM or time, there are three to five levels of E/M services available for reporting purposes. Levels of E/M services are **not** interchangeable among the different categories or subcategories of service. For example, the first level of E/M services in the subcategory of office visit, new patient, does not have the same definition as the first level of E/M services in the subcategory of office visit, established patient. Each level of E/M services may be used by all physicians or other qualified health care professionals.

Guidelines for Selecting Level of Service Based on Medical Decision Making

Four types of MDM are recognized: straightforward, low, moderate, and high. The concept of the level of MDM does not apply to 99211, 99281.

MDM includes establishing diagnoses, assessing the status of a condition, and/or selecting a management option. MDM is defined by three elements. The elements are:

- *The number and complexity of problem(s) that are addressed during the encounter.*

- *The amount and/or complexity of data to be reviewed and analyzed.* These data include medical records, tests, and/or other information that must be obtained, ordered, reviewed, and analyzed for the encounter. This includes information obtained from multiple sources or interprofessional communications that are not reported separately and interpretation of tests that are not reported separately. Ordering a test is included in the category of test result(s) and the review of the test result is part of the encounter and not a subsequent encounter. Ordering a test may include those considered but not selected after shared decision making. For example, a patient may request diagnostic imaging that is not necessary for their condition and discussion of the lack of benefit may be required. Alternatively, a test may normally be performed, but due to the risk for a specific patient it is not ordered. These considerations must be documented. Data are divided into three categories:

  - Tests, documents, orders, or independent historian(s). (Each unique test, order, or document is counted to meet a threshold number.)

  - Independent interpretation of tests (not separately reported).

  - Discussion of management or test interpretation with external physician or other qualified health care professional or appropriate source (not separately reported).

- *The risk of complications and/or morbidity or mortality of patient management.* This includes decisions made at the encounter associated with diagnostic procedure(s) and treatment(s). This includes the possible management options selected and those considered but not selected after shared decision making with the patient and/or family. For example, a decision about hospitalization includes consideration of alternative levels of care. Examples may include a psychiatric patient with a sufficient degree of support in the outpatient setting or the decision to not hospitalize a patient with advanced dementia with an acute condition that would generally warrant inpatient care, but for whom the goal is palliative treatment.

Shared decision making involves eliciting patient and/or family preferences, patient and/or family education, and explaining risks and benefits of management options.

MDM may be impacted by role and management responsibility.

When the physician or other qualified health care professional is reporting a separate CPT code that includes interpretation and/or report, the interpretation and/or report is not counted toward the MDM when selecting a level of E/M services. When the physician or other qualified health care professional is reporting a separate service for discussion of management with a physician or another qualified health care professional, the discussion is not counted toward the MDM when selecting a level of E/M services.

The Levels of Medical Decision Making (MDM) table (Table 1) is a guide to assist in selecting the level of MDM for reporting an E/M services code. The table includes the four levels of MDM (ie, straightforward, low, moderate, high) and the three elements of MDM (ie, number and complexity of problems addressed at the encounter, amount and/or complexity of data reviewed and analyzed, and risk of complications and/or morbidity or mortality of patient management). To qualify for a particular level of MDM, two of the three elements for that level of MDM must be met or exceeded.

Examples in the table may be more or less applicable to specific settings of care. For example, the decision to hospitalize applies to the outpatient or nursing facility encounters, whereas the decision to escalate hospital level of care (eg, transfer to ICU) applies to the hospitalized or observation care patient. See also the introductory guidelines of each code family section.

The elements listed in Table 1, Levels of Medical Decision Making, are defined in the guidelines for number and complexity of problems addressed at the encounter, amount and/or complexity of data to be reviewed and analyzed, and risk of complications and/or morbidity or mortality of patient management.

Number and Complexity of Problems Addressed at the Encounter

One element used in selecting the level of service is the number and complexity of the problems that are addressed at the encounter. Multiple new or established conditions may be addressed at the same time and may affect MDM. Symptoms may cluster around a specific diagnosis and each symptom is not necessarily a unique condition. Comorbidities and underlying diseases, in and of themselves, are not considered in selecting a level of E/M services **unless** they are addressed, and their presence increases the amount and/or complexity of data to be reviewed and analyzed or the risk of complications and/or morbidity or mortality of patient management. The final diagnosis for a condition does not, in and of itself, determine the complexity or risk, as extensive evaluation may be required to reach the conclusion that the signs or symptoms do not represent a highly morbid condition. Therefore, presenting symptoms that are likely to represent a highly morbid condition may "drive"

MDM even when the ultimate diagnosis is not highly morbid. The evaluation and/or treatment should be consistent with the likely nature of the condition. Multiple problems of a lower severity may, in the aggregate, create higher risk due to interaction.

The term "risk" as used in the definition of this element relates to risk from the condition. While condition risk and management risk may often correlate, the risk from the condition is distinct from the risk of the management.

Problem: A problem is a disease, condition, illness, injury, symptom, sign, finding, complaint, or other matter addressed at the encounter, with or without a diagnosis being established at the time of the encounter.

Problem addressed: A problem is addressed or managed when it is evaluated or treated at the encounter by the physician or other qualified health care professional reporting the service. This includes consideration of further testing or treatment that may not be elected by virtue of risk/benefit analysis or patient/parent/guardian/surrogate choice. Notation in the patient's medical record that another professional is managing the problem without additional assessment or care coordination documented does not qualify as being addressed or managed by the physician or other qualified health care professional reporting the service. Referral without evaluation (by history, examination, or diagnostic

(continued on page 11)

Table 1: Levels of Medical Decision Making (MDM)

	Elements of Medical Decision Making		
Level of MDM (Based on 2 out of 3 Elements of MDM)	**Number and Complexity of Problems Addressed at the Encounter**	**Amount and/or Complexity of Data to Be Reviewed and Analyzed** **Each unique test, order, or document contributes to the combination of 2 or combination of 3 in Category 1 below.*	**Risk of Complications and/or Morbidity or Mortality of Patient Management**
Straightforward	**Minimal** ▪ **1** self-limited or minor problem	**Minimal or none**	**Minimal risk of morbidity from additional diagnostic testing or treatment**
Low	**Low** ▪ **2** or more self-limited or minor problems; or ▪ **1** stable, chronic illness; or ▪ **1** acute, uncomplicated illness or injury; or ▪ **1** stable, acute illness; or ▪ **1** acute, uncomplicated illness or injury requiring hospital inpatient or observation level of care	**Limited** *(Must meet the requirements of at least 1 out of 2 categories)* **Category 1: Tests and documents** ▪ **Any combination of 2 from the following:** • Review of prior external note(s) from each unique source*; • Review of the result(s) of each unique test*; • Ordering of each unique test* **or** **Category 2: Assessment requiring an independent historian(s)** *(For the categories of independent interpretation of tests and discussion of management or test interpretation, see moderate or high)*	**Low risk of morbidity from additional diagnostic testing or treatment**

(continued)

Elements of Medical Decision Making

Level of MDM (Based on 2 out of 3 Elements of MDM)	Number and Complexity of Problems Addressed at the Encounter	Amount and/or Complexity of Data to Be Reviewed and Analyzed *Each unique test, order, or document contributes to the combination of 2 or combination of 3 in Category 1 below.*	Risk of Complications and/or Morbidity or Mortality of Patient Management
Moderate	**Moderate** ■ **1** or more chronic illnesses with exacerbation, progression, or side effects of treatment; **or** ■ **2** or more stable, chronic illnesses; **or** ■ **1** undiagnosed new problem with uncertain prognosis; **or** ■ **1** acute illness with systemic symptoms; **or** ■ **1** acute, complicated injury	**Moderate** *(Must meet the requirements of at least 1 out of 3 categories)* **Category 1: Tests, documents, or independent historian(s)** ■ **Any combination of 3 from the following:** • Review of prior external note(s) from each unique source*; • Review of the result(s) of each unique test*; • Ordering of each unique test*; • Assessment requiring an independent historian(s) **or** **Category 2: Independent interpretation of tests** ■ Independent interpretation of a test performed by another physician/other qualified health care professional (not separately reported); **or** **Category 3: Discussion of management or test interpretation** ■ Discussion of management or test interpretation with external physician/other qualified health care professional/appropriate source (not separately reported)	**Moderate risk of morbidity from additional diagnostic testing or treatment** *Examples only:* ■ Prescription drug management ■ Decision regarding minor surgery with identified patient or procedure risk factors ■ Decision regarding elective major surgery without identified patient or procedure risk factors ■ Diagnosis or treatment significantly limited by social determinants of health
High	**High** ■ **1** or more chronic illnesses with severe exacerbation, progression, or side effects of treatment; **or** ■ **1** acute or chronic illness or injury that poses a threat to life or bodily function	**Extensive** *(Must meet the requirements of at least 2 out of 3 categories)* **Category 1: Tests, documents, or independent historian(s)** ■ **Any combination of 3 from the following:** • Review of prior external note(s) from each unique source*; • Review of the result(s) of each unique test*; • Ordering of each unique test*; • Assessment requiring an independent historian(s) **or** **Category 2: Independent interpretation of tests** ■ Independent interpretation of a test performed by another physician/other qualified health care professional (not separately reported); **or** **Category 3: Discussion of management or test interpretation** ■ Discussion of management or test interpretation with external physician/other qualified health care professional/appropriate source (not separately reported)	**High risk of morbidity from additional diagnostic testing or treatment** *Examples only:* ■ Drug therapy requiring intensive monitoring for toxicity ■ Decision regarding elective major surgery with identified patient or procedure risk factors ■ Decision regarding emergency major surgery ■ Decision regarding hospitalization or escalation of hospital-level care ■ Decision not to resuscitate or to de-escalate care because of poor prognosis ■ Decision regarding parenteral controlled substances

(continued from page 9)

study[ies]) or consideration of treatment does not qualify as being addressed or managed by the physician or other qualified health care professional reporting the service. For hospital inpatient and observation care services, the problem addressed is the problem status on the date of the encounter, which may be significantly different than on admission. It is the problem being managed or co-managed by the reporting physician or other qualified health care professional and may not be the cause of admission or continued stay.

Minimal problem: A problem that may not require the presence of the physician or other qualified health care professional, but the service is provided under the physician's or other qualified health care professional's supervision (see 99211, 99281).

Self-limited or minor problem: A problem that runs a definite and prescribed course, is transient in nature, and is not likely to permanently alter health status.

Stable, chronic illness: A problem with an expected duration of at least one year or until the death of the patient. For the purpose of defining chronicity, conditions are treated as chronic whether or not stage or severity changes (eg, uncontrolled diabetes and controlled diabetes are a single chronic condition). "Stable" for the purposes of categorizing MDM is defined by the specific treatment goals for an individual patient. A patient who is not at his or her treatment goal is not stable, even if the condition has not changed and there is no short-term threat to life or function. For example, a patient with persistently poorly controlled blood pressure for whom better control is a goal is not stable, even if the pressures are not changing and the patient is asymptomatic. The risk of morbidity **without** treatment is significant.

Acute, uncomplicated illness or injury: A recent or new short-term problem with low risk of morbidity for which treatment is considered. There is little to no risk of mortality with treatment, and full recovery without functional impairment is expected. A problem that is normally self-limited or minor but is not resolving consistent with a definite and prescribed course is an acute, uncomplicated illness.

Acute, uncomplicated illness or injury requiring hospital inpatient or observation level care: A recent or new short-term problem with low risk of morbidity for which treatment is required. There is little to no risk of mortality with treatment, and full recovery without functional impairment is expected. The treatment required is delivered in a hospital inpatient or observation level setting.

Stable, acute illness: A problem that is new or recent for which treatment has been initiated. The patient is improved and, while resolution may not be complete, is stable with respect to this condition.

Chronic illness with exacerbation, progression, or side effects of treatment: A chronic illness that is acutely worsening, poorly controlled, or progressing with an intent to control progression and requiring additional supportive care or requiring attention to treatment for side effects.

Undiagnosed new problem with uncertain prognosis: A problem in the differential diagnosis that represents a condition likely to result in a high risk of morbidity without treatment.

Acute illness with systemic symptoms: An illness that causes systemic symptoms and has a high risk of morbidity without treatment. For systemic general symptoms, such as fever, body aches, or fatigue in a minor illness that may be treated to alleviate symptoms, see the definitions for **self-limited or minor problem** or **acute, uncomplicated illness or injury.** Systemic symptoms may not be general but may be single system.

Acute, complicated injury: An injury which requires treatment that includes evaluation of body systems that are not directly part of the injured organ, the injury is extensive, or the treatment options are multiple and/or associated with risk of morbidity.

Chronic illness with severe exacerbation, progression, or side effects of treatment: The severe exacerbation or progression of a chronic illness or severe side effects of treatment that have significant risk of morbidity and may require escalation in level of care.

Acute or chronic illness or injury that poses a threat to life or bodily function: An acute illness with systemic symptoms, an acute complicated injury, or a chronic illness or injury with exacerbation and/or progression or side effects of treatment, that poses a threat to life or bodily function in the near term without treatment. Some symptoms may represent a condition that is significantly probable and poses a potential threat to life or bodily function. These may be included in this category when the evaluation and treatment are consistent with this degree of potential severity.

Amount and/or Complexity of Data to Be Reviewed and Analyzed

One element used in selecting the level of services is the amount and/or complexity of data to be reviewed or analyzed at an encounter.

Analyzed: The process of using the data as part of the MDM. The data element itself may not be subject to analysis (eg, glucose), but it is instead included in the thought processes for diagnosis, evaluation, or treatment. Tests ordered are presumed to be analyzed when the results are reported. Therefore, when they are ordered during an encounter, they are counted in that encounter. Tests that are ordered outside of an encounter may be counted in the encounter in which they are analyzed. In the case of a recurring order, each new result may be counted in the encounter in which it is analyzed. For example, an encounter that includes an order for monthly prothrombin times would count for one prothrombin time ordered and reviewed. Additional future results, if analyzed in a subsequent encounter, may be counted as a single test in that subsequent encounter. Any service for which the professional component is separately reported by the physician or other qualified health care professional reporting the E/M services is not counted as a data element ordered, reviewed, analyzed, or independently interpreted for the purposes of determining the level of MDM.

Test: Tests are imaging, laboratory, psychometric, or physiologic data. A clinical laboratory panel (eg, basic metabolic panel [80047]) is a single test. The differentiation between single or multiple tests is defined in accordance with the CPT code set. For the purpose of data reviewed and analyzed, pulse oximetry is not a test.

Unique: A unique test is defined by the CPT code set. When multiple results of the same unique test (eg, serial blood glucose values) are compared during an E/M service, count it as one unique test. Tests that have overlapping elements are not unique, even if they are identified with distinct CPT codes. For example, a CBC with differential would incorporate the set of hemoglobin, CBC without differential, and platelet count. A unique source is defined as a physician or other qualified health care professional in a distinct group or different specialty or subspecialty, or a unique entity. Review of all materials from any unique source counts as one element toward MDM.

Combination of data elements: A combination of different data elements, for example, a combination of notes reviewed, tests ordered, tests reviewed, or independent historian, allows these elements to be summed. It does not require each item type or category to be represented. A unique test ordered, plus a note reviewed and an independent historian would be a combination of three elements.

External: External records, communications and/or test results are from an external physician, other qualified health care professional, facility, or health care organization.

External physician or other qualified health care professional: An external physician or other qualified health care professional who is not in the same group practice or is of a different specialty or subspecialty. This includes licensed professionals who are practicing independently. The individual may also be a facility or organizational provider such as from a hospital, nursing facility, or home health care agency.

Discussion: Discussion requires an interactive exchange. The exchange must be direct and not through intermediaries (eg, clinical staff or trainees). Sending chart notes or written exchanges that are within progress notes does not qualify as an interactive exchange. The discussion does not need to be on the date of the encounter, but it is counted only once and only when it is used in the decision making of the encounter. It may be asynchronous (ie, does not need to be in person), but it must be initiated and completed within a short time period (eg, within a day or two).

Independent historian(s): An individual (eg, parent, guardian, surrogate, spouse, witness) who provides a history in addition to a history provided by the patient who is unable to provide a complete or reliable history (eg, due to developmental stage, dementia, or psychosis) or because a confirmatory history is judged to be necessary. In the case where there may be conflict or poor communication between multiple historians and more than one historian is needed, the independent historian requirement is met. It does not include translation services. The independent history does not need to be obtained in person but does need to be obtained directly from the historian providing the independent information.

Independent interpretation: The interpretation of a test for which there is a CPT code, and an interpretation or report is customary. This does not apply when the physician or other qualified health care professional who reports the E/M service is reporting or has previously reported the test. A form of interpretation should be documented but need not conform to the usual standards of a complete report for the test. A test that is ordered and independently interpreted may count both as a test ordered and interpreted.

Appropriate source: For the purpose of the **discussion of management** data element (see Table 1, Levels of Medical Decision Making), an appropriate source includes professionals who are not health care professionals but may be involved in the management of the patient (eg, lawyer, parole officer, case manager, teacher). It does not include discussion with family or informal caregivers. For the purpose of *documents reviewed,* documents from an appropriate source may be counted.

Risk of Complications and/or Morbidity or Mortality of Patient Management

One element used in selecting the level of service is the risk of complications and/or morbidity or mortality of patient management at an encounter. This is distinct from the risk of the condition itself.

Risk: The probability and/or consequences of an event. The assessment of the level of risk is affected by the nature of the event under consideration. For example, a low probability of death may be high risk, whereas a high chance of a minor, self-limited adverse effect of treatment may be low risk. Definitions of risk are based upon the usual behavior and thought processes of a physician or other qualified health care professional in the same specialty. Trained clinicians apply common language usage meanings to terms such as *high, medium, low,* or *minimal* risk and do not require quantification for these definitions (though quantification may be provided when evidence-based medicine has established probabilities). For the purpose of MDM, level of risk is based upon consequences of the problem(s) addressed at the encounter when appropriately treated. Risk also includes MDM related to the need to initiate or forego further testing, treatment, and/or hospitalization. The risk of patient management criteria applies to the patient management decisions made by the reporting physician or other qualified health care professional as part of the reported encounter.

Morbidity: A state of illness or functional impairment that is expected to be of substantial duration during which function is limited, quality of life is impaired, or there is organ damage that may not be transient despite treatment.

Social determinants of health: Economic and social conditions that influence the health of people and communities. Examples may include food or housing insecurity.

Surgery (minor or major, elective, emergency, procedure or patient risk):

Surgery—Minor or Major: The classification of surgery into minor or major is based on the common meaning of such terms when used by trained clinicians, similar to the use of the term "risk." These terms are not defined by a surgical package classification.

Surgery—Elective or Emergency: Elective procedures and emergent or urgent procedures describe the timing of a procedure when the timing is related to the patient's condition. An elective procedure is typically planned in advance (eg, scheduled for weeks later), while an emergent procedure is typically performed immediately or with minimal delay to allow for patient stabilization. Both elective and emergent procedures may be minor or major procedures.

Surgery—Risk Factors, Patient or Procedure: Risk factors are those that are relevant to the patient and procedure. Evidence-based risk calculators may be used, but are not required, in assessing patient and procedure risk.

Drug therapy requiring intensive monitoring for toxicity: A drug that requires intensive monitoring is a therapeutic agent that has the potential to cause serious morbidity or death. The monitoring is performed for assessment of these adverse effects and not primarily for assessment of therapeutic efficacy. The monitoring should be that which is generally accepted practice for the agent but may be patient-specific in some cases. Intensive monitoring may be long-term or short-term. Long-term intensive monitoring is not performed less than quarterly. The monitoring may be performed with a laboratory test, a physiologic test, or imaging. Monitoring by history or examination does not qualify. The monitoring affects the level of MDM in an encounter in which it is considered in the management of the patient. An example may be monitoring for cytopenia in the use of an antineoplastic agent between dose cycles. Examples of monitoring that do not qualify include monitoring glucose levels during insulin therapy, as the primary reason is the therapeutic effect (unless severe hypoglycemia is a current, significant concern); or annual electrolytes and renal function for a patient on a diuretic, as the frequency does not meet the threshold.

Parenteral controlled substances: The level of risk is based on the usual behavior and thought processes of a physician or other qualified health care professional in the same specialty and subspecialty and not simply based on the presence of an order for parenteral controlled substances.

Guidelines for Selecting Level of Service Based on Time

Certain categories of time-based E/M codes that do not have levels of services based on MDM (eg, Critical Care Services) in the E/M section use time differently. It is important to review the instructions for each category.

Time is **not** a descriptive component for the emergency department levels of E/M services because emergency department services are typically provided on a variable intensity basis, often involving multiple encounters with several patients over an extended period of time.

When time is used for reporting E/M services codes, the time defined in the service descriptors is used for selecting the appropriate level of services. The E/M services for which these guidelines apply require a face-to-face encounter with the physician or other qualified health care professional and the patient and/or family/caregiver. For office or other outpatient services, if the physician's or other qualified health care professional's time is spent in the supervision of clinical staff who perform the face-to-face services of the encounter, use 99211.

For coding purposes, time for these services is the total time on the date of the encounter. It includes both the face-to-face time with the patient and/or family/caregiver and non-face-to-face time personally spent by the physician and/or other qualified health care professional(s) on the day of the encounter (includes time in activities that require the physician or other qualified health care professional and does not include time in activities normally performed by clinical staff). It includes time regardless of the location of the physician or other qualified health care professional (eg, whether on or off the inpatient unit or in or out of the outpatient office). It does not include any time spent in the performance of other separately reported service(s).

Each service that may be reported using time for code level selection has a required time threshold. The concept of attaining a mid-point between levels does not apply. A full 15 minutes is required to report any unit of prolonged services codes 99417, 99418.

Physician(s) and other qualified health care professional(s) may each provide a portion of the face-to-face and non-face-to-face work related to the service. When time is being used to select the appropriate level of services for which time-based reporting is allowed, the time personally spent by the physician(s) and other qualified health care professional(s) assessing and managing the patient and/or counseling, educating, communicating results to the patient/family/caregiver on the date of the encounter is summed to define total time. Only distinct time should be summed (ie, when two or more individuals jointly meet with or discuss the patient, only the time of one individual should be counted).

When prolonged time occurs, the appropriate prolonged services code may be reported. The total time on the date of the encounter spent caring for the patient should be documented in the medical record when it is used as the basis for code selection.

Physician or other qualified health care professional time includes the following activities, when performed:

- preparing to see the patient (eg, review of tests)

- obtaining and/or reviewing separately obtained history

- performing a medically appropriate examination and/or evaluation

- counseling and educating the patient/family/caregiver

- ordering medications, tests, or procedures

- referring and communicating with other health care professionals (when not separately reported)

- documenting clinical information in the electronic or other health record

- independently interpreting results (not separately reported) and communicating results to the patient/family/caregiver

- care coordination (not separately reported)

Do not count time spent on the following:

- the performance of other services that are reported separately

- travel

- teaching that is general and not limited to discussion that is required for the management of a specific patient

For split or shared visits, see the split or shared visits guidelines.

Unlisted Service

An E/M service may be provided that is not listed in this section of the CPT codebook. When reporting such a service, the appropriate unlisted code may be used to indicate the service, identifying it by "Special Report," as discussed in the following paragraph. The "Unlisted Services" and accompanying codes for the E/M section are as follows:

99429   **Unlisted preventive** medicine service

99499   **Unlisted evaluation and management** service

Special Report

An unlisted service or one that is unusual, variable, or new may require a special report demonstrating the medical appropriateness of the service. Pertinent information should include an adequate definition or description of the nature, extent, and need for the procedure and the time, effort, and equipment necessary to provide the service. Additional items that may be included are complexity of symptoms, final diagnosis, pertinent physical findings, diagnostic and therapeutic procedures, concurrent problems, and follow-up care.

Evaluation and Management

Office or Other Outpatient Services

The following codes are used to report evaluation and management services provided in the office or in an outpatient or other ambulatory facility.

To report services provided to a patient who is admitted to a hospital or nursing facility in the course of an encounter in the office or other ambulatory facility, see the notes for initial hospital inpatient or observation care or initial nursing facility care.

For services provided in the emergency department, see 99281-99285.

For observation care, see 99221-99239.

For hospital inpatient or observation care services (including admission and discharge services), see 99234-99236.

─── *Coding Tip* ───────

Determination of Patient Status as New or Established Patient

Solely for the purposes of distinguishing between new and established patients, **professional services** are those face-to-face services rendered by physicians and other qualified health care professionals who may report evaluation and management services. A new patient is one who has not received any professional services from the physician or other qualified health care professional or another physician or other qualified health care professional of the **exact** same specialty and subspecialty who belongs to the same group practice, within the past three years.

An established patient is one who has received professional services from the physician or other qualified health care professional or another physician or other qualified health care professional of the **exact** same specialty **and subspecialty** who belongs to the same group practice, within the past three years.

In the instance where a physician or other qualified health care professional is on call for or covering for another physician or other qualified health care professional, the patient's encounter will be classified as it would have been by the physician or other qualified health care professional who is not available. When advanced practice nurses and physician assistants are working with physicians they are considered as working in the **exact** same specialty and **subspecialty** as the physician.

CPT Coding Guidelines, Evaluation and Management, Classification of Evaluation and Management (E/M) Services, New and Established Patients

New Patient

99202   **Office or other outpatient visit** for the evaluation and management of a new patient, which requires a medically appropriate history and/or examination and straightforward medical decision making.

When using total time on the date of the encounter for code selection, 15 minutes must be met or exceeded.

➲ *CPT Changes: An Insider's View* 2013, 2017, 2021, 2024

➲ *CPT Assistant* Winter 91:11, Spring 92:13, 24, Summer 92:1, 24, Spring 93:34, Summer 93:2, Fall 93:9, Spring 95:1, Summer 95:4, Fall 95:9, Jul 98:9, Sep 98:5, Feb 00:11, Aug 01:2, Apr 02:14, Oct 04:10, Apr 05:1, 3, Jun 05:11, Dec 05:10, May 06:1, Jun 06:1, Oct 06:15, Apr 07:11, Sep 07:1, Mar 09:3, Aug 09:5, Dec 09:9, Jan 11:3, Mar 12:4, 8, Jan 13:9, Jun 13:3, Aug 13:13-14, Jan 15:12, Mar 16:11, Sep 16:6, Apr 18:10, Sep 18:14, Jan 19:3, Jan 20:3, Feb 20:3, Mar 20:3, May 20:3, Jun 20:3, Sep 20:13, Oct 20:15, Nov 20:3, Dec 20:11, Jan 21:3, Feb 21:8, Jun 21:13, Jul 21:8, Aug 21:13, Sep 21:3, 14, Nov 21:12, Jan 22:3, 17, Feb 22:13, Jun 22:19, Jul 22:17, Aug 22:3-7, Sep 22:6, Oct 22:7, Nov 22:1, Dec 22:15, Mar 23:1, Oct 23:18, Dec 23:49, Jan 24:1

➲ *Clinical Examples in Radiology* Winter 12:9

99203   **Office or other outpatient visit** for the evaluation and management of a new patient, which requires a medically appropriate history and/or examination and low level of medical decision making.

When using total time on the date of the encounter for code selection, 30 minutes must be met or exceeded.

➲ *CPT Changes: An Insider's View* 2013, 2017, 2021, 2024

➲ *CPT Assistant* Winter 91:11, Spring 92:14, 24, Summer 92:1, 24, Spring 93:34, Summer 93:2, Fall 93:9, Spring 95:1, Summer 95:4, Fall 95:9, Jul 98:9, Sep 98:5, Feb 00:11, Aug 01:2, Apr 02:14, Oct 04:10, Feb 05:9, Apr 05:1, 3, Jun 05:11, Dec 05:10, May 06:1, Jun 06:1, Oct 06:15, Apr 07:11, Sep 07:1, Mar 09:3, Aug 09:5, Dec 09:9, Jan 11:3, Mar 12:4, 8, Jan 13:9, Jun 13:3, Aug 13:13-14, Jan 15:12, Mar 16:11, Sep 16:6, Apr 18:10, Sep 18:14, Jan 19:3, Jan 20:3, Feb 20:3, Mar 20:3, May 20:3, Jun 20:3, Sep 20:14, Oct 20:15, Nov 20:3, Jan 21:3, Feb 21:8, Jun 21:13, Jul 21:8, Aug 21:13, Sep 21:3, 14, Nov 21:12, Jan 22:3, 17, Feb 22:13, Jun 22:19, Jul 22:17, Aug 22:3-7, Sep 22:6, Nov 22:19, Dec 22:15, Mar 23:1, Oct 23:18, Jan 24:1

➲ *Clinical Examples in Radiology* Winter 12:9

99204 **Office or other outpatient visit** for the evaluation and management of a new patient, which requires a medically appropriate history and/or examination and moderate level of medical decision making.

When using total time on the date of the encounter for code selection, 45 minutes must be met or exceeded.

➔ *CPT Changes: An Insider's View* 2013, 2017, 2021, 2024

➔ *CPT Assistant* Winter 91:11, Spring 92:14, 24, Summer 92:1, 24, Spring 93:34, Summer 93:2, Fall 93:9, Spring 95:1, Summer 95:4, Fall 95:9, Jul 98:9, Sep 98:5, Feb 00:11, Aug 01:2, Apr 02:14, May 02:1, Oct 04:10, Apr 05:1, 3, Jun 05:11, Dec 05:10, May 06:1, Jun 06:1, Oct 06:15, Apr 07:11, Sep 07:1, Mar 09:3, Aug 09:5, Dec 09:9, Jan 11:3, Mar 12:4, 8, Jan 13:9, Jun 13:3, Aug 13:13-14, Jan 15:12, Mar 16:11, Sep 16:6, Apr 18:10, Sep 18:14, Jan 19:3, Jan 20:3, Feb 20:3, Mar 20:3, May 20:3, Jun 20:3, Sep 20:14, Oct 20:15, Nov 20:12, Jan 21:3, Feb 21:8, Jun 21:13, Jul 21:8, Aug 21:13, Sep 21:3, 14, Nov 21:12, Jan 22:3, 17, Feb 22:13, Jun 22:19, Jul 22:17, Aug 22:3-7, Sep 22:6, Nov 22:19, Dec 22:15, Mar 23:1, Oct 23:18, Jan 24:1

➔ *Clinical Examples in Radiology* Winter 12:9

99205 **Office or other outpatient visit** for the evaluation and management of a new patient, which requires a medically appropriate history and/or examination and high level of medical decision making.

When using total time on the date of the encounter for code selection, 60 minutes must be met or exceeded.

➔ *CPT Changes: An Insider's View* 2013, 2017, 2021, 2024

➔ *CPT Assistant* Winter 91:11, Spring 92:14, 24, Summer 92:1, 24, Spring 93:34, Summer 93:2, Fall 93:9, Spring 95:1, Summer 95:4, Fall 95:9, Jul 98:9, Sep 98:5, Feb 00:11, Aug 01:2, Apr 02:2, May 02:1, Oct 04:10, Apr 05:1, 3, Jun 05:11, Dec 05:10, May 06:1, Jun 06:1, Oct 06:15, Apr 07:11, Sep 07:1, Mar 09:3, Aug 09:5, Dec 09:9, Jul 10:4, Jan 11:3, Jan 12:3, Mar 12:4, 8, Jan 13:9, Jun 13:3, Aug 13:13-14, Jan 15:12, Mar 16:11, Sep 16:6, Apr 18:10, Sep 18:14, Jan 19:3, Jan 20:3, Feb 20:3, Mar 20:3, May 20:3, Jun 20:3, Sep 20:14, Oct 20:15, Nov 20:12, Jan 21:3, Feb 21:8, Jun 21:13, Jul 21:8, Aug 21:13, Sep 21:3, 14, Nov 21:12, Jan 22:3, 17, Feb 22:13, Jun 22:19, Jul 22:17, Aug 22:3-7, Sep 22:6, Nov 22:1, Dec 22:15, Mar 23:1, Oct 23:18, Jan 24:1, Mar 24:24

➔ *Clinical Examples in Radiology* Winter 12:9

(For services 75 minutes or longer, use prolonged services code 99417)

Established Patient

★ **99211** **Office or other outpatient visit** for the evaluation and management of an established patient that may not require the presence of a physician or other qualified health care professional

➔ *CPT Changes: An Insider's View* 2013, 2021, 2022

➔ *CPT Assistant* Winter 91:11, Spring 92:14, 24, Summer 92:1, 24, Spring 93:34, Summer 93:2, Fall 93:9, Spring 95:1, Summer 95:4, Fall 95:9, Oct 96:10, Feb 97:9, May 97:4, Jul 98:9, Sep 98:5, Oct 99:9, Feb 00:11, Aug 01:2, Jan 02:2, Oct 04:10, Feb 05:15, Mar 05:11, Apr 05:1, 3, May 05:1, Jun 05:11, Nov 05:1, Dec 05:10, Feb 06:14, May 06:1, Jun 06:1, Jul 06:19, Oct 06:15, Nov 06:21, Apr 07:11, Jul 07:1, Sep 07:1, Dec 07:9, Mar 08:3, Aug 08:13, Mar 09:3, Aug 09:5, Apr 10:10, Jan 11:3, Jan 12:3, Mar 12:4, 8, Apr 12:10, Jan 13:9, Mar 13:13, Jun 13:3, Aug 13:13-14, Nov 13:3, Mar 14:14, Jan 15:12, Mar 16:11, Sep 16:6, Mar 17:10, Apr 18:10, Sep 18:14, Jan 19:3, Jan 20:3, Feb 20:3, Mar 20:3, May 20:3, Jun 20:3, Sep 20:14, Oct 20:14, Nov 20:12, Jan 21:3, Feb 21:8, Jan 22:3, 17, Jan 22:3, Jun 22:19, Sep 22:6, Jan 24:1

99212 **Office or other outpatient visit** for the evaluation and management of an established patient, which requires a medically appropriate history and/or examination and straightforward medical decision making.

When using total time on the date of the encounter for code selection, 10 minutes must be met or exceeded.

➔ *CPT Changes: An Insider's View* 2013, 2017, 2021, 2024

➔ *CPT Assistant* Winter 91:11, Spring 92:14, 24, Summer 92:1, 24, Spring 93:34, Summer 93:2, Fall 93:9, Spring 95:1, Summer 95:4, Fall 95:9, Jul 98:9, Sep 98:5, Feb 00:11, Jun 00:11, Aug 01:2, Jan 02:2, May 02:3, Apr 04:14, Oct 04:10, Apr 05:1, 3, Jun 05:11, Dec 05:10, May 06:1, Jun 06:1, 11, Sep 06:8, Oct 06:15, Apr 07:11, Jul 07:1, Sep 07:1, Mar 08:3, Mar 09:3, Aug 09:5, Feb 10:13, Jul 10:4, Sep 10:4, Jan 11:3, Jun 11:3, Mar 12:4, 8, Apr 12:17, Jan 13:9, Mar 13:13, Jun 13:3, Aug 13:13-14, Feb 14:11, Jan 15:12, Mar 16:11, Sep 16:6, Dec 16:12, Oct 17:6, Apr 18:10, Sep 18:14, Jan 19:3, Jan 20:3, Feb 20:3, Mar 20:3, May 20:3, Jun 20:3, Sep 20:13, Oct 20:14, Nov 20:3, Jan 21:3, Feb 21:8, Jun 21:13, Aug 21:13, Sep 21:3, 14, Nov 21:12, Jan 22:3, 17, Feb 22:13, Jun 22:19, Jul 22:17, Aug 22:3-7, Sep 22:6, Nov 22:1, Mar 23:1, Jun 23:25, Oct 23:18, Jan 24:1

99213 **Office or other outpatient visit** for the evaluation and management of an established patient, which requires a medically appropriate history and/or examination and low level of medical decision making.

When using total time on the date of the encounter for code selection, 20 minutes must be met or exceeded.

➔ *CPT Changes: An Insider's View* 2013, 2017, 2021, 2024

➔ *CPT Assistant* Winter 91:11, Spring 92:14, 24, Summer 92:1, 24, Spring 93:34, Summer 93:2, Fall 93:9, Spring 95:1, Summer 95:4, Fall 95:9, Jan 97:10, Jul 98:9, Sep 98:5, Aug 01:2, May 02:3, Oct 03:5, Apr 04:14, Oct 04:10, Mar 05:11, Apr 05:1, 3, Jun 05:11, Dec 05:10, May 06:1, Jun 06:1, 11, Sep 06:8, Oct 06:15, Apr 07:11, Jul 07:1, Sep 07:1, Mar 08:3, Mar 09:3, Aug 09:5, Sep 10:4, Jan 11:3, Jun 11:3, Mar 12:4, 8, Jan 13:9, Mar 13:13, Jun 13:3, Aug 13:13-14, Jan 15:12, Mar 16:11, Sep 16:6, Apr 18:10, Sep 18:14, Jan 19:3, Jan 20:3, Feb 20:3, Mar 20:3, May 20:3, Jun 20:3, Sep 20:14, Oct 20:14, Nov 20:3, Jan 21:3, Feb 21:8, Apr 21:13, Jun 21:13, Aug 21:13, Sep 21:3, 14, Nov 21:12, Jan 22:3, 17, Feb 22:13, Jun 22:19, Jul 22:17, Aug 22:3-7, Sep 22:6, Nov 22:19, Dec 22:19, Mar 23:1, Jun 23:25, Oct 23:18, Jan 24:1

Evaluation / Management 99202-99499

99214　**Office or other outpatient visit** for the evaluation and management of an established patient, which requires a medically appropriate history and/or examination and moderate level of medical decision making.

When using total time on the date of the encounter for code selection, 30 minutes must be met or exceeded.

➔ *CPT Changes: An Insider's View* 2013, 2017, 2021, 2024

➔ *CPT Assistant* Winter 91:11, Spring 92:15, 24, Summer 92:1, 24, Spring 93:34, Summer 93:2, Fall 93:9, Spring 95:1, Summer 95:4, Fall 95:9, May 97:4, Jul 98:9, Sep 98:5, Aug 01:2, Jan 02:2, May 02:1-2, Oct 03:5, Apr 04:14, Oct 04:10, Apr 05:1, 3, Jun 05:11, Dec 05:10, May 06:1, Jun 06:1, 11, Sep 06:8, Oct 06:15, Apr 07:11, Jul 07:1, Sep 07:1, Mar 08:3, Mar 09:3, Aug 09:5, Sep 10:4, Jan 11:3, Jun 11:3, Mar 12:4, 8, Jan 13:9, Mar 13:13, Jun 13:3, Aug 13:13-14, Jan 15:12, Oct 15:3, Mar 16:11, Sep 16:6, Apr 18:10, Sep 18:14, Jan 19:3, Jan 20:3, Feb 20:3, Mar 20:3, May 20:3, Jun 20:3, Sep 20:14, Oct 20:14, Nov 20:12, Jan 21:3, Feb 21:8, Apr 21:13, Jun 21:13, Aug 21:13, Sep 21:3, 14, Nov 21:12, Jan 22:3, 17, Feb 22:13, Jun 22:19, Jul 22:17, Aug 22:3-7, Sep 22:6, Nov 22:19, Mar 23:1, Jun 23:25, Oct 23:18, Jan 24:1

99215　**Office or other outpatient visit** for the evaluation and management of an established patient, which requires a medically appropriate history and/or examination and high level of medical decision making.

When using total time on the date of the encounter for code selection, 40 minutes must be met or exceeded.

➔ *CPT Changes: An Insider's View* 2013, 2017, 2021, 2024

➔ *CPT Assistant* Winter 91:11, Spring 92:15, 24, Summer 92:1, 24, Spring 93:34, Summer 93:2, Fall 93:9, Spring 95:1, Summer 95:4, Fall 95:9, Jan 97:10, Jul 98:9, Sep 98:5, Aug 01:2, Jan 02:2, May 02:1, 3, Apr 04:14, Oct 04:10, Mar 05:11, Apr 05:1, 3, Jun 05:11, Dec 05:10, May 06:1, Jun 06:1, 11, Sep 06:8, Oct 06:15, Apr 07:11, Jul 07:1, Sep 07:1, Mar 08:3, Mar 09:3, Aug 09:5, Jul 10:4, Sep 10:4, Jan 11:3, Jun 11:3, Jan 12:3, Mar 12:4, 8, Apr 12:10, Jan 13:9, Mar 13:13, Jun 13:3, Aug 13:13-14, Nov 13:3, Aug 14:3, Oct 14:3, Nov 14:14, Jan 15:12, Mar 16:11, Sep 16:6, Apr 18:10, Sep 18:14, Jan 19:3, Oct 19:10, Jan 20:3, Feb 20:3, Mar 20:3, May 20:3, Jun 20:3, Sep 20:14, Oct 20:14, Nov 20:12, Jan 21:3, Feb 21:8, Jun 21:13, Aug 21:13, Sep 21:3, 14, Nov 21:12, Jan 22:3, 17, Feb 22:13, Jun 22:19, Jul 22:17, Aug 22:3-7, Sep 22:6, Oct 22:7, Nov 22:1, Dec 22:15, Mar 23:1, Jun 23:25, Oct 23:18, Jan 24:1

(For services 55 minutes or longer, use prolonged services code 99417)

▶Telemedicine Services◀

▶Telemedicine services are synchronous, real-time, interactive encounters between a physician or other qualified health care professional (QHP) and a patient utilizing either combined audio-video or audio-only telecommunication. Unless specifically stated in the code descriptor, level selection for telemedicine services is based on either the level of medical decision making (MDM) or the total time for E/M services performed on the date of the encounter, as defined for each service. Telemedicine services are used in lieu of an in-person service when medically appropriate to address the care of the patient and when the patient and/or family/caregiver agree to this format of care. Telemedicine services are not used to report routine telecommunications related to a previous encounter (eg, to communicate laboratory results). They may be used for follow-up of a previous encounter, when a follow-up E/M service is required, in the same manner as in-person E/M services are used. For example, telemedicine services may be used for a patient requiring re-assessment for response or complications related to the treatment plan of a previous visit. Except for 98016, these services do not require a specific time interval from the last in-person or telemedicine visit and may be initiated by a physician or other QHP as well as by a patient and/or family/caregiver. However, the telemedicine services must be performed on a separate calendar date from another E/M service. When performed on the same date as another E/M service, the elements and time of these services are summed and reported in aggregate, ensuring that any overlapping time is only counted once. If the minimum time for reporting a telemedicine service has not been achieved, time spent with the patient may still count toward the total time on the date of the encounter of an in-person E/M service.

For audio-only telemedicine services for established patients with 5 to 10 minutes of medical discussion, report brief communication technology service (eg, virtual check-in) code 98016. Code 98016 is reported for established patients only. The service is patient-initiated and intended to evaluate whether a more extensive visit type is required (eg, an office or other outpatient E/M service [99212, 99213, 99214, 99215]). Video technology is not required for audio-only visits. When the patient-initiated check-in leads to an E/M service on the same calendar date, and when time is used to select the level of that E/M service, the time from 98016 may be added to the time of the E/M service for the total time on the date of the encounter.

For services that are asynchronous (ie, not live in real-time), see **Online Digital Evaluation and Management Services** (99421, 99422, 99423). Do not report telemedicine services for oversight of clinical staff (eg, chronic care management [CCM]). Do not count the time performing telemedicine services toward time performing CCM (99437, 99491) or principal care management services (99424, 99425). See Table 2, Telemedicine and Non-Face-to-Face Services.

For 98000-98015, the level of service is selected based on MDM or total time on the date of the encounter. For audio-only codes 98008, 98009, 98010, 98011, 98012, 98013, 98014, 98015, the service must exceed 10 minutes of medical discussion. Code 98016 describes services for established patients with 5 to 10 minutes of medical discussion and is based only on the time of

Copying, photographing, or sharing this CPT® book violates AMA's copyright.

medical discussion and not MDM. Do not count time for establishing the connection or arranging the appointment, even when performed by the physician or other QHP. Services of less than five minutes are not reported.

For audio-only codes 98008, 98009, 98010, 98011, 98012, 98013, 98014, 98015, medical discussion is synchronous (real-time) interactive verbal communication and does not include online digital communication (except when via a telecommunication technology device for the deaf). The meaning of MDM has the meaning used in the E/M Guidelines and is a cognitive process by the physician or other QHP.

If during the encounter, audio-video connections are lost and only audio is restored, report the service that accounted for the majority of the time of the interactive portion of the service. Ten minutes of medical discussion or patient observation must be exceeded in order to report the audio-only service.◄

►Synchronous Audio-Video Evaluation and Management Services◄

►Codes 98000, 98001, 98002, 98003, 98004, 98005, 98006, 98007 may be reported for new or established patients. Synchronous audio and video telecommunication is required. These services may be reported based on total time on the date of the encounter or MDM.◄

►New Patient◄

#● **98000**   **Synchronous audio-video visit** for the evaluation and management of a new patient, which requires a medically appropriate history and/or examination and straightforward medical decision making.

When using total time on the date of the encounter for code selection, 15 minutes must be met or exceeded.

➔ *CPT Changes: An Insider's View* 2025

►Table 2: Telemedicine and Non-Face-to-Face Services

Service	New/Established	Synchronous	Level/Unit Reported	Service Reported	Other E/M Notations
Synchronous audio-video (98000-98007)	Both	Yes	MDM or total time on the date of the service. No minimum required time, unless level selected by time.	Per single calendar date	Do not report with same-day in-person E/M
Synchronous audio-only (98008-98015)	Both	Yes	MDM or total time on the date of the service. Must be more than 10 minutes of medical discussion.	Per single calendar date	Do not report with same-day in-person E/M
Brief synchronous communication technology service (98016)	Established	Yes	A single 5- to 10-minute medical discussion	Per single calendar date	Not related to E/M in prior 7 days or leading to E/M in next 24 hours
Online digital E/M (99421-99423)	Established	No	Minutes during 7-day period	Per 7 days	Not related to E/M in prior 7 days or leading to E/M in next 24 hours
Interprofessional telephone/Internet/EHR consultations (99446-99451)	Both	Not required	Minutes during 7-day period	Per 7 days	No in-person encounter within 14 days
Interprofessional telephone/Internet/EHR consultations (99452)	Both	Not required	Minutes during a single day	Per 14 days	No in-person encounter within 14 days
Care management and remote treatment management (99424, 99425, 99437, 99484, 99491)	Established	Not required	Minutes	Per calendar month	Physician or QHP time excluded on date of other E/M
All services (98000-98016, 99421-99425, 99437, 99446-99452, 99484, 99491)			Same time is not counted twice◄		

#● **98001**   **Synchronous audio-video visit** for the evaluation and management of a new patient, which requires a medically appropriate history and/or examination and low medical decision making.

When using total time on the date of the encounter for code selection, 30 minutes must be met or exceeded.

➔ *CPT Changes: An Insider's View* 2025

#● **98002**   **Synchronous audio-video visit** for the evaluation and management of a new patient, which requires a medically appropriate history and/or examination and moderate medical decision making.

When using total time on the date of the encounter for code selection, 45 minutes must be met or exceeded.

➔ *CPT Changes: An Insider's View* 2025

#● **98003**   **Synchronous audio-video visit** for the evaluation and management of a new patient, which requires a medically appropriate history and/or examination and high medical decision making.

When using total time on the date of the encounter for code selection, 60 minutes must be met or exceeded.

➔ *CPT Changes: An Insider's View* 2025

▶(For services 75 minutes or longer, use prolonged services code 99417)◀

▶Established Patient◀

#● **98004**   **Synchronous audio-video visit** for the evaluation and management of an established patient, which requires a medically appropriate history and/or examination and straightforward medical decision making.

When using total time on the date of the encounter for code selection, 10 minutes must be met or exceeded.

➔ *CPT Changes: An Insider's View* 2025

#● **98005**   **Synchronous audio-video visit** for the evaluation and management of an established patient, which requires a medically appropriate history and/or examination and low medical decision making.

When using total time on the date of the encounter for code selection, 20 minutes must be met or exceeded.

➔ *CPT Changes: An Insider's View* 2025

#● **98006**   **Synchronous audio-video visit** for the evaluation and management of an established patient, which requires a medically appropriate history and/or examination and moderate medical decision making.

When using total time on the date of the encounter for code selection, 30 minutes must be met or exceeded.

➔ *CPT Changes: An Insider's View* 2025

#● **98007**   **Synchronous audio-video visit** for the evaluation and management of an established patient, which requires a medically appropriate history and/or examination and high medical decision making.

When using total time on the date of the encounter for code selection, 40 minutes must be met or exceeded.

➔ *CPT Changes: An Insider's View* 2025

▶(For services 55 minutes or longer, use prolonged services code 99417)◀

▶Synchronous Audio-Only Evaluation and Management Services◀

▶Codes 98008, 98009, 98010, 98011, 98012, 98013, 98014, 98015 may be reported for new or established patients. They require more than 10 minutes of medical discussion. For services of 5 to 10 minutes of medical discussion, report 98016, if appropriate. If 10 minutes of medical discussion is exceeded, total time on the date of the encounter or MDM may be used for code level selection.◀

▶New Patient◀

#● **98008**   **Synchronous audio-only visit** for the evaluation and management of a new patient, which requires a medically appropriate history and/or examination, straightforward medical decision making, and more than 10 minutes of medical discussion.

When using total time on the date of the encounter for code selection, 15 minutes must be met or exceeded.

➔ *CPT Changes: An Insider's View* 2025

#● **98009**   **Synchronous audio-only visit** for the evaluation and management of a new patient, which requires a medically appropriate history and/or examination, low medical decision making, and more than 10 minutes of medical discussion.

When using total time on the date of the encounter for code selection, 30 minutes must be met or exceeded.

➔ *CPT Changes: An Insider's View* 2025

#● **98010**   **Synchronous audio-only visit** for the evaluation and management of a new patient, which requires a medically appropriate history and/or examination, moderate medical decision making, and more than 10 minutes of medical discussion.

When using total time on the date of the encounter for code selection, 45 minutes must be met or exceeded.

➔ *CPT Changes: An Insider's View* 2025

#● 98011 **Synchronous audio-only visit** for the evaluation and management of a new patient, which requires a medically appropriate history and/or examination, high medical decision making, and more than 10 minutes of medical discussion.

When using total time on the date of the encounter for code selection, 60 minutes must be met or exceeded.

➔ *CPT Changes: An Insider's View* 2025

▶(For services 75 minutes or longer, use prolonged services code 99417)◀

▶Established Patient◀

#● 98012 **Synchronous audio-only visit** for the evaluation and management of an established patient, which requires a medically appropriate history and/or examination, straightforward medical decision making, and more than 10 minutes of medical discussion.

When using total time on the date of the encounter for code selection, 10 minutes must be exceeded.

➔ *CPT Changes: An Insider's View* 2025

▶(Do not report 98012 for home and outpatient INR monitoring when reporting 93792, 93793)◀

▶(Do not report 98012 when using 99374, 99375, 99377, 99378, 99379, 99380 for the same call[s])◀

▶(Do not report 98012 during the same month with 99487, 99489)◀

▶(Do not report 98012 when performed during the service time of 99495, 99496)◀

#● 98013 **Synchronous audio-only visit** for the evaluation and management of an established patient, which requires a medically appropriate history and/or examination, low medical decision making, and more than 10 minutes of medical discussion.

When using total time on the date of the encounter for code selection, 20 minutes must be met or exceeded.

➔ *CPT Changes: An Insider's View* 2025

▶(Do not report 98013 for home and outpatient INR monitoring when reporting 93792, 93793)◀

▶(Do not report 98013 when using 99374, 99375, 99377, 99378, 99379, 99380 for the same call[s])◀

▶(Do not report 98013 during the same month with 99487, 99489)◀

▶(Do not report 98013 when performed during the service time of 99495, 99496)◀

#● 98014 **Synchronous audio-only visit** for the evaluation and management of an established patient, which requires a medically appropriate history and/or examination, moderate medical decision making, and more than 10 minutes of medical discussion.

When using total time on the date of the encounter for code selection, 30 minutes must be met or exceeded.

➔ *CPT Changes: An Insider's View* 2025

▶(Do not report 98014 for home and outpatient INR monitoring when reporting 93792, 93793)◀

▶(Do not report 98014 when using 99374, 99375, 99377, 99378, 99379, 99380 for the same call[s])◀

▶(Do not report 98014 during the same month with 99487, 99489)◀

▶(Do not report 98014 when performed during the service time of 99495, 99496)◀

#● 98015 **Synchronous audio-only visit** for the evaluation and management of an established patient, which requires a medically appropriate history and/or examination, high medical decision making, and more than 10 minutes of medical discussion.

When using total time on the date of the encounter for code selection, 40 minutes must be met or exceeded.

➔ *CPT Changes: An Insider's View* 2025

▶(Do not report 98015 for home and outpatient INR monitoring when reporting 93792, 93793)◀

▶(Do not report 98015 when using 99374, 99375, 99377, 99378, 99379, 99380 for the same call[s])◀

▶(Do not report 98015 during the same month with 99487, 99489)◀

▶(Do not report 98015 when performed during the service time of 99495, 99496)◀

▶(For services 55 minutes or longer, use prolonged services code 99417)◀

▶Brief Synchronous Communication Technology Service (eg, Virtual Check-In)◀

▶Code 98016 is reported for established patients only. The service is patient-initiated and intended to evaluate whether a more extensive visit type is required (eg, an office or other outpatient E/M service [99212, 99213, 99214, 99215]). Video technology is not required. Code 98016 describes a service of shorter duration than the audio-only services and has other restrictions that are related to the intended use as a "virtual check-in" or triage to determine if another E/M service is necessary. When the patient-initiated check-in leads to an E/M service on the same calendar date, and when time is used to select the level of that E/M service, the time from 98016 may be added to the time of the E/M service for total time on the date of the encounter.◀

#● **98016** **Brief communication technology-based service** (eg, virtual check-in) by a physician or other qualified health care professional who can report evaluation and management services, provided to an established patient, not originating from a related evaluation and management service provided within the previous 7 days nor leading to an evaluation and management service or procedure within the next 24 hours or soonest available appointment, 5-10 minutes of medical discussion

➔ *CPT Changes: An Insider's View* 2025

▶(Do not report 98016 in conjunction with 98000-98015)◀

▶(Do not report services of less than 5 minutes of medical discussion)◀

Hospital Observation Services

Observation Care Discharge Services

(99217 has been deleted. To report observation care discharge services, see 99238, 99239)

Initial Observation Care

New or Established Patient

(99218, 99219, 99220 have been deleted. To report initial observation care, new or established patient, see 99221, 99222, 99223)

Subsequent Observation Care

(99224, 99225, 99226 have been deleted. To report subsequent observation care, see 99231, 99232, 99233)

Hospital Inpatient and Observation Care Services

The following codes are used to report initial and subsequent evaluation and management services provided to hospital inpatients and to patients designated as hospital outpatient "observation status." Hospital inpatient or observation care codes are also used to report partial hospitalization services.

For patients designated/admitted as "observation status" in a hospital, it is not necessary that the patient be located in an observation area designated by the hospital. If such an area does exist in a hospital (as a separate unit in the hospital, in the emergency department, etc), these codes may be utilized if the patient is placed in such an area.

For a patient admitted and discharged from hospital inpatient or observation status on the same date, report 99234, 99235, 99236, as appropriate.

Total time on the date of the encounter is by calendar date. When using MDM or total time for code selection, a continuous visit that spans the transition of two calendar dates is a single service and is reported on one calendar date. If the service is continuous before and through midnight, all the time may be applied to the reported date of the service.

Initial Hospital Inpatient or Observation Care

New or Established Patient

The following codes are used to report the first hospital inpatient or observation status encounter with the patient.

An initial service may be reported when the patient has not received any professional services from the physician or other qualified health care professional or another physician or other qualified health care professional of the exact same specialty and subspecialty who belongs to the same group practice during the stay. When advanced practice nurses and physician assistants are working with physicians, they are considered as working in the exact same specialty and subspecialty as the physician.

For admission services for the neonate (28 days of age or younger) requiring intensive observation, frequent interventions, and other intensive care services, see 99477.

When the patient is admitted to the hospital as an inpatient or to observation status in the course of an encounter in another site of service (eg, hospital emergency department, office, nursing facility), the services in the initial site may be separately reported. Modifier 25 may be added to the other evaluation and management service to indicate a significant, separately identifiable service by the same physician or other qualified health care professional was performed on the same date.

In the case when the services in a separate site are reported and the initial inpatient or observation care service is a consultation service, do not report 99221, 99222, 99223, 99252, 99253, 99254, 99255. The consultant reports the subsequent hospital inpatient or observation care codes 99231, 99232, 99233 for the second service on the same date.

If a consultation is performed in anticipation of, or related to, an admission by another physician or other qualified health care professional, and then the same consultant performs an encounter once the patient is admitted by the other physician or other qualified health care professional, report the consultant's inpatient encounter with the appropriate subsequent care code (99231, 99232, 99233). It applies for consultations reported with any appropriate code (eg, office or other outpatient visit or office or other outpatient consultation).

For a patient admitted and discharged from hospital inpatient or observation status on the same date, report 99234, 99235, 99236, as appropriate.

For the purpose of reporting an initial hospital inpatient or observation care service, a transition from observation level to inpatient does not constitute a new stay.

99221 **Initial hospital inpatient or observation care,** per day, for the evaluation and management of a patient, which requires a medically appropriate history and/or examination and straightforward or low level medical decision making.

When using total time on the date of the encounter for code selection, 40 minutes must be met or exceeded.

➤ *CPT Changes: An Insider's View* 2013, 2023
➤ *CPT Assistant* Winter 91:11, Spring 92:14, 24, Summer 92:10, 24, Fall 92:1, Spring 93:34, Spring 95:1, Fall 95:9, Jul 96:11, Sep 96:10, Nov 97:2, Mar 98:1, Sep 98:5, Jan 02:2-3, Apr 03:26, Apr 04:14, Aug 04:11, May 05:1, Sep 06:8, Jul 07:12, Jul 12:12, Jan 13:9, Jun 13:3, Aug 13:13, Feb 14:11, May 14:4, Nov 14:14, Dec 15:16, Mar 16:11, Dec 18:8, Oct 20:15, Aug 22:3-7, Sep 22:6, Oct 22:7, Jan 23:20, Feb 23:12, May 23:23, Oct 23:16

99222 **Initial hospital inpatient or observation care,** per day, for the evaluation and management of a patient, which requires a medically appropriate history and/or examination and moderate level of medical decision making.

When using total time on the date of the encounter for code selection, 55 minutes must be met or exceeded.

➤ *CPT Changes: An Insider's View* 2013, 2023
➤ *CPT Assistant* Winter 91:11, Spring 92:14, 24, Summer 92:10, 24, Fall 92:1, Spring 93:34, Spring 95:1, Fall 95:9, Jul 96:11, Sep 96:10, Nov 97:2, Mar 98:1, Sep 98:5, Jan 02:2-3, Apr 03:26, Apr 04:14, Aug 04:11, Sep 06:8, Jul 07:12, Jul 12:12, Jan 13:9, Jun 13:3, Aug 13:13, Mar 15:3, Dec 15:16, Mar 16:11, Dec 18:8, Oct 20:15, Aug 22:3-7, Sep 22:6, Oct 22:7, Jan 23:20, Feb 23:12, May 23:23, Oct 23:16

99223 **Initial hospital inpatient or observation care,** per day, for the evaluation and management of a patient, which requires a medically appropriate history and/or examination and high level of medical decision making.

When using total time on the date of the encounter for code selection, 75 minutes must be met or exceeded.

➤ *CPT Changes: An Insider's View* 2013, 2023
➤ *CPT Assistant* Winter 91:11, Spring 92:14, 24, Summer 92:10, 24, Fall 92:1, Spring 93:34, Spring 95:1, Fall 95:9, Jul 96:11, Sep 96:10, Nov 97:2, Mar 98:1, Sep 98:5, Jan 02:2-3, Apr 03:26, Apr 04:14, Aug 04:11, Sep 06:8, Jul 07:12, Jul 12:12, Jan 13:9, Jun 13:3, Aug 13:13, May 14:4, Nov 14:14, Dec 15:16, Mar 16:11, Dec 18:8, Oct 20:15, Sep 21:12, Aug 22:3-7, Sep 22:6, Oct 22:7, Nov 22:1, Jan 23:20, Feb 23:12, May 23:23, Jul 23:14, Oct 23:16, Mar 24:24

(For services of 90 minutes or longer, use prolonged services code 99418)

Subsequent Hospital Inpatient or Observation Care

★ **99231** **Subsequent hospital inpatient or observation care,** per day, for the evaluation and management of a patient, which requires a medically appropriate history and/or examination and straightforward or low level of medical decision making.

When using total time on the date of the encounter for code selection, 25 minutes must be met or exceeded.

➤ *CPT Changes: An Insider's View* 2013, 2017, 2023
➤ *CPT Assistant* Winter 91:11, Spring 92:14, 24, Summer 92:10, 24, Fall 92:1, Spring 93:34, Spring 95:1, Fall 95:16, Nov 97:2, Sep 98:5, Jan 99:10, Nov 99:5, Aug 01:2, Jan 02:2-3, Apr 04:14, Aug 04:11, Mar 05:11, May 05:1, May 06:1, 16, Jul 06:4, Mar 07:9, Jul 07:1, Mar 09:3, Dec 09:9, Jun 11:3, Jul 12:12, Jan 13:9, Jun 13:3, Aug 13:14, Sep 13:18, May 14:4, Nov 14:14, Dec 18:8, Jun 21:13, Dec 21:19, Aug 22:3-7, Oct 22:7, Dec 22:15, Jan 23:20, Feb 23:12, May 23:23, Oct 23:16

★ **99232** **Subsequent hospital inpatient or observation care,** per day, for the evaluation and management of a patient, which requires a medically appropriate history and/or examination and moderate level of medical decision making.

When using total time on the date of the encounter for code selection, 35 minutes must be met or exceeded.

➤ *CPT Changes: An Insider's View* 2013, 2017, 2023
➤ *CPT Assistant* Winter 91:11, Spring 92:14, 24, Summer 92:10, 24, Fall 92:1, Spring 93:34, Spring 95:1, Fall 95:16, Nov 97:2, Sep 98:5, Jan 99:10, Nov 99:5, Jan 00:11, Aug 01:2, Apr 04:14, Aug 04:11, May 06:1, 16, Jul 06:4, Mar 07:9, Jul 07:1, Mar 09:3, Dec 09:9, Jun 11:3, Jul 12:12, Jan 13:9, Jun 13:3, Aug 13:14, Oct 16:8, Dec 18:8, Jun 21:13, Dec 21:19, Aug 22:3-7, Oct 22:7, Jan 23:20, Feb 23:12, May 23:23, Oct 23:16, Jan 24:36

★ **99233**   **Subsequent hospital inpatient or observation care,** per day, for the evaluation and management of a patient, which requires a medically appropriate history and/or examination and high level of medical decision making.

When using total time on the date of the encounter for code selection, 50 minutes must be met or exceeded.

➔ *CPT Changes: An Insider's View* 2013, 2017, 2023

➔ *CPT Assistant* Winter 91:11, Spring 92:14, 24, Summer 92:10, 24, Fall 92:1, Spring 93:34, Spring 95:1, Fall 95:16, Nov 97:2, Sep 98:5, Jan 99:10, Nov 99:5, Aug 01:2, Apr 04:14, Aug 04:11, May 06:1, 16, Jul 06:4, Mar 07:9, Jul 07:1, Mar 09:3, Dec 09:9, Jun 11:3, Jul 12:12, Jan 13:9, Jun 13:3, Aug 13:13-14, May 14:4, Nov 14:14, Oct 16:8, Dec 18:8, Jun 21:13, Dec 21:19, Aug 22:3-7, Oct 22:7, Nov 22:1, Jan 23:20, Feb 23:12, May 23:23, Jul 23:14, Oct 23:16

(For services of 65 minutes or longer, use prolonged services code 99418)

Hospital Inpatient or Observation Care Services (Including Admission and Discharge Services)

The following codes are used to report hospital inpatient or observation care services provided to patients admitted and discharged on the same date of service when the stay is more than eight hours. These services are only used by the physician or other qualified health care professional team who performs both the initial and discharge services. Other physicians and other qualified health care professionals may report 99221, 99222, 99223, as appropriate.

When a patient receives hospital inpatient or observation care for fewer than eight hours, only the initial hospital inpatient or observation care codes (99221, 99222, 99223) may be reported for the date of admission. Hospital or observation discharge day management codes (99238, 99239) may not be reported. When a patient receives hospital inpatient or observation care for a minimum of eight hours and is discharged on the same calendar date, observation or inpatient care services (including admission and discharge services) codes (99234, 99235, 99236) may be reported. Codes 99238, 99239 are not reported.

For patients admitted to hospital inpatient or observation care and discharged on a different date, see 99221, 99222, 99223, 99231, 99232, 99233, 99238, 99239.

Codes 99234, 99235, 99236 require two or more visits on the same date of which one of these visits is an initial admission and another being a discharge. For a patient admitted and discharged at the same visit (ie, one visit), see 99221, 99222, 99223. Do not report 99238, 99239 in conjunction with 99221, 99222, 99223 for admission and discharge services performed on the same date.

Length of Stay	Discharged On	Report Codes
<8 hours	Same calendar date as initial hospital inpatient or observation care service	99221, 99222, 99223
8 or more hours	Same calendar date as initial hospital inpatient or observation care service	99234, 99235, 99236
<8 hours	Different calendar date as initial hospital inpatient or observation care service	99221, 99222, 99223
8 or more hours	Different calendar date as initial hospital inpatient or observation care service	99221, 99222, 99223 and 99238, 99239

(For discharge services provided to newborns admitted and discharged on the same date, use 99463)

99234   **Hospital inpatient or observation care,** for the evaluation and management of a patient including admission and discharge on the same date, which requires a medically appropriate history and/or examination and straightforward or low level of medical decision making.

When using total time on the date of the encounter for code selection, 45 minutes must be met or exceeded.

➔ *CPT Changes: An Insider's View* 2013, 2023

➔ *CPT Assistant* Nov 97:2, Mar 98:2, May 98:1, Sep 98:5, Jan 00:11, Sep 00:3, Jan 02:2, Jun 02:10, Jan 03:10, May 05:1, Nov 05:10, Sep 06:8, Dec 06:14, Sep 10:4, Jun 11:3, Jul 12:14, Jun 13:3, Apr 18:10, Dec 18:8, Aug 22:3-7, Jan 23:20

99235   **Hospital inpatient or observation care,** for the evaluation and management of a patient including admission and discharge on the same date, which requires a medically appropriate history and/or examination and moderate level of medical decision making.

When using total time on the date of the encounter for code selection, 70 minutes must be met or exceeded.

➡ *CPT Changes: An Insider's View* 2013, 2023

➡ *CPT Assistant* Nov 97:2, Mar 98:2, May 98:1, Sep 98:5, Jan 00:11, Sep 00:3, Jan 02:2, Jun 02:10, Jan 03:10, Nov 05:10, Sep 06:8, Dec 06:14, Sep 10:4, Jun 11:3, Jul 12:14, Jun 13:3, Apr 18:10, Dec 18:8, Aug 22:3-7, Jan 23:20

99236   **Hospital inpatient or observation care,** for the evaluation and management of a patient including admission and discharge on the same date, which requires a medically appropriate history and/or examination and high level of medical decision making.

When using total time on the date of the encounter for code selection, 85 minutes must be met or exceeded.

➡ *CPT Changes: An Insider's View* 2013, 2023

➡ *CPT Assistant* Nov 97:2, Mar 98:2, May 98:1, Sep 98:5, Jan 00:11, Sep 00:3, Jan 02:2, Jun 02:10, Jan 03:10, Nov 05:10, Sep 06:8, Dec 06:14, Sep 10:4, Jun 11:3, Jul 12:14, Jun 13:3, Apr 18:10, Dec 18:8, Aug 22:3-7, Nov 22:1, Dec 22:15, Jan 23:20

(For services of 100 minutes or longer, use prolonged services code 99418)

Hospital Inpatient or Observation Discharge Services

The hospital inpatient or observation discharge day management codes are to be used to report the total duration of time on the date of the encounter spent by a physician or other qualified health care professional for final hospital or observation discharge of a patient, even if the time spent by the physician or other qualified health care professional on that date is not continuous. The codes include, as appropriate, final examination of the patient, discussion of the hospital stay, instructions for continuing care to all relevant caregivers, and preparation of discharge records, prescriptions, and referral forms. These codes are to be utilized to report all services provided to a patient on the date of discharge, if other than the initial date of inpatient or observation status. For a patient admitted and discharged from hospital inpatient or observation status on the same date, report 99234, 99235, 99236, as appropriate.

Codes 99238, 99239 are to be used by the physician or other qualified health care professional who is responsible for discharge services. Services by other physicians or other qualified health care professionals that may include instructions to the patient and/or family/caregiver and coordination of post-discharge services may be reported with 99231, 99232, 99233.

99238   **Hospital inpatient or observation discharge day management;** 30 minutes or less on the date of the encounter

➡ *CPT Changes: An Insider's View* 2023

➡ *CPT Assistant* Fall 92:1, Spring 93:4, Nov 97:4, Mar 98:3, 11, May 98:2, Jan 99:10, Jan 02:2, Aug 04:11, May 05:1, Sep 06:8, Nov 09:10, Dec 09:9, Jul 11:16, Jul 12:10, 12, Jun 13:3, Aug 13:13, Dec 18:8, Aug 22:3-7, Dec 22:15, Jan 23:20

99239   more than 30 minutes on the date of the encounter

➡ *CPT Changes: An Insider's View* 2023

➡ *CPT Assistant* Nov 97:4, Mar 98:3, 11, May 98:2, Jan 99:10, Jan 02:2, Aug 04:11, Sep 06:8, Nov 09:10, Dec 09:9, Jul 11:16, Jul 12:12, Jun 13:3, Aug 13:13, Dec 18:8, Aug 22:3-7, Dec 22:15, Jan 23:20

(For hospital inpatient or observation care including the admission and discharge of the patient on the same date, see 99234, 99235, 99236)

(For discharge services provided to newborns admitted and discharged on the same date, use 99463)

(Do not report 99238, 99239 in conjunction with 99221, 99222, 99223 for admission and discharge services performed on the same date)

Consultations

A consultation is a type of evaluation and management service provided at the request of another physician, other qualified health care professional, or appropriate source to recommend care for a specific condition or problem.

A physician or other qualified health care professional consultant may initiate diagnostic and/or therapeutic services at the same or subsequent visit.

A "consultation" initiated by a patient and/or family, and not requested by a physician, other qualified health care professional, or other appropriate source (eg, non-clinical social worker, educator, lawyer, or insurance company), is not reported using the consultation codes.

The consultant's opinion and any services that were ordered or performed must also be communicated by written report to the requesting physician, other qualified health care professional, or other appropriate source.

If a consultation is mandated (eg, by a third-party payer) modifier 32 should also be reported.

To report services when a patient is admitted to hospital inpatient, or observation status, or to a nursing facility in the course of an encounter in another setting, see **Initial Hospital Inpatient or Observation Care** or **Initial Nursing Facility Care.**

★=Telemedicine   ◀=Audio-only   ✚=Add-on code   ✗=FDA approval pending   #=Resequenced code   ⊘=Modifier 51 exempt   ➡➡➡=See p xxi for details

Office or Other Outpatient Consultations

New or Established Patient

The following codes may be used to report consultations that are provided in the office or other outpatient site, including the home or residence, or emergency department. Follow-up visits in the consultant's office or other outpatient facility that are initiated by the consultant or patient are reported using the appropriate codes for established patients in the office (99212, 99213, 99214, 99215) or home or residence (99347, 99348, 99349, 99350). Services that constitute transfer of care (ie, are provided for the management of the patient's entire care or for the care of a specific condition or problem) are reported with the appropriate new or established patient codes for office or other outpatient visits or home or residence services.

> (For an outpatient consultation requiring prolonged services, use 99417)

> (99241 has been deleted. To report, use 99242)

★ **99242**   **Office or other outpatient consultation** for a new or established patient, which requires a medically appropriate history and/or examination and straightforward medical decision making.

When using total time on the date of the encounter for code selection, 20 minutes must be met or exceeded.

➔ *CPT Changes: An Insider's View* 2000, 2013, 2017, 2023

➔ *CPT Assistant* Winter 91:11, Spring 92:4, 23-24, Summer 92:12, Spring 93:2, 34, Spring 95:1, Oct 97:1, Sep 98:5, Aug 01:3, Jan 02:2, Jul 02:2, Sep 02:11, Dec 05:10, May 06:1, 16, Jun 06:1, Sep 06:8, Apr 07:11, Jul 07:1, Jan 10:3, Jun 11:3, Jan 13:9, Jun 13:3, Sep 14:13, Jan 15:12, Sep 16:6, Apr 18:10, Nov 20:3, Feb 22:4, Aug 22:3-7, Oct 22:7, Feb 23:12, Mar 23:14, Oct 23:16,18

➔ *Clinical Examples in Radiology* Summer 09:3

★ **99243**   **Office or other outpatient consultation** for a new or established patient, which requires a medically appropriate history and/or examination and low level of medical decision making.

When using total time on the date of the encounter for code selection, 30 minutes must be met or exceeded.

➔ *CPT Changes: An Insider's View* 2013, 2017, 2023

➔ *CPT Assistant* Winter 91:11, Spring 92:4, 23-24, Summer 92:12, Spring 93:2, 34, Spring 95:1, Oct 97:1, Sep 98:5, Aug 01:3, Jan 02:2, Jul 02:2, Sep 02:11, Oct 03:5, Dec 05:10, May 06:1, 16, Jun 06:1, Sep 06:8, Apr 07:11, Jul 07:1, Jan 10:3, Jun 11:3, Jan 13:9, Jun 13:3, Sep 14:13, Jan 15:12, Sep 16:6, Apr 18:10, Nov 20:3, Feb 22:4, Aug 22:3-7, Oct 22:7, Feb 23:12, Mar 23:14, Oct 23:16,18

➔ *Clinical Examples in Radiology* Summer 09:3

★ **99244**   **Office or other outpatient consultation** for a new or established patient, which requires a medically appropriate history and/or examination and moderate level of medical decision making.

When using total time on the date of the encounter for code selection, 40 minutes must be met or exceeded.

➔ *CPT Changes: An Insider's View* 2013, 2017, 2023

➔ *CPT Assistant* Winter 91:11, Spring 92:3, 23-24, Summer 92:12, Spring 93:2, 34, Spring 95:1, Oct 97:1, Sep 98:5, Aug 01:3, Jan 02:2, Jul 02:2, Sep 02:11, Oct 03:5, Dec 05:10, May 06:1, 16, Jun 06:1, Sep 06:8, Apr 07:11, Jul 07:1, Jan 10:3, Jun 11:3, Jan 13:9, Jun 13:3, Aug 13:12, Sep 14:13, Jan 15:12, Sep 16:6, Apr 18:10, Nov 20:3, Feb 22:4, Aug 22:3-7, Oct 22:7, Feb 23:12, Mar 23:14, Oct 23:16,18

➔ *Clinical Examples in Radiology* Summer 09:2-3

★ **99245**   **Office or other outpatient consultation** for a new or established patient, which requires a medically appropriate history and/or examination and high level of medical decision making.

When using total time on the date of the encounter for code selection, 55 minutes must be met or exceeded.

➔ *CPT Changes: An Insider's View* 2013, 2017, 2023

➔ *CPT Assistant* Winter 91:11, Spring 92:4, 23-24, Summer 92:12, Spring 93:2, 34, Spring 95:1, Oct 97:1, Sep 98:5, Aug 01:2, Jan 02:2, Jul 02:2, Sep 02:11, Dec 05:10, May 06:1, 16, Jun 06:1, Sep 06:8, Apr 07:11, Jul 07:1, Jan 10:3, Jul 10:4, Jun 11:3, Apr 12:10, Jan 13:9, Jun 13:3, Aug 14:3, Sep 14:13, Jan 15:12, Sep 16:6, Apr 18:10, Nov 20:3, Feb 22:4, Aug 22:3-7, Oct 22:7, Nov 22:1, Dec 22:15, Feb 23:12, Mar 23:14, Oct 23:16,18

➔ *Clinical Examples in Radiology* Summer 09:3

> (For services 70 minutes or longer, use prolonged services code 99417)

Inpatient or Observation Consultations

New or Established Patient

Codes 99252, 99253, 99254, 99255 are used to report physician or other qualified health care professional consultations provided to hospital inpatients, observation-level patients, residents of nursing facilities, or patients in a partial hospital setting, and when the patient has not received any face-to-face professional services from the physician or other qualified health care professional or another physician or other qualified health care professional of the exact same specialty and subspecialty who belongs to the same group practice during the stay. When advanced practice nurses and physician assistants are working with physicians, they are considered as working in the exact same specialty and subspecialty as the physician. Only one consultation may be reported by a consultant per admission. Subsequent consultation services during the same admission are reported using subsequent inpatient or observation hospital care codes (99231-99233) or subsequent nursing facility care codes (99307-99310).

(For an inpatient or observation consultation requiring prolonged services, use 99418)

(99251 has been deleted. To report, use 99252)

★ **99252**   **Inpatient or observation consultation** for a new or established patient, which requires a medically appropriate history and/or examination and straightforward medical decision making.

When using total time on the date of the encounter for code selection, 35 minutes must be met or exceeded.

➡ *CPT Changes: An Insider's View* 2007, 2013, 2017, 2023

➡ *CPT Assistant* Winter 91:11, Spring 92:16, 23-24, Summer 92:12, Summer 93:34, Spring 95:1, Oct 97:1, Sep 98:5, Aug 01:4, Sep 02:11, May 06:1, 16, Jun 06:1, Jul 06:19, Jul 07:1, Jan 10:3, Jan 13:9, Jun 13:3, Feb 22:4, Aug 22:3-7, Oct 22:1,7, Mar 23:14, May 23:23, Jul 23:14, Oct 23:16

➡ *Clinical Examples in Radiology* Summer 09:3

★ **99253**   **Inpatient or observation consultation** for a new or established patient, which requires a medically appropriate history and/or examination and low level of medical decision making.

When using total time on the date of the encounter for code selection, 45 minutes must be met or exceeded.

➡ *CPT Changes: An Insider's View* 2007, 2013, 2017, 2023

➡ *CPT Assistant* Winter 91:11, Spring 92:16, 23-24, Summer 92:12, Summer 93:34, Spring 95:1, Oct 97:1, Sep 98:5, Aug 01:4, Sep 02:11, May 06:1, 16, Jun 06:1, Jul 06:19, Jul 07:1, Jan 10:3, Jan 13:9, Jun 13:3, Sep 21:12, Feb 22:4, Aug 22:3-7, Oct 22:1,7, Mar 23:14, May 23:23, Jul 23:14, Oct 23:16

➡ *Clinical Examples in Radiology* Summer 09:3

★ **99254**   **Inpatient or observation consultation** for a new or established patient, which requires a medically appropriate history and/or examination and moderate level of medical decision making.

When using total time on the date of the encounter for code selection, 60 minutes must be met or exceeded.

➡ *CPT Changes: An Insider's View* 2007, 2013, 2017, 2023

➡ *CPT Assistant* Winter 91:11, Spring 92:16, 23-24, Summer 92:12, Summer 93:34, Spring 95:1, Oct 97:1, Sep 98:5, Aug 01:4, Sep 02:11, May 06:1, 16, Jun 06:1, Jul 06:19, Jul 07:1, Jan 10:3, Jan 13:9, Jun 13:3, Feb 22:4, Aug 22:3-7, Oct 22:1,7, Mar 23:14, May 23:23, Jul 23:14, Oct 23:16

➡ *Clinical Examples in Radiology* Summer 09:3

★ **99255**   **Inpatient or observation consultation** for a new or established patient, which requires a medically appropriate history and/or examination and high level of medical decision making.

When using total time on the date of the encounter for code selection, 80 minutes must be met or exceeded.

➡ *CPT Changes: An Insider's View* 2007, 2013, 2017, 2023

➡ *CPT Assistant* Winter 91:11, Spring 92:16, 23-24, Summer 92:12, Summer 93:34, Spring 95:1, Oct 97:1, Sep 98:5, Aug 01:4, Sep 02:11, May 06:1, 16, Jun 06:1, Jul 06:19, Jul 07:1, Jan 10:3, Jan 13:9, Jun 13:3, Nov 14:14, Feb 22:4, Aug 22:3-7, Oct 22:1,7, Dec 22:15, Mar 23:14, May 23:23, Jul 23:14, Oct 23:16, Dec 23:49, Mar 24:24

➡ *Clinical Examples in Radiology* Summer 09:3

(For services 95 minutes or longer, use prolonged services code 99418)

Emergency Department Services

New or Established Patient

The following codes are used to report evaluation and management services provided in the emergency department. No distinction is made between new and established patients in the emergency department.

An emergency department is defined as an organized hospital-based facility for the provision of unscheduled episodic services to patients who present for immediate medical attention. The facility must be available 24 hours a day.

For critical care services provided in the emergency department, see Critical Care guidelines and 99291, 99292. Critical care and emergency department services may both be reported on the same day when after completion of the emergency department service, the condition of the patient changes and critical care services are provided.

For evaluation and management services provided to a patient in observation status, see 99221, 99222, 99223 for the initial observation encounter and 99231, 99232, 99233, 99238, 99239 for subsequent or discharge hospital inpatient or observation encounters.

For hospital inpatient or observation care services (including admission and discharge services), see 99234, 99235, 99236.

To report services when a patient is admitted to hospital inpatient or observation status, or to a nursing facility in the course of an encounter in another setting, see **Initial Hospital Inpatient or Observation Care** or **Initial Nursing Facility Care**.

For procedures or services identified by a CPT code that may be separately reported on the same date, use the appropriate CPT code. Use the appropriate modifier(s) to report separately identifiable evaluation and management services and the extent of services provided in a surgical package.

If a patient is seen in the emergency department for the convenience of a physician or other qualified health care professional, use office or other outpatient services codes (99202-99215).

— *Coding Tip* —

Time as a Factor in the Emergency Department Setting

Time is **not** a descriptive component for the emergency department levels of E/M services because emergency department services are typically provided on a variable intensity basis, often involving multiple encounters with several patients over an extended period of time.

CPT Coding Guidelines, Evaluation and Management, Guidelines for Selecting Level of Service Based on Time

99281   **Emergency department visit** for the evaluation and management of a patient that may not require the presence of a physician or other qualified health care professional

   ➡ *CPT Changes: An Insider's View* 2013, 2023

   ➡ *CPT Assistant* Winter 91:11, Spring 92:24, Summer 92:18, Spring 93:34, Spring 95:1, Feb 96:3, Sep 98:5, Jan 00:11, Feb 00:11, Sep 00:3, Apr 02:14, Jul 02:2, Nov 05:10, Feb 06:14, Dec 06:14, Dec 07:13, Jan 13:9, Jun 13:3, Nov 14:14, Jan 15:12, Jul 19:10, Jul 20:13, Oct 20:13, Aug 22:3-7, Sep 22:6, Oct 22:7, Dec 22:15, May 23:23, Jul 23:1

99282   **Emergency department visit** for the evaluation and management of a patient, which requires a medically appropriate history and/or examination and straightforward medical decision making

   ➡ *CPT Changes: An Insider's View* 2013, 2023

   ➡ *CPT Assistant* Winter 91:11, Spring 92:24, Summer 92:18, Spring 93:34, Spring 95:1, Summer 95:1, Feb 96:3, Sep 98:5, Jan 00:11, Feb 00:11, Sep 00:3, Apr 02:14, Jul 02:2, Nov 05:10, Feb 06:14, Dec 06:14, Dec 07:13, Jan 13:9, Jun 13:3, Jan 15:12, Jul 19:10, Jul 20:13, Oct 20:13, Aug 22:3-7, Sep 22:6, Oct 22:7, Mar 23:1, Jul 23:1, Apr 24:33

99283   **Emergency department visit** for the evaluation and management of a patient, which requires a medically appropriate history and/or examination and low level of medical decision making

   ➡ *CPT Changes: An Insider's View* 2013, 2023

   ➡ *CPT Assistant* Winter 91:11, Spring 92:24, Summer 92:18, Spring 93:34, Spring 95:1, Summer 95:1, Feb 96:3, Sep 98:5, Jan 00:11, Feb 00:11, Sep 00:3, Apr 02:14, Jul 02:2, Nov 05:10, Feb 06:14, Dec 06:14, Dec 07:13, Jan 13:9, Jun 13:3, Jan 15:12, Jul 19:10, Jul 20:13, Oct 20:13, Aug 22:3-7, Sep 22:6, Oct 22:7, Mar 23:1, Jul 23:1, Apr 24:33

99284   **Emergency department visit** for the evaluation and management of a patient, which requires a medically appropriate history and/or examination and moderate level of medical decision making

   ➡ *CPT Changes: An Insider's View* 2013, 2023

   ➡ *CPT Assistant* Winter 91:11, Spring 92:24, Summer 92:18, Spring 93:34, Spring 95:1, Summer 95:1, Feb 96:3, Sep 98:5, Jan 00:11, Feb 00:11, Sep 00:3, Apr 02:14, Jul 02:2, Nov 05:10, Feb 06:14, Dec 06:14, Dec 07:13, Jan 13:9, Jun 13:3, Jan 15:12, Jul 19:10, Jul 20:13, Oct 20:13, Aug 22:3-7, Sep 22:6, Oct 22:7, Mar 23:1, Jul 23:1, Apr 24:33

99285   **Emergency department visit** for the evaluation and management of a patient, which requires a medically appropriate history and/or examination and high level of medical decision making

   ➡ *CPT Changes: An Insider's View* 2000, 2013, 2023

   ➡ *CPT Assistant* Winter 91:11, Spring 92:24, Summer 92:18, Spring 93:34, Spring 95:1, Summer 95:1, Feb 96:3, Aug 98:8, Sep 98:5, Nov 99:23, Jan 00:11, Feb 00:11, Sep 00:3, Apr 02:14, Jul 02:2, Sep 02:11, Mar 05:11, Nov 05:10, Feb 06:14, Dec 06:14, Dec 07:13, Jan 13:9, Jun 13:3, Nov 14:14, Jan 15:12, Jul 19:10, Jan 20:12, Jul 20:13, Oct 20:13, Aug 22:3-7, Sep 22:6, Oct 22:7, Dec 22:15, Mar 23:1, Jul 23:1, Apr 24:33

— *Coding Tip* —

Emergency Department Classification of New vs Established Patient

No distinction is made between new and established patients in the emergency department. E/M services in the emergency department category may be reported for any new or established patient who presents for treatment in the emergency department.

CPT Coding Guidelines, Evaluation and Management, Classification of E/M Services, New and Established Patients

Other Emergency Services

In directed emergency care, advanced life support, the physician or other qualified health care professional is located in a hospital emergency or critical care department, and is in two-way voice communication with ambulance or rescue personnel outside the hospital. Direction of the performance of necessary medical procedures includes but is not limited to: telemetry of cardiac rhythm; cardiac and/or pulmonary resuscitation; endotracheal or esophageal obturator airway intubation; administration of intravenous fluids and/or administration of intramuscular, intratracheal or subcutaneous drugs; and/or electrical conversion of arrhythmia.

99288 **Physician or other qualified health care professional direction of** emergency medical systems (EMS) emergency care, advanced life support

➡ *CPT Changes: An Insider's View* 2013

➡ *CPT Assistant* Summer 92:18, May 05:1, Nov 07:5, May 13:6

Critical Care Services

Critical care is the direct delivery by a physician(s) or other qualified health care professional of medical care for a critically ill or critically injured patient. A critical illness or injury acutely impairs one or more vital organ systems such that there is a high probability of imminent or life threatening deterioration in the patient's condition. Critical care involves high complexity decision making to assess, manipulate, and support vital system function(s) to treat single or multiple vital organ system failure and/or to prevent further life threatening deterioration of the patient's condition. Examples of vital organ system failure include, but are not limited to: central nervous system failure, circulatory failure, shock, renal, hepatic, metabolic, and/or respiratory failure. Although critical care typically requires interpretation of multiple physiologic parameters and/or application of advanced technology(s), critical care may be provided in life threatening situations when these elements are not present. Critical care may be provided on multiple days, even if no changes are made in the treatment rendered to the patient, provided that the patient's condition continues to require the level of attention described above.

Providing medical care to a critically ill, injured, or post-operative patient qualifies as a critical care service only if both the illness or injury and the treatment being provided meet the above requirements. Critical care is usually, but not always, given in a critical care area, such as the coronary care unit, intensive care unit, pediatric intensive care unit, respiratory care unit, or the emergency care facility.

Inpatient critical care services provided to infants 29 days through 71 months of age are reported with pediatric critical care codes 99471-99476. The pediatric critical care codes are reported as long as the infant/young child qualifies for critical care services during the hospital stay through 71 months of age. Inpatient critical care services provided to neonates (28 days of age or younger) are reported with the neonatal critical care codes 99468 and

99469. The neonatal critical care codes are reported as long as the neonate qualifies for critical care services during the hospital stay through the 28th postnatal day. The reporting of the pediatric and neonatal critical care services is not based on time or the type of unit (eg, pediatric or neonatal critical care unit) and it is not dependent upon the type of physician or other qualified health care professional delivering the care. To report critical care services provided in the outpatient setting (eg, emergency department or office), for neonates and pediatric patients up through 71 months of age, see the critical care codes 99291, 99292. If the same individual provides critical care services for a neonatal or pediatric patient in both the outpatient and inpatient settings on the same day, report only the appropriate neonatal or pediatric critical care code 99468-99472 for all critical care services provided on that day. Also report 99291-99292 for neonatal or pediatric critical care services provided by the individual providing critical care at one facility but transferring the patient to another facility. Critical care services provided by a second individual of a different specialty not reporting a per day neonatal or pediatric critical care code can be reported with codes 99291, 99292. For additional instructions on reporting these services, see the Neonatal and Pediatric Critical Care section and codes 99468-99476.

Services for a patient who is not critically ill but happens to be in a critical care unit are reported using other appropriate E/M codes.

Critical care and other E/M services may be provided to the same patient on the same date by the same individual.

For reporting by professionals, the following services are included in critical care when performed during the critical period by the physician(s) providing critical care: the interpretation of cardiac output measurements (93598), chest X rays (71045, 71046), pulse oximetry (94760, 94761, 94762), blood gases, and collection and interpretation of physiologic data (eg, ECGs, blood pressures, hematologic data); gastric intubation (43752, 43753); temporary transcutaneous pacing (92953); ventilatory management (94002-94004, 94660, 94662); and vascular access procedures (36000, 36410, 36415, 36591, 36600). Any services performed that are not included in this listing should be reported separately. Facilities may report the above services separately.

Codes 99291, 99292 should be reported for the attendance during the transport of critically ill or critically injured patients older than 24 months of age to or from a facility or hospital. For transport services of critically ill or critically injured pediatric patients 24 months of age or younger, see 99466, 99467.

Codes 99291, 99292 are used to report the total duration of time spent in provision of critical care services to a critically ill or critically injured patient, even if the time spent providing care on that date is not continuous. For any given period of time spent providing critical care services, the individual must devote his or her full attention to the patient and, therefore, cannot provide services to any other patient during the same period of time.

Time spent with the individual patient should be recorded in the patient's record. The time that can be reported as critical care is the time spent engaged in work directly related to the individual patient's care whether that time was spent at the immediate bedside or elsewhere on the floor or unit. For example, time spent on the unit or at the nursing station on the floor reviewing test results or imaging studies, discussing the critically ill patient's care with other medical staff or documenting critical care services in the medical record would be reported as critical care, even though it does not occur at the bedside. Also, when the patient is unable or lacks capacity to participate in discussions, time spent on the floor or unit with family members or surrogate decision makers obtaining a medical history, reviewing the patient's condition or prognosis, or discussing treatment or limitation(s) of treatment may be reported as critical care, provided that the conversation bears directly on the management of the patient.

Time spent in activities that occur outside of the unit or off the floor (eg, telephone calls whether taken at home, in the office, or elsewhere in the hospital) may not be reported as critical care since the individual is not immediately available to the patient. Time spent in activities that do not directly contribute to the treatment of the patient may not be reported as critical care, even if they are performed in the critical care unit (eg, participation in administrative meetings or telephone calls to discuss other patients). Time spent performing separately reportable procedures or services should not be included in the time reported as critical care time.

Code 99291 is used to report the first 30-74 minutes of critical care on a given date. It should be used only once per date even if the time spent by the individual is not continuous on that date. Critical care of less than 30 minutes total duration on a given date should be reported with the appropriate E/M code.

Code 99292 is used to report additional block(s) of time, of up to 30 minutes each beyond the first 74 minutes. (See the following table.)

The following examples illustrate the correct reporting of critical care services:

Total Duration of Critical Care	Codes
less than 30 minutes	appropriate E/M codes
30-74 minutes (30 minutes - 1 hr. 14 min.)	99291 X 1
75-104 minutes (1 hr. 15 min. - 1 hr. 44 min.)	99291 X 1 AND 99292 X 1
105-134 minutes (1 hr. 45 min. - 2 hr. 14 min.)	99291 X 1 AND 99292 X 2
135-164 minutes (2 hr. 15 min. - 2 hr. 44 min.)	99291 X 1 AND 99292 X 3
165-194 minutes (2 hr. 45 min. - 3 hr. 14 min.)	99291 X 1 AND 99292 X 4
195 minutes or longer (3 hr. 15 min. - etc.)	99291 and 99292 as appropriate (see illustrated reporting examples above)

99291   **Critical care, evaluation and management** of the critically ill or critically injured patient; first 30-74 minutes

➔ *CPT Assistant* Summer 92:18, Summer 93:1, Summer 95:1, Jan 96:7, Apr 97:3, Dec 98:6, Nov 99:3, Apr 00:6, Sep 00:1, Dec 00:15, Jul 02:2, Feb 03:15, Oct 03:2, Aug 04:7, 10, Oct 04:14, May 05:1, Jul 05:15, Nov 05:10, Jul 06:4, Dec 06:13, Nov 07:5, Jan 09:5, Mar 09:3, Jul 09:10, Aug 11:10, Sep 11:3, Jul 12:13, Feb 13:17, May 13:6, May 14:4, Aug 14:5, Oct 14:14, Feb 15:10, May 16:3, Aug 16:9, Oct 16:8, Jun 18:9, Dec 18:8, Jul 19:10, Aug 19:8, Dec 19:14, Jan 20:12, Feb 20:7, Jun 21:13, Sep 21:13, Jan 22:3, 14, Mar 22:12, Sep 22:6, Dec 22:15, Feb 23:12, Mar 23:1

+ **99292**   each additional 30 minutes (List separately in addition to code for primary service)

➔ *CPT Assistant* Summer 92:18, Summer 93:1, Summer 95:1, Jan 96:7, Apr 97:3, Dec 98:6, Nov 99:3, Apr 00:6, Sep 00:1, Dec 00:15, Feb 03:15, Oct 03:2, Aug 04:10, Oct 04:14, Jul 05:15, Nov 05:10, Jul 06:4, Dec 06:13, Nov 07:5, Jan 09:5, Mar 09:3, Aug 11:10, Sep 11:3, Feb 13:17, May 13:6, May 14:4, Aug 14:5, Oct 14:14, Feb 15:10, May 16:3, Aug 16:9, Jun 18:9, Dec 18:8, Jul 19:10, Aug 19:8, Dec 19:14, Feb 20:7, Jan 22:3, 14, Mar 22:12, Sep 22:6, Dec 22:15, Feb 23:12

(Use 99292 in conjunction with 99291)

Evaluation / Management 99202-99499

Coding Tip

Services Included in Critical Care Services

For reporting by professionals, the following services are included in critical care when performed during the critical period by the physician(s) providing critical care: the interpretation of cardiac output measurements (93598), chest X rays (71045, 71046), pulse oximetry (94760, 94761, 94762), blood gases, and collection and interpretation of physiologic data (eg, ECGs, blood pressures, hematologic data); gastric intubation (43752, 43753); temporary transcutaneous pacing (92953); ventilatory management (94002-94004, 94660, 94662); and vascular access procedures (36000, 36410, 36415, 36591, 36600). Any services performed that are not listed above should be reported separately. Facilities may report the above services separately.

CPT Coding Guidelines, Critical Care Services

Nursing Facility Services

The following codes are used to report evaluation and management services to patients in nursing facilities and skilled nursing facilities. These codes should also be used to report evaluation and management services provided to a patient in a psychiatric residential treatment center and intermediate care facility for individuals with intellectual disabilities.

Regulations pertaining to the care of nursing facility residents govern the nature and minimum frequency of assessments and visits. These regulations also govern who may perform the initial comprehensive visit.

These services are performed by the principal physician(s) and other qualified health care professional(s) overseeing the care of the patient in the facility. The principal physician is sometimes referred to as the admitting physician and is the physician who oversees the patient's care as opposed to other physicians or other qualified health care professionals who may be furnishing specialty care. These services are also performed by physicians or other qualified health care professionals in the role of a specialist performing a consultation or concurrent care. Modifiers may be required to identify the role of the individual performing the service.

Two major subcategories of nursing facility services are recognized: Initial Nursing Facility Care and Subsequent Nursing Facility Care. Both subcategories apply to new or established patients.

The types of care (eg, skilled nursing facility and nursing facility care) are reported with the same codes. Place of service codes should be reported to specify the type of facility (and care) where the service(s) is performed.

When selecting a level of medical decision making (MDM) for nursing facility services, the number and complexity of problems addressed at the encounter is considered. For this determination, a high-level MDM-type specific to initial nursing facility care by the principal physician or other qualified health care professional is recognized. This type is:

Multiple morbidities requiring intensive management: A set of conditions, syndromes, or functional impairments that are likely to require frequent medication changes or other treatment changes and/or re-evaluations. The patient is at significant risk of worsening medical (including behavioral) status and risk for (re)admission to a hospital.

The definitions and requirements related to the amount and/or complexity of data to be reviewed and analyzed and the risk of complications and/or morbidity or mortality of patient management are unchanged.

Initial Nursing Facility Care

New or Established Patient

When the patient is admitted to the nursing facility in the course of an encounter in another site of service (eg, hospital emergency department, office), the services in the initial site may be separately reported. Modifier 25 may be added to the other evaluation and management service to indicate a significant, separately identifiable service by the same physician or other qualified health care professional was performed on the same date.

In the case when services in a separate site are reported and the initial nursing facility care service is a consultation service performed by the same physician or other qualified health care professional and reported on the same date, do not report 99252, 99253, 99254, 99255, 99304, 99305, 99306. The consultant reports the subsequent nursing facility care codes 99307, 99308, 99309, 99310 for the second service on the same date.

Hospital inpatient or observation discharge services performed on the same date of nursing facility admission or readmission may be reported separately. For a patient discharged from inpatient or observation status on the same date of nursing facility admission or readmission, the hospital or observation discharge services may be reported with codes 99238, 99239, as appropriate. For a patient admitted and discharged from hospital inpatient

---

or observation status on the same date, see 99234, 99235, 99236. Time related to hospital inpatient or observation care services may not be used for code selection of any nursing facility service.

Initial nursing facility care codes 99304, 99305, 99306 may be used once per admission, per physician or other qualified health care professional, regardless of length of stay. They may be used for the initial comprehensive visit performed by the principal physician or other qualified health care professional. Skilled nursing facility initial comprehensive visits must be performed by a physician. Qualified health care professionals may report initial comprehensive nursing facility visits for nursing facility level of care patients, if allowed by state law or regulation. The principal physician or other qualified health care professional may work with others (who may not always be in the same group) but are overseeing the overall medical care of the patient, in order to provide timely care to the patient. Medically necessary assessments conducted by these professionals prior to the initial comprehensive visit are reported using subsequent care codes (99307, 99308, 99309, 99310).

Initial services by other physicians and other qualified health care professionals who are performing consultations may be reported using initial nursing facility care codes (99304, 99305, 99306) or inpatient or observation consultation codes (99252, 99253, 99254, 99255). This is not dependent upon the principal care professional's completion of the initial comprehensive services first.

An initial service may be reported when the patient has not received any face-to-face professional services from the physician or other qualified health care professional or another physician or other qualified health care professional of the exact same specialty and subspecialty who belongs to the same group practice during the stay. When advanced practice nurses or physician assistants are working with physicians, they are considered as working in the exact same specialty and subspecialty as the physician. An initial service may also be reported if the patient is a new patient as defined in the Evaluation and Management Guidelines.

For reporting initial nursing facility care, transitions between skilled nursing facility level of care and nursing facility level of care do not constitute a new stay.

99304   **Initial nursing facility care,** per day, for the evaluation and management of a patient, which requires a medically appropriate history and/or examination and straightforward or low level of medical decision making.

When using total time on the date of the encounter for code selection, 25 minutes must be met or exceeded.

➧ *CPT Changes: An Insider's View* 2006, 2008, 2010, 2013, 2023

➧ *CPT Assistant* Jul 10:4, Jan 11:3, Jun 11:3, Jan 12:3, Jul 12:12, Jan 13:9, Jun 13:3, Nov 14:14, Nov 20:3, Aug 22:3-7, Oct 22:1,7, Dec 22:15, Jan 23:28, Dec 23:49

99305   **Initial nursing facility care,** per day, for the evaluation and management of a patient, which requires a medically appropriate history and/or examination and moderate level of medical decision making.

When using total time on the date of the encounter for code selection, 35 minutes must be met or exceeded.

➧ *CPT Changes: An Insider's View* 2006, 2008, 2010, 2013, 2023

➧ *CPT Assistant* Jan 11:3, Jun 11:3, Jul 12:12, Jan 13:9, Jun 13:3, Nov 20:3, Aug 22:3-7, Oct 22:1, Jan 23:28

99306   **Initial nursing facility care,** per day, for the evaluation and management of a patient, which requires a medically appropriate history and/or examination and high level of medical decision making.

When using total time on the date of the encounter for code selection, 50 minutes must be met or exceeded.

➧ *CPT Changes: An Insider's View* 2006, 2008, 2010, 2013, 2023, 2024

➧ *CPT Assistant* Jan 11:3, Jun 11:3, Jan 12:3, Jul 12:12, Jan 13:9, Jun 13:3, Nov 20:3, Aug 22:3-7, Oct 22:1, Nov 22:1, Jan 23:28

(For services 65 minutes or longer, use prolonged services code 99418)

Subsequent Nursing Facility Care

★ **99307**   **Subsequent nursing facility care,** per day, for the evaluation and management of a patient, which requires a medically appropriate history and/or examination and straightforward medical decision making.

When using total time on the date of the encounter for code selection, 10 minutes must be met or exceeded.

➧ *CPT Changes: An Insider's View* 2006, 2008, 2010, 2013, 2017, 2023

➧ *CPT Assistant* May 06:1, 16, Jun 06:1, 19, Mar 07:9, Jul 07:1, Jul 09:3, 8, Jan 11:3, Jan 12:3, Jul 12:12, Jan 13:9, Jun 13:3, Nov 20:3, Aug 22:3-7, Oct 22:1

★ **99308**   **Subsequent nursing facility care,** per day, for the evaluation and management of a patient, which requires a medically appropriate history and/or examination and low level of medical decision making.

When using total time on the date of the encounter for code selection, 20 minutes must be met or exceeded.

➧ *CPT Changes: An Insider's View* 2006, 2008, 2010, 2013, 2017, 2023, 2024

➧ *CPT Assistant* May 06:1, 16, Jun 06:1, 19, Mar 07:9, Jul 07:1, Jul 09:3, 8, Jan 11:3, Jul 12:12, Jan 13:9, Jun 13:3, May 20:12, Nov 20:3, Aug 22:3-7, Oct 22:1

★ **99309** **Subsequent nursing facility care,** per day, for the evaluation and management of a patient, which requires a medically appropriate history and/or examination and moderate level of medical decision making.

When using total time on the date of the encounter for code selection, 30 minutes must be met or exceeded.

➔ *CPT Changes: An Insider's View* 2006, 2008, 2010, 2013, 2017, 2023

➔ *CPT Assistant* May 06:1, 16, Jun 06:1, 19, Mar 07:9, Jul 07:1, Jul 09:3, 8, Jan 11:3, Jul 12:12, Jan 13:9, Jun 13:3, Nov 20:3, Aug 22:3-7, Oct 22:1

★ **99310** **Subsequent nursing facility care,** per day, for the evaluation and management of a patient, which requires a medically appropriate history and/or examination and high level of medical decision making.

When using total time on the date of the encounter for code selection, 45 minutes must be met or exceeded.

➔ *CPT Changes: An Insider's View* 2006, 2008, 2010, 2013, 2017, 2023

➔ *CPT Assistant* May 06:1, 16, Jun 06:1, 19, Mar 07:9, Jul 07:1, Jul 09:3, 8, Jul 10:4, Jan 11:3, Jan 12:3, Jul 12:12, Jan 13:9, Jun 13:3, Nov 20:3, Aug 22:3-7, Oct 22:1, Nov 22:1, Dec 22:15

(For services 60 minutes or longer, use prolonged services code 99418)

Nursing Facility Discharge Services

The nursing facility discharge management codes are to be used to report the total duration of time spent by a physician or other qualified health care professional for the final nursing facility discharge of a patient. The codes include, as appropriate, final examination of the patient, discussion of the nursing facility stay, even if the time spent on that date is not continuous. Instructions are given for continuing care to all relevant caregivers, and preparation of discharge records, prescriptions, and referral forms. These services require a face-to-face encounter with the patient and/or family/caregiver that may be performed on a date prior to the date the patient leaves the facility. Code selection is based on the total time on the date of the discharge management face-to-face encounter.

99315 **Nursing facility discharge management;** 30 minutes or less total time on the date of the encounter

➔ *CPT Changes: An Insider's View* 2023

➔ *CPT Assistant* Nov 97:5-6, Sep 98:5, May 02:19, Nov 02:11, May 05:1, Jul 09:3, Jan 11:3, Jan 12:3, Jul 12:12, Jan 13:9, Jun 13:3, Nov 20:3, Aug 22:3-7, Oct 22:1, Dec 22:15

99316 more than 30 minutes total time on the date of the encounter

➔ *CPT Changes: An Insider's View* 2023

➔ *CPT Assistant* Nov 97:5-6, Sep 98:5, May 02:19, Nov 02:11, Jul 09:3, Jan 11:3, Jul 12:12, Jan 13:9, Jun 13:3, Nov 20:3, Aug 22:3-7, Oct 22:1, Dec 22:15, Dec 23:49

Other Nursing Facility Services

(99318 has been deleted. To report, see 99307, 99308, 99309, 99310)

Domiciliary, Rest Home (eg, Boarding Home), or Custodial Care Services

New Patient

(99324, 99325, 99326, 99327, 99328 have been deleted. For domiciliary, rest home [eg, boarding home], or custodial care services, new patient, see home or residence services codes 99341, 99342, 99344, 99345)

Established Patient

(99334, 99335, 99336, 99337 have been deleted. For domiciliary, rest home [eg, boarding home], or custodial care services, established patient, see home or residence services codes 99347, 99348, 99349, 99350)

Domiciliary, Rest Home (eg, Assisted Living Facility), or Home Care Plan Oversight Services

(99339, 99340 have been deleted. For domiciliary, rest home [eg, assisted living facility], or home care plan oversight services, see care management services codes 99437, 99491, or principal care management codes 99424, 99425)

Home or Residence Services

The following codes are used to report evaluation and management services provided in a home or residence. Home may be defined as a private residence, temporary lodging, or short-term accommodation (eg, hotel, campground, hostel, or cruise ship).

These codes are also used when the residence is an assisted living facility, group home (that is not licensed as an intermediate care facility for individuals with intellectual disabilities), custodial care facility, or residential substance abuse treatment facility.

For services in an intermediate care facility for individuals with intellectual disabilities and services provided in a psychiatric residential treatment center, see **Nursing Facility Services**.

When selecting code level using time, do not count any travel time.

To report services when a patient is admitted to hospital inpatient, observation status, or to a nursing facility in the course of an encounter in another setting, see **Initial Hospital Inpatient and Observation Care** or **Initial Nursing Facility Care**.

New Patient

99341   **Home or residence visit** for the evaluation and management of a new patient, which requires a medically appropriate history and/or examination and straightforward medical decision making.

When using total time on the date of the encounter for code selection, 15 minutes must be met or exceeded.

➲ *CPT Changes: An Insider's View* 2013, 2023

➲ *CPT Assistant* Winter 91:11, Spring 92:24, Summer 92:12, Spring 93:34, Spring 95:1, Jun 97:6, Nov 97:6, 8, Oct 98:6, Oct 03:7, May 05:1, Jan 06:1, Jul 09:8, Aug 09:5, Jan 11:3, Jan 12:3, Apr 12:10, Jan 13:9, Jun 13:3, Oct 14:3, Nov 14:14, Nov 20:3, Oct 22:7, Dec 22:3,15, Dec 23:49

99342   **Home or residence visit** for the evaluation and management of a new patient, which requires a medically appropriate history and/or examination and low level of medical decision making.

When using total time on the date of the encounter for code selection, 30 minutes must be met or exceeded.

➲ *CPT Changes: An Insider's View* 2013, 2023

➲ *CPT Assistant* Winter 91:11, Spring 92:24, Summer 92:12, Spring 93:34, Spring 95:1, Jun 97:6, Nov 97:6, 8, Oct 98:6, Jan 06:1, Jul 09:8, Aug 09:5, Jan 11:3, Jan 13:9, Jun 13:3, Nov 20:3, Dec 22:3

(99343 has been deleted. To report, see 99341, 99342, 99344, 99345)

99344   **Home or residence visit** for the evaluation and management of a new patient, which requires a medically appropriate history and/or examination and moderate level of medical decision making.

When using total time on the date of the encounter for code selection, 60 minutes must be met or exceeded.

➲ *CPT Changes: An Insider's View* 2013, 2023

➲ *CPT Assistant* Nov 97:6, 8, Oct 98:6, Jan 06:1, Jul 09:8, Aug 09:5, Jan 11:3, Jan 13:9, Jun 13:3, Nov 20:3, Dec 22:3

99345   **Home or residence visit** for the evaluation and management of a new patient, which requires a medically appropriate history and/or examination and high level of medical decision making.

When using total time on the date of the encounter for code selection, 75 minutes must be met or exceeded.

➲ *CPT Changes: An Insider's View* 2013, 2023

➲ *CPT Assistant* Nov 97:6, 8, Oct 98:6, Jan 06:1, Jul 09:8, Aug 09:5, Jan 11:3, Jan 12:3, Jan 13:9, Jun 13:3, Nov 20:3, Nov 22:1, Dec 22:3,15

(For services 90 minutes or longer, see prolonged services code 99417)

Established Patient

99347   **Home or residence visit** for the evaluation and management of an established patient, which requires a medically appropriate history and/or examination and straightforward medical decision making.

When using total time on the date of the encounter for code selection, 20 minutes must be met or exceeded.

➲ *CPT Changes: An Insider's View* 2013, 2023

➲ *CPT Assistant* Nov 97:6, 8, Oct 98:6, May 05:1, Jan 06:1, Jul 07:1, Jul 09:8, Aug 09:5, Jan 11:3, Jan 12:3, Jan 13:9, Jun 13:3, Nov 13:3, Nov 20:3, Dec 22:3,15

99348   **Home or residence visit** for the evaluation and management of an established patient, which requires a medically appropriate history and/or examination and low level of medical decision making.

When using total time on the date of the encounter for code selection, 30 minutes must be met or exceeded.

➲ *CPT Changes: An Insider's View* 2013, 2023

➲ *CPT Assistant* Nov 97:6, 8, Oct 98:6, Jan 06:1, Jul 07:1, Jul 09:8, Aug 09:5, Jan 11:3, Jan 13:9, Jun 13:3, Nov 20:3, Dec 22:3

99349   **Home or residence visit** for the evaluation and management of an established patient, which requires a medically appropriate history and/or examination and moderate level of medical decision making.

When using total time on the date of the encounter for code selection, 40 minutes must be met or exceeded.

➲ *CPT Changes: An Insider's View* 2013, 2023

➲ *CPT Assistant* Nov 97:6, 8, Oct 98:6, Jan 06:1, Jul 07:1, Jul 09:8, Aug 09:5, Jan 13:9, Jun 13:3, Nov 20:3, Dec 22:3

99350   **Home or residence visit** for the evaluation and management of an established patient, which requires a medically appropriate history and/or examination and high level of medical decision making.

When using total time on the date of the encounter for code selection, 60 minutes must be met or exceeded.

➲ *CPT Changes: An Insider's View* 2013, 2023

➲ *CPT Assistant* Nov 97:6, 8, Oct 98:6, Oct 03:7, Jan 06:1, Jul 07:1, Jul 09:8, Aug 09:5, Jan 12:3, Apr 12:10, Jan 13:9, Jun 13:3, Nov 13:3, Oct 14:3, Nov 14:14, Nov 20:3, Oct 22:7, Nov 22:1, Dec 22:3,15, Dec 23:49

(For services 75 minutes or longer, see prolonged services code 99417)

Prolonged Services

Prolonged Service With Direct Patient Contact (Except with Office or Other Outpatient Services)

(99354, 99355 have been deleted. For prolonged evaluation and management services on the date of an outpatient service, home or residence service, or cognitive assessment and care plan, use 99417)

(99356, 99357 have been deleted. For prolonged evaluation and management services on the date of an inpatient or observation or nursing facility service, use 99418)

Prolonged Service Without Direct Patient Contact on Date Other Than the Face-to-Face Evaluation and Management Service

Codes 99358 and 99359 are used when a prolonged service is provided on a date other than the date of a face-to-face evaluation and management encounter with the patient and/or family/caregiver. Codes 99358, 99359 may be reported for prolonged services in relation to any evaluation and management service on a date other than the face-to-face service, whether or not time was used to select the level of the face-to-face service.

This service is to be reported in relation to other physician or other qualified health care professional services, including evaluation and management services at any level, on a date other than the face-to-face service to which it is related. Prolonged service without direct patient contact may only be reported when it occurs on a **date other than** the date of the evaluation and management service. For example, extensive record review may relate to a previous evaluation and management service performed at an earlier date. However, it must relate to a service or patient in which (face-to-face) patient care has occurred or will occur and relate to ongoing patient management.

Codes 99358 and 99359 are used to report the total duration of non-face-to-face time spent by a physician or other qualified health care professional on a given date providing prolonged service, even if the time spent by the physician or other qualified health care professional on that date is not continuous. Code 99358 is used to report the first hour of prolonged service on a given date regardless of the place of service. It should be used only once per date.

Prolonged service of less than 30 minutes total duration on a given date is not separately reported.

Code 99359 is used to report each additional 30 minutes beyond the first hour. It may also be used to report the final 15 to 30 minutes of prolonged service on a given date.

Prolonged service of less than 15 minutes beyond the first hour or less than 15 minutes beyond the final 30 minutes is not reported separately.

Do not report 99358, 99359 for time without direct patient contact reported in other services, such as care plan oversight services (99374-99380), chronic care management by a physician or other qualified health care professional (99437, 99491), principal care management by a physician or other qualified health care professional (99424, 99425, 99426, 99427), home and outpatient INR monitoring (93792, 93793), medical team conferences (99366-99368), interprofessional telephone/Internet/electronic health record consultations (99446, 99447, 99448, 99449, 99451, 99452), or online digital evaluation and management services (99421, 99422, 99423).

99358 **Prolonged evaluation and management service** before and/or after direct patient care; first hour

➔ *CPT Changes: An Insider's View* 2010, 2012

➔ *CPT Assistant* Spring 94:34, Nov 98:3, Sep 00:3, Nov 05:10, Jun 08:12, Sep 08:3, Aug 12:3-5, Apr 13:3, Oct 13:11, Nov 13:3, Oct 14:3, Oct 18:9, Jan 19:13, Jun 19:7, Sep 21:13, Jun 22:20, Nov 22:1, Dec 22:19, Mar 23:20

+ 99359 each additional 30 minutes (List separately in addition to code for prolonged service)

➔ *CPT Changes: An Insider's View* 2010, 2012

➔ *CPT Assistant* Spring 94:34, Sep 00:3, Nov 05:10, Jun 08:12, Sep 08:3, Aug 12:3-5, Apr 13:3, Oct 13:11, Nov 13:3, Oct 14:3, Oct 18:9, Jan 19:13, Jun 19:7, Sep 21:13, Nov 22:1, Dec 22:19, Mar 23:20

(Use 99359 in conjunction with 99358)

(Do not report 99358, 99359 on the same date of service as 99202, 99203, 99204, 99205, 99212, 99213, 99214, 99215, 99221, 99222, 99223, 99231, 99232, 99233, 99234, 99235, 99236, 99242, 99243, 99244, 99245, 99252, 99253, 99254, 99255, 99281, 99282, 99283, 99284, 99285, 99304, 99305, 99306, 99307, 99308, 99309, 99310, 99341, 99342, 99344, 99345, 99347, 99348, 99349, 99350, 99417, 99418, 99483)

Total Duration of Prolonged Services Without Direct Face-to-Face Contact	Code(s)
less than 30 minutes	Not reported separately
30-74 minutes (30 minutes - 1 hr. 14 min.)	99358 X 1
75-104 minutes (1 hr. 15 min. - 1 hr. 44 min.)	99358 X 1 AND 99359 X 1
105 minutes or more (1 hr. 45 min. or more)	99358 X 1 AND 99359 X 2 or more for each additional 30 minutes

Prolonged Clinical Staff Services With Physician or Other Qualified Health Care Professional Supervision

Codes 99415, 99416 are used when an evaluation and management (E/M) service is provided in the office or outpatient setting that involves prolonged clinical staff face-to-face time with the patient and/or family/caregiver. The physician or other qualified health care professional is present to provide direct supervision of the clinical staff. This service is reported in addition to the designated E/M services and any other services provided at the same session as E/M services.

Codes 99415, 99416 are used to report the total duration of face-to-face time with the patient and/or family/caregiver spent by clinical staff on a given date providing prolonged service in the office or other outpatient setting, even if the time spent by the clinical staff on that date is not continuous. Time spent performing separately reported services other than the E/M service is not counted toward the prolonged services time.

Code 99415 is used to report the first hour of prolonged clinical staff service on a given date. Code 99415 should be used only once per date, even if the time spent by the clinical staff is not continuous on that date. Prolonged service of less than 30 minutes total duration on a given date is not separately reported. When face-to-face time is noncontinuous, use only the face-to-face time provided to the patient and/or family/caregiver by the clinical staff.

Code 99416 is used to report each additional 30 minutes of prolonged clinical staff service beyond the first hour. Code 99416 may also be used to report the final 15-30 minutes of prolonged service on a given date. Prolonged service of less than 15 minutes beyond the first hour or less than 15 minutes beyond the final 30 minutes is not reported separately.

Codes 99415, 99416 may be reported for no more than two simultaneous patients and the time reported is the time devoted only to a single patient.

For prolonged services by the physician or other qualified health care professional on the date of an office or other outpatient evaluation and management service (with or without direct patient contact), use 99417. Do not report 99415, 99416 in conjunction with 99417.

Facilities may not report 99415, 99416.

#+ 99415   **Prolonged clinical staff service** (the service beyond the highest time in the range of total time of the service) during an evaluation and management service in the office or outpatient setting, direct patient contact with physician supervision; first hour (List separately in addition to code for outpatient **Evaluation and Management** service)

➔ *CPT Changes: An Insider's View* 2016, 2021
➔ *CPT Assistant* Oct 15:3, Feb 16:13, Oct 19:10, Nov 20:12, Nov 22:1

(Use 99415 in conjunction with 99202, 99203, 99204, 99205, 99212, 99213, 99214, 99215)

(Do not report 99415 in conjunction with 99417)

#+ 99416   each additional 30 minutes (List separately in addition to code for prolonged service)

➔ *CPT Changes: An Insider's View* 2016, 2021
➔ *CPT Assistant* Oct 15:3, Feb 16:13, Oct 19:10, Nov 20:12, Nov 22:1

(Use 99416 in conjunction with 99415)

(Do not report 99416 in conjunction with 99417)

The starting point for 99415 is 30 minutes beyond the typical clinical staff time for ongoing assessment of the patient during the office visit. The Reporting Prolonged Clinical Staff Time table provides the typical clinical staff times for the office or other outpatient primary codes, the range of time beyond the clinical staff time for which 99415 may be reported, and the starting point at which 99416 may be reported.

Reporting Prolonged Clinical Staff Time

Code	Typical Clinical Staff Time	99415 Time Range (Minutes)	99416 Start Point (Minutes)
99202	29	59-103	104
99203	34	64-108	109
99204	41	71-115	116
99205	46	76-120	121
99211	16	46-90	91
99212	24	54-98	99
99213	27	57-101	102
99214	40	70-114	115
99215	45	75-119	120

Prolonged Service With or Without Direct Patient Contact on the Date of an Evaluation and Management Service

Code 99417 is used to report prolonged total time (ie, combined time with and without direct patient contact) provided by the physician or other qualified health care professional on the date of office or other outpatient services, office consultation, or other outpatient evaluation and management services (ie, 99205, 99215, 99245, 99345, 99350, 99483). Code 99418 is used to report prolonged total time (ie, combined time with and without direct patient contact) provided by the physician or other qualified health care professional on the date of an inpatient evaluation and management service (ie, 99223, 99233, 99236, 99255, 99306, 99310). Prolonged total time is time that is 15 minutes beyond the time threshold required to report the highest-level primary service. Codes 99417, 99418 are only used when the primary service has been selected using time alone as the basis and only after the time required to report the highest-level service has been exceeded by 15 minutes. Cognitive assessment and care plan services code 99483 does not have a required time threshold, and 99417 may be reported when the typical time has been exceeded by 15 minutes. To report a unit of 99417, 99418, 15 minutes of prolonged services time must have been attained. Do not report 99417, 99418 for any time increment of less than 15 minutes.

When reporting 99417, 99418, the initial time unit of 15 minutes may be added once the time threshold required for the primary E/M code has been surpassed by 15 minutes. For example, to report the initial unit of 99417 for a new patient encounter (99205), do not report 99417 until at least 15 minutes of time have been accumulated beyond 60 minutes (ie, 75 minutes) on the

date of the encounter. For an established patient encounter (99215), do not report 99417 until at least 15 minutes of time have been accumulated beyond 40 minutes (ie, 55 minutes) on the date of the encounter.

Time spent performing separately reported services other than the primary E/M service and prolonged E/M service is not counted toward the primary E/M and prolonged services time.

For prolonged services on a date other than the date of a face-to-face evaluation and management encounter with the patient and/or family/caregiver, see 99358, 99359. For E/M services that require prolonged clinical staff time and may include face-to-face services by the physician or other qualified health care professional, see 99415, 99416. Do not report 99417, 99418 in conjunction with 99358, 99359, 99415, 99416.

#★+ 99417   **Prolonged outpatient evaluation and management service(s)** time with or without direct patient contact beyond the required time of the primary service when the primary service level has been selected using total time, each 15 minutes of total time (List separately in addition to the code of the outpatient **Evaluation and Management** service)

➔ *CPT Changes: An Insider's View* 2021, 2023

➔ *CPT Assistant* Nov 20:3, Jan 21:4, Aug 22:3-7, Nov 22:1, Dec 22:3, Mar 23:14

▶(Use 99417 in conjunction with 98003, 98007, 98011, 98015, 99205, 99215, 99245, 99345, 99350, 99483)◀

(Use 99417 in conjunction with 99483, when the total time on the date of the encounter exceeds the typical time of 99483 by 15 minutes or more)

(Do not report 99417 on the same date of service as 90833, 90836, 90838, 99358, 99359, 99415, 99416)

(Do not report 99417 for any time unit less than 15 minutes)

#★+ 99418   **Prolonged inpatient or observation evaluation and management service(s)** time with or without direct patient contact beyond the required time of the primary service when the primary service level has been selected using total time, each 15 minutes of total time (List separately in addition to the code of the inpatient and observation **Evaluation and Management** service)

➔ *CPT Changes: An Insider's View* 2023

➔ *CPT Assistant* Aug 22:3-7, Oct 22:1, Nov 22:1, Jan 23:20, Mar 23:14

(Use 99418 in conjunction with 99223, 99233, 99236, 99255, 99306, 99310)

(Do not report 99418 on the same date of service as 90833, 90836, 90838, 99358, 99359)

(Do not report 99418 for any time unit less than 15 minutes)

Example of initial and multiple units of prolonged service(s)

Total Duration of New Patient Office or Other Outpatient Services (use with 99205)	Code(s)
less than 75 minutes	Not reported separately
75-89 minutes	99205 X 1 and 99417 X 1
90-104 minutes	99205 X 1 and 99417 X 2
105 minutes or more	99205 X 1 and 99417 X 3 or more for each additional 15 minutes

Reporting Prolonged Services

Primary Code	Prolonged Services Code	Total Time to Report Initial Unit of Prolonged Services	Total Time to Report Second Unit of Prolonged Services
99205	99417	75	90
99215	99417	55	70
99223	99418	90	105
99233	99418	65	80
99236	99418	100	115
99245	99417	70	85
99255	99418	95	110
99306	99418	65	80
99310	99418	60	75
99345	99417	90	105
99350	99417	75	90
99483	99417	75	90

Standby Services

Code 99360 is used to report physician or other qualified health care professional standby services that are requested by another individual and that involve prolonged attendance without direct (face-to-face) patient contact. Care or services may not be provided to other patients during this period. This code is not used to report time spent proctoring another individual. It is also not used if the period of standby ends with the performance of a procedure, subject to a surgical package by the individual who was on standby.

Code 99360 is used to report the total duration of time spent on a given date on standby. Standby service of less than 30 minutes total duration on a given date is not reported separately.

Second and subsequent periods of standby beyond the first 30 minutes may be reported only if a full 30 minutes of standby was provided for each unit of service reported.

99360   **Standby service,** requiring prolonged attendance, each 30 minutes (eg, operative standby, standby for frozen section, for cesarean/high risk delivery, for monitoring EEG)

➔ *CPT Changes: An Insider's View* 2013

➔ *CPT Assistant* Spring 94:32, Apr 97:10, Aug 97:18, Nov 97:8, Nov 99:5-6, Aug 00:3, Sep 00:3, May 05:1, Nov 05:10, Nov 06:23, Mar 08:14, Feb 11:3, May 13:8, Apr 14:5, 11

(For hospital mandated on call services, see 99026, 99027)

(99360 may be reported in addition to 99460, 99465 as appropriate)

(Do not report 99360 in conjunction with 99464)

Case Management Services

Case management is a process in which a physician or another qualified health care professional is responsible for direct care of a patient and, additionally, for coordinating, managing access to, initiating, and/or supervising other health care services needed by the patient.

Medical Team Conferences

Medical team conferences include face-to-face participation by a minimum of three qualified health care professionals from different specialties or disciplines (each of whom provide direct care to the patient), with or without the presence of the patient, family member(s), community agencies, surrogate decision maker(s) (eg, legal guardian), and/or caregiver(s). The participants are actively involved in the development, revision, coordination, and implementation of health care services needed by the patient. Reporting participants shall have performed face-to-face evaluations or treatments of the patient, independent of any team conference, within the previous 60 days.

Physicians or other qualified health care professionals who may report evaluation and management services should report their time spent in a team conference with the patient and/or family/caregiver present using evaluation and management (E/M) codes. These introductory guidelines do not apply to services reported using E/M codes (see E/M Services Guidelines). However, the individual must be directly involved with the patient, providing face-to-face services outside of the conference visit with other physicians, and qualified health care professionals, or agencies.

Reporting participants shall document their participation in the team conference as well as their contributed information and subsequent treatment recommendations.

No more than one individual from the same specialty may report 99366-99368 at the same encounter.

Individuals should not report 99366-99368 when their participation in the medical team conference is part of a facility or organizational service contractually provided by the organization or facility.

▶The team conference starts at the beginning of the review of an individual patient and ends at the conclusion of the review. Time related to record keeping and report generation is not reported. The reporting participant shall be present for all time reported. The time reported is not limited to the time that the participant is communicating to the other team members or patient and/or family/caregiver. Time reported for medical team conferences may not be used in the determination of time for other services such as care plan oversight (99374-99380), prolonged services (99358, 99359), psychotherapy, or any E/M service. For team conferences where the patient is present for any part of the duration of the conference, nonphysician qualified health care professionals report the team conference face-to-face code 99366.◀

Medical Team Conference, Direct (Face-to-Face) Contact With Patient and/or Family

99366 **Medical team conference** with interdisciplinary team of health care professionals, face-to-face with patient and/or family, 30 minutes or more, participation by nonphysician qualified health care professional
→ *CPT Changes: An Insider's View* 2008
→ *CPT Assistant* Apr 13:3, Jun 14:3, Oct 14:3

(Team conference services of less than 30 minutes duration are not reported separately)

(For team conference services by a physician with patient and/or family present, see Evaluation and Management services)

(Do not report 99366 for the same time reported for 99424, 99425, 99426, 99427, 99437, 99439, 99487, 99489, 99490, 99491)

Medical Team Conference, Without Direct (Face-to-Face) Contact With Patient and/or Family

99367 **Medical team conference** with interdisciplinary team of health care professionals, patient and/or family not present, 30 minutes or more; participation by physician
→ *CPT Changes: An Insider's View* 2008
→ *CPT Assistant* Apr 13:3, Jun 14:3, Dec 19:14

99368 participation by nonphysician qualified health care professional
→ *CPT Changes: An Insider's View* 2008
→ *CPT Assistant* Apr 13:3, Jun 14:3, Oct 14:3

(Team conference services of less than 30 minutes duration are not reported separately)

(Do not report 99367, 99368 during the same month with 99437, 99439, 99487, 99489, 99490, 99491)

Care Plan Oversight Services

Care plan oversight services are reported separately from codes for office/outpatient, hospital, home or residence (including assisted living facility, group home, custodial care facility, residential substance abuse treatment facility, rest home), nursing facility, or non-face-to-face services. The complexity and approximate time of the care plan oversight services provided within a 30-day period determine code selection. Only one individual may report services for a given period of time to reflect the sole or predominant supervisory role with a particular patient. These codes should not be reported for supervision of patients in nursing facilities or under the care of home health agencies, unless they require recurrent supervision of therapy.

The work involved in providing very low intensity or infrequent supervision services is included in the pre- and post-encounter work for home, office/outpatient and nursing facility or domiciliary visit codes.

(For care plan oversight services provided in rest home [eg, assisted living facility] or home, see care management services codes 99437, 99491, or principal care management codes 99424, 99425, and for hospice agency, see 99377, 99378)

▶(Do not report 99374-99380 for time reported with 98012, 98013, 98014, 98015, 98016, 98966, 98967, 98968, 99421, 99422, 99423)◀

(Do not report 99374-99378 during the same month with 99487, 99489)

★=Telemedicine ◀=Audio-only ✛=Add-on code ✗=FDA approval pending #=Resequenced code ⊘=Modifier 51 exempt →→→=See p xxi for details

99374 **Supervision** of a patient under care of home health agency (patient not present) in home, domiciliary or equivalent environment (eg, Alzheimer's facility) requiring complex and multidisciplinary care modalities involving regular development and/or revision of care plans by that individual, review of subsequent reports of patient status, review of related laboratory and other studies, communication (including telephone calls) for purposes of assessment or care decisions with health care professional(s), family member(s), surrogate decision maker(s) (eg, legal guardian) and/or key caregiver(s) involved in patient's care, integration of new information into the medical treatment plan and/or adjustment of medical therapy, within a calendar month; 15-29 minutes

➲ *CPT Changes: An Insider's View* 2002, 2013

➲ *CPT Assistant* Summer 94:9, Nov 97:8-9, May 05:1, Dec 06:4, Mar 07:11, Mar 08:6, Sep 08:3, Jul 09:5, 10, Apr 13:3, Jul 13:11, Sep 13:15, Nov 13:3, Feb 14:11, Oct 14:3, Jan 22:6

99375 30 minutes or more

➲ *CPT Changes: An Insider's View* 2013

➲ *CPT Assistant* Summer 94:9, Nov 97:8-9, Dec 06:4, Mar 07:11, Mar 08:6, Sep 08:3, Jul 09:5, 10, Apr 13:3, Jul 13:11, Sep 13:15, Jan 22:6

99377 **Supervision** of a hospice patient (patient not present) requiring complex and multidisciplinary care modalities involving regular development and/or revision of care plans by that individual, review of subsequent reports of patient status, review of related laboratory and other studies, communication (including telephone calls) for purposes of assessment or care decisions with health care professional(s), family member(s), surrogate decision maker(s) (eg, legal guardian) and/or key caregiver(s) involved in patient's care, integration of new information into the medical treatment plan and/or adjustment of medical therapy, within a calendar month; 15-29 minutes

➲ *CPT Changes: An Insider's View* 2001, 2002, 2013

➲ *CPT Assistant* Nov 97:8-9, Dec 06:4, Mar 07:11, Sep 08:3, Jul 09:5, 10, Apr 13:3, Jul 13:11, Sep 13:15, Jan 22:6

99378 30 minutes or more

➲ *CPT Changes: An Insider's View* 2013

➲ *CPT Assistant* Nov 97:8-9, Dec 06:4, Mar 07:11, Mar 08:6, Sep 08:3, Jul 09:5, 10, Apr 13:3, Jul 13:11, Sep 13:15, Jan 22:6

99379 **Supervision** of a nursing facility patient (patient not present) requiring complex and multidisciplinary care modalities involving regular development and/or revision of care plans by that individual, review of subsequent reports of patient status, review of related laboratory and other studies, communication (including telephone calls) for purposes of assessment or care decisions with health care professional(s), family member(s), surrogate decision maker(s) (eg, legal guardian) and/or key caregiver(s) involved in patient's care, integration of new information into the medical treatment plan and/or adjustment of medical therapy, within a calendar month; 15-29 minutes

➲ *CPT Changes: An Insider's View* 2002, 2013

➲ *CPT Assistant* Dec 06:4, Mar 08:6, Sep 08:3, Jul 09:5, Apr 13:3, Jul 13:11, Sep 13:15

99380 30 minutes or more

➲ *CPT Changes: An Insider's View* 2013

➲ *CPT Assistant* Nov 97:8-9, Dec 06:4, Mar 08:6, Sep 08:3, Jul 09:5, Apr 13:3, Jul 13:11, Sep 13:15, Nov 13:3, Oct 14:3

Preventive Medicine Services

The following codes are used to report the preventive medicine evaluation and management of infants, children, adolescents, and adults.

The extent and focus of the services will largely depend on the age of the patient.

If an abnormality is encountered or a preexisting problem is addressed in the process of performing this preventive medicine evaluation and management service, and if the problem or abnormality is significant enough to require additional work to perform the key components of a problem-oriented evaluation and management service, then the appropriate office/outpatient code 99202, 99203, 99204, 99205, 99211, 99212, 99213, 99214, 99215 should also be reported. Modifier 25 should be added to the office/outpatient code to indicate that a significant, separately identifiable evaluation and management service was provided on the same day as the preventive medicine service. The appropriate preventive medicine service is additionally reported.

An insignificant or trivial problem/abnormality that is encountered in the process of performing the preventive medicine evaluation and management service and which does not require additional work and the performance of the key components of a problem-oriented E/M service should not be reported.

The "comprehensive" nature of the preventive medicine services codes 99381-99397 reflects an age- and gender-appropriate history/exam and is **not** synonymous with the "comprehensive" examination required in evaluation and management codes 99202-99350.

Codes 99381-99397 include counseling/anticipatory guidance/risk factor reduction interventions which are provided at the time of the initial or periodic comprehensive preventive medicine examination. (Refer to 99401, 99402, 99403, 99404, 99411, and 99412 for reporting those counseling/anticipatory guidance/risk factor reduction interventions that are provided at an encounter separate from the preventive medicine examination.)

(For behavior change intervention, see 99406, 99407, 99408, 99409)

►Immunization/vaccine/toxoid products, immunization administrations, ancillary studies involving laboratory, radiology, other procedures, or screening tests (eg, vision, hearing, developmental) identified with a specific CPT code are reported separately. For immunization administration and immunization risk/benefit counseling, see 90460, 90461, 90471-90474, 90480, 96380, 96381. For immunization/vaccine/toxoid products, see 90380, 90381, 90476-90759, 91304, 91318, 91319, 91320, 91321, 91322.◄

New Patient

99381 **Initial comprehensive preventive medicine** evaluation and management of an individual including an age and gender appropriate history, examination, counseling/anticipatory guidance/risk factor reduction interventions, and the ordering of laboratory/diagnostic procedures, new patient; infant (age younger than 1 year)
➔ *CPT Changes: An Insider's View* 2002, 2009
➔ *CPT Assistant* Winter 91:11, Spring 93:14, 34, Spring 95:1, Aug 97:1, Jul 98:9, Sep 98:5, Nov 98:3-4, May 02:1, May 05:1, Aug 05:15, Oct 06:15, Mar 09:3, Jul 09:7, Aug 09:5, Jan 13:9, Dec 14:18, Mar 16:7, Feb 21:8, Nov 21:12, Dec 22:15

99382 early childhood (age 1 through 4 years)
➔ *CPT Changes: An Insider's View* 2009
➔ *CPT Assistant* Winter 91:11, Spring 93:14, 34, Spring 95:1, Aug 97:1, Jul 98:9, Sep 98:5, Nov 98:3-4, May 02:1, Aug 05:15, Oct 06:15, Jul 09:5, Aug 09:5, Jan 13:9, Dec 14:18, Mar 16:7, Feb 21:8

99383 late childhood (age 5 through 11 years)
➔ *CPT Changes: An Insider's View* 2009
➔ *CPT Assistant* Winter 91:11, Spring 93:14, 34, Spring 95:1, Aug 97:1, Jul 98:9, Sep 98:5, Nov 98:3-4, May 02:1, Aug 05:15, Oct 06:15, Jul 09:7, Aug 09:5, Jan 13:9, Dec 14:18, Mar 16:7, Feb 21:8

99384 adolescent (age 12 through 17 years)
➔ *CPT Changes: An Insider's View* 2009
➔ *CPT Assistant* Winter 91:11, Spring 93:14, 34, Spring 95:1, Aug 97:1, Jul 98:9, Sep 98:5, Nov 98:3-4, May 02:1, Aug 05:15, Oct 06:15, Jul 09:7, Aug 09:5, Jan 13:9, Dec 14:18, Jan 15:12, Mar 16:7, Feb 21:8

99385 18-39 years
➔ *CPT Changes: An Insider's View* 2009
➔ *CPT Assistant* Winter 91:11, Spring 93:14, 34, Spring 95:1, Aug 97:7, Jul 98:9, Sep 98:5, Nov 98:3-4, May 02:1, Aug 05:15, Oct 06:15, Jul 09:5, Aug 09:5, Jan 13:9, Dec 14:18, Jan 15:12, Mar 16:7, Feb 21:8

99386 40-64 years
➔ *CPT Changes: An Insider's View* 2009
➔ *CPT Assistant* Winter 91:11, Spring 93:14, 34, Spring 95:1, Aug 97:1, Jul 98:9, Sep 98:5, Nov 98:3-4, May 02:1, Aug 05:15, Oct 06:15, Jul 09:7, Aug 09:5, Jan 13:9, Dec 14:18, Jan 15:12, Mar 16:7, Feb 21:8

99387 65 years and older
➔ *CPT Changes: An Insider's View* 2009
➔ *CPT Assistant* Winter 91:11, Spring 93:14, 34, Spring 95:1, Aug 97:1, Jul 98:9, Sep 98:5, Nov 98:3-4, May 02:1, Aug 05:15, Oct 06:15, Jul 09:7, Aug 09:5, Jan 13:9, Dec 14:18, Mar 16:7, Feb 21:8, Nov 21:12

Established Patient

99391 **Periodic comprehensive preventive medicine** reevaluation and management of an individual including an age and gender appropriate history, examination, counseling/anticipatory guidance/risk factor reduction interventions, and the ordering of laboratory/diagnostic procedures, established patient; infant (age younger than 1 year)
➔ *CPT Changes: An Insider's View* 2002, 2009
➔ *CPT Assistant* Winter 91:11, Spring 93:14, 34, Spring 95:1, Aug 97:1, Jul 98:9, Sep 98:5, Nov 98:3-4, May 02:1, May 05:1, Aug 05:15, Oct 06:15, Mar 09:3, Jul 09:7, Aug 09:5, Jan 13:9, Dec 14:18, Mar 16:7, Feb 21:8

99392 early childhood (age 1 through 4 years)
➔ *CPT Changes: An Insider's View* 2009
➔ *CPT Assistant* Winter 91:11, Spring 93:14, 34, Spring 95:1, Aug 97:1, Jul 98:9, Sep 98:5, Nov 98:3-4, May 02:1, Aug 05:15, Oct 06:15, Jul 09:7, Jan 13:9, Dec 14:18, Mar 16:7, Feb 21:8, Mar 23:1

99393 late childhood (age 5 through 11 years)
➔ *CPT Changes: An Insider's View* 2009
➔ *CPT Assistant* Winter 91:11, Spring 93:14, 34, Spring 95:1, Aug 97:1, Jul 98:9, Sep 98:5, Nov 98:3-4, May 02:1, Aug 05:15, Oct 06:15, Jul 09:7, Jan 13:9, Dec 14:18, Mar 16:7, Feb 21:8

99394 adolescent (age 12 through 17 years)
➔ *CPT Changes: An Insider's View* 2009
➔ *CPT Assistant* Winter 91:11, Spring 93:14, 34, Spring 95:1, Aug 97:1, Jul 98:9, Sep 98:5, Nov 98:3-4, May 02:1, Aug 05:15, Oct 06:15, Jul 09:7, Jan 13:9, Dec 14:18, Jan 15:12, Mar 16:7, Feb 21:8, Jul 23:1

99395 18-39 years
➔ *CPT Changes: An Insider's View* 2009
➔ *CPT Assistant* Winter 91:11, Spring 93:14, 34, Spring 95:1, Aug 97:1, Jul 98:9, Sep 98:5, Nov 98:3-4, May 02:1, Aug 05:15, Oct 06:15, Mar 08:3, Jul 09:7, Jan 13:9, Dec 14:18, Jan 15:12, Mar 16:7, Feb 21:8

99396 40-64 years
➔ *CPT Changes: An Insider's View* 2009
➔ *CPT Assistant* Winter 91:11, Spring 93:14, 34, Spring 95:1, Aug 97:1, Jul 98:9, Sep 98:5, Nov 98:3-4, May 02:1, Aug 05:15, Oct 06:15, Jul 09:7, Mar 12:4, Jan 13:9, Dec 14:18, Jan 15:12, Mar 16:7, Sep 17:11, Feb 21:8

99397 65 years and older
➔ *CPT Changes: An Insider's View* 2009
➔ *CPT Assistant* Winter 91:11, Spring 93:14, 34, Spring 95:1, Aug 97:1, Jul 98:9, Sep 98:5, Nov 98:3-4, May 02:1, Aug 05:15, Oct 06:15, Jul 09:7, Jan 13:9, Dec 14:18, Mar 16:7, Feb 21:8, Dec 22:15

Counseling Risk Factor Reduction and Behavior Change Intervention

New or Established Patient

These codes are used to report services provided face-to-face by a physician or other qualified health care professional for the purpose of promoting health and preventing illness or injury. They are distinct from evaluation and management (E/M) services that may be reported separately with modifier 25 when performed. Risk factor reduction services are used for persons without a specific illness for which the counseling might otherwise be used as part of treatment.

Preventive medicine counseling and risk factor reduction interventions will vary with age and should address such issues as family problems, diet and exercise, substance use, sexual practices, injury prevention, dental health, and diagnostic and laboratory test results available at the time of the encounter.

Behavior change interventions are for persons who have a behavior that is often considered an illness itself, such as tobacco use and addiction, substance abuse/misuse, or obesity. Behavior change services may be reported when performed as part of the treatment of condition(s) related to or potentially exacerbated by the behavior or when performed to change the harmful behavior that has not yet resulted in illness. Any E/M services reported on the same day must be distinct and reported with modifier 25, and time spent providing these services may not be used as a basis for the E/M code selection. Behavior change services involve specific validated interventions of assessing readiness for change and barriers to change, advising a change in behavior, assisting by providing specific suggested actions and motivational counseling, and arranging for services and follow-up.

For counseling groups of patients with symptoms or established illness, use 99078.

Health behavior assessment and intervention services (96156, 96158, 96159, 96164, 96165, 96167, 96168, 96170, 96171) should not be reported on the same day as codes 99401-99412.

Preventive Medicine, Individual Counseling

99401   **Preventive medicine counseling** and/or risk factor reduction intervention(s) provided to an individual (separate procedure); approximately 15 minutes

➔ *CPT Assistant* Aug 97:1, Jan 98:12, May 05:1, Aug 07:9, Oct 10:3, Dec 10:3, Jan 13:9, Aug 14:5, Mar 16:7, Aug 20:3, Jan 22:17, Apr 22:13, Oct 22:7

99402   approximately 30 minutes

➔ *CPT Assistant* Aug 97:1, Jan 98:12, May 05:1, Oct 10:3, Dec 10:3, Jan 13:9, Mar 16:7, Aug 20:3, Jan 22:17, Apr 22:13

99403   approximately 45 minutes

➔ *CPT Assistant* Aug 97:1, Jan 98:12, May 05:1, Oct 10:3, Dec 10:3, Jan 13:9, Mar 16:7, Aug 20:3, Jan 22:17, Apr 22:13

99404   approximately 60 minutes

➔ *CPT Assistant* Aug 97:1, Jan 98:12, May 05:1, Oct 10:3, Dec 10:3, Jan 13:9, Aug 14:5, Mar 16:7, Aug 20:3, Jan 22:17, Apr 22:13

Behavior Change Interventions, Individual

★◀ **99406**   **Smoking and tobacco use cessation counseling visit;** intermediate, greater than 3 minutes up to 10 minutes

➔ *CPT Changes: An Insider's View* 2008, 2017

➔ *CPT Assistant* Jan 08:1, Sep 09:11, Oct 10:3, Dec 10:3, Jan 13:9, Mar 16:7, Aug 20:3, Sep 20:14, Apr 24:33

★◀ **99407**   intensive, greater than 10 minutes

➔ *CPT Changes: An Insider's View* 2008, 2017

➔ *CPT Assistant* Jan 08:1, Sep 09:11, Oct 10:3, Dec 10:3, Jan 13:9, Mar 16:7, Aug 20:3

(Do not report 99407 in conjunction with 99406)

★◀ **99408**   **Alcohol and/or substance (other than tobacco) abuse structured screening** (eg, AUDIT, DAST), and brief intervention (SBI) services; 15 to 30 minutes

➔ *CPT Changes: An Insider's View* 2008, 2017

➔ *CPT Assistant* Oct 10:3, Dec 10:3, Jan 13:9, Mar 16:7, Nov 16:5, Aug 20:3

(Do not report services of less than 15 minutes with 99408)

★◀ **99409**   greater than 30 minutes

➔ *CPT Changes: An Insider's View* 2008, 2017

➔ *CPT Assistant* Oct 10:3, Dec 10:3, Jan 13:9, Mar 16:7, Nov 16:5, Aug 20:3

(Do not report 99409 in conjunction with 99408)

(Do not report 99408, 99409 in conjunction with 96160, 96161)

(Use 99408, 99409 only for initial screening and brief intervention)

Preventive Medicine, Group Counseling

99411   **Preventive medicine counseling** and/or risk factor reduction intervention(s) provided to individuals in a group setting (separate procedure); approximately 30 minutes

➔ *CPT Assistant* Aug 97:1, Jan 98:12, Sep 98:5, May 05:1, Oct 10:3, Dec 10:3, Jan 13:9, Mar 16:7, Aug 20:3

99412 approximately 60 minutes

➔ *CPT Assistant* Aug 97:1, Jan 98:12, Sep 98:5, May 05:1, Aug 07:9, Oct 10:3, Dec 10:3, Jan 13:9, Mar 16:7, Aug 20:3, Oct 22:7

99415 Code is out of numerical sequence. See 99358-99366

99416 Code is out of numerical sequence. See 99358-99366

99417 Code is out of numerical sequence. See 99358-99366

99418 Code is out of numerical sequence. See 99358-99366

Other Preventive Medicine Services

99421 Code is out of numerical sequence. See 99412-99447

99422 Code is out of numerical sequence. See 99412-99447

99423 Code is out of numerical sequence. See 99412-99447

99424 Code is out of numerical sequence. See 99487-99493

99425 Code is out of numerical sequence. See 99487-99493

99426 Code is out of numerical sequence. See 99487-99493

99427 Code is out of numerical sequence. See 99487-99493

99429 **Unlisted preventive** medicine service

➔ *CPT Assistant* Sep 98:5, May 05:1, Oct 10:3, Dec 10:3, Jan 13:9, Mar 16:7, Oct 22:7

Non-Face-to-Face Services

Telephone Services

99437 Code is out of numerical sequence. See 99480-99489

99439 Code is out of numerical sequence. See 99480-99489

▶(99441, 99442, 99443 have been deleted. To report, see 98008, 98009, 98010, 98011, 98012, 98013, 98014, 98015, 98016)◀

Online Digital Evaluation and Management Services

Online digital evaluation and management (E/M) services (99421, 99422, 99423) are patient-initiated services with physicians or other qualified health care professionals (QHPs). Online digital E/M services require physician or other QHP's evaluation, assessment, and management of the patient. These services are not for the nonevaluative electronic communication of test results, scheduling of appointments, or other communication that does not include E/M. While the patient's problem may be new to the physician or other QHP, the patient is an established patient. Patients initiate these services through Health Insurance Portability and Accountability Act (HIPAA)-compliant secure platforms, such as electronic health record (EHR) portals, secure email, or other digital applications, which allow digital communication with the physician or other QHP.

Online digital E/M services are reported once for the physician's or other QHP's cumulative time devoted to the service during a seven-day period. The seven-day period begins with the physician's or other QHP's initial, personal review of the patient-generated inquiry. Physician's or other QHP's cumulative service time includes review of the initial inquiry, review of patient records or data pertinent to assessment of the patient's problem, personal physician or other QHP interaction with clinical staff focused on the patient's problem, development of management plans, including physician- or other QHP generation of prescriptions or ordering of tests, and subsequent communication with the patient through online, telephone, email, or other digitally supported communication, which does not otherwise represent a separately reported E/M service. All professional decision making, assessment, and subsequent management by physicians or other QHPs in the same group practice contribute to the cumulative service time of the patient's online digital E/M service. Online digital E/M services require permanent documentation storage (electronic or hard copy) of the encounter.

▶If within seven days of the initiation of an online digital E/M service, a separately reported E/M visit occurs, then the physician or other QHP work devoted to the online digital E/M service is incorporated into the separately reported E/M visit. This includes E/M services that are provided through synchronous telemedicine visits using interactive audio and video telecommunication equipment. To report synchronous audio-video E/M services, see 98000, 98001, 98002, 98003, 98004, 98005, 98006, 98007. To report synchronous audio-only E/M services, see 98008, 98009, 98010, 98011, 98012, 98013, 98014, 98015, 98016.◀

If the patient initiates an online digital inquiry for the same or a related problem within seven days of a previous E/M service, then the online digital visit is not reported. If the online digital inquiry is related to a surgical procedure and occurs during the postoperative period of a previously completed procedure, then the online digital E/M service is not reported separately.

If the patient generates the initial online digital inquiry for a new problem within seven days of a previous E/M visit that addressed a different problem, then the online digital E/M service may be reported separately.

If the patient presents a new, unrelated problem during the seven-day period of an online digital E/M service, then the physician's or other QHP's time spent on evaluation, assessment, and management of the additional problem is added to the cumulative service time of the online digital E/M service for that seven-day period.

> ►(For online digital assessment and management services provided by a nonphysician qualified health care professional who may not report E/M services, see 98970, 98971, 98972)◄

 # 99421   **Online digital evaluation and management service,** for an established patient, for up to 7 days, cumulative time during the 7 days; 5-10 minutes

➲ *CPT Changes: An Insider's View* 2020
➲ *CPT Assistant* Jan 20:3, Mar 20:6, Sep 21:3, Nov 23:22

 # 99422   11-20 minutes

➲ *CPT Changes: An Insider's View* 2020
➲ *CPT Assistant* Jan 20:3, Mar 20:6, Sep 21:3, Nov 23:22

 # 99423   21 or more minutes

➲ *CPT Changes: An Insider's View* 2020
➲ *CPT Assistant* Jan 20:3, Mar 20:6, Sep 21:3, Nov 23:22

(Report 99421, 99422, 99423 once per 7-day period)

(Clinical staff time is not calculated as part of cumulative time for 99421, 99422, 99423)

(Do not report online digital E/M services for cumulative service time less than 5 minutes)

(Do not count 99421, 99422, 99423 time otherwise reported with other services)

(Do not report 99421, 99422, 99423 on a day when the physician or other qualified health care professional reports E/M services [99202, 99203, 99204, 99205, 99212, 99213, 99214, 99215, 99242, 99243, 99244, 99245])

(Do not report 99421, 99422, 99423 when using 99091, 99374, 99375, 99377, 99378, 99379, 99380, 99424, 99425, 99426, 99427, 99437, 99487, 99489, 99491, 99495, 99496, for the same communication[s])

(Do not report 99421, 99422, 99423 for home and outpatient INR monitoring when reporting 93792, 93793)

Interprofessional Telephone/Internet/Electronic Health Record Consultations

The consultant should use codes 99446, 99447, 99448, 99449, 99451 to report interprofessional telephone/Internet/electronic health record consultations. An interprofessional telephone/Internet/electronic health record consultation is an assessment and management service in which a patient's treating (eg, attending or primary) physician or other qualified health care professional requests the opinion and/or treatment advice of a physician or other qualified health care professional with specific specialty expertise (the consultant) to assist the treating physician or other qualified health care professional in the diagnosis and/or management of the patient's problem without patient face-to-face contact with the consultant.

The patient for whom the interprofessional telephone/Internet/electronic health record consultation is requested may be either a new patient to the consultant or an established patient with a new problem or an exacerbation of an existing problem. However, the consultant should not have seen the patient in a face-to-face encounter within the last 14 days. When the telephone/Internet/electronic health record consultation leads to a transfer of care or other face-to-face service (eg, a surgery, a hospital visit, or a scheduled office evaluation of the patient) within the next 14 days or next available appointment date of the consultant, these codes are not reported.

Review of pertinent medical records, laboratory studies, imaging studies, medication profile, pathology specimens, etc is included in the telephone/Internet/electronic health record consultation service and should not be reported separately when reporting 99446, 99447, 99448, 99449, 99451. The majority of the service time reported (greater than 50%) must be devoted to the medical consultative verbal or Internet discussion. If greater than 50% of the time for the service is devoted to data review and/or analysis, 99446, 99447, 99448, 99449 should not be reported. However, the service time for 99451 is based on total review and interprofessional-communication time.

If more than one telephone/Internet/electronic health record contact(s) is required to complete the consultation request (eg, discussion of test results), the entirety of the service and the cumulative discussion and information review time should be reported with a single code. Codes 99446, 99447, 99448, 99449, 99451 should not be reported more than once within a seven-day interval.

The written or verbal request for telephone/Internet/electronic health record advice by the treating/requesting physician or other qualified health care professional should be documented in the patient's medical record, including the reason for the request. Codes 99446, 99447, 99448, 99449 conclude with a verbal opinion report and written report from the consultant to the treating/requesting physician or other qualified health care professional. Code 99451 concludes with only a written report.

> ►Telephone/Internet/electronic health record consultations of less than five minutes should not be reported. Consultant communications with the patient and/or family may be reported using 98012, 98013, 98014, 98015, 98016, 98966, 98967, 98968, 99421, 99422, 99423, and the time related to these services is not used in reporting 99446, 99447, 99448, 99449. Do not report 99358, 99359 for any time within the service period, if reporting 99446, 99447, 99448, 99449, 99451.◄

When the sole purpose of the telephone/Internet/electronic health record communication is to arrange a transfer of care or other face-to-face service, these codes are not reported.

The treating/requesting physician or other qualified health care professional may report 99452, if spending 16-30 minutes in a service day preparing for the referral and/or communicating with the consultant. Do not report 99452 more than once in a 14-day period. If the telephone/Internet/electronic health record referral service(s) and an E/M service are performed on the same day by the treating/requesting physician or other qualified health care professional and total time is used to select the level of E/M service, the time spent providing the referral service is added to the time spent on the day of the encounter performing the E/M service. If MDM is used to select the level of E/M service, the work of performing the referral service is considered part of the MDM. Do not report 99452 separately on the same date an E/M service is reported.

▶(For telephone services provided by a physician or other qualified health care professional to a patient, see 98008, 98009, 98010, 98011, 98012, 98013, 98014, 98015, 98016)◀

▶(For telephone services provided by a nonphysician qualified health care professional who may not report evaluation and management services, see 98966, 98967, 98968)◀

(For online digital E/M services provided by a physician or other qualified health care professional to a patient, see 99421, 99422, 99423)

99446 **Interprofessional telephone/Internet/electronic health record assessment and management service** provided by a consultative physician or other qualified health care professional, including a verbal and written report to the patient's treating/requesting physician or other qualified health care professional; 5-10 minutes of medical consultative discussion and review
→ *CPT Changes: An Insider's View* 2014, 2019, 2023
→ *CPT Assistant* Jun 14:14, Jan 19:3, Jun 19:7, Sep 21:4, Mar 23:20

99447 11-20 minutes of medical consultative discussion and review
→ *CPT Changes: An Insider's View* 2014, 2019, 2023
→ *CPT Assistant* Jun 14:14, Jan 19:3, Jun 19:7, Mar 23:20

99448 21-30 minutes of medical consultative discussion and review
→ *CPT Changes: An Insider's View* 2014, 2019, 2023
→ *CPT Assistant* Jun 14:14, Jan 19:3, Jun 19:7, Mar 23:20

99449 31 minutes or more of medical consultative discussion and review
→ *CPT Changes: An Insider's View* 2014, 2019, 2023
→ *CPT Assistant* Jun 14:14, Jan 19:3, Jun 19:7, Mar 23:20

 # 99451 **Interprofessional telephone/Internet/electronic health record assessment and management service** provided by a consultative physician or other qualified

health care professional, including a written report to the patient's treating/requesting physician or other qualified health care professional, 5 minutes or more of medical consultative time
→ *CPT Changes: An Insider's View* 2019, 2023
→ *CPT Assistant* Jan 19:3, Jun 19:7, Mar 23:20

 # 99452 **Interprofessional telephone/Internet/electronic health record referral service(s)** provided by a treating/requesting physician or other qualified health care professional, 30 minutes
→ *CPT Changes: An Insider's View* 2019
→ *CPT Assistant* Jan 19:3, Jun 19:7, Jun 20:3, Sep 21:4, Mar 23:20

Digitally Stored Data Services/ Remote Physiologic Monitoring

Codes 99453 and 99454 are used to report remote physiologic monitoring services (eg, weight, blood pressure, pulse oximetry) during a 30-day period. To report 99453, 99454, the device used must be a medical device as defined by the FDA, and the service must be ordered by a physician or other qualified health care professional. Code 99453 may be used to report the set-up and patient education on use of the device(s). Code 99454 may be used to report supply of the device for daily recording or programmed alert transmissions. Codes 99453, 99454 are not reported if monitoring is less than 16 days. Do not report 99453, 99454 when these services are included in other codes for the duration of time of the physiologic monitoring service (eg, 95250 for continuous glucose monitoring requires a minimum of 72 hours of monitoring).

Code 99091 should be reported no more than once in a 30-day period to include the physician or other qualified health care professional time involved with data accession, review and interpretation, modification of care plan as necessary (including communication to patient and/or caregiver), and associated documentation.

If the services described by 99091 or 99474 are provided on the same day the patient presents for an evaluation and management (E/M) service to the same provider, these services should be considered part of the E/M service and not reported separately.

Do not report 99091 for time in the same calendar month when used to meet the criteria for care plan oversight services (99374, 99375, 99377, 99378, 99379, 99380), remote physiologic monitoring services (99457, 99458), or personally performed chronic or principal care management (99424, 99425, 99426, 99427, 99437, 99491). Do not report 99091 if other more specific codes exist (eg, 93227, 93272 for cardiographic services; 95250 for continuous glucose monitoring). Do not report 99091 for transfer and interpretation of data from hospital or clinical laboratory computers.

Code 99453 is reported for each episode of care. For coding remote monitoring of physiologic parameters, an episode of care is defined as beginning when the remote monitoring physiologic service is initiated, and ends with attainment of targeted treatment goals.

 # 99453   **Remote monitoring of physiologic parameter(s)** (eg, weight, blood pressure, pulse oximetry, respiratory flow rate), initial; set-up and patient education on use of equipment

➔ *CPT Changes: An Insider's View* 2019

➔ *CPT Assistant* Jan 19:3, Mar 19:10, Feb 21:13, Feb 22:7-8, Oct 22:14, Feb 24:28

(Do not report 99453 more than once per episode of care)

(Do not report 99453 for monitoring of less than 16 days)

(Do not report 99453 in conjunction with 0811T)

 # 99454   device(s) supply with daily recording(s) or programmed alert(s) transmission, each 30 days

➔ *CPT Changes: An Insider's View* 2019

➔ *CPT Assistant* Jan 19:3, Mar 19:10, Feb 22:7-8, Oct 22:14, Feb 23:3, Feb 24:28

(For physiologic monitoring treatment management services, use 99457)

(Do not report 99454 for monitoring of less than 16 days)

(Do not report 99453, 99454 in conjunction with codes for more specific physiologic parameters [eg, 93296, 94760])

(Do not report 99454 in conjunction with 0812T)

(For remote therapeutic monitoring, see 98975, 98976, 98977, 98978)

(For self-measured blood pressure monitoring, see 99473, 99474)

 # 99091   **Collection and interpretation of physiologic data** (eg, ECG, blood pressure, glucose monitoring) digitally stored and/or transmitted by the patient and/or caregiver to the physician or other qualified health care professional, qualified by education, training, licensure/ regulation (when applicable) requiring a minimum of 30 minutes of time, each 30 days

➔ *CPT Changes: An Insider's View* 2002, 2013, 2019

➔ *CPT Assistant* May 02:19, Jun 03:10, Aug 06:6, Sep 06:15, Jan 07:30, Apr 09:7, Dec 09:6, Apr 13:3, Nov 13:3, Oct 14:3, Feb 18:7, Mar 18:5, Dec 18:11, Feb 20:7, Apr 20:5, May 21:12

(Do not report 99091 in conjunction with 99457, 99458)

(Do not report 99091 for time in a calendar month when used to meet the criteria for 99374, 99375, 99377, 99378, 99379, 99380, 99424, 99425, 99426, 99427, 99437, 99457, 99487, 99491)

 # 99473   **Self-measured blood pressure** using a device validated for clinical accuracy; patient education/training and device calibration

➔ *CPT Changes: An Insider's View* 2020

➔ *CPT Assistant* Jan 20:3, Feb 20:7, Apr 20:5

(Do not report 99473 more than once per device)

(For ambulatory blood pressure monitoring, see 93784, 93786, 93788, 93790)

 # 99474   separate self-measurements of two readings one minute apart, twice daily over a 30-day period (minimum of 12 readings), collection of data reported by the patient and/or caregiver to the physician or other qualified health care professional, with report of average systolic and diastolic pressures and subsequent communication of a treatment plan to the patient

➔ *CPT Changes: An Insider's View* 2020

➔ *CPT Assistant* Jan 20:3, Feb 20:7, Apr 20:5

(Do not report 99473, 99474 in the same calendar month as 93784, 93786, 93788, 93790, 99091, 99424, 99425, 99426, 99427, 99437, 99439, 99453, 99454, 99457, 99487, 99489, 99490, 99491)

(Do not report 99474 more than once per calendar month)

Remote Physiologic Monitoring Treatment Management Services

Remote physiologic monitoring treatment management services are provided when clinical staff/physician/other qualified health care professional use the results of remote physiological monitoring to manage a patient under a specific treatment plan. To report remote physiological monitoring, the device used must be a medical device as defined by the FDA, and the service must be ordered by a physician or other qualified health care professional. Do not use 99457, 99458 for time that can be reported using codes for more specific monitoring services. Codes 99457, 99458 may be reported during the same service period as chronic care management services (99437, 99439, 99487, 99489, 99490, 99491), principal care management services (99424, 99425, 99426, 99427), transitional care management services (99495, 99496), and behavioral health integration services (99484, 99492, 99493, 99494). However, time spent performing these services should remain separate and no time should be counted twice toward the required time for any services in a single month. Codes 99457, 99458 require a live, interactive communication with the patient/caregiver. The interactive communication contributes to the total time, but it does not need to represent the entire cumulative reported time of the treatment management service. For the first completed 20 minutes of clinical staff/physician/other qualified health care professional time in a calendar month report 99457, and report 99458 for each additional completed 20 minutes. Do not report 99457, 99458 for services of less than 20 minutes. Report 99457 one time regardless of the number of physiologic monitoring modalities performed in a given calendar month.

To report remote therapeutic monitoring treatment management services provided by physician or other qualified health care professional, see 98980, 98981.

Do not count any time on a day when the physician or other qualified health care professional reports an E/M service (office or other outpatient services 99202, 99203, 99204, 99205, 99211, 99212, 99213, 99214, 99215, home or residence services 99341, 99342, 99344, 99345, 99347, 99348, 99349, 99350, initial or subsequent hospital inpatient or observation services 99221, 99222, 99223, 99231, 99232, 99233, inpatient or observation consultations 99252, 99253, 99254, 99255). Do not count any time related to other reported services (eg, 93290, 93793, 99291, 99292).

 # 99457 **Remote physiologic monitoring treatment management services,** clinical staff/physician/other qualified health care professional time in a calendar month requiring interactive communication with the patient/caregiver during the month; first 20 minutes

➔ *CPT Changes: An Insider's View* 2019, 2020

➔ *CPT Assistant* Jan 19:3, Jun 19:3, Feb 20:7, Apr 20:5, Jan 22:3-4, Feb 22:7-8, Oct 22:14

(Report 99457 once each 30 days, regardless of the number of parameters monitored)

(Do not report 99457 for services of less than 20 minutes)

(Do not report 99457 in conjunction with 93264, 99091)

(Do not report 99457 in the same month as 99473, 99474)

#+ 99458 each additional 20 minutes (List separately in addition to code for primary procedure)

➔ *CPT Changes: An Insider's View* 2020

➔ *CPT Assistant* Feb 20:7, Jan 22:3, Feb 22:7-8, Oct 22:14

(Use 99458 in conjunction with 99457)

(For remote therapeutic monitoring treatment management services, see 98980, 98981)

(Do not report 99458 for services of less than an additional increment of 20 minutes)

Special Evaluation and Management Services

The following codes are used to report evaluations performed to establish baseline information prior to life or disability insurance certificates being issued. This service is performed in the office or other setting, and applies to both new and established patients. When using these codes, no active management of the problem(s) is undertaken during the encounter.

If other evaluation and management services and/or procedures are performed on the same date, the appropriate E/M or procedure code(s) should be reported in addition to these codes.

Basic Life and/or Disability Evaluation Services

99450 **Basic life** and/or disability examination that includes:

- **Measurement of height, weight, and blood pressure;**
- **Completion of a medical history following a life insurance pro forma;**
- **Collection of blood sample and/or urinalysis complying with "chain of custody" protocols; and**
- **Completion of necessary documentation/ certificates.**

➔ *CPT Assistant* Summer 95:14, Sep 98:5, May 05:1, Jun 19:7

99451 Code is out of numerical sequence. See 99448-99455

99452 Code is out of numerical sequence. See 99448-99455

99453 Code is out of numerical sequence. See 99448-99455

99454 Code is out of numerical sequence. See 99448-99455

Evaluation / Management 99202-99499

Work Related or Medical Disability Evaluation Services

99455   **Work related** or medical disability examination by the treating physician that includes:

- **Completion of a medical history commensurate with the patient's condition;**
- **Performance of an examination commensurate with the patient's condition;**
- **Formulation of a diagnosis, assessment of capabilities and stability, and calculation of impairment;**
- **Development of future medical treatment plan; and**
- **Completion of necessary documentation/ certificates and report.**

➔ *CPT Assistant* Summer 95:14, Sep 98:5, May 05:1, Aug 13:13

99456   **Work related** or medical disability examination by other than the treating physician that includes:

- **Completion of a medical history commensurate with the patient's condition;**
- **Performance of an examination commensurate with the patient's condition;**
- **Formulation of a diagnosis, assessment of capabilities and stability, and calculation of impairment;**
- **Development of future medical treatment plan; and**
- **Completion of necessary documentation/ certificates and report.**

➔ *CPT Assistant* Summer 95:14, Sep 98:5, Aug 13:13

(Do not report 99455, 99456 in conjunction with 99080 for the completion of Workman's Compensation forms)

99457   Code is out of numerical sequence. See 99448-99455

99458   Code is out of numerical sequence. See 99448-99455

99459   Code is out of numerical sequence. See 99497-99499

Newborn Care Services

The following codes are used to report the services provided to newborns (birth through the first 28 days) in several different settings. Use of the normal newborn codes is limited to the initial care of the newborn in the first days after birth prior to home discharge.

Evaluation and Management (E/M) services for the newborn include maternal and/or fetal and newborn history, newborn physical examination(s), ordering of diagnostic tests and treatments, meetings with the family, and documentation in the medical record.

When delivery room attendance services (99464) or delivery room resuscitation services (99465) are required, report these in addition to normal newborn services Evaluation and Management codes.

For E/M services provided to newborns who are other than normal, see codes for hospital inpatient or observation services (99221-99233) and neonatal intensive and critical care services (99466-99469, 99477-99480). When normal newborn services are provided by the same individual on the same date that the newborn later becomes ill and receives additional intensive or critical care services, report the appropriate E/M code with modifier 25 for these services in addition to the normal newborn code.

Procedures (eg, 54150, newborn circumcision) are not included with the normal newborn codes, and when performed, should be reported in addition to the newborn services.

When newborns are seen in follow-up after the date of discharge in the office or other outpatient setting, see 99202-99215, 99381, 99391, as appropriate.

99460   **Initial hospital or birthing center care,** per day, for evaluation and management of normal newborn infant

➔ *CPT Changes: An Insider's View* 2009

99461   **Initial care,** per day, for evaluation and management of normal newborn infant seen in other than hospital or birthing center

➔ *CPT Changes: An Insider's View* 2009

99462   **Subsequent hospital care,** per day, for evaluation and management of normal newborn

➔ *CPT Changes: An Insider's View* 2009

99463   **Initial hospital or birthing center care,** per day, for evaluation and management of normal newborn infant admitted and discharged on the same date

➔ *CPT Changes: An Insider's View* 2009

➔ *CPT Assistant* Jan 23:20

(For newborn hospital discharge services provided on a date subsequent to the admission date, see 99238, 99239)

Delivery/Birthing Room Attendance and Resuscitation Services

99464   **Attendance at delivery** (when requested by the delivering physician or other qualified health care professional) and initial stabilization of newborn

➔ *CPT Changes: An Insider's View* 2009, 2013

(99464 may be reported in conjunction with 99221, 99222, 99223, 99291, 99460, 99468, 99477)

(Do not report 99464 in conjunction with 99465)

99465 **Delivery/birthing room resuscitation,** provision of positive pressure ventilation and/or chest compressions in the presence of acute inadequate ventilation and/or cardiac output

➔ *CPT Changes: An Insider's View* 2009
➔ *CPT Assistant* Nov 23:23

(99465 may be reported in conjunction with 99221, 99222, 99223, 99291, 99460, 99468, 99477)

(Do not report 99465 in conjunction with 99464)

(Procedures that are performed as a necessary part of the resuscitation [eg, intubation, vascular lines] are reported separately in addition to 99465. In order to report these procedures, they must be performed as a necessary component of the resuscitation and not as a convenience before admission to the neonatal intensive care unit)

Inpatient Neonatal Intensive Care Services and Pediatric and Neonatal Critical Care Services

Pediatric Critical Care Patient Transport

Codes 99466, 99467 are used to report the physical attendance and direct face-to-face care by a physician during the interfacility transport of a critically ill or critically injured pediatric patient 24 months of age or younger. Codes 99485, 99486 are used to report the control physician's non-face-to-face supervision of interfacility transport of a critically ill or critically injured pediatric patient 24 months of age or younger. These codes are not reported together for the same patient by the same physician. For the purpose of reporting 99466 and 99467, face-to-face care begins when the physician assumes primary responsibility of the pediatric patient at the referring facility, and ends when the receiving facility accepts responsibility for the pediatric patient's care. Only the time the physician spends in direct face-to-face contact with the patient during the transport should be reported. Pediatric patient transport services involving less than 30 minutes of face-to-face physician care should not be reported using 99466, 99467. Procedure(s) or service(s) performed by other members of the transporting team may not be reported by the supervising physician.

Codes 99485, 99486 may be used to report control physician's non-face-to-face supervision of interfacility pediatric critical care transport, which includes all two-way communication between the control physician and the specialized transport team prior to transport, at the referring facility and during transport of the patient back to the receiving facility. The "control" physician is the physician directing transport services. These codes do not include pretransport communication between the control physician and the referring facility before or following patient transport. These codes may only be reported for patients 24 months of age or younger who are critically ill or critically injured. The control physician provides treatment advice to a specialized transport team who are present and delivering the hands-on patient care. The control physician does not report any services provided by the specialized transport team. The control physician's non-face-to-face time begins with the first contact by the control physician with the specialized transport team and ends when the patient's care is handed over to the receiving facility team. Refer to 99466 and 99467 for face-to-face transport care of the critically ill/injured patient. Time spent with the individual patient's transport team and reviewing data submissions should be recorded. Code 99485 is used to report the first 16-45 minutes of direction on a given date and should only be used once even if time spent by the physician is discontinuous. Do not report services of 15 minutes or less or any time when another physician is reporting 99466, 99467. Do not report 99485 or 99486 in conjunction with 99466, 99467 when performed by the same physician.

For the definition of the critically injured pediatric patient, see the **Neonatal and Pediatric Critical Care Services** section.

The non-face-to-face direction of emergency care to a patient's transporting staff by a physician located in a hospital or other facility by two-way communication is not considered direct face-to-face care and should not be reported with 99466, 99467. Physician-directed non-face-to-face emergency care through outside voice communication to transporting staff personnel is reported with 99288 or 99485, 99486 based upon the age and clinical condition of the patient.

Emergency department services (99281-99285), initial hospital inpatient or observation care (99221-99223), critical care (99291, 99292), initial date neonatal intensive (99477), or critical care (99468) may only be reported after the patient has been admitted to the emergency department, the hospital inpatient or observation floor, or the critical care unit of the receiving facility. If inpatient critical care services are reported in the referring facility prior to transfer to the receiving hospital, use the critical care codes (99291, 99292).

The following services are included when performed during the pediatric patient transport by the physician providing critical care and may not be reported separately: routine monitoring evaluations (eg, heart rate, respiratory rate, blood pressure, and pulse oximetry), the

Evaluation / Management 99202-99499

interpretation of cardiac output measurements (93598), chest X rays (71045, 71046), pulse oximetry (94760, 94761, 94762), blood gases and information data stored in computers (eg, ECGs, blood pressures, hematologic data), gastric intubation (43752, 43753), temporary transcutaneous pacing (92953), ventilatory management (94002, 94003, 94660, 94662), and vascular access procedures (36000, 36400, 36405, 36406, 36415, 36591, 36600). Any services performed which are not listed above should be reported separately.

Services provided by the specialized transport team during non-face-to-face transport supervision are not reported by the control physician.

Code 99466 is used to report the first 30 to 74 minutes of direct face-to-face time with the transport pediatric patient and should be reported only once on a given date. Code 99467 is used to report each additional 30 minutes provided on a given date. Face-to-face services of less than 30 minutes should not be reported with these codes.

Code 99485 is used to report the first 30 minutes of non-face-to-face supervision of an interfacility transport of a critically ill or critically injured pediatric patient and should be reported only once per date of service. Only the communication time spent by the supervising physician with the specialty transport team members during an interfacility transport should be reported. Code 99486 is used to report each additional 30 minutes beyond the initial 30 minutes. Non-face-to-face interfacility transport of 15 minutes or less is not reported.

(For total body and selective head cooling of neonates, use 99184)

99466   **Critical care** face-to-face services, during an interfacility transport of critically ill or critically injured pediatric patient, 24 months of age or younger; first 30-74 minutes of hands-on care during transport

➔ *CPT Changes: An Insider's View* 2009, 2013

➔ *CPT Assistant* Sep 11:3, May 13:6, May 14:4, Jun 18:9, Sep 22:6

+ 99467   each additional 30 minutes (List separately in addition to code for primary service)

➔ *CPT Changes: An Insider's View* 2009, 2013

➔ *CPT Assistant* Sep 11:3, May 13:6, May 14:4, Jun 18:9, Sep 22:6

(Use 99467 in conjunction with 99466)

(Critical care of less than 30 minutes total duration should be reported with the appropriate E/M code)

 # 99485   **Supervision** by a control physician of interfacility transport care of the critically ill or critically injured pediatric patient, 24 months of age or younger, includes two-way communication with transport team before transport, at the referring facility and during the transport, including data interpretation and report; first 30 minutes

➔ *CPT Changes: An Insider's View* 2013

➔ *CPT Assistant* May 13:6, May 14:4, Jun 18:9, Sep 22:6

#+ 99486   each additional 30 minutes (List separately in addition to code for primary procedure)

➔ *CPT Changes: An Insider's View* 2013

➔ *CPT Assistant* May 13:6, May 14:4, Jun 18:9, Sep 22:6

(Use 99486 in conjunction with 99485)

(For physician direction of emergency medical systems supervision for a pediatric patient older than 24 months of age, or at any age if not critically ill or injured, use 99288)

(Do not report 99485, 99486 with any other services reported by the control physician for the same period)

(Do not report 99485, 99486 in conjunction with 99466, 99467 when performed by the same physician)

Inpatient Neonatal and Pediatric Critical Care

The same definitions for critical care services apply for the adult, child, and neonate.

Codes 99468, 99469 may be used to report the services of directing the inpatient care of a critically ill neonate or infant 28 days of age or younger. They represent care starting with the date of admission (99468) for critical care services and all subsequent day(s) (99469) that the neonate remains in critical care. These codes may be reported only by a single individual and only once per calendar day, per patient. Initial inpatient neonatal critical care (99468) may only be reported once per hospital admission. If readmitted for neonatal critical care services during the same hospital stay, then report the subsequent inpatient neonatal critical care code (99469) for the first day of readmission to critical care, and 99469 for each day of critical care following readmission.

The initial inpatient neonatal critical care code (99468) can be used in addition to 99464 or 99465 as appropriate, when the physician or other qualified health care professional is present for the delivery (99464) or resuscitation (99465) is required. Other procedures performed as a necessary part of the resuscitation (eg, endotracheal intubation [31500]) may also be reported separately, when performed as part of the pre-admission delivery room care. In order to report these procedures separately, they must be performed as a necessary component of the resuscitation and not simply as a convenience before admission to the neonatal intensive care unit.

Codes 99471-99476 may be used to report the services of directing the inpatient care of a critically ill infant or young child from 29 days of postnatal age through 5 years of age. They represent care starting with the date of admission (99471, 99475) for pediatric critical care services and all subsequent day(s) (99472, 99476) that the infant or child remains in critical condition. These codes may only be reported by a single individual and only once per calendar day, per patient. Services for the critically ill or critically injured child 6 years of age or older would be reported with the time-based critical care codes (99291, 99292). Initial inpatient critical care (99471, 99475) may only be reported once per hospital admission. If readmitted to the pediatric critical care unit during the same hospital stay, then report the subsequent inpatient pediatric critical care code 99472 or 99476 for the first day of readmission to critical care and 99472 or 99476 for each day of critical care following readmission.

The pediatric and neonatal critical care codes include those procedures listed for the critical care codes (99291, 99292). In addition, the following procedures are also included (and are not separately reported by professionals, but may be reported by facilities) in the pediatric and neonatal critical care service codes (99468-99472, 99475, 99476) and the intensive care services codes (99477-99480).

Any services performed that are not included in these listings may be reported separately. For initiation of selective head or total body hypothermia in the critically ill neonate, report 99184. Facilities may report the included services separately.

Invasive or non-invasive electronic monitoring of vital signs

Vascular access procedures

Peripheral vessel catheterization (36000)

Other arterial catheters (36140, 36620)

Umbilical venous catheters (36510)

Central vessel catheterization (36555)

Vascular access procedures (36400, 36405, 36406)

Vascular punctures (36420, 36600)

Umbilical arterial catheters (36660)

Airway and ventilation management

Endotracheal intubation (31500)

Ventilatory management (94002-94004)

Bedside pulmonary function testing (94375)

Surfactant administration (94610)

Continuous positive airway pressure (CPAP) (94660)

Monitoring or interpretation of blood gases or oxygen saturation (94760-94762)

Car Seat Evaluation (94780-94781)

Transfusion of blood components (36430, 36440)

Oral or nasogastric tube placement (43752)

Suprapubic bladder aspiration (51100)

Bladder catheterization (51701, 51702)

Lumbar puncture (62270)

Any services performed which are not listed above may be reported separately.

When a neonate or infant is not critically ill but requires intensive observation, frequent interventions, and other intensive care services, the Continuing Intensive Care Services codes (99477-99480) should be used to report these services.

To report critical care services provided in the outpatient setting (eg, emergency department or office) for neonates and pediatric patients of any age, see the Critical Care codes 99291, 99292. If the same individual provides critical care services for a neonatal or pediatric patient less than 6 years of age in both the outpatient and inpatient settings on the same day, report only the appropriate Neonatal or Pediatric Critical Care codes 99468-99476 for all critical care services provided on that day. Critical care services provided by a second individual of a different specialty not reporting a per-day neonatal or pediatric critical care code can be reported with 99291, 99292.

When critical care services are provided to neonates or pediatric patients less than 6 years of age at two separate institutions by an individual from a different group on the same date of service, the individual from the referring institution should report their critical care services with the time-based critical care codes (99291, 99292) and the receiving institution should report the appropriate initial day of care code 99468, 99471, 99475 for the same date of service.

Critical care services to a pediatric patient 6 years of age or older are reported with the time based critical care codes 99291, 99292.

When the critically ill neonate or pediatric patient improves and is transferred to a lower level of care to another individual in another group within the same facility, the transferring individual does not report a per day critical care service. Subsequent hospital inpatient or observation care (99231-99233) or time-based critical care services (99291-99292) is reported, as appropriate, based upon the condition of the neonate or child. The

★=Telemedicine ◀=Audio-only ✚=Add-on code ✔=FDA approval pending #=Resequenced code ⊘=Modifier 51 exempt ➌➌➌=See p xxi for details

receiving individual reports subsequent intensive care (99478-99480) or subsequent hospital inpatient or observation care (99231-99233) services, as appropriate, based upon the condition of the neonate or child.

When the neonate or infant becomes critically ill on a day when initial or subsequent intensive care services (99477-99480), hospital inpatient or observation services (99221-99233), or normal newborn services (99460, 99461, 99462) have been performed by one individual and is transferred to a critical care level of care provided by a different individual in a different group, the transferring individual reports either the time-based critical care services (99291, 99292) performed for the time spent providing critical care to the patient, the intensive care service (99477-99480), hospital inpatient or observation care services (99221-99233), or normal newborn service (99460, 99461, 99462) performed, but only one service. The receiving individual reports initial or subsequent inpatient neonatal or pediatric critical care (99468-99476), as appropriate, based upon the patient's age and whether this is the first or subsequent admission to the critical care unit for the hospital stay.

When a newborn becomes critically ill on the same day they have already received normal newborn care (99460, 99461, 99462), and the same individual or group assumes critical care, report initial critical care service (99468) with modifier 25 in addition to the normal newborn code.

When a neonate, infant, or child requires initial critical care services on the same day the patient already has received hospital care or intensive care services by the same individual or group, only the initial critical care service code (99468, 99471, 99475) is reported.

Time-based critical care services (99291, 99292) are not reportable by the same individual or different individual of the same specialty and same group, when neonatal or pediatric critical care services (99468-99476) may be reported for the same patient on the same day. Time-based critical care services (99291, 99292) may be reported by an individual of a different specialty from either the same or different group on the same day that neonatal or pediatric critical care services are reported. Critical care interfacility transport face-to-face (99466, 99467) or supervisory (99485, 99486) services may be reported by the same or different individual of the same specialty and same group, when neonatal or pediatric critical care services (99468-99476) are reported for the same patient on the same day.

99468   **Initial inpatient neonatal critical care,** per day, for the evaluation and management of a critically ill neonate, 28 days of age or younger

➲ *CPT Changes: An Insider's View* 2009

➲ *CPT Assistant* Nov 11:5, May 14:4, Feb 15:10, Oct 15:8, May 16:3, Jun 18:9, Dec 18:8, Sep 22:6, Dec 22:15, Feb 23:12

99469   **Subsequent inpatient neonatal critical care,** per day, for the evaluation and management of a critically ill neonate, 28 days of age or younger

➲ *CPT Changes: An Insider's View* 2009

➲ *CPT Assistant* Nov 11:5, May 14:4, Feb 15:10, Oct 15:8, May 16:4, Jun 18:9, Dec 18:8, Sep 22:6, Dec 22:15, Feb 23:12

99471   **Initial inpatient pediatric critical care,** per day, for the evaluation and management of a critically ill infant or young child, 29 days through 24 months of age

➲ *CPT Changes: An Insider's View* 2009

➲ *CPT Assistant* Nov 11:5, Feb 15:10, May 16:3, Jun 18:9, Dec 18:8, Sep 22:6, Dec 22:15, Jan 23:28, Feb 23:12

99472   **Subsequent inpatient pediatric critical care,** per day, for the evaluation and management of a critically ill infant or young child, 29 days through 24 months of age

➲ *CPT Changes: An Insider's View* 2009

➲ *CPT Assistant* Nov 11:5, Feb 15:10, May 16:4, Jun 18:9, Dec 18:8, Sep 22:6, Dec 22:15, Jan 23:28, Feb 23:12

99473   Code is out of numerical sequence. See 99448-99455

99474   Code is out of numerical sequence. See 99448-99455

99475   **Initial inpatient pediatric critical care,** per day, for the evaluation and management of a critically ill infant or young child, 2 through 5 years of age

➲ *CPT Changes: An Insider's View* 2009

➲ *CPT Assistant* Feb 15:10, May 16:3, Jun 18:9, Dec 18:8, Sep 22:6, Dec 22:15, Jan 23:28, Feb 23:12

99476   **Subsequent inpatient pediatric critical care,** per day, for the evaluation and management of a critically ill infant or young child, 2 through 5 years of age

➲ *CPT Changes: An Insider's View* 2009

➲ *CPT Assistant* Feb 15:10, May 16:4, Jun 18:9, Dec 18:8, Sep 22:6, Jan 23:28, Feb 23:12

Initial and Continuing Intensive Care Services

Code 99477 represents the initial day of inpatient care for the child who is not critically ill but requires intensive observation, frequent interventions, and other intensive care services. Codes 99478-99480 are used to report the subsequent day services of directing the continuing intensive care of the low birth weight (LBW 1500-2500 grams) present body weight infant, very low birth weight (VLBW less than 1500 grams) present body weight infant, or normal (2501-5000 grams) present body weight newborn who does not meet the definition of critically ill but continues to require intensive observation, frequent interventions, and other intensive care services. These services are for infants and neonates who are not critically ill but continue to require intensive cardiac and respiratory monitoring, continuous and/or frequent vital sign monitoring, heat maintenance, enteral and/or parenteral nutritional adjustments, laboratory and oxygen monitoring, and constant observation by the health care team under direct supervision of the physician or other qualified health care professional. Codes 99477-99480 may be reported by a single individual and only once per day, per patient in a given facility. If readmitted to the intensive care unit during the same hospital stay, report 99478-99480 for the first day of intensive care and for each successive day that the child requires intensive care services.

These codes include the same procedures that are outlined in the **Neonatal and Pediatric Critical Care Services** section and these services should not be separately reported.

The initial day neonatal intensive care code (99477) can be used in addition to 99464 or 99465 as appropriate, when the physician or other qualified health care professional is present for the delivery (99464) or resuscitation (99465) is required. In this situation, report 99477 with modifier 25. Other procedures performed as a necessary part of the resuscitation (eg, endotracheal intubation [31500]) are also reported separately when performed as part of the pre-admission delivery room care. In order to report these procedures separately, they must be performed as a necessary component of the resuscitation and not simply as a convenience before admission to the neonatal intensive care unit.

The same procedures are included as bundled services with the neonatal intensive care codes as those listed for the neonatal (99468, 99469) and pediatric (99471-99476) critical care codes.

When the neonate or infant improves after the initial day and no longer requires intensive care services and is transferred to a lower level of care, the transferring individual does not report a per day intensive care service. Subsequent hospital inpatient or observation care (99231-99233) or subsequent normal newborn care (99460, 99462) is reported, as appropriate, based upon the condition of the neonate or infant. If the transfer to a lower level of care occurs on the same day as initial intensive care services were provided by the transferring individual, 99477 may be reported.

When the neonate or infant is transferred after the initial day within the same facility to the care of another individual in a different group, both individuals report subsequent hospital inpatient or observation care (99231-99233) services. The receiving individual reports subsequent hospital inpatient or observation care (99231-99233) or subsequent normal newborn care (99462).

When the neonate or infant becomes critically ill on a day when initial or subsequent intensive care services (99477-99480) have been reported by one individual and is transferred to a critical care level of care provided by a different individual from a different group, the transferring individual reports either the time-based critical care services performed (99291, 99292) for the time spent providing critical care to the patient or the initial or subsequent intensive care (99477-99480) service, but not both. The receiving individual reports initial or subsequent inpatient neonatal or pediatric critical care (99468-99476) based upon the patient's age and whether this is the first or subsequent admission to critical care for the same hospital stay.

When the neonate or infant becomes critically ill on a day when initial or subsequent intensive care services (99477-99480) have been performed by the same individual or group, report only initial or subsequent inpatient neonatal or pediatric critical care (99468-99476) based upon the patient's age and whether this is the first or subsequent admission to critical care for the same hospital stay.

For the subsequent care of the sick neonate younger than 28 days of age but more than 5000 grams who does not require intensive or critical care services, use codes 99231-99233.

99477   **Initial hospital care,** per day, for the evaluation and management of the neonate, 28 days of age or younger, who requires intensive observation, frequent interventions, and other intensive care services

➤ *CPT Changes: An Insider's View* 2008

➤ *CPT Assistant* Jan 08:8, Jul 08:10, Mar 09:3, Nov 11:5, May 14:4, Dec 18:8, Sep 22:6

(For the initiation of inpatient care of the normal newborn, use 99460)

(For the initiation of care of the critically ill neonate, use 99468)

(For initiation of hospital inpatient or observation care of the ill neonate not requiring intensive observation, frequent interventions, and other intensive care services, see 99221-99223)

99478　**Subsequent intensive care,** per day, for the evaluation and management of the recovering very low birth weight infant (present body weight less than 1500 grams)

➔ *CPT Changes: An Insider's View* 2009

➔ *CPT Assistant* Jun 18:11, Dec 18:8

99479　**Subsequent intensive care,** per day, for the evaluation and management of the recovering low birth weight infant (present body weight of 1500-2500 grams)

➔ *CPT Changes: An Insider's View* 2009

➔ *CPT Assistant* Jun 18:11, Dec 18:8

99480　**Subsequent intensive care,** per day, for the evaluation and management of the recovering infant (present body weight of 2501-5000 grams)

➔ *CPT Changes: An Insider's View* 2009

➔ *CPT Assistant* May 14:4, Jul 15:3, Jun 18:11, Dec 18:8, Dec 21:19, Dec 22:15

Cognitive Assessment and Care Plan Services

Cognitive assessment and care plan services are provided when a comprehensive evaluation of a new or existing patient, who exhibits signs and/or symptoms of cognitive impairment, is required to establish or confirm a diagnosis, etiology and severity for the condition. This service includes a thorough evaluation of medical and psychosocial factors, potentially contributing to increased morbidity. Do not report cognitive assessment and care plan services if any of the required elements are not performed or are deemed unnecessary for the patient's condition. For these services, see the appropriate evaluation and management code. A single physician or other qualified health care professional should not report 99483 more than once every 180 days.

Services for cognitive assessment and care plan include a cognition-relevant history, as well as an assessment of factors that could be contributing to cognitive impairment, including, but not limited to, psychoactive medication, chronic pain syndromes, infection, depression and other brain disease (eg, tumor, stroke, normal pressure hydrocephalus). Medical decision making includes current and likely progression of the disease, assessing the need for referral for rehabilitative, social, legal, financial, or community-based services, meal, transportation, and other personal assistance services.

99483　**Assessment of and care planning** for a patient with cognitive impairment, requiring an independent historian, in the office or other outpatient, home or domiciliary or rest home, with all of the following required elements:

■ Cognition-focused evaluation including a pertinent history and examination,

■ Medical decision making of moderate or high complexity,

■ Functional assessment (eg, basic and instrumental activities of daily living), including decision-making capacity,

■ Use of standardized instruments for staging of dementia (eg, functional assessment staging test [FAST], clinical dementia rating [CDR]),

■ Medication reconciliation and review for high-risk medications,

■ Evaluation for neuropsychiatric and behavioral symptoms, including depression, including use of standardized screening instrument(s),

■ Evaluation of safety (eg, home), including motor vehicle operation,

■ Identification of caregiver(s), caregiver knowledge, caregiver needs, social supports, and the willingness of caregiver to take on caregiving tasks,

■ Development, updating or revision, or review of an Advance Care Plan,

■ Creation of a written care plan, including initial plans to address any neuropsychiatric symptoms, neuro-cognitive symptoms, functional limitations, and referral to community resources as needed (eg, rehabilitation services, adult day programs, support groups) shared with the patient and/or caregiver with initial education and support.

Typically, 60 minutes of total time is spent on the date of the encounter.

➔ *CPT Changes: An Insider's View* 2018, 2022, 2023

➔ *CPT Assistant* Apr 18:9, Jul 18:12, Nov 22:1, Dec 22:15

(For services of 75 minutes or longer, use 99417)

(Do not report 99483 in conjunction with E/M services [99202, 99203, 99204, 99205, 99211, 99212, 99213, 99214, 99215, 99242, 99243, 99244, 99245, 99341, 99342, 99344, 99345, 99347, 99348, 99349, 99350, 99366, 99367, 99368, 99497, 99498]; psychiatric diagnostic procedures [90785, 90791, 90792]; brief emotional/behavioral assessment [96127]; psychological or neuropsychological test administration [96146]; health risk assessment administration [96160, 96161]; medication therapy management services [99605, 99606, 99607])

99484	Code is out of numerical sequence. See 99497-99499
99485	Code is out of numerical sequence. See 99466-99469
99486	Code is out of numerical sequence. See 99466-99469

Care Management Services

Care management services are management and support services provided by clinical staff, under the direction of a physician or other qualified health care professional, or may be provided personally by a physician or other qualified health care professional to a patient residing at home or in a domiciliary, rest home, or assisted living facility. Care management services improve care coordination, reduce avoidable hospital services, improve patient engagement, and decrease care fragmentation. The physician or other qualified health care professional provides or oversees the management and/or coordination of care management services, which include establishing, implementing, revising, or monitoring the care plan, coordinating the care of other professionals and agencies, and educating the patient or caregiver about the patient's condition, care plan, and prognosis.

There are three general categories of care management services: chronic care management (99437, 99439, 99490, 99491), complex chronic care management (99487, 99489), and principal care management (99424, 99425, 99426, 99427). Complex chronic care management addresses all of the patient's medical conditions, and principal care management services address a single condition. Each of the three categories is further subdivided into those services that are personally performed by the physician or other qualified health care professional and those services that are performed by the clinical staff and overseen by the physician or other qualified health care professional. Code selection for these services is based on time in a calendar month, and time used in reporting these services may not represent time spent in another reported service. Chronic care management services do not require moderate or high-level medical decision making and may be reported for a shorter time threshold than complex chronic care management services. Both chronic care and complex chronic care management address, as needed, all medical conditions, psychosocial needs, and activities of daily living. Principal care management services are disease-specific management services. A patient may have multiple chronic conditions of sufficient severity to warrant complex chronic care management but may receive principal care management if the reporting physician or other qualified health care professional is providing single disease rather than comprehensive care management.

── *Coding Tip* ────────────

If the treating physician or other qualified health care professional personally performs any of the care management services and those activities are not used to meet the criteria for a separately reported code (99424, 99491), then his or her time may be counted toward the required clinical staff time to meet the elements of 99426, 99487, 99490, as applicable.

Care Planning

A plan of care for health problems is based on a physical, mental, cognitive, social, functional, and environmental evaluation. It is intended to provide a simple and concise overview of the patient, and his or her medical condition(s) and be a useful resource for patients, caregivers, health care professionals, and others, as necessary.

A typical plan of care is not limited to, but may include:

- Problem list
- Expected outcome and prognosis
- Measurable treatment goals
- Cognitive assessment
- Functional assessment
- Symptom management
- Planned interventions
- Medical management
- Environmental evaluation
- Caregiver assessment
- Interaction and coordination with outside resources and health care professionals and others, as necessary
- Summary of advance directives

The above elements are intended to be a guide for creating a meaningful plan of care rather than a strict set of requirements, so each should be addressed only as appropriate for the individual.

The plan of care should include specific and achievable goals for each condition and be relevant to the patient's well-being and lifestyle. When possible, the treatment goals should also be measurable and time bound. The plan should be updated periodically based on status or goal changes. The entire care plan should be reviewed, or revised as needed, but at least annually.

An electronic and/or printed plan of care must be documented and shared with the patient and/or caregiver.

Codes 99424, 99426, 99487, 99490, 99491 are reported only once per calendar month. Codes 99427, 99439 are reported no more than twice per calendar month. Codes

99437, 99439, 99487, 99489, 99490, 99491 may only be reported by the single physician or other qualified health care professional who assumes the care management role with a particular patient for the calendar month. Codes 99424, 99425, 99426, 99427 may be reported by different physicians or qualified health care professionals in the same calendar month for the same patient, and documentation in the patient's medical record should reflect coordination among relevant managing clinicians.

For 99426, 99427, 99439, 99487, 99489, 99490, the face-to-face and non-face-to-face time spent by the clinical staff in communicating with the patient and/or family, caregivers, other professionals, and agencies; creating, revising, documenting, and implementing the care plan; or teaching self-management is used in determining the care management clinical staff time for the month. Only the time of the clinical staff of the reporting professional is counted, and the reporting professional's time is additionally included only if he or she is not otherwise reporting his or her care management time with another service (see Coding Tip in column one). Only count the time of one clinical staff member or physician or other qualified health care professional when two or more are meeting about the patient at the same time. For 99424, 99425, 99437, 99491, only count the time personally spent by the physician or other qualified health care professional. Time spent by the physician or other qualified health care professional that does not meet the threshold to report 99424, 99425, 99437, 99491 may be used toward the time necessary to report 99426, 99427, 99439, 99487, 99489, 99490. Do not count clinical staff time spent as part of a separately reported service.

Care management activities performed by clinical staff, or personally by the physician or other qualified health care professional, typically include:

- communication and engagement with patient, family members, guardian or caretaker, surrogate decision makers, and/or other professionals regarding aspects of care;
- communication with home health agencies and other community services utilized by the patient;
- collection of health outcomes data and registry documentation;
- patient and/or family/caregiver education to support self-management, independent living, and activities of daily living;
- assessment and support for treatment regimen adherence and medication management;
- identification of available community and health resources;
- facilitating access to care and services needed by the patient and/or family;
- management of care transitions not reported as part of transitional care management (99495, 99496);
- ongoing review of patient status, including review of laboratory and other studies not reported as part of an E/M service, noted above;
- development, communication, and maintenance of a comprehensive or disease-specific (as applicable) care plan.

The care management office/practice must have the following capabilities:

- provide 24/7 access to physicians or other qualified health care professionals or clinical staff including providing patients/caregivers with a means to make contact with health care professionals in the practice to address urgent needs regardless of the time of day or day of week;
- provide continuity of care with a designated member of the care team with whom the patient is able to schedule successive routine appointments;
- provide timely access and management for follow-up after an emergency department visit or facility discharge;
- utilize an electronic health record system for timely access to clinical information;
- be able to engage and educate patients and caregivers as well as coordinate and integrate care among all service professionals, as appropriate for each patient;
- reporting physician or other qualified health care professional oversees activities of the care team;
- all care team members providing services are clinically integrated.

Each minute of service time is counted toward only one service. Do not count any time and activities used to meet criteria for another reported service. However, time of clinical staff and time of a physician or other qualified health care professional are reported separately when each provides distinct services to the same patient at different times during the same calendar month. A list of services not reported in the same calendar month as 99439, 99487, 99489, 99490 is provided in the parenthetical instructions following the care management codes. If the care management services are performed within the postoperative period of a reported surgery, the same individual may not report 99439, 99487, 99489, 99490, 99491.

When behavioral or psychiatric collaborative care management services are also provided, 99484, 99492, 99493, 99494 may be reported in addition.

Chronic Care Management Services

Chronic care management services are provided when medical and/or psychosocial needs of the patient require establishing, implementing, revising, or monitoring the care plan. Patients who receive chronic care management services have two or more chronic continuous or episodic health conditions that are expected to last at least 12 months, or until the death of the patient, and that place the patient at significant risk of death, acute exacerbation/decompensation, or functional decline. Code 99490 is reported when, during the calendar month, at least 20 minutes of clinical staff time is spent in care management activities. Code 99439 is reported in conjunction with 99490 for each additional 20 minutes of clinical staff time spent in care management activities during the calendar month up to a maximum of 60 minutes total time (ie, 99439 may only be reported twice per calendar month). Code 99491 is reported for at least 30 minutes of physician or other qualified health care professional time personally spent in care management during the calendar month. Code 99437 is reported in conjunction with 99491 for each additional minimum 30 minutes of physician or other qualified health care professional time. If reporting 99437, 99491 do not include any time devoted to the patient and/or family on the date that the reporting physician or other qualified health care professional also performed a face-to-face E/M encounter.

 # 99490   **Chronic care management services** with the following required elements:

- multiple (two or more) chronic conditions expected to last at least 12 months, or until the death of the patient,

- chronic conditions that place the patient at significant risk of death, acute exacerbation/decompensation, or functional decline,

- comprehensive care plan established, implemented, revised, or monitored;

first 20 minutes of clinical staff time directed by a physician or other qualified health care professional, per calendar month.

➔ *CPT Changes: An Insider's View* 2015, 2021, 2022
➔ *CPT Assistant* Oct 14:3, Feb 15:3, Feb 18:7, Mar 18:5, Oct 18:9, Feb 20:7, Jan 21:5, Jan 22:3-4, 8

#+ 99439   each additional 20 minutes of clinical staff time directed by a physician or other qualified health care professional, per calendar month (List separately in addition to code for primary procedure)

➔ *CPT Changes: An Insider's View* 2021, 2022
➔ *CPT Assistant* Jan 21:5, Jan 22:3-4, 8

(Use 99439 in conjunction with 99490)

(Chronic care management services of less than 20 minutes duration in a calendar month are not reported separately)

(Chronic care management services of 60 minutes or more and requiring moderate or high complexity medical decision making may be reported using 99487, 99489)

(Do not report 99439 more than twice per calendar month)

(Do not report 99439, 99490 in the same calendar month with 90951-90970, 99374, 99375, 99377, 99378, 99379, 99380, 99424, 99425, 99426, 99427, 99437, 99487, 99489, 99491, 99605, 99606, 99607)

▶(Do not report 99439, 99490 for service time reported with 93792, 93793, 98012, 98013, 98014, 98015, 98016, 98960, 98961, 98962, 98966, 98967, 98968, 98970, 98971, 98972, 99071, 99078, 99080, 99091, 99358, 99359, 99366, 99367, 99368, 99421, 99422, 99423, 99605, 99606, 99607)◀

 # 99491   **Chronic care management services** with the following required elements:

- multiple (two or more) chronic conditions expected to last at least 12 months, or until the death of the patient,

- chronic conditions that place the patient at significant risk of death, acute exacerbation/decompensation, or functional decline,

- comprehensive care plan established, implemented, revised, or monitored;

first 30 minutes provided personally by a physician or other qualified health care professional, per calendar month.

➔ *CPT Changes: An Insider's View* 2019, 2022
➔ *CPT Assistant* Oct 18:9, Jan 22:3-4, 8, Dec 22:3

#+ 99437   each additional 30 minutes by a physician or other qualified health care professional, per calendar month (List separately in addition to code for primary procedure)

➔ *CPT Changes: An Insider's View* 2022
➔ *CPT Assistant* Jan 22:3-4, 8, Dec 22:3

(Use 99437 in conjunction with 99491)

(Do not report 99437 for less than 30 minutes)

(Do not report 99437, 99491 in the same calendar month with 90951-90970, 99374, 99375, 99377, 99378, 99379, 99380, 99424, 99425, 99426, 99427, 99439, 99487, 99489, 99490, 99605, 99606, 99607)

►(Do not report 99437, 99491 for service time reported with 93792, 93793, 98012, 98013, 98014, 98015, 98016, 98960, 98961, 98962, 98966, 98967, 98968, 98970, 98971, 98972, 99071, 99078, 99080, 99091, 99358, 99359, 99366, 99367, 99368, 99421, 99422, 99423, 99495, 99496, 99605, 99606, 99607)◄

Table for Reporting Chronic Care Management Services

Total Duration Care Management Services	Staff Type	Chronic Care Management
Less than 20 minutes	Not reported separately	Not reported separately
Less than 30 minutes	Physician or other qualified health care professional	Not reported separately or see 99490
20-39 minutes	Clinical staff	99490 X 1
30-59 minutes	Physician or other qualified health care professional	99491 X 1
40-59 minutes	Clinical staff	99490 X 1 and 99439 X 1
60-89 minutes	Physician or other qualified health care professional	99491 X 1 and 99437 X 1
60 minutes or more	Clinical staff	99490 X 1 and 99439 X 2
90 minutes or more	Physician or other qualified health care professional	99491 X 1 and 99437 X 2 as appropriate (see illustrated reporting examples above)

Complex Chronic Care Management Services

Complex chronic care management services are services that require at least 60 minutes of clinical staff time, under the direction of a physician or other qualified health care professional. Complex chronic care management services require moderate or high medical decision making as defined in the Evaluation and Management (E/M) guidelines.

Patients who require complex chronic care management services may be identified by practice-specific or other published algorithms that recognize multiple illnesses, multiple medication use, inability to perform activities of daily living, requirement for a caregiver, and/or repeat admissions or emergency department visits. Typical adult patients who receive complex chronic care management

services are treated with three or more prescription medications and may be receiving other types of therapeutic interventions (eg, physical therapy, occupational therapy). Typical pediatric patients receive three or more therapeutic interventions (eg, medications, nutritional support, respiratory therapy). All patients have two or more chronic continuous or episodic health conditions that are expected to last at least 12 months, or until the death of the patient, and that place the patient at significant risk of death, acute exacerbation/ decompensation, or functional decline. Typical patients have complex diseases and morbidities and, as a result, demonstrate one or more of the following:

- need for the coordination of a number of specialties and services;
- inability to perform activities of daily living and/or cognitive impairment resulting in poor adherence to the treatment plan without substantial assistance from a caregiver;
- psychiatric and other medical comorbidities (eg, dementia and chronic obstructive pulmonary disease or substance abuse and diabetes) that complicate their care; and/or
- social support requirements or difficulty with access to care.

Total Duration of Staff Care Management Services	Complex Chronic Care Management
less than 60 minutes	Not reported separately
60 to 89 minutes (1 hour - 1 hr. 29 min.)	99487 X 1
90 - 119 minutes (1 hr. 30 min. - 1 hr. 59 min.)	99487 X 1 and 99489 X 1
120 minutes or more (2 hours or more)	99487 X 1 and 99489 X 2 and 99489 for each additional 30 minutes

99487   **Complex chronic care management services** with the following required elements:

- multiple (two or more) chronic conditions expected to last at least 12 months, or until the death of the patient,

- chronic conditions that place the patient at significant risk of death, acute exacerbation/decompensation, or functional decline,

- comprehensive care plan established, implemented, revised, or monitored,

- moderate or high complexity medical decision making;

first 60 minutes of clinical staff time directed by a physician or other qualified health care professional, per calendar month.

➲ *CPT Changes: An Insider's View* 2013, 2015, 2021, 2022

➲ *CPT Assistant* Apr 13:3, Sep 13:15, Nov 13:3, Feb 14:3, Jun 14:3, 5, Oct 14:3, Apr 17:9, Feb 18:7, Mar 18:5, Oct 18:9, Feb 20:7, Jan 22:3-4, 6, 8

(Complex chronic care management services of less than 60 minutes duration in a calendar month are not reported separately)

+ **99489**   each additional 30 minutes of clinical staff time directed by a physician or other qualified health care professional, per calendar month (List separately in addition to code for primary procedure)

➲ *CPT Changes: An Insider's View* 2013, 2015, 2021, 2022

➲ *CPT Assistant* Apr 13:3, Sep 13:15, Nov 13:3, Jun 14:5, Oct 14:3, Apr 17:9, Feb 18:7, Mar 18:5, Oct 18:9, Feb 20:7, Jan 22:3-4, 6, 8

(Report 99489 in conjunction with 99487)

(Do not report 99489 for care management service of less than 30 minutes)

(Do not report 99487, 99489 during the same calendar month with 90951-90970, 99374, 99375, 99377, 99378, 99379, 99380, 99424, 99425, 99426, 99427, 99437, 99439, 99490, 99491)

▶(Do not report 99487, 99489 for service time reported with 93792, 93793, 98012, 98013, 98014, 98015, 98016, 98960, 98961, 98962, 98966, 98967, 98968, 98970, 98971, 98972, 99071, 99078, 99080, 99091, 99358, 99359, 99366, 99367, 99368, 99421, 99422, 99423, 99605, 99606, 99607)◀

—— *Coding Tip* ——

If the physician personally performs the clinical staff activities, his or her time may be counted toward the required clinical staff time to meet the elements of the code.

99490   Code is out of numerical sequence. See 99480-99489

99491   Code is out of numerical sequence. See 99480-99489

Principal Care Management Services

Principal care management represents services that focus on the medical and/or psychological needs manifested by a single, complex chronic condition expected to last at least 3 months and includes establishing, implementing, revising, or monitoring a care plan specific to that single disease. Code 99424 is reported for at least 30 minutes of physician or other qualified health care professional personal time in care management activities during a calendar month. Code 99425 is reported in conjunction with 99424, when at least an additional 30 minutes of physician or other qualified health care professional personal time is spent in care management activities during the calendar month. Code 99426 is reported for the first 30 minutes of clinical staff time spent in care management activities during the calendar month. Code 99427 is reported in conjunction with 99426, when at least an additional 30 minutes of clinical staff time is spent in care management activities during the calendar month.

99424   **Principal care management services,** for a single high-risk disease, with the following required elements:

- one complex chronic condition expected to last at least 3 months, and that places the patient at significant risk of hospitalization, acute exacerbation/ decompensation, functional decline, or death,

- the condition requires development, monitoring, or revision of disease-specific care plan,

- the condition requires frequent adjustments in the medication regimen and/or the management of the condition is unusually complex due to comorbidities,

- ongoing communication and care coordination between relevant practitioners furnishing care;

first 30 minutes provided personally by a physician or other qualified health care professional, per calendar month.

➲ *CPT Changes: An Insider's View* 2022

➲ *CPT Assistant* Jan 22:3-4, 8-9, Nov 22:16, Dec 22:3

Table for Reporting Principal Care Management Services

Total Duration Principal Care Management Services	Staff Type	Principal Care Management
Less than 30 minutes	Not separately reported	Not separately reported
30-59 minutes	Physician or other qualified health care professional	99424 X 1
	Clinical staff	99426 X 1
60-89 minutes	Physician or other qualified health care professional	99424 X 1 and 99425 X 1
	Clinical staff	99426 X 1 and 99427 X 1
90-119 minutes	Physician or other qualified health care professional	99424 X 1 and 99425 X 2
	Clinical staff	99426 X 1 and 99427 X 2
120 minutes or more	Physician or other qualified health care professional	99424 X 1 and 99425 X 3, as appropriate (see illustrated reporting examples above)
	Clinical staff	99426 X 1 and 99427 X 2

Care Management Services

Code	Service	Staff Type	Unit Duration (Time Span)	Unit Max Per Month
99490	Chronic care management	Clinical staff	20 minutes (20-39 minutes)	1
+99439	Chronic care management	Clinical staff	40-59 minutes X 1 60 or more minutes X 2)	2
99491	Chronic care management	Physician or other qualified health care professional	30 minutes (30-59 minutes)	1
+99437	Chronic care management	Physician or other qualified health care professional	30 minutes (60 minutes or more)	No limit
99487	Complex chronic care management	Clinical staff	60 minutes (60-89 minutes)	1
+99489	Complex chronic care management	Clinical staff	30 minutes (≥90 minutes X 1) (≥120 minutes X 2, etc)	No limit
99424	Principal care management	Physician or other qualified health care professional	30 minutes (30-59 minutes)	1
+99425	Principal care management	Physician or other qualified health care professional	30 minutes (60 minutes or more)	No limit
99426	Principal care management	Clinical staff	30 minutes (30-59 minutes)	1
+99427	Principal care management	Clinical staff	30 minutes (60 minutes or more)	2

#+ 99425   each additional 30 minutes provided personally by a physician or other qualified health care professional, per calendar month (List separately in addition to code for primary procedure)

➔ *CPT Changes: An Insider's View* 2022

➔ *CPT Assistant* Jan 22:3-4, 8-9, Nov 22:16, Dec 22:3

(Use 99425 in conjunction with 99424)

(Principal care management services of less than 30 minutes duration in a calendar month are not reported separately)

(Do not report 99424, 99425 in the same calendar month with 90951-90970, 99374, 99375, 99377, 99378, 99379, 99380, 99426, 99427, 99437, 99439, 99473, 99474, 99487, 99489, 99490, 99491)

▶(Do not report 99424, 99425 for service time reported with 93792, 93793, 98012, 98013, 98014, 98015, 98016, 98960, 98961, 98962, 98966, 98967, 98968, 98970, 98971, 98972, 99071, 99078, 99080, 99091, 99358, 99359, 99366, 99367, 99368, 99421, 99422, 99423, 99605, 99606, 99607)◀

 # 99426   **Principal care management services,** for a single high-risk disease, with the following required elements:

- one complex chronic condition expected to last at least 3 months, and that places the patient at significant risk of hospitalization, acute exacerbation/decompensation, functional decline, or death,

- the condition requires development, monitoring, or revision of disease-specific care plan,

- the condition requires frequent adjustments in the medication regimen and/or the management of the condition is unusually complex due to comorbidities,

- ongoing communication and care coordination between relevant practitioners furnishing care;

first 30 minutes of clinical staff time directed by physician or other qualified health care professional, per calendar month.

➔ *CPT Changes: An Insider's View* 2022

➔ *CPT Assistant* Jan 22:3-4, 8-9, Nov 22:16

#+ 99427   each additional 30 minutes of clinical staff time directed by a physician or other qualified health care professional, per calendar month (List separately in addition to code for primary procedure)

➔ *CPT Changes: An Insider's View* 2022

➔ *CPT Assistant* Jan 22:3-4, 8-9, Nov 22:16

(Use 99427 in conjunction with 99426)

(Principal care management services of less than 30 minutes duration in a calendar month are not reported separately)

(Do not report 99427 more than twice per calendar month)

(Do not report 99426, 99427 in the same calendar month with 90951-90970, 99374, 99375, 99377, 99378, 99379, 99380, 99424, 99425, 99437, 99439, 99473, 99474, 99487, 99489, 99490, 99491)

▶(Do not report 99426, 99427 for service time reported with 93792, 93793, 98012, 98013, 98014, 98015, 98016, 98960, 98961, 98962, 98966, 98967, 98968, 98970, 98971, 98972, 99071, 99078, 99080, 99091, 99358, 99359, 99366, 99367, 99368, 99421, 99422, 99423, 99605, 99606, 99607)◀

Psychiatric Collaborative Care Management Services

Psychiatric collaborative care services are provided under the direction of a treating physician or other qualified health care professional (see definitions below) during a calendar month. These services are reported by the treating physician or other qualified health care professional and include the services of the treating physician or other qualified health care professional, the behavioral health care manager (see definition below), and the psychiatric consultant (see definition below), who has contracted directly with the treating physician or other qualified health care professional, to provide consultation. Patients directed to the behavioral health care manager typically have behavioral health signs and/or symptoms or a newly diagnosed behavioral health condition, may need help in engaging in treatment, have not responded to standard care delivered in a nonpsychiatric setting, or require further assessment and engagement, prior to consideration of referral to a psychiatric care setting.

These services are provided when a patient requires a behavioral health care assessment; establishing, implementing, revising, or monitoring a care plan; and provision of brief interventions.

The following definitions apply to this section:

Definitions

Episode of care patients are treated for an episode of care, which is defined as beginning when the patient is directed by the treating physician or other qualified health care professional to the behavioral health care manager and ending with:

- the attainment of targeted treatment goals, which typically results in the discontinuation of care management services and continuation of usual follow-up with the treating physician or other qualified health care professional; or

- failure to attain targeted treatment goals culminating in referral to a psychiatric care provider for ongoing treatment of the behavioral health condition; or

- lack of continued engagement with no psychiatric collaborative care management services provided over a consecutive six month calendar period (break in episode).

A new episode of care starts after a break in episode of six calendar months or more.

Health care professionals refers to the treating physician or other qualified health care professional who directs the behavioral health care manager and continues to oversee the patient's care, including prescribing medications, providing treatments for medical conditions, and making referrals to specialty care when needed. Evaluation and management (E/M) and other services may be reported separately by the same physician or other qualified health care professional during the same calendar month.

Behavioral health care manager refers to clinical staff with a masters-/doctoral-level education or specialized training in behavioral health who provides care management services as well as an assessment of needs, including the administration of validated rating scales, the development of a care plan, provision of brief interventions, ongoing collaboration with the treating physician or other qualified health care professional, maintenance of a registry, all in consultation with a psychiatric consultant. Services are provided both face-to-face and non-face-to-face and psychiatric consultation is provided minimally on a weekly basis, typically non-face-to-face.

The behavioral health care manager providing other services in the same calendar month, such as psychiatric evaluation (90791, 90792), psychotherapy (90832, 90833, 90834, 90836, 90837, 90838), psychotherapy for crisis (90839, 90840), family psychotherapy (90846, 90847), multiple family group psychotherapy (90849), group psychotherapy (90853), smoking and tobacco use cessation counseling (99406, 99407), and alcohol and/or substance abuse structured screening and brief intervention services (99408, 99409), may report these services separately. Activities for services reported separately are not included in the time applied to 99492, 99493, 99494.

Psychiatric consultant refers to a medical professional, who is trained in psychiatry or behavioral health, and qualified to prescribe the full range of medications. The psychiatric consultant advises and makes recommendations, as needed, for psychiatric and other medical care, including psychiatric and other medical differential diagnosis, treatment strategies regarding appropriate therapies, medication management, medical

management of complications associated with treatment of psychiatric disorders, and referral for specialty services, which are typically communicated to the treating physician or other qualified health care professional through the behavioral health care manager. The psychiatric consultant typically does not see the patient or prescribe medications, except in rare circumstances.

The psychiatric consultant may provide services in the calendar month described by other codes, such as evaluation and management (E/M) services and psychiatric evaluation (90791, 90792). These services may be reported separately by the psychiatric consultant. Activities for services reported separately are not included in the services reported using 99492, 99493, 99494.

Do not report 99492 and 99493 in the same calendar month.

99492   **Initial psychiatric collaborative care management,** first 70 minutes in the first calendar month of behavioral health care manager activities, in consultation with a psychiatric consultant, and directed by the treating physician or other qualified health care professional, with the following required elements:

- outreach to and engagement in treatment of a patient directed by the treating physician or other qualified health care professional,

- initial assessment of the patient, including administration of validated rating scales, with the development of an individualized treatment plan,

- review by the psychiatric consultant with modifications of the plan if recommended,

- entering patient in a registry and tracking patient follow-up and progress using the registry, with appropriate documentation, and participation in weekly caseload consultation with the psychiatric consultant, and

- provision of brief interventions using evidence-based techniques such as behavioral activation, motivational interviewing, and other focused treatment strategies.

➲ *CPT Changes: An Insider's View* 2018, 2022

➲ *CPT Assistant* Nov 17:3, Feb 18:7, Mar 18:5, Jul 18:12, Feb 20:7, Jan 22:3

Type of Service	Total Duration of Collaborative Care Management Over Calendar Month	Code(s)
Initial - 70 minutes	Less than 36 minutes	Not reported separately
	36-85 minutes (36 minutes - 1 hr. 25 minutes)	99492 X 1
Initial plus each additional increment up to 30 minutes	86-115 minutes (1 hr. 26 minutes - 1 hr. 55 minutes)	99492 X 1 AND 99494 X 1
Subsequent - 60 minutes	Less than 31 minutes	Not reported separately
	31-75 minutes (31 minutes - 1 hr. 15 minutes)	99493 X 1
Subsequent plus each additional increment up to 30 minutes	76-105 minutes (1 hr. 16 minutes - 1 hr. 45 minutes)	99493 X 1 AND 99494 X 1

99493 **Subsequent psychiatric collaborative care management,** first 60 minutes in a subsequent month of behavioral health care manager activities, in consultation with a psychiatric consultant, and directed by the treating physician or other qualified health care professional, with the following required elements:

- tracking patient follow-up and progress using the registry, with appropriate documentation,

- participation in weekly caseload consultation with the psychiatric consultant,

- ongoing collaboration with and coordination of the patient's mental health care with the treating physician or other qualified health care professional and any other treating mental health providers,

- additional review of progress and recommendations for changes in treatment, as indicated, including medications, based on recommendations provided by the psychiatric consultant,

- provision of brief interventions using evidence-based techniques such as behavioral activation, motivational interviewing, and other focused treatment strategies,

- monitoring of patient outcomes using validated rating scales, and

- relapse prevention planning with patients as they achieve remission of symptoms and/or other treatment goals and are prepared for discharge from active treatment.

➔ *CPT Changes: An Insider's View* 2018, 2022

➔ *CPT Assistant* Nov 17:3, Feb 18:7, Mar 18:5, Jul 18:12, Feb 20:7, Jan 22:3

+ 99494 **Initial or subsequent psychiatric collaborative care management,** each additional 30 minutes in a calendar month of behavioral health care manager activities, in consultation with a psychiatric consultant, and directed by the treating physician or other qualified health care professional (List separately in addition to code for primary procedure)

➔ *CPT Changes: An Insider's View* 2018

➔ *CPT Assistant* Nov 17:3, Feb 18:7, Mar 18:5, Jul 18:12, Feb 20:7, Jan 22:3

(Use 99494 in conjunction with 99492, 99493)

─── *Coding Tip* ───

If the treating physician or other qualified health care professional personally performs behavioral health care manager activities and those activities are not used to meet criteria for a separately reported code, his or her time may be counted toward the required behavioral health care manager time to meet the elements of 99492, 99493, 99494.

Transitional Care Management Services

Codes 99495 and 99496 are used to report transitional care management (TCM) services. These services are for a new or established patient whose medical and/or psychosocial problems require a moderate or high level of medical decision making during transitions in care from an inpatient hospital setting (including acute hospital, rehabilitation hospital, long-term acute care hospital), partial hospital, observation status in a hospital, or skilled nursing facility/nursing facility to the patient's community setting (eg, home, rest home, or assisted living). Home may be defined as a private residence, temporary lodging, or short-term accommodation (eg, hotel, campground, hostel, or cruise ship).

These codes are also used when the residence is an assisted living facility, group home (that is not licensed as an intermediate care facility for individuals with intellectual disabilities), custodial care facility, or residential substance abuse treatment facility.

TCM commences upon the date of discharge and continues for the next 29 days.

TCM is comprised of one face-to-face visit within the specified timeframes, in combination with non-face-to-face services that may be performed by the physician or other qualified health care professional and/or licensed clinical staff under his/her direction.

Non-face-to-face services provided by clinical staff, under the direction of the physician or other qualified health care professional, may include:

- communication (with patient, family members, guardian or caretaker, surrogate decision makers, and/or other professionals) regarding aspects of care,
- communication with home health agencies and other community services utilized by the patient,
- patient and/or family/caretaker education to support self-management, independent living, and activities of daily living,
- assessment and support for treatment regimen adherence and medication management,
- identification of available community and health resources,
- facilitating access to care and services needed by the patient and/or family

Non-face-to-face services provided by the physician or other qualified health care provider may include:

- obtaining and reviewing the discharge information (eg, discharge summary, as available, or continuity of care documents);
- reviewing need for or follow-up on pending diagnostic tests and treatments;
- interaction with other qualified health care professionals who will assume or reassume care of the patient's system-specific problems;
- education of patient, family, guardian, and/or caregiver;
- establishment or reestablishment of referrals and arranging for needed community resources;
- assistance in scheduling any required follow-up with community providers and services.

TCM requires a face-to-face visit, initial patient contact, and medication reconciliation within specified time frames. The first face-to-face visit is part of the TCM service and not reported separately. Additional E/M services provided on subsequent dates after the first face-to-face visit may be reported separately. TCM requires an interactive contact with the patient or caregiver, as appropriate, within two business days of discharge. The contact may be direct (face-to-face), telephonic, or by electronic means. Medication reconciliation and management must occur no later than the date of the face-to-face visit.

These services address any needed coordination of care performed by multiple disciplines and community service agencies. The reporting individual provides or oversees the management and/or coordination of services, as needed, for all medical conditions, psychosocial needs and activity of daily living support by providing first contact and continuous access.

Medical decision making and the date of the first face-to-face visit are used to select and report the appropriate TCM code. For 99496, the face-to-face visit must occur within 7 calendar days of the date of discharge and there must be a high level of medical decision making. For 99495, the face-to-face visit must occur within 14 calendar days of the date of discharge and there must be at least a moderate level of medical decision making.

Level of Medical Decision Making	Face-to-Face Visit Within 7 Days	Face-to-Face Visit Within 8 to 14 Days
Moderate	99495	99495
High	99496	99495

Medical decision making is defined by the E/M Services Guidelines. The medical decision making over the service period reported is used to define the medical decision making of TCM. Documentation includes the timing of the initial post-discharge communication with the patient or caregivers, date of the face-to-face visit, and the level of medical decision making.

Only one individual may report these services and only once per patient within 30 days of discharge. Another TCM may not be reported by the same individual or group for any subsequent discharge(s) within the 30 days. The same individual may report hospital or observation discharge services and TCM. However, the discharge service may not constitute the required face-to-face visit. The same individual should not report TCM services provided in the postoperative period of a service that the individual reported.

★ **99495**   **Transitional care management services** with the following required elements:

- Communication (direct contact, telephone, electronic) with the patient and/or caregiver within 2 business days of discharge
- At least moderate level of medical decision making during the service period
- Face-to-face visit, within 14 calendar days of discharge

➔ *CPT Changes: An Insider's View* 2013, 2017, 2023

➔ *CPT Assistant* Apr 13:3, Jul 13:11, Aug 13:13, Sep 13:15, Nov 13:3, Dec 13:11, Mar 14:13, Oct 14:3, Feb 18:7, Mar 18:5, Jan 20:3, Feb 20:7, Jan 22:3, 8, Dec 22:15

★ **99496** **Transitional care management services** with the following required elements:

- Communication (direct contact, telephone, electronic) with the patient and/or caregiver within 2 business days of discharge

- High level of medical decision making during the service period

- Face-to-face visit, within 7 calendar days of discharge

➜ *CPT Changes: An Insider's View* 2013, 2017, 2023

➜ *CPT Assistant* Apr 13:3, Jul 13:11, Aug 13:13, Sep 13:15, Nov 13:3, Mar 14:13, Oct 14:3, Feb 18:7, Mar 18:5, Jan 20:3, Feb 20:7, Jan 22:3, 8, Dec 22:15

── *Coding Tip* ──────────────

If another individual provides TCM services within the postoperative period of a surgical package, modifier 54 is not required.

The required contact with the patient or caregiver, as appropriate, may be by the physician or qualified health care professional or clinical staff and must occur before the end of the second business day after discharge. A business day is Monday through Friday except holidays without respect to normal practice hours or date of notification of discharge. However, the contact may occur on weekends and holidays. The contact must include capacity for prompt interactive communication addressing patient status and needs beyond scheduling follow-up care. If two or more separate attempts are made in a timely manner, but are unsuccessful and other transitional care management criteria are met, the service may be reported.

Advance Care Planning

Codes 99497, 99498 are used to report the face-to-face service between a physician or other qualified health care professional and a patient, family member, or surrogate in counseling and discussing advance directives, with or without completing relevant legal forms. An advance directive is a document appointing an agent and/or recording the wishes of a patient pertaining to his/her medical treatment at a future time should he/she lack decisional capacity at that time. Examples of written advance directives include, but are not limited to, Health Care Proxy, Durable Power of Attorney for Health Care, Living Will, and Medical Orders for Life-Sustaining Treatment (MOLST).

When using codes 99497, 99498, no active management of the problem(s) is undertaken during the time period reported.

Codes 99497, 99498 may be reported separately if these services are performed on the same day as another evaluation and management service (99202-99215, 99221, 99222, 99223, 99231, 99232, 99233, 99234, 99235, 99236, 99238, 99239, 99242, 99243, 99244, 99245, 99252, 99253, 99254, 99255, 99281, 99282,

99283, 99284, 99285, 99304, 99305, 99306, 99307, 99308, 99309, 99310, 99315, 99316, 99341, 99342, 99344, 99345, 99347, 99348, 99349, 99350, 99381-99397, 99495, 99496).

★◀ **99497** **Advance care planning** including the explanation and discussion of advance directives such as standard forms (with completion of such forms, when performed), by the physician or other qualified health care professional; first 30 minutes, face-to-face with the patient, family member(s), and/or surrogate

➜ *CPT Changes: An Insider's View* 2015

➜ *CPT Assistant* Dec 14:11, Feb 16:7, Dec 22:15

★+◀ **99498** each additional 30 minutes (List separately in addition to code for primary procedure)

➜ *CPT Changes: An Insider's View* 2015

➜ *CPT Assistant* Dec 14:11, Feb 16:7, Dec 22:15

(Use 99498 in conjunction with 99497)

(Do not report 99497 and 99498 on the same date of service as 99291, 99292, 99468, 99469, 99471, 99472, 99475, 99476, 99477, 99478, 99479, 99480, 99483)

General Behavioral Health Integration Care Management

General behavioral health integration care management services (99484) are reported by the supervising physician or other qualified health care professional. The services are performed by clinical staff for a patient with a behavioral health (including substance use) condition that requires care management services (face-to-face or non-face-to-face) of 20 or more minutes in a calendar month. A treatment plan as well as the specified elements of the service description is required. The assessment and treatment plan is not required to be comprehensive and the office/practice is not required to have all the functions of chronic care management (99439, 99487, 99489, 99490). Code 99484 may be used in any outpatient setting, as long as the reporting professional has an ongoing relationship with the patient and clinical staff and as long as the clinical staff is available for face-to-face services with the patient.

The reporting professional must be able to perform the evaluation and management (E/M) services of an initiating visit. General behavioral integration care management (99484) and chronic care management services may be reported by the same professional in the same month, as long as distinct care management services are performed. Behavioral health integration care management (99484) and psychiatric collaborative care management (99492, 99493, 99494) may not be reported by the same professional in the same month. Behavioral health care integration clinical staff are not required to have qualifications that would permit them to separately report services (eg, psychotherapy), but, if qualified and they perform such services, they may report such services separately, as long as the time of the service is not used in reporting 99484.

 # 99484   Care management services for behavioral health conditions, at least 20 minutes of clinical staff time, directed by a physician or other qualified health care professional, per calendar month, with the following required elements:

- initial assessment or follow-up monitoring, including the use of applicable validated rating scales,

- behavioral health care planning in relation to behavioral/psychiatric health problems, including revision for patients who are not progressing or whose status changes,

- facilitating and coordinating treatment such as psychotherapy, pharmacotherapy, counseling and/or psychiatric consultation, and

- continuity of care with a designated member of the care team.

➲ CPT Changes: An Insider's View 2018, 2022

➲ CPT Assistant Feb 18:7, Mar 18:5, Jul 18:12, Feb 20:7, Jan 22:3, 8

(Do not report 99484 in conjunction with 99492, 99493, 99494 in the same calendar month)

(E/M services, including care management services [99424, 99425, 99426, 99427, 99437, 99439, 99487, 99489, 99490, 99491, 99495, 99496], and psychiatric services [90785-90899] may be reported separately by the same physician or other qualified health care professional on the same day or during the same calendar month, but time and activities used to meet criteria for another reported service do not count toward meeting criteria for 99484.)

—— *Coding Tip* ——

If the treating physician or other qualified health care professional personally performs behavioral health care manager activities and those activities are not used to meet the criteria for a separately reported code, his or her time may be counted toward the required behavioral health care manager time to meet the elements of 99484, 99492, 99493, 99494.

Clinical staff time spent coordinating care with the emergency department may be reported using 99484, but time spent while the patient is inpatient or admitted to observation status may not be reported using 99484.

Other Evaluation and Management Services

#+ 99459   Pelvic examination (List separately in addition to code for primary procedure)

➲ CPT Changes: An Insider's View 2024

➲ CPT Assistant Jan 24:1

(Use 99459 in conjunction with 99202, 99203, 99204, 99205, 99212, 99213, 99214, 99215, 99242, 99243, 99244, 99245, 99383, 99384, 99385, 99386, 99387, 99393, 99394, 99395, 99396, 99397)

99499   Unlisted evaluation and management service

➲ CPT Assistant Apr 96:11, Mar 05:11, May 05:1, Jan 06:46, Sep 06:8, Jan 07:30, May 11:7, Apr 12:10, Jul 12:10-11, Nov 12:13, Oct 14:9, Aug 19:8, Feb 21:13, Jul 22:17

Notes

Anesthesia Guidelines

The following is a listing of headings and subheadings that appear within the Anesthesia section of the CPT codebook. The subheadings or subsections denoted with asterisks (*) below have special instructions unique to that subsection. Where these are indicated, special notes or guidelines will be presented preceding those procedural terminology listings, referring to that subsection specifically. Note that all code ranges in each subsection are listed as they appear in the subsection, even if the code numbers are out of numerical sequence and/or repeated in the next subsection.

Anesthesia

Anesthesia Guidelines

Services involving administration of anesthesia are reported by the use of the anesthesia five-digit procedure code (00100-01999) plus modifier codes (defined under "Anesthesia Modifiers" later in these Guidelines).

The reporting of anesthesia services is appropriate by or under the responsible supervision of a physician. These services may include but are not limited to general, regional, supplementation of local anesthesia, or other supportive services in order to afford the patient the anesthesia care deemed optimal by the anesthesiologist during any procedure. These services include the usual preoperative and postoperative visits, the anesthesia care during the procedure, the administration of fluids and/or blood and the usual monitoring services (eg, ECG, temperature, blood pressure, oximetry, capnography, and mass spectrometry). Unusual forms of monitoring (eg, intra-arterial, central venous, and Swan-Ganz) are not included.

Items used by all physicians in reporting their services are presented in the **Introduction.** Some of the commonalities are repeated in this section for the convenience of those physicians referring to this section on **Anesthesia.** Other definitions and items unique to anesthesia are also listed.

To report moderate (conscious) sedation provided by a physician also performing the service for which conscious sedation is being provided, see codes 99151, 99152, 99153.

When a second physician other than the health care professional performing the diagnostic or therapeutic services provides moderate (conscious) sedation in the facility setting (eg, hospital, outpatient hospital/ambulatory surgery center, skilled nursing facility), the second physician reports the associated moderate sedation procedure/service 99155, 99156, 99157; when these services are performed by the second physician in the nonfacility setting (eg, physician office, freestanding imaging center), codes 99155, 99156, 99157 would not be reported. Moderate sedation does not include minimal sedation (anxiolysis), deep sedation, or monitored anesthesia care (00100-01999).

To report regional or general anesthesia provided by a physician also performing the services for which the anesthesia is being provided, see modifier 47 in Appendix A.

Time Reporting

Time for anesthesia procedures may be reported as is customary in the local area. Anesthesia time begins when the anesthesiologist begins to prepare the patient for the induction of anesthesia in the operating room (or in an equivalent area) and ends when the anesthesiologist is no longer in personal attendance, that is, when the patient may be safely placed under postoperative supervision.

Anesthesia Services

►Services rendered in the office, home, or hospital; consultation; and other medical services are listed in the **Evaluation and Management Services** section (98000-98016, 99202-99499 series) on page 15. "Special Services, Procedures and Reports" (99000-99082 series) are listed in the **Medicine** section.◄

Supplied Materials

Supplies and materials provided (eg, sterile trays, drugs) over and above those usually included with the office visit or other services rendered may be listed separately. Drugs, tray supplies, and materials provided should be listed and identified with 99070 or the appropriate supply code.

Separate or Multiple Procedures

When multiple surgical procedures are performed during a single anesthetic administration, the anesthesia code representing the most complex procedure is reported. The time reported is the combined total for all procedures.

Unlisted Service or Procedure

A service or procedure may be provided that is not listed in this edition of the CPT codebook. When reporting such a service, the appropriate "Unlisted Procedure" code may be used to indicate the service, identifying it by "Special Report" as discussed in the section below. The "Unlisted Procedures" and accompanying code for **Anesthesia** is as follows:

01999   Unlisted anesthesia procedure(s)

Special Report

A service that is rarely provided, unusual, variable, or new may require a special report. Pertinent information should include an adequate definition or description of the nature, extent, and need for the procedure and the time, effort, and equipment necessary to provide the service.

Anesthesia Modifiers

All anesthesia services are reported by use of the anesthesia five-digit procedure code (00100-01999) plus the addition of a physical status modifier. The use of other optional modifiers may be appropriate.

Physical Status Modifiers

Physical Status modifiers are represented by the initial letter 'P' followed by a single digit from 1 to 6 as defined in the following list:

P1: A normal healthy patient

P2: A patient with mild systemic disease

P3: A patient with severe systemic disease

P4: A patient with severe systemic disease that is a constant threat to life

P5: A moribund patient who is not expected to survive without the operation

P6: A declared brain-dead patient whose organs are being removed for donor purposes

These six levels are consistent with the American Society of Anesthesiologists (ASA) ranking of patient physical status. Physical status is included in the CPT codebook to distinguish among various levels of complexity of the anesthesia service provided.

Example: 00100-P1

Qualifying Circumstances

More than one qualifying circumstance may be selected.

Many anesthesia services are provided under particularly difficult circumstances, depending on factors such as extraordinary condition of patient, notable operative conditions, and/or unusual risk factors. This section includes a list of important qualifying circumstances that significantly affect the character of the anesthesia service provided. These procedures would not be reported alone but would be reported as additional procedure numbers qualifying an anesthesia procedure or service.

+ 99100 Anesthesia for patient of extreme age, younger than 1 year and older than 70 (List separately in addition to code for primary anesthesia procedure)

(For procedure performed on infants younger than 1 year of age at time of surgery, see 00326, 00561, 00834, 00836)

+ 99116 Anesthesia complicated by utilization of total body hypothermia (List separately in addition to code for primary anesthesia procedure)

+ 99135 Anesthesia complicated by utilization of controlled hypotension (List separately in addition to code for primary anesthesia procedure)

+ 99140 Anesthesia complicated by emergency conditions (specify) (List separately in addition to code for primary anesthesia procedure)

(An emergency is defined as existing when delay in treatment of the patient would lead to a significant increase in the threat to life or body part)

Anesthesia 00100-01999

Anesthesia

Head

00100 Anesthesia for procedures on salivary glands, including biopsy
> *CPT Assistant* Feb 97:4, Nov 99:6, Feb 06:9, Mar 06:15, Nov 07:8, Oct 11:3, Jul 12:13, Aug 14:6, Dec 17:8, Oct 19:10, Jul 21:9
> *Clinical Examples in Radiology* Summer 11:2, Winter 13:5, Spring 13:5, Summer 13:5, Spring 14:7, Winter 16:4

00102 Anesthesia for procedures involving plastic repair of cleft lip
> *CPT Changes: An Insider's View* 2000
> *CPT Assistant* Nov 99:6

00103 Anesthesia for reconstructive procedures of eyelid (eg, blepharoplasty, ptosis surgery)
> *CPT Changes: An Insider's View* 2000
> *CPT Assistant* Nov 99:6

00104 Anesthesia for electroconvulsive therapy

00120 Anesthesia for procedures on external, middle, and inner ear including biopsy; not otherwise specified

00124 otoscopy
> *CPT Assistant* Nov 99:7

00126 tympanotomy

00140 Anesthesia for procedures on eye; not otherwise specified

00142 lens surgery

00144 corneal transplant

00145 vitreoretinal surgery
> *CPT Changes: An Insider's View* 2001

00147 iridectomy

00148 ophthalmoscopy

00160 Anesthesia for procedures on nose and accessory sinuses; not otherwise specified

00162 radical surgery

00164 biopsy, soft tissue

00170 Anesthesia for intraoral procedures, including biopsy; not otherwise specified

00172 repair of cleft palate

00174 excision of retropharyngeal tumor

00176 radical surgery

00190 Anesthesia for procedures on facial bones or skull; not otherwise specified
> *CPT Changes: An Insider's View* 2001

00192 radical surgery (including prognathism)

00210 Anesthesia for intracranial procedures; not otherwise specified

00211 craniotomy or craniectomy for evacuation of hematoma
> *CPT Changes: An Insider's View* 2009

00212 subdural taps

00214 burr holes, including ventriculography
> *CPT Changes: An Insider's View* 2000
> *CPT Assistant* Nov 99:7

00215 cranioplasty or elevation of depressed skull fracture, extradural (simple or compound)
> *CPT Changes: An Insider's View* 2001

00216 vascular procedures

00218 procedures in sitting position

00220 cerebrospinal fluid shunting procedures

00222 electrocoagulation of intracranial nerve
> *CPT Assistant* Jul 12:13

Neck

00300 Anesthesia for all procedures on the integumentary system, muscles and nerves of head, neck, and posterior trunk, not otherwise specified
> *CPT Assistant* Nov 99:7, Mar 06:15, Oct 11:3, Jul 12:13

00320 Anesthesia for all procedures on esophagus, thyroid, larynx, trachea and lymphatic system of neck; not otherwise specified, age 1 year or older
> *CPT Changes: An Insider's View* 2003

00322 needle biopsy of thyroid

(For procedures on cervical spine and cord, see 00600, 00604, 00670)

00326 Anesthesia for all procedures on the larynx and trachea in children younger than 1 year of age
> *CPT Changes: An Insider's View* 2003
> *CPT Assistant* Dec 17:8

(Do not report 00326 in conjunction with 99100)

00350 Anesthesia for procedures on major vessels of neck; not otherwise specified

00352 simple ligation
> *CPT Assistant* Nov 07:8, Jul 12:13

(For arteriography, use 01916)

Thorax (Chest Wall and Shoulder Girdle)

00400   Anesthesia for procedures on the integumentary system on the extremities, anterior trunk and perineum; not otherwise specified
➡ *CPT Assistant* Mar 06:15, Nov 07:8, Oct 11:3, Jul 12:13

00402   reconstructive procedures on breast (eg, reduction or augmentation mammoplasty, muscle flaps)

00404   radical or modified radical procedures on breast

00406   radical or modified radical procedures on breast with internal mammary node dissection

00410   electrical conversion of arrhythmias

00450   Anesthesia for procedures on clavicle and scapula; not otherwise specified

00454   biopsy of clavicle

00470   Anesthesia for partial rib resection; not otherwise specified

00472   thoracoplasty (any type)

00474   radical procedures (eg, pectus excavatum)
➡ *CPT Assistant* Nov 07:8, Jul 12:13

Intrathoracic

00500   Anesthesia for all procedures on esophagus
➡ *CPT Assistant* Mar 06:15, Nov 07:8, Oct 11:3, Jul 12:13

00520   Anesthesia for closed chest procedures; (including bronchoscopy) not otherwise specified
➡ *CPT Changes: An Insider's View* 2000
➡ *CPT Assistant* Nov 99:7

00522   needle biopsy of pleura

00524   pneumocentesis

00528   mediastinoscopy and diagnostic thoracoscopy not utilizing 1 lung ventilation
➡ *CPT Changes: An Insider's View* 2000, 2003, 2004
➡ *CPT Assistant* Nov 99:7

(For tracheobronchial reconstruction, use 00539)

00529   mediastinoscopy and diagnostic thoracoscopy utilizing 1 lung ventilation
➡ *CPT Changes: An Insider's View* 2004
➡ *CPT Assistant* Jun 04:3

00530   Anesthesia for permanent transvenous pacemaker insertion
➡ *CPT Changes: An Insider's View* 2001

00532   Anesthesia for access to central venous circulation

00534   Anesthesia for transvenous insertion or replacement of pacing cardioverter-defibrillator
➡ *CPT Changes: An Insider's View* 2001

(For transthoracic approach, use 00560)

00537   Anesthesia for cardiac electrophysiologic procedures including radiofrequency ablation
➡ *CPT Changes: An Insider's View* 2001

00539   Anesthesia for tracheobronchial reconstruction
➡ *CPT Changes: An Insider's View* 2003

00540   Anesthesia for thoracotomy procedures involving lungs, pleura, diaphragm, and mediastinum (including surgical thoracoscopy); not otherwise specified

00541   utilizing 1 lung ventilation
➡ *CPT Changes: An Insider's View* 2003

(For thoracic spine and cord anesthesia procedures via an anterior transthoracic approach, see 00625-00626)

00542   decortication

00546   pulmonary resection with thoracoplasty

00548   intrathoracic procedures on the trachea and bronchi
➡ *CPT Assistant* Nov 97:10

00550   Anesthesia for sternal debridement
➡ *CPT Changes: An Insider's View* 2001

00560   Anesthesia for procedures on heart, pericardial sac, and great vessels of chest; without pump oxygenator
➡ *CPT Changes: An Insider's View* 2002

00561   with pump oxygenator, younger than 1 year of age
➡ *CPT Changes: An Insider's View* 2005
➡ *CPT Assistant* Dec 17:8

(Do not report 00561 in conjunction with 99100, 99116, and 99135)

00562   with pump oxygenator, age 1 year or older, for all noncoronary bypass procedures (eg, valve procedures) or for re-operation for coronary bypass more than 1 month after original operation
➡ *CPT Changes: An Insider's View* 2009

00563   with pump oxygenator with hypothermic circulatory arrest
➡ *CPT Changes: An Insider's View* 2001

00566   Anesthesia for direct coronary artery bypass grafting; without pump oxygenator
➡ *CPT Changes: An Insider's View* 2001, 2009

00567   with pump oxygenator
➡ *CPT Changes: An Insider's View* 2009

00580   Anesthesia for heart transplant or heart/lung transplant
➡ *CPT Assistant* Nov 07:8, Jul 12:13

Spine and Spinal Cord

00600 Anesthesia for procedures on cervical spine and cord; not otherwise specified

➔ *CPT Assistant* Mar 06:15, May 07:9, Nov 07:8, Oct 11:3, Jul 12:13

(For percutaneous image-guided spine and spinal cord anesthesia procedures, see 01937, 01938, 01939, 01940, 01941, 01942)

00604 procedures with patient in the sitting position

➔ *CPT Changes: An Insider's View* 2001

00620 Anesthesia for procedures on thoracic spine and cord, not otherwise specified

➔ *CPT Assistant* Mar 07:9

00625 Anesthesia for procedures on the thoracic spine and cord, via an anterior transthoracic approach; not utilizing 1 lung ventilation

➔ *CPT Changes: An Insider's View* 2007

➔ *CPT Assistant* Mar 07:9

00626 utilizing 1 lung ventilation

➔ *CPT Changes: An Insider's View* 2007

➔ *CPT Assistant* Mar 07:9

(For anesthesia for thoracotomy procedures other than spinal, see 00540-00541)

00630 Anesthesia for procedures in lumbar region; not otherwise specified

00632 lumbar sympathectomy

00635 diagnostic or therapeutic lumbar puncture

➔ *CPT Changes: An Insider's View* 2001

00640 Anesthesia for manipulation of the spine or for closed procedures on the cervical, thoracic or lumbar spine

➔ *CPT Changes: An Insider's View* 2003

➔ *CPT Assistant* Jul 21:8

00670 Anesthesia for extensive spine and spinal cord procedures (eg, spinal instrumentation or vascular procedures)

➔ *CPT Changes: An Insider's View* 2001

➔ *CPT Assistant* Nov 07:8, Jul 12:13

Upper Abdomen

00700 Anesthesia for procedures on upper anterior abdominal wall; not otherwise specified

➔ *CPT Assistant* Mar 06:15, Nov 07:8, Oct 11:3, Jul 12:13, Jan 24:36

00702 percutaneous liver biopsy

00730 Anesthesia for procedures on upper posterior abdominal wall

➔ *CPT Assistant* Jan 24:36

00731 Anesthesia for upper gastrointestinal endoscopic procedures, endoscope introduced proximal to duodenum; not otherwise specified

➔ *CPT Changes: An Insider's View* 2018

➔ *CPT Assistant* Dec 17:8

00732 endoscopic retrograde cholangiopancreatography (ERCP)

➔ *CPT Changes: An Insider's View* 2018

➔ *CPT Assistant* Dec 17:8

(For combined upper and lower gastrointestinal endoscopic procedures, use 00813)

00750 Anesthesia for hernia repairs in upper abdomen; not otherwise specified

00752 lumbar and ventral (incisional) hernias and/or wound dehiscence

00754 omphalocele

00756 transabdominal repair of diaphragmatic hernia

00770 Anesthesia for all procedures on major abdominal blood vessels

00790 Anesthesia for intraperitoneal procedures in upper abdomen including laparoscopy; not otherwise specified

00792 partial hepatectomy or management of liver hemorrhage (excluding liver biopsy)

➔ *CPT Changes: An Insider's View* 2001

00794 pancreatectomy, partial or total (eg, Whipple procedure)

00796 liver transplant (recipient)

(For harvesting of liver, use 01990)

00797 gastric restrictive procedure for morbid obesity

➔ *CPT Changes: An Insider's View* 2002

➔ *CPT Assistant* Nov 07:8, Jul 12:13

Lower Abdomen

00800 Anesthesia for procedures on lower anterior abdominal wall; not otherwise specified

➔ *CPT Assistant* Mar 06:15, Nov 07:8, Oct 11:3, Jul 12:13

00802 panniculectomy

00811 Anesthesia for lower intestinal endoscopic procedures, endoscope introduced distal to duodenum; not otherwise specified

➔ *CPT Changes: An Insider's View* 2018

➔ *CPT Assistant* Dec 17:8

00812   screening colonoscopy

➡ *CPT Changes: An Insider's View* 2018

➡ *CPT Assistant* Dec 17:8

(Report 00812 to describe anesthesia for any screening colonoscopy regardless of ultimate findings)

00813   Anesthesia for combined upper and lower gastrointestinal endoscopic procedures, endoscope introduced both proximal to and distal to the duodenum

➡ *CPT Changes: An Insider's View* 2018

➡ *CPT Assistant* Dec 17:8

00820   Anesthesia for procedures on lower posterior abdominal wall

00830   Anesthesia for hernia repairs in lower abdomen; not otherwise specified

00832   ventral and incisional hernias

(For hernia repairs in the infant 1 year of age or younger, see 00834, 00836)

00834   Anesthesia for hernia repairs in the lower abdomen not otherwise specified, younger than 1 year of age

➡ *CPT Changes: An Insider's View* 2003

➡ *CPT Assistant* Dec 17:8

(Do not report 00834 in conjunction with 99100)

00836   Anesthesia for hernia repairs in the lower abdomen not otherwise specified, infants younger than 37 weeks gestational age at birth and younger than 50 weeks gestational age at time of surgery

➡ *CPT Changes: An Insider's View* 2003

➡ *CPT Assistant* Dec 17:8

(Do not report 00836 in conjunction with 99100)

00840   Anesthesia for intraperitoneal procedures in lower abdomen including laparoscopy; not otherwise specified

00842   amniocentesis

00844   abdominoperineal resection

00846   radical hysterectomy

00848   pelvic exenteration

00851   tubal ligation/transection

➡ *CPT Changes: An Insider's View* 2002

➡ *CPT Assistant* Oct 14:14

00860   Anesthesia for extraperitoneal procedures in lower abdomen, including urinary tract; not otherwise specified

00862   renal procedures, including upper one-third of ureter, or donor nephrectomy

00864   total cystectomy

00865   radical prostatectomy (suprapubic, retropubic)

00866   adrenalectomy

00868   renal transplant (recipient)

(For donor nephrectomy, use 00862)

(For harvesting kidney from brain-dead patient, use 01990)

00870   cystolithotomy

00872   Anesthesia for lithotripsy, extracorporeal shock wave; with water bath

00873   without water bath

00880   Anesthesia for procedures on major lower abdominal vessels; not otherwise specified

00882   inferior vena cava ligation

Perineum

(For perineal procedures on integumentary system, muscles and nerves, see 00300, 00400)

00902   Anesthesia for; anorectal procedure

➡ *CPT Changes: An Insider's View* 2001

➡ *CPT Assistant* Mar 06:15, Oct 11:3, Jul 12:13

00904   radical perineal procedure

00906   vulvectomy

00908   perineal prostatectomy

00910   Anesthesia for transurethral procedures (including urethrocystoscopy); not otherwise specified

00912   transurethral resection of bladder tumor(s)

00914   transurethral resection of prostate

00916   post-transurethral resection bleeding

00918   with fragmentation, manipulation and/or removal of ureteral calculus

➡ *CPT Changes: An Insider's View* 2000

➡ *CPT Assistant* Nov 99:8, Apr 09:8

00920   Anesthesia for procedures on male genitalia (including open urethral procedures); not otherwise specified

➡ *CPT Changes: An Insider's View* 2001

➡ *CPT Assistant* Sep 12:16

00921   vasectomy, unilateral or bilateral

➡ *CPT Changes: An Insider's View* 2003

00922   seminal vesicles

00924   undescended testis, unilateral or bilateral

00926   radical orchiectomy, inguinal

00928   radical orchiectomy, abdominal

00930   orchiopexy, unilateral or bilateral

00932   complete amputation of penis

00934   radical amputation of penis with bilateral inguinal lymphadenectomy

Anesthesia 00100-01999

Copying, photographing, or sharing this CPT® book violates AMA's copyright.

00936 radical amputation of penis with bilateral inguinal and iliac lymphadenectomy

00938 insertion of penile prosthesis (perineal approach)

00940 Anesthesia for vaginal procedures (including biopsy of labia, vagina, cervix or endometrium); not otherwise specified

00942 colpotomy, vaginectomy, colporrhaphy, and open urethral procedures
➔ *CPT Changes: An Insider's View* 2001, 2002

00944 vaginal hysterectomy

00948 cervical cerclage

00950 culdoscopy

00952 hysteroscopy and/or hysterosalpingography
➔ *CPT Changes: An Insider's View* 2000
➔ *CPT Assistant* Nov 99:8, Jul 12:13

Pelvis (Except Hip)

01112 Anesthesia for bone marrow aspiration and/or biopsy, anterior or posterior iliac crest
➔ *CPT Changes: An Insider's View* 2001
➔ *CPT Assistant* Mar 06:15, Oct 11:3, Jul 12:13

01120 Anesthesia for procedures on bony pelvis

01130 Anesthesia for body cast application or revision

01140 Anesthesia for interpelviabdominal (hindquarter) amputation

01150 Anesthesia for radical procedures for tumor of pelvis, except hindquarter amputation

01160 Anesthesia for closed procedures involving symphysis pubis or sacroiliac joint

01170 Anesthesia for open procedures involving symphysis pubis or sacroiliac joint

01173 Anesthesia for open repair of fracture disruption of pelvis or column fracture involving acetabulum
➔ *CPT Changes: An Insider's View* 2004
➔ *CPT Assistant* Jun 04:3-4

Upper Leg (Except Knee)

01200 Anesthesia for all closed procedures involving hip joint
➔ *CPT Assistant* Mar 06:15, Nov 07:8, Jul 12:13

01202 Anesthesia for arthroscopic procedures of hip joint

01210 Anesthesia for open procedures involving hip joint; not otherwise specified

01212 hip disarticulation

01214 total hip arthroplasty
➔ *CPT Changes: An Insider's View* 2001, 2002

01215 revision of total hip arthroplasty
➔ *CPT Changes: An Insider's View* 2001, 2002

01220 Anesthesia for all closed procedures involving upper two-thirds of femur

01230 Anesthesia for open procedures involving upper two-thirds of femur; not otherwise specified

01232 amputation

01234 radical resection

01250 Anesthesia for all procedures on nerves, muscles, tendons, fascia, and bursae of upper leg

01260 Anesthesia for all procedures involving veins of upper leg, including exploration

01270 Anesthesia for procedures involving arteries of upper leg, including bypass graft; not otherwise specified

01272 femoral artery ligation

01274 femoral artery embolectomy
➔ *CPT Assistant* Nov 07:8, Jul 12:13

Knee and Popliteal Area

01320 Anesthesia for all procedures on nerves, muscles, tendons, fascia, and bursae of knee and/or popliteal area
➔ *CPT Assistant* Mar 06:15, Nov 07:8, Oct 11:3, Jul 12:13

01340 Anesthesia for all closed procedures on lower one-third of femur

01360 Anesthesia for all open procedures on lower one-third of femur

01380 Anesthesia for all closed procedures on knee joint

01382 Anesthesia for diagnostic arthroscopic procedures of knee joint
➔ *CPT Changes: An Insider's View* 2003

01390 Anesthesia for all closed procedures on upper ends of tibia, fibula, and/or patella

01392 Anesthesia for all open procedures on upper ends of tibia, fibula, and/or patella

01400 Anesthesia for open or surgical arthroscopic procedures on knee joint; not otherwise specified
➔ *CPT Changes: An Insider's View* 2003

01402 total knee arthroplasty
➔ *CPT Changes: An Insider's View* 2002

01404 disarticulation at knee

01420 Anesthesia for all cast applications, removal, or repair involving knee joint

01430 Anesthesia for procedures on veins of knee and popliteal area; not otherwise specified

01432   arteriovenous fistula

01440   Anesthesia for procedures on arteries of knee and popliteal area; not otherwise specified

01442   popliteal thromboendarterectomy, with or without patch graft

01444   popliteal excision and graft or repair for occlusion or aneurysm
> *CPT Assistant* Nov 07:8, Jul 12:13

Lower Leg (Below Knee, Includes Ankle and Foot)

01462   Anesthesia for all closed procedures on lower leg, ankle, and foot
> *CPT Assistant* Mar 06:15, Nov 07:8, Oct 11:3, Jul 12:13

01464   Anesthesia for arthroscopic procedures of ankle and/or foot
> *CPT Changes: An Insider's View* 2003

01470   Anesthesia for procedures on nerves, muscles, tendons, and fascia of lower leg, ankle, and foot; not otherwise specified

01472   repair of ruptured Achilles tendon, with or without graft

01474   gastrocnemius recession (eg, Strayer procedure)

01480   Anesthesia for open procedures on bones of lower leg, ankle, and foot; not otherwise specified

01482   radical resection (including below knee amputation)
> *CPT Changes: An Insider's View* 2001

01484   osteotomy or osteoplasty of tibia and/or fibula

01486   total ankle replacement

01490   Anesthesia for lower leg cast application, removal, or repair

01500   Anesthesia for procedures on arteries of lower leg, including bypass graft; not otherwise specified

01502   embolectomy, direct or with catheter

01520   Anesthesia for procedures on veins of lower leg; not otherwise specified

01522   venous thrombectomy, direct or with catheter
> *CPT Assistant* Nov 07:8, Jul 12:13

Shoulder and Axilla

Includes humeral head and neck, sternoclavicular joint, acromioclavicular joint, and shoulder joint.

01610   Anesthesia for all procedures on nerves, muscles, tendons, fascia, and bursae of shoulder and axilla
> *CPT Assistant* Mar 06:15, Nov 07:8, Oct 11:3, Jul 12:13

01620   Anesthesia for all closed procedures on humeral head and neck, sternoclavicular joint, acromioclavicular joint, and shoulder joint

01622   Anesthesia for diagnostic arthroscopic procedures of shoulder joint
> *CPT Changes: An Insider's View* 2003

01630   Anesthesia for open or surgical arthroscopic procedures on humeral head and neck, sternoclavicular joint, acromioclavicular joint, and shoulder joint; not otherwise specified
> *CPT Changes: An Insider's View* 2003

01634   shoulder disarticulation

01636   interthoracoscapular (forequarter) amputation

01638   total shoulder replacement

01650   Anesthesia for procedures on arteries of shoulder and axilla; not otherwise specified

01652   axillary-brachial aneurysm

01654   bypass graft

01656   axillary-femoral bypass graft

01670   Anesthesia for all procedures on veins of shoulder and axilla

01680   Anesthesia for shoulder cast application, removal or repair, not otherwise specified

Upper Arm and Elbow

01710   Anesthesia for procedures on nerves, muscles, tendons, fascia, and bursae of upper arm and elbow; not otherwise specified
> *CPT Assistant* Mar 06:15, Nov 07:8, Oct 11:3, Jul 12:13

01712   tenotomy, elbow to shoulder, open

01714   tenoplasty, elbow to shoulder

01716   tenodesis, rupture of long tendon of biceps

01730   Anesthesia for all closed procedures on humerus and elbow

01732   Anesthesia for diagnostic arthroscopic procedures of elbow joint
> *CPT Changes: An Insider's View* 2003

01740   Anesthesia for open or surgical arthroscopic procedures of the elbow; not otherwise specified
> *CPT Changes: An Insider's View* 2003

01742   osteotomy of humerus

01744   repair of nonunion or malunion of humerus

01756   radical procedures

01758   excision of cyst or tumor of humerus

01760   total elbow replacement

01770   Anesthesia for procedures on arteries of upper arm and elbow; not otherwise specified

01772   embolectomy

01780   Anesthesia for procedures on veins of upper arm and elbow; not otherwise specified

01782   phleborrhaphy
➔ *CPT Assistant* Nov 07:8, Jul 12:13

Forearm, Wrist, and Hand

01810   Anesthesia for all procedures on nerves, muscles, tendons, fascia, and bursae of forearm, wrist, and hand
➔ *CPT Assistant* Mar 06:15, Nov 07:8, Oct 11:3, Jul 12:13

01820   Anesthesia for all closed procedures on radius, ulna, wrist, or hand bones

01829   Anesthesia for diagnostic arthroscopic procedures on the wrist
➔ *CPT Changes: An Insider's View* 2003

01830   Anesthesia for open or surgical arthroscopic/endoscopic procedures on distal radius, distal ulna, wrist, or hand joints; not otherwise specified
➔ *CPT Changes: An Insider's View* 2003

01832   total wrist replacement

01840   Anesthesia for procedures on arteries of forearm, wrist, and hand; not otherwise specified

01842   embolectomy

01844   Anesthesia for vascular shunt, or shunt revision, any type (eg, dialysis)

01850   Anesthesia for procedures on veins of forearm, wrist, and hand; not otherwise specified

01852   phleborrhaphy

01860   Anesthesia for forearm, wrist, or hand cast application, removal, or repair
➔ *CPT Assistant* Nov 07:8, Jul 12:13

Radiological Procedures

01916   Anesthesia for diagnostic arteriography/venography
➔ *CPT Changes: An Insider's View* 2002
➔ *CPT Assistant* Nov 07:8, Oct 11:3, Jul 12:13

(Do not report 01916 in conjunction with therapeutic codes 01924-01926, 01930-01933)

01920   Anesthesia for cardiac catheterization including coronary angiography and ventriculography (not to include Swan-Ganz catheter)

01922   Anesthesia for non-invasive imaging or radiation therapy

01924   Anesthesia for therapeutic interventional radiological procedures involving the arterial system; not otherwise specified
➔ *CPT Changes: An Insider's View* 2002

01925   carotid or coronary
➔ *CPT Changes: An Insider's View* 2002

01926   intracranial, intracardiac, or aortic
➔ *CPT Changes: An Insider's View* 2002

01930   Anesthesia for therapeutic interventional radiological procedures involving the venous/lymphatic system (not to include access to the central circulation); not otherwise specified
➔ *CPT Changes: An Insider's View* 2002

01931   intrahepatic or portal circulation (eg, transvenous intrahepatic portosystemic shunt[s] [TIPS])
➔ *CPT Changes: An Insider's View* 2002, 2008
➔ *CPT Assistant* Apr 08:3

01932   intrathoracic or jugular
➔ *CPT Changes: An Insider's View* 2002

01933   intracranial
➔ *CPT Changes: An Insider's View* 2002

01937   Anesthesia for percutaneous image-guided injection, drainage or aspiration procedures on the spine or spinal cord; cervical or thoracic
➔ *CPT Changes: An Insider's View* 2022
➔ *CPT Assistant* Nov 21:10, Jun 22:11-12

01938   lumbar or sacral
➔ *CPT Changes: An Insider's View* 2022
➔ *CPT Assistant* Nov 21:10, Jun 22:11-12

(For anesthesia for percutaneous image-guided destruction procedures on the spine or spinal cord, see 01939, 01940)

01939   Anesthesia for percutaneous image-guided destruction procedures by neurolytic agent on the spine or spinal cord; cervical or thoracic
➔ *CPT Changes: An Insider's View* 2022
➔ *CPT Assistant* Nov 21:10, Jun 22:11-12

01940   lumbar or sacral
➔ *CPT Changes: An Insider's View* 2022
➔ *CPT Assistant* Nov 21:10, Jun 22:11-12

(For anesthesia for percutaneous image-guided injection, drainage or aspiration procedures on the spine or spinal cord, see 01937, 01938)

01941 Anesthesia for percutaneous image-guided neuromodulation or intravertebral procedures (eg, kyphoplasty, vertebroplasty) on the spine or spinal cord; cervical or thoracic
➜ *CPT Changes: An Insider's View* 2022
➜ *CPT Assistant* Nov 21:10, Jun 22:11-12

01942 lumbar or sacral
➜ *CPT Changes: An Insider's View* 2022
➜ *CPT Assistant* Nov 21:10, Jun 22:11-12

Burn Excisions or Debridement

01951 Anesthesia for second- and third-degree burn excision or debridement with or without skin grafting, any site, for total body surface area (TBSA) treated during anesthesia and surgery; less than 4% total body surface area
➜ *CPT Changes: An Insider's View* 2001, 2002
➜ *CPT Assistant* Mar 06:15, Oct 11:3, Jul 12:13

01952 between 4% and 9% of total body surface area
➜ *CPT Changes: An Insider's View* 2001, 2002

+ 01953 each additional 9% total body surface area or part thereof (List separately in addition to code for primary procedure)
➜ *CPT Changes: An Insider's View* 2001
➜ *CPT Assistant* Jun 11:13, Jul 12:13

(Use 01953 in conjunction with 01952)

Obstetric

01958 Anesthesia for external cephalic version procedure
➜ *CPT Changes: An Insider's View* 2004
➜ *CPT Assistant* Jun 04:5-6, Oct 11:3, Jul 12:13

01960 Anesthesia for vaginal delivery only
➜ *CPT Changes: An Insider's View* 2002
➜ *CPT Assistant* Dec 01:3

01961 Anesthesia for cesarean delivery only
➜ *CPT Changes: An Insider's View* 2002, 2003

01962 Anesthesia for urgent hysterectomy following delivery
➜ *CPT Changes: An Insider's View* 2002, 2003

01963 Anesthesia for cesarean hysterectomy without any labor analgesia/anesthesia care
➜ *CPT Changes: An Insider's View* 2002, 2003

01965 Anesthesia for incomplete or missed abortion procedures
➜ *CPT Changes: An Insider's View* 2006

01966 Anesthesia for induced abortion procedures
➜ *CPT Changes: An Insider's View* 2006

01967 Neuraxial labor analgesia/anesthesia for planned vaginal delivery (this includes any repeat subarachnoid needle placement and drug injection and/or any necessary replacement of an epidural catheter during labor)
➜ *CPT Changes: An Insider's View* 2002
➜ *CPT Assistant* Dec 01:3, Oct 14:14

+ 01968 Anesthesia for cesarean delivery following neuraxial labor analgesia/anesthesia (List separately in addition to code for primary procedure performed)
➜ *CPT Changes: An Insider's View* 2002, 2003
➜ *CPT Assistant* Dec 01:3, Jun 11:13, Oct 14:14

(Use 01968 in conjunction with 01967)

+ 01969 Anesthesia for cesarean hysterectomy following neuraxial labor analgesia/anesthesia (List separately in addition to code for primary procedure performed)
➜ *CPT Changes: An Insider's View* 2002, 2003
➜ *CPT Assistant* Dec 01:3, Jun 11:13, Jul 12:13

(Use 01969 in conjunction with 01967)

Other Procedures

01990 Physiological support for harvesting of organ(s) from brain-dead patient
➜ *CPT Assistant* Mar 06:15, Nov 07:8, Oct 11:3, Jul 12:13

01991 Anesthesia for diagnostic or therapeutic nerve blocks and injections (when block or injection is performed by a different physician or other qualified health care professional); other than the prone position
➜ *CPT Changes: An Insider's View* 2003, 2013

01992 prone position
➜ *CPT Changes: An Insider's View* 2003, 2013

(Do not report 01991 or 01992 in conjunction with 99151, 99152, 99153, 99155, 99156, 99157)

(When regional intravenous administration of local anesthetic agent or other medication in the upper or lower extremity is used as the anesthetic for a surgical procedure, report the appropriate anesthesia code. To report a Bier block for pain management, use 64999)

(For intra-arterial or intravenous therapy for pain management, see 96373, 96374)

01996   Daily hospital management of epidural or subarachnoid continuous drug administration

➡ *CPT Changes: An Insider's View* 2003

➡ *CPT Assistant* Feb 97:5, Nov 97:10, May 99:6, Jul 12:5, Oct 12:14, May 15:10

(Report code 01996 for daily hospital management of continuous epidural or subarachnoid drug administration performed after insertion of an epidural or subarachnoid catheter)

01999   Unlisted anesthesia procedure(s)

➡ *CPT Assistant* Feb 97:4, Feb 06:9, Mar 06:15, Jan 07:30, Nov 07:8, Oct 11:3, Jul 12:13, Aug 14:6, 14, May 15:10, Dec 17:8, Oct 19:10, Jul 21:9

➡ *Clinical Examples in Radiology* Summer 11:2, Winter 13:5, Spring 13:5, Summer 13:5, Spring 14:7, Winter 16:4

Surgery Guidelines

Surgery Guidelines

Guidelines to direct general reporting of services are presented in the **Introduction.** Some of the commonalities are repeated here for the convenience of those referring to this section on **Surgery.** Other definitions and items unique to Surgery are also listed.

Services

▶Services rendered in the office, home, or hospital, consultations, and other medical services are listed in the **Evaluation and Management Services** section (98000-98016, 99202-99499) beginning on page 15. "Special Services, Procedures and Reports" (99000-99082) are listed in the **Medicine** section.◄

CPT Surgical Package Definition

By their very nature, the services to any patient are variable. The CPT codes that represent a readily identifiable surgical procedure thereby include, on a procedure-by-procedure basis, a variety of services. In defining the specific services "included" in a given CPT surgical code, the following services related to the surgery when furnished by the physician or other qualified health care professional who performs the surgery are included in addition to the operation per se:

- Evaluation and Management (E/M) service(s) subsequent to the decision for surgery on the day before and/or day of surgery (including history and physical)
- Local infiltration, metacarpal/metatarsal/digital block or topical anesthesia
- Immediate postoperative care, including dictating operative notes, talking with the family and other physicians or other qualified health care professionals
- Writing orders
- Evaluating the patient in the postanesthesia recovery area
- Typical postoperative follow-up care

Follow-Up Care for Diagnostic Procedures

Follow-up care for diagnostic procedures (eg, endoscopy, arthroscopy, injection procedures for radiography) includes only that care related to recovery from the diagnostic procedure itself. Care of the condition for which the diagnostic procedure was performed or of other concomitant conditions is not included and may be listed separately.

Follow-Up Care for Therapeutic Surgical Procedures

Follow-up care for therapeutic surgical procedures includes only that care which is usually a part of the surgical service. Complications, exacerbations, recurrence, or the presence of other diseases or injuries requiring additional services should be separately reported.

Supplied Materials

Supplies and materials (eg, sterile trays/drugs), over and above those usually included with the procedure(s) rendered are reported separately. List drugs, trays, supplies, and materials provided. Identify as 99070 or specific supply code.

Reporting More Than One Procedure/Service

When more than one procedure/service is performed on the same date, same session or during a post-operative period (subject to the "surgical package" concept), several CPT modifiers may apply (see Appendix A for definition).

Separate Procedure

Some of the procedures or services listed in the CPT codebook that are commonly carried out as an integral component of a total service or procedure have been identified by the inclusion of the term "separate procedure." The codes designated as "separate procedure" should not be reported in addition to the code for the total procedure or service of which it is considered an integral component.

However, when a procedure or service that is designated as a "separate procedure" is carried out independently or considered to be unrelated or distinct from other procedures/services provided at that time, it may be reported by itself, or in addition to other procedures/services by appending modifier 59 to the specific "separate procedure" code to indicate that the procedure is not considered to be a component of another procedure, but is a distinct, independent procedure. This may represent a different session, different procedure or surgery, different site or organ system, separate incision/excision, separate lesion, or separate injury (or area of injury in extensive injuries).

Unlisted Service or Procedure

A service or procedure may be provided that is not listed in this edition of the CPT codebook. When reporting such a service, the appropriate "Unlisted Procedure" code may be used to indicate the service, identifying it by "Special Report" as discussed in the section below. The "Unlisted Procedures" and accompanying codes for **Surgery** are as follows:

15999	Unlisted procedure, excision pressure ulcer
17999	Unlisted procedure, skin, mucous membrane and subcutaneous tissue
19499	Unlisted procedure, breast
20999	Unlisted procedure, musculoskeletal system, general
21089	Unlisted maxillofacial prosthetic procedure
21299	Unlisted craniofacial and maxillofacial procedure
21499	Unlisted musculoskeletal procedure, head
21899	Unlisted procedure, neck or thorax
22899	Unlisted procedure, spine
22999	Unlisted procedure, abdomen, musculoskeletal system
23929	Unlisted procedure, shoulder
24999	Unlisted procedure, humerus or elbow
25999	Unlisted procedure, forearm or wrist
26989	Unlisted procedure, hands or fingers
27299	Unlisted procedure, pelvis or hip joint
27599	Unlisted procedure, femur or knee
27899	Unlisted procedure, leg or ankle
28899	Unlisted procedure, foot or toes
29799	Unlisted procedure, casting or strapping
29999	Unlisted procedure, arthroscopy
30999	Unlisted procedure, nose
31299	Unlisted procedure, accessory sinuses
31599	Unlisted procedure, larynx
31899	Unlisted procedure, trachea, bronchi

32999	Unlisted procedure, lungs and pleura
33999	Unlisted procedure, cardiac surgery
36299	Unlisted procedure, vascular injection
37501	Unlisted vascular endoscopy procedure
37799	Unlisted procedure, vascular surgery
38129	Unlisted laparoscopy procedure, spleen
38589	Unlisted laparoscopy procedure, lymphatic system
38999	Unlisted procedure, hemic or lymphatic system
39499	Unlisted procedure, mediastinum
39599	Unlisted procedure, diaphragm
40799	Unlisted procedure, lips
40899	Unlisted procedure, vestibule of mouth
41599	Unlisted procedure, tongue, floor of mouth
41899	Unlisted procedure, dentoalveolar structures
42299	Unlisted procedure, palate, uvula
42699	Unlisted procedure, salivary glands or ducts
42999	Unlisted procedure, pharynx, adenoids, or tonsils
43289	Unlisted laparoscopy procedure, esophagus
43499	Unlisted procedure, esophagus
43659	Unlisted laparoscopy procedure, stomach
43999	Unlisted procedure, stomach
44238	Unlisted laparoscopy procedure, intestine (except rectum)
44799	Unlisted procedure, small intestine
44899	Unlisted procedure, Meckel's diverticulum and the mesentery
44979	Unlisted laparoscopy procedure, appendix
45399	Unlisted procedure, colon
45499	Unlisted laparoscopy procedure, rectum
45999	Unlisted procedure, rectum
46999	Unlisted procedure, anus
47379	Unlisted laparoscopic procedure, liver
47399	Unlisted procedure, liver
47579	Unlisted laparoscopy procedure, biliary tract
47999	Unlisted procedure, biliary tract
48999	Unlisted procedure, pancreas
49329	Unlisted laparoscopy procedure, abdomen, peritoneum and omentum
49659	Unlisted laparoscopy procedure, hernioplasty, herniorrhaphy, herniotomy
49999	Unlisted procedure, abdomen, peritoneum and omentum
50549	Unlisted laparoscopy procedure, renal
50949	Unlisted laparoscopy procedure, ureter

51999	Unlisted laparoscopy procedure, bladder
53899	Unlisted procedure, urinary system
54699	Unlisted laparoscopy procedure, testis
55559	Unlisted laparoscopy procedure, spermatic cord
55899	Unlisted procedure, male genital system
58578	Unlisted laparoscopy procedure, uterus
58579	Unlisted hysteroscopy procedure, uterus
58679	Unlisted laparoscopy procedure, oviduct, ovary
58999	Unlisted procedure, female genital system (nonobstetrical)
59897	Unlisted fetal invasive procedure, including ultrasound guidance, when performed
59898	Unlisted laparoscopy procedure, maternity care and delivery
59899	Unlisted procedure, maternity care and delivery
60659	Unlisted laparoscopy procedure, endocrine system
60699	Unlisted procedure, endocrine system
64999	Unlisted procedure, nervous system
66999	Unlisted procedure, anterior segment of eye
67299	Unlisted procedure, posterior segment
67399	Unlisted procedure, extraocular muscle
67599	Unlisted procedure, orbit
67999	Unlisted procedure, eyelids
68399	Unlisted procedure, conjunctiva
68899	Unlisted procedure, lacrimal system
69399	Unlisted procedure, external ear
69799	Unlisted procedure, middle ear
69949	Unlisted procedure, inner ear
69979	Unlisted procedure, temporal bone, middle fossa approach

Special Report

A service that is rarely provided, unusual, variable, or new may require a special report. Pertinent information should include an adequate definition or description of the nature, extent, and need for the procedure, and the time, effort, and equipment necessary to provide the service.

Imaging Guidance

When imaging guidance or imaging supervision and interpretation is included in a surgical procedure, guidelines for image documentation and report, included in the guidelines for Radiology (Including Nuclear Medicine and Diagnostic Ultrasound), will apply. Imaging guidance should not be reported for use of a nonimaging-guided tracking or localizing system (eg, radar signals, electromagnetic signals). Imaging guidance should only be reported when an imaging modality (eg, radiography, fluoroscopy, ultrasonography, magnetic resonance imaging, computed tomography, or nuclear medicine) is used and is appropriately documented.

Surgical Destruction

Surgical destruction is a part of a surgical procedure and different methods of destruction are not ordinarily listed separately unless the technique substantially alters the standard management of a problem or condition. Exceptions under special circumstances are provided for by separate code numbers.

Foreign Body/Implant Definition

An object intentionally placed by a physician or other qualified health care professional for any purpose (eg, diagnostic or therapeutic) is considered an implant. An object that is unintentionally placed (eg, trauma or ingestion) is considered a foreign body. If an implant (or part thereof) has moved from its original position or is structurally broken and no longer serves its intended purpose or presents a hazard to the patient, it qualifies as a foreign body for coding purposes, unless CPT coding instructions direct otherwise or a specific CPT code exists to describe the removal of that broken/moved implant.

★ =Telemedicine   ◀ =Audio-only   ✚ =Add-on code   ⊁ =FDA approval pending   # =Resequenced code   ⊘ =Modifier 51 exempt   ➲➲➲ =See p xxi for details

Surgery

The following is a listing of headings and subheadings that appear within the Integumentary System section of the CPT codebook. The subheadings or subsections denoted with asterisks (*) below have special instructions unique to that subsection. Where these are indicated, special notes or guidelines will be presented preceding those procedural terminology listings, referring to that subsection specifically. Note that all code ranges in each subsection are listed as they appear in the subsection, even if the code numbers are out of numerical sequence and/or repeated in the next subsection.

Structure of Skin

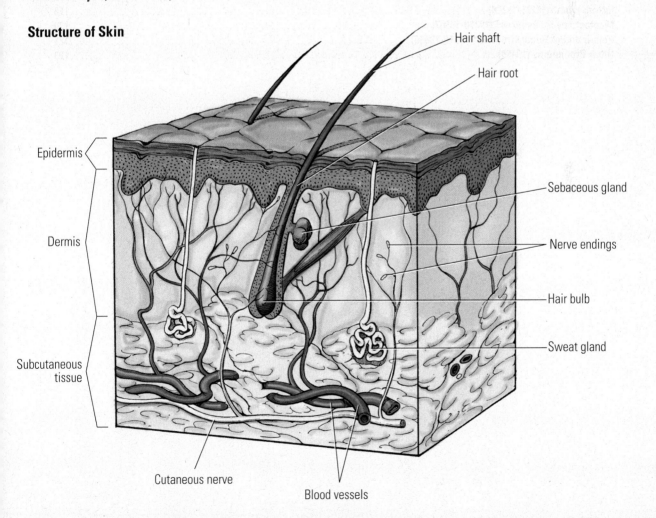

Epidermis

Dermis

Subcutaneous tissue

Hair shaft

Hair root

Sebaceous gland

Nerve endings

Hair bulb

Sweat gland

Cutaneous nerve

Blood vessels

Surgery

General

Fine Needle Aspiration (FNA) Biopsy

A **fine needle aspiration** (FNA) biopsy is performed when material is aspirated with a fine needle and the cells are examined cytologically. A **core needle biopsy** is typically performed with a larger bore needle to obtain a core sample of tissue for histopathologic evaluation. FNA biopsy procedures are performed with or without imaging guidance. Imaging guidance codes (eg, 76942, 77002, 77012, 77021) may not be reported separately with 10004, 10005, 10006, 10007, 10008, 10009, 10010, 10011, 10012, 10021. Codes 10004, 10005, 10006, 10007, 10008, 10009, 10010, 10011, 10012, 10021 are reported once per lesion sampled in a single session. When more than one FNA biopsy is performed on separate lesions at the same session, same day, same imaging modality, use the appropriate imaging modality add-on code for the second and subsequent lesion(s). When more than one FNA biopsy is performed on separate lesions, same session, same day, using different imaging modalities, report the corresponding primary code with modifier 59 for each additional imaging modality and corresponding add-on codes for subsequent lesions sampled. This instruction applies regardless of whether the lesions are ipsilateral or contralateral to each other, and/or whether they are in the same or different organs/structures. When FNA biopsy and core needle biopsy both are performed on the same lesion, same session, same day using the same type of imaging guidance, do not separately report the imaging guidance for the core needle biopsy. When FNA biopsy is performed on one lesion and core needle biopsy is performed on a separate lesion, same session, same day using the same type of imaging guidance, both the core needle biopsy and the imaging guidance for the core needle biopsy may be reported separately with modifier 59. When FNA biopsy is performed on one lesion and core needle biopsy is performed on a separate lesion, same session, same day using different types of imaging guidance, both the core needle biopsy and the imaging guidance for the core needle biopsy may be reported with modifier 59.

10004 Code is out of numerical sequence. See 10021-10035

10005 Code is out of numerical sequence. See 10021-10035

10006 Code is out of numerical sequence. See 10021-10035

10007 Code is out of numerical sequence. See 10021-10035

10008 Code is out of numerical sequence. See 10021-10035

10009 Code is out of numerical sequence. See 10021-10035

10010 Code is out of numerical sequence. See 10021-10035

10011 Code is out of numerical sequence. See 10021-10035

10012 Code is out of numerical sequence. See 10021-10035

10021 Fine needle aspiration biopsy, without imaging guidance; first lesion
➔ *CPT Changes: An Insider's View* 2002, 2019
➔ *CPT Assistant* Aug 02:10, Mar 05:11, Apr 19:4, May 19:10
➔ *Clinical Examples in Radiology* Fall 08:4, Fall 10:3, 8, Spring 14:3, Winter 17:4

#+ 10004 each additional lesion (List separately in addition to code for primary procedure)
➔ *CPT Changes: An Insider's View* 2019
➔ *CPT Assistant* Feb 19:8, Apr 19:4, Feb 22:13
➔ *Clinical Examples in Radiology* Winter 19:2

(Use 10004 in conjunction with 10021)

(Do not report 10004, 10021 in conjunction with 10005, 10006, 10007, 10008, 10009, 10010, 10011, 10012 for the same lesion)

(For evaluation of fine needle aspirate, see 88172, 88173, 88177)

 # 10005 Fine needle aspiration biopsy, including ultrasound guidance; first lesion
➔ *CPT Changes: An Insider's View* 2019
➔ *CPT Assistant* Feb 19:8, Apr 19:4, May 19:10, Mar 23:1
➔ *Clinical Examples in Radiology* Winter 19:2, Summer 19:10

#+ 10006 each additional lesion (List separately in addition to code for primary procedure)
➔ *CPT Changes: An Insider's View* 2019
➔ *CPT Assistant* Feb 19:8, Apr 19:4
➔ *Clinical Examples in Radiology* Winter 19:2

(Use 10006 in conjunction with 10005)

(Do not report 10005, 10006 in conjunction with 76942)

(For evaluation of fine needle aspirate, see 88172, 88173, 88177)

 # 10007 Fine needle aspiration biopsy, including fluoroscopic guidance; first lesion
➔ *CPT Changes: An Insider's View* 2019
➔ *CPT Assistant* Feb 19:8, Apr 19:4
➔ *Clinical Examples in Radiology* Spring 22:10

#+ 10008   each additional lesion (List separately in addition to code for primary procedure)

➜ *CPT Changes: An Insider's View* 2019

➜ *CPT Assistant* Feb 19:8, Apr 19:4

➜ *Clinical Examples in Radiology* Winter 19:2

(Use 10008 in conjunction with 10007)

(Do not report 10007, 10008 in conjunction with 77002)

(For evaluation of fine needle aspirate, see 88172, 88173, 88177)

 # 10009   Fine needle aspiration biopsy, including CT guidance; first lesion

➜ *CPT Changes: An Insider's View* 2019

➜ *CPT Assistant* Feb 19:8, Apr 19:4

➜ *Clinical Examples in Radiology* Spring 22:10

#+ 10010   each additional lesion (List separately in addition to code for primary procedure)

➜ *CPT Changes: An Insider's View* 2019

➜ *CPT Assistant* Feb 19:8, Apr 19:4

➜ *Clinical Examples in Radiology* Winter 19:2

(Use 10010 in conjunction with 10009)

(Do not report 10009, 10010 in conjunction with 77012)

(For evaluation of fine needle aspirate, see 88172, 88173, 88177)

 # 10011   Fine needle aspiration biopsy, including MR guidance; first lesion

➜ *CPT Changes: An Insider's View* 2019

➜ *CPT Assistant* Feb 19:8, Apr 19:4

➜ *Clinical Examples in Radiology* Winter 19:2

#+ 10012   each additional lesion (List separately in addition to code for primary procedure)

➜ *CPT Changes: An Insider's View* 2019

➜ *CPT Assistant* Feb 19:8, Apr 19:4

➜ *Clinical Examples in Radiology* Winter 19:2

(Use 10012 in conjunction with 10011)

(Do not report 10011, 10012 in conjunction with 77021)

(For evaluation of fine needle aspirate, see 88172, 88173, 88177)

(For percutaneous needle biopsy other than fine needle aspiration, see 19081-19086 for breast, 20206 for muscle, 32400 for pleura, 32408 for lung or mediastinum, 42400 for salivary gland, 47000 for liver, 48102 for pancreas, 49180 for abdominal or retroperitoneal mass, 50200 for kidney, 54500 for testis, 54800 for epididymis, 60100 for thyroid, 62267 for nucleus pulposus, intervertebral disc, or paravertebral tissue, 62269 for spinal cord)

(For percutaneous image-guided fluid collection drainage by catheter of soft tissue [eg, extremity, abdominal wall, neck], use 10030)

Integumentary System

Skin, Subcutaneous, and Accessory Structures

Introduction and Removal

10030   Image-guided fluid collection drainage by catheter (eg, abscess, hematoma, seroma, lymphocele, cyst), soft tissue (eg, extremity, abdominal wall, neck), percutaneous

➜ *CPT Changes: An Insider's View* 2014, 2017

➜ *CPT Assistant* May 14:3, 9, Aug 17:9, Mar 24:26

➜ *Clinical Examples in Radiology* Fall 13:6, Summer 14:9, Spring 15:8, Winter 16:10, Fall 18:15

(Report 10030 for each individual collection drained with a separate catheter)

(Do not report 10030 in conjunction with 75989, 76942, 77002, 77003, 77012, 77021)

(For image-guided fluid collection drainage, percutaneous or transvaginal/transrectal of visceral, peritoneal, or retroperitoneal collections, see 49405-49407)

Soft tissue-marker placement with imaging guidance is reported with 10035 and 10036. If a more specific site descriptor than soft tissue is applicable (eg, breast), use the site-specific codes for marker placement at that site. Report 10035 and 10036 only once per target, regardless of how many markers (eg, clips, wires, pellets, radioactive seeds) are used to mark that target.

10035   Placement of soft tissue localization device(s) (eg, clip, metallic pellet, wire/needle, radioactive seeds), percutaneous, including imaging guidance; first lesion

➜ *CPT Changes: An Insider's View* 2016

➜ *CPT Assistant* Jun 16:3

➜ *Clinical Examples in Radiology* Winter 16:4, Summer 19:10, Winter 23:16

+ 10036   each additional lesion (List separately in addition to code for primary procedure)

➜ *CPT Changes: An Insider's View* 2016

➜ *CPT Assistant* Jun 16:3

➜ *Clinical Examples in Radiology* Winter 16:5, Summer 19:10, Winter 23:16

(Use 10036 in conjunction with 10035)

(Do not report 10035, 10036 in conjunction with 76942, 77002, 77012, 77021)

(To report a second procedure on the same side or contralateral side, use 10036)

Incision and Drainage

(For excision, see 11400, et seq)

10040   Acne surgery (eg, marsupialization, opening or removal of multiple milia, comedones, cysts, pustules)
➔ *CPT Assistant* Fall 92:10, Feb 08:8

10060   Incision and drainage of abscess (eg, carbuncle, suppurative hidradenitis, cutaneous or subcutaneous abscess, cyst, furuncle, or paronychia); simple or single
➔ *CPT Assistant* Sep 12:10, Oct 21:13, Apr 23:25, Jan 24:37

10061   complicated or multiple
➔ *CPT Assistant* Sep 12:10, Oct 21:13, Apr 23:25

10080   Incision and drainage of pilonidal cyst; simple
➔ *CPT Assistant* Fall 92:13, Dec 06:15, May 07:5

10081   complicated
➔ *CPT Assistant* Fall 92:13, Dec 06:15, May 07:5

(For excision of pilonidal cyst, see 11770-11772)

10120   Incision and removal of foreign body, subcutaneous tissues; simple
➔ *CPT Assistant* Sep 12:10, Apr 13:10, Dec 13:16

10121   complicated
➔ *CPT Assistant* Spring 91:7, Dec 06:15, Sep 12:10, Dec 13:16, Apr 21:6

(To report wound exploration due to penetrating trauma without laparotomy or thoracotomy, see 20100-20103, as appropriate)

(To report debridement associated with open fracture(s) and/or dislocation(s), use 11010-11012, as appropriate)

10140   Incision and drainage of hematoma, seroma or fluid collection
➔ *CPT Changes: An Insider's View* 2002
➔ *CPT Assistant* Nov 14:5

10160   Puncture aspiration of abscess, hematoma, bulla, or cyst
➔ *CPT Changes: An Insider's View* 2002
➔ *CPT Assistant* Aug 17:9, Aug 21:14, Mar 24:26
➔ *Clinical Examples in Radiology* Fall 09:8, Summer 14:9, Spring 15:8, Winter 16:10

(If imaging guidance is performed, see 76942, 77002, 77012, 77021)

10180   Incision and drainage, complex, postoperative wound infection
➔ *CPT Assistant* Nov 14:5

(For secondary closure of surgical wound, see 12020, 12021, 13160)

Debridement

Wound debridements (11042-11047) are reported by depth of tissue that is removed and by surface area of the wound. These services may be reported for injuries, infections, wounds and chronic ulcers. When performing debridement of a single wound, report depth using the deepest level of tissue removed. In multiple wounds, sum the surface area of those wounds that are at the same depth, but do not combine sums from different depths. For example: When bone is debrided from a 4 sq cm heel ulcer and from a 10 sq cm ischial ulcer, report the work with a single code, 11044. When subcutaneous tissue is debrided from a 16 sq cm dehisced abdominal wound and a 10 sq cm thigh wound, report the work with 11042 for the first 20 sq cm and 11045 for the second 6 sq cm. If all four wounds were debrided on the same day, use modifier 59 with either 11042, or 11044 as appropriate.

(For dermabrasions, see 15780-15783)

(For nail debridement, see 11720-11721)

(For burn(s), see 16000-16035)

(For pressure ulcers, see 15920-15999)

—— *Coding Tip* ——

Use of Depth and Surface Area For Reporting Debridement of Wounds

When performing debridement of a single wound, report depth using the deepest level of tissue removed. In multiple wounds, sum the surface area of those wounds that are at the same depth, but do not combine sums from different depths.

CPT Coding Guidelines, Debridement

11000   Debridement of extensive eczematous or infected skin; up to 10% of body surface
➔ *CPT Assistant* May 99:10, Oct 12:3, Feb 18:10

(For abdominal wall or genitalia debridement for necrotizing soft tissue infection, see 11004-11006)

+ 11001   each additional 10% of the body surface, or part thereof (List separately in addition to code for primary procedure)
➔ *CPT Changes: An Insider's View* 2009
➔ *CPT Assistant* May 99:10, Oct 12:3, Feb 18:10

(Use 11001 in conjunction with 11000)

11004   Debridement of skin, subcutaneous tissue, muscle and fascia for necrotizing soft tissue infection; external genitalia and perineum
➔ *CPT Changes: An Insider's View* 2005
➔ *CPT Assistant* Jan 12:6, Oct 12:3, Oct 13:15, Feb 18:10, Nov 19:14, Jun 23:25

11005   abdominal wall, with or without fascial closure
➔ *CPT Changes: An Insider's View* 2005
➔ *CPT Assistant* Jan 12:6, Oct 12:3, Oct 13:15, Feb 18:10, Nov 19:14

Debridement of Abdominal Wall
11005

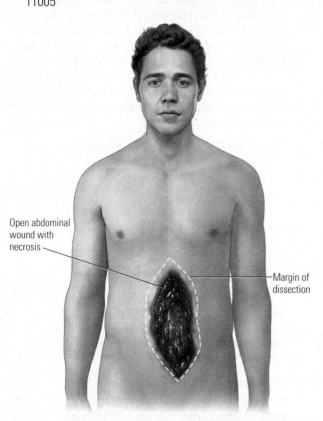

Open abdominal wound with necrosis

Margin of dissection

11006 external genitalia, perineum and abdominal wall, with or without fascial closure

➔ *CPT Changes: An Insider's View* 2005

➔ *CPT Assistant* Jan 12:6, Oct 12:3, Oct 13:15, Nov 19:14

(If orchiectomy is performed, use 54520)

(If testicular transplantation is performed, use 54680)

+ 11008 Removal of prosthetic material or mesh, abdominal wall for infection (eg, for chronic or recurrent mesh infection or necrotizing soft tissue infection) (List separately in addition to code for primary procedure)

➔ *CPT Changes: An Insider's View* 2005, 2008

➔ *CPT Assistant* Jan 12:6, Oct 12:3

(Use 11008 in conjunction with 10180, 11004-11006)

(Report skin grafts or flaps separately when performed for closure at the same session as 11004-11008)

(For implantation of absorbable mesh or other prosthesis for delayed closure of external genitalia, perineum, and/or abdominal wall defect[s] due to soft tissue infection or trauma, use 15778)

11010 Debridement including removal of foreign material at the site of an open fracture and/or an open dislocation (eg, excisional debridement); skin and subcutaneous tissues

➔ *CPT Changes: An Insider's View* 2011

➔ *CPT Assistant* Mar 97:2, Apr 97:10, Aug 97:6, Oct 03:10, May 11:3, Oct 12:13

11011 skin, subcutaneous tissue, muscle fascia, and muscle

➔ *CPT Changes: An Insider's View* 2011

➔ *CPT Assistant* Mar 97:2, Apr 97:10, Aug 97:6, May 11:3, Oct 12:13

11012 skin, subcutaneous tissue, muscle fascia, muscle, and bone

➔ *CPT Changes: An Insider's View* 2011

➔ *CPT Assistant* Mar 97:2, Apr 97:10, Aug 97:6, Oct 03:10, May 11:3, Oct 12:13

(For debridement of skin [ie, epidermis and/or dermis only], see 97597, 97598)

(For active wound care management, see 97597, 97598)

(For debridement of burn wounds, see 16020-16030)

11042 Debridement, subcutaneous tissue (includes epidermis and dermis, if performed); first 20 sq cm or less

➔ *CPT Changes: An Insider's View* 2011

➔ *CPT Assistant* Winter 92:10, May 96:6, Feb 97:7, Aug 97:6, Jun 05:1, 10, Oct 07:15, Nov 10:9, May 11:3, Sep 11:11, Jan 12:6, Mar 12:3, Oct 12:13, Feb 13:16, Sep 13:17, Oct 13:15, Nov 14:5, Feb 16:14, Aug 16:9, Oct 16:3, Aug 22:16

(For debridement of skin [ie, epidermis and/or dermis only], see 97597, 97598)

#+ 11045 each additional 20 sq cm, or part thereof (List separately in addition to code for primary procedure)

➔ *CPT Changes: An Insider's View* 2011

➔ *CPT Assistant* May 11:3, Sep 11:11, Jan 12:6, Mar 12:3, Oct 12:13, Nov 14:5, Aug 16:9, Oct 16:3

(Use 11045 in conjunction with 11042)

11043 Debridement, muscle and/or fascia (includes epidermis, dermis, and subcutaneous tissue, if performed); first 20 sq cm or less

➔ *CPT Changes: An Insider's View* 2011

➔ *CPT Assistant* May 96:6, Feb 97:7, Apr 97:11, Aug 97:6, Dec 99:10, Jun 05:1, 10, Oct 07:15, Nov 10:9, May 11:3, Sep 11:11, Jan 12:6, Mar 12:3, Oct 12:13, Feb 13:16, Nov 14:5, Aug 16:9, Oct 16:3, Mar 20:14

#+ 11046 each additional 20 sq cm, or part thereof (List separately in addition to code for primary procedure)

➔ *CPT Changes: An Insider's View* 2011

➔ *CPT Assistant* May 11:3, Sep 11:11, Jan 12:6, Mar 12:3, Oct 12:13, Feb 13:16, Nov 14:5, Aug 16:9, Oct 16:3

(Use 11046 in conjunction with 11043)

11044   Debridement, bone (includes epidermis, dermis,
              subcutaneous tissue, muscle and/or fascia, if performed);
              first 20 sq cm or less
              ➲ *CPT Changes: An Insider's View* 2011
              ➲ *CPT Assistant* Fall 93:21, Mar 96:10, May 96:6, Feb 97:7,
                 Apr 97:11, Aug 97:6, Jun 05:1, 10, Oct 07:15, Nov 10:9,
                 May 11:3, Sep 11:11, Jan 12:6, Mar 12:3, Oct 12:13, Feb 13:16,
                 Nov 14:5, Aug 16:9, Oct 16:3

11045   Code is out of numerical sequence. See 11012-11047

11046   Code is out of numerical sequence. See 11012-11047

+ 11047   each additional 20 sq cm, or part thereof (List
              separately in addition to code for primary procedure)
              ➲ *CPT Changes: An Insider's View* 2011
              ➲ *CPT Assistant* May 11:3, Sep 11:11, Jan 12:6, Mar 12:3,
                 Oct 12:13, Nov 14:5, Aug 16:9, Oct 16:3, Aug 22:16

              (Do not report 11042-11047 in conjunction with 97597-
              97602 for the same wound)

              (Use 11047 in conjunction with 11044)

Paring or Cutting

              (To report destruction of benign lesions other than skin
              tags or cutaneous vascular proliferative lesions, see
              17110, 17111)

11055   Paring or cutting of benign hyperkeratotic lesion (eg, corn
              or callus); single lesion
              ➲ *CPT Assistant* Nov 97:11, Jan 99:11

11056   2 to 4 lesions
              ➲ *CPT Assistant* Nov 97:11, Jan 99:11, Sep 10:9

11057   more than 4 lesions
              ➲ *CPT Assistant* Nov 97:11, Jan 99:11, May 99:10

Biopsy

The use of a biopsy procedure code (eg, 11102, 11103, 11104, 11105, 11106, 11107) indicates that the procedure to obtain tissue solely for diagnostic histopathologic examination was performed independently, or was unrelated or distinct from other procedures/services provided at that time. Biopsies performed on different lesions or different sites on the same date of service may be reported separately, as they are not considered components of other procedures.

During certain surgical procedures in the integumentary system, such as excision, destruction, or shave removals, the removed tissue is often submitted for pathologic examination. The obtaining of tissue for pathology during the course of these procedures is a routine component of such procedures. This obtaining of tissue is not considered a separate biopsy procedure and is not separately reported.

Partial-thickness biopsies are those that sample a portion of the thickness of skin or mucous membrane and do not penetrate below the dermis or lamina propria. Full-thickness biopsies penetrate into tissue deep to the dermis or lamina propria, into the subcutaneous or submucosal space.

Sampling of stratum corneum only, by any modality (eg, skin scraping, tape stripping) does not constitute a skin biopsy procedure and is not separately reportable.

An appropriate biopsy technique is selected based on optimal tissue-sampling considerations for the type of neoplastic, inflammatory, or other lesion requiring a tissue diagnosis. Biopsy of the skin is reported under three distinct techniques:

Tangential biopsy **(eg, shave, scoop, saucerize, curette)** is performed with a sharp blade, such as a flexible biopsy blade, obliquely oriented scalpel or curette to remove a sample of epidermal tissue with or without portions of underlying dermis. The intent of a tangential biopsy (11102, 11103) is to obtain a tissue sample from a lesion for the purpose of diagnostic pathologic examination. Biopsy of lesions by tangential technique (11102, 11103) is not considered an excision. Tangential biopsy technique may be represented by a superficial sample and does not involve the full thickness of the dermis, which could result in portions of the lesion remaining in the deeper layers of the dermis.

For therapeutic removal of epidermal or dermal lesion(s) using shave technique, see 11300-11313.

An indication for a shave removal (11300-11313) procedure may include a symptomatic lesion that rubs on waistband or bra, or any other reason why an elevated lesion is being completely removed with the shave technique, suggesting a therapeutic intent. It is the responsibility of the physician or qualified health care professional performing the procedure to clearly indicate the purpose of the procedure.

Punch biopsy requires a punch tool to remove a full-thickness cylindrical sample of skin. The intent of a punch biopsy (11104, 11105) is to obtain a cylindrical tissue sample of a cutaneous lesion for the purpose of diagnostic pathologic examination. Simple closure of the defect is included in the service. Manipulation of the biopsy defect to improve wound approximation is included in simple closure.

Incisional biopsy requires the use of a sharp blade (not a punch tool) to remove a full-thickness sample of tissue via a vertical incision or wedge, penetrating deep to the dermis, into the subcutaneous space. The intent of an incisional biopsy (11106, 11107) is to obtain a full-thickness tissue sample of a skin lesion for the purpose of diagnostic pathologic examination. This type of biopsy may sample subcutaneous fat, such as those performed for the evaluation of panniculitis. Although closure is usually performed on incisional biopsies, simple closure is not separately reported.

(For complete lesion excision with margins, see 11400-11646)

When multiple biopsy techniques are performed during the same encounter, only one primary lesion biopsy code (11102, 11104, 11106) is reported. Additional biopsy codes should be selected based on the following convention:

If multiple biopsies of the same type are performed, the primary code for that biopsy should be used along with the corresponding add-on code(s).

If an incisional biopsy is performed, report 11106 in combination with a tangential (11103), punch (11105), or incisional biopsy (11107) for the additional biopsy procedures.

If a punch biopsy is performed, report 11104 in combination with a tangential (11103), or punch (11105), for the additional biopsy procedures.

If multiple tangential biopsies are performed, report tangential biopsy (11102) in combination with 11103 for the additional tangential biopsy procedures.

When two or more biopsies of the same technique (ie, tangential, punch, or incisional) are performed on separate/additional lesions, use the appropriate add-on code (11103, 11105, 11107) to specify each additional biopsy. When two or three different biopsy techniques (ie, tangential, punch, or incisional) are performed to sample separate/additional lesions, select the appropriate biopsy code (11102, 11104, 11106) plus an additional add-on code (11103, 11105, 11107) for each additional biopsy performed.

The following table provides an illustration of the appropriate use of these codes for multiple biopsies:

Procedures Performed	CPT Code(s) Reported
2 tangential biopsies	11102 X 1, 11103 X 1
3 punch biopsies	11104 X 1, 11105 X 2
2 incisional biopsies	11106 X 1, 11107 X 1
1 incisional biopsy, 1 tangential biopsy and 1 punch biopsy	11106 X 1, 11103 X 1, 11105 X 1
1 punch biopsy and 2 tangential biopsies	11104 X 1, 11103 X 2

(For biopsy of nail unit, use 11755)

(For biopsy, intranasal, use 30100)

(For biopsy of lip, use 40490)

(For biopsy of vestibule of mouth, use 40808)

(For biopsy of tongue, anterior two-thirds, use 41100)

(For biopsy of floor of mouth, use 41108)

(For biopsy of penis, use 54100)

(For biopsy of vulva or perineum, see 56605, 56606)

(For biopsy of eyelid skin including lid margin, use 67810)

(For biopsy of conjunctiva, use 68100)

(For biopsy of ear, use 69100)

11102 Tangential biopsy of skin (eg, shave, scoop, saucerize, curette); single lesion

➲ *CPT Changes: An Insider's View* 2019
➲ *CPT Assistant* Jan 19:9, Dec 19:9, May 20:13, Aug 21:3, Mar 23:1

+ 11103 each separate/additional lesion (List separately in addition to code for primary procedure)

➲ *CPT Changes: An Insider's View* 2019
➲ *CPT Assistant* Jan 19:9, Dec 19:9, May 20:13

(Report 11103 in conjunction with 11102, 11104, 11106, when different biopsy techniques are performed to sample separate/additional lesions for each type of biopsy technique used)

Tangential Biopsy of Skin
11102, 11103

Tangential biopsy of skin shown with scalpel blade.

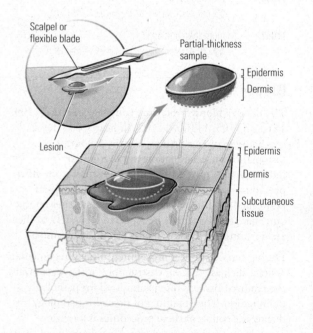

Scalpel or flexible blade

Partial-thickness sample

Epidermis
Dermis

Lesion

Epidermis

Dermis

Subcutaneous tissue

11104 Punch biopsy of skin (including simple closure, when performed); single lesion

➜ *CPT Changes: An Insider's View* 2019

➜ *CPT Assistant* Jan 19:9, Dec 19:9

+ 11105 each separate/additional lesion (List separately in addition to code for primary procedure)

➜ *CPT Changes: An Insider's View* 2019

➜ *CPT Assistant* Jan 19:9, Dec 19:9

(Report 11105 in conjunction with 11104, 11106, when different biopsy techniques are performed to sample separate/additional lesions for each type of biopsy technique used)

Punch Biopsy of Skin
11104, 11105

Punch biopsy of skin shown with punch device.

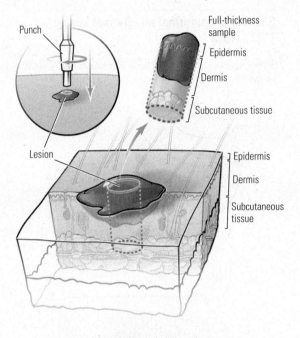

11106 Incisional biopsy of skin (eg, wedge) (including simple closure, when performed); single lesion

➜ *CPT Changes: An Insider's View* 2019

➜ *CPT Assistant* Jan 19:9, Dec 19:9, Jan 22:17

+ 11107 each separate/additional lesion (List separately in addition to code for primary procedure)

➜ *CPT Changes: An Insider's View* 2019

➜ *CPT Assistant* Jan 19:9, Dec 19:9, Aug 21:3

(Report 11107 in conjunction with 11106)

Incisional Biopsy of Skin
11106, 11107

Incisional biopsy of skin shown with scalpel.

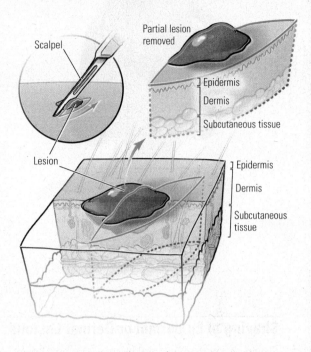

Removal of Skin Tags

Removal by scissoring or any sharp method, ligature strangulation, electrosurgical destruction or combination of treatment modalities, including chemical destruction or electrocauterization of wound, with or without local anesthesia.

11200 Removal of skin tags, multiple fibrocutaneous tags, any area; up to and including 15 lesions

➜ *CPT Assistant* Winter 90:3, Nov 97:11-12, Nov 02:11, Aug 09:7, Jun 11:13

+ 11201 each additional 10 lesions, or part thereof (List separately in addition to code for primary procedure)

➜ *CPT Changes: An Insider's View* 2009

➜ *CPT Assistant* Winter 90:3, Nov 97:11-12, Nov 02:11, Jun 11:13

(Use 11201 in conjunction with 11200)

Removal of Skin Tags
11200, 11201

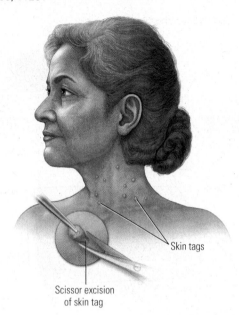

Skin tags

Scissor excision
of skin tag

Shaving of Epidermal or Dermal Lesions

Shaving is the sharp removal by transverse incision or
horizontal slicing to remove epidermal and dermal lesions
without a full-thickness dermal excision. This includes
local anesthesia, chemical or electrocauterization of the
wound. The wound does not require suture closure.

11300 Shaving of epidermal or dermal lesion, single lesion,
trunk, arms or legs; lesion diameter 0.5 cm or less
➡ *CPT Assistant* Feb 00:11, Nov 02:11, Feb 08:1, Dec 17:14,
Feb 18:10, Jan 19:9, Jun 21:6

11301 lesion diameter 0.6 to 1.0 cm
➡ *CPT Assistant* Feb 00:11, Feb 08:1, Dec 17:14, Feb 18:10,
Jan 19:9, Jun 21:6

11302 lesion diameter 1.1 to 2.0 cm
➡ *CPT Assistant* Feb 00:11, Feb 08:1, Dec 17:14, Feb 18:10,
Jan 19:9, Jun 21:6

11303 lesion diameter over 2.0 cm
➡ *CPT Assistant* Feb 00:11, Feb 08:1, Dec 17:14, Feb 18:10,
Jan 19:9, Jun 21:6

11305 Shaving of epidermal or dermal lesion, single lesion,
scalp, neck, hands, feet, genitalia; lesion diameter 0.5 cm
or less
➡ *CPT Assistant* Feb 00:11, Feb 08:1, Dec 17:14, Feb 18:10,
Jan 19:9, Jun 21:6

11306 lesion diameter 0.6 to 1.0 cm
➡ *CPT Assistant* Feb 00:11, Feb 08:1, Dec 17:14, Feb 18:10,
Jan 19:9, Jun 21:6

11307 lesion diameter 1.1 to 2.0 cm
➡ *CPT Assistant* Feb 00:11, Feb 08:1, Dec 17:14, Feb 18:10,
Jan 19:9, Jun 21:6

11308 lesion diameter over 2.0 cm
➡ *CPT Assistant* Feb 00:11, Feb 08:1, Dec 17:14, Feb 18:10,
Jan 19:9, Jun 21:6

11310 Shaving of epidermal or dermal lesion, single lesion,
face, ears, eyelids, nose, lips, mucous membrane; lesion
diameter 0.5 cm or less
➡ *CPT Assistant* Feb 00:11, Feb 08:1, Feb 13:16, Mar 13:6,
Dec 17:14, Feb 18:10, Jan 19:9, Jun 21:6

11311 lesion diameter 0.6 to 1.0 cm
➡ *CPT Assistant* Feb 00:11, Feb 08:1, Feb 13:16, Mar 13:6,
Feb 18:10, Jan 19:9, Jun 21:6

11312 lesion diameter 1.1 to 2.0 cm
➡ *CPT Assistant* Feb 00:11, Feb 08:1, Feb 13:16, Mar 13:6,
Feb 18:10, Jan 19:9, Jun 21:6

11313 lesion diameter over 2.0 cm
➡ *CPT Assistant* Feb 00:11, Feb 08:1, Feb 13:16, Mar 13:6,
Feb 18:10, Jan 19:9, Jun 21:6

Shaving of Epidermal and Dermal Lesion
11300-11313

Shaving of epidermal and dermal lesion with flexible blade and entire lesion
removed.

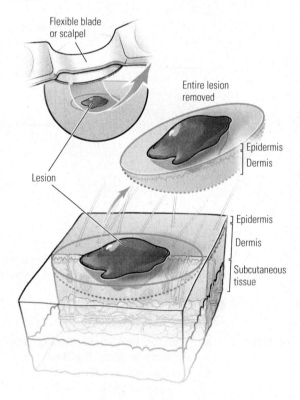

Flexible blade
or scalpel

Entire lesion
removed

Lesion

Epidermis
Dermis

Epidermis

Dermis

Subcutaneous
tissue

Measuring and Coding the Removal of a Lesion

Measuring lesion removal.

A. Example: Excision, malignant lesion of the back, 1.0 cm. Code 11606.

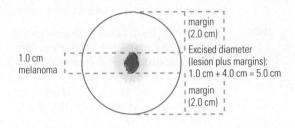

B. Example: Excision of benign lesion of the neck, 1.0 cm by 2.0 cm. Code 11423.

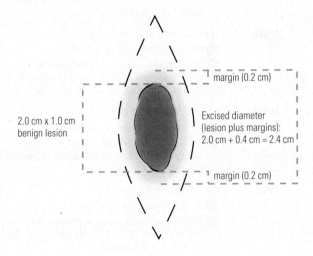

C. Example: Excision, malignant lesion of the nose, 0.9 cm. Code 11642.

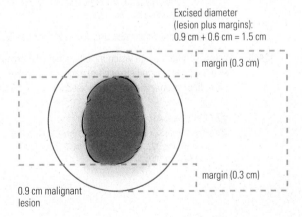

Excision—Benign Lesions

Excision (including simple closure) of benign lesions of skin (eg, neoplasm, cicatricial, fibrous, inflammatory, congenital, cystic lesions), includes local anesthesia. See appropriate size and area below. For shave removal, see 11300 et seq, and for electrosurgical and other methods see 17000 et seq.

Excision is defined as full-thickness (through the dermis) removal of a lesion, including margins, and includes simple (non-layered) closure when performed. Report separately each benign lesion excised. Code selection is determined by measuring the greatest clinical diameter of the apparent lesion plus that margin required for complete excision (lesion diameter plus the most narrow margins required equals the excised diameter). The margins refer to the most narrow margin required to adequately excise the lesion, based on individual judgment. The measurement of lesion plus margin is made prior to excision. The excised diameter is the same whether the surgical defect is repaired in a linear fashion, or reconstructed (eg, with a skin graft).

The closure of defects created by incision, excision, or trauma may require intermediate or complex closure. Repair by intermediate or complex closure should be reported separately. For excision of benign lesions requiring more than simple closure, ie, requiring intermediate or complex closure, report 11400-11446 in addition to appropriate intermediate (12031-12057) or complex closure (13100-13153) codes. For reconstructive closure, see 15002-15261, 15570-15770. For excision performed in conjunction with adjacent tissue transfer, report only the adjacent tissue transfer code (14000-14302). Excision of lesion (11400-11446) is not separately reportable with adjacent tissue transfer. See pages 98 and 99 for the definition of *intermediate* or *complex* closure.

> (For destruction [eg, laser surgery, electrosurgery, cryosurgery, chemosurgery, surgical curette] of benign lesions other than skin tags or cutaneous vascular proliferative lesions, see 17110, 17111; premalignant lesions, see 17000, 17003, 17004; cutaneous vascular proliferative lesions, see 17106, 17107, 17108; malignant lesions, see 17260-17286)
>
> (For excision of cicatricial lesion[s] [eg, full thickness excision, through the dermis], see 11400-11446)
>
> (For incisional removal of burn scar, see 16035, 16036)
>
> (For fractional ablative laser fenestration for functional improvement of traumatic or burn scars, see 0479T, 0480T)

11400 Excision, benign lesion including margins, except skin tag (unless listed elsewhere), trunk, arms or legs; excised diameter 0.5 cm or less

➜ *CPT Changes: An Insider's View* 2003

➜ *CPT Assistant* Summer 92:22, Fall 93:7, Fall 95:3, May 96:11, Aug 00:5, Nov 02:5, 7, Aug 06:10, Jul 08:5, Apr 10:3, Jul 10:10, Jan 11:9, May 12:13, Mar 14:4, 12, Apr 14:10, Apr 16:3, Feb 18:10, Sep 18:7, Nov 19:3, Aug 21:3, May 23:24, Jan 24:37

11401 excised diameter 0.6 to 1.0 cm

➜ *CPT Changes: An Insider's View* 2003

➜ *CPT Assistant* Summer 92:22, Fall 93:7, Fall 95:3, May 96:11, Nov 02:5, 7, Jul 10:10, Jan 11:9, May 12:13, Mar 14:4, 12, Apr 16:3, Feb 18:10, Sep 18:7, Nov 19:3, May 23:24

11402 excised diameter 1.1 to 2.0 cm

➜ *CPT Changes: An Insider's View* 2003

➜ *CPT Assistant* Summer 92:22, Fall 93:7, Fall 95:3, May 96:11, Nov 02:5, 7, Jul 10:10, Jan 11:9, May 12:13, Mar 14:4, 12, Apr 16:3, Feb 18:10, Sep 18:7, Nov 19:3

11403 excised diameter 2.1 to 3.0 cm

➜ *CPT Changes: An Insider's View* 2003

➜ *CPT Assistant* Summer 92:22, Fall 93:7, Fall 95:3, May 96:11, Nov 02:5, 7, Jul 10:10, Jan 11:9, May 12:13, Mar 14:4, 12, Apr 16:3, Feb 18:10, Sep 18:7, Nov 19:3, May 23:24, Dec 23:44

11404 excised diameter 3.1 to 4.0 cm

➜ *CPT Changes: An Insider's View* 2003

➜ *CPT Assistant* Summer 92:22, Fall 93:7, Fall 95:3, May 96:11, Nov 02:5, 7, Jul 10:10, Jan 11:9, May 12:13, Mar 14:4, 12, Apr 16:3, Feb 18:10, Sep 18:7, Nov 19:3

Excision of Lesion
11400 and 11600 series

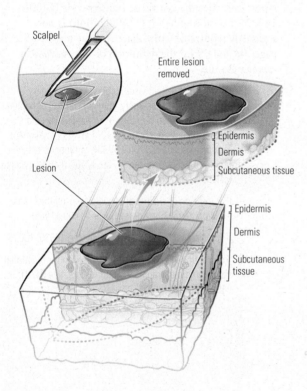

Scalpel

Entire lesion removed

Lesion

Epidermis
Dermis
Subcutaneous tissue

Epidermis
Dermis
Subcutaneous tissue

11406 excised diameter over 4.0 cm

➜ *CPT Changes: An Insider's View* 2003

➜ *CPT Assistant* Summer 92:22, Fall 93:7, Fall 95:3, May 96:11, Nov 02:5, 7, Jul 10:10, Jan 11:9, May 12:13, Mar 14:4, 12, Apr 14:10, Apr 16:3, Feb 18:10, Sep 18:7, Nov 19:3, Aug 21:3

(For unusual or complicated excision, add modifier 22)

11420 Excision, benign lesion including margins, except skin tag (unless listed elsewhere), scalp, neck, hands, feet, genitalia; excised diameter 0.5 cm or less

➜ *CPT Changes: An Insider's View* 2003

➜ *CPT Assistant* Summer 92:22, Fall 95:3, Jul 08:5, Jul 10:10, May 12:13, Jan 13:15, Mar 14:4, 12, Apr 16:3, Feb 18:10, Sep 18:7, Nov 19:3

11421 excised diameter 0.6 to 1.0 cm

➜ *CPT Changes: An Insider's View* 2003

➜ *CPT Assistant* Summer 92:22, Fall 95:3, May 96:11, Jul 10:10, May 12:13, Jan 13:15, Mar 14:4, 12, Apr 16:3, Feb 18:10, Sep 18:7, Nov 19:3

11422 excised diameter 1.1 to 2.0 cm

➜ *CPT Changes: An Insider's View* 2003

➜ *CPT Assistant* Summer 92:22, Fall 95:3, May 96:11, Aug 00:5, Jul 10:10, Mar 12:4, May 12:13, Jan 13:15, Mar 14:4, 12, Apr 16:3, Feb 18:10, Sep 18:7, Nov 19:3

11423 excised diameter 2.1 to 3.0 cm

➜ *CPT Changes: An Insider's View* 2003

➜ *CPT Assistant* Summer 92:22, Fall 95:3, May 96:11, Jul 10:10, May 12:13, Jan 13:15, Mar 14:4, 12, Apr 16:3, Feb 18:10, Sep 18:7, Nov 19:3

11424 excised diameter 3.1 to 4.0 cm

➜ *CPT Changes: An Insider's View* 2003

➜ *CPT Assistant* Summer 92:22, Fall 95:3, May 96:11, Jul 10:10, May 12:13, Jan 13:15, Mar 14:4, 12, Apr 16:3, Feb 18:10, Sep 18:7, Nov 19:3

11426 excised diameter over 4.0 cm

➜ *CPT Changes: An Insider's View* 2003

➜ *CPT Assistant* Summer 92:22, Fall 95:3, May 96:11, Jul 10:10, May 12:13, Jan 13:15, Mar 14:4, 12, Apr 16:3, Feb 18:10, Sep 18:7, Nov 19:3

(For unusual or complicated excision, add modifier 22)

11440 Excision, other benign lesion including margins, except skin tag (unless listed elsewhere), face, ears, eyelids, nose, lips, mucous membrane; excised diameter 0.5 cm or less

➜ *CPT Changes: An Insider's View* 2003

➜ *CPT Assistant* Summer 92:22, Fall 95:3, May 96:11, Jul 08:5, Jul 10:10, May 12:13, Mar 14:4, 12, Apr 16:3, Feb 18:10, Sep 18:7, Nov 19:3, Jun 22:20

11441   excised diameter 0.6 to 1.0 cm
> *CPT Changes: An Insider's View* 2003
> *CPT Assistant* Summer 92:22, Fall 95:3, May 96:11,
>   Jul 10:10, May 12:13, Mar 14:4, 12, Apr 16:3, Feb 18:10,
>   Sep 18:7, Nov 19:3

11442   excised diameter 1.1 to 2.0 cm
> *CPT Changes: An Insider's View* 2003
> *CPT Assistant* Summer 92:22, Fall 95:3, May 96:11,
>   Aug 00:5, Jun 08:14, Jul 10:10, May 12:13, Mar 14:4, 12,
>   Apr 16:3, Feb 18:10, Sep 18:7, Nov 19:3, Nov 22:21

11443   excised diameter 2.1 to 3.0 cm
> *CPT Changes: An Insider's View* 2003
> *CPT Assistant* Summer 92:22, Fall 95:3, May 96:11,
>   Jul 10:10, May 12:13, Mar 14:4, 12, Apr 16:3, Feb 18:10,
>   Sep 18:7, Nov 19:3

11444   excised diameter 3.1 to 4.0 cm
> *CPT Changes: An Insider's View* 2003
> *CPT Assistant* Summer 92:22, Fall 95:3, May 96:11,
>   Jul 10:10, May 12:13, Mar 14:4, 12, Apr 16:3, Feb 18:10,
>   Sep 18:7, Nov 19:3

11446   excised diameter over 4.0 cm
> *CPT Changes: An Insider's View* 2003
> *CPT Assistant* Summer 92:22, Fall 95:3, May 96:11,
>   Aug 06:10, Jul 08:5, Apr 10:3, Jul 10:10, May 12:13,
>   Mar 14:4, 12, Apr 16:3, Feb 18:10, Sep 18:7, Nov 19:3,
>   Jan 24:37

(For unusual or complicated excision, add modifier 22)

(For eyelids involving more than skin, see also 67800 et seq)

11450   Excision of skin and subcutaneous tissue for hidradenitis, axillary; with simple or intermediate repair
> *CPT Assistant* May 12:13, Aug 16:9, Feb 18:10, Sep 18:7

11451   with complex repair
> *CPT Assistant* May 12:13, Aug 16:9, Feb 18:10, Sep 18:7

11462   Excision of skin and subcutaneous tissue for hidradenitis, inguinal; with simple or intermediate repair
> *CPT Assistant* May 12:13, Aug 16:9, Feb 18:10, Sep 18:7

11463   with complex repair
> *CPT Assistant* May 12:13, Aug 16:9, Feb 18:10, Sep 18:7

11470   Excision of skin and subcutaneous tissue for hidradenitis, perianal, perineal, or umbilical; with simple or intermediate repair
> *CPT Assistant* May 12:13, Aug 16:9, Feb 18:10

11471   with complex repair
> *CPT Assistant* May 12:13, Aug 16:9, Feb 18:10, Sep 18:7,
>   Aug 21:3

(When skin graft or flap is used for closure, use appropriate procedure code in addition)

(For bilateral procedure, add modifier 50)

Excision—Malignant Lesions

Excision (including simple closure) of malignant lesions of skin (eg, basal cell carcinoma, squamous cell carcinoma, melanoma) includes local anesthesia. (See appropriate size and body area below.) For destruction of malignant lesions of skin, see destruction codes 17260-17286.

Excision is defined as full-thickness (through the dermis) removal of a lesion including margins, and includes simple (non-layered) closure when performed. Report separately each malignant lesion excised. Code selection is determined by measuring the greatest clinical diameter of the apparent lesion plus that margin required for complete excision (lesion diameter plus the most narrow margins required equals the excised diameter). The margins refer to the most narrow margin required to adequately excise the lesion, based on the physician's judgment. The measurement of lesion plus margin is made prior to excision. The excised diameter is the same whether the surgical defect is repaired in a linear fashion, or reconstructed (eg, with a skin graft).

The closure of defects created by incision, excision, or trauma may require intermediate or complex closure. Repair by intermediate or complex closure should be reported separately. For excision of malignant lesions requiring more than simple closure, ie, requiring intermediate or complex closure, report 11600-11646 in addition to appropriate intermediate (12031-12057) or complex closure (13100-13153) codes. For reconstructive closure, see 15002-15261, 15570-15770. For excision performed in conjunction with adjacent tissue transfer, report only the adjacent tissue transfer code (14000-14302). Excision of lesion (11600-11646) is not separately reportable with adjacent tissue transfer. See pages 98 and 99 for the definition of *intermediate* or *complex* closure.

When frozen section pathology shows the margins of excision were not adequate, an additional excision may be necessary for complete tumor removal. Use only one code to report the additional excision and re-excision(s) based on the final widest excised diameter required for complete tumor removal at the same operative session. To report a re-excision procedure performed to widen margins at a subsequent operative session, see codes 11600-11646, as appropriate. Append modifier 58 if the re-excision procedure is performed during the postoperative period of the primary excision procedure.

11600 Excision, malignant lesion including margins, trunk, arms, or legs; excised diameter 0.5 cm or less

➜ *CPT Changes: An Insider's View* 2003

➜ *CPT Assistant* Fall 95:3, May 96:11, Nov 02:5, Oct 04:4, Feb 08:8, Feb 10:3, Apr 10:3, May 12:13, Jul 12:12, Mar 14:4, 12, Sep 18:7, Nov 19:3, Jan 24:37

11601 excised diameter 0.6 to 1.0 cm

➜ *CPT Changes: An Insider's View* 2003

➜ *CPT Assistant* Fall 95:3, May 96:11, Nov 02:5, Feb 10:3, Mar 12:7, May 12:13, Jul 12:12, Mar 14:4, 12, Sep 18:7, Nov 19:3

11602 excised diameter 1.1 to 2.0 cm

➜ *CPT Changes: An Insider's View* 2003

➜ *CPT Assistant* Fall 95:3, May 96:11, Nov 02:5, Feb 08:8, Feb 10:3, Apr 10:3, Mar 12:4, May 12:13, Jul 12:12, Mar 14:4, 12, Sep 18:7, Nov 19:3, Jul 23:1

11603 excised diameter 2.1 to 3.0 cm

➜ *CPT Changes: An Insider's View* 2003

➜ *CPT Assistant* Fall 95:3, May 96:11, Nov 02:5, Feb 08:8, Feb 10:3, May 12:13, Jul 12:12, Mar 14:4, 12, Sep 18:7, Nov 19:3, Aug 21:3, Nov 22:21, Jul 23:1, Dec 23:44

11604 excised diameter 3.1 to 4.0 cm

➜ *CPT Changes: An Insider's View* 2003

➜ *CPT Assistant* Fall 95:3, May 96:11, Nov 02:5, Feb 08:8, Feb 10:3, May 12:13, Jul 12:12, Mar 14:4, 12, Sep 18:7, Nov 19:3

11606 excised diameter over 4.0 cm

➜ *CPT Changes: An Insider's View* 2003

➜ *CPT Assistant* Fall 91:6, Fall 95:3, May 96:11, Nov 02:5, Feb 08:8, Feb 10:3, May 12:13, Jul 12:12, Mar 14:4, 12, Sep 18:7, Nov 19:3

Measuring and Coding the Removal of a Lesion
11600

Example: Excision, malignant lesion, 0.4 cm. Code 11600.

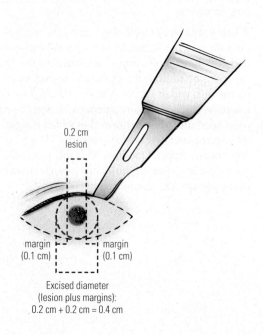

0.2 cm
lesion

margin
(0.1 cm)

margin
(0.1 cm)

Excised diameter
(lesion plus margins):
0.2 cm + 0.2 cm = 0.4 cm

11620 Excision, malignant lesion including margins, scalp, neck, hands, feet, genitalia; excised diameter 0.5 cm or less

➜ *CPT Changes: An Insider's View* 2003

➜ *CPT Assistant* Fall 95:3, Nov 02:5, Oct 04:4, Feb 08:8, Feb 10:3, May 12:13, Jul 12:12, Mar 14:4, 12, Sep 18:7, Nov 19:3

11621 excised diameter 0.6 to 1.0 cm

➜ *CPT Changes: An Insider's View* 2003

➜ *CPT Assistant* Fall 95:3, May 96:11, Nov 02:5, Feb 08:8, Feb 10:3, May 12:13, Mar 14:4, 12, Sep 18:7, Nov 19:3

11622 excised diameter 1.1 to 2.0 cm

➜ *CPT Changes: An Insider's View* 2003

➜ *CPT Assistant* Fall 95:3, May 96:11, Nov 02:5, Feb 08:8, Feb 10:3, May 12:13, Mar 14:4, 12, Sep 18:7, Nov 19:3

11623 excised diameter 2.1 to 3.0 cm

➜ *CPT Changes: An Insider's View* 2003

➜ *CPT Assistant* Fall 95:3, May 96:11, Nov 02:5, Feb 08:8, Feb 10:3, May 12:13, Mar 14:4, 12, Sep 18:7, Nov 19:3

11624 excised diameter 3.1 to 4.0 cm

➜ *CPT Changes: An Insider's View* 2003

➜ *CPT Assistant* Fall 95:3, May 96:11, Nov 02:5, Feb 08:8, Feb 10:3, May 12:13, Mar 14:4, 12, Sep 18:7, Nov 19:3

11626 excised diameter over 4.0 cm

➜ *CPT Changes: An Insider's View* 2003

➜ *CPT Assistant* Fall 95:3, May 96:11, Nov 02:5, Feb 08:8, Feb 10:3, May 12:13, Mar 14:4, 12, Sep 18:7, Nov 19:3

11640 Excision, malignant lesion including margins, face, ears, eyelids, nose, lips; excised diameter 0.5 cm or less

➜ *CPT Changes: An Insider's View* 2003

➜ *CPT Assistant* Fall 95:3, May 96:11, Nov 02:5, Oct 04:4, Feb 08:8, Feb 10:3, May 12:13, Mar 14:4, 12, Sep 18:7, Nov 19:3

11641 excised diameter 0.6 to 1.0 cm

➜ *CPT Changes: An Insider's View* 2003

➜ *CPT Assistant* Fall 95:3, May 96:11, Feb 08:8, Feb 10:3, May 12:13, Mar 14:4, 12, Sep 18:7, Nov 19:3

11642 excised diameter 1.1 to 2.0 cm

➜ *CPT Changes: An Insider's View* 2003

➜ *CPT Assistant* Fall 95:3, May 96:11, Feb 08:8, Feb 10:3, May 12:13, Mar 14:4, 12, Sep 18:7, Nov 19:3

11643 excised diameter 2.1 to 3.0 cm

➜ *CPT Changes: An Insider's View* 2003

➜ *CPT Assistant* Fall 95:3, May 96:11, Feb 08:8, Feb 10:3, May 12:13, Mar 14:4, 12, Sep 18:7, Nov 19:3

11644 excised diameter 3.1 to 4.0 cm

➜ *CPT Changes: An Insider's View* 2003

➜ *CPT Assistant* Fall 95:3, May 96:11, Feb 08:8, Feb 10:3, May 12:13, Mar 14:4, 12, Sep 18:7, Nov 19:3

11646   excised diameter over 4.0 cm
> *CPT Changes: An Insider's View* 2003
> *CPT Assistant* Fall 95:3, May 96:11, Feb 08:8, Feb 10:3,
> Apr 10:3, May 12:13, Mar 14:4, 12, Sep 18:7, Nov 19:3,
> Aug 21:3, Jan 24:37

(For eyelids involving more than skin, see also 67800 et seq)

Nails

(For drainage of paronychia or onychia, see 10060, 10061)

11719   Trimming of nondystrophic nails, any number
> *CPT Assistant* Nov 97:12, Dec 02:4

Lateral Nail View
11719-11765

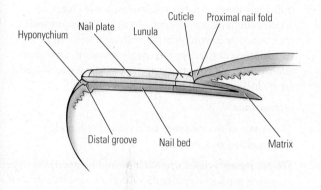

11720   Debridement of nail(s) by any method(s); 1 to 5
> *CPT Assistant* Nov 96:3, Dec 02:4

11721   6 or more
> *CPT Assistant* Nov 96:3, Dec 02:4

11730   Avulsion of nail plate, partial or complete, simple; single
> *CPT Assistant* Mar 96:10, Dec 02:4, Dec 03:11

+ 11732   each additional nail plate (List separately in addition to code for primary procedure)
> *CPT Assistant* Dec 02:4

(Use 11732 in conjunction with 11730)

11740   Evacuation of subungual hematoma
> *CPT Assistant* Dec 02:4

11750   Excision of nail and nail matrix, partial or complete (eg, ingrown or deformed nail), for permanent removal
> *CPT Assistant* Dec 02:4

(For pinch graft, use 15050)

11755   Biopsy of nail unit (eg, plate, bed, matrix, hyponychium, proximal and lateral nail folds) (separate procedure)
> *CPT Changes: An Insider's View* 2002
> *CPT Assistant* Mar 96:11, Dec 02:4, Oct 04:14

11760   Repair of nail bed
> *CPT Assistant* Dec 02:4

11762   Reconstruction of nail bed with graft
> *CPT Assistant* Dec 02:4

11765   Wedge excision of skin of nail fold (eg, for ingrown toenail)
> *CPT Assistant* Dec 02:4

Dorsal Nail View
11719-11765

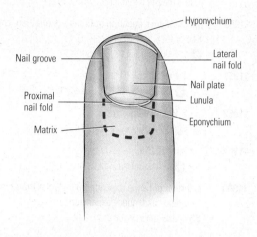

Pilonidal Cyst

11770   Excision of pilonidal cyst or sinus; simple

11771   extensive

11772   complicated
> *CPT Assistant* Sep 15:12

(For incision of pilonidal cyst, see 10080, 10081)

Introduction

11900   Injection, intralesional; up to and including 7 lesions
> *CPT Assistant* Sep 96:5, May 98:10, Nov 99:8, Feb 00:11,
> Sep 04:12, Nov 13:14, Aug 22:16

11901   more than 7 lesions
> *CPT Assistant* Sep 96:5, May 98:10, Nov 99:8, Feb 00:11,
> Sep 04:12

(11900, 11901 are not to be used for preoperative local anesthetic injection)

(For veins, see 36470, 36471)

(For intralesional chemotherapy administration, see 96405, 96406)

11920   Tattooing, intradermal introduction of insoluble opaque pigments to correct color defects of skin, including micropigmentation; 6.0 sq cm or less
> *CPT Assistant* Aug 16:9

11921 6.1 to 20.0 sq cm
➡️ *CPT Assistant* Aug 16:9

+ 11922 each additional 20.0 sq cm, or part thereof (List separately in addition to code for primary procedure)
➡️ *CPT Changes: An Insider's View* 2009

(Use 11922 in conjunction with 11921)

11950 Subcutaneous injection of filling material (eg, collagen); 1 cc or less
➡️ *CPT Assistant* Jun 12:15, Aug 19:10

11951 1.1 to 5.0 cc
➡️ *CPT Assistant* Jun 12:15, Aug 19:10

11952 5.1 to 10.0 cc
➡️ *CPT Assistant* Jun 12:15, Aug 19:10

11954 over 10.0 cc
➡️ *CPT Assistant* Jun 12:15, Aug 19:10

11960 Insertion of tissue expander(s) for other than breast, including subsequent expansion
➡️ *CPT Assistant* Winter 91:2

(Do not report 11960 in conjunction with 11971, 13160, 29848, 64702-64726)

(For insertion of tissue expander in breast reconstruction, use 19357)

11970 Replacement of tissue expander with permanent implant
➡️ *CPT Changes: An Insider's View* 2021
➡️ *CPT Assistant* Aug 05:1, Jan 13:15, Apr 21:3, Sep 21:13-14, Sep 22:18

11971 Removal of tissue expander without insertion of implant
➡️ *CPT Changes: An Insider's View* 2021
➡️ *CPT Assistant* Jun 05:11, Apr 21:3

(Do not report 11971 in conjunction with 11960, 11970)

(For removal of breast-tissue expander and replacement with breast implant, use 11970)

11976 Removal, implantable contraceptive capsules

11980 Subcutaneous hormone pellet implantation (implantation of estradiol and/or testosterone pellets beneath the skin)
➡️ *CPT Changes: An Insider's View* 2000
➡️ *CPT Assistant* Nov 99:8

11981 Insertion, drug-delivery implant (ie, bioresorbable, biodegradable, non-biodegradable)
➡️ *CPT Changes: An Insider's View* 2002, 2022
➡️ *CPT Assistant* Apr 11:12, Mar 20:14, Sep 21:6

(For manual preparation and insertion of deep [eg, subfascial], intramedullary, or intra-articular drug-delivery device, see 20700, 20702, 20704)

(For removal of biodegradable or bioresorbable implant, use 17999)

(Do not report 11981 in conjunction with 20700, 20702, 20704)

11982 Removal, non-biodegradable drug delivery implant
➡️ *CPT Changes: An Insider's View* 2002
➡️ *CPT Assistant* Sep 21:6

(For removal of deep [eg, subfascial], intramedullary, or intra-articular drug-delivery device, see 20701, 20703, 20705)

(Do not report 11982 in conjunction with 20701, 20703, 20705)

11983 Removal with reinsertion, non-biodegradable drug delivery implant
➡️ *CPT Changes: An Insider's View* 2002
➡️ *CPT Assistant* Sep 21:6, Mar 22:12

Repair (Closure)

Use the codes in this section to designate wound closure utilizing sutures, staples, or tissue adhesives (eg, 2-cyanoacrylate), either singly or in combination with each other, or in combination with adhesive strips. Chemical cauterization, electrocauterization, or wound closure utilizing adhesive strips as the sole repair material are included in the appropriate E/M code.

Definitions

The repair of wounds may be classified as Simple, Intermediate, or Complex.

Simple repair is used when the wound is superficial (eg, involving primarily epidermis or dermis, or subcutaneous tissues without significant involvement of deeper structures) and requires simple one-layer closure. Hemostasis and local or topical anesthesia, when performed, are not reported separately.

Intermediate repair includes the repair of wounds that, in addition to the above, require layered closure of one or more of the deeper layers of subcutaneous tissue and superficial (non-muscle) fascia, in addition to the skin (epidermal and dermal) closure. It includes limited undermining (defined as a distance less than the maximum width of the defect, measured perpendicular to the closure line, along at least one entire edge of the defect). Single-layer closure of heavily contaminated wounds that have required extensive cleaning or removal of particulate matter also constitutes intermediate repair.

Complex repair includes the repair of wounds that, in addition to the requirements for intermediate repair, require at least one of the following: exposure of bone, cartilage, tendon, or named neurovascular structure; debridement of wound edges (eg, traumatic lacerations or avulsions); extensive undermining (defined as a distance greater than or equal to the maximum width of the defect, measured perpendicular to the closure line along at least one entire edge of the defect); involvement of free margins of helical rim, vermilion border, or nostril rim; placement of retention sutures. Necessary preparation includes creation of a limited defect for repairs or the debridement of complicated lacerations or avulsions. Complex repair does not include excision of benign (11400-11446) or malignant (11600-11646) lesions, excisional preparation of a wound bed (15002-15005) or debridement of an open fracture or open dislocation.

Extensive Undermining

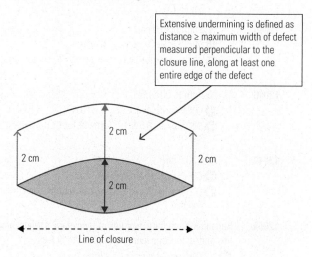

Extensive undermining is defined as distance ≥ maximum width of defect measured perpendicular to the closure line, along at least one entire edge of the defect

2 cm

2 cm   2 cm   2 cm

2 cm

Line of closure

Instructions for listing services at time of wound repair:

1. The repaired wound(s) should be measured and recorded in centimeters, whether curved, angular, or stellate.

2. When multiple wounds are repaired, add together the lengths of those in the same classification (see above) and from all anatomic sites that are grouped together into the same code descriptor. For example, add together the lengths of intermediate repairs to the trunk and extremities. Do not add lengths of repairs from different groupings of anatomic sites (eg, face and extremities). Also, do not add together lengths of different classifications (eg, intermediate and complex repairs).

   When more than one classification of wounds is repaired, list the more complicated as the primary procedure and the less complicated as the secondary procedure, using modifier 59.

3. Decontamination and/or debridement: Debridement is considered a separate procedure only when gross contamination requires prolonged cleansing, when appreciable amounts of devitalized or contaminated tissue are removed, or when debridement is carried out separately without immediate primary closure.

   (For extensive debridement of soft tissue and/or bone, not associated with open fracture(s) and/or dislocation(s) resulting from penetrating and/or blunt trauma, see 11042-11047.)

(For extensive debridement of subcutaneous tissue, muscle fascia, muscle, and/or bone associated with open fracture(s) and/or dislocation(s), see 11010-11012.)

4. Involvement of nerves, blood vessels and tendons: Report under appropriate system (Nervous, Cardiovascular, Musculoskeletal) for repair of these structures. The repair of these associated wounds is included in the primary procedure unless it qualifies as a complex repair, in which case modifier 59 applies.

Simple ligation of vessels in an open wound is considered as part of any wound closure.

Simple "exploration" of nerves, blood vessels or tendons exposed in an open wound is also considered part of the essential treatment of the wound and is not a separate procedure unless appreciable dissection is required. If the wound requires enlargement, extension of dissection (to determine penetration), debridement, removal of foreign body(s), ligation or coagulation of minor subcutaneous and/or muscular blood vessel(s) of the subcutaneous tissue, muscle fascia, and/or muscle, not requiring thoracotomy or laparotomy, use codes 20100-20103, as appropriate.

Repair—Simple

Sum of lengths of repairs for each group of anatomic sites.

12001   Simple repair of superficial wounds of scalp, neck, axillae, external genitalia, trunk and/or extremities (including hands and feet); 2.5 cm or less

➔ *CPT Assistant* Jun 96:7, Feb 98:11, Jan 00:11, Feb 00:10, Apr 00:8, Jul 00:10, Jan 02:10, Feb 07:10, Feb 08:8, Mar 12:5, Dec 17:15, Sep 18:7, Aug 22:16, Mar 23:1

12002   2.6 cm to 7.5 cm

➔ *CPT Assistant* Feb 00:10, Jan 02:10, Feb 08:8, Oct 14:14, Sep 18:7, Jul 23:1

12004   7.6 cm to 12.5 cm

➔ *CPT Assistant* Feb 00:10, Jan 02:10, Feb 08:8, Sep 18:7

12005   12.6 cm to 20.0 cm

➔ *CPT Assistant* Feb 00:10, Jan 02:10, Feb 08:8, Sep 18:7

12006   20.1 cm to 30.0 cm

➔ *CPT Assistant* Feb 98:11, Feb 00:10, Jan 02:10, Feb 08:8, Sep 18:7

12007   over 30.0 cm

➔ *CPT Assistant* Feb 00:10, Jan 02:10, Feb 08:8, Sep 18:7

12011   Simple repair of superficial wounds of face, ears, eyelids, nose, lips and/or mucous membranes; 2.5 cm or less

➔ *CPT Assistant* Feb 00:10, May 00:8, Jan 02:10, Feb 08:8, May 14:5, Sep 18:7

12013   2.6 cm to 5.0 cm

➔ *CPT Assistant* Feb 00:10, Jan 02:10, Feb 08:8, Sep 18:7

12014   5.1 cm to 7.5 cm

➔ *CPT Assistant* Feb 00:10, Jan 02:10, Feb 08:8, Sep 18:7

12015   7.6 cm to 12.5 cm

➔ *CPT Assistant* Feb 00:10, Jan 02:10, Feb 08:8, Sep 18:7, Aug 23:16-19

12016   12.6 cm to 20.0 cm

➔ *CPT Assistant* Feb 00:10, Jan 02:10, Feb 08:8, Sep 18:7

12017   20.1 cm to 30.0 cm

➔ *CPT Assistant* Feb 00:10, Jan 02:10, Feb 08:8, Sep 18:7

12018   over 30.0 cm

➔ *CPT Assistant* Feb 00:10, Jan 02:10, Feb 07:10, Feb 08:8, May 14:5, Sep 18:7

12020   Treatment of superficial wound dehiscence; simple closure

➔ *CPT Assistant* Feb 00:10, Jan 02:10, Feb 08:8

12021   with packing

➔ *CPT Assistant* Feb 00:10, Jan 02:10, Feb 08:8, Aug 22:16

(For extensive or complicated secondary wound closure, use 13160)

Repair—Intermediate

Sum of lengths of repairs for each group of anatomic sites.

12031   Repair, intermediate, wounds of scalp, axillae, trunk and/or extremities (excluding hands and feet); 2.5 cm or less

➔ *CPT Changes: An Insider's View* 2009

➔ *CPT Assistant* Sep 97:11, Feb 00:10, Apr 00:8, Jan 02:10, Aug 06:1, Feb 07:10, Apr 10:3, Sep 18:7, Aug 22:16, May 23:24

12032   2.6 cm to 7.5 cm

➔ *CPT Changes: An Insider's View* 2009

➔ *CPT Assistant* May 96:6, Jun 96:8, Feb 00:10, Jan 02:10, Feb 07:10, Sep 18:7, May 23:24, Jul 23:1, Aug 23:16-19, Dec 23:44

12034   7.6 cm to 12.5 cm

➔ *CPT Changes: An Insider's View* 2009

➔ *CPT Assistant* Fall 91:6, Feb 00:10, Jan 02:10, Feb 07:10, Sep 18:7

12035   12.6 cm to 20.0 cm

➔ *CPT Changes: An Insider's View* 2009

➔ *CPT Assistant* Feb 00:10, Jan 02:10, Feb 07:10, Sep 18:7, Aug 23:16-19

12036   20.1 cm to 30.0 cm

➔ *CPT Changes: An Insider's View* 2009

➔ *CPT Assistant* Feb 00:10, Jan 02:10, Feb 07:10, Sep 18:7

12037   over 30.0 cm

➔ *CPT Changes: An Insider's View* 2009

➔ *CPT Assistant* Feb 00:10, Jan 02:10, Feb 07:10, Sep 18:7

12041   Repair, intermediate, wounds of neck, hands, feet and/or external genitalia; 2.5 cm or less

➔ *CPT Changes: An Insider's View* 2009

➔ *CPT Assistant* Sep 97:11, Feb 00:10, Apr 00:8, Jan 02:10, Feb 07:10, Jan 13:15, Sep 18:7

12042   2.6 cm to 7.5 cm

➔ *CPT Changes: An Insider's View* 2009

➔ *CPT Assistant* Feb 00:10, Apr 00:9, Jan 02:10, Feb 07:10, Jan 13:15, Sep 18:7

12044   7.6 cm to 12.5 cm

➔ *CPT Changes: An Insider's View* 2009

➔ *CPT Assistant* Feb 00:10, Jan 02:10, Feb 07:10, Jan 13:15, Sep 18:7

12045   12.6 cm to 20.0 cm

➔ *CPT Changes: An Insider's View* 2009

➔ *CPT Assistant* Feb 00:10, Jan 02:10, Feb 07:10, Jan 13:15, Sep 18:7

12046   20.1 cm to 30.0 cm

➔ *CPT Changes: An Insider's View* 2009

➔ *CPT Assistant* Feb 00:10, Jan 02:10, Feb 07:10, Jan 13:15, Sep 18:7

12047   over 30.0 cm

➔ *CPT Changes: An Insider's View* 2009

➔ *CPT Assistant* Feb 00:10, Jan 02:10, Feb 07:10, Jan 13:15, Sep 18:7

12051   Repair, intermediate, wounds of face, ears, eyelids, nose, lips and/or mucous membranes; 2.5 cm or less

➔ *CPT Changes: An Insider's View* 2009

➔ *CPT Assistant* Sep 97:11, Feb 00:10, Apr 00:8, Jan 02:10, Feb 07:10, May 14:5, Sep 18:7

12052   2.6 cm to 5.0 cm

➔ *CPT Changes: An Insider's View* 2009

➔ *CPT Assistant* Feb 00:10, Aug 00:9, Jan 02:10, Feb 07:10, Jul 08:5, Sep 18:7

12053   5.1 cm to 7.5 cm

➔ *CPT Changes: An Insider's View* 2009

➔ *CPT Assistant* Feb 00:10, Jan 02:10, Feb 07:10, Sep 18:7

12054   7.6 cm to 12.5 cm

➔ *CPT Changes: An Insider's View* 2009

➔ *CPT Assistant* Feb 00:10, Jan 02:10, Feb 07:10, Sep 18:7

12055   12.6 cm to 20.0 cm

➔ *CPT Changes: An Insider's View* 2009

➔ *CPT Assistant* Feb 00:10, Jan 02:10, Feb 07:10, Sep 18:7

12056   20.1 cm to 30.0 cm

➔ *CPT Changes: An Insider's View* 2009

➔ *CPT Assistant* Feb 00:10, Jan 02:10, Feb 07:10, Sep 18:7

12057   over 30.0 cm
➔ *CPT Changes: An Insider's View* 2009
➔ *CPT Assistant* Feb 00:10, Jan 02:10, Feb 07:10, Apr 10:3, May 14:5, Sep 18:7, Aug 22:16

Repair—Complex

Reconstructive procedures, complicated wound closure.

Sum of lengths of repairs for each group of anatomic sites.

> (For full thickness repair of lip or eyelid, see respective anatomical subsections)

13100   Repair, complex, trunk; 1.1 cm to 2.5 cm
➔ *CPT Assistant* Sep 97:11, Dec 98:5, Nov 99:9-10, Feb 00:10, Apr 00:8, Feb 10:3, Apr 10:3, May 11:4, Jan 12:8, Dec 12:6, Apr 17:9, Sep 18:7, Nov 19:14, Aug 22:16, Nov 22:21, May 23:24

> (For 1.0 cm or less, see simple or intermediate repairs)

13101   2.6 cm to 7.5 cm
➔ *CPT Assistant* Dec 98:5, Nov 99:9-10, Feb 00:10, Apr 00:9, Feb 10:3, May 11:4, Jan 12:8, Dec 12:6, Apr 17:9, Sep 18:7, Dec 19:14, May 23:24

+ 13102   each additional 5 cm or less (List separately in addition to code for primary procedure)
➔ *CPT Changes: An Insider's View* 2000
➔ *CPT Assistant* Nov 99:9-10, Feb 00:10, Apr 00:9, Feb 10:3, May 11:4, Jan 12:8, Dec 12:6, Apr 17:9, Sep 18:7, Nov 19:14

> (Use 13102 in conjunction with 13101)

13120   Repair, complex, scalp, arms, and/or legs; 1.1 cm to 2.5 cm
➔ *CPT Assistant* Sep 97:11, Apr 99:11, Nov 99:9-10, Feb 00:10, Apr 00:8, Feb 10:3, May 11:4, Jan 12:8, Dec 12:6, Sep 18:7, Aug 23:16-19

> (For 1.0 cm or less, see simple or intermediate repairs)

13121   2.6 cm to 7.5 cm
➔ *CPT Assistant* Dec 98:5, Nov 99:9-10, Feb 00:10, Feb 10:3, Apr 10:3, May 11:4, Jan 12:8, Dec 12:6, Sep 18:7, Nov 22:21

+ 13122   each additional 5 cm or less (List separately in addition to code for primary procedure)
➔ *CPT Changes: An Insider's View* 2000
➔ *CPT Assistant* Nov 99:10, Feb 10:3, May 11:4, Jan 12:8, Dec 12:6, Sep 18:7

> (Use 13122 in conjunction with 13121)

13131   Repair, complex, forehead, cheeks, chin, mouth, neck, axillae, genitalia, hands and/or feet; 1.1 cm to 2.5 cm
➔ *CPT Assistant* Fall 93:7, Sep 97:11, Dec 98:5, Nov 99:10, Feb 00:10, Apr 00:8, Feb 10:3, May 11:4, Jan 12:8, Dec 12:6, Jan 13:15, Apr 17:9, Sep 18:7, Apr 23:24

> (For 1.0 cm or less, see simple or intermediate repairs)

13132   2.6 cm to 7.5 cm
➔ *CPT Assistant* Fall 93:7, Dec 98:5, Nov 99:10, Dec 99:10, Feb 00:10, Apr 00:9, Aug 00:9, Feb 10:3, May 11:4, Jan 12:8, Dec 12:6, Jan 13:15, Oct 14:14, Apr 17:9, Sep 18:7, Apr 23:24, Aug 23:16-19

+ 13133   each additional 5 cm or less (List separately in addition to code for primary procedure)
➔ *CPT Changes: An Insider's View* 2000
➔ *CPT Assistant* Fall 93:7, Feb 00:10, Apr 00:9, Feb 10:3, May 11:4, Jan 12:8, Dec 12:6, Jan 13:15, Apr 17:9, Sep 18:7

> (Use 13133 in conjunction with 13132)

> (For 1.0 cm or less, see simple or intermediate repairs)

13151   Repair, complex, eyelids, nose, ears and/or lips; 1.1 cm to 2.5 cm
➔ *CPT Changes: An Insider's View* 2014
➔ *CPT Assistant* Dec 98:5, Nov 99:10, Feb 00:10, Feb 10:3, May 11:4, Jan 12:8, Dec 12:6, Mar 14:12, May 14:3, 5, Sep 18:7, Jun 22:20, Aug 23:16-19, Dec 23:42

13152   2.6 cm to 7.5 cm
➔ *CPT Changes: An Insider's View* 2014
➔ *CPT Assistant* Dec 98:5, Nov 99:10, Feb 00:10, Feb 10:3, May 11:4, Jan 12:8, Dec 12:6, May 14:3, Oct 14:14, Sep 18:7

+ 13153   each additional 5 cm or less (List separately in addition to code for primary procedure)
➔ *CPT Changes: An Insider's View* 2000, 2014
➔ *CPT Assistant* Nov 99:10, Feb 00:10, Feb 10:3, Apr 10:3, May 11:4, Jan 12:8, Dec 12:6, May 14:3, 5, Sep 18:7, Aug 22:16

> (Use 13153 in conjunction with 13152)

13160   Secondary closure of surgical wound or dehiscence, extensive or complicated
➔ *CPT Assistant* Sep 97:11, Dec 98:5, Apr 00:8, May 11:4, Dec 12:6, Nov 22:21

> (Do not report 13160 in conjunction with 11960)

> (For packing or simple secondary wound closure, see 12020, 12021)

Adjacent Tissue Transfer or Rearrangement

For full thickness repair of lip or eyelid, see respective anatomical subsections.

Codes 14000-14302 are used for excision (including lesion) and/or repair by adjacent tissue transfer or rearrangement (eg, Z-plasty, W-plasty, V-Y plasty, rotation flap, random island flap, advancement flap). When applied in repairing lacerations, the procedures listed must be performed by the surgeon to accomplish the repair. They do not apply to direct closure or rearrangement of traumatic wounds incidentally resulting in these configurations. Undermining alone of adjacent tissues to achieve closure, without additional incisions, does not constitute adjacent tissue transfer, see complex repair codes 13100-13160. The excision of a benign lesion (11400-11446) or a malignant lesion (11600-11646) is not separately reportable with codes 14000-14302.

Skin graft necessary to close secondary defect is considered an additional procedure. For purposes of code selection, the term "defect" includes the primary and secondary defects. The primary defect resulting from the excision and the secondary defect resulting from flap design to perform the reconstruction are measured together to determine the code.

14000 Adjacent tissue transfer or rearrangement, trunk; defect 10 sq cm or less
→ *CPT Assistant* Sep 96:11, Jul 99:3, Jul 00:10, Jan 06:47, Dec 06:15, Jul 08:5, Mar 10:4, Apr 10:3, Jan 12:8, May 12:13, Nov 12:13, Dec 12:6, Apr 14:10, Feb 15:10, Sep 15:12, Oct 17:9, Apr 21:5, Mar 23:34, Jan 24:37

14001 defect 10.1 sq cm to 30.0 sq cm
→ *CPT Assistant* Aug 96:8, Jul 99:3, Jan 06:47, Dec 06:15, Jul 08:5, Mar 10:4, Jan 12:8, May 12:13, Nov 12:13, Dec 12:6, Apr 14:10, Feb 15:10, Oct 17:9, Jan 24:37

14020 Adjacent tissue transfer or rearrangement, scalp, arms and/or legs; defect 10 sq cm or less
→ *CPT Assistant* Jul 99:3, Jan 06:47, Dec 06:15, Jul 08:5, Mar 10:4, Jan 12:8, May 12:13, Nov 12:13, Dec 12:6

14021 defect 10.1 sq cm to 30.0 sq cm
→ *CPT Assistant* Jul 99:3, Jan 06:47, Dec 06:15, Jul 08:5, Mar 10:4, Jan 12:8, May 12:13, Nov 12:13, Dec 12:6

14040 Adjacent tissue transfer or rearrangement, forehead, cheeks, chin, mouth, neck, axillae, genitalia, hands and/or feet; defect 10 sq cm or less
→ *CPT Assistant* Jul 99:3, Jul 00:10, Jan 06:47, Dec 06:15, Jul 08:5, Mar 10:4, Jan 12:8, May 12:13, Nov 12:13, Dec 12:6, Mar 21:9

14041 defect 10.1 sq cm to 30.0 sq cm
→ *CPT Assistant* Jul 99:3, Jan 06:47, Dec 06:15, Jul 08:5, Mar 10:4, Jan 12:8, May 12:13, Nov 12:13, Dec 12:6

14060 Adjacent tissue transfer or rearrangement, eyelids, nose, ears and/or lips; defect 10 sq cm or less
→ *CPT Assistant* Fall 93:7, Jul 99:3, Jan 06:47, Dec 06:15, Jul 08:5, Mar 10:4, Jan 12:8, May 12:13, Aug 12:13, Nov 12:13, Dec 12:6, Mar 20:14, Dec 22:21

14061 defect 10.1 sq cm to 30.0 sq cm
→ *CPT Assistant* Jul 99:3, Jan 06:47, Dec 06:15, Jul 08:5, Mar 10:4, Jan 12:8, May 12:13, Nov 12:13, Dec 12:6

(For eyelid, full thickness, see 67961 et seq)

14301 Adjacent tissue transfer or rearrangement, any area; defect 30.1 sq cm to 60.0 sq cm
→ *CPT Changes: An Insider's View* 2010
→ *CPT Assistant* May 12:13, Nov 12:13, Dec 12:6, Apr 17:9, Jan 24:37

+ 14302 each additional 30.0 sq cm, or part thereof (List separately in addition to code for primary procedure)
→ *CPT Changes: An Insider's View* 2010
→ *CPT Assistant* May 12:13, Nov 12:13, Dec 12:6, Mar 23:34, Jan 24:37

(Use 14302 in conjunction with 14301)

14350 Filleted finger or toe flap, including preparation of recipient site
→ *CPT Assistant* Jan 06:47, Jul 08:5, Mar 10:4, May 12:13, Dec 12:6, Apr 21:5

Skin Replacement Surgery

▶Skin replacement surgery consists of *surgical preparation* and topical placement of an *autograft* (including tissue cultured autograft and skin cell suspension autograft [SCSA]) or *skin substitute graft* (ie, homograft, allograft, xenograft). The graft is anchored using the individual's choice of fixation. When services are performed in the office, routine dressing supplies are not reported separately.◀

The following definition should be applied to those codes that reference "100 sq cm or 1% of body area of infants and children" when determining the involvement of body size: The measurement of 100 sq cm is applicable to adults and children 10 years of age and older; and percentages of body surface area apply to infants and children younger than 10 years of age. The measurements apply to the size of the recipient area.

Procedures involving wrist and/or ankle are reported with codes that include arm or leg in the descriptor.

When a primary procedure requires a skin substitute or skin autograft for definitive skin closure (eg, orbitectomy, radical mastectomy, deep tumor removal), use 15100-15278 in conjunction with primary procedure.

For biological implant for soft tissue reinforcement, use 15777 in conjunction with primary procedure.

The supply of skin substitute graft(s) should be reported separately in conjunction with 15271-15278.

★ = Telemedicine   ◀ = Audio-only   + = Add-on code   ⚡ = FDA approval pending   # = Resequenced code   ⊘ = Modifier 51 exempt   →→→ = See p xxi for details

Adjacent Tissue Repairs
14000-14061

Repair of primary and secondary defects requires assignment of a code based upon the location and the approximate description (as demonstrated below) of the area required.

A. Advancement Flap

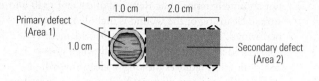

Area 1: 1.0 cm x 1.0 cm = 1.0 sq cm
Area 2: 1.0 cm x 2.0 cm = 2.0 sq cm
(Area 1) + (Area 2) = 1.0 sq cm + 2.0 sq cm = 3.0 sq cm

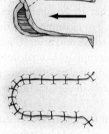

B. Rotation Flap

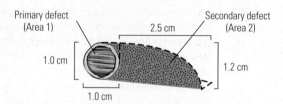

Area 1: 1.0 cm x 1.0 cm = 1.0 sq cm
Area 2: 2.5 cm x 1.2 cm = 3.0 sq cm
(Area 1) + (Area 2) = 1.0 sq cm + 3.0 sq cm = 4.0 sq cm

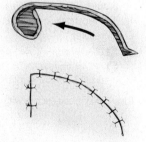

Definitions

Surgical preparation codes 15002-15005 for skin replacement surgery describe the initial services related to preparing a clean and viable wound surface for placement of an autograft, flap, skin substitute graft or for negative pressure wound therapy. In some cases, closure may be possible using adjacent tissue transfer (14000-14061) or complex repair (13100-13153). In all cases, appreciable nonviable tissue is removed to treat a burn, traumatic wound or a necrotizing infection. The clean wound bed may also be created by incisional release of a scar contracture resulting in a surface defect from separation of tissues. The intent is to heal the wound by primary intention, or by the use of negative pressure wound therapy. Patient conditions may require the closure or application of graft, flap, or skin substitute to be delayed, but in all cases the intent is to include these treatments or negative pressure wound therapy to heal the wound. Do not report 15002-15005 for removal of nonviable tissue/ debris in a chronic wound (eg, venous or diabetic) when the wound is left to heal by secondary intention. See active wound management codes (97597, 97598) and debridement codes (11042-11047) for this service. For necrotizing soft tissue infections in specific anatomic locations, see 11004-11008.

Select the appropriate code from 15002-15005 based upon location and size of the resultant defect. For multiple wounds, sum the surface area of all wounds from all anatomic sites that are grouped together into the same code descriptor. For example, sum the surface area of all wounds on the trunk and arms. Do not sum wounds from different groupings of anatomic sites (eg, face and arms). Use 15002 or 15004, as appropriate, for excisions and incisional releases resulting in wounds up to and including 100 sq cm of surface area. Use 15003 or 15005 for each additional 100 sq cm or part thereof. For example: Surgical preparation of a 20 sq cm wound on the right hand and a 15 sq cm wound on the left hand would be reported with a single code, 15004. Surgical preparation of a 75 sq cm wound on the right thigh and a 75 sq cm wound on the left thigh would be reported with 15002 for the first 100 sq cm and 15003 for the second 50 sq cm. If all four wounds required surgical preparation on the same day, use modifier 59 with 15002, and 15004.

▶ *Skin Cell Suspension Autograft (SCSA)* involves harvesting of skin and preparing a suspension of autologous skin cells for direct spray-on application for treatment of conditions such as thermal burn wounds, traumatic avulsion (eg, degloving), surgical excision (eg, necrotizing tissue infection), or resection (eg, skin cancer).

Codes 15011, 15012 are used to report the harvest of epidermal and dermal skin (eg, 0.006-0.008 inch depth). The harvested skin may be divided into smaller portions for processing. The expansion ratio of harvested skin to prepare a SCSA is typically 1:80. For example, 25 sq cm of harvested skin will produce a quantity of skin cells sufficient to cover a defect measuring up to 2000 sq cm.

Codes 15013, 15014 are used to report the preparation of the SCSA, which requires enzymatic processing, manual mechanical disaggregation of skin cells, and filtration of the final suspension.

Codes 15013, 15014 are not reported if the harvested skin is nonmanually processed (ie, using automation).

Codes 15015, 15016, 15017, 15018 are used to report the spray-on application of the SCSA to the wound and the donor site when performed. Application of a primary dressing with choice of fixation (eg, surgical glue, sutures, staples) is included in 15015, 15016, 15017, 15018.

For surgical preparation of the recipient site prior to application of the SCSA, see 15002, 15003, 15004, 15005.

Placement of a separate additional autograft (eg, split-thickness, full-thickness autograft) prior to application of SCSA is separately reportable with 15040-15261, as appropriate.

Repair of donor site requiring skin graft or local flaps is considered a separate procedure.

Autografts/tissue cultured autografts (other than SCSA) include the harvest and/or application of an autologous skin graft. Repair of donor sites requiring skin graft or local flaps is reported separately. Removal of current graft and/or simple cleansing of the wound is included, when performed. Do not report 97602. Debridement is considered a separate procedure only when gross contamination requires prolonged cleansing, when appreciable amounts of devitalized or contaminated tissue are removed, or when debridement is carried out separately without immediate primary closure. ◄

Select the appropriate code from 15040-15261 based upon type of autograft and location and size of the defect. The measurements apply to the size of the recipient area. For multiple wounds, sum the surface area of all wounds from all anatomic sites that are grouped together into the same code descriptor. For example, sum the surface area of all wounds on the trunk and arms. Do not sum wounds from different groupings of anatomic sites (eg, face and arms).

Skin substitute grafts include non-autologous human skin (dermal or epidermal, cellular and acellular) grafts (eg, homograft, allograft), non-human skin substitute grafts (ie, xenograft), and biological products that form a sheet scaffolding for skin growth. These codes are not to be reported for application of non-graft wound dressings (eg, gel, powder, ointment, foam, liquid) or injected skin substitutes. Application of non-graft wound dressings is not separately reportable. Removal of current graft and/or simple cleansing of the wound is included, when performed. Do not report 97602. Debridement is considered a separate procedure only when gross contamination requires prolonged cleansing, when appreciable amounts of devitalized or contaminated tissue are removed, or when debridement is carried out separately without immediate primary closure.

Select the appropriate code from 15271-15278 based upon location and size of the defect. For multiple wounds, sum the surface area of all wounds from all anatomic sites that are grouped together into the same code descriptor. For example, sum the surface area of all wounds on the trunk and arms. Do not sum wounds from different groupings of anatomic sites (eg, face and arms). The supply of skin substitute graft(s) should be reported separately in conjunction with 15271, 15272, 15273, 15274, 15275, 15276, 15277, 15278. For biologic implant for soft tissue reinforcement, use 15777 in conjunction with code for primary procedure.

Surgical Preparation

15002　Surgical preparation or creation of recipient site by excision of open wounds, burn eschar, or scar (including subcutaneous tissues), or incisional release of scar contracture, trunk, arms, legs; first 100 sq cm or 1% of body area of infants and children

➲ *CPT Changes: An Insider's View* 2007

➲ *CPT Assistant* Jan 12:6, Oct 12:13, Dec 12:6, Feb 13:16, Mar 14:12, Oct 16:3, Nov 19:3, Aug 22:16

(For linear scar revision, see 13100-13153)

+ 15003　each additional 100 sq cm, or part thereof, or each additional 1% of body area of infants and children (List separately in addition to code for primary procedure)

➲ *CPT Changes: An Insider's View* 2007, 2009

➲ *CPT Assistant* Jan 12:6, Oct 12:13, Feb 13:16, Mar 14:12, Oct 16:3, Nov 19:3, Aug 22:16

(Use 15003 in conjunction with 15002)

15004   Surgical preparation or creation of recipient site by excision of open wounds, burn eschar, or scar (including subcutaneous tissues), or incisional release of scar contracture, face, scalp, eyelids, mouth, neck, ears, orbits, genitalia, hands, feet and/or multiple digits; first 100 sq cm or 1% of body area of infants and children

➔ *CPT Changes: An Insider's View* 2007

➔ *CPT Assistant* Jan 12:6, Oct 12:13, Feb 13:16, Mar 14:12, Oct 16:3, Nov 19:3, Aug 22:16

+ 15005   each additional 100 sq cm, or part thereof, or each additional 1% of body area of infants and children (List separately in addition to code for primary procedure)

➔ *CPT Changes: An Insider's View* 2007, 2009

➔ *CPT Assistant* Jan 12:6, Oct 12:13, Feb 13:16, Mar 14:12, Oct 16:3, Nov 19:3, Aug 22:16

(Use 15005 in conjunction with 15004)

▶ *Skin Cell Suspension Autograft* ◀

● **15011**   Harvest of skin for skin cell suspension autograft; first 25 sq cm or less

➔ *CPT Changes: An Insider's View* 2025

+● **15012**   each additional 25 sq cm or part thereof (List separately in addition to code for primary procedure)

➔ *CPT Changes: An Insider's View* 2025

▶(Use 15012 in conjunction with 15011)◀

● **15013**   Preparation of skin cell suspension autograft, requiring enzymatic processing, manual mechanical disaggregation of skin cells, and filtration; first 25 sq cm or less of harvested skin

➔ *CPT Changes: An Insider's View* 2025

+● **15014**   each additional 25 sq cm of harvested skin or part thereof (List separately in addition to code for primary procedure)

➔ *CPT Changes: An Insider's View* 2025

▶(Use 15014 in conjunction with 15013)◀

● **15015**   Application of skin cell suspension autograft to wound and donor sites, including application of primary dressing, trunk, arms, legs; first 480 sq cm or less

➔ *CPT Changes: An Insider's View* 2025

+● **15016**   each additional 480 sq cm or part thereof (List separately in addition to code for primary procedure)

➔ *CPT Changes: An Insider's View* 2025

▶(Use 15016 in conjunction with 15015)◀

● **15017**   Application of skin cell suspension autograft to wound and donor sites, including application of primary dressing, face, scalp, eyelids, mouth, neck, ears, orbits, genitalia, hands, feet, and/or multiple digits; first 480 sq cm or less

➔ *CPT Changes: An Insider's View* 2025

+● **15018**   each additional 480 sq cm or part thereof (List separately in addition to code for primary procedure)

➔ *CPT Changes: An Insider's View* 2025

▶(Use 15018 in conjunction with 15017)◀

Autografts/Tissue Cultured Autograft

15040   Harvest of skin for tissue cultured skin autograft, 100 sq cm or less

➔ *CPT Changes: An Insider's View* 2006

➔ *CPT Assistant* Aug 06:10, Oct 06:1, Feb 08:3, Apr 10:3, Jan 12:6

15050   Pinch graft, single or multiple, to cover small ulcer, tip of digit, or other minimal open area (except on face), up to defect size 2 cm diameter

➔ *CPT Assistant* Apr 97:4, Sep 97:2, Nov 98:6, Jan 12:6, Jun 16:8

15100   Split-thickness autograft, trunk, arms, legs; first 100 sq cm or less, or 1% of body area of infants and children (except 15050)

➔ *CPT Changes: An Insider's View* 2002, 2006

➔ *CPT Assistant* Fall 93:7, Apr 97:4, Aug 97:6, Sep 97:3, Nov 98:6, Sep 02:3, Oct 06:1, Feb 08:3, Mar 11:9, Jan 12:6, Oct 12:3, Jun 16:8

+ 15101   each additional 100 sq cm, or each additional 1% of body area of infants and children, or part thereof (List separately in addition to code for primary procedure)

➔ *CPT Changes: An Insider's View* 2002

➔ *CPT Assistant* Apr 97:4, Nov 98:6, Sep 02:3, Feb 08:3, Mar 11:9, Jan 12:6, Oct 12:3, Jun 16:8

(Use 15101 in conjunction with 15100)

15110   Epidermal autograft, trunk, arms, legs; first 100 sq cm or less, or 1% of body area of infants and children

➔ *CPT Changes: An Insider's View* 2006

➔ *CPT Assistant* Feb 08:3, Mar 11:9, Jan 12:6, Oct 12:3

+ 15111   each additional 100 sq cm, or each additional 1% of body area of infants and children, or part thereof (List separately in addition to code for primary procedure)

➔ *CPT Changes: An Insider's View* 2006

➔ *CPT Assistant* Feb 08:3, Mar 11:9, Jan 12:6, Oct 12:3

(Use 15111 in conjunction with 15110)

15115   Epidermal autograft, face, scalp, eyelids, mouth, neck, ears, orbits, genitalia, hands, feet, and/or multiple digits; first 100 sq cm or less, or 1% of body area of infants and children

➔ *CPT Changes: An Insider's View* 2006

➔ *CPT Assistant* Feb 08:3, Mar 11:9, Jan 12:6, Oct 12:3

+ 15116   each additional 100 sq cm, or each additional 1% of body area of infants and children, or part thereof (List separately in addition to code for primary procedure)

➔ *CPT Changes: An Insider's View* 2006

➔ *CPT Assistant* Feb 08:3, Mar 11:9, Jan 12:6, Oct 12:3

(Use 15116 in conjunction with 15115)

15120 Split-thickness autograft, face, scalp, eyelids, mouth, neck, ears, orbits, genitalia, hands, feet, and/or multiple digits; first 100 sq cm or less, or 1% of body area of infants and children (except 15050)

➔ *CPT Changes: An Insider's View* 2002, 2006

➔ *CPT Assistant* Apr 97:4, Aug 97:6, Sep 97:3, Nov 98:6, Jan 99:4, Sep 02:3, Feb 08:3, Jul 08:5, Mar 11:9, Jan 12:6, Oct 12:3, Jun 16:8

+ 15121 each additional 100 sq cm, or each additional 1% of body area of infants and children, or part thereof (List separately in addition to code for primary procedure)

➔ *CPT Changes: An Insider's View* 2002

➔ *CPT Assistant* Apr 97:4, Aug 97:6, Sep 97:3, Nov 98:6, Jan 99:4, Sep 02:3, Feb 08:3, Mar 11:9, Jan 12:6, Oct 12:3, Jun 16:8

(Use 15121 in conjunction with 15120)

(For eyelids, see also 67961-67975)

15130 Dermal autograft, trunk, arms, legs; first 100 sq cm or less, or 1% of body area of infants and children

➔ *CPT Changes: An Insider's View* 2006

➔ *CPT Assistant* Feb 08:3, Mar 11:9, Jan 12:6, Oct 12:3

+ 15131 each additional 100 sq cm, or each additional 1% of body area of infants and children, or part thereof (List separately in addition to code for primary procedure)

➔ *CPT Changes: An Insider's View* 2006

➔ *CPT Assistant* Feb 08:3, Mar 11:9, Jan 12:6, Oct 12:3

(Use 15131 in conjunction with 15130)

15135 Dermal autograft, face, scalp, eyelids, mouth, neck, ears, orbits, genitalia, hands, feet, and/or multiple digits; first 100 sq cm or less, or 1% of body area of infants and children

➔ *CPT Changes: An Insider's View* 2006

➔ *CPT Assistant* Feb 08:3, Mar 11:9, Jan 12:6, Oct 12:3

+ 15136 each additional 100 sq cm, or each additional 1% of body area of infants and children, or part thereof (List separately in addition to code for primary procedure)

➔ *CPT Changes: An Insider's View* 2006

➔ *CPT Assistant* Mar 11:9, Jan 12:6, Oct 12:3

(Use 15136 in conjunction with 15135)

15150 Tissue cultured skin autograft, trunk, arms, legs; first 25 sq cm or less

➔ *CPT Changes: An Insider's View* 2006, 2012

➔ *CPT Assistant* Oct 06:1, Feb 08:3, Mar 11:9, Jan 12:6, Oct 12:3

+ 15151 additional 1 sq cm to 75 sq cm (List separately in addition to code for primary procedure)

➔ *CPT Changes: An Insider's View* 2006, 2012

➔ *CPT Assistant* Oct 06:1, Feb 08:3, Mar 11:9, Jan 12:6, Oct 12:3

(Do not report 15151 more than once per session)

(Use 15151 in conjunction with 15150)

+ 15152 each additional 100 sq cm, or each additional 1% of body area of infants and children, or part thereof (List separately in addition to code for primary procedure)

➔ *CPT Changes: An Insider's View* 2006, 2012

➔ *CPT Assistant* Oct 06:1, Feb 08:3, Mar 11:9, Jan 12:6, Oct 12:3

(Use 15152 in conjunction with 15151)

15155 Tissue cultured skin autograft, face, scalp, eyelids, mouth, neck, ears, orbits, genitalia, hands, feet, and/or multiple digits; first 25 sq cm or less

➔ *CPT Changes: An Insider's View* 2006, 2012

➔ *CPT Assistant* Oct 06:1, Feb 08:3, Mar 11:9, Jan 12:6, Oct 12:3

+ 15156 additional 1 sq cm to 75 sq cm (List separately in addition to code for primary procedure)

➔ *CPT Changes: An Insider's View* 2006, 2012

➔ *CPT Assistant* Oct 06:1, Feb 08:3, Mar 11:9, Jan 12:6, Oct 12:3

(Do not report 15156 more than once per session)

(Use 15156 in conjunction with 15155)

+ 15157 each additional 100 sq cm, or each additional 1% of body area of infants and children, or part thereof (List separately in addition to code for primary procedure)

➔ *CPT Changes: An Insider's View* 2006, 2012

➔ *CPT Assistant* Oct 06:1, Feb 08:3, Apr 10:3, Mar 11:9, Jan 12:6, Oct 12:3

(Use 15157 in conjunction with 15156)

15200 Full thickness graft, free, including direct closure of donor site, trunk; 20 sq cm or less

➔ *CPT Changes: An Insider's View* 2002

➔ *CPT Assistant* Aug 96:11, Aug 97:6, Sep 97:3, Feb 08:3, Mar 08:14, Jan 12:6, Oct 12:3, Jun 16:8

+ 15201 each additional 20 sq cm, or part thereof (List separately in addition to code for primary procedure)

➔ *CPT Changes: An Insider's View* 2002, 2009

➔ *CPT Assistant* Apr 97:4, Aug 97:6, Sep 97:3, Feb 08:3, Mar 08:14, Jan 12:6, Oct 12:3, Jun 16:8

(Use 15201 in conjunction with 15200)

15220 Full thickness graft, free, including direct closure of donor site, scalp, arms, and/or legs; 20 sq cm or less

➔ *CPT Changes: An Insider's View* 2002

➔ *CPT Assistant* Apr 97:4, Aug 97:6, Sep 97:3, Aug 98:9, Feb 08:3, Mar 08:14, Jan 12:6, Oct 12:3, Jun 16:8

+ 15221 each additional 20 sq cm, or part thereof (List separately in addition to code for primary procedure)

➔ *CPT Changes: An Insider's View* 2002, 2009

➔ *CPT Assistant* Apr 97:4, Aug 97:6, Sep 97:3, Aug 98:9, Feb 08:3, Mar 08:14, Jan 12:6, Oct 12:3, Jun 16:8

(Use 15221 in conjunction with 15220)

★ = Telemedicine ◀ = Audio-only ✚ = Add-on code ✗ = FDA approval pending # = Resequenced code ⊘ = Modifier 51 exempt ➔➔➔ = See p xxi for details

15240   Full thickness graft, free, including direct closure of donor site, forehead, cheeks, chin, mouth, neck, axillae, genitalia, hands, and/or feet; 20 sq cm or less
➔ *CPT Changes: An Insider's View* 2002
➔ *CPT Assistant* Apr 97:4, Aug 97:6, Sep 97:3, Nov 00:10, Feb 08:3, Mar 08:14, Jan 12:6, Oct 12:3, Jun 16:8

(For fingertip graft, use 15050)

(For repair of syndactyly, fingers, see 26560-26562)

+ **15241**   each additional 20 sq cm, or part thereof (List separately in addition to code for primary procedure)
➔ *CPT Changes: An Insider's View* 2002, 2009
➔ *CPT Assistant* Apr 97:4, Aug 97:6, Sep 97:3, Feb 08:3, Mar 08:14, Jan 12:6, Oct 12:3, Jun 16:8

(Use 15241 in conjunction with 15240)

15260   Full thickness graft, free, including direct closure of donor site, nose, ears, eyelids, and/or lips; 20 sq cm or less
➔ *CPT Changes: An Insider's View* 2002
➔ *CPT Assistant* Fall 91:7, Fall 93:7, Apr 97:4, Aug 97:6, Sep 97:3, Jul 99:3, Feb 08:3, Mar 08:14, Jan 12:6, Oct 12:3, Jun 16:8

+ **15261**   each additional 20 sq cm, or part thereof (List separately in addition to code for primary procedure)
➔ *CPT Changes: An Insider's View* 2002, 2009
➔ *CPT Assistant* Fall 91:7, Apr 97:4, Aug 97:6, Sep 97:3, Feb 08:3, Mar 08:14, Apr 10:3, Jan 12:6, Oct 12:3, Jun 16:8

(Use 15261 in conjunction with 15260)

(For eyelids, see also 67961-67975)

(Repair of donor site requiring skin graft or local flaps is considered a separate procedure)

Skin Substitute Grafts

The supply of skin substitute graft(s) should be reported separately in conjunction with 15271-15278. For biologic implant for soft tissue reinforcement, use 15777 in conjunction with code for primary procedure.

15271   Application of skin substitute graft to trunk, arms, legs, total wound surface area up to 100 sq cm; first 25 sq cm or less wound surface area
➔ *CPT Changes: An Insider's View* 2012
➔ *CPT Assistant* Jan 12:6, Oct 12:3, Jun 14:14, Oct 17:9, Aug 22:16, Feb 24:32

+ **15272**   each additional 25 sq cm wound surface area, or part thereof (List separately in addition to code for primary procedure)
➔ *CPT Changes: An Insider's View* 2012
➔ *CPT Assistant* Jan 12:6, Oct 12:3, Oct 13:15, Jun 14:14

(Use 15272 in conjunction with 15271)

(For total wound surface area greater than or equal to 100 sq cm, see 15273, 15274)

(Do not report 15271, 15272 in conjunction with 15273, 15274)

15273   Application of skin substitute graft to trunk, arms, legs, total wound surface area greater than or equal to 100 sq cm; first 100 sq cm wound surface area, or 1% of body area of infants and children
➔ *CPT Changes: An Insider's View* 2012
➔ *CPT Assistant* Jan 12:6, Oct 12:3, Oct 13:15, Nov 13:14, Jun 14:14

+ **15274**   each additional 100 sq cm wound surface area, or part thereof, or each additional 1% of body area of infants and children, or part thereof (List separately in addition to code for primary procedure)
➔ *CPT Changes: An Insider's View* 2012
➔ *CPT Assistant* Jan 12:6, Oct 12:3, Oct 13:15, Nov 13:14, Jun 14:14

(Use 15274 in conjunction with 15273)

(For total wound surface area up to 100 sq cm, see 15271, 15272)

15275   Application of skin substitute graft to face, scalp, eyelids, mouth, neck, ears, orbits, genitalia, hands, feet, and/or multiple digits, total wound surface area up to 100 sq cm; first 25 sq cm or less wound surface area
➔ *CPT Changes: An Insider's View* 2012
➔ *CPT Assistant* Jan 12:6, Oct 12:3, Oct 13:15, Jun 14:14

+ **15276**   each additional 25 sq cm wound surface area, or part thereof (List separately in addition to code for primary procedure)
➔ *CPT Changes: An Insider's View* 2012
➔ *CPT Assistant* Jan 12:6, Oct 12:3, Oct 13:15, Jun 14:14

(Use 15276 in conjunction with 15275)

(For total wound surface area greater than or equal to 100 sq cm, see 15277, 15278)

(Do not report 15275, 15276 in conjunction with 15277, 15278)

15277   Application of skin substitute graft to face, scalp, eyelids, mouth, neck, ears, orbits, genitalia, hands, feet, and/or multiple digits, total wound surface area greater than or equal to 100 sq cm; first 100 sq cm wound surface area, or 1% of body area of infants and children
➔ *CPT Changes: An Insider's View* 2012
➔ *CPT Assistant* Jan 12:6, Oct 12:3, Oct 13:15, Nov 13:14, Jun 14:14

+ **15278**   each additional 100 sq cm wound surface area, or part thereof, or each additional 1% of body area of infants and children, or part thereof (List separately in addition to code for primary procedure)
➔ *CPT Changes: An Insider's View* 2012
➔ *CPT Assistant* Jan 12:6, Oct 12:3, Oct 13:15, Nov 13:14, Jun 14:14, Aug 22:16

(Use 15278 in conjunction with 15277)

(For total wound surface area up to 100 sq cm, see 15275, 15276)

(Do not report 15271-15278 in conjunction with 97602)

Flaps (Skin and/or Deep Tissues)

The regions listed refer to the recipient area (not the donor site) when a flap is being attached in a transfer or to a final site.

The regions listed refer to a donor site when a tube is formed for later transfer or when a "delay" of flap occurs prior to the transfer. Codes 15733-15738 are described by donor site of the muscle, myocutaneous, or fasciocutaneous flap.

Codes 15570-15738 do not include extensive immobilization (eg, large plaster casts and other immobilizing devices are considered additional separate procedures).

A repair of a donor site requiring a skin graft or local flaps is considered an additional separate procedure.

(For microvascular flaps, see 15756-15758)

(For flaps without inclusion of a vascular pedicle, see 15570-15576)

(For adjacent tissue transfer flaps, see 14000-14302)

15570 Formation of direct or tubed pedicle, with or without transfer; trunk
➔ *CPT Assistant* Nov 02:7, Mar 10:4, Apr 10:3, Dec 12:6

15572 scalp, arms, or legs
➔ *CPT Assistant* Mar 10:4, Dec 12:6

15574 forehead, cheeks, chin, mouth, neck, axillae, genitalia, hands or feet
➔ *CPT Assistant* Mar 10:4, Dec 12:6

15576 eyelids, nose, ears, lips, or intraoral
➔ *CPT Assistant* Mar 10:4, Dec 12:6

15600 Delay of flap or sectioning of flap (division and inset); at trunk
➔ *CPT Assistant* Nov 99:10, Mar 10:4, Dec 12:6; Jun 19:14

15610 at scalp, arms, or legs
➔ *CPT Assistant* Mar 10:4, Dec 12:6

15620 at forehead, cheeks, chin, neck, axillae, genitalia, hands, or feet
➔ *CPT Assistant* Mar 10:4, Dec 12:6

15630 at eyelids, nose, ears, or lips
➔ *CPT Assistant* Mar 10:4, Dec 12:6

15650 Transfer, intermediate, of any pedicle flap (eg, abdomen to wrist, Walking tube), any location
➔ *CPT Assistant* Mar 10:4, Dec 12:6

(For eyelids, nose, ears, or lips, see also anatomical area)

(For revision, defatting or rearranging of transferred pedicle flap or skin graft, see 13100-14302)

15730 Midface flap (ie, zygomaticofacial flap) with preservation of vascular pedicle(s)
➔ *CPT Changes: An Insider's View* 2018
➔ *CPT Assistant* Nov 17:6, Apr 18:10

Midface Flap Surgery
15730

Midface muscles surrounding eye [skin and muscle flap procedures]

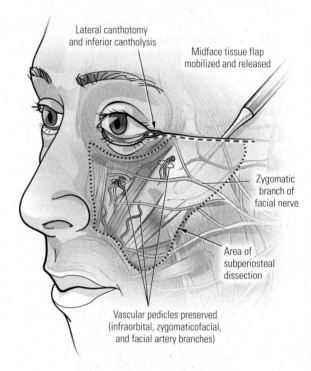

Lateral canthotomy and inferior cantholysis

Midface tissue flap mobilized and released

Zygomatic branch of facial nerve

Area of subperiosteal dissection

Vascular pedicles preserved (infraorbital, zygomaticofacial, and facial artery branches)

15731 Forehead flap with preservation of vascular pedicle (eg, axial pattern flap, paramedian forehead flap)
➔ *CPT Changes: An Insider's View* 2007
➔ *CPT Assistant* Dec 12:6, Nov 17:6

(For muscle, myocutaneous, or fasciocutaneous flap of the head or neck, use 15733)

15733 Muscle, myocutaneous, or fasciocutaneous flap; head and neck with named vascular pedicle (ie, buccinators, genioglossus, temporalis, masseter, sternocleidomastoid, levator scapulae)
➔ *CPT Changes: An Insider's View* 2018
➔ *CPT Assistant* Nov 17:6, Apr 18:10

(For forehead flap with preservation of vascular pedicle, use 15731)

(For anterior pericranial flap on named vascular pedicle, for repair of extracranial defect, use 15731)

(For repair of head and neck defects using non-axial pattern advancement flaps [including lesion] and/or repair by adjacent tissue transfer or rearrangement [eg, Z-plasty, W-plasty, V-Y plasty, rotation flap, random island flap, advancement flap], see 14040, 14041, 14060, 14061, 14301, 14302)

Axial Pattern Forehead Flap

15731

Reconstruction of a nasal defect with a forehead flap based on the left supratrochlear vessels

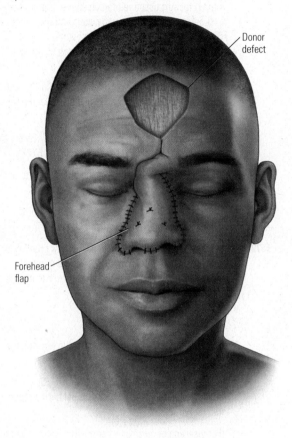

Donor defect

Forehead flap

15734   trunk
> *CPT Changes: An Insider's View* 2018
> *CPT Assistant* Dec 12:6, Oct 13:15, Apr 14:10, Nov 17:6, Aug 18:10, Jul 21:8, Jul 23:18

15736   upper extremity
> *CPT Changes: An Insider's View* 2018
> *CPT Assistant* Dec 12:6, Mar 13:13, Nov 17:6

15738   lower extremity
> *CPT Changes: An Insider's View* 2018
> *CPT Assistant* Sep 03:15, Apr 10:3, Dec 12:6, Nov 17:6

Other Flaps and Grafts

Code 15740 describes a cutaneous flap, transposed into a nearby but not immediately adjacent defect, with a pedicle that incorporates an anatomically named axial vessel into its design. The flap is typically transferred through a tunnel underneath the skin and sutured into its new position. The donor site is closed directly.

Neurovascular pedicle procedures are reported with 15750. This code includes not only skin but also a functional motor or sensory nerve(s). The flap serves to reinnervate a damaged portion of the body dependent on touch or movement (eg, thumb).

Repair of donor site requiring skin graft or local flaps should be reported as an additional procedure.

For random island flaps, V-Y subcutaneous flaps, advancement flaps, and other flaps from adjacent areas without clearly defined anatomically named axial vessels, see 14000-14302.

Code 15769 may be used to report autologous soft tissue grafts, such as fat, dermis, fascia, or other soft tissues, which are harvested from the patient using an excisional technique. The autologous soft tissue grafts are then placed into a defect during the same operation. Autologous grafts that are already defined in the CPT code set, including skin, bone, nerve, tendon, fascia lata or vessels, should be reported with the specific codes for each tissue type. For harvesting, preparation or injection(s) of platelet-rich plasma, use 0232T.

Codes 15771, 15772, 15773, 15774 may be used to report autologous fat grafting when the adipose cells are harvested via a liposuction technique, prepared with minimal manipulation, and then injected via cannula in multiple small aliquots to the defect. The regions listed refer to the recipient area (not the donor site). Volumes are based on total injectate. For multiple sites of injection, sum the total volume of injectate to anatomic sites that are grouped together into the same code descriptor. Do not report 11950, 11951, 11952, 11954 in conjunction with 15771, 15772, 15773, 15774, for the same anatomic site.

15740   Flap; island pedicle requiring identification and dissection of an anatomically named axial vessel
> *CPT Changes: An Insider's View* 2013
> *CPT Assistant* Mar 04:11, Sep 04:12, Oct 04:15, Apr 10:3, Dec 12:6, Dec 17:14, Mar 21:9

15750   neurovascular pedicle
> *CPT Assistant* Dec 17:14

15756 Free muscle or myocutaneous flap with microvascular anastomosis
➲ *CPT Changes: An Insider's View* 2003
➲ *CPT Assistant* Apr 97:5, Nov 97:12, Nov 98:6

(Do not report code 69990 in addition to code 15756)

15757 Free skin flap with microvascular anastomosis
➲ *CPT Assistant* Apr 97:5, Nov 98:6, Apr 16:8

(Do not report code 69990 in addition to code 15757)

15758 Free fascial flap with microvascular anastomosis
➲ *CPT Assistant* Apr 97:5, Nov 98:6

(Do not report code 69990 in addition to code 15758)

15760 Graft; composite (eg, full thickness of external ear or nasal ala), including primary closure, donor area
➲ *CPT Assistant* Sep 97:3

15769 Code is out of numerical sequence. See 15760-15772

15770 derma-fat-fascia
➲ *CPT Assistant* Sep 97:3, Apr 10:3, Oct 19:5, Jul 23:11

 # 15769 Grafting of autologous soft tissue, other, harvested by direct excision (eg, fat, dermis, fascia)
➲ *CPT Changes: An Insider's View* 2020
➲ *CPT Assistant* Oct 19:5, Dec 22:1, Jul 23:11

(For injection[s] of platelet-rich plasma, use 0232T)

15771 Grafting of autologous fat harvested by liposuction technique to trunk, breasts, scalp, arms, and/or legs; 50 cc or less injectate
➲ *CPT Changes: An Insider's View* 2020
➲ *CPT Assistant* Oct 19:5, Apr 20:10, Apr 21:5, Dec 22:1, Jul 23:11, Dec 23:37

(Report 15771 only once per session)

+ 15772 each additional 50 cc injectate, or part thereof (List separately in addition to code for primary procedure)
➲ *CPT Changes: An Insider's View* 2020
➲ *CPT Assistant* Oct 19:5, Apr 20:10, Apr 21:5, Dec 22:1, Jul 23:11, Dec 23:37

(Use 15772 in conjunction with 15771)

15773 Grafting of autologous fat harvested by liposuction technique to face, eyelids, mouth, neck, ears, orbits, genitalia, hands, and/or feet; 25 cc or less injectate
➲ *CPT Changes: An Insider's View* 2020
➲ *CPT Assistant* Oct 19:5, Dec 22:1, Jul 23:11, Dec 23:37

(Report 15773 only once per session)

+ 15774 each additional 25 cc injectate, or part thereof (List separately in addition to code for primary procedure)
➲ *CPT Changes: An Insider's View* 2020
➲ *CPT Assistant* Oct 19:5, Dec 22:1, Jul 23:11, Dec 23:37

(Use 15774 in conjunction with 15773)

(Do not report 15769, 15771, 15772, 15773, 15774 in conjunction with 15876, 15877, 15878, 15879, 0232T, 0481T, 0489T, 0490T)

(For injection[s], autologous white blood cell concentrate [autologous protein solution], any site, including image guidance, harvesting and preparation, when performed, use 0481T)

15775 Punch graft for hair transplant; 1 to 15 punch grafts
➲ *CPT Assistant* Sep 97:3

15776 more than 15 punch grafts
➲ *CPT Assistant* Sep 97:3

(For strip transplant, use 15220)

+ 15777 Implantation of biologic implant (eg, acellular dermal matrix) for soft tissue reinforcement (ie, breast, trunk) (List separately in addition to code for primary procedure)
➲ *CPT Changes: An Insider's View* 2012, 2014
➲ *CPT Assistant* Jan 12:10, Oct 13:15, Nov 19:14, Apr 21:5, Jan 22:17, Feb 22:13, Feb 23:13, Dec 23:37

(For implantation of biologic implants for soft tissue reinforcement in tissues other than breast and trunk, use 17999)

(For bilateral breast procedure, report 15777 twice. Do not report modifier 50 in conjunction with 15777)

(For topical application of skin substitute graft to a wound surface, see 15271-15278)

(The supply of biologic implant should be reported separately in conjunction with 15777)

15778 Implantation of absorbable mesh or other prosthesis for delayed closure of defect(s) (ie, external genitalia, perineum, abdominal wall) due to soft tissue infection or trauma
➲ *CPT Changes: An Insider's View* 2023
➲ *CPT Assistant* Sep 23:1

(For repair of anorectal fistula with plug [eg, porcine small intestine submucosa {SIS}], use 46707)

(For implantation of mesh or other prosthesis for anterior abdominal hernia repair or parastomal hernia repair, see 49591-49622)

(For insertion of mesh or other prosthesis for repair of pelvic floor defect, use 57267)

(For implantation of non-biologic or synthetic implant for fascial reinforcement of the abdominal wall, use 0437T)

Other Procedures

15780 Dermabrasion; total face (eg, for acne scarring, fine wrinkling, rhytids, general keratosis)
➲ *CPT Assistant* Apr 03:27

15781 segmental, face

15782   regional, other than face

15783   superficial, any site (eg, tattoo removal)
↪ *CPT Assistant* Apr 03:27

15786   Abrasion; single lesion (eg, keratosis, scar)

+ 15787   each additional 4 lesions or less (List separately in addition to code for primary procedure)

(Use 15787 in conjunction with 15786)

15788   Chemical peel, facial; epidermal

15789   dermal

15792   Chemical peel, nonfacial; epidermal

15793   dermal

▶(15819 has been deleted)◀

15820   Blepharoplasty, lower eyelid;
↪ *CPT Assistant* Feb 04:11, May 04:12, Feb 05:16

15821   with extensive herniated fat pad
↪ *CPT Assistant* Feb 04:11, May 04:12, Feb 05:16

15822   Blepharoplasty, upper eyelid;
↪ *CPT Assistant* Feb 04:11, May 04:12, Feb 05:16

15823   with excessive skin weighting down lid
↪ *CPT Assistant* Sep 00:7, Feb 04:11, May 04:12, Feb 05:16, Aug 11:8, Mar 21:11

(For bilateral blepharoplasty, add modifier 50)

15824   Rhytidectomy; forehead
↪ *CPT Assistant* Apr 17:9

(For repair of brow ptosis, use 67900)

15825   neck with platysmal tightening (platysmal flap, P-flap)
↪ *CPT Assistant* Apr 17:9

15826   glabellar frown lines

15828   cheek, chin, and neck

15829   superficial musculoaponeurotic system (SMAS) flap

(For bilateral rhytidectomy, add modifier 50)

15830   Excision, excessive skin and subcutaneous tissue (includes lipectomy); abdomen, infraumbilical panniculectomy
↪ *CPT Changes: An Insider's View* 2007

(Do not report 15830 in conjunction with 12031-12037, 13100-13102, 14000, 14001, 14302 for the same wound)

15832   thigh
↪ *CPT Assistant* May 22:15

15833   leg

15834   hip

15835   buttock

15836   arm

15837   forearm or hand

15838   submental fat pad

15839   other area

(For bilateral procedure, add modifier 50)

15840   Graft for facial nerve paralysis; free fascia graft (including obtaining fascia)
↪ *CPT Assistant* May 21:13

(For bilateral procedure, add modifier 50)

15841   free muscle graft (including obtaining graft)

15842   free muscle flap by microsurgical technique
↪ *CPT Changes: An Insider's View* 2001

(Do not report code 69990 in addition to code 15842)

15845   regional muscle transfer

(For intravenous fluorescein examination of blood flow in graft or flap, use 15860)

(For nerve transfers, decompression, or repair, see 64831-64876, 64905, 64907, 69720, 69725, 69740, 69745, 69955)

+ 15847   Excision, excessive skin and subcutaneous tissue (includes lipectomy), abdomen (eg, abdominoplasty) (includes umbilical transposition and fascial plication) (List separately in addition to code for primary procedure)
↪ *CPT Changes: An Insider's View* 2007

(Use 15847 in conjunction with 15830)

(For other abdominoplasty, use 17999)

(For inguinal hernia repair, see 49491-49525)

(For anterior abdominal hernia[s] repair, see 49591-49618)

(15850 has been deleted. To report, use 15851)

15851   Removal of sutures **or** staples requiring anesthesia (ie, general anesthesia, moderate sedation)
↪ *CPT Changes: An Insider's View* 2023
↪ *CPT Assistant* Spring 93:34, Nov 97:22, Mar 23:28

(Do not report 15851 for suture and/or staple removal to re-open a wound prior to performing another procedure through the same incision)

#+ 15853   Removal of sutures **or** staples not requiring anesthesia (List separately in addition to E/M code)
↪ *CPT Changes: An Insider's View* 2023
↪ *CPT Assistant* Mar 23:28, May 23:24, Jul 23:14

(Use 15853 in conjunction with 99202, 99203, 99204, 99205, 99211, 99212, 99213, 99214, 99215, 99281, 99282, 99283, 99284, 99285, 99341, 99342, 99344, 99345, 99347, 99348, 99349, 99350)

(Do not report 15853 in conjunction with 15854)

#+ 15854 Removal of sutures **and** staples not requiring anesthesia (List separately in addition to E/M code)

→ *CPT Changes: An Insider's View* 2023

→ *CPT Assistant* Mar 23:28, Jul 23:14

(Use 15854 in conjunction with 99202, 99203, 99204, 99205, 99211, 99212, 99213, 99214, 99215, 99281, 99282, 99283, 99284, 99285, 99341, 99342, 99344, 99345, 99347, 99348, 99349, 99350)

(Do not report 15854 in conjunction with 15853)

15852 Dressing change (for other than burns) under anesthesia (other than local)

15853 Code is out of numerical sequence. See 15851-15860

15854 Code is out of numerical sequence. See 15851-15860

15860 Intravenous injection of agent (eg, fluorescein) to test vascular flow in flap or graft

→ *CPT Changes: An Insider's View* 2002

→ *CPT Assistant* Oct 23:18, Dec 23:44

15876 Suction assisted lipectomy; head and neck

→ *CPT Assistant* Aug 19:10, May 22:15, Dec 22:1

15877 trunk

→ *CPT Assistant* Oct 99:10, Feb 05:14, Aug 19:10, May 22:15, Dec 22:1

15878 upper extremity

→ *CPT Assistant* Aug 19:10, May 22:15, Dec 22:1

15879 lower extremity

→ *CPT Assistant* Aug 19:10, May 22:15, Dec 22:1

(Do not report 15876, 15877, 15878, 15879 in conjunction with 15771, 15772, 15773, 15774, 0489T, 0490T)

(For harvesting of adipose tissue for autologous adipose-derived regenerative cell therapy, use 0489T)

(For autologous fat grafting harvested by liposuction technique, see 15771, 15772, 15773, 15774)

Pressure Ulcers (Decubitus Ulcers)

15920 Excision, coccygeal pressure ulcer, with coccygectomy; with primary suture

15922 with flap closure

15931 Excision, sacral pressure ulcer, with primary suture;

15933 with ostectomy

15934 Excision, sacral pressure ulcer, with skin flap closure;

15935 with ostectomy

15936 Excision, sacral pressure ulcer, in preparation for muscle or myocutaneous flap or skin graft closure;

→ *CPT Assistant* Nov 98:6-7

15937 with ostectomy

(For repair of defect using muscle or myocutaneous flap, use code(s) 15734 and/or 15738 in addition to 15936, 15937. For repair of defect using split skin graft, use codes 15100 and/or 15101 in addition to 15936, 15937)

15940 Excision, ischial pressure ulcer, with primary suture;

15941 with ostectomy (ischiectomy)

15944 Excision, ischial pressure ulcer, with skin flap closure;

15945 with ostectomy

15946 Excision, ischial pressure ulcer, with ostectomy, in preparation for muscle or myocutaneous flap or skin graft closure

→ *CPT Assistant* Nov 98:6-7, Jun 02:10, Jan 03:23

(For repair of defect using muscle or myocutaneous flap, use code(s) 15734 and/or 15738 in addition to 15946. For repair of defect using split skin graft, use codes 15100 and/or 15101 in addition to 15946)

15950 Excision, trochanteric pressure ulcer, with primary suture;

15951 with ostectomy

15952 Excision, trochanteric pressure ulcer, with skin flap closure;

15953 with ostectomy

15956 Excision, trochanteric pressure ulcer, in preparation for muscle or myocutaneous flap or skin graft closure;

→ *CPT Assistant* Nov 98:6-7

15958 with ostectomy

→ *CPT Assistant* Nov 98:6-7

(For repair of defect using muscle or myocutaneous flap, use code(s) 15734 and/or 15738 in addition to 15956, 15958. For repair of defect using split skin graft, use codes 15100 and/or 15101 in addition to 15956, 15958)

15999 Unlisted procedure, excision pressure ulcer

(For free skin graft to close ulcer or donor site, see 15002 et seq)

Burns, Local Treatment

Procedures 16000-16036 refer to local treatment of burned surface only. Codes 16020-16030 include the application of materials (eg, dressings) not described in codes 15100-15278.

List percentage of body surface involved and depth of burn.

For necessary related medical services (eg, hospital visits, detention) in management of burned patients, see appropriate services in **Evaluation and Management** and **Medicine** sections.

For the application of skin grafts or skin substitutes, see codes 15100-15777.

(For fractional ablative laser fenestration for functional improvement of traumatic or burn scars, see 0479T, 0480T)

16000 Initial treatment, first degree burn, when no more than local treatment is required

➔ *CPT Assistant* Aug 97:6, Oct 12:3

16020 Dressings and/or debridement of partial-thickness burns, initial or subsequent; small (less than 5% total body surface area)

➔ *CPT Changes: An Insider's View* 2006

➔ *CPT Assistant* Aug 97:6, Oct 12:3, Jan 24:37

16025 medium (eg, whole face or whole extremity, or 5% to 10% total body surface area)

➔ *CPT Changes: An Insider's View* 2006

➔ *CPT Assistant* Aug 97:6, Jun 08:14, Oct 12:3

16030 large (eg, more than 1 extremity, or greater than 10% total body surface area)

➔ *CPT Changes: An Insider's View* 2006

➔ *CPT Assistant* Aug 97:6, Jun 08:14, Oct 12:3

16035 Escharotomy; initial incision

➔ *CPT Changes: An Insider's View* 2001

➔ *CPT Assistant* Aug 97:6, Oct 12:3

+ 16036 each additional incision (List separately in addition to code for primary procedure)

➔ *CPT Changes: An Insider's View* 2001

➔ *CPT Assistant* Oct 12:3

(Use 16036 in conjunction with 16035)

(For debridement, curettement of burn wound, see 16020-16030)

Destruction

Destruction means the ablation of benign, premalignant or malignant tissues by any method, with or without curettement, including local anesthesia, and not usually requiring closure.

Any method includes electrosurgery, cryosurgery, laser and chemical treatment. Lesions include condylomata, papillomata, molluscum contagiosum, herpetic lesions, warts (ie, common, plantar, flat), milia, or other benign, premalignant (eg, actinic keratoses), or malignant lesions.

(For destruction of lesion(s) in specific anatomic sites, see 40820, 46900-46917, 46924, 54050-54057, 54065, 56501, 56515, 57061, 57065, 67850, 68135)

(For laser treatment for inflammatory skin disease, see 96920-96922)

(For paring or cutting of benign hyperkeratotic lesions (eg, corns or calluses), see 11055-11057)

(For sharp removal or electrosurgical destruction of skin tags and fibrocutaneous tags, see 11200, 11201)

(For cryotherapy of acne, use 17340)

(For initiation or follow-up care of topical chemotherapy (eg, 5-FU or similar agents), see appropriate office visits)

(For shaving of epidermal or dermal lesions, see 11300-11313)

(For excision of cicatricial lesion[s] [eg, full thickness excision, through the dermis], see 11400-11446)

(For incisional removal of burn scar, see 16035, 16036)

(For fractional ablative laser fenestration for functional improvement of traumatic or burn scars, see 0479T, 0480T)

Destruction, Benign or Premalignant Lesions

17000 Destruction (eg, laser surgery, electrosurgery, cryosurgery, chemosurgery, surgical curettement), premalignant lesions (eg, actinic keratoses); first lesion

➔ *CPT Changes: An Insider's View* 2002, 2007

➔ *CPT Assistant* Winter 90:3, Nov 97:12, Jun 99:10, May 06:19, Feb 07:10, Aug 09:7, Mar 10:10, Mar 12:7, May 12:13, Dec 17:14, Aug 21:3, Mar 22:14, Jan 24:37

+ 17003 second through 14 lesions, each (List separately in addition to code for first lesion)

➔ *CPT Assistant* Nov 97:12, Jun 99:10, May 06:19, Feb 07:10, Aug 09:7, Mar 10:10, Dec 17:14, Jan 24:37

(Use 17003 in conjunction with 17000)

(For destruction of common or plantar warts, see 17110, 17111)

17004 Destruction (eg, laser surgery, electrosurgery, cryosurgery, chemosurgery, surgical curettement), premalignant lesions (eg, actinic keratoses), 15 or more lesions

➔ *CPT Changes: An Insider's View* 2002, 2007, 2020

➔ *CPT Assistant* Nov 97:12, Nov 98:7, Jun 99:10, Mar 03:21, Feb 07:10, Aug 09:7, Mar 10:10, Dec 17:14

(Do not report 17004 in conjunction with 17000-17003)

17106 Destruction of cutaneous vascular proliferative lesions (eg, laser technique); less than 10 sq cm

➔ *CPT Assistant* Winter 90:3, Apr 07:11, Jun 08:14, Aug 09:7, Dec 17:14, Sep 19:10

17107 10.0 to 50.0 sq cm

➔ *CPT Assistant* Winter 90:3, Apr 07:11, Jun 08:14, Aug 09:7, Dec 17:14, Jan 23:29

17108 over 50.0 sq cm

➔ *CPT Assistant* Winter 90:3, Apr 07:11, Jun 08:14, Aug 09:7, Dec 17:14

Lund-Browder Diagram and Classification Method Table for Burn Estimations

The Lund-Browder Classification Method is used for estimating the extent, depth, and percentage of burns, allowing for the varying proportion of body surface in persons of different ages.

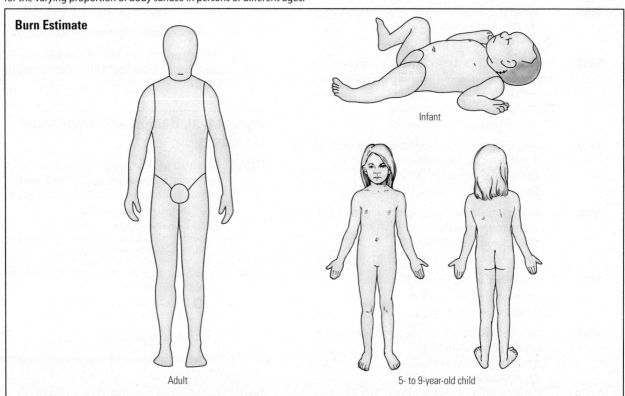

Burn Estimate

Adult

Infant

5- to 9-year-old child

Area	Birth 1 year	1-4 years	5-9 years	10-14 years	15 years	Adult	2 degrees	3 degrees	Total	Donor areas
Head	19	17	13	11	9	7				
Neck	2	2	2	2	2	2				
Ant. trunk	13	13	13	13	13	13				
Post. trunk	13	13	13	13	13	13				
R. buttock	2 1/2	2 1/2	2 1/2	2 1/2	2 1/2	2 1/2				
L. buttock	2 1/2	2 1/2	2 1/2	2 1/2	2 1/2	2 1/2				
Genitalia	1	1	1	1	1	1				
R. U. arm	4	4	4	4	4	4				
L. U. arm	4	4	4	4	4	4				
R. L. arm	3	3	3	3	3	3				
L. L. arm	3	3	3	3	3	3				
R. hand	2 1/2	2 1/2	2 1/2	2 1/2	2 1/2	2 1/2				
L. hand	2 1/2	2 1/2	2 1/2	2 1/2	2 1/2	2 1/2				
R. thigh	5 1/2	6 1/2	8	8 1/2	9	9 1/2				
L. thigh	5 1/2	6 1/2	8	8 1/2	9	9 1/2				
R. leg	5	5	5 1/2	6	6 1/2	7				
L. leg	5	5	5 1/2	6	6 1/2	7				
R. foot	3 1/2	3 1/2	3 1/2	3 1/2	3 1/2	3 1/2				
L. foot	3 1/2	3 1/2	3 1/2	3 1/2	3 1/2	3 1/2				
Total										

Destruction, Benign or Premalignant Lesions
17004

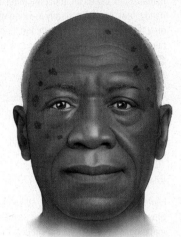

The lesions, seen as rough scaling patches scattered over the face, scalp, and ears, are destroyed by cryosurgery or other surgical means.

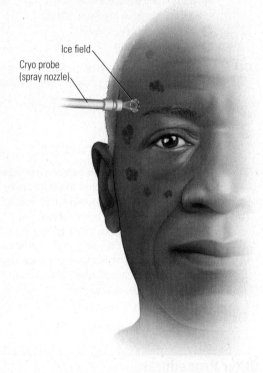

Ice field

Cryo probe (spray nozzle)

17110   Destruction (eg, laser surgery, electrosurgery, cryosurgery, chemosurgery, surgical curettement), of benign lesions other than skin tags or cutaneous vascular proliferative lesions; up to 14 lesions
➔ *CPT Changes: An Insider's View* 2002, 2007, 2008
➔ *CPT Assistant* Nov 97:13, Feb 07:10, Apr 07:11, Nov 08:10, Aug 09:7, Apr 16:3, Dec 17:14, Apr 20:10, Aug 22:16, Jan 23:29

17111   15 or more lesions
➔ *CPT Assistant* Nov 97:13, Feb 07:10, Apr 07:11, Nov 08:10, Aug 09:7, Apr 16:3, Dec 17:14, Aug 22:16

(For destruction of extensive cutaneous neurofibroma over 50-100 lesions, see 0419T, 0420T)

17250   Chemical cauterization of granulation tissue (ie, proud flesh)
➔ *CPT Changes: An Insider's View* 2018
➔ *CPT Assistant* May 12:13, Dec 12:15, Dec 17:14

(Do not report 17250 with removal or excision codes for the same lesion)

(Do not report 17250 when chemical cauterization is used to achieve wound hemostasis)

(Do not report 17250 in conjunction with 97597, 97598, 97602 for the same lesion)

Destruction, Malignant Lesions, Any Method

17260   Destruction, malignant lesion (eg, laser surgery, electrosurgery, cryosurgery, chemosurgery, surgical curettement), trunk, arms or legs; lesion diameter 0.5 cm or less
➔ *CPT Changes: An Insider's View* 2002
➔ *CPT Assistant* May 12:13, Dec 17:14

17261   lesion diameter 0.6 to 1.0 cm
➔ *CPT Assistant* Dec 17:14, Aug 21:3

17262   lesion diameter 1.1 to 2.0 cm
➔ *CPT Assistant* Dec 17:14

17263   lesion diameter 2.1 to 3.0 cm
➔ *CPT Assistant* Dec 17:14, Aug 23:16-19

17264   lesion diameter 3.1 to 4.0 cm
➔ *CPT Assistant* Dec 17:14

17266   lesion diameter over 4.0 cm
➔ *CPT Assistant* Dec 17:14

17270   Destruction, malignant lesion (eg, laser surgery, electrosurgery, cryosurgery, chemosurgery, surgical curettement), scalp, neck, hands, feet, genitalia; lesion diameter 0.5 cm or less
➔ *CPT Changes: An Insider's View* 2002
➔ *CPT Assistant* Dec 17:14

17271   lesion diameter 0.6 to 1.0 cm
➔ *CPT Assistant* Dec 17:14

17272   lesion diameter 1.1 to 2.0 cm
➔ *CPT Assistant* Dec 17:14

17273   lesion diameter 2.1 to 3.0 cm
➔ *CPT Assistant* Dec 17:14

17274   lesion diameter 3.1 to 4.0 cm
➔ *CPT Assistant* Dec 17:14

17276   lesion diameter over 4.0 cm
➔ *CPT Assistant* Dec 17:14

17280   Destruction, malignant lesion (eg, laser surgery, electrosurgery, cryosurgery, chemosurgery, surgical curettement), face, ears, eyelids, nose, lips, mucous membrane; lesion diameter 0.5 cm or less

> ➜ CPT Changes: An Insider's View 2002
> ➜ CPT Assistant Dec 17:14

17281   lesion diameter 0.6 to 1.0 cm

> ➜ CPT Assistant Dec 17:14, Aug 23:16-19

17282   lesion diameter 1.1 to 2.0 cm

> ➜ CPT Assistant Dec 17:14, Aug 23:16-19

17283   lesion diameter 2.1 to 3.0 cm

> ➜ CPT Assistant Dec 17:14

17284   lesion diameter 3.1 to 4.0 cm

> ➜ CPT Assistant Dec 17:14

17286   lesion diameter over 4.0 cm

> ➜ CPT Assistant Dec 17:14, Aug 21:3

Mohs Micrographic Surgery

Mohs micrographic surgery is a technique for the removal of complex or ill-defined skin cancer with histologic examination of 100% of the surgical margins. It requires the integration of an individual functioning in two separate and distinct capacities: surgeon and pathologist. If either of these responsibilities is delegated to another physician or other qualified health care professional who reports the services separately, these codes should not be reported. The Mohs surgeon removes the tumor tissue and maps and divides the tumor specimen into pieces, and each piece is embedded into an individual tissue block for histopathologic examination. Thus a tissue block in Mohs surgery is defined as an individual tissue piece embedded in a mounting medium for sectioning.

If repair is performed, use separate repair, flap, or graft codes. If a biopsy of a suspected skin cancer is performed on the same day as Mohs surgery because there was no prior pathology confirmation of a diagnosis, then report a diagnostic skin biopsy (11102, 11104, 11106) and frozen section pathology (88331) with modifier 59 to distinguish from the subsequent definitive surgical procedure of Mohs surgery.

> (If additional special pathology procedures, stains or immunostains are required, see 88311-88314, 88342)

> (Do not report 88314 in conjunction with 17311-17315 for routine frozen section stain (eg, hematoxylin and eosin, toluidine blue) performed during Mohs surgery. When a nonroutine histochemical stain on frozen tissue is utilized, report 88314 with modifier 59)

> (Do not report 88302-88309 on the same specimen as part of the Mohs surgery)

17311   Mohs micrographic technique, including removal of all gross tumor, surgical excision of tissue specimens, mapping, color coding of specimens, microscopic examination of specimens by the surgeon, and histopathologic preparation including routine stain(s) (eg, hematoxylin and eosin, toluidine blue), head, neck, hands, feet, genitalia, or any location with surgery directly involving muscle, cartilage, bone, tendon, major nerves, or vessels; first stage, up to 5 tissue blocks

> ➜ CPT Changes: An Insider's View 2007
> ➜ CPT Assistant Feb 14:10, Oct 14:14, Apr 23:24

+ 17312   each additional stage after the first stage, up to 5 tissue blocks (List separately in addition to code for primary procedure)

> ➜ CPT Changes: An Insider's View 2007
> ➜ CPT Assistant Apr 23:24

(Use 17312 in conjunction with 17311)

17313   Mohs micrographic technique, including removal of all gross tumor, surgical excision of tissue specimens, mapping, color coding of specimens, microscopic examination of specimens by the surgeon, and histopathologic preparation including routine stain(s) (eg, hematoxylin and eosin, toluidine blue), of the trunk, arms, or legs; first stage, up to 5 tissue blocks

> ➜ CPT Changes: An Insider's View 2007
> ➜ CPT Assistant Apr 23:24

+ 17314   each additional stage after the first stage, up to 5 tissue blocks (List separately in addition to code for primary procedure)

> ➜ CPT Changes: An Insider's View 2007
> ➜ CPT Assistant Apr 23:24

(Use 17314 in conjunction with 17313)

+ 17315   Mohs micrographic technique, including removal of all gross tumor, surgical excision of tissue specimens, mapping, color coding of specimens, microscopic examination of specimens by the surgeon, and histopathologic preparation including routine stain(s) (eg, hematoxylin and eosin, toluidine blue), each additional block after the first 5 tissue blocks, any stage (List separately in addition to code for primary procedure)

> ➜ CPT Changes: An Insider's View 2007
> ➜ CPT Assistant May 12:13, Feb 14:10, Oct 14:14, Apr 23:24

(Use 17315 in conjunction with 17311-17314)

Other Procedures

17340   Cryotherapy (CO_2 slush, liquid N_2) for acne

> ➜ CPT Assistant May 12:13

17360   Chemical exfoliation for acne (eg, acne paste, acid)

17380   Electrolysis epilation, each 30 minutes

(For actinotherapy, use 96900)

★ = Telemedicine   ◀ = Audio-only   + = Add-on code   ✗ = FDA approval pending   # = Resequenced code   ⊘ = Modifier 51 exempt   ➜➜➜ = See p xxi for details

17999   Unlisted procedure, skin, mucous membrane and subcutaneous tissue
➔ *CPT Assistant* Dec 98:9, May 99:11, Jun 05:11, Nov 08:10, Mar 11:9, May 12:13, Oct 13:15, May 16:13, Dec 17:13, Mar 19:10, Sep 19:10, May 21:13, Feb 22:13, Mar 22:12, Dec 23:37, Apr 24:34
➔ *Clinical Examples in Radiology* Winter 10:15

Breast

19000   Puncture aspiration of cyst of breast;
➔ *CPT Assistant* Fall 94:18, Apr 05:6, Nov 08:10, Dec 13:17, Apr 24:34

+ 19001   each additional cyst (List separately in addition to code for primary procedure)
➔ *CPT Assistant* Fall 94:18, Apr 05:6, Dec 13:17, Apr 24:34

(Use 19001 in conjunction with 19000)

(If imaging guidance is performed, see 76942, 77021)

19020   Mastotomy with exploration or drainage of abscess, deep
➔ *CPT Assistant* Apr 05:6, Dec 14:16, May 21:13

19030   Injection procedure only for mammary ductogram or galactogram
➔ *CPT Assistant* Jul 04:8, Apr 05:6
➔ *Clinical Examples in Radiology* Fall 22:6

(For radiological supervision and interpretation, see 77053, 77054)

Breast biopsy procedures may be performed via a percutaneous or open approach and with or without imaging guidance.

Percutaneous image-guided breast biopsies, including the placement of breast localization device(s), when performed, are reported with 19081, 19082, 19083, 19084, 19085, 19086. Imaging codes 76098, 76942, 77002, 77021 may not be separately reported for the same lesion. When more than one percutaneous breast biopsy with or without localization device placement is performed using the same imaging modality, use an add-on code whether the additional service(s) is on the same or contralateral breast. If additional percutaneous biopsies with or without localization device placements are performed using different imaging modalities, report another primary code for each additional biopsy with or without localization device placement performed using a different image guidance modality.

To report bilateral image-guided breast biopsies, report 19081, 19083, 19085 for the initial biopsy. The contralateral and each additional breast image-guided biopsy are then reported with 19082, 19084, 19086.

Percutaneous breast biopsies without imaging guidance are reported with 19100.

Open incisional breast biopsy (19101) does not include imaging guidance. However, if an open incisional biopsy is performed after image-guided placement of a localization device, the appropriate image-guided localization device placement code (19281, 19282, 19283, 19284, 19285, 19286, 19287, 19288) may also be reported.

Percutaneous cryosurgical ablation of a fibroadenoma (19105) includes ultrasound guidance and, therefore, 76940, 76942 may not be separately reported. Code 19105 may only be reported once per cryoprobe insertion site, even if several adjacent lesions are ablated.

Open excision of a breast lesion (eg, lesions of breast duct[s], cyst[s], benign or malignant tumor[s]), without specific attention to adequate surgical margins, with or without the preoperative placement of radiological markers are reported with 19110, 19112, 19120, 19125, 19126. If an open excision of a breast lesion is performed after image-guided placement of a localization device, the appropriate image-guided localization device placement code (19281, 19282, 19283, 19284, 19285, 19286, 19287, 19288) may also be reported.

To report bilateral procedures for 19100, 19101, 19105, 19110, 19112, 19120, report modifier 50 with the procedure code.

19081   Biopsy, breast, with placement of breast localization device(s) (eg, clip, metallic pellet), when performed, and imaging of the biopsy specimen, when performed, percutaneous; first lesion, including stereotactic guidance
➔ *CPT Changes: An Insider's View* 2014
➔ *CPT Assistant* May 14:3, Jun 14:14, Mar 15:5, May 15:8, Jun 16:3
➔ *Clinical Examples in Radiology* Spring 14:4, 10, Winter 17:5, Summer 21:12, Spring 23:10

+ 19082   each additional lesion, including stereotactic guidance (List separately in addition to code for primary procedure)
➔ *CPT Changes: An Insider's View* 2014
➔ *CPT Assistant* May 14:3, Jun 14:14, Mar 15:5, May 15:8, Jun 16:3
➔ *Clinical Examples in Radiology* Winter 17:5, Spring 23:10

(Use 19082 in conjunction with 19081)

19083 Biopsy, breast, with placement of breast localization device(s) (eg, clip, metallic pellet), when performed, and imaging of the biopsy specimen, when performed, percutaneous; first lesion, including ultrasound guidance

➜ *CPT Changes: An Insider's View* 2014

➜ *CPT Assistant* May 14:3, Jun 14:14, Mar 15:5, May 15:8, Jun 16:3

➜ *Clinical Examples in Radiology* Spring 14:2-3, Winter 17:5, Spring 18:13, Spring 23:10

+ 19084 each additional lesion, including ultrasound guidance (List separately in addition to code for primary procedure)

➜ *CPT Changes: An Insider's View* 2014

➜ *CPT Assistant* May 14:3, Jun 14:14, Mar 15:5, May 15:8, Jun 16:3

➜ *Clinical Examples in Radiology* Spring 14:10, Winter 17:5, Spring 23:10

(Use 19084 in conjunction with 19083)

19085 Biopsy, breast, with placement of breast localization device(s) (eg, clip, metallic pellet), when performed, and imaging of the biopsy specimen, when performed, percutaneous; first lesion, including magnetic resonance guidance

➜ *CPT Changes: An Insider's View* 2014

➜ *CPT Assistant* May 14:3, Jun 14:14, Mar 15:5, May 15:8, Jun 16:3

➜ *Clinical Examples in Radiology* Winter 17:5, Spring 23:10

+ 19086 each additional lesion, including magnetic resonance guidance (List separately in addition to code for primary procedure)

➜ *CPT Changes: An Insider's View* 2014

➜ *CPT Assistant* May 14:3, Jun 14:14, Mar 15:5, May 15:8, Jun 16:3

➜ *Clinical Examples in Radiology* Spring 14:4, Winter 17:5

(Use 19086 in conjunction with 19085)

(Do not report 19081-19086 in conjunction with 19281-19288, 76098, 76942, 77002, 77021 for same lesion)

19100 Biopsy of breast; percutaneous, needle core, not using imaging guidance (separate procedure)

➜ *CPT Changes: An Insider's View* 2001

➜ *CPT Assistant* Spring 93:35, Fall 94:18, Apr 96:8, Mar 97:4, Nov 97:24, Nov 98:7, Jan 01:10, May 02:18, Apr 05:6, Dec 06:10, Nov 08:10, May 14:3

➜ *Clinical Examples in Radiology* Fall 10:3, Spring 14:10, Winter 17:5, Spring 23:11

(For fine needle aspiration biopsy, see 10004, 10005, 10006, 10007, 10008, 10009, 10010, 10011, 10012, 10021)

19101 open, incisional

➜ *CPT Changes: An Insider's View* 2001

➜ *CPT Assistant* Spring 93:35, Fall 94:19, Nov 97:24, Jan 01:8, May 02:18, Apr 05:6, May 14:3, May 21:13

➜ *Clinical Examples in Radiology* Spring 14:10

(For placement of percutaneous localization clip with imaging guidance, see 19281-19288)

19105 Ablation, cryosurgical, of fibroadenoma, including ultrasound guidance, each fibroadenoma

➜ *CPT Changes: An Insider's View* 2007

(Do not report 19105 in conjunction with 76940, 76942)

(For cryoablation of malignant breast tumor[s], use 0581T)

(For adjacent lesions treated with 1 cryoprobe insertion, report once)

19110 Nipple exploration, with or without excision of a solitary lactiferous duct or a papilloma lactiferous duct

➜ *CPT Assistant* Apr 05:6

19112 Excision of lactiferous duct fistula

➜ *CPT Assistant* Apr 05:6

19120 Excision of cyst, fibroadenoma, or other benign or malignant tumor, aberrant breast tissue, duct lesion, nipple or areolar lesion (except 19300), open, male or female, 1 or more lesions

➜ *CPT Changes: An Insider's View* 2001, 2007

➜ *CPT Assistant* Feb 96:9, Nov 97:14, Jan 01:8, May 01:10, Apr 05:6, 13, Mar 14:13, Mar 15:5

19125 Excision of breast lesion identified by preoperative placement of radiological marker, open; single lesion

➜ *CPT Changes: An Insider's View* 2001

➜ *CPT Assistant* Fall 94:18, Mar 98:10, Jan 01:8, Apr 05:6, Mar 09:10, Mar 15:5

+ 19126 each additional lesion separately identified by a preoperative radiological marker (List separately in addition to code for primary procedure)

➜ *CPT Changes: An Insider's View* 2001

➜ *CPT Assistant* Fall 94:18, Mar 98:10, Jan 01:8, Apr 05:6

(Use 19126 in conjunction with 19125)

(Intraoperative placement of clip[s] is not separately reported)

Introduction

Percutaneous image-guided placement of breast localization device(s) without image-guided breast biopsy(ies) is reported with 19281, 19282, 19283, 19284, 19285, 19286, 19287, 19288. When more than one localization device placement without image-guided biopsy is performed using the same imaging modality, report an add-on code whether the additional service(s) is on the same or contralateral breast. If additional localization device placements without image-guided biopsy(ies) are performed using different imaging modalities, report another primary code for each additional localization device placement without image-guided biopsy performed using a different image guidance modality.

To report bilateral image-guided placement of localization devices report 19281, 19283, 19285, or 19287 for the initial lesion localized. The contra-lateral and each additional breast image-guided localization device placement is reported with code 19282, 19284, 19286 or 19288.

When an open breast biopsy or open excision of a breast lesion is performed after image-guided percutaneous placement of a localization device, the appropriate image-guided localization device placement code (19281, 19282, 19283, 19284, 19285, 19286, 19287, 19288) may also be reported.

Code 19294 is used to report the preparation of the tumor cavity with placement of an intraoperative radiation therapy applicator concurrent with partial mastectomy (19301, 19302).

Codes 19296, 19297, 19298 describe placement of radiotherapy catheters (afterloading expandable or afterloading brachytherapy) into the breast for interstitial radioelement application either concurrent or on a separate date from a partial mastectomy procedure. Imaging guidance is included and may not be separately reported.

19281   Placement of breast localization device(s) (eg, clip, metallic pellet, wire/needle, radioactive seeds), percutaneous; first lesion, including mammographic guidance

➔ *CPT Changes: An Insider's View* 2014

➔ *CPT Assistant* May 14:3, Jun 14:14, May 15:8, Jun 16:3, May 21:11

➔ *Clinical Examples in Radiology* Spring 14:8, Spring 18:3

+ 19282   each additional lesion, including mammographic guidance (List separately in addition to code for primary procedure)

➔ *CPT Changes: An Insider's View* 2014

➔ *CPT Assistant* May 14:3, Jun 14:14, May 15:8, Jun 16:3, May 21:11

➔ *Clinical Examples in Radiology* Spring 18:3

(Use 19282 in conjunction with 19281)

19283   Placement of breast localization device(s) (eg, clip, metallic pellet, wire/needle, radioactive seeds), percutaneous; first lesion, including stereotactic guidance

➔ *CPT Changes: An Insider's View* 2014

➔ *CPT Assistant* May 14:3, May 15:8, May 16:13, Jun 16:3, May 21:11

➔ *Clinical Examples in Radiology* Spring 18:3

+ 19284   each additional lesion, including stereotactic guidance (List separately in addition to code for primary procedure)

➔ *CPT Changes: An Insider's View* 2014

➔ *CPT Assistant* May 14:3, May 15:8, May 16:13, Jun 16:3, May 21:11

➔ *Clinical Examples in Radiology* Spring 18:3

(Use 19284 in conjunction with 19283)

19285   Placement of breast localization device(s) (eg, clip, metallic pellet, wire/needle, radioactive seeds), percutaneous; first lesion, including ultrasound guidance

➔ *CPT Changes: An Insider's View* 2014

➔ *CPT Assistant* May 14:3, May 15:8, May 16:13, Jun 16:3, May 21:11

➔ *Clinical Examples in Radiology* Spring 18:3

+ 19286   each additional lesion, including ultrasound guidance (List separately in addition to code for primary procedure)

➔ *CPT Changes: An Insider's View* 2014

➔ *CPT Assistant* May 14:3, May 15:8, May 16:13, Jun 16:3, May 21:11

➔ *Clinical Examples in Radiology* Spring 18:3

(Use 19286 in conjunction with 19285)

19287   Placement of breast localization device(s) (eg clip, metallic pellet, wire/needle, radioactive seeds), percutaneous; first lesion, including magnetic resonance guidance

➔ *CPT Changes: An Insider's View* 2014

➔ *CPT Assistant* May 14:3, May 16:13, Jun 16:3, May 21:11

➔ *Clinical Examples in Radiology* Spring 18:3

+ 19288   each additional lesion, including magnetic resonance guidance (List separately in addition to code for primary procedure)

➔ *CPT Changes: An Insider's View* 2014

➔ *CPT Assistant* May 14:3, May 16:13, Jun 16:3, May 21:11

➔ *Clinical Examples in Radiology* Spring 14:8, Spring 18:3

(Use 19288 in conjunction with 19287)

(Do not report 19281-19288 in conjunction with 19081-19086, 76942, 77002, 77021 for same lesion)

(For surgical specimen radiography, use 76098)

(To report image-guided placement of breast localization devices during image-guided biopsy, see 19081-19086. To report image-guided placement of breast localization devices without image-guided biopsy, see 19281-19288)

Integumentary 10004-19499

+ 19294   Preparation of tumor cavity, with placement of a radiation therapy applicator for intraoperative radiation therapy (IORT) concurrent with partial mastectomy (List separately in addition to code for primary procedure)

➔ *CPT Changes: An Insider's View* 2018

(Use 19294 in conjunction with 19301, 19302)

19296   Placement of radiotherapy afterloading expandable catheter (single or multichannel) into the breast for interstitial radioelement application following partial mastectomy, includes imaging guidance; on date separate from partial mastectomy

➔ *CPT Changes: An Insider's View* 2005, 2009

➔ *CPT Assistant* Apr 05:6, 8, Nov 05:15, Apr 09:3, Dec 09:9, Mar 10:10

+ 19297   concurrent with partial mastectomy (List separately in addition to code for primary procedure)

➔ *CPT Changes: An Insider's View* 2005, 2009

➔ *CPT Assistant* Apr 05:6, 8, Nov 05:15, Apr 09:3, Mar 10:10, Apr 19:10

(Use 19297 in conjunction with 19301 or 19302)

19298   Placement of radiotherapy after loading brachytherapy catheters (multiple tube and button type) into the breast for interstitial radioelement application following (at the time of or subsequent to) partial mastectomy, includes imaging guidance

➔ *CPT Changes: An Insider's View* 2005, 2017

➔ *CPT Assistant* Apr 05:6-7, 9, 16, Nov 05:15, Apr 09:3, Mar 10:10

Mastectomy Procedures

Mastectomy procedures (with the exception of gynecomastia [19300]) are performed either for treatment or prevention of breast cancer.

Code 19301 describes a partial mastectomy where only a portion of the ipsilateral breast tissue is removed (eg, lumpectomy, tylectomy, quadrantectomy, segmentectomy). When a complete axillary lymphadenectomy is performed in addition to a partial mastectomy, report 19302. When breast tissue is removed for breast-size reduction and not for treatment or prevention of breast cancer, report 19318 (reduction mammaplasty).

Code 19303 describes total removal of ipsilateral breast tissue with or without removal of skin and/or nipples (eg, nipple-sparing), for treatment or prevention of breast cancer. Code 19303 does not include excision of pectoral muscle(s) and/or axillary and internal mammary lymph nodes. When a total mastectomy is performed for gynecomastia, report 19300.

Codes 19305, 19306, 19307 describe radical procedures that include total removal of the ipsilateral breast tissue, including the nipple for treatment of breast cancer and excision of pectoral muscle(s) and/or axillary lymph nodes and/or internal mammary lymph nodes.

To report bilateral procedures for 19300, 19301, 19302, 19303, 19305, 19306, 19307, report modifier 50 with the procedure code.

19300   Mastectomy for gynecomastia

➔ *CPT Changes: An Insider's View* 2007

➔ *CPT Assistant* Feb 07:4, Mar 14:13, May 20:9

(For breast tissue removed for breast-size reduction for other than gynecomastia, use 19318)

19301   Mastectomy, partial (eg, lumpectomy, tylectomy, quadrantectomy, segmentectomy);

➔ *CPT Changes: An Insider's View* 2007

➔ *CPT Assistant* Feb 07:4, Dec 07:8, Sep 08:5, Mar 10:10, Nov 13:14, Mar 15:5, Oct 17:9, May 20:9, May 21:11

▶(For intraoperative assessment for abnormal [tumor] tissue, in-vivo, following partial mastectomy using computer-aided fluorescence imaging, use 19301 in conjunction with 0945T)◀

19302   with axillary lymphadenectomy

➔ *CPT Changes: An Insider's View* 2007

➔ *CPT Assistant* Feb 07:4, Dec 07:8, Sep 08:5, Mar 10:10, Mar 15:5, May 20:9, Nov 20:12, May 21:11

(For placement of radiotherapy afterloading balloon/ brachytherapy catheters, see 19296-19298)

(Intraoperative placement of clip[s] is not separately reported)

(For the preparation of tumor cavity with placement of an intraoperative radiation therapy applicator concurrent with partial mastectomy, use 19294)

(For radiofrequency spectroscopy, real time, intraoperative margin assessment, at the time of partial mastectomy, with report, use 0546T)

(For 3-dimensional volumetric specimen imaging, use 0694T)

19303   Mastectomy, simple, complete

➔ *CPT Changes: An Insider's View* 2007

➔ *CPT Assistant* Feb 07:4, Mar 15:5, Dec 19:4, May 20:9, May 21:11

(Intraoperative placement of clip[s] is not separately reported)

(For immediate or delayed insertion of implant, see 19340, 19342)

(For gynecomastia, use 19300)

(For breast tissue removed for breast-size reduction for gynecomastia, use 19300)

(For breast tissue removed for breast-size reduction for other than gynecomastia, use 19318)

19305 Mastectomy, radical, including pectoral muscles, axillary lymph nodes

➔ *CPT Changes: An Insider's View* 2007

➔ *CPT Assistant* Feb 07:4, Sep 08:5, May 20:9, May 21:11

(Intraoperative placement of clip[s] is not separately reported)

(For immediate or delayed insertion of implant, see 19340, 19342)

19306 Mastectomy, radical, including pectoral muscles, axillary and internal mammary lymph nodes (Urban type operation)

➔ *CPT Changes: An Insider's View* 2007

➔ *CPT Assistant* Feb 07:4, Sep 08:5, May 20:9, May 21:11

(Intraoperative placement of clip[s] is not separately reported)

(For immediate or delayed insertion of implant, see 19340, 19342)

19307 Mastectomy, modified radical, including axillary lymph nodes, with or without pectoralis minor muscle, but excluding pectoralis major muscle

➔ *CPT Changes: An Insider's View* 2007

➔ *CPT Assistant* Feb 07:4, Sep 08:5, Mar 15:5, May 20:9, May 21:11

(Intraoperative placement of clip[s] is not separately reported)

(For immediate or delayed insertion of implant, see 19340, 19342)

Repair and/or Reconstruction

Breast reconstruction is performed to repair defects due to congenital anomaly or loss of breast tissue after a surgical excision. The goal of breast reconstruction is to correct the anatomic defect and to restore form and breast symmetry. A breast can be reconstructed using a single technique or a combination of techniques, and each technique can stand alone. In addition, both breasts may be reconstructed at the same time, but may use different techniques or a combination of techniques. In many instances breast reconstruction requires more than one planned procedure or may require revisions.

The native breast may be altered using different techniques. The breast and breast mound can be lifted with a mastopexy (19316), reduced in volume with a breast reduction (19318), or augmented with a breast implant (19325).

Post-mastectomy breast reconstruction may be performed using a variety of techniques. An implant-based reconstruction involves placement of a device filled with fluid (eg, saline, silicone gel) to provide volume to the breast. In immediate reconstruction, an implant is primarily placed at the time of a mastectomy (19340). In delayed reconstruction, an implant is placed at any date separate from the mastectomy (19342). This includes

placement of any new implant or replacement of an existing implant within the mastectomy defect or reconstructed breast. The removal of an intact breast implant for replacement is included in 19342.

A breast implant cannot always be placed due to the lack of an adequate skin envelope. Code 19357 describes insertion of a tissue expander, which is a device that is surgically implanted to create an adequately sized pocket for subsequent insertion of a permanent implant. A tissue expander is an inflatable device placed beneath the skin and chest muscle, into which saline is injected over a period of weeks in the office to create the implant pocket. The tissue expander is eventually removed and may be replaced with a permanent breast implant (11970). Placement of either a breast implant (19340, 19342) or tissue expander (19357) may be reported separately when performed with flap reconstruction (19361, 19364, 19367, 19368, 19369).

Code 11970 describes the removal of a tissue expander with concurrent insertion of a permanent breast implant. Code 11970 includes removal of the expander, minor revisions to the breast capsule and placement of the new breast implant. Code 19370 may be reported in addition to 11970 if more extensive capsular revision is performed. Code 11971 describes the removal of a tissue expander without the replacement of an expander or implant.

Autologous breast reconstruction involves harvesting a flap of skin, subcutaneous fat and/or muscle from one area of the body and relocating the tissue to the anterior chest to create a new breast mound. Flap reconstruction may be performed at the time of mastectomy or in a delayed fashion depending on patient preference and other oncologic treatments.

Code 19361 describes breast reconstruction with a flap composed of the latissimus dorsi muscle including some of the overlying skin and subcutaneous fat to reconstruct the breast mound. This flap is left on its vascular pedicle and tunneled beneath the armpit skin to the anterior chest to rebuild the breast. The blood supply to the flap is left attached to its origin in the axilla. To give the breast mound additional volume, a tissue expander or permanent breast implant may be placed beneath the latissimus flap. Placement of either a breast implant (19340, 19342) or tissue expander (19357) may be reported separately.

Code 19364 describes a microsurgical free tissue transfer of skin and subcutaneous fat and/or muscle for breast reconstruction. This code includes the flap harvest, microsurgical anastomosis of one artery and two veins with use of an operating microscope, flap inset as a breast mound, and donor-site closure. Typical free flaps include free transverse rectus abdominis myocutaneous (fTRAM), deep inferior epigastric perforator (DIEP), superficial inferior epigastric artery (SIEA), or gluteal artery perforator (GAP) flaps.

Code 19367 describes a single-pedicled transverse rectus abdominis myocutaneous (TRAM) flap, in which skin, subcutaneous fat, and a large portion of the rectus abdominis muscle from the lower abdomen is moved beneath the upper abdominal wall skin up to the chest to rebuild the breast. The blood supply to the flap is left attached to its origin in the abdomen.

Code 19368 describes "supercharging" of a single-pedicled TRAM flap. This is typically performed to increase blood flow in TRAM flaps with marginal circulation to ensure flap survival. In addition to the standard unipedicle TRAM procedure, the inferior epigastric artery and/or veins are also anastomosed to recipient vessels in the chest using microsurgical techniques.

Code 19369 describes a bipedicled TRAM flap in which skin, subcutaneous fat, and both rectus muscles are harvested for the reconstruction of a single breast. The dual-blood supply to the flap is left attached to its origins in the abdomen.

Secondary and ancillary breast-reconstruction procedures include nipple reconstruction (19350), implant adjustments through revisions to the breast capsule (19370), or removal of the entire breast capsule via a complete capsulectomy (19371) to achieve correct breast tissue positioning. In addition, procedures may be performed on the contralateral breast to create symmetry (19316, 19318, 19325). Removal of an intact breast implant without replacement is reported with 19328. Removal of a ruptured breast implant, including the implant contents, is reported with 19330. A complete capsulectomy (19371) includes removal of the breast implant and all intracapsular contents.

Code 19380 describes a revision of a reconstructed breast, including significant excision of tissue re-advancement or re-inset of flaps. For autologous reconstruction, 19380 includes revisions of the flap position on the chest wall, removal of portions of the flap (via direct excision or liposuction), re-shaping of the flap, or scar revisions. However, if a limited procedure is performed with a defined code (eg, scar revision) then the more specific code should be used. The placement of a new implant (19342) or autologous fat grafting for increased volume (15771, 15772) may be separately reportable. For implant-based reconstruction, 19380 includes revisions to the skin and capsule when performed together. The exchange for a new or different size/shape/type of implant (19342) or autologous fat grafting for increased volume/contour irregularities (15771, 15772) may be reported

separately. Nipple reconstruction is reported with 19350 and includes local flaps (14000, 14001), areolar skin grafting (15100, 15200, 15201), and subsequent tattooing (11920, 11921, 11922).

Code 19396 describes the formation of a moulage cast of a patient's chest defect. The mold is used to fabricate a specific, custom-made implant that fits the patient's defect.

(To report bilateral procedure, report modifier 50 with the procedure code)

(For biologic implant for soft tissue reinforcement, use 15777 in conjunction with primary procedure)

19316 Mastopexy
➡ *CPT Assistant* Jan 03:7, Apr 05:6, Feb 12:11

19318 Breast reduction
➡ *CPT Changes: An Insider's View* 2021
➡ *CPT Assistant* Jan 03:7, Apr 05:6, Apr 14:10, Apr 21:3

19325 Breast augmentation with implant
➡ *CPT Changes: An Insider's View* 2021
➡ *CPT Assistant* Apr 05:6, Apr 21:3, Sep 22:18

(For fat grafting performed in conjunction with 19325, see 15771, 15772)

19328 Removal of intact breast implant
➡ *CPT Changes: An Insider's View* 2021
➡ *CPT Assistant* Apr 05:6, Apr 21:3

(Do not report 19328 for removal of tissue expander)

(Do not report 19328 in conjunction with 19370)

(For removal of tissue expander with placement of breast implant, use 11970)

(For removal of tissue expander without replacement, use 11971)

19330 Removal of ruptured breast implant, including implant contents (eg, saline, silicone gel)
➡ *CPT Changes: An Insider's View* 2021
➡ *CPT Assistant* Nov 01:11, Apr 05:6, Apr 21:3

(Do not report 19330 for removal of ruptured tissue expander)

(For removal of ruptured tissue expander with placement of breast implant, use 11970)

(For removal of ruptured tissue expander without replacement, use 11971)

(For placement of new breast implant during same operative session, use 19342)

19340   Insertion of breast implant on same day of mastectomy (ie, immediate)
→ *CPT Changes: An Insider's View* 2021
→ *CPT Assistant* Aug 96:8, Apr 05:6, Aug 05:1, Mar 10:9, Dec 15:18, Apr 21:3

19342   Insertion or replacement of breast implant on separate day from mastectomy
→ *CPT Changes: An Insider's View* 2021
→ *CPT Assistant* Aug 96:8, Apr 05:6, Aug 05:1, Jan 13:15, Nov 15:10, Apr 21:3, Sep 21:13-14, Sep 22:18, May 23:24

(Do not report 19342 in conjunction with 19328 for removal of implant in same breast)

(For removal of tissue expander and replacement with breast implant, use 11970)

(For supply of implant, use 99070)

19350   Nipple/areola reconstruction
→ *CPT Assistant* Aug 96:11, Apr 05:6, Jan 13:15, Aug 16:9

(Do not report 19350 in conjunction with 11920, 11921, 11922, 14000, 14001, 15100, 15200, 15201)

19355   Correction of inverted nipples
→ *CPT Assistant* Apr 05:6

19357   Tissue expander placement in breast reconstruction, including subsequent expansion(s)
→ *CPT Changes: An Insider's View* 2021
→ *CPT Assistant* Winter 91:2, Apr 05:6, Aug 05:1, Mar 10:9, Oct 13:15, Feb 15:10, Apr 21:3, Sep 22:18

19361   Breast reconstruction; with latissimus dorsi flap
→ *CPT Changes: An Insider's View* 2007, 2021
→ *CPT Assistant* Apr 05:6, Aug 05:1, Mar 10:9, Feb 15:10, Nov 19:14, Apr 21:3

(For insertion of breast implant with latissimus dorsi flap on same day of mastectomy, use 19340)

(For insertion of breast implant with latissimus dorsi flap on day separate from mastectomy, use 19342)

(For insertion of tissue expander with latissimus dorsi flap, use 19357)

19364   with free flap (eg, fTRAM, DIEP, SIEA, GAP flap)
→ *CPT Changes: An Insider's View* 2021
→ *CPT Assistant* Aug 96:8, Nov 98:7, Apr 05:6, Aug 05:1, Jun 10:8, Dec 11:14, Jul 12:12, Mar 13:13, Apr 14:10, Feb 15:10, Nov 19:14, Dec 20:11, Jun 21:13

(Do not report code 69990 in addition to code 19364)

19367   with single-pedicled transverse rectus abdominis myocutaneous (TRAM) flap
→ *CPT Changes: An Insider's View* 2021
→ *CPT Assistant* Nov 98:7, Apr 05:6, Aug 05:1, Feb 15:10, Nov 19:14, Apr 21:4

19368   with single-pedicled transverse rectus abdominis myocutaneous (TRAM) flap, requiring separate microvascular anastomosis (supercharging)
→ *CPT Changes: An Insider's View* 2021
→ *CPT Assistant* Nov 98:7, Apr 05:6, Aug 05:1, Feb 15:10, Nov 19:14, Apr 21:4

(Do not report code 69990 in addition to code 19368)

19369   with bipedicled transverse rectus abdominis myocutaneous (TRAM) flap
→ *CPT Changes: An Insider's View* 2021
→ *CPT Assistant* Oct 00:3, Apr 05:6, Aug 05:1, Feb 15:10, Nov 19:14, Apr 21:4

(19361, 19364, 19367, 19368, 19369 include harvesting of the flap, closure of the donor site, insetting and shaping the flap)

19370   Revision of peri-implant capsule, breast, including capsulotomy, capsulorrhaphy, and/or partial capsulectomy
→ *CPT Changes: An Insider's View* 2021
→ *CPT Assistant* Aug 96:8, Apr 05:6, Dec 15:18, Apr 21:4, Sep 21:13, Sep 22:18

(Do not report 19370 in conjunction with 19328 for removal and replacement of same implant to access capsule)

(For removal and replacement with new implant, use 19342)

19371   Peri-implant capsulectomy, breast, complete, including removal of all intracapsular contents
→ *CPT Changes: An Insider's View* 2021
→ *CPT Assistant* Aug 96:8, Nov 01:11, Apr 05:6, Jan 13:15, Apr 21:5

(Do not report 19371 in conjunction with 19328, 19330)

(Do not report 19371 in conjunction with 19370 in same breast)

(For removal and replacement with new implant, use 19342)

19380   Revision of reconstructed breast (eg, significant removal of tissue, re-advancement and/or re-inset of flaps in autologous reconstruction or significant capsular revision combined with soft tissue excision in implant-based reconstruction)
→ *CPT Changes: An Insider's View* 2021
→ *CPT Assistant* Apr 05:6, Dec 15:18, Dec 17:13, Nov 19:14, Apr 21:4, Sep 21:13-14, Sep 22:18, May 23:24

(Do not report 19380 in conjunction with 12031, 12032, 12034, 12035, 12036, 12037, 13100, 13101, 13102, 15877, 19316, 19318, 19370, for the same breast)

19396   Preparation of moulage for custom breast implant
→ *CPT Assistant* Jan 03:7, Apr 05:6

Other Procedures

19499   Unlisted procedure, breast
→ *CPT Assistant* Apr 05:6, Dec 09:9, Nov 13:14, Dec 14:16, Dec 16:16, Apr 19:10, Aug 19:10, Feb 22:13, Oct 23:18
→ *Clinical Examples in Radiology* Fall 08:4, Summer 09:15

Notes

Surgery

The following is a listing of headings and subheadings that appear within the Musculoskeletal System section of the CPT codebook. The subheadings or subsections denoted with asterisks (*) below have special instructions unique to that subsection. Where these are indicated, special notes or guidelines will be presented preceding those procedural terminology listings, referring to that subsection specifically. Note that all code ranges in each subsection are listed as they appear in the subsection, even if the code numbers are out of numerical sequence and/or repeated in the next subsection.

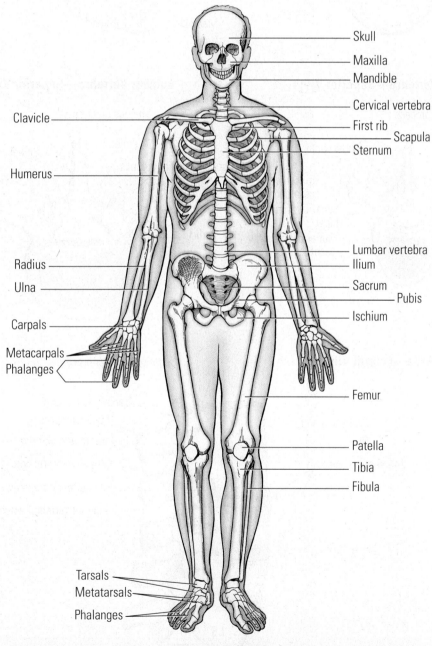

Skeletal System

Skull, Frontal View

Parietal bone

Temporal bone

Sphenoid bone

Zygomatic bone

Maxilla

Mandible

Frontal bone

Nasal bone

Skull, Lateral View

Frontal bone

Nasal bone

Zygomatic bone

Maxilla bone

Mandible

Parietal bone

Occipital bone

Temporal bone

Temporomandibul joint

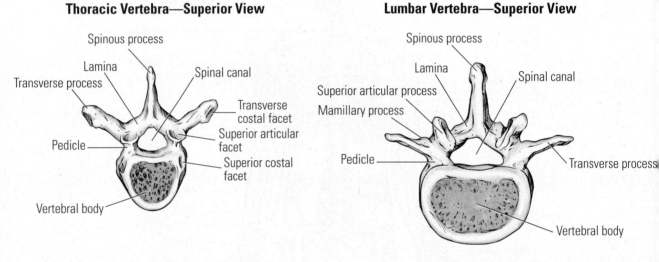

Thoracic Vertebra—Superior View

Spinous process

Lamina

Transverse process

Pedicle

Vertebral body

Spinal canal

Transverse costal facet

Superior articular facet

Superior costal facet

Lumbar Vertebra—Superior View

Spinous process

Lamina

Superior articular process

Mamillary process

Pedicle

Spinal canal

Transverse process

Vertebral body

Lumbar Vertebrae—Lateral View

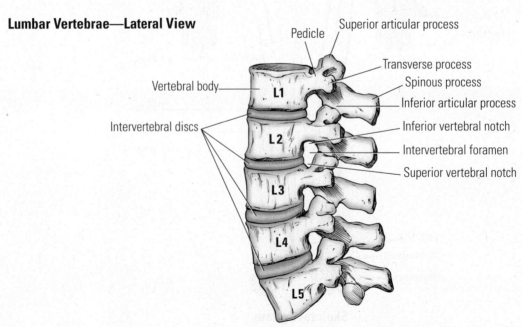

Pedicle

Superior articular process

Vertebral body

Intervertebral discs

L 1

L 2

L 3

L 4

L 5

Transverse process

Spinous process

Inferior articular process

Inferior vertebral notch

Intervertebral foramen

Superior vertebral notch

Bones, Muscles, and Tendons of Hand

Musculoskeletal 20100-29999

Bones and Muscles of Foot

Musculoskeletal 20100-29999

Musculoskeletal 20100-29999

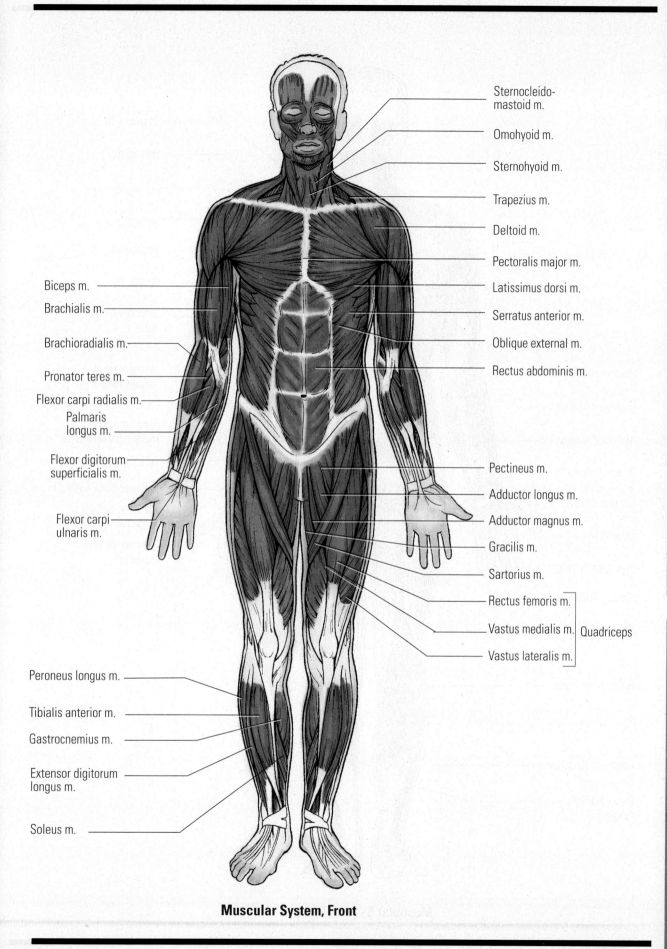

Sternocleido-
mastoid m.

Omohyoid m.

Sternohyoid m.

Trapezius m.

Deltoid m.

Pectoralis major m.

Biceps m.

Brachialis m.

Latissimus dorsi m.

Serratus anterior m.

Brachioradialis m.

Oblique external m.

Pronator teres m.

Rectus abdominis m.

Flexor carpi radialis m.

Palmaris
longus m.

Flexor digitorum
superficialis m.

Pectineus m.

Adductor longus m.

Adductor magnus m.

Flexor carpi
ulnaris m.

Gracilis m.

Sartorius m.

Rectus femoris m.

Vastus medialis m.   Quadriceps

Vastus lateralis m.

Peroneus longus m.

Tibialis anterior m.

Gastrocnemius m.

Extensor digitorum
longus m.

Soleus m.

Muscular System, Front

Trapezius m.

Deltoid m.

Infraspinatus m.

Teres minor m.

Teres major m.

Triceps m.

Latissimus dorsi m.

Anconeus m.

Extensor carpi radialis longus m.

Flexor carpi ulnaris m.

Extensor carpi radialis brevis m.

Extensor digitorum m.

Extensor carpi ulnaris m.

Abductor pollicis longus m.

Extensor pollicis brevis m.

Gluteus medius m.

Gluteus maximus m.

Adductor magnus m.

Biceps femoris m.

Semitendinosus m.

Gracilis m.

Semimembranosus m.

Vastus lateralis m.

Sartorius m.

Gastrocnemius m.

Peroneus longus m.

Flexor hallucis longus m.

Muscular System, Back

Musculoskeletal System

All services that appear in the Musculoskeletal System section include the application and removal of the first cast, splint, or traction device, when performed. Supplies may be reported separately. If a cast is removed by someone other than the physician or other qualified health care professional who applied the cast, report a cast removal code (29700, 29705, 29710).

Subsequent replacement of cast, splint, or strapping (29000-29750) and/or traction device (eg, 20690, 20692) during or after the global period may be reported separately.

A cast, splint, or strapping is not considered part of the preoperative care; therefore, the use of modifier 56 for preoperative management only is not applicable.

Codes for obtaining autogenous bone grafts, cartilage, tendon, fascia lata grafts or other tissues through separate incisions are to be used only when the graft is not already listed as part of the basic procedure.

Fracture and/or Dislocation Treatment

Fracture and dislocation treatment codes appear throughout the Musculoskeletal System section. These codes are categorized by the type of treatment (closed, percutaneous, open) and type of stabilization (fixation, immobilization). There is no coding correlation between the type of fracture/dislocation (eg, open [compound], closed) and the type of treatment (eg, closed, percutaneous, open) provided. For example, a closed fracture may require open treatment.

Fracture/Dislocation Treatment Definitions

Manipulation: Reduction by the application of manually applied forces or traction to achieve satisfactory alignment of the fracture or dislocation. If satisfactory alignment (reduction) is not maintained and requires subsequent re-reduction of a fracture or dislocation by the same physician or same qualified health care professional, append modifier 76 to the fracture/dislocation treatment code.

Traction: The application of a distracting or traction force to the spine or a limb. *Skeletal traction* includes a wire, pin, screw, or clamp that is attached to (penetrates) bone. *Skin traction* is the application of force to a limb using strapping or a device that is applied directly to the skin only.

Closed treatment: The treatment site is not surgically opened (ie, not exposed to the external environment nor directly visualized). Closed treatment of a fracture/dislocation may be performed without manipulation (eg, application of cast, splint, or strapping), with manipulation, with skeletal traction, and/or with skin traction.

Casting, splinting, or strapping used solely to temporarily stabilize the fracture for patient comfort is not considered closed treatment.

Percutaneous skeletal fixation: Treatment that is neither open nor closed. In this procedure, the fracture fragments are not visualized, but fixation (eg, pins, screws) is placed across the fracture site, typically with imaging guidance.

Open treatment: The site is opened surgically to expose the fracture/dislocation to the external environment for treatment, or the fracture/dislocation is treated through the traumatic wound or an extension thereof or is treated with an intramedullary nail or other internal fixation device placed through a surgical exposure that is remote from the fracture site with or without direct visualization of the fracture site.

External fixation: The use of pins and/or wires that penetrate the bone(s) and interconnection devices (eg, clamps, bars, rings) for fracture/dislocation treatment. External fixation may be used for temporary or long-term fracture/dislocation treatment. *Uniplanar external fixation* places all the pins in approximately the same plane but may also include triangular fixation across a joint. *Multiplanar external fixation* uses transosseous wires and threaded pins placed in several planes that are held with interconnected stabilizing and/or tensioning rings and/or half rings. External fixation may be used for all types of fracture/dislocation treatment (ie, closed, percutaneous, open). Codes for external fixation are reported separately only when external fixation is not listed in the code descriptor as inherent to the procedure.

Reporting Fracture and/or Dislocation Treatment Codes

The physician or other qualified health care professional providing fracture/dislocation treatment should report the appropriate fracture/dislocation treatment codes for the service he or she provided. If the person providing the initial treatment will **not** be providing subsequent treatment, modifier 54 should be appended to the fracture/dislocation treatment codes. If treatment of a fracture as defined above is not performed, report an evaluation and management code.

Excision/Resection Soft Tissue Tumors Definitions

Excision of subcutaneous soft connective tissue tumors (including simple or intermediate repair) involves the simple or marginal resection of tumors confined to subcutaneous tissue below the skin but above the deep fascia. These tumors are usually benign and are resected without removing a significant amount of surrounding normal tissue. Code selection is based on the location and size of the tumor. Code selection is determined by measuring the greatest diameter of the tumor plus that margin required for complete excision of the tumor. The margins refer to the most narrow margin required to adequately excise the tumor, based on the physician's judgment. The measurement of the tumor plus margin is made at the time of the excision. Appreciable vessel exploration and/or neuroplasty should be reported separately. Extensive undermining or other techniques to close a defect created by skin excision may require a complex repair which should be reported separately. Dissection or elevation of tissue planes to permit resection of the tumor is included in the excision. For excision of benign lesions of cutaneous origin (eg, sebaceous cyst), see 11400-11446.

Excision of fascial or subfascial soft tissue tumors (including simple or intermediate repair) involves the resection of tumors confined to the tissue within or below the deep fascia, but not involving the bone. These tumors are usually benign, are often intramuscular, and are resected without removing a significant amount of surrounding normal tissue. Code selection is based on size and location of the tumor. Code selection is determined by measuring the greatest diameter of the tumor plus that margin required for complete excision of the tumor. The margins refer to the most narrow margin required to adequately excise the tumor, based on individual judgment. The measurement of the tumor plus margin is made at the time of the excision. Appreciable vessel exploration and/or neuroplasty should be reported separately. Extensive undermining or other techniques to close a defect created by skin excision may require a complex repair which should be reported separately. Dissection or elevation of tissue planes to permit resection of the tumor is included in the excision.

Digital (ie, fingers and toes) subfascial tumors are defined as those tumors involving the tendons, tendon sheaths, or joints of the digit. Tumors which simply abut but do not breach the tendon, tendon sheath, or joint capsule are considered subcutaneous soft tissue tumors.

Radical resection of soft connective tissue tumors (including simple or intermediate repair) involves the resection of the tumor with wide margins of normal tissue. Appreciable vessel exploration and/or neuroplasty repair or reconstruction (eg, adjacent tissue transfer[s], flap[s]) should be reported separately. Extensive undermining or other techniques to close a defect created by skin excision may require a complex repair which should be reported separately. Dissection or elevation of tissue planes to permit resection of the tumor is included in the excision. Although these tumors may be confined to a specific layer (eg, subcutaneous, subfascial), radical resection may involve removal of tissue from one or more layers. Radical resection of soft tissue tumors is most commonly used for malignant connective tissue tumors or very aggressive benign connective tissue tumors. Code selection is based on size and location of the tumor. Code

selection is determined by measuring the greatest diameter of the tumor plus that margin required for complete excision of the tumor. The margins refer to the most narrow margin required to adequately excise the tumor, based on individual judgment. The measurement of the tumor plus margin is made at the time of the excision. For radical resection of tumor(s) of cutaneous origin (eg, melanoma), see 11600-11646.

Radical resection of bone tumors (including simple or intermediate repair) involves the resection of the tumor with wide margins of normal tissue. Appreciable vessel exploration and/or neuroplasty and complex bone repair or reconstruction (eg, adjacent tissue transfer[s], flap[s]) should be reported separately. Extensive undermining or other techniques to close a defect created by skin excision may require a complex repair which should be reported separately. Dissection or elevation of tissue planes to permit resection of the tumor is included in the excision. It may require removal of the entire bone if tumor growth is extensive (eg, clavicle). Radical resection of bone tumors is usually performed for malignant tumors or very aggressive benign tumors. If surrounding soft tissue is removed during these procedures, the radical resection of soft tissue tumor codes should not be reported separately. Code selection is based solely on the location of the tumor, **not** on the size of the tumor or whether the tumor is benign or malignant, primary or metastatic.

General

Incision

(For incision and drainage of subfascial soft tissue abscess, see appropriate incision and drainage for specific anatomic sites)

Wound Exploration—Trauma (eg, Penetrating Gunshot, Stab Wound)

20100-20103 relate to wound(s) resulting from penetrating trauma. These codes describe surgical exploration and enlargement of the wound, extension of dissection (to determine penetration), debridement, removal of foreign body(s), ligation or coagulation of minor subcutaneous and/or muscular blood vessel(s), of the subcutaneous tissue, muscle fascia, and/or muscle, not requiring thoracotomy or laparotomy. If a repair is done to major structure(s) or major blood vessel(s) requiring thoracotomy or laparotomy, then those specific code(s) would supersede the use of codes 20100-20103. To report

★ = Telemedicine   ◀ = Audio-only   + = Add-on code   ✗ = FDA approval pending   # = Resequenced code   ⊘ = Modifier 51 exempt   ➋➋➋ = See p xxi for details

simple, intermediate, or complex repair of wound(s) that do not require enlargement of the wound, extension of dissection, etc, as stated above, use specific Repair code(s) in the **Integumentary System** section.

20100   Exploration of penetrating wound (separate procedure); neck
> *CPT Assistant* Jun 96:7, Aug 96:10, Sep 06:13

20101   chest
> *CPT Assistant* Jun 96:7, Sep 06:13

20102   abdomen/flank/back
> *CPT Assistant* Jun 96:7, Sep 06:13

20103   extremity
> *CPT Assistant* Jun 96:7, Aug 96:10, Sep 06:13, Oct 23:19

Excision

20150   Excision of epiphyseal bar, with or without autogenous soft tissue graft obtained through same fascial incision

20200   Biopsy, muscle; superficial

20205   deep

20206   Biopsy, muscle, percutaneous needle
> *Clinical Examples in Radiology* Summer 08:5, Fall 10:7, Winter 17:5, Spring 22:9

(If imaging guidance is performed, see 76942, 77002, 77012, 77021)

(For fine needle aspiration biopsy, see 10004, 10005, 10006, 10007, 10008, 10009, 10010, 10011, 10012, 10021)

(For evaluation of fine needle aspirate, see 88172-88173)

(For excision of muscle tumor, deep, see specific anatomic section)

20220   Biopsy, bone, trocar, or needle; superficial (eg, ilium, sternum, spinous process, ribs)
> *CPT Assistant* Winter 92:17, Jul 98:4
> *Clinical Examples in Radiology* Summer 08:5, Fall 10:7, Winter 17:5, Winter 20:6, Spring 22:9

20225   deep (eg, vertebral body, femur)
> *CPT Changes: An Insider's View* 2002
> *CPT Assistant* Winter 92:17, Jul 98:4, Jun 12:10, Jan 15:8
> *Clinical Examples in Radiology* Fall 10:8, Winter 17:5, Winter 20:6, Spring 22:10, Fall 22:21

(Do not report 20225 in conjunction with 22510, 22511, 22512, 22513, 22514, 22515, 0200T, 0201T, when performed at the same level)

(For bone marrow biopsy[ies] and/or aspiration[s], see 38220, 38221, 38222)

(For radiologic supervision and interpretation, see 77002, 77012, 77021)

20240   Biopsy, bone, open; superficial (eg, sternum, spinous process, rib, patella, olecranon process, calcaneus, tarsal, metatarsal, carpal, metacarpal, phalanx)
> *CPT Changes: An Insider's View* 2004, 2017
> *CPT Assistant* Winter 92:17, Jul 98:4, Aug 04:11, Aug 05:13, May 23:26

20245   deep (eg, humeral shaft, ischium, femoral shaft)
> *CPT Changes: An Insider's View* 2017
> *CPT Assistant* Winter 92:17, Jul 98:4

20250   Biopsy, vertebral body, open; thoracic
> *CPT Assistant* Winter 92:17, Jul 98:4

20251   lumbar or cervical
> *CPT Assistant* Winter 92:17, Jul 98:4

(For sequestrectomy, osteomyelitis or drainage of bone abscess, see anatomical area)

Introduction or Removal

(For injection procedure for arthrography, see anatomical area)

(For injection of autologous adipose-derived regenerative cells, use 0490T)

20500   Injection of sinus tract; therapeutic (separate procedure)
> *Clinical Examples in Radiology* Summer 15:8

20501   diagnostic (sinogram)

(For radiological supervision and interpretation, use 76080)

(For contrast injection[s] and radiological assessment of gastrostomy, duodenostomy, jejunostomy, gastro-jejunostomy, or cecostomy [or other colonic] tube including fluoroscopic imaging guidance, use 49465)

20520   Removal of foreign body in muscle or tendon sheath; simple

20525   deep or complicated

20526   Injection, therapeutic (eg, local anesthetic, corticosteroid), carpal tunnel
> *CPT Changes: An Insider's View* 2002
> *CPT Assistant* Mar 02:7

20527   Injection, enzyme (eg, collagenase), palmar fascial cord (ie, Dupuytren's contracture)
> *CPT Changes: An Insider's View* 2012
> *CPT Assistant* Jul 12:8, 14

(For manipulation of palmar fascial cord (ie, Dupuytren's cord) post enzyme injection (eg, collagenase), use 26341)

Musculoskeletal 20100-29999

20550 Injection(s); single tendon sheath, or ligament, aponeurosis (eg, plantar "fascia")

➔ *CPT Changes: An Insider's View* 2002, 2003, 2004

➔ *CPT Assistant* Jan 96:7, Jun 98:10, Mar 02:7, Aug 03:14, Sep 03:13, Dec 03:11, Jan 09:6, Jul 12:14, Oct 14:9, Feb 23:13

➔ *Clinical Examples in Radiology* Winter 10:14

(For injection of Morton's neuroma, see 64455, 64632)

20551 single tendon origin/insertion

➔ *CPT Changes: An Insider's View* 2002, 2004

➔ *CPT Assistant* Mar 02:7, Sep 03:13, Oct 14:9, Dec 17:16

➔ *Clinical Examples in Radiology* Winter 10:14, Fall 10:10, Spring 21:12

(Do not report 20550, 20551 in conjunction with 0232T, 0481T)

(For harvesting, preparation, and injection[s] of platelet-rich plasma, use 0232T)

20552 Injection(s); single or multiple trigger point(s), 1 or 2 muscle(s)

➔ *CPT Changes: An Insider's View* 2002, 2003, 2004

➔ *CPT Assistant* Mar 02:7, May 03:19, Sep 03:11, Feb 10:9, Feb 11:5, Jul 11:16, Apr 12:19, Oct 14:9, Jun 17:10, Dec 17:16, Feb 20:9, Oct 21:8, Jul 22:17

➔ *Clinical Examples in Radiology* Winter 10:14, Fall 11:10

20553 single or multiple trigger point(s), 3 or more muscles

➔ *CPT Changes: An Insider's View* 2002, 2003

➔ *CPT Assistant* Mar 02:7, May 03:19, Sep 03:11, Jun 08:8, Feb 10:9, Feb 11:5, Jul 11:16, Oct 14:9, Jun 17:10, Dec 18:8, Feb 20:9, Oct 21:8

➔ *Clinical Examples in Radiology* Winter 10:14

(Do not report 20552, 20553 in conjunction with 20560, 20561 for the same muscle[s])

(If imaging guidance is performed, see 76942, 77002, 77021)

 # 20560 Needle insertion(s) without injection(s); 1 or 2 muscle(s)

➔ *CPT Changes: An Insider's View* 2020

➔ *CPT Assistant* Feb 20:9

 # 20561 3 or more muscles

➔ *CPT Changes: An Insider's View* 2020

➔ *CPT Assistant* Feb 20:9

20555 Placement of needles or catheters into muscle and/or soft tissue for subsequent interstitial radioelement application (at the time of or subsequent to the procedure)

➔ *CPT Changes: An Insider's View* 2008

➔ *CPT Assistant* Feb 08:8

(For placement of devices into the breast for interstitial radioelement application, see 19296-19298)

(For placement of needles, catheters, or devices into muscle or soft tissue of the head and neck, for interstitial radioelement application, use 41019)

(For placement of needles or catheters for interstitial radioelement application into prostate, use 55875)

(For placement of needles or catheters into the pelvic organs or genitalia [except prostate] for interstitial radioelement application, use 55920)

(For interstitial radioelement application, see 77770, 77771, 77772, 77778)

(For imaging guidance, see 76942, 77002, 77012, 77021)

20560 Code is out of numerical sequence. See 20552-20600

20561 Code is out of numerical sequence. See 20552-20600

Trigger Point Injection
20552, 20553

Insertion of needle into muscle trigger point for injection of therapeutic agent

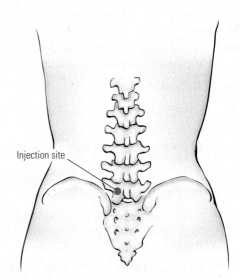

Injection site

Cross section through the body wall at level of lumbar vertebra

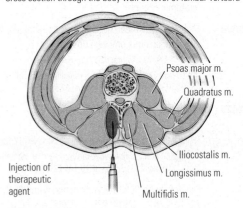

Psoas major m.

Quadratus m.

Iliocostalis m.

Injection of therapeutic agent

Longissimus m.

Multifidis m.

Musculoskeletal 20100-29999

20600   Arthrocentesis, aspiration and/or injection, small joint or bursa (eg, fingers, toes); without ultrasound guidance
> *CPT Changes: An Insider's View* 2003, 2015
> *CPT Assistant* Dec 07:10, Feb 15:6, Nov 15:10, Aug 17:9
> *Clinical Examples in Radiology* Spring 15:6, Spring 21:13

20604   with ultrasound guidance, with permanent recording and reporting
> *CPT Changes: An Insider's View* 2015
> *CPT Assistant* Feb 15:6, Jul 15:10
> *Clinical Examples in Radiology* Spring 15:6

(Do not report 20600, 20604 in conjunction with 76942, 0489T, 0490T)

(If fluoroscopic, CT, or MRI guidance is performed, see 77002, 77012, 77021)

20605   Arthrocentesis, aspiration and/or injection, intermediate joint or bursa (eg, temporomandibular, acromioclavicular, wrist, elbow or ankle, olecranon bursa); without ultrasound guidance
> *CPT Changes: An Insider's View* 2003, 2015
> *CPT Assistant* Dec 07:10, Feb 15:6, Nov 15:10, Aug 17:9
> *Clinical Examples in Radiology* Spring 15:6, Winter 23:12

20606   with ultrasound guidance, with permanent recording and reporting
> *CPT Changes: An Insider's View* 2015
> *CPT Assistant* Feb 15:6, Jul 15:10
> *Clinical Examples in Radiology* Spring 15:6, Winter 23:12

(Do not report 20605, 20606 in conjunction with 76942)

(If fluoroscopic, CT, or MRI guidance is performed, see 77002, 77012, 77021)

20610   Arthrocentesis, aspiration and/or injection, major joint or bursa (eg, shoulder, hip, knee, subacromial bursa); without ultrasound guidance
> *CPT Changes: An Insider's View* 2015
> *CPT Assistant* Spring 92:8, Mar 01:10, Apr 04:15, Jul 06:1, Dec 07:10, Jul 08:9, Mar 12:6, Jun 12:14, Dec 14:18, Feb 15:6, Aug 15:6, Nov 15:10, Apr 17:10, Aug 19:7, Dec 22:1
> *Clinical Examples in Radiology* Spring 13:11, Spring 15:7, Summer 18:15, Winter 19:14, Spring 21:7

20611   with ultrasound guidance, with permanent recording and reporting
> *CPT Changes: An Insider's View* 2015
> *CPT Assistant* Feb 15:6, Jul 15:10, Aug 15:6, Nov 15:10, Aug 19:7, Dec 22:1
> *Clinical Examples in Radiology* Spring 15:7, Winter 19:14, Spring 21:12,13

(Do not report 20610, 20611 in conjunction with 27369, 76942)

(If fluoroscopic, CT, or MRI guidance is performed, see 77002, 77012, 77021)

20612   Aspiration and/or injection of ganglion cyst(s) any location
> *CPT Changes: An Insider's View* 2003

(To report multiple ganglion cyst aspirations/injections, use 20612 and append modifier 59)

Arthrocentesis, Aspiration, or Injection of Major Joint or Bursa
20610

Insertion of needle into major joint or bursa for injection of therapeutic or diagnostic agent, aspiration, or arthrocentesis

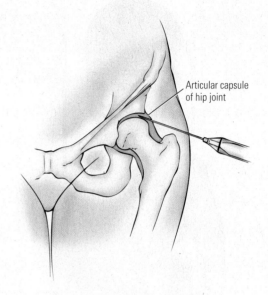

Articular capsule of hip joint

20615   Aspiration and injection for treatment of bone cyst

(For injection of bone-substitute material for bone marrow lesions, use 0707T)

20650   Insertion of wire or pin with application of skeletal traction, including removal (separate procedure)

20660   Application of cranial tongs, caliper, or stereotactic frame, including removal (separate procedure)
> *CPT Changes: An Insider's View* 2008
> *CPT Assistant* Jun 96:10, Nov 97:14, Jan 06:46, Dec 06:10, Feb 08:8, Jul 08:10, Nov 09:6, Apr 12:11, Aug 12:14

20661   Application of halo, including removal; cranial
> *CPT Assistant* Nov 97:14, Aug 12:14

20662   pelvic

20663   femoral

20664   Application of halo, including removal, cranial, 6 or more pins placed, for thin skull osteology (eg, pediatric patients, hydrocephalus, osteogenesis imperfecta)
> *CPT Changes: An Insider's View* 2011
> *CPT Assistant* Nov 97:14, Aug 12:5, Aug 13:12

Halo Application for Thin Skull Osteology
20664

A cranial halo is placed on the head of a child whose skull is unusually thin due to congenital or developmental problems.

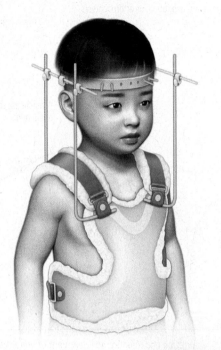

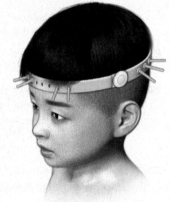

20665   Removal of tongs or halo applied by another individual

➔ *CPT Changes: An Insider's View* 2013

➔ *CPT Assistant* Apr 12:12

20670   Removal of implant; superficial (eg, buried wire, pin or rod) (separate procedure)

➔ *CPT Assistant* Dec 07:7-8, Jun 09:7, Apr 12:17

20680   deep (eg, buried wire, pin, screw, metal band, nail, rod or plate)

➔ *CPT Assistant* Spring 92:11, Jun 09:7, Sep 12:16, Mar 14:4, Nov 15:10, Nov 16:9, Jan 18:3, Sep 21:7, Apr 23:1

(For removal of sinus tarsi implant, use 0510T)

(For removal and reinsertion of sinus tarsi implant, use 0511T)

20690   Application of a uniplane (pins or wires in 1 plane), unilateral, external fixation system

➔ *CPT Changes: An Insider's View* 2008

➔ *CPT Assistant* Winter 90:4, Winter 92:11, Fall 93:21, Oct 99:5, Jan 04:27, Jun 05:12, Oct 07:7, Jan 08:4, Feb 08:9, Jun 09:7, Jan 18:3

Uniplane External Fixation System
20690

The following figures are examples of types of stabilization devices. Codes 20690 and 20692 describe the placement of types of external fixation devices. The method of stabilization depends upon fracture grade (degree of soft tissue injury/skin integrity disruption), type (eg, comminuted, spiral, impacted), and location (eg, extremity, pelvis).

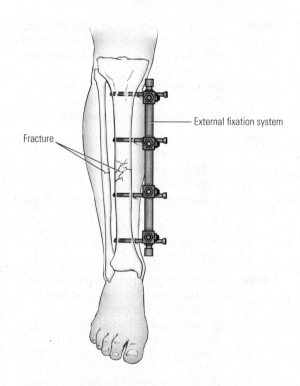

External fixation system

Fracture

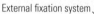

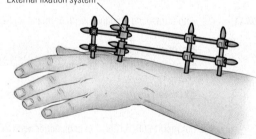

External fixation system

20692   Application of a multiplane (pins or wires in more than 1 plane), unilateral, external fixation system (eg, Ilizarov, Monticelli type)

➔ *CPT Changes: An Insider's View* 2008

➔ *CPT Assistant* Winter 90:4, Fall 93:21, Oct 99:5, Jul 00:11, Feb 08:9, Jun 09:7, Jan 18:3, May 19:10

Multiplane External Fixation System
20692

The following figure is an example of a type of multiplane stabilization device. Codes 20690 and 20692 describe the placement of types of external fixation devices. The method of stabilization depends upon fracture grade (degree of soft tissue injury/skin integrity disruption), type (eg, comminuted, spiral, impacted), and location (eg, extremity, pelvis).

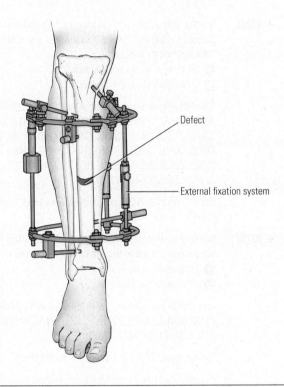

Defect

External fixation system

20693   Adjustment or revision of external fixation system requiring anesthesia (eg, new pin[s] or wire[s] and/or new ring[s] or bar[s])

➔ *CPT Assistant* Fall 93:21, Oct 99:5, Jul 00:11, Jun 09:7, Jan 18:3

20694   Removal, under anesthesia, of external fixation system

➔ *CPT Assistant* Winter 92:10, Fall 93:21, Oct 99:5, Jul 00:11, Jan 18:3

20696   Application of multiplane (pins or wires in more than 1 plane), unilateral, external fixation with stereotactic computer-assisted adjustment (eg, spatial frame), including imaging; initial and subsequent alignment(s), assessment(s), and computation(s) of adjustment schedule(s)

➔ *CPT Changes: An Insider's View* 2009

➔ *CPT Assistant* Jan 18:3

(Do not report 20696 in conjunction with 20692, 20697)

⊘ **20697**   exchange (ie, removal and replacement) of strut, each

➔ *CPT Changes: An Insider's View* 2009

➔ *CPT Assistant* Jan 18:3

(Do not report 20697 in conjunction with 20692, 20696)

Manual preparation involves the mixing and preparation of antibiotics or other therapeutic agent(s) with a carrier substance by the physician or other qualified health care professional during the surgical procedure and then shaping the mixture into a drug-delivery device(s) (eg, beads, nails, spacers) for placement in the deep (eg, subfascial), intramedullary, or intra-articular space(s). Codes 20700, 20702, 20704 are add-on codes for the manual preparation and insertion of the drug-delivery device(s). They may be used with any open procedure code except those that include the placement of a "spacer" (eg, 27091, 27488). The add-on codes may be used when infection is present, suspected, or anticipated during the surgery. The location of the primary service determines which of the insertion codes may be selected. If the primary surgery is in the deep (subfascial) region, add-on code 20700 may be reported. If the primary surgery is within the bone or "intramedullary," add-on code 20702 may be reported. If the primary surgery is within the joint, add-on code 20704 may be reported.

Codes 20701, 20703, 20705 are add-on codes used to report removal of drug-delivery device(s). These codes may be typically associated with specific surgeries if the infection has been eradicated. For removal of a drug-delivery device from a deep (subfascial) space performed in conjunction with a primary procedure (ie, complex wound closure [13100-13160], adjacent tissue transfer [14000-14350], or a flap closure [15570-15758]), add-on code 20701 may be reported. For infection that has not been eradicated, see the tissue debridement codes (eg, 11011, 11012, 11042, 11043, 11044, 11045, 11046, 11047) for the primary procedure. If a subsequent new drug-delivery device is placed, 20700 may be additionally reported.

Similarly, for add-on code 20703, removal of drug delivery device from the bone may be associated with different procedures. If the infection has been eradicated and the drug delivery device removal is the only procedure being performed, report 20680 (removal of deep hardware). Bony reconstruction performed in conjunction with eradication of infection may be reported using the reconstruction as the primary procedure. Persistent infection that is treated using an additional bony debridement procedure (eg, 11012, 23180, 23182, 23184, 24140, 24145, 25150, 25151, 26230, 26235, 26236, 27070, 27071, 27360, 27640,

Musculoskeletal 20100-29999

27641, 28122, 28124) may be reported using the debridement as the primary procedure. Amputation (eg, 27290, 27590, 27598) performed in conjunction with delivery of a new, manually prepared drug delivery device may be reported with add-on code 20702.

When joint infection is present, suspected, or anticipated, add-on code 20704 (for manual preparation of an intra-articular drug delivery device) may be reported. Code 20704 may not be reported when the placement of a spacer is included in the code (eg, 27091, 27488) or when antibiotic cement is used for implant fixation.

Add-on code 20705 (for removal of a manually prepared intra-articular drug delivery device) may be typically used in conjunction with a joint stabilization procedure such as arthrodesis (eg, 22532, 22533, 22534, 22548, 22551, 22552, 22554, 22556, 22558, 22585, 22586, 22590, 22595, 22600, 22610, 22614, 22634, 22800, 22802, 22804, 22808, 22810, 22812, 22830, 22853, 22854, 22899, 24800, 24802, 25800, 25805, 25810, 25825, 25830, 26841, 26842, 26843, 26844, 26850, 26852, 26860, 26861, 26862, 26863, 27279, 27280, 27282, 27284, 27286, 27580, 27870, 27871, 28295, 28296, 28298, 28299, 28705, 28715, 28725, 28730, 28735, 28737, 28740, 28750, 28755, 28760, 29907) and revision joint arthroplasties (eg, 23473, 23474 [shoulder], 24370, 24371 [elbow], 25449 [wrist], 27134 [hip], 27487 [knee], and 27703 [ankle]). In the rare circumstance in which only part of the joint is destroyed by infection, a partial arthroplasty may be reported (eg, 23470, 24360, 24361, 24362, 24365, 24366, 25441, 25442, 25443, 25444, 25445, 27125, 27236, 27438, 27440, 27441, 27442, 27443, and 27446).

If no primary service is associated with add-on code 20705 and the joint is left without remaining cartilage or stabilization (ie, flail joint), only 20680 may be reported.

Insertion of a prefabricated drug device(s) may not be reported with 20700, 20702, 20704. Report 20680, if removal of drug-delivery device(s) is performed alone. Report 20700, 20701, 20702, 20703, 20704, 20705 once per anatomic location.

+ 20700 Manual preparation and insertion of drug-delivery device(s), deep (eg, subfascial) (List separately in addition to code for primary procedure)

➔ *CPT Changes: An Insider's View* 2020
➔ *CPT Assistant* Sep 21:6-7, Apr 23:1

(Use 20700 in conjunction with 11010, 11011, 11012, 11043, 11044, 11046, 11047, 20240, 20245, 20250, 20251, 21010, 21025, 21026, 21501, 21502, 21510, 21627, 21630, 22010, 22015, 23030, 23031, 23035, 23040, 23044, 23170, 23172, 23174, 23180, 23182, 23184, 23334, 23335, 23930, 23931, 23935, 24000, 24134, 24136, 24138, 24140, 24147, 24160, 25031, 25035, 25040, 25145, 25150, 25151, 26070, 26230, 26235, 26236, 26990, 26991, 26992, 27030, 27070, 27071, 27090, 27301, 27303, 27310, 27360, 27603, 27604, 27610, 27640, 27641, 28001, 28002, 28003, 28020, 28120, 28122)

(Do not report 20700 in conjunction with any services that include placement of a spacer [eg, 11981, 27091, 27488])

+ 20701 Removal of drug-delivery device(s), deep (eg, subfascial) (List separately in addition to code for primary procedure)

➔ *CPT Changes: An Insider's View* 2020
➔ *CPT Assistant* Sep 21:6-7, Apr 23:1

(Use 20701 in conjunction with 11010, 11011, 11012, 11043, 11044, 11046, 11047, 13100-13160, 14000-14350, 15570, 15572, 15574, 15576, 15736, 15738, 15740, 15750, 15756, 15757, 15758)

(Do not report 20701 in conjunction with 11982)

(For removal of a deep drug-delivery device only, use 20680)

+ 20702 Manual preparation and insertion of drug-delivery device(s), intramedullary (List separately in addition to code for primary procedure)

➔ *CPT Changes: An Insider's View* 2020
➔ *CPT Assistant* Sep 21:6-7, Apr 23:1

(Use 20702 in conjunction with 20680, 20690, 20692, 20694, 20802, 20805, 20838, 21510, 23035, 23170, 23180, 23184, 23515, 23615, 23935, 24134, 24138, 24140, 24147, 24430, 24516, 25035, 25145, 25150, 25151, 25400, 25515, 25525, 25526, 25545, 25574, 25575, 27245, 27259, 27360, 27470, 27506, 27640, 27720)

(Do not report 20702 in conjunction with 11981, 27091, 27488)

+ 20703 Removal of drug-delivery device(s), intramedullary (List separately in addition to code for primary procedure)

➔ *CPT Changes: An Insider's View* 2020
➔ *CPT Assistant* Sep 21:6-7, Apr 23:1

(Use 20703 in conjunction with 23485, 24430, 24435, 25400, 25405, 25415, 25420, 25425, 27470, 27472, 27720, 27722, 27724, 27725)

(Do not report 20703 in conjunction with 11982)

(For removal of an intramedullary drug-delivery device as a stand-alone procedure, use 20680)

+ 20704 Manual preparation and insertion of drug-delivery device(s), intra-articular (List separately in addition to code for primary procedure)

➔ *CPT Changes: An Insider's View* 2020
➔ *CPT Assistant* Mar 20:14, Sep 21:6-9, Apr 23:1

(Use 20704 in conjunction with 22864, 22865, 23040, 23044, 23334, 23335, 23473, 23474, 24000, 24160, 24370, 24371, 25040, 25250, 25251, 25449, 26070, 26990, 27030, 27090, 27132, 27134, 27137, 27138, 27301, 27310, 27487, 27603, 27610, 27703, 28020)

(Do not report 20704 in conjunction with 11981, 27091, 27488)

+ 20705 Removal of drug-delivery device(s), intra-articular (List separately in addition to code for primary procedure)

➔ *CPT Changes: An Insider's View* 2020

➔ *CPT Assistant* Sep 21:6-7, Apr 23:1

(Use 20705 in conjunction with 22864, 22865, 23040, 23044, 23334, 23473, 23474, 24000, 24160, 24370, 24371, 25040, 25250, 25251, 25449, 26070, 26075, 26080, 26990, 27030, 27090, 27132, 27134, 27137, 27138, 27301, 27310, 27487, 27603, 27610, 27703, 28020)

(Do not report 20705 in conjunction with 11982, 27130, 27447, 27486)

(For arthrodesis after eradicated infection, see 22532, 22533, 22534, 22548, 22551, 22552, 22554, 22556, 22558, 22585, 22586, 22590, 22595, 22600, 22610, 22614, 22634, 22800, 22802, 22804, 22808, 22810, 22812, 22830, 22853, 22854, 22899, 24800, 24802, 25800, 25805, 25810, 25825, 25830, 26841, 26842, 26843, 26844, 26850, 26852, 26860, 26861, 26862, 26863, 27279, 27280, 27282, 27284, 27286, 27580, 27870, 27871, 28295, 28296, 28298, 28299, 28705, 28715, 28725, 28730, 28735, 28737, 28740, 28750, 28755, 28760, 29907)

(For implant removal after failed drug delivery device placement, see 22862, 22864, 23334, 23335, 24160, 25250, 25251, 27090, 27091, 27488, 27704)

(For partial replacement after successful eradication of infection with removal of drug delivery implant, see 23470, 24360, 24361, 24362, 24365, 24366, 25441, 25442, 25443, 25444, 25445, 27125, 27236, 27438, 27440, 27441, 27442, 27443, 27446)

Replantation

(For repair of incomplete amputation of the arm, forearm, hand, digit, thumb, thigh, leg, foot, or toe, report the specific code[s] for repair of bone[s], ligament[s], tendon[s], nerve[s], and/or blood vessel[s] and append modifier 51 or 59 as appropriate)

(For replantation of complete amputation of the lower extremity, except foot, report the specific code[s] for repair of bone[s], ligament[s], tendon[s], nerve[s], and/or blood vessel[s] and append modifier 51 or 59 as appropriate)

20802 Replantation, arm (includes surgical neck of humerus through elbow joint), complete amputation

20805 Replantation, forearm (includes radius and ulna to radial carpal joint), complete amputation

20808 Replantation, hand (includes hand through metacarpophalangeal joints), complete amputation

20816 Replantation, digit, excluding thumb (includes metacarpophalangeal joint to insertion of flexor sublimis tendon), complete amputation

➔ *CPT Assistant* Oct 96:11

20822 Replantation, digit, excluding thumb (includes distal tip to sublimis tendon insertion), complete amputation

20824 Replantation, thumb (includes carpometacarpal joint to MP joint), complete amputation

20827 Replantation, thumb (includes distal tip to MP joint), complete amputation

➔ *CPT Assistant* Aug 23:19-20

20838 Replantation, foot, complete amputation

Grafts (or Implants)

Codes for obtaining autogenous bone, cartilage, tendon, fascia lata grafts, bone marrow, or other tissues through separate skin/fascial incisions should be reported separately, unless the code descriptor references the harvesting of the graft or implant (eg, includes obtaining graft). Autologous grafts that are already defined in the CPT code set, including skin, bone, nerve, tendon, fascia lata, or vessels, should be reported with the more specific codes for each tissue type. Code 15769 may be used for other autologous soft tissue grafts harvested by direct excision. See 15771, 15772, 15773, 15774 for autologous fat grafting harvested by liposuction technique.

Do not append modifier 62 to bone graft codes 20900-20938.

(For spinal surgery bone graft[s] see codes 20930-20938)

20900 Bone graft, any donor area; minor or small (eg, dowel or button)

➔ *CPT Changes: An Insider's View* 2008

➔ *CPT Assistant* Dec 00:15, Jul 11:18, Jul 18:14, May 20:14, Jul 21:7, Dec 21:5-6, 22

20902   major or large

➔ *CPT Changes: An Insider's View* 2008

➔ *CPT Assistant* Dec 00:15, Jul 11:18, Jul 18:14, Dec 21:5-6, 22

20910 Cartilage graft; costochondral

➔ *CPT Changes: An Insider's View* 2008

➔ *CPT Assistant* Jan 13:15, Jul 18:14, Dec 21:5-6, 22

20912   nasal septum

➔ *CPT Changes: An Insider's View* 2008

➔ *CPT Assistant* Jul 18:14, Dec 21:5-6, 22

(For ear cartilage, use 21235)

20920 Fascia lata graft; by stripper

➔ *CPT Changes: An Insider's View* 2008

➔ *CPT Assistant* Aug 99:5, Jan 05:8, Jul 18:14, Dec 21:5-6, 22

20922   by incision and area exposure, complex or sheet

➔ *CPT Changes: An Insider's View* 2008

➔ *CPT Assistant* Jan 05:8, Jul 18:14, Dec 21:5-6, 22

20924 Tendon graft, from a distance (eg, palmaris, toe extensor, plantaris)

➜ *CPT Changes: An Insider's View* 2008

➜ *CPT Assistant* Jul 18:14, Dec 21:5-6, 22

(To report autologous soft tissue grafts harvested by direct excision, use 15769)

(To report autologous fat grafting harvested by liposuction technique, see 15771, 15772, 15773, 15774)

+ 20930 Allograft, morselized, or placement of osteopromotive material, for spine surgery only (List separately in addition to code for primary procedure)

➜ *CPT Changes: An Insider's View* 2008, 2011

➜ *CPT Assistant* Feb 96:6, Mar 96:4, Sep 97:8, Nov 99:10, Feb 02:6, Jan 04:27, Dec 07:1, Feb 08:8, Nov 10:8, Jul 11:18, Dec 11:15, Apr 12:14, Jun 12:11, Jul 13:3, Jul 18:14, May 19:7, Dec 21:5-6, 22

(Use 20930 in conjunction with 22319, 22532, 22533, 22548-22558, 22590-22612, 22630, 22633, 22634, 22800-22812)

+ 20931 Allograft, structural, for spine surgery only (List separately in addition to code for primary procedure)

➜ *CPT Changes: An Insider's View* 2008, 2011

➜ *CPT Assistant* Feb 96:6, Feb 02:6, Feb 05:15, Feb 08:8, Nov 10:8, Jul 11:18, Sep 11:12, Dec 11:15, Apr 12:14, Jun 12:11, Jul 13:3, Jul 18:14, May 19:7, Dec 21:5-6, 22

(Use 20931 in conjunction with 22319, 22532-22533, 22548-22558, 22590-22612, 22630, 22633, 22634, 22800-22812)

+ 20932 Allograft, includes templating, cutting, placement and internal fixation, when performed; osteoarticular, including articular surface and contiguous bone (List separately in addition to code for primary procedure)

➜ *CPT Changes: An Insider's View* 2019

➜ *CPT Assistant* May 19:7, Dec 21:5-6, 22

(Do not report 20932 in conjunction with 20933, 20934, 23200, 24152, 27078, 27090, 27091, 27448, 27646, 27647, 27648)

+ 20933 hemicortical intercalary, partial (ie, hemicylindrical) (List separately in addition to code for primary procedure)

➜ *CPT Changes: An Insider's View* 2019

➜ *CPT Assistant* May 19:7, Dec 21:5-6, 22

(Do not report 20933 in conjunction with 20932, 20934, 20955, 20956, 20957, 20962, 23146, 23156, 23200, 24116, 24126, 24152, 25126, 25136, 27078, 27090, 27091, 27130, 27132, 27134, 27138, 27236, 27244, 27356, 27448, 27638, 27646, 27647, 27648, 28103, 28107)

+ 20934 intercalary, complete (ie, cylindrical) (List separately in addition to code for primary procedure)

➜ *CPT Changes: An Insider's View* 2019

➜ *CPT Assistant* May 19:7, Dec 21:5-6, 22

(Do not report 20934 in conjunction with 20932, 20933, 23200, 24152, 27078, 27090, 27091, 27448, 27646, 27647, 27648)

(Insertion of joint prosthesis may be separately reported)

(Use 20932, 20933, 20934 in conjunction with 23210, 23220, 24150, 25170, 27075, 27076, 27077, 27365, 27645, 27704)

Postoperative Osteoarticular Allograft Left Humerus Fixed with Plates
20932

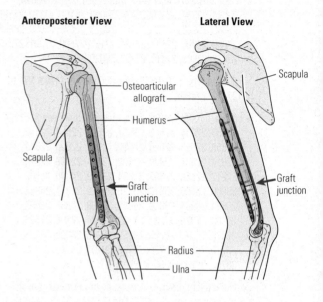

Anteroposterior View — Lateral View

Parosteal Osteosarcoma Replaced with Hemicortical Intercalary Allograft
20933

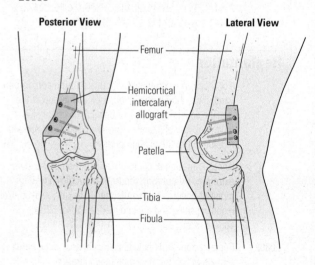

Posterior View — Lateral View

Osteosarcoma Femur with Complete Intercalary Allograft with Plate Fixation
20934

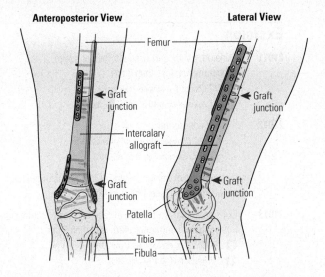

Anteroposterior View — Femur — Graft junction — Intercalary allograft — Graft junction — Patella — Tibia — Fibula — **Lateral View** — Graft junction — Graft junction

+ 20936   Autograft for spine surgery only (includes harvesting the graft); local (eg, ribs, spinous process, or laminar fragments) obtained from same incision (List separately in addition to code for primary procedure)

➔ *CPT Changes: An Insider's View* 2008

➔ *CPT Assistant* Feb 96:6, Sep 97:8, Feb 02:6, Feb 08:8, Dec 11:15, Apr 12:14, Jun 12:11, Jul 13:3, Jul 18:14, Dec 21:5-6, 22

(Use 20936 in conjunction with 22319, 22532, 22533, 22548-22558, 22590-22612, 22630, 22633, 22634, 22800-22812)

+ 20937   morselized (through separate skin or fascial incision) (List separately in addition to code for primary procedure)

➔ *CPT Changes: An Insider's View* 2008

➔ *CPT Assistant* Feb 96:6, Sep 97:8, Dec 99:2, Feb 02:6, Feb 08:8, Dec 11:15, Apr 12:11, Jun 12:11, Jul 13:3, Jul 18:14, Dec 21:5-6, 22

(Use 20937 in conjunction with 22319, 22532, 22533, 22548-22558, 22590-22612, 22630, 22633, 22634, 22800-22812)

+ 20938   structural, bicortical or tricortical (through separate skin or fascial incision) (List separately in addition to code for primary procedure)

➔ *CPT Changes: An Insider's View* 2008

➔ *CPT Assistant* Feb 96:6, Mar 96:5, Sep 97:8, Feb 02:6, Feb 08:8, Jul 11:18, Dec 11:15, Apr 12:12, May 12:11, Jun 12:11, Jul 13:3, May 20:14, Jul 21:7, Dec 21:5-6, 22

(Use 20938 in conjunction with 22319, 22532, 22533, 22548-22558, 22590-22612, 22630, 22633, 22634, 22800-22812)

(For aspiration of bone marrow for bone grafting, spine surgery only, use 20939)

+ 20939   Bone marrow aspiration for bone grafting, spine surgery only, through separate skin or fascial incision (List separately in addition to code for primary procedure)

➔ *CPT Changes: An Insider's View* 2018

➔ *CPT Assistant* May 18:3

➔ *Clinical Examples in Radiology* Spring 18:6

(Use 20939 in conjunction with 22319, 22532, 22533, 22534, 22548, 22551, 22552, 22554, 22556, 22558, 22590, 22595, 22600, 22610, 22612, 22630, 22633, 22634, 22800, 22802, 22804, 22808, 22810, 22812)

(For bilateral procedure, report 20939 twice. Do not report modifier 50 in conjunction with 20939)

(For aspiration of bone marrow for the purpose of bone grafting, other than spine surgery and other therapeutic musculoskeletal applications, use 20999)

(For bone marrow aspiration[s] for platelet-rich stem cell injection, use 0232T)

(For diagnostic bone marrow aspiration[s], see 38220, 38222)

Other Procedures

20950   Monitoring of interstitial fluid pressure (includes insertion of device, eg, wick catheter technique, needle manometer technique) in detection of muscle compartment syndrome

➔ *CPT Assistant* Sep 07:10, Mar 23:32

20955   Bone graft with microvascular anastomosis; fibula

➔ *CPT Assistant* Apr 97:4

20956   iliac crest

➔ *CPT Assistant* Apr 97:4

20957   metatarsal

➔ *CPT Assistant* Apr 97:4

20962   other than fibula, iliac crest, or metatarsal

➔ *CPT Assistant* Apr 97:4

(Do not report code 69990 in addition to codes 20955-20962)

20969   Free osteocutaneous flap with microvascular anastomosis; other than iliac crest, metatarsal, or great toe

➔ *CPT Assistant* Apr 97:4, Oct 19:10

20970   iliac crest

➔ *CPT Assistant* Apr 97:4

20972   metatarsal

➔ *CPT Assistant* Apr 97:4

20973   great toe with web space
> *CPT Assistant* Apr 97:4

(Do not report code 69990 in addition to codes 20969-20973)

(For great toe, wrap-around procedure, use 26551)

⊘ **20974** Electrical stimulation to aid bone healing; noninvasive (nonoperative)
> *CPT Assistant* Sep 96:11, Nov 00:8

⊘ **20975**   invasive (operative)
> *CPT Assistant* Nov 00:8

20979 Low intensity ultrasound stimulation to aid bone healing, noninvasive (nonoperative)
> *CPT Changes: An Insider's View* 2000
> *CPT Assistant* Nov 99:10, Nov 00:8

20982 Ablation therapy for reduction or eradication of 1 or more bone tumors (eg, metastasis) including adjacent soft tissue when involved by tumor extension, percutaneous, including imaging guidance when performed; radiofrequency
> *CPT Changes: An Insider's View* 2004, 2015, 2017
> *CPT Assistant* Jul 15:8, Sep 15:12
> *Clinical Examples in Radiology* Spring 15:3

20983   cryoablation
> *CPT Changes: An Insider's View* 2015, 2017
> *CPT Assistant* Jul 15:8
> *Clinical Examples in Radiology* Spring 15:2

(Do not report 20982, 20983 in conjunction with 76940, 77002, 77013, 77022)

+ **20985** Computer-assisted surgical navigational procedure for musculoskeletal procedures, image-less (List separately in addition to code for primary procedure)
> *CPT Changes: An Insider's View* 2008, 2009
> *CPT Assistant* Jul 11:12

(Do not report 20985 in conjunction with 61781-61783)

(20986, 20987 have been deleted)

(For computer-assisted navigational procedures with image guidance based on pre-operative and intraoperatively obtained images, see 0054T, 0055T)

20999 Unlisted procedure, musculoskeletal system, general
> *CPT Assistant* Sep 03:13, Jul 15:8, May 18:3, Feb 23:13
> *Clinical Examples in Radiology* Spring 15:3

Head

Skull, facial bones, and temporomandibular joint.

Incision

(For incision and drainage procedures, cutaneous/subcutaneous, see 10060, 10061)

(For removal of embedded foreign body from dentoalveolar structure, see 41805, 41806)

21010 Arthrotomy, temporomandibular joint

(To report bilateral procedure, report 21010 with modifier 50)

Excision

21011 Excision, tumor, soft tissue of face or scalp, subcutaneous; less than 2 cm
> *CPT Changes: An Insider's View* 2010
> *CPT Assistant* Feb 10:3, Apr 10:3, Sep 18:7

21012   2 cm or greater
> *CPT Changes: An Insider's View* 2010
> *CPT Assistant* Feb 10:3, Apr 10:3

(For excision of benign lesions of cutaneous origin [eg, sebaceous cyst], see 11420-11426)

21013 Excision, tumor, soft tissue of face and scalp, subfascial (eg, subgaleal, intramuscular); less than 2 cm
> *CPT Changes: An Insider's View* 2010
> *CPT Assistant* Feb 10:3, Apr 10:3

21014   2 cm or greater
> *CPT Changes: An Insider's View* 2010
> *CPT Assistant* Feb 10:3, Apr 10:3

21015 Radical resection of tumor (eg, sarcoma), soft tissue of face or scalp; less than 2 cm
> *CPT Changes: An Insider's View* 2010, 2014
> *CPT Assistant* Feb 10:3, Apr 10:3

(To report excision of skull tumor for osteomyelitis, use 61501)

21016   2 cm or greater
> *CPT Changes: An Insider's View* 2010, 2014
> *CPT Assistant* Feb 10:3, Apr 10:3

(For radical resection of tumor[s] of cutaneous origin [eg, melanoma], see 11620-11646)

21025 Excision of bone (eg, for osteomyelitis or bone abscess); mandible
> *CPT Assistant* Oct 11:10

21026   facial bone(s)

21029 Removal by contouring of benign tumor of facial bone (eg, fibrous dysplasia)

21030 Excision of benign tumor or cyst of maxilla or zygoma by enucleation and curettage
> *CPT Changes: An Insider's View* 2003
> *CPT Assistant* Nov 03:9

21031 Excision of torus mandibularis

21032 Excision of maxillary torus palatinus

21034　Excision of malignant tumor of maxilla or zygoma

➔ *CPT Changes: An Insider's View* 2003

➔ *CPT Assistant* Nov 03:9

21040　Excision of benign tumor or cyst of mandible, by enucleation and/or curettage

➔ *CPT Changes: An Insider's View* 2003

➔ *CPT Assistant* Nov 03:9

(For enucleation and/or curettage of benign cysts or tumors of mandible not requiring osteotomy, use 21040)

(For excision of benign tumor or cyst of mandible requiring osteotomy, see 21046-21047)

21044　Excision of malignant tumor of mandible;

21045　　radical resection

(For bone graft, use 21215)

21046　Excision of benign tumor or cyst of mandible; requiring intra-oral osteotomy (eg, locally aggressive or destructive lesion[s])

➔ *CPT Changes: An Insider's View* 2003

➔ *CPT Assistant* Nov 03:9

21047　　requiring extra-oral osteotomy and partial mandibulectomy (eg, locally aggressive or destructive lesion[s])

➔ *CPT Changes: An Insider's View* 2003

➔ *CPT Assistant* Nov 03:9

21048　Excision of benign tumor or cyst of maxilla; requiring intra-oral osteotomy (eg, locally aggressive or destructive lesion[s])

➔ *CPT Changes: An Insider's View* 2003

➔ *CPT Assistant* Nov 03:9

21049　　requiring extra-oral osteotomy and partial maxillectomy (eg, locally aggressive or destructive lesion[s])

➔ *CPT Changes: An Insider's View* 2003

➔ *CPT Assistant* Nov 03:9

21050　Condylectomy, temporomandibular joint (separate procedure)

(For bilateral procedures, report 21050 with modifier 50)

21060　Meniscectomy, partial or complete, temporomandibular joint (separate procedure)

(For bilateral procedures, report 21060 with modifier 50)

21070　Coronoidectomy (separate procedure)

(For bilateral procedures, report 21070 with modifier 50)

Manipulation

21073　Manipulation of temporomandibular joint(s) (TMJ), therapeutic, requiring an anesthesia service (ie, general or monitored anesthesia care)

➔ *CPT Changes: An Insider's View* 2008

➔ *CPT Assistant* Feb 08:9, Jan 18:3

(For TMJ manipulation without an anesthesia service [ie, general or monitored anesthesia care], see 97140, 98925-98929, 98943)

(For closed treatment of temporomandibular dislocation, see 21480, 21485)

Head Prosthesis

Codes 21076-21089 describe professional services for the rehabilitation of patients with oral, facial, or other anatomical deficiencies by means of prostheses such as an artificial eye, ear, or nose or intraoral obturator to close a cleft. Codes 21076-21089 should only be used when the physician or other qualified health care professional actually designs and prepares the prosthesis (ie, not prepared by an outside laboratory).

(For application or removal of caliper or tongs, see 20660, 20665)

21076　Impression and custom preparation; surgical obturator prosthesis

21077　　orbital prosthesis

➔ *CPT Assistant* Apr 23:25

21079　　interim obturator prosthesis

➔ *CPT Assistant* Winter 90:5, Sep 06:13, Dec 06:10

21080　　definitive obturator prosthesis

➔ *CPT Assistant* Winter 90:5, Sep 06:13, Dec 06:10

21081　　mandibular resection prosthesis

➔ *CPT Assistant* Winter 90:5, Sep 06:13, Dec 06:10

21082　　palatal augmentation prosthesis

➔ *CPT Assistant* Winter 90:5, Sep 06:13, Dec 06:10

21083　　palatal lift prosthesis

➔ *CPT Assistant* Winter 90:5, Sep 06:13, Dec 06:10

21084　　speech aid prosthesis

➔ *CPT Assistant* Winter 90:5, Sep 06:13, Dec 06:10

21085　　oral surgical splint

➔ *CPT Assistant* Winter 90:5, Sep 06:13, Dec 06:10, Sep 17:14

21086　　auricular prosthesis

➔ *CPT Assistant* Winter 90:5, Sep 06:13, Dec 06:10

21087　　nasal prosthesis

➔ *CPT Assistant* Winter 90:5, Sep 06:13, Dec 06:10

21088　　facial prosthesis

➔ *CPT Assistant* Winter 90:5, Sep 06:13, Dec 06:10, Apr 23:25

Other Procedures

21089　Unlisted maxillofacial prosthetic procedure

➔ *CPT Assistant* Winter 90:5, Sep 06:13, Dec 06:10

Introduction or Removal

21100 Application of halo type appliance for maxillofacial fixation, includes removal (separate procedure)

21110 Application of interdental fixation device for conditions other than fracture or dislocation, includes removal
➜ *CPT Assistant* Mar 97:10, Dec 13:16

(For removal of interdental fixation by another individual, see 20670-20680)

21116 Injection procedure for temporomandibular joint arthrography
➜ *CPT Assistant* Aug 15:6, May 16:13
➜ *Clinical Examples in Radiology* Summer 18:15

(For radiological supervision and interpretation, use 70332. Do not report 77002 in conjunction with 70332)

Repair, Revision, and/or Reconstruction

(For cranioplasty, see 21179, 21180 and 62120, 62140-62147)

21120 Genioplasty; augmentation (autograft, allograft, prosthetic material)

21121 sliding osteotomy, single piece

21122 sliding osteotomies, 2 or more osteotomies (eg, wedge excision or bone wedge reversal for asymmetrical chin)

21123 sliding, augmentation with interpositional bone grafts (includes obtaining autografts)

21125 Augmentation, mandibular body or angle; prosthetic material

21127 with bone graft, onlay or interpositional (includes obtaining autograft)

21137 Reduction forehead; contouring only

21138 contouring and application of prosthetic material or bone graft (includes obtaining autograft)

21139 contouring and setback of anterior frontal sinus wall

21141 Reconstruction midface, LeFort I; single piece, segment movement in any direction (eg, for Long Face Syndrome), without bone graft

21142 2 pieces, segment movement in any direction, without bone graft

21143 3 or more pieces, segment movement in any direction, without bone graft

21145 single piece, segment movement in any direction, requiring bone grafts (includes obtaining autografts)

21146 2 pieces, segment movement in any direction, requiring bone grafts (includes obtaining autografts) (eg, ungrafted unilateral alveolar cleft)

21147 3 or more pieces, segment movement in any direction, requiring bone grafts (includes obtaining autografts) (eg, ungrafted bilateral alveolar cleft or multiple osteotomies)

21150 Reconstruction midface, LeFort II; anterior intrusion (eg, Treacher-Collins Syndrome)

21151 any direction, requiring bone grafts (includes obtaining autografts)

21154 Reconstruction midface, LeFort III (extracranial), any type, requiring bone grafts (includes obtaining autografts); without LeFort I

21155 with LeFort I

21159 Reconstruction midface, LeFort III (extra and intracranial) with forehead advancement (eg, mono bloc), requiring bone grafts (includes obtaining autografts); without LeFort I

21160 with LeFort I

21172 Reconstruction superior-lateral orbital rim and lower forehead, advancement or alteration, with or without grafts (includes obtaining autografts)

(For frontal or parietal craniotomy performed for craniosynostosis, use 61556)

21175 Reconstruction, bifrontal, superior-lateral orbital rims and lower forehead, advancement or alteration (eg, plagiocephaly, trigonocephaly, brachycephaly), with or without grafts (includes obtaining autografts)

(For bifrontal craniotomy performed for craniosynostosis, use 61557)

21179 Reconstruction, entire or majority of forehead and/or supraorbital rims; with grafts (allograft or prosthetic material)

21180 with autograft (includes obtaining grafts)

(For extensive craniectomy for multiple suture craniosynostosis, use only 61558 or 61559)

21181 Reconstruction by contouring of benign tumor of cranial bones (eg, fibrous dysplasia), extracranial

21182 Reconstruction of orbital walls, rims, forehead, nasoethmoid complex following intra- and extracranial excision of benign tumor of cranial bone (eg, fibrous dysplasia), with multiple autografts (includes obtaining grafts); total area of bone grafting less than 40 sq cm

21183 total area of bone grafting greater than 40 sq cm but less than 80 sq cm
➜ *CPT Changes: An Insider's View* 2002

21184 total area of bone grafting greater than 80 sq cm
➜ *CPT Changes: An Insider's View* 2002

(For excision of benign tumor of cranial bones, see 61563, 61564)

★=Telemedicine ◀=Audio-only ✛=Add-on code ⊬=FDA approval pending #=Resequenced code ⊘=Modifier 51 exempt ➜➜➜=See p xxi for details

21188 Reconstruction midface, osteotomies (other than LeFort type) and bone grafts (includes obtaining autografts)

21193 Reconstruction of mandibular rami, horizontal, vertical, C, or L osteotomy; without bone graft
> *CPT Assistant* Apr 96:11

21194   with bone graft (includes obtaining graft)
> *CPT Assistant* Apr 96:11

21195 Reconstruction of mandibular rami and/or body, sagittal split; without internal rigid fixation
> *CPT Assistant* Apr 96:11

21196   with internal rigid fixation
> *CPT Assistant* Apr 96:11, Mar 97:11

Reconstruction of Mandibular Rami
21196

The mandibular ramus is reconstructed to lengthen, set back, or rotate the mandible.

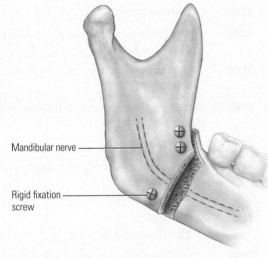

Mandibular nerve

Rigid fixation screw

21198 Osteotomy, mandible, segmental;
> *CPT Changes: An Insider's View* 2001
> *CPT Assistant* Dec 13:16

21199   with genioglossus advancement
> *CPT Changes: An Insider's View* 2001

(To report total osteotomy of the maxilla, see 21141-21160)

21206 Osteotomy, maxilla, segmental (eg, Wassmund or Schuchard)

21208 Osteoplasty, facial bones; augmentation (autograft, allograft, or prosthetic implant)

21209   reduction

21210 Graft, bone; nasal, maxillary or malar areas (includes obtaining graft)

(For cleft palate repair, see 42200-42225)

21215   mandible (includes obtaining graft)

21230 Graft; rib cartilage, autogenous, to face, chin, nose or ear (includes obtaining graft)

21235   ear cartilage, autogenous, to nose or ear (includes obtaining graft)

(To report graft augmentation of facial bones, use 21208)

21240 Arthroplasty, temporomandibular joint, with or without autograft (includes obtaining graft)

21242 Arthroplasty, temporomandibular joint, with allograft

21243 Arthroplasty, temporomandibular joint, with prosthetic joint replacement

21244 Reconstruction of mandible, extraoral, with transosteal bone plate (eg, mandibular staple bone plate)

21245 Reconstruction of mandible or maxilla, subperiosteal implant; partial

21246   complete

21247 Reconstruction of mandibular condyle with bone and cartilage autografts (includes obtaining grafts) (eg, for hemifacial microsomia)

21248 Reconstruction of mandible or maxilla, endosteal implant (eg, blade, cylinder); partial

21249   complete

(To report midface reconstruction, see 21141-21160)

21255 Reconstruction of zygomatic arch and glenoid fossa with bone and cartilage (includes obtaining autografts)

21256 Reconstruction of orbit with osteotomies (extracranial) and with bone grafts (includes obtaining autografts) (eg, micro-ophthalmia)

21260 Periorbital osteotomies for orbital hypertelorism, with bone grafts; extracranial approach

21261   combined intra- and extracranial approach

21263   with forehead advancement

21267 Orbital repositioning, periorbital osteotomies, unilateral, with bone grafts; extracranial approach

21268   combined intra- and extracranial approach

21270 Malar augmentation, prosthetic material

(For malar augmentation with bone graft, use 21210)

21275 Secondary revision of orbitocraniofacial reconstruction

21280 Medial canthopexy (separate procedure)

(For medial canthoplasty, use 67950)

21282 Lateral canthopexy

21295 Reduction of masseter muscle and bone (eg, for treatment of benign masseteric hypertrophy); extraoral approach

21296   intraoral approach

Other Procedures

21299 Unlisted craniofacial and maxillofacial procedure

Fracture and/or Dislocation

(For operative repair of skull fracture, see 62000-62010)

(To report closed treatment of skull fracture, use the appropriate Evaluation and Management code)

21315 Closed treatment of nasal bone fracture with manipulation; without stabilization
➔ *CPT Changes: An Insider's View* 2022
➔ *CPT Assistant* Jan 18:3, Sep 19:3, May 22:5,6

(For closed treatment of nasal bone fracture without manipulation or stabilization, use appropriate E/M code)

21320   with stabilization
➔ *CPT Changes: An Insider's View* 2022
➔ *CPT Assistant* Sep 19:3, May 22:5,6

21325 Open treatment of nasal fracture; uncomplicated
➔ *CPT Assistant* Jan 21:13

21330   complicated, with internal and/or external skeletal fixation
➔ *CPT Assistant* Jan 21:13

21335   with concomitant open treatment of fractured septum

21336 Open treatment of nasal septal fracture, with or without stabilization

21337 Closed treatment of nasal septal fracture, with or without stabilization
➔ *CPT Assistant* Sep 19:3

21338 Open treatment of nasoethmoid fracture; without external fixation

21339   with external fixation

21340 Percutaneous treatment of nasoethmoid complex fracture, with splint, wire or headcap fixation, including repair of canthal ligaments and/or the nasolacrimal apparatus

21343 Open treatment of depressed frontal sinus fracture

21344 Open treatment of complicated (eg, comminuted or involving posterior wall) frontal sinus fracture, via coronal or multiple approaches

21345 Closed treatment of nasomaxillary complex fracture (LeFort II type), with interdental wire fixation or fixation of denture or splint

21346 Open treatment of nasomaxillary complex fracture (LeFort II type); with wiring and/or local fixation

21347   requiring multiple open approaches

21348   with bone grafting (includes obtaining graft)

21355 Percutaneous treatment of fracture of malar area, including zygomatic arch and malar tripod, with manipulation

21356 Open treatment of depressed zygomatic arch fracture (eg, Gillies approach)

21360 Open treatment of depressed malar fracture, including zygomatic arch and malar tripod

21365 Open treatment of complicated (eg, comminuted or involving cranial nerve foramina) fracture(s) of malar area, including zygomatic arch and malar tripod; with internal fixation and multiple surgical approaches

21366   with bone grafting (includes obtaining graft)

21385 Open treatment of orbital floor blowout fracture; transantral approach (Caldwell-Luc type operation)

21386   periorbital approach

21387   combined approach

21390   periorbital approach, with alloplastic or other implant
➔ *CPT Assistant* Dec 20:11

21395   periorbital approach with bone graft (includes obtaining graft)

21400 Closed treatment of fracture of orbit, except blowout; without manipulation

21401   with manipulation

21406 Open treatment of fracture of orbit, except blowout; without implant
➔ *CPT Assistant* Dec 20:11

21407   with implant
➔ *CPT Assistant* Dec 20:11

21408   with bone grafting (includes obtaining graft)

21421 Closed treatment of palatal or maxillary fracture (LeFort I type), with interdental wire fixation or fixation of denture or splint

21422 Open treatment of palatal or maxillary fracture (LeFort I type);

21423   complicated (comminuted or involving cranial nerve foramina), multiple approaches

21431 Closed treatment of craniofacial separation (LeFort III type) using interdental wire fixation of denture or splint

21432 Open treatment of craniofacial separation (LeFort III type); with wiring and/or internal fixation

★ = Telemedicine   ◀ = Audio-only   ✚ = Add-on code   ✔ = FDA approval pending   # = Resequenced code   ⊘ = Modifier 51 exempt   ➔➔➔ = See p xxi for details

21433   complicated (eg, comminuted or involving cranial nerve foramina), multiple surgical approaches

21435   complicated, utilizing internal and/or external fixation techniques (eg, head cap, halo device, and/or intermaxillary fixation)

(For removal of internal or external fixation device, use 20670)

21436   complicated, multiple surgical approaches, internal fixation, with bone grafting (includes obtaining graft)

21440   Closed treatment of mandibular or maxillary alveolar ridge fracture (separate procedure)

21445   Open treatment of mandibular or maxillary alveolar ridge fracture (separate procedure)

21450   Closed treatment of mandibular fracture; without manipulation

21451   with manipulation

21452   Percutaneous treatment of mandibular fracture, with external fixation

21453   Closed treatment of mandibular fracture with interdental fixation
➔ *CPT Assistant* Dec 07:7-8

21454   Open treatment of mandibular fracture with external fixation

21461   Open treatment of mandibular fracture; without interdental fixation

21462   with interdental fixation

21465   Open treatment of mandibular condylar fracture

21470   Open treatment of complicated mandibular fracture by multiple surgical approaches including internal fixation, interdental fixation, and/or wiring of dentures or splints
➔ *CPT Assistant* Nov 02:10

21480   Closed treatment of temporomandibular dislocation; initial or subsequent

21485   complicated (eg, recurrent requiring intermaxillary fixation or splinting), initial or subsequent

21490   Open treatment of temporomandibular dislocation

(For interdental wire fixation, use 21497)

(To report treatment of closed fracture of larynx, use the applicable Evaluation and Management codes)

21497   Interdental wiring, for condition other than fracture
➔ *CPT Assistant* Mar 97:10

Other Procedures

21499   Unlisted musculoskeletal procedure, head

(For unlisted craniofacial or maxillofacial procedure, use 21299)

Neck (Soft Tissues) and Thorax

(For cervical spine and back, see 21920 et seq)

(For injection of fracture site or trigger point, use 20550)

Incision

(For incision and drainage of abscess or hematoma, superficial, see 10060, 10140)

21501   Incision and drainage, deep abscess or hematoma, soft tissues of neck or thorax;
➔ *CPT Assistant* Dec 14:16

(For posterior spine subfascial incision and drainage, see 22010-22015)

21502   with partial rib ostectomy

21510   Incision, deep, with opening of bone cortex (eg, for osteomyelitis or bone abscess), thorax

Excision

(For bone biopsy, see 20220-20251)

21550   Biopsy, soft tissue of neck or thorax

(For needle biopsy of soft tissue, use 20206)

21552   Code is out of numerical sequence. See 21550-21558

21554   Code is out of numerical sequence. See 21550-21558

21555   Excision, tumor, soft tissue of neck or anterior thorax, subcutaneous; less than 3 cm
➔ *CPT Changes: An Insider's View* 2010
➔ *CPT Assistant* Oct 02:11

 # 21552   3 cm or greater
➔ *CPT Changes: An Insider's View* 2010

(For excision of benign lesions of cutaneous origin [eg, sebaceous cyst], see 11420-11426)

21556   Excision, tumor, soft tissue of neck or anterior thorax, subfascial (eg, intramuscular); less than 5 cm
➔ *CPT Changes: An Insider's View* 2010

 # 21554   5 cm or greater
➔ *CPT Changes: An Insider's View* 2010

21557   Radical resection of tumor (eg, sarcoma), soft tissue of neck or anterior thorax; less than 5 cm
➔ *CPT Changes: An Insider's View* 2010, 2014
➔ *CPT Assistant* Apr 10:11, Apr 20:10

21558   5 cm or greater

➔ *CPT Changes: An Insider's View* 2010, 2014

➔ *CPT Assistant* Apr 20:10

(For radical resection of tumor[s] of cutaneous origin [eg, melanoma], see 11600-11620)

21600   Excision of rib, partial

➔ *CPT Assistant* Jul 12:12, Mar 13:13

(For radical resection of chest wall and rib cage for tumor, use 21601)

(For radical debridement of chest wall and rib cage for injury, see 11044, 11047)

21601   Excision of chest wall tumor including rib(s)

➔ *CPT Changes: An Insider's View* 2020

➔ *CPT Assistant* Dec 19:4

21602   Excision of chest wall tumor involving rib(s), with plastic reconstruction; without mediastinal lymphadenectomy

➔ *CPT Changes: An Insider's View* 2020

➔ *CPT Assistant* Dec 19:4

21603   with mediastinal lymphadenectomy

➔ *CPT Changes: An Insider's View* 2020

➔ *CPT Assistant* Dec 19:4

(Do not report 21601, 21602, 21603 in conjunction with 32100, 32503, 32504, 32551, 32554, 32555)

21610   Costotransversectomy (separate procedure)

21615   Excision first and/or cervical rib;

➔ *CPT Assistant* Mar 14:13

21616   with sympathectomy

21620   Ostectomy of sternum, partial

21627   Sternal debridement

➔ *CPT Assistant* May 11:3

(For debridement and closure, use 21750)

▲ **21630**   Radical resection of sternum

➔ *CPT Changes: An Insider's View* 2025

▶(21632 has been deleted)◀

Repair, Revision, and/or Reconstruction

(For superficial wound, see **Integumentary System** section under Repair—Simple)

21685   Hyoid myotomy and suspension

➔ *CPT Changes: An Insider's View* 2004

➔ *CPT Assistant* Aug 04:11

21700   Division of scalenus anticus; without resection of cervical rib

21705   with resection of cervical rib

➔ *CPT Assistant* Mar 14:13

21720   Division of sternocleidomastoid for torticollis, open operation; without cast application

(For transection of spinal accessory and cervical nerves, see 63191, 64722)

21725   with cast application

21740   Reconstructive repair of pectus excavatum or carinatum; open

➔ *CPT Changes: An Insider's View* 2003

21742   minimally invasive approach (Nuss procedure), without thoracoscopy

➔ *CPT Changes: An Insider's View* 2003

21743   minimally invasive approach (Nuss procedure), with thoracoscopy

➔ *CPT Changes: An Insider's View* 2003

➔ *CPT Assistant* Nov 19:15

21750   Closure of median sternotomy separation with or without debridement (separate procedure)

➔ *CPT Changes: An Insider's View* 2002

➔ *CPT Assistant* May 11:3

Fracture and/or Dislocation

(To report closed treatment of an uncomplicated rib fracture, use the Evaluation and Management codes)

21811   Open treatment of rib fracture(s) with internal fixation, includes thoracoscopic visualization when performed, unilateral; 1-3 ribs

➔ *CPT Changes: An Insider's View* 2015

➔ *CPT Assistant* Aug 15:3

(For bilateral procedure, report 21811 with modifier 50)

21812   4-6 ribs

➔ *CPT Changes: An Insider's View* 2015

➔ *CPT Assistant* Aug 15:3

(For bilateral procedure, report 21812 with modifier 50)

21813   7 or more ribs

➔ *CPT Changes: An Insider's View* 2015

➔ *CPT Assistant* Aug 15:3

(For bilateral procedure, report 21813 with modifier 50)

21820   Closed treatment of sternum fracture

21825   Open treatment of sternum fracture with or without skeletal fixation

(For sternoclavicular dislocation, see 23520-23532)

Other Procedures

21899   Unlisted procedure, neck or thorax

➔ *CPT Assistant* Aug 15:3

Back and Flank

Excision

21920 Biopsy, soft tissue of back or flank; superficial

21925   deep

(For needle biopsy of soft tissue, use 20206)

21930 Excision, tumor, soft tissue of back or flank, subcutaneous; less than 3 cm
➜ *CPT Changes: An Insider's View* 2010

21931   3 cm or greater
➜ *CPT Changes: An Insider's View* 2010

(For excision of benign lesions of cutaneous origin [eg, sebaceous cyst], see 11400-11406)

21932 Excision, tumor, soft tissue of back or flank, subfascial (eg, intramuscular); less than 5 cm
➜ *CPT Changes: An Insider's View* 2010

21933   5 cm or greater
➜ *CPT Changes: An Insider's View* 2010

21935 Radical resection of tumor (eg, sarcoma), soft tissue of back or flank; less than 5 cm
➜ *CPT Changes: An Insider's View* 2010, 2014

21936   5 cm or greater
➜ *CPT Changes: An Insider's View* 2010, 2014

(For radical resection of tumor[s] of cutaneous origin [eg, melanoma], see 11600-11606)

Spine (Vertebral Column)

Cervical, thoracic, and lumbar spine.

Within the spine section, bone grafting procedures are reported separately and in addition to arthrodesis. For bone grafts in other Musculoskeletal sections, see specific code(s) descriptor(s) and/or accompanying guidelines.

To report bone grafts performed after arthrodesis, see 20930-20938. Do not append modifier 62 to bone graft codes 20900-20938.

Example:

Posterior arthrodesis of L5-S1 for degenerative disc disease utilizing morselized autogenous iliac bone graft harvested through a separate fascial incision.

Report as 22612 and 20937.

Within the spine section, instrumentation is reported separately and in addition to arthrodesis. To report instrumentation procedures performed with definitive vertebral procedure(s), see 22840-22855, 22859. Instrumentation procedure codes 22840-22848, 22853, 22854, 22859 are reported in addition to the definitive procedure(s). Modifier 62 may not be appended to the definitive or add-on spinal instrumentation procedure code(s) 22840-22848, 22850, 22852, 22853, 22854, 22859.

Example:

Posterior arthrodesis of L4-S1, utilizing morselized autogenous iliac bone graft harvested through separate fascial incision, and pedicle screw fixation.

Report as 22612, 22614, 22842, and 20937.

Vertebral procedures are sometimes followed by arthrodesis and in addition may include bone grafts and instrumentation.

When arthrodesis is performed in addition to another procedure, the arthrodesis should be reported in addition to the original procedure with modifier 51 (multiple procedures). Examples are after osteotomy, fracture care, vertebral corpectomy, and laminectomy. Bone grafts and instrumentation are never performed without arthrodesis.

Example:

Treatment of a burst fracture of L2 by corpectomy followed by arthrodesis of L1-L3, utilizing anterior instrumentation L1-L3 and structural allograft.

Report as 63090, 22558-51, 22585, 22845, and 20931.

When two surgeons work together as primary surgeons performing distinct part(s) of a single reportable procedure, each surgeon should report his/her distinct operative work by appending modifier 62 to the single definitive procedure code. If additional procedure(s) (including add-on procedure[s]) are performed during the same surgical session, separate code(s) may be reported by each co-surgeon, with modifier 62 appended (see Appendix A).

Example:

A 42-year-old male with a history of posttraumatic degenerative disc disease at L3-4 and L4-5 (internal disc disruption) underwent surgical repair. Surgeon A performed an anterior exposure of the spine with mobilization of the great vessels. Surgeon B performed anterior (minimal) discectomy and fusion at L3-4 and L4-5 using anterior interbody technique.

Report surgeon A: 22558 append modifier 62, 22585 append modifier 62

Report surgeon B: 22558 append modifier 62, 22585 append modifier 62, 20931

(Do not append modifier 62 to bone graft code 20931)

(For injection procedure for myelography, use 62284)

(For injection procedure for discography, see 62290, 62291)

Musculoskeletal 20100-29999

(For injection procedure, chemonucleolysis, single or multiple levels, use 62292)

(For injection procedure for facet joints, see 64490-64495, 64633-64636)

(For needle or trocar biopsy, see 20220-20225)

Incision

22010 Incision and drainage, open, of deep abscess (subfascial), posterior spine; cervical, thoracic, or cervicothoracic
➔ *CPT Changes: An Insider's View* 2006

22015 lumbar, sacral, or lumbosacral
➔ *CPT Changes: An Insider's View* 2006

(Do not report 22015 in conjunction with 22010)

(Do not report 22015 in conjunction with instrumentation removal, 10180, 22850, 22852)

(For incision and drainage of abscess or hematoma, superficial, see 10060, 10140)

Excision

For the following codes, when two surgeons work together as primary surgeons performing distinct part(s) of partial vertebral body excision, each surgeon should report his/her distinct operative work by appending modifier 62 to the procedure code. In this situation, modifier 62 may be appended to the procedure code(s) 22100-22102, 22110-22114 and, as appropriate, to the associated additional vertebral segment add-on code(s) 22103, 22116 as long as both surgeons continue to work together as primary surgeons.

(For bone biopsy, see 20220-20251)

(To report soft tissue biopsy of back or flank, see 21920-21925)

(For needle biopsy of soft tissue, use 20206)

(To report excision of soft tissue tumor of back or flank, use 21930)

22100 Partial excision of posterior vertebral component (eg, spinous process, lamina or facet) for intrinsic bony lesion, single vertebral segment; cervical
➔ *CPT Assistant* Jul 13:3, Dec 21:3

22101 thoracic
➔ *CPT Assistant* Jul 13:3, Dec 21:3

22102 lumbar
➔ *CPT Assistant* Jul 13:3, Dec 21:3

(For insertion of posterior spinous process distraction devices, see 22867, 22868, 22869, 22870)

+ 22103 each additional segment (List separately in addition to code for primary procedure)
➔ *CPT Assistant* Feb 96:6, Dec 21:3

(Use 22103 in conjunction with 22100, 22101, 22102)

22110 Partial excision of vertebral body, for intrinsic bony lesion, without decompression of spinal cord or nerve root(s), single vertebral segment; cervical
➔ *CPT Assistant* Jul 13:3

22112 thoracic
➔ *CPT Assistant* Jul 13:3

22114 lumbar
➔ *CPT Assistant* Jul 13:3

+ 22116 each additional vertebral segment (List separately in addition to code for primary procedure)
➔ *CPT Assistant* Feb 96:6

(Use 22116 in conjunction with 22110, 22112, 22114)

(For complete or near complete resection of vertebral body, see vertebral corpectomy, 63081-63091)

(For spinal reconstruction with bone graft [autograft, allograft] and/or methylmethacrylate of cervical vertebral body, use 63081 and 22554 and 20931 or 20938)

(For spinal reconstruction with bone graft [autograft, allograft] and/or methylmethacrylate of thoracic vertebral body, use 63085 or 63087 and 22556 and 20931 or 20938)

(For spinal reconstruction with bone graft [autograft, allograft] and/or methylmethacrylate of lumbar vertebral body, use 63087 or 63090 and 22558 and 20931 or 20938)

(For spinal reconstruction following vertebral body resection, use 63082 or 63086 or 63088 or 63091, and 22585)

(For harvest of bone autograft for vertebral reconstruction, see 20931 or 20938)

(For cervical spinal reconstruction with prosthetic replacement of resected vertebral bodies, see codes 63081 and 22554 and 20931 or 20938 and 22853, 22854, 22859)

(For thoracic spinal reconstruction with prosthetic replacement of resected vertebral bodies, see codes 63085 or 63087 and 22556 and 20931 or 20938 and 22853, 22854, 22859)

(For lumbar spinal reconstruction with prosthetic replacement of resected vertebral bodies, see codes 63087 or 63090 and 22558 and 20931 or 20938 and 22853, 22854, 22859)

(For osteotomy of spine, see 22210-22226)

Osteotomy

To report arthrodesis, see codes 22590-22632. (Report in addition to code[s] for the definitive procedure with modifier 51.)

To report instrumentation procedures, see 22840-22855, 22859. (Report in addition to code[s] for the definitive procedure[s].) Do not append modifier 62 to spinal instrumentation codes 22840-22848, 22850, 22852, 22853, 22854, 22859.

To report bone graft procedures, see 20930-20938. (Report in addition to code[s] for the definitive procedure[s].) Do not append modifier 62 to bone graft codes 20900-20938.

For the following codes, when two surgeons work together as primary surgeons performing distinct part(s) of an anterior spine osteotomy, each surgeon should report his/her distinct operative work by appending modifier 62 to the procedure code. In this situation, modifier 62 may be appended to the procedure code(s) 22210-22214, 22220-22224 and, as appropriate, to associated additional segment add-on code(s) 22216, 22226 as long as both surgeons continue to work together as primary surgeons.

Spinal osteotomy procedures are reported when a portion(s) of the vertebral segment(s) is cut and removed in preparation for re-aligning the spine as part of a spinal deformity correction. For excision of an intrinsic lesion of the vertebra without deformity correction, see 22100-22116. For decompression of the spinal cord and/or nerve roots, see 63001-63308.

The three columns are defined as anterior (anterior two-thirds of the vertebral body), middle (posterior third of the vertebral body and the pedicle), and posterior (articular facets, lamina, and spinous process).

22206   Osteotomy of spine, posterior or posterolateral approach, 3 columns, 1 vertebral segment (eg, pedicle/vertebral body subtraction); thoracic
➜ *CPT Changes: An Insider's View* 2008
➜ *CPT Assistant* Feb 08:9, Jul 13:3, Dec 21:5-6

(Do not report 22206 in conjunction with 22207)

22207   lumbar
➜ *CPT Changes: An Insider's View* 2008
➜ *CPT Assistant* Feb 08:9, Jul 13:3, Dec 21:5-6

(Do not report 22207 in conjunction with 22206)

+ 22208   each additional vertebral segment (List separately in addition to code for primary procedure)
➜ *CPT Changes: An Insider's View* 2008
➜ *CPT Assistant* Feb 08:9, Dec 21:5-6

(Use 22208 in conjunction with 22206, 22207)

(Do not report 22206, 22207, 22208 in conjunction with 22210-22226, 22830, 63001-63048, 63055-63066, 63075-63091, 63101-63103, when performed at the same level)

22210   Osteotomy of spine, posterior or posterolateral approach, 1 vertebral segment; cervical
➜ *CPT Assistant* Jul 13:3, Dec 21:4-5

22212   thoracic
➜ *CPT Assistant* Dec 07:1, Jul 13:3, Dec 21:4-5

22214   lumbar
➜ *CPT Assistant* Dec 07:1, Jul 13:3, Dec 14:16, Dec 21:4-5

+ 22216   each additional vertebral segment (List separately in addition to primary procedure)
➜ *CPT Assistant* Dec 07:1, Dec 21:4-5

(Use 22216 in conjunction with 22210, 22212, 22214)

22220   Osteotomy of spine, including discectomy, anterior approach, single vertebral segment; cervical
➜ *CPT Assistant* Feb 02:4, Jul 13:3, Dec 21:5-6

22222   thoracic
➜ *CPT Assistant* Feb 02:4, Dec 21:5-6

22224   lumbar
➜ *CPT Assistant* Feb 02:4, Jul 13:3, Dec 21:5-6

+ 22226   each additional vertebral segment (List separately in addition to code for primary procedure)
➜ *CPT Assistant* Feb 96:6, Feb 02:4, Dec 21:5-6

(Use 22226 in conjunction with 22220, 22222, 22224)

(For vertebral corpectomy, see 63081-63091)

Fracture and/or Dislocation

To report arthrodesis, see codes 22590-22632. (Report in addition to code[s] for the definitive procedure with modifier 51.)

To report instrumentation procedures, see 22840-22855, 22859. (Report in addition to code[s] for the definitive procedure[s].) Do not append modifier 62 to spinal instrumentation codes 22840-22848, 22850, 22852, 22853, 22854, 22859.

To report bone graft procedures, see 20930-20938. (Report in addition to code[s] for the definitive procedure[s].) Do not append modifier 62 to bone graft codes 20900-20938.

For the following codes, when two surgeons work together as primary surgeons performing distinct part(s) of open fracture and/or dislocation procedure(s), each surgeon should report his/her distinct operative work by appending modifier 62 to the procedure code. In this situation, modifier 62 may be appended to the procedure code(s) 22318-22327 and, as appropriate, the associated additional fracture vertebrae or dislocated segment add-on code 22328 as long as both surgeons continue to work together as primary surgeons.

Musculoskeletal 20100-29999

22310 Closed treatment of vertebral body fracture(s), without manipulation, requiring and including casting or bracing
➔ *CPT Assistant* Jun 12:10, Jul 13:3, Jul 14:8

(Do not report 22310 in conjunction with 22510, 22511, 22512, 22513, 22514, 22515, when performed at the same level)

22315 Closed treatment of vertebral fracture(s) and/or dislocation(s) requiring casting or bracing, with and including casting and/or bracing by manipulation or traction
➔ *CPT Changes: An Insider's View* 2011
➔ *CPT Assistant* Apr 12:11, Jun 12:10, Jul 13:3

(Do not report 22315 in conjunction with 22510, 22511, 22512, 22513, 22514, 22515, when performed at the same level)

(For spinal subluxation, use 97140)

22318 Open treatment and/or reduction of odontoid fracture(s) and or dislocation(s) (including os odontoideum), anterior approach, including placement of internal fixation; without grafting
➔ *CPT Changes: An Insider's View* 2000
➔ *CPT Assistant* Nov 99:11, Apr 12:13, Jul 13:3

22319 with grafting
➔ *CPT Changes: An Insider's View* 2000
➔ *CPT Assistant* Nov 99:11, Apr 12:16, Jul 13:3

22325 Open treatment and/or reduction of vertebral fracture(s) and/or dislocation(s), posterior approach, 1 fractured vertebra or dislocated segment; lumbar
➔ *CPT Assistant* Sep 97:8, Jun 12:10, Jul 13:3, Aug 17:9

(Do not report 22325 in conjunction with 22511, 22512, 22514, 22515 when performed at the same level)

22326 cervical
➔ *CPT Assistant* Sep 97:8, Jul 13:3

(Do not report 22326 in conjunction with 22510, 22512, when performed at the same level)

22327 thoracic
➔ *CPT Assistant* Sep 97:8, Jun 12:10, Jul 13:3

(Do not report 22327 in conjunction with 22510, 22512, 22513, 22515 when performed at the same level)

+ 22328 each additional fractured vertebra or dislocated segment (List separately in addition to code for primary procedure)
➔ *CPT Assistant* Feb 96:6

(Use 22328 in conjunction with 22325-22327)

(For treatment of vertebral fracture by the anterior approach, see corpectomy 63081-63091, and appropriate arthrodesis, bone graft and instrument codes)

(For decompression of spine following fracture, see 63001-63091; for arthrodesis of spine following fracture, see 22548-22632)

Manipulation

(For spinal manipulation without anesthesia, use 97140)

22505 Manipulation of spine requiring anesthesia, any region
➔ *CPT Assistant* Mar 97:11, Jan 99:11

Percutaneous Vertebroplasty and Vertebral Augmentation

Codes 22510, 22511, 22512, 22513, 22514, 22515 describe procedures for percutaneous vertebral augmentation that include vertebroplasty of the cervical, thoracic, lumbar, and sacral spine and vertebral augmentation of the thoracic and lumbar spine.

For the purposes of reporting 22510, 22511, 22512, 22513, 22514, 22515, "vertebroplasty" is the process of injecting a material (cement) into the vertebral body to reinforce the structure of the body using image guidance. "Vertebral augmentation" is the process of cavity creation followed by the injection of the material (cement) under image guidance. For 0200T and 0201T, "sacral augmentation (sacroplasty)" refers to the creation of a cavity within a sacral vertebral body followed by injection of a material to fill that cavity.

The procedure codes are inclusive of bone biopsy, when performed, and imaging guidance necessary to perform the procedure. Use one primary procedure code and an add-on code for additional levels. When treating the sacrum, sacral procedures are reported only once per encounter.

(For thermal destruction of intraosseous basivertebral nerve, see 64628, 64629)

22510 Percutaneous vertebroplasty (bone biopsy included when performed), 1 vertebral body, unilateral or bilateral injection, inclusive of all imaging guidance; cervicothoracic
➔ *CPT Changes: An Insider's View* 2015, 2017
➔ *CPT Assistant* Jan 15:8
➔ *Clinical Examples in Radiology* Fall 14:3, Summer 15:14, Summer 20:10

22511 lumbosacral
➔ *CPT Changes: An Insider's View* 2015, 2017
➔ *CPT Assistant* Jan 15:8, Apr 15:8
➔ *Clinical Examples in Radiology* Fall 14:3-4, Summer 20:10, Fall 22:20

+ 22512   each additional cervicothoracic or lumbosacral vertebral body (List separately in addition to code for primary procedure)

➲ *CPT Changes: An Insider's View* 2015, 2017

➲ *CPT Assistant* Jan 15:8

➲ *Clinical Examples in Radiology* Fall 14:3-4, Summer 15:14, Summer 20:10

(Use 22512 in conjunction with 22510, 22511)

(Do not report 22510, 22511, 22512 in conjunction with 20225, 22310, 22315, 22325, 22327, when performed at the same level as 22510, 22511, 22512)

Percutaneous Vertebroplasty

22510

Augmentation of a vertebral fracture is achieved by percutaneous injections of polymethylmethacrylate under fluoroscopic guidance.

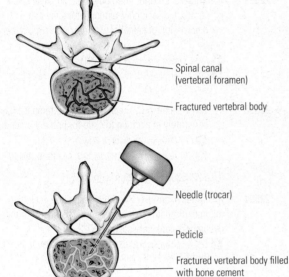

Spinal canal (vertebral foramen)

Fractured vertebral body

Needle (trocar)

Pedicle

Fractured vertebral body filled with bone cement

22513   Percutaneous vertebral augmentation, including cavity creation (fracture reduction and bone biopsy included when performed) using mechanical device (eg, kyphoplasty), 1 vertebral body, unilateral or bilateral cannulation, inclusive of all imaging guidance; thoracic

➲ *CPT Changes: An Insider's View* 2015, 2017

➲ *CPT Assistant* Jan 15:8

➲ *Clinical Examples in Radiology* Fall 14:3, Summer 20:10

22514   lumbar

➲ *CPT Changes: An Insider's View* 2015, 2017

➲ *CPT Assistant* Jan 15:8

➲ *Clinical Examples in Radiology* Fall 14:3-4

+ 22515   each additional thoracic or lumbar vertebral body (List separately in addition to code for primary procedure)

➲ *CPT Changes: An Insider's View* 2015, 2017

➲ *CPT Assistant* Jan 15:8

➲ *Clinical Examples in Radiology* Fall 14:3

(Use 22515 in conjunction with 22513, 22514)

(Do not report 22513, 22514, 22515 in conjunction with 20225, 22310, 22315, 22325, 22327, when performed at the same level as 22513, 22514, 22515)

Percutaneous Augmentation and Annuloplasty

22526   Percutaneous intradiscal electrothermal annuloplasty, unilateral or bilateral including fluoroscopic guidance; single level

➲ *CPT Changes: An Insider's View* 2007, 2017

➲ *CPT Assistant* Sep 07:10, Nov 10:3, Jan 11:8, Jan 15:8, Feb 21:13, Dec 23:46

+ 22527   1 or more additional levels (List separately in addition to code for primary procedure)

➲ *CPT Changes: An Insider's View* 2007, 2017

➲ *CPT Assistant* Sep 07:10, Nov 10:3, Jan 11:8, Jan 15:8

(Use 22527 in conjunction with 22526)

(Do not report codes 22526, 22527 in conjunction with 77002, 77003)

(For percutaneous intradiscal annuloplasty using method other than electrothermal, use 22899)

Arthrodesis

Arthrodesis may be performed in the absence of other procedures and therefore when it is combined with another definitive procedure (eg, osteotomy, fracture care, vertebral corpectomy or laminectomy), modifier 51 is appropriate. However, arthrodesis codes 22585, 22614, and 22632 are considered add-on procedure codes and should not be used with modifier 51.

To report instrumentation procedures, see 22840-22855, 22859. (Codes 22840-22848, 22853, 22854, 22859 are reported in conjunction with code[s] for the definitive procedure[s]. When instrumentation reinsertion or removal is reported in conjunction with other definitive procedures, including arthrodesis, decompression, and exploration of fusion, append modifier 51 to 22849, 22850, 22852, and 22855.) To report exploration of fusion, use 22830. (When exploration is reported in conjunction with other definitive procedures, including arthrodesis and decompression, append modifier 51 to 22830.) Do not append modifier 62 to spinal instrumentation codes 22840-22848, 22850, 22852, 22853, 22854, 22859.

To report bone graft procedures, see 20930-20938. (Report in addition to code[s] for the definitive procedure[s].) Do not append modifier 62 to bone graft codes 20900-20938.

Lateral Extracavitary Approach Technique

22532 Arthrodesis, lateral extracavitary technique, including minimal discectomy to prepare interspace (other than for decompression); thoracic

➔ *CPT Changes: An Insider's View* 2004

➔ *CPT Assistant* Apr 12:16, Jul 13:3, May 20:14, Jul 21:7

22533 lumbar

➔ *CPT Changes: An Insider's View* 2004

➔ *CPT Assistant* Apr 12:16, Jul 13:3

+ 22534 thoracic or lumbar, each additional vertebral segment (List separately in addition to code for primary procedure)

➔ *CPT Changes: An Insider's View* 2004

(Use 22534 in conjunction with 22532 and 22533)

Anterior or Anterolateral Approach Technique

Procedure codes 22554-22558 are for SINGLE interspace; for additional interspaces, use 22585. A vertebral interspace is the non-bony compartment between two adjacent vertebral bodies, which contains the intervertebral disc, and includes the nucleus pulposus, annulus fibrosus, and two cartilaginous endplates.

For the following codes, when two surgeons work together as primary surgeons performing distinct part(s) of an anterior interbody arthrodesis, each surgeon should report his/her distinct operative work by appending modifier 62 to the procedure code. In this situation, modifier 62 may be appended to the procedure code(s) 22548-22558 and, as appropriate, to the associated additional interspace add-on code 22585 as long as both surgeons continue to work together as primary surgeons.

22548 Arthrodesis, anterior transoral or extraoral technique, clivus-C1-C2 (atlas-axis), with or without excision of odontoid process

➔ *CPT Assistant* Spring 93:36, Feb 96:7, Sep 97:8, Sep 00:10, Feb 02:4, Apr 12:16, Jul 13:3

(For intervertebral disc excision by laminotomy or laminectomy, see 63020-63042)

Arthrodesis (Anterior Transoral Technique)
22548

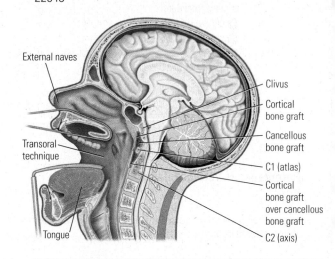

22551 Arthrodesis, anterior interbody, including disc space preparation, discectomy, osteophytectomy and decompression of spinal cord and/or nerve roots; cervical below C2

➔ *CPT Changes: An Insider's View* 2011

➔ *CPT Assistant* Apr 12:16, Jul 13:3, Jan 15:13, May 16:13, Aug 18:10, Aug 23:11

+ 22552 cervical below C2, each additional interspace (List separately in addition to code for primary procedure)

➔ *CPT Changes: An Insider's View* 2011

➔ *CPT Assistant* Apr 12:16, Jul 13:3, Aug 18:10, Aug 23:11

(Use 22552 in conjunction with 22551)

22554 Arthrodesis, anterior interbody technique, including minimal discectomy to prepare interspace (other than for decompression); cervical below C2

➔ *CPT Assistant* Spring 93:36, Sep 97:8, Sep 00:10, Jan 01:12, Feb 02:4, Apr 12:16, Jul 13:3, Apr 15:7, Aug 23:11

(Do not report 22554 in conjunction with 63075, even if performed by a separate individual. To report anterior cervical discectomy and interbody fusion at the same level during the same session, use 22551)

22556 thoracic

➔ *CPT Assistant* Spring 93:36, Jul 96:7, Sep 97:8, Sep 00:10, Feb 02:4, Apr 12:16, Jul 13:3

22558 lumbar

➔ *CPT Assistant* Spring 93:36, Mar 96:6, Jul 96:7, Sep 97:8, Sep 00:10, Feb 02:4, Oct 09:9, Apr 12:16, Jul 13:3, Mar 15:9

(For arthrodesis using pre-sacral interbody technique, use 22586)

Anterior Approach for Cervical Fusion
22554

An example of an exposure technique used to reach anterior cervical vertebrae for spinal procedures (eg, discectomy, arthrodesis, spinal instrumentation)

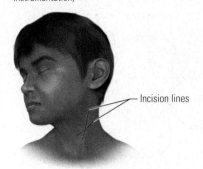

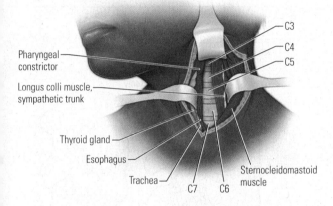

Incision lines

Pharyngeal constrictor

Longus colli muscle, sympathetic trunk

Thyroid gland

Esophagus

Trachea

C3
C4
C5

Sternocleidomastoid muscle

C7   C6

+ 22585   each additional interspace (List separately in addition to code for primary procedure)
  → *CPT Changes: An Insider's View* 2011
  → *CPT Assistant* Spring 93:36, Feb 96:6, Mar 96:6, Sep 97:8, Sep 00:10, Feb 02:4, Apr 08:11

  (Use 22585 in conjunction with 22554, 22556, 22558)

  (Do not report 22585 in conjunction with 63075, even if performed by a separate individual. To report anterior cervical discectomy and interbody fusion at the same level during the same session, use 22552)

22586   Arthrodesis, pre-sacral interbody technique, including disc space preparation, discectomy, with posterior instrumentation, with image guidance, includes bone graft when performed, L5-S1 interspace
  → *CPT Changes: An Insider's View* 2013

  (Do not report 22586 in conjunction with 20930-20938, 22840, 22848, 77002, 77003, 77011, 77012)

Posterior, Posterolateral or Lateral Transverse Process Technique

To report instrumentation procedures, see 22840-22855, 22859. (Report in addition to code[s] for the definitive procedure[s].) Do not append modifier 62 to spinal instrumentation codes 22840-22848, 22850, 22852, 22853, 22854, 22859.

Anterior Approach for Lumbar Fusion (Anterior Retroperitoneal Exposure)
22558

An example of an exposure technique used to reach anterior lumbar vertebrae for spinal procedures (eg, discectomy, arthrodesis, spinal instrumentation)

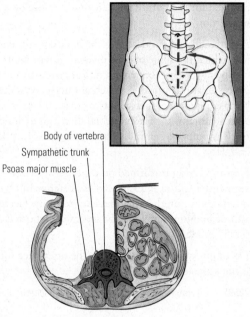

Incision line and approach to lumbar spine

Body of vertebra
Sympathetic trunk
Psoas major muscle

To report bone graft procedures, see 20930-20938. (Report in addition to code[s] for the definitive procedure[s].) Do not append modifier 62 to bone graft codes 20900-20938.

Definitions

Corpectomy: Identifies removal of a vertebral body during spinal surgery.

Facetectomy: The excision of the facet joint between two vertebral bodies. There are two facet joints at each vertebral segment (see below).

Foraminotomy: The excision of bone to widen the intervertebral foramen. The intervertebral foramen is bordered by the superior notch of the adjacent vertebra, the inferior notch of the vertebra, the facet joint, and the intervertebral disc.

Hemilaminectomy: Removal of a portion of a vertebral lamina, usually performed for exploration of, access to, or decompression of the intraspinal contents.

Musculoskeletal 20100-29999

Lamina: Pertains to the vertebral arch, the flattened posterior portion of the vertebral arch extending between the pedicles and the midline, forming the dorsal wall of the vertebral forameny, and from the midline junction of which the spinous process extends.

Laminectomy: Excision of a vertebral lamina, commonly used to denote removal of the posterior arch.

Laminotomy: Excision of a portion of the vertebral lamina, resulting in enlargement of the intervertebral foramen for the purpose of relieving pressure on a spinal nerve root.

A vertebral segment describes the basic constituent part into which the spine may be divided. It represents a single complete vertebral bone with its associated articular processes and laminae. A vertebral interspace is the non-bony compartment between two adjacent vertebral bodies which contains the intervertebral disc, and includes the nucleus pulposus, annulus fibrosus, and two cartilaginous endplates.

Decompression performed on the same vertebral segment(s) and/or interspace(s) as posterior lumbar interbody fusion that includes laminectomy, facetectomy, and/or foraminotomy may be separately reported using 63052, 63053.

Decompression solely to prepare the interspace for fusion is not separately reported.

22590 Arthrodesis, posterior technique, craniocervical (occiput-C2)

> *CPT Assistant* Spring 93:36, Sep 97:8, Apr 12:16, Jul 13:3, Dec 21:5-6

22595 Arthrodesis, posterior technique, atlas-axis (C1-C2)

> *CPT Assistant* Spring 93:36, Sep 97:8, Apr 12:12, Jul 13:3, Dec 21:5-6

22600 Arthrodesis, posterior or posterolateral technique, single interspace; cervical below C2 segment

> *CPT Changes: An Insider's View* 2022
> *CPT Assistant* Spring 93:36, Sep 97:8, Nov 10:8, Apr 12:16, Jun 12:11, Jul 13:3, Dec 21:5-6, Oct 23:19

22610 thoracic (with lateral transverse technique, when performed)

> *CPT Changes: An Insider's View* 2012, 2022
> *CPT Assistant* Spring 93:36, Sep 97:8, Nov 10:8, Apr 12:16, Jun 12:10, Jul 13:3, Dec 21:5-6, Oct 23:19

22612 lumbar (with lateral transverse technique, when performed)

> *CPT Changes: An Insider's View* 2012, 2022
> *CPT Assistant* Spring 93:36, Mar 96:7, Sep 97:8, 11, Apr 08:11, Jul 08:7, Oct 09:9, Nov 10:8, Dec 11:14, Jan 12:3, Apr 12:16, Jun 12:10, Jul 13:3, Dec 13:14, Dec 21:5-6, 22, Jun 23:26, Oct 23:19

(Do not report 22612 in conjunction with 22630 for the same interspace; use 22633)

Visual Definitions of Spinal Anatomy and Procedures

A. Vertebral interspace (non-bony) and segment (bony)

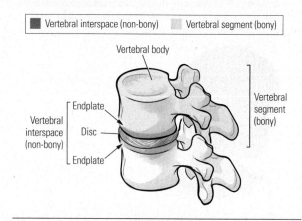

B. Foraminotomy and facetectomy

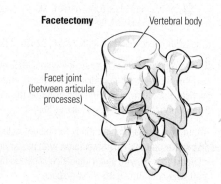

C. Laminotomy, hemilaminectomy, and laminectomy

☐ = Area of bone removed during procedure

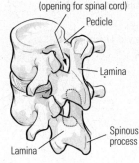

Laminotomy

Vertebral foramen (opening for spinal cord)

Pedicle

Lamina

Spinous process

Lamina

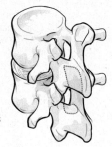

Hemilaminectomy

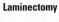

Laminectomy

D. Corpectomy

☐ = Area of bone removed during procedure

Corpectomy *(expanded views)*

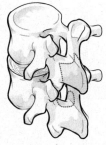

Cervical (≥50%)   Thoracic (≥33%)   Lumbar (≥33%)

Vertebral body

+ 22614   each additional interspace (List separately in addition to code for primary procedure)

⊘ *CPT Changes: An Insider's View* 2022

⊘ *CPT Assistant* Feb 96:6, Mar 96:7, Nov 10:8, Jun 12:11, Jul 13:3, Dec 21:5-6, 22

(Use 22614 in conjunction with 22600, 22610, 22612, 22630, or 22633, when performed for arthrodesis at a different interspace. When performing a posterior or posterolateral technique for fusion/arthrodesis at an additional interspace, use 22614. When performing a posterior interbody fusion arthrodesis at an additional interspace, use 22632. When performing a combined posterior or posterolateral technique with posterior interbody arthrodesis at an additional interspace, use 22634)

(For facet joint fusion, see 0219T-0222T)

(For placement of a posterior intrafacet implant, see 0219T-0222T)

22630   Arthrodesis, posterior interbody technique, including laminectomy and/or discectomy to prepare interspace (other than for decompression), single interspace, lumbar;

⊘ *CPT Changes: An Insider's View* 2000

⊘ *CPT Assistant* Spring 93:36, Sep 97:8, Nov 99:11, Dec 99:2, Jan 01:12, Oct 09:9, Nov 11:10, Dec 11:14, Jan 12:3, Apr 12:16, Jun 12:11, Jul 13:3, Dec 21:22, Mar 22:4-5

(Do not report 22630 in conjunction with 22612 for the same interspace and segment, use 22633)

+ 22632   each additional interspace (List separately in addition to code for primary procedure)

⊘ *CPT Assistant* Feb 96:6, Sep 97:8, Dec 99:2, Jun 12:11, Jul 13:3, Dec 21:22, Mar 22:4

(Use 22632 in conjunction with 22612, 22630, or 22633, when performed at a different interspace. When performing a posterior interbody fusion arthrodesis at an additional interspace, use 22632. When performing a posterior or posterolateral technique for fusion/ arthrodesis at an additional interspace, use 22614. When performing a combined posterior or posterolateral technique with posterior interbody arthrodesis at an additional interspace, use 22634)

(Do not report 22630, 22632 in conjunction with 63030, 63040, 63042, 63047, 63052, 63053, 63056, for laminectomy performed to prepare the interspace on the same spinal interspace[s])

22633   Arthrodesis, combined posterior or posterolateral technique with posterior interbody technique including laminectomy and/or discectomy sufficient to prepare interspace (other than for decompression), single interspace, lumbar;

⊘ *CPT Changes: An Insider's View* 2012, 2022

⊘ *CPT Assistant* Dec 11:14, Jan 12:3, Jun 12:10, Jul 13:3, Oct 16:11, May 18:9, Jul 18:14, Dec 21:6, 22, Feb 22:14, Mar 22:3, 5

(Do not report with 22612 or 22630 for the same interspace)

Examples of TLIF, PLIF, and Laminectomy Techniques and Procedures
22630, 63052

A. Examples of posterior interbody fusion techniques (22630)

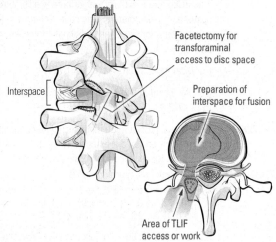

Transforaminal lumbar interbody fusion (TLIF)

Facetectomy for transforaminal access to disc space

Interspace

Preparation of interspace for fusion

Area of TLIF access or work

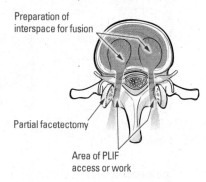

Posterior lumbar interbody fusion (PLIF)

Preparation of interspace for fusion

Partial facetectomy

Area of PLIF access or work

B. Examples of posterior interbody fusion techniques and laminectomy at same interspace (22630, 63052)

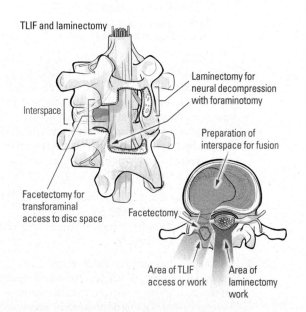

TLIF and laminectomy

Laminectomy for neural decompression with foraminotomy

Interspace

Preparation of interspace for fusion

Facetectomy for transforaminal access to disc space

Facetectomy

Area of TLIF access or work

Area of laminectomy work

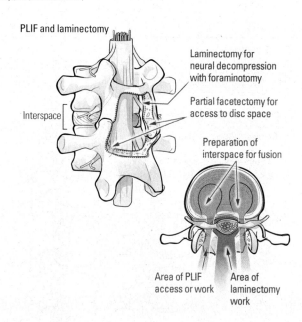

PLIF and laminectomy

Laminectomy for neural decompression with foraminotomy

Partial facetectomy for access to disc space

Interspace

Preparation of interspace for fusion

Area of PLIF access or work

Area of laminectomy work

+ 22634   each additional interspace (List separately in addition to code for primary procedure)

➜ *CPT Changes: An Insider's View* 2012, 2022

➜ *CPT Assistant* Dec 11:14, Jan 12:3, Jun 12:10, Jul 13:3, Jul 18:14, Dec 21:6, 22, Feb 22:14, Mar 22:3

(Use 22634 in conjunction with 22633)

(Do not report 22633, 22634 in conjunction with 63030, 63040, 63042, 63047, 63052, 63053, 63056, for laminectomy performed to prepare the interspace on the same spinal interspace[s] and vertebral segment[s])

(For decompression performed on the same interspace[s] and vertebral segment[s] as posterior interbody fusion that includes laminectomy, removal of facets, and/or opening/widening of the foramen for decompression of nerves or spinal components, such as spinal cord, cauda equina, or nerve roots, see 63052, 63053)

Spine Deformity (eg, Scoliosis, Kyphosis)

To report instrumentation procedures, see 22840-22855, 22859. (Report in addition to code[s] for the definitive procedure[s].) Do not append modifier 62 to spinal instrumentation codes 22840-22848, 22850, 22852, 22853, 22854, 22859.

To report bone graft procedures, see 20930-20938. (Report in addition to code[s] for the definitive procedure[s].) Do not append modifier 62 to bone graft codes 20900-20938.

A vertebral segment describes the basic constituent part into which the spine may be divided. It represents a single complete vertebral bone with its associated articular processes and laminae.

For the following codes, when two surgeons work together as primary surgeons performing distinct part(s) of an arthrodesis for spinal deformity, each surgeon should report his or her distinct operative work by appending modifier 62 to the procedure code. In this situation, modifier 62 may be appended to procedure code(s) 22800-22819 as long as both surgeons continue to work together as primary surgeons. The spinal deformity arthrodesis codes (22800, 22802, 22804, 22808, 22810, 22812) and kyphectomy codes (22818, 22819) should not be reported in conjunction with thoracic vertebral body tethering codes (22836, 22837, 22838) or lumbar or thoracolumbar vertebral body tethering codes (0656T, 0657T, 0790T).

When two surgeons work together as primary surgeons performing distinct part(s) of the thoracic vertebral body tethering, each surgeon should report his or her distinct operative work by appending modifier 62 to the procedure code. Modifier 62 may be appended to procedure code(s) 22836, 22837, 22838, as long as both surgeons continue to work together as primary surgeons.

22800   Arthrodesis, posterior, for spinal deformity, with or without cast; up to 6 vertebral segments
➔ *CPT Assistant* Apr 12:16, Jul 13:3, Sep 17:14, Dec 21:22, Jan 24:26

22802   7 to 12 vertebral segments
➔ *CPT Assistant* Mar 96:10, Apr 12:16, Jul 13:3, Sep 17:14, Jul 18:14, Dec 21:22, Dec 21:6, Jan 24:26

22804   13 or more vertebral segments
➔ *CPT Assistant* Apr 12:16, Jul 13:3, Sep 17:14, Dec 21:22, Jan 24:26

(Do not report 22800, 22802, 22804 in conjunction with 0656T, 0657T)

22808   Arthrodesis, anterior, for spinal deformity, with or without cast; 2 to 3 vertebral segments
➔ *CPT Assistant* Feb 02:4, Apr 12:16, Jul 13:3, Sep 17:14, Jan 24:26

22810   4 to 7 vertebral segments
➔ *CPT Assistant* Mar 96:10, Sep 97:8, Feb 02:4, Apr 12:16, Jul 13:3, Sep 17:14, Jan 24:26

22812   8 or more vertebral segments
➔ *CPT Assistant* Feb 02:4, Apr 12:16, Jul 13:3, Sep 17:14, Jan 24:26

(Do not report 22808, 22810, 22812 in conjunction with 0656T, 0657T)

22818   Kyphectomy, circumferential exposure of spine and resection of vertebral segment(s) (including body and posterior elements); single or 2 segments
➔ *CPT Assistant* Nov 97:14, Sep 17:14, Jan 24:26

22819   3 or more segments
➔ *CPT Assistant* Nov 97:14, Sep 17:14, May 20:14, Jul 21:7, Jan 24:26

(Do not report 22818, 22819 in conjunction with 0656T, 0657T)

(To report arthrodesis, see 22800-22804 and add modifier 51)

Exploration

To report instrumentation procedures, see 22840-22855, 22859. (Codes 22840-22848, 22853, 22854, 22859 are reported in conjunction with code[s] for the definitive procedure[s]. When instrumentation reinsertion or removal is reported in conjunction with other definitive procedures, including arthrodesis, decompression, and exploration of fusion, append modifier 51 to 22849, 22850, 22852, and 22855.) Code 22849 should not be reported with 22850, 22852, and 22855 at the same spinal levels. To report exploration of fusion, see 22830. (When exploration is reported in conjunction with other definitive procedures, including arthrodesis and decompression, append modifier 51 to 22830.)

(To report bone graft procedures, see 20930-20938)

22830   Exploration of spinal fusion
➔ *CPT Assistant* Sep 97:11, Mar 10:9, Mar 20:14

22836   Code is out of numerical sequence. See 22846-22849

22837   Code is out of numerical sequence. See 22846-22849

22838   Code is out of numerical sequence. See 22846-22849

Spinal Instrumentation

Segmental instrumentation is defined as fixation at each end of the construct and at least one additional interposed bony attachment.

Non-segmental instrumentation is defined as fixation at each end of the construct and may span several vertebral segments without attachment to the intervening segments.

Insertion of spinal instrumentation is reported separately and in addition to arthrodesis. Instrumentation procedure codes 22840-22848, 22853, 22854, 22859 are reported in addition to the definitive procedure(s). Do not append modifier 62 to spinal instrumentation codes 22840-22848, 22850, 22852, 22853, 22854, 22859.

To report bone graft procedures, see 20930-20938. (Report in addition to code[s] for definitive procedure[s].) Do not append modifier 62 to bone graft codes 20900-20938.

A vertebral segment describes the basic constituent part into which the spine may be divided. It represents a single complete vertebral bone with its associated articular processes and laminae. A vertebral interspace is the non-bony compartment between two adjacent vertebral bodies, which contains the intervertebral disc, and includes the nucleus pulposus, annulus fibrosus, and two cartilaginous endplates.

Codes 22849, 22850, 22852, and 22855 are subject to modifier 51 if reported with other definitive procedure(s), including arthrodesis, decompression, and exploration of fusion. Code 22849 should not be reported in conjunction with 22850, 22852, and 22855 at the same spinal levels. Only the appropriate insertion code (22840-22848) should be reported when previously placed spinal instrumentation is being removed or revised during the same session where new instrumentation is inserted at levels including all or part of the previously instrumented segments. Do not report the reinsertion (22849) or removal (22850, 22852, 22855) procedures in addition to the insertion of the new instrumentation (22840-22848).

Codes 22836, 22837, 22838 describe anterior thoracic vertebral body tethering, which corrects scoliosis without fusion using a tether (cord) to compress the vertebral growth plates on the convex side of the curve to inhibit their growth, while allowing the growth plates on the concave side of the curve to continue to grow. Codes 22836, 22837 may not be reported with anterior instrumentation codes 22845, 22846, 22847.

For the following codes, when two surgeons work together as primary surgeons performing distinct part(s) of the thoracic vertebral body tethering, each surgeon should report his or her distinct operative work by appending modifier 62 to the procedure code. Modifier 62 may be appended to procedure code(s) 22836, 22837, 22838, as long as both surgeons continue to work together as primary surgeons.

Regions of the spine include cervical, cervicothoracic, thoracic, thoracolumbar, lumbar, lumbosacral, sacral, and coccygeal.

+ **22840** Posterior non-segmental instrumentation (eg, Harrington rod technique, pedicle fixation across 1 interspace, atlantoaxial transarticular screw fixation, sublaminar wiring at C1, facet screw fixation) (List separately in addition to code for primary procedure)

➜ *CPT Changes: An Insider's View* 2000, 2008

➜ *CPT Assistant* Feb 96:6, Jul 96:10, Sep 97:8, Nov 99:12, Feb 02:6, Nov 10:8, Jan 11:9, Dec 11:15, Apr 12:12, Jun 12:11, Jul 13:3, Dec 13:17, Oct 14:15, Jun 17:10, May 20:14, Jul 21:7, Dec 21:5-6, 22, Oct 23:19

(Use 22840 in conjunction with 22100-22102, 22110-22114, 22206, 22207, 22210-22214, 22220-22224, 22310-22327, 22532, 22533, 22548-22558, 22590-22612, 22630, 22633, 22634, 22800-22812, 63001-63030, 63040-63042, 63045-63047, 63050-63056, 63064, 63075, 63077, 63081, 63085, 63087, 63090, 63101, 63102, 63170-63290, 63300-63307)

Non-Segmental Spinal Instrumentation
22840

Fixation at each end of the construct

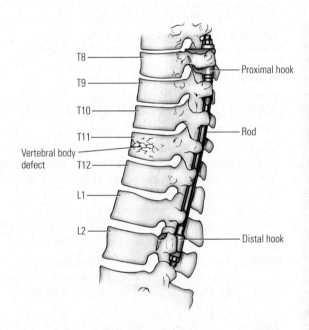

+ **22841** Internal spinal fixation by wiring of spinous processes (List separately in addition to code for primary procedure)

➜ *CPT Changes: An Insider's View* 2008

➜ *CPT Assistant* Feb 96:6, Sep 97:8, Feb 02:6, Jun 12:11, Jul 13:3, Dec 21:5-6, 22

(Use 22841 in conjunction with 22100-22102, 22110-22114, 22206, 22207, 22210-22214, 22220-22224, 22310-22327, 22532, 22533, 22548-22558, 22590-22612, 22630, 22633, 22634, 22800-22812, 63001-63030, 63040-63042, 63045-63047, 63050-63056, 63064, 63075, 63077, 63081, 63085, 63087, 63090, 63101, 63102, 63170-63290, 63300-63307)

+ **22842** Posterior segmental instrumentation (eg, pedicle fixation, dual rods with multiple hooks and sublaminar wires); 3 to 6 vertebral segments (List separately in addition to code for primary procedure)

➲ *CPT Changes: An Insider's View* 2008

➲ *CPT Assistant* Feb 96:6, Mar 96:7, Sep 97:8, Feb 02:6, Dec 11:15, Jun 12:11, Jul 13:3, Dec 21:5-6, 22, Oct 23:19

(Use 22842 in conjunction with 22100-22102, 22110-22114, 22206, 22207, 22210-22214, 22220-22224, 22310-22327, 22532, 22533, 22548-22558, 22590-22612, 22630, 22633, 22634, 22800-22812, 63001-63030, 63040-63042, 63045-63047, 63050-63056, 63064, 63075, 63077, 63081, 63085, 63087, 63090, 63101, 63102, 63170-63290, 63300-63307)

+ **22843** 7 to 12 vertebral segments (List separately in addition to code for primary procedure)

➲ *CPT Changes: An Insider's View* 2008

➲ *CPT Assistant* Feb 96:6, Sep 97:8, Feb 02:6, Dec 11:15, Jun 12:11, Jul 13:3, Jul 18:14, Dec 21:5-6, 22

(Use 22843 in conjunction with 22100-22102, 22110-22114, 22206, 22207, 22210-22214, 22220-22224, 22310-22327, 22532, 22533, 22548-22558, 22590-22612, 22630, 22633, 22634, 22800-22812, 63001-63030, 63040-63042, 63045-63047, 63050-63056, 63064, 63075, 63077, 63081, 63085, 63087, 63090, 63101, 63102, 63170-63290, 63300-63307)

+ **22844** 13 or more vertebral segments (List separately in addition to code for primary procedure)

➲ *CPT Changes: An Insider's View* 2008

➲ *CPT Assistant* Feb 96:6, Sep 97:8, Feb 02:6, Dec 11:15, Jun 12:11, Jul 13:3, Dec 21:5-6, 22

(Use 22844 in conjunction with 22100-22102, 22110-22114, 22206, 22207, 22210-22214, 22220-22224, 22310-22327, 22532, 22533, 22548-22558, 22590-22612, 22630, 22633, 22634, 22800-22812, 63001-63030, 63040-63042, 63045-63047, 63050-63056, 63064, 63075, 63077, 63081, 63085, 63087, 63090, 63101, 63102, 63170-63290, 63300-63307)

+ **22845** Anterior instrumentation; 2 to 3 vertebral segments (List separately in addition to code for primary procedure)

➲ *CPT Changes: An Insider's View* 2008

➲ *CPT Assistant* Feb 96:6, Mar 96:10, Jul 96:7, 10, Sep 97:8, Feb 02:6, Jun 12:11, Jul 13:3, Nov 14:14, Jan 15:13, Mar 15:9, Apr 15:7, May 16:13, Mar 17:7, Dec 21:5-6, 22

(Use 22845 in conjunction with 22100-22102, 22110-22114, 22206, 22207, 22210-22214, 22220-22224, 22310-22327, 22532, 22533, 22548-22558, 22590-22612, 22630, 22633, 22634, 22800-22812, 63001-63030, 63040-63042, 63045-63047, 63050-63056, 63064, 63075, 63077, 63081, 63085, 63087, 63090, 63101, 63102, 63170-63290, 63300-63307)

(For vertebral body tethering of the thoracic spine, see 22836, 22837, 22838)

(For vertebral body tethering of the lumbar or thoracolumbar spine, see 0656T, 0657T, 0790T)

Segmental Spinal Instrumentation
22842-22844

Fixation at each end of the construct and at least one additional interposed bony attachment

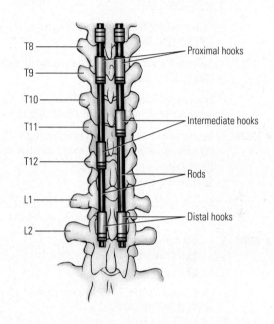

+ **22846** 4 to 7 vertebral segments (List separately in addition to code for primary procedure)

➲ *CPT Changes: An Insider's View* 2008

➲ *CPT Assistant* Feb 96:6, Sep 97:8, Feb 02:6, Jun 12:11, Jul 13:3, May 16:13, Dec 21:5-6, 22

(Use 22846 in conjunction with 22100-22102, 22110-22114, 22206, 22207, 22210-22214, 22220-22224, 22310-22327, 22532, 22533, 22548-22558, 22590-22612, 22630, 22633, 22634, 22800-22812, 63001-63030, 63040-63042, 63045-63047, 63050-63056, 63064, 63075, 63077, 63081, 63085, 63087, 63090, 63101, 63102, 63170-63290, 63300-63307)

(For vertebral body tethering of the thoracic spine, see 22836, 22837, 22838)

(For vertebral body tethering of the lumbar or thoracolumbar spine, see 0656T, 0657T, 0790T)

+ 22847 8 or more vertebral segments (List separately in addition to code for primary procedure)

→ *CPT Changes: An Insider's View* 2008

→ *CPT Assistant* Feb 96:6, Sep 97:8, Feb 02:6, Jun 12:11, Jul 13:3, May 16:13, Dec 21:5-6, 22

(Use 22847 in conjunction with 22100-22102, 22110-22114, 22206, 22207, 22210-22214, 22220-22224, 22310-22327, 22532, 22533, 22548-22558, 22590-22612, 22630, 22633, 22634, 22800-22812, 63001-63030, 63040-63042, 63045-63047, 63050-63056, 63064, 63075, 63077, 63081, 63085, 63087, 63090, 63101, 63102, 63170-63290, 63300-63307)

(Do not report 22845, 22846, 22847 in conjunction with 22836, 22837, 22838)

(For vertebral body tethering of the thoracic spine, see 22836, 22837, 22838)

(For vertebral body tethering of the lumbar or thoracolumbar spine, see 0656T, 0657T, 0790T)

 # 22836 Anterior thoracic vertebral body tethering, including thoracoscopy, when performed; up to 7 vertebral segments

→ *CPT Changes: An Insider's View* 2024

→ *CPT Assistant* Jan 24:26

(For anterior lumbar or thoracolumbar vertebral body tethering, up to 7 vertebral segments, use 0656T)

 # 22837 8 or more vertebral segments

→ *CPT Changes: An Insider's View* 2024

→ *CPT Assistant* Jan 24:26

(Do not report 22836, 22837 in conjunction with 22845, 22846, 22847, 32601)

(For anterior lumbar or thoracolumbar vertebral body tethering, 8 or more vertebral segments, use 0657T)

 # 22838 Revision (eg, augmentation, division of tether), replacement, or removal of thoracic vertebral body tethering, including thoracoscopy, when performed

→ *CPT Changes: An Insider's View* 2024

→ *CPT Assistant* Jan 24:26

(Do not report 22838 in conjunction with 22849, 22855, 32601)

+ 22848 Pelvic fixation (attachment of caudal end of instrumentation to pelvic bony structures) other than sacrum (List separately in addition to code for primary procedure)

→ *CPT Changes: An Insider's View* 2008

→ *CPT Assistant* Feb 96:6, Sep 97:8, Feb 02:6, Jun 12:11, Jul 13:3, Dec 21:5-6

(Use 22848 in conjunction with 22100-22102, 22110-22114, 22206, 22207, 22210-22214, 22220-22224, 22310-22327, 22532, 22533, 22548-22558, 22590-22612, 22630, 22633, 22634, 22800-22812, 63001-63030, 63040-63042, 63045-63047, 63050-63056, 63064, 63075, 63077, 63081, 63085, 63087, 63090, 63101, 63102, 63170-63290, 63300-63307)

22849 Reinsertion of spinal fixation device

→ *CPT Assistant* Feb 96:6, Sep 97:8, Feb 02:6, Nov 02:3, Oct 11:10, Jun 12:11, Jul 13:3, May 16:13, Jun 17:10

22850 Removal of posterior nonsegmental instrumentation (eg, Harrington rod)

→ *CPT Assistant* Feb 96:6, Sep 97:8, Feb 02:6, Jun 12:11, Jul 13:3, May 16:13, Jun 17:10

22852 Removal of posterior segmental instrumentation

→ *CPT Assistant* Feb 96:6, Sep 97:8, Feb 02:6, May 06:16, Jun 12:11, Jun 17:10

+ 22853 Insertion of interbody biomechanical device(s) (eg, synthetic cage, mesh) with integral anterior instrumentation for device anchoring (eg, screws, flanges), when performed, to intervertebral disc space in conjunction with interbody arthrodesis, each interspace (List separately in addition to code for primary procedure)

→ *CPT Changes: An Insider's View* 2017

→ *CPT Assistant* Mar 17:7, Aug 17:9, Jul 18:14, Dec 21:5-6, 22

(Use 22853 in conjunction with 22100-22102, 22110-22114, 22206, 22207, 22210-22214, 22220-22224, 22310-22327, 22532, 22533, 22548-22558, 22590-22612, 22630, 22633, 22634, 22800-22812, 63001-63030, 63040-63042, 63045-63047, 63050-63056, 63064, 63075, 63077, 63081, 63085, 63087, 63090, 63101, 63102, 63170-63290, 63300-63307)

(Report 22853 for each treated intervertebral disc space)

+ 22854 Insertion of intervertebral biomechanical device(s) (eg, synthetic cage, mesh) with integral anterior instrumentation for device anchoring (eg, screws, flanges), when performed, to vertebral corpectomy(ies) (vertebral body resection, partial or complete) defect, in conjunction with interbody arthrodesis, each contiguous defect (List separately in addition to code for primary procedure)

→ *CPT Changes: An Insider's View* 2017

→ *CPT Assistant* Mar 17:7, Dec 21:5-6

(Use 22854 in conjunction with 22100-22102, 22110-22114, 22206, 22207, 22210-22214, 22220-22224, 22310-22327, 22532, 22533, 22548-22558, 22590-22612, 22630, 22633, 22634, 22800-22812, 63001-63030, 63040-63042, 63045-63047, 63050-63056, 63064, 63075, 63077, 63081, 63085, 63087, 63090, 63101, 63102, 63170-63290, 63300-63307)

#+ 22859 Insertion of intervertebral biomechanical device(s) (eg, synthetic cage, mesh, methylmethacrylate) to intervertebral disc space or vertebral body defect without interbody arthrodesis, each contiguous defect (List separately in addition to code for primary procedure)

→ *CPT Changes: An Insider's View* 2017

→ *CPT Assistant* Mar 17:7, Dec 21:5-6

(Use 22859 in conjunction with 22100-22102, 22110-22114, 22206, 22207, 22210-22214, 22220-22224, 22310-22327, 22532, 22533, 22548-22558, 22590-22612, 22630, 22633, 22634, 22800-22812, 63001-63030, 63040-63042,

★ = Telemedicine   ◄ = Audio-only   + = Add-on code   ✗ = FDA approval pending   # = Resequenced code   ⊘ = Modifier 51 exempt   ➡➡➡ = See p xxi for details

63045-63047, 63050-63056, 63064, 63075, 63077, 63081, 63085, 63087, 63090, 63101, 63102, 63170-63290, 63300-63307)

(22853, 22854, 22859 may be reported more than once for noncontiguous defects)

(For application of an intervertebral bone device/graft, see 20930, 20931, 20936, 20937, 20938)

Spinal Prosthetic Devices
22853, 22854, 22859

Application of prosthetic device

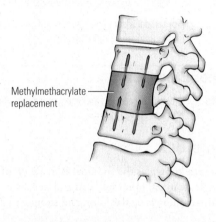

Methylmethacrylate replacement

22855   Removal of anterior instrumentation
➔ CPT Assistant Feb 96:6, Sep 97:8, Feb 02:6, Nov 02:2, Jun 12:11, Jun 17:10

22856   Total disc arthroplasty (artificial disc), anterior approach, including discectomy with end plate preparation (includes osteophytectomy for nerve root or spinal cord decompression and microdissection); single interspace, cervical
➔ CPT Changes: An Insider's View 2009, 2015
➔ CPT Assistant Apr 15:7

(Do not report 22856 in conjunction with 22554, 22845, 22853, 22854, 22859, 63075, when performed at the same level)

(Do not report 22856 in conjunction with 69990)

(For additional interspace cervical total disc arthroplasty, use 22858)

#+ 22858   second level, cervical (List separately in addition to code for primary procedure)
➔ CPT Changes: An Insider's View 2015
➔ CPT Assistant Apr 15:7

(Use 22858 in conjunction with 22856)

22857   Total disc arthroplasty (artificial disc), anterior approach, including discectomy to prepare interspace (other than for decompression); single interspace, lumbar
➔ CPT Changes: An Insider's View 2007, 2009, 2023
➔ CPT Assistant Jun 23:16

(Do not report 22857 in conjunction with 22558, 22845, 22853, 22854, 22859, 49010 when performed at the same level)

22858   Code is out of numerical sequence. See 22853-22861

22859   Code is out of numerical sequence. See 22853-22861

+ 22860   second interspace, lumbar (List separately in addition to code for primary procedure)
➔ CPT Changes: An Insider's View 2023
➔ CPT Assistant Jun 23:16

(Use 22860 in conjunction with 22857)

(For total disc arthroplasty, anterior approach, lumbar, more than two interspaces, use 22899)

22861   Revision including replacement of total disc arthroplasty (artificial disc), anterior approach, single interspace; cervical
➔ CPT Changes: An Insider's View 2009

(Do not report 22861 in conjunction with 22845, 22853, 22854, 22859, 22864, 63075 when performed at the same level)

(Do not report 22861 in conjunction with 69990)

(For additional interspace revision of cervical total disc arthroplasty, use 0098T)

22862   lumbar
➔ CPT Changes: An Insider's View 2007, 2009
➔ CPT Assistant Jun 07:1

(Do not report 22862 in conjunction with 22558, 22845, 22853, 22854, 22859, 22865, 49010 when performed at the same level)

(For additional interspace, use Category III code 0165T)

22864   Removal of total disc arthroplasty (artificial disc), anterior approach, single interspace; cervical
➔ CPT Changes: An Insider's View 2009
➔ CPT Assistant Mar 20:14

(Do not report 22864 in conjunction with 22861, 69990)

(For additional interspace removal of cervical total disc arthroplasty, use 0095T)

22865   lumbar
➔ CPT Changes: An Insider's View 2007, 2009
➔ CPT Assistant Jun 07:1, Mar 20:14

(Do not report 22865 in conjunction with 49010)

(For additional interspace, see Category III code 0164T)

(22856-22865 include fluoroscopy when performed)

(For decompression, see 63001-63048)

Musculoskeletal 20100-29999

22867   Insertion of interlaminar/interspinous process stabilization/distraction device, without fusion, including image guidance when performed, with open decompression, lumbar; single level
➜ *CPT Changes: An Insider's View* 2017
➜ *CPT Assistant* Feb 17:9

+ 22868   second level (List separately in addition to code for primary procedure)
➜ *CPT Changes: An Insider's View* 2017
➜ *CPT Assistant* Feb 17:9

(Use 22868 in conjunction with 22867)

(Do not report 22867, 22868 in conjunction with 22532, 22533, 22534, 22558, 22612, 22614, 22630, 22632, 22633, 22634, 22800, 22802, 22804, 22840, 22841, 22842, 22869, 22870, 63005, 63012, 63017, 63030, 63035, 63042, 63044, 63047, 63048, 77003 for the same level)

(For insertion of interlaminar/interspinous process stabilization/distraction device, without open decompression or fusion, see 22869, 22870)

22869   Insertion of interlaminar/interspinous process stabilization/distraction device, without open decompression or fusion, including image guidance when performed, lumbar; single level
➜ *CPT Changes: An Insider's View* 2017
➜ *CPT Assistant* Feb 17:9

+ 22870   second level (List separately in addition to code for primary procedure)
➜ *CPT Changes: An Insider's View* 2017
➜ *CPT Assistant* Feb 17:9, May 20:14, Jul 21:7

(Use 22870 in conjunction with 22869)

(Do not report 22869, 22870 in conjunction with 22532, 22533, 22534, 22558, 22612, 22614, 22630, 22632, 22633, 22634, 22800, 22802, 22804, 22840, 22841, 22842, 63005, 63012, 63017, 63030, 63035, 63042, 63044, 63047, 63048, 77003)

Other Procedures

22899   Unlisted procedure, spine
➜ *CPT Assistant* May 00:11, Sep 00:10, Jul 06:19, Feb 10:13, Nov 10:4, Jan 12:14, Sep 12:16, Dec 12:13, Dec 13:14, 17, Oct 14:15, Jan 15:8, Feb 17:9, May 18:10, Oct 21:10, Feb 22:14, Apr 22:13, Dec 22:16, Apr 23:16, Jun 23:16, 26
➜ *Clinical Examples in Radiology* Fall 14:3

Abdomen

Excision

22900   Excision, tumor, soft tissue of abdominal wall, subfascial (eg, intramuscular); less than 5 cm
➜ *CPT Changes: An Insider's View* 2010

22901   5 cm or greater
➜ *CPT Changes: An Insider's View* 2010

22902   Excision, tumor, soft tissue of abdominal wall, subcutaneous; less than 3 cm
➜ *CPT Changes: An Insider's View* 2010

22903   3 cm or greater
➜ *CPT Changes: An Insider's View* 2010

(For excision of benign lesions of cutaneous origin [eg, sebaceous cyst], see 11400-11406)

22904   Radical resection of tumor (eg, sarcoma), soft tissue of abdominal wall; less than 5 cm
➜ *CPT Changes: An Insider's View* 2010, 2014

22905   5 cm or greater
➜ *CPT Changes: An Insider's View* 2010, 2014

(For radical resection of tumor[s] of cutaneous origin [eg, melanoma], see 11600-11606)

Other Procedures

22999   Unlisted procedure, abdomen, musculoskeletal system
➜ *CPT Assistant* Apr 23:25

Shoulder

The area known as the shoulder is made up of the clavicle, scapula, humerus head and neck, sternoclavicular joint, acromioclavicular joint, and shoulder joint.

Incision

23000   Removal of subdeltoid calcareous deposits, open
➜ *CPT Changes: An Insider's View* 2002, 2003

(For arthroscopic removal of bursal deposits, use 29999)

23020   Capsular contracture release (eg, Sever type procedure)

(For incision and drainage procedures, superficial, see 10040-10160)

23030   Incision and drainage, shoulder area; deep abscess or hematoma

23031   infected bursa

23035   Incision, bone cortex (eg, osteomyelitis or bone abscess), shoulder area

23040   Arthrotomy, glenohumeral joint, including exploration, drainage, or removal of foreign body
➜ *CPT Assistant* Nov 98:8, Mar 20:14

23044   Arthrotomy, acromioclavicular, sternoclavicular joint, including exploration, drainage, or removal of foreign body
➜ *CPT Assistant* Nov 98:8, Mar 20:14

Excision

23065　Biopsy, soft tissue of shoulder area; superficial

23066　　　deep

（For needle biopsy of soft tissue, use 20206）

23071　Code is out of numerical sequence. See 23066-23078

23073　Code is out of numerical sequence. See 23066-23078

23075　Excision, tumor, soft tissue of shoulder area, subcutaneous; less than 3 cm
➲ *CPT Changes: An Insider's View* 2010
➲ *CPT Assistant* Summer 92:22, Nov 98:8, Sep 18:7

 # 23071　　　3 cm or greater
➲ *CPT Changes: An Insider's View* 2010
➲ *CPT Assistant* Sep 18:7

（For excision of benign lesions of cutaneous origin [eg, sebaceous cyst], see 11400-11406）

23076　Excision, tumor, soft tissue of shoulder area, subfascial (eg, intramuscular); less than 5 cm
➲ *CPT Changes: An Insider's View* 2010
➲ *CPT Assistant* Summer 92:22, Oct 09:7, Sep 18:7

 # 23073　　　5 cm or greater
➲ *CPT Changes: An Insider's View* 2010
➲ *CPT Assistant* Sep 18:7

23077　Radical resection of tumor (eg, sarcoma), soft tissue of shoulder area; less than 5 cm
➲ *CPT Changes: An Insider's View* 2010, 2014

23078　　　5 cm or greater
➲ *CPT Changes: An Insider's View* 2010, 2014
➲ *CPT Assistant* Sep 18:7

（For radical resection of tumor[s] of cutaneous origin [eg, melanoma], see 11600-11606）

23100　Arthrotomy, glenohumeral joint, including biopsy
➲ *CPT Assistant* Nov 98:8

23101　Arthrotomy, acromioclavicular joint or sternoclavicular joint, including biopsy and/or excision of torn cartilage
➲ *CPT Assistant* Nov 98:8

23105　Arthrotomy; glenohumeral joint, with synovectomy, with or without biopsy
➲ *CPT Assistant* Nov 98:8

23106　　　sternoclavicular joint, with synovectomy, with or without biopsy

23107　Arthrotomy, glenohumeral joint, with joint exploration, with or without removal of loose or foreign body

23120　Claviculectomy; partial
➲ *CPT Assistant* Sep 12:16

（For arthroscopic procedure, use 29824）

23125　　　total

23130　Acromioplasty or acromionectomy, partial, with or without coracoacromial ligament release
➲ *CPT Assistant* Aug 01:11, Feb 15:10, Mar 15:7

23140　Excision or curettage of bone cyst or benign tumor of clavicle or scapula;

23145　　　with autograft (includes obtaining graft)

23146　　　with allograft

23150　Excision or curettage of bone cyst or benign tumor of proximal humerus;

23155　　　with autograft (includes obtaining graft)

23156　　　with allograft

23170　Sequestrectomy (eg, for osteomyelitis or bone abscess), clavicle

23172　Sequestrectomy (eg, for osteomyelitis or bone abscess), scapula

23174　Sequestrectomy (eg, for osteomyelitis or bone abscess), humeral head to surgical neck

23180　Partial excision (craterization, saucerization, or diaphysectomy) bone (eg, osteomyelitis), clavicle
➲ *CPT Assistant* Nov 98:9

23182　Partial excision (craterization, saucerization, or diaphysectomy) bone (eg, osteomyelitis), scapula
➲ *CPT Assistant* Nov 98:9

23184　Partial excision (craterization, saucerization, or diaphysectomy) bone (eg, osteomyelitis), proximal humerus
➲ *CPT Assistant* Nov 98:9

23190　Ostectomy of scapula, partial (eg, superior medial angle)

23195　Resection, humeral head

（For replacement with implant, use 23470）

23200　Radical resection of tumor; clavicle
➲ *CPT Changes: An Insider's View* 2010

23210　　　scapula
➲ *CPT Changes: An Insider's View* 2010

23220　Radical resection of tumor, proximal humerus
➲ *CPT Changes: An Insider's View* 2010
➲ *CPT Assistant* Nov 98:8

Introduction or Removal

（For arthrocentesis or needling of bursa, use 20610）

（For K-wire or pin insertion or removal, see 20650, 20670, 20680）

23330　Removal of foreign body, shoulder; subcutaneous
➲ *CPT Assistant* Aug 99:3, Mar 14:4

（To report removal of foreign body, see 23330, 23333）

Musculoskeletal 20100-29999

23333   deep (subfascial or intramuscular)

➔ *CPT Changes: An Insider's View* 2014

➔ *CPT Assistant* Mar 14:4

23334   Removal of prosthesis, includes debridement and synovectomy when performed; humeral **or** glenoid component

➔ *CPT Changes: An Insider's View* 2014

➔ *CPT Assistant* Mar 14:4, Mar 20:14

23335   humeral **and** glenoid components (eg, total shoulder)

➔ *CPT Changes: An Insider's View* 2014

➔ *CPT Assistant* Mar 14:4

(Do not report 23334, 23335 in conjunction with 23473, 23474 if a prosthesis [ie, humeral and/or glenoid component(s)] is being removed and replaced in the same shoulder during the same surgical session)

(To report removal of hardware, other than humeral and/or glenoid prosthesis, use 20680)

23350   Injection procedure for shoulder arthrography or enhanced CT/MRI shoulder arthrography

➔ *CPT Changes: An Insider's View* 2002

➔ *CPT Assistant* Jul 01:3, Aug 15:6, May 16:13

➔ *Clinical Examples in Radiology* Spring 05:5, Spring 09:6-7, Summer 18:14

(For radiographic arthrography, radiological supervision and interpretation, use 73040. Fluoroscopy [77002] is inclusive of radiographic arthrography)

(When fluoroscopic guided injection is performed for enhanced CT arthrography, use 23350, 77002, and 73201 or 73202)

(When fluoroscopic guided injection is performed for enhanced MR arthrography, use 23350, 77002, and 73222 or 73223)

(For enhanced CT or enhanced MRI arthrography, use 77002 and either 73201, 73202, 73222, or 73223)

(To report biopsy of the shoulder and joint, see 29805-29826)

Repair, Revision, and/or Reconstruction

23395   Muscle transfer, any type, shoulder or upper arm; single

23397   multiple

23400   Scapulopexy (eg, Sprengels deformity or for paralysis)

23405   Tenotomy, shoulder area; single tendon

➔ *CPT Assistant* Nov 98:8

23406   multiple tendons through same incision

➔ *CPT Assistant* Nov 98:8

23410   Repair of ruptured musculotendinous cuff (eg, rotator cuff) open; acute

➔ *CPT Changes: An Insider's View* 2003

➔ *CPT Assistant* Aug 01:11, Feb 02:11

23412   chronic

➔ *CPT Assistant* Feb 02:11, Sep 12:16, Feb 15:10, Jun 15:10, May 22:15

(For arthroscopic procedure, use 29827)

23415   Coracoacromial ligament release, with or without acromioplasty

➔ *CPT Assistant* Mar 15:7

(For arthroscopic procedure, use 29826)

23420   Reconstruction of complete shoulder (rotator) cuff avulsion, chronic (includes acromioplasty)

➔ *CPT Assistant* Feb 02:11, Oct 05:23

23430   Tenodesis of long tendon of biceps

(For arthroscopic biceps tenodesis, use 29828)

23440   Resection or transplantation of long tendon of biceps

23450   Capsulorrhaphy, anterior; Putti-Platt procedure or Magnuson type operation

(To report arthroscopic thermal capsulorrhaphy, use 29999)

23455   with labral repair (eg, Bankart procedure)

➔ *CPT Assistant* Nov 98:8

(For arthroscopic procedure, use 29806)

23460   Capsulorrhaphy, anterior, any type; with bone block

23462   with coracoid process transfer

(To report open thermal capsulorrhaphy, use 23929)

23465   Capsulorrhaphy, glenohumeral joint, posterior, with or without bone block

➔ *CPT Assistant* Nov 98:8

(For sternoclavicular and acromioclavicular reconstruction, see 23530, 23550)

23466   Capsulorrhaphy, glenohumeral joint, any type multidirectional instability

➔ *CPT Assistant* Nov 98:8

23470   Arthroplasty, glenohumeral joint; hemiarthroplasty

➔ *CPT Assistant* Nov 98:8, Mar 14:4

23472   total shoulder (glenoid and proximal humeral replacement (eg, total shoulder))

➔ *CPT Assistant* Jun 96:10, Nov 98:8, Mar 13:12, Mar 14:4

(For removal of total shoulder implants, see 23334, 23335)

(For osteotomy, proximal humerus, use 24400)

23473   Revision of total shoulder arthroplasty, including allograft when performed; humeral **or** glenoid component

➔ *CPT Changes: An Insider's View* 2013

➔ *CPT Assistant* Feb 13:11, Mar 13:12, Mar 14:4

★ = Telemedicine   ◀ = Audio-only   ✛ = Add-on code   ⁄ = FDA approval pending   # = Resequenced code   ⊘ = Modifier 51 exempt   ➔➔➔ = See p xxi for details

23474   humeral **and** glenoid component
→ *CPT Changes: An Insider's View* 2013
→ *CPT Assistant* Feb 13:11, Mar 13:12, Mar 14:4

(Do not report 23473, 23474 in conjunction with 23334, 23335 if a prosthesis [ie, humeral and/or glenoid component(s)] is being removed and replaced in the same shoulder during the same surgical session)

23480   Osteotomy, clavicle, with or without internal fixation;

23485   with bone graft for nonunion or malunion (includes obtaining graft and/or necessary fixation)

23490   Prophylactic treatment (nailing, pinning, plating or wiring) with or without methylmethacrylate; clavicle

23491   proximal humerus
→ *CPT Assistant* Nov 98:8

Fracture and/or Dislocation

―― *Coding Tip* ――

Reporting for Categories of Manipulation and/or Fracture

The codes for treatment of fractures and joint injuries (dislocations) are categorized by the type of manipulation (reduction) and stabilization (fixation or immobilization). These codes can apply to either open (compound) or closed fractures or joint injuries.

CPT Coding Guidelines, Musculoskeletal System

23500   Closed treatment of clavicular fracture; without manipulation

23505   with manipulation

23515   Open treatment of clavicular fracture, includes internal fixation, when performed
→ *CPT Changes: An Insider's View* 2008
→ *CPT Assistant* Jan 08:4

23520   Closed treatment of sternoclavicular dislocation; without manipulation

23525   with manipulation

23530   Open treatment of sternoclavicular dislocation, acute or chronic;

23532   with fascial graft (includes obtaining graft)

23540   Closed treatment of acromioclavicular dislocation; without manipulation

23545   with manipulation

23550   Open treatment of acromioclavicular dislocation, acute or chronic;

23552   with fascial graft (includes obtaining graft)
→ *CPT Assistant* Nov 19:14

23570   Closed treatment of scapular fracture; without manipulation

23575   with manipulation, with or without skeletal traction (with or without shoulder joint involvement)

23585   Open treatment of scapular fracture (body, glenoid or acromion) includes internal fixation, when performed
→ *CPT Changes: An Insider's View* 2009
→ *CPT Assistant* Oct 04:10

23600   Closed treatment of proximal humeral (surgical or anatomical neck) fracture; without manipulation

23605   with manipulation, with or without skeletal traction

23615   Open treatment of proximal humeral (surgical or anatomical neck) fracture, includes internal fixation, when performed, includes repair of tuberosity(s), when performed;
→ *CPT Changes: An Insider's View* 2008
→ *CPT Assistant* Jan 08:4

23616   with proximal humeral prosthetic replacement
→ *CPT Changes: An Insider's View* 2008

23620   Closed treatment of greater humeral tuberosity fracture; without manipulation
→ *CPT Assistant* Nov 98:8

23625   with manipulation

23630   Open treatment of greater humeral tuberosity fracture, includes internal fixation, when performed
→ *CPT Changes: An Insider's View* 2008
→ *CPT Assistant* Nov 98:8

23650   Closed treatment of shoulder dislocation, with manipulation; without anesthesia

23655   requiring anesthesia

23660   Open treatment of acute shoulder dislocation
→ *CPT Assistant* Feb 96:5

(Repairs for recurrent dislocations, see 23450-23466)

23665   Closed treatment of shoulder dislocation, with fracture of greater humeral tuberosity, with manipulation
→ *CPT Assistant* Nov 98:8

23670   Open treatment of shoulder dislocation, with fracture of greater humeral tuberosity, includes internal fixation, when performed
→ *CPT Changes: An Insider's View* 2008
→ *CPT Assistant* Nov 98:8

23675   Closed treatment of shoulder dislocation, with surgical or anatomical neck fracture, with manipulation

23680   Open treatment of shoulder dislocation, with surgical or anatomical neck fracture, includes internal fixation, when performed
→ *CPT Changes: An Insider's View* 2008

Musculoskeletal 20100-29999

Manipulation

23700   Manipulation under anesthesia, shoulder joint, including application of fixation apparatus (dislocation excluded)

⮕ *CPT Assistant* Jan 99:10, Apr 05:14, May 09:8, Jun 15:10

Arthrodesis

23800   Arthrodesis, glenohumeral joint;

⮕ *CPT Assistant* Nov 98:8, May 20:14, Jul 21:7

23802   with autogenous graft (includes obtaining graft)

⮕ *CPT Assistant* May 20:14, Jul 21:7

Amputation

23900   Interthoracoscapular amputation (forequarter)

23920   Disarticulation of shoulder;

23921   secondary closure or scar revision

Other Procedures

23929   Unlisted procedure, shoulder

Humerus (Upper Arm) and Elbow

The elbow area includes the head and neck of the radius and olecranon process.

Incision

(For incision and drainage procedures, superficial, see 10040-10160)

23930   Incision and drainage, upper arm or elbow area; deep abscess or hematoma

23931   bursa

⮕ *CPT Assistant* Nov 98:8

23935   Incision, deep, with opening of bone cortex (eg, for osteomyelitis or bone abscess), humerus or elbow

24000   Arthrotomy, elbow, including exploration, drainage, or removal of foreign body

⮕ *CPT Assistant* Nov 98:8-9, Mar 20:14

24006   Arthrotomy of the elbow, with capsular excision for capsular release (separate procedure)

⮕ *CPT Assistant* May 22:15

Excision

24065   Biopsy, soft tissue of upper arm or elbow area; superficial

24066   deep (subfascial or intramuscular)

(For needle biopsy of soft tissue, use 20206)

24071   Code is out of numerical sequence. See 24066-24079

24073   Code is out of numerical sequence. See 24066-24079

24075   Excision, tumor, soft tissue of upper arm or elbow area, subcutaneous; less than 3 cm

⮕ *CPT Changes: An Insider's View* 2002, 2010

 # 24071   3 cm or greater

⮕ *CPT Changes: An Insider's View* 2010

(For excision of benign lesions of cutaneous origin [eg, sebaceous cyst], see 11400-11406)

24076   Excision, tumor, soft tissue of upper arm or elbow area, subfascial (eg, intramuscular); less than 5 cm

⮕ *CPT Changes: An Insider's View* 2010

 # 24073   5 cm or greater

⮕ *CPT Changes: An Insider's View* 2010

24077   Radical resection of tumor (eg, sarcoma), soft tissue of upper arm or elbow area; less than 5 cm

⮕ *CPT Changes: An Insider's View* 2010, 2014

24079   5 cm or greater

⮕ *CPT Changes: An Insider's View* 2010, 2014

(For radical resection of tumor[s] of cutaneous origin [eg, melanoma], see 11600-11606)

24100   Arthrotomy, elbow; with synovial biopsy only

24101   with joint exploration, with or without biopsy, with or without removal of loose or foreign body

24102   with synovectomy

24105   Excision, olecranon bursa

24110   Excision or curettage of bone cyst or benign tumor, humerus;

24115   with autograft (includes obtaining graft)

24116   with allograft

24120   Excision or curettage of bone cyst or benign tumor of head or neck of radius or olecranon process;

24125   with autograft (includes obtaining graft)

24126   with allograft

24130   Excision, radial head

(For replacement with implant, use 24366)

24134   Sequestrectomy (eg, for osteomyelitis or bone abscess), shaft or distal humerus

24136   Sequestrectomy (eg, for osteomyelitis or bone abscess), radial head or neck

24138   Sequestrectomy (eg, for osteomyelitis or bone abscess), olecranon process

24140 Partial excision (craterization, saucerization, or diaphysectomy) bone (eg, osteomyelitis), humerus
➜ *CPT Assistant* Nov 98:9

24145 Partial excision (craterization, saucerization, or diaphysectomy) bone (eg, osteomyelitis), radial head or neck
➜ *CPT Assistant* Nov 98:9

24147 Partial excision (craterization, saucerization, or diaphysectomy) bone (eg, osteomyelitis), olecranon process
➜ *CPT Assistant* Nov 98:9

24149 Radical resection of capsule, soft tissue, and heterotopic bone, elbow, with contracture release (separate procedure)
➜ *CPT Assistant* Nov 96:4

(For capsular and soft tissue release only, use 24006)

24150 Radical resection of tumor, shaft or distal humerus
➜ *CPT Changes: An Insider's View* 2010

24152 Radical resection of tumor, radial head or neck
➜ *CPT Changes: An Insider's View* 2010

24155 Resection of elbow joint (arthrectomy)

Introduction or Removal

(For K-wire or pin insertion or removal, see 20650, 20670, 20680)

(For arthrocentesis or needling of bursa or joint, use 20605)

24160 Removal of prosthesis, includes debridement and synovectomy when performed; humeral **and** ulnar components
➜ *CPT Changes: An Insider's View* 2014
➜ *CPT Assistant* Feb 13:11, Mar 14:4, Mar 20:14

(To report removal of foreign body, elbow, see 24200, 24201)

(To report removal of hardware from the distal humerus or proximal ulna, other than humeral and ulnar prosthesis, use 20680)

(Do not report 24160 in conjunction with 24370 or 24371 if a prosthesis [ie, humeral and/or ulnar component(s)] is being removed and replaced in the same elbow during the same surgical session)

24164   radial head
➜ *CPT Changes: An Insider's View* 2014
➜ *CPT Assistant* Mar 14:4

(To report removal of foreign body, elbow, see 24200, 24201)

(To report removal of hardware from proximal radius, other than radial head prosthesis, use 20680)

24200 Removal of foreign body, upper arm or elbow area; subcutaneous
➜ *CPT Assistant* Mar 14:4

24201   deep (subfascial or intramuscular)
➜ *CPT Assistant* Nov 98:8, Mar 14:4

24220 Injection procedure for elbow arthrography
➜ *CPT Assistant* Aug 15:6, May 16:13
➜ *Clinical Examples in Radiology* Summer 18:15

(For radiological supervision and interpretation, use 73085. Do not report 77002 in conjunction with 73085)

(For injection for tennis elbow, use 20550)

Repair, Revision, and/or Reconstruction

24300 Manipulation, elbow, under anesthesia
➜ *CPT Changes: An Insider's View* 2002

(For application of external fixation, see 20690 or 20692)

24301 Muscle or tendon transfer, any type, upper arm or elbow, single (excluding 24320-24331)

24305 Tendon lengthening, upper arm or elbow, each tendon
➜ *CPT Assistant* Nov 98:8

24310 Tenotomy, open, elbow to shoulder, each tendon
➜ *CPT Assistant* Nov 98:8

24320 Tenoplasty, with muscle transfer, with or without free graft, elbow to shoulder, single (Seddon-Brookes type procedure)

24330 Flexor-plasty, elbow (eg, Steindler type advancement);

24331   with extensor advancement

24332 Tenolysis, triceps
➜ *CPT Changes: An Insider's View* 2002

24340 Tenodesis of biceps tendon at elbow (separate procedure)

24341 Repair, tendon or muscle, upper arm or elbow, each tendon or muscle, primary or secondary (excludes rotator cuff)
➜ *CPT Assistant* Nov 96:4, May 23:24

24342 Reinsertion of ruptured biceps or triceps tendon, distal, with or without tendon graft
➜ *CPT Assistant* Nov 96:4, Apr 17:9

24343 Repair lateral collateral ligament, elbow, with local tissue
➜ *CPT Changes: An Insider's View* 2002

24344 Reconstruction lateral collateral ligament, elbow, with tendon graft (includes harvesting of graft)
➜ *CPT Changes: An Insider's View* 2002

24345 Repair medial collateral ligament, elbow, with local tissue
➜ *CPT Changes: An Insider's View* 2002

24346   Reconstruction medial collateral ligament, elbow, with tendon graft (includes harvesting of graft)
➔ *CPT Changes: An Insider's View* 2002

24357   Tenotomy, elbow, lateral or medial (eg, epicondylitis, tennis elbow, golfer's elbow); percutaneous
➔ *CPT Changes: An Insider's View* 2008
➔ *CPT Assistant* Jan 08:4

24358   debridement, soft tissue and/or bone, open
➔ *CPT Changes: An Insider's View* 2008
➔ *CPT Assistant* Jan 08:4

24359   debridement, soft tissue and/or bone, open with tendon repair or reattachment
➔ *CPT Changes: An Insider's View* 2008
➔ *CPT Assistant* Jan 08:4

(Do not report 24357-24359 in conjunction with 29837, 29838)

24360   Arthroplasty, elbow; with membrane (eg, fascial)
➔ *CPT Assistant* Nov 98:8

24361   with distal humeral prosthetic replacement

24362   with implant and fascia lata ligament reconstruction

24363   with distal humerus and proximal ulnar prosthetic replacement (eg, total elbow)
➔ *CPT Assistant* Feb 13:11

(For revision of total elbow implant, see 24370, 24371)

24365   Arthroplasty, radial head;

24366   with implant

24370   Revision of total elbow arthroplasty, including allograft when performed; humeral **or** ulnar component
➔ *CPT Changes: An Insider's View* 2013
➔ *CPT Assistant* Feb 13:11, Mar 14:4

24371   humeral **and** ulnar component
➔ *CPT Changes: An Insider's View* 2013
➔ *CPT Assistant* Feb 13:11, Mar 14:4

(Do not report 24370, 24371 in conjunction with 24160 if a prosthesis [ie, humeral and/or ulnar component(s)] is being removed and replaced in the same elbow)

24400   Osteotomy, humerus, with or without internal fixation
➔ *CPT Assistant* Mar 14:4

24410   Multiple osteotomies with realignment on intramedullary rod, humeral shaft (Sofield type procedure)

24420   Osteoplasty, humerus (eg, shortening or lengthening) (excluding 64876)

24430   Repair of nonunion or malunion, humerus; without graft (eg, compression technique)

24435   with iliac or other autograft (includes obtaining graft)

(For proximal radius and/or ulna, see 25400-25420)

24470   Hemiepiphyseal arrest (eg, cubitus varus or valgus, distal humerus)

24495   Decompression fasciotomy, forearm, with brachial artery exploration

24498   Prophylactic treatment (nailing, pinning, plating or wiring), with or without methylmethacrylate, humeral shaft
➔ *CPT Assistant* Nov 98:8

Fracture and/or Dislocation

—— *Coding Tip* ——

Reporting for Categories of Manipulation and/or Fracture

The codes for treatment of fractures and joint injuries (dislocations) are categorized by the type of manipulation (reduction) and stabilization (fixation or immobilization). These codes can apply to either open (compound) or closed fractures or joint injuries.

CPT Coding Guidelines, Musculoskeletal System

24500   Closed treatment of humeral shaft fracture; without manipulation

24505   with manipulation, with or without skeletal traction

24515   Open treatment of humeral shaft fracture with plate/screws, with or without cerclage

24516   Treatment of humeral shaft fracture, with insertion of intramedullary implant, with or without cerclage and/or locking screws
➔ *CPT Changes: An Insider's View* 2003
➔ *CPT Assistant* Feb 96:4, Jun 09:7, Jan 18:3

24530   Closed treatment of supracondylar or transcondylar humeral fracture, with or without intercondylar extension; without manipulation

24535   with manipulation, with or without skin or skeletal traction

24538   Percutaneous skeletal fixation of supracondylar or transcondylar humeral fracture, with or without intercondylar extension
➔ *CPT Assistant* Winter 92:10

24545   Open treatment of humeral supracondylar or transcondylar fracture, includes internal fixation, when performed; without intercondylar extension
➔ *CPT Changes: An Insider's View* 2008

24546   with intercondylar extension
➔ *CPT Changes: An Insider's View* 2008

24560   Closed treatment of humeral epicondylar fracture, medial or lateral; without manipulation

24565   with manipulation

24566   Percutaneous skeletal fixation of humeral epicondylar fracture, medial or lateral, with manipulation

24575   Open treatment of humeral epicondylar fracture, medial or lateral, includes internal fixation, when performed
→ *CPT Changes: An Insider's View* 2008

24576   Closed treatment of humeral condylar fracture, medial or lateral; without manipulation

24577   with manipulation

24579   Open treatment of humeral condylar fracture, medial or lateral, includes internal fixation, when performed
→ *CPT Changes: An Insider's View* 2008

(To report closed treatment of fractures without manipulation, see 24530, 24560, 24576, 24650, 24670)

(To report closed treatment of fractures with manipulation, see 24535, 24565, 24577, 24675)

24582   Percutaneous skeletal fixation of humeral condylar fracture, medial or lateral, with manipulation

24586   Open treatment of periarticular fracture and/or dislocation of the elbow (fracture distal humerus and proximal ulna and/or proximal radius);

24587   with implant arthroplasty

(See also 24361)

24600   Treatment of closed elbow dislocation; without anesthesia

24605   requiring anesthesia

24615   Open treatment of acute or chronic elbow dislocation

24620   Closed treatment of Monteggia type of fracture dislocation at elbow (fracture proximal end of ulna with dislocation of radial head), with manipulation

24635   Open treatment of Monteggia type of fracture dislocation at elbow (fracture proximal end of ulna with dislocation of radial head), includes internal fixation, when performed
→ *CPT Changes: An Insider's View* 2008

24640   Closed treatment of radial head subluxation in child, nursemaid elbow, with manipulation

24650   Closed treatment of radial head or neck fracture; without manipulation

24655   with manipulation

24665   Open treatment of radial head or neck fracture, includes internal fixation or radial head excision, when performed;
→ *CPT Changes: An Insider's View* 2008

24666   with radial head prosthetic replacement
→ *CPT Changes: An Insider's View* 2008

24670   Closed treatment of ulnar fracture, proximal end (eg, olecranon or coronoid process[es]); without manipulation
→ *CPT Changes: An Insider's View* 2008

24675   with manipulation
→ *CPT Changes: An Insider's View* 2008

24685   Open treatment of ulnar fracture, proximal end (eg, olecranon or coronoid process[es]), includes internal fixation, when performed
→ *CPT Changes: An Insider's View* 2008
→ *CPT Assistant* Jan 18:3

(Do not report 24685 in conjunction with 24100-24102)

Arthrodesis

24800   Arthrodesis, elbow joint; local
→ *CPT Assistant* May 20:14, Jul 21:7

24802   with autogenous graft (includes obtaining graft)
→ *CPT Assistant* May 20:14, Jul 21:7

Amputation

24900   Amputation, arm through humerus; with primary closure

24920   open, circular (guillotine)

24925   secondary closure or scar revision

24930   re-amputation

24931   with implant

24935   Stump elongation, upper extremity

24940   Cineplasty, upper extremity, complete procedure

Other Procedures

24999   Unlisted procedure, humerus or elbow
→ *CPT Assistant* May 22:15

Forearm and Wrist

Radius, ulna, carpal bones, and joints.

Incision

25000   Incision, extensor tendon sheath, wrist (eg, de Quervains disease)
→ *CPT Assistant* Nov 98:8

(For decompression median nerve or for carpal tunnel syndrome, use 64721)

25001   Incision, flexor tendon sheath, wrist (eg, flexor carpi radialis)
→ *CPT Changes: An Insider's View* 2002

25020   Decompression fasciotomy, forearm and/or wrist, flexor OR extensor compartment; without debridement of nonviable muscle and/or nerve
→ *CPT Changes: An Insider's View* 2002

Musculoskeletal 20100-29999

25023   with debridement of nonviable muscle and/or nerve

(For decompression fasciotomy with brachial artery exploration, use 24495)

(For incision and drainage procedures, superficial, see 10060-10160)

(For debridement, see also 11000-11044)

25024   Decompression fasciotomy, forearm and/or wrist, flexor AND extensor compartment; without debridement of nonviable muscle and/or nerve
➡ *CPT Changes: An Insider's View* 2002

25025   with debridement of nonviable muscle and/or nerve
➡ *CPT Changes: An Insider's View* 2002

25028   Incision and drainage, forearm and/or wrist; deep abscess or hematoma

25031   bursa
➡ *CPT Assistant* Nov 98:9

25035   Incision, deep, bone cortex, forearm and/or wrist (eg, osteomyelitis or bone abscess)

25040   Arthrotomy, radiocarpal or midcarpal joint, with exploration, drainage, or removal of foreign body
➡ *CPT Assistant* Mar 20:14

Excision

25065   Biopsy, soft tissue of forearm and/or wrist; superficial

25066   deep (subfascial or intramuscular)
➡ *CPT Assistant* Nov 98:8, Apr 10:3

(For needle biopsy of soft tissue, use 20206)

25071   Code is out of numerical sequence. See 25066-25078

25073   Code is out of numerical sequence. See 25066-25078

25075   Excision, tumor, soft tissue of forearm and/or wrist area, subcutaneous; less than 3 cm
➡ *CPT Changes: An Insider's View* 2002, 2010

 # 25071   3 cm or greater
➡ *CPT Changes: An Insider's View* 2010

(For excision of benign lesions of cutaneous origin [eg, sebaceous cyst], see 11400-11406)

25076   Excision, tumor, soft tissue of forearm and/or wrist area, subfascial (eg, intramuscular); less than 3 cm
➡ *CPT Changes: An Insider's View* 2010

 # 25073   3 cm or greater
➡ *CPT Changes: An Insider's View* 2010

25077   Radical resection of tumor (eg, sarcoma), soft tissue of forearm and/or wrist area; less than 3 cm
➡ *CPT Changes: An Insider's View* 2010, 2014

25078   3 cm or greater
➡ *CPT Changes: An Insider's View* 2010, 2014

(For radical resection of tumor[s] of cutaneous origin [eg, melanoma], see 11600-11606)

25085   Capsulotomy, wrist (eg, contracture)

25100   Arthrotomy, wrist joint; with biopsy

25101   with joint exploration, with or without biopsy, with or without removal of loose or foreign body

25105   with synovectomy

25107   Arthrotomy, distal radioulnar joint including repair of triangular cartilage, complex

25109   Excision of tendon, forearm and/or wrist, flexor or extensor, each
➡ *CPT Changes: An Insider's View* 2007

25110   Excision, lesion of tendon sheath, forearm and/or wrist

25111   Excision of ganglion, wrist (dorsal or volar); primary

25112   recurrent

(For hand or finger, use 26160)

25115   Radical excision of bursa, synovia of wrist, or forearm tendon sheaths (eg, tenosynovitis, fungus, Tbc, or other granulomas, rheumatoid arthritis); flexors
➡ *CPT Assistant* Jun 12:15

25116   extensors, with or without transposition of dorsal retinaculum

(For finger synovectomies, use 26145)

25118   Synovectomy, extensor tendon sheath, wrist, single compartment;
➡ *CPT Assistant* Apr 12:17, Jun 15:10

25119   with resection of distal ulna

25120   Excision or curettage of bone cyst or benign tumor of radius or ulna (excluding head or neck of radius and olecranon process);

(For head or neck of radius or olecranon process, see 24120-24126)

25125   with autograft (includes obtaining graft)

25126   with allograft

25130   Excision or curettage of bone cyst or benign tumor of carpal bones;

25135   with autograft (includes obtaining graft)

25136   with allograft

25145   Sequestrectomy (eg, for osteomyelitis or bone abscess), forearm and/or wrist

25150   Partial excision (craterization, saucerization, or diaphysectomy) of bone (eg, for osteomyelitis); ulna

25151   radius

(For head or neck of radius or olecranon process, see 24145, 24147)

25170 Radical resection of tumor, radius or ulna
➔ *CPT Changes: An Insider's View* 2010

25210 Carpectomy; 1 bone
➔ *CPT Assistant* Oct 22:16

(For carpectomy with implant, see 25441-25445)

25215 all bones of proximal row
➔ *CPT Assistant* Dec 19:14

25230 Radial styloidectomy (separate procedure)

25240 Excision distal ulna partial or complete (eg, Darrach type or matched resection)

(For implant replacement, distal ulna, use 25442)

(For obtaining fascia for interposition, see 20920, 20922)

Introduction or Removal

(For K-wire, pin or rod insertion or removal, see 20650, 20670, 20680)

25246 Injection procedure for wrist arthrography
➔ *CPT Assistant* Aug 15:6
➔ *Clinical Examples in Radiology* Summer 18:15

(For radiological supervision and interpretation, use 73115. Do not report 77002 in conjunction with 73115)

(For foreign body removal, superficial use 20520)

25248 Exploration with removal of deep foreign body, forearm or wrist

25250 Removal of wrist prosthesis; (separate procedure)
➔ *CPT Assistant* Mar 20:14

25251 complicated, including total wrist
➔ *CPT Assistant* Mar 20:14

25259 Manipulation, wrist, under anesthesia
➔ *CPT Changes: An Insider's View* 2002
➔ *CPT Assistant* Jan 04:27, Jun 05:12

(For application of external fixation, see 20690 or 20692)

Repair, Revision, and/or Reconstruction

25260 Repair, tendon or muscle, flexor, forearm and/or wrist; primary, single, each tendon or muscle

25263 secondary, single, each tendon or muscle

25265 secondary, with free graft (includes obtaining graft), each tendon or muscle

25270 Repair, tendon or muscle, extensor, forearm and/or wrist; primary, single, each tendon or muscle

25272 secondary, single, each tendon or muscle

25274 secondary, with free graft (includes obtaining graft), each tendon or muscle
➔ *CPT Changes: An Insider's View* 2002

25275 Repair, tendon sheath, extensor, forearm and/or wrist, with free graft (includes obtaining graft) (eg, for extensor carpi ulnaris subluxation)
➔ *CPT Changes: An Insider's View* 2002

25280 Lengthening or shortening of flexor or extensor tendon, forearm and/or wrist, single, each tendon

25290 Tenotomy, open, flexor or extensor tendon, forearm and/or wrist, single, each tendon

25295 Tenolysis, flexor or extensor tendon, forearm and/or wrist, single, each tendon
➔ *CPT Assistant* Apr 97:11, Aug 98:10

25300 Tenodesis at wrist; flexors of fingers

25301 extensors of fingers

25310 Tendon transplantation or transfer, flexor or extensor, forearm and/or wrist, single; each tendon
➔ *CPT Assistant* Jun 02:11

▶(Do not report 25310 in conjunction with 25447, 25448, when performed for intercarpal or carpometacarpal joint arthroplasty)◀

25312 with tendon graft(s) (includes obtaining graft), each tendon

25315 Flexor origin slide (eg, for cerebral palsy, Volkmann contracture), forearm and/or wrist;

25316 with tendon(s) transfer

25320 Capsulorrhaphy or reconstruction, wrist, open (eg, capsulodesis, ligament repair, tendon transfer or graft) (includes synovectomy, capsulotomy and open reduction) for carpal instability
➔ *CPT Changes: An Insider's View* 2003

25332 Arthroplasty, wrist, with or without interposition, with or without external or internal fixation
➔ *CPT Assistant* Nov 96:5, Jan 05:8

(For obtaining fascia for interposition, see 20920, 20922)

(For prosthetic replacement arthroplasty, see 25441-25446)

25335 Centralization of wrist on ulna (eg, radial club hand)
➔ *CPT Assistant* May 18:10

25337 Reconstruction for stabilization of unstable distal ulna or distal radioulnar joint, secondary by soft tissue stabilization (eg, tendon transfer, tendon graft or weave, or tenodesis) with or without open reduction of distal radioulnar joint

(For harvesting of fascia lata graft, see 20920, 20922)

25350 Osteotomy, radius; distal third

Musculoskeletal 20100-29999

25355   middle or proximal third

25360 Osteotomy; ulna

25365   radius AND ulna

25370 Multiple osteotomies, with realignment on intramedullary rod (Sofield type procedure); radius OR ulna

25375   radius AND ulna

25390 Osteoplasty, radius OR ulna; shortening

25391   lengthening with autograft

25392 Osteoplasty, radius AND ulna; shortening (excluding 64876)

25393   lengthening with autograft

25394 Osteoplasty, carpal bone, shortening
➲ *CPT Changes: An Insider's View* 2002

25400 Repair of nonunion or malunion, radius OR ulna; without graft (eg, compression technique)

25405   with autograft (includes obtaining graft)
➲ *CPT Changes: An Insider's View* 2002

25415 Repair of nonunion or malunion, radius AND ulna; without graft (eg, compression technique)

25420   with autograft (includes obtaining graft)
➲ *CPT Changes: An Insider's View* 2002

25425 Repair of defect with autograft; radius OR ulna

25426   radius AND ulna

25430 Insertion of vascular pedicle into carpal bone (eg, Hori procedure)
➲ *CPT Changes: An Insider's View* 2002

25431 Repair of nonunion of carpal bone (excluding carpal scaphoid (navicular)) (includes obtaining graft and necessary fixation), each bone
➲ *CPT Changes: An Insider's View* 2002

25440 Repair of nonunion, scaphoid carpal (navicular) bone, with or without radial styloidectomy (includes obtaining graft and necessary fixation)
➲ *CPT Changes: An Insider's View* 2002

25441 Arthroplasty with prosthetic replacement; distal radius
➲ *CPT Assistant* Jan 05:8-9, Aug 17:9

25442   distal ulna
➲ *CPT Assistant* Jan 05:8-9, Aug 17:9

25443   scaphoid carpal (navicular)
➲ *CPT Changes: An Insider's View* 2002
➲ *CPT Assistant* Jan 05:8-9

25444   lunate
➲ *CPT Assistant* Jan 05:8, 10

25445   trapezium
➲ *CPT Assistant* Jan 05:8, 10, Aug 21:14

25446   distal radius and partial or entire carpus (total wrist)
➲ *CPT Assistant* Jan 05:8, 11

▲ **25447** Arthroplasty, intercarpal or carpometacarpal joints; interposition (eg, tendon)
➲ *CPT Changes: An Insider's View* 2025
➲ *CPT Assistant* Nov 98:8, Jan 05:8, 11-12, Aug 21:14

▶(Do not report 25447 in conjunction with 25448)◀

▶(Do not report 25447 in conjunction with 25310, 26480, when performed for intercarpal or carpometacarpal joint arthroplasty)◀

(For wrist arthroplasty, use 25332)

● **25448**   suspension, including transfer or transplant of tendon, with interposition, when performed
➲ *CPT Changes: An Insider's View* 2025

▶(Do not report 25448 in conjunction with 25447)◀

▶(Do not report 25448 in conjunction with 25310, 26480, when performed for intercarpal or carpometacarpal joint arthroplasty)◀

25449 Revision of arthroplasty, including removal of implant, wrist joint

25450 Epiphyseal arrest by epiphysiodesis or stapling; distal radius OR ulna

25455   distal radius AND ulna

25490 Prophylactic treatment (nailing, pinning, plating or wiring) with or without methylmethacrylate; radius

25491   ulna

25492   radius AND ulna

Fracture and/or Dislocation

(For application of external fixation in addition to internal fixation, use 20690 and the appropriate internal fixation code)

25500 Closed treatment of radial shaft fracture; without manipulation

25505   with manipulation

25515 Open treatment of radial shaft fracture, includes internal fixation, when performed
➲ *CPT Changes: An Insider's View* 2008

25520 Closed treatment of radial shaft fracture and closed treatment of dislocation of distal radioulnar joint (Galeazzi fracture/dislocation)
➲ *CPT Changes: An Insider's View* 2002

25525 Open treatment of radial shaft fracture, includes internal fixation, when performed, and closed treatment of distal radioulnar joint dislocation (Galeazzi fracture/dislocation), includes percutaneous skeletal fixation, when performed
➔ *CPT Changes: An Insider's View* 2008

25526 Open treatment of radial shaft fracture, includes internal fixation, when performed, and open treatment of distal radioulnar joint dislocation (Galeazzi fracture/dislocation), includes internal fixation, when performed, includes repair of triangular fibrocartilage complex
➔ *CPT Changes: An Insider's View* 2002, 2008

25530 Closed treatment of ulnar shaft fracture; without manipulation
➔ *CPT Assistant* Apr 02:14

25535   with manipulation
➔ *CPT Assistant* Sep 10:7

25545 Open treatment of ulnar shaft fracture, includes internal fixation, when performed
➔ *CPT Changes: An Insider's View* 2008
➔ *CPT Assistant* Fall 93:23, Oct 99:5

25560 Closed treatment of radial and ulnar shaft fractures; without manipulation

25565   with manipulation

25574 Open treatment of radial AND ulnar shaft fractures, with internal fixation, when performed; of radius OR ulna
➔ *CPT Changes: An Insider's View* 2008
➔ *CPT Assistant* Fall 93:23, Oct 99:5

25575   of radius AND ulna
➔ *CPT Changes: An Insider's View* 2008

25600 Closed treatment of distal radial fracture (eg, Colles or Smith type) or epiphyseal separation, includes closed treatment of fracture of ulnar styloid, when performed; without manipulation
➔ *CPT Changes: An Insider's View* 2007
➔ *CPT Assistant* Oct 07:7, Apr 13:10

25605   with manipulation
➔ *CPT Assistant* Oct 07:7, Apr 13:10

(Do not report 25600, 25605 in conjunction with 25650)

25606 Percutaneous skeletal fixation of distal radial fracture or epiphyseal separation
➔ *CPT Changes: An Insider's View* 2007

(Do not report 25606 in conjunction with 25650)

(For percutaneous treatment of ulnar styloid fracture, use 25651)

(For open treatment of ulnar styloid fracture, use 25652)

25607 Open treatment of distal radial extra-articular fracture or epiphyseal separation, with internal fixation
➔ *CPT Changes: An Insider's View* 2007
➔ *CPT Assistant* Oct 07:7, Nov 12:13

(Do not report 25607 in conjunction with 25650)

(For percutaneous treatment of ulnar styloid fracture, use 25651)

(For open treatment of ulnar styloid fracture, use 25652)

25608 Open treatment of distal radial intra-articular fracture or epiphyseal separation; with internal fixation of 2 fragments
➔ *CPT Changes: An Insider's View* 2007
➔ *CPT Assistant* Oct 07:7

(Do not report 25608 in conjunction with 25609)

25609   with internal fixation of 3 or more fragments
➔ *CPT Changes: An Insider's View* 2007
➔ *CPT Assistant* Oct 07:7, Mar 13:13, Dec 13:14, Oct 22:16

(Do not report 25608, 25609 in conjunction with 25650)

(For percutaneous treatment of ulnar styloid fracture, use 25651)

(For open treatment of ulnar styloid fracture, use 25652)

25622 Closed treatment of carpal scaphoid (navicular) fracture; without manipulation

25624   with manipulation

25628 Open treatment of carpal scaphoid (navicular) fracture, includes internal fixation, when performed
➔ *CPT Changes: An Insider's View* 2008

25630 Closed treatment of carpal bone fracture (excluding carpal scaphoid [navicular]); without manipulation, each bone

25635   with manipulation, each bone

25645 Open treatment of carpal bone fracture (other than carpal scaphoid [navicular]), each bone
➔ *CPT Changes: An Insider's View* 2002

25650 Closed treatment of ulnar styloid fracture
➔ *CPT Assistant* Oct 07:7, Apr 13:10

(Do not report 25650 in conjunction with 25600, 25605, 25607-25609)

25651 Percutaneous skeletal fixation of ulnar styloid fracture
➔ *CPT Changes: An Insider's View* 2002

25652 Open treatment of ulnar styloid fracture
➔ *CPT Changes: An Insider's View* 2002
➔ *CPT Assistant* Oct 07:7

25660 Closed treatment of radiocarpal or intercarpal dislocation, 1 or more bones, with manipulation

25670 Open treatment of radiocarpal or intercarpal dislocation, 1 or more bones

25671 Percutaneous skeletal fixation of distal radioulnar dislocation
> *CPT Changes: An Insider's View* 2002

25675 Closed treatment of distal radioulnar dislocation with manipulation

25676 Open treatment of distal radioulnar dislocation, acute or chronic

25680 Closed treatment of trans-scaphoperilunar type of fracture dislocation, with manipulation

25685 Open treatment of trans-scaphoperilunar type of fracture dislocation

25690 Closed treatment of lunate dislocation, with manipulation

25695 Open treatment of lunate dislocation

Arthrodesis

25800 Arthrodesis, wrist; complete, without bone graft (includes radiocarpal and/or intercarpal and/or carpometacarpal joints)
> *CPT Assistant* Nov 98:8, May 20:14, Jul 21:7

25805 with sliding graft

25810 with iliac or other autograft (includes obtaining graft)

25820 Arthrodesis, wrist; limited, without bone graft (eg, intercarpal or radiocarpal)
> *CPT Assistant* Nov 98:8

25825 with autograft (includes obtaining graft)
> *CPT Assistant* Jul 12:12

25830 Arthrodesis, distal radioulnar joint with segmental resection of ulna, with or without bone graft (eg, Sauve-Kapandji procedure)
> *CPT Assistant* Nov 98:8, May 20:14, Jul 21:7

Amputation

25900 Amputation, forearm, through radius and ulna;

25905 open, circular (guillotine)

25907 secondary closure or scar revision

25909 re-amputation

25915 Krukenberg procedure

25920 Disarticulation through wrist;

25922 secondary closure or scar revision

25924 re-amputation

25927 Transmetacarpal amputation;

25929 secondary closure or scar revision

25931 re-amputation

Other Procedures

25999 Unlisted procedure, forearm or wrist
> *CPT Assistant* Sep 19:10, Oct 22:16

Hand and Fingers

Incision

26010 Drainage of finger abscess; simple
> *CPT Assistant* Oct 21:13

26011 complicated (eg, felon)

26020 Drainage of tendon sheath, digit and/or palm, each

26025 Drainage of palmar bursa; single, bursa
> *CPT Assistant* Nov 98:8

26030 multiple bursa
> *CPT Assistant* Nov 98:8

26034 Incision, bone cortex, hand or finger (eg, osteomyelitis or bone abscess)
> *CPT Assistant* Nov 98:8

26035 Decompression fingers and/or hand, injection injury (eg, grease gun)

26037 Decompressive fasciotomy, hand (excludes 26035)

(For injection injury, use 26035)

26040 Fasciotomy, palmar (eg, Dupuytren's contracture); percutaneous
> *CPT Assistant* Nov 98:8, Apr 10:10, Oct 10:10

26045 open, partial

(For palmar fasciotomy by enzyme injection (eg, collagenase), see 20527, 26341)

(For fasciectomy, see 26121-26125)

26055 Tendon sheath incision (eg, for trigger finger)
> *CPT Assistant* Jan 22:17, Apr 22:11

26060 Tenotomy, percutaneous, single, each digit

26070 Arthrotomy, with exploration, drainage, or removal of loose or foreign body; carpometacarpal joint
> *CPT Assistant* Nov 98:10, Mar 20:14

26075 metacarpophalangeal joint, each
> *CPT Assistant* Sep 12:10, Mar 20:14

26080 interphalangeal joint, each
> *CPT Assistant* Sep 12:10, Mar 20:14

Excision

26100 Arthrotomy with biopsy; carpometacarpal joint, each

26105 metacarpophalangeal joint, each

26110 interphalangeal joint, each

26111   Code is out of numerical sequence. See 26110-26118

26113   Code is out of numerical sequence. See 26110-26118

26115   Excision, tumor or vascular malformation, soft tissue of hand or finger, subcutaneous; less than 1.5 cm
> *CPT Changes: An Insider's View* 2002, 2010
> *CPT Assistant* Apr 21:13, Aug 23:19-20

 # 26111   1.5 cm or greater
> *CPT Changes: An Insider's View* 2010
> *CPT Assistant* Aug 23:19-20

(For excision of benign lesions of cutaneous origin [eg, sebaceous cyst], see 11420-11426)

26116   Excision, tumor, soft tissue, or vascular malformation, of hand or finger, subfascial (eg, intramuscular); less than 1.5 cm
> *CPT Changes: An Insider's View* 2002, 2010
> *CPT Assistant* Apr 10:3, Apr 21:13, Aug 23:19-20

 # 26113   1.5 cm or greater
> *CPT Changes: An Insider's View* 2010
> *CPT Assistant* Apr 10:3, Aug 23:19-20

26117   Radical resection of tumor (eg, sarcoma), soft tissue of hand or finger; less than 3 cm
> *CPT Changes: An Insider's View* 2010, 2014

26118   3 cm or greater
> *CPT Changes: An Insider's View* 2010, 2014

(For radical resection of tumor[s] of cutaneous origin [eg, melanoma], see 11620-11626)

26121   Fasciectomy, palm only, with or without Z-plasty, other local tissue rearrangement, or skin grafting (includes obtaining graft)
> *CPT Assistant* Oct 10:10, Jun 11:13

26123   Fasciectomy, partial palmar with release of single digit including proximal interphalangeal joint, with or without Z-plasty, other local tissue rearrangement, or skin grafting (includes obtaining graft);
> *CPT Assistant* Jan 05:8, Oct 10:10, Jun 11:13, May 21:13

+ 26125   each additional digit (List separately in addition to code for primary procedure)
> *CPT Assistant* Jan 05:8, Oct 10:10, Jun 11:13

(Use 26125 in conjunction with 26123)

(For palmar fasciotomy by enzyme injection (eg, collagenase), see 20527, 26341)

(For fasciotomy, see 26040, 26045)

26130   Synovectomy, carpometacarpal joint

26135   Synovectomy, metacarpophalangeal joint including intrinsic release and extensor hood reconstruction, each digit

26140   Synovectomy, proximal interphalangeal joint, including extensor reconstruction, each interphalangeal joint

26145   Synovectomy, tendon sheath, radical (tenosynovectomy), flexor tendon, palm and/or finger, each tendon
> *CPT Assistant* Nov 98:8

(For tendon sheath synovectomies at wrist, see 25115, 25116)

26160   Excision of lesion of tendon sheath or joint capsule (eg, cyst, mucous cyst, or ganglion), hand or finger
> *CPT Changes: An Insider's View* 2002
> *CPT Assistant* Jul 19:10, Aug 21:14

(For wrist ganglion, see 25111, 25112)

(For trigger digit, use 26055)

26170   Excision of tendon, palm, flexor or extensor, single, each tendon
> *CPT Changes: An Insider's View* 2007
> *CPT Assistant* Jun 13:13

(Do not report 26170 in conjunction with 26390, 26415)

26180   Excision of tendon, finger, flexor or extensor, each tendon
> *CPT Changes: An Insider's View* 2007
> *CPT Assistant* Nov 98:8

(Do not report 26180 in conjunction with 26390, 26415)

26185   Sesamoidectomy, thumb or finger (separate procedure)

26200   Excision or curettage of bone cyst or benign tumor of metacarpal;

26205   with autograft (includes obtaining graft)

26210   Excision or curettage of bone cyst or benign tumor of proximal, middle, or distal phalanx of finger;
> *CPT Assistant* Aug 21:14

26215   with autograft (includes obtaining graft)

26230   Partial excision (craterization, saucerization, or diaphysectomy) bone (eg, osteomyelitis); metacarpal

26235   proximal or middle phalanx of finger
> *CPT Assistant* Jul 19:10, Aug 21:14

26236   distal phalanx of finger
> *CPT Assistant* Jul 19:10, Aug 21:14

26250   Radical resection of tumor, metacarpal
> *CPT Changes: An Insider's View* 2010
> *CPT Assistant* Nov 98:8

26260   Radical resection of tumor, proximal or middle phalanx of finger
> *CPT Changes: An Insider's View* 2010
> *CPT Assistant* Nov 98:8

26262   Radical resection of tumor, distal phalanx of finger
> *CPT Changes: An Insider's View* 2010
> *CPT Assistant* Nov 98:8

Introduction or Removal

26320 Removal of implant from finger or hand

(For removal of foreign body in hand or finger, see 20520, 20525)

Repair, Revision, and/or Reconstruction

26340 Manipulation, finger joint, under anesthesia, each joint
➔ *CPT Changes: An Insider's View* 2002
➔ *CPT Assistant* Nov 02:10

(For application of external fixation, see 20690 or 20692)

26341 Manipulation, palmar fascial cord (ie, Dupuytren's cord), post enzyme injection (eg, collagenase), single cord
➔ *CPT Changes: An Insider's View* 2012
➔ *CPT Assistant* Jul 12:8, 14

(For enzyme injection (eg, collagenase), palmar fascial cord (eg, Dupuytren's contracture), use 20527)

(Report custom orthotic fabrication/application separately)

26350 Repair or advancement, flexor tendon, not in zone 2 digital flexor tendon sheath (eg, no man's land); primary or secondary without free graft, each tendon
➔ *CPT Changes: An Insider's View* 2002
➔ *CPT Assistant* Nov 98:8

26352 secondary with free graft (includes obtaining graft), each tendon

26356 Repair or advancement, flexor tendon, in zone 2 digital flexor tendon sheath (eg, no man's land); primary, without free graft, each tendon
➔ *CPT Changes: An Insider's View* 2002, 2004
➔ *CPT Assistant* Nov 98:8, Dec 98:9, Dec 08:6, Sep 14:13, Dec 17:15

26357 secondary, without free graft, each tendon
➔ *CPT Changes: An Insider's View* 2004

26358 secondary, with free graft (includes obtaining graft), each tendon

26370 Repair or advancement of profundus tendon, with intact superficialis tendon; primary, each tendon
➔ *CPT Assistant* Nov 98:8, Dec 08:6

26372 secondary with free graft (includes obtaining graft), each tendon
➔ *CPT Assistant* Nov 98:8

26373 secondary without free graft, each tendon
➔ *CPT Assistant* Nov 98:8

26390 Excision flexor tendon, with implantation of synthetic rod for delayed tendon graft, hand or finger, each rod
➔ *CPT Changes: An Insider's View* 2002
➔ *CPT Assistant* Nov 98:8

26392 Removal of synthetic rod and insertion of flexor tendon graft, hand or finger (includes obtaining graft), each rod
➔ *CPT Changes: An Insider's View* 2002
➔ *CPT Assistant* Nov 98:8

26410 Repair, extensor tendon, hand, primary or secondary; without free graft, each tendon
➔ *CPT Assistant* Nov 98:8

26412 with free graft (includes obtaining graft), each tendon
➔ *CPT Assistant* Nov 98:8

26415 Excision of extensor tendon, with implantation of synthetic rod for delayed tendon graft, hand or finger, each rod
➔ *CPT Changes: An Insider's View* 2002
➔ *CPT Assistant* Nov 98:8

26416 Removal of synthetic rod and insertion of extensor tendon graft (includes obtaining graft), hand or finger, each rod
➔ *CPT Changes: An Insider's View* 2000, 2002
➔ *CPT Assistant* Nov 99:12

26418 Repair, extensor tendon, finger, primary or secondary; without free graft, each tendon
➔ *CPT Assistant* Nov 98:8, Dec 99:10, Dec 00:14

26420 with free graft (includes obtaining graft) each tendon

26426 Repair of extensor tendon, central slip, secondary (eg, boutonniere deformity); using local tissue(s), including lateral band(s), each finger
➔ *CPT Changes: An Insider's View* 2002
➔ *CPT Assistant* Nov 98:8

26428 with free graft (includes obtaining graft), each finger
➔ *CPT Changes: An Insider's View* 2002

26432 Closed treatment of distal extensor tendon insertion, with or without percutaneous pinning (eg, mallet finger)
➔ *CPT Assistant* Nov 98:8

26433 Repair of extensor tendon, distal insertion, primary or secondary; without graft (eg, mallet finger)
➔ *CPT Assistant* Nov 98:8

26434 with free graft (includes obtaining graft)

(For tenovaginotomy for trigger finger, use 26055)

26437 Realignment of extensor tendon, hand, each tendon
➔ *CPT Assistant* Nov 98:8

26440 Tenolysis, flexor tendon; palm OR finger, each tendon
➔ *CPT Changes: An Insider's View* 2003
➔ *CPT Assistant* Apr 02:18, Jun 15:10

26442 palm AND finger, each tendon
➔ *CPT Assistant* Feb 22:14, Jul 22:17

26445 Tenolysis, extensor tendon, hand OR finger, each tendon
➔ *CPT Changes: An Insider's View* 2002
➔ *CPT Assistant* Nov 98:8, Dec 02:11, Mar 03:20

26449 Tenolysis, complex, extensor tendon, finger, including forearm, each tendon
↪ *CPT Assistant* Nov 98:8

26450 Tenotomy, flexor, palm, open, each tendon
↪ *CPT Assistant* Nov 98:8, Jul 23:15

26455 Tenotomy, flexor, finger, open, each tendon
↪ *CPT Assistant* Nov 98:8

26460 Tenotomy, extensor, hand or finger, open, each tendon
↪ *CPT Assistant* Nov 98:8

26471 Tenodesis; of proximal interphalangeal joint, each joint
↪ *CPT Assistant* Nov 98:8

26474   of distal joint, each joint
↪ *CPT Assistant* Nov 98:8

26476 Lengthening of tendon, extensor, hand or finger, each tendon
↪ *CPT Assistant* Nov 98:8

26477 Shortening of tendon, extensor, hand or finger, each tendon
↪ *CPT Assistant* Nov 98:8

26478 Lengthening of tendon, flexor, hand or finger, each tendon
↪ *CPT Assistant* Nov 98:8, Dec 13:16

26479 Shortening of tendon, flexor, hand or finger, each tendon
↪ *CPT Assistant* Nov 98:8

26480 Transfer or transplant of tendon, carpometacarpal area or dorsum of hand; without free graft, each tendon
↪ *CPT Assistant* Nov 98:8, Dec 13:16

▶(Do not report 26480 in conjunction with 25447, 25448, when performed for intercarpal or carpometacarpal joint arthroplasty)◀

26483   with free tendon graft (includes obtaining graft), each tendon

26485 Transfer or transplant of tendon, palmar; without free tendon graft, each tendon
↪ *CPT Assistant* Nov 98:8

26489   with free tendon graft (includes obtaining graft), each tendon

26490 Opponensplasty; superficialis tendon transfer type, each tendon

26492   tendon transfer with graft (includes obtaining graft), each tendon

26494   hypothenar muscle transfer

26496   other methods

(For thumb fusion in opposition, use 26820)

26497 Transfer of tendon to restore intrinsic function; ring and small finger
↪ *CPT Assistant* Nov 98:8

26498   all 4 fingers

26499 Correction claw finger, other methods

26500 Reconstruction of tendon pulley, each tendon; with local tissues (separate procedure)
↪ *CPT Assistant* Nov 98:8

26502   with tendon or fascial graft (includes obtaining graft) (separate procedure)

26508 Release of thenar muscle(s) (eg, thumb contracture)
↪ *CPT Assistant* Nov 98:8

26510 Cross intrinsic transfer, each tendon
↪ *CPT Changes: An Insider's View* 2002

26516 Capsulodesis, metacarpophalangeal joint; single digit
↪ *CPT Assistant* Nov 98:8

26517   2 digits

26518   3 or 4 digits

26520 Capsulectomy or capsulotomy; metacarpophalangeal joint, each joint
↪ *CPT Assistant* Nov 98:8

26525   interphalangeal joint, each joint
↪ *CPT Assistant* Nov 98:8, Apr 02:18, Mar 03:20, Jun 15:10

26530 Arthroplasty, metacarpophalangeal joint; each joint
↪ *CPT Assistant* Nov 98:8

(To report carpometacarpal joint arthroplasty, use 25447)

26531   with prosthetic implant, each joint
↪ *CPT Assistant* Nov 98:8, Sep 11:12

26535 Arthroplasty, interphalangeal joint; each joint
↪ *CPT Assistant* Nov 98:8

26536   with prosthetic implant, each joint
↪ *CPT Assistant* Nov 98:8, Jul 23:15

26540 Repair of collateral ligament, metacarpophalangeal or interphalangeal joint
↪ *CPT Assistant* Nov 96:6

26541 Reconstruction, collateral ligament, metacarpophalangeal joint, single; with tendon or fascial graft (includes obtaining graft)
↪ *CPT Assistant* Jan 97:3

26542   with local tissue (eg, adductor advancement)
↪ *CPT Assistant* Jan 97:3

26545 Reconstruction, collateral ligament, interphalangeal joint, single, including graft, each joint

26546 Repair non-union, metacarpal or phalanx (includes obtaining bone graft with or without external or internal fixation)
↪ *CPT Assistant* Nov 96:6

26548 Repair and reconstruction, finger, volar plate, interphalangeal joint

26550	Pollicization of a digit
26551	Transfer, toe-to-hand with microvascular anastomosis; great toe wrap-around with bone graft

↪ *CPT Assistant* Nov 96:6, Apr 97:7, Jun 97:9, Nov 98:8, 10-11

(For great toe with web space, use 20973)

26553	other than great toe, single

↪ *CPT Assistant* Nov 96:6, Apr 97:7, Jun 97:9, Nov 98:8, 10-11

26554	other than great toe, double

↪ *CPT Assistant* Nov 96:6, Apr 97:7, Jun 97:9, Nov 98:8, 10-11

(Do not report code 69990 in addition to codes 26551-26554)

26555	Transfer, finger to another position without microvascular anastomosis

↪ *CPT Assistant* Nov 98:8, 10-11

26556	Transfer, free toe joint, with microvascular anastomosis

↪ *CPT Assistant* Nov 96:6, Apr 97:7, Jun 97:9, Nov 98:8

(Do not report code 69990 in addition to code 26556)

(To report great toe-to-hand transfer, use 20973)

26560	Repair of syndactyly (web finger) each web space; with skin flaps
26561	with skin flaps and grafts
26562	complex (eg, involving bone, nails)
26565	Osteotomy; metacarpal, each

↪ *CPT Assistant* Nov 98:9

26567	phalanx of finger, each

↪ *CPT Assistant* Apr 12:17

26568	Osteoplasty, lengthening, metacarpal or phalanx
26580	Repair cleft hand
26587	Reconstruction of polydactylous digit, soft tissue and bone

↪ *CPT Changes: An Insider's View* 2002
↪ *CPT Assistant* Oct 01:10, Aug 03:14, May 04:16

(For excision of polydactylous digit, soft tissue only, use 11200)

26590	Repair macrodactylia, each digit

↪ *CPT Changes: An Insider's View* 2002
↪ *CPT Assistant* Oct 01:10, Aug 03:14, May 04:16

26591	Repair, intrinsic muscles of hand, each muscle

↪ *CPT Assistant* May 98:11, Jul 98:11, Nov 98:8, 11

26593	Release, intrinsic muscles of hand, each muscle

↪ *CPT Assistant* Nov 98:8, 11

26596	Excision of constricting ring of finger, with multiple Z-plasties

(To report release of scar contracture or graft repairs see 11042, 14040-14041, or 15120, 15240)

Fracture and/or Dislocation

— *Coding Tip* —

Reporting for Categories of Manipulation and/or Fracture

The codes for treatment of fractures and joint injuries (dislocations) are categorized by the type of manipulation (reduction) and stabilization (fixation or immobilization). These codes can apply to either open (compound) or closed fractures or joint injuries.

CPT Coding Guidelines, Musculoskeletal System

26600	Closed treatment of metacarpal fracture, single; without manipulation, each bone
26605	with manipulation, each bone
26607	Closed treatment of metacarpal fracture, with manipulation, with external fixation, each bone

↪ *CPT Changes: An Insider's View* 2002

26608	Percutaneous skeletal fixation of metacarpal fracture, each bone
26615	Open treatment of metacarpal fracture, single, includes internal fixation, when performed, each bone

↪ *CPT Changes: An Insider's View* 2008

26641	Closed treatment of carpometacarpal dislocation, thumb, with manipulation
26645	Closed treatment of carpometacarpal fracture dislocation, thumb (Bennett fracture), with manipulation
26650	Percutaneous skeletal fixation of carpometacarpal fracture dislocation, thumb (Bennett fracture), with manipulation

↪ *CPT Changes: An Insider's View* 2008

26665	Open treatment of carpometacarpal fracture dislocation, thumb (Bennett fracture), includes internal fixation, when performed

↪ *CPT Changes: An Insider's View* 2008

26670	Closed treatment of carpometacarpal dislocation, other than thumb, with manipulation, each joint; without anesthesia

↪ *CPT Changes: An Insider's View* 2002

26675	requiring anesthesia
26676	Percutaneous skeletal fixation of carpometacarpal dislocation, other than thumb, with manipulation, each joint

↪ *CPT Changes: An Insider's View* 2002

26685   Open treatment of carpometacarpal dislocation, other than thumb; includes internal fixation, when performed, each joint
➔ *CPT Changes: An Insider's View* 2002, 2008

26686   complex, multiple, or delayed reduction

26700   Closed treatment of metacarpophalangeal dislocation, single, with manipulation; without anesthesia
➔ *CPT Assistant* May 14:10

26705   requiring anesthesia

26706   Percutaneous skeletal fixation of metacarpophalangeal dislocation, single, with manipulation

26715   Open treatment of metacarpophalangeal dislocation, single, includes internal fixation, when performed
➔ *CPT Changes: An Insider's View* 2008

26720   Closed treatment of phalangeal shaft fracture, proximal or middle phalanx, finger or thumb; without manipulation, each

26725   with manipulation, with or without skin or skeletal traction, each

26727   Percutaneous skeletal fixation of unstable phalangeal shaft fracture, proximal or middle phalanx, finger or thumb, with manipulation, each

26735   Open treatment of phalangeal shaft fracture, proximal or middle phalanx, finger or thumb, includes internal fixation, when performed, each
➔ *CPT Changes: An Insider's View* 2008

26740   Closed treatment of articular fracture, involving metacarpophalangeal or interphalangeal joint; without manipulation, each

26742   with manipulation, each

26746   Open treatment of articular fracture, involving metacarpophalangeal or interphalangeal joint, includes internal fixation, when performed, each
➔ *CPT Changes: An Insider's View* 2008

26750   Closed treatment of distal phalangeal fracture, finger or thumb; without manipulation, each

26755   with manipulation, each

26756   Percutaneous skeletal fixation of distal phalangeal fracture, finger or thumb, each

26765   Open treatment of distal phalangeal fracture, finger or thumb, includes internal fixation, when performed, each
➔ *CPT Changes: An Insider's View* 2008

26770   Closed treatment of interphalangeal joint dislocation, single, with manipulation; without anesthesia
➔ *CPT Assistant* Mar 23:1

26775   requiring anesthesia

26776   Percutaneous skeletal fixation of interphalangeal joint dislocation, single, with manipulation

26785   Open treatment of interphalangeal joint dislocation, includes internal fixation, when performed, single
➔ *CPT Changes: An Insider's View* 2008

Arthrodesis

26820   Fusion in opposition, thumb, with autogenous graft (includes obtaining graft)
➔ *CPT Assistant* May 20:14, Jul 21:7

26841   Arthrodesis, carpometacarpal joint, thumb, with or without internal fixation;

26842   with autograft (includes obtaining graft)

26843   Arthrodesis, carpometacarpal joint, digit, other than thumb, each;
➔ *CPT Changes: An Insider's View* 2002

26844   with autograft (includes obtaining graft)

26850   Arthrodesis, metacarpophalangeal joint, with or without internal fixation;

26852   with autograft (includes obtaining graft)

26860   Arthrodesis, interphalangeal joint, with or without internal fixation;

+ **26861**   each additional interphalangeal joint (List separately in addition to code for primary procedure)

(Use 26861 in conjunction with 26860)

26862   with autograft (includes obtaining graft)

+ **26863**   with autograft (includes obtaining graft), each additional joint (List separately in addition to code for primary procedure)
➔ *CPT Assistant* May 20:14, Jul 21:7

(Use 26863 in conjunction with 26862)

Amputation

(For hand through metacarpal bones, use 25927)

26910   Amputation, metacarpal, with finger or thumb (ray amputation), single, with or without interosseous transfer

(For repositioning, see 26550, 26555)

26951   Amputation, finger or thumb, primary or secondary, any joint or phalanx, single, including neurectomies; with direct closure

26952   with local advancement flaps (V-Y, hood)

(For repair of soft tissue defect requiring split or full thickness graft or other pedicle flaps, see 15050-15758)

Other Procedures

26989   Unlisted procedure, hands or fingers
➔ *CPT Assistant* Jan 22:17, Apr 22:11, Feb 23:13

Musculoskeletal 20100-29999

Pelvis and Hip Joint

Including head and neck of femur.

Incision

(For incision and drainage procedures, superficial, see 10040-10160)

26990   Incision and drainage, pelvis or hip joint area; deep abscess or hematoma
➔ *CPT Assistant* Mar 20:14

26991   infected bursa

26992   Incision, bone cortex, pelvis and/or hip joint (eg, osteomyelitis or bone abscess)
➔ *CPT Assistant* Jan 02:10, Oct 12:14

27000   Tenotomy, adductor of hip, percutaneous (separate procedure)

27001   Tenotomy, adductor of hip, open

(To report bilateral procedure, report 27001 with modifier 50)

27003   Tenotomy, adductor, subcutaneous, open, with obturator neurectomy

(To report bilateral procedure, report 27003 with modifier 50)

27005   Tenotomy, hip flexor(s), open (separate procedure)

27006   Tenotomy, abductors and/or extensor(s) of hip, open (separate procedure)

27025   Fasciotomy, hip or thigh, any type

(To report bilateral procedure, report 27025 with modifier 50)

27027   Decompression fasciotomy(ies), pelvic (buttock) compartment(s) (eg, gluteus medius-minimus, gluteus maximus, iliopsoas, and/or tensor fascia lata muscle), unilateral
➔ *CPT Changes: An Insider's View* 2009

(To report bilateral procedure, report 27027 with modifier 50)

27030   Arthrotomy, hip, with drainage (eg, infection)
➔ *CPT Assistant* Nov 98:8, Mar 20:14, Sep 21:8

27033   Arthrotomy, hip, including exploration or removal of loose or foreign body
➔ *CPT Assistant* Spring 92:11

27035   Denervation, hip joint, intrapelvic or extrapelvic intra-articular branches of sciatic, femoral, or obturator nerves
➔ *CPT Assistant* Nov 98:8, Mar 14:13

(For obturator neurectomy, see 64763, 64766)

27036   Capsulectomy or capsulotomy, hip, with or without excision of heterotopic bone, with release of hip flexor muscles (ie, gluteus medius, gluteus minimus, tensor fascia latae, rectus femoris, sartorius, iliopsoas)
➔ *CPT Assistant* Jan 05:8

Excision

27040   Biopsy, soft tissue of pelvis and hip area; superficial
➔ *CPT Assistant* May 23:26

27041   deep, subfascial or intramuscular
➔ *CPT Assistant* Nov 98:8, May 23:26

(For needle biopsy of soft tissue, use 20206)

27043   Code is out of numerical sequence. See 27041-27052

27045   Code is out of numerical sequence. See 27041-27052

27047   Excision, tumor, soft tissue of pelvis and hip area, subcutaneous; less than 3 cm
➔ *CPT Changes: An Insider's View* 2010
➔ *CPT Assistant* Nov 98:8

27043   3 cm or greater
➔ *CPT Changes: An Insider's View* 2010

(For excision of benign lesions of cutaneous origin [eg, sebaceous cyst], see 11400-11406)

27048   Excision, tumor, soft tissue of pelvis and hip area, subfascial (eg, intramuscular); less than 5 cm
➔ *CPT Changes: An Insider's View* 2010

27045   5 cm or greater
➔ *CPT Changes: An Insider's View* 2010

27049   Radical resection of tumor (eg, sarcoma), soft tissue of pelvis and hip area; less than 5 cm
➔ *CPT Changes: An Insider's View* 2010, 2014
➔ *CPT Assistant* Nov 98:8

27059   5 cm or greater
➔ *CPT Changes: An Insider's View* 2010, 2014

(For radical resection of tumor[s] of cutaneous origin [eg, melanoma], see 11600-11606)

27050   Arthrotomy, with biopsy; sacroiliac joint

27052   hip joint

27054   Arthrotomy with synovectomy, hip joint

27057   Decompression fasciotomy(ies), pelvic (buttock) compartment(s) (eg, gluteus medius-minimus, gluteus maximus, iliopsoas, and/or tensor fascia lata muscle) with debridement of nonviable muscle, unilateral
➔ *CPT Changes: An Insider's View* 2009

(To report bilateral procedure, report 27057 with modifier 50)

27059   Code is out of numerical sequence. See 27041-27052

27060   Excision; ischial bursa

27062   trochanteric bursa or calcification

(For arthrocentesis or needling of bursa, use 20610)

27065   Excision of bone cyst or benign tumor, wing of ilium, symphysis pubis, or greater trochanter of femur; superficial, includes autograft, when performed
➲ *CPT Changes: An Insider's View* 2011

27066   deep (subfascial), includes autograft, when performed
➲ *CPT Changes: An Insider's View* 2011
➲ *CPT Assistant* Dec 21:19

27067   with autograft requiring separate incision
➲ *CPT Changes: An Insider's View* 2011

27070   Partial excision, wing of ilium, symphysis pubis, or greater trochanter of femur, (craterization, saucerization) (eg, osteomyelitis or bone abscess); superficial
➲ *CPT Changes: An Insider's View* 2011

27071   deep (subfascial or intramuscular)
➲ *CPT Changes: An Insider's View* 2011
➲ *CPT Assistant* Sep 21:7

27075   Radical resection of tumor; wing of ilium, 1 pubic or ischial ramus or symphysis pubis
➲ *CPT Changes: An Insider's View* 2010

27076   ilium, including acetabulum, both pubic rami, or ischium and acetabulum
➲ *CPT Changes: An Insider's View* 2010

27077   innominate bone, total
➲ *CPT Changes: An Insider's View* 2010

27078   ischial tuberosity and greater trochanter of femur
➲ *CPT Changes: An Insider's View* 2010

27080   Coccygectomy, primary

(For pressure (decubitus) ulcer, see 15920, 15922 and 15931-15958)

Introduction or Removal

27086   Removal of foreign body, pelvis or hip; subcutaneous tissue
➲ *CPT Assistant* Jul 98:8

27087   deep (subfascial or intramuscular)
➲ *CPT Assistant* Nov 98:8

27090   Removal of hip prosthesis; (separate procedure)
➲ *CPT Assistant* Mar 20:14

27091   complicated, including total hip prosthesis, methylmethacrylate with or without insertion of spacer
➲ *CPT Assistant* Mar 20:14, Sep 21:7-8

27093   Injection procedure for hip arthrography; without anesthesia
➲ *CPT Assistant* Jun 12:14, Aug 15:6
➲ *Clinical Examples in Radiology* Fall 07:7, Spring 13:11, Summer 18:15, Spring 21:7

(For radiological supervision and interpretation, use 73525. Do not report 77002 in conjunction with 73525)

27095   with anesthesia
➲ *CPT Assistant* Jun 12:14, Aug 15:6, Jan 16:11
➲ *Clinical Examples in Radiology* Fall 07:7, Summer 18:15, Spring 21:7

(For radiological supervision and interpretation, use 73525. Do not report 77002 in conjunction with 73525)

27096   Injection procedure for sacroiliac joint, anesthetic/steroid, with image guidance (fluoroscopy or CT) including arthrography when performed
➲ *CPT Changes: An Insider's View* 2000, 2012
➲ *CPT Assistant* Nov 99:12, Apr 03:8, Apr 04:15, Jul 08:9, Jan 12:3, Aug 15:6
➲ *Clinical Examples in Radiology* Fall 11:10, Summer 18:15

(27096 is to be used only with CT or fluoroscopic imaging confirmation of intra-articular needle positioning)

(If CT or fluoroscopy imaging is not performed, use 20552)

(Code 27096 is a unilateral procedure. For bilateral procedure, use modifier 50)

Repair, Revision, and/or Reconstruction

27097   Release or recession, hamstring, proximal
➲ *CPT Assistant* Nov 98:8

27098   Transfer, adductor to ischium
➲ *CPT Assistant* Nov 98:8

27100   Transfer external oblique muscle to greater trochanter including fascial or tendon extension (graft)

27105   Transfer paraspinal muscle to hip (includes fascial or tendon extension graft)

27110   Transfer iliopsoas; to greater trochanter of femur
➲ *CPT Changes: An Insider's View* 2002

27111   to femoral neck

27120   Acetabuloplasty; (eg, Whitman, Colonna, Haygroves, or cup type)

27122   resection, femoral head (eg, Girdlestone procedure)

27125   Hemiarthroplasty, hip, partial (eg, femoral stem prosthesis, bipolar arthroplasty)
➲ *CPT Assistant* Spring 92:8, Feb 98:11, Nov 98:8

(For prosthetic replacement following fracture of the hip, use 27236)

27130   Arthroplasty, acetabular and proximal femoral prosthetic replacement (total hip arthroplasty), with or without autograft or allograft
➲ *CPT Changes: An Insider's View* 2002
➲ *CPT Assistant* Spring 92:8, Jan 07:1, Dec 11:14

Musculoskeletal 20100-29999

Partial Hip Replacement With or Without Bipolar Prosthesis
27125

The femoral neck is excised so the physician can measure and then replace the femoral stem.

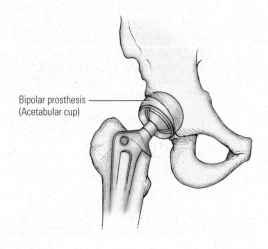

Bipolar prosthesis (Acetabular cup)

Total Hip Replacement
27130

The femoral head is excised, osteophytes are removed, and acetabulum is reamed out before replacement is inserted in the femoral shaft.

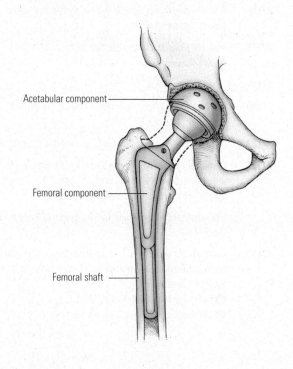

Acetabular component

Femoral component

Femoral shaft

27132 Conversion of previous hip surgery to total hip arthroplasty, with or without autograft or allograft

⮕ *CPT Changes: An Insider's View* 2002

⮕ *CPT Assistant* Spring 92:11, Dec 08:3, May 17:10, Sep 17:14

27134 Revision of total hip arthroplasty; both components, with or without autograft or allograft

⮕ *CPT Assistant* Spring 92:7, Dec 08:3, Sep 21:8-9

27137 acetabular component only, with or without autograft or allograft

⮕ *CPT Assistant* Spring 92:7, Sep 21:8

27138 femoral component only, with or without allograft

⮕ *CPT Assistant* Spring 92:7, Sep 21:8

27140 Osteotomy and transfer of greater trochanter of femur (separate procedure)

⮕ *CPT Changes: An Insider's View* 2002

27146 Osteotomy, iliac, acetabular or innominate bone;

⮕ *CPT Assistant* Feb 99:10

27147 with open reduction of hip

27151 with femoral osteotomy

27156 with femoral osteotomy and with open reduction of hip

27158 Osteotomy, pelvis, bilateral (eg, congenital malformation)

27161 Osteotomy, femoral neck (separate procedure)

27165 Osteotomy, intertrochanteric or subtrochanteric including internal or external fixation and/or cast

⮕ *CPT Assistant* Spring 92:11

27170 Bone graft, femoral head, neck, intertrochanteric or subtrochanteric area (includes obtaining bone graft)

⮕ *CPT Assistant* Spring 92:11

27175 Treatment of slipped femoral epiphysis; by traction, without reduction

27176 by single or multiple pinning, in situ

27177 Open treatment of slipped femoral epiphysis; single or multiple pinning or bone graft (includes obtaining graft)

27178 closed manipulation with single or multiple pinning

27179 osteoplasty of femoral neck (Heyman type procedure)

27181 osteotomy and internal fixation

27185 Epiphyseal arrest by epiphysiodesis or stapling, greater trochanter of femur

⮕ *CPT Changes: An Insider's View* 2002

27187 Prophylactic treatment (nailing, pinning, plating or wiring) with or without methylmethacrylate, femoral neck and proximal femur

Fracture and/or Dislocation

─── *Coding Tip* ───

Reporting for Categories of Manipulation and/or Fracture

The codes for treatment of fractures and joint injuries (dislocations) are categorized by the type of manipulation (reduction) and stabilization (fixation or immobilization). These codes can apply to either open (compound) or closed fractures or joint injuries.

CPT Coding Guidelines, Musculoskeletal System

27197   Closed treatment of posterior pelvic ring fracture(s), dislocation(s), diastasis or subluxation of the ilium, sacroiliac joint, and/or sacrum, with or without anterior pelvic ring fracture(s) and/or dislocation(s) of the pubic symphysis and/or superior/inferior rami, unilateral or bilateral; without manipulation
➔ *CPT Changes: An Insider's View* 2017
➔ *CPT Assistant* Jun 17:9

27198   with manipulation, requiring more than local anesthesia (ie, general anesthesia, moderate sedation, spinal/epidural)
➔ *CPT Changes: An Insider's View* 2017
➔ *CPT Assistant* Jun 17:9, Jan 18:3

(To report closed treatment of **only** anterior pelvic ring fracture(s) and/or dislocation(s) of the pubic symphysis and/or superior/inferior rami, unilateral or bilateral, use the appropriate evaluation and management services codes)

27200   Closed treatment of coccygeal fracture

27202   Open treatment of coccygeal fracture

27215   Open treatment of iliac spine(s), tuberosity avulsion, or iliac wing fracture(s), unilateral, for pelvic bone fracture patterns that do not disrupt the pelvic ring, includes internal fixation, when performed
➔ *CPT Changes: An Insider's View* 2009

(To report bilateral procedure, report 27215 with modifier 50)

27216   Percutaneous skeletal fixation of posterior pelvic bone fracture and/or dislocation, for fracture patterns that disrupt the pelvic ring, unilateral (includes ipsilateral ilium, sacroiliac joint and/or sacrum)
➔ *CPT Changes: An Insider's View* 2009
➔ *CPT Assistant* Sep 13:19, Mar 14:4

(To report bilateral procedure, report 27216 with modifier 50)

(For percutaneous/minimally invasive arthrodesis of the sacroiliac joint without fracture and/or dislocation, use 27279)

27217   Open treatment of anterior pelvic bone fracture and/or dislocation for fracture patterns that disrupt the pelvic ring, unilateral, includes internal fixation, when performed (includes pubic symphysis and/or ipsilateral superior/inferior rami)
➔ *CPT Changes: An Insider's View* 2009

(To report bilateral procedure, report 27217 with modifier 50)

27218   Open treatment of posterior pelvic bone fracture and/or dislocation, for fracture patterns that disrupt the pelvic ring, unilateral, includes internal fixation, when performed (includes ipsilateral ilium, sacroiliac joint and/or sacrum)
➔ *CPT Changes: An Insider's View* 2009
➔ *CPT Assistant* Mar 14:4

(To report bilateral procedure, report 27218 with modifier 50)

(For percutaneous/minimally invasive arthrodesis of the sacroiliac joint without fracture and/or dislocation, use 27279)

27220   Closed treatment of acetabulum (hip socket) fracture(s); without manipulation

27222   with manipulation, with or without skeletal traction

27226   Open treatment of posterior or anterior acetabular wall fracture, with internal fixation

27227   Open treatment of acetabular fracture(s) involving anterior or posterior (one) column, or a fracture running transversely across the acetabulum, with internal fixation

27228   Open treatment of acetabular fracture(s) involving anterior and posterior (two) columns, includes T-fracture and both column fracture with complete articular detachment, or single column or transverse fracture with associated acetabular wall fracture, with internal fixation

27230   Closed treatment of femoral fracture, proximal end, neck; without manipulation

27232   with manipulation, with or without skeletal traction

27235   Percutaneous skeletal fixation of femoral fracture, proximal end, neck
➔ *CPT Changes: An Insider's View* 2003

(For percutaneous injection of calcium-based biodegradable osteoconductive material, use 0814T)

Musculoskeletal 20100-29999

Percutaneous Treatment of Femoral Fracture
27235

Femoral fracture treatment without fracture exposure

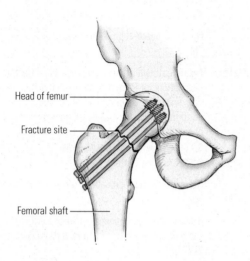

Head of femur

Fracture site

Femoral shaft

Open Treatment of Femoral Fracture
27236

A. Femoral fracture treatment by internal fixation device (with fracture exposure)

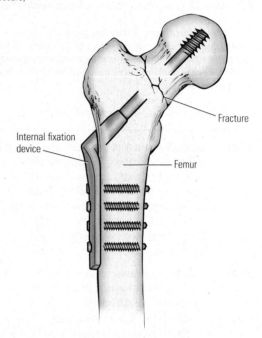

Fracture

Internal fixation device

Femur

B. Femoral fracture treatment by prosthetic replacement

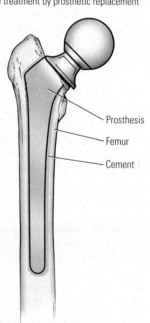

Prosthesis

Femur

Cement

27236   Open treatment of femoral fracture, proximal end, neck, internal fixation or prosthetic replacement

    ➲ *CPT Changes: An Insider's View* 2000

    ➲ *CPT Assistant* Spring 92:10, Feb 98:11, Jan 07:1, Nov 16:9

27238   Closed treatment of intertrochanteric, peritrochanteric, or subtrochanteric femoral fracture; without manipulation

    ➲ *CPT Assistant* Summer 93:12

27240   with manipulation, with or without skin or skeletal traction

    ➲ *CPT Assistant* Summer 93:12

27244   Treatment of intertrochanteric, peritrochanteric, or subtrochanteric femoral fracture; with plate/screw type implant, with or without cerclage

    ➲ *CPT Changes: An Insider's View* 2003

    ➲ *CPT Assistant* Summer 93:12

27245   with intramedullary implant, with or without interlocking screws and/or cerclage

    ➲ *CPT Assistant* Summer 93:12, Sep 13:17

27246   Closed treatment of greater trochanteric fracture, without manipulation

27248   Open treatment of greater trochanteric fracture, includes internal fixation, when performed

    ➲ *CPT Changes: An Insider's View* 2008

27250   Closed treatment of hip dislocation, traumatic; without anesthesia

27252   requiring anesthesia

27253   Open treatment of hip dislocation, traumatic, without internal fixation

27254 Open treatment of hip dislocation, traumatic, with acetabular wall and femoral head fracture, with or without internal or external fixation

(For treatment of acetabular fracture with fixation, see 27226, 27227)

27256 Treatment of spontaneous hip dislocation (developmental, including congenital or pathological), by abduction, splint or traction; without anesthesia, without manipulation

27257   with manipulation, requiring anesthesia

27258 Open treatment of spontaneous hip dislocation (developmental, including congenital or pathological), replacement of femoral head in acetabulum (including tenotomy, etc);

27259   with femoral shaft shortening

27265 Closed treatment of post hip arthroplasty dislocation; without anesthesia

27266   requiring regional or general anesthesia

27267 Closed treatment of femoral fracture, proximal end, head; without manipulation
➡ *CPT Changes: An Insider's View* 2008
➡ *CPT Assistant* Jan 08:4

27268   with manipulation
➡ *CPT Changes: An Insider's View* 2008
➡ *CPT Assistant* Jan 08:4

27269 Open treatment of femoral fracture, proximal end, head, includes internal fixation, when performed
➡ *CPT Changes: An Insider's View* 2008
➡ *CPT Assistant* Jan 08:4, Dec 08:3

(Do not report 27269 in conjunction with 27033, 27253)

Manipulation

27275 Manipulation, hip joint, requiring general anesthesia
➡ *CPT Assistant* Jan 16:11, May 16:13

Arthrodesis

Code 27279 describes percutaneous arthrodesis of the sacroiliac joint using a minimally invasive technique to place an internal fixation device(s) that passes through the ilium, across the sacroiliac joint and into the sacrum, thus transfixing the sacroiliac joint. Report 27278 for the percutaneous placement of an intra-articular stabilization device into the sacroiliac joint using a minimally invasive technique that does not transfix the sacroiliac joint.

27278 Arthrodesis, sacroiliac joint, percutaneous, with image guidance, including placement of intra-articular implant(s) (eg, bone allograft[s], synthetic device[s]), without placement of transfixation device
➡ *CPT Changes: An Insider's View* 2024

(For arthrodesis, sacroiliac joint, with placement of a percutaneous transfixation device, use 27279)

(For bilateral procedure, report 27278 with modifier 50)

27279 Arthrodesis, sacroiliac joint, percutaneous or minimally invasive (indirect visualization), with image guidance, includes obtaining bone graft when performed, and placement of transfixation device
➡ *CPT Changes: An Insider's View* 2015
➡ *CPT Assistant* May 20:14, Jul 21:7, Feb 22:14, Apr 23:16

(For percutaneous arthrodesis of the sacroiliac joint by intra-articular implant[s], use 27278)

(For bilateral procedure, report 27279 with modifier 50)

27280 Arthrodesis, sacroiliac joint, open, includes obtaining bone graft, including instrumentation, when performed
➡ *CPT Changes: An Insider's View* 2015, 2023
➡ *CPT Assistant* Sep 13:19, Mar 14:4

(For percutaneous/minimally invasive arthrodesis of the sacroiliac joint without fracture and/or dislocation, utilizing a transfixation device, use 27279)

(To report bilateral procedure, report 27280 with modifier 50)

27282 Arthrodesis, symphysis pubis (including obtaining graft)

27284 Arthrodesis, hip joint (including obtaining graft);

27286   with subtrochanteric osteotomy
➡ *CPT Assistant* May 20:14, Jul 21:7

Amputation

27290 Interpelviabdominal amputation (hindquarter amputation)

27295 Disarticulation of hip

Other Procedures

27299 Unlisted procedure, pelvis or hip joint
➡ *CPT Assistant* Jan 02:10, Dec 05:9, Dec 08:3, Oct 12:14, Nov 12:13, Mar 14:13, Jun 16:8

Femur (Thigh Region) and Knee Joint

Including tibial plateaus.

Incision

(For incision and drainage of abscess or hematoma, superficial, see 10040-10160)

27301 Incision and drainage, deep abscess, bursa, or hematoma, thigh or knee region
➡ *CPT Assistant* Nov 98:9, Dec 08:3, Mar 20:14

Musculoskeletal 20100-29999

27303 Incision, deep, with opening of bone cortex, femur or knee (eg, osteomyelitis or bone abscess)
➲ *CPT Assistant* Nov 98:8

27305 Fasciotomy, iliotibial (tenotomy), open

(For combined Ober-Yount fasciotomy, use 27025)

27306 Tenotomy, percutaneous, adductor or hamstring; single tendon (separate procedure)
➲ *CPT Assistant* Nov 98:8, Aug 17:9

27307   multiple tendons
➲ *CPT Assistant* Nov 98:8, Aug 17:9

27310 Arthrotomy, knee, with exploration, drainage, or removal of foreign body (eg, infection)
➲ *CPT Assistant* Nov 98:8, Dec 08:3, Mar 20:14, Sep 21:8

Excision

27323 Biopsy, soft tissue of thigh or knee area; superficial
➲ *CPT Assistant* Jun 97:12

27324   deep (subfascial or intramuscular)
➲ *CPT Assistant* Mar 97:4, Nov 98:8

(For needle biopsy of soft tissue, use 20206)

27325 Neurectomy, hamstring muscle
➲ *CPT Changes: An Insider's View* 2007

27326 Neurectomy, popliteal (gastrocnemius)
➲ *CPT Changes: An Insider's View* 2007

27327 Excision, tumor, soft tissue of thigh or knee area, subcutaneous; less than 3 cm
➲ *CPT Changes: An Insider's View* 2010

 # 27337   3 cm or greater
➲ *CPT Changes: An Insider's View* 2010

(For excision of benign lesions of cutaneous origin [eg, sebaceous cyst], see 11400-11406)

27328 Excision, tumor, soft tissue of thigh or knee area, subfascial (eg, intramuscular); less than 5 cm
➲ *CPT Changes: An Insider's View* 2010
➲ *CPT Assistant* Nov 16:9

27329 Code is out of numerical sequence. See 27358-27365

 # 27339   5 cm or greater
➲ *CPT Changes: An Insider's View* 2010

27330 Arthrotomy, knee; with synovial biopsy only
➲ *CPT Assistant* Mar 12:9

27331   including joint exploration, biopsy, or removal of loose or foreign bodies
➲ *CPT Assistant* May 96:6, Nov 98:8, Nov 12:13

27332 Arthrotomy, with excision of semilunar cartilage (meniscectomy) knee; medial OR lateral
➲ *CPT Assistant* Nov 98:8

27333   medial AND lateral
➲ *CPT Assistant* Mar 12:9

27334 Arthrotomy, with synovectomy, knee; anterior OR posterior
➲ *CPT Assistant* Nov 98:8

27335   anterior AND posterior including popliteal area

27337 Code is out of numerical sequence. See 27326-27331

27339 Code is out of numerical sequence. See 27326-27331

27340 Excision, prepatellar bursa

27345 Excision of synovial cyst of popliteal space (eg, Baker's cyst)

27347 Excision of lesion of meniscus or capsule (eg, cyst, ganglion), knee
➲ *CPT Assistant* Nov 98:11

27350 Patellectomy or hemipatellectomy

27355 Excision or curettage of bone cyst or benign tumor of femur;

27356   with allograft

27357   with autograft (includes obtaining graft)
➲ *CPT Assistant* Dec 02:11

+ 27358   with internal fixation (List in addition to code for primary procedure)

(Use 27358 in conjunction with 27355, 27356, or 27357)

27360 Partial excision (craterization, saucerization, or diaphysectomy) bone, femur, proximal tibia and/or fibula (eg, osteomyelitis or bone abscess)
➲ *CPT Assistant* Nov 98:8, Sep 21:7

 # 27329 Radical resection of tumor (eg, sarcoma), soft tissue of thigh or knee area; less than 5 cm
➲ *CPT Changes: An Insider's View* 2010, 2014

27364   5 cm or greater
➲ *CPT Changes: An Insider's View* 2010, 2014

(For radical resection of tumor[s] of cutaneous origin [eg, melanoma], see 11600-11606)

27365 Radical resection of tumor, femur or knee
➲ *CPT Changes: An Insider's View* 2010

(For radical resection of tumor, soft tissue of thigh or knee area, see 27329, 27364)

Introduction or Removal

27369 Injection procedure for contrast knee arthrography or contrast enhanced CT/MRI knee arthrography
➲ *CPT Changes: An Insider's View* 2019
➲ *CPT Assistant* Aug 19:7
➲ *Clinical Examples in Radiology* Winter 19:15

(Use 27369 in conjunction with 73580, 73701, 73702, 73722, 73723)

(Do not report 27369 in conjunction with 20610, 20611, 29871)

(For arthrocentesis of the knee or injection of any material other than contrast for subsequent arthrography, see 20610, 20611)

(When fluoroscopic guided injection is performed for enhanced CT arthrography, use 27369, 77002, and 73701 or 73702)

(When fluoroscopic guided injection is performed for enhanced MR arthrography, use 27369, 77002, and 73722 or 73723)

(For arthroscopic lavage and drainage of the knee, use 29871)

(For radiographic arthrography, radiological supervision and interpretation, use 73580)

(For arthrocentesis of the knee or injection of any material other than contrast for subsequent arthrography, see 20610, 20611)

(For injection procedure for contrast knee arthrography or contrast enhanced CT/MRI knee arthrography, use 27369)

27372   Removal of foreign body, deep, thigh region or knee area

(For removal of knee prosthesis including "total knee," use 27488)

(For surgical arthroscopic knee procedures, see 29870-29887)

Repair, Revision, and/or Reconstruction

27380   Suture of infrapatellar tendon; primary

27381   secondary reconstruction, including fascial or tendon graft

27385   Suture of quadriceps or hamstring muscle rupture; primary
➲ *CPT Assistant* Aug 17:9, Dec 23:38

27386   secondary reconstruction, including fascial or tendon graft
➲ *CPT Assistant* Apr 20:10

27390   Tenotomy, open, hamstring, knee to hip; single tendon
➲ *CPT Assistant* Nov 98:8

27391   multiple tendons, 1 leg
➲ *CPT Assistant* Nov 98:8

27392   multiple tendons, bilateral
➲ *CPT Assistant* Nov 98:8

27393   Lengthening of hamstring tendon; single tendon
➲ *CPT Assistant* Nov 98:8

27394   multiple tendons, 1 leg
➲ *CPT Assistant* Nov 98:8

27395   multiple tendons, bilateral
➲ *CPT Assistant* Nov 98:8

27396   Transplant or transfer (with muscle redirection or rerouting), thigh (eg, extensor to flexor); single tendon
➲ *CPT Changes: An Insider's View* 2009
➲ *CPT Assistant* Nov 98:8

27397   multiple tendons
➲ *CPT Changes: An Insider's View* 2009
➲ *CPT Assistant* Nov 98:8

27400   Transfer, tendon or muscle, hamstrings to femur (eg, Egger's type procedure)
➲ *CPT Assistant* Nov 98:8

27403   Arthrotomy with meniscus repair, knee
➲ *CPT Assistant* Nov 98:8, May 19:10

(For arthroscopic repair, use 29882)

27405   Repair, primary, torn ligament and/or capsule, knee; collateral
➲ *CPT Assistant* Dec 12:12

27407   cruciate

(For cruciate ligament reconstruction, use 27427)

27409   collateral and cruciate ligaments

(For ligament reconstruction, see 27427-27429)

27412   Autologous chondrocyte implantation, knee
➲ *CPT Changes: An Insider's View* 2005

(Do not report 27412 in conjunction with 15769, 15771, 15772, 15773, 15774, 27331, 27570)

(For harvesting of chondrocytes, use 29870)

27415   Osteochondral allograft, knee, open
➲ *CPT Changes: An Insider's View* 2005
➲ *CPT Assistant* Apr 19:10

(For arthroscopic implant of osteochondral allograft, use 29867)

(Do not report 27415 in conjunction with 27416)

(For osteochondral xenograft scaffold, use 0737T)

27416   Osteochondral autograft(s), knee, open (eg, mosaicplasty) (includes harvesting of autograft[s])
➲ *CPT Changes: An Insider's View* 2008
➲ *CPT Assistant* Jan 08:4

(Do not report 27416 in conjunction with 27415, 29870, 29871, 29875, 29884 when performed at the same session and/or 29874, 29877, 29879, 29885-29887 when performed in the same compartment)

(For arthroscopic osteochondral autograft of knee, use 29866)

(For osteochondral xenograft scaffold, use 0737T)

27418   Anterior tibial tubercleplasty (eg, Maquet type procedure)
⮕ *CPT Assistant* Feb 10:13

27420   Reconstruction of dislocating patella; (eg, Hauser type procedure)
⮕ *CPT Assistant* Nov 12:13

27422   with extensor realignment and/or muscle advancement or release (eg, Campbell, Goldwaite type procedure)
⮕ *CPT Assistant* Mar 11:9, Oct 22:16

27424   with patellectomy

27425   Lateral retinacular release, open
⮕ *CPT Changes: An Insider's View* 2002, 2003
⮕ *CPT Assistant* Nov 00:11, Mar 11:9, Nov 15:7

(For arthroscopic lateral release, use 29873)

Posterolateral Corner of the Knee
27405, 27427

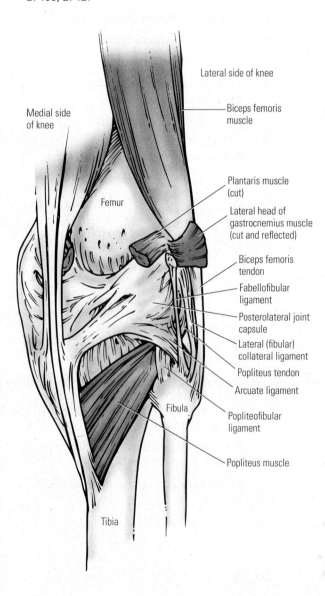

Lateral side of knee

Medial side of knee

Biceps femoris muscle

Femur

Plantaris muscle (cut)

Lateral head of gastrocnemius muscle (cut and reflected)

Biceps femoris tendon

Fabellofibular ligament

Posterolateral joint capsule

Lateral (fibular) collateral ligament

Popliteus tendon

Arcuate ligament

Fibula

Popliteofibular ligament

Popliteus muscle

Tibia

27427   Ligamentous reconstruction (augmentation), knee; extra-articular
⮕ *CPT Changes: An Insider's View* 2000
⮕ *CPT Assistant* Nov 99:13, Dec 12:12, May 17:10, Mar 24:25

27428   intra-articular (open)
⮕ *CPT Changes: An Insider's View* 2000
⮕ *CPT Assistant* Nov 99:13, Apr 09:8

27429   intra-articular (open) and extra-articular
⮕ *CPT Changes: An Insider's View* 2000
⮕ *CPT Assistant* Nov 99:13, Apr 09:8

(For primary repair of ligament(s) performed in conjunction with reconstruction, report 27405, 27407 or 27409 in conjunction with 27427, 27428 or 27429)

27430   Quadricepsplasty (eg, Bennett or Thompson type)

27435   Capsulotomy, posterior capsular release, knee
⮕ *CPT Assistant* Nov 98:8

27437   Arthroplasty, patella; without prosthesis

27438   with prosthesis
⮕ *CPT Assistant* Feb 21:12

27440   Arthroplasty, knee, tibial plateau;

27441   with debridement and partial synovectomy

27442   Arthroplasty, femoral condyles or tibial plateau(s), knee;
⮕ *CPT Assistant* Nov 99:13, Jun 16:8, Feb 21:12

27443   with debridement and partial synovectomy

27445   Arthroplasty, knee, hinge prosthesis (eg, Walldius type)
⮕ *CPT Assistant* Nov 98:8

27446   Arthroplasty, knee, condyle and plateau; medial OR lateral compartment
⮕ *CPT Assistant* Dec 17:13, Feb 21:12

27447   medial AND lateral compartments with or without patella resurfacing (total knee arthroplasty)
⮕ *CPT Changes: An Insider's View* 2002
⮕ *CPT Assistant* Jan 07:1

(For revision of total knee arthroplasty, use 27487)

(For removal of total knee prosthesis, use 27488)

27448   Osteotomy, femur, shaft or supracondylar; without fixation

(To report bilateral procedure, report 27448 with modifier 50)

27450   with fixation

(To report bilateral procedure, report 27450 with modifier 50)

27454   Osteotomy, multiple, with realignment on intramedullary rod, femoral shaft (eg, Sofield type procedure)
➜ *CPT Assistant* Nov 98:8

27455   Osteotomy, proximal tibia, including fibular excision or osteotomy (includes correction of genu varus [bowleg] or genu valgus [knock-knee]); before epiphyseal closure

(To report bilateral procedure, report 27455 with modifier 50)

27457   after epiphyseal closure

(To report bilateral procedure, report 27457 with modifier 50)

27465   Osteoplasty, femur; shortening (excluding 64876)

27466   lengthening

27468   combined, lengthening and shortening with femoral segment transfer

27470   Repair, nonunion or malunion, femur, distal to head and neck; without graft (eg, compression technique)

27472   with iliac or other autogenous bone graft (includes obtaining graft)

27475   Arrest, epiphyseal, any method (eg, epiphysiodesis); distal femur
➜ *CPT Assistant* Nov 98:8

27477   tibia and fibula, proximal

27479   combined distal femur, proximal tibia and fibula

27485   Arrest, hemiepiphyseal, distal femur or proximal tibia or fibula (eg, genu varus or valgus)
➜ *CPT Assistant* Nov 98:8

27486   Revision of total knee arthroplasty, with or without allograft; 1 component
➜ *CPT Assistant* Dec 13:16, Jul 15:10, Apr 18:10, Sep 21:8, Nov 21:12-13

27487   femoral and entire tibial component
➜ *CPT Assistant* Nov 98:8, Jul 13:6, Sep 21:8-9, Nov 21:12-13

27488   Removal of prosthesis, including total knee prosthesis, methylmethacrylate with or without insertion of spacer, knee
➜ *CPT Assistant* Nov 98:8, Jul 13:6, Mar 20:14, Sep 21:7-8

27495   Prophylactic treatment (nailing, pinning, plating, or wiring) with or without methylmethacrylate, femur

27496   Decompression fasciotomy, thigh and/or knee, 1 compartment (flexor or extensor or adductor);

27497   with debridement of nonviable muscle and/or nerve

27498   Decompression fasciotomy, thigh and/or knee, multiple compartments;

27499   with debridement of nonviable muscle and/or nerve

Fracture and/or Dislocation

--- *Coding Tip* ---

Reporting for Categories of Manipulation and/or Fracture

The codes for treatment of fractures and joint injuries (dislocations) are categorized by the type of manipulation (reduction) and stabilization (fixation or immobilization). These codes can apply to either open (compound) or closed fractures or joint injuries.

CPT Coding Guidelines, Musculoskeletal System

(For arthroscopic treatment of intercondylar spine[s] and tuberosity fracture[s] of the knee, see 29850, 29851)

(For arthroscopic treatment of tibial fracture, see 29855, 29856)

27500   Closed treatment of femoral shaft fracture, without manipulation

27501   Closed treatment of supracondylar or transcondylar femoral fracture with or without intercondylar extension, without manipulation

27502   Closed treatment of femoral shaft fracture, with manipulation, with or without skin or skeletal traction
➜ *CPT Assistant* Fall 93:22, Oct 99:5

27503   Closed treatment of supracondylar or transcondylar femoral fracture with or without intercondylar extension, with manipulation, with or without skin or skeletal traction

27506   Open treatment of femoral shaft fracture, with or without external fixation, with insertion of intramedullary implant, with or without cerclage and/or locking screws
➜ *CPT Assistant* Winter 92:10, Jun 09:7

27507   Open treatment of femoral shaft fracture with plate/screws, with or without cerclage

27508   Closed treatment of femoral fracture, distal end, medial or lateral condyle, without manipulation

27509   Percutaneous skeletal fixation of femoral fracture, distal end, medial or lateral condyle, or supracondylar or transcondylar, with or without intercondylar extension, or distal femoral epiphyseal separation
➜ *CPT Assistant* Dec 18:10

27510   Closed treatment of femoral fracture, distal end, medial or lateral condyle, with manipulation

Musculoskeletal 20100-29999

27511   Open treatment of femoral supracondylar or transcondylar fracture without intercondylar extension, includes internal fixation, when performed
➔ *CPT Changes: An Insider's View* 2008
➔ *CPT Assistant* May 96:6

27513   Open treatment of femoral supracondylar or transcondylar fracture with intercondylar extension, includes internal fixation, when performed
➔ *CPT Changes: An Insider's View* 2008

27514   Open treatment of femoral fracture, distal end, medial or lateral condyle, includes internal fixation, when performed
➔ *CPT Changes: An Insider's View* 2008

27516   Closed treatment of distal femoral epiphyseal separation; without manipulation

27517   with manipulation, with or without skin or skeletal traction

27519   Open treatment of distal femoral epiphyseal separation, includes internal fixation, when performed
➔ *CPT Changes: An Insider's View* 2008

27520   Closed treatment of patellar fracture, without manipulation

27524   Open treatment of patellar fracture, with internal fixation and/or partial or complete patellectomy and soft tissue repair

27530   Closed treatment of tibial fracture, proximal (plateau); without manipulation

27532   with or without manipulation, with skeletal traction

(For arthroscopic treatment, see 29855, 29856)

27535   Open treatment of tibial fracture, proximal (plateau); unicondylar, includes internal fixation, when performed
➔ *CPT Changes: An Insider's View* 2008

27536   bicondylar, with or without internal fixation

(For arthroscopic treatment, see 29855, 29856)

27538   Closed treatment of intercondylar spine(s) and/or tuberosity fracture(s) of knee, with or without manipulation

(For arthroscopic treatment, see 29850, 29851)

27540   Open treatment of intercondylar spine(s) and/or tuberosity fracture(s) of the knee, includes internal fixation, when performed
➔ *CPT Changes: An Insider's View* 2008

27550   Closed treatment of knee dislocation; without anesthesia

27552   requiring anesthesia

27556   Open treatment of knee dislocation, includes internal fixation, when performed; without primary ligamentous repair or augmentation/reconstruction
➔ *CPT Changes: An Insider's View* 2008

27557   with primary ligamentous repair
➔ *CPT Changes: An Insider's View* 2008

27558   with primary ligamentous repair, with augmentation/reconstruction
➔ *CPT Changes: An Insider's View* 2008

27560   Closed treatment of patellar dislocation; without anesthesia
➔ *CPT Assistant* Apr 02:15

(For recurrent dislocation, see 27420-27424)

27562   requiring anesthesia

27566   Open treatment of patellar dislocation, with or without partial or total patellectomy
➔ *CPT Assistant* Oct 22:16

Manipulation

27570   Manipulation of knee joint under general anesthesia (includes application of traction or other fixation devices)
➔ *CPT Assistant* Mar 11:9

Arthrodesis

27580   Arthrodesis, knee, any technique
➔ *CPT Assistant* May 20:14, Jul 21:7

Amputation

27590   Amputation, thigh, through femur, any level;
➔ *CPT Assistant* Dec 17:13

27591   immediate fitting technique including first cast

27592   open, circular (guillotine)

27594   secondary closure or scar revision

27596   re-amputation

27598   Disarticulation at knee

Other Procedures

27599   Unlisted procedure, femur or knee
➔ *CPT Assistant* Mar 08:14, Dec 12:13, Jan 14:9, Jan 15:13, Jun 16:8, Nov 16:9, Mar 17:10, Aug 17:9, Apr 18:10, Dec 18:10, Apr 19:10, Feb 21:12, Dec 23:50, Mar 24:25

Leg (Tibia and Fibula) and Ankle Joint

Incision

27600   Decompression fasciotomy, leg; anterior and/or lateral compartments only

27601   posterior compartment(s) only

27602   anterior and/or lateral, and posterior compartment(s)

(For incision and drainage procedures, superficial, see 10040-10160)

(For decompression fasciotomy with debridement, see 27892-27894)

27603   Incision and drainage, leg or ankle; deep abscess or hematoma
⮑ *CPT Assistant* Mar 20:14

27604   infected bursa

27605   Tenotomy, percutaneous, Achilles tendon (separate procedure); local anesthesia
⮑ *CPT Assistant* Sep 18:14

27606   general anesthesia
⮑ *CPT Assistant* Sep 18:14

27607   Incision (eg, osteomyelitis or bone abscess), leg or ankle

27610   Arthrotomy, ankle, including exploration, drainage, or removal of foreign body
⮑ *CPT Assistant* Nov 98:9, Mar 20:14

27612   Arthrotomy, posterior capsular release, ankle, with or without Achilles tendon lengthening
⮑ *CPT Assistant* Nov 98:8

(See also 27685)

Excision

27613   Biopsy, soft tissue of leg or ankle area; superficial

27614   deep (subfascial or intramuscular)
⮑ *CPT Assistant* Nov 98:8

(For needle biopsy of soft tissue, use 20206)

27615   Radical resection of tumor (eg, sarcoma), soft tissue of leg or ankle area; less than 5 cm
⮑ *CPT Changes: An Insider's View* 2010, 2014

27616   5 cm or greater
⮑ *CPT Changes: An Insider's View* 2010, 2014

(For radical resection of tumor[s] of cutaneous origin [eg, melanoma], see 11600-11606)

27618   Excision, tumor, soft tissue of leg or ankle area, subcutaneous; less than 3 cm
⮑ *CPT Changes: An Insider's View* 2010
⮑ *CPT Assistant* Sep 18:7

 # 27632   3 cm or greater
⮑ *CPT Changes: An Insider's View* 2010
⮑ *CPT Assistant* Apr 10:3

(For excision of benign lesions of cutaneous origin [eg, sebaceous cyst], see 11400-11406)

27619   Excision, tumor, soft tissue of leg or ankle area, subfascial (eg, intramuscular); less than 5 cm
⮑ *CPT Changes: An Insider's View* 2010
⮑ *CPT Assistant* Oct 22:16

 # 27634   5 cm or greater
⮑ *CPT Changes: An Insider's View* 2010
⮑ *CPT Assistant* Oct 22:16

27620   Arthrotomy, ankle, with joint exploration, with or without biopsy, with or without removal of loose or foreign body

27625   Arthrotomy, with synovectomy, ankle;
⮑ *CPT Assistant* Nov 98:8

27626   including tenosynovectomy

27630   Excision of lesion of tendon sheath or capsule (eg, cyst or ganglion), leg and/or ankle

27632   Code is out of numerical sequence. See 27616-27625

27634   Code is out of numerical sequence. See 27616-27625

27635   Excision or curettage of bone cyst or benign tumor, tibia or fibula;
⮑ *CPT Assistant* Apr 12:17

27637   with autograft (includes obtaining graft)

27638   with allograft

27640   Partial excision (craterization, saucerization, or diaphysectomy), bone (eg, osteomyelitis); tibia
⮑ *CPT Changes: An Insider's View* 2010
⮑ *CPT Assistant* Apr 12:17

(For exostosis excision, use 27635)

27641   fibula
⮑ *CPT Changes: An Insider's View* 2010

(For exostosis excision, use 27635)

27645   Radical resection of tumor; tibia
⮑ *CPT Changes: An Insider's View* 2010

27646   fibula
⮑ *CPT Changes: An Insider's View* 2010

27647   talus or calcaneus
⮑ *CPT Changes: An Insider's View* 2010

Introduction or Removal

27648   Injection procedure for ankle arthrography
⮑ *CPT Assistant* Aug 15:6
⮑ *Clinical Examples in Radiology* Summer 18:15

(For radiological supervision and interpretation, use 73615. Do not report 77002 in conjunction with 73615)

(For ankle arthroscopy, see 29894-29898)

Repair, Revision, and/or Reconstruction

27650 Repair, primary, open or percutaneous, ruptured Achilles tendon;
> *CPT Assistant* Jul 14:5

27652   with graft (includes obtaining graft)
> *CPT Assistant* Jul 14:5

27654 Repair, secondary, Achilles tendon, with or without graft
> *CPT Assistant* Jul 14:5, Dec 16:16, Mar 20:14

27656 Repair, fascial defect of leg

27658 Repair, flexor tendon, leg; primary, without graft, each tendon
> *CPT Assistant* Nov 98:8

27659   secondary, with or without graft, each tendon
> *CPT Assistant* Jan 15:13

27664 Repair, extensor tendon, leg; primary, without graft, each tendon
> *CPT Assistant* Nov 98:8, Jan 15:13

27665   secondary, with or without graft, each tendon
> *CPT Assistant* Nov 98:8

27675 Repair, dislocating peroneal tendons; without fibular osteotomy

27676   with fibular osteotomy

27680 Tenolysis, flexor or extensor tendon, leg and/or ankle; single, each tendon
> *CPT Assistant* Nov 98:8

27681   multiple tendons (through separate incision[s])
> *CPT Assistant* Nov 98:8

27685 Lengthening or shortening of tendon, leg or ankle; single tendon (separate procedure)
> *CPT Assistant* Nov 98:8, Sep 09:11, Sep 18:14

27686   multiple tendons (through same incision), each
> *CPT Assistant* Nov 98:8, Sep 09:11

27687 Gastrocnemius recession (eg, Strayer procedure)

(Toe extensors are considered as a group to be a single tendon when transplanted into midfoot)

27690 Transfer or transplant of single tendon (with muscle redirection or rerouting); superficial (eg, anterior tibial extensors into midfoot)
> *CPT Assistant* May 21:13

27691   deep (eg, anterior tibial or posterior tibial through interosseous space, flexor digitorum longus, flexor hallucis longus, or peroneal tendon to midfoot or hindfoot)
> *CPT Assistant* May 21:13

+ 27692   each additional tendon (List separately in addition to code for primary procedure)

(Use 27692 in conjunction with 27690, 27691)

27695 Repair, primary, disrupted ligament, ankle; collateral
> *CPT Assistant* Mar 14:14, Nov 18:11

27696   both collateral ligaments
> *CPT Assistant* Mar 14:14, Nov 18:11

27698 Repair, secondary, disrupted ligament, ankle, collateral (eg, Watson-Jones procedure)
> *CPT Assistant* Mar 14:14

27700 Arthroplasty, ankle;

27702   with implant (total ankle)

27703   revision, total ankle

27704 Removal of ankle implant

27705 Osteotomy; tibia

27707   fibula

27709   tibia and fibula

27712   multiple, with realignment on intramedullary rod (eg, Sofield type procedure)

(For osteotomy to correct genu varus [bowleg] or genu valgus [knock-knee], see 27455-27457)

27715 Osteoplasty, tibia and fibula, lengthening or shortening

27720 Repair of nonunion or malunion, tibia; without graft, (eg, compression technique)

27722   with sliding graft

27724   with iliac or other autograft (includes obtaining graft)
> *CPT Assistant* May 12:11

27725   by synostosis, with fibula, any method

27726 Repair of fibula nonunion and/or malunion with internal fixation
> *CPT Changes: An Insider's View* 2008
> *CPT Assistant* Jan 08:4, Apr 09:9

(Do not report 27726 in conjunction with 27707)

27727 Repair of congenital pseudarthrosis, tibia

27730 Arrest, epiphyseal (epiphysiodesis), open; distal tibia
> *CPT Changes: An Insider's View* 2003
> *CPT Assistant* Nov 98:8

27732   distal fibula

27734   distal tibia and fibula

27740 Arrest, epiphyseal (epiphysiodesis), any method, combined, proximal and distal tibia and fibula;
> *CPT Assistant* Nov 98:8

27742   and distal femur

(For epiphyseal arrest of proximal tibia and fibula, use 27477)

27745 Prophylactic treatment (nailing, pinning, plating or wiring) with or without methylmethacrylate, tibia

Fracture and/or Dislocation

—— *Coding Tip* ——

Reporting for Categories of Manipulation and/or Fracture

The codes for treatment of fractures and joint injuries (dislocations) are categorized by the type of manipulation (reduction) and stabilization (fixation or immobilization). These codes can apply to either open (compound) or closed fractures or joint injuries.

CPT Coding Guidelines, Musculoskeletal System

27750 Closed treatment of tibial shaft fracture (with or without fibular fracture); without manipulation
➔ *CPT Assistant* Winter 92:10, Fall 93:21, Mar 96:10

27752 with manipulation, with or without skeletal traction
➔ *CPT Assistant* Winter 92:10, Fall 93:21, Feb 96:3, Mar 96:10, Jan 18:3

27756 Percutaneous skeletal fixation of tibial shaft fracture (with or without fibular fracture) (eg, pins or screws)
➔ *CPT Assistant* Winter 92:10

27758 Open treatment of tibial shaft fracture (with or without fibular fracture), with plate/screws, with or without cerclage
➔ *CPT Assistant* Winter 92:10, Mar 00:11

27759 Treatment of tibial shaft fracture (with or without fibular fracture) by intramedullary implant, with or without interlocking screws and/or cerclage
➔ *CPT Changes: An Insider's View* 2003
➔ *CPT Assistant* Winter 92:10

27760 Closed treatment of medial malleolus fracture; without manipulation

27762 with manipulation, with or without skin or skeletal traction

27766 Open treatment of medial malleolus fracture, includes internal fixation, when performed
➔ *CPT Changes: An Insider's View* 2008

27767 Closed treatment of posterior malleolus fracture; without manipulation
➔ *CPT Changes: An Insider's View* 2008

27768 with manipulation
➔ *CPT Changes: An Insider's View* 2008

27769 Open treatment of posterior malleolus fracture, includes internal fixation, when performed
➔ *CPT Changes: An Insider's View* 2008

(Do not report 27767-27769 in conjunction with 27808-27823)

27780 Closed treatment of proximal fibula or shaft fracture; without manipulation
➔ *CPT Assistant* Winter 92:11

27781 with manipulation

27784 Open treatment of proximal fibula or shaft fracture, includes internal fixation, when performed
➔ *CPT Changes: An Insider's View* 2008
➔ *CPT Assistant* Mar 00:11

27786 Closed treatment of distal fibular fracture (lateral malleolus); without manipulation

27788 with manipulation

27792 Open treatment of distal fibular fracture (lateral malleolus), includes internal fixation, when performed
➔ *CPT Changes: An Insider's View* 2008

(For treatment of tibia and fibula shaft fractures, see 27750-27759)

27808 Closed treatment of bimalleolar ankle fracture (eg, lateral and medial malleoli, or lateral and posterior malleoli or medial and posterior malleoli); without manipulation
➔ *CPT Changes: An Insider's View* 2008

27810 with manipulation
➔ *CPT Changes: An Insider's View* 2008

27814 Open treatment of bimalleolar ankle fracture (eg, lateral and medial malleoli, or lateral and posterior malleoli, or medial and posterior malleoli), includes internal fixation, when performed
➔ *CPT Changes: An Insider's View* 2008
➔ *CPT Assistant* Feb 16:13

27816 Closed treatment of trimalleolar ankle fracture; without manipulation

27818 with manipulation

27822 Open treatment of trimalleolar ankle fracture, includes internal fixation, when performed, medial and/or lateral malleolus; without fixation of posterior lip
➔ *CPT Changes: An Insider's View* 2008

27823 with fixation of posterior lip
➔ *CPT Changes: An Insider's View* 2008

27824 Closed treatment of fracture of weight bearing articular portion of distal tibia (eg, pilon or tibial plafond), with or without anesthesia; without manipulation

27825 with skeletal traction and/or requiring manipulation

27826 Open treatment of fracture of weight bearing articular surface/portion of distal tibia (eg, pilon or tibial plafond), with internal fixation, when performed; of fibula only
➔ *CPT Changes: An Insider's View* 2008

27827 of tibia only
➔ *CPT Changes: An Insider's View* 2008

27828 of both tibia and fibula
➔ *CPT Changes: An Insider's View* 2008
➔ *CPT Assistant* Apr 14:10

27829 Open treatment of distal tibiofibular joint (syndesmosis) disruption, includes internal fixation, when performed
➔ *CPT Changes: An Insider's View* 2008
➔ *CPT Assistant* Winter 92:11, Mar 09:10, Feb 16:13

27830 Closed treatment of proximal tibiofibular joint dislocation; without anesthesia

27831 requiring anesthesia

27832 Open treatment of proximal tibiofibular joint dislocation, includes internal fixation, when performed, or with excision of proximal fibula
➔ *CPT Changes: An Insider's View* 2008

27840 Closed treatment of ankle dislocation; without anesthesia

27842 requiring anesthesia, with or without percutaneous skeletal fixation

27846 Open treatment of ankle dislocation, with or without percutaneous skeletal fixation; without repair or internal fixation

27848 with repair or internal or external fixation

(For surgical or diagnostic arthroscopic procedures, see 29894-29898)

Manipulation

27860 Manipulation of ankle under general anesthesia (includes application of traction or other fixation apparatus)

Arthrodesis

27870 Arthrodesis, ankle, open
➔ *CPT Changes: An Insider's View* 2003
➔ *CPT Assistant* May 20:14, Jul 21:7

(For arthroscopic ankle arthrodesis, use 29899)

27871 Arthrodesis, tibiofibular joint, proximal or distal
➔ *CPT Assistant* May 20:14, Jul 21:7

Amputation

27880 Amputation, leg, through tibia and fibula;

27881 with immediate fitting technique including application of first cast

27882 open, circular (guillotine)

27884 secondary closure or scar revision

27886 re-amputation

27888 Amputation, ankle, through malleoli of tibia and fibula (eg, Syme, Pirogoff type procedures), with plastic closure and resection of nerves

27889 Ankle disarticulation

Other Procedures

27892 Decompression fasciotomy, leg; anterior and/or lateral compartments only, with debridement of nonviable muscle and/or nerve

(For decompression fasciotomy of the leg without debridement, use 27600)

27893 posterior compartment(s) only, with debridement of nonviable muscle and/or nerve

(For decompression fasciotomy of the leg without debridement, use 27601)

27894 anterior and/or lateral, and posterior compartment(s), with debridement of nonviable muscle and/or nerve

(For decompression fasciotomy of the leg without debridement, use 27602)

27899 Unlisted procedure, leg or ankle
➔ *CPT Assistant* Aug 00:11, Dec 16:16, Mar 20:14, Mar 21:9

Foot and Toes

Incision

(For incision and drainage procedures, superficial, see 10040-10160)

28001 Incision and drainage, bursa, foot
➔ *CPT Assistant* Nov 98:9

28002 Incision and drainage below fascia, with or without tendon sheath involvement, foot; single bursal space
➔ *CPT Assistant* Nov 98:8, Feb 24:32

28003 multiple areas
➔ *CPT Assistant* Nov 98:9

28005 Incision, bone cortex (eg, osteomyelitis or bone abscess), foot
➔ *CPT Assistant* Nov 98:9

28008 Fasciotomy, foot and/or toe

(See also 28060, 28062, 28250)

28010 Tenotomy, percutaneous, toe; single tendon
➔ *CPT Assistant* Nov 98:8

28011 multiple tendons
➔ *CPT Assistant* Nov 98:8

(For open tenotomy, see 28230-28234)

28020   Arthrotomy, including exploration, drainage, or removal of loose or foreign body; intertarsal or tarsometatarsal joint

➡ *CPT Assistant* Mar 20:14

28022   metatarsophalangeal joint

28024   interphalangeal joint

28035   Release, tarsal tunnel (posterior tibial nerve decompression)

➡ *CPT Assistant* Nov 98:8

(For other nerve entrapments, see 64704, 64722)

Excision

28039   Code is out of numerical sequence. See 28035-28047

28041   Code is out of numerical sequence. See 28035-28047

28043   Excision, tumor, soft tissue of foot or toe, subcutaneous; less than 1.5 cm

➡ *CPT Changes: An Insider's View* 2010

➡ *CPT Assistant* Aug 23:19-20

 # 28039   1.5 cm or greater

➡ *CPT Changes: An Insider's View* 2010

➡ *CPT Assistant* Aug 23:19-20

(For excision of benign lesions of cutaneous origin [eg, sebaceous cyst], see 11420-11426)

28045   Excision, tumor, soft tissue of foot or toe, subfascial (eg, intramuscular); less than 1.5 cm

➡ *CPT Changes: An Insider's View* 2010

➡ *CPT Assistant* Aug 23:19-20

 # 28041   1.5 cm or greater

➡ *CPT Changes: An Insider's View* 2010

➡ *CPT Assistant* Aug 23:19-20

28046   Radical resection of tumor (eg, sarcoma), soft tissue of foot or toe; less than 3 cm

➡ *CPT Changes: An Insider's View* 2010, 2014

28047   3 cm or greater

➡ *CPT Changes: An Insider's View* 2010, 2014

➡ *CPT Assistant* Sep 18:7

(For radical resection of tumor[s] of cutaneous origin [eg, melanoma], see 11620-11626)

28050   Arthrotomy with biopsy; intertarsal or tarsometatarsal joint

28052   metatarsophalangeal joint

28054   interphalangeal joint

28055   Neurectomy, intrinsic musculature of foot

➡ *CPT Changes: An Insider's View* 2007

28060   Fasciectomy, plantar fascia; partial (separate procedure)

➡ *CPT Assistant* Mar 08:14

28062   radical (separate procedure)

(For plantar fasciotomy, see 28008, 28250)

28070   Synovectomy; intertarsal or tarsometatarsal joint, each

28072   metatarsophalangeal joint, each

28080   Excision, interdigital (Morton) neuroma, single, each

28086   Synovectomy, tendon sheath, foot; flexor

28088   extensor

28090   Excision of lesion, tendon, tendon sheath, or capsule (including synovectomy) (eg, cyst or ganglion); foot

➡ *CPT Assistant* Nov 98:8

28092   toe(s), each

28100   Excision or curettage of bone cyst or benign tumor, talus or calcaneus;

➡ *CPT Assistant* Mar 21:9

28102   with iliac or other autograft (includes obtaining graft)

28103   with allograft

28104   Excision or curettage of bone cyst or benign tumor, tarsal or metatarsal, except talus or calcaneus;

➡ *CPT Changes: An Insider's View* 2002

28106   with iliac or other autograft (includes obtaining graft)

28107   with allograft

28108   Excision or curettage of bone cyst or benign tumor, phalanges of foot

(For partial excision of bossing or exostosis for phalanx in the foot, use 28124)

28110   Ostectomy, partial excision, fifth metatarsal head (bunionette) (separate procedure)

➡ *CPT Assistant* Oct 98:10, Sep 00:9, Dec 10:17, Oct 21:13-14

28111   Ostectomy, complete excision; first metatarsal head

28112   other metatarsal head (second, third or fourth)

28113   fifth metatarsal head

28114   all metatarsal heads, with partial proximal phalangectomy, excluding first metatarsal (eg, Clayton type procedure)

28116   Ostectomy, excision of tarsal coalition

28118   Ostectomy, calcaneus;

➡ *CPT Assistant* May 11:9, Jan 15:13

28119   for spur, with or without plantar fascial release

➡ *CPT Assistant* May 11:9

28120   Partial excision (craterization, saucerization, sequestrectomy, or diaphysectomy) bone (eg, osteomyelitis or bossing); talus or calcaneus

➡ *CPT Assistant* May 11:9

Musculoskeletal 20100-29999

28122   tarsal or metatarsal bone, except talus or calcaneus
➔ *CPT Assistant* Nov 98:11, Aug 20:14

(For partial excision of talus or calcaneus, use 28120)

(For cheilectomy for hallux rigidus, use 28289)

28124   phalanx of toe

28126   Resection, partial or complete, phalangeal base, each toe
➔ *CPT Assistant* Nov 98:8, Mar 15:9

28130   Talectomy (astragalectomy)

(For calcanectomy, use 28118)

28140   Metatarsectomy

28150   Phalangectomy, toe, each toe
➔ *CPT Assistant* Nov 98:8

28153   Resection, condyle(s), distal end of phalanx, each toe
➔ *CPT Assistant* Nov 98:8, Dec 11:15

28160   Hemiphalangectomy or interphalangeal joint excision, toe, proximal end of phalanx, each
➔ *CPT Assistant* Nov 98:8

28171   Radical resection of tumor; tarsal (except talus or calcaneus)
➔ *CPT Changes: An Insider's View* 2010

28173   metatarsal
➔ *CPT Changes: An Insider's View* 2010

28175   phalanx of toe
➔ *CPT Changes: An Insider's View* 2010

(For talus or calcaneus, use 27647)

Introduction or Removal

28190   Removal of foreign body, foot; subcutaneous
➔ *CPT Assistant* Dec 13:16

28192   deep
➔ *CPT Assistant* Dec 13:16

28193   complicated

Repair, Revision, and/or Reconstruction

28200   Repair, tendon, flexor, foot; primary or secondary, without free graft, each tendon
➔ *CPT Assistant* Nov 98:8, Jul 14:5, Feb 16:15

28202   secondary with free graft, each tendon (includes obtaining graft)

28208   Repair, tendon, extensor, foot; primary or secondary, each tendon
➔ *CPT Assistant* Nov 98:8

28210   secondary with free graft, each tendon (includes obtaining graft)

28220   Tenolysis, flexor, foot; single tendon
➔ *CPT Assistant* Nov 98:8

28222   multiple tendons
➔ *CPT Assistant* Nov 98:8

28225   Tenolysis, extensor, foot; single tendon
➔ *CPT Assistant* Nov 98:8

28226   multiple tendons
➔ *CPT Assistant* Nov 98:8

28230   Tenotomy, open, tendon flexor; foot, single or multiple tendon(s) (separate procedure)
➔ *CPT Assistant* Nov 98:8

28232   toe, single tendon (separate procedure)
➔ *CPT Assistant* Nov 98:8, Mar 15:9, Apr 20:10

28234   Tenotomy, open, extensor, foot or toe, each tendon
➔ *CPT Assistant* Nov 98:8, Sep 10:9

(For tendon transfer to midfoot or hindfoot, see 27690, 27691)

28238   Reconstruction (advancement), posterior tibial tendon with excision of accessory tarsal navicular bone (eg, Kidner type procedure)
➔ *CPT Changes: An Insider's View* 2002

(For subcutaneous tenotomy, see 28010, 28011)

(For transfer or transplant of tendon with muscle redirection or rerouting, see 27690-27692)

(For extensor hallucis longus transfer with great toe IP fusion (Jones procedure), use 28760)

28240   Tenotomy, lengthening, or release, abductor hallucis muscle

28250   Division of plantar fascia and muscle (eg, Steindler stripping) (separate procedure)

28260   Capsulotomy, midfoot; medial release only (separate procedure)

28261   with tendon lengthening

28262   extensive, including posterior talotibial capsulotomy and tendon(s) lengthening (eg, resistant clubfoot deformity)

28264   Capsulotomy, midtarsal (eg, Heyman type procedure)

28270   Capsulotomy; metatarsophalangeal joint, with or without tenorrhaphy, each joint (separate procedure)
➔ *CPT Assistant* Sep 10:9, Sep 11:11, Sep 14:13

28272   interphalangeal joint, each joint (separate procedure)
➔ *CPT Assistant* Dec 02:11

28280   Syndactylization, toes (eg, webbing or Kelikian type procedure)
➔ *CPT Assistant* Nov 98:8

28285   Correction, hammertoe (eg, interphalangeal fusion, partial or total phalangectomy)
➔ *CPT Assistant* Nov 98:8, May 06:18, Sep 10:9, Sep 11:11, Mar 15:9, Jun 16:8

★ = Telemedicine   ◀ = Audio-only   ✛ = Add-on code   ✗ = FDA approval pending   # = Resequenced code   ⊘ = Modifier 51 exempt   ➔➔➔ = See p xxi for details

28286   Correction, cock-up fifth toe, with plastic skin closure (eg, Ruiz-Mora type procedure)

➜ *CPT Assistant* Nov 98:8

28288   Ostectomy, partial, exostectomy or condylectomy, metatarsal head, each metatarsal head

28289   Hallux rigidus correction with cheilectomy, debridement and capsular release of the first metatarsophalangeal joint; without implant

➜ *CPT Changes: An Insider's View* 2017

➜ *CPT Assistant* Nov 98:11, May 11:3, Sep 15:12, Dec 16:7, Jul 20:13, Aug 20:14

Hallux Rigidus Correction
28289

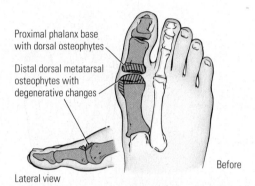

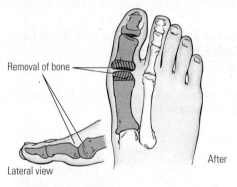

28291   with implant

➜ *CPT Changes: An Insider's View* 2017

➜ *CPT Assistant* Dec 16:7, Nov 17:10, Aug 20:14

28292   Correction, hallux valgus with bunionectomy, with sesamoidectomy when performed; with resection of proximal phalanx base, when performed, any method

➜ *CPT Changes: An Insider's View* 2017, 2024

➜ *CPT Assistant* Dec 96:5, Sep 00:9, Jan 07:31, May 10:9, Dec 10:12, Dec 16:3

28295   Code is out of numerical sequence. See 28292-28298

28296   with distal metatarsal osteotomy, any method

➜ *CPT Changes: An Insider's View* 2017, 2024

➜ *CPT Assistant* Dec 96:6, Jan 97:10, Jan 07:31, May 10:9, Sep 13:17, Dec 16:4, Sep 18:14, Jul 20:13, Apr 24:35

Hallux Rigidus Correction with Implant
28291

A single- or double-stem implant may be used

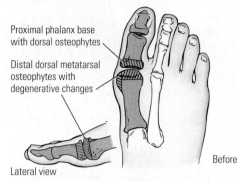

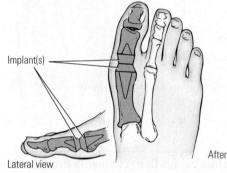

 # 28295   with proximal metatarsal osteotomy, any method

➜ *CPT Changes: An Insider's View* 2017, 2024

➜ *CPT Assistant* Dec 16:5

28297   with first metatarsal and medial cuneiform joint arthrodesis, any method

➜ *CPT Changes: An Insider's View* 2017, 2024

➜ *CPT Assistant* Dec 96:6, Jan 07:31, May 10:9, Dec 16:5, Apr 21:14

(For first metatarsal-cuneiform joint fusion without concomitant removal of the distal medial prominence of the first metatarsal for hallux valgus correction, use 28740)

28298   with proximal phalanx osteotomy, any method

➜ *CPT Changes: An Insider's View* 2017, 2024

➜ *CPT Assistant* Dec 96:7, Jan 07:31, May 10:9, Oct 13:18, Dec 16:6

28299   with double osteotomy, any method

➜ *CPT Changes: An Insider's View* 2002, 2017, 2024

➜ *CPT Assistant* Dec 96:7, Jan 07:31, May 10:9, Sep 13:17, Oct 13:18, Apr 16:8, Dec 16:6

Hallux Valgus Correction
28292

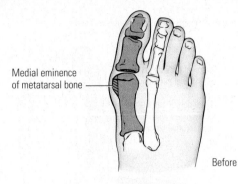

Medial eminence
of metatarsal bone

Before

After

Hallux Valgus Correction with Proximal Phalanx Base Resection
28292

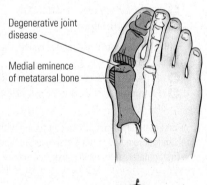

Degenerative joint
disease

Medial eminence
of metatarsal bone

Before

Kirschner wire
holding joint

After

Hallux Valgus Correction with Proximal First Metatarsal Osteotomy
28295

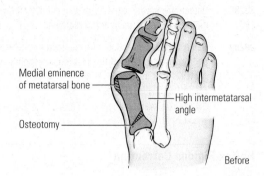

Medial eminence
of metatarsal bone

High intermetatarsal
angle

Osteotomy

Before

After

Hallux Valgus Correction with Distal First Metatarsal Osteotomy
28296

A single or multiple plane osteotomy originating through the distal aspect of the first metatarsal

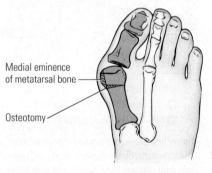

Medial eminence
of metatarsal bone

Osteotomy

Before

After

Hallux Valgus Correction with Metatarsal-Medial Cuneiform Joint Arthrodesis
28297

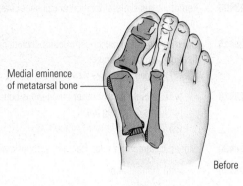

Medial eminence of metatarsal bone

Before

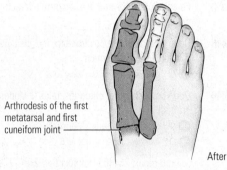

Arthrodesis of the first metatarsal and first cuneiform joint

After

Hallux Valgus Correction with Proximal Phalanx Osteotomy
28298

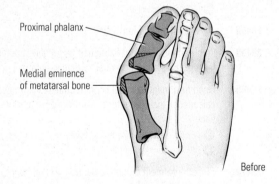

Proximal phalanx

Medial eminence of metatarsal bone

Before

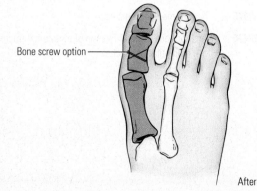

Bone screw option

After

Hallux Valgus Correction with Double Osteotomy
28299

These illustrations depict medial resection of the first metatarsal along with several first ray double osteotomy options for hallux valgus and metatarsus primus adductus (high intermetatarsal angle) correction.

Surgical Option 1
PREOP

POSTOP

Angular deformity of proximal phalanx

Medial eminence of metatarsal bone

Osteotomy proximal phalanx

Osteotomy distal first metatarsal

Note: Internal fixation is not depicted, but would include screw(s), pin(s), wire(s), as needed.

Surgical Option 2
PREOP

POSTOP

Medial eminence of metatarsal bone

Double osteotomy of the metatarsal with internal fixation

Note: Internal fixation is not depicted, but would include screw(s), pin(s), wire(s), as needed.

Surgical Option 3
PREOP

POSTOP

Angular deformity of proximal phalanx

Medial eminence of metatarsal bone

Angular deformity at the first metatarsal base

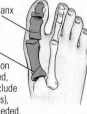

Osteotomy proximal phalanx

Osteotomy proximal first metatarsal

Note: Internal fixation is not depicted, but would include screw(s), pin(s), wire(s), as needed.

Musculoskeletal 20100-29999

28300 Osteotomy; calcaneus (eg, Dwyer or Chambers type procedure), with or without internal fixation

28302 talus
⊃ *CPT Assistant* Mar 21:9

28304 Osteotomy, tarsal bones, other than calcaneus or talus;
⊃ *CPT Assistant* Nov 98:8

28305 with autograft (includes obtaining graft) (eg, Fowler type)

28306 Osteotomy, with or without lengthening, shortening or angular correction, metatarsal; first metatarsal
⊃ *CPT Assistant* Nov 98:8, Dec 99:7, Dec 10:12

28307 first metatarsal with autograft (other than first toe)
⊃ *CPT Assistant* Nov 98:9

28308 other than first metatarsal, each
⊃ *CPT Assistant* Oct 21:13-14

28309 multiple (eg, Swanson type cavus foot procedure)
⊃ *CPT Assistant* Nov 98:8, Dec 99:7

28310 Osteotomy, shortening, angular or rotational correction; proximal phalanx, first toe (separate procedure)
⊃ *CPT Assistant* Sep 13:17

28312 other phalanges, any toe

28313 Reconstruction, angular deformity of toe, soft tissue procedures only (eg, overlapping second toe, fifth toe, curly toes)
⊃ *CPT Assistant* Nov 98:8

28315 Sesamoidectomy, first toe (separate procedure)

28320 Repair, nonunion or malunion; tarsal bones
⊃ *CPT Assistant* Nov 98:9

28322 metatarsal, with or without bone graft (includes obtaining graft)

28340 Reconstruction, toe, macrodactyly; soft tissue resection

28341 requiring bone resection

28344 Reconstruction, toe(s); polydactyly

28345 syndactyly, with or without skin graft(s), each web

28360 Reconstruction, cleft foot

Fracture and/or Dislocation

—— *Coding Tip* ——

Reporting for Categories of Manipulation and/or Fracture

The codes for treatment of fractures and joint injuries (dislocations) are categorized by the type of manipulation (reduction) and stabilization (fixation or immobilization). These codes can apply to either open (compound) or closed fractures or joint injuries.

CPT Coding Guidelines, Musculoskeletal System

28400 Closed treatment of calcaneal fracture; without manipulation

28405 with manipulation

28406 Percutaneous skeletal fixation of calcaneal fracture, with manipulation

28415 Open treatment of calcaneal fracture, includes internal fixation, when performed;
⊃ *CPT Changes: An Insider's View* 2008

28420 with primary iliac or other autogenous bone graft (includes obtaining graft)
⊃ *CPT Changes: An Insider's View* 2008

28430 Closed treatment of talus fracture; without manipulation

28435 with manipulation

28436 Percutaneous skeletal fixation of talus fracture, with manipulation

28445 Open treatment of talus fracture, includes internal fixation, when performed
⊃ *CPT Changes: An Insider's View* 2008

28446 Open osteochondral autograft, talus (includes obtaining graft[s])
⊃ *CPT Changes: An Insider's View* 2008
⊃ *CPT Assistant* Jan 08:4, Dec 08:6

(Do not report 28446 in conjunction with 27705, 27707)

(For arthroscopic osteochondral talus graft, use 29892)

(For open osteochondral allograft or repairs with industrial grafts, use 28899)

28450 Treatment of tarsal bone fracture (except talus and calcaneus); without manipulation, each
⊃ *CPT Assistant* Dec 01:7

28455 with manipulation, each

28456 Percutaneous skeletal fixation of tarsal bone fracture (except talus and calcaneus), with manipulation, each

28465 Open treatment of tarsal bone fracture (except talus and calcaneus), includes internal fixation, when performed, each
⊃ *CPT Changes: An Insider's View* 2008
⊃ *CPT Assistant* Aug 19:10

28470 Closed treatment of metatarsal fracture; without manipulation, each

28475 with manipulation, each

28476 Percutaneous skeletal fixation of metatarsal fracture, with manipulation, each

28485   Open treatment of metatarsal fracture, includes internal fixation, when performed, each
→ *CPT Changes: An Insider's View 2008*
→ *CPT Assistant Aug 19:10*

28490   Closed treatment of fracture great toe, phalanx or phalanges; without manipulation

28495   with manipulation

28496   Percutaneous skeletal fixation of fracture great toe, phalanx or phalanges, with manipulation

28505   Open treatment of fracture, great toe, phalanx or phalanges, includes internal fixation, when performed
→ *CPT Changes: An Insider's View 2008*

28510   Closed treatment of fracture, phalanx or phalanges, other than great toe; without manipulation, each

28515   with manipulation, each

28525   Open treatment of fracture, phalanx or phalanges, other than great toe, includes internal fixation, when performed, each
→ *CPT Changes: An Insider's View 2008*

28530   Closed treatment of sesamoid fracture

28531   Open treatment of sesamoid fracture, with or without internal fixation

28540   Closed treatment of tarsal bone dislocation, other than talotarsal; without anesthesia

28545   requiring anesthesia

28546   Percutaneous skeletal fixation of tarsal bone dislocation, other than talotarsal, with manipulation

28555   Open treatment of tarsal bone dislocation, includes internal fixation, when performed
→ *CPT Changes: An Insider's View 2008*

28570   Closed treatment of talotarsal joint dislocation; without anesthesia

28575   requiring anesthesia

28576   Percutaneous skeletal fixation of talotarsal joint dislocation, with manipulation

28585   Open treatment of talotarsal joint dislocation, includes internal fixation, when performed
→ *CPT Changes: An Insider's View 2008*
→ *CPT Assistant Sep 11:12*

28600   Closed treatment of tarsometatarsal joint dislocation; without anesthesia

28605   requiring anesthesia

28606   Percutaneous skeletal fixation of tarsometatarsal joint dislocation, with manipulation

28615   Open treatment of tarsometatarsal joint dislocation, includes internal fixation, when performed
→ *CPT Changes: An Insider's View 2008*
→ *CPT Assistant Dec 21:19*

28630   Closed treatment of metatarsophalangeal joint dislocation; without anesthesia

28635   requiring anesthesia

28636   Percutaneous skeletal fixation of metatarsophalangeal joint dislocation, with manipulation

28645   Open treatment of metatarsophalangeal joint dislocation, includes internal fixation, when performed
→ *CPT Changes: An Insider's View 2008*
→ *CPT Assistant Sep 14:13*

28660   Closed treatment of interphalangeal joint dislocation; without anesthesia

28665   requiring anesthesia

28666   Percutaneous skeletal fixation of interphalangeal joint dislocation, with manipulation

28675   Open treatment of interphalangeal joint dislocation, includes internal fixation, when performed
→ *CPT Changes: An Insider's View 2008*

Arthrodesis

28705   Arthrodesis; pantalar
→ *CPT Assistant May 20:14, Jul 21:7*

28715   triple

28725   subtalar
→ *CPT Assistant Sep 11:11*

28730   Arthrodesis, midtarsal or tarsometatarsal, multiple or transverse;

28735   with osteotomy (eg, flatfoot correction)
→ *CPT Assistant May 19:10*

28737   Arthrodesis, with tendon lengthening and advancement, midtarsal, tarsal navicular-cuneiform (eg, Miller type procedure)
→ *CPT Changes: An Insider's View 2002*

28740   Arthrodesis, midtarsal or tarsometatarsal, single joint
→ *CPT Assistant Dec 21:19*

(For first metatarsal-cuneiform joint fusion without concomitant removal of the distal medial prominence of the first metatarsal for hallux valgus correction, use 28740)

28750   Arthrodesis, great toe; metatarsophalangeal joint
→ *CPT Assistant Dec 96:7, Dec 16:8*

28755   interphalangeal joint

28760   Arthrodesis, with extensor hallucis longus transfer to first metatarsal neck, great toe, interphalangeal joint (eg, Jones type procedure)
→ *CPT Assistant Nov 98:8, May 20:14, Jul 21:7*

(For hammertoe operation or interphalangeal fusion, use 28285)

Amputation

28800 Amputation, foot; midtarsal (eg, Chopart type procedure)

28805 transmetatarsal
➔ *CPT Assistant* May 97:8, Mar 21:9

28810 Amputation, metatarsal, with toe, single

28820 Amputation, toe; metatarsophalangeal joint
➔ *CPT Assistant* May 97:8

28825 interphalangeal joint

Other Procedures

28890 Extracorporeal shock wave, high energy, performed by a physician or other qualified health care professional, requiring anesthesia other than local, including ultrasound guidance, involving the plantar fascia
➔ *CPT Changes: An Insider's View* 2006, 2013
➔ *CPT Assistant* Dec 05:10, Mar 06:1, Dec 18:5

(For extracorporeal shock wave therapy involving musculoskeletal system not otherwise specified, see 0101T, 0102T)

(For extracorporeal shock wave therapy involving integumentary system not otherwise specified, see 0512T, 0513T)

(Do not report 28890 in conjunction with 0512T, 0513T, when treating the same area)

28899 Unlisted procedure, foot or toes
➔ *CPT Assistant* Sep 11:12, Nov 15:10, Jun 16:8, Sep 17:14, Nov 17:10, Oct 18:11

Application of Casts and Strapping

All services that appear in the Musculoskeletal System section include the application and removal of the first cast, splint, or traction device, when performed. Supplies are reported separately. If a cast is removed by someone other than the physician or other qualified health care professional who applied the cast, report the cast removal code (29700, 29705, 29710).

Subsequent replacement of cast, splint, or strapping (29000-29750) and/or traction device (eg, 20690, 20692) during or after the global period may be reported separately.

A cast, splint, or strapping is not considered part of the preoperative care; therefore, the use of modifier 56 for preoperative management only is not applicable.

(For orthotics management and training, see 97760, 97761, 97763)

Body and Upper Extremity

Casts

29000 Application of halo type body cast (see 20661-20663 for insertion)
➔ *CPT Assistant* Feb 96:3, 5, Apr 02:13, Jan 18:3

29010 Application of Risser jacket, localizer, body; only
➔ *CPT Assistant* Feb 96:3, Apr 02:13

29015 including head
➔ *CPT Assistant* Feb 96:3, Apr 02:13

29035 Application of body cast, shoulder to hips;
➔ *CPT Assistant* Feb 96:3, Apr 02:13

29040 including head, Minerva type
➔ *CPT Assistant* Feb 96:3, Apr 02:13

29044 including 1 thigh
➔ *CPT Assistant* Feb 96:3, Apr 02:13

29046 including both thighs
➔ *CPT Assistant* Feb 96:3, Apr 02:13

29049 Application, cast; figure-of-eight
➔ *CPT Changes: An Insider's View* 2002
➔ *CPT Assistant* Feb 96:3, Apr 02:13

29055 shoulder spica
➔ *CPT Assistant* Feb 96:3, Apr 02:13

29058 plaster Velpeau
➔ *CPT Assistant* Feb 96:3, Apr 02:13

29065 shoulder to hand (long arm)
➔ *CPT Assistant* Feb 96:3, Apr 02:13

29075 elbow to finger (short arm)
➔ *CPT Assistant* Feb 96:3-4, Apr 02:13

29085 hand and lower forearm (gauntlet)
➔ *CPT Assistant* Feb 96:3, Apr 02:13, Dec 02:11

29086 finger (eg, contracture)
➔ *CPT Changes: An Insider's View* 2002
➔ *CPT Assistant* Apr 02:13

Splints

29105 Application of long arm splint (shoulder to hand)
➔ *CPT Assistant* Feb 96:3, Apr 02:13, May 09:8, Jan 18:3

29125 Application of short arm splint (forearm to hand); static
➔ *CPT Assistant* Feb 96:3-4, Apr 02:13, Jan 18:3

29126 dynamic
➔ *CPT Assistant* Feb 96:3, Apr 02:13

29130   Application of finger splint; static
     CPT Assistant Feb 96:3, Apr 02:13

29131   dynamic
     CPT Assistant Feb 96:3, Apr 02:13

Strapping—Any Age

29200   Strapping; thorax
     CPT Assistant Feb 96:3, Apr 02:13

(To report low back strapping, use 29799)

29240   shoulder (eg, Velpeau)
     CPT Assistant Feb 96:3, Apr 02:13, Jun 10:8

29260   elbow or wrist
     CPT Assistant Feb 96:3, Apr 02:13

29280   hand or finger
     CPT Assistant Feb 96:3, Apr 02:13

Lower Extremity

Casts

29305   Application of hip spica cast; 1 leg
     CPT Assistant Feb 96:3, Apr 02:13

29325   1 and one-half spica or both legs
     CPT Assistant Feb 96:3, Apr 02:13

(For hip spica (body) cast, including thighs only, use 29046)

29345   Application of long leg cast (thigh to toes);
     CPT Assistant Feb 96:3, Apr 02:13, Sep 11:11

29355   walker or ambulatory type
     CPT Assistant Feb 96:3, Apr 02:13, Sep 11:11, Jan 18:3

29358   Application of long leg cast brace
     CPT Assistant Feb 96:3, Apr 02:13, Sep 11:11

29365   Application of cylinder cast (thigh to ankle)
     CPT Assistant Feb 96:3, Apr 02:13, Sep 11:11

29405   Application of short leg cast (below knee to toes);
     CPT Assistant Feb 96:3, Apr 02:13, Mar 03:17, Sep 11:11, Jan 18:3

29425   walking or ambulatory type
     CPT Assistant Feb 96:3, Apr 02:13, Sep 11:11

29435   Application of patellar tendon bearing (PTB) cast
     CPT Assistant Feb 96:3, Apr 02:13, Sep 11:11

29440   Adding walker to previously applied cast
     CPT Assistant Feb 96:3, Apr 02:13

29445   Application of rigid total contact leg cast
     CPT Assistant Feb 96:3, Apr 02:13, Sep 11:11

29450   Application of clubfoot cast with molding or manipulation, long or short leg
     CPT Assistant Feb 96:3, Apr 02:13

(To report bilateral procedure, use 29450 with modifier 50)

Splints

29505   Application of long leg splint (thigh to ankle or toes)
     CPT Assistant Feb 96:3, Apr 02:13, May 09:8

29515   Application of short leg splint (calf to foot)
     CPT Assistant Feb 96:3, Apr 02:13, Mar 03:18, Jan 18:3, Oct 19:10

Strapping—Any Age

29520   Strapping; hip
     CPT Assistant Feb 96:3, Apr 02:13

29530   knee
     CPT Assistant Feb 96:3, Apr 02:13, Jun 10:8, Aug 10:15

29540   ankle and/or foot
     CPT Changes: An Insider's View 2003
     CPT Assistant Feb 96:3, Apr 02:13, Mar 03:17, Jun 10:8, Aug 10:15, Mar 14:4

(Do not report 29540 in conjunction with 29580, 29581, for the same extremity)

29550   toes
     CPT Assistant Feb 96:3, Apr 02:13

29580   Unna boot
     CPT Assistant Feb 96:3, Jul 99:10, Apr 02:13, Mar 14:4

(Do not report 29580 in conjunction with 29540, 29581, for the same extremity)

29581   Application of multi-layer compression system; leg (below knee), including ankle and foot
     CPT Changes: An Insider's View 2010, 2012
     CPT Assistant May 11:11, Sep 12:16, Sep 13:17, Mar 14:4, Oct 14:6, Mar 15:10, Aug 16:3

(Do not report 29581 in conjunction with 29540, 29580, for the same extremity)

(Do not report 29520, 29530, 29540, 29550, 29580, 29581 in conjunction with 36465, 36466, 36468, 36470, 36471, 36473, 36474, 36475, 36476, 36478, 36479, 36482, 36483, for the same extremity)

29584   upper arm, forearm, hand, and fingers
     CPT Changes: An Insider's View 2012
     CPT Assistant Mar 15:10, Aug 16:3

(Do not report 29584 in conjunction with 36465, 36466, 36468, 36470, 36471, 36473, 36474, 36475, 36476, 36478, 36479, 36482, 36483, for the same extremity)

Removal or Repair

Codes for cast removals should be employed only for casts applied by another individual.

29700   Removal or bivalving; gauntlet, boot or body cast
➔ *CPT Assistant* Apr 02:13, May 22:2

29705   full arm or full leg cast
➔ *CPT Assistant* Apr 02:13, May 22:2

29710   shoulder or hip spica, Minerva, or Risser jacket, etc.
➔ *CPT Assistant* Apr 02:13, May 22:2

29720   Repair of spica, body cast or jacket
➔ *CPT Assistant* Apr 02:13

29730   Windowing of cast
➔ *CPT Assistant* Apr 02:13

29740   Wedging of cast (except clubfoot casts)
➔ *CPT Assistant* Apr 02:13

29750   Wedging of clubfoot cast
➔ *CPT Assistant* Apr 02:13, Jan 18:3

(To report bilateral procedure, use 29750 with modifier 50)

Other Procedures

29799   Unlisted procedure, casting or strapping
➔ *CPT Assistant* Sep 12:16, Aug 16:11, Jan 18:3

Endoscopy/Arthroscopy

Surgical endoscopy/arthroscopy always includes a diagnostic endoscopy/arthroscopy.

When arthroscopy is performed in conjunction with arthrotomy, add modifier 51.

Arthroscopic removal of loose body(ies) or foreign body(ies) (ie, 29819, 29834, 29861, 29874, 29894, 29904) may be reported only when the loose body(ies) or foreign body(ies) is equal to or larger than the diameter of the arthroscopic cannula(s) used for the specific procedure, and can only be removed through a cannula larger than that used for the specific procedure or through a separate incision or through a portal that has been enlarged to allow removal of the loose or foreign body(ies).

29800   Arthroscopy, temporomandibular joint, diagnostic, with or without synovial biopsy (separate procedure)
➔ *CPT Assistant* May 13:12

29804   Arthroscopy, temporomandibular joint, surgical
➔ *CPT Assistant* May 13:12

(For open procedure, use 21010)

29805   Arthroscopy, shoulder, diagnostic, with or without synovial biopsy (separate procedure)
➔ *CPT Changes: An Insider's View* 2002
➔ *CPT Assistant* May 13:12, Jun 15:10

(For open procedure, see 23065-23066, 23100-23101)

29806   Arthroscopy, shoulder, surgical; capsulorrhaphy
➔ *CPT Changes: An Insider's View* 2002
➔ *CPT Assistant* May 13:12, Mar 15:7, Jul 15:10, Jun 18:11

(For open procedure, see 23450-23466)

(To report thermal capsulorrhaphy, use 29999)

29807   repair of SLAP lesion
➔ *CPT Changes: An Insider's View* 2002
➔ *CPT Assistant* May 13:12, Mar 15:7

29819   with removal of loose body or foreign body
➔ *CPT Changes: An Insider's View* 2002
➔ *CPT Assistant* May 13:12, Mar 15:7, Jun 18:11, Dec 20:8

(For open procedure, see 23040-23044, 23107)

29820   synovectomy, partial
➔ *CPT Assistant* May 13:12, Jun 13:13, Mar 15:7

(For open procedure, see 23105)

29821   synovectomy, complete
➔ *CPT Assistant* May 13:12, Jun 13:13, Mar 15:7

(For open procedure, see 23105)

29822   debridement, limited, 1 or 2 discrete structures (eg, humeral bone, humeral articular cartilage, glenoid bone, glenoid articular cartilage, biceps tendon, biceps anchor complex, labrum, articular capsule, articular side of the rotator cuff, bursal side of the rotator cuff, subacromial bursa, foreign body[ies])
➔ *CPT Changes: An Insider's View* 2021
➔ *CPT Assistant* May 01:9, Apr 12:17, Sep 12:16, May 13:12, Mar 15:7, Jan 18:7, Dec 20:8

(For open procedure, see specific open shoulder procedure performed)

29823   debridement, extensive, 3 or more discrete structures (eg, humeral bone, humeral articular cartilage, glenoid bone, glenoid articular cartilage, biceps tendon, biceps anchor complex, labrum, articular capsule, articular side of the rotator cuff, bursal side of the rotator cuff, subacromial bursa, foreign body[ies])
➔ *CPT Changes: An Insider's View* 2021
➔ *CPT Assistant* Apr 12:17, Sep 12:16, May 13:12, Mar 15:7, Dec 16:16, Jan 18:7, Dec 20:8

(For open procedure, see specific open shoulder procedure performed)

29824   distal claviculectomy including distal articular surface (Mumford procedure)
➔ *CPT Changes: An Insider's View* 2002
➔ *CPT Assistant* May 13:12, Mar 15:7, Sep 23:47

(For open procedure, use 23120)

Arthroscopy, Shoulder, Distal Claviculectomy (Mumford Procedure)
29824

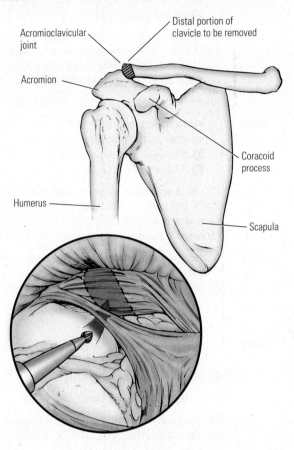

Acromioclavicular joint

Distal portion of clavicle to be removed

Acromion

Coracoid process

Humerus

Scapula

29825   with lysis and resection of adhesions, with or without manipulation
> *CPT Assistant* May 13:12, Mar 15:7

(For open procedure, see specific open shoulder procedure performed)

+ 29826   decompression of subacromial space with partial acromioplasty, with coracoacromial ligament (ie, arch) release, when performed (List separately in addition to code for primary procedure)
> *CPT Changes: An Insider's View* 2012
> *CPT Assistant* May 01:9, Aug 02:10, May 13:12, Mar 15:7

(For open procedure, use 23130 or 23415)

(Use 29826 in conjunction with 29806-29825, 29827, 29828)

29827   with rotator cuff repair
> *CPT Changes: An Insider's View* 2003
> *CPT Assistant* Mar 08:14, May 13:12, Mar 15:7, Jul 16:8, May 22:15

(For open or mini-open rotator cuff repair, use 23412)

(When arthroscopic distal clavicle resection is performed at the same setting, use 29824 and append modifier 51)

29828   biceps tenodesis
> *CPT Changes: An Insider's View* 2008
> *CPT Assistant* Feb 08:9, May 13:12, Mar 15:7, Jul 16:8

(Do not report 29828 in conjunction with 29805, 29820, 29822)

(For open biceps tenodesis, use 23430)

29830   Arthroscopy, elbow, diagnostic, with or without synovial biopsy (separate procedure)
> *CPT Assistant* May 13:12

29834   Arthroscopy, elbow, surgical; with removal of loose body or foreign body
> *CPT Assistant* May 13:12, Dec 20:8

29835   synovectomy, partial
> *CPT Assistant* May 13:12

29836   synovectomy, complete
> *CPT Assistant* May 13:12

29837   debridement, limited
> *CPT Assistant* May 13:12

29838   debridement, extensive
> *CPT Assistant* May 13:12

29840   Arthroscopy, wrist, diagnostic, with or without synovial biopsy (separate procedure)
> *CPT Assistant* May 13:12

29843   Arthroscopy, wrist, surgical; for infection, lavage and drainage
> *CPT Assistant* May 13:12

29844   synovectomy, partial
> *CPT Assistant* May 13:12

29845   synovectomy, complete
> *CPT Assistant* Dec 03:11, May 13:12

29846   excision and/or repair of triangular fibrocartilage and/or joint debridement
> *CPT Assistant* Dec 03:11, May 13:12

29847   internal fixation for fracture or instability
> *CPT Assistant* May 13:12

29848   Endoscopy, wrist, surgical, with release of transverse carpal ligament
> *CPT Assistant* Dec 99:7, May 13:12, Jul 15:10, Jan 17:6, Apr 18:10

(Do not report 29848 in conjunction with 11960)

(For open procedure, use 64721)

29850 Arthroscopically aided treatment of intercondylar spine(s) and/or tuberosity fracture(s) of the knee, with or without manipulation; without internal or external fixation (includes arthroscopy)
➔ *CPT Assistant* May 13:12

29851 with internal or external fixation (includes arthroscopy)
➔ *CPT Assistant* May 13:12

(For bone graft, use 20900, 20902)

29855 Arthroscopically aided treatment of tibial fracture, proximal (plateau); unicondylar, includes internal fixation, when performed (includes arthroscopy)
➔ *CPT Changes: An Insider's View* 2008
➔ *CPT Assistant* May 13:12, Sep 18:14, Nov 19:13

29856 bicondylar, includes internal fixation, when performed (includes arthroscopy)
➔ *CPT Changes: An Insider's View* 2008
➔ *CPT Assistant* May 13:12

(For bone graft, use 20900, 20902)

29860 Arthroscopy, hip, diagnostic with or without synovial biopsy (separate procedure)
➔ *CPT Assistant* Nov 97:15, Jul 98:8, Sep 11:6, May 13:12

29861 Arthroscopy, hip, surgical; with removal of loose body or foreign body
➔ *CPT Assistant* Nov 97:15, Jul 98:8, Sep 11:5, May 13:12, Dec 20:8

29862 with debridement/shaving of articular cartilage (chondroplasty), abrasion arthroplasty, and/or resection of labrum
➔ *CPT Assistant* Nov 97:15, Jul 98:8, Sep 11:5, May 13:12

29863 with synovectomy
➔ *CPT Assistant* Nov 97:15, Jul 98:8, Sep 11:5, May 13:12

 # 29914 with femoroplasty (ie, treatment of cam lesion)
➔ *CPT Changes: An Insider's View* 2011
➔ *CPT Assistant* Sep 11:5

 # 29915 with acetabuloplasty (ie, treatment of pincer lesion)
➔ *CPT Changes: An Insider's View* 2011
➔ *CPT Assistant* Sep 11:5

(Do not report 29914, 29915 in conjunction with 29862, 29863)

 # 29916 with labral repair
➔ *CPT Changes: An Insider's View* 2011
➔ *CPT Assistant* Sep 11:5

(Do not report 29916 in conjunction with 29915, 29862, 29863)

29866 Arthroscopy, knee, surgical; osteochondral autograft(s) (eg, mosaicplasty) (includes harvesting of the autograft[s])
➔ *CPT Changes: An Insider's View* 2005, 2008
➔ *CPT Assistant* May 13:12

(Do not report 29866 in conjunction with 29870, 29871, 29875, 29884 when performed at the same session and/or 29874, 29877, 29879, 29885-29887 when performed in the same compartment)

(For open osteochondral autograft of knee, use 27416)

29867 osteochondral allograft (eg, mosaicplasty)
➔ *CPT Changes: An Insider's View* 2005
➔ *CPT Assistant* May 13:12

(Do not report 29867 in conjunction with 27570, 29870, 29871, 29875, 29884 when performed at the same session and/or 29874, 29877, 29879, 29885-29887 when performed in the same compartment)

(Do not report 29867 in conjunction with 27415)

29868 meniscal transplantation (includes arthrotomy for meniscal insertion), medial or lateral
➔ *CPT Changes: An Insider's View* 2005
➔ *CPT Assistant* May 13:12

(Do not report 29868 in conjunction with 29870, 29871, 29875, 29880, 29883, 29884 when performed at the same session or 29874, 29877, 29881, 29882 when performed in the same compartment)

29870 Arthroscopy, knee, diagnostic, with or without synovial biopsy (separate procedure)
➔ *CPT Assistant* Dec 07:10, Mar 11:9, May 13:12, Nov 19:14

(For open autologous chondrocyte implantation of the knee, use 27412)

29871 Arthroscopy, knee, surgical; for infection, lavage and drainage
➔ *CPT Assistant* Aug 01:6, May 13:12, Aug 19:7

(Do not report 29871 in conjunction with 27369)

(For implantation of osteochondral graft for treatment of articular surface defect, see 27412, 27415, 29866, 29867)

29873 with lateral release
➔ *CPT Changes: An Insider's View* 2003
➔ *CPT Assistant* Dec 07:10, Aug 09:11, May 13:12, Nov 15:7

(For open lateral release, use 27425)

29874 for removal of loose body or foreign body (eg, osteochondritis dissecans fragmentation, chondral fragmentation)
➔ *CPT Assistant* Aug 01:6, Apr 03:12, May 13:12, Dec 20:8

29875 synovectomy, limited (eg, plica or shelf resection) (separate procedure)
➔ *CPT Assistant* Aug 01:6, May 13:12, May 14:10, Jan 16:11, Aug 21:14

29876 synovectomy, major, 2 or more compartments (eg, medial or lateral)
➔ *CPT Assistant* Aug 01:6, May 13:12, Aug 21:14

★=Telemedicine ◀=Audio-only ✚=Add-on code ✗=FDA approval pending #=Resequenced code ⊘=Modifier 51 exempt ➔➔➔=See p xxi for details

29877   debridement/shaving of articular cartilage (chondroplasty)

     🔁 *CPT Assistant* Feb 96:9, Jun 99:11, Aug 01:7, Apr 03:7, Apr 05:14, Dec 07:10, May 13:12, May 20:13, Jun 21:12

(When performed with arthroscopic meniscectomy, see 29880 or 29881)

29879   abrasion arthroplasty (includes chondroplasty where necessary) or multiple drilling or microfracture

     🔁 *CPT Changes: An Insider's View* 2000

     🔁 *CPT Assistant* Nov 99:13, Aug 01:7, May 13:12

29880   with meniscectomy (medial AND lateral, including any meniscal shaving) including debridement/shaving of articular cartilage (chondroplasty), same or separate compartment(s), when performed

     🔁 *CPT Changes: An Insider's View* 2012

     🔁 *CPT Assistant* Jun 99:11, Aug 01:7, Jan 12:3, May 13:12

29881   with meniscectomy (medial OR lateral, including any meniscal shaving) including debridement/shaving of articular cartilage (chondroplasty), same or separate compartment(s), when performed

     🔁 *CPT Changes: An Insider's View* 2012

     🔁 *CPT Assistant* Feb 96:9, Jun 99:11, Aug 01:7, Oct 03:11, Apr 05:14, Dec 07:10, Jan 12:3, May 13:12, May 14:10, Jan 16:11, Nov 19:14, May 20:13, Sep 20:14, Jun 21:12

29882   with meniscus repair (medial OR lateral)

     🔁 *CPT Assistant* Aug 01:7, Sep 04:12, Dec 07:10, Dec 11:15, May 13:12, May 19:10

29883   with meniscus repair (medial AND lateral)

     🔁 *CPT Assistant* Aug 01:7, Sep 04:12, Dec 07:10, Dec 11:15, May 13:12

(For meniscal transplantation, medial or lateral, knee, use 29868)

29884   with lysis of adhesions, with or without manipulation (separate procedure)

     🔁 *CPT Assistant* Aug 01:7, Mar 11:9, May 13:12

29885   drilling for osteochondritis dissecans with bone grafting, with or without internal fixation (including debridement of base of lesion)

     🔁 *CPT Assistant* Aug 01:7, May 13:12

29886   drilling for intact osteochondritis dissecans lesion

     🔁 *CPT Assistant* Aug 01:12, May 13:12

29887   drilling for intact osteochondritis dissecans lesion with internal fixation

     🔁 *CPT Assistant* Aug 01:12, May 13:12

29888   Arthroscopically aided anterior cruciate ligament repair/augmentation or reconstruction

     🔁 *CPT Assistant* Oct 03:11, Dec 07:10, May 13:12, Nov 16:9, May 17:10

29889   Arthroscopically aided posterior cruciate ligament repair/augmentation or reconstruction

     🔁 *CPT Assistant* Sep 96:9, Oct 98:11, Aug 01:8, Dec 07:10, May 13:12

Arthroscopy of the Knee
29866-29887

Portal incisions are made on either side of the patellar tendon and compartments of the knee are examined using the arthroscope and a probe. Additional treatment is performed as needed.

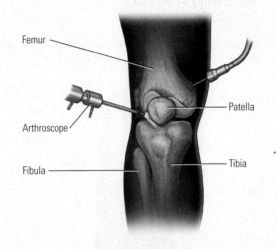

Femur

Patella

Arthroscope

Tibia

Fibula

29891   Arthroscopy, ankle, surgical, excision of osteochondral defect of talus and/or tibia, including drilling of the defect

     🔁 *CPT Assistant* Nov 97:15, May 13:12

29892   Arthroscopically aided repair of large osteochondritis dissecans lesion, talar dome fracture, or tibial plafond fracture, with or without internal fixation (includes arthroscopy)

     🔁 *CPT Assistant* Nov 97:15, Dec 08:6, May 13:12

29893   Endoscopic plantar fasciotomy

     🔁 *CPT Assistant* Nov 97:15, May 13:12

29894   Arthroscopy, ankle (tibiotalar and fibulotalar joints), surgical; with removal of loose body or foreign body

     🔁 *CPT Assistant* May 13:12, Dec 20:8

29895   synovectomy, partial

     🔁 *CPT Assistant* May 13:12

29897   debridement, limited

     🔁 *CPT Assistant* May 13:12

29898   debridement, extensive

     🔁 *CPT Assistant* May 13:12

29899   with ankle arthrodesis

➔ *CPT Changes: An Insider's View* 2003

➔ *CPT Assistant* May 13:12

(For open ankle arthrodesis, use 27870)

Arthroscopy of the Ankle
29894-29899

Incisions are made allowing the ankle to be examined using the arthroscope and a probe. Additional treatment is performed as needed.

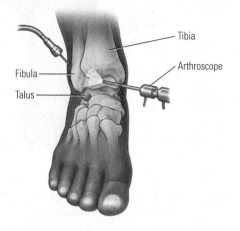

29900   Arthroscopy, metacarpophalangeal joint, diagnostic, includes synovial biopsy

➔ *CPT Changes: An Insider's View* 2002

➔ *CPT Assistant* May 13:12

(Do not report 29900 with 29901, 29902)

29901   Arthroscopy, metacarpophalangeal joint, surgical; with debridement

➔ *CPT Changes: An Insider's View* 2002

➔ *CPT Assistant* May 13:12

29902   with reduction of displaced ulnar collateral ligament (eg, Stener lesion)

➔ *CPT Changes: An Insider's View* 2002

➔ *CPT Assistant* May 13:12

29904   Arthroscopy, subtalar joint, surgical; with removal of loose body or foreign body

➔ *CPT Changes: An Insider's View* 2008

➔ *CPT Assistant* May 13:12, Dec 20:8

29905   with synovectomy

➔ *CPT Changes: An Insider's View* 2008

➔ *CPT Assistant* May 13:12

29906   with debridement

➔ *CPT Changes: An Insider's View* 2008

➔ *CPT Assistant* May 13:12

29907   with subtalar arthrodesis

➔ *CPT Changes: An Insider's View* 2008

➔ *CPT Assistant* May 13:12

29914   Code is out of numerical sequence. See 29862-29867

29915   Code is out of numerical sequence. See 29862-29867

29916   Code is out of numerical sequence. See 29862-29867

29999   Unlisted procedure, arthroscopy

➔ *CPT Changes: An Insider's View* 2002

➔ *CPT Assistant* Aug 02:10, Sep 04:12, Nov 08:10, Mar 09:10, Dec 11:15, Apr 12:17, May 13:12, Dec 15:18, Dec 16:16, Apr 17:9, Nov 19:13, Dec 19:12, Dec 23:38

Musculoskeletal 20100-29999

Surgery

The following is a listing of headings and subheadings that appear within the Respiratory System section of the CPT codebook. The subheadings or subsections denoted with asterisks (*) below have special instructions unique to that subsection. Where these are indicated, special notes or guidelines will be presented preceding those procedural terminology listings, referring to that subsection specifically. Note that all code ranges in each subsection are listed as they appear in the subsection, even if the code numbers are out of numerical sequence and/or repeated in the next subsection.

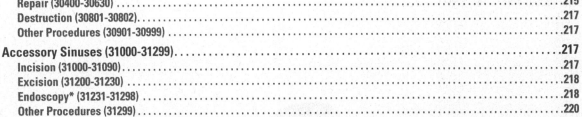

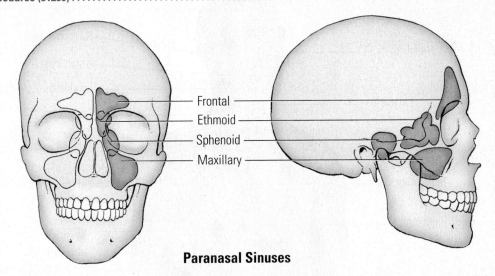

Paranasal Sinuses

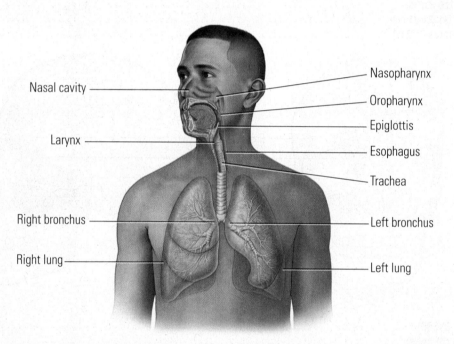

Respiratory System

Nasal cavity

Larynx

Right bronchus

Right lung

Nasopharynx

Oropharynx

Epiglottis

Esophagus

Trachea

Left bronchus

Left lung

Respiratory System

Nose

Incision

30000 Drainage abscess or hematoma, nasal, internal approach

(For external approach, see 10060, 10140)

30020 Drainage abscess or hematoma, nasal septum

(For lateral rhinotomy, see specific application [eg, 30118, 30320])

Excision

30100 Biopsy, intranasal

(For biopsy skin of nose, see 11102, 11103, 11104, 11105, 11106, 11107)

30110 Excision, nasal polyp(s), simple

(30110 would normally be completed in an office setting)

(To report bilateral procedure, use 30110 with modifier 50)

30115 Excision, nasal polyp(s), extensive

(30115 would normally require the facilities available in a hospital setting)

(To report bilateral procedure, use 30115 with modifier 50)

30117 Excision or destruction (eg, laser), intranasal lesion; internal approach
→ *CPT Changes: An Insider's View* 2002
→ *CPT Assistant* Jul 19:10, Nov 19:14, Sep 20:14, Jan 22:18, Feb 23:6, Dec 23:23

30118   external approach (lateral rhinotomy)
→ *CPT Changes: An Insider's View* 2002
→ *CPT Assistant* Dec 23:23

(For surgical nasal/sinus endoscopy with destruction by radiofrequency ablation of posterior nasal nerve, use 31242)

(For surgical nasal/sinus endoscopy with destruction by cryoablation of posterior nasal nerve, use 31243)

30120 Excision or surgical planing of skin of nose for rhinophyma
→ *CPT Assistant* May 07:9

30124 Excision dermoid cyst, nose; simple, skin, subcutaneous

30125   complex, under bone or cartilage

30130 Excision inferior turbinate, partial or complete, any method
→ *CPT Changes: An Insider's View* 2006
→ *CPT Assistant* Feb 98:11, Nov 98:11, Sep 01:10, May 03:5

(For excision of superior or middle turbinate, use 30999)

30140 Submucous resection inferior turbinate, partial or complete, any method
→ *CPT Changes: An Insider's View* 2006
→ *CPT Assistant* Nov 98:11, Dec 02:10, Apr 03:26, May 03:5, Dec 04:18, Mar 08:14, Jan 20:12

(Do not report 30130 or 30140 in conjunction with 30801, 30802, 30930)

(For submucous resection of superior or middle turbinate, use 30999)

(For endoscopic resection of concha bullosa of middle turbinate, use 31240)

(For submucous resection of nasal septum, use 30520)

30150 Rhinectomy; partial

30160   total

(For closure and/or reconstruction, primary or delayed, see **Integumentary System,** 13151-13160, 14060-14302, 15120, 15121, 15260, 15261, 15760, 20900-20912)

Introduction

30200 Injection into turbinate(s), therapeutic
→ *CPT Assistant* Dec 04:19

30210 Displacement therapy (Proetz type)

30220 Insertion, nasal septal prosthesis (button)

Removal of Foreign Body

30300 Removal foreign body, intranasal; office type procedure
→ *CPT Assistant* Jan 12:13

30310   requiring general anesthesia

30320   by lateral rhinotomy

Repair

(For obtaining tissues for graft, see 15769, 20900, 20902, 20910, 20912, 20920, 20922, 20924, 21210)

(For correction of nasal defects using fat harvested via liposuction technique, see 15773, 15774)

30400 Rhinoplasty, primary; lateral and alar cartilages and/or elevation of nasal tip

(For columellar reconstruction, see 13151 et seq)

30410   complete, external parts including bony pyramid, lateral and alar cartilages, and/or elevation of nasal tip
→ *CPT Assistant* Jan 21:13

Respiratory 30000-32999

30420   including major septal repair

➔ *CPT Assistant* Jul 16:8

30430   Rhinoplasty, secondary; minor revision (small amount of nasal tip work)

30435   intermediate revision (bony work with osteotomies)

30450   major revision (nasal tip work and osteotomies)

30460   Rhinoplasty for nasal deformity secondary to congenital cleft lip and/or palate, including columellar lengthening; tip only

➔ *CPT Assistant* Dec 14:18

30462   tip, septum, osteotomies

➔ *CPT Assistant* Dec 14:18

30465   Repair of nasal vestibular stenosis (eg, spreader grafting, lateral nasal wall reconstruction)

➔ *CPT Changes: An Insider's View* 2001

➔ *CPT Assistant* Sep 20:14, Feb 23:6, Mar 24:26

(Do not report 30465 in conjunction with 30468, 30469, when performed on the ipsilateral side)

(30465 excludes obtaining graft. For graft procedure, see 15769, 20900, 20902, 20910, 20912, 20920, 20922, 20924, 21210, 21235)

(For repair of nasal vestibular lateral wall collapse with subcutaneous/submucosal lateral wall implant[s], use 30468)

(For repair of nasal valve collapse with low energy, temperature-controlled [ie, radiofrequency] subcutaneous/submucosal remodeling, use 30469)

(30465 is used to report a bilateral procedure. For unilateral procedure, use modifier 52)

30468   Repair of nasal valve collapse with subcutaneous/ submucosal lateral wall implant(s)

➔ *CPT Changes: An Insider's View* 2021

➔ *CPT Assistant* Feb 23:6, Mar 24:26

(Do not report 30468 in conjunction with 30465, 30469, when performed on the ipsilateral side)

(For repair of nasal vestibular stenosis [eg, spreader grafting, lateral nasal wall reconstruction], use 30465)

(For repair of nasal vestibular stenosis or collapse without cartilage graft, lateral wall reconstruction, or subcutaneous/submucosal implant [eg, lateral wall suspension, or stenting without graft or subcutaneous/ submucosal implant], use 30999)

(30468 is used to report a bilateral procedure. For unilateral procedure, use modifier 52)

30469   Repair of nasal valve collapse with low energy, temperature-controlled (ie, radiofrequency) subcutaneous/submucosal remodeling

➔ *CPT Changes: An Insider's View* 2023

➔ *CPT Assistant* Feb 23:6

(Do not report 30469 in conjunction with 30465, 30468, when performed on the ipsilateral side)

(For repair of nasal vestibular stenosis [eg, spreader grafting, lateral nasal wall reconstruction], use 30465)

(For repair of nasal vestibular lateral wall collapse with subcutaneous/submucosal lateral wall implant[s], use 30468)

(For repair of nasal vestibular stenosis or collapse without cartilage graft, lateral wall reconstruction, or subcutaneous/submucosal implant [eg, lateral wall suspension or stenting without graft or subcutaneous/ submucosal implant], use 30999)

(30469 is used to report a bilateral procedure. For unilateral procedure, use modifier 52)

Surgical Repair of Vestibular Stenosis
30465

An incision is made in the upper lateral cartilage and continued as an osteotomy of the medial aspect of the nasal bones. The spreader graft is placed to widen the nasal vestibule.

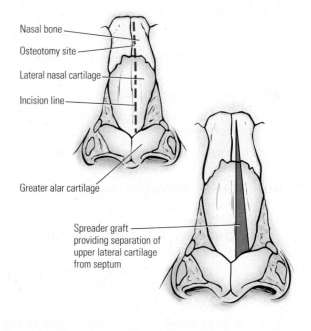

Nasal bone

Osteotomy site

Lateral nasal cartilage

Incision line

Greater alar cartilage

Spreader graft providing separation of upper lateral cartilage from septum

30520   Septoplasty or submucous resection, with or without cartilage scoring, contouring or replacement with graft

➔ *CPT Assistant* Oct 97:11, Dec 02:10, Mar 12:9, Jul 15:10, Jul 19:10, Jan 21:13, Feb 23:6, Jul 23:15

(For submucous resection of turbinates, use 30140)

30540   Repair choanal atresia; intranasal

30545   transpalatine

(Do not report modifier 63 in conjunction with 30540, 30545)

30560   Lysis intranasal synechia

30580   Repair fistula; oromaxillary (combine with 31030 if antrotomy is included)

30600   oronasal

30620   Septal or other intranasal dermatoplasty (does not include obtaining graft)

30630   Repair nasal septal perforations
→ *CPT Assistant* Aug 12:13

Destruction

30801   Ablation, soft tissue of inferior turbinates, unilateral or bilateral, any method (eg, electrocautery, radiofrequency ablation, or tissue volume reduction); superficial
→ *CPT Changes: An Insider's View* 2002, 2006, 2010
→ *CPT Assistant* Jul 19:10

(For ablation of superior or middle turbinates, use 30999)

30802   intramural (ie, submucosal)
→ *CPT Changes: An Insider's View* 2010
→ *CPT Assistant* Mar 08:14, Sep 10:10, Jul 19:10, Feb 23:6

(Do not report 30801 in conjunction with 30802)

(Do not report 30801, 30802, 30930 in conjunction with 30130 or 30140)

(For cautery performed for control of nasal hemorrhage, see 30901-30906)

Other Procedures

30901   Control nasal hemorrhage, anterior, simple (limited cautery and/or packing) any method
→ *CPT Assistant* Jul 20:13, Oct 20:13

(To report bilateral procedure, use 30901 with modifier 50)

30903   Control nasal hemorrhage, anterior, complex (extensive cautery and/or packing) any method

(To report bilateral procedure, use 30903 with modifier 50)

30905   Control nasal hemorrhage, posterior, with posterior nasal packs and/or cautery, any method; initial
→ *CPT Changes: An Insider's View* 2002
→ *CPT Assistant* Sep 10:7

30906   subsequent

30915   Ligation arteries; ethmoidal

30920   internal maxillary artery, transantral

(For ligation external carotid artery, use 37600)

30930   Fracture nasal inferior turbinate(s), therapeutic
→ *CPT Changes: An Insider's View* 2006
→ *CPT Assistant* Jul 01:11, Dec 02:10, Jul 03:15, Aug 03:14, Dec 04:18, Sep 10:10, Jul 16:8

(Do not report 30801, 30802, 30930 in conjunction with 30130 or 30140)

(For fracture of superior or middle turbinate[s], use 30999)

30999   Unlisted procedure, nose
→ *CPT Assistant* Feb 13:13, Nov 19:14, Sep 20:14, Jan 21:13, Jan 22:18, Feb 23:6

Accessory Sinuses

Incision

31000   Lavage by cannulation; maxillary sinus (antrum puncture or natural ostium)
→ *CPT Assistant* Apr 14:10

(To report bilateral procedure, use 31000 with modifier 50)

31002   sphenoid sinus

31020   Sinusotomy, maxillary (antrotomy); intranasal

(To report bilateral procedure, use 31020 with modifier 50)

31030   radical (Caldwell-Luc) without removal of antrochoanal polyps

(To report bilateral procedure, use 31030 with modifier 50)

31032   radical (Caldwell-Luc) with removal of antrochoanal polyps

(To report bilateral procedure, use 31032 with modifier 50)

31040   Pterygomaxillary fossa surgery, any approach

(For transantral ligation of internal maxillary artery, use 30920)

31050   Sinusotomy, sphenoid, with or without biopsy;

31051   with mucosal stripping or removal of polyp(s)

31070   Sinusotomy frontal; external, simple (trephine operation)

(For frontal intranasal sinusotomy, use 31276)

31075   transorbital, unilateral (for mucocele or osteoma, Lynch type)

31080   obliterative without osteoplastic flap, brow incision (includes ablation)

31081   obliterative, without osteoplastic flap, coronal incision (includes ablation)

31084   obliterative, with osteoplastic flap, brow incision

31085   obliterative, with osteoplastic flap, coronal incision

31086   nonobliterative, with osteoplastic flap, brow incision

31087   nonobliterative, with osteoplastic flap, coronal incision

Sinusotomy, Frontal
31070

A trephine is used to access the frontal sinus.

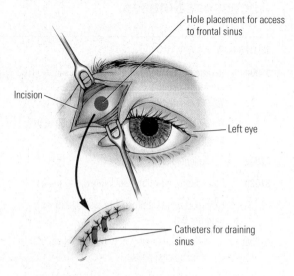

- Hole placement for access to frontal sinus
- Incision
- Left eye
- Catheters for draining sinus

31090 Sinusotomy, unilateral, 3 or more paranasal sinuses (frontal, maxillary, ethmoid, sphenoid)

➡ *CPT Assistant* Nov 97:15, Nov 98:11

Excision

31200 Ethmoidectomy; intranasal, anterior

➡ *CPT Assistant* Feb 16:10

31201 intranasal, total

➡ *CPT Assistant* Feb 16:10

31205 extranasal, total

➡ *CPT Assistant* Feb 16:10

31225 Maxillectomy; without orbital exenteration

31230 with orbital exenteration (en bloc)

(For orbital exenteration only, see 65110 et seq)

(For skin grafts, see 15120 et seq)

Endoscopy

A surgical sinus endoscopy includes a sinusotomy (when appropriate) and diagnostic endoscopy.

Codes 31295-31298 describe dilation of sinus ostia by displacement of tissue, any method, and include fluoroscopy if performed.

Stereotactic computer-assisted navigation may be used to facilitate the performance of endoscopic sinus surgery, and may be reported with 61782.

Codes 31233-31298 are used to report unilateral procedures unless otherwise specified.

Codes 31231-31235 for diagnostic evaluation refer to employing a nasal/sinus endoscope to inspect the interior of the nasal cavity and the middle and superior meatus, the turbinates, and the spheno-ethmoid recess. Any time a diagnostic evaluation is performed all these areas would be inspected and a separate code is not reported for each area. To report these services when all of the elements are not fully examined (eg, judged not clinically pertinent), or because the clinical situation precludes such exam (eg, technically unable, altered anatomy), append modifier 52 if repeat examination is not planned, or modifier 53 if repeat examination is planned.

31231 Nasal endoscopy, diagnostic, unilateral or bilateral (separate procedure)

➡ *CPT Assistant* Winter 93:22, Jan 97:4, Feb 16:10, Jan 17:6, Apr 18:3, Apr 21:12, Jul 21:3, Dec 23:23

31233 Nasal/sinus endoscopy, diagnostic; with maxillary sinusoscopy (via inferior meatus or canine fossa puncture)

➡ *CPT Changes: An Insider's View* 2020

➡ *CPT Assistant* Winter 93:22, Jan 97:4, Jun 11:11, Apr 18:3

(Do not report 31233 in conjunction with 31256, 31267, 31295, when performed on the ipsilateral side)

31235 with sphenoid sinusoscopy (via puncture of sphenoidal face or cannulation of ostium)

➡ *CPT Changes: An Insider's View* 2020

➡ *CPT Assistant* Winter 93:22, Jan 97:4, Apr 18:3

(Do not report 31235 in conjunction with 31257, 31259, 31287, 31288, 31297, 31298, when performed on the ipsilateral side)

(To report endoscopic placement of a drug-eluting implant in the ethmoid sinus without any other nasal/sinus endoscopic surgical service, use 31299. To report endoscopic placement of a drug-eluting implant in the ethmoid sinus in conjunction with biopsy, polypectomy, or debridement, use 31237)

31237 Nasal/sinus endoscopy, surgical; with biopsy, polypectomy or debridement (separate procedure)

➡ *CPT Assistant* Winter 93:23, Jan 97:4, Dec 01:6, May 03:5, Dec 11:13, Jan 15:13, Feb 16:10, Apr 18:3, Apr 19:10, Jul 19:7, Jan 20:12, Jul 21:3, Nov 21:13, Feb 23:6, Jul 23:15

(Do not report 31237 in conjunction with 31238, 31253, 31254, 31255, 31256, 31257, 31259, 31267, 31276, 31287, 31288, 31290, 31291, 31292, 31293, 31294, when performed on the ipsilateral side)

 # 31242 with destruction by radiofrequency ablation, posterior nasal nerve

➡ *CPT Changes: An Insider's View* 2024

➡ *CPT Assistant* Dec 23:39, Dec 23:23

Sinus Endoscopy
31231-31294

The physician uses an endoscope for visualizing and magnifying the internal structure of the sinuses.

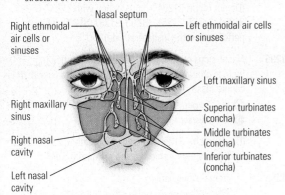

Right ethmoidal air cells or sinuses — Nasal septum — Left ethmoidal air cells or sinuses

Right maxillary sinus — Left maxillary sinus

Superior turbinates (concha)

Middle turbinates (concha)

Right nasal cavity — Inferior turbinates (concha)

Left nasal cavity

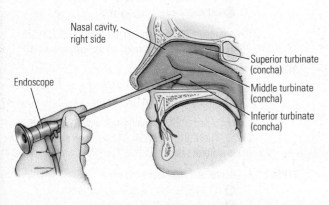

Nasal cavity, right side

Endoscope

Superior turbinate (concha)

Middle turbinate (concha)

Inferior turbinate (concha)

 # 31243 with destruction by cryoablation, posterior nasal nerve

→ *CPT Changes: An Insider's View* 2024

→ *CPT Assistant* Dec 23:23

(Do not report 31242, 31243 in conjunction with 31231, 92511)

(31242, 31243 are used to report bilateral procedures. For unilateral procedure, use modifier 52)

31238 with control of nasal hemorrhage

→ *CPT Changes: An Insider's View* 2002

→ *CPT Assistant* Winter 93:23, Jan 97:4, Apr 18:3

(Do not report 31238 in conjunction with 31237, 31241, when performed on the ipsilateral side)

31239 with dacryocystorhinostomy

→ *CPT Assistant* Winter 93:23, Jan 97:4, Apr 18:3

31240 with concha bullosa resection

→ *CPT Assistant* Winter 93:23, Jan 97:4, May 03:5, Feb 16:10, Apr 18:3

31241 with ligation of sphenopalatine artery

→ *CPT Changes: An Insider's View* 2018

→ *CPT Assistant* Apr 18:3

(Do not report 31241 in conjunction with 31238, when performed on the ipsilateral side)

31242 Code is out of numerical sequence. See 31235-31239

31243 Code is out of numerical sequence. See 31235-31239

31253 Code is out of numerical sequence. See 31254-31267

31254 Nasal/sinus endoscopy, surgical with ethmoidectomy; partial (anterior)

→ *CPT Changes: An Insider's View* 2018

→ *CPT Assistant* Winter 93:23, Jan 97:4, Sep 97:10, Oct 97:5, Dec 01:6, May 03:5, Jul 11:13, Feb 16:10, Apr 18:3

(Do not report 31254 in conjunction with 31237, 31253, 31255, 31257, 31259, 31290, 31291, 31292, 31293, 31294, when performed on the ipsilateral side)

31255   total (anterior and posterior)

→ *CPT Changes: An Insider's View* 2018

→ *CPT Assistant* Winter 93:23, Jan 97:4, Dec 02:10, May 03:5, Jul 11:13, Feb 16:10, Apr 18:4

(Do not report 31255 in conjunction with 31237, 31253, 31254, 31257, 31259, 31276, 31287, 31288, 31290, 31291, 31292, 31293, 31294, when performed on the ipsilateral side)

 # 31253   total (anterior and posterior), including frontal sinus exploration, with removal of tissue from frontal sinus, when performed

→ *CPT Changes: An Insider's View* 2018

→ *CPT Assistant* Apr 18:4, Apr 19:10, Dec 21:19

(Do not report 31253 in conjunction with 31237, 31254, 31255, 31276, 31290, 31291, 31292, 31293, 31294, 31296, 31298, when performed on the ipsilateral side)

 # 31257   total (anterior and posterior), including sphenoidotomy

→ *CPT Changes: An Insider's View* 2018

→ *CPT Assistant* Apr 18:4, Apr 19:10

(Do not report 31257 in conjunction with 31235, 31237, 31254, 31255, 31259, 31287, 31288, 31290, 31291, 31292, 31293, 31294, 31297, 31298, when performed on the ipsilateral side)

 # 31259   total (anterior and posterior), including sphenoidotomy, with removal of tissue from the sphenoid sinus

→ *CPT Changes: An Insider's View* 2018

→ *CPT Assistant* Apr 18:3, Apr 19:10, Dec 21:19

(Do not report 31259 in conjunction with 31235, 31237, 31254, 31255, 31257, 31287, 31288, 31290, 31291, 31292, 31293, 31294, 31297, 31298, when performed on the ipsilateral side)

31256 Nasal/sinus endoscopy, surgical, with maxillary antrostomy;

→ *CPT Assistant* Winter 93:23, Jan 97:4, Jun 11:11, Jul 11:13, Jun 13:13, Apr 18:11, Apr 19:10

(Do not report 31256 in conjunction with 31233, 31237, 31267, 31295, when performed on the ipsilateral side)

31257   Code is out of numerical sequence. See 31254-31267

31259   Code is out of numerical sequence. See 31254-31267

31267   with removal of tissue from maxillary sinus
> *CPT Assistant* Jan 97:4, Dec 01:6, Jun 11:11, Jul 11:13, Apr 18:3, Apr 19:10

(Do not report 31267 in conjunction with 31233, 31237, 31256, 31295, when performed on the ipsilateral side)

31276   Nasal/sinus endoscopy, surgical, with frontal sinus exploration, including removal of tissue from frontal sinus, when performed
> *CPT Changes: An Insider's View* 2018

> *CPT Assistant* Winter 93:24, Jan 97:4, Jan 10:11, Jun 11:13, Apr 18:4, Apr 19:10, Dec 21:19

(Do not report 31276 in conjunction with 31237, 31253, 31255, 31296, 31298, when performed on the ipsilateral side)

31287   Nasal/sinus endoscopy, surgical, with sphenoidotomy;
> *CPT Assistant* Winter 93:24, Jan 97:4, Jun 11:11, Apr 18:3, Apr 19:10

(Do not report 31287 in conjunction with 31235, 31237, 31255, 31257, 31259, 31288, 31291, 31294, 31297, 31298, when performed on the ipsilateral side)

31288   with removal of tissue from the sphenoid sinus
> *CPT Assistant* Winter 93:24, Jan 97:4, Jun 11:11, Feb 16:10, Apr 18:3, Apr 19:10

(Do not report 31288 in conjunction with 31235, 31237, 31255, 31257, 31259, 31287, 31291, 31294, 31297, 31298, when performed on the ipsilateral side)

31290   Nasal/sinus endoscopy, surgical, with repair of cerebrospinal fluid leak; ethmoid region
> *CPT Assistant* Winter 93:24, Jan 97:4, Jul 11:13, Feb 16:10, Apr 18:3

(Do not report 31290 in conjunction with 31237, 31253, 31254, 31255, 31257, 31259, when performed on the ipsilateral side)

31291   sphenoid region
> *CPT Assistant* Winter 93:24, Jan 97:4, Jul 11:13, Apr 18:3

(Do not report 31291 in conjunction with 31237, 31253, 31254, 31255, 31257, 31259, 31287, 31288, when performed on the ipsilateral side)

31292   Nasal/sinus endoscopy, surgical, with orbital decompression; medial or inferior wall
> *CPT Changes: An Insider's View* 2020

> *CPT Assistant* Winter 93:24, Jan 97:4, Jul 11:3, Apr 18:3

(Do not report 31292 in conjunction with 31237, 31253, 31254, 31255, 31257, 31259, 31293, 31296, when performed on the ipsilateral side)

31293   medial and inferior wall
> *CPT Changes: An Insider's View* 2020

> *CPT Assistant* Winter 93:24, Jan 97:4, Jul 11:13, Apr 18:3

(Do not report 31293 in conjunction with 31237, 31253, 31254, 31255, 31257, 31259, 31292, when performed on the ipsilateral side)

31294   Nasal/sinus endoscopy, surgical, with optic nerve decompression
> *CPT Changes: An Insider's View* 2020

> *CPT Assistant* Winter 93:24, Jan 97:4, Jul 11:13, Apr 18:3

(Do not report 31294 in conjunction with 31237, 31253, 31254, 31255, 31257, 31259, 31287, 31288, when performed on the ipsilateral side)

31295   Nasal/sinus endoscopy, surgical, with dilation (eg, balloon dilation); maxillary sinus ostium, transnasal or via canine fossa
> *CPT Changes: An Insider's View* 2011, 2020

> *CPT Assistant* Jun 11:11, Apr 18:3

(Do not report 31295 in conjunction with 31233, 31256, 31267, when performed on the ipsilateral side)

31296   frontal sinus ostium
> *CPT Changes: An Insider's View* 2011, 2020

> *CPT Assistant* Jun 11:11, Apr 18:3

(Do not report 31296 in conjunction with 31253, 31276, 31297, 31298, when performed on the ipsilateral side)

31297   sphenoid sinus ostium
> *CPT Changes: An Insider's View* 2011, 2020

> *CPT Assistant* Jun 11:11, Apr 18:3

(Do not report 31297 in conjunction with 31235, 31257, 31259, 31287, 31288, 31296, 31298, when performed on the ipsilateral side)

31298   frontal and sphenoid sinus ostia
> *CPT Changes: An Insider's View* 2018, 2020

> *CPT Assistant* Apr 18:3, Feb 23:6

(Do not report 31298 in conjunction with 31235, 31253, 31257, 31259, 31276, 31287, 31288, 31296, 31297, when performed on the ipsilateral side)

Other Procedures

(For hypophysectomy, transantral or transeptal approach, use 61548)

(For transcranial hypophysectomy, use 61546)

31299   Unlisted procedure, accessory sinuses
> *CPT Assistant* Jan 10:11, Jun 11:11, Jun 13:13, Jul 15:10, Feb 16:10, Apr 19:10, Jul 19:7, Dec 23:39

Respiratory 30000-32999

Larynx

Excision

31300 Laryngotomy (thyrotomy, laryngofissure), with removal of tumor or laryngocele, cordectomy

31360 Laryngectomy; total, without radical neck dissection
➔ *CPT Assistant* Aug 10:4

31365   total, with radical neck dissection
➔ *CPT Assistant* Oct 01:10, Aug 10:4

31367   subtotal supraglottic, without radical neck dissection
➔ *CPT Assistant* Aug 10:4

31368   subtotal supraglottic, with radical neck dissection

31370 Partial laryngectomy (hemilaryngectomy); horizontal

31375   laterovertical

31380   anterovertical

31382   antero-latero-vertical

31390 Pharyngolaryngectomy, with radical neck dissection; without reconstruction

31395   with reconstruction

31400 Arytenoidectomy or arytenoidopexy, external approach

(For endoscopic arytenoidectomy, use 31560)

31420 Epiglottidectomy

Introduction

31500 Intubation, endotracheal, emergency procedure
➔ *CPT Assistant* Nov 99:32-33, Oct 03:2, Aug 04:8, Jul 06:4, Jul 07:1, Dec 09:10, May 16:3, Oct 16:8, Jul 21:8

31502 Tracheotomy tube change prior to establishment of fistula tract
➔ *CPT Assistant* Winter 90:6, Dec 20:11

Endoscopy

For endoscopic procedures, report appropriate endoscopy of each anatomic site examined. Laryngoscopy includes examination of the tongue base, larynx, and hypopharynx. The anatomic structures examined with this procedure include both midline (single anatomic sites) and paired structures. Midline, single anatomic sites include tongue base, vallecula, epiglottis, subglottis, and posterior pharyngeal wall. Paired structures include true vocal cords, arytenoids, false vocal cords, ventricles, pyriform sinuses, and aryepiglottic folds. For the purposes of reporting therapeutic interventions, all paired structures contained within one side of the larynx/pharynx are considered unilateral. If using operating microscope, telescope, or both, use the applicable code only once per operative session.

31505 Laryngoscopy, indirect; diagnostic (separate procedure)
➔ *CPT Changes: An Insider's View* 2000
➔ *CPT Assistant* Nov 99:13

31510   with biopsy
➔ *CPT Assistant* Nov 99:13

31511   with removal of foreign body
➔ *CPT Assistant* Nov 99:13

31512   with removal of lesion
➔ *CPT Assistant* Nov 99:13

31513   with vocal cord injection
➔ *CPT Assistant* Nov 99:13

31515 Laryngoscopy direct, with or without tracheoscopy; for aspiration

31520   diagnostic, newborn

(Do not report modifier 63 in conjunction with 31520)

31525   diagnostic, except newborn
➔ *CPT Assistant* Aug 10:3

31526   diagnostic, with operating microscope or telescope
➔ *CPT Changes: An Insider's View* 2006
➔ *CPT Assistant* Nov 98:11-12, Jun 17:10

(Do not report 31526 in conjunction with 69990)

31527   with insertion of obturator

31528   with dilation, initial
➔ *CPT Changes: An Insider's View* 2002
➔ *CPT Assistant* May 21:14, Nov 23:24

31529   with dilation, subsequent
➔ *CPT Changes: An Insider's View* 2002
➔ *CPT Assistant* Nov 23:24

31530 Laryngoscopy, direct, operative, with foreign body removal;

31531   with operating microscope or telescope
➔ *CPT Changes: An Insider's View* 2006
➔ *CPT Assistant* Nov 98:11-12, Jun 17:10

(Do not report code 69990 in addition to code 31531)

31535 Laryngoscopy, direct, operative, with biopsy;

31536   with operating microscope or telescope
➔ *CPT Changes: An Insider's View* 2006
➔ *CPT Assistant* Nov 98:11-12, Jun 17:10, May 21:14

(Do not report code 69990 in addition to code 31536)

31540 Laryngoscopy, direct, operative, with excision of tumor and/or stripping of vocal cords or epiglottis;
➔ *CPT Assistant* Apr 22:13

31541 with operating microscope or telescope

➔ *CPT Changes: An Insider's View* 2006

➔ *CPT Assistant* Nov 98:11-12, Jun 17:10, Jul 19:10, Sep 19:10, Apr 22:13

(Do not report code 69990 in addition to code 31541)

31545 Laryngoscopy, direct, operative, with operating microscope or telescope, with submucosal removal of non-neoplastic lesion(s) of vocal cord; reconstruction with local tissue flap(s)

➔ *CPT Changes: An Insider's View* 2005

31546 reconstruction with graft(s) (includes obtaining autograft)

➔ *CPT Changes: An Insider's View* 2005

(Do not report 31546 in conjunction with 15769, 15771, 15772, 15773, 15774 for graft harvest)

(For reconstruction of vocal cord with allograft, use 31599)

(Do not report 31545 or 31546 in conjunction with 31540, 31541, 69990)

31551 Code is out of numerical sequence. See 31579-31587

31552 Code is out of numerical sequence. See 31579-31587

31553 Code is out of numerical sequence. See 31579-31587

31554 Code is out of numerical sequence. See 31579-31587

31560 Laryngoscopy, direct, operative, with arytenoidectomy;

➔ *CPT Assistant* Apr 22:13

31561 with operating microscope or telescope

➔ *CPT Changes: An Insider's View* 2006

➔ *CPT Assistant* Nov 98:11-12, Jun 17:10, Apr 22:13

(Do not report code 69990 in addition to code 31561)

31570 Laryngoscopy, direct, with injection into vocal cord(s), therapeutic;

➔ *CPT Assistant* Jan 14:6, Jan 17:6

31571 with operating microscope or telescope

➔ *CPT Changes: An Insider's View* 2006

➔ *CPT Assistant* Nov 98:11-12, Nov 12:14, Jan 14:6, Jan 17:6, Jun 17:10, May 21:14

(Do not report 31571 in conjunction with 69990)

31572 Code is out of numerical sequence. See 31577-31580

31573 Code is out of numerical sequence. See 31577-31580

31574 Code is out of numerical sequence. See 31577-31580

31575 Laryngoscopy, flexible; diagnostic

➔ *CPT Changes: An Insider's View* 2017

➔ *CPT Assistant* Dec 16:13, Apr 17:8, Jul 17:7, Dec 20:11, Dec 21:20, Mar 23:1

(Do not report 31575 in conjunction with 31231, unless performed for a separate condition using a separate endoscope)

(Do not report 31575 in conjunction with 31572, 31573, 31574, 31576, 31577, 31578, 42975, 43197, 43198, 92511, 92612, 92614, 92616)

31576 with biopsy(ies)

➔ *CPT Changes: An Insider's View* 2017

➔ *CPT Assistant* Dec 16:13, Apr 17:8, Jul 17:7

(Do not report 31576 in conjunction with 31572, 31578)

31577 with removal of foreign body(s)

➔ *CPT Changes: An Insider's View* 2017

➔ *CPT Assistant* Dec 16:13, Apr 17:8, Jul 17:7, Aug 23:20

31578 with removal of lesion(s), non-laser

➔ *CPT Changes: An Insider's View* 2017

➔ *CPT Assistant* Dec 16:13, Apr 17:8, Jul 17:7

 # 31572 with ablation or destruction of lesion(s) with laser, unilateral

➔ *CPT Changes: An Insider's View* 2017

➔ *CPT Assistant* Dec 16:13, Apr 17:8, Jul 17:7, Sep 19:10

(Do not report 31572 in conjunction with 31576, 31578)

(To report flexible endoscopic evaluation of swallowing, see 92612-92613)

(To report flexible endoscopic evaluation with sensory testing, see 92614-92615)

(To report flexible endoscopic evaluation of swallowing with sensory testing, see 92616-92617)

(For flexible laryngoscopy as part of flexible endoscopic evaluation of swallowing and/or laryngeal sensory testing by cine or video recording, see 92612-92617)

 # 31573 with therapeutic injection(s) (eg, chemodenervation agent or corticosteroid, injected percutaneous, transoral, or via endoscope channel), unilateral

➔ *CPT Changes: An Insider's View* 2017

➔ *CPT Assistant* Dec 16:13, Apr 17:8, Jul 17:7, May 18:7

 # 31574 with injection(s) for augmentation (eg, percutaneous, transoral), unilateral

➔ *CPT Changes: An Insider's View* 2017

➔ *CPT Assistant* Dec 16:13, Apr 17:8, Jul 17:7, May 18:7

31579 Laryngoscopy, flexible or rigid telescopic, with stroboscopy

➔ *CPT Changes: An Insider's View* 2017

➔ *CPT Assistant* Dec 16:13, Apr 17:8, Jul 17:7

Repair

31580 Laryngoplasty; for laryngeal web, with indwelling keel or stent insertion

➔ *CPT Changes: An Insider's View* 2017

➔ *CPT Assistant* Mar 17:10, Apr 17:5

(Do not report 31580 in conjunction with 31551, 31552, 31553, 31554)

★ = Telemedicine ◀ = Audio-only ✚ = Add-on code ⁄ = FDA approval pending # = Resequenced code ⊘ = Modifier 51 exempt ➔➔➔ = See p xxi for details

(To report tracheostomy, see 31600, 31601, 31603, 31605, 31610)

(To report removal of the keel or stent, use 31599)

 # 31551   for laryngeal stenosis, with graft, without indwelling stent placement, younger than 12 years of age
➔ *CPT Changes: An Insider's View* 2017
➔ *CPT Assistant* Mar 17:10, Apr 17:5, Jul 17:7

(Do not report graft separately if harvested through the laryngoplasty incision [eg, thyroid cartilage graft])

(Do not report 31551 in conjunction with 31552, 31553, 31554, 31580)

(To report tracheostomy, see 31600, 31601, 31603, 31605, 31610)

 # 31552   for laryngeal stenosis, with graft, without indwelling stent placement, age 12 years or older
➔ *CPT Changes: An insider's View* 2017
➔ *CPT Assistant* Mar 17:10, Apr 17:5, Jul 17:7

(Do not report graft separately if harvested through the laryngoplasty incision [eg, thyroid cartilage graft])

(Do not report 31552 in conjunction with 31551, 31553, 31554, 31580)

(To report tracheostomy, see 31600, 31601, 31603, 31605, 31610)

 # 31553   for laryngeal stenosis, with graft, with indwelling stent placement, younger than 12 years of age
➔ *CPT Changes: An Insider's View* 2017
➔ *CPT Assistant* Mar 17:10, Apr 17:5, Jul 17:7

(Do not report graft separately if harvested through the laryngoplasty incision [eg, thyroid cartilage graft])

(Do not report 31553 in conjunction with 31551, 31552, 31554, 31580)

(To report tracheostomy, see 31600, 31601, 31603, 31605, 31610)

(To report removal of the stent, use 31599)

 # 31554   for laryngeal stenosis, with graft, with indwelling stent placement, age 12 years or older
➔ *CPT Changes: An Insider's View* 2017
➔ *CPT Assistant* Mar 17:10, Apr 17:5, Jul 17:7

(Do not report graft separately if harvested through the laryngoplasty incision [eg, thyroid cartilage graft])

(Do not report 31554 in conjunction with 31551, 31552, 31553, 31580)

(To report tracheostomy, see 31600, 31601, 31603, 31605, 31610)

(To report removal of the stent, use 31599)

31584   with open reduction and fixation of (eg, plating) fracture, includes tracheostomy, if performed
➔ *CPT Changes: An Insider's View* 2017
➔ *CPT Assistant* Mar 17:10, Apr 17:5

(Do not report graft separately if harvested through the laryngoplasty incision [eg, thyroid cartilage graft])

31587   Laryngoplasty, cricoid split, without graft placement
➔ *CPT Changes: An Insider's View* 2017
➔ *CPT Assistant* Mar 17:10, Apr 17:5

(To report tracheostomy, see 31600, 31601, 31603, 31605, 31610)

31590   Laryngeal reinnervation by neuromuscular pedicle
➔ *CPT Assistant* Mar 17:10

31591   Laryngoplasty, medialization, unilateral
➔ *CPT Changes: An Insider's View* 2017
➔ *CPT Assistant* Mar 17:10, Apr 17:5, Jul 17:7

31592   Cricotracheal resection
➔ *CPT Changes: An Insider's View* 2017
➔ *CPT Assistant* Feb 17:14, Mar 17:10, Apr 17:5, Jul 17:7

(Do not report graft separately if harvested through cricotracheal resection incision [eg, trachealis muscle])

(Do not report local advancement and rotational flaps separately if performed through the same incision)

(To report tracheostomy, see 31600, 31601, 31603, 31605, 31610)

(To report excision of tracheal stenosis and anastomosis, see 31780, 31781)

Other Procedures

31599   Unlisted procedure, larynx
➔ *CPT Assistant* Nov 12:14, Jan 17:6, Apr 22:13, Jul 22:18

Trachea and Bronchi

Incision

31600   Tracheostomy, planned (separate procedure);
➔ *CPT Assistant* Aug 10:5, Sep 19:10, Dec 20:12, Jul 23:1

31601   younger than 2 years
➔ *CPT Assistant* Dec 20:12

31603   Tracheostomy, emergency procedure; transtracheal
➔ *CPT Assistant* Dec 20:12

31605   cricothyroid membrane

31610   Tracheostomy, fenestration procedure with skin flaps
➔ *CPT Assistant* Dec 20:12

(For endotracheal intubation, use 31500)

(For tracheal aspiration under direct vision, use 31515)

31611   Construction of tracheoesophageal fistula and subsequent insertion of an alaryngeal speech prosthesis (eg, voice button, Blom-Singer prosthesis)

31612 Tracheal puncture, percutaneous with transtracheal aspiration and/or injection

31613 Tracheostoma revision; simple, without flap rotation

31614 complex, with flap rotation

Endoscopy

For endoscopy procedures, code appropriate endoscopy of each anatomic site examined. Surgical bronchoscopy always includes diagnostic bronchoscopy when performed by the same physician. Codes 31622-31651, 31660, 31661 include fluoroscopic guidance, when performed.

Codes 31652 and 31653 are complete services used for sampling (eg, aspiration/biopsy) lymph node(s) or adjacent structure(s) utilizing endobronchial ultrasound (EBUS) and are reported separately. Code 31654 is an add-on code and should be reported for identifying one or more peripheral lesion(s) with transendoscopic ultrasound.

31615 Tracheobronchoscopy through established tracheostomy incision

➤ *CPT Changes: An Insider's View* 2017

➤ *CPT Assistant* Feb 10:6, Nov 12:14, Dec 20:11, Aug 21:14

(For tracheoscopy, see laryngoscopy codes 31515-31574)

(For bronchoscopy with endobronchial ultrasound [EBUS] guided transtracheal/transbronchial sampling of mediastinal and/or hilar lymph node stations or structures, see 31652, 31653. For transendoscopic ultrasound during bronchoscopic diagnostic or therapeutic intervention[s] for peripheral lesion[s], use 31654)

31622 Bronchoscopy, rigid or flexible, including fluoroscopic guidance, when performed; diagnostic, with cell washing, when performed (separate procedure)

➤ *CPT Changes: An Insider's View* 2004, 2010, 2017

➤ *CPT Assistant* Jul 96:11, Nov 98:12, Dec 98:8, Mar 99:3, Apr 00:10, Jun 01:10, Jan 02:10, Sep 04:8, 12, Aug 05:4, Dec 09:10, Feb 10:6, Apr 10:5, Feb 11:8, Jun 23:21

31623 with brushing or protected brushings

➤ *CPT Changes: An Insider's View* 2017

➤ *CPT Assistant* Nov 98:12, Mar 99:3, Nov 99:13, Jan 02:10, Sep 04:8, Aug 05:4, May 08:15, Apr 10:5, Mar 13:8, Apr 21:8, Jun 23:21

31624 with bronchial alveolar lavage

➤ *CPT Changes: An Insider's View* 2017

➤ *CPT Assistant* Nov 98:12, Feb 99:9, Mar 99:3, 11, Jan 02:10, Sep 04:8, Aug 05:4, May 08:15, Feb 10:6, Apr 10:5, Mar 13:8, Jun 17:10, Aug 21:14, Jun 23:21

31625 with bronchial or endobronchial biopsy(s), single or multiple sites

➤ *CPT Changes: An Insider's View* 2004, 2017

➤ *CPT Assistant* Spring 91:2, Jan 02:10, Jun 02:10, Sep 03:15, Sep 04:9, Aug 05:4, Feb 10:6, Apr 10:5, Mar 13:8, Apr 21:8, Sep 21:14, Jun 23:21

31626 with placement of fiducial markers, single or multiple

➤ *CPT Changes: An Insider's View* 2010, 2017

➤ *CPT Assistant* Feb 10:6, Apr 10:5, Jan 11:6, Mar 13:8, Jun 15:6, Jun 17:10, Jun 23:21, Oct 23:21

(Report supply of device separately)

+ 31627 with computer-assisted, image-guided navigation (List separately in addition to code for primary procedure[s])

➤ *CPT Changes: An Insider's View* 2010, 2017

➤ *CPT Assistant* Feb 10:6, Apr 10:5, Jan 11:6, Mar 13:8, Jun 23:21

(31627 includes 3D reconstruction. Do not report 31627 in conjunction with 76376, 76377)

(Use 31627 in conjunction with 31615, 31622-31626, 31628-31631, 31635, 31636, 31638-31643)

31628 with transbronchial lung biopsy(s), single lobe

➤ *CPT Changes: An Insider's View* 2004, 2017

➤ *CPT Assistant* Jun 01:10, Jan 02:10, Sep 04:9, Aug 05:4, May 08:15, Feb 10:6, Apr 10:5, Mar 13:8, Jun 17:10, Mar 21:10, Apr 21:9, Sep 21:14, Jun 23:21, Dec 23:39

(31628 should be reported only once regardless of how many transbronchial lung biopsies are performed in a lobe)

(To report transbronchial lung biopsies performed on additional lobe, use 31632)

31629 with transbronchial needle aspiration biopsy(s), trachea, main stem and/or lobar bronchus(i)

➤ *CPT Changes: An Insider's View* 2004, 2017

➤ *CPT Assistant* Apr 00:10, Jan 02:10, Sep 03:15, May 04:15, Jul 04:13, Aug 05:4, Nov 09:8, Feb 10:6, Apr 10:5, Apr 11:12, Mar 13:8, Mar 21:10, Apr 21:9, Sep 21:14, Jun 23:21

(31629 should be reported only once for upper airway biopsies regardless of how many transbronchial needle aspiration biopsies are performed in the upper airway or in a lobe)

(To report transbronchial needle aspiration biopsies performed on additional lobe[s], use 31633)

31630 with tracheal/bronchial dilation or closed reduction of fracture

➤ *CPT Changes: An Insider's View* 2005

➤ *CPT Assistant* Jan 02:10, Aug 05:4, Feb 10:6, Apr 10:5, Mar 13:8, Jun 23:21

31631 with placement of tracheal stent(s) (includes tracheal/bronchial dilation as required)

➤ *CPT Changes: An Insider's View* 2005

➤ *CPT Assistant* Jan 02:10, Aug 05:4, Feb 10:6, Apr 10:5, Mar 13:8, Jun 23:21

(For placement of bronchial stent, see 31636, 31637)

(For revision of tracheal/bronchial stent, use 31638)

224 ★ = Telemedicine ◀ = Audio-only + = Add-on code ✔ = FDA approval pending # = Resequenced code ⊘ = Modifier 51 exempt ➤➤➤ = See p xxi for details

Respiratory 30000-32999

+ 31632   with transbronchial lung biopsy(s), each additional lobe (List separately in addition to code for primary procedure)

➔ *CPT Changes: An Insider's View* 2004, 2016, 2017

➔ *CPT Assistant* Jan 02:10, Sep 04:9, Aug 05:4, Mar 13:8, Apr 21:8, Sep 21:14, Jun 23:21, Dec 23:39

(Use 31632 in conjunction with 31628)

(31632 should be reported only once regardless of how many transbronchial lung biopsies are performed in a lobe)

+ 31633   with transbronchial needle aspiration biopsy(s), each additional lobe (List separately in addition to code for primary procedure)

➔ *CPT Changes: An Insider's View* 2004, 2016, 2017

➔ *CPT Assistant* Jan 02:10, May 04:15, Jul 04:13, Sep 04:10, Aug 05:4, Nov 09:8, Apr 11:12, Mar 13:8, Apr 21:8, Sep 21:14, Jun 23:21

(Use 31633 in conjunction with 31629)

(31633 should be reported only once regardless of how many transbronchial needle aspiration biopsies are performed in the trachea or the additional lobe)

31634   with balloon occlusion, with assessment of air leak, with administration of occlusive substance (eg, fibrin glue), if performed

➔ *CPT Changes: An Insider's View* 2011, 2017

➔ *CPT Assistant* Jan 11:6, Mar 13:8, Jun 23:21, Dec 23:39

(Do not report 31634 in conjunction with 31647, 31651 at the same session)

31635   with removal of foreign body

➔ *CPT Changes: An Insider's View* 2017

➔ *CPT Assistant* Jan 02:10, Jun 02:10, Feb 10:6, Apr 10:5, Jan 11:6, Mar 13:8, Jun 23:21

(For removal of implanted bronchial valves, see 31648-31649)

31636   with placement of bronchial stent(s) (includes tracheal/bronchial dilation as required), initial bronchus

➔ *CPT Changes: An Insider's View* 2005

➔ *CPT Assistant* Aug 05:4, Apr 10:5, Mar 13:8, Jun 23:21

+ 31637   each additional major bronchus stented (List separately in addition to code for primary procedure)

➔ *CPT Changes: An Insider's View* 2005

➔ *CPT Assistant* Aug 05:4, Mar 13:8, Jun 23:21

(Use 31637 in conjunction with 31636)

31638   with revision of tracheal or bronchial stent inserted at previous session (includes tracheal/bronchial dilation as required)

➔ *CPT Changes: An Insider's View* 2005

➔ *CPT Assistant* Aug 05:4, Apr 10:5, Mar 13:8, Jun 23:21

31640   with excision of tumor

➔ *CPT Assistant* Jan 02:10, Aug 05:4, Apr 10:5, Mar 13:8, Jun 23:21

31641   with destruction of tumor or relief of stenosis by any method other than excision (eg, laser therapy, cryotherapy)

➔ *CPT Changes: An Insider's View* 2002, 2010

➔ *CPT Assistant* Nov 99:13, Sep 00:5, Jan 02:10, Aug 05:4, Apr 10:5, Oct 11:11, Mar 13:8, Apr 13:8, Jun 23:21

(For bronchoscopic photodynamic therapy, report 31641 in addition to 96570, 96571 as appropriate)

31643   with placement of catheter(s) for intracavitary radioelement application

➔ *CPT Changes: An Insider's View* 2010

➔ *CPT Assistant* Nov 98:12, Mar 99:3, Jan 02:10, Aug 05:4, Apr 09:3, Mar 13:8, Jun 23:21

(For intracavitary radioelement application, see 77761-77763, 77770, 77771, 77772)

31645   with therapeutic aspiration of tracheobronchial tree, initial

➔ *CPT Changes: An Insider's View* 2010, 2017, 2018

➔ *CPT Assistant* Jan 02:10, Aug 05:4, Mar 13:8, Jun 23:21

31646   with therapeutic aspiration of tracheobronchial tree, subsequent, same hospital stay

➔ *CPT Changes: An Insider's View* 2010, 2017, 2018

➔ *CPT Assistant* Jan 02:10, Aug 05:4, Mar 13:8, Jun 23:21, 27

(For catheter aspiration of tracheobronchial tree with fiberscope at bedside, use 31725)

31647   with balloon occlusion, when performed, assessment of air leak, airway sizing, and insertion of bronchial valve(s), initial lobe

➔ *CPT Changes: An Insider's View* 2013, 2017

➔ *CPT Assistant* Mar 13:8, Jun 23:21

#+ 31651   with balloon occlusion, when performed, assessment of air leak, airway sizing, and insertion of bronchial valve(s), each additional lobe (List separately in addition to code for primary procedure[s])

➔ *CPT Changes: An Insider's View* 2013, 2017

➔ *CPT Assistant* Mar 13:8, Sep 18:3, Jun 23:21

(Use 31651 in conjunction with 31647)

31648   with removal of bronchial valve(s), initial lobe

➔ *CPT Changes: An Insider's View* 2013, 2017

➔ *CPT Assistant* Mar 13:8, Sep 18:3, Jun 23:21

(For removal and insertion of a bronchial valve at the same session, see 31647, 31648, and 31651)

Respiratory 30000-32999

+ 31649   with removal of bronchial valve(s), each additional lobe (List separately in addition to code for primary procedure)

> *CPT Changes: An Insider's View* 2013, 2017

> *CPT Assistant* Mar 13:8, Sep 18:3, Jun 23:21

(Use 31649 in conjunction with 31648)

31651   Code is out of numerical sequence. See 31646-31649

31652   with endobronchial ultrasound (EBUS) guided transtracheal and/or transbronchial sampling (eg, aspiration[s]/biopsy[ies]), one or two mediastinal and/or hilar lymph node stations or structures

> *CPT Changes: An Insider's View* 2016, 2017

> *CPT Assistant* Apr 16:5, Apr 21:7, Sep 21:14, Jun 23:21

31653   with endobronchial ultrasound (EBUS) guided transtracheal and/or transbronchial sampling (eg, aspiration[s]/biopsy[ies]), 3 or more mediastinal and/or hilar lymph node stations or structures

> *CPT Changes: An Insider's View* 2016, 2017

> *CPT Assistant* Apr 16:5, Apr 21:8, Sep 21:14, Jun 23:21

+ 31654   with transendoscopic endobronchial ultrasound (EBUS) during bronchoscopic diagnostic or therapeutic intervention(s) for peripheral lesion(s) (List separately in addition to code for primary procedure[s])

> *CPT Changes: An Insider's View* 2016, 2017

> *CPT Assistant* Apr 16:5, Apr 21:8, Sep 21:14, Jun 23:21

(Use 31654 in conjunction with 31622, 31623, 31624, 31625, 31626, 31628, 31629, 31640, 31643, 31645, 31646)

(For EBUS to access mediastinal or hilar lymph node station[s] or adjacent structure[s], see 31652, 31653)

(Report 31652, 31653, 31654 only once per session)

Bronchial Thermoplasty

31660   Bronchoscopy, rigid or flexible, including fluoroscopic guidance, when performed; with bronchial thermoplasty, 1 lobe

> *CPT Changes: An Insider's View* 2013, 2017

> *CPT Assistant* Mar 13:8, Jun 23:21

31661   with bronchial thermoplasty, 2 or more lobes

> *CPT Changes: An Insider's View* 2013, 2017

> *CPT Assistant* Mar 13:8, Jun 23:21

(For radiofrequency destruction of pulmonary nerves of the bronchi, see 0781T, 0782T)

Bronchoscopy
31622-31661

A rigid or flexible bronchoscope is inserted through the oropharynx and vocal cords and beyond the trachea into the right or left bronchi.

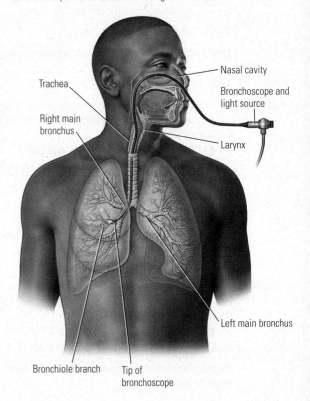

Nasal cavity

Bronchoscope and light source

Trachea

Right main bronchus

Larynx

Left main bronchus

Bronchiole branch   Tip of bronchoscope

Introduction

(For endotracheal intubation, use 31500)

(For tracheal aspiration under direct vision, see 31515)

31717   Catheterization with bronchial brush biopsy

> *CPT Assistant* Feb 01:11

31720   Catheter aspiration (separate procedure); nasotracheal

31725   tracheobronchial with fiberscope, bedside

> *CPT Changes: An Insider's View* 2017

31730   Transtracheal (percutaneous) introduction of needle wire dilator/stent or indwelling tube for oxygen therapy

Excision, Repair

31750   Tracheoplasty; cervical

> *CPT Assistant* Jul 11:12

31755   tracheopharyngeal fistulization, each stage

31760	intrathoracic
31766	Carinal reconstruction
31770	Bronchoplasty; graft repair
31775	excision stenosis and anastomosis

(For lobectomy and bronchoplasty, use 32501)

31780	Excision tracheal stenosis and anastomosis; cervical

➲ *CPT Assistant* Feb 17:14

31781	cervicothoracic

➲ *CPT Assistant* Feb 17:14

31785	Excision of tracheal tumor or carcinoma; cervical
31786	thoracic
31800	Suture of tracheal wound or injury; cervical
31805	intrathoracic
31820	Surgical closure tracheostomy or fistula; without plastic repair
31825	with plastic repair

(For repair tracheoesophageal fistula, see 43305, 43312)

31830	Revision of tracheostomy scar

Other Procedures

31899	Unlisted procedure, trachea, bronchi

➲ *CPT Assistant* Jan 10:11, May 14:10, Dec 20:11, Jun 23:21

Lungs and Pleura

Pleural cavity or lung biopsy procedures may be accomplished using a percutaneous, thoracoscopic (Video-Assisted Thoracoscopic Surgery [VATS]), or thoracotomy approach. They involve the removal of differing amounts of tissue for diagnosis. A biopsy may be performed using different techniques such as incision or wedge. Lung resection procedures include diagnostic and therapeutic procedures, including the removal of blebs, bullae, cysts, and benign or malignant tumors or lesions. These procedures may involve the removal of small portions of the lung or even an entire lung. Additionally, lung resection procedures may require the removal of adjacent structures. Both diagnostic lung biopsies and therapeutic lung resections can be performed utilizing a wedge technique. However, a diagnostic biopsy of a lung nodule using a wedge technique requires only that a tissue sample be obtained without particular attention to resection margins. A therapeutic wedge resection requires attention to margins and complete resection even when the wedge resection is ultimately followed by a more extensive resection. In the case of a wedge resection in which intraoperative pathology consultation determines that a more extensive resection is required in the same anatomic location, it becomes classified as a diagnostic wedge resection (32507, 32668). When no more extensive resection is required, the same procedure is a therapeutic wedge resection (32505, 32666).

Pleural or lung biopsies or diagnostic wedge resections should be reported using codes 32096, 32097, 32098, 32400, 32408, 32507, 32607, 32608, 32609, or 32668. The open or thoracoscopic (VATS) therapeutic resection of lung mass or nodules via a wedge resection is reported using codes 32505, 32506, 32666, and 32667. More extensive anatomic lung resection procedures, which can be performed with either thoracotomy or thoracoscopic (VATS) approaches, include: segmentectomy, lobectomy, bilobectomy, and pneumonectomy.

When diagnostic biopsy(ies) of the lung are performed, regardless of the approach (ie, open or thoracoscopic [VATS]) or technique (eg, incisional resection, cautery resection, or stapled wedge), and the specimen is sent for intraoperative pathology consultation, and during that same operative session the surgeon uses these results to determine the extent of the necessary surgical resection that includes the anatomical location biopsied, only the most extensive procedure performed (eg, segmentectomy, lobectomy, thoracoscopic [VATS] lobectomy) should be reported.

The therapeutic wedge resection codes (32505, 32506, 32666, or 32667) should not be reported in addition to the more extensive lung procedure (eg, lobectomy) unless the therapeutic wedge resection was performed on a different lobe or on the contralateral lung, whether or not an intraoperative pathology consultation is used to determine the extent of lung resection. When a diagnostic wedge resection is followed by a more extensive procedure in the same anatomical location, report add-on codes 32507 or 32668 with the more extensive procedure(s). When a therapeutic wedge resection (32505, 32506, 32666, or 32667) is performed in a different lobe than the more extensive lung resection (eg, lobectomy), report the therapeutic wedge resection with modifier 59.

Incision

32035	Thoracostomy; with rib resection for empyema
32036	with open flap drainage for empyema

(To report wound exploration due to penetrating trauma without thoracotomy, use 20101)

32096	Thoracotomy, with diagnostic biopsy(ies) of lung infiltrate(s) (eg, wedge, incisional), unilateral

➲ *CPT Changes: An Insider's View* 2012

➲ *CPT Assistant* Sep 12:3

(Do not report 32096 more than once per lung)

(Do not report 32096 in conjunction with 32440, 32442, 32445, 32488)

Respiratory 30000-32999

32097 Thoracotomy, with diagnostic biopsy(ies) of lung nodule(s) or mass(es) (eg, wedge, incisional), unilateral

➡ *CPT Changes: An Insider's View* 2012
➡ *CPT Assistant* Sep 12:3

(Do not report 32097 more than once per lung)

(Do not report 32097 in conjunction with 32440, 32442, 32445, 32488)

32098 Thoracotomy, with biopsy(ies) of pleura

➡ *CPT Changes: An Insider's View* 2012
➡ *CPT Assistant* Sep 12:3

32100 Thoracotomy; with exploration

➡ *CPT Changes: An Insider's View* 2012
➡ *CPT Assistant* Mar 07:1, Sep 12:3, Jan 13:6

(Do not report 32100 in conjunction with 21601, 21602, 21603, 32503, 32504, 33955, 33956, 33957, 33963, 33964)

32110 with control of traumatic hemorrhage and/or repair of lung tear

➡ *CPT Changes: An Insider's View* 2012
➡ *CPT Assistant* Sep 12:3

32120 for postoperative complications

➡ *CPT Changes: An Insider's View* 2012

32124 with open intrapleural pneumonolysis

➡ *CPT Changes: An Insider's View* 2012
➡ *CPT Assistant* Sep 12:3

32140 with cyst(s) removal, includes pleural procedure when performed

➡ *CPT Changes: An Insider's View* 2012
➡ *CPT Assistant* Sep 12:3

32141 with resection-plication of bullae, includes any pleural procedure when performed

➡ *CPT Changes: An Insider's View* 2012
➡ *CPT Assistant* Sep 12:3

(For lung volume reduction, use 32491)

32150 with removal of intrapleural foreign body or fibrin deposit

➡ *CPT Changes: An Insider's View* 2012
➡ *CPT Assistant* Sep 12:3

32151 with removal of intrapulmonary foreign body

➡ *CPT Changes: An Insider's View* 2012

32160 with cardiac massage

➡ *CPT Changes: An Insider's View* 2012

(For segmental or other resections of lung, see 32480-32504)

32200 Pneumonostomy, with open drainage of abscess or cyst

➡ *CPT Assistant* Nov 97:15

(For percutaneous image-guided drainage of abscess or cyst of lungs or mediastinum by catheter placement, use 49405)

32215 Pleural scarification for repeat pneumothorax

32220 Decortication, pulmonary (separate procedure); total

32225 partial

Excision/Resection

32310 Pleurectomy, parietal (separate procedure)

32320 Decortication and parietal pleurectomy

32400 Biopsy, pleura, percutaneous needle

➡ *CPT Assistant* Fall 94:1-2
➡ *Clinical Examples in Radiology* Summer 08:5-6, Winter 17:5

(If imaging guidance is performed, see 76942, 77002, 77012, 77021)

(For fine needle aspiration biopsy, see 10004, 10005, 10006, 10007, 10008, 10009, 10010, 10011, 10012, 10021)

A **core needle biopsy** is typically performed with a needle that is designed to obtain a core sample of tissue for histopathologic evaluation. A **fine needle aspiration** (FNA) biopsy is performed when material is aspirated with a fine needle and the cells are examined cytologically.

A core needle biopsy of the lung or mediastinum is most commonly performed with imaging guidance (ie, ultrasound, fluoroscopy, CT, MRI). Imaging guidance codes (ie, 76942, 77002, 77012, 77021) may not be reported separately with 32408. Code 32408 is reported once per lesion sampled in a single session.

Code 32408 includes all imaging guidance regardless of the number of imaging modalities used on the same lesion during the same session.

When more than one core needle biopsy of the lung or mediastinum with imaging guidance is performed on separate lesions at the same session on the same day, use 32408 once for each lesion with modifier 59 for the second and each additional core needle lung or mediastinal biopsy.

When a core needle biopsy of the lung or mediastinum with imaging guidance is performed at the same session as a core biopsy of a site other than the lung or mediastinum (eg, liver), both the core needle biopsy for the other site (eg, 47000) and the imaging guidance for that additional core needle biopsy may be reported separately with modifier 59.

When FNA biopsy and core needle biopsy of the lung or mediastinum are performed on the same lesion at the same session on the same day using the same type of imaging guidance, modifier 52 should be used with either the FNA biopsy code or the core lung or mediastinal biopsy code.

Respiratory 30000-32999

When FNA biopsy and core needle biopsy of the lung or mediastinum are performed on the same lesion at the same session on the same day using different types of imaging guidance, both image-guided biopsy codes may be reported separately and one of them should be appended with modifier 59.

When FNA biopsy is performed on one lesion and core needle biopsy of the lung or mediastinum is performed on a separate lesion at the same session on the same day using the same type of imaging guidance, both the modality-specific image-guided FNA biopsy code and 32408 may be reported separately and one of the codes should be appended with modifier 59.

When FNA biopsy is performed on one lesion and core needle biopsy of the lung or mediastinum is performed on a separate lesion at the same session on the same day using different types of imaging guidance, both the modality-specific image-guided FNA biopsy code and 32408 may be reported separately and one of the codes should be appended with modifier 59.

32408 Core needle biopsy, lung or mediastinum, percutaneous, including imaging guidance, when performed

➔ *CPT Changes: An Insider's View* 2021

➔ *CPT Assistant* Apr 21:10, Sep 21:14

➔ *Clinical Examples in Radiology* Fall 20:3-4, Summer 21:12

(Do not report 32408 in conjunction with 76942, 77002, 77012, 77021)

(For open biopsy of lung, see 32096, 32097. For open biopsy of mediastinum, see 39000 or 39010. For thoracoscopic [VATS] biopsy of lung, pleura, pericardium, or mediastinal space structure, see 32604, 32606, 32607, 32608, 32609)

(For fine needle aspiration biopsy, see 10004, 10005, 10006, 10007, 10008, 10009, 10010, 10011, 10012, 10021)

Removal

32440 Removal of lung, pneumonectomy;

➔ *CPT Changes: An Insider's View* 2012

➔ *CPT Assistant* Fall 94:1, Sep 12:3

32442 with resection of segment of trachea followed by broncho-tracheal anastomosis (sleeve pneumonectomy)

➔ *CPT Changes: An Insider's View* 2012

➔ *CPT Assistant* Fall 94:1, 3, Jun 17:10

32445 extrapleural

➔ *CPT Changes: An Insider's View* 2012

➔ *CPT Assistant* Fall 94:1, 3, Sep 12:3

(For extrapleural pneumonectomy, with empyemectomy, use 32445 and 32540)

(If lung resection is performed with chest wall tumor resection, report the appropriate chest wall tumor resection code [21601, 21602, 21603], in addition to lung resection code [32440-32445])

32480 Removal of lung, other than pneumonectomy; single lobe (lobectomy)

➔ *CPT Changes: An Insider's View* 2012

➔ *CPT Assistant* Spring 91:5, Fall 94:1, 4, Sep 12:3

32482 2 lobes (bilobectomy)

➔ *CPT Changes: An Insider's View* 2012

➔ *CPT Assistant* Fall 94:1, 4, Jan 07:31, Sep 12:3

32484 single segment (segmentectomy)

➔ *CPT Changes: An Insider's View* 2012

➔ *CPT Assistant* Fall 94:1, 4, Sep 12:3

(For removal of lung with bronchoplasty, use 32501)

32486 with circumferential resection of segment of bronchus followed by broncho-bronchial anastomosis (sleeve lobectomy)

➔ *CPT Changes: An Insider's View* 2012

➔ *CPT Assistant* Fall 94:1, 4, Jun 17:10

32488 with all remaining lung following previous removal of a portion of lung (completion pneumonectomy)

➔ *CPT Changes: An Insider's View* 2012

➔ *CPT Assistant* Fall 94:1, 4, Sep 12:3

(For lobectomy or segmentectomy, with concomitant decortication, use 32320 and the appropriate removal of lung code)

32491 with resection-plication of emphysematous lung(s) (bullous or non-bullous) for lung volume reduction, sternal split or transthoracic approach, includes any pleural procedure, when performed

➔ *CPT Changes: An Insider's View* 2012

➔ *CPT Assistant* Nov 96:7, Sep 12:3

(If lung resection is performed with chest wall tumor resection, report the appropriate chest wall tumor resection code [21601, 21602, 21603] in addition to lung resection code [32480, 32482, 32484, 32486, 32488, 32505, 32506, 32507])

+ 32501 Resection and repair of portion of bronchus (bronchoplasty) when performed at time of lobectomy or segmentectomy (List separately in addition to code for primary procedure)

(Use 32501 in conjunction with 32480, 32482, 32484)

(32501 is to be used when a portion of the bronchus to preserved lung is removed and requires plastic closure to preserve function of that preserved lung. It is not to be used for closure for the proximal end of a resected bronchus)

32503 Resection of apical lung tumor (eg, Pancoast tumor), including chest wall resection, rib(s) resection(s), neurovascular dissection, when performed; without chest wall reconstruction(s)

➔ CPT Changes: An Insider's View 2006

32504 with chest wall reconstruction

➔ CPT Changes: An Insider's View 2006

(Do not report 32503, 32504 in conjunction with 21601, 21602, 21603, 32100, 32551, 32554, 32555)

32505 Thoracotomy; with therapeutic wedge resection (eg, mass, nodule), initial

➔ CPT Changes: An Insider's View 2012
➔ CPT Assistant Sep 12:3

(Do not report 32505 in conjunction with 32440, 32442, 32445, 32488)

+ 32506 with therapeutic wedge resection (eg, mass or nodule), each additional resection, ipsilateral (List separately in addition to code for primary procedure)

➔ CPT Changes: An Insider's View 2012
➔ CPT Assistant Sep 12:3

(Report 32506 only in conjunction with 32505)

(If lung resection is performed with chest wall tumor resection, report the appropriate chest wall tumor resection code [21601, 21602, 21603], in addition to lung resection code [32480, 32482, 32484, 32486, 32488, 32505, 32506, 32507])

+ 32507 with diagnostic wedge resection followed by anatomic lung resection (List separately in addition to code for primary procedure)

➔ CPT Changes: An Insider's View 2012
➔ CPT Assistant Sep 12:3

(Report 32507 in conjunction with 32440, 32442, 32445, 32480, 32482, 32484, 32486, 32488, 32503, 32504)

32540 Extrapleural enucleation of empyema (empyemectomy)

(For extrapleural enucleation of empyema [empyemectomy] with lobectomy, use 32540 and the appropriate removal of lung code)

Introduction and Removal

32550 Insertion of indwelling tunneled pleural catheter with cuff

➔ CPT Changes: An Insider's View 2008, 2017
➔ CPT Assistant Jul 10:10, Mar 14:14, May 14:3

(Do not report 32550 in conjunction with 32554, 32555, 32556, 32557 when performed on the same side of the chest)

(If imaging guidance is performed, use 75989)

32551 Tube thoracostomy, includes connection to drainage system (eg, water seal), when performed, open (separate procedure)

➔ CPT Changes: An Insider's View 2008, 2013, 2017
➔ CPT Assistant Feb 09:7, Sep 10:6, Aug 11:4, Nov 12:3, May 14:3, Jun 17:10, Jul 18:7, Nov 21:13, Mar 23:1
➔ Clinical Examples in Radiology Fall 10:10, Winter 13:5

(Do not report 32551 in conjunction with 33020, 33025, if pleural drain/chest tube is placed on the ipsilateral side)

32552 Removal of indwelling tunneled pleural catheter with cuff

➔ CPT Changes: An Insider's View 2010
➔ CPT Assistant Feb 10:6

32553 Placement of interstitial device(s) for radiation therapy guidance (eg, fiducial markers, dosimeter), percutaneous, intra-thoracic, single or multiple

➔ CPT Changes: An Insider's View 2010, 2017
➔ CPT Assistant Feb 10:6-7, Jun 15:6, Jun 16:3
➔ Clinical Examples in Radiology Winter 23:16

(Report supply of device separately)

(For imaging guidance, see 76942, 77002, 77012, 77021)

(For percutaneous placement of interstitial device[s] for intra-abdominal, intrapelvic, and/or retroperitoneal radiation therapy guidance, use 49411)

32554 Thoracentesis, needle or catheter, aspiration of the pleural space; without imaging guidance

➔ CPT Changes: An Insider's View 2013
➔ CPT Assistant Nov 12:3, May 14:3
➔ Clinical Examples in Radiology Winter 13:5-6, Summer 13:6

32555 with imaging guidance

➔ CPT Changes: An Insider's View 2013
➔ CPT Assistant Nov 12:3
➔ Clinical Examples in Radiology Winter 13:6, Summer 13:6

32556 Pleural drainage, percutaneous, with insertion of indwelling catheter; without imaging guidance

➔ CPT Changes: An Insider's View 2013
➔ Clinical Examples in Radiology Winter 13:6, Summer 13:6

32557 with imaging guidance

➔ CPT Changes: An Insider's View 2013
➔ CPT Assistant Nov 12:3, May 14:3
➔ Clinical Examples in Radiology Winter 13:5-6, Summer 13:5-6

(For insertion of indwelling tunneled pleural catheter with cuff, use 32550)

(For open procedure, use 32551)

(Do not report 32554-32557 in conjunction with 32550, 32551 when performed on the same side of the chest)

(Do not report 32554-32557 in conjunction with 75989, 76942, 77002, 77012, 77021)

Respiratory 30000-32999

Thoracentesis
32554, 32555

Accumulated fluid or air is removed from the pleural space by puncturing space between the ribs. In 32555, a tube is inserted and a syringe attached to the catheter for the removal of fluid and/or air.

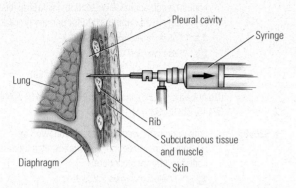

Thoracoscopy
32601-32665

The inside of the chest cavity is examined through a fiberoptic endoscope.

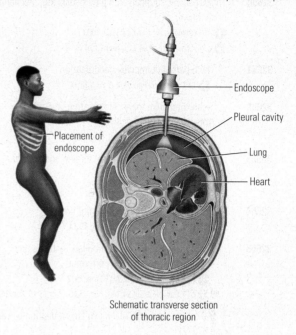

Schematic transverse section
of thoracic region

Destruction

The instillation of a fibrinolytic agent may be performed multiple times per day over the course of several days. Code 32561 should be reported only once on the initial day treatment. Code 32562 should be reported only once on each subsequent day of treatment.

32560   Instillation, via chest tube/catheter, agent for pleurodesis (eg, talc for recurrent or persistent pneumothorax)
> *CPT Changes: An Insider's View* 2008, 2010

> *CPT Assistant* Feb 10:6

(For chest tube insertion, use 32551)

32561   Instillation(s), via chest tube/catheter, agent for fibrinolysis (eg, fibrinolytic agent for break up of multiloculated effusion); initial day
> *CPT Changes: An Insider's View* 2010

> *CPT Assistant* Feb 10:6

(For chest tube insertion, use 32551)

32562   subsequent day
> *CPT Changes: An Insider's View* 2010

> *CPT Assistant* Feb 10:6

(For chest tube insertion, use 32551)

Thoracoscopy (Video-assisted thoracic surgery [VATS])

Surgical thoracoscopy (video-assisted thoracic surgery [VATS]) always includes diagnostic thoracoscopy.

32601   Thoracoscopy, diagnostic (separate procedure); lungs, pericardial sac, mediastinal or pleural space, without biopsy
> *CPT Changes: An Insider's View* 2012

> *CPT Assistant* Fall 94:1, 4, Sep 12:3, Aug 13:14

(Do not report 32601 in conjunction with 22836, 22837, 22838)

32604   pericardial sac, with biopsy
> *CPT Assistant* Fall 94:1, 4, Aug 13:14

(For open pericardial biopsy, use 39010)

32606   mediastinal space, with biopsy
> *CPT Assistant* Fall 94:1, 5, Aug 13:14

32607   Thoracoscopy; with diagnostic biopsy(ies) of lung infiltrate(s) (eg, wedge, incisional), unilateral
> *CPT Changes: An Insider's View* 2012

> *CPT Assistant* Sep 12:3, Aug 13:14

(Do not report 32607 more than once per lung)

(Do not report 32607 in conjunction with 32440, 32442, 32445, 32488, 32671)

32608   with diagnostic biopsy(ies) of lung nodule(s) or mass(es) (eg, wedge, incisional), unilateral
> *CPT Changes: An Insider's View* 2012

> *CPT Assistant* Sep 12:3, Aug 13:14

(Do not report 32608 more than once per lung)

(Do not report 32608 in conjunction with 32440, 32442, 32445, 32488, 32671)

Respiratory 30000-32999

32609   with biopsy(ies) of pleura

➔ *CPT Changes: An Insider's View* 2012

➔ *CPT Assistant* Sep 12:3, Aug 13:14

32650   Thoracoscopy, surgical; with pleurodesis (eg, mechanical or chemical)

➔ *CPT Changes: An Insider's View* 2002

➔ *CPT Assistant* Fall 94:1, 6, Aug 13:14

32651   with partial pulmonary decortication

➔ *CPT Assistant* Fall 94:1, 6, Aug 13:14

32652   with total pulmonary decortication, including intrapleural pneumonolysis

➔ *CPT Assistant* Fall 94:1, 6, Aug 13:14

32653   with removal of intrapleural foreign body or fibrin deposit

➔ *CPT Assistant* Fall 94:1, 6, Aug 13:14

32654   with control of traumatic hemorrhage

➔ *CPT Assistant* Fall 94:1, 6, Aug 13:14

32655   with resection-plication of bullae, includes any pleural procedure when performed

➔ *CPT Changes: An Insider's View* 2012

➔ *CPT Assistant* Fall 94:1, 6, Aug 05:15, Aug 13:14, Feb 24:33

(For thoracoscopic [VATS] lung volume reduction surgery, use 32672)

32656   with parietal pleurectomy

➔ *CPT Assistant* Fall 94:1, 6, Aug 13:14, Feb 24:33

32658   with removal of clot or foreign body from pericardial sac

➔ *CPT Assistant* Fall 94:1, 6, Aug 13:14

32659   with creation of pericardial window or partial resection of pericardial sac for drainage

➔ *CPT Assistant* Fall 94:1, 6, Aug 13:14

32661   with excision of pericardial cyst, tumor, or mass

➔ *CPT Assistant* Fall 94:1, 6, Aug 13:14

32662   with excision of mediastinal cyst, tumor, or mass

➔ *CPT Assistant* Fall 94:1, 6, Aug 13:14

32663   with lobectomy (single lobe)

➔ *CPT Changes: An Insider's View* 2012

➔ *CPT Assistant* Fall 94:1, 6, Sep 12:3, Aug 13:14

(For thoracoscopic [VATS] segmentectomy, use 32669)

32664   with thoracic sympathectomy

➔ *CPT Assistant* Fall 94:1, Oct 99:10, Aug 13:14, Dec 15:16, Apr 24:36

32665   with esophagomyotomy (Heller type)

➔ *CPT Assistant* Fall 94:1, 6, Aug 13:14

(Do not report 32665 in conjunction with 43497)

(For exploratory thoracoscopy, and exploratory thoracoscopy with biopsy, see 32601-32609)

32666   with therapeutic wedge resection (eg, mass, nodule), initial unilateral

➔ *CPT Changes: An Insider's View* 2012

➔ *CPT Assistant* Sep 12:3, Aug 13:14

(To report bilateral procedure, report 32666 with modifier 50)

(Do not report 32666 in conjunction with 32440, 32442, 32445, 32488, 32671)

+ 32667   with therapeutic wedge resection (eg, mass or nodule), each additional resection, ipsilateral (List separately in addition to code for primary procedure)

➔ *CPT Changes: An Insider's View* 2012

➔ *CPT Assistant* Sep 12:3, Aug 13:14

(Report 32667 only in conjunction with 32666)

(Do not report 32667 in conjunction with 32440, 32442, 32445, 32488, 32671)

+ 32668   with diagnostic wedge resection followed by anatomic lung resection (List separately in addition to code for primary procedure)

➔ *CPT Changes: An Insider's View* 2012

➔ *CPT Assistant* Sep 12:3, Aug 13:14

(Report 32668 in conjunction with 32440, 32442, 32445, 32480, 32482, 32484, 32486, 32488, 32503, 32504, 32663, 32669, 32670, 32671)

32669   with removal of a single lung segment (segmentectomy)

➔ *CPT Changes: An Insider's View* 2012

➔ *CPT Assistant* Sep 12:3, Aug 13:14

32670   with removal of two lobes (bilobectomy)

➔ *CPT Changes: An Insider's View* 2012

➔ *CPT Assistant* Sep 12:3, Aug 13:14

32671   with removal of lung (pneumonectomy)

➔ *CPT Changes: An Insider's View* 2012

➔ *CPT Assistant* Sep 12:3, Aug 13:14

32672   with resection-plication for emphysematous lung (bullous or non-bullous) for lung volume reduction (LVRS), unilateral includes any pleural procedure, when performed

➔ *CPT Changes: An Insider's View* 2012

➔ *CPT Assistant* Sep 12:3, Aug 13:14

32673   with resection of thymus, unilateral or bilateral

➔ *CPT Changes: An Insider's View* 2012

➔ *CPT Assistant* Sep 12:3, Aug 13:14

(For open thymectomy see 60520, 60521, 60522)

(For open excision mediastinal cyst, see 39200; for open excision mediastinal tumor, use 39220)

(For exploratory thoracoscopy, and exploratory thoracoscopy with biopsy, see 32601-32609)

★ = Telemedicine   ◀ = Audio-only   + = Add-on code   ⚡ = FDA approval pending   # = Resequenced code   ⊘ = Modifier 51 exempt   ➔➔➔ = See p xxi for details

+ 32674   with mediastinal and regional lymphadenectomy (List separately in addition to code for primary procedure)

> *CPT Changes: An Insider's View* 2012

> *CPT Assistant* Sep 12:3, Aug 13:14, May 14:3

(On the right, mediastinal lymph nodes include the paratracheal, subcarinal, paraesophageal, and inferior pulmonary ligament)

(On the left, mediastinal lymph nodes include the aortopulmonary window, subcarinal, paraesophageal, and inferior pulmonary ligament)

(Report 32674 in conjunction with 21601, 31760, 31766, 31786, 32096-32200, 32220-32320, 32440-32491, 32503-32505, 32601-32663, 32666, 32669-32673, 32815, 33025, 33030, 33050-33130, 39200-39220, 39560, 39561, 43101, 43112, 43117, 43118, 43122, 43123, 43287, 43288, 43351, 60270, 60505)

(To report mediastinal and regional lymphadenectomy via thoracotomy, use 38746)

Stereotactic Radiation Therapy

Thoracic stereotactic body radiation therapy (SRS/SBRT) is a distinct procedure which may involve collaboration between a surgeon and radiation oncologist. The surgeon identifies and delineates the target for therapy. The radiation oncologist reports the appropriate code(s) for clinical treatment planning, physics and dosimetry, treatment delivery and management from the Radiation Oncology section (see 77295, 77331, 77370, 77373, 77435). The same physician should not report target delineation services with radiation treatment management codes (77427-77499).

Target delineation involves specific determination of tumor borders to identify tumor volume and relationship with adjacent structures (eg, chest wall, intraparenchymal vasculature and atelectatic lung) and previously placed fiducial markers, when present. Target delineation also includes availability to identify and validate the thoracic target prior to treatment delivery when a fiducial-less tracking system is utilized.

Do not report target delineation more than once per entire course of treatment when the treatment requires greater than one session.

32701   Thoracic target(s) delineation for stereotactic body radiation therapy (SRS/SBRT), (photon or particle beam), entire course of treatment

> *CPT Changes: An Insider's View* 2013

> *CPT Assistant* Jun 15:6

(Do not report 32701 in conjunction with 77261-77799)

(For placement of fiducial markers, see 31626, 32553)

Mediastinal Lymph Nodes: Station Number and Descriptions
32674

Relevant mediastinal lymph nodes typically removed with procedures described by code 38746, and sampled removal described with code 39402.

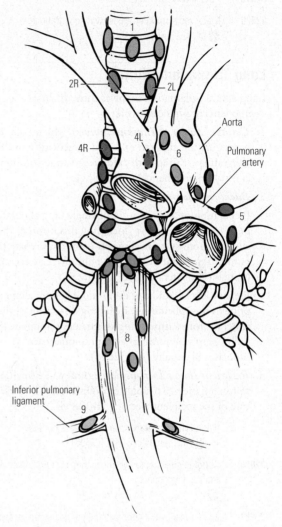

Station #	Lymph Node Descriptions
1	Low cervical, supraclavicular, and sternal notch
2	Upper paratracheal (R & L)
4	Lower paratracheal (R & L)
5	Subaortic or aortopulmonary window
6	Para-aortic
7	Subcarinal
8	Paraesophageal (below the carina)
9	Inferior pulmonary ligament

*Station #3 is not depicted as it is not applicable to the use of codes 32674, 38746, or 39402.

Repair

32800   Repair lung hernia through chest wall

32810   Closure of chest wall following open flap drainage for empyema (Clagett type procedure)

32815   Open closure of major bronchial fistula

32820   Major reconstruction, chest wall (posttraumatic)
→ *CPT Assistant* Mar 23:33

Lung Transplantation

Lung allotransplantation involves three distinct components of physician work:

1. ***Cadaver donor pneumonectomy(s)***, which include(s) harvesting the allograft and cold preservation of the allograft (perfusing with cold preservation solution and cold maintenance) (use 32850).

2. ***Backbench work:***

   Preparation of a cadaver donor single lung allograft prior to transplantation, including dissection of the allograft from surrounding soft tissues to prepare the pulmonary venous/atrial cuff, pulmonary artery, and bronchus unilaterally (use 32855).

   Preparation of a cadaver donor double lung allograft prior to transplantation, including dissection of the allograft from surrounding soft tissues to prepare the pulmonary venous/atrial cuff, pulmonary artery, and bronchus bilaterally (use 32856).

3. ***Recipient lung allotransplantation***, which includes transplantation of a single or double lung allograft and care of the recipient (see 32851-32854).

(For ex-vivo assessment of marginal donor lung transplant, see 0494T, 0495T, 0496T)

32850   Donor pneumonectomy(s) (including cold preservation), from cadaver donor
→ *CPT Changes: An Insider's View* 2005

32851   Lung transplant, single; without cardiopulmonary bypass

32852   with cardiopulmonary bypass

32853   Lung transplant, double (bilateral sequential or en bloc); without cardiopulmonary bypass

32854   with cardiopulmonary bypass

32855   Backbench standard preparation of cadaver donor lung allograft prior to transplantation, including dissection of allograft from surrounding soft tissues to prepare pulmonary venous/atrial cuff, pulmonary artery, and bronchus; unilateral
→ *CPT Changes: An Insider's View* 2005

32856   bilateral
→ *CPT Changes: An Insider's View* 2005

(For repair or resection procedures on the donor lung, see 32491, 32505, 32506, 32507, 35216, 35276)

Surgical Collapse Therapy; Thoracoplasty

(See also 32503, 32504)

32900   Resection of ribs, extrapleural, all stages

32905   Thoracoplasty, Schede type or extrapleural (all stages);

32906   with closure of bronchopleural fistula

(For open closure of major bronchial fistula, use 32815)

(For resection of first rib for thoracic outlet compression, see 21615, 21616)

32940   Pneumonolysis, extraperiosteal, including filling or packing procedures

32960   Pneumothorax, therapeutic, intrapleural injection of air

Other Procedures

32994   Code is out of numerical sequence. See 32997-32999

32997   Total lung lavage (unilateral)
→ *CPT Changes: An Insider's View* 2000, 2002
→ *CPT Assistant* Nov 98:13, Nov 99:14

(For bronchoscopic bronchial alveolar lavage, use 31624)

32998   Ablation therapy for reduction or eradication of 1 or more pulmonary tumor(s) including pleura or chest wall when involved by tumor extension, percutaneous, including imaging guidance when performed, unilateral; radiofrequency
→ *CPT Changes: An Insider's View* 2007, 2018
→ *CPT Assistant* Nov 17:8
→ *Clinical Examples in Radiology* Summer 12:11

 # 32994   cryoablation
→ *CPT Changes: An Insider's View* 2018
→ *CPT Assistant* Nov 17:8
→ *Clinical Examples in Radiology* Fall 17:4

(For bilateral procedure, report 32994, 32998 with modifier 50)

32999   Unlisted procedure, lungs and pleura
→ *CPT Assistant* Jan 02:11, Feb 02:11, Jul 08:10, Apr 10:10, Aug 11:9, Jun 15:6, Dec 15:16
→ *Clinical Examples in Radiology* Spring 06:8-9, Winter 23:16

Respiratory 30000-32999

Cryoablation Therapy of Pulmonary Tumors
32994

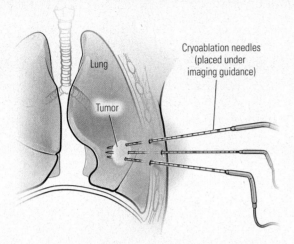

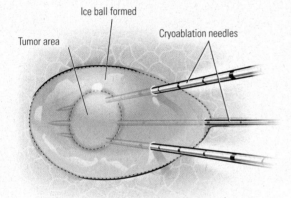

Notes

Surgery

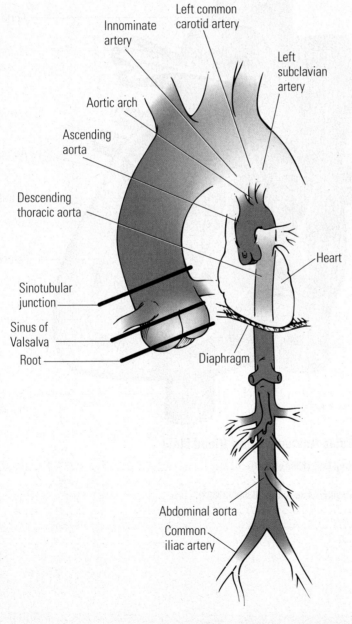

Aortic Anatomy

Cardiac Anatomy, Heart Blood Flow

Cardiovascular 33016-39599

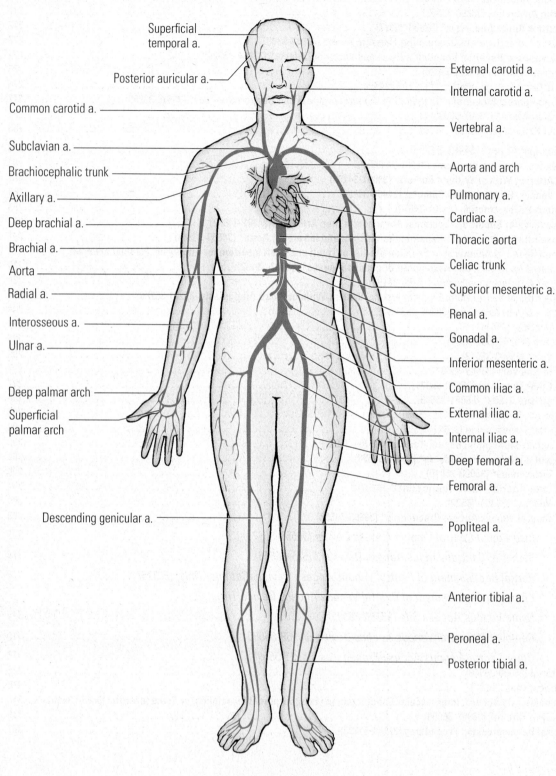

Superficial temporal a.

Posterior auricular a.

Common carotid a.

Subclavian a.

Brachiocephalic trunk

Axillary a.

Deep brachial a.

Brachial a.

Aorta

Radial a.

Interosseous a.

Ulnar a.

Deep palmar arch

Superficial palmar arch

Descending genicular a.

External carotid a.

Internal carotid a.

Vertebral a.

Aorta and arch

Pulmonary a.

Cardiac a.

Thoracic aorta

Celiac trunk

Superior mesenteric a.

Renal a.

Gonadal a.

Inferior mesenteric a.

Common iliac a.

External iliac a.

Internal iliac a.

Deep femoral a.

Femoral a.

Popliteal a.

Anterior tibial a.

Peroneal a.

Posterior tibial a.

Circulatory System, Arteries

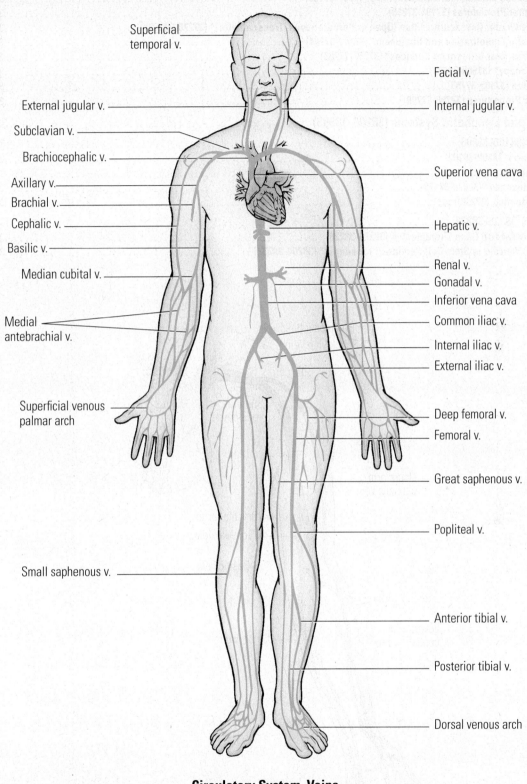

Superficial temporal v.

Facial v.

External jugular v.

Internal jugular v.

Subclavian v.

Brachiocephalic v.

Superior vena cava

Axillary v.

Brachial v.

Cephalic v.

Hepatic v.

Basilic v.

Median cubital v.

Renal v.

Gonadal v.

Inferior vena cava

Medial antebrachial v.

Common iliac v.

Internal iliac v.

External iliac v.

Superficial venous palmar arch

Deep femoral v.

Femoral v.

Great saphenous v.

Popliteal v.

Small saphenous v.

Anterior tibial v.

Posterior tibial v.

Dorsal venous arch

Circulatory System, Veins

Cardiovascular 33016-39599

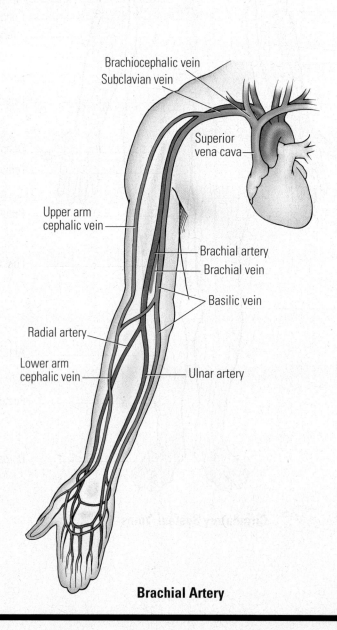

Brachial Artery

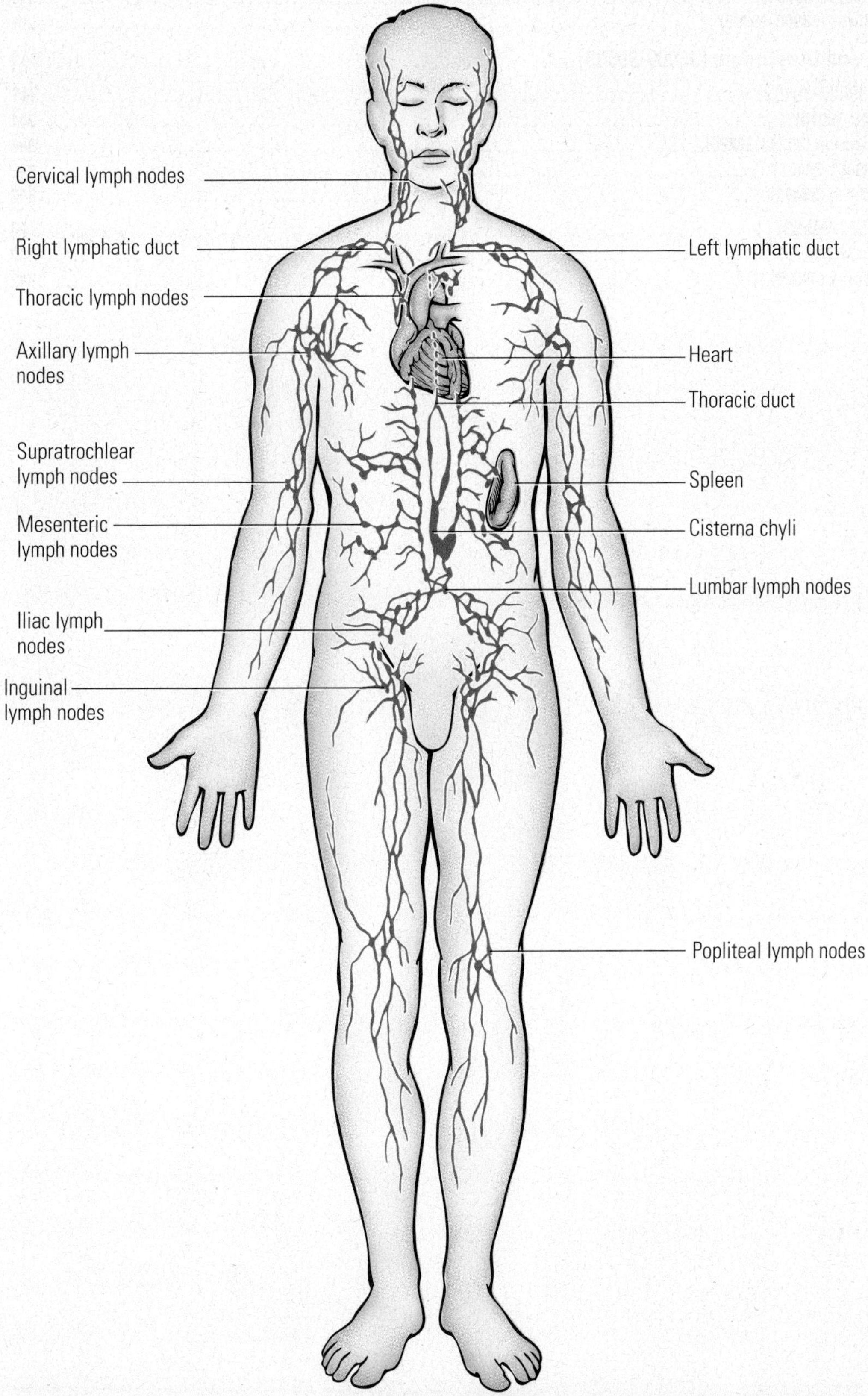

Cervical lymph nodes

Right lymphatic duct

Thoracic lymph nodes

Axillary lymph nodes

Supratrochlear lymph nodes

Mesenteric lymph nodes

Iliac lymph nodes

Inguinal lymph nodes

Left lymphatic duct

Heart

Thoracic duct

Spleen

Cisterna chyli

Lumbar lymph nodes

Popliteal lymph nodes

Lymphatic System

Cardiovascular 33016-39599

Cardiovascular 33016-39599

Cardiovascular System

Selective vascular catheterizations should be coded to include introduction and all lesser order selective catheterizations used in the approach (eg, the description for a selective right middle cerebral artery catheterization includes the introduction and placement catheterization of the right common and internal carotid arteries).

Additional second and/or third order arterial catheterizations within the same family of arteries supplied by a single first order artery should be expressed by 36218 or 36248. Additional first order or higher catheterizations in vascular families supplied by a first order vessel different from a previously selected and coded family should be separately coded using the conventions described above.

> (For monitoring, operation of pump and other nonsurgical services, see 99190-99192, 99291, 99292, 99358, 99359, 99360)

> (For other medical or laboratory related services, see appropriate section)

> (For radiological supervision and interpretation, see 75600-75970)

> (For anatomic guidance of arterial and venous anatomy, see Appendix L)

Heart and Pericardium

Pericardium

In order to report pericardial drainage with insertion of indwelling catheter (33017, 33018, 33019), the catheter needs to remain in place when the procedure is completed. Codes 33017, 33018, 33019 should not be reported when a catheter is placed to aspirate fluid and then removed at the conclusion of the procedure.

Congenital cardiac anomaly for reporting percutaneous pericardial drainage with insertion of indwelling catheter is defined as abnormal situs (heterotaxy, dextrocardia, mesocardia), single ventricle anomaly/physiology, or any patient in the first 90-day postoperative period after repair of a congenital cardiac anomaly.

> (For thoracoscopic (VATS) pericardial procedures, see 32601, 32604, 32658, 32659, 32661)

33016   Pericardiocentesis, including imaging guidance, when performed
➔ *CPT Changes: An Insider's View* 2020
➔ *CPT Assistant* Jan 20:7, Aug 22:18
➔ *Clinical Examples in Radiology* Winter 20:11

> (Do not report 33016 in conjunction with 76942, 77002, 77012, 77021)

33017   Pericardial drainage with insertion of indwelling catheter, percutaneous, including fluoroscopy and/or ultrasound guidance, when performed; 6 years and older without congenital cardiac anomaly
➔ *CPT Changes: An Insider's View* 2020
➔ *CPT Assistant* Jan 20:7, Mar 20:14, Aug 22:18

33018   birth through 5 years of age or any age with congenital cardiac anomaly
➔ *CPT Changes: An Insider's View* 2020
➔ *CPT Assistant* Jan 20:7, Mar 20:14

> (Do not report 33017, 33018 in conjunction with 75989, 76942, 77002, 77012, 77021)

> (Do not report 33016, 33017, 33018 in conjunction with 93303-93325 when echocardiography is performed solely for the purpose of pericardiocentesis guidance)

> (For CT-guided pericardial drainage, use 33019)

33019   Pericardial drainage with insertion of indwelling catheter, percutaneous, including CT guidance
➔ *CPT Changes: An Insider's View* 2020
➔ *CPT Assistant* Jan 20:7

> (Do not report 33019 in conjunction with 75989, 76942, 77002, 77012, 77021)

33020   Pericardiotomy for removal of clot or foreign body (primary procedure)
➔ *CPT Assistant* Nov 21:13

33025   Creation of pericardial window or partial resection for drainage
➔ *CPT Assistant* Nov 21:13

> (Do not report 33020, 33025 in conjunction with 32551, if pleural drain/chest tube is placed on the ipsilateral side)

> (For thoracoscopic (VATS) pericardial window, use 32659)

33030   Pericardiectomy, subtotal or complete; without cardiopulmonary bypass

33031   with cardiopulmonary bypass

33050   Resection of pericardial cyst or tumor
➔ *CPT Changes: An Insider's View* 2012

> (For open pericardial biopsy, use 39010)

> (For thoracoscopic (VATS) resection of pericardial cyst, tumor or mass, use 32661)

Cardiac Tumor

33120   Excision of intracardiac tumor, resection with cardiopulmonary bypass
➔ *CPT Assistant* Mar 07:1

33130   Resection of external cardiac tumor
➔ *CPT Assistant* Mar 07:1

Transmyocardial Revascularization

33140 Transmyocardial laser revascularization, by thoracotomy; (separate procedure)

➔ *CPT Changes: An Insider's View* 2000, 2001, 2002

➔ *CPT Assistant* Nov 99:14, Nov 00:5, Apr 01:7

+ 33141 performed at the time of other open cardiac procedure(s) (List separately in addition to code for primary procedure)

➔ *CPT Changes: An Insider's View* 2001

➔ *CPT Assistant* Apr 01:7

(Use 33141 in conjunction with 33390, 33391, 33404-33496, 33510-33536, 33542)

Pacemaker or Implantable Defibrillator

A pacemaker system with lead(s) includes a pulse generator containing electronics, a battery, and one or more leads. A lead consists of one or more electrodes, as well as conductor wires, insulation, and a fixation mechanism. Pulse generators are placed in a subcutaneous "pocket" created in either a subclavicular site or just above the abdominal muscles just below the ribcage. Leads may be inserted through a vein (transvenous) or they may be placed on the surface of the heart (epicardial). The epicardial location of leads requires a thoracotomy for insertion.

A single chamber pacemaker system with lead includes a pulse generator and one electrode inserted in either the atrium or ventricle. A dual chamber pacemaker system with two leads includes a pulse generator and one lead inserted in the right atrium and one lead inserted in the right ventricle. In certain circumstances, an additional lead may be required to achieve pacing of the left ventricle (bi-ventricular pacing). In this event, transvenous (cardiac vein) placement of the lead should be separately reported using code 33224 or 33225. For body surface–activation mapping to optimize electrical synchrony of a biventricular pacing or biventricular pacing-defibrillator system at the time of implant, also report 0695T with the appropriate code (ie, 33224, 33225, 33226). Epicardial placement of the lead should be separately reported using 33202, 33203.

A leadless cardiac pacemaker system includes a pulse generator with built-in battery and electrode for implantation in a cardiac chamber via a transvenous transcatheter approach. For implantation of a right ventricular leadless pacemaker system, use 33274. Insertion, replacement, or removal of a right ventricular leadless pacemaker system includes insertion of a catheter via transvenous access under fluoroscopic guidance into the right ventricle. For a complete dual-chamber leadless cardiac pacemaker system which is implanted in both the right ventricle and right atrium, or individual components of a dual-chamber leadless pacemaker system, see 0795T, 0796T, 0797T, 0798T, 0799T, 0800T, 0801T, 0802T, 0803T. Device evaluation at the time of leadless pacemaker insertion, replacement, or removal is included in 33274, 33275, 0795T, 0796T, 0797T, 0798T, 0799T, 0800T, 0801T, 0802T, 0803T, 0823T, 0824T, 0825T and is not separately reported. For subsequent leadless pacemaker device evaluation, see 93279, 93286, 93288, 93294, 93296, 0804T, 0826T.

For a single-chamber leadless cardiac pacemaker implanted in the right atrium that is not a component of a dual-chamber leadless pacemaker system, see 0823T, 0824T, 0825T.

Right heart catheterization (93451, 93453, 93456, 93457, 93460, 93461, 93593, 93594, 93596, 93597) may not be reported in conjunction with leadless pacemaker insertion and removal codes 33274, 33275, 0795T, 0796T, 0797T, 0798T, 0799T, 0800T, 0801T, 0802T, 0803T, 0823T, 0824T, 0825T, unless complete right heart catheterization is performed for an indication distinct from the leadless pacemaker procedure.

Like a pacemaker system, an implantable defibrillator system includes a pulse generator and electrodes. Three general categories of implantable defibrillators exist: transvenous implantable pacing cardioverter-defibrillator (ICD), subcutaneous implantable defibrillator (S-ICD), and substernal implantable cardioverter-defibrillator. Implantable pacing cardioverter-defibrillator devices use a combination of antitachycardia pacing, low-energy cardioversion or defibrillating shocks to treat ventricular tachycardia or ventricular fibrillation. The subcutaneous implantable defibrillator uses a single subcutaneous electrode to treat ventricular tachyarrhythmias. The substernal implantable cardioverter-defibrillator uses at least one substernal electrode to perform defibrillation, cardioversion, and antitachycardia pacing. Subcutaneous implantable defibrillators differ from transvenous implantable pacing cardioverter-defibrillators in that subcutaneous defibrillators do not provide antitachycardia pacing or chronic pacing. Substernal implantable defibrillators differ from both subcutaneous and transvenous implantable pacing cardioverter-defibrillators in that they provide antitachycardia pacing, but not chronic pacing.

Implantable defibrillator pulse generators may be implanted in a subcutaneous infraclavicular, axillary, or abdominal pocket. Removal of an implantable defibrillator pulse generator requires opening of the existing subcutaneous pocket and disconnection of the pulse generator from its electrode(s). A thoracotomy (or laparotomy in the case of abdominally placed pulse generators) is not required to remove the pulse generator.

Cardiovascular 33016-39599

The electrodes (leads) of an implantable defibrillator system may be positioned within the atrial and/or ventricular chambers of the heart via the venous system (transvenously), or placed on the surface of the heart (epicardial), or positioned under the skin overlying the heart (subcutaneous). Electrode positioning on the epicardial surface of the heart requires a thoracotomy or thoracoscopic placement of the leads. Epicardial placement of electrode(s) may be separately reported using 33202, 33203. The electrode (lead) of a subcutaneous implantable defibrillator system is tunneled under the skin to the left parasternal margin. Subcutaneous placement of electrode may be reported using 33270 or 33271. The electrode (lead) of a substernal implantable defibrillator system is tunneled subcutaneously and placed into the substernal anterior mediastinum without entering the pericardial cavity and may be reported using 0571T, 0572T. In certain circumstances, an additional electrode may be required to achieve pacing of the left ventricle (bi-ventricular pacing). In this event, transvenous (cardiac vein) placement of the electrode may be separately reported using 33224 or 33225.

Removal of a transvenous electrode(s) may first be attempted by transvenous extraction (33234, 33235, or 33244). However, if transvenous extraction is unsuccessful, a thoracotomy may be required to remove the electrodes (33238 or 33243). Use 33212, 33213, 33221, 33230, 33231, 33240 as appropriate, in addition to the thoracotomy or endoscopic epicardial lead placement codes (33202 or 33203) to report the insertion of the generator if done by the same physician during the same session. Removal of a subcutaneous implantable defibrillator electrode may be separately reported using 33272. For removal of a leadless pacemaker system without replacement, use 33275. For removal and replacement of a leadless pacemaker system during the same session, use 33274.

►When the "battery" of a pacemaker system with lead(s) or implantable defibrillator is changed, it is actually the pulse generator that is changed. Removal of only the pacemaker or implantable defibrillator pulse generator is reported with 33233 or 33241. If only a pulse generator is inserted or replaced without any right atrial and/or right ventricular lead(s) inserted or replaced, report the appropriate code for only pulse generator insertion or replacement based on the number of final existing lead(s) (33227, 33228, 33229 and 33262, 33263, 33264). Do not report removal of a pulse generator (33233 or 33241) separately for this service. Insertion of a new pulse generator, when existing lead(s) are already in place and when no prior pulse generator is removed, is reported with 33212, 33213, 33221, 33230, 33231, 33240. When a pulse generator insertion involves the insertion or replacement of one or more right atrial and/or right ventricular lead(s) or subcutaneous lead(s), use system codes 33206, 33207, 33208 for pacemaker, 33249 for implantable pacing cardioverter-defibrillator, or 33270

for subcutaneous implantable defibrillator. When reporting the system insertion or replacement codes, removal of a pulse generator (33233 or 33241) may be reported separately, when performed. In addition, extraction of leads 33234, 33235 or 33244 for transvenous or 33272 for subcutaneous may be reported separately, when performed. An exception involves a pacemaker upgrade from single to dual system that includes removal of pulse generator, replacement of new pulse generator, and insertion of new lead, reported with 33214. For insertion, removal, relocation, and repositioning of cardiac contractility modulation-defibrillation codes, see 0915T-0925T.◄

Revision of a skin pocket is included in 33206-33249, 33262, 33263, 33264, 33270, 33271, 33272, 33273. When revision of a skin pocket involves incision and drainage of a hematoma or complex wound infection, see 10140, 10180, 11042, 11043, 11044, 11045, 11046, 11047, as appropriate.

Relocation of a skin pocket for a pacemaker (33222) or implantable defibrillator (33223) is necessary for various clinical situations such as infection or erosion. Relocation of an existing pulse generator may be performed as a stand-alone procedure or at the time of a pulse generator or electrode insertion, replacement, or repositioning. When skin pocket relocation is performed as part of an explant of an existing generator followed by replacement with a new generator, the pocket relocation is reported separately. Skin pocket relocation includes all work associated with the initial pocket (eg, opening the pocket, incision and drainage of hematoma or abscess if performed, and any closure performed), in addition to the creation of a new pocket for the new generator to be placed.

Repositioning of a pacemaker electrode, implantable defibrillator electrode(s), or a left ventricular pacing electrode is reported using 33215, 33226, or 33273, as appropriate.

Device evaluation codes 93260, 93261, 93279-93298 for pacemaker system with lead(s) may not be reported in conjunction with pulse generator and lead insertion or revision codes 33206-33249, 33262, 33263, 33264, 33270, 33271, 33272, 33273. For leadless pacemaker systems, device evaluation codes 93279, 93286, 93288, 93294, 93296 may not be reported in conjunction with leadless pacemaker insertion and removal codes 33274, 33275. Defibrillator threshold testing (DFT) during transvenous implantable defibrillator insertion or replacement may be separately reported using 93640, 93641. DFT testing during subcutaneous implantable

Procedure	System	
	Pacemaker	**Implantable Defibrillator**
Insert transvenous single lead only without pulse generator	33216	33216
Insert transvenous dual leads without pulse generator	33217	33217
Insert transvenous multiple leads without pulse generator	33217 + 33224	33217 + 33224
Insert subcutaneous defibrillator electrode only without pulse generator	N/A	33271
Initial pulse generator insertion only with existing single lead, includes transvenous or subcutaneous defibrillator lead	33212	33240
Initial pulse generator insertion only with existing dual leads	33213	33230
Initial pulse generator insertion only with existing multiple leads	33221	33231
Initial pulse generator insertion or replacement plus insertion of transvenous single lead	33206 (atrial) or 33207 (ventricular)	33249
Initial pulse generator insertion or replacement plus insertion of transvenous dual leads	33208	33249
Initial pulse generator insertion or replacement plus insertion of transvenous multiple leads	33208 + 33225	33249 + 33225
Initial pulse generator insertion or replacement plus insertion of subcutaneous defibrillator electrode	N/A	33270
Insertion, replacement, or removal and replacement of permanent single-chamber leadless ventricular pacemaker	33274	N/A
Insertion permanent single-chamber leadless pacemaker, right atrial	0823T	N/A
Insertion permanent dual-chamber leadless pacemaker, right atrial and right ventricular components	0795T	N/A
Insertion permanent dual-chamber leadless pacemaker, right atrial component	0796T	N/A
Insertion permanent dual-chamber leadless pacemaker, right ventricular component (when part of a dual-chamber leadless pacemaker system)	0797T	N/A
Upgrade single chamber system to dual chamber system	33214 (includes removal of existing pulse generator)	33241 + 33249
Removal pulse generator only (without replacement)	33233	33241
Removal pulse generator with replacement pulse generator only single lead system (applies to transvenous or subcutaneous defibrillator lead systems)	33227	33262
Removal pulse generator with replacement pulse generator only dual lead system (transvenous)	33228	33263
Removal pulse generator with replacement pulse generator only multiple lead system (transvenous)	33229	33264
Removal transvenous electrode only single lead system	33234	33244
Removal transvenous electrode only dual lead system	33235	33244
Removal subcutaneous defibrillator lead only	N/A	33272
Removal and replacement of pulse generator and transvenous electrodes	33233 + (33234 or 33235) + (33206, 33207 or 33208) and 33225, when appropriate	33241 + 33244 + 33249 and 33225, when appropriate

★=Telemedicine ◀=Audio-only ✛=Add-on code ✗=FDA approval pending #=Resequenced code ⊘=Modifier 51 exempt ➲➲➲=See p xxi for details

Procedure	System	
	Pacemaker	**Implantable Defibrillator**
Removal and replacement of implantable defibrillator pulse generator and subcutaneous electrode	N/A	33272 + 33241 + 33270
Removal and replacement permanent single-chamber leadless pacemaker, right atrial	0825T	N/A
Removal and replacement permanent dual-chamber leadless pacemaker, right atrial and right ventricular components	0801T	N/A
Removal and replacement permanent dual-chamber leadless pacemaker, right atrial component	0802T	N/A
Removal and replacement permanent dual-chamber leadless pacemaker, right ventricular component (when part of a dual-chamber leadless pacemaker system)	0803T	N/A
Removal of permanent single-chamber leadless ventricular pacemaker	33275	N/A
Removal permanent single-chamber leadless right atrial pacemaker	0824T	N/A
Removal permanent dual-chamber leadless pacemaker, right atrial and right ventricular components	0798T	N/A
Removal permanent dual-chamber leadless pacemaker, right atrial component	0799T	N/A
Removal permanent dual-chamber leadless pacemaker, right ventricular component (when part of a dual-chamber leadless pacemaker system)	0800T	N/A
Conversion of existing system to bi-ventricular system (addition of LV lead and removal of current pulse generator with insertion of new pulse generator with bi-ventricular pacing capabilities)	33225 + 33228 or 33229	33225 + 33263 or 33264

defibrillator system insertion is not separately reportable. DFT testing for transvenous or subcutaneous implantable defibrillator in follow-up or at the time of replacement may be separately reported using 93642 or 93644.

Radiological supervision and interpretation related to the pacemaker or implantable defibrillator procedure is included in 33206-33249, 33262, 33263, 33264, 33270, 33271, 33272, 33273, 33274, 33275. Fluoroscopy (76000, 77002), ultrasound guidance for vascular access (76937), right ventriculography (93566), and femoral venography (75820) are included in 33274, 33275, when performed). To report fluoroscopic guidance for diagnostic lead evaluation without lead insertion, replacement, or revision procedures, use 76000.

The following definitions apply to 33206-33249, 33262, 33263, 33264, 33270, 33271, 33272, 33273.

Single lead: a pacemaker or implantable defibrillator with pacing and sensing function in only one chamber of the heart or a subcutaneous electrode.

Dual lead: a pacemaker or implantable defibrillator with pacing and sensing function in only two chambers of the heart.

Multiple lead: a pacemaker or implantable defibrillator with pacing and sensing function in three or more chambers of the heart.

33202   Insertion of epicardial electrode(s); open incision (eg, thoracotomy, median sternotomy, subxiphoid approach)
➲ *CPT Changes: An Insider's View* 2007
➲ *CPT Assistant* Jun 12:5, Nov 14:5, May 15:3, Aug 16:5, Mar 19:6

33203   endoscopic approach (eg, thoracoscopy, pericardioscopy)
➲ *CPT Changes: An Insider's View* 2007
➲ *CPT Assistant* Jun 12:4, Nov 14:5, May 15:3, Aug 16:5

(When epicardial lead placement is performed with insertion of the generator, report 33202, 33203 in conjunction with 33212, 33213, 33221, 33230, 33231, 33240)

33206   Insertion of new or replacement of permanent pacemaker with transvenous electrode(s); atrial
➲ *CPT Changes: An Insider's View* 2012, 2017
➲ *CPT Assistant* Summer 94:10, 17, Oct 96:9, Nov 99:15, Jun 08:14, Jun 12:3, Apr 13:10, Nov 14:5, May 15:3, Aug 16:5

Cardiovascular 33016-39599

33207   ventricular

➲ *CPT Changes: An Insider's View* 2012, 2017

➲ *CPT Assistant* Summer 94:10, 17, Oct 96:9, Nov 99:15, Jun 08:14, Jun 12:3, Apr 13:10, May 15:3, Aug 16:5

33208   atrial and ventricular

➲ *CPT Changes: An Insider's View* 2012, 2017

➲ *CPT Assistant* Summer 94:10, 17, Jul 96:10, Nov 99:15, Jun 08:14, Jun 12:3, Apr 13:10, Nov 14:5, May 15:3, Aug 16:5

(Do not report 33206-33208 in conjunction with 33227-33229)

(Do not report 33206, 33207, 33208 in conjunction with 33216, 33217)

(Codes 33206-33208 include subcutaneous insertion of the pulse generator and transvenous placement of electrode[s])

(For removal and replacement of pacemaker pulse generator and transvenous electrode(s), use 33233 in conjunction with either 33234 or 33235 and 33206-33208)

33210   Insertion or replacement of temporary transvenous single chamber cardiac electrode or pacemaker catheter (separate procedure)

➲ *CPT Changes: An Insider's View* 2017

➲ *CPT Assistant* Summer 94:10, 17, Mar 07:1, Aug 11:4, Jun 12:3, Jan 13:6, May 15:3, Aug 16:5

33211   Insertion or replacement of temporary transvenous dual chamber pacing electrodes (separate procedure)

➲ *CPT Changes: An Insider's View* 2017

➲ *CPT Assistant* Summer 94:10, 17, Mar 07:1, Aug 11:4, Jun 12:3, May 15:3, Aug 16:5

33212   Insertion of pacemaker pulse generator only; with existing single lead

➲ *CPT Changes: An Insider's View* 2012, 2017

➲ *CPT Assistant* Summer 94:10, 18, Fall 94:24, May 04:15, Jun 08:14, Jun 12:3, Nov 14:5, May 15:3, Aug 16:5

33213   with existing dual leads

➲ *CPT Changes: An Insider's View* 2012, 2017

➲ *CPT Assistant* Summer 94:10, 18, Oct 96:10, Feb 98:11, Jun 12:3, Nov 14:5, May 15:3, Aug 16:5

 # 33221   with existing multiple leads

➲ *CPT Changes: An Insider's View* 2012, 2017

➲ *CPT Assistant* Jun 12:3, Nov 14:5, May 15:3, Aug 16:5

(Do not report 33212, 33213, 33221 in conjunction with 33216, 33217)

(Do not report 33212, 33213, 33221 in conjunction with 33233 for removal and replacement of the pacemaker pulse generator. Use 33227-33229, as appropriate, when pulse generator replacement is indicated)

(When epicardial lead placement is performed with insertion of generator, report 33202, 33203 in conjunction with 33212, 33213, 33221)

Temporary Pacemaker
33210

The pacemaker pulse generator with the electrodes transvenously placed

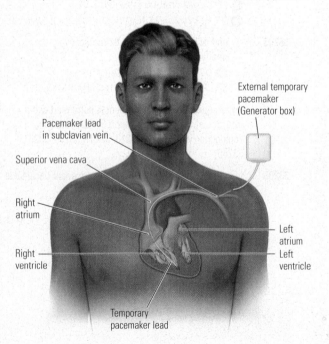

External temporary pacemaker (Generator box)

Pacemaker lead in subclavian vein

Superior vena cava

Right atrium

Right ventricle

Left atrium

Left ventricle

Temporary pacemaker lead

Implanted Pacemaker
33212

In 33212, a pacemaker pulse generator is inserted with an existing single lead.

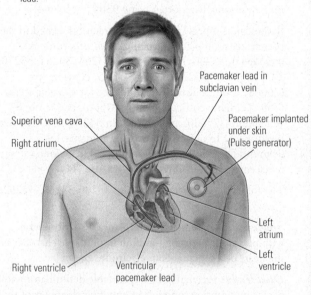

Pacemaker lead in subclavian vein

Superior vena cava

Right atrium

Pacemaker implanted under skin (Pulse generator)

Left atrium

Left ventricle

Right ventricle

Ventricular pacemaker lead

33214 Upgrade of implanted pacemaker system, conversion of single chamber system to dual chamber system (includes removal of previously placed pulse generator, testing of existing lead, insertion of new lead, insertion of new pulse generator)

➡ *CPT Changes: An Insider's View* 2017

➡ *CPT Assistant* Summer 94:10, 18, Fall 94:24, Jun 08:14, Jun 12:3, Nov 14:5, Aug 16:5

(Do not report 33214 in conjunction with 33216, 33217, 33227, 33228, 33229)

Implanted Pacemaker
33213, 33214

In 33213, a pacemaker pulse generator is inserted with existing dual leads. In 33214, an upgrade to an existing pacemaker system is done.

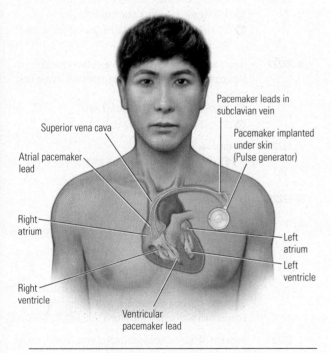

Superior vena cava

Atrial pacemaker lead

Pacemaker leads in subclavian vein

Pacemaker implanted under skin (Pulse generator)

Right atrium

Left atrium

Left ventricle

Right ventricle

Ventricular pacemaker lead

33215 Repositioning of previously implanted transvenous pacemaker or implantable defibrillator (right atrial or right ventricular) electrode

➡ *CPT Changes: An Insider's View* 2003, 2015

➡ *CPT Assistant* Jun 12:3, Nov 14:5, Aug 16:5

33216 Insertion of a single transvenous electrode, permanent pacemaker or implantable defibrillator

➡ *CPT Changes: An Insider's View* 2000, 2003, 2010, 2015, 2017

➡ *CPT Assistant* Summer 94:10, 18, Jul 96:10, Nov 99:15-16, Aug 16:5

(Do not report 33216 in conjunction with 33206, 33207, 33208, 33212, 33213, 33214, 33221, 33227, 33228, 33229, 33230, 33231, 33240, 33249, 33262, 33263, 33264)

33217 Insertion of 2 transvenous electrodes, permanent pacemaker or implantable defibrillator

➡ *CPT Changes: An Insider's View* 2000, 2010, 2015, 2017

➡ *CPT Assistant* Summer 94:10, 18, Jul 96:10, Nov 99:15-16, Jul 00:5, Apr 09:8, Jun 12:3, Aug 16:5

(Do not report 33217 in conjunction with 33206, 33207, 33208, 33212, 33213, 33214, 33221, 33227, 33228, 33229, 33230, 33231, 33240, 33249, 33262, 33263, 33264)

(For insertion or replacement of a cardiac venous system lead, see 33224, 33225)

33218 Repair of single transvenous electrode, permanent pacemaker or implantable defibrillator

➡ *CPT Changes: An Insider's View* 2000, 2012, 2015, 2017

➡ *CPT Assistant* Summer 94:10, 19, Oct 96:9, Nov 99:15-16, Jun 12:3, Aug 16:5

(For repair of single permanent pacemaker or implantable defibrillator electrode with replacement of pulse generator, see 33227, 33228, 33229 or 33262, 33263, 33264 and 33218)

33220 Repair of 2 transvenous electrodes for permanent pacemaker or implantable defibrillator

➡ *CPT Changes: An Insider's View* 2000, 2012, 2015, 2017

➡ *CPT Assistant* Summer 94:10, 19, Oct 96:9, Nov 99:15-16, Jun 08:14, Jun 12:3, Aug 16:5

(For repair of 2 transvenous electrodes for permanent pacemaker or implantable defibrillator with replacement of pulse generator, use 33220 in conjunction with 33228, 33229, 33263, 33264)

33221 Code is out of numerical sequence. See 33212-33215

33222 Relocation of skin pocket for pacemaker

➡ *CPT Changes: An Insider's View* 2000, 2014, 2017

➡ *CPT Assistant* Spring 94:30, Summer 94:10, Nov 99:15-16, Jun 08:14, Jun 12:3, Nov 14:5, May 15:3, Aug 16:5

(Do not report 33222 in conjunction with 10140, 10180, 11042, 11043, 11044, 11045, 11046, 11047, 13100, 13101, 13102)

33223 Relocation of skin pocket for implantable defibrillator

➡ *CPT Changes: An Insider's View* 2000, 2010, 2014, 2015, 2017

➡ *CPT Assistant* Summer 94:10, 19, Nov 99:15-16, Jun 08:14, Jun 12:3, Nov 14:5, Aug 16:5

(Do not report 33223 in conjunction with 10140, 10180, 11042, 11043, 11044, 11045, 11046, 11047, 13100, 13101, 13102)

Cardiovascular 33016-39599

33224 Insertion of pacing electrode, cardiac venous system, for left ventricular pacing, with attachment to previously placed pacemaker or implantable defibrillator pulse generator (including revision of pocket, removal, insertion, and/or replacement of existing generator)

➔ CPT Changes: An Insider's View 2003, 2012, 2015

➔ CPT Assistant Dec 07:16, Jun 12:3, Nov 14:5, May 15:3, Aug 16:5

(When epicardial electrode placement is performed, report 33224 in conjunction with 33202, 33203)

(Use 33224 in conjunction with 0695T when body surface–activation mapping to optimize electrical synchrony is also performed)

Biventricular Pacing
33224-33226

Insertion or repositioning of venous pacing electrode

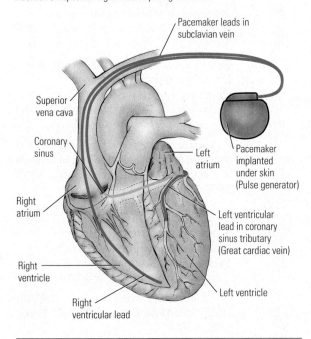

Pacemaker leads in subclavian vein

Superior vena cava

Coronary sinus

Left atrium

Pacemaker implanted under skin (Pulse generator)

Right atrium

Left ventricular lead in coronary sinus tributary (Great cardiac vein)

Right ventricle

Left ventricle

Right ventricular lead

+ 33225 Insertion of pacing electrode, cardiac venous system, for left ventricular pacing, at time of insertion of implantable defibrillator or pacemaker pulse generator (eg, for upgrade to dual chamber system) (List separately in addition to code for primary procedure)

➔ CPT Changes: An Insider's View 2003, 2012, 2013, 2015

➔ CPT Assistant Dec 07:16, Jun 12:3, Nov 14:5, May 15:3, Aug 16:5

(Use 33225 in conjunction with 33206, 33207, 33208, 33212, 33213, 33214, 33216, 33217, 33221, 33223, 33228, 33229, 33230, 33231, 33233, 33234, 33235, 33240, 33249, 33263, 33264)

(Use 33225 in conjunction with 33222 only with pacemaker pulse generator pocket relocation and with 33223 only with implantable defibrillator [ICD] pocket relocation)

(Use 33225 in conjunction with 0695T when body surface–activation mapping to optimize electrical synchrony is also performed)

33226 Repositioning of previously implanted cardiac venous system (left ventricular) electrode (including removal, insertion and/or replacement of existing generator)

➔ CPT Changes: An Insider's View 2003, 2012

➔ CPT Assistant Jun 12:3, Nov 14:5, May 15:3, Aug 16:5

(Use 33226 in conjunction with 0695T when body surface–activation mapping to optimize electrical synchrony is also performed)

33227 Code is out of numerical sequence. See 33226-33244

33228 Code is out of numerical sequence. See 33226-33244

33229 Code is out of numerical sequence. See 33226-33244

33230 Code is out of numerical sequence. See 33226-33244

33231 Code is out of numerical sequence. See 33226-33244

33233 Removal of permanent pacemaker pulse generator only

➔ CPT Changes: An Insider's View 2000, 2012, 2017

➔ CPT Assistant Summer 94:10, 19, Fall 94:24, Oct 96:10, Jun 12:3, Nov 14:5, Aug 16:5

 # 33227 Removal of permanent pacemaker pulse generator with replacement of pacemaker pulse generator; single lead system

➔ CPT Changes: An Insider's View 2012, 2017

➔ CPT Assistant Jun 12:3, Apr 13:10, Nov 14:5, Aug 16:5

 # 33228 dual lead system

➔ CPT Changes: An Insider's View 2012, 2017

➔ CPT Assistant Jun 12:3, Apr 13:10, Aug 16:5

 # 33229 multiple lead system

➔ CPT Changes: An Insider's View 2012, 2017

➔ CPT Assistant Jun 12:3, Apr 13:10, Nov 14:5, Aug 16:5

(Do not report 33227, 33228, 33229 in conjunction with 33214, 33216, 33217, 33233)

(For removal and replacement of pacemaker pulse generator and transvenous electrode[s], use 33233 in conjunction with either 33234 or 33235 and 33206-33208)

33234 Removal of transvenous pacemaker electrode(s); single lead system, atrial or ventricular

➔ CPT Changes: An Insider's View 2000, 2017

➔ CPT Assistant Summer 94:10, 19, Nov 99:16, Jun 12:3, Oct 12:15, Nov 14:5, Aug 16:5

33235 dual lead system

➔ CPT Changes: An Insider's View 2000, 2017

➔ CPT Assistant Summer 94:10, 19, Nov 99:16, Jun 12:3, Oct 12:15, Dec 13:14, Nov 14:5, Aug 16:5

33236 Removal of permanent epicardial pacemaker and electrodes by thoracotomy; single lead system, atrial or ventricular

➔ CPT Changes: An Insider's View 2000

➔ CPT Assistant Summer 94:10, 19, Nov 99:16, Jun 12:3, Aug 16:5

33237   dual lead system

➔ *CPT Changes: An Insider's View* 2000

➔ *CPT Assistant* Summer 94:10, 19, Nov 99:16, Jun 12:3, Aug 16:5, Mar 19:6

33238   Removal of permanent transvenous electrode(s) by thoracotomy

➔ *CPT Changes: An Insider's View* 2000

➔ *CPT Assistant* Summer 94:10, 19, Nov 99:16, Jun 12:3, Nov 14:5, Aug 16:5

33240   Insertion of implantable defibrillator pulse generator only; with existing single lead

➔ *CPT Changes: An Insider's View* 2000, 2012, 2015, 2017

➔ *CPT Assistant* Summer 94:40, Jun 96:10, Nov 99:16-17, Jul 00:5, Apr 04:6, Jun 08:14, Jun 12:3, Nov 14:5, Aug 16:5

(Do not report 33240 in conjunction with 33271, 93260, 93261)

(Use 33240, as appropriate, in addition to the epicardial lead placement codes to report the insertion of the generator when done by the same physician during the same session)

 # 33230   with existing dual leads

➔ *CPT Changes: An Insider's View* 2012, 2015, 2017

➔ *CPT Assistant* Jun 12:3, Nov 14:5, Aug 16:5

 # 33231   with existing multiple leads

➔ *CPT Changes: An Insider's View* 2012, 2015, 2017

➔ *CPT Assistant* Jun 12:3, Nov 14:5, Aug 16:5

(Do not report 33230, 33231, 33240 in conjunction with 33216, 33217)

(Do not report 33230, 33231, 33240 in conjunction with 33241 for removal and replacement of the implantable defibrillator pulse generator. Use 33262, 33263, 33264, as appropriate, when pulse generator replacement is indicated)

(When epicardial lead placement is performed with insertion of generator, report 33202, 33203 in conjunction with 33230, 33231, 33240)

33241   Removal of implantable defibrillator pulse generator only

➔ *CPT Changes: An Insider's View* 2000, 2012, 2015, 2017

➔ *CPT Assistant* Summer 94:40, Nov 99:16-17, Jun 12:3, Nov 14:5, Aug 16:5

(Do not report 33241 in conjunction with 93260, 93261)

(Do not report 33241 in conjunction with 33230, 33231, 33240 for removal and replacement of the implantable defibrillator pulse generator. Use 33262, 33263, 33264, as appropriate, when pulse generator replacement is indicated)

(For removal and replacement of an implantable defibrillator pulse generator and electrode[s], use 33241 in conjunction with either 33243 or 33244 and 33249 for transvenous electrode[s] or 33270 and 33272 for subcutaneous electrode)

(For removal of implantable defibrillator with substernal lead, generator only, use 0580T)

 # 33262   Removal of implantable defibrillator pulse generator with replacement of implantable defibrillator pulse generator; single lead system

➔ *CPT Changes: An Insider's View* 2012, 2015, 2017

➔ *CPT Assistant* Jun 12:3, Nov 14:5, Aug 16:5

(Do not report 33262 in conjunction with 33271, 93260, 93261, 0614T)

(For removal and replacement of substernal implantable pulse generator, use 0614T)

 # 33263   dual lead system

➔ *CPT Changes: An Insider's View* 2012, 2015, 2017

➔ *CPT Assistant* Jun 12:3, Dec 13:17, Nov 14:5, Aug 16:5

 # 33264   multiple lead system

➔ *CPT Changes: An Insider's View* 2012, 2015, 2017

➔ *CPT Assistant* Jun 12:3, Dec 13:17, Nov 14:5, Aug 16:5

(Do not report 33262, 33263, 33264 in conjunction with 33216, 33217, 33241)

(For removal of electrode[s] by thoracotomy in conjunction with pulse generator removal or replacement, use 33243 in conjunction with 33241 or 33262, 33263, 33264)

(For removal of electrode[s] by transvenous extraction in conjunction with pulse generator removal or replacement, use 33244 in conjunction with 33241 or 33262, 33263, 33264)

(For repair of implantable defibrillator pulse generator and/or leads, see 33218, 33220)

(For removal of subcutaneous electrode in conjunction with implantable defibrillator pulse generator removal or replacement, use 33272 in conjunction with 33241 or 33262)

— *Coding Tip* —

Reporting for Electrode Removal and Lead Placement

Removal of electrode(s) may first be attempted by transvenous extraction (code 33244). However, if transvenous extraction is unsuccessful, a thoracotomy may be required to remove the electrodes (code 33243). Use codes 33212, 33213, 33240 as appropriate in addition to the thoracotomy or endoscopic epicardial lead placement codes to report the insertion of the generator if done by the same physician during the same session.

CPT Coding Guidelines, Pacemaker or Pacing Cardioverter-Defibrillator

---

33243 Removal of single or dual chamber implantable defibrillator electrode(s); by thoracotomy

➲ *CPT Changes: An Insider's View* 2000, 2015

➲ *CPT Assistant* Summer 94:40, Nov 99:16-17, Jun 12:3, Nov 14:5, Aug 16:5

33244 by transvenous extraction

➲ *CPT Changes: An Insider's View* 2000, 2012, 2015, 2017

➲ *CPT Assistant* Summer 94:40, Nov 99:16-17, Jul 00:5, Jun 12:3, Nov 14:5, Aug 16:5

33249 Insertion or replacement of permanent implantable defibrillator system, with transvenous lead(s), single or dual chamber

➲ *CPT Changes: An Insider's View* 2000, 2012, 2015, 2017

➲ *CPT Assistant* Summer 94:21, Nov 99:16-17, Apr 04:6, May 08:14, Jun 08:14, Jun 12:3, Nov 14:5, Aug 16:5

(Do not report 33249 in conjunction with 33216, 33217)

(For removal and replacement of an implantable defibrillator pulse generator and transvenous electrode[s], use 33241 in conjunction with either 33243 or 33244 and 33249)

(For insertion of transvenous implantable defibrillator lead(s), without thoracotomy, use 33216 or 33217)

 # 33270 Insertion or replacement of permanent subcutaneous implantable defibrillator system, with subcutaneous electrode, including defibrillation threshold evaluation, induction of arrhythmia, evaluation of sensing for arrhythmia termination, and programming or reprogramming of sensing or therapeutic parameters, when performed

➲ *CPT Changes: An Insider's View* 2015

➲ *CPT Assistant* Nov 14:5, Aug 16:5

(Do not report 33270 in conjunction with 33271, 93260, 93261, 93644)

(For removal and replacement of an implantable defibrillator pulse generator and subcutaneous electrode, use 33241 in conjunction with 33270 and 33272)

(For insertion of subcutaneous implantable defibrillator lead[s], use 33271)

(For insertion or replacement of permanent implantable defibrillator system with substernal electrode, use 0571T)

 # 33271 Insertion of subcutaneous implantable defibrillator electrode

➲ *CPT Changes: An Insider's View* 2015

➲ *CPT Assistant* Nov 14:5, Aug 16:5

(Do not report 33271 in conjunction with 33240, 33262, 33270, 93260, 93261)

(For insertion or replacement of a cardiac venous system lead, see 33224, 33225)

(For insertion of substernal defibrillator electrode, use 0572T)

 # 33272 Removal of subcutaneous implantable defibrillator electrode

➲ *CPT Changes: An Insider's View* 2015

➲ *CPT Assistant* Nov 14:5, Aug 16:5

(For removal of substernal defibrillator electrode, use 0573T)

 # 33273 Repositioning of previously implanted subcutaneous implantable defibrillator electrode

➲ *CPT Changes: An Insider's View* 2015

➲ *CPT Assistant* Nov 14:5, Aug 16:5

(Do not report 33272, 33273 in conjunction with 93260, 93261)

(For repositioning of substernal defibrillator electrode, use 0574T)

 # 33274 Transcatheter insertion or replacement of permanent leadless pacemaker, right ventricular, including imaging guidance (eg, fluoroscopy, venous ultrasound, ventriculography, femoral venography) and device evaluation (eg, interrogation or programming), when performed

➲ *CPT Changes: An Insider's View* 2019

➲ *CPT Assistant* Mar 19:6, Mar 24:1

 # 33275 Transcatheter removal of permanent leadless pacemaker, right ventricular, including imaging guidance (eg, fluoroscopy, venous ultrasound, ventriculography, femoral venography), when performed

➲ *CPT Changes: An Insider's View* 2019, 2020

➲ *CPT Assistant* Mar 19:6

(Do not report 33275 in conjunction with 33274)

(Do not report 33274, 33275 in conjunction with femoral venography [75820], fluoroscopy [76000, 77002], ultrasound guidance for vascular access [76937], right ventriculography [93566])

(Do not report 33274, 33275 in conjunction with 93451, 93453, 93456, 93457, 93460, 93461, 93593, 93594, 93596, 93597, 93598, unless complete right heart catheterization is performed for indications distinct from the leadless pacemaker procedure)

(Do not report 33274, 33275 in conjunction with dual-chamber leadless pacemaker codes 0795T, 0796T, 0797T, 0798T, 0799T, 0800T, 0801T, 0802T, 0803T)

(Do not report 33274, 33275 in conjunction with 0823T, 0824T, 0825T, for right atrial single-chamber leadless pacemaker)

(Do not report 33274, 33275 when the right ventricular single-chamber leadless pacemaker is part of a complete dual-chamber leadless pacemaker system)

(For insertion, replacement, repositioning, and removal of pacemaker systems with leads, see 33202, 33203, 33206, 33207, 33208, 33212, 33213, 33214, 33215, 33216, 33217, 33218, 33220, 33221, 33227, 33228, 33229, 33233, 33234, 33235, 33236, 33237)

(For subsequent leadless pacemaker device evaluation, see 93279, 93286, 93288, 93294, 93296, 0804T, 0826T)

(For dual-chamber leadless pacemaker, see 0795T, 0796T, 0797T, 0798T, 0799T, 0800T, 0801T, 0802T, 0803T)

(For insertion or replacement of a leadless pacemaker into the right ventricle as part of a complete dual-chamber leadless pacemaker system, use 0797T)

(For removal of right ventricular pacemaker component of a complete dual-chamber leadless pacemaker system, use 0800T)

Phrenic Nerve Stimulation System

Insertion of a phrenic nerve stimulation system includes a pulse generator (containing electronics and a battery) and one stimulation lead and is reported with 33276. Pulse generators are placed in a submuscular or subcutaneous "pocket" in the pectoral region. The stimulation lead is placed transvenously into the right brachiocephalic vein or left pericardiophrenic vein. Rarely, a separate sensing lead may be needed to augment system function and, when performed at time of system insertion, is reported with 33277. This sensing lead is placed transvenously into the azygos vein. Initial system placement includes initiation of diagnostic mode and associated system evaluation. Codes 33276, 33277, 33278, 33279, 33280, 33281, 33287, 33288 include vessel catheterization and all imaging guidance required for the procedure, when performed. For therapeutic activation of the phrenic nerve stimulation system, see 93150, 93151, 93152, 93153.

 # 33276   Insertion of phrenic nerve stimulator system (pulse generator and stimulating lead[s]), including vessel catheterization, all imaging guidance, and pulse generator initial analysis with diagnostic mode activation, when performed

➔ *CPT Changes: An Insider's View 2024*
➔ *CPT Assistant Apr 24:9*

(Do not report 33276 in conjunction with 93150, 93151, 93152, 93153)

#+ 33277   Insertion of phrenic nerve stimulator transvenous sensing lead (List separately in addition to code for primary procedure)

➔ *CPT Changes: An Insider's View 2024*
➔ *CPT Assistant Apr 24:9*

(Use 33277 in conjunction with 33276, 33287)

(For insertion of a phrenic nerve sensing lead other than at initial insertion of the phrenic nerve stimulator system, use 33999)

 # 33278   Removal of phrenic nerve stimulator, including vessel catheterization, all imaging guidance, and interrogation and programming, when performed; system, including pulse generator and lead(s)

➔ *CPT Changes: An Insider's View 2024*
➔ *CPT Assistant Apr 24:9*

 # 33279   transvenous stimulation or sensing lead(s) only

➔ *CPT Changes: An Insider's View 2024*
➔ *CPT Assistant Apr 24:9*

(Use 33279 once for removal of one or more lead[s])

 # 33280   pulse generator only

➔ *CPT Changes: An Insider's View 2024*
➔ *CPT Assistant Apr 24:9*

(Do not report 33278, 33279, 33280 in conjunction with 33276, 33277, 33281, 33287, 33288)

 # 33281   Repositioning of phrenic nerve stimulator transvenous lead(s)

➔ *CPT Changes: An Insider's View 2024*
➔ *CPT Assistant Apr 24:9*

(Do not report 33281 in conjunction with 33276, 33277)

(Report 33281 only once per patient per day)

 # 33287   Removal and replacement of phrenic nerve stimulator, including vessel catheterization, all imaging guidance, and interrogation and programming, when performed; pulse generator

➔ *CPT Changes: An Insider's View 2024*
➔ *CPT Assistant Apr 24:9*

(Do not report 33287 in conjunction with 33276, 33278)

 # 33288   transvenous stimulation or sensing lead(s)

➔ *CPT Changes: An Insider's View 2024*
➔ *CPT Assistant Apr 24:9*

(Use 33288 once for removal of one or more lead[s])

(Do not report 33288 in conjunction with 33277, 33279, 33281)

Electrophysiologic Operative Procedures

This family of codes describes the surgical treatment of supraventricular dysrhythmias. Tissue ablation, disruption, and reconstruction can be accomplished by many methods including surgical incision or through the use of a variety of energy sources (eg, radiofrequency, cryotherapy, microwave, ultrasound, laser). If excision or isolation of the left atrial appendage by any method, including stapling, oversewing, ligation, or plication, is performed in conjunction with any of the atrial tissue ablation and reconstruction (maze) procedures (33254-

Cardiovascular 33016-39599

33259, 33265-33266), it is considered part of the procedure. Codes 33254-33256 are only to be reported when there is no concurrently performed procedure that requires median sternotomy or cardiopulmonary bypass. The appropriate atrial tissue ablation add-on code, 33257, 33258, 33259 should be reported in addition to an open cardiac procedure requiring sternotomy or cardiopulmonary bypass if performed concurrently.

Definitions

Limited operative ablation and reconstruction includes:

Surgical isolation of triggers of supraventricular dysrhythmias by operative ablation that isolates the pulmonary veins or other anatomically defined triggers in the left or right atrium.

Extensive operative ablation and reconstruction includes:

1. The services included in *"limited"*
2. Additional ablation of atrial tissue to eliminate sustained supraventricular dysrhythmias. This must include operative ablation that involves either the right atrium, the atrial septum, or left atrium in continuity with the atrioventricular annulus.

Codes 33267, 33268, 33269 describe surgical left atrial appendage (LAA) exclusion (eg, excision, isolation via stapling, oversewing, ligation, plication, clip) performed to treat atrial fibrillation and mitigate postoperative thromboembolic complications. Surgical LAA exclusion may be performed as a stand-alone procedure via a sternotomy, thoracotomy, or thoracoscopic approach. It is most commonly performed in conjunction with other procedures requiring a sternotomy or thoracotomy approach. Surgical LAA exclusion is inherent to maze procedures (33254, 33255, 33256, 33257, 33258, 33259, 33265, 33266) and mitral valve repair/replacement procedures (33420, 33422, 33425, 33426, 33427, 33430) and may not be reported separately when performed in the same operative session.

Code 33267 may only be reported when there is no concurrently performed procedure that requires a sternotomy or thoracotomy approach.

Add-on code 33268, if performed concurrently, may be reported in conjunction with a primary procedure performed via a sternotomy or thoracotomy.

Code 33269 may be reported for thoracoscopic LAA exclusion, other than with maze or mitral valve procedures (33254, 33255, 33256, 33257, 33258, 33259, 33265, 33266, 33420, 33422, 33425, 33426, 33427, 33430), when performed during the same operative session.

Incision

33250 Operative ablation of supraventricular arrhythmogenic focus or pathway (eg, Wolff-Parkinson-White, atrioventricular node re-entry), tract(s) and/or focus (foci); without cardiopulmonary bypass

➔ *CPT Changes: An Insider's View* 2000, 2002

➔ *CPT Assistant* Summer 94:16, Nov 99:17-18

(For intraoperative pacing and mapping by a separate provider, use 93631)

33251 with cardiopulmonary bypass

➔ *CPT Changes: An Insider's View* 2000

➔ *CPT Assistant* Summer 94:16, Nov 99:17-18

— *Coding Tip* —

Reporting Restriction for Operative Tissue Ablation

Codes 33254-33256 are only to be reported when there is no concurrently performed procedure that requires median sternotomy or cardiopulmonary bypass.

CPT Coding Guidelines, Electrophysiologic Operative Procedures

33254 Operative tissue ablation and reconstruction of atria, limited (eg, modified maze procedure)

➔ *CPT Changes: An Insider's View* 2007

➔ *CPT Assistant* Mar 07:1

33255 Operative tissue ablation and reconstruction of atria, extensive (eg, maze procedure); without cardiopulmonary bypass

➔ *CPT Changes: An Insider's View* 2007

➔ *CPT Assistant* Mar 07:1

33256 with cardiopulmonary bypass

➔ *CPT Changes: An Insider's View* 2007

➔ *CPT Assistant* Mar 07:1

(Do not report 33254-33256 in conjunction with 32100, 32551, 33120, 33130, 33210, 33211, 33390, 33391, 33404-33507, 33510-33523, 33533-33548, 33600-33853, 33858, 33859, 33863, 33864, 33910-33920)

+ 33257 Operative tissue ablation and reconstruction of atria, performed at the time of other cardiac procedure(s), limited (eg, modified maze procedure) (List separately in addition to code for primary procedure)

➔ *CPT Changes: An Insider's View* 2008

(Use 33257 in conjunction with 33120-33130, 33250, 33251, 33261, 33300-33335, 33365, 33390, 33391, 33404-33417, 33420-33476, 33478, 33496, 33500-33507, 33510-33516, 33533-33548, 33600-33619, 33641-33697, 33702-33732, 33735-33767, 33770-33877, 33910-33922, 33925, 33926, 33975, 33976, 33977, 33978, 33979, 33980, 33981, 33982, 33983)

+ 33258   Operative tissue ablation and reconstruction of atria, performed at the time of other cardiac procedure(s), extensive (eg, maze procedure), without cardiopulmonary bypass (List separately in addition to code for primary procedure)

➔ *CPT Changes: An Insider's View* 2008

▶(Use 33258 in conjunction with 33130, 33250, 33300, 33310, 33320, 33321, 33330, 33365, 33420, 33501-33503, 33510-33516, 33533-33536, 33690, 33735, 33750, 33755, 33762, 33764, 33766, 33800-33803, 33820, 33822, 33824, 33840, 33845, 33851, 33852, 33875, 33877, 33915, 33925, 33981, 33982, when the procedure is performed without cardiopulmonary bypass)◀

+ 33259   Operative tissue ablation and reconstruction of atria, performed at the time of other cardiac procedure(s), extensive (eg, maze procedure), with cardiopulmonary bypass (List separately in addition to code for primary procedure)

➔ *CPT Changes: An Insider's View* 2008

(Use 33259 in conjunction with 33120, 33251, 33261, 33305, 33315, 33322, 33335, 33390, 33391, 33404, 33405, 33406, 33410, 33411, 33412, 33413, 33414, 33415, 33416, 33417, 33422-33468, 33474, 33475, 33476, 33478, 33496, 33500, 33504-33507, 33510-33516, 33533-33548, 33600-33688, 33692-33726, 33730, 33732, 33736, 33767, 33770, 33783, 33786-33788, 33814, 33853, 33858-33877, 33910, 33916-33922, 33926, 33975-33980, 33983, when the procedure is performed with cardiopulmonary bypass)

(Do not report 33257, 33258 and 33259 in conjunction with 32551, 33210, 33211, 33254-33256, 33265, 33266)

33261   Operative ablation of ventricular arrhythmogenic focus with cardiopulmonary bypass

➔ *CPT Assistant* Summer 94:16

 # 33267   Exclusion of left atrial appendage, open, any method (eg, excision, isolation via stapling, oversewing, ligation, plication, clip)

➔ *CPT Changes: An Insider's View* 2022
➔ *CPT Assistant* Nov 21:3-4

(Do not report 33267 in conjunction with 33254, 33255, 33256, 33257, 33258, 33259, 33265, 33266, 33420, 33422, 33425, 33426, 33427, 33430)

(Do not report 33267 in conjunction with other sternotomy or thoracotomy procedures performed during the same session)

#+ 33268   Exclusion of left atrial appendage, open, performed at the time of other sternotomy or thoracotomy procedure(s), any method (eg, excision, isolation via stapling, oversewing, ligation, plication, clip) (List separately in addition to code for primary procedure)

➔ *CPT Changes: An Insider's View* 2022
➔ *CPT Assistant* Nov 21:3-4

(Use 33268 in conjunction with primary procedures performed via sternotomy or thoracotomy approach)

(Do not report 33268 in conjunction with 33254, 33255, 33256, 33257, 33258, 33259, 33265, 33266, 33420, 33422, 33425, 33426, 33427, 33430)

33262   Code is out of numerical sequence. See 33226-33244

33263   Code is out of numerical sequence. See 33226-33244

33264   Code is out of numerical sequence. See 33226-33244

Endoscopy

 # 33269   Exclusion of left atrial appendage, thoracoscopic, any method (eg, excision, isolation via stapling, oversewing, ligation, plication, clip)

➔ *CPT Changes: An Insider's View* 2022
➔ *CPT Assistant* Nov 21:3-4

(Do not report 33269 in conjunction with 33254, 33255, 33256, 33257, 33258, 33259, 33265, 33266, 33420, 33422, 33425, 33426, 33427, 33430)

33265   Endoscopy, surgical; operative tissue ablation and reconstruction of atria, limited (eg, modified maze procedure), without cardiopulmonary bypass

➔ *CPT Changes: An Insider's View* 2007
➔ *CPT Assistant* Mar 07:1

33266   operative tissue ablation and reconstruction of atria, extensive (eg, maze procedure), without cardiopulmonary bypass

➔ *CPT Changes: An Insider's View* 2007
➔ *CPT Assistant* Mar 07:1

(Do not report 33265-33266 in conjunction with 32551, 33210, 33211)

33267   Code is out of numerical sequence. See 33259-33266

33268   Code is out of numerical sequence. See 33259-33266

33269   Code is out of numerical sequence. See 33259-33266

33270   Code is out of numerical sequence. See 33244-33251

33271   Code is out of numerical sequence. See 33244-33251

33272   Code is out of numerical sequence. See 33244-33251

33273   Code is out of numerical sequence. See 33244-33251

33274   Code is out of numerical sequence. See 33244-33251

33275   Code is out of numerical sequence. See 33244-33251

33276   Code is out of numerical sequence. See 33244-33251

33277   Code is out of numerical sequence. See 33244-33251

33278   Code is out of numerical sequence. See 33244-33251

33279   Code is out of numerical sequence. See 33244-33251

33280   Code is out of numerical sequence. See 33244-33251

33281   Code is out of numerical sequence. See 33244-33251

Subcutaneous Cardiac Rhythm Monitor

A subcutaneous cardiac rhythm monitor, also known as a cardiac event recorder or implantable/insertable loop recorder (ILR), is a subcutaneously placed device that continuously records the electrocardiographic rhythm, triggered automatically by rapid, irregular and/or slow heart rates or by the patient during a symptomatic episode. A subcutaneous cardiac rhythm monitor is placed using a small parasternal incision followed by insertion of the monitor into a small subcutaneous pre-pectoral pocket, followed by closure of the incision.

33285 Insertion, subcutaneous cardiac rhythm monitor, including programming
➜ *CPT Changes: An Insider's View* 2019
➜ *CPT Assistant* Apr 19:3, Sep 22:1

33286 Removal, subcutaneous cardiac rhythm monitor
➜ *CPT Changes: An Insider's View* 2019
➜ *CPT Assistant* Apr 19:3

(Initial insertion includes programming. For subsequent electronic analysis and/or reprogramming, see 93285, 93291, 93298)

33287 Code is out of numerical sequence. See 33244-33251

33288 Code is out of numerical sequence. See 33244-33251

Implantable Hemodynamic Monitors

Transcatheter implantation of a wireless pulmonary artery pressure sensor (33289) establishes an intravascular device used for long-term remote monitoring of pulmonary artery pressures (93264). The hemodynamic data derived from this device is used to guide management of patients with heart failure. Code 33289 includes deployment and calibration of the sensor, right heart catheterization, selective pulmonary artery catheterization, radiological supervision and interpretation, and pulmonary artery angiography, when performed.

33289 Transcatheter implantation of wireless pulmonary artery pressure sensor for long-term hemodynamic monitoring, including deployment and calibration of the sensor, right heart catheterization, selective pulmonary catheterization, radiological supervision and interpretation, and pulmonary artery angiography, when performed
➜ *CPT Changes: An Insider's View* 2019
➜ *CPT Assistant* Jun 19:3, May 23:1

(Do not report 33289 in conjunction with 36013, 36014, 36015, 75741, 75743, 75746, 76000, 93451, 93453, 93456, 93457, 93460, 93461, 93568, 93569, 93573, 93593, 93594, 93596, 93597, 93598)

(For remote monitoring of an implantable wireless pulmonary artery pressure sensor, use 93264)

▶(For implantation of a wireless left atrial pressure sensor, use 0933T)◀

Heart (Including Valves) and Great Vessels

Patients receiving major cardiac procedures may require simultaneous cardiopulmonary bypass insertion of cannulae into the venous and arterial vasculatures with support of circulation and oxygenation by a heart-lung machine. Most services are described by codes in dyad arrangements to allow distinct reporting of procedures with or without cardiopulmonary bypass. Cardio-pulmonary bypass is distinct from support of cardiac output using devices (eg, ventricular assist or intra-aortic balloon). For cardiac assist services, see 33946, 33947, 33948, 33949, 33967-33983, 33990, 33991, 33992, 33993, 33995, 33997.

33300 Repair of cardiac wound; without bypass

33305 with cardiopulmonary bypass

33310 Cardiotomy, exploratory (includes removal of foreign body, atrial or ventricular thrombus); without bypass
➜ *CPT Changes: An Insider's View* 2004

33315 with cardiopulmonary bypass
➜ *CPT Assistant* Oct 10:12, Dec 10:12

(Do not report removal of thrombus [33310-33315] in conjunction with other cardiac procedures unless a separate incision in the heart is required to remove the atrial or ventricular thrombus)

(If removal of thrombus with cardiopulmonary bypass [33315] is reported in conjunction with 33120, 33130, 33420-33430, 33460-33468, 33496, 33542, 33545, 33641-33647, 33670, 33681, 33975-33980 which requires a separate heart incision, report 33315 with modifier 59)

33320 Suture repair of aorta or great vessels; without shunt or cardiopulmonary bypass
➜ *CPT Assistant* Fall 91:7, Jun 18:11

33321 with shunt bypass
➜ *CPT Assistant* Fall 91:7, Jun 18:11

33322 with cardiopulmonary bypass
➜ *CPT Assistant* Fall 91:7, Jun 18:11

33330 Insertion of graft, aorta or great vessels; without shunt, or cardiopulmonary bypass
➜ *CPT Assistant* Jun 18:11

33335 with cardiopulmonary bypass
➜ *CPT Assistant* Jun 18:11

33340   Percutaneous transcatheter closure of the left atrial appendage with endocardial implant, including fluoroscopy, transseptal puncture, catheter placement(s), left atrial angiography, left atrial appendage angiography, when performed, and radiological supervision and interpretation

→ *CPT Changes: An Insider's View* 2017

→ *CPT Assistant* Jul 17:3, Nov 21:3

(Do not report 33340 in conjunction with 93462)

(Do not report 33340 in conjunction with 93452, 93453, 93458, 93459, 93460, 93461, 93595, 93596, 93597, 93598, unless catheterization of the left ventricle is performed by a non-transseptal approach for indications distinct from the left atrial appendage closure procedure)

(Do not report 33340 in conjunction with 93451, 93453, 93456, 93460, 93461, 93593, 93594, 93596, 93597, 93598, unless complete right heart catheterization is performed for indications distinct from the left atrial appendage closure procedure)

Cardiac Valves

(For multiple valve procedures, see 33390, 33391, 33404-33478 and add modifier 51 to the secondary valve procedure code)

Aortic Valve

Codes 33361, 33362, 33363, 33364, 33365, 33366 are used to report transcatheter aortic valve replacement (TAVR)/transcatheter aortic valve implantation (TAVI). TAVR/TAVI requires two physician operators and all components of the procedure are reported using modifier 62.

Codes 33361, 33362, 33363, 33364, 33365, 33366 include the work, when performed, of percutaneous access, placing the access sheath, balloon aortic valvuloplasty, advancing the valve delivery system into position, repositioning the valve as needed, deploying the valve, temporary pacemaker insertion for rapid pacing (33210), and closure of the arteriotomy when performed. Codes 33361, 33362, 33363, 33364, 33365, 33366 include open arterial or cardiac approach.

Angiography, radiological supervision, and interpretation performed to guide TAVR/TAVI (eg, guiding valve placement, documenting completion of the intervention, assessing the vascular access site for closure) are included in these codes.

Add-on code 33370 may be reported for cerebral embolic protection in conjunction with TAVR/TAVI codes 33361, 33362, 33363, 33364, 33365, 33366. Code 33370 includes percutaneous arterial (eg, right radial or femoral) access, placement of a guiding catheter, and delivery of the embolic protection filter(s) prior to the procedure. Placement of additional/multiple filters is not separately reportable. Code 33370 includes removal of

the filter(s) and debris, removal of the arterial sheath, and closure of the arteriotomy by pressure and application of an arterial closure device or standard closure of the puncture by suture. Extensive repair or replacement of an artery may be additionally reported. Code 33370 includes all imaging guidance and radiological supervision and interpretation associated with performing cerebral embolic protection (eg, 75600, 75710, 76937).

Diagnostic left heart catheterization codes (93452, 93453, 93458-93461) and the supravalvular aortography code (93567) should **not** be used with TAVR/TAVI services (33361, 33362, 33363, 33364, 33365, 33366) to report:

1. Contrast injections, angiography, roadmapping, and/or fluoroscopic guidance for the TAVR/TAVI,

2. Aorta/left ventricular outflow tract measurement for the TAVR/TAVI, or

3. Post-TAVR/TAVI aortic or left ventricular angiography, as this work is captured in the TAVR/TAVI services codes (33361, 33362, 33363, 33364, 33365, 33366).

Diagnostic coronary angiography performed at the time of TAVR/TAVI may be separately reportable if:

1. No prior catheter-based coronary angiography study is available and a full diagnostic study is performed, or

2. A prior study is available, but as documented in the medical record:

   a. The patient's condition with respect to the clinical indication has changed since the prior study, or

   b. There is inadequate visualization of the anatomy and/or pathology, or

   c. There is a clinical change during the procedure that requires new evaluation.

   d. For same session/same day diagnostic coronary angiography services, report the appropriate diagnostic cardiac catheterization code(s) appended with modifier 59 indicating separate and distinct procedural service from TAVR/TAVI.

Diagnostic coronary angiography performed at a separate session from an interventional procedure may be separately reportable.

Other cardiac catheterization services may be reported separately when performed for diagnostic purposes not intrinsic to TAVR/TAVI.

Percutaneous coronary interventional procedures are reported separately, when performed.

When transcatheter ventricular support is required in conjunction with TAVR/TAVI, the appropriate code may be reported with the appropriate ventricular assist device (VAD) procedure code (33975, 33976, 33990, 33991, 33992, 33993, 33995, 33997) or balloon pump insertion code (33967, 33970, 33973).

The TAVR/TAVI cardiovascular access and delivery procedures are reported with 33361, 33362, 33363, 33364, 33365, 33366. When cardiopulmonary bypass is performed in conjunction with TAVR/TAVI, codes 33361, 33362, 33363, 33364, 33365, 33366 should be reported with the appropriate add-on code for percutaneous peripheral bypass (33367), open peripheral bypass (33368), or central bypass (33369).

33361   Transcatheter aortic valve replacement (TAVR/TAVI) with prosthetic valve; percutaneous femoral artery approach
➔ *CPT Changes: An Insider's View* 2013
➔ *CPT Assistant* Jan 13:6, Jan 14:5, Jul 14:8, Mar 15:9, Jan 22:16, Apr 22:13

33362   open femoral artery approach
➔ *CPT Changes: An Insider's View* 2013
➔ *CPT Assistant* Jan 13:6, Jan 14:5, Mar 15:9, Jan 22:16, Apr 22:13

33363   open axillary artery approach
➔ *CPT Changes: An Insider's View* 2013
➔ *CPT Assistant* Jan 13:6, Jan 14:5, Mar 15:9, Jan 22:16, Apr 22:13

33364   open iliac artery approach
➔ *CPT Changes: An Insider's View* 2013
➔ *CPT Assistant* Jan 13:6, Jan 14:5, Mar 15:9, Jan 22:16, Apr 22:13

33365   transaortic approach (eg, median sternotomy, mediastinotomy)
➔ *CPT Changes: An Insider's View* 2013
➔ *CPT Assistant* Jan 13:6, Jan 14:5, Mar 15:9, Jan 22:16, Apr 22:13

33366   transapical exposure (eg, left thoracotomy)
➔ *CPT Changes: An Insider's View* 2014
➔ *CPT Assistant* Jan 14:5, Jul 14:8, Mar 15:9, Jan 22:16, Apr 22:13

+ 33367   cardiopulmonary bypass support with percutaneous peripheral arterial and venous cannulation (eg, femoral vessels) (List separately in addition to code for primary procedure)
➔ *CPT Changes: An Insider's View* 2013
➔ *CPT Assistant* Jan 13:6, Sep 15:3, Mar 16:5

(Use 33367 in conjunction with 33361, 33362, 33363, 33364, 33365, 33366, 33418, 33477, 0483T, 0484T, 0544T, 0545T, 0569T, 0570T, 0643T, 0644T)

(Do not report 33367 in conjunction with 33368, 33369)

(For cerebral embolic protection, use 33370)

+ 33368   cardiopulmonary bypass support with open peripheral arterial and venous cannulation (eg, femoral, iliac, axillary vessels) (List separately in addition to code for primary procedure)
➔ *CPT Changes: An Insider's View* 2013
➔ *CPT Assistant* Jan 13:6, Sep 15:3, Mar 16:5

(Use 33368 in conjunction with 33361, 33362, 33363, 33364, 33365, 33366, 33418, 33477, 0483T, 0484T, 0544T, 0545T, 0569T, 0570T, 0643T, 0644T)

(Do not report 33368 in conjunction with 33367, 33369)

+ 33369   cardiopulmonary bypass support with central arterial and venous cannulation (eg, aorta, right atrium, pulmonary artery) (List separately in addition to code for primary procedure)
➔ *CPT Changes: An Insider's View* 2013
➔ *CPT Assistant* Jan 13:6, Sep 15:3, Mar 16:5

(Use 33369 in conjunction with 33361, 33362, 33363, 33364, 33365, 33366, 33418, 33477, 0483T, 0484T, 0544T, 0545T, 0569T, 0570T, 0643T, 0644T)

(Do not report 33369 in conjunction with 33367, 33368)

+ 33370   Transcatheter placement and subsequent removal of cerebral embolic protection device(s), including arterial access, catheterization, imaging, and radiological supervision and interpretation, percutaneous (List separately in addition to code for primary procedure)
➔ *CPT Changes: An Insider's View* 2022
➔ *CPT Assistant* Jan 22:16, Apr 22:13

(Use 33370 in conjunction with 33361, 33362, 33363, 33364, 33365, 33366)

33390   Valvuloplasty, aortic valve, open, with cardiopulmonary bypass; simple (ie, valvotomy, debridement, debulking, and/or simple commissural resuspension)
➔ *CPT Changes: An Insider's View* 2017
➔ *CPT Assistant* May 17:9

33391   complex (eg, leaflet extension, leaflet resection, leaflet reconstruction, or annuloplasty)
➔ *CPT Changes: An Insider's View* 2017
➔ *CPT Assistant* May 17:9

(Do not report 33391 in conjunction with 33390)

33404   Construction of apical-aortic conduit
➔ *CPT Assistant* Jan 04:28, Feb 05:14

33405   Replacement, aortic valve, open, with cardiopulmonary bypass; with prosthetic valve other than homograft or stentless valve
➔ *CPT Changes: An Insider's View* 2000, 2017
➔ *CPT Assistant* Nov 99:18, Feb 05:14, Aug 11:3, Jan 13:6, May 17:9, Apr 19:6

33406   with allograft valve (freehand)

➡ *CPT Changes: An Insider's View* 2002, 2017

➡ *CPT Assistant* Nov 99:18, Feb 05:14, Aug 11:3, May 17:9, Apr 19:6

33410   with stentless tissue valve

➡ *CPT Changes: An Insider's View* 2000, 2017

➡ *CPT Assistant* Nov 99:18, Feb 05:14, Aug 11:3, May 17:9, Apr 19:6

 # 33440   Replacement, aortic valve; by translocation of autologous pulmonary valve and transventricular aortic annulus enlargement of the left ventricular outflow tract with valved conduit replacement of pulmonary valve (Ross-Konno procedure)

➡ *CPT Changes: An Insider's View* 2019

➡ *CPT Assistant* Apr 19:6

(Do not report 33440 in conjunction with 33405, 33406, 33410, 33411, 33412, 33413, 33414, 33416, 33417, 33475, 33608, 33920)

33411   with aortic annulus enlargement, noncoronary sinus

➡ *CPT Changes: An Insider's View* 2011

➡ *CPT Assistant* Feb 05:14, Aug 11:3, Apr 19:6, Mar 23:33

33412   with transventricular aortic annulus enlargement (Konno procedure)

➡ *CPT Assistant* Feb 05:14, Aug 11:3, Apr 19:6

(Do not report 33412 in conjunction with 33413, 33440)

(For replacement of aortic valve with transventricular aortic annulus enlargement [Konno procedure] in conjunction with translocation of autologous pulmonary valve with allograft replacement of pulmonary valve [Ross procedure], use 33440)

33413   by translocation of autologous pulmonary valve with allograft replacement of pulmonary valve (Ross procedure)

➡ *CPT Changes: An Insider's View* 2002

➡ *CPT Assistant* Feb 05:14, Aug 11:3, Apr 19:6

(Do not report 33413 in conjunction with 33412, 33440)

(For replacement of aortic valve with transventricular aortic annulus enlargement [Konno procedure] in conjunction with translocation of autologous pulmonary valve with allograft replacement of pulmonary valve [Ross procedure], use 33440)

33414   Repair of left ventricular outflow tract obstruction by patch enlargement of the outflow tract

➡ *CPT Assistant* Feb 05:14, Apr 19:6, Mar 23:33

33415   Resection or incision of subvalvular tissue for discrete subvalvular aortic stenosis

➡ *CPT Assistant* Feb 05:14

33416   Ventriculomyotomy (-myectomy) for idiopathic hypertrophic subaortic stenosis (eg, asymmetric septal hypertrophy)

➡ *CPT Assistant* Feb 05:14, Apr 19:6

(For percutaneous transcatheter septal reduction therapy, use 93583)

33417   Aortoplasty (gusset) for supravalvular stenosis

➡ *CPT Assistant* Feb 05:14, Apr 19:6

Mitral Valve

Codes 33418 and 33419 are used to report transcatheter mitral valve repair (TMVR). Code 33419 should only be reported once per session.

Codes 33418 and 33419 include the work, when performed, of percutaneous access, placing the access sheath, transseptal puncture, advancing the repair device delivery system into position, repositioning the device as needed, and deploying the device(s).

Angiography, radiological supervision, and interpretation performed to guide TMVR (eg, guiding device placement and documenting completion of the intervention) are included in these codes.

Diagnostic right and left heart catheterization codes (93451, 93452, 93453, 93456, 93457, 93458, 93459, 93460, 93461, 93593, 93594, 93595, 93596, 93597, 93598) should **not** be used with 33418, 33419 to report:

1. Contrast injections, angiography, road-mapping, and/or fluoroscopic guidance for the transcatheter mitral valve repair (TMVR),

2. Left ventricular angiography to assess mitral regurgitation for guidance of TMVR, or

3. Right and left heart catheterization for hemodynamic measurements before, during, and after TMVR for guidance of TMVR.

Diagnostic right and left heart catheterization codes (93451, 93452, 93453, 93456, 93457, 93458, 93459, 93460, 93461, 93593, 93594, 93595, 93596, 93597, 93598) and diagnostic coronary angiography codes (93454, 93455, 93456, 93457, 93458, 93459, 93460, 93461, 93563, 93564) may be reported with 33418, 33419, representing separate and distinct services from TMVR, if:

1. No prior study is available and a full diagnostic study is performed, or

2. A prior study is available, but as documented in the medical record:

   a. There is inadequate visualization of the anatomy and/or pathology, or

   b. The patient's condition with respect to the clinical indication has changed since the prior study, or

   c. There is a clinical change during the procedure that requires new evaluation.

Other cardiac catheterization services may be reported separately when performed for diagnostic purposes not intrinsic to TMVR.

For same session/same day diagnostic cardiac catheterization services, report the appropriate diagnostic cardiac catheterization code(s) appended with modifier 59 indicating separate and distinct procedural service from TMVR.

Diagnostic coronary angiography performed at a separate session from an interventional procedure may be separately reportable.

Percutaneous coronary interventional procedures may be reported separately, when performed.

When transcatheter ventricular support is required in conjunction with TMVR, the appropriate code may be reported with the appropriate ventricular assist device (VAD) procedure code (33990, 33991, 33992, 33993, 33995, 33997) or balloon pump insertion code (33967, 33970, 33973).

When cardiopulmonary bypass is performed in conjunction with TMVR, 33418, 33419 may be reported with the appropriate add-on code for percutaneous peripheral bypass (33367), open peripheral bypass (33368), or central bypass (33369).

33418 Transcatheter mitral valve repair, percutaneous approach, including transseptal puncture when performed; initial prosthesis
➔ *CPT Changes: An Insider's View* 2015
➔ *CPT Assistant* Sep 15:3

(Do not report 33418 in conjunction with 93462 unless transapical puncture is performed)

+ 33419 additional prosthesis(es) during same session (List separately in addition to code for primary procedure)
➔ *CPT Changes: An Insider's View* 2015
➔ *CPT Assistant* Sep 15:3

(Use 33419 in conjunction with 33418)

(For transcatheter mitral valve repair, percutaneous approach via the coronary sinus, use 0345T)

(For transcatheter mitral valve implantation/replacement [TMVI], see 0483T, 0484T)

(For transcatheter mitral valve annulus reconstruction, use 0544T)

33420 Valvotomy, mitral valve; closed heart
➔ *CPT Assistant* Feb 05:14

33422 open heart, with cardiopulmonary bypass
➔ *CPT Assistant* Feb 05:14

33425 Valvuloplasty, mitral valve, with cardiopulmonary bypass;
➔ *CPT Assistant* May 03:19, Feb 05:14

33426 with prosthetic ring
➔ *CPT Assistant* Feb 05:14, Apr 21:14

33427 radical reconstruction, with or without ring
➔ *CPT Assistant* Feb 05:14, Apr 21:14

33430 Replacement, mitral valve, with cardiopulmonary bypass
➔ *CPT Assistant* Feb 05:14

33440 Code is out of numerical sequence. See 33406-33412

Tricuspid Valve

(For transcatheter tricuspid valve implantation [TTVI]/replacement, use 0646T)

(For transcatheter tricuspid valve repair [TTVr], see 0569T, 0570T)

33460 Valvectomy, tricuspid valve, with cardiopulmonary bypass
➔ *CPT Assistant* Feb 05:14

33463 Valvuloplasty, tricuspid valve; without ring insertion
➔ *CPT Assistant* Feb 05:14

33464 with ring insertion
➔ *CPT Assistant* Feb 05:14

33465 Replacement, tricuspid valve, with cardiopulmonary bypass
➔ *CPT Assistant* Feb 05:14

33468 Tricuspid valve repositioning and plication for Ebstein anomaly
➔ *CPT Assistant* Feb 05:14

(For transcatheter tricuspid valve annulus reconstruction, use 0545T)

Pulmonary Valve

Code 33477 is used to report transcatheter pulmonary valve implantation (TPVI). Code 33477 should only be reported once per session.

Code 33477 includes the work, when performed, of percutaneous access, placing the access sheath, advancing the repair device delivery system into position, repositioning the device as needed, and deploying the device(s). Angiography, radiological supervision, and interpretation performed to guide TPVI (eg, guiding device placement and documenting completion of the intervention) are included in the code.

Code 33477 includes all cardiac catheterization(s), intraprocedural contrast injection(s), fluoroscopic radiological supervision and interpretation, and imaging guidance performed to complete the pulmonary valve procedure. Do not report 33477 in conjunction with 76000, 93451, 93453, 93454, 93455, 93456, 93457, 93458, 93459, 93460, 93461, 93563, 93566, 93567, 93568, 93569, 93573, 93593, 93594, 93596, 93597, 93598, for angiography intrinsic to the procedure.

Code 33477 includes percutaneous balloon angioplasty of the conduit/treatment zone, valvuloplasty of the pulmonary valve conduit, and stent deployment within the pulmonary conduit or an existing bioprosthetic pulmonary valve, when performed. Do not report 33477 in conjunction with 37236, 37237, 92997, 92998 for pulmonary artery angioplasty/valvuloplasty or stenting within the prosthetic valve delivery site.

Codes 92997, 92998 may be reported separately when pulmonary artery angioplasty is performed at a site separate from the prosthetic valve delivery site. Codes 37236, 37237 may be reported separately when pulmonary artery stenting is performed at a site separate from the prosthetic valve delivery site.

Diagnostic right heart catheterization and diagnostic angiography codes (93451, 93453, 93454, 93455, 93456, 93457, 93458, 93459, 93460, 93461, 93563, 93566, 93567, 93568, 93569, 93573, 93593, 93594, 93596, 93597, 93598) should **not** be used with 33477 to report:

1. Contrast injections, angiography, roadmapping, and/or fluoroscopic guidance for the TPVI,

2. Pulmonary conduit angiography for guidance of TPVI, or

3. Right heart catheterization for hemodynamic measurements before, during, and after TPVI for guidance of TPVI.

Diagnostic right and left heart catheterization codes (93451, 93452, 93453, 93456, 93457, 93458, 93459, 93460, 93461, 93593, 93594, 93595, 93596, 93597, 93598), diagnostic coronary angiography codes (93454, 93455, 93456, 93457, 93458, 93459, 93460, 93461, 93563, 93564), and diagnostic pulmonary angiography codes (93568, 93569, 93573, 93574, 93575) may be reported with 33477, representing separate and distinct services from TPVI, if:

1. No prior study is available and a full diagnostic study is performed, or

2. A prior study is available, but as documented in the medical record:

   a. There is inadequate visualization of the anatomy and/or pathology, or

   b. The patient's condition with respect to the clinical indication has changed since the prior study, or

   c. There is a clinical change during the procedure that requires new evaluation.

Other cardiac catheterization services may be reported separately when performed for diagnostic purposes not intrinsic to TPVI.

For same session/same day diagnostic cardiac catheterization services, report the appropriate diagnostic cardiac catheterization code(s) appended with modifier 59 to indicate separate and distinct procedural services from TPVI.

Diagnostic coronary angiography performed at a separate session from an interventional procedure may be separately reportable, when performed.

Percutaneous coronary interventional procedures may be reported separately, when performed.

Percutaneous pulmonary artery branch interventions may be reported separately, when performed.

When transcatheter ventricular support is required in conjunction with TPVI, the appropriate code may be reported with the appropriate percutaneous ventricular assist device (VAD) procedure codes (33990, 33991, 33992, 33993, 33995, 33997), extracorporeal membrane oxygenation (ECMO) or extracorporeal life support services (ECLS) procedure codes (33946-33989), or balloon pump insertion codes (33967, 33970, 33973).

When cardiopulmonary bypass is performed in conjunction with TPVI, code 33477 may be reported with the appropriate add-on code for percutaneous peripheral bypass (33367), open peripheral bypass (33368), or central bypass (33369).

▶(33471 has been deleted)◀

33474   Valvotomy, pulmonary valve, open heart, with cardiopulmonary bypass
➲ *CPT Assistant* Feb 05:14

33475   Replacement, pulmonary valve
➲ *CPT Assistant* Feb 05:14, Apr 19:6

33476   Right ventricular resection for infundibular stenosis, with or without commissurotomy
➲ *CPT Assistant* Feb 05:14

33477   Transcatheter pulmonary valve implantation, percutaneous approach, including pre-stenting of the valve delivery site, when performed
➲ *CPT Changes: An Insider's View* 2016
➲ *CPT Assistant* Mar 16:5, Aug 16:10

33478   Outflow tract augmentation (gusset), with or without commissurotomy or infundibular resection
➲ *CPT Assistant* Feb 05:14

(Use 33478 in conjunction with 33768 when a cavopulmonary anastomosis to a second superior vena cava is performed)

Other Valvular Procedures

33496   Repair of non-structural prosthetic valve dysfunction with cardiopulmonary bypass (separate procedure)
➲ *CPT Assistant* Nov 97:16, Feb 05:14

(For reoperation, use 33530 in addition to 33496)

Coronary Artery Anomalies

Basic procedures include endarterectomy or angioplasty.

33500 Repair of coronary arteriovenous or arteriocardiac chamber fistula; with cardiopulmonary bypass

➔ *CPT Assistant* Dec 21:18

33501 without cardiopulmonary bypass

33502 Repair of anomalous coronary artery from pulmonary artery origin; by ligation

➔ *CPT Changes: An Insider's View* 2006

33503 by graft, without cardiopulmonary bypass

(Do not report modifier 63 in conjunction with 33502, 33503)

33504 by graft, with cardiopulmonary bypass

33505 with construction of intrapulmonary artery tunnel (Takeuchi procedure)

33506 by translocation from pulmonary artery to aorta

(Do not report modifier 63 in conjunction with 33505, 33506)

33507 Repair of anomalous (eg, intramural) aortic origin of coronary artery by unroofing or translocation

➔ *CPT Changes: An Insider's View* 2006

➔ *CPT Assistant* Mar 07:1

Endoscopy

To report endoscopic harvesting of a vein for coronary artery bypass procedure, use 33508 in addition to the code for the associated bypass procedure. To report endoscopic harvesting of an upper extremity artery for a bypass procedure, use 33509.

Surgical vascular endoscopy always includes diagnostic endoscopy.

+ 33508 Endoscopy, surgical, including video-assisted harvest of vein(s) for coronary artery bypass procedure (List separately in addition to code for primary procedure)

➔ *CPT Changes: An Insider's View* 2003

➔ *CPT Assistant* Dec 21:18

(Use 33508 in conjunction with 33510-33523)

(For open harvest of upper extremity vein procedure, use 35500)

⊘ 33509 Harvest of upper extremity artery, 1 segment, for coronary artery bypass procedure, endoscopic

➔ *CPT Changes: An Insider's View* 2022

➔ *CPT Assistant* Dec 21:17

(For open harvest of upper extremity artery, use 35600)

(For bilateral procedure, report 33509 with modifier 50)

Venous Grafting Only for Coronary Artery Bypass

The following codes are used to report coronary artery bypass procedures using venous grafts only. These codes should NOT be used to report the performance of coronary artery bypass procedures using arterial grafts and venous grafts during the same procedure. See 33517-33523 and 33533-33536 for reporting combined arterial-venous grafts.

Procurement of the saphenous vein graft is included in the description of the work for 33510-33516 and should not be reported as a separate service or co-surgery. To report harvesting of an upper extremity vein, use 35500 in addition to the bypass procedure. To report harvesting of a femoropopliteal vein segment, report 35572 in addition to the bypass procedure. When surgical assistant performs graft procurement, add modifier 80 to 33510-33516. For percutaneous ventricular assist device insertion, removal, repositioning, see 33990, 33991, 33992, 33993, 33995, 33997.

33510 Coronary artery bypass, vein only; single coronary venous graft

➔ *CPT Assistant* Fall 91:5, Winter 92:12, Jul 99:11, Apr 01:7, Feb 05:14, Jan 07:7, Mar 07:1, Aug 14:14

33511 2 coronary venous grafts

➔ *CPT Assistant* Fall 91:5, Winter 92:12, Jul 99:11, Apr 01:7, Feb 05:14, Jan 07:7, Mar 07:1

33512 3 coronary venous grafts

➔ *CPT Assistant* Fall 91:5, Winter 92:12, Apr 01:7, Feb 05:14, Jan 07:7, Mar 07:1

33513 4 coronary venous grafts

➔ *CPT Assistant* Fall 91:5, Winter 92:12, Apr 01:7, Feb 05:14, Jan 07:7, Mar 07:1

33514 5 coronary venous grafts

➔ *CPT Assistant* Fall 91:5, Winter 92:12, Apr 01:7, Feb 05:14, Jan 07:7, Mar 07:1

33516 6 or more coronary venous grafts

➔ *CPT Assistant* Fall 91:5, Winter 92:12, Jul 99:11, Apr 01:7, Feb 05:14, Jan 07:7, Mar 07:1, Aug 14:14

Coronary Artery Bypass-Venous Grafting Only
33510-33516

A. Use 33510 to report a single coronary venous graft.

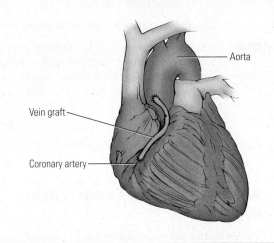

B. Report 33512 when 3 coronary venous grafts are performed.

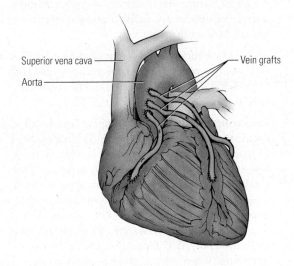

Combined Arterial-Venous Grafting for Coronary Bypass

The following codes are used to report coronary artery bypass procedures using venous grafts and arterial grafts during the same procedure. These codes may NOT be used alone.

To report combined arterial-venous grafts it is necessary to report two codes: (1) the appropriate combined arterial-venous graft code (33517-33523); and (2) the appropriate arterial graft code (33533-33536).

Procurement of the saphenous vein graft is included in the description of the work for 33517-33523 and should not be reported as a separate service or co-surgery. Procurement of the artery for grafting is included in the description of the work for 33533-33536 and should not be reported as a separate service or co-surgery, except

when an upper extremity artery (eg, radial artery) is procured. To report harvesting of an upper extremity artery, use 33509 or 35600. To report harvesting of an upper extremity vein, use 35500 in addition to the bypass procedure. To report harvesting of a femoropopliteal vein segment, report 35572 in addition to the bypass procedure. When surgical assistant performs arterial and/or venous graft procurement, add modifier 80 to 33517-33523, 33533-33536, as appropriate. For percutaneous ventricular assist device insertion, removal, repositioning, see 33990, 33991, 33992, 33993, 33995, 33997.

+ 33517   Coronary artery bypass, using venous graft(s) and arterial graft(s); single vein graft (List separately in addition to code for primary procedure)

➔ *CPT Changes: An Insider's View* 2000, 2008

➔ *CPT Assistant* Fall 91:5, Winter 92:13, Nov 99:18, Apr 01:7, Feb 05:14, Dec 21:18

(Use 33517 in conjunction with 33533-33536)

+ 33518   2 venous grafts (List separately in addition to code for primary procedure)

➔ *CPT Changes: An Insider's View* 2008

➔ *CPT Assistant* Fall 91:5, Winter 92:13, Apr 01:7, Feb 05:14, Jan 07:7, Mar 07:1, Dec 21:18

(Use 33518 in conjunction with 33533-33536)

+ 33519   3 venous grafts (List separately in addition to code for primary procedure)

➔ *CPT Changes: An Insider's View* 2008

➔ *CPT Assistant* Fall 91:5, Winter 92:13, Apr 01:7, Feb 05:14, Jan 07:7, Mar 07:1, Dec 21:18

(Use 33519 in conjunction with 33533-33536)

+ 33521   4 venous grafts (List separately in addition to code for primary procedure)

➔ *CPT Changes: An Insider's View* 2008

➔ *CPT Assistant* Fall 91:5, Winter 92:13, Apr 01:7, Feb 05:14, Jan 07:7, Mar 07:1, Dec 21:18

(Use 33521 in conjunction with 33533-33536)

+ 33522   5 venous grafts (List separately in addition to code for primary procedure)

➔ *CPT Changes: An Insider's View* 2008

➔ *CPT Assistant* Fall 91:5, Winter 92:13, Apr 01:7, Feb 05:14, Jan 07:7, Mar 07:1, Dec 21:18

(Use 33522 in conjunction with 33533-33536)

Cardiovascular 33016-39599

Coronary Artery Bypass Combined Arterial-Venous Grafting
33517-33530

Both venous and arterial grafts are used in these bypass procedures. The appropriate arterial graft codes (33533-33536) must also be reported in conjunction with codes 33517-33530.

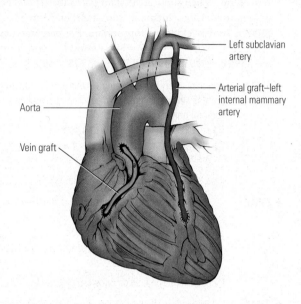

Left subclavian artery

Arterial graft—left internal mammary artery

Aorta

Vein graft

Coronary Artery Bypass-Sequential Combined Arterial-Venous Grafting
33517-33530

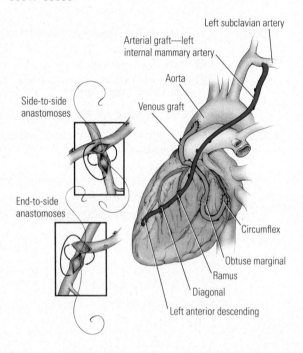

Left subclavian artery

Arterial graft—left internal mammary artery

Aorta

Side-to-side anastomoses

Venous graft

End-to-side anastomoses

Circumflex

Obtuse marginal

Ramus

Diagonal

Left anterior descending

Note: To determine the number of bypass grafts in a coronary artery bypass (CABG), count the number of distal anastomoses (contact point[s]) where the bypass graft artery or vein is sutured to the diseased coronary artery(s).

+ 33523 6 or more venous grafts (List separately in addition to code for primary procedure)

➡ *CPT Changes: An Insider's View* 2008

➡ *CPT Assistant* Fall 91:5, Winter 92:13, Apr 01:7, Feb 05:14, Jan 07:7, Mar 07:1, Dec 21:18

(Use 33523 in conjunction with 33533-33536)

+ 33530 Reoperation, coronary artery bypass procedure or valve procedure, more than 1 month after original operation (List separately in addition to code for primary procedure)

➡ *CPT Assistant* Winter 90:6, Fall 91:5, Winter 92:13, Apr 01:7, Jul 01:11, Feb 05:13-14, Jan 07:7, Feb 11:8

(Use 33530 in conjunction with 33390, 33391, 33404-33496, 33510-33523, 33533, 33534, 33535, 33536, 33863)

Arterial Grafting for Coronary Artery Bypass

The following codes are used to report coronary artery bypass procedures using either arterial grafts only or a combination of arterial-venous grafts. The codes include the use of the internal mammary artery, gastroepiploic artery, epigastric artery, radial artery, and arterial conduits procured from other sites.

To report combined arterial-venous grafts it is necessary to report two codes: (1) the appropriate arterial graft code (33533-33536); and (2) the appropriate combined arterial-venous graft code (33517-33523).

Procurement of the artery for grafting is included in the description of the work for 33533-33536 and should not be reported as a separate service or co-surgery, except when an upper extremity artery (eg, radial artery) is procured. To report harvesting of an upper extremity artery, use 33509 or 35600. To report harvesting of an upper extremity vein, use 35500 in addition to the bypass procedure. To report harvesting of a femoropopliteal vein segment, report 35572 in addition to the bypass procedure. When surgical assistant performs arterial and/or venous graft procurement, add modifier 80 to 33517-33523, 33533-33536, as appropriate. For percutaneous ventricular assist device insertion, removal, repositioning, see 33990, 33991, 33992, 33993, 33995, 33997.

33533 Coronary artery bypass, using arterial graft(s); single arterial graft

➡ *CPT Changes: An Insider's View* 2000

➡ *CPT Assistant* Winter 92:12, Nov 99:18, Apr 01:7, Feb 05:14, Jan 07:7, Mar 07:1, Nov 14:14, Dec 21:18

33534 2 coronary arterial grafts

➡ *CPT Assistant* Winter 92:12, Apr 01:7, Feb 05:14, Jan 07:7, Mar 07:1, Dec 21:18

Cardiovascular 33016-39599

33535   3 coronary arterial grafts

> *CPT Assistant* Winter 92:12, Apr 01:7, Feb 05:14, Jan 07:7, Mar 07:1, Dec 21:18

33536   4 or more coronary arterial grafts

> *CPT Assistant* Winter 92:12, Apr 01:7, Feb 05:14, Jan 07:7, Mar 07:1, Nov 14:14, Dec 21:18

33542   Myocardial resection (eg, ventricular aneurysmectomy)

> *CPT Assistant* Winter 92:12, Mar 07:1

33545   Repair of postinfarction ventricular septal defect, with or without myocardial resection

> *CPT Assistant* Winter 92:12, Mar 07:1

33548   Surgical ventricular restoration procedure, includes prosthetic patch, when performed (eg, ventricular remodeling, SVR, SAVER, Dor procedures)

> *CPT Changes: An Insider's View* 2006

> *CPT Assistant* Nov 06:21, Dec 06:10, Mar 07:1

(Do not report 33548 in conjunction with 32551, 33210, 33211, 33310, 33315)

(For Batista procedure or pachopexy, use 33999)

(For transcatheter left ventricular restoration device implantation, use 0643T)

Coronary Endarterectomy

+ 33572   Coronary endarterectomy, open, any method, of left anterior descending, circumflex, or right coronary artery performed in conjunction with coronary artery bypass graft procedure, each vessel (List separately in addition to primary procedure)

(Use 33572 in conjunction with 33510-33516, 33533-33536)

Single Ventricle and Other Complex Cardiac Anomalies

33600   Closure of atrioventricular valve (mitral or tricuspid) by suture or patch

> *CPT Assistant* Mar 07:1, Dec 21:17

33602   Closure of semilunar valve (aortic or pulmonary) by suture or patch

33606   Anastomosis of pulmonary artery to aorta (Damus-Kaye-Stansel procedure)

33608   Repair of complex cardiac anomaly other than pulmonary atresia with ventricular septal defect by construction or replacement of conduit from right or left ventricle to pulmonary artery

> *CPT Assistant* Apr 19:6

(For repair of pulmonary artery arborization anomalies by unifocalization, see 33925-33926)

33610   Repair of complex cardiac anomalies (eg, single ventricle with subaortic obstruction) by surgical enlargement of ventricular septal defect

> *CPT Changes: An Insider's View* 2002

(Do not report modifier 63 in conjunction with 33610)

33611   Repair of double outlet right ventricle with intraventricular tunnel repair;

(Do not report modifier 63 in conjunction with 33611)

33612   with repair of right ventricular outflow tract obstruction

33615   Repair of complex cardiac anomalies (eg, tricuspid atresia) by closure of atrial septal defect and anastomosis of atria or vena cava to pulmonary artery (simple Fontan procedure)

33617   Repair of complex cardiac anomalies (eg, single ventricle) by modified Fontan procedure

(Use 33617 in conjunction with 33768 when a cavopulmonary anastomosis to a second superior vena cava is performed)

33619   Repair of single ventricle with aortic outflow obstruction and aortic arch hypoplasia (hypoplastic left heart syndrome) (eg, Norwood procedure)

> *CPT Assistant* Mar 07:1, Apr 11:6, May 12:14, Jul 16:3

(Do not report modifier 63 in conjunction with 33619)

33620   Application of right and left pulmonary artery bands (eg, hybrid approach stage 1)

> *CPT Changes: An Insider's View* 2011

> *CPT Assistant* Apr 11:3, May 12:14, Jul 16:3

(For banding of the main pulmonary artery related to septal defect, use 33690)

33621   Transthoracic insertion of catheter for stent placement with catheter removal and closure (eg, hybrid approach stage 1)

> *CPT Changes: An Insider's View* 2011

> *CPT Assistant* Apr 11:3, Jul 16:3

(For placement of stent, use 37236)

(Report both 33620, 33621 if performed in same session)

33622   Reconstruction of complex cardiac anomaly (eg, single ventricle or hypoplastic left heart) with palliation of single ventricle with aortic outflow obstruction and aortic arch hypoplasia, creation of cavopulmonary anastomosis, and removal of right and left pulmonary bands (eg, hybrid approach stage 2, Norwood, bidirectional Glenn, pulmonary artery debanding)

> *CPT Changes: An Insider's View* 2011

> *CPT Assistant* Apr 11:3, May 12:14, Jul 16:3

(Do not report 33622 in conjunction with 33619, 33767, 33822, 33840, 33845, 33851, 33853, 33917)

(For bilateral, bidirectional Glenn procedure, use 33622 in conjunction with 33768)

Cardiovascular 33016-39599

Initial Hybrid Palliation
33621

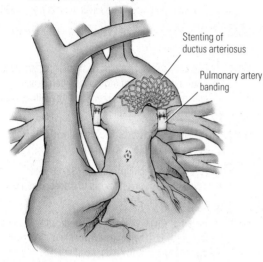

Initial Hybrid Palliation, Stage I

Stenting of ductus arteriosus

Pulmonary artery banding

Hybrid Reconstruction
33622

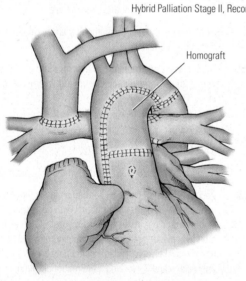

Hybrid Palliation Stage II, Reconstruction

Homograft

Septal Defect

33641 Repair atrial septal defect, secundum, with cardiopulmonary bypass, with or without patch
> *CPT Assistant* Mar 07:1, Dec 10:12

33645 Direct or patch closure, sinus venosus, with or without anomalous pulmonary venous drainage

(Do not report 33645 in conjunction with 33724, 33726)

33647 Repair of atrial septal defect and ventricular septal defect, with direct or patch closure

(Do not report modifier 63 in conjunction with 33647)

(For repair of tricuspid atresia (eg, Fontan, Gago procedures), use 33615)

33660 Repair of incomplete or partial atrioventricular canal (ostium primum atrial septal defect), with or without atrioventricular valve repair

33665 Repair of intermediate or transitional atrioventricular canal, with or without atrioventricular valve repair

33670 Repair of complete atrioventricular canal, with or without prosthetic valve

(Do not report modifier 63 in conjunction with 33670)

33675 Closure of multiple ventricular septal defects;
> *CPT Changes: An Insider's View* 2007
> *CPT Assistant* Mar 07:1

33676 with pulmonary valvotomy or infundibular resection (acyanotic)
> *CPT Changes: An Insider's View* 2007
> *CPT Assistant* Mar 07:1

33677 with removal of pulmonary artery band, with or without gusset
> *CPT Changes: An Insider's View* 2007
> *CPT Assistant* Mar 07:1

(Do not report 33675-33677 in conjunction with 32100, 32551, 32554, 32555, 33210, 33681, 33684, 33688)

(For percutaneous closure, use 93581)

33681 Closure of single ventricular septal defect, with or without patch;
> *CPT Changes: An Insider's View* 2007
> *CPT Assistant* Mar 07:1

33684 with pulmonary valvotomy or infundibular resection (acyanotic)

33688 with removal of pulmonary artery band, with or without gusset

(For pulmonary vein repair requiring creation of atrial septal defect, use 33724)

33690 Banding of pulmonary artery
> *CPT Assistant* Apr 11:4, May 12:14

(For right and left pulmonary artery banding in a single ventricle [eg, hybrid approach stage 1], use 33620)

(Do not report modifier 63 in conjunction with 33690)

33692   Complete repair tetralogy of Fallot without pulmonary atresia;

33694   with transannular patch

(Do not report modifier 63 in conjunction with 33694)

(For ligation and takedown of a systemic-to-pulmonary artery shunt, performed in conjunction with a congenital heart procedure; see 33924)

33697   Complete repair tetralogy of Fallot with pulmonary atresia including construction of conduit from right ventricle to pulmonary artery and closure of ventricular septal defect

→ *CPT Assistant* Mar 07:1

(For ligation and takedown of a systemic-to-pulmonary artery shunt, performed in conjunction with a congenital heart procedure; see 33924)

Sinus of Valsalva

33702   Repair sinus of Valsalva fistula, with cardiopulmonary bypass;

→ *CPT Assistant* Mar 07:1

33710   with repair of ventricular septal defect

33720   Repair sinus of Valsalva aneurysm, with cardiopulmonary bypass

Venous Anomalies

33724   Repair of isolated partial anomalous pulmonary venous return (eg, Scimitar Syndrome)

→ *CPT Changes: An Insider's View* 2007

→ *CPT Assistant* Mar 07:1

(Do not report 33724 in conjunction with 32551, 33210, 33211)

33726   Repair of pulmonary venous stenosis

→ *CPT Changes: An Insider's View* 2007

→ *CPT Assistant* Mar 07:1

(Do not report 33726 in conjunction with 32551, 33210, 33211)

33730   Complete repair of anomalous pulmonary venous return (supracardiac, intracardiac, or infracardiac types)

→ *CPT Assistant* Mar 07:1

(Do not report modifier 63 in conjunction with 33730)

(For partial anomalous pulmonary venous return, use 33724; for repair of pulmonary venous stenosis, use 33726)

33732   Repair of cor triatriatum or supravalvular mitral ring by resection of left atrial membrane

→ *CPT Assistant* Mar 07:1

(Do not report modifier 63 in conjunction with 33732)

Shunting Procedures

Codes 33741, 33745 are typically used to report creation of effective intracardiac blood flow in the setting of congenital heart defects. Code 33741 (transcatheter atrial septostomy) involves the percutaneous creation of improved atrial blood flow (eg, balloon/blade method), typically in infants ≤4 kg with congenital heart disease. Code 33745 is typically used for intracardiac shunt creation by stent placement to establish improved intracardiac blood flow (eg, atrial septum, Fontan fenestration, right ventricular outflow tract, Mustard/Senning/Warden baffles). Code 33746 is used to describe each additional intracardiac shunt creation by stent placement at a separate location during the same session as the primary intervention (33745).

Code 33741 includes percutaneous access, placing the access sheath(s), advancement of the transcatheter delivery system, and creation of effective intracardiac atrial blood flow. Codes 33741, 33745 include, when performed, ultrasound guidance for vascular access and fluoroscopic guidance for the intervention. Code 33745 additionally includes intracardiac stent placement, target zone angioplasty preceding or after stent implantation, and complete diagnostic right and left heart catheterization, when performed.

Diagnostic cardiac catheterization is not typically performed at the same session as transcatheter atrial septostomy (33741) and, when performed, may be separately reported. Diagnostic cardiac catheterization is typically performed at the same session with 33745 and the code descriptor includes this work, when performed.

Cardiovascular injection procedures for diagnostic angiography reported using 93563, 93565, 93566, 93567, 93568, 93569, 93573, 93574, 93575 are not typically performed at the same session as 33741. Although diagnostic angiography is typically performed during 33745, target vessels and chambers are highly variable and, when performed for an evaluation separate and distinct from the shunt creation, may be reported separately.

Codes 33745, 33746 are used to describe intracardiac stent placement. Multiple stents placed in a single location may only be reported with a single code. When additional, different intracardiac locations are treated in the same session, 33746 may be reported. Codes 33745, 33746 include all balloon angioplasty(ies) performed in the target lesion, including any pre-dilation (whether performed as a primary or secondary dilation), post-dilation following stent placement, or use of larger/

smaller balloon, to achieve therapeutic result. Angioplasty in a separate and distinct intracardiac lesion may be reported separately. Use 33746 in conjunction with 33745.

Diagnostic right and left heart catheterization codes (93451, 93452, 93453, 93456, 93457, 93458, 93459, 93460, 93461, 93593, 93594, 93595, 93596, 93597) should not be used in conjunction with 33741, 33745 to report:

1. Fluoroscopic guidance for the intervention, or

2. Limited hemodynamic and angiographic data used solely for purposes of accomplishing the intervention (eg, measurement of atrial pressures before and after septostomy, atrial injections to determine appropriate catheter position).

Diagnostic right and left heart catheterization (93451, 93452, 93453, 93456, 93457, 93458, 93459, 93460, 93461, 93593, 93594, 93595, 93596, 93597) performed at the same session as 33741 may be separately reported, if:

1. No prior study is available, and a full diagnostic study is performed, or

2. A prior study is available, but as documented in the medical record:

   a. There is inadequate visualization of the anatomy and/or pathology, or

   b. The patient's condition with respect to the clinical indication has changed since the prior study, or

   c. There is a clinical change during the procedure that requires a more thorough evaluation.

For same-session diagnostic cardiac angiography for an evaluation separate and distinct from 33741 or 33745, the appropriate contrast injection(s) performed (93563, 93565, 93566, 93567, 93568, 93569, 93573, 93574, 93575) may be reported.

33735 Atrial septectomy or septostomy; closed heart (Blalock-Hanlon type operation)
➔ *CPT Assistant* Mar 07:1

33736 open heart with cardiopulmonary bypass

(Do not report modifier 63 in conjunction with 33735, 33736)

▶(33737 has been deleted)◀

33741 Transcatheter atrial septostomy (TAS) for congenital cardiac anomalies to create effective atrial flow, including all imaging guidance by the proceduralist, when performed, any method (eg, Rashkind, Sang-Park, balloon, cutting balloon, blade)
➔ *CPT Changes: An Insider's View* 2021
➔ *CPT Assistant* Nov 20:7, Dec 21:20-21, May 23:1, Dec 23:47

(Do not report modifier 63 in conjunction with 33741)

(For transseptal puncture, use 93462)

33745 Transcatheter intracardiac shunt (TIS) creation by stent placement for congenital cardiac anomalies to establish effective intracardiac flow, including all imaging guidance by the proceduralist, when performed, left and right heart diagnostic cardiac catheterization for congenital cardiac anomalies, and target zone angioplasty, when performed (eg, atrial septum, Fontan fenestration, right ventricular outflow tract, Mustard/Senning/Warden baffles); initial intracardiac shunt
➔ *CPT Changes: An Insider's View* 2021, 2022
➔ *CPT Assistant* Nov 20:7, Dec 21:19-20, May 23:1, Dec 23:47

+ 33746 each additional intracardiac shunt location (List separately in addition to code for primary procedure)
➔ *CPT Changes: An Insider's View* 2021
➔ *CPT Assistant* Nov 20:7, Dec 21:19-20, May 23:1

(Use 33746 in conjunction with 33745)

(Do not report 33745, 33746 in conjunction with 93593, 93594, 93595, 93596, 93597)

33750 Shunt; subclavian to pulmonary artery (Blalock-Taussig type operation)

33755 ascending aorta to pulmonary artery (Waterston type operation)

33762 descending aorta to pulmonary artery (Potts-Smith type operation)

(Do not report modifier 63 in conjunction with 33750, 33755, 33762)

33764 central, with prosthetic graft

33766 superior vena cava to pulmonary artery for flow to 1 lung (classical Glenn procedure)

33767 superior vena cava to pulmonary artery for flow to both lungs (bidirectional Glenn procedure)
➔ *CPT Assistant* Apr 11:6, Jul 16:3

+ 33768 Anastomosis, cavopulmonary, second superior vena cava (List separately in addition to primary procedure)
➔ *CPT Changes: An Insider's View* 2006
➔ *CPT Assistant* Mar 07:1, Apr 11:6, Jul 16:3

(Use 33768 in conjunction with 33478, 33617, 33622, 33767)

(Do not report 33768 in conjunction with 32551, 33210, 33211)

Transposition of the Great Vessels

33770 Repair of transposition of the great arteries with ventricular septal defect and subpulmonary stenosis; without surgical enlargement of ventricular septal defect
➔ *CPT Assistant* Mar 07:1

33771   with surgical enlargement of ventricular septal defect

33774   Repair of transposition of the great arteries, atrial baffle procedure (eg, Mustard or Senning type) with cardiopulmonary bypass;

33775   with removal of pulmonary band

33776   with closure of ventricular septal defect

33777   with repair of subpulmonic obstruction

33778   Repair of transposition of the great arteries, aortic pulmonary artery reconstruction (eg, Jatene type);

(Do not report modifier 63 in conjunction with 33778)

33779   with removal of pulmonary band

33780   with closure of ventricular septal defect

33781   with repair of subpulmonic obstruction
→ *CPT Assistant* Mar 07:1

33782   Aortic root translocation with ventricular septal defect and pulmonary stenosis repair (ie, Nikaidoh procedure); without coronary ostium reimplantation
→ *CPT Changes: An Insider's View* 2010

(Do not report 33782 in conjunction with 33412, 33413, 33608, 33681, 33770, 33771, 33778, 33780, 33920)

33783   with reimplantation of 1 or both coronary ostia
→ *CPT Changes: An Insider's View* 2010 ·

Truncus Arteriosus

33786   Total repair, truncus arteriosus (Rastelli type operation)
→ *CPT Assistant* Mar 07:1

(Do not report modifier 63 in conjunction with 33786)

33788   Reimplantation of an anomalous pulmonary artery
→ *CPT Assistant* Mar 07:1

(For pulmonary artery band, use 33690)

Aortic Anomalies

33800   Aortic suspension (aortopexy) for tracheal decompression (eg, for tracheomalacia) (separate procedure)
→ *CPT Assistant* Mar 07:1

33802   Division of aberrant vessel (vascular ring);

33803   with reanastomosis

▶(33813 has been deleted)◀

▲ **33814**   Obliteration of aortopulmonary septal defect, with cardiopulmonary bypass
→ *CPT Changes: An Insider's View* 2025

33820   Repair of patent ductus arteriosus; by ligation
→ *CPT Assistant* Mar 07:1

33822   by division, younger than 18 years
→ *CPT Assistant* Mar 07:1, Apr 11:6, Jul 16:3

Patent Ductus Arteriosus
33820

The tissues surrounding the ductus are dissected away and then several heavy ligatures are passed around the ductus and tied off on both ends.

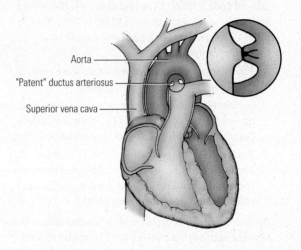

Aorta

"Patent" ductus arteriosus

Superior vena cava

33824   by division, 18 years and older

(For percutaneous transcatheter closure of patent ductus arteriosus, use 93582)

33840   Excision of coarctation of aorta, with or without associated patent ductus arteriosus; with direct anastomosis
→ *CPT Assistant* Apr 11:6, Jul 16:3, Dec 21:8

33845   with graft
→ *CPT Assistant* Apr 11:6, Jul 16:3, Dec 21:8

33851   repair using either left subclavian artery or prosthetic material as gusset for enlargement
→ *CPT Assistant* Apr 11:6, Jul 16:3, Dec 21:8

33852   Repair of hypoplastic or interrupted aortic arch using autogenous or prosthetic material; without cardiopulmonary bypass

33853   with cardiopulmonary bypass
→ *CPT Assistant* Mar 07:1, Apr 11:6, Jul 16:3

(For repair of hypoplastic left heart syndrome (eg, Norwood type), via excision of coarctation of aorta, use 33619)

Thoracic Aortic Aneurysm

When ascending aortic disease involves the aortic arch, an aortic hemiarch graft may be necessary in conjunction with the ascending aortic graft and may be reported with add-on code 33866 in conjunction with the appropriate ascending aortic graft code (33858, 33859, 33863, 33864). Aortic hemiarch graft requires all of the following components:

1. Either total circulatory arrest or isolated cerebral perfusion (retrograde or antegrade);

2. Incision into the transverse arch extending under one or more of the arch vessels (eg, innominate, left common carotid, or left subclavian arteries); and

3. Extension of the ascending aortic graft under the aortic arch by construction of a beveled anastomosis to the distal ascending aorta and aortic arch without a cross-clamp (an open anastomosis).

An ascending aortic repair with a beveled anastomosis into the arch with a cross-clamp cannot be reported separately as a hemiarch graft using 33866. Use 33866 for aortic hemiarch graft when performed in conjunction with the ascending aortic graft codes 33858, 33859, 33863, 33864. Code 33871 describes a complete transverse arch graft placement, and is not used to report an aortic hemiarch graft procedure.

33858   Ascending aorta graft, with cardiopulmonary bypass, includes valve suspension, when performed; for aortic dissection

➔ *CPT Changes: An Insider's View* 2020

➔ *CPT Assistant* Nov 19:9

33859   for aortic disease other than dissection (eg, aneurysm)

➔ *CPT Changes: An Insider's View* 2020

➔ *CPT Assistant* Nov 19:9

33863   Ascending aorta graft, with cardiopulmonary bypass, with aortic root replacement using valved conduit and coronary reconstruction (eg, Bentall)

➔ *CPT Changes: An Insider's View* 2011

➔ *CPT Assistant* Feb 05:14, Mar 07:1, Aug 11:3, Nov 19:9

(Do not report 33863 in conjunction with 33405, 33406, 33410, 33411, 33412, 33413, 33858, 33859)

33864   Ascending aorta graft, with cardiopulmonary bypass with valve suspension, with coronary reconstruction and valve-sparing aortic root remodeling (eg, David Procedure, Yacoub Procedure)

➔ *CPT Changes: An Insider's View* 2008, 2011

➔ *CPT Assistant* Aug 11:3, Nov 19:9

(Do not report 33864 in conjunction with 33858, 33859, 33863)

+ 33866   Aortic hemiarch graft including isolation and control of the arch vessels, beveled open distal aortic anastomosis extending under one or more of the arch vessels, and total circulatory arrest or isolated cerebral perfusion (List separately in addition to code for primary procedure)

➔ *CPT Changes: An Insider's View* 2019

➔ *CPT Assistant* Nov 19:9

(Use 33866 for aortic hemiarch graft performed in conjunction with ascending aortic graft [33858, 33859, 33863, 33864])

(Do not report 33866 in conjunction with 33871)

Aortic Root Remodeling: Coronary Arteries Reimplanted
33864

Valve-sparing aortic root replacement (code 33864)

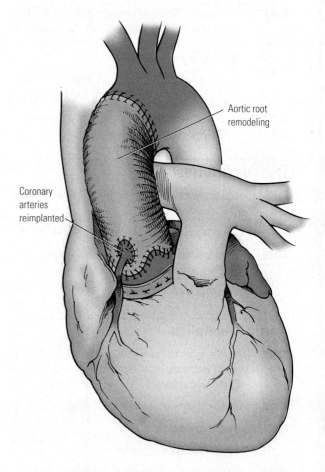

Aortic root remodeling

Coronary arteries reimplanted

33871   Transverse aortic arch graft, with cardiopulmonary bypass, with profound hypothermia, total circulatory arrest and isolated cerebral perfusion with reimplantation of arch vessel(s) (eg, island pedicle or individual arch vessel reimplantation)

➔ *CPT Changes: An Insider's View* 2020

➔ *CPT Assistant* Nov 19:9

(Do not report 33871 for aortic hemiarch graft)

(Do not report 33871 in conjunction with 33866)

(For aortic hemiarch graft performed in conjunction with ascending aortic graft [33858, 33859, 33863, 33864], use 33866)

33875   Descending thoracic aorta graft, with or without bypass

33877   Repair of thoracoabdominal aortic aneurysm with graft, with or without cardiopulmonary bypass

Endovascular Repair of Descending Thoracic Aorta

Codes 33880-33891 represent a family of procedures to report placement of an endovascular graft for repair of the descending thoracic aorta. These codes include all device introduction, manipulation, positioning, and deployment. All balloon angioplasty and/or stent deployment within the target treatment zone for the endoprosthesis, either before or after endograft deployment, are not separately reportable.

Open arterial exposure and associated closure of the arteriotomy sites (eg, 34714, 34715, 34716, 34812, 34820, 34833, 34834), introduction of guidewires and catheters (eg, 36140, 36200-36218), and extensive repair or replacement of an artery (eg, 35226, 35286) may be additionally reported. Transposition of subclavian artery to carotid, and carotid-carotid bypass performed in conjunction with endovascular repair of the descending thoracic aorta (eg, 33889, 33891) may be separately reported. The primary codes, 33880 and 33881, include placement of all distal extensions, if required, in the distal thoracic aorta, while proximal extensions, if needed, may be reported separately.

For fluoroscopic guidance in conjunction with endovascular repair of the thoracic aorta, see codes 75956-75959 as appropriate. Codes 75956 and 75957 include all angiography of the thoracic aorta and its branches for diagnostic imaging prior to deployment of the primary endovascular devices (including all routine components of modular devices), fluoroscopic guidance in the delivery of the endovascular components, and intraprocedural arterial angiography (eg, confirm position, detect endoleak, evaluate runoff). Code 75958 includes the analogous services for placement of each proximal thoracic endovascular extension. Code 75959 includes the analogous services for placement of a distal thoracic endovascular extension(s) placed during a procedure after the primary repair.

Other interventional procedures performed at the time of endovascular repair of the descending thoracic aorta should be additionally reported (eg, innominate, carotid, subclavian, visceral, or iliac artery transluminal angioplasty or stenting, arterial embolization, intravascular ultrasound) when performed before or after deployment of the aortic prostheses.

For endovascular stenting or balloon angioplasty of congenital coarctation or postsurgical recoarctation of the ascending, transverse, or descending thoracic or abdominal aorta, see 33894, 33895, 33897.

33880   Endovascular repair of descending thoracic aorta (eg, aneurysm, pseudoaneurysm, dissection, penetrating ulcer, intramural hematoma, or traumatic disruption); involving coverage of left subclavian artery origin, initial endoprosthesis plus descending thoracic aortic extension(s), if required, to level of celiac artery origin

➔ *CPT Changes: An Insider's View* 2006

➔ *CPT Assistant* Dec 17:3

➔ *Clinical Examples in Radiology* Winter 06:14

(For radiological supervision and interpretation, use 75956 in conjunction with 33880)

33881   not involving coverage of left subclavian artery origin, initial endoprosthesis plus descending thoracic aortic extension(s), if required, to level of celiac artery origin

➔ *CPT Changes: An Insider's View* 2006

➔ *CPT Assistant* Dec 17:3

➔ *Clinical Examples in Radiology* Winter 06:14

(For radiological supervision and interpretation, use 75957 in conjunction with 33881)

33883   Placement of proximal extension prosthesis for endovascular repair of descending thoracic aorta (eg, aneurysm, pseudoaneurysm, dissection, penetrating ulcer, intramural hematoma, or traumatic disruption); initial extension

➔ *CPT Changes: An Insider's View* 2006

➔ *CPT Assistant* Dec 17:3

➔ *Clinical Examples in Radiology* Winter 06:14

(For radiological supervision and interpretation, use 75958 in conjunction with 33883)

(Do not report 33881, 33883 when extension placement converts repair to cover left subclavian origin. Use only 33880)

+ 33884   each additional proximal extension (List separately in addition to code for primary procedure)

➔ *CPT Changes: An Insider's View* 2006

➔ *CPT Assistant* Dec 17:3

➔ *Clinical Examples in Radiology* Winter 06:14

(Use 33884 in conjunction with 33883)

(For radiological supervision and interpretation, use 75958 in conjunction with 33884)

33886 Placement of distal extension prosthesis(s) delayed after endovascular repair of descending thoracic aorta

➡ *CPT Changes: An Insider's View* 2006

➡ *CPT Assistant* Dec 17:3

➡ *Clinical Examples in Radiology* Winter 06:14

(Do not report 33886 in conjunction with 33880, 33881)

(Report 33886 once, regardless of number of modules deployed)

(For radiological supervision and interpretation, use 75959 in conjunction with 33886)

33889 Open subclavian to carotid artery transposition performed in conjunction with endovascular repair of descending thoracic aorta, by neck incision, unilateral

➡ *CPT Changes: An Insider's View* 2006

➡ *Clinical Examples in Radiology* Winter 06:15

(Do not report 33889 in conjunction with 35694)

33891 Bypass graft, with other than vein, transcervical retropharyngeal carotid-carotid, performed in conjunction with endovascular repair of descending thoracic aorta, by neck incision

➡ *CPT Changes: An Insider's View* 2006

➡ *Clinical Examples in Radiology* Winter 06:15

(Do not report 33891 in conjunction with 35509, 35601)

Endovascular Repair of Congenital Heart and Vascular Defects

Codes 33894, 33895, 33897 describe transcatheter interventions for revascularization or repair for coarctation of the aorta. Code 33897 describes dilation of the coarctation using balloon angioplasty without stent placement. Codes 33894, 33895 describe stent placement to treat the coarctation. The procedure described in 33894 involves stent placement across one or more major side branches of the aorta. For reporting purposes, the major side branches of the thoracic aorta are the brachiocephalic, carotid, and subclavian arteries, and the major side branches of the abdominal aorta are the celiac, superior mesenteric, inferior mesenteric, and renal arteries.

Codes 33894, 33895, 33897 include all fluoroscopic guidance of the intervention, diagnostic congenital left heart catheterization, all catheter and wire introductions and manipulation, and angiography of the target lesion.

Codes 33894, 33895 include stent introduction, manipulation, positioning, and deployment, temporary pacemaker insertion for rapid pacing (33210) to facilitate stent positioning, when performed, as well as any additional stent delivery in tandem with the initial stent for extension purposes. Balloon angioplasty within the target-treatment zone, either before or after stent deployment, is not separately reportable. For balloon angioplasty of an additional coarctation of the aorta in a

segment separate from the treatment zone for the coarctation stent, use 33897.

▶For balloon angioplasty or stenting of the aorta for lesions other than coarctation (eg, atherosclerosis) of the aorta in a segment separate from the coarctation treatment zone, see 37236, 37246.◀

For additional diagnostic right heart catheterization in the same setting as 33894, 33895, see 93593, 93594.

Other interventional procedures performed at the time of endovascular repair of coarctation of the aorta (33894, 33895) may be reported separately (eg, innominate, carotid, subclavian, visceral, iliac, or pulmonary artery balloon angioplasty or stenting, arterial or venous embolization), when performed before or after coarctation stent deployment.

33894 Endovascular stent repair of coarctation of the ascending, transverse, or descending thoracic or abdominal aorta, involving stent placement; across major side branches

➡ *CPT Changes: An Insider's View* 2022

➡ *CPT Assistant* Dec 21:7-8

33895 not crossing major side branches

➡ *CPT Changes: An Insider's View* 2022

➡ *CPT Assistant* Dec 21:7-8

(Do not report 33894, 33895 in conjunction with 33210, 34701, 34702, 34703, 34704, 34705, 34706, 36200, 75600, 75605, 75625, 93567, 93595, 93596, 93597)

▶(Do not report 33894, 33895 in conjunction with 33897, 37236, 37246, for balloon angioplasty or stenting of the aorta within the coarctation stent treatment zone)◀

▶(For balloon angioplasty or stenting of the aorta for lesions other than coarctation [eg, atherosclerosis] of the aorta in a segment separate from the coarctation treatment zone, see 37236, 37246)◀

(For additional atrial, ventricular, pulmonary, coronary, or bypass graft angiography in the same setting, see 93563, 93564, 93565, 93566, 93568)

(For additional congenital right heart catheterization at same setting as 33894, 33895, see 93593, 93594)

(For angiography of other vascular structures, use the appropriate code from the Radiology/Diagnostic Radiology section)

33897 Percutaneous transluminal angioplasty of native or recurrent coarctation of the aorta

➡ *CPT Changes: An Insider's View* 2022

➡ *CPT Assistant* Dec 21:7-8

▶(Do not report 33897 in conjunction with 33210, 34701, 34702, 34703, 34704, 34705, 34706, 36200, 75600, 75605, 75625, 93567, 93595, 93596, 93597)◀

(Do not report 33897 in conjunction with 33894, 33895 for balloon angioplasty of the aorta within the coarctation stent treatment zone)

▶(Do not report 33897 in conjunction with 37236, 37246 for stenting or additional balloon angioplasty of the aorta within the coarctation treatment zone)◀

▶(For balloon angioplasty or stenting of the aorta for lesions other than coarctation [eg, atherosclerosis] of the aorta in a segment separate from the coarctation treatment zone, see 37236, 37246)◀

(For additional congenital right heart diagnostic catheterization performed in same setting as 33897, see 93593, 93594)

(For angioplasty and other transcatheter revascularization interventions of additional upper or lower extremity vessels in same setting, use the appropriate code from the Surgery/Cardiovascular System section)

Coarctation of the Aorta and Its Repair
33894, 33895

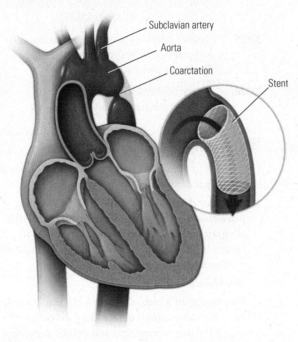

Subclavian artery

Aorta

Coarctation

Stent

Codes 33900, 33901, 33902, 33903, 33904 describe endovascular repair of pulmonary artery stenosis by stent placement. Codes 33900, 33901 describe stent placement within the pulmonary arteries via normal native connections, defined as superior vena cava/inferior vena cava to right atrium, then right ventricle, then pulmonary arteries. Codes 33902, 33903 describe stent placement within the pulmonary arteries, ductus arteriosus, or within a surgical shunt, via abnormal connections or through post-surgical shunts (eg, Blalock-Taussig shunt, Sano shunt, or post Glenn or Fontan procedures). Code 33904 is an add-on code that describes placement of stent(s) in additional vessels or lesions beyond the primary vessel or lesion treated whether access is via normal or abnormal connection.

Codes 33900, 33901, 33902, 33903, 33904 include vascular access and all catheter and guidewire manipulation, fluoroscopy to guide the intervention, any post-diagnostic angiography for roadmapping purposes and post-implant evaluation, stent positioning and balloon inflation for stent delivery, and radiologic supervision and interpretation of the intervention. Angiography at the same session, as part of a diagnostic cardiac catheterization, may be reported with the appropriate angiographic codes from the Radiology or Medicine/Cardiovascular/Cardiac Catheterization/Injection Procedures sections.

Diagnostic cardiac catheterization and diagnostic angiography codes (93451, 93452, 93453, 93454, 93455, 93456, 93457, 93458, 93459, 93460, 93461, 93563, 93566, 93567, 93568, 93593, 93594, 93596, 93597, 93598) should **not** be used with 33900, 33901, 33902, 33903, 33904 to report:

1. Contrast injections, angiography, roadmapping, and/or fluoroscopic guidance for the percutaneous pulmonary artery revascularization by stent placement,

2. Pulmonary conduit angiography for guidance of percutaneous pulmonary artery revascularization by stent placement, or

3. Right heart catheterization for hemodynamic measurements before, during, and after percutaneous pulmonary artery revascularization by stent placement for guidance of percutaneous pulmonary artery revascularization by stent placement.

Diagnostic right and left heart catheterization codes (93451, 93452, 93453, 93456, 93457, 93458, 93459, 93460, 93461, 93593, 93594, 93595, 93596, 93597, 93598), diagnostic coronary angiography codes (93454, 93455, 93456, 93457, 93458, 93459, 93460, 93461, 93563, 93564), and diagnostic angiography codes 93565, 93566, 93567, 93568 may be separately reported in conjunction with 33900, 33901, 33902, 33903, 33904, representing separate and distinct services from pulmonary artery revascularization, if:

1. No prior study is available and a full diagnostic study is performed, or

2. A prior study is available, but as documented in the medical record:

   a. There is inadequate visualization of the anatomy and/or pathology, or

   b. The patient's condition with respect to the clinical indication has changed since the prior study, or

   c. There is a clinical change during the procedure that requires new evaluation.

▲=Revised code   ●=New code   ▶◀=Contains new or revised text   ✖=Duplicate PLA test   ↑↓=Category I PLA   American Medical Association   **275**

Cardiovascular 33016-39599

Do not report 33900, 33901, 33902, 33903, 33904 in conjunction with 76000, 93451, 93452, 93453, 93454, 93455, 93456, 93457, 93458, 93459, 93460, 93461, 93563, 93564, 93565, 93566, 93567, 93568, 93593, 93594, 93596, 93597, 93598 for catheterization and angiography services intrinsic to the procedure.

Balloon angioplasty (92997, 92998) within the same target lesion as stent implant, either before or after stent deployment, is not separately reported.

For balloon angioplasty at the same session as 33900, 33901, 33902, 33903, 33904, but for a distinct lesion or in a different artery, see 92997, 92998.

To report percutaneous pulmonary artery revascularization by stent placement in conjunction with diagnostic congenital cardiac catheterization, see 33900, 33901, 33902, 33903, 33904.

For transcatheter intracardiac shunt (TIS) creation by stent placement for congenital cardiac anomalies to establish effective intracardiac flow, see 33745, 33746.

33900 Percutaneous pulmonary artery revascularization by stent placement, initial; normal native connections, unilateral
➡ *CPT Changes: An Insider's View* 2023
➡ *CPT Assistant* Jun 23:1

33901 normal native connections, bilateral
➡ *CPT Changes: An Insider's View* 2023
➡ *CPT Assistant* Jun 23:1

33902 abnormal connections, unilateral
➡ *CPT Changes: An Insider's View* 2023
➡ *CPT Assistant* Jun 23:1

33903 abnormal connections, bilateral
➡ *CPT Changes: An Insider's View* 2023
➡ *CPT Assistant* Jun 23:1

+ 33904 Percutaneous pulmonary artery revascularization by stent placement, each additional vessel or separate lesion, normal or abnormal connections (List separately in addition to code for primary procedure)
➡ *CPT Changes: An Insider's View* 2023
➡ *CPT Assistant* Jun 23:1

(Use 33904 in conjunction with 33900, 33901, 33902, 33903)

Pulmonary Artery

33910 Pulmonary artery embolectomy; with cardiopulmonary bypass
➡ *CPT Assistant* Mar 07:1, Jan 23:30

33915 without cardiopulmonary bypass
➡ *CPT Assistant* Mar 07:1, Jan 23:30

33916 Pulmonary endarterectomy, with or without embolectomy, with cardiopulmonary bypass
➡ *CPT Assistant* Mar 07:1, Jan 23:30

33917 Repair of pulmonary artery stenosis by reconstruction with patch or graft
➡ *CPT Assistant* Mar 07:1, Apr 11:6, Jul 16:3

33920 Repair of pulmonary atresia with ventricular septal defect, by construction or replacement of conduit from right or left ventricle to pulmonary artery
➡ *CPT Assistant* Mar 07:1, Apr 19:6

(For repair of other complex cardiac anomalies by construction or replacement of right or left ventricle to pulmonary artery conduit, use 33608)

33922 Transection of pulmonary artery with cardiopulmonary bypass

(Do not report modifier 63 in conjunction with 33922)

+ 33924 Ligation and takedown of a systemic-to-pulmonary artery shunt, performed in conjunction with a congenital heart procedure (List separately in addition to code for primary procedure)

▶(Use 33924 in conjunction with 33474, 33475, 33476, 33477, 33478, 33600-33617, 33622, 33684-33688, 33692-33697, 33735-33767, 33770-33783, 33786, 33917, 33920, 33922, 33925, 33926, 33935, 33945)◀

33925 Repair of pulmonary artery arborization anomalies by unifocalization; without cardiopulmonary bypass
➡ *CPT Changes: An Insider's View* 2006

33926 with cardiopulmonary bypass
➡ *CPT Changes: An Insider's View* 2006

Heart/Lung Transplantation

Heart with or without lung allotransplantation involves three distinct components of physician work:

1. **Cadaver donor cardiectomy with or without pneumonectomy,** which includes harvesting the allograft and cold preservation of the allograft (perfusing with cold preservation solution and cold maintenance) (see 33930, 33940).

2. **Backbench work:**

   Preparation of a cadaver donor heart and lung allograft prior to transplantation, including dissection of the allograft from surrounding soft tissues to prepare the aorta, superior vena cava, inferior vena cava, and trachea for implantation (use 33933).

   Preparation of a cadaver donor heart allograft prior to transplantation, including dissection of the allograft from surrounding soft tissues to prepare aorta, superior vena cava, inferior vena cava, pulmonary artery, and left atrium for implantation (use 33944).

★ = Telemedicine   ◀ = Audio-only   + = Add-on code   ✚ = FDA approval pending   # = Resequenced code   ⊘ = Modifier 51 exempt   ➡➡➡ = See p xxi for details

3. ***Recipient heart with or without lung
allotransplantation,*** which includes transplantation
of allograft and care of the recipient (see 33935,
33945).

> (For implantation of a total replacement heart system
> [artificial heart] with recipient cardiectomy, use 33927)

33927   Implantation of a total replacement heart system
(artificial heart) with recipient cardiectomy

> ➔ *CPT Changes: An Insider's View* 2018
> ➔ *CPT Assistant* Jun 18:3

> (For implantation of ventricular assist device, see 33975,
> 33976, 33979, 33990, 33991, 33995)

33928   Removal and replacement of total replacement heart
system (artificial heart)

> ➔ *CPT Changes: An Insider's View* 2018
> ➔ *CPT Assistant* Jun 18:3

> (For revision or replacement of components only of a
> replacement heart system [artificial heart], use 33999)

+ 33929   Removal of a total replacement heart system (artificial
heart) for heart transplantation (List separately in
addition to code for primary procedure)

> ➔ *CPT Changes: An Insider's View* 2018
> ➔ *CPT Assistant* Jun 18:3

> (Use 33929 in conjunction with 33945)

Total Heart Implantation Device
33927, 33928, 33929

Total heart implantation device in place after cardiectomy

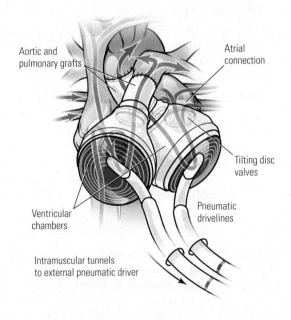

Aortic and
pulmonary grafts

Atrial
connection

Tilting disc
valves

Ventricular
chambers

Pneumatic
drivelines

Intramuscular tunnels
to external pneumatic driver

33930   Donor cardiectomy-pneumonectomy (including cold
preservation)

> ➔ *CPT Changes: An Insider's View* 2005

33933   Backbench standard preparation of cadaver donor heart/
lung allograft prior to transplantation, including
dissection of allograft from surrounding soft tissues to
prepare aorta, superior vena cava, inferior vena cava, and
trachea for implantation

> ➔ *CPT Changes: An Insider's View* 2005

33935   Heart-lung transplant with recipient cardiectomy-
pneumonectomy

33940   Donor cardiectomy (including cold preservation)

> ➔ *CPT Changes: An Insider's View* 2005
> ➔ *CPT Assistant* Apr 05:10-11

33944   Backbench standard preparation of cadaver donor heart
allograft prior to transplantation, including dissection of
allograft from surrounding soft tissues to prepare aorta,
superior vena cava, inferior vena cava, pulmonary artery,
and left atrium for implantation

> ➔ *CPT Changes: An Insider's View* 2005

> (For repair or resection procedures on the donor heart,
> see 33300, 33310, 33320, 33390, 33463, 33464, 33510,
> 33641, 35216, 35276, 35685)

33945   Heart transplant, with or without recipient cardiectomy

> ➔ *CPT Assistant* Fall 92:20, Jun 18:3

Extracorporeal Membrane Oxygenation or Extracorporeal Life Support Services

Prolonged extracorporeal membrane oxygenation
(ECMO) or extracorporeal life support (ECLS) is a
procedure that provides cardiac and/or respiratory
support to the heart and/or lungs, which allows them to
rest and recover when sick or injured. ECMO/ECLS
supports the function of the heart and/or lungs by
continuously pumping some of the patient's blood out of
the body to an oxygenator (membrane lung) where
oxygen is added to the blood, carbon dioxide (CO_2) is
removed, and the blood is warmed before it is returned to
the patient. There are two methods that can be used to
accomplish ECMO/ECLS. One method is veno-arterial
extracorporeal life support, which will support both the
heart and lungs. Veno-arterial ECMO/ECLS requires
that two cannula(e) are placed—one in a large vein and
one in a large artery. The other method is veno-venous
extracorporeal life support. Veno-venous ECMO/ECLS is
used for lung support only and requires one or two
cannula(e), which are placed in a vein.

Services directly related to the cannulation, initiation,
management, and discontinuation of the ECMO/ECLS
circuit and parameters (33946, 33947, 33948, 33949) are
distinct from the daily overall management of the patient.
The daily overall management of the patient is a factor

that will vary greatly depending on the patient's age, disease process, and condition. Daily overall management of the patient may be separately reported using the relevant hospital inpatient or observation care services (99221, 99222, 99223, 99231, 99232, 99233, 99234, 99235, 99236) or critical care or intensive care evaluation and management codes (99291, 99292, 99468, 99469, 99471, 99472, 99475, 99476, 99477, 99478, 99479, 99480).

Services directly related to the ECMO/ECLS involve the initial cannulation and repositioning, removing, or adding cannula(e) while the patient is being supported by the ECMO/ECLS. Initiation of the ECMO/ECLS circuit and setting parameters (33946, 33947) is performed by the physician and involves determining the necessary ECMO/ECLS device components, blood flow, gas exchange, and other necessary parameters to manage the circuit. The daily management of the ECMO/ECLS circuit and monitoring parameters (33948, 33949) requires physician oversight to ensure that specific features of the interaction of the circuit with the patient are met. Daily management of the circuit and parameters includes management of blood flow, oxygenation, CO_2 clearance by the membrane lung, systemic response, anticoagulation and treatment of bleeding, and cannula(e) positioning, alarms and safety. Once the patient's heart and/or lung function has sufficiently recovered, the physician will wean the patient from the ECMO/ECLS circuit and finally decannulate the patient. The basic management of the ECMO/ECLS circuit and parameters are similar, regardless of the patient's condition.

ECMO/ECLS commonly involves multiple physicians and supporting nonphysician personnel to manage each patient. Different physicians may insert the cannula(e) and initiate ECMO/ECLS, manage the ECMO/ECLS circuit, and decannulate the patient. In addition, it would be common for one physician to manage the ECMO/ECLS circuit and patient-related issues (eg, anticoagulation, complications related to the ECMO/ECLS devices), while another physician manages the overall patient medical condition and underlying disorders, all on a daily basis. The physicians involved in the patient's care are commonly of different specialties, and significant physician team interaction may be required. Depending on the type of circuit and the patient's condition, there is substantial nonphysician work by ECMO/ECLS specialists, cardiac perfusionists, respiratory therapists, and specially trained nurses who provide long periods of constant attention.

If the same physician provides any or all of the services for placing a patient on an ECMO/ECLS circuit, they may report the appropriate codes for the services they performed, which may include codes for the cannula(e) insertion (33951, 33952, 33953, 33954, 33955, 33956), ECMO/ECLS initiation (33946 or 33947), and overall

patient management (99221, 99222, 99223, 99231, 99232, 99233, 99234, 99235, 99236, 99291, 99292, 99468, 99469, 99471, 99472, 99475, 99476, 99477, 99478, 99479, 99480).

ECMO/ECLS daily management (33948, 33949) and repositioning services (33957, 33958, 33959, 33962, 33963, 33964) may not be reported on the same day as initiation services (33946, 33947) by the same or different individuals.

If different physicians provide parts of the service, each physician may report the correct code(s) for the service(s) they provided, except as noted.

Repositioning of the ECMO/ECLS cannula(e) (33957, 33958, 33959, 33962, 33963, 33964) at the same session as insertion (33951, 33952, 33953, 33954, 33955, 33956) is not separately reportable. Replacement of ECMO/ECLS cannula(e) in the same vessel should only be reported using the insertion code (33951, 33952, 33953, 33954, 33955, 33956). If cannula(e) are removed from one vessel and new cannula(e) are placed in a different vessel, report the appropriate cannula(e) removal (33965, 33966, 33969, 33984, 33985, 33986) and insertion (33951, 33952, 33953, 33954, 33955, 33956) codes. Extensive repair or replacement of an artery may be additionally reported (eg, 35266, 35286, 35371, and 35665). Fluoroscopic guidance used for cannula(e) repositioning (33957, 33958, 33959, 33962, 33963, 33964) is included in the procedure when performed and should not be separately reported.

Daily management codes (33948 and 33949) should not be reported on the same day as initiation of ECMO (33946 or 33947).

Initiation codes (33946 or 33947) should not be reported on the same day as repositioning codes (33957, 33958, 33959, 33962, 33963, 33964). See the CPT codes for ECMO/ECLS Procedure Chart.

33946 Extracorporeal membrane oxygenation (ECMO)/extracorporeal life support (ECLS) provided by physician; initiation, veno-venous

➡ *CPT Changes: An Insider's View* 2015

➡ *CPT Assistant* Jul 15:3, Mar 16:5

(Do not report modifier 63 in conjunction with 33946, 33947, 33948, 33949)

(For insertion of cannula[e] for extracorporeal circulation, see 33951, 33952, 33953, 33954, 33955, 33956)

33947 initiation, veno-arterial

➡ *CPT Changes: An Insider's View* 2015

➡ *CPT Assistant* Jul 15:3, Mar 16:5

CPT Codes For ECMO/ECLS Procedures

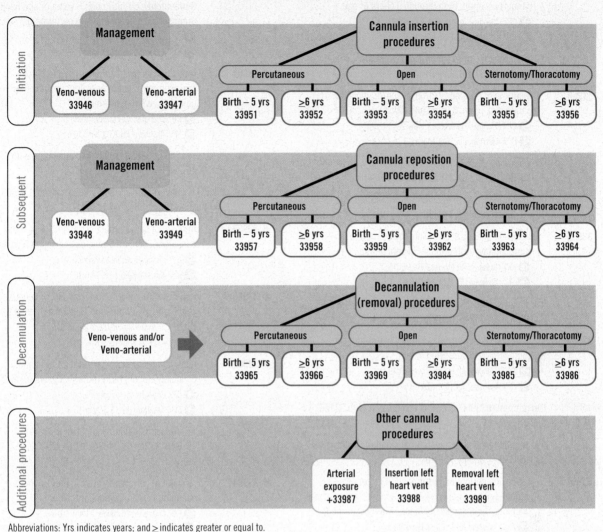

Abbreviations: Yrs indicates years; and ≥ indicates greater or equal to.

(Do not report modifier 63 in conjunction with 33946, 33947, 33948, 33949)

(Do not report 33946, 33947 in conjunction with 33948, 33949, 33957, 33958, 33959, 33962, 33963, 33964)

33948   daily management, each day, veno-venous
> *CPT Changes: An Insider's View* 2015
> *CPT Assistant* Jul 15:3, Mar 16:5

(Do not report modifier 63 in conjunction with 33946, 33947, 33948, 33949)

33949   daily management, each day, veno-arterial
> *CPT Changes: An Insider's View* 2015
> *CPT Assistant* Jul 15:3, Mar 16:5

(Do not report modifier 63 in conjunction with 33946, 33947, 33948, 33949)

(Do not report 33948, 33949 in conjunction with 33946, 33947)

33951   insertion of peripheral (arterial and/or venous) cannula(e), percutaneous, birth through 5 years of age (includes fluoroscopic guidance, when performed)
> *CPT Changes: An Insider's View* 2015
> *CPT Assistant* Jul 15:3, Mar 16:5

(For initiation and daily management of extracorporeal circulation, see 33946, 33947, 33948, 33949)

33952   insertion of peripheral (arterial and/or venous) cannula(e), percutaneous, 6 years and older (includes fluoroscopic guidance, when performed)
> *CPT Changes: An Insider's View* 2015
> *CPT Assistant* Jul 15:3, Mar 16:5

(For maintenance of extracorporeal circulation, see 33946, 33947, 33948, 33949)

Cardiovascular 33016-39599

33953   insertion of peripheral (arterial and/or venous) cannula(e), open, birth through 5 years of age

➔ *CPT Changes: An Insider's View* 2015

➔ *CPT Assistant* Jul 15:3, Mar 16:5

(For maintenance of extracorporeal circulation, see 33946, 33947, 33948, 33949)

33954   insertion of peripheral (arterial and/or venous) cannula(e), open, 6 years and older

➔ *CPT Changes: An Insider's View* 2015

➔ *CPT Assistant* Jul 15:3, Mar 16:5

(Do not report 33953, 33954 in conjunction with 34714, 34715, 34716, 34812, 34820, 34833, 34834)

(For maintenance of extracorporeal circulation, see 33946, 33947, 33948, 33949)

33955   insertion of central cannula(e) by sternotomy or thoracotomy, birth through 5 years of age

➔ *CPT Changes: An Insider's View* 2015

➔ *CPT Assistant* Jul 15:3, Mar 16:5

(For maintenance of extracorporeal circulation, see 33946, 33947, 33948, 33949)

33956   insertion of central cannula(e) by sternotomy or thoracotomy, 6 years and older

➔ *CPT Changes: An Insider's View* 2015

➔ *CPT Assistant* Jul 15:3, Mar 16:5

(Do not report 33955, 33956 in conjunction with 32100, 39010)

(For maintenance of extracorporeal circulation, see 33946, 33947, 33948, 33949)

33957   reposition peripheral (arterial and/or venous) cannula(e), percutaneous, birth through 5 years of age (includes fluoroscopic guidance, when performed)

➔ *CPT Changes: An Insider's View* 2015

➔ *CPT Assistant* Jul 15:3, Mar 16:5

33958   reposition peripheral (arterial and/or venous) cannula(e), percutaneous, 6 years and older (includes fluoroscopic guidance, when performed)

➔ *CPT Changes: An Insider's View* 2015

➔ *CPT Assistant* Jul 15:3, Mar 16:5

(Do not report 33957, 33958 in conjunction with 34713)

33959   reposition peripheral (arterial and/or venous) cannula(e), open, birth through 5 years of age (includes fluoroscopic guidance, when performed)

➔ *CPT Changes: An Insider's View* 2015

➔ *CPT Assistant* Jul 15:3, Mar 16:5

 # 33962   reposition peripheral (arterial and/or venous) cannula(e), open, 6 years and older (includes fluoroscopic guidance, when performed)

➔ *CPT Changes: An Insider's View* 2015

➔ *CPT Assistant* Jul 15:3, Mar 16:5

(Do not report 33959, 33962 in conjunction with 34714, 34715, 34716, 34812, 34820, 34834)

 # 33963   reposition of central cannula(e) by sternotomy or thoracotomy, birth through 5 years of age (includes fluoroscopic guidance, when performed)

➔ *CPT Changes: An Insider's View* 2015

➔ *CPT Assistant* Jul 15:3, Mar 16:5

 # 33964   reposition central cannula(e) by sternotomy or thoracotomy, 6 years and older (includes fluoroscopic guidance, when performed)

➔ *CPT Changes: An Insider's View* 2015

➔ *CPT Assistant* Jul 15:3, Mar 16:5

(Do not report 33963, 33964 in conjunction with 32100, 39010)

(Do not report 33957, 33958, 33959, 33962, 33963, 33964 in conjunction with 33946, 33947)

 # 33965   removal of peripheral (arterial and/or venous) cannula(e), percutaneous, birth through 5 years of age

➔ *CPT Changes: An Insider's View* 2015

➔ *CPT Assistant* Jul 15:3, Mar 16:5

 # 33966   removal of peripheral (arterial and/or venous) cannula(e), percutaneous, 6 years and older

➔ *CPT Changes: An Insider's View* 2015

➔ *CPT Assistant* Jul 15:3, Mar 16:5

 # 33969   removal of peripheral (arterial and/or venous) cannula(e), open, birth through 5 years of age

➔ *CPT Changes: An Insider's View* 2015

➔ *CPT Assistant* Jul 15:3, Mar 16:5

(Do not report 33969 in conjunction with 34714, 34715, 34716, 34812, 34820, 34834, 35201, 35206, 35211, 35226)

 # 33984   removal of peripheral (arterial and/or venous) cannula(e), open, 6 years and older

➔ *CPT Changes: An Insider's View* 2015

➔ *CPT Assistant* Jul 15:3, Mar 16:5

(Do not report 33984 in conjunction with 34714, 34715, 34716, 34812, 34820, 34834, 35201, 35206, 35211, 35226)

 # 33985   removal of central cannula(e) by sternotomy or thoracotomy, birth through 5 years of age

➔ *CPT Changes: An Insider's View* 2015

➔ *CPT Assistant* Jul 15:3, Mar 16:5

(Do not report 33985 in conjunction with 35211)

 # 33986   removal of central cannula(e) by sternotomy or thoracotomy, 6 years and older

➔ *CPT Changes: An Insider's View* 2015

➔ *CPT Assistant* Jul 15:3, Mar 16:5

(Do not report 33986 in conjunction with 35211)

#+ 33987 Arterial exposure with creation of graft conduit (eg, chimney graft) to facilitate arterial perfusion for ECMO/ECLS (List separately in addition to code for primary procedure)
➔ *CPT Changes: An Insider's View* 2015
➔ *CPT Assistant* Jul 15:3, Mar 16:5

(Use 33987 in conjunction with 33953, 33954, 33955, 33956)

(Do not report 33987 in conjunction with 34714, 34716, 34833)

 # 33988 Insertion of left heart vent by thoracic incision (eg, sternotomy, thoracotomy) for ECMO/ECLS
➔ *CPT Changes: An Insider's View* 2015
➔ *CPT Assistant* Jul 15:3, Mar 16:5

 # 33989 Removal of left heart vent by thoracic incision (eg, sternotomy, thoracotomy) for ECMO/ECLS
➔ *CPT Changes: An Insider's View* 2015
➔ *CPT Assistant* Jul 15:3, Mar 16:5

Cardiac Assist

A ventricular assist device is placed to provide hemodynamic support to the right heart, left heart, or both. The insertion of a ventricular assist device (VAD) can be performed via percutaneous (33990, 33991, 33995) or transthoracic (33975, 33976, 33979) approach. The location of the ventricular assist device may be intracorporeal or extracorporeal.

Removal of a transthoracic ventricular assist device (33977, 33978, 33980) or percutaneous ventricular assist device (33992, 33997) includes removal of the entire device, including the cannulas. Removal of a percutaneous ventricular assist device at the same session as insertion is not separately reportable. For removal of a percutaneous ventricular assist device at a separate and distinct session, but on the same day as insertion, report 33992, 33997 appended with modifier 59 indicating a distinct procedural service.

Repositioning of a percutaneous ventricular assist device at the same session as insertion is not separately reportable. Repositioning of percutaneous ventricular assist device not necessitating imaging guidance is not a reportable service. For repositioning of a percutaneous ventricular assist device necessitating imaging guidance at a separate and distinct session, but on the same day as insertion, report 33993 with modifier 59 indicating a distinct procedural service.

Replacement of a ventricular assist device pump (ie, 33981-33983) includes the removal of the pump and insertion of a new pump, connection, de-airing, and initiation of the new pump.

Replacement of the entire implantable ventricular assist device system, ie, pump(s) and cannulas, is reported using the insertion codes (ie, 33975, 33976, 33979). Removal (ie, 33977, 33978, 33980) of the ventricular assist device system being replaced is not separately reported. Replacement of a percutaneous ventricular assist device is reported using implantation codes (ie, 33990, 33991, 33995). Removal (ie, 33992, 33997) is not reported separately when a device is replaced.

33962 Code is out of numerical sequence. See 33958-33968

33963 Code is out of numerical sequence. See 33958-33968

33964 Code is out of numerical sequence. See 33958-33968

33965 Code is out of numerical sequence. See 33958-33968

33966 Code is out of numerical sequence. See 33958-33968

33967 Insertion of intra-aortic balloon assist device, percutaneous
➔ *CPT Changes: An Insider's View* 2002
➔ *CPT Assistant* Feb 02:2, Nov 11:8, Mar 13:10, Sep 15:3, Mar 16:5

33968 Removal of intra-aortic balloon assist device, percutaneous
➔ *CPT Changes: An Insider's View* 2000
➔ *CPT Assistant* Nov 99:19, Jan 00:10, Nov 11:8

33969 Code is out of numerical sequence. See 33958-33968

33970 Insertion of intra-aortic balloon assist device through the femoral artery, open approach
➔ *CPT Changes: An Insider's View* 2000
➔ *CPT Assistant* Nov 99:19, Nov 11:8, Mar 13:10, Sep 15:3, Mar 16:5

33971 Removal of intra-aortic balloon assist device including repair of femoral artery, with or without graft
➔ *CPT Assistant* Nov 11:8

33973 Insertion of intra-aortic balloon assist device through the ascending aorta
➔ *CPT Assistant* Nov 11:8, Mar 13:10, Sep 15:3, Mar 16:5

33974 Removal of intra-aortic balloon assist device from the ascending aorta, including repair of the ascending aorta, with or without graft
➔ *CPT Assistant* Nov 11:8

33975 Insertion of ventricular assist device; extracorporeal, single ventricle
➔ *CPT Changes: An Insider's View* 2002
➔ *CPT Assistant* Feb 92:2, Jan 04:28, Nov 09:10, Jan 10:11, Apr 10:6, Mar 13:10

33976 extracorporeal, biventricular
➔ *CPT Changes: An Insider's View* 2002
➔ *CPT Assistant* Feb 02:2, Nov 09:10, Jan 10:11, Apr 10:6, Mar 13:10

Cardiovascular 33016-39599

33977 Removal of ventricular assist device; extracorporeal, single ventricle

➔ *CPT Changes: An Insider's View* 2002

➔ *CPT Assistant* Feb 02:2, Nov 09:10, Jan 10:11, Apr 10:6, Mar 13:10

33978 extracorporeal, biventricular

➔ *CPT Changes: An Insider's View* 2002

➔ *CPT Assistant* Feb 02:2, Nov 09:10, Jan 10:11, Apr 10:6, Mar 13:10

33979 Insertion of ventricular assist device, implantable intracorporeal, single ventricle

➔ *CPT Changes: An Insider's View* 2002

➔ *CPT Assistant* Feb 02:3, Jan 04:28, Nov 09:10, Jan 10:11, Apr 10:6, Mar 13:10

Insertion of Implantable Single Ventricle Assist Device
33979

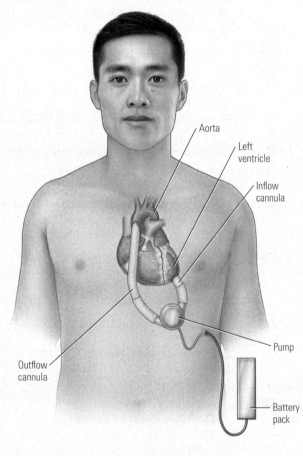

Aorta

Left ventricle

Inflow cannula

Pump

Outflow cannula

Battery pack

33980 Removal of ventricular assist device, implantable intracorporeal, single ventricle

➔ *CPT Changes: An Insider's View* 2002

➔ *CPT Assistant* Feb 02:3, Nov 09:10, Apr 10:6, Mar 13:10

33981 Replacement of extracorporeal ventricular assist device, single or biventricular, pump(s), single or each pump

➔ *CPT Changes: An Insider's View* 2010

➔ *CPT Assistant* Apr 10:6

33982 Replacement of ventricular assist device pump(s); implantable intracorporeal, single ventricle, without cardiopulmonary bypass

➔ *CPT Changes: An Insider's View* 2010

➔ *CPT Assistant* Apr 10:6

33983 implantable intracorporeal, single ventricle, with cardiopulmonary bypass

➔ *CPT Changes: An Insider's View* 2010

➔ *CPT Assistant* Apr 10:6

33984 Code is out of numerical sequence. See 33958-33968

33985 Code is out of numerical sequence. See 33958-33968

33986 Code is out of numerical sequence. See 33958-33968

33987 Code is out of numerical sequence. See 33958-33968

33988 Code is out of numerical sequence. See 33958-33968

33989 Code is out of numerical sequence. See 33958-33968

 # 33995 Insertion of ventricular assist device, percutaneous, including radiological supervision and interpretation; right heart, venous access only

➔ *CPT Changes: An Insider's View* 2021

➔ *CPT Assistant* Dec 20:4, Dec 21:18

33990 left heart, arterial access only

➔ *CPT Changes: An Insider's View* 2013, 2017, 2021

➔ *CPT Assistant* Mar 13:10, Oct 14:15, Sep 15:3, Mar 16:5, Dec 20:4, Dec 21:18

33991 left heart, both arterial and venous access, with transseptal puncture

➔ *CPT Changes: An Insider's View* 2013, 2017, 2021

➔ *CPT Assistant* Mar 13:10, Sep 15:3, Mar 16:5, Dec 20:4, Dec 21:18

33992 Removal of percutaneous left heart ventricular assist device, arterial or arterial and venous cannula(s), at separate and distinct session from insertion

➔ *CPT Changes: An Insider's View* 2013, 2017, 2021

➔ *CPT Assistant* Mar 13:10, Sep 15:3, Mar 16:5, Dec 20:4, Dec 21:18

 # 33997 Removal of percutaneous right heart ventricular assist device, venous cannula, at separate and distinct session from insertion

➔ *CPT Changes: An Insider's View* 2021

➔ *CPT Assistant* Dec 20:4, Dec 21:18

(For removal of left or right heart ventricular assist device via open approach, see appropriate vessel repair code [eg, 35206, 35226, 35286, 35371])

33993 Repositioning of percutaneous right or left heart ventricular assist device with imaging guidance at separate and distinct session from insertion

> *CPT Changes: An Insider's View* 2013, 2017, 2021

> *CPT Assistant* Mar 13:10, Sep 15:3, Mar 16:5, Dec 20:4, Dec 21:18

33995 Code is out of numerical sequence. See 33982-33991

33997 Code is out of numerical sequence. See 33991-33993

Other Procedures

33999 Unlisted procedure, cardiac surgery

> *CPT Assistant* Oct 99:11, Jan 04:7, Mar 07:1, Nov 09:10, Jan 10:11, Apr 10:6, Feb 13:13, Mar 13:10, Dec 13:14, Dec 14:17, Apr 19:10, Nov 21:3, Apr 24:9

Arteries and Veins

Primary vascular procedure listings include establishing both inflow and outflow by whatever procedures necessary. Also included is that portion of the operative arteriogram performed by the surgeon, as indicated. Sympathectomy, when done, is included in the listed aortic procedures. For unlisted vascular procedure, use 37799.

Embolectomy/Thrombectomy

Arterial, With or Without Catheter

34001 Embolectomy or thrombectomy, with or without catheter; carotid, subclavian or innominate artery, by neck incision

> *CPT Assistant* Jun 22:22

34051 innominate, subclavian artery, by thoracic incision

34101 axillary, brachial, innominate, subclavian artery, by arm incision

34111 radial or ulnar artery, by arm incision

34151 renal, celiac, mesentery, aortoiliac artery, by abdominal incision

34201 femoropopliteal, aortoiliac artery, by leg incision

> *CPT Assistant* Aug 11:9

34203 popliteal-tibio-peroneal artery, by leg incision

Venous, Direct or With Catheter

34401 Thrombectomy, direct or with catheter; vena cava, iliac vein, by abdominal incision

34421 vena cava, iliac, femoropopliteal vein, by leg incision

> *CPT Assistant* Spring 94:30

34451 vena cava, iliac, femoropopliteal vein, by abdominal and leg incision

34471 subclavian vein, by neck incision

34490 axillary and subclavian vein, by arm incision

> *CPT Assistant* Jun 22:22

Venous Reconstruction

34501 Valvuloplasty, femoral vein

> (For insertion of bioprosthetic valve into femoral vein, use 0744T)

34502 Reconstruction of vena cava, any method

34510 Venous valve transposition, any vein donor

> (For insertion of bioprosthetic valve into femoral vein, use 0744T)

34520 Cross-over vein graft to venous system

> *CPT Assistant* Mar 23:33

34530 Saphenopopliteal vein anastomosis

Endovascular Repair of Abdominal Aorta and/or Iliac Arteries

Codes 34701, 34702, 34703, 34704, 34705, 34706 describe introduction, positioning, and deployment of an endograft for treatment of abdominal aortic pathology (with or without rupture), such as aneurysm, pseudoaneurysm, dissection, penetrating ulcer, or traumatic disruption in the infrarenal abdominal aorta with or without extension into the iliac artery(ies). The terms, endovascular graft, endoprosthesis, endograft, and stentgraft, refer to a covered stent. The infrarenal aortic endograft may be an aortic tube device, a bifurcated unibody device, a modular bifurcated docking system with docking limb(s), or an aorto-uni-iliac device. Codes 34707 and 34708 describe introduction, positioning, and deployment of an ilio-iliac endograft for treatment of isolated arterial pathology (with or without rupture), such as aneurysm, pseudoaneurysm, arteriovenous malformation, or trauma involving the iliac artery. For treatment of atherosclerotic occlusive disease in the iliac artery(ies) with a covered stent(s), see 37221, 37223. For covered stent placement for atherosclerotic occlusive disease in the aorta, see 37236, 37237.

Add-on code 34717 is reported at the time of aorto-iliac artery endograft placement (34703, 34704, 34705, 34706) for deployment of a bifurcated endograft in the common iliac artery with extension(s) into both the internal iliac and external iliac arteries, when performed, to maintain perfusion in both vessels for treatment of iliac artery pathology (with or without rupture), such as aneurysm, pseudoaneurysm, dissection, penetrating ulcer, arteriovenous malformation, or traumatic disruption. The iliac branched endograft is a multi-piece system consisting of a bifurcated device that is placed in the common iliac artery and then additional extension(s) are placed into

Cardiovascular 33016-39599

both the internal iliac artery and external iliac/common femoral arteries as needed, as well as a proximal extension that overlaps with an aorto-iliac endograft, when performed. All additional extensions proximally into the common iliac artery or distally into the external iliac and/or common femoral arteries are inherent to these codes.

Report 34705 or 34706 for simultaneous bilateral iliac artery aneurysm repairs with aorto-bi-iliac endograft. For isolated bilateral iliac artery repair using iliac artery tube endografts, report 34707 or 34708 with modifier 50 appended.

Decompressive laparotomy for abdominal compartment syndrome after ruptured abdominal aortic and/or iliac artery aneurysm repair may be separately reported with 49000 in addition to 34702, 34704, 34706, or 34708.

The treatment zone for endograft procedures is defined by those vessels that contain an endograft(s) (main body, docking limb[s], and/or extension[s]) deployed during that operative session. Adjunctive procedures outside the treatment zone may be separately reported (eg, angioplasty, endovascular stent placement, embolization). For example, when an endograft terminates in the common iliac artery, any additional treatment performed in the external and/or internal iliac artery may be separately reportable. Placement of a docking limb is inherent to a modular endograft(s), and, therefore, 34709 may not be reported separately if the docking limb extends into the external iliac artery. In addition, any interventions (eg, angioplasty, stenting, additional stent graft extension[s]) in the external iliac artery where the docking limb terminates may not be reported separately. Any catheterization or treatment of the internal iliac artery, such as embolization, may be separately reported. For 34701 and 34702, the abdominal aortic treatment zone is defined as the infrarenal aorta. For 34703 and 34704, the abdominal aortic treatment zone is typically defined as the infrarenal aorta and ipsilateral common iliac artery. For 34705 and 34706, the abdominal aortic treatment zone is typically defined as the infrarenal aorta and both common iliac arteries. For 34707, 34708, 34717, 34718, the treatment zone is defined as the portion of the iliac artery(ies) (eg, common, internal, external iliac arteries) that contains the endograft.

Codes 34702, 34704, 34706, 34708 are reported when endovascular repair is performed on ruptured aneurysm in the aorta or iliac artery(ies). Rupture is defined as clinical and/or radiographic evidence of acute hemorrhage for purposes of reporting these codes. A chronic, contained rupture is considered a pseudoaneurysm, and endovascular treatment of a chronic, contained rupture is reported with 34701, 34703, 34705, or 34707.

Code 34709 is reported for placement of extension prosthesis(es) that terminate(s) either in the internal iliac, external iliac, or common femoral artery(ies) or in the abdominal aorta proximal to the renal artery(ies) in conjunction with 34701, 34702, 34703, 34704, 34705, 34706, 34707, 34708. Code 34709 may only be reported once per vessel treated (ie, multiple endograft extensions placed in a single vessel may only be reported once). Endograft extension(s) that terminate(s) in the common iliac arteries are included in 34703, 34704, 34705, 34706, 34707, 34708 and are not separately reported. Treatment zone angioplasty/stenting, when performed, is included in 34709. In addition, proximal infrarenal abdominal aortic extension prosthesis(es) that terminate(s) in the aorta below the renal artery(ies) are also included in 34701, 34702, 34703, 34704, 34705, 34706 and are not separately reportable.

Codes 34710, 34711 are reported for delayed placement of distal or proximal extension prosthesis(es) for endovascular repair of infrarenal abdominal aortic or iliac aneurysm, false aneurysm, dissection, endoleak, or endograft migration. Pre-procedure sizing and device selection, all nonselective catheterization(s), all associated radiological supervision and interpretation, and treatment zone angioplasty/stenting, when performed, are included in 34710 and 34711. Codes 34710 and 34711 may only be reported once per vessel treated (ie, multiple endograft extensions placed in a single vessel may only be reported once).

If an aorto-iliac artery endograft (34703, 34704, 34705, 34706) is not being placed during the same operative session, 34718 may be reported for placement of a bifurcated endograft in the common iliac artery with extension(s) into both the internal iliac and external iliac arteries, to maintain perfusion in both vessels for treatment of iliac artery pathology (without rupture), such as aneurysm, pseudoaneurysm, dissection, arteriovenous malformation. The iliac branched endograft is a multi-piece system consisting of a bifurcated device that is placed in the common iliac artery and then additional extension(s) are placed into both the internal iliac artery and external iliac/common femoral arteries as needed as well as a proximal extension that overlaps with an aorto-iliac endograft, when performed. All additional extensions placed proximally into the common iliac artery or distally into the external iliac and/or common femoral arteries are inherent to these codes. For isolated bilateral iliac artery repair using iliac artery branched endografts, use 34718 with modifier 50 appended.

Codes 34709, 34710, 34711 may not be separately reported with 34717, 34718 for ipsilateral extension prosthesis(es). However, 34709, 34710, 34711 may be reported separately for extension prosthesis(es) in the iliac/femoral arteries contralateral to the iliac branched endograft.

Nonselective catheterization is included in 34701, 34702, 34703, 34704, 34705, 34706, 34707, 34708 and is not separately reported. However, selective catheterization of the hypogastric artery(ies), renal artery(ies), and/or arterial families outside the treatment zone of the endograft may be separately reported. Intravascular ultrasound (37252, 37253) performed during endovascular aneurysm repair may be separately reported. Balloon angioplasty and/or stenting within the treatment zone of the endograft, either before or after endograft deployment, is not separately reported. Fluoroscopic guidance and radiological supervision and interpretation in conjunction with endograft repair is not separately reported, and includes all intraprocedural imaging (eg, angiography, rotational CT) of the aorta and its branches prior to deployment of the endovascular device, fluoroscopic guidance and roadmapping used in the delivery of the endovascular components, and intraprocedural and completion angiography (eg, confirm position, detect endoleak, evaluate runoff) performed at the time of the endovascular infrarenal aorta and/or iliac repair.

Selective arterial catheterization of the internal and external iliac arteries (eg, 36245, 36246, 36247, 36248) ipsilateral to an iliac branched endograft is included in 34717, 34718 and not separately reported. However, selective catheterization of the renal artery(ies), the contralateral hypogastric artery, and/or arterial families outside the treatment zone of the graft may be separately reported. Intravascular ultrasound (37252, 37253) performed during endovascular aneurysm repair may be separately reported. Balloon angioplasty within the target treatment zone of the endograft, either before or after endograft deployment, is not separately reported. Fluoroscopic guidance and radiological supervision and interpretation performed in conjunction with endovascular iliac branched repair is not separately reported. Endovascular iliac branched repair includes all intraprocedural imaging (eg, angiography, rotational CT) of the aorta and its branches prior to deployment of the endovascular device, fluoroscopic guidance in the delivery of the endovascular components, and intraprocedural arterial angiography (eg, confirm position, detect endoleak, evaluate runoff) performed at the time of the endovascular aorto-iliac repair).

Codes 34709, 34710, 34711 include nonselective introduction of guidewires and catheters into the treatment zone from peripheral artery access(es). However, selective catheterization of the hypogastric artery(ies), renal artery(ies), and/or arterial families outside the treatment zone may be separately reported. Codes 34709, 34710, 34711 also include balloon angioplasty and/or stenting within the treatment zone of the endograft extension, either before or after deployment of the endograft, fluoroscopic guidance, and all associated radiological supervision and interpretation performed in conjunction with endovascular endograft extension (eg, angiographic diagnostic imaging of the aorta and its

branches prior to deployment of the endovascular device, fluoroscopic guidance in the delivery of the endovascular components, and intraprocedural and completion angiography to confirm endograft position, detect endoleak, and evaluate runoff).

Code 34712 describes transcatheter delivery of accessory-enhanced fixation devices to the endograft (eg, anchor, screw, tack), including all associated radiological supervision and interpretation. Code 34712 may only be reported once per operative session.

Vascular access requiring use of closure devices for large sheaths (ie, 12 French or larger) or access requiring open surgical arterial exposure may be separately reported (eg, 34713, 34714, 34715, 34716, 34812, 34820, 34833, 34834). Code 34713 describes percutaneous access and closure of a femoral arteriotomy for delivery of endovascular prosthesis through a large arterial sheath (ie, 12 French or larger). Ultrasound guidance (ie, 76937), when performed, is included in 34713. (Percutaneous access using a sheath smaller than 12 French is included in 34701-34712 and is not separately reported.)

Code 34812 describes open repair and closure of the femoral artery. Extensive repair of an artery (eg, 35226, 35286, 35371) may also be reported separately. Iliac exposure for device delivery through a retroperitoneal incision, open brachial exposure, or axillary or subclavian exposure through an infraclavicular, or supraclavicular or sternotomy incision during endovascular aneurysm repair may be separately reported (eg, 34715, 34812, 34820, 34834). Endovascular device delivery or establishment of cardiopulmonary bypass that requires creation of a prosthetic conduit utilizing a femoral artery, iliac artery with a retroperitoneal incision, or axillary or subclavian artery exposure through an infraclavicular, supraclavicular, or sternotomy incision (34714, 34716, 34833) and oversewing of the conduit at the time of procedure completion may be separately reported during endovascular aneurysm repair or cardiac procedures requiring cardiopulmonary bypass. If a conduit is converted to a bypass, report the bypass (eg, 35665) and not the arterial exposure with conduit (34714, 34716, 34833). Arterial embolization(s) of renal, lumbar, inferior mesenteric, hypogastric or external iliac arteries to facilitate complete endovascular aneurysm exclusion may be separately reported (eg, 37242).

Cardiovascular 33016-39599

Balloon angioplasty and/or stenting at the sealing zone(s) of an endograft is an integral part of the procedure and is not separately reported. However, balloon angioplasty and/or stent deployment in vessels that do not contain endograft (outside the treatment zone for the endograft), either before or after endograft deployment, may be separately reported (eg, 37220, 37221, 37222, 37223).

Other interventional procedures performed at the time of endovascular abdominal aortic aneurysm repair may be additionally reported (eg, renal transluminal angioplasty, arterial embolization, intravascular ultrasound, balloon angioplasty or stenting of native artery[s] outside the endograft treatment zone, when done before or after deployment of endograft).

(For fenestrated endovascular repair of the visceral aorta, see 34841-34844. For fenestrated endovascular repair of the visceral aorta and concomitant infrarenal abdominal aorta, see 34845-34848)

34701 Endovascular repair of infrarenal aorta by deployment of an aorto-aortic tube endograft including pre-procedure sizing and device selection, all nonselective catheterization(s), all associated radiological supervision and interpretation, all endograft extension(s) placed in the aorta from the level of the renal arteries to the aortic bifurcation, and all angioplasty/stenting performed from the level of the renal arteries to the aortic bifurcation; for other than rupture (eg, for aneurysm, pseudoaneurysm, dissection, penetrating ulcer)

➲ *CPT Changes: An Insider's View* 2018
➲ *CPT Assistant* Dec 17:3

(For covered stent placement[s] for atherosclerotic occlusive disease isolated to the aorta, see 37236, 37237)

34702 for rupture including temporary aortic and/or iliac balloon occlusion, when performed (eg, for aneurysm, pseudoaneurysm, dissection, penetrating ulcer, traumatic disruption)

➲ *CPT Changes: An Insider's View* 2018
➲ *CPT Assistant* Dec 17:3

34703 Endovascular repair of infrarenal aorta and/or iliac artery(ies) by deployment of an aorto-uni-iliac endograft including pre-procedure sizing and device selection, all nonselective catheterization(s), all associated radiological supervision and interpretation, all endograft extension(s) placed in the aorta from the level of the renal arteries to the iliac bifurcation, and all angioplasty/stenting performed from the level of the renal arteries to the iliac bifurcation; for other than rupture (eg, for aneurysm, pseudoaneurysm, dissection, penetrating ulcer)

➲ *CPT Changes: An Insider's View* 2018
➲ *CPT Assistant* Dec 17:3, Nov 19:6

34704 for rupture including temporary aortic and/or iliac balloon occlusion, when performed (eg, for aneurysm, pseudoaneurysm, dissection, penetrating ulcer, traumatic disruption)

➲ *CPT Changes: An Insider's View* 2018
➲ *CPT Assistant* Dec 17:3, Nov 19:6

34705 Endovascular repair of infrarenal aorta and/or iliac artery(ies) by deployment of an aorto-bi-iliac endograft including pre-procedure sizing and device selection, all nonselective catheterization(s), all associated radiological supervision and interpretation, all endograft extension(s) placed in the aorta from the level of the renal arteries to the iliac bifurcation, and all angioplasty/stenting performed from the level of the renal arteries to the iliac bifurcation; for other than rupture (eg, for aneurysm, pseudoaneurysm, dissection, penetrating ulcer)

➲ *CPT Changes: An Insider's View* 2018
➲ *CPT Assistant* Dec 17:3, Nov 19:6

34706 for rupture including temporary aortic and/or iliac balloon occlusion, when performed (eg, for aneurysm, pseudoaneurysm, dissection, penetrating ulcer, traumatic disruption)

➲ *CPT Changes: An Insider's View* 2018
➲ *CPT Assistant* Dec 17:3, Nov 19:6

34707 Endovascular repair of iliac artery by deployment of an ilio-iliac tube endograft including pre-procedure sizing and device selection, all nonselective catheterization(s), all associated radiological supervision and interpretation, and all endograft extension(s) proximally to the aortic bifurcation and distally to the iliac bifurcation, and treatment zone angioplasty/stenting, when performed, unilateral; for other than rupture (eg, for aneurysm, pseudoaneurysm, dissection, arteriovenous malformation)

➲ *CPT Changes: An Insider's View* 2018
➲ *CPT Assistant* Dec 17:3

(For covered stent placement[s] for atherosclerotic occlusive disease of the abdominal aorta, see 37236, 37237)

(For covered stent placement[s] for atherosclerotic occlusive disease of the iliac artery, see 37221, 37223)

34708 for rupture including temporary aortic and/or iliac balloon occlusion, when performed (eg, for aneurysm, pseudoaneurysm, dissection, arteriovenous malformation, traumatic disruption)

➲ *CPT Changes: An Insider's View* 2018
➲ *CPT Assistant* Dec 17:3

(For endovascular repair of iliac artery by deployment of an iliac branched endograft, see 34717, 34718)

★ = Telemedicine ◀ = Audio-only ✚ = Add-on code ✗ = FDA approval pending # = Resequenced code ⊘ = Modifier 51 exempt ➲➲➲ = See p xxi for details

Endovascular Repair
34705, 34706, 34709, 34710, 34711

Endovascular repair of abdominal aorta and/or iliac arteries

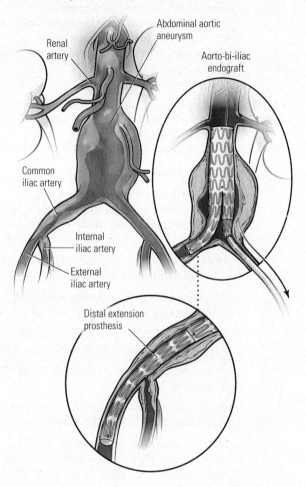

Endovascular Repair
34717, 34718

A. Placement of iliac branch endoprosthesis (IBE) associated with placement of aorto-bi-iliac artery endoprosthesis (same session)

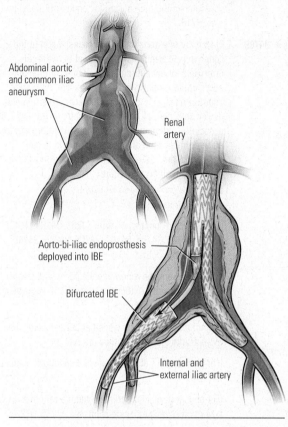

B. Placement of IBE, not associated with placement of aorto-bi-iliac endoprosthesis (different session)

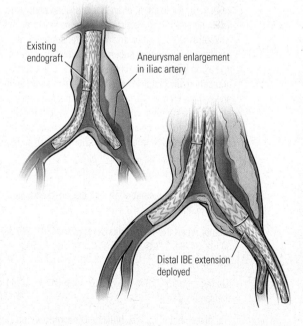

#+ 34717 Endovascular repair of iliac artery at the time of aorto-iliac artery endograft placement by deployment of an iliac branched endograft including pre-procedure sizing and device selection, all ipsilateral selective iliac artery catheterization(s), all associated radiological supervision and interpretation, and all endograft extension(s) proximally to the aortic bifurcation and distally in the internal iliac, external iliac, and common femoral artery(ies), and treatment zone angioplasty/stenting, when performed, for rupture or other than rupture (eg, for aneurysm, pseudoaneurysm, dissection, arteriovenous malformation, penetrating ulcer, traumatic disruption), unilateral (List separately in addition to code for primary procedure)

➔ *CPT Changes: An Insider's View* 2020

➔ *CPT Assistant* Nov 19:6

(Use 34717 in conjunction with 34703, 34704, 34705, 34706)

(34717 may only be reported once per side. For bilateral procedure, report 34717 twice. Do not report modifier 50 in conjunction with 34717)

Cardiovascular 33016-39599

(Do not report 34717 in conjunction with 34709 on the same side)

(Do not report 34717 in conjunction with 34710, 34711)

(For placement of an iliac branched endograft at a separate setting than aorto-iliac endograft placement, use 34718)

+ **34709** Placement of extension prosthesis(es) distal to the common iliac artery(ies) or proximal to the renal artery(ies) for endovascular repair of infrarenal abdominal aortic or iliac aneurysm, false aneurysm, dissection, penetrating ulcer, including pre-procedure sizing and device selection, all nonselective catheterization(s), all associated radiological supervision and interpretation, and treatment zone angioplasty/stenting, when performed, per vessel treated (List separately in addition to code for primary procedure)

➔ *CPT Changes: An Insider's View* 2018
➔ *CPT Assistant* Dec 17:3

(Use 34709 in conjunction with 34701, 34702, 34703, 34704, 34705, 34706, 34707, 34708, 34845, 34846, 34847, 34848)

(34709 may only be reported once per vessel treated [ie, multiple endograft extensions placed in a single vessel may only be reported once])

(Do not report 34709 for placement of a docking limb that extends into the external iliac artery)

(For placement of an iliac branched endograft, see 34717, 34718)

(For endograft placement into a renal artery that is being covered by a proximal extension, see 37236, 37237)

\# **34718** Endovascular repair of iliac artery, not associated with placement of an aorto-iliac artery endograft at the same session, by deployment of an iliac branched endograft, including pre-procedure sizing and device selection, all ipsilateral selective iliac artery catheterization(s), all associated radiological supervision and interpretation, and all endograft extension(s) proximally to the aortic bifurcation and distally in the internal iliac, external iliac, and common femoral artery(ies), and treatment zone angioplasty/stenting, when performed, for other than rupture (eg, for aneurysm, pseudoaneurysm, dissection, arteriovenous malformation, penetrating ulcer), unilateral

➔ *CPT Changes: An Insider's View* 2020
➔ *CPT Assistant* Nov 19:6

(For bilateral placement of an iliac branched endograft, report modifier 50)

(Do not report 34718 in conjunction with 34701, 34702, 34703, 34704, 34705, 34706, 34707, 34708, 34709, 34717)

(Do not report 34718 in conjunction with 34710, 34711 on the same side)

(For placement of an iliac branched endograft in the same setting as aorto-iliac endograft placement, use 34717)

(For placement of an isolated iliac branched endograft for rupture, use 37799)

34710 Delayed placement of distal or proximal extension prosthesis for endovascular repair of infrarenal abdominal aortic or iliac aneurysm, false aneurysm, dissection, endoleak, or endograft migration, including pre-procedure sizing and device selection, all nonselective catheterization(s), all associated radiological supervision and interpretation, and treatment zone angioplasty/stenting, when performed; initial vessel treated

➔ *CPT Changes: An Insider's View* 2018
➔ *CPT Assistant* Dec 17:3

+ **34711** each additional vessel treated (List separately in addition to code for primary procedure)

➔ *CPT Changes: An Insider's View* 2018
➔ *CPT Assistant* Dec 17:3

(Use 34711 in conjunction with 34710)

(34710, 34711 may each be reported only once per operative session [ie, multiple endograft extensions placed in a single vessel may only be reported with a single code])

(For decompressive laparotomy, use 49000 in conjunction with 34702, 34704, 34706, 34708, 34710)

(If the delayed revision is a transcatheter enhanced fixation device [eg, anchors, screws], report 34712)

(Do not report 34710, 34711 in conjunction with 34701, 34702, 34703, 34704, 34705, 34706, 34707, 34708, 34709)

(Do not report 34710, 34711 in conjunction with 34718 on the same side)

(Do not report 34701-34711 in conjunction with 34841, 34842, 34843, 34844, 34845, 34846, 34847, 34848)

(For endovascular repair of iliac artery bifurcation [eg, aneurysm, pseudoaneurysm, arteriovenous malformation, trauma] using bifurcated endograft, see 34717, 34718)

(Report 37252, 37253 for intravascular ultrasound when performed during endovascular aneurysm repair)

(For isolated bilateral iliac artery repair using iliac artery tube endografts, report 34707 or 34708 with modifier 50)

(For open arterial exposure, report 34714, 34715, 34716, 34812, 34820, 34833, 34834 as appropriate, in conjunction with 34701, 34702, 34703, 34704, 34705, 34706, 34707, 34708, 34710, 34712, 34718)

(For percutaneous arterial closure, report 34713 as appropriate, in conjunction with 34701, 34702, 34703, 34704, 34705, 34706, 34707, 34708, 34710, 34712, 34718)

(For simultaneous bilateral iliac artery aneurysm repairs with aorto-biiliac endograft, see 34705, 34706, as appropriate)

34712 Transcatheter delivery of enhanced fixation device(s) to the endograft (eg, anchor, screw, tack) and all associated radiological supervision and interpretation
➔ *CPT Changes: An Insider's View* 2018
➔ *CPT Assistant* Dec 17:3

(Report 34712 only once per operative session)

+ 34713 Percutaneous access and closure of femoral artery for delivery of endograft through a large sheath (12 French or larger), including ultrasound guidance, when performed, unilateral (List separately in addition to code for primary procedure)
➔ *CPT Changes: An Insider's View* 2018
➔ *CPT Assistant* Dec 17:3, Oct 22:17

(Use 34713 in conjunction with 33880, 33881, 33883, 33884, 33886, 34701, 34702, 34703, 34704, 34705, 34706, 34707, 34708, 34710, 34712, 34718, 34841, 34842, 34843, 34844, 34845, 34846, 34847, 34848, as appropriate. Do not report 34713 in conjunction with 33880, 33881, 33883, 33884, 33886, 34701, 34702, 34703, 34704, 34705, 34706, 34707, 34708, 34710, 34712, 34718, 34841, 34842, 34843, 34844, 34845, 34846, 34847, 34848, for percutaneous closure of femoral artery after delivery of endovascular prosthesis if a sheath smaller than 12 French was used)

(34713 may only be reported once per side. For bilateral procedure, report 34713 twice. Do not report modifier 50 in conjunction with 34713)

(Do not report ultrasound guidance [ie, 76937] for percutaneous vascular access in conjunction with 34713 for the same access)

(Do not report 34713 for percutaneous access and closure of the femoral artery in conjunction with 37221, 37223, 37236, 37237)

(Do not report 34713 in conjunction with 37221, 37223 for covered stent placement[s] for atherosclerotic occlusive disease of the iliac artery[ies])

#+ 34812 Open femoral artery exposure for delivery of endovascular prosthesis, by groin incision, unilateral (List separately in addition to code for primary procedure)
➔ *CPT Changes: An Insider's View* 2001, 2003, 2018
➔ *CPT Assistant* Dec 00:6, Sep 02:3, Feb 03:2, Mar 04:10, Jul 06:7, Mar 13:10, Dec 13:8, Dec 17:3
➔ *Clinical Examples in Radiology* Summer 14:2-3

(Use 34812 in conjunction with 33880, 33881, 33883, 33884, 33886, 33990, 33991, 34701, 34702, 34703, 34704, 34705, 34706, 34707, 34708, 34710, 34712, 34718, 34841, 34842, 34843, 34844, 34845, 34846, 34847, 34848)

(34812 may only be reported once per side. For bilateral procedure, report 34812 twice. Do not report modifier 50 in conjunction with 34812)

(Do not report 34812 in conjunction with 33953, 33954, 33959, 33962, 33969, 33984, 33987)

+ 34714 Open femoral artery exposure with creation of conduit for delivery of endovascular prosthesis or for establishment of cardiopulmonary bypass, by groin incision, unilateral (List separately in addition to code for primary procedure)
➔ *CPT Changes: An Insider's View* 2018
➔ *CPT Assistant* Dec 17:3

(Use 34714 in conjunction with 32852, 32854, 33031, 33120, 33251, 33256, 33259, 33261, 33305, 33315, 33322, 33335, 33390, 33391, 33404, 33405, 33406, 33410, 33411, 33412, 33413, 33414, 33415, 33416, 33417, 33422, 33425, 33426, 33427, 33430, 33440, 33460, 33463, 33464, 33465, 33468, 33474, 33475, 33476, 33478, 33496, 33500, 33502, 33504, 33505, 33506, 33507, 33510, 33511, 33512, 33513, 33514, 33516, 33533, 33534, 33535, 33536, 33542, 33545, 33548, 33600-33688, 33692, 33694, 33697, 33702, 33710, 33720, 33724, 33726, 33730, 33732, 33736, 33750, 33755, 33762, 33764, 33766, 33767, 33770-33783, 33786, 33788, 33802, 33803, 33814, 33820, 33822, 33824, 33840, 33845, 33851, 33853, 33858, 33859, 33863, 33864, 33871, 33875, 33877, 33880, 33881, 33883, 33884, 33886, 33910, 33916, 33917, 33920, 33922, 33926, 33935, 33945, 33975, 33976, 33977, 33978, 33979, 33980, 33983, 33990, 33991, 34701, 34702, 34703, 34704, 34705, 34706, 34707, 34708, 34710, 34712, 34718, 34841, 34842, 34843, 34844, 34845, 34846, 34847, 34848)

(34714 may only be reported once per side. For bilateral procedure, report 34714 twice. Do not report modifier 50 in conjunction with 34714)

(Do not report 34714 in conjunction with 33362, 33953, 33954, 33959, 33962, 33969, 33984, 34812 when performed on the same side)

#+ 34820 Open iliac artery exposure for delivery of endovascular prosthesis or iliac occlusion during endovascular therapy, by abdominal or retroperitoneal incision, unilateral (List separately in addition to code for primary procedure)
➔ *CPT Changes: An Insider's View* 2001, 2018
➔ *CPT Assistant* Dec 00:7-8, Sep 02:3, Feb 03:4, Aug 04:10, Jul 06:7, Dec 17:3

(Use 34820 in conjunction with 33880, 33881, 33883, 33884, 33886, 33990, 33991, 34701, 34702, 34703, 34704, 34705, 34706, 34707, 34708, 34710, 34712, 34718, 34841, 34842, 34843, 34844, 34845, 34846, 34847, 34848)

(34820 may only be reported once per side. For bilateral procedure, report 34820 twice. Do not report modifier 50 in conjunction with 34820)

(Do not report 34820 in conjunction with 33953, 33954, 33959, 33962, 33969, 33984)

Cardiovascular 33016-39599

#+ 34833 Open iliac artery exposure with creation of conduit for delivery of endovascular prosthesis or for establishment of cardiopulmonary bypass, by abdominal or retroperitoneal incision, unilateral (List separately in addition to code for primary procedure)

➲ *CPT Changes: An Insider's View* 2003, 2006, 2018
➲ *CPT Assistant* Feb 03:4, Aug 04:10, Jul 06:7, Dec 17:3
➲ *Clinical Examples in Radiology* Winter 06:19

(Use 34833 in conjunction with 32852, 32854, 33031, 33120, 33251, 33256, 33259, 33261, 33305, 33315, 33322, 33335, 33390, 33391, 33404, 33405, 33406, 33410, 33411, 33412, 33413, 33414, 33415, 33416, 33417, 33422, 33425, 33426, 33427, 33430, 33440, 33460, 33463, 33464, 33465, 33468, 33474, 33475, 33476, 33478, 33496, 33500, 33502, 33504, 33505, 33506, 33507, 33510, 33511, 33512, 33513, 33514, 33516, 33533, 33534, 33535, 33536, 33542, 33545, 33548, 33600-33688, 33692, 33694, 33697, 33702, 33710, 33720, 33724, 33726, 33730, 33732, 33736, 33750, 33755, 33762, 33764, 33766, 33767, 33770-33783, 33786, 33788, 33802, 33803, 33814, 33820, 33822, 33824, 33840, 33845, 33851, 33853, 33858, 33859, 33863, 33864, 33871, 33875, 33877, 33880, 33881, 33883, 33884, 33886, 33910, 33916, 33917, 33920, 33922, 33926, 33935, 33945, 33975, 33976, 33977, 33978, 33979, 33980, 33983, 33990, 33991, 34701, 34702, 34703, 34704, 34705, 34706, 34707, 34708, 34710, 34712, 34718, 34841, 34842, 34843, 34844, 34845, 34846, 34847, 34848)

(34833 may only be reported once per side. For bilateral procedure, report 34833 twice. Do not report modifier 50 in conjunction with 34833)

(Do not report 34833 in conjunction with 33364, 33953, 33954, 33959, 33962, 33969, 33984, 34820 when performed on the same side)

#+ 34834 Open brachial artery exposure for delivery of endovascular prosthesis, unilateral (List separately in addition to code for primary procedure)

➲ *CPT Changes: An Insider's View* 2003, 2006, 2018
➲ *CPT Assistant* Feb 03:4, Jul 06:7, Dec 17:3
➲ *Clinical Examples in Radiology* Winter 06:19

(Use 34834 in conjunction with 33880, 33881, 33883, 33884, 33886, 33990, 33991, 34701, 34702, 34703, 34704, 34705, 34706, 34707, 34708, 34710, 34712, 34718, 34841, 34842, 34843, 34844, 34845, 34846, 34847, 34848)

(34834 may only be reported once per side. For bilateral procedure, report 34834 twice. Do not report modifier 50 in conjunction with 34834)

(Do not report 34834 in conjunction with 33953, 33954, 33959, 33962, 33969, 33984)

+ 34715 Open axillary/subclavian artery exposure for delivery of endovascular prosthesis by infraclavicular or supraclavicular incision, unilateral (List separately in addition to code for primary procedure)

➲ *CPT Changes: An Insider's View* 2018
➲ *CPT Assistant* Dec 17:3

(Use 34715 in conjunction with 33880, 33881, 33883, 33884, 33886, 33990, 33991, 34701, 34702, 34703, 34704, 34705, 34706, 34707, 34708, 34710, 34712, 34718, 34841, 34842, 34843, 34844, 34845, 34846, 34847, 34848)

(34715 may only be reported once per side. For bilateral procedure, report 34715 twice. Do not report modifier 50 in conjunction with 34715)

(Do not report 34715 in conjunction with 33363, 33953, 33954, 33959, 33962, 33969, 33984)

+ 34716 Open axillary/subclavian artery exposure with creation of conduit for delivery of endovascular prosthesis or for establishment of cardiopulmonary bypass, by infraclavicular or supraclavicular incision, unilateral (List separately in addition to code for primary procedure)

➲ *CPT Changes: An Insider's View* 2018
➲ *CPT Assistant* Dec 17:3

(Use 34716 in conjunction with 32852, 32854, 33031, 33120, 33251, 33256, 33259-33261, 33305, 33315, 33322, 33335, 33390, 33391, 33404, 33405, 33406, 33410, 33411, 33412, 33413, 33414, 33415, 33416, 33417, 33422, 33425, 33426, 33427, 33430, 33440, 33460, 33463, 33464, 33465, 33468, 33474, 33475, 33476, 33478, 33496, 33500, 33502, 33504, 33505, 33506, 33507, 33510, 33511, 33512, 33513, 33514, 33516, 33533, 33534, 33535, 33536, 33542, 33545, 33548, 33600-33688, 33692, 33694, 33697, 33702, 33710, 33720, 33724, 33726, 33730, 33732, 33736, 33750, 33755, 33762, 33764, 33766, 33767, 33770-33783, 33786, 33788, 33802, 33803, 33814, 33820, 33822, 33824, 33840, 33845, 33851, 33853, 33858, 33859, 33863, 33864, 33871, 33875, 33877, 33880, 33881, 33883, 33884, 33886, 33910, 33916, 33917, 33920, 33922, 33926, 33935, 33945, 33975, 33976, 33977, 33978, 33979, 33980, 33983, 33990, 33991, 34701, 34702, 34703, 34704, 34705, 34706, 34707, 34708, 34710, 34712, 34718, 34841, 34842, 34843, 34844, 34845, 34846, 34847, 34848)

(34716 may only be reported once per side. For bilateral procedure, report 34716 twice. Do not report modifier 50 in conjunction with 34716)

34717 Code is out of numerical sequence. See 34707-34711

34718 Code is out of numerical sequence. See 34707-34711

+ 34808 Endovascular placement of iliac artery occlusion device (List separately in addition to code for primary procedure)

➲ *CPT Changes: An Insider's View* 2001
➲ *CPT Assistant* Dec 00:6, Sep 02:3, Apr 12:3

(Use 34808 in conjunction with 34701, 34702, 34703, 34704, 34707, 34708, 34709, 34710, 34813, 34841, 34842, 34843, 34844)

★=Telemedicine ◀=Audio-only +=Add-on code ✔=FDA approval pending #=Resequenced code ⊘=Modifier 51 exempt ➲➲➲=See p xxi for details

34812   Code is out of numerical sequence. See 34712-34716

+ 34813   Placement of femoral-femoral prosthetic graft during
                endovascular aortic aneurysm repair (List separately in
                addition to code for primary procedure)
                ➲ *CPT Changes: An Insider's View* 2001
                ➲ *CPT Assistant* Dec 00:6, Sep 02:3, Apr 12:3   .

                (Use 34813 in conjunction with 34812)

                (For femoral artery grafting, see 35521, 35533, 35539,
                35540, 35556, 35558, 35566, 35621, 35646, 35654-
                35661, 35666, 35700)

34820   Code is out of numerical sequence. See 34712-34716

34830   Open repair of infrarenal aortic aneurysm or dissection,
                plus repair of associated arterial trauma, following
                unsuccessful endovascular repair; tube prosthesis
                ➲ *CPT Changes: An Insider's View* 2001
                ➲ *CPT Assistant* Dec 00:6, Sep 02:3, Oct 08:10

34831   aorto-bi-iliac prosthesis
                ➲ *CPT Changes: An Insider's View* 2001
                ➲ *CPT Assistant* Dec 00:6, Sep 02:3, Oct 08:10

34832   aorto-bifemoral prosthesis
                ➲ *CPT Changes: An Insider's View* 2001
                ➲ *CPT Assistant* Dec 00:6, Sep 02:3, Oct 08:10

34833   Code is out of numerical sequence. See 34712-34716

34834   Code is out of numerical sequence. See 34712-34716

Fenestrated Endovascular Repair of the Visceral and Infrarenal Aorta

The upper abdominal aorta that contains the celiac,
superior mesenteric, and renal arteries is termed the
visceral aorta. For reporting purposes, the thoracic aorta
extends from the aortic valve to the aortic segment just
proximal to the celiac artery.

Code 34839 is used to report the physician planning and
sizing for a patient-specific fenestrated visceral aortic
endograft. The planning includes review of high-
resolution cross-sectional images (eg, CT, CTA, MRI)
and utilization of 3D software for iterative modeling of
the aorta and device in multiplanar views and center line
of flow analysis. Code 34839 may only be reported when
the physician spends a minimum of 90 total minutes
performing patient-specific fenestrated endograft
planning. Physician planning time does not need to be
continuous and should be clearly documented in the
patient record. Code 34839 is reported on the date that
planning work is complete and may not include time
spent on the day before or the day of the fenestrated
endovascular repair procedure (34841, 34842, 34843,
34844, 34845, 34846, 34847, 34848) nor be reported on
the day before or the day of the fenestrated endovascular
repair procedure.

Codes 34841, 34842, 34843, 34844, 34845,
34847, 34848 are used to report placement of a
fenestrated endovascular graft in the visceral aorta, either
alone or in combination with the infrarenal aorta for
aneurysm, pseudoaneurysm, dissection, penetrating ulcer,
intramural hematoma, or traumatic disruption. The
fenestrated main body endoprosthesis is deployed within
the visceral aorta. Fenestrations within the fabric allow for
selective catheterization of the visceral and/or renal
arteries and subsequent placement of an endoprosthesis
(ie, bare metal or covered stent) to maintain flow to the
visceral artery. Patient variation in the location and
relative orientation of the renal and visceral artery origins
requires use of a patient-specific fenestrated endograft for
endovascular repair that preserves flow to essential visceral
arteries and allows proximal seal and fixation to be
achieved above the renal level as well as in the distal aorta
or iliac vessel(s).

Fenestrated aortic repair is reported based on the extent
of aorta treated. Codes 34841, 34842, 34843, 34844
describe repair using proximal endoprostheses that span
from the visceral aortic component to one, two, three, or
four visceral artery origins and distal extent limited to the
infrarenal aorta. These devices do not extend into the
common iliac arteries. Codes 34845, 34846, 34847,
34848 are used to report deployment of a fenestrated
endograft that spans from the visceral aorta (including
one, two, three, or four visceral artery origins) through
the infrarenal aorta into the common iliac arteries. The
infrarenal component may be a bifurcated unibody
device, a modular bifurcated docking system with
docking limb(s), or an aorto-uniiliac device. Codes
34845, 34846, 34847, 34848 include placement of
unilateral or bilateral docking limbs (depending on the
device). Any additional endograft extensions that
terminate in the common iliac arteries are included in
34845, 34846, 34847, 34848. Codes 34709, 34710,
34711 may not be separately reported for proximal
abdominal aortic extension prosthesis(es) or for distal
extension prosthesis(es) that terminate(s) in the aorta or
the common iliac arteries. However, 34709, 34710,
34711 may be reported for distal extension prosthesis(es)
that terminate(s) in the internal iliac, external iliac, or
common femoral artery(ies).

Codes 34841-34844 and 34845-34848 define the total
number of visceral and/or renal arteries (ie, celiac,
superior mesenteric, and/or unilateral or bilateral renal
artery[s]) requiring placement of an endoprosthesis (ie,
bare metal or covered stent) through an aortic endograft
fenestration.

Introduction of guide wires and catheters in the aorta and visceral and/or renal arteries is included in the work of 34841-34848 and is not separately reportable. However, catheterization of the hypogastric artery(s) and/or arterial families outside the treatment zone of the graft may be separately reported. Balloon angioplasty within the target treatment zone of the endograft, either before or after endograft deployment, is not separately reportable. Fluoroscopic guidance and radiological supervision and interpretation in conjunction with fenestrated endovascular aortic repair is not separately reportable and includes angiographic diagnostic imaging of the aorta and its branches prior to deployment of the fenestrated endovascular device, fluoroscopic guidance in the delivery of the fenestrated endovascular components, and intraprocedural arterial angiography (eg, confirm position, detect endoleak, evaluate runoff) done at the time of the endovascular aortic repair.

Exposure of the access vessels (eg, 34713, 34714, 34715, 34716, 34812, 34820, 34833, 34834) may be reported separately. Extensive repair of an artery (eg, 35226, 35286) may be reported separately. For concomitant endovascular treatment of the descending thoracic aorta, 33880-33886 and 75956-75959 may be reported with 34841, 34842, 34843, 34844, 34845, 34846, 34847, 34848. For isolated endovascular infrarenal abdominal aortic aneurysm repair that does not require placement of a fenestrated graft to preserve flow to the visceral branch(es), see 34701, 34702, 34703, 34704, 34705, 34706.

Other interventional procedures performed at the time of fenestrated endovascular abdominal aortic aneurysm repair may be reported separately (eg, arterial embolization, intravascular ultrasound, balloon angioplasty or stenting of native artery[s] outside the endoprosthesis target zone, when done before or after deployment of endoprosthesis).

34839 Physician planning of a patient-specific fenestrated visceral aortic endograft requiring a minimum of 90 minutes of physician time

➔ *CPT Changes: An Insider's View* 2015

(Do not report 34839 in conjunction with 76376, 76377)

(Do not report 34839 in conjunction with 34841, 34842, 34843, 34844, 34845, 34846, 34847, 34848, when performed on the day before or the day of the fenestrated endovascular repair procedure)

34841 Endovascular repair of visceral aorta (eg, aneurysm, pseudoaneurysm, dissection, penetrating ulcer, intramural hematoma, or traumatic disruption) by deployment of a fenestrated visceral aortic endograft and all associated radiological supervision and interpretation, including target zone angioplasty, when performed; including one visceral artery endoprosthesis (superior mesenteric, celiac or renal artery)

➔ *CPT Changes: An Insider's View* 2014
➔ *CPT Assistant* Dec 13:8, Dec 17:3

34842 including two visceral artery endoprostheses (superior mesenteric, celiac and/or renal artery[s])

➔ *CPT Changes: An Insider's View* 2014
➔ *CPT Assistant* Dec 13:8, Dec 17:3

34843 including three visceral artery endoprostheses (superior mesenteric, celiac and/or renal artery[s])

➔ *CPT Changes: An Insider's View* 2014
➔ *CPT Assistant* Dec 13:8, Dec 17:3

34844 including four or more visceral artery endoprostheses (superior mesenteric, celiac and/or renal artery[s])

➔ *CPT Changes: An Insider's View* 2014
➔ *CPT Assistant* Dec 13:8, Dec 17:3

(Do not report 34841, 34842, 34843, 34844 in conjunction with 34701, 34702, 34703, 34704, 34705, 34706, 34845, 34846, 34847, 34848)

(Do not report 34841, 34842, 34843, 34844 in conjunction with 34839, when planning services are performed on the day before or the day of the fenestrated endovascular repair procedure)

34845 Endovascular repair of visceral aorta and infrarenal abdominal aorta (eg, aneurysm, pseudoaneurysm, dissection, penetrating ulcer, intramural hematoma, or traumatic disruption) with a fenestrated visceral aortic endograft and concomitant unibody or modular infrarenal aortic endograft and all associated radiological supervision and interpretation, including target zone angioplasty, when performed; including one visceral artery endoprosthesis (superior mesenteric, celiac or renal artery)

➔ *CPT Changes: An Insider's View* 2014
➔ *CPT Assistant* Dec 13:8, Dec 17:3

34846 including two visceral artery endoprostheses (superior mesenteric, celiac and/or renal artery[s])

➔ *CPT Changes: An Insider's View* 2014
➔ *CPT Assistant* Dec 13:8, Dec 17:3

34847 including three visceral artery endoprostheses (superior mesenteric, celiac and/or renal artery[s])

➔ *CPT Changes: An Insider's View* 2014
➔ *CPT Assistant* Dec 13:8, Dec 17:3

34848 including four or more visceral artery endoprostheses (superior mesenteric, celiac and/or renal artery[s])

➔ *CPT Changes: An Insider's View* 2014
➔ *CPT Assistant* Dec 13:8, Jul 16:6, Aug 17:10, Dec 17:3, Oct 22:17

(Do not report 34845, 34846, 34847, 34848 in conjunction with 34701, 34702, 34703, 34704, 34705, 34706, 34841, 34842, 34843, 34844, 35081, 35102)

(Do not report 34845, 34846, 34847, 34848 in conjunction with 34839, when planning services are performed on the day before or the day of the fenestrated endovascular repair procedure)

(Do not report 34841-34848 in conjunction with 37236, 37237 for bare metal or covered stents placed into the visceral branches within the endoprosthesis target zone)

(For placement of distal extension prosthesis[es] terminating in the internal iliac, external iliac, or common femoral artery[ies], see 34709, 34710, 34711, 34718)

(Use 34845, 34846, 34847, 34848 in conjunction with 37220, 37221, 37222, 37223, only when 37220, 37221, 37222, 37223 are performed outside the target treatment zone of the endoprosthesis)

Direct Repair of Aneurysm or Excision (Partial or Total) and Graft Insertion for Aneurysm, Pseudoaneurysm, Ruptured Aneurysm, and Associated Occlusive Disease

Procedures 35001-35152 include preparation of artery for anastomosis including endarterectomy.

(For direct repairs associated with occlusive disease only, see 35201-35286)

(For intracranial aneurysm, see 61700 et seq)

(For endovascular repair of abdominal aortic and/or iliac artery aneurysm, see 34701-34716)

(For thoracic aortic aneurysm, see 33858-33875)

(For endovascular repair of descending thoracic aorta, involving coverage of left subclavian artery origin, use 33880)

35001 Direct repair of aneurysm, pseudoaneurysm, or excision (partial or total) and graft insertion, with or without patch graft; for aneurysm and associated occlusive disease, carotid, subclavian artery, by neck incision
> *CPT Changes: An Insider's View* 2002

35002 for ruptured aneurysm, carotid, subclavian artery, by neck incision

35005 for aneurysm, pseudoaneurysm, and associated occlusive disease, vertebral artery
> *CPT Changes: An Insider's View* 2002

35011 for aneurysm and associated occlusive disease, axillary-brachial artery, by arm incision

35013 for ruptured aneurysm, axillary-brachial artery, by arm incision

35021 for aneurysm, pseudoaneurysm, and associated occlusive disease, innominate, subclavian artery, by thoracic incision
> *CPT Changes: An Insider's View* 2002

35022 for ruptured aneurysm, innominate, subclavian artery, by thoracic incision

35045 for aneurysm, pseudoaneurysm, and associated occlusive disease, radial or ulnar artery
> *CPT Changes: An Insider's View* 2002

35081 for aneurysm, pseudoaneurysm, and associated occlusive disease, abdominal aorta
> *CPT Changes: An Insider's View* 2002
> *CPT Assistant* Dec 00:2, Dec 01:7, Dec 13:8

35082 for ruptured aneurysm, abdominal aorta

35091 for aneurysm, pseudoaneurysm, and associated occlusive disease, abdominal aorta involving visceral vessels (mesenteric, celiac, renal)
> *CPT Changes: An Insider's View* 2002
> *CPT Assistant* Dec 00:2

35092 for ruptured aneurysm, abdominal aorta involving visceral vessels (mesenteric, celiac, renal)

35102 for aneurysm, pseudoaneurysm, and associated occlusive disease, abdominal aorta involving iliac vessels (common, hypogastric, external)
> *CPT Changes: An Insider's View* 2002
> *CPT Assistant* Dec 13:8

35103 for ruptured aneurysm, abdominal aorta involving iliac vessels (common, hypogastric, external)

35111 for aneurysm, pseudoaneurysm, and associated occlusive disease, splenic artery
> *CPT Changes: An Insider's View* 2002

35112 for ruptured aneurysm, splenic artery

35121 for aneurysm, pseudoaneurysm, and associated occlusive disease, hepatic, celiac, renal, or mesenteric artery
> *CPT Changes: An Insider's View* 2002

35122 for ruptured aneurysm, hepatic, celiac, renal, or mesenteric artery

35131 for aneurysm, pseudoaneurysm, and associated occlusive disease, iliac artery (common, hypogastric, external)
> *CPT Changes: An Insider's View* 2002
> *CPT Assistant* Feb 03:2

35132 for ruptured aneurysm, iliac artery (common, hypogastric, external)

35141 for aneurysm, pseudoaneurysm, and associated occlusive disease, common femoral artery (profunda femoris, superficial femoral)
> *CPT Changes: An Insider's View* 2002

35142 for ruptured aneurysm, common femoral artery (profunda femoris, superficial femoral)

35151   for aneurysm, pseudoaneurysm, and associated occlusive disease, popliteal artery
➜ *CPT Changes: An Insider's View* 2002

35152   for ruptured aneurysm, popliteal artery

Repair Arteriovenous Fistula

35180   Repair, congenital arteriovenous fistula; head and neck
➜ *CPT Assistant* Aug 11:9

35182   thorax and abdomen
➜ *CPT Assistant* Apr 11:9

35184   extremities
➜ *CPT Assistant* Apr 11:9

35188   Repair, acquired or traumatic arteriovenous fistula; head and neck
➜ *CPT Assistant* Apr 11:9

35189   thorax and abdomen
➜ *CPT Assistant* Apr 11:9

35190   extremities
➜ *CPT Assistant* Aug 11:9

Repair Blood Vessel Other Than for Fistula, With or Without Patch Angioplasty

(For AV fistula repair, see 35180-35190)

35201   Repair blood vessel, direct; neck
➜ *CPT Assistant* Mar 14:8, Apr 14:10

(Do not report 35201 in conjunction with 33969, 33984, 33985, 33986)

35206   upper extremity
➜ *CPT Assistant* Oct 00:3, Nov 03:5, Apr 12:4, Apr 14:10

(Do not report 35206 in conjunction with 33969, 33984, 33985, 33986)

35207   hand, finger

35211   intrathoracic, with bypass

(Do not report 35211 in conjunction with 33969, 33984, 33985, 33986)

35216   intrathoracic, without bypass
➜ *CPT Assistant* Apr 05:10-11

(Do not report 35216 in conjunction with 33969, 33984, 33985, 33986)

35221   intra-abdominal

35226   lower extremity
➜ *CPT Assistant* Apr 12:8-9, Mar 13:10, Dec 13:8, Jul 17:5, Jul 19:11

(Do not report 35226 in conjunction with 33969, 33984, 33985, 33986)

35231   Repair blood vessel with vein graft; neck

35236   upper extremity
➜ *CPT Assistant* Oct 04:8

35241   intrathoracic, with bypass

35246   intrathoracic, without bypass

35251   intra-abdominal

35256   lower extremity

35261   Repair blood vessel with graft other than vein; neck

35266   upper extremity

35271   intrathoracic, with bypass

35276   intrathoracic, without bypass

35281   intra-abdominal

35286   lower extremity
➜ *CPT Assistant* Apr 12:8-9, Mar 13:10, Dec 13:8, Apr 14:10, Jul 17:5, Jul 19:11

Thromboendarterectomy

(For coronary artery, see 33510-33536 and 33572)

(35301-35372 include harvest of saphenous or upper extremity vein when performed)

35301   Thromboendarterectomy, including patch graft, if performed; carotid, vertebral, subclavian, by neck incision
➜ *CPT Changes: An Insider's View* 2007
➜ *CPT Assistant* Jan 07:7, Sep 10:7

35302   superficial femoral artery
➜ *CPT Changes: An Insider's View* 2007
➜ *CPT Assistant* Jan 07:7, May 07:9

35303   popliteal artery
➜ *CPT Changes: An Insider's View* 2007
➜ *CPT Assistant* Jan 07:7, May 07:9

(Do not report 35302, 35303 in conjunction with 37225, 37227 when performed in the same vessel)

35304   tibioperoneal trunk artery
➜ *CPT Changes: An Insider's View* 2007
➜ *CPT Assistant* Jan 07:7, May 07:9

35305   tibial or peroneal artery, initial vessel
➜ *CPT Changes: An Insider's View* 2007
➜ *CPT Assistant* May 07:9

+ 35306   each additional tibial or peroneal artery (List separately in addition to code for primary procedure)
➜ *CPT Changes: An Insider's View* 2007
➜ *CPT Assistant* Jan 07:7, May 07:9

(Use 35306 in conjunction with 35305)

(Do not report 35304, 35305, 35306 in conjunction with 37229, 37231, 37233, 37235 when performed in the same vessel)

35311	subclavian, innominate, by thoracic incision
35321	axillary-brachial
35331	abdominal aorta
35341	mesenteric, celiac, or renal
35351	iliac
35355	iliofemoral
35361	combined aortoiliac
35363	combined aortoiliofemoral
35371	common femoral

> *CPT Assistant* Jan 07:7, Jul 17:5

35372	deep (profunda) femoral

> *CPT Assistant* Jan 07:7

Thromboendarterectomy
35371-35372

The common femoral artery (35371) or the deep (profunda) femoral artery (35372) is incised and the plaque and lining are removed, enlarging the diameter of the artery.

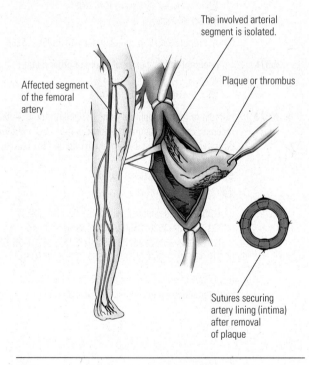

The involved arterial segment is isolated.

Plaque or thrombus

Affected segment of the femoral artery

Sutures securing artery lining (intima) after removal of plaque

+ 35390 Reoperation, carotid, thromboendarterectomy, more than 1 month after original operation (List separately in addition to code for primary procedure)

> *CPT Assistant* Nov 97:16

(Use 35390 in conjunction with 35301)

Angioscopy

+ 35400 Angioscopy (noncoronary vessels or grafts) during therapeutic intervention (List separately in addition to code for primary procedure)

> *CPT Assistant* Nov 97:16

Bypass Graft

Vein

Procurement of the saphenous vein graft is included in the description of the work for 35501-35587 and should not be reported as a separate service or co-surgery. To report harvesting of an upper extremity vein, use 35500 in addition to the bypass procedure. To report harvesting of a femoropopliteal vein segment, use 35572 in addition to the bypass procedure. To report harvesting and construction of an autogenous composite graft of two segments from two distant locations, report 35682 in addition to the bypass procedure, for autogenous composite of three or more segments from distant sites, report 35683.

+ 35500 Harvest of upper extremity vein, 1 segment, for lower extremity or coronary artery bypass procedure (List separately in addition to code for primary procedure)

> *CPT Changes: An Insider's View* 2000

> *CPT Assistant* Nov 98:13, Mar 99:6, Nov 99:19, Jan 07:7, Apr 12:4

(Use 35500 in conjunction with 33510-33536, 35556, 35566, 35570, 35571, 35583-35587)

(For harvest of more than one vein segment, see 35682, 35683)

(For endoscopic procedure, use 33508)

35501 Bypass graft, with vein; common carotid-ipsilateral internal carotid

> *CPT Changes: An Insider's View* 2007

> *CPT Assistant* Apr 99:11

35506 carotid-subclavian or subclavian-carotid

> *CPT Changes: An Insider's View* 2007

> *CPT Assistant* Oct 04:6, Jan 07:7

35508 carotid-vertebral

35509 carotid-contralateral carotid

> *CPT Changes: An Insider's View* 2007

> *CPT Assistant* Jan 07:7, May 07:9

35510 carotid-brachial

> *CPT Changes: An Insider's View* 2004

> *CPT Assistant* Oct 04:6, Nov 07:8

35511 subclavian-subclavian

35512 subclavian-brachial

> *CPT Changes: An Insider's View* 2004

> *CPT Assistant* Oct 04:7

35515 subclavian-vertebral

35516 subclavian-axillary

35518   axillary-axillary
   ➡ *CPT Assistant* Oct 04:9

35521   axillary-femoral

   (For bypass graft performed with synthetic graft, use 35621)

35522   axillary-brachial
   ➡ *CPT Changes: An Insider's View* 2004
   ➡ *CPT Assistant* Oct 04:9

35523   brachial-ulnar or -radial
   ➡ *CPT Changes: An Insider's View* 2008

   (Do not report 35523 in conjunction with 35206, 35500, 35525, 36838)

   (For bypass graft performed with synthetic conduit, use 37799)

35525   brachial-brachial
   ➡ *CPT Changes: An Insider's View* 2004
   ➡ *CPT Assistant* Oct 04:10

35526   aortosubclavian, aortoinnominate, or aortocarotid
   ➡ *CPT Changes: An Insider's View* 2011

   (For bypass graft performed with synthetic graft, use 35626)

35531   aortoceliac or aortomesenteric

35533   axillary-femoral-femoral

   (For bypass graft performed with synthetic graft, use 35654)

35535   hepatorenal
   ➡ *CPT Changes: An Insider's View* 2009

   (Do not report 35535 in conjunction with 35221, 35251, 35281, 35500, 35536, 35560, 35631, 35636)

35536   splenorenal
   ➡ *CPT Assistant* Jun 99:10

35537   aortoiliac
   ➡ *CPT Changes: An Insider's View* 2007
   ➡ *CPT Assistant* Jan 07:7

   (For bypass graft performed with synthetic graft, use 35637)

   (Do not report 35537 in conjunction with 35538)

35538   aortobi-iliac
   ➡ *CPT Changes: An Insider's View* 2007
   ➡ *CPT Assistant* Jan 07:7

   (For bypass graft performed with synthetic graft, use 35638)

   (Do not report 35538 in conjunction with 35537)

35539   aortofemoral
   ➡ *CPT Changes: An Insider's View* 2007
   ➡ *CPT Assistant* Jan 07:7

   (For bypass graft performed with synthetic graft, use 35647)

   (Do not report 35539 in conjunction with 35540)

35540   aortobifemoral
   ➡ *CPT Changes: An Insider's View* 2007
   ➡ *CPT Assistant* Jan 07:7

   (For bypass graft performed with synthetic graft, use 35646)

   (Do not report 35540 in conjunction with 35539)

35556   femoral-popliteal
   ➡ *CPT Assistant* Fall 92:20, May 97:10, Jan 07:7, Nov 07:8

35558   femoral-femoral

35560   aortorenal
   ➡ *CPT Assistant* Jun 99:10

35563   ilioiliac

35565   iliofemoral
   ➡ *CPT Assistant* Oct 04:8

35566   femoral-anterior tibial, posterior tibial, peroneal artery or other distal vessels
   ➡ *CPT Assistant* Jan 07:7, Nov 07:8

35570   tibial-tibial, peroneal-tibial, or tibial/peroneal trunk-tibial
   ➡ *CPT Changes: An Insider's View* 2009
   ➡ *CPT Assistant* Apr 12:4

   (Do not report 35570 in conjunction with 35256, 35286)

35571   popliteal-tibial, -peroneal artery or other distal vessels
   ➡ *CPT Assistant* Jan 07:7, Nov 07:8

+ 35572   Harvest of femoropopliteal vein, 1 segment, for vascular reconstruction procedure (eg, aortic, vena caval, coronary, peripheral artery) (List separately in addition to code for primary procedure)
   ➡ *CPT Changes: An Insider's View* 2003
   ➡ *CPT Assistant* Jan 07:28

   (Use 35572 in conjunction with 33510-33516, 33517-33523, 33533-33536, 34502, 34520, 35001, 35002, 35011-35022, 35102, 35103, 35121-35152, 35231-35256, 35501-35571, 35583, 35585, 35587, 35879-35907)

   (For bilateral procedure, report 35572 twice. Do not report modifier 50 in conjunction with 35572)

Bypass Graft, Vein
35571

The physician creates a bypass around the popliteal artery, using a harvested vein that is sutured to the tibial artery.

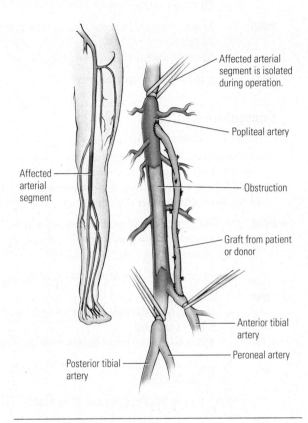

Affected arterial segment is isolated during operation.

Popliteal artery

Affected arterial segment

Obstruction

Graft from patient or donor

Anterior tibial artery

Peroneal artery

Posterior tibial artery

In-Situ Vein

(To report aortobifemoral bypass using synthetic conduit, and femoral-popliteal bypass with vein conduit in-situ, use 35646 and 35583. To report aorto[uni]femoral bypass with synthetic conduit, and femoral-popliteal bypass with vein conduit in-situ, use 35647 and 35583. To report aortofemoral bypass using vein conduit, and femoral-popliteal bypass with vein conduit in-situ, use 35539 and 35583)

35583   In-situ vein bypass; femoral-popliteal
> *CPT Assistant* Jan 07:7, Nov 07:8

35585   femoral-anterior tibial, posterior tibial, or peroneal artery
> *CPT Assistant* Jan 07:7, Nov 07:8

35587   popliteal-tibial, peroneal
> *CPT Assistant* Apr 99:11, Jan 07:7, Nov 07:8

Other Than Vein

(For arterial transposition and/or reimplantation, see 35691-35695)

⊘ **35600**   Harvest of upper extremity artery, 1 segment, for coronary artery bypass procedure, open
> *CPT Changes: An Insider's View* 2001, 2008, 2022
> *CPT Assistant* Apr 07:12

(For endoscopic approach, see 33508, 33509, 37500)

(For bilateral procedure, report 35600 with modifier 50)

Harvest of Upper Extremity Artery
35600

Open procurement of a radial artery to secure conduit for construction of a coronary artery bypass graft

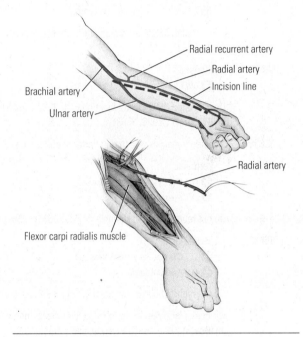

Radial recurrent artery

Radial artery

Incision line

Brachial artery

Ulnar artery

Radial artery

Flexor carpi radialis muscle

35601   Bypass graft, with other than vein; common carotid-ipsilateral internal carotid
> *CPT Changes: An Insider's View* 2007
> *CPT Assistant* Jul 06:7, Jan 07:7

35606   carotid-subclavian

(For open transcervical common carotid-common carotid bypass performed in conjunction with endovascular repair of descending thoracic aorta, use 33891)

(For open subclavian to carotid artery transposition performed in conjunction with endovascular thoracic aneurysm repair by neck incision, use 33889)

35612   subclavian-subclavian

35616   subclavian-axillary

35621	axillary-femoral
	➲ *CPT Assistant* Jan 07:7

35623	axillary-popliteal or -tibial

35626	aortosubclavian, aortoinnominate, or aortocarotid
	➲ *CPT Changes: An Insider's View* 2011

35631	aortoceliac, aortomesenteric, aortorenal

35632	ilio-celiac
	➲ *CPT Changes: An Insider's View* 2009

(Do not report 35632 in conjunction with 35221, 35251, 35281, 35531, 35631)

35633	ilio-mesenteric
	➲ *CPT Changes: An Insider's View* 2009

(Do not report 35633 in conjunction with 35221, 35251, 35281, 35531, 35631)

35634	iliorenal
	➲ *CPT Changes: An Insider's View* 2009

(Do not report 35634 in conjunction with 35221, 35251, 35281, 35560, 35536, 35631)

35636	splenorenal (splenic to renal arterial anastomosis)

35637	aortoiliac
	➲ *CPT Changes: An Insider's View* 2007
	➲ *CPT Assistant* Jan 07:7

(Do not report 35637 in conjunction with 35638, 35646)

35638	aortobi-iliac
	➲ *CPT Changes: An Insider's View* 2007
	➲ *CPT Assistant* Jan 07:7

(Do not report 35638 in conjunction with 35637, 35646)

(For open placement of aortobi-iliac prosthesis following unsuccessful endovascular repair, use 34831)

35642	carotid-vertebral

35645	subclavian-vertebral

35646	aortobifemoral
	➲ *CPT Changes: An Insider's View* 2002
	➲ *CPT Assistant* Jan 07:7

(For bypass graft performed with vein graft, use 35540)

(For open placement of aortobifemoral prosthesis following unsuccessful endovascular repair, use 34832)

35647	aortofemoral
	➲ *CPT Changes: An Insider's View* 2002
	➲ *CPT Assistant* Jan 07:7

(For bypass graft performed with vein graft, use 35539)

35650	axillary-axillary

35654	axillary-femoral-femoral
	➲ *CPT Assistant* Jan 07:7

35656	femoral-popliteal
	➲ *CPT Assistant* Nov 07:8

35661	femoral-femoral
	➲ *CPT Assistant* Dec 04:6, Jan 07:7

35663	ilioiliac

35665	iliofemoral
	➲ *CPT Assistant* Jan 07:7

35666	femoral-anterior tibial, posterior tibial, or peroneal artery
	➲ *CPT Assistant* Nov 07:8

35671	popliteal-tibial or -peroneal artery

Composite Grafts

Codes 35682-35683 are used to report harvest and anastomosis of multiple vein segments from distant sites for use as arterial bypass graft conduits. These codes are intended for use when the two or more vein segments are harvested from a limb other than that undergoing bypass.

+ 35681	Bypass graft; composite, prosthetic and vein (List separately in addition to code for primary procedure)
	➲ *CPT Assistant* Nov 98:13-14, Mar 99:6, Apr 99:11

(Do not report 35681 in addition to 35682, 35683)

+ 35682	autogenous composite, 2 segments of veins from 2 locations (List separately in addition to code for primary procedure)
	➲ *CPT Assistant* Nov 98:13-14, Mar 99:6, Apr 99:11, Sep 02:4

(Use 35682 in conjunction with 35556, 35566, 35570, 35571, 35583-35587)

(Do not report 35682 in addition to 35681, 35683)

+ 35683	autogenous composite, 3 or more segments of vein from 2 or more locations (List separately in addition to code for primary procedure)
	➲ *CPT Assistant* Nov 98:13-14, Mar 99:6, Apr 99:11, Sep 02:4

(Use 35683 in conjunction with 35556, 35566, 35570, 35571, 35583-35587)

(Do not report 35683 in addition to 35681, 35682)

Adjuvant Techniques

Adjuvant (additional) technique(s) may be required at the time a bypass graft is created to improve patency of the lower extremity autogenous or synthetic bypass graft (eg, femoral-popliteal, femoral-tibial, or popliteal-tibial arteries). Code 35685 should be reported in addition to the primary synthetic bypass graft procedure, when an interposition of venous tissue (vein patch or cuff) is placed at the anastomosis between the synthetic bypass conduit and the involved artery (includes harvest).

Code 35686 should be reported in addition to the primary bypass graft procedure, when autogenous vein is used to create a fistula between the tibial or peroneal artery and vein at or beyond the distal bypass anastomosis site of the involved artery.

(For composite graft(s), see 35681-35683)

+ 35685 Placement of vein patch or cuff at distal anastomosis of bypass graft, synthetic conduit (List separately in addition to code for primary procedure)

➜ *CPT Changes: An Insider's View* 2002

➜ *CPT Assistant* Sep 02:3

(Use 35685 in conjunction with 35656, 35666, or 35671)

+ 35686 Creation of distal arteriovenous fistula during lower extremity bypass surgery (non-hemodialysis) (List separately in addition to code for primary procedure)

➜ *CPT Changes: An Insider's View* 2002

➜ *CPT Assistant* Sep 02:3, Apr 12:4

(Use 35686 in conjunction with 35556, 35566, 35570, 35571, 35583-35587, 35623, 35656, 35666, 35671)

Arterial Transposition

35691 Transposition and/or reimplantation; vertebral to carotid artery

35693 vertebral to subclavian artery

35694 subclavian to carotid artery

(For open subclavian to carotid artery transposition performed in conjunction with endovascular repair of descending thoracic aorta, use 33889)

35695 carotid to subclavian artery

+ 35697 Reimplantation, visceral artery to infrarenal aortic prosthesis, each artery (List separately in addition to code for primary procedure)

➜ *CPT Changes: An Insider's View* 2004

(Do not report 35697 in conjunction with 33877)

Excision, Exploration, Repair, Revision

+ 35700 Reoperation, femoral-popliteal or femoral (popliteal)-anterior tibial, posterior tibial, peroneal artery, or other distal vessels, more than 1 month after original operation (List separately in addition to code for primary procedure)

➜ *CPT Assistant* Apr 12:4

(Use 35700 in conjunction with 35556, 35566, 35570, 35571, 35583, 35585, 35587, 35656, 35666, 35671)

35701 Exploration not followed by surgical repair, artery; neck (eg, carotid, subclavian)

➜ *CPT Changes: An Insider's View* 2020

➜ *CPT Assistant* Dec 19:5

(Do not report 35701 in conjunction with 35201, 35231, 35261, 35800, when performed on the same side of the neck)

35702 upper extremity (eg, axillary, brachial, radial, ulnar)

➜ *CPT Changes: An Insider's View* 2020

➜ *CPT Assistant* Dec 19:5

35703 lower extremity (eg, common femoral, deep femoral, superficial femoral, popliteal, tibial, peroneal)

➜ *CPT Changes: An Insider's View* 2020

➜ *CPT Assistant* Dec 19:5

(When additional surgical procedures are performed at the same setting by the same surgeon, 35701, 35702, 35703 may only be reported when a nonvascular surgical procedure is performed and only when the artery exploration is performed through a separate incision)

(Do not report 35702, 35703 in conjunction with 35206, 35207, 35236, 35256, 35266, 35286, 35860 in the same extremity)

(Do not report 35701, 35702, 35703 to explore and identify a recipient artery [eg, external carotid artery] when performed in conjunction with 15756, 15757, 15758, 20955, 20956, 20957, 20962, 20969, 20970, 20972, 20973, 43496, 49906)

(To report exploration of lower extremity artery, use 35703)

(To report vascular exploration not followed by surgical repair, other than neck artery, upper extremity artery, lower extremity artery, chest, abdomen, or retroperitoneal area, use 37799)

(For vascular exploration of the chest not followed by surgical repair, use 32100)

(For vascular exploration of the abdomen not followed by surgical repair, use 49000)

(For vascular exploration of the retroperitoneal area not followed by surgical repair, use 49010)

35800 Exploration for postoperative hemorrhage, thrombosis or infection; neck

35820 chest

35840 abdomen

➜ *CPT Assistant* May 97:8

35860 extremity

➜ *CPT Assistant* Fall 92:21, Apr 14:10

35870 Repair of graft-enteric fistula

35875 Thrombectomy of arterial or venous graft (other than hemodialysis graft or fistula);

➜ *CPT Assistant* Nov 98:14, Feb 99:6, Mar 99:6, Apr 00:10

35876 with revision of arterial or venous graft

➜ *CPT Assistant* Nov 98:14

(For thrombectomy of hemodialysis graft or fistula, see 36831, 36833)

Codes 35879 and 35881 describe open revision of graft-threatening stenoses of lower extremity arterial bypass graft(s) (previously constructed with autogenous vein conduit) using vein patch angioplasty or segmental vein interposition techniques. For thrombectomy with revision of any noncoronary arterial or venous graft, including those of the lower extremity, (other than hemodialysis graft or fistula), use 35876. For direct repair (other than for fistula) of a lower extremity blood vessel (with or without patch angioplasty), use 35226. For repair (other than for fistula) of a lower extremity blood vessel using a vein graft, use 35256.

35879 Revision, lower extremity arterial bypass, without thrombectomy, open; with vein patch angioplasty
➜ *CPT Changes: An Insider's View* 2000
➜ *CPT Assistant* Nov 99:19

35881 with segmental vein interposition
➜ *CPT Changes: An Insider's View* 2000
➜ *CPT Assistant* Nov 99:19

(For revision of femoral anastomosis of synthetic arterial bypass graft, see 35883, 35884)

(For excision of infected graft, see 35901-35907 and appropriate revascularization code)

35883 Revision, femoral anastomosis of synthetic arterial bypass graft in groin, open; with nonautogenous patch graft (eg, polyester, ePTFE, bovine pericardium)
➜ *CPT Changes: An Insider's View* 2007, 2023
➜ *CPT Assistant* Jan 07:7

(For bilateral procedure, use modifier 50)

(Do not report 35883 in conjunction with 35700, 35875, 35876, 35884)

35884 with autogenous vein patch graft
➜ *CPT Changes: An Insider's View* 2007
➜ *CPT Assistant* Jan 07:7

(For bilateral procedure, use modifier 50)

(Do not report 35884 in conjunction with 35700, 35875, 35876, 35883)

35901 Excision of infected graft; neck

35903 extremity
➜ *CPT Assistant* Aug 18:10

35905 thorax

35907 abdomen

Vascular Injection Procedures

Listed services for injection procedures include necessary local anesthesia, introduction of needles or catheter, injection of contrast media with or without automatic power injection, and/or necessary pre- and postinjection care specifically related to the injection procedure.

Selective vascular catheterization should be coded to include introduction and all lesser order selective catheterization used in the approach (eg, the description for a selective right middle cerebral artery catheterization includes the introduction and placement catheterization of the right common and internal carotid arteries).

Additional second and/or third order arterial catheterization within the same family of arteries or veins supplied by a single first order vessel should be expressed by 36012, 36218, or 36248.

Additional first order or higher catheterization in vascular families supplied by a first order vessel different from a previously selected and coded family should be separately coded using the conventions described above.

(For radiological supervision and interpretation, see **Radiology**)

(For injection procedures in conjunction with cardiac catheterization, see 93452, 93453, 93454, 93455, 93456, 93457, 93458, 93459, 93460, 93461, 93563, 93564, 93565, 93566, 93567, 93568, 93569, 93573, 93574, 93575)

(For chemotherapy of malignant disease, see 96401-96549)

Intravenous

An intracatheter is a sheathed combination of needle and short catheter.

36000 Introduction of needle or intracatheter, vein
➜ *CPT Assistant* Summer 95:2, Apr 98:1, 3, 7, Jul 98:1, Apr 03:26, Oct 03:2, Jul 06:4, Feb 07:10, Jul 07:1, Dec 08:7, May 14:4, Sep 14:13, Oct 14:6, Aug 19:8, Jan 22:3

36002 Injection procedures (eg, thrombin) for percutaneous treatment of extremity pseudoaneurysm
➜ *CPT Changes: An Insider's View* 2002
➜ *CPT Assistant* Nov 13:6, Oct 14:6

(For imaging guidance, see 76942, 77002, 77012, 77021)

(For ultrasound guided compression repair of pseudoaneurysms, use 76936)

(Do not report 36002 for vascular sealant of an arteriotomy site)

★ = Telemedicine   ◀ = Audio-only   ✛ = Add-on code   ✗ = FDA approval pending   # = Resequenced code   ⊘ = Modifier 51 exempt   ➜➜➜ = See p xxi for details

Injection Procedure (eg, Thrombin) for Percutaneous Treatment of Extremity Pseudoaneurysm
36002

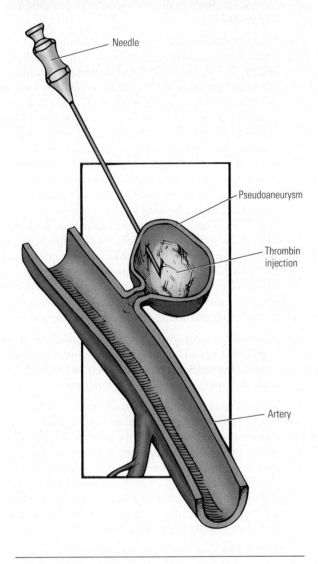

Needle

Pseudoaneurysm

Thrombin injection

Artery

36005   Injection procedure for extremity venography (including introduction of needle or intracatheter)

➔ *CPT Changes: An Insider's View* 2002

➔ *CPT Assistant* Oct 14:6

➔ *Clinical Examples in Radiology* Spring 14:7

(Do not report 36005 in conjunction with 36836, 36837)

(For radiological supervision and interpretation, see 75820, 75822)

36010   Introduction of catheter, superior or inferior vena cava

➔ *CPT Changes: An Insider's View* 2013, 2017

➔ *CPT Assistant* Aug 96:2, Apr 98:7, Sep 00:11, May 01:10, Jul 03:12, Oct 08:11, Jan 09:7, Apr 12:4, Feb 17:14

➔ *Clinical Examples in Radiology* Winter 05:5-6, Spring 08:7-8, Winter 12:3, Spring 13:3, Winter 16:2

36011   Selective catheter placement, venous system; first order branch (eg, renal vein, jugular vein)

➔ *CPT Assistant* Aug 96:11, Apr 98:7, Jul 03:12, Dec 03:2, Apr 12:5

➔ *Clinical Examples in Radiology* Winter 12:3, Summer 16:3

36012   second order, or more selective, branch (eg, left adrenal vein, petrosal sinus)

➔ *CPT Assistant* Aug 96:11, Sep 98:7, Jul 03:12, Apr 12:5, Oct 18:3

➔ *Clinical Examples in Radiology* Winter 12:3

36013   Introduction of catheter, right heart or main pulmonary artery

➔ *CPT Assistant* Aug 96:11, Oct 08:11, Jan 09:7, Jun 19:3

➔ *Clinical Examples in Radiology* Winter 23:8

36014   Selective catheter placement, left or right pulmonary artery

➔ *CPT Assistant* Aug 96:11, Apr 98:7, Jun 19:3

➔ *Clinical Examples in Radiology* Winter 23:8

36015   Selective catheter placement, segmental or subsegmental pulmonary artery

➔ *CPT Assistant* Aug 96:11, Sep 00:11, Mar 12:10, Jun 19:3

➔ *Clinical Examples in Radiology* Summer 12:1-2, Spring 13:1-2, Winter 23:8

(For insertion of flow directed catheter (eg, Swan-Ganz), use 93503)

(For venous catheterization for selective organ blood sampling, use 36500)

Intra-Arterial—Intra-Aortic

(For radiological supervision and interpretation, see **Radiology**)

36100   Introduction of needle or intracatheter, carotid or vertebral artery

➔ *CPT Assistant* Aug 96:11

(For bilateral procedure, report 36100 with modifier 50)

36140   Introduction of needle or intracatheter, upper or lower extremity artery

➔ *CPT Changes: An Insider's View* 2013, 2017, 2018

➔ *CPT Assistant* Fall 93:16, Aug 96:3, Nov 99:32-33, Oct 03:2, Jul 06:4, 7, Jul 07:1, Dec 07:10-11, Jun 09:10, Jul 11:5

(Do not report 36140 in conjunction with 36836, 36837)

(For insertion of arteriovenous cannula, see 36810-36821)

36160   Introduction of needle or intracatheter, aortic, translumbar

➔ *CPT Assistant* Aug 96:3

Cardiovascular 33016-39599

Diagnostic Studies of Cervicocerebral Arteries: Codes 36221-36228 describe non-selective and selective arterial catheter placement and diagnostic imaging of the aortic arch, carotid, and vertebral arteries. Codes 36221-36226 include the work of accessing the vessel, placement of catheter(s), contrast injection(s), fluoroscopy, radiological supervision and interpretation, and closure of the arteriotomy by pressure, or application of an arterial closure device. Codes 36221-36228 describe arterial contrast injections with arterial, capillary, and venous phase imaging, when performed.

Code 36227 is an add-on code to report unilateral selective arterial catheter placement and diagnostic imaging of the ipsilateral external carotid circulation and includes all the work of accessing the additional vessel, placement of catheter(s), contrast injection(s), fluoroscopy, radiological supervision and interpretation. Code 36227 is reported in conjunction with 36222, 36223, or 36224.

Code 36228 is an add-on code to report unilateral selective arterial catheter placement and diagnostic imaging of the initial and each additional intracranial branch of the internal carotid or vertebral arteries. Code 36228 is reported in conjunction with 36223, 36224, 36225 or 36226. This includes any additional second or third order catheter selective placement in the same primary branch of the internal carotid, vertebral, or basilar artery and includes all the work of accessing the additional vessel, placement of catheter(s), contrast injection(s), fluoroscopy, radiological supervision and interpretation. It is not reported more than twice per side, regardless of the number of additional branches selectively catheterized.

Codes 36221-36226 are built on progressive hierarchies with more intensive services inclusive of less intensive services. The code inclusive of all of the services provided for that vessel should be reported (ie, use the code inclusive of the most intensive services provided). Only one code in the range 36222-36224 may be reported for each ipsilateral carotid territory. Only one code in the range 36225-36226 may be reported for each ipsilateral vertebral territory.

Code 36221 is reported for non-selective arterial catheter placement in the thoracic aorta and diagnostic imaging of the aortic arch and great vessel origins. Codes 36222-36228 are reported for unilateral artery catheterization. Do not report 36221 in conjunction with 36222-36226 as these selective codes include the work of 36221 when performed.

Do not report 36222, 36223, or 36224 together for ipsilateral angiography. Instead, select the code that represents the most comprehensive service using the following hierarchy of complexity (listed in descending order of complexity): 36224>36223>36222.

Do not report 36225 and 36226 together for ipsilateral angiography. Select the code that represents the more comprehensive service using the following hierarchy of complexity (listed in descending order of complexity): 36226>36225.

When bilateral carotid and/or vertebral arterial catheterization and imaging is performed, report 36222, 36223, 36224, 36225, 36226 with modifier 50, and report add-on codes 36227, 36228 twice (do not report modifier 50 in conjunction with 36227, 36228) if the same procedure is performed on both sides. For example, bilateral extracranial carotid angiography with selective catheterization of each common carotid artery would be reported with 36222 and modifier 50. However, when different territory(ies) is studied in the same session on both sides of the body, modifiers may be required to report the imaging performed. Use modifier 59 to denote that different carotid and/or vertebral arteries are being studied. For example, when selective right internal carotid artery catheterization accompanied by right extracranial and intracranial carotid angiography is followed by selective left common carotid artery catheterization with left extracranial carotid angiography, use 36224 to report the right side and 36222-59 to report the left side.

Diagnostic angiography of the cervicocerebral vessels may be followed by an interventional procedure at the same session. Interventional procedures may be separately reportable using standard coding conventions.

Do not report 36218 or 75774 as part of diagnostic angiography of the extracranial and intracranial cervicocerebral vessels. It may be appropriate to report 36218 and 75774 for diagnostic angiography of upper extremities and other vascular beds of the neck and/or shoulder girdle performed in the same session as vertebral angiography (eg, workup of a neck tumor that requires catheterization and angiography of the vertebral artery as well as other brachiocephalic arteries).

Report 76376 or 76377 for 3D rendering when performed in conjunction with 36221-36228.

Report 76937 for ultrasound guidance for vascular access, when performed in conjunction with 36221-36228.

36200   Introduction of catheter, aorta
> *CPT Changes: An Insider's View* 2012, 2017
> *CPT Assistant* Fall 93:16, Aug 96:3, Jul 06:7, Dec 07:10, 14, Apr 08:11, Dec 09:13, Jul 11:5, Oct 11:9, Apr 12:4, Feb 13:16, Mar 17:4, Jul 21:4
> *Clinical Examples in Radiology* Spring 12:6, Winter 14:5-6, Summer 14:2-3

★=Telemedicine ◀=Audio-only ╋=Add-on code ✗=FDA approval pending #=Resequenced code ⊘=Modifier 51 exempt ➲➲➲=See p xxi for details

(For non-selective angiography of the extracranial carotid and/or cerebral vessels and cervicocerebral arch, when performed, use 36221)

36215 Selective catheter placement, arterial system; each first order thoracic or brachiocephalic branch, within a vascular family

➔ *CPT Assistant* Fall 93:15, Aug 96:3, Nov 97:16, Apr 98:9, Sep 00:11, Oct 00:4, Feb 03:3, Apr 12:4, Mar 17:4, May 17:8, Jul 21:4, Oct 23:21

➔ *Clinical Examples in Radiology* Spring 12:4, Spring 13:4-6, Winter 18:2

(For catheter placement for coronary angiography, see 93454-93461)

36216 initial second order thoracic or brachiocephalic branch, within a vascular family

➔ *CPT Assistant* Fall 93:15, Aug 96:3, Oct 00:4, Dec 07:10, Dec 11:12, Apr 12:4, Nov 13:14, Oct 23:21

➔ *Clinical Examples in Radiology* Spring 13:4-6, Winter 18:2

36217 initial third order or more selective thoracic or brachiocephalic branch, within a vascular family

➔ *CPT Assistant* Fall 93:15, Aug 96:3, Oct 00:4, Dec 07:10, Dec 11:12, Apr 12:5

➔ *Clinical Examples in Radiology* Summer 07:1-2

+ 36218 additional second order, third order, and beyond, thoracic or brachiocephalic branch, within a vascular family (List in addition to code for initial second or third order vessel as appropriate)

➔ *CPT Assistant* Fall 93:15, Aug 96:3, Oct 00:4, Jul 06:7, Dec 07:10, Apr 12:5, May 13:3, Oct 18:3

➔ *Clinical Examples in Radiology* Winter 15:4-6, Winter 18:2

(Use 36218 in conjunction with 36216, 36217, 36225, 36226)

(Do not report 36215, 36216, 36217, 36218 in conjunction with 36836, 36837)

(For angiography, see 36222-36228, 75600-75774)

(For transluminal balloon angioplasty [except lower extremity artery[ies] for occlusive disease, intracranial, coronary, pulmonary, or dialysis circuit], see 37246, 37247)

(For transcatheter therapies, see 37200, 37211, 37213, 37214, 37236, 37237, 37238, 37239, 37241, 37242, 37243, 37244, 61624, 61626)

(When arterial [eg, internal mammary, inferior epigastric or free radial artery] or venous bypass graft angiography is performed in conjunction with cardiac catheterization, see the appropriate cardiac catheterization, injection procedure, and imaging supervision code[s] [93454, 93455, 93456, 93457, 93458, 93459, 93460, 93461, 93564, 93593, 93594, 93595, 93596, 93597] in the **Medicine** section. When internal mammary artery angiography only is performed without a concomitant cardiac catheterization, use 36216 or 36217 as appropriate)

36221 Non-selective catheter placement, thoracic aorta, with angiography of the extracranial carotid, vertebral, and/or intracranial vessels, unilateral or bilateral, and all associated radiological supervision and interpretation, includes angiography of the cervicocerebral arch, when performed

➔ *CPT Changes: An Insider's View* 2013, 2017

➔ *CPT Assistant* Feb 13:16, May 13:3, Jun 13:12, Oct 13:18, Mar 14:8, May 15:7, Dec 21:19

➔ *Clinical Examples in Radiology* Winter 15:6

(Do not report 36221 with 36222-36226)

36222 Selective catheter placement, common carotid or innominate artery, unilateral, any approach, with angiography of the ipsilateral extracranial carotid circulation and all associated radiological supervision and interpretation, includes angiography of the cervicocerebral arch, when performed

➔ *CPT Changes: An Insider's View* 2013, 2017

➔ *CPT Assistant* Feb 13:17, May 13:3, Jun 13:12, Oct 13:18, Nov 13:14, Mar 14:8, May 15:7, Nov 15:10

➔ *Clinical Examples in Radiology* Winter 15:6, Spring 16:6

(Do not report 36222 in conjunction with 37215, 37216, 37218 for the treated carotid artery)

36223 Selective catheter placement, common carotid or innominate artery, unilateral, any approach, with angiography of the ipsilateral intracranial carotid circulation and all associated radiological supervision and interpretation, includes angiography of the extracranial carotid and cervicocerebral arch, when performed

➔ *CPT Changes: An Insider's View* 2013, 2017

➔ *CPT Assistant* Feb 13:17, May 13:3, Jun 13:12, Oct 13:18, Mar 14:8

➔ *Clinical Examples in Radiology* Winter 15:6, Spring 16:6

(Do not report 36223 in conjunction with 37215, 37216, 37218 for the treated carotid artery)

36224 Selective catheter placement, internal carotid artery, unilateral, with angiography of the ipsilateral intracranial carotid circulation and all associated radiological supervision and interpretation, includes angiography of the extracranial carotid and cervicocerebral arch, when performed

➔ *CPT Changes: An Insider's View* 2013, 2017

➔ *CPT Assistant* Feb 13:17, May 13:3, Jun 13:12, Oct 13:18, Mar 14:8

➔ *Clinical Examples in Radiology* Winter 15:5-6, Spring 16:5

(Do not report 36224 in conjunction with 37215, 37216, 37218 for the treated carotid artery)

36225 Selective catheter placement, subclavian or innominate artery, unilateral, with angiography of the ipsilateral vertebral circulation and all associated radiological supervision and interpretation, includes angiography of the cervicocerebral arch, when performed

➲ *CPT Changes: An Insider's View* 2013, 2017

➲ *CPT Assistant* May 13:3, Jun 13:12, Oct 13:18, Nov 13:14, Mar 14:8

➲ *Clinical Examples in Radiology* Spring 13:6, Winter 15:6

36226 Selective catheter placement, vertebral artery, unilateral, with angiography of the ipsilateral vertebral circulation and all associated radiological supervision and interpretation, includes angiography of the cervicocerebral arch, when performed

➲ *CPT Changes: An Insider's View* 2013, 2017

➲ *CPT Assistant* May 13:3, Jun 13:12, Oct 13:18, Mar 14:8

➲ *Clinical Examples in Radiology* Winter 15:4-6, Winter 18:2

+ 36227 Selective catheter placement, external carotid artery, unilateral, with angiography of the ipsilateral external carotid circulation and all associated radiological supervision and interpretation (List separately in addition to code for primary procedure)

➲ *CPT Changes: An Insider's View* 2013, 2017

➲ *CPT Assistant* Feb 13:17, May 13:3, Jun 13:12, Oct 13:18, Mar 14:8, Nov 15:10

➲ *Clinical Examples in Radiology* Winter 15:5-6, Spring 16:5

(Use 36227 in conjunction with 36222, 36223, or 36224)

(Do not report 36221-36227 in conjunction with 37217 for ipsilateral services)

+ 36228 Selective catheter placement, each intracranial branch of the internal carotid or vertebral arteries, unilateral, with angiography of the selected vessel circulation and all associated radiological supervision and interpretation (eg, middle cerebral artery, posterior inferior cerebellar artery) (List separately in addition to code for primary procedure)

➲ *CPT Changes: An Insider's View* 2013, 2017

➲ *CPT Assistant* Feb 13:17, May 13:3, Jun 13:12, Oct 13:18

(Use 36228 in conjunction with 36223, 36224, 36225 or 36226)

(Do not report 36228 more than twice per side)

36245 Selective catheter placement, arterial system; each first order abdominal, pelvic, or lower extremity artery branch, within a vascular family

➲ *CPT Changes: An Insider's View* 2012, 2017

➲ *CPT Assistant* Fall 93:15, Aug 96:3, Jan 01:14, Jan 07:7, Dec 07:10, Jul 11:5, Oct 11:9, Apr 12:4, Nov 13:14

➲ *Clinical Examples in Radiology* Summer 08:1, 3, Fall 11:3, Winter 14:2-3, Winter 18:2, Spring 19:2, Fall 21:16

Angiography, Carotid Artery
36222-36228

A radiologic contrast study is performed on the carotid artery vascular family.

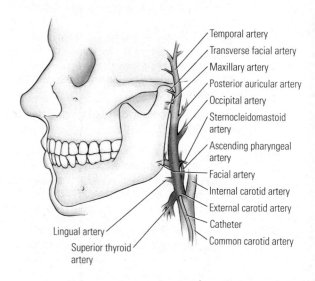

36246 initial second order abdominal, pelvic, or lower extremity artery branch, within a vascular family

➲ *CPT Changes: An Insider's View* 2012, 2017

➲ *CPT Assistant* Fall 93:15, Aug 96:3, Jan 01:14, Jan 07:7, Dec 07:10-11, Jul 11:5, Oct 11:9, Apr 12:4, Nov 13:14

➲ *Clinical Examples in Radiology* Winter 13:2-3, Winter 14:1, 3, Winter 18:11, Spring 19:3, Fall 21:16

36247 initial third order or more selective abdominal, pelvic, or lower extremity artery branch, within a vascular family

➲ *CPT Changes: An Insider's View* 2012, 2017

➲ *CPT Assistant* Fall 93:15, Aug 96:3, Jan 01:14, Jan 07:7, Dec 07:10, Jul 11:5, Apr 12:4, Nov 13:14, Sep 20:14

➲ *Clinical Examples in Radiology* Winter 08:1, Summer 08:1, 3, Winter 13:1, 3, Fall 13:2-4, Summer 15:2, Winter 18:11, Summer 18:2, Summer 19:4, Fall 21:16

+ 36248 additional second order, third order, and beyond, abdominal, pelvic, or lower extremity artery branch, within a vascular family (List in addition to code for initial second or third order vessel as appropriate)

➲ *CPT Changes: An Insider's View* 2012, 2017

➲ *CPT Assistant* Fall 93:15, Aug 96:3, Apr 98:1, 7, Oct 00:4, Jan 01:14, Jan 07:7, Jul 11:5, Apr 12:4, Oct 18:3

➲ *Clinical Examples in Radiology* Winter 10:7, Fall 21:16

(Use 36248 in conjunction with 36246, 36247)

(Do not report 36245, 36246, 36247, 36248 in conjunction with 36836, 36837)

36251 Selective catheter placement (first-order), main renal artery and any accessory renal artery(s) for renal angiography, including arterial puncture and catheter placement(s), fluoroscopy, contrast injection(s), image postprocessing, permanent recording of images, and radiological supervision and interpretation, including pressure gradient measurements when performed, and flush aortogram when performed; unilateral

➔ *CPT Changes: An Insider's View* 2012, 2017

➔ *CPT Assistant* Apr 12:6, Aug 12:13, Nov 13:14

➔ *Clinical Examples in Radiology* Fall 11:2, Spring 19:2

36252 bilateral

➔ *CPT Changes: An Insider's View* 2012, 2017

➔ *CPT Assistant* Apr 12:6

➔ *Clinical Examples in Radiology* Fall 11:2

36253 Superselective catheter placement (one or more second order or higher renal artery branches) renal artery and any accessory renal artery(s) for renal angiography, including arterial puncture, catheterization, fluoroscopy, contrast injection(s), image postprocessing, permanent recording of images, and radiological supervision and interpretation, including pressure gradient measurements when performed, and flush aortogram when performed; unilateral

➔ *CPT Changes: An Insider's View* 2012, 2017

➔ *CPT Assistant* Apr 12:6, Aug 12:13, Nov 13:14

➔ *Clinical Examples in Radiology* Fall 11:2

(Do not report 36253 in conjunction with 36251 when performed for the same kidney)

36254 bilateral

➔ *CPT Changes: An Insider's View* 2012, 2017

➔ *CPT Assistant* Apr 12:6, Aug 12:13

➔ *Clinical Examples in Radiology* Fall 11:2

(Do not report 36254 in conjunction with 36252)

(Placement of closure device at the vascular access site is not separately reported with 36251-36254)

(Do not report 36251, 36252, 36253, 36254 in conjunction with 0338T, 0339T)

36260 Insertion of implantable intra-arterial infusion pump (eg, for chemotherapy of liver)

➔ *CPT Assistant* Fall 95:5

36261 Revision of implanted intra-arterial infusion pump

36262 Removal of implanted intra-arterial infusion pump

36299 Unlisted procedure, vascular injection

Venous

Venipuncture, needle or catheter for diagnostic study or intravenous therapy, percutaneous. These codes are also used to report the therapy as specified. For collection of a specimen from an established catheter, use 36592. For collection of a specimen from a completely implantable venous access device, use 36591.

36400 Venipuncture, younger than age 3 years, necessitating the skill of a physician or other qualified health care professional, not to be used for routine venipuncture; femoral or jugular vein

➔ *CPT Changes: An Insider's View* 2002, 2004, 2013

➔ *CPT Assistant* Jul 06:4, Jul 07:1, Dec 08:7, May 14:4

➔ *Clinical Examples in Radiology* Fall 18:9, Winter 19:12

36405 scalp vein

➔ *CPT Changes: An Insider's View* 2013

➔ *CPT Assistant* Jul 06:4, Jul 07:1, Dec 08:7, May 14:4

➔ *Clinical Examples in Radiology* Fall 18:9, Winter 19:12

36406 other vein

➔ *CPT Changes: An Insider's View* 2013

➔ *CPT Assistant* Jul 06:4, Jul 07:1, May 14:4

➔ *Clinical Examples in Radiology* Fall 18:9, Winter 19:12

36410 Venipuncture, age 3 years or older, necessitating the skill of a physician or other qualified health care professional (separate procedure), for diagnostic or therapeutic purposes (not to be used for routine venipuncture)

➔ *CPT Changes: An Insider's View* 2004, 2013

➔ *CPT Assistant* Jun 96:10, May 01:11, Aug 02:2, Oct 03:10, Feb 07:10, Jul 07:1, Dec 08:7, Sep 13:18, Oct 14:6, Aug 19:8, Jan 22:3

➔ *Clinical Examples in Radiology* Spring 09:8, Fall 18:9, Winter 19:12

— *Coding Tip* —

Instructions for Use of the CPT Codebook

When advanced practice nurses and physician assistants are working with physicians they are considered as working in the exact same specialty and exact same subspecialties as the physician. A "physician or other qualified health care professional" is an individual who is qualified by education, training, licensure/regulation (when applicable), and facility privileging (when applicable) who performs a professional service within his or her scope of practice and independently reports that professional service. The professionals are distinct from "clinical staff." A clinical staff member is a person who works under the supervison of a physician or other qualified health care professional, and who is allowed by law, regulation, and facility policy to perform or assist in the performance of a specific professional service, but does not individually report that professional service. Other policies may also affect who may report specific services.

CPT Coding Guidelines, Introduction, Instructions for Use of the CPT Codebook

36415 Collection of venous blood by venipuncture

➔ *CPT Changes: An Insider's View* 2003

➔ *CPT Assistant* Jun 96:10, Mar 98:10, Oct 99:11, Aug 00:2, Feb 07:10, Jul 07:1, Dec 08:7, May 14:4, Aug 19:8, Jan 22:3

(Do not report modifier 63 in conjunction with 36415)

36416   Collection of capillary blood specimen (eg, finger, heel, ear stick)
➡ *CPT Changes: An Insider's View* 2003

36420   Venipuncture, cutdown; younger than age 1 year
➡ *CPT Assistant* Nov 99:32-33, Aug 00:2, Oct 03:2, Jul 06:4

(Do not report modifier 63 in conjunction with 36420)

36425   age 1 or over
➡ *CPT Assistant* Oct 14:6
➡ *Clinical Examples in Radiology* Summer 08:1

(Do not report 36425 in conjunction with 36475, 36476, 36478)

36430   Transfusion, blood or blood components
➡ *CPT Assistant* Aug 97:18, Nov 99:32-33, Aug 00:2, Mar 01:10, Oct 03:2, Jul 06:4, Jul 07:1, Jul 17:4

(When a partial exchange transfusion is performed in a newborn, use 36456)

36440   Push transfusion, blood, 2 years or younger
➡ *CPT Assistant* Aug 00:2, Oct 03:2, Jul 06:4, Jul 07:1, Jul 17:4

(When a partial exchange transfusion is performed in a newborn, use 36456)

36450   Exchange transfusion, blood; newborn
➡ *CPT Assistant* Jul 17:3, Oct 21:12

(When a partial exchange transfusion is performed in a newborn, use 36456)

(Do not report modifier 63 in conjunction with 36450)

(For manual red cell exchange, see 36450, 36455, 36456)

(For automated red cell exchange, use 36512)

36455   other than newborn
➡ *CPT Assistant* Oct 21:12

36456   Partial exchange transfusion, blood, plasma or crystalloid necessitating the skill of a physician or other qualified health care professional, newborn
➡ *CPT Changes: An Insider's View* 2017, 2018
➡ *CPT Assistant* Jul 17:3, Oct 21:12

(Do not report 36456 in conjunction with 36430, 36440, 36450)

(Do not report modifier 63 in conjunction with 36456)

36460   Transfusion, intrauterine, fetal

(Do not report modifier 63 in conjunction with 36460)

(For radiological supervision and interpretation, use 76941)

Codes 36468, 36470, 36471 describe injection(s) of a sclerosant for sclerotherapy of telangiectasia and/or incompetent vein(s). Code 36468 may only be reported once per extremity per session, regardless of the number of needle injections performed. Codes 36466, 36471 may only be reported once per extremity, regardless of the number of veins treated. Ultrasound guidance (76942), when performed, is not included in 36468, 36470, 36471 and may be reported separately.

Codes 36465, 36466 describe injection(s) of a non-compounded foam sclerosant into an extremity truncal vein (eg, great saphenous vein, accessory saphenous vein) using ultrasound-guided compression of the junction of the central vein (saphenofemoral junction or saphenopopliteal junction) to limit the dispersion of injectate. Do not report 36465, 36466 for injection of compounded foam sclerosant(s).

Compounding is a practice in which a qualified health care professional (eg, pharmacist, physician) combines, mixes, or alters ingredients of a drug to create a medication tailored to the needs of an individual patient.

When performed in the office setting, all required supplies and equipment are included in 36465, 36466, 36468, 36470, 36471 and may not be separately reported. In addition, application of compression dressing(s) (eg, compression bandages/stockings) is included in 36465, 36466, 36468, 36470, 36471, when performed, and may not be reported separately.

36465   Code is out of numerical sequence. See 36470-36474

36466   Code is out of numerical sequence. See 36470-36474

36468   Injection(s) of sclerosant for spider veins (telangiectasia), limb or trunk
➡ *CPT Changes: An Insider's View* 2018
➡ *CPT Assistant* Aug 14:14, Oct 14:6, Apr 15:10, Nov 16:3, Mar 18:3
➡ *Clinical Examples in Radiology* Summer 15:8, Spring 17:3

(For ultrasound imaging guidance performed in conjunction with 36468, use 76942)

(Do not report 36468 in conjunction with 29520, 29530, 29540, 29550, 29580, 29581, 29584, for the same extremity)

(Do not report 36468 more than once per extremity)

(Do not report 36468 in conjunction with 37241 in the same surgical field)

36470   Injection of sclerosant; single incompetent vein (other than telangiectasia)
➡ *CPT Changes: An Insider's View* 2018
➡ *CPT Assistant* Oct 14:6, Apr 15:10, Nov 15:10, Nov 16:3, Mar 18:3, Dec 18:10
➡ *Clinical Examples in Radiology* Summer 15:8, Spring 17:3

36471   multiple incompetent veins (other than telangiectasia), same leg
➡ *CPT Changes: An Insider's View* 2018
➡ *CPT Assistant* Oct 14:6, Apr 15:10, Aug 15:8, Nov 15:10, Nov 16:3, Mar 18:3, Dec 18:10
➡ *Clinical Examples in Radiology* Summer 15:8, Spring 17:3

(For ultrasound imaging guidance performed in conjunction with 36470, 36471, use 76942)

(Do not report 36470, 36471 in conjunction with 29520, 29530, 29540, 29550, 29580, 29581, 29584, for the same extremity)

(Do not report 36471 more than once per extremity)

(If the targeted vein is an extremity truncal vein and injection of non-compounded foam sclerosant with ultrasound guided compression maneuvers to guide dispersion of the injectate is performed, see 36465, 36466)

(Do not report 36470, 36471 in conjunction with 37241 in the same surgical field)

 # 36465   Injection of non-compounded foam sclerosant with ultrasound compression maneuvers to guide dispersion of the injectate, inclusive of all imaging guidance and monitoring; single incompetent extremity truncal vein (eg, great saphenous vein, accessory saphenous vein)
> *CPT Changes: An Insider's View* 2018
> *CPT Assistant* Mar 18:3, Dec 18:10, Feb 19:9

 # 36466   multiple incompetent truncal veins (eg, great saphenous vein, accessory saphenous vein), same leg
> *CPT Changes: An Insider's View* 2018
> *CPT Assistant* Mar 18:3, Dec 18:10, Feb 19:9

(Do not report 36465, 36466 in conjunction with 29520, 29530, 29540, 29550, 29580, 29581, 29584, for the same extremity)

(Do not report 36465, 36466 in conjunction with 37241 in the same surgical field)

(For extremity truncal vein injection of compounded foam sclerosant[s], see 36470, 36471)

(For injection of a sclerosant into an incompetent vein without compression maneuvers to guide dispersion of the injectate, see 36470, 36471)

(For endovenous ablation therapy of incompetent vein[s] by transcatheter delivery of a chemical adhesive, see 36482, 36483)

(For vascular embolization and occlusion procedures, see 37241, 37242, 37243, 37244)

Codes 36473, 36474, 36475, 36476, 36478, 36479, 36482, 36483 describe endovascular ablation therapy of incompetent extremity vein(s), including all necessary imaging guidance and monitoring. Sclerosant injection(s) of vein(s) by needle or mini-catheter (36468, 36470, 36471) followed by a compression technique is not endovascular ablation therapy. Codes 36473, 36474, 36482, 36483 can be performed under local anesthesia without the need for tumescent (peri-saphenous) anesthesia. Codes 36475, 36476, 36478, 36479 are performed using adjunctive tumescent anesthesia.

Codes 36473, 36474 involve concomitant use of an intraluminal device that mechanically disrupts/abrades the venous intima and infusion of a physician-specified medication in the target vein(s).

Codes 36482, 36483 involve positioning an intravenous catheter the length of an incompetent vein, remote from the percutaneous access site, with subsequent delivery of a chemical adhesive to ablate the incompetent vein. This often includes ultrasound compression of the outflow vein to limit the dispersion of the injected solution.

Codes 36475, 36476 involve advancing a radiofrequency device the length of an incompetent vein, with subsequent delivery of radiofrequency energy to ablate the incompetent vein.

Codes 36478, 36479 involve advancing a laser device the length of an incompetent vein, with subsequent delivery of thermal energy to ablate the incompetent vein.

Codes 36474, 36476, 36479, 36483 for subsequent vein(s) treated in the same extremity may only be reported once per extremity, regardless of the number of additional vein(s) treated.

When performed in the office setting, all required supplies and equipment are included in 36473, 36474, 36475, 36476, 36478, 36479, 36482, 36483 and may not be separately reported. In addition, application of compression dressing(s) (eg, compression bandages/ stockings) is included in 36473, 36474, 36475, 36476, 36478, 36479, 36482, 36483, when performed, and may not be reported separately.

36473   Endovenous ablation therapy of incompetent vein, extremity, inclusive of all imaging guidance and monitoring, percutaneous, mechanochemical; first vein treated
> *CPT Changes: An Insider's View* 2017
> *CPT Assistant* Nov 16:3, May 17:3, Mar 18:3, Feb 19:9
> *Clinical Examples in Radiology* Spring 17:2

+ 36474   subsequent vein(s) treated in a single extremity, each through separate access sites (List separately in addition to code for primary procedure)
> *CPT Changes: An Insider's View* 2017
> *CPT Assistant* Nov 16:3, May 17:3, Mar 18:3, Feb 19:9
> *Clinical Examples in Radiology* Spring 17:3

(Use 36474 in conjunction with 36473)

(Do not report 36474 more than once per extremity)

(Do not report 36473, 36474 in conjunction with 29520, 29530, 29540, 29550, 29580, 29581, 29584, for the same extremity)

Cardiovascular 33016-39599

(Do not report 36473, 36474 in conjunction with 36000, 36002, 36005, 36410, 36425, 36475, 36476, 36478, 36479, 37241, 75894, 76000, 76937, 76942, 76998, 77022, 93970, 93971, in the same surgical field)

36475   Endovenous ablation therapy of incompetent vein, extremity, inclusive of all imaging guidance and monitoring, percutaneous, radiofrequency; first vein treated

➔ *CPT Changes: An Insider's View* 2005

➔ *CPT Assistant* Jul 10:11, Mar 14:4, Oct 14:6, Apr 15:10, Nov 16:3, Mar 18:3

➔ *Clinical Examples in Radiology* Fall 08:10, Spring 17:3

+ 36476   subsequent vein(s) treated in a single extremity, each through separate access sites (List separately in addition to code for primary procedure)

➔ *CPT Changes: An Insider's View* 2005, 2017

➔ *CPT Assistant* Jul 10:11, Mar 14:4, Oct 14:6, Apr 15:10, Nov 16:3, Mar 18:3

➔ *Clinical Examples in Radiology* Spring 17:3

(Use 36476 in conjunction with 36475)

(Do not report 36476 more than once per extremity)

(Do not report 36475, 36476 in conjunction with 29520, 29530, 29540, 29550, 29580, 29581, 29584, for the same extremity)

(Do not report 36475, 36476 in conjunction with 36000, 36002, 36005, 36410, 36425, 36478, 36479, 36482, 36483, 37241-37244, 75894, 76000, 76937, 76942, 76998, 77022, 93970, 93971, in the same surgical field)

36478   Endovenous ablation therapy of incompetent vein, extremity, inclusive of all imaging guidance and monitoring, percutaneous, laser; first vein treated

➔ *CPT Changes: An Insider's View* 2005

➔ *CPT Assistant* Jul 12:12, Mar 14:4, Oct 14:6, Apr 15:10, Nov 16:3, Mar 18:3, May 20:13

➔ *Clinical Examples in Radiology* Spring 17:3

+ 36479   subsequent vein(s) treated in a single extremity, each through separate access sites (List separately in addition to code for primary procedure)

➔ *CPT Changes: An Insider's View* 2005, 2017

➔ *CPT Assistant* Jul 10:11, Jul 12:12, Mar 14:4, Aug 14:14, Oct 14:6, Apr 15:10, Nov 16:3, Mar 18:3, May 20:13

➔ *Clinical Examples in Radiology* Spring 17:3

(Use 36479 in conjunction with 36478)

(Do not report 36479 more than once per extremity)

(Do not report 36478, 36479 in conjunction with 29520, 29530, 29540, 29550, 29580, 29581, 29584, for the same extremity)

(Do not report 36478, 36479 in conjunction with 36000, 36002, 36005, 36410, 36425, 36475, 36476, 36482, 36483, 37241, 75894, 76000, 76937, 76942, 76998, 77022, 93970, 93971, in the same surgical field)

 # 36482   Endovenous ablation therapy of incompetent vein, extremity, by transcatheter delivery of a chemical adhesive (eg, cyanoacrylate) remote from the access site, inclusive of all imaging guidance and monitoring, percutaneous; first vein treated

➔ *CPT Changes: An Insider's View* 2018

➔ *CPT Assistant* Mar 18:3, Feb 19:9

#+ 36483   subsequent vein(s) treated in a single extremity, each through separate access sites (List separately in addition to code for primary procedure)

➔ *CPT Changes: An Insider's View* 2018

➔ *CPT Assistant* Mar 18:3, Feb 19:9

(Use 36483 in conjunction with 36482)

(Do not report 36483 more than once per extremity)

(Do not report 36482, 36483 in conjunction with 29520, 29530, 29540, 29550, 29580, 29581, 29584, for the same extremity)

(Do not report 36482, 36483 in conjunction with 36000, 36002, 36005, 36410, 36425, 36475, 36476, 36478, 36479, 37241, 75894, 76000, 76937, 76942, 76998, 77022, 93970, 93971, in the same surgical field)

36481   Percutaneous portal vein catheterization by any method

➔ *CPT Changes: An Insider's View* 2010, 2017

➔ *CPT Assistant* Oct 96:1, Mar 02:10, Dec 03:2

➔ *Clinical Examples in Radiology* Winter 18:11

36482   Code is out of numerical sequence. See 36478-36500

36483   Code is out of numerical sequence. See 36478-36500

(For radiological supervision and interpretation, see 75885, 75887)

36500   Venous catheterization for selective organ blood sampling

➔ *Clinical Examples in Radiology* Summer 16:2

(For catheterization in superior or inferior vena cava, use 36010)

(For radiological supervision and interpretation, use 75893)

36510   Catheterization of umbilical vein for diagnosis or therapy, newborn

➔ *CPT Assistant* Nov 99:5-6, Aug 00:2, Oct 03:2, Jul 06:4, Jul 07:1, May 16:3

(Do not report modifier 63 in conjunction with 36510)

36511   Therapeutic apheresis; for white blood cells

➔ *CPT Changes: An Insider's View* 2003

➔ *CPT Assistant* Oct 13:3

Cardiovascular 33016-39599

36512   for red blood cells
➔ *CPT Changes: An Insider's View* 2003
➔ *CPT Assistant* Oct 13:3, Oct 21:12

(For manual red cell exchange, see 36450, 36455, 36456)

(For automated red cell exchange, use 36512)

36513   for platelets
➔ *CPT Changes: An Insider's View* 2003
➔ *CPT Assistant* Oct 13:3

(Report 36513 only when platelets are removed by apheresis for treatment of the patient. Do not report 36513 for donor platelet collections)

36514   for plasma pheresis
➔ *CPT Changes: An Insider's View* 2003
➔ *CPT Assistant* Oct 13:3, May 18:10

36516   with extracorporeal immunoadsorption, selective adsorption or selective filtration and plasma reinfusion
➔ *CPT Changes: An Insider's View* 2003, 2018
➔ *CPT Assistant* Oct 13:3

(For professional evaluation, use modifier 26)

36522   Photopheresis, extracorporeal
➔ *CPT Assistant* Fall 93:25, Jun 09:3, Sep 09:3, Aug 10:12, Oct 13:3, May 18:10

(For dialysis services, see 90935-90999)

(For therapeutic ultrafiltration, use 0692T)

(For therapeutic apheresis for white blood cells, red blood cells, platelets and plasma pheresis, see 36511, 36512, 36513, 36514)

(For therapeutic apheresis extracorporeal adsorption procedures, use 36516)

Central Venous Access Procedures

To qualify as a central venous access catheter or device, the tip of the catheter/device must terminate in the subclavian, brachiocephalic (innominate) or iliac veins, the superior or inferior vena cava, or the right atrium. The venous access device may be either centrally inserted (jugular, subclavian, femoral vein or inferior vena cava catheter entry site) or peripherally inserted (eg, basilic, cephalic, or saphenous vein entry site). The device may be accessed for use either via exposed catheter (external to the skin), via a subcutaneous port or via a subcutaneous pump.

The procedures involving these types of devices fall into five categories:

1. *Insertion* (placement of catheter through a newly established venous access)

2. *Repair* (fixing device without replacement of either catheter or port/pump, other than pharmacologic or mechanical correction of intracatheter or pericatheter occlusion [see 36595 or 36596])

3. *Partial replacement* of only the catheter component associated with a port/pump device, but not entire device

4. *Complete replacement* of entire device via same venous access site (complete exchange)

5. *Removal* of entire device.

There is no coding distinction between venous access achieved percutaneously versus by cutdown or based on catheter size.

For the repair, partial (catheter only) replacement, complete replacement, or removal of both catheters (placed from separate venous access sites) of a multi-catheter device, with or without subcutaneous ports/pumps, use the appropriate code describing the service with a frequency of two.

If an existing central venous access device is removed and a new one placed via a separate venous access site, appropriate codes for both procedures (removal of old, if code exists, and insertion of new device) should be reported.

When imaging guidance is used for centrally inserted central venous catheters, for gaining access to the venous entry site and/or for manipulating the catheter into final central position, imaging guidance codes (eg, 76937, 77001) may be reported separately. Do not use 76937, 77001 in conjunction with 36568, 36569, 36572, 36573, 36584.

(For refilling and maintenance of an implantable pump or reservoir for intravenous or intra-arterial drug delivery, use 96522)

Insertion of Central Venous Access Device

36555   Insertion of non-tunneled centrally inserted central venous catheter; younger than 5 years of age
➔ *CPT Changes: An Insider's View* 2004, 2017
➔ *CPT Assistant* Dec 04:7, Jul 06:4, Jul 07:1, Jun 08:8, Sep 23:47
➔ *Clinical Examples in Radiology* Summer 06:8-9, Winter 09:9, Spring 09:10, Winter 17:8

(For peripherally inserted non-tunneled central venous catheter, younger than 5 years of age, use 36568)

36556   age 5 years or older
➔ *CPT Changes: An Insider's View* 2004
➔ *CPT Assistant* Dec 04:7, Jun 08:8, Nov 18:11, Sep 23:47
➔ *Clinical Examples in Radiology* Summer 06:8-9, Spring 08:7-8, Winter 09:8-9, Spring 09:10, Winter 17:8

(For peripherally inserted non-tunneled central venous catheter, age 5 years or older, use 36569)

Insertion of Non-Tunneled Centrally Inserted Central Venous Catheter
36555

During placement of a central venous catheter, a short tract is developed as the catheter is advanced from the skin entry site to the point of venous cannulation. The catheter tip must reside in the subclavian, innominate or iliac veins, the inferior or superior vena cava, or right atrium to be considered a "central venous" catheter.

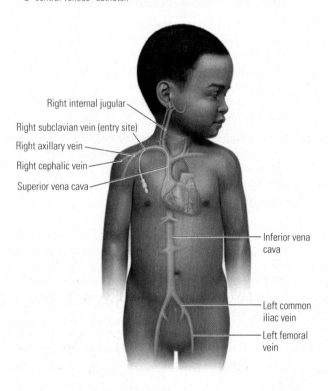

Right internal jugular
Right subclavian vein (entry site)
Right axillary vein
Right cephalic vein
Superior vena cava
Inferior vena cava
Left common iliac vein
Left femoral vein

Insertion of Non-Tunneled Centrally Inserted Central Venous Catheter
36556

During placement of a central venous catheter, a short tract is developed as the catheter is advanced from the skin entry site to the point of venous cannulation. The catheter tip must reside in the subclavian, innominate or iliac veins, the inferior or superior vena cava, or right atrium, to be considered a "central venous" catheter.

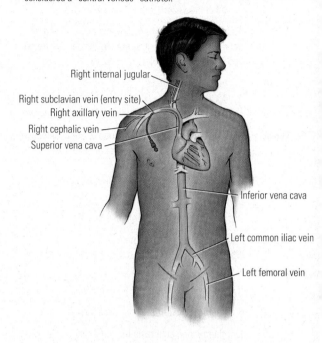

Right internal jugular
Right subclavian vein (entry site)
Right axillary vein
Right cephalic vein
Superior vena cava
Inferior vena cava
Left common iliac vein
Left femoral vein

Insertion of Tunneled Central Venous Catheter
36557-36558

36557   Insertion of tunneled centrally inserted central venous catheter, without subcutaneous port or pump; younger than 5 years of age

> ➔ *CPT Changes: An Insider's View* 2004, 2017
> ➔ *CPT Assistant* Dec 04:7, Jun 08:8
> ➔ *Clinical Examples in Radiology* Winter 09:9, Spring 09:10, Winter 17:10

36558   age 5 years or older

> ➔ *CPT Changes: An Insider's View* 2004, 2017
> ➔ *CPT Assistant* Dec 04:7, Jun 08:8, Jan 15:13
> ➔ *Clinical Examples in Radiology* Winter 09:9, Spring 09:10, Winter 17:10

(For peripherally inserted central venous catheter with port, 5 years or older, use 36571)

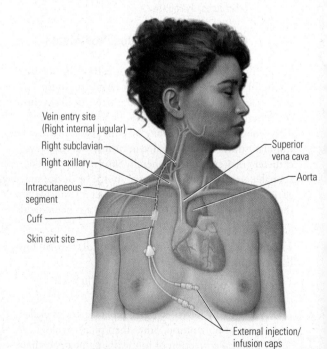

Vein entry site (Right internal jugular)
Right subclavian
Right axillary
Intracutaneous segment
Cuff
Skin exit site
Superior vena cava
Aorta
External injection/ infusion caps

The Central Venous Access Procedures Table

	Non-tunneled	Tunneled Without Port or Pump (w/out port or pump)	Central Tunneled	Tunneled With Port (w/port)	Tunneled With Pump (w/pump)	Peripheral	<5 years	≥5 years	Any Age
Insertion									
Catheter (without imaging guidance)	36555						36555		
	36556							36556	
		36557	36557				36557		
		36558	36558					36558	
	36568 (w/o port or pump)					36568 (w/o port or pump)	36568 (w/o port or pump)		
	36569 (w/o port or pump)					36569 (w/o port or pump)		36569 (w/o port or pump)	
Catheter (with bundled imaging guidance)						36572 (w/o port or pump)	36572 (w/o port or pump)		
						36573 (w/o port or pump)		36573 (w/o port or pump)	
Device			36560	36560			36560		
			36561	36561				36561	
			36563		36563				36563
		36565	36565						36565
			36566	36566					
	36570 (w/port)			36570 (w/port)		36570 (w/port)	36570 (w/port)		
	36571 (w/port)			36571 (w/port)		36571 (w/port)		36571 (w/port)	
Repair									
Catheter	36575 (w/o port or pump)	36575 (w/o port or pump)	36575 (w/o port or pump)			36575 (w/o port or pump)			36575
Device	36576 (w/port or pump)					36576 (w/port or pump)			36576
Partial Replacement - Central Venous Access Device (Catheter only)									
			36578	36578	36578	36578			36578
Complete Replacement - Central Venous Access Device (Through Same Venous Access Site)									
Catheter (without imaging guidance)	36580 (w/o port or pump)								36580
		36581	36581						36581
Catheter (with bundled imaging guidance)	36584 (w/o port or pump)					36584 (w/o port or pump)			36584 (w/o port or pump)
Device			36582	36582					36582
			36583		36583				36583
				36585 (w/port)		36585 (w/port)			36585
Removal									
Catheter		36589							36589
Device			36590	36590	36590	36590			36590
Removal of Obstructive Material from Device									
	36595 (pericatheter)	36595 (pericatheter)	36595 (pericatheter)	36595 (pericatheter)	36595 (pericatheter)	36595 (pericatheter)			36595 (pericatheter)
	36596 (intraluminal)	36596 (intraluminal)	36596 (intraluminal)	36596 (intraluminal)	36596 (intraluminal)	36596 (intraluminal)			36596 (intraluminal)
Repositioning of Catheter									
	36597	36597	36597	36597	36597	36597	36597	36597	36597

Cardiovascular 33016-39599

36560 Insertion of tunneled centrally inserted central venous access device, with subcutaneous port; younger than 5 years of age

➔ *CPT Changes: An Insider's View* 2004, 2017

➔ *CPT Assistant* Dec 04:7, Jun 08:8, Dec 09:11

➔ *Clinical Examples in Radiology* Winter 09:9, Spring 09:10, Winter 17:10

(For peripherally inserted central venous access device with subcutaneous port, younger than 5 years of age, use 36570)

36561 age 5 years or older

➔ *CPT Changes: An Insider's View* 2004, 2017

➔ *CPT Assistant* Dec 04:7, Jun 08:8, Dec 09:11, Jan 22:18

➔ *Clinical Examples in Radiology* Winter 09:9, Spring 09:10, Winter 17:10

(For peripherally inserted central venous catheter with subcutaneous port, 5 years or older, use 36571)

36563 Insertion of tunneled centrally inserted central venous access device with subcutaneous pump

➔ *CPT Changes: An Insider's View* 2004, 2017

➔ *CPT Assistant* Dec 04:8, Jun 08:8

➔ *Clinical Examples in Radiology* Winter 09:9, Spring 09:10, Winter 17:10

36565 Insertion of tunneled centrally inserted central venous access device, requiring 2 catheters via 2 separate venous access sites; without subcutaneous port or pump (eg, Tesio type catheter)

➔ *CPT Changes: An Insider's View* 2004, 2017

➔ *CPT Assistant* Dec 04:8, Jun 08:8

➔ *Clinical Examples in Radiology* Winter 09:9, Spring 09:10, Winter 17:10

36566 with subcutaneous port(s)

➔ *CPT Changes: An Insider's View* 2004, 2017

➔ *CPT Assistant* Dec 04:8, Jun 08:8

➔ *Clinical Examples in Radiology* Winter 09:9, Spring 09:10, Winter 17:10

Peripherally inserted central venous catheters (PICCs) may be placed or replaced with or without imaging guidance. When performed without imaging guidance, report using 36568 or 36569. When imaging guidance (eg, ultrasound, fluoroscopy) is used for PICC placement or complete replacement, bundled service codes 36572, 36573, 36584 include all imaging necessary to complete the procedure, image documentation (representative images from all modalities used are stored to patient's permanent record), associated radiological supervision and interpretation, venography performed through the same venous puncture, and documentation of final central position of the catheter with imaging. Ultrasound guidance for PICC placement should include documentation of evaluation of the potential puncture sites, patency of the entry vein, and real-time ultrasound visualization of needle entry into the vein.

Codes 71045, 71046, 71047, 71048 should not be reported for the purpose of documenting the final catheter position on the same day of service as 36572, 36573, 36584. Codes 36572, 36573, 36584 include confirmation of catheter tip location. The physician or other qualified health care professional reporting image-guided PICC insertion cannot report confirmation of catheter tip location separately (eg, via X ray, ultrasound). Report 36572, 36573, 36584 with modifier 52 when performed without confirmation of catheter tip location.

"Midline" catheters by definition terminate in the peripheral venous system. They are **not** central venous access devices and may not be reported as a PICC service. Midline catheter placement may be reported with 36400, 36406, or 36410. PICCs placed using magnetic guidance or any other guidance modality that does not include imaging or image documentation are reported with 36568, 36569.

36568 Insertion of peripherally inserted central venous catheter (PICC), without subcutaneous port or pump, without imaging guidance; younger than 5 years of age

➔ *CPT Changes: An Insider's View* 2004, 2017, 2019

➔ *CPT Assistant* Oct 04:14, Dec 04:8, May 05:13, Jun 08:8, Nov 12:14, May 19:3

➔ *Clinical Examples in Radiology* Winter 09:9, Spring 09:10, Winter 17:10, Fall 18:7, Winter 19:12, Fall 19:12

(For placement of centrally inserted non-tunneled central venous catheter, without subcutaneous port or pump, younger than 5 years of age, use 36555)

(For placement of peripherally inserted non-tunneled central venous catheter, without subcutaneous port or pump, with imaging guidance, younger than 5 years of age, use 36572)

36569 age 5 years or older

➔ *CPT Changes: An Insider's View* 2004, 2019

➔ *CPT Assistant* Oct 04:14, Dec 04:8, May 05:13, Jun 08:8, Nov 12:14, Sep 13:18, Sep 14:13, May 19:3

➔ *Clinical Examples in Radiology* Inaugural 04:1-2, Spring 08:7, Fall 08:5-6, Winter 09:9, Spring 09:10, Winter 17:10, Fall 18:7, Winter 19:12, Fall 19:12

(Do not report 36568, 36569 in conjunction with 76937, 77001)

(For placement of centrally inserted non-tunneled central venous catheter, without subcutaneous port or pump, age 5 years or older, use 36556)

(For placement of peripherally inserted non-tunneled central venous catheter, without subcutaneous port or pump, with imaging guidance, age 5 years or older, use 36573)

36572   Insertion of peripherally inserted central venous catheter (PICC), without subcutaneous port or pump, including all imaging guidance, image documentation, and all associated radiological supervision and interpretation required to perform the insertion; younger than 5 years of age
➔ *CPT Changes: An Insider's View* 2019
➔ *CPT Assistant* Mar 19:10, May 19:3
➔ *Clinical Examples in Radiology* Fall 18:7, Winter 19:12, Fall 19:11

(For placement of centrally inserted non-tunneled central venous catheter, without subcutaneous port or pump, younger than 5 years of age, use 36555)

(For placement of peripherally inserted non-tunneled central venous catheter, without subcutaneous port or pump, without imaging guidance, younger than 5 years of age, use 36568)

36573   age 5 years or older
➔ *CPT Changes: An Insider's View* 2019
➔ *CPT Assistant* Mar 19:10, May 19:3
➔ *Clinical Examples in Radiology* Fall 18:7, Winter 19:13, Fall 19:11

(For placement of centrally inserted non-tunneled central venous catheter, without subcutaneous port or pump, age 5 years or older, use 36556)

(For placement of peripherally inserted non-tunneled central venous catheter, without subcutaneous port or pump, without imaging guidance, age 5 years or older, use 36569)

(Do not report 36572, 36573 in conjunction with 76937, 77001)

36570   Insertion of peripherally inserted central venous access device, with subcutaneous port; younger than 5 years of age
➔ *CPT Changes: An Insider's View* 2004, 2017
➔ *CPT Assistant* Dec 04:8, Jun 08:8, Dec 09:11
➔ *Clinical Examples in Radiology* Winter 09:9, Spring 09:10, Winter 17:10

(For insertion of tunneled centrally inserted central venous access device with subcutaneous port, younger than 5 years of age, use 36560)

36571   age 5 years or older
➔ *CPT Changes: An Insider's View* 2004, 2017
➔ *CPT Assistant* Dec 04:9, Jun 08:8, Dec 09:11
➔ *Clinical Examples in Radiology* Winter 09:9, Spring 09:10, Winter 17:10

(For insertion of tunneled centrally inserted central venous access device with subcutaneous port, age 5 years or older, use 36561)

36572   Code is out of numerical sequence. See 36568-36571

36573   Code is out of numerical sequence. See 36568-36571

Peripherally Inserted Central Catheter
36572

A peripherally inserted central catheter, which is non-tunneled and without a subcutaneous port/pump, is placed in a child younger than 5 years of age.

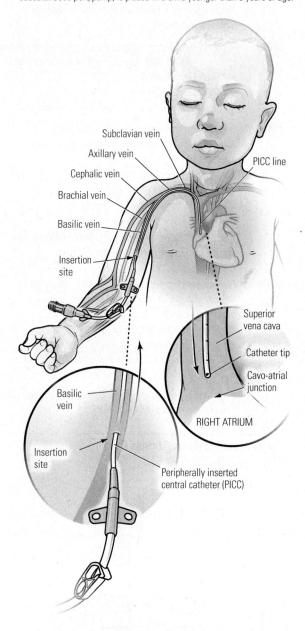

Subclavian vein
Axillary vein
Cephalic vein
Brachial vein
Basilic vein
PICC line
Insertion site
Superior vena cava
Catheter tip
Cavo-atrial junction
Basilic vein
RIGHT ATRIUM
Insertion site
Peripherally inserted central catheter (PICC)

Repair of Central Venous Access Device

(For mechanical removal of pericatheter obstructive material, use 36595)

(For mechanical removal of intracatheter obstructive material, use 36596)

36575 Repair of tunneled or non-tunneled central venous access catheter, without subcutaneous port or pump, central or peripheral insertion site
➲ *CPT Changes: An Insider's View* 2004
➲ *Clinical Examples in Radiology* Spring 09:10, Summer 10:11

36576 Repair of central venous access device, with subcutaneous port or pump, central or peripheral insertion site
➲ *CPT Changes: An Insider's View* 2004, 2017
➲ *CPT Assistant* Dec 04:9, Jun 08:8
➲ *Clinical Examples in Radiology* Spring 09:10

Partial Replacement of Central Venous Access Device (Catheter Only)

36578 Replacement, catheter only, of central venous access device, with subcutaneous port or pump, central or peripheral insertion site
➲ *CPT Changes: An Insider's View* 2004, 2017
➲ *CPT Assistant* Dec 04:10, Jun 08:8
➲ *Clinical Examples in Radiology* Winter 09:9, Spring 09:10, Winter 17:10

(For complete replacement of entire device through same venous access, use 36582 or 36583)

Implantable Venous Access Port
36570, 36571, 36576, 36578

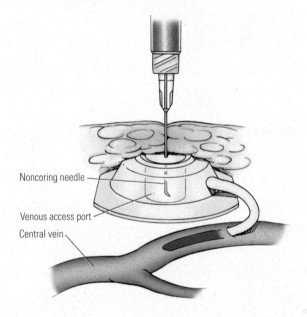

Noncoring needle

Venous access port

Central vein

Complete Replacement of Central Venous Access Device Through Same Venous Access Site

36580 Replacement, complete, of a non-tunneled centrally inserted central venous catheter, without subcutaneous port or pump, through same venous access
➲ *CPT Changes: An Insider's View* 2004
➲ *CPT Assistant* Dec 04:10, Jun 08:8
➲ *Clinical Examples in Radiology* Winter 09:9, Spring 09:10, Winter 17:10

36581 Replacement, complete, of a tunneled centrally inserted central venous catheter, without subcutaneous port or pump, through same venous access
➲ *CPT Changes: An Insider's View* 2004, 2017
➲ *CPT Assistant* Dec 04:10, Jun 08:8, Jul 23:17
➲ *Clinical Examples in Radiology* Winter 09:9, Spring 09:10, Winter 17:10, Fall 23:28

36582 Replacement, complete, of a tunneled centrally inserted central venous access device, with subcutaneous port, through same venous access
➲ *CPT Changes: An Insider's View* 2004, 2017
➲ *CPT Assistant* Dec 04:10, Jun 08:8
➲ *Clinical Examples in Radiology* Winter 09:9, Spring 09:10, Winter 17:10

36583 Replacement, complete, of a tunneled centrally inserted central venous access device, with subcutaneous pump, through same venous access
➲ *CPT Changes: An Insider's View* 2004, 2017
➲ *CPT Assistant* Dec 04:10-11, Jun 08:8
➲ *Clinical Examples in Radiology* Winter 09:9, Spring 09:10, Winter 17:10

36584 Replacement, complete, of a peripherally inserted central venous catheter (PICC), without subcutaneous port or pump, through same venous access, including all imaging guidance, image documentation, and all associated radiological supervision and interpretation required to perform the replacement
➲ *CPT Changes: An Insider's View* 2004, 2019
➲ *CPT Assistant* Dec 04:11, Jun 08:8, Mar 19:10, May 19:3
➲ *Clinical Examples in Radiology* Winter 09:9, Spring 09:10, Winter 17:10, Fall 18:8

(For replacement of a peripherally inserted central venous catheter [PICC] without subcutaneous port or pump, through same venous access, without imaging guidance, use 37799)

(Do not report 36584 in conjunction with 76937, 77001)

★=Telemedicine ◀=Audio-only ✚=Add-on code ✗=FDA approval pending #=Resequenced code ⊘=Modifier 51 exempt ➲➲➲=See p xxi for details

36585   Replacement, complete, of a peripherally inserted central venous access device, with subcutaneous port, through same venous access

➔ *CPT Changes: An Insider's View* 2004, 2017

➔ *CPT Assistant* Dec 04:11, Jun 08:8

➔ *Clinical Examples in Radiology* Winter 09:9, Spring 09:10, Winter 17:10

Removal of Central Venous Access Device

36589   Removal of tunneled central venous catheter, without subcutaneous port or pump

➔ *CPT Changes: An Insider's View* 2004

➔ *CPT Assistant* Dec 04:11, Jun 08:8, Nov 15:10

36590   Removal of tunneled central venous access device, with subcutaneous port or pump, central or peripheral insertion

➔ *CPT Changes: An Insider's View* 2004, 2017

➔ *CPT Assistant* Dec 04:11, Jun 08:8, Jul 10:10

➔ *Clinical Examples in Radiology* Spring 08:7

(Do not report 36589 or 36590 for removal of non-tunneled central venous catheters)

Other Central Venous Access Procedures

36591   Collection of blood specimen from a completely implantable venous access device

➔ *CPT Changes: An Insider's View* 2008

➔ *CPT Assistant* Apr 08:9, Jul 11:16, May 14:4, Aug 19:8, Jan 22:3

(Do not report 36591 in conjunction with other services except a laboratory service)

(For collection of venous blood specimen by venipuncture, use 36415)

(For collection of capillary blood specimen, use 36416)

36592   Collection of blood specimen using established central or peripheral catheter, venous, not otherwise specified

➔ *CPT Changes: An Insider's View* 2008

➔ *CPT Assistant* Apr 08:9, Jul 11:16

(For blood collection from an established arterial catheter, use 37799)

(Do not report 36592 in conjunction with other services except a laboratory service)

36593   Declotting by thrombolytic agent of implanted vascular access device or catheter

➔ *CPT Changes: An Insider's View* 2008

➔ *CPT Assistant* Apr 08:9, Dec 09:11, Aug 11:9, Feb 13:3

➔ *Clinical Examples in Radiology* Summer 12:4-5

36595   Mechanical removal of pericatheter obstructive material (eg, fibrin sheath) from central venous device via separate venous access

➔ *CPT Changes: An Insider's View* 2004

➔ *CPT Assistant* Dec 04:9, 12

(Do not report 36595 in conjunction with 36593)

(For venous catheterization, see 36010-36012)

(For radiological supervision and interpretation, use 75901)

36596   Mechanical removal of intraluminal (intracatheter) obstructive material from central venous device through device lumen

➔ *CPT Changes: An Insider's View* 2004

➔ *CPT Assistant* Dec 04:9, 12

(Do not report 36596 in conjunction with 36593)

(For venous catheterization, see 36010-36012)

(For radiological supervision and interpretation, use 75902)

36597   Repositioning of previously placed central venous catheter under fluoroscopic guidance

➔ *CPT Changes: An Insider's View* 2004

➔ *CPT Assistant* Dec 04:12, Sep 14:5

(For fluoroscopic guidance, use 76000)

36598   Contrast injection(s) for radiologic evaluation of existing central venous access device, including fluoroscopy, image documentation and report

➔ *CPT Changes: An Insider's View* 2006

➔ *Clinical Examples in Radiology* Winter 06:15, Spring 08:7, Summer 12:4

(Do not report 36598 in conjunction with 76000)

(Do not report 36598 in conjunction with 36595, 36596)

(For complete diagnostic studies, see 75820, 75825, 75827)

Arterial

36600   Arterial puncture, withdrawal of blood for diagnosis

➔ *CPT Assistant* Fall 95:7, Aug 00:2, Oct 03:2, Jul 05:11, Jul 06:4, Feb 07:10, Jul 07:1, May 14:4, Aug 19:8, Jan 22:3

36620   Arterial catheterization or cannulation for sampling, monitoring or transfusion (separate procedure); percutaneous

➔ *CPT Assistant* Fall 95:7, Apr 98:3, Nov 99:32-33, Aug 00:2, Oct 03:2, Jul 06:4, Jul 07:1

36625   cutdown

➔ *CPT Assistant* Fall 95:7

36640   Arterial catheterization for prolonged infusion therapy (chemotherapy), cutdown

➔ *CPT Assistant* Fall 95:7

(See also 96420-96425)

(For arterial catheterization for occlusion therapy, see 75894)

36660 Catheterization, umbilical artery, newborn, for diagnosis or therapy

➲ *CPT Changes: An Insider's View* 2008

➲ *CPT Assistant* Fall 95:8, Oct 03:2, Jul 06:4, Jul 07:1

(Do not report modifier 63 in conjunction with 36660)

Intraosseous

36680 Placement of needle for intraosseous infusion

Hemodialysis Access, Intervascular Cannulation for Extracorporeal Circulation, or Shunt Insertion

36800 Insertion of cannula for hemodialysis, other purpose (separate procedure); vein to vein

➲ *CPT Assistant* Fall 93:3, Mar 23:23

36810 arteriovenous, external (Scribner type)

➲ *CPT Assistant* Fall 93:3, May 97:10

36815 arteriovenous, external revision, or closure

➲ *CPT Assistant* Fall 93:3, Mar 23:23

36818 Arteriovenous anastomosis, open; by upper arm cephalic vein transposition

➲ *CPT Changes: An Insider's View* 2005

➲ *CPT Assistant* Jul 05:9, Mar 16:10, Mar 17:5, Mar 23:23

(Do not report 36818 in conjunction with 36819, 36820, 36821, 36830 during a unilateral upper extremity procedure. For bilateral upper extremity open arteriovenous anastomoses performed at the same operative session, use modifier 50 or 59 as appropriate)

36819 by upper arm basilic vein transposition

➲ *CPT Changes: An Insider's View* 2000, 2002

➲ *CPT Assistant* Nov 99:20, Jul 05:9, Mar 17:5, Mar 23:23

(Do not report 36819 in conjunction with 36818, 36820, 36821, 36830 during a unilateral upper extremity procedure. For bilateral upper extremity open arteriovenous anastomoses performed at the same operative session, use modifier 50 or 59 as appropriate)

36820 by forearm vein transposition

➲ *CPT Changes: An Insider's View* 2002

➲ *CPT Assistant* Fall 93:4, Jul 05:9, Mar 17:5, Mar 23:23

36821 direct, any site (eg, Cimino type) (separate procedure)

➲ *CPT Changes: An Insider's View* 2000

➲ *CPT Assistant* Fall 93:3, Feb 97:2, Nov 99:20, Jul 05:9, Aug 15:8, Mar 17:5, Mar 23:23

Arteriovenous Anastomosis, Direct
36821

A section of artery and a neighboring vein are joined, allowing blood to flow down the artery and into the vein for the purpose of increasing blood flow, usually in hemodialysis.

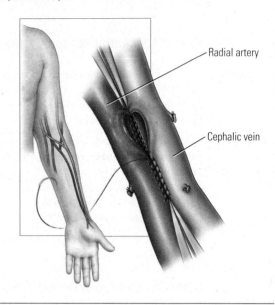

Radial artery

Cephalic vein

36823 Insertion of arterial and venous cannula(s) for isolated extracorporeal circulation including regional chemotherapy perfusion to an extremity, with or without hyperthermia, with removal of cannula(s) and repair of arteriotomy and venotomy sites

➲ *CPT Changes: An Insider's View* 2002

➲ *CPT Assistant* Nov 98:14-15, Mar 17:5

(36823 includes chemotherapy perfusion supported by a membrane oxygenator/perfusion pump. Do not report 96409-96425 in conjunction with 36823)

36825 Creation of arteriovenous fistula by other than direct arteriovenous anastomosis (separate procedure); autogenous graft

➲ *CPT Assistant* Fall 93:3, Feb 97:2, Jul 05:9, Mar 17:5

(For direct arteriovenous anastomosis, use 36821)

36830 nonautogenous graft (eg, biological collagen, thermoplastic graft)

➲ *CPT Changes: An Insider's View* 2003

➲ *CPT Assistant* Fall 93:3, Feb 97:2, Jul 05:9, Jan 15:13, Mar 17:5, Nov 23:25

(For direct arteriovenous anastomosis, use 36821)

Arteriovenous Fistula
36825-36830

A donor's vein (36825) or a synthetic vein (36830) is used to connect an artery and vein.

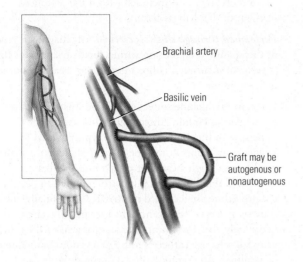

- Brachial artery
- Basilic vein
- Graft may be autogenous or nonautogenous

36831   Thrombectomy, open, arteriovenous fistula without revision, autogenous or nonautogenous dialysis graft (separate procedure)

➜ *CPT Changes: An Insider's View* 2001

➜ *CPT Assistant* Nov 98:14-15, Feb 99:6, Mar 99:6, Apr 99:11, Mar 17:5

36832   Revision, open, arteriovenous fistula; without thrombectomy, autogenous or nonautogenous dialysis graft (separate procedure)

➜ *CPT Changes: An Insider's View* 2000, 2001

➜ *CPT Assistant* Fall 93:3, Feb 97:2, Nov 98:15, Feb 99:6, Mar 99:6, Apr 99:11, Nov 99:20-21, Mar 17:5, May 22:16

36833   with thrombectomy, autogenous or nonautogenous dialysis graft (separate procedure)

➜ *CPT Assistant* Nov 98:15, Feb 99:6, Apr 99:11, Mar 17:5

(For percutaneous thrombectomy within the dialysis circuit, see 36904, 36905, 36906)

(For central dialysis segment angioplasty in conjunction with 36818-36833, use 36907)

(For central dialysis segment stent placement in conjunction with 36818-36833, use 36908)

(Do not report 36832, 36833 in conjunction with 36901, 36902, 36903, 36904, 36905, 36906 for revision of the dialysis circuit)

Codes 36836, 36837 describe percutaneous arteriovenous fistula creation in the upper extremity for hemodialysis access, including image-guided percutaneous access into a peripheral artery and peripheral vein via single access (36836) or two separate access sites (36837). The artery and vein are approximated and then energy (eg, thermal) is applied to establish the fistulous communication between the two vessels. Fistula maturation procedures promote blood flow through the newly created fistula by augmentation (eg, angioplasty) or redirection (eg, coil embolization of collateral pathways) of blood flow. Codes 36836, 36837 include all vascular access, angiography, imaging guidance, and blood flow redirection or maturation techniques (eg, transluminal balloon angioplasty, coil embolization) performed for fistula creation. These procedures may not be reported separately with 36836, 36837, when performed at the same operative session.

 # 36836   Percutaneous arteriovenous fistula creation, upper extremity, single access of both the peripheral artery and peripheral vein, including fistula maturation procedures (eg, transluminal balloon angioplasty, coil embolization) when performed, including all vascular access, imaging guidance and radiologic supervision and interpretation

➜ *CPT Changes: An Insider's View* 2023

➜ *CPT Assistant* Oct 22:11, Mar 23:23

(Do not report 36836 in conjunction with 36005, 36140, 36215, 36216, 36217, 36218, 36245, 36246, 36247, 36837, 36901, 36902, 36903, 36904, 36905, 36906, 36907, 36908, 36909, 37236, 37238, 37241, 37242, 37246, 37248, 37252, 75710, 75716, 75820, 75822, 75894, 75898, 76937, 77001)

(For arteriovenous fistula creation via an open approach, see 36800, 36810, 36815, 36818, 36819, 36820, 36821)

(For percutaneous arteriovenous fistula creation in any location other than the upper extremity, use 37799)

 # 36837   Percutaneous arteriovenous fistula creation, upper extremity, separate access sites of the peripheral artery and peripheral vein, including fistula maturation procedures (eg, transluminal balloon angioplasty, coil embolization) when performed, including all vascular access, imaging guidance and radiologic supervision and interpretation

➜ *CPT Changes: An Insider's View* 2023

➜ *CPT Assistant* Oct 22:11, Mar 23:23

(Do not report 36837 in conjunction with 36005, 36140, 36215, 36216, 36217, 36218, 36245, 36246, 36247, 36836, 36901, 36902, 36903, 36904, 36905, 36906, 36907, 36908, 36909, 37236, 37238, 37241, 37242, 37246, 37248, 37252, 75710, 75716, 75820, 75822, 75894, 75898, 76937, 77001)

(For arteriovenous fistula creation via an open approach, see 36800, 36810, 36815, 36818, 36819, 36820, 36821)

(For percutaneous arteriovenous fistula creation in any location other than the upper extremity, use 37799)

36835   Insertion of Thomas shunt (separate procedure)

36836   Code is out of numerical sequence. See 36832-36838

36837   Code is out of numerical sequence. See 36832-36838

36838   Distal revascularization and interval ligation (DRIL), upper extremity hemodialysis access (steal syndrome)

➔ *CPT Changes: An Insider's View* 2004

(Do not report 36838 in conjunction with 35512, 35522, 35523, 36832, 37607, 37618)

36860   External cannula declotting (separate procedure); without balloon catheter

➔ *CPT Assistant* Fall 93:3, Feb 97:2, Nov 98:15, Feb 99:6, May 01:3

36861   with balloon catheter

➔ *CPT Assistant* Fall 93:3, Feb 97:2, May 01:3

(If imaging guidance is performed, use 76000)

Dialysis Circuit

Definitions

Dialysis circuit: The arteriovenous (AV) dialysis circuit is designed for easy and repetitive access to perform hemodialysis. It begins at the arterial anastomosis and extends to the right atrium. The circuit may be created using either an arterial-venous anastomosis, known as an arteriovenous fistula (AVF), or a prosthetic graft placed between an artery and vein, known as an arteriovenous graft (AVG). The dialysis circuit is comprised of two segments, termed the (1) peripheral dialysis segment and (2) central dialysis segment. Both are defined as follows.

Peripheral dialysis segment: The peripheral dialysis segment is the portion of the dialysis circuit that begins at the arterial anastomosis and extends to the central dialysis segment. In the upper extremity, the peripheral dialysis segment extends through the axillary vein (or entire cephalic vein in the case of cephalic venous outflow). In the lower extremity, the peripheral dialysis segment extends through the common femoral vein. The peripheral dialysis segment includes the historic "peri-anastomotic region" (defined below).

Central dialysis segment: The central dialysis segment includes all draining veins central to the peripheral dialysis segment. In the upper extremity, the central dialysis segment includes the veins central to the axillary and cephalic veins, including the subclavian and innominate veins through the superior vena cava. In the lower extremity, the central dialysis segment includes the veins central to the common femoral vein, including the external iliac and common iliac veins through the inferior vena cava.

Peri-anastomotic region: A historic term referring to the region of a dialysis circuit near the arterial anastomosis encompassing a short segment of the parent artery, the anastomosis, and a short segment of the dialysis circuit immediately adjacent to the anastomosis. The peri-anastomotic region is included within the peripheral segment of the dialysis circuit.

Performed through dialysis circuit: Any diagnostic study or therapeutic intervention within the dialysis circuit that is performed through a direct percutaneous access to the dialysis circuit.

Code 36901 includes direct access and imaging of the entire dialysis circuit. Antegrade and/or retrograde punctures of the dialysis circuit are typically used for imaging, and contrast may be injected directly through a needle or through a catheter placed into the dialysis circuit. All dialysis circuit punctures required to perform the procedure are included in 36901. Occasionally, the catheter needs to be advanced further into the circuit to adequately visualize the arterial anastomosis or the central veins, or selective catheterization of a venous branch may be required. All manipulation(s) of the catheter for diagnostic imaging of the dialysis circuit is included in 36901. Advancement of the catheter to the vena cava to adequately image that segment of the dialysis circuit is included in 36901 and is not separately reported. Code 36901 also includes catheterization of additional venous side branches communicating with the dialysis circuit, known as accessory veins. Advancement of the catheter tip through the arterial anastomosis to adequately visualize the anastomosis is also included in the service described by 36901 and is not separately reported. Evaluation of the peri-anastomotic portion of the inflow is an integral part of the dialysis circuit angiogram and is included in 36901.

For the purposes of reporting dialysis access maintenance services, the arterial inflow to the dialysis circuit is considered a separate vessel. If a more proximal arterial inflow problem separate from the peripheral dialysis segment is suspected, additional catheter placement and imaging required for adequate evaluation of the artery may be separately reported. If a catheter is selectively advanced from the dialysis circuit puncture beyond the peri-anastomotic segment into the inflow artery, an additional catheterization code may be reported. For example, 36215 may be used to report image-guided retrograde catheter placement into the inflow artery and into the aorta, if necessary (36200 is not reported in addition to 36215 in this example). Note that 75710 may

Cardiovascular 33016-39599

also be reported if contrast injection for diagnostic arteriography is performed through this catheter and radiological supervision and interpretation and imaging documentation is performed.

Ultrasound guidance for puncture of the dialysis circuit access is not typically performed and is not included in 36901, 36902, 36903, 36904, 36905, 36906. However, in the case of a new (immature) or failing AVF, ultrasound may be necessary to safely and effectively puncture the dialysis circuit for evaluation, and this may be reported separately with 76937, if all the appropriate elements for reporting 76937 are performed and documented.

For radiological supervision and interpretation of dialysis circuit angiography performed through existing access(es) or catheter-based arterial access, report 36901 with modifier 52.

Dialysis Circuit Interventions (AV Grafts and AV Fistulae): For the purposes of coding interventional procedures in the dialysis circuit (both AVF and AVG), the dialysis circuit is artificially divided into two distinct segments: peripheral dialysis segment and central dialysis segment (see definitions).

Codes 36901, 36902, 36903 and 36904, 36905, 36906 are built on progressive hierarchies that have more intensive services, which include less intensive services. Report only one code (36901, 36902, 36903, 36904, 36905, 36906) for services provided in a dialysis circuit.

Code 36901 describes the diagnostic evaluation of the dialysis circuit, and this service is included in the services described by 36901, 36902, 36903, 36904, 36905, 36906. All catheterizations required to perform diagnostic fistulography are included in 36901. All catheterizations required to perform additional interventional services are included in codes 36902, 36903, 36904, 36905, 36906, 36907, 36908, 36909 and not separately reported. All angiography, fluoroscopic image guidance, roadmapping, and radiological supervision and interpretation required to perform each service are included in each code. Closure of the puncture(s) by any method is included in the service of each individual code.

Code 36902 includes the services in 36901 plus transluminal balloon angioplasty in the peripheral segment of the dialysis circuit. Code 36902 would be reported only once per session to describe all angioplasty services performed in the peripheral segment of the dialysis circuit, regardless of the number of distinct lesions treated within that segment, the number of times the balloon is inflated, or the number of balloon catheters or sizes required to open all lesions, and includes angioplasty of the peri-anastomotic segment when performed. Code 36903 includes the services in 36902 plus transcatheter stent placement in the peripheral segment of the dialysis circuit. Code 36903 is reported only once per session to describe placing stent(s) within

the peripheral segment, regardless of the number of stent(s) placed or the number of discrete lesion(s) treated within the peripheral segment. If both angioplasty and stenting are performed in the peripheral segment, including treatment of separate lesions, report 36903 only once.

Code 36904 describes percutaneous transluminal mechanical thrombectomy and/or infusion for thrombolysis in the dialysis circuit (all thrombus treated in both the peripheral and central dialysis circuit segments) and includes diagnostic angiography (36901), fluoroscopic image guidance, catheter placement(s), and all maneuvers required to remove thrombus from the peripheral and/or central segments, including all intraprocedural pharmacological thrombolytic injection(s)/infusion(s). It is never appropriate to report removal of the arterial plug during a declot/thrombectomy procedure as an angioplasty (36905). Removal of the arterial plug is included in a fistula thrombectomy, even if a balloon catheter is used to mechanically dislodge the resistant thrombus. Codes 36905 (angioplasty) and 36906 (stent) describe services in the peripheral circuit when performed in conjunction with thrombolysis/thrombectomy. Code 36905 includes the services in 36904 plus transluminal balloon angioplasty in the peripheral segment of the dialysis circuit. Code 36905 may be reported only once per session to describe all angioplasty performed in the peripheral segment of the dialysis circuit, regardless of the number of distinct lesions treated within that segment, the number of times the balloon is inflated, or the number of balloon catheters required to open all lesions. Code 36906 includes the services in 36905 plus transcatheter stent placement in the peripheral segment of the dialysis circuit. Code 36906 is reported only once per session to describe placing stent(s) within the peripheral segment, regardless of the number of stent(s) placed or the number of discrete lesion(s) treated within the peripheral segment.

Codes 36907 and 36908 describe procedures performed through puncture(s) in the dialysis circuit. Similar procedures performed from a different access (eg, common femoral vein) may be reported using 37248, 37249 or 37238, 37239. Code 36907 is an add-on code used in conjunction with 36901, 36902, 36903, 36904, 36905, 36906 to report angioplasty within the central dialysis segment when performed through puncture of the dialysis circuit, and is reported once per session independent of the number of discrete lesions treated, the number of balloon inflations, and number of balloon catheters or sizes required. These additional services should be clearly documented in the patient record, including the recorded images. Code 36907 may be reported only once per session with 36901, 36902, 36903, 36904, 36905, 36906, as appropriate. Report 36907 once for all angioplasty performed within the central dialysis segment.

Code 36908 is an add-on code used in conjunction with 36901, 36902, 36903, 36904, 36905, 36906 to report stenting lesion(s) in the central dialysis segment when performed through puncture of the dialysis circuit. It is reported once, regardless of the number of discrete lesions treated or the number of stents placed. Code 36908 includes the services in 36907; therefore, 36908 may not be reported with 36907 in the same session. Code 36908 may be reported only once per session with 36901, 36902, 36903, 36904, 36905, 36906, as appropriate.

Code 36909 is an add-on code used to report endovascular embolization or occlusion of the main vessel or side branches arising from (emptying into) the dialysis circuit. Code 36909 may only be reported once per therapeutic session, irrespective of the number of branches embolized or occluded. Embolization or occlusion of the main vessel or these side branches may not be reported with 37241.

If open dialysis circuit creation, revision, and/or thrombectomy (36818-36833) are performed, completion angiography is bundled, as is peripheral segment angioplasty and/or stent placement (36901, 36902, 36903) and, therefore, not separately reported. However, dialysis circuit central segment angioplasty and/or stent placement may be separately reported (36907, 36908).

36901　Introduction of needle(s) and/or catheter(s), dialysis circuit, with diagnostic angiography of the dialysis circuit, including all direct puncture(s) and catheter placement(s), injection(s) of contrast, all necessary imaging from the arterial anastomosis and adjacent artery through entire venous outflow including the inferior or superior vena cava, fluoroscopic guidance, radiological supervision and interpretation and image documentation and report;

➔ *CPT Changes: An Insider's View* 2017
➔ *CPT Assistant* Mar 17:3, May 17:3, Jul 21:4
➔ *Clinical Examples in Radiology* Spring 18:8

(Do not report 36901 in conjunction with 36833, 36836, 36837, 36902, 36903, 36904, 36905, 36906)

36902　with transluminal balloon angioplasty, peripheral dialysis segment, including all imaging and radiological supervision and interpretation necessary to perform the angioplasty

➔ *CPT Changes: An Insider's View* 2017
➔ *CPT Assistant* Mar 17:3, May 17:3
➔ *Clinical Examples in Radiology* Spring 18:8

(Do not report 36902 in conjunction with 36836, 36837, 36903)

36903　with transcatheter placement of intravascular stent(s), peripheral dialysis segment, including all imaging and radiological supervision and interpretation necessary to perform the stenting, and all angioplasty within the peripheral dialysis segment

➔ *CPT Changes: An Insider's View* 2017
➔ *CPT Assistant* Mar 17:3, May 17:3
➔ *Clinical Examples in Radiology* Spring 18:9

(Do not report 36902, 36903 in conjunction with 36833, 36836, 36837, 36904, 36905, 36906)

(Do not report 36901, 36902, 36903 more than once per operative session)

(For transluminal balloon angioplasty within central vein(s) when performed through dialysis circuit, use 36907)

(For transcatheter placement of intravascular stent(s) within central vein(s) when performed through dialysis circuit, use 36908)

36904　Percutaneous transluminal mechanical thrombectomy and/or infusion for thrombolysis, dialysis circuit, any method, including all imaging and radiological supervision and interpretation, diagnostic angiography, fluoroscopic guidance, catheter placement(s), and intraprocedural pharmacological thrombolytic injection(s);

➔ *CPT Changes: An Insider's View* 2017
➔ *CPT Assistant* Mar 17:3, May 17:3, Jun 22:22
➔ *Clinical Examples in Radiology* Spring 18:9

(Do not report 36904 in conjunction with 36836, 36837)

(For open thrombectomy within the dialysis circuit, see 36831, 36833)

36905　with transluminal balloon angioplasty, peripheral dialysis segment, including all imaging and radiological supervision and interpretation necessary to perform the angioplasty

➔ *CPT Changes: An Insider's View* 2017
➔ *CPT Assistant* Mar 17:3, May 17:3, Jun 22:22
➔ *Clinical Examples in Radiology* Spring 18:9

(Do not report 36905 in conjunction with 36836, 36837, 36904)

36906　with transcatheter placement of intravascular stent(s), peripheral dialysis segment, including all imaging and radiological supervision and interpretation necessary to perform the stenting, and all angioplasty within the peripheral dialysis circuit

➔ *CPT Changes: An Insider's View* 2017
➔ *CPT Assistant* Mar 17:3, May 17:3, Jul 21:4, Jun 22:22
➔ *Clinical Examples in Radiology* Spring 18:9

(Do not report 36906 in conjunction with 36836, 36837, 36901, 36902, 36903, 36904, 36905)

(Do not report 36904, 36905, 36906 more than once per operative session)

(For transluminal balloon angioplasty within central vein(s) when performed through dialysis circuit, use 36907)

(For transcatheter placement of intravascular stent(s) within central vein(s) when performed through dialysis circuit, use 36908)

+ 36907 Transluminal balloon angioplasty, central dialysis segment, performed through dialysis circuit, including all imaging and radiological supervision and interpretation required to perform the angioplasty (List separately in addition to code for primary procedure)
➔ CPT Changes: An Insider's View 2017
➔ CPT Assistant Mar 17:3, May 17:3
➔ Clinical Examples in Radiology Spring 18:8

(Use 36907 in conjunction with 36818-36833, 36901, 36902, 36903, 36904, 36905, 36906)

(Do not report 36907 in conjunction with 36836, 36837, 36908)

(Report 36907 once for all angioplasty performed within the central dialysis segment)

+ 36908 Transcatheter placement of intravascular stent(s), central dialysis segment, performed through dialysis circuit, including all imaging and radiological supervision and interpretation required to perform the stenting, and all angioplasty in the central dialysis segment (List separately in addition to code for primary procedure)
➔ CPT Changes: An Insider's View 2017, 2018
➔ CPT Assistant Mar 17:3, May 17:3

(Use 36908 in conjunction with 36818-36833, 36901, 36902, 36903, 36904, 36905, 36906)

(Do not report 36908 in conjunction with 36836, 36837, 36907)

(Report 36908 once for all stenting performed within the central dialysis segment)

+ 36909 Dialysis circuit permanent vascular embolization or occlusion (including main circuit or any accessory veins), endovascular, including all imaging and radiological supervision and interpretation necessary to complete the intervention (List separately in addition to primary procedure)
➔ CPT Changes: An Insider's View 2017
➔ CPT Assistant Mar 17:3, May 17:3, Jul 21:4, Jun 22:22

(Use 36909 in conjunction with 36901, 36902, 36903, 36904, 36905, 36906)

(Do not report 36909 in conjunction with 36836, 36837)

(For open ligation/occlusion in dialysis access, use 37607)

(36909 includes all permanent vascular occlusions within the dialysis circuit and may only be reported once per encounter per day)

Portal Decompression Procedures

37140 Venous anastomosis, open; portocaval
➔ CPT Changes: An Insider's View 2003

(For peritoneal-venous shunt, use 49425)

37145 renoportal

37160 caval-mesenteric

37180 splenorenal, proximal

37181 splenorenal, distal (selective decompression of esophagogastric varices, any technique)

(For percutaneous procedure, use 37182)

37182 Insertion of transvenous intrahepatic portosystemic shunt(s) (TIPS) (includes venous access, hepatic and portal vein catheterization, portography with hemodynamic evaluation, intrahepatic tract formation/dilatation, stent placement and all associated imaging guidance and documentation)
➔ CPT Changes: An Insider's View 2003
➔ CPT Assistant Dec 03:2, Sep 13:17, Jan 23:32
➔ Clinical Examples in Radiology Summer 10:2

(Do not report 75885 or 75887 in conjunction with 37182)

(For open procedure, use 37140)

37183 Revision of transvenous intrahepatic portosystemic shunt(s) (TIPS) (includes venous access, hepatic and portal vein catheterization, portography with hemodynamic evaluation, intrahepatic tract recannulization/dilatation, stent placement and all associated imaging guidance and documentation)
➔ CPT Changes: An Insider's View 2003, 2010, 2017
➔ CPT Assistant Dec 03:2, Jan 23:32
➔ Clinical Examples in Radiology Fall 09:9, Summer 10:3

(Do not report 75885 or 75887 in conjunction with 37183)

(For repair of arteriovenous aneurysm, use 36832)

Cardiovascular 33016-39599

Transcatheter Procedures

Codes for catheter placement and the radiologic supervision and interpretation should also be reported, in addition to the code(s) for the therapeutic aspect of the procedure.

Mechanical Thrombectomy

Code(s) for catheter placement(s), diagnostic studies, and other percutaneous interventions (eg, transluminal balloon angioplasty, stent placement) provided are separately reportable.

Codes 37184-37188 specifically include intraprocedural fluoroscopic radiological supervision and interpretation services for guidance of the procedure.

Intraprocedural injection(s) of a thrombolytic agent is an included service and not separately reportable in conjunction with mechanical thrombectomy. However, subsequent or prior continuous infusion of a thrombolytic is not an included service and is separately reportable (see 37211-37214).

For coronary mechanical thrombectomy, use 92973.

For intracranial arterial mechanical thrombectomy, use 61645.

Transcatheter Thrombolytic Infusion

Codes 37211 or 37212 are used to report the initial day of transcatheter thrombolytic infusion(s) including follow-up arteriography/venography, and catheter position change or exchange, when performed. To report bilateral thrombolytic infusion through a separate access site(s), use modifier 50 in conjunction with 37211, 37212. Code 37213 is used to report continued transcatheter thrombolytic infusion(s) on subsequent day(s), other than initial day and final day of treatment. Code 37214 is used to report final day of transcatheter thrombolytic infusion(s). When initiation and completion of thrombolysis occur on the same day, report only 37211 or 37212.

Code(s) for catheter placement(s), diagnostic studies, and other percutaneous interventions (eg, transluminal balloon angioplasty, stent placement) provided may be separately reportable.

Codes 37211-37214 include fluoroscopic guidance and associated radiological supervision and interpretation.

Ongoing evaluation and management services on the day of the procedure related to thrombolysis are included in 37211-37214. If a significant, separately identifiable E/M service is performed by the same physician on the same day of the procedure, report the appropriate level of E/M service and append modifier 25.

Ultrasound guidance for vascular access is not included in 37211-37214. Code 76937 may be reported separately when performed if all the required elements are performed.

For intracranial arterial mechanical thrombectomy and/or infusion for thrombolysis, use 61645.

Arterial Mechanical Thrombectomy

Arterial mechanical thrombectomy may be performed as a "primary" transcatheter procedure with pretreatment planning, performance of the procedure, and postprocedure evaluation focused on providing this service. Typically, the diagnosis of thrombus has been made prior to the procedure, and a mechanical thrombectomy is planned preoperatively. Primary mechanical thrombectomy is reported per vascular family using 37184 for the initial vessel treated and 37185 for second or all subsequent vessel(s) within the same vascular family. To report mechanical thrombectomy of an additional vascular family treated through a separate access site, use modifier 59 in conjunction with the primary service code (37184) for the mechanical transluminal thrombectomy.

Primary mechanical thrombectomy may precede or follow another percutaneous intervention. Most commonly primary mechanical thrombectomy will precede another percutaneous intervention with the decision regarding the need for other services not made until after mechanical thrombectomy has been performed. Occasionally, the performance of primary mechanical thrombectomy may follow another percutaneous intervention.

Do **NOT** report 37184-37185 for mechanical thrombectomy performed for the retrieval of short segments of thrombus or embolus evident during other percutaneous interventional procedures. See 37186 for these procedures.

Arterial mechanical thrombectomy is considered a "secondary" transcatheter procedure for removal or retrieval of short segments of thrombus or embolus when performed either before or after another percutaneous intervention (eg, percutaneous transluminal balloon angioplasty, stent placement). Secondary mechanical thrombectomy is reported using 37186. Do **NOT** report 37186 in conjunction with 37184-37185.

Venous Mechanical Thrombectomy

Use 37187 to report the initial application of venous mechanical thrombectomy. To report bilateral venous mechanical thrombectomy performed through a separate access site(s), use modifier 50 in conjunction with 37187. For repeat treatment on a subsequent day during a course of thrombolytic therapy, use 37188.

Cardiovascular 33016-39599

322 ★=Telemedicine ◀=Audio-only ✛=Add-on code ⚡=FDA approval pending #=Resequenced code ⊘=Modifier 51 exempt ⟳⟳⟳=See p xxi for details

Arterial Mechanical Thrombectomy

37184 Primary percutaneous transluminal mechanical thrombectomy, noncoronary, non-intracranial, arterial or arterial bypass graft, including fluoroscopic guidance and intraprocedural pharmacological thrombolytic injection(s); initial vessel

➔ *CPT Changes: An Insider's View* 2006, 2016, 2017

➔ *CPT Assistant* Nov 11:11, Feb 13:3, Apr 15:10, Nov 15:3, Sep 19:5, Jun 22:22, Jan 23:30

➔ *Clinical Examples in Radiology* Winter 06:15, Summer 10:4, Winter 13:2-4, Spring 16:3, Winter 23:8

(Do not report 37184 in conjunction with 61645, 76000, 96374)

+ 37185 second and all subsequent vessel(s) within the same vascular family (List separately in addition to code for primary mechanical thrombectomy procedure)

➔ *CPT Changes: An Insider's View* 2006, 2016, 2017

➔ *CPT Assistant* Nov 11:11, Feb 13:3, Apr 15:10, Nov 15:3, Sep 19:5, Jan 23:30

➔ *Clinical Examples in Radiology* Winter 06:15, Winter 13:2-3, Spring 16:3, Winter 23:8

(Do not report 37185 in conjunction with 76000, 96375)

(Do not report 37185 in conjunction with 61645 for treatment of the same vascular territory. See Nervous System Endovascular Therapy)

+ 37186 Secondary percutaneous transluminal thrombectomy (eg, nonprimary mechanical, snare basket, suction technique), noncoronary, non-intracranial, arterial or arterial bypass graft, including fluoroscopic guidance and intraprocedural pharmacological thrombolytic injections, provided in conjunction with another percutaneous intervention other than primary mechanical thrombectomy (List separately in addition to code for primary procedure)

➔ *CPT Changes: An Insider's View* 2006, 2016, 2017

➔ *CPT Assistant* Jul 11:11, Nov 11:9, Feb 13:3, Nov 15:3, Sep 19:5

➔ *Clinical Examples in Radiology* Winter 06:15, Winter 13:4, Spring 16:3, Winter 23:8

(Do not report 37186 in conjunction with 76000, 96375)

(Do not report 37186 in conjunction with 61645 for treatment of the same vascular territory. See Nervous System Endovascular Therapy)

Venous Mechanical Thrombectomy

37187 Percutaneous transluminal mechanical thrombectomy, vein(s), including intraprocedural pharmacological thrombolytic injections and fluoroscopic guidance

➔ *CPT Changes: An Insider's View* 2006, 2017

➔ *CPT Assistant* Nov 11:11, Feb 13:3

➔ *Clinical Examples in Radiology* Winter 06:15, Winter 12:3, Winter 13:4, Summer 13:1-4, Winter 23:8

(Do not report 37187 in conjunction with 76000, 96375)

37188 Percutaneous transluminal mechanical thrombectomy, vein(s), including intraprocedural pharmacological thrombolytic injections and fluoroscopic guidance, repeat treatment on subsequent day during course of thrombolytic therapy

➔ *CPT Changes: An Insider's View* 2006, 2017

➔ *CPT Assistant* Nov 11:11, Feb 13:3, Jun 22:22

➔ *Clinical Examples in Radiology* Winter 06:15, Winter 12:3, Winter 13:4, Summer 13:4, Winter 23:8

(Do not report 37188 in conjunction with 76000, 96375)

Other Procedures

37191 Insertion of intravascular vena cava filter, endovascular approach including vascular access, vessel selection, and radiological supervision and interpretation, intraprocedural roadmapping, and imaging guidance (ultrasound and fluoroscopy), when performed

➔ *CPT Changes: An Insider's View* 2012, 2017

➔ *CPT Assistant* Apr 12:8, Feb 13:3, May 16:11, Feb 17:14

➔ *Clinical Examples in Radiology* Winter 12:1, Winter 16:4

(For open surgical interruption of the inferior vena cava through a laparotomy or retroperitoneal exposure, use 37619)

37192 Repositioning of intravascular vena cava filter, endovascular approach including vascular access, vessel selection, and radiological supervision and interpretation, intraprocedural roadmapping, and imaging guidance (ultrasound and fluoroscopy), when performed

➔ *CPT Changes: An Insider's View* 2012, 2017

➔ *CPT Assistant* Apr 12:8, Feb 13:3, May 16:11

➔ *Clinical Examples in Radiology* Winter 12:2, Winter 16:4

(Do not report 37192 in conjunction with 37191)

37193 Retrieval (removal) of intravascular vena cava filter, endovascular approach including vascular access, vessel selection, and radiological supervision and interpretation, intraprocedural roadmapping, and imaging guidance (ultrasound and fluoroscopy), when performed

➔ *CPT Changes: An Insider's View* 2012, 2017

➔ *CPT Assistant* Apr 12:8, Feb 13:3, May 16:11

➔ *Clinical Examples in Radiology* Winter 12:2, Winter 16:4, Summer 16:12, Summer 18:13

(Do not report 37193 in conjunction with 37197)

37195 Thrombolysis, cerebral, by intravenous infusion

➔ *CPT Assistant* Nov 97:16, Jan 20:12

Vena Cava Filter
37191

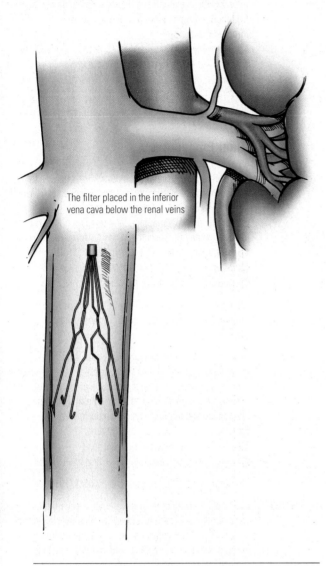

The filter placed in the inferior vena cava below the renal veins

37197 Transcatheter retrieval, percutaneous, of intravascular foreign body (eg, fractured venous or arterial catheter), includes radiological supervision and interpretation, and imaging guidance (ultrasound or fluoroscopy), when performed

➲ *CPT Changes: An Insider's View* 2013, 2017

➲ *CPT Assistant* Feb 13:3, May 16:11, Feb 17:14, Dec 21:21

➲ *Clinical Examples in Radiology* Spring 13:2-3, Winter 16:4

(For percutaneous retrieval of a vena cava filter, use 37193)

(For transcatheter removal of permanent leadless pacemaker, use 33275)

37200 Transcatheter biopsy

(For radiological supervision and interpretation, use 75970)

37211 Transcatheter therapy, arterial infusion for thrombolysis other than coronary or intracranial, any method, including radiological supervision and interpretation, initial treatment day

➲ *CPT Changes: An Insider's View* 2013, 2016, 2017

➲ *CPT Assistant* Feb 13:3, Nov 15:3, Mar 16:3, Sep 19:6, Jun 22:22

➲ *Clinical Examples in Radiology* Winter 13:2-4, Spring 13:11, Summer 13:3-4, Spring 16:3

(For intracranial arterial mechanical thrombectomy and/or infusion for thrombolysis, use 61645)

37212 Transcatheter therapy, venous infusion for thrombolysis, any method, including radiological supervision and interpretation, initial treatment day

➲ *CPT Changes: An Insider's View* 2013, 2017

➲ *CPT Assistant* Feb 13:3, Nov 15:3, Mar 16:3, Sep 19:6

➲ *Clinical Examples in Radiology* Winter 13:4, Spring 13:11, Summer 13:4, Spring 16:4

37213 Transcatheter therapy, arterial or venous infusion for thrombolysis other than coronary, any method, including radiological supervision and interpretation, continued treatment on subsequent day during course of thrombolytic therapy, including follow-up catheter contrast injection, position change, or exchange, when performed;

➲ *CPT Changes: An Insider's View* 2013, 2017

➲ *CPT Assistant* Feb 13:3, Nov 15:3, Mar 16:3, Sep 19:6

➲ *Clinical Examples in Radiology* Winter 13:4, Spring 13:11, Summer 13:1-4, Spring 16:4

37214 cessation of thrombolysis including removal of catheter and vessel closure by any method

➲ *CPT Changes: An Insider's View* 2013, 2017

➲ *CPT Assistant* Feb 13:3, Nov 15:3, Mar 16:3, Sep 19:6, Jun 22:22

➲ *Clinical Examples in Radiology* Winter 13:4, Spring 13:11, Summer 13:2-4, Spring 16:4

(Report 37211-37214 once per date of treatment)

(For declotting by thrombolytic agent of implanted vascular access device or catheter, use 36593)

(Do not report 37211-37214 in conjunction with 75898)

37215 Transcatheter placement of intravascular stent(s), cervical carotid artery, open or percutaneous, including angioplasty, when performed, and radiological supervision and interpretation; with distal embolic protection

➲ *CPT Changes: An Insider's View* 2005, 2015, 2017

➲ *CPT Assistant* May 05:7, Feb 13:3, Mar 14:8

➲ *Clinical Examples in Radiology* Winter 15:2-3

Cardiovascular 33016-39599

324 ★=Telemedicine ◀=Audio-only ✦=Add-on code ✗=FDA approval pending #=Resequenced code ⊘=Modifier 51 exempt ➲➲➲=See p xxi for details

37216 without distal embolic protection

➲ *CPT Changes: An Insider's View* 2005, 2015, 2017
➲ *CPT Assistant* May 05:7, Feb 13:3, Mar 14:8
➲ *Clinical Examples in Radiology* Winter 15:3

(37215 and 37216 include all ipsilateral selective carotid catheterization, all diagnostic imaging for ipsilateral, cervical and cerebral carotid arteriography, and all related radiological supervision and interpretation. When ipsilateral carotid arteriogram (including imaging and selective catheterization) confirms the need for carotid stenting, 37215 and 37216 are inclusive of these services. If carotid stenting is not indicated, then the appropriate codes for carotid catheterization and imaging should be reported in lieu of 37215 and 37216)

(Do not report 37215, 37216 in conjunction with 36222-36224 for the treated carotid artery)

(For open or percutaneous transcatheter placement of extracranial vertebral artery stent[s], see Category III codes 0075T, 0076T)

37217 Transcatheter placement of intravascular stent(s), intrathoracic common carotid artery or innominate artery by retrograde treatment, open ipsilateral cervical carotid artery exposure, including angioplasty, when performed, and radiological supervision and interpretation

➲ *CPT Changes: An Insider's View* 2014, 2015
➲ *CPT Assistant* Mar 14:8, May 15:7

(37217 includes open vessel exposure and vascular access closure, all access and selective catheterization of the vessel, traversing the lesion, and any radiological supervision and interpretation directly related to the intervention when performed, standard closure of arteriotomy by suture, and imaging performed to document completion of the intervention in addition to the intervention[s] performed. Carotid artery revascularization services [eg, 33891, 35301, 35509, 35510, 35601, 35606] performed during the same session may be reported separately, when performed)

(Do not report 37217 in conjunction with 35201, 36221-36227, 37246, 37247 for ipsilateral services)

(For open or percutaneous transcatheter placement of intravascular cervical carotid artery stent[s], see 37215, 37216)

(For open or percutaneous antegrade transcatheter placement of innominate and/or intrathoracic carotid artery stent[s], use 37218)

(For open or percutaneous transcatheter placement of extracranial vertebral artery stent[s], see 0075T, 0076T)

(For transcatheter placement of intracranial stent[s], use 61635)

37218 Transcatheter placement of intravascular stent(s), intrathoracic common carotid artery or innominate artery, open or percutaneous antegrade approach, including angioplasty, when performed, and radiological supervision and interpretation

➲ *CPT Changes: An Insider's View* 2015, 2017
➲ *CPT Assistant* May 15:7

(37218 includes all ipsilateral extracranial intrathoracic selective innominate and carotid catheterization, all diagnostic imaging for ipsilateral extracranial intrathoracic innominate and/or carotid artery stenting, and all related radiologic supervision and interpretation. Report 37218 when the ipsilateral extracranial intrathoracic carotid arteriogram (including imaging and selective catheterization) confirms the need for stenting. If stenting is not indicated, report the appropriate codes for selective catheterization and imaging)

(Do not report 37218 in conjunction with 36222, 36223, 36224 for the treated carotid artery)

(For open or percutaneous transcatheter placement of intravascular cervical carotid artery stent[s], see 37215, 37216)

(For open or percutaneous transcatheter placement of extracranial vertebral artery stent[s], see 0075T, 0076T)

(For transcatheter placement of intracranial stent[s], use 61635)

Endovascular Revascularization (Open or Percutaneous, Transcatheter)

Codes 37220-37235 are to be used to describe lower extremity endovascular revascularization services performed for occlusive disease. These lower extremity codes are built on progressive hierarchies with more intensive services inclusive of lesser intensive services. The code inclusive of all of the services provided for that vessel should be reported (ie, use the code inclusive of the most intensive services provided). Only one code from this family (37220-37235) should be reported for each lower extremity vessel treated.

These lower extremity endovascular revascularization codes all include the work of accessing and selectively catheterizing the vessel, traversing the lesion, radiological supervision and interpretation directly related to the intervention(s) performed, embolic protection if used, closure of the arteriotomy by pressure and application of an arterial closure device or standard closure of the puncture by suture, and imaging performed to document completion of the intervention in addition to the intervention(s) performed. Extensive repair or replacement of an artery may be additionally reported (eg, 35226 or 35286). These codes describe endovascular procedures performed percutaneously and/or through an open surgical exposure. These codes include balloon angioplasty (eg, low-profile, cutting balloon, cryoplasty), atherectomy (eg, directional, rotational, laser), and stenting (eg, balloon-expandable, self-expanding, bare metal, covered, drug-eluting). Each code in this family (37220-37235) includes balloon angioplasty, when performed.

These codes describe revascularization therapies (ie, transluminal angioplasty, atherectomy, and stent placement) provided in three arterial vascular territories: iliac, femoral/popliteal, and tibial/peroneal.

When treating multiple vessels within a territory, report each additional vessel using an add-on code, as applicable. Select the base code that represents the most complex service using the following hierarchy of complexity (in descending order of complexity): atherectomy and stent> atherectomy>stent>angioplasty. When treating multiple lesions within the same vessel, report one service that reflects the combined procedures, whether done on one lesion or different lesions, using the same hierarchy.

1. **Iliac Vascular Territory**—The iliac territory is divided into 3 vessels: common iliac, internal iliac, and external iliac.

2. **Femoral/Popliteal Vascular Territory**—The entire femoral/popliteal territory in 1 lower extremity is considered a single vessel for CPT reporting specifically for the endovascular lower extremity revascularization codes 37224-37227.

3. **Tibial/Peroneal Territory**—The tibial/peroneal territory is divided into 3 vessels: anterior tibial, posterior tibial, and peroneal arteries.

There are specific coding guidelines for each of the 3 vascular territories.

1. **Iliac Vascular Territory**—A single primary code is used for the initial iliac artery treated in each leg (37220 or 37221). If other iliac vessels are also treated in that leg, these interventions are reported with the appropriate add-on code(s) (37222, 37223). Up to 2 add-on codes can be used in a unilateral iliac vascular territory since there are 3 vessels which could be treated. Add-on codes are used for different vessels, not distinct lesions within the same vessel.

2. **Femoral/Popliteal Territory**—A single interventional code is used no matter what combination of angioplasty/stent/atherectomy is applied to all segments, including the common, deep and superficial femoral arteries as well as the popliteal artery (37224, 37225, 37226, or 37227). There are no add-on codes for additional vessels treated within the femoral/

popliteal territory. Because only 1 service is reported when 2 lesions are treated in this territory, report the most complex service (eg, use 37227 if a stent is placed for 1 lesion and an atherectomy is performed on a second lesion).

3. **Tibial/Peroneal Territory**—A single primary code is used for the initial tibial/peroneal artery treated in each leg (37228, 37229, 37230, or 37231). If other tibial/peroneal vessels are also treated in the same leg, these interventions are reported with the appropriate add-on code(s) (37232-37235). Up to 2 add-on codes could be used to describe services provided in a single leg since there are 3 tibial/peroneal vessels which could be treated. Add-on codes are used for different vessels, not distinct lesions within the same vessel. The common tibio-peroneal trunk is considered part of the tibial/peroneal territory, but is not considered a separate, fourth segment of vessel in the tibio-peroneal family for CPT reporting of endovascular lower extremity interventions. For instance, if lesions in the common tibio-peroneal trunk are treated in conjunction with lesions in the posterior tibial artery, a single code would be reported for treatment of this segment.

When treating multiple territories in the same leg, one primary lower extremity revascularization code is used for each territory treated. When second or third vessel(s) are treated in the iliac and/or tibial/peroneal territories, add-on code(s) are used to report the additional service(s). When more than one stent is placed in the same vessel, the code should be reported only once.

When multiple vessels in multiple territories in a single leg are treated at the same setting, the primary code for the treatment in the initial vessel in each vascular territory is reported. Add-on code(s) are reported when second and third iliac or tibial/peroneal arteries are treated in addition to the initial vessel in that vascular territory.

If a lesion extends across the margins of one vessel vascular territory into another, but can be opened with a single therapy, this intervention should be reported with a single code despite treating more than one vessel and/or vascular territory. For instance, if a stenosis extends from the common iliac artery into the proximal external iliac artery, and a single stent is placed to open the entire lesion, this therapy should be coded as a single stent placement in the iliac artery (37221). In this example, a code for an additional vessel treatment would not be used (do not report both 37221 and 37223).

For bifurcation lesions distal to the common iliac origins which require therapy of 2 distinct branches of the iliac or tibial/peroneal vascular territories, a primary code and an add-on code would be used to describe the intervention. In the femoral/popliteal territory, all branches are included in the primary code, so treatment of a bifurcation lesion would be reported as a single code.

When the same territory(ies) of both legs are treated in the same session, modifiers may be required to describe the interventions. Use modifier 59 to denote that different legs are being treated, even if the mode of therapy is different.

Mechanical thrombectomy and/or thrombolysis in the lower extremity vessels are sometimes necessary to aid in restoring flow to areas of occlusive disease, and are reported separately.

37220   Revascularization, endovascular, open or percutaneous, iliac artery, unilateral, initial vessel; with transluminal angioplasty

➲ *CPT Changes: An Insider's View* 2011, 2017

➲ *CPT Assistant* Jul 11:3, Oct 11:9, Dec 13:8, Jul 16:8, Jun 19:14

➲ *Clinical Examples in Radiology* Winter 11:3, Spring 14:9

37221   with transluminal stent placement(s), includes angioplasty within the same vessel, when performed

➲ *CPT Changes: An Insider's View* 2011, 2017

➲ *CPT Assistant* Jul 11:3, Oct 11:9, Jan 15:13, Jul 16:8, Jun 19:14

➲ *Clinical Examples in Radiology* Winter 11:2, Spring 16:13

(Use 37220, 37221 in conjunction with 34701-34711, 34718, 34845, 34846, 34847, 34848, only when 37220 or 37221 is performed outside the treatment zone of the endograft)

+ 37222   Revascularization, endovascular, open or percutaneous, iliac artery, each additional ipsilateral iliac vessel; with transluminal angioplasty (List separately in addition to code for primary procedure)

➲ *CPT Changes: An Insider's View* 2011, 2017

➲ *CPT Assistant* Jul 11:3, Oct 11:9, Jul 16:8, Jun 19:14

➲ *Clinical Examples in Radiology* Winter 11:2, Spring 16:13

(Use 37222 in conjunction with 37220, 37221)

+ 37223   with transluminal stent placement(s), includes angioplasty within the same vessel, when performed (List separately in addition to code for primary procedure)

➲ *CPT Changes: An Insider's View* 2011, 2017

➲ *CPT Assistant* Jul 11:3, Oct 11:9, Apr 12:8, Dec 13:8, Jul 16:8, Jun 19:14

➲ *Clinical Examples in Radiology* Winter 11:3, Spring 16:13

(Use 37223 in conjunction with 37221)

(Use 37222, 37223 in conjunction with 34701-34711, 34718, 34845, 34846, 34847, 34848 only when 37222 or 37223 are performed outside the treatment zone of the endograft)

Transluminal Balloon Angioplasty
37220 and 37222

A balloon catheter is passed into the iliac artery and inflated to stretch the blood vessel to a larger diameter.

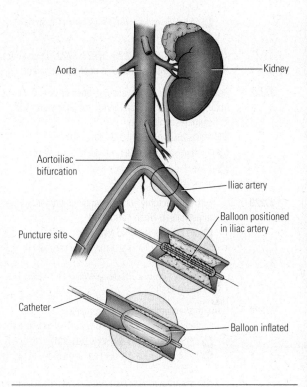

37224   Revascularization, endovascular, open or percutaneous, femoral, popliteal artery(s), unilateral; with transluminal angioplasty

➲ *CPT Changes: An Insider's View* 2011, 2017

➲ *CPT Assistant* Jul 11:3, Oct 11:9, Dec 11:15, Jul 16:8, Jun 19:14

➲ *Clinical Examples in Radiology* Winter 11:3, Summer 11:10, Spring 16:13

37225   with atherectomy, includes angioplasty within the same vessel, when performed

➲ *CPT Changes: An Insider's View* 2011, 2017

➲ *CPT Assistant* Jul 11:3, Oct 11:9, Nov 11:9, Jul 16:8, Jun 19:14

➲ *Clinical Examples in Radiology* Winter 11:3, Spring 11:3, Spring 16:13

37226   with transluminal stent placement(s), includes angioplasty within the same vessel, when performed

➲ *CPT Changes: An Insider's View* 2011, 2017

➲ *CPT Assistant* Jul 11:3, Oct 11:9, Dec 11:15, Jul 16:8, Jun 19:14, Dec 23:40

➲ *Clinical Examples in Radiology* Winter 11:2, Spring 16:13

Cardiovasciar 33016-39599

37227 with transluminal stent placement(s) and atherectomy, includes angioplasty within the same vessel, when performed

> ➡ *CPT Changes: An Insider's View* 2011, 2017
> ➡ *CPT Assistant* Jul 11:3, Oct 11:9, Nov 11:9, Jul 16:8, Jun 19:14
> ➡ *Clinical Examples in Radiology* Winter 11:3, Spring 11:2, Spring 16:13

(Do not report 37224, 37225, 37226, 37227 in conjunction with 0505T, within the femoral-popliteal segment)

37228 Revascularization, endovascular, open or percutaneous, tibial, peroneal artery, unilateral, initial vessel; with transluminal angioplasty

> ➡ *CPT Changes: An Insider's View* 2011, 2017
> ➡ *CPT Assistant* Jul 11:3, Oct 11:9, Jul 16:8, Jun 19:14
> ➡ *Clinical Examples in Radiology* Winter 11:2, Spring 11:2, Spring 16:13

37229 with atherectomy, includes angioplasty within the same vessel, when performed

> ➡ *CPT Changes: An Insider's View* 2011, 2017
> ➡ *CPT Assistant* Jul 11:3, Oct 11:9, Nov 11:9, Jul 16:8, Jun 19:14
> ➡ *Clinical Examples in Radiology* Winter 11:3, Spring 11:3, Spring 16:13

37230 with transluminal stent placement(s), includes angioplasty within the same vessel, when performed

> ➡ *CPT Changes: An Insider's View* 2011, 2017
> ➡ *CPT Assistant* Jul 11:3, Oct 11:9, Jul 16:8, Jun 19:14, Jul 20:13
> ➡ *Clinical Examples in Radiology* Winter 11:3, Spring 16:13

37231 with transluminal stent placement(s) and atherectomy, includes angioplasty within the same vessel, when performed

> ➡ *CPT Changes: An Insider's View* 2011, 2017
> ➡ *CPT Assistant* Jul 11:3, Oct 11:9, Nov 11:9, Jul 16:8, Jun 19:14
> ➡ *Clinical Examples in Radiology* Winter 11:3, Spring 11:3, Spring 16:13

+ 37232 Revascularization, endovascular, open or percutaneous, tibial/peroneal artery, unilateral, each additional vessel; with transluminal angioplasty (List separately in addition to code for primary procedure)

> ➡ *CPT Changes: An Insider's View* 2011, 2017
> ➡ *CPT Assistant* Jul 11:3, Oct 11:9, Apr 12:8, Jul 16:8, Jun 19:14
> ➡ *Clinical Examples in Radiology* Winter 11:3, Spring 16:13

(Use 37232 in conjunction with 37228-37231)

+ 37233 with atherectomy, includes angioplasty within the same vessel, when performed (List separately in addition to code for primary procedure)

> ➡ *CPT Changes: An Insider's View* 2011, 2017
> ➡ *CPT Assistant* Jul 11:3, Oct 11:9, Nov 11:9, Apr 12:8, Jul 16:8, Jun 19:14
> ➡ *Clinical Examples in Radiology* Winter 11:3, Spring 11:3, Spring 16:13

(Use 37233 in conjunction with 37229, 37231)

+ 37234 with transluminal stent placement(s), includes angioplasty within the same vessel, when performed (List separately in addition to code for primary procedure)

> ➡ *CPT Changes: An Insider's View* 2011, 2017
> ➡ *CPT Assistant* Jul 11:3, Oct 11:9, Apr 12:9, Jul 16:8, Jun 19:14
> ➡ *Clinical Examples in Radiology* Winter 11:3, Spring 11:11, Spring 16:13

(Use 37234 in conjunction with 37229, 37230, 37231)

Iliac and Lower Extremity Arterial Anatomy Territory
37220-37235

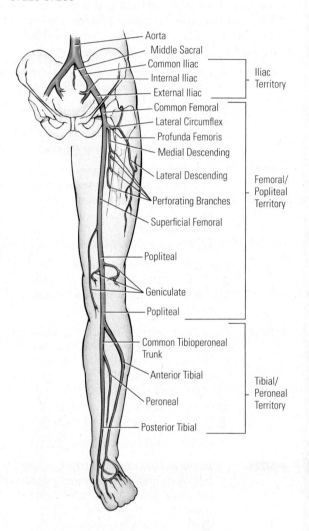

Aorta
Middle Sacral
Common Iliac
Internal Iliac
External Iliac

Iliac Territory

Common Femoral
Lateral Circumflex
Profunda Femoris
Medial Descending
Lateral Descending
Perforating Branches
Superficial Femoral
Popliteal
Geniculate
Popliteal

Femoral/ Popliteal Territory

Common Tibioperoneal Trunk
Anterior Tibial
Peroneal
Posterior Tibial

Tibial/ Peroneal Territory

+ 37235   with transluminal stent placement(s) and atherectomy, includes angioplasty within the same vessel, when performed (List separately in addition to code for primary procedure)

⮕ *CPT Changes: An Insider's View* 2011, 2017

⮕ *CPT Assistant* Jul 11:3, Oct 11:9, Nov 11:9, Jul 16:8, Jun 19:14

⮕ *Clinical Examples in Radiology* Winter 11:3, Spring 11:3, Spring 14:9, Spring 16:13

(Use 37235 in conjunction with 37231)

►Codes 37246, 37247, 37248, 37249 describe open or percutaneous transluminal balloon angioplasty (eg, conventional, low profile, cutting, drug-coated balloon). Codes 37246, 37247 describe transluminal balloon angioplasty in an artery, excluding the central nervous system (61630, 61635), coronary (92920-92944, 0913T), pulmonary (92997, 92998), and lower extremities for occlusive disease (37220-37235). Codes 37248 and 37249 describe transluminal balloon angioplasty in a vein excluding the dialysis circuit (36902, 36905, 36907) when approached through the ipsilateral dialysis access. Transluminal balloon angioplasty is inherent to stenting in the extracranial carotid and innominate arteries (37215, 37216, 37217, 37218), peripheral arteries (37220-37237), and in peripheral veins (37238, 37239) and, therefore, is not separately reportable. Multiple angioplasties performed in a single vessel, including treatment of separate and distinct lesions within a single vessel, are reported with a single code. If a lesion extends across the margins of one vessel into another, but can be treated with a single therapy, the intervention should be reported only once. When additional, separate and distinct ipsilateral or contralateral vessels are treated in the same session, 37247 and/or 37249 may be reported as appropriate.◄

Non-selective and/or selective catheterization (eg, 36005, 36010, 36011, 36012, 36200, 36215, 36216, 36217, 36218, 36245, 36246, 36247, 36248) is reported separately. Codes 37246, 37247, 37248, 37249 include radiological supervision and interpretation directly related to the intervention performed and imaging performed to document completion of the intervention. Extensive repair or replacement of an artery may be reported separately (eg, 35226, 35286). Intravascular ultrasound may be reported separately (ie, 37252, 37253). Mechanical thrombectomy and/or thrombolytic therapy, when performed, may be reported separately (eg, 37184, 37185, 37186, 37187, 37188, 37211, 37212, 37213, 37214).

 # 37246   Transluminal balloon angioplasty (except lower extremity artery(ies) for occlusive disease, intracranial, coronary, pulmonary, or dialysis circuit), open or percutaneous, including all imaging and radiological supervision and interpretation necessary to perform the angioplasty within the same artery; initial artery

⮕ *CPT Changes: An Insider's View* 2017

⮕ *CPT Assistant* May 17:3, Jul 17:3

Transluminal Balloon Angioplasty
37246

A balloon catheter is inserted and advanced across the lesion into the narrowed portion of the vessel. The balloon is inflated to enlarge the diameter and restore normal blood flow.

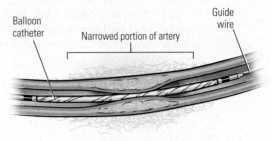

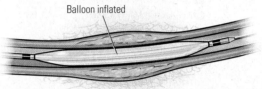

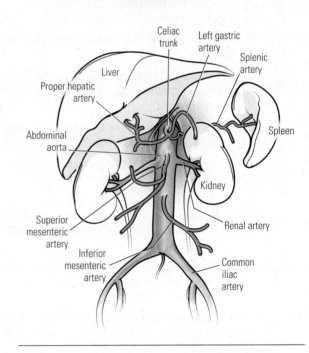

#+ 37247   each additional artery (List separately in addition to code for primary procedure)

⮕ *CPT Changes: An Insider's View* 2017

⮕ *CPT Assistant* May 17:3, Jul 17:3

(Use 37247 in conjunction with 37246)

Cardiovascular 33016-39599

(Do not report 37246, 37247 in conjunction with 36836, 36837)

(Do not report 37246, 37247 in conjunction with 37215, 37216, 37217, 37218, 37220-37237 when performed in the same artery during the same operative session)

(Do not report 37246, 37247 in conjunction with 34841, 34842, 34843, 34844, 34845, 34846, 34847, 34848 for angioplasty[ies] performed, when placing bare metal or covered stents into the visceral branches within the endoprosthesis target zone)

\# **37248**　Transluminal balloon angioplasty (except dialysis circuit), open or percutaneous, including all imaging and radiological supervision and interpretation necessary to perform the angioplasty within the same vein; initial vein

➲ *CPT Changes: An Insider's View* 2017

➲ *CPT Assistant* Mar 17:4, May 17:3, Jul 17:3, Oct 22:17, Nov 23:25

\#+ **37249**　　each additional vein (List separately in addition to code for primary procedure)

➲ *CPT Changes: An Insider's View* 2017

➲ *CPT Assistant* Mar 17:4, May 17:3, Jul 17:3

(Use 37249 in conjunction with 37248)

(Do not report 37248, 37249 in conjunction with 36836, 36837)

(Do not report 37248, 37249 in conjunction with 37238, 37239 when performed in the same vein during the same operative session)

(Do not report 37248, 37249 in conjunction with 0505T, within the femoral-popliteal segment)

(Do not report 37248, 37249 in conjunction with 0620T within the tibial-peroneal segment)

(For transluminal balloon angioplasty in aorta/visceral artery[ies] in conjunction with fenestrated endovascular repair, see 34841, 34842, 34843, 34844, 34845, 34846, 34847, 34848)

(For transluminal balloon angioplasty in iliac, femoral, popliteal, or tibial/peroneal artery[ies] for occlusive disease, see 37220-37235)

(For transluminal balloon angioplasty in a dialysis circuit performed through the circuit, see 36902, 36903, 36904, 36905, 36906, 36907, 36908)

(For transluminal balloon angioplasty in an intracranial artery, see 61630, 61635)

(For transluminal balloon angioplasty in a coronary artery, see 92920-92944)

(For transluminal balloon angioplasty in a pulmonary artery, see 92997, 92998)

Codes 37236-37239 are used to report endovascular revascularization for vessels other than lower extremity artery(ies) for occlusive disease (ie, 37221, 37223, 37226, 37227, 37230, 37231, 37234, 37235), cervical carotid (ie, 37215, 37216), intracranial (ie, 61635), intracoronary (ie, 92928, 92929, 92933, 92934, 92937, 92938, 92941, 92943, 92944), innominate and/or intrathoracic carotid artery through an antegrade approach (37218), extracranial vertebral (ie, 0075T, 0076T) performed percutaneously and/or through an open surgical exposure, open retrograde intrathoracic common carotid or innominate (37217), or dialysis circuit when performed through the dialysis circuit (36903, 36905, 36908).

Codes 37236, 37237 describe transluminal intravascular stent insertion in an artery while 37238, 37239 describe transluminal intravascular stent insertion in a vein. Multiple stents placed in a single vessel may only be reported with a single code. If a lesion extends across the margins of one vessel into another, but can be treated with a single therapy, the intervention should be reported only once. When additional, different vessels are treated in the same session, report 37237 and/or 37239 as appropriate. Each code in this family (37236-37239) includes any and all balloon angioplasty(s) performed in the treated vessel, including any pre-dilation (whether performed as a primary or secondary angioplasty), post-dilation following stent placement, treatment of a lesion outside the stented segment but in the same vessel, or use of larger/smaller balloon to achieve therapeutic result. Angioplasty in a separate and distinct vessel may be reported separately. Non-selective and/or selective catheterization(s) (eg, 36005, 36010-36015, 36200, 36215-36218, 36245-36248) is reported separately.

Codes 37236-37239 include radiological supervision and interpretation directly related to the intervention(s) performed, closure of the arteriotomy by pressure, application of an arterial closure device or standard closure of the puncture by suture, and imaging performed to document completion of the intervention in addition to the intervention(s) performed. Extensive repair or replacement of an artery may be reported separately (eg, 35226 or 35286). Report 76937 for ultrasound guidance for vascular access, when performed in conjunction with 37236-37239. Intravascular ultrasound may be reported separately (ie, 37252, 37253). For mechanical thrombectomy and/or thrombolytic therapy, when performed, see 37184-37188, 37211-37214.

Intravascular stents, both covered and uncovered, are a class of devices that may be used as part of an embolization procedure. As such, there is the potential for overlap among codes used for placement of vascular stents and those used for embolization. When a stent is placed for the purpose of providing a latticework for deployment of embolization coils, such as for embolization of an aneurysm, the embolization code is reported and not the stent code. If a covered stent is deployed as the sole management of an aneurysm, pseudoaneurysm, or vascular extravasation, then the stent deployment code should be reported and not the embolization code.

37236   Transcatheter placement of an intravascular stent(s) (except lower extremity artery(s) for occlusive disease, cervical carotid, extracranial vertebral or intrathoracic carotid, intracranial, or coronary), open or percutaneous, including radiological supervision and interpretation and including all angioplasty within the same vessel, when performed; initial artery

➜ *CPT Changes: An Insider's View* 2014, 2015, 2017

➜ *CPT Assistant* Dec 13:8, May 15:7, Mar 16:5, Jul 16:3

➜ *Clinical Examples in Radiology* Winter 14:5-6, Spring 14:9, Spring 16:13

+ 37237   each additional artery (List separately in addition to code for primary procedure)

➜ *CPT Changes: An Insider's View* 2014, 2015, 2017

➜ *CPT Assistant* Dec 13:8, Mar 16:5, Jul 16:6

➜ *Clinical Examples in Radiology* Winter 14:6, Spring 16:13

(Use 37237 in conjunction with 37236)

(Do not report 37236, 37237 in conjunction with 36836, 36837)

(Do not report 37236, 37237 in conjunction with 34841-34848 for bare metal or covered stents placed into the visceral branches within the endoprosthesis target zone)

(For stent placement(s) in iliac, femoral, popliteal, or tibial/peroneal artery(s) for occlusive disease, see 37221, 37223, 37226, 37227, 37230, 37231, 37234, 37235)

(For transcatheter placement of intravascular cervical carotid artery stent(s), see 37215, 37216)

(For transcatheter placement of intracranial stent(s), use 61635)

(For transcatheter placement of intracoronary stent(s), see 92928, 92929, 92933, 92934, 92937, 92938, 92941, 92943, 92944)

(For stenting of visceral arteries in conjunction with fenestrated endovascular repair, see 34841-34848)

(For open or percutaneous antegrade transcatheter placement of intrathoracic carotid/innominate artery stent(s), use 37218)

(For open or percutaneous transcatheter placement of extracranial vertebral artery stent(s), see Category III codes 0075T, 0076T)

(For open retrograde transcatheter placement of intrathoracic common carotid/innominate artery stent(s), use 37217)

(For placement of a stent at the arterial anastomosis of a dialysis circuit with or without transluminal mechanical thrombectomy and/or infusion for thrombolysis, see 36903, 36906)

37238   Transcatheter placement of an intravascular stent(s), open or percutaneous, including radiological supervision and interpretation and including angioplasty within the same vessel, when performed; initial vein

➜ *CPT Changes: An Insider's View* 2014, 2017

➜ *CPT Assistant* Jun 16:8, Jul 16:6, Mar 17:4

➜ *Clinical Examples in Radiology* Winter 14:6, Spring 16:13

+ 37239   each additional vein (List separately in addition to code for primary procedure)

➜ *CPT Changes: An Insider's View* 2014, 2017

➜ *CPT Assistant* Jul 16:6, Mar 17:4

➜ *Clinical Examples in Radiology* Winter 14:6, Spring 14:9, Spring 16:13

(Use 37239 in conjunction with 37238)

(Do not report 37238, 37239 in conjunction with 36836, 36837)

(Do not report 37238, 37239 in conjunction with 0505T, within the femoral-popliteal segment)

(Do not report 37238, 37239 in conjunction with 0620T within the tibial-peroneal segment)

(For placement of a stent[s] within the peripheral segment of the dialysis circuit, see 36903, 36906)

(For transcatheter placement of an intravascular stent[s] within central dialysis segment when performed through the dialysis circuit, use 36908)

Vascular Embolization and Occlusion

Codes 37241-37244 are used to describe vascular embolization and occlusion procedures, excluding the central nervous system and the head and neck, which are reported using 61624, 61626, 61710, and 75894, and excluding the ablation/sclerotherapy procedures for venous insufficiency/telangiectasia of the extremities/skin, which are reported using 36468, 36470, and 36471. Embolization and occlusion procedures are performed for a wide variety of clinical indications and in a range of vascular territories. Arteries, veins, and lymphatics may all be the target of embolization.

The embolization codes include all associated radiological supervision and interpretation, intra-procedural guidance and road-mapping, and imaging necessary to document completion of the procedure. They do not include diagnostic angiography and all necessary catheter placement(s). Code(s) for catheter placement(s) may be separately reported using selective catheter placement code(s), if used consistent with guidelines. Code(s) for diagnostic angiography may also be separately reported, when performed according to guidelines for diagnostic

Cardiovascular 33016-39599

angiography during endovascular procedures, using the appropriate diagnostic angiography codes. Report these services with an appropriate modifier (eg, modifier 59). Please see the guidelines on the reporting of diagnostic angiography preceding 75600 in the **Vascular Procedures, Aorta and Arteries** section.

Code 37241 is used to report endovascular embolization or occlusion procedures performed for venous conditions other than hemorrhage or hemodialysis access. Examples include embolization of venous malformations, capillary hemangiomas, varicoceles, and visceral varices. (For endovascular embolization or occlusion of side branch[es] of an outflow vein[s] from a hemodialysis access, use 36909.)

Code 37242 is used to report vascular embolization or occlusion performed for arterial conditions other than hemorrhage or tumor such as arteriovenous malformations and arteriovenous fistulas whether congenital or acquired. Embolizations of aneurysms and pseudoaneurysms are also reported with 37242. Tumor embolization is reported with 37243. Note that injection to treat an extremity pseudoaneurysm is correctly reported with 36002. Sometimes, embolization and occlusion of an artery are performed prior to another planned interventional procedure; an example is embolization of the left gastric artery prior to planned implantation of a hepatic artery chemotherapy port. The artery embolization is reported with 37242.

Code 37243 is used to report embolization for the purpose of tissue ablation and organ infarction or ischemia. This can be performed in many clinical circumstances, including embolization of benign or malignant tumors of the liver, kidney, uterus, or other organs. When chemotherapy is given as part of an embolization procedure, additional codes (eg, 96420) may be separately reported. When a radioisotope (eg, Yttrium-90) is injected as part of an embolization, then additional codes (eg, 79445) may be separately reported. Uterine fibroid embolization is reported with 37243.

Code 37244 is used to report embolization for treatment of hemorrhage or vascular or lymphatic extravasation. Examples include embolization for management of gastrointestinal bleed, trauma-induced hemorrhage of the viscera or pelvis, embolization of the thoracic duct for chylous effusion and bronchial artery embolization for hemoptysis. Embolization of the uterine arteries for management of hemorrhage (eg, postpartum hemorrhage) is also reported with 37244.

Intravascular stents, both covered and uncovered, are a class of devices that may be used as part of an embolization procedure. As such, there is the potential for overlap among codes used for placement of vascular stents and those used for embolization. When a stent is placed for the purpose of providing a latticework for deployment of embolization coils, such as for embolization of an aneurysm, the embolization code is reported and not the

stent code. If a stent is deployed as the sole management of an aneurysm, pseudoaneurysm, or vascular extravasation, then the stent deployment code should be reported and not the embolization code.

Only one embolization code should be reported for each surgical field (ie, the area immediately surrounding and directly involved in a treatment/procedure). Embolization procedures performed at a single setting and including multiple surgical fields (eg, a patient with multiple trauma and bleeding from the pelvis and the spleen) may be reported with multiple embolization codes with the appropriate modifier (eg, modifier 59).

There may be overlapping indications for an embolization procedure. The code for the immediate indication for the embolization should be used. For instance, if the immediate cause for embolization is bleeding in a patient with an aneurysm, report 37244.

37241 Vascular embolization or occlusion, inclusive of all radiological supervision and interpretation, intraprocedural roadmapping, and imaging guidance necessary to complete the intervention; venous, other than hemorrhage (eg, congenital or acquired venous malformations, venous and capillary hemangiomas, varices, varicoceles)

➔ *CPT Changes: An Insider's View* 2014, 2017

➔ *CPT Assistant* Nov 13:6, Aug 14:14, Oct 14:6, Apr 15:10, Aug 15:8, Nov 15:3, Mar 18:3, Sep 19:6

➔ *Clinical Examples in Radiology* Spring 14:7, Spring 16:4, Winter 18:10, Summer 18:4, Spring 19:4, Summer 19:6, Spring 20:14

(Do not report 37241 in conjunction with 36468, 36470, 36471, 36473, 36474, 36475-36479, 75894, 75898 in the same surgical field)

(For sclerosis of veins or endovenous ablation of incompetent extremity veins, see 36468-36479)

(For dialysis circuit permanent endovascular embolization or occlusion, use 36909)

37242 arterial, other than hemorrhage or tumor (eg, congenital or acquired arterial malformations, arteriovenous malformations, arteriovenous fistulas, aneurysms, pseudoaneurysms)

➔ *CPT Changes: An Insider's View* 2014, 2017

➔ *CPT Assistant* Nov 13:6, Oct 14:6, Nov 15:3, Jul 18:14, Sep 19:6

➔ *Clinical Examples in Radiology* Spring 14:8, Summer 15:8, Spring 16:4, Winter 18:10, Summer 18:2, Spring 19:4, Summer 19:6, Spring 20:15, Fall 21:16

(Do not report 37241, 37242 in conjunction with 36836, 36837)

★ = Telemedicine   ◀ = Audio-only   ✚ = Add-on code   ✔ = FDA approval pending   # = Resequenced code   ⊘ = Modifier 51 exempt   ➔➔➔ = See p xxi for details

Cardiovascular 33016-39599

(For percutaneous treatment of extremity pseudoaneurysm, use 36002)

37243   for tumors, organ ischemia, or infarction

➲ *CPT Changes: An Insider's View* 2014, 2017

➲ *CPT Assistant* Nov 13:7, Oct 14:6, Nov 15:3, Sep 19:6

➲ *Clinical Examples in Radiology* Winter 14:4, Summer 15:2, Spring 16:4, Winter 18:10, Summer 18:4, Spring 19:4, Summer 19:4, Spring 20:15

37244   for arterial or venous hemorrhage or lymphatic extravasation

➲ *CPT Changes: An Insider's View* 2014, 2017

➲ *CPT Assistant* Nov 13:7, Aug 14:14, Oct 14:6, Nov 15:3, Oct 17:9, Jul 18:14, Sep 19:6

➲ *Clinical Examples in Radiology* Winter 14:2, 4, Spring 14:7, Summer 15:8, Spring 16:4, Winter 18:11, Summer 18:4, Spring 19:2, Summer 19:6, Spring 20:15

(Do not report 37242-37244 in conjunction with 75894, 75898 in the same surgical field)

(For embolization procedures of the central nervous system or head and neck, see 61624, 61626, 61710)

37246   Code is out of numerical sequence. See 37234-37237

37247   Code is out of numerical sequence. See 37234-37237

37248   Code is out of numerical sequence. See 37234-37237

37249   Code is out of numerical sequence. See 37234-37237

Intravascular Ultrasound Services

Intravascular ultrasound (IVUS) services include all transducer manipulations and repositioning within the specific vessel being examined during a diagnostic procedure or before, during, and/or after therapeutic intervention (eg, stent or stent graft placement, angioplasty, atherectomy, embolization, thrombolysis, transcatheter biopsy).

IVUS is included in the work described by codes 37191, 37192, 37193, 37197 (intravascular vena cava [IVC] filter placement, repositioning and removal, and intravascular foreign body retrieval) and should not be separately reported with those procedures. If a lesion extends across the margins of one vessel into another, this should be reported with a single code despite imaging more than one vessel.

Non-selective and/or selective vascular catheterization may be separately reportable (eg, 36005-36248).

+ 37252   Intravascular ultrasound (noncoronary vessel) during diagnostic evaluation and/or therapeutic intervention, including radiological supervision and interpretation; initial noncoronary vessel (List separately in addition to code for primary procedure)

➲ *CPT Changes: An Insider's View* 2016, 2017

➲ *CPT Assistant* May 16:11, Mar 17:4, Nov 19:6, Jun 21:14, Feb 23:14

➲ *Clinical Examples in Radiology* Winter 16:2

+ 37253   each additional noncoronary vessel (List separately in addition to code for primary procedure)

➲ *CPT Changes: An Insider's View* 2016, 2017

➲ *CPT Assistant* May 16:11, Mar 17:4, Nov 19:6, Jun 21:14, Feb 23:14

➲ *Clinical Examples in Radiology* Winter 16:2

(Use 37253 in conjunction with 37252)

(Use 37252, 37253 in conjunction with 33361, 33362, 33363, 33364, 33365, 33366, 33367, 33368, 33369, 33477, 33880, 33881, 33883, 33884, 33886, 34701, 34702, 34703, 34704, 34705, 34706, 34707, 34708, 34709, 34710, 34711, 34712, 34718, 34841, 34842, 34843, 34844, 34845, 34846, 34847, 34848, 36010, 36011, 36012, 36013, 36014, 36015, 36100, 36140, 36160, 36200, 36215, 36216, 36217, 36218, 36221, 36222, 36223, 36224, 36225, 36226, 36227, 36228, 36245, 36246, 36247, 36248, 36251, 36252, 36253, 36254, 36481, 36555-36571, 36578, 36580, 36581, 36582, 36583, 36584, 36585, 36595, 36901, 36902, 36903, 36904, 36905, 36906, 36907, 36908, 36909, 37184, 37185, 37186, 37187, 37188, 37200, 37211, 37212, 37213, 37214, 37215, 37216, 37218, 37220, 37221, 37222, 37223, 37224, 37225, 37226, 37227, 37228, 37229, 37230, 37231, 37232, 37233, 37234, 37235, 37236, 37237, 37238, 37239, 37241, 37242, 37243, 37244, 37246, 37247, 37248, 37249, 61623, 75600, 75605, 75625, 75630, 75635, 75705, 75710, 75716, 75726, 75731, 75733, 75736, 75741, 75743, 75746, 75756, 75774, 75805, 75807, 75810, 75820, 75822, 75825, 75827, 75831, 75833, 75860, 75870, 75872, 75885, 75887, 75889, 75891, 75893, 75894, 75898, 75901, 75902, 75956, 75957, 75958, 75959, 75970, 76000, 77001, 0075T, 0076T, 0234T, 0235T, 0236T, 0237T, 0238T, 0338T)

(Do not report 37252, 37253 in conjunction with 36836, 36837, 37191, 37192, 37193, 37197)

Endoscopy

Surgical vascular endoscopy always includes diagnostic endoscopy.

37500   Vascular endoscopy, surgical, with ligation of perforator veins, subfascial (SEPS)

➲ *CPT Changes: An Insider's View* 2003

➲ *CPT Assistant* Jul 10:6

(For open procedure, use 37760)

37501   Unlisted vascular endoscopy procedure

➲ *CPT Changes: An Insider's View* 2003

Cardiovascular 33016-39599

Ligation

(For phleborrhaphy and arteriorrhaphy, see 35201-35286)

37565 Ligation, internal jugular vein

37600 Ligation; external carotid artery

37605 internal or common carotid artery

37606 internal or common carotid artery, with gradual occlusion, as with Selverstone or Crutchfield clamp

(For transcatheter permanent arterial occlusion or embolization, see 61624-61626)

(For endovascular temporary arterial balloon occlusion, use 61623)

(For ligation treatment of intracranial aneurysm, use 61703)

37607 Ligation or banding of angioaccess arteriovenous fistula
➔ *CPT Assistant* May 22:16

37609 Ligation or biopsy, temporal artery

37615 Ligation, major artery (eg, post-traumatic, rupture); neck

37616 chest

37617 abdomen
➔ *CPT Assistant* Aug 13:14

37618 extremity

37619 Ligation of inferior vena cava
➔ *CPT Changes: An Insider's View* 2012
➔ *CPT Assistant* Apr 12:8

(For endovascular delivery of an inferior vena cava filter, use 37191)

37650 Ligation of femoral vein

(For bilateral procedure, report 37650 with modifier 50)

37660 Ligation of common iliac vein

37700 Ligation and division of long saphenous vein at saphenofemoral junction, or distal interruptions
➔ *CPT Assistant* Aug 96:10, Nov 16:3, Mar 18:3
➔ *Clinical Examples in Radiology* Spring 17:3

(Do not report 37700 in conjunction with 37718, 37722)

(For bilateral procedure, report 37700 with modifier 50)

37718 Ligation, division, and stripping, short saphenous vein
➔ *CPT Changes: An Insider's View* 2006
➔ *CPT Assistant* Nov 16:3, Mar 18:3
➔ *Clinical Examples in Radiology* Spring 17:3

(For bilateral procedure, use modifier 50)

(Do not report 37718 in conjunction with 37735, 37780)

Ligation and Division of Long Saphenous Vein
37700

The physician ligates sections of the saphenous vein along the leg.

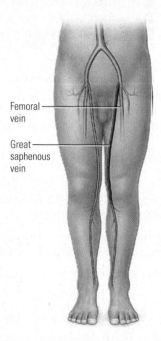

Femoral vein

Great saphenous vein

37722 Ligation, division, and stripping, long (greater) saphenous veins from saphenofemoral junction to knee or below
➔ *CPT Changes: An Insider's View* 2006
➔ *CPT Assistant* Nov 16:3, Mar 18:3
➔ *Clinical Examples in Radiology* Spring 17:3

(For ligation and stripping of the short saphenous vein, use 37718)

(For bilateral procedure, report 37722 with modifier 50)

(Do not report 37722 in conjunction with 37700, 37735)

(For ligation, division, and stripping of the greater saphenous vein, use 37722. For ligation, division, and stripping of the short saphenous vein, use 37718)

37735 Ligation and division and complete stripping of long or short saphenous veins with radical excision of ulcer and skin graft and/or interruption of communicating veins of lower leg, with excision of deep fascia
➔ *CPT Assistant* Nov 16:3, Mar 18:3
➔ *Clinical Examples in Radiology* Spring 17:3

(Do not report 37735 in conjunction with 37700, 37718, 37722, 37780)

(For bilateral procedure, report 37735 with modifier 50)

Cardiovascular 33016-39599

37760   Ligation of perforator veins, subfascial, radical (Linton type), including skin graft, when performed, open, 1 leg
- ➲ *CPT Changes: An Insider's View* 2003, 2010
- ➲ *CPT Assistant* Jul 10:6, Nov 16:3, Mar 18:3
- ➲ *Clinical Examples in Radiology* Spring 17:3

(For endoscopic procedure, use 37500)

37761   Ligation of perforator vein(s), subfascial, open, including ultrasound guidance, when performed, 1 leg
- ➲ *CPT Changes: An Insider's View* 2010
- ➲ *CPT Assistant* Jul 10:6, Nov 16:3, Mar 18:3
- ➲ *Clinical Examples in Radiology* Spring 17:3

(For bilateral procedure, report 37761 with modifier 50)

(Do not report 37760, 37761 in conjunction with 76937, 76942, 76998, 93971)

(For endoscopic ligation of subfascial perforator veins, use 37500)

37765   Stab phlebectomy of varicose veins, 1 extremity; 10-20 stab incisions
- ➲ *CPT Changes: An Insider's View* 2004
- ➲ *CPT Assistant* Aug 04:6, Nov 10:9, Oct 14:6, Nov 16:3, Mar 18:3
- ➲ *Clinical Examples in Radiology* Spring 17:3

(For less than 10 incisions, use 37799)

(For more than 20 incisions, use 37766)

37766   more than 20 incisions
- ➲ *CPT Changes: An Insider's View* 2004
- ➲ *CPT Assistant* Aug 04:6, Sep 13:17, Oct 14:6, Nov 16:3, Mar 18:3
- ➲ *Clinical Examples in Radiology* Spring 17:3

37780   Ligation and division of short saphenous vein at saphenopopliteal junction (separate procedure)
- ➲ *CPT Assistant* Aug 96:10, Nov 16:3
- ➲ *Clinical Examples in Radiology* Spring 17:3

(For bilateral procedure, report 37780 with modifier 50)

37785   Ligation, division, and/or excision of varicose vein cluster(s), 1 leg
- ➲ *CPT Changes: An Insider's View* 2004
- ➲ *CPT Assistant* Aug 04:5, Nov 10:9, Nov 16:3
- ➲ *Clinical Examples in Radiology* Spring 17:3

(For bilateral procedure, report 37785 with modifier 50)

Other Procedures

37788   Penile revascularization, artery, with or without vein graft

37790   Penile venous occlusive procedure

37799   Unlisted procedure, vascular surgery
- ➲ *CPT Assistant* Spring 93:12, Fall 93:3, Feb 97:10, Sep 97:10, May 01:11, Oct 04:16, Nov 10:9, Aug 11:9, Nov 13:14, Mar 14:8, Aug 14:14, Oct 14:6, Apr 15:10, Nov 16:3, Nov 18:11, Jun 22:22, Mar 23:23,33, Jul 23:17
- ➲ *Clinical Examples in Radiology* Summer 15:7, Spring 17:3, Fall 18:8, Fall 23:28

Hemic and Lymphatic Systems

Spleen

Excision

38100   Splenectomy; total (separate procedure)
- ➲ *CPT Assistant* July 93:9, Summer 93:10, Sep 12:11

38101   partial (separate procedure)
- ➲ *CPT Assistant* Summer 93:10, Sep 12:11

+ 38102   total, en bloc for extensive disease, in conjunction with other procedure (List in addition to code for primary procedure)
- ➲ *CPT Assistant* Summer 93:10, Sep 12:11

Repair

38115   Repair of ruptured spleen (splenorrhaphy) with or without partial splenectomy
- ➲ *CPT Assistant* Summer 93:10, Sep 12:11

Laparoscopy

Surgical laparoscopy always includes diagnostic laparoscopy. To report a diagnostic laparoscopy (peritoneoscopy) (separate procedure), use 49320.

38120   Laparoscopy, surgical, splenectomy
- ➲ *CPT Changes: An Insider's View* 2000
- ➲ *CPT Assistant* Nov 99:20-21, Mar 00:8, Sep 12:11

38129   Unlisted laparoscopy procedure, spleen
- ➲ *CPT Changes: An Insider's View* 2000
- ➲ *CPT Assistant* Nov 99:20-21, Mar 00:8, Sep 12:11

Introduction

38200   Injection procedure for splenoportography

(For radiological supervision and interpretation, use 75810)

Hemic and Lymphatic Systems   38100-38999

General

▶Cellular and Gene Therapies◀

▶Cellular and gene therapies involve the collection, processing and handling of cells or other tissues, genetic modification of those cells or tissues, and administration of the genetically modified cells or tissues with the intent to treat, modify, reverse, or cure a serious or life-threatening disease or condition.

Codes 38225, 38226, 38227, 38228 describe the various steps required to collect, prepare, transport, receive, and administer genetically modified T cells. The collection and handling code (38225) may be reported only once per day, regardless of the number of collections or quantity of cells collected. Similarly, the administration code (38228) may only be reported once per day, regardless of the number of units administered. The development of genetically modified cells is not reported with this family of codes.

Chimeric antigen receptor therapy (CAR-T) with genetically modified T cells begins with the collection of cells from the patient by peripheral blood leukocyte cell harvesting. The cells are then cryopreserved and/or otherwise prepared for processing or shipping to a manufacturing or cell-processing facility, if applicable, where gene modification and expansion of the cells are performed. When gene modification and expansion of the cells by the manufacturer are complete, the genetically modified cells are returned to the physician or other qualified health care professional when additional preparation occurs, including thawing of the cryopreserved CAR-T cells, if necessary, before the cells are administered to the patient.

The procedure to administer CAR-T cells includes physician or other qualified health care professional monitoring of multiple physiologic parameters, verification of cell processing, evaluation of the patient during, as well as immediately before and after the administration of the CAR-T cells, direct supervision of clinical staff, and management of any adverse events during the administration. Care on the same date of service that is not directly related to the service of administration of the CAR-T cells (eg, care provided after the administration is complete, care for the patient's underlying condition or other medical problems) may be separately reported using the appropriate evaluation and management code with modifier 25. Management of uncomplicated adverse events (eg, nausea, urticaria) during the infusion is not reported separately.

The fluid used to administer the cells and other infusions for incidental hydration (eg, 96360, 96361) are not reported separately. Similarly, infusion(s) of any supportive medication(s) (eg, steroids) concurrently with the CAR-T cell administration are not reported separately. However, hydration or administration of medications (eg, antibiotics, opioids) unrelated to the

CAR-T administration may be reported separately with modifier 59.◀

▶(For administration of drugs, agents and biologic response modifiers, see Chemotherapy and Other Highly Complex Drug or Highly Complex Biologic Agent Administration)◀

▶(For transplant services/procedures, see Bone Marrow or Stem Cell Services/Procedures)◀

#● **38225**   Chimeric antigen receptor T-cell (CAR-T) therapy; harvesting of blood-derived T lymphocytes for development of genetically modified autologous CAR-T cells, per day
> *CPT Changes: An Insider's View* 2025

#● **38226**   preparation of blood-derived T lymphocytes for transportation (eg, cryopreservation, storage)
> *CPT Changes: An Insider's View* 2025

#● **38227**   receipt and preparation of CAR-T cells for administration
> *CPT Changes: An Insider's View* 2025

#● **38228**   CAR-T cell administration, autologous
> *CPT Changes: An Insider's View* 2025

Bone Marrow or Stem Cell Services/ Procedures

Codes 38207-38215 describe various steps used to preserve, prepare and purify bone marrow/stem cells prior to transplantation or reinfusion. Each code may be reported only once per day regardless of the quantity of bone marrow/stem cells manipulated.

38204   Management of recipient hematopoietic progenitor cell donor search and cell acquisition
> *CPT Changes: An Insider's View* 2003
> *CPT Assistant* Oct 13:3

38205   Blood-derived hematopoietic progenitor cell harvesting for transplantation, per collection; allogeneic
> *CPT Changes: An Insider's View* 2003, 2012
> *CPT Assistant* Oct 13:3, May 18:3

38206   autologous
> *CPT Changes: An Insider's View* 2003
> *CPT Assistant* Oct 13:3, May 18:3

38207   Transplant preparation of hematopoietic progenitor cells; cryopreservation and storage
> *CPT Changes: An Insider's View* 2003
> *CPT Assistant* Jul 03:9, Jun 09:3, Oct 13:3

(For diagnostic cryopreservation and storage, use 88240)

38208   thawing of previously frozen harvest, without washing, per donor

➔ *CPT Changes: An Insider's View* 2003, 2004, 2012

➔ *CPT Assistant* Jul 03:9, Jun 09:3, Oct 13:3

(For diagnostic thawing and expansion of frozen cells, use 88241)

38209   thawing of previously frozen harvest, with washing, per donor

➔ *CPT Changes: An Insider's View* 2003, 2004, 2012

➔ *CPT Assistant* Oct 13:3

38210   specific cell depletion within harvest, T-cell depletion

➔ *CPT Changes: An Insider's View* 2003

➔ *CPT Assistant* Oct 13:3

38211   tumor cell depletion

➔ *CPT Changes: An Insider's View* 2003

➔ *CPT Assistant* Oct 13:3

38212   red blood cell removal

➔ *CPT Changes: An Insider's View* 2003

➔ *CPT Assistant* Oct 13:3

38213   platelet depletion

➔ *CPT Changes: An Insider's View* 2003

➔ *CPT Assistant* Oct 13:3

38214   plasma (volume) depletion

➔ *CPT Changes: An Insider's View* 2003

➔ *CPT Assistant* Oct 13:3

38215   cell concentration in plasma, mononuclear, or buffy coat layer

➔ *CPT Changes: An Insider's View* 2003

➔ *CPT Assistant* Oct 13:3

(Do not report 38207-38215 in conjunction with 88182, 88184-88189)

38220   Diagnostic bone marrow; aspiration(s)

➔ *CPT Changes: An Insider's View* 2002, 2003, 2018

➔ *CPT Assistant* Jan 04:26, Jun 07:10, Apr 12:15, May 12:11, Oct 13:3, Mar 15:9, May 18:3

➔ *Clinical Examples in Radiology* Spring 18:5

(Do not report 38220 in conjunction with 38221)

(For diagnostic bone marrow biopsy[ies] and aspiration[s] performed at the same session, use 38222)

(For aspiration of bone marrow for bone graft, spine surgery only, use 20939)

(For bone marrow aspiration[s] for platelet-rich stem cell injection, use 0232T)

38221   biopsy(ies)

➔ *CPT Changes: An Insider's View* 2002, 2003, 2018

➔ *CPT Assistant* Mar 15:9, May 18:3

➔ *Clinical Examples in Radiology* Winter 17:5, Spring 18:5

(Do not report 38221 in conjunction with 38220)

(For diagnostic bone marrow biopsy[ies] and aspiration[s] performed at the same session, use 38222)

38222   biopsy(ies) and aspiration(s)

➔ *CPT Changes: An Insider's View* 2018

➔ *CPT Assistant* May 18:3

➔ *Clinical Examples in Radiology* Spring 18:4, Fall 18:12

(Do not report 38222 in conjunction with 38220 and 38221)

(For bilateral procedure, report 38220, 38221, 38222 with modifier 50)

(For bone marrow biopsy interpretation, use 88305)

38225   Code is out of numerical sequence. See 38129-38205

38226   Code is out of numerical sequence. See 38129-38205

38227   Code is out of numerical sequence. See 38129-38205

38228   Code is out of numerical sequence. See 38129-38205

38230   Bone marrow harvesting for transplantation; allogeneic

➔ *CPT Changes: An Insider's View* 2012

➔ *CPT Assistant* Apr 96:1, Jun 09:3, May 12:11, Oct 13:3

Bone Marrow Harvesting for Transplantation
38230

A biopsy needle is inserted into the marrow cavity of the iliac crest and bone marrow is removed from the donor.

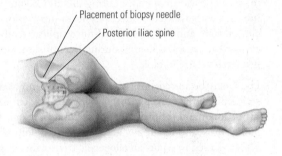

Placement of biopsy needle

Posterior iliac spine

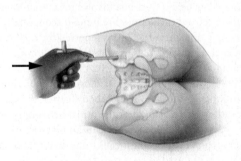

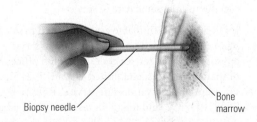

Biopsy needle

Bone marrow

38232 autologous

➡ *CPT Changes: An Insider's View* 2012

➡ *CPT Assistant* Oct 13:3

(For autologous and allogeneic blood-derived peripheral stem cell harvesting for transplantation, see 38205, 38206)

(For diagnostic bone marrow aspiration[s], see 38220, 38222)

(For aspiration of bone marrow for bone graft, spine surgery only, use 20939)

(For bone marrow aspiration[s] for platelet-rich stem cell injection, use 0232T)

Transplantation and Post-Transplantation Cellular Infusions

Hematopoietic cell transplantation (HCT) refers to the infusion of hematopoietic progenitor cells (HPC) obtained from bone marrow, peripheral blood apheresis, and/or umbilical cord blood. These procedure codes (38240-38243) include physician monitoring of multiple physiologic parameters, physician verification of cell processing, evaluation of the patient during as well as immediately before and after the HPC/lymphocyte infusion, physician presence during the HPC/lymphocyte infusion with associated direct physician supervision of clinical staff, and management of uncomplicated adverse events (eg, nausea, urticaria) during the infusion, which is not separately reportable.

HCT may be autologous (when the HPC donor and recipient are the same person) or allogeneic (when the HPC donor and recipient are not the same person). Code 38241 is used to report any autologous transplant while 38240 is used to report an allogeneic transplant. In some cases allogeneic transplants involve more than one donor and cells from each donor are infused sequentially whereby one unit of 38240 is reported for each donor infused. Code 38242 is used to report a donor lymphocyte infusion. Code 38243 is used to report a HPC boost from the original allogeneic HPC donor. A lymphocyte infusion or HPC boost can occur days, months or even years after the initial hematopoietic cell transplant. HPC boost represents an infusion of hematopoietic progenitor cells from the original donor that is being used to treat post-transplant cytopenia(s). Codes 38240, 38242, and 38243 should not be reported together on the same date of service.

If a separately identifiable evaluation and management service is performed on the same date of service, the appropriate E/M service code, including office or other outpatient services, established (99211-99215), hospital inpatient or observation care services (99221-99223, 99231-99239), and inpatient neonatal and pediatric critical care (99471, 99472, 99475, 99476), may be reported using modifier 25 in addition to 38240, 38242 or 38243. Post-transplant infusion management of

adverse reactions is reported separately using the appropriate E/M, prolonged service or critical care code(s). In accordance with place of service and facility reporting guidelines, the fluid used to administer the cells and other infusions for incidental hydration (eg, 96360, 96361) are not separately reportable. Similarly, infusion(s) of any medication(s) concurrently with the transplant infusion are not separately reportable. However, hydration or administration of medications (eg, antibiotics, narcotics) unrelated to the transplant are separately reportable using modifier 59.

38240 Hematopoietic progenitor cell (HPC); allogeneic transplantation per donor

➡ *CPT Changes: An Insider's View* 2000, 2012, 2013

➡ *CPT Assistant* Apr 96:2, Nov 98:15, Nov 99:21, Jun 09:3, Oct 13:3

38241 autologous transplantation

➡ *CPT Changes: An Insider's View* 2000, 2013

➡ *CPT Assistant* Apr 96:2, Nov 98:15, Nov 99:21, Jun 09:3, Oct 13:3, Feb 15:10

38243 HPC boost

➡ *CPT Changes: An Insider's View* 2013

➡ *CPT Assistant* Jun 13:13, Oct 13:3, Feb 15:10

38242 Allogeneic lymphocyte infusions

➡ *CPT Changes: An Insider's View* 2003, 2013

➡ *CPT Assistant* Jun 13:13, Oct 13:3

(For diagnostic bone marrow aspiration[s], see 38220, 38222)

(For aspiration of bone marrow for bone graft, spine surgery only, use 20939)

(For bone marrow aspiration[s] for platelet-rich stem cell injection, use 0232T)

(For modification, treatment, and processing of hematopoietic progenitor cell specimens for transplantation, see 38210-38215)

(For cryopreservation, freezing, and storage of hematopoietic progenitor cells for transplantation, use 38207)

(For thawing and expansion of hematopoietic progenitor cells for transplantation, see 38208, 38209)

(For compatibility studies, see 81379-81383, 86812, 86813, 86816, 86817, 86821)

38243 Code is out of numerical sequence. See 38240-38300

Lymph Nodes and Lymphatic Channels

Incision

38300 Drainage of lymph node abscess or lymphadenitis; simple

38305   extensive

38308 Lymphangiotomy or other operations on lymphatic channels

38380 Suture and/or ligation of thoracic duct; cervical approach

38381   thoracic approach

38382   abdominal approach

Excision

(For injection for sentinel node identification, use 38792)

38500 Biopsy or excision of lymph node(s); open, superficial
> *CPT Changes: An Insider's View* 2001
> *CPT Assistant* Jun 97:5, Jul 99:7, Oct 05:23, Dec 07:8, Sep 08:5, Jan 09:7, Jun 12:15

(Do not report 38500 with 38700-38780)

38505   by needle, superficial (eg, cervical, inguinal, axillary)
> *CPT Assistant* Jul 99:6, Jan 09:7, Feb 19:8
> *Clinical Examples in Radiology* Winter 17:5

(If imaging guidance is performed, see 76942, 77002, 77012, 77021)

(For fine needle aspiration biopsy, see 10004, 10005, 10006, 10007, 10008, 10009, 10010, 10011, 10012, 10021)

(For evaluation of fine needle aspirate, see 88172, 88173)

38510   open, deep cervical node(s)
> *CPT Changes: An Insider's View* 2001
> *CPT Assistant* May 98:10, Jul 99:6, Jun 12:15

38520   open, deep cervical node(s) with excision scalene fat pad
> *CPT Changes: An Insider's View* 2001
> *CPT Assistant* May 98:10, Jul 99:6

38525   open, deep axillary node(s)
> *CPT Changes: An Insider's View* 2001
> *CPT Assistant* May 98:10, Jul 99:7, Oct 05:23, Dec 07:8, Sep 08:5, Apr 14:11, Mar 15:5

38530   open, internal mammary node(s)
> *CPT Changes: An Insider's View* 2001
> *CPT Assistant* May 98:10, Jul 99:6, Aug 10:6, Apr 14:11, Feb 19:8, Feb 22:13-14

(Do not report 38530 with 38720-38746)

(For percutaneous needle biopsy, retroperitoneal lymph node or mass, use 49180)

(For fine needle aspiration biopsy, retroperitoneal lymph node or mass, see 10005, 10006, 10007, 10008, 10009, 10010, 10011, 10012)

38531   open, inguinofemoral node(s)
> *CPT Changes: An Insider's View* 2019
> *CPT Assistant* Feb 19:8

(For bilateral procedure, report 38531 with modifier 50)

38542 Dissection, deep jugular node(s)
> *CPT Assistant* Jul 99:7, Aug 10:6

(For radical cervical neck dissection, use 38720)

38550 Excision of cystic hygroma, axillary or cervical; without deep neurovascular dissection

38555   with deep neurovascular dissection

Limited Lymphadenectomy for Staging

38562 Limited lymphadenectomy for staging (separate procedure); pelvic and para-aortic
> *CPT Assistant* Mar 01:10

(When combined with prostatectomy, use 55812 or 55842)

(When combined with insertion of radioactive substance into prostate, use 55862)

38564   retroperitoneal (aortic and/or splenic)

Laparoscopy

Surgical laparoscopy always includes diagnostic laparoscopy. To report a diagnostic laparoscopy (peritoneoscopy) (separate procedure), use 49320.

38570 Laparoscopy, surgical; with retroperitoneal lymph node sampling (biopsy), single or multiple
> *CPT Changes: An Insider's View* 2000
> *CPT Assistant* Nov 99:21, Mar 00:8

38571   with bilateral total pelvic lymphadenectomy
> *CPT Changes: An Insider's View* 2000
> *CPT Assistant* Nov 99:21, Mar 00:8

38572   with bilateral total pelvic lymphadenectomy and peri-aortic lymph node sampling (biopsy), single or multiple
> *CPT Changes: An Insider's View* 2000
> *CPT Assistant* Nov 99:21, Jan 15:14

(For drainage of lymphocele to peritoneal cavity, use 49323)

38573 with bilateral total pelvic lymphadenectomy and peri-aortic lymph node sampling, peritoneal washings, peritoneal biopsy(ies), omentectomy, and diaphragmatic washings, including diaphragmatic and other serosal biopsy(ies), when performed

➲ *CPT Changes: An Insider's View* 2018

➲ *CPT Assistant* Apr 18:11, Mar 19:5

(Do not report 38573 in conjunction with 38562, 38564, 38570, 38571, 38572, 38589, 38770, 38780, 49255, 49320, 49326, 58541, 58542, 58543, 58544, 58548, 58550, 58552, 58553, 58554)

38589 Unlisted laparoscopy procedure, lymphatic system

➲ *CPT Changes: An Insider's View* 2000

➲ *CPT Assistant* Nov 99:21, Mar 00:8, Apr 18:11

Radical Lymphadenectomy (Radical Resection of Lymph Nodes)

(For limited pelvic and retroperitoneal lymphadenectomies, see 38562, 38564)

38700 Suprahyoid lymphadenectomy

➲ *CPT Assistant* Aug 02:8, Aug 10:3

(For bilateral procedure, report 38700 with modifier 50)

38720 Cervical lymphadenectomy (complete)

➲ *CPT Assistant* Oct 01:10, Aug 02:8, Aug 10:4, Apr 20:10

(For bilateral procedure, report 38720 with modifier 50)

38724 Cervical lymphadenectomy (modified radical neck dissection)

➲ *CPT Assistant* Jan 01:13, Aug 02:8, Aug 10:4, Dec 12:3, Mar 19:11

38740 Axillary lymphadenectomy; superficial

➲ *CPT Assistant* Apr 14:11

38745 complete

+ 38746 Thoracic lymphadenectomy by thoracotomy, mediastinal and regional lymphadenectomy (List separately in addition to code for primary procedure)

➲ *CPT Changes: An Insider's View* 2012

➲ *CPT Assistant* Sep 12:3, May 14:3

(On the right, mediastinal lymph nodes include the paratracheal, subcarinal, paraesophageal, and inferior pulmonary ligament)

(On the left, mediastinal lymph nodes include the aortopulmonary window, subcarinal, paraesophageal, and inferior pulmonary ligament)

(Report 38746 in conjunction with 21601, 31760, 31766, 31786, 32096-32200, 32220-32320, 32440-32491, 32503-32505, 33025, 33030, 33050-33130, 39200-39220, 39560, 39561, 43101, 43112, 43117, 43118, 43122, 43123, 43351, 60270, 60505)

(To report mediastinal and regional lymphadenectomy via thoracoscopy [VATS], see 32674)

Mediastinal Lymph Nodes: Station Number and Descriptions
38746

Relevant mediastinal lymph nodes typically removed with procedures described by code 38746, and sampled removal described with code 39402.

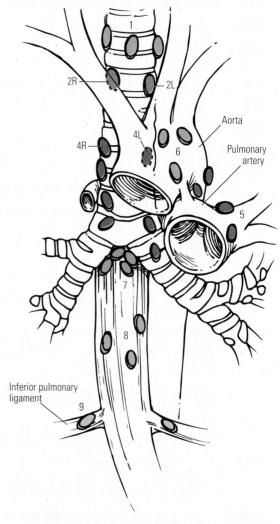

Station #	Lymph Node Descriptions
1	Low cervical, supraclavicular, and sternal notch
2	Upper paratracheal (R & L)
4	Lower paratracheal (R & L)
5	Subaortic or aortopulmonary window
6	Para-aortic
7	Subcarinal
8	Paraesophageal (below the carina)
9	Inferior pulmonary ligament

*Station #3 is not depicted as it is not applicable to the use of codes 32674, 38746, or 39402.

Hemic and Lymphatic Systems 38100-38999

+ 38747　Abdominal lymphadenectomy, regional, including celiac, gastric, portal, peripancreatic, with or without para-aortic and vena caval nodes (List separately in addition to code for primary procedure)

➔ *CPT Assistant* Nov 98:15, Apr 20:10

38760　Inguinofemoral lymphadenectomy, superficial, including Cloquet's node (separate procedure)

(For bilateral procedure, report 38760 with modifier 50)

38765　Inguinofemoral lymphadenectomy, superficial, in continuity with pelvic lymphadenectomy, including external iliac, hypogastric, and obturator nodes (separate procedure)

(For bilateral procedure, report 38765 with modifier 50)

38770　Pelvic lymphadenectomy, including external iliac, hypogastric, and obturator nodes (separate procedure)

(For bilateral procedure, report 38770 with modifier 50)

38780　Retroperitoneal transabdominal lymphadenectomy, extensive, including pelvic, aortic, and renal nodes (separate procedure)

(For excision and repair of lymphedematous skin and subcutaneous tissue, see 15004-15005, 15570-15650)

Introduction

38790　Injection procedure; lymphangiography

➔ *CPT Assistant* Jul 99:6, Apr 21:14

➔ *Clinical Examples in Radiology* Summer 15:8, Winter 21:12, Winter 23:19

(For bilateral procedure, report 38790 with modifier 50)

(For radiological supervision and interpretation, see 75801-75807)

38792　　radioactive tracer for identification of sentinel node

➔ *CPT Changes: An Insider's View* 2008, 2012

➔ *CPT Assistant* Nov 98:15, Jul 99:6, Dec 99:8, Sep 08:5, Mar 15:5

(For excision of sentinel node, see 38500-38542)

(For nuclear medicine lymphatics and lymph gland imaging, use 78195)

(For intraoperative identification (eg, mapping) of sentinel lymph node(s) including injection of non-radioactive dye, see 38900)

38794　Cannulation, thoracic duct

Other Procedures

+ 38900　Intraoperative identification (eg, mapping) of sentinel lymph node(s) includes injection of non-radioactive dye, when performed (List separately in addition to code for primary procedure)

➔ *CPT Changes: An Insider's View* 2011

➔ *CPT Assistant* Mar 15:5, Feb 19:8

(Use 38900 in conjunction with 19302, 19307, 38500, 38510, 38520, 38525, 38530, 38531, 38542, 38562, 38564, 38570, 38571, 38572, 38740, 38745, 38760, 38765, 38770, 38780, 56630, 56631, 56632, 56633, 56634, 56637, 56640)

(For injection of radioactive tracer for identification of sentinel node, use 38792)

38999　Unlisted procedure, hemic or lymphatic system

➔ *CPT Assistant* May 98:10, Oct 21:14, Sep 23:51

Mediastinum and Diaphragm

Mediastinum

Incision

39000　Mediastinotomy with exploration, drainage, removal of foreign body, or biopsy; cervical approach

39010　　transthoracic approach, including either transthoracic or median sternotomy

➔ *CPT Assistant* Jan 13:6, Jan 14:5

(Do not report 39010 in conjunction with 33955, 33956, 33963, 33964)

(For VATS pericardial biopsy, use 32604)

Excision/Resection

39200　Resection of mediastinal cyst

➔ *CPT Changes: An Insider's View* 2012

39220　Resection of mediastinal tumor

➔ *CPT Changes: An Insider's View* 2012

(For substernal thyroidectomy, use 60270)

(For thymectomy, use 60520)

(For thoracoscopic [VATS] resection of mediastinal cyst, tumor, or mass, use 32662)

Endoscopy

39401 Mediastinoscopy; includes biopsy(ies) of mediastinal mass (eg, lymphoma), when performed

➔ *CPT Changes: An Insider's View* 2016

➔ *CPT Assistant* Jun 16:4

39402 with lymph node biopsy(ies) (eg, lung cancer staging)

➔ *CPT Changes: An Insider's View* 2016

➔ *CPT Assistant* Jun 16:4

Other Procedures

39499 Unlisted procedure, mediastinum

Diaphragm

Repair

(For transabdominal repair of diaphragmatic [esophageal hiatal] hernia, use 43325)

(For laparoscopic repair of diaphragmatic [esophageal hiatal] hernias and fundoplication, see 43280, 43281, 43282)

39501 Repair, laceration of diaphragm, any approach

➔ *CPT Assistant* Nov 00:3, Dec 14:16

(For laparoscopic paraesophageal hernia repair, see 43281, 43282)

39503 Repair, neonatal diaphragmatic hernia, with or without chest tube insertion and with or without creation of ventral hernia

➔ *CPT Assistant* Feb 12:3

(Do not report modifier 63 in conjunction with 39503)

(For laparoscopic paraesophageal hernia repair, see 43281, 43282)

39540 Repair, diaphragmatic hernia (other than neonatal), traumatic; acute

➔ *CPT Assistant* Nov 00:9, Jun 08:3

39541 chronic

39545 Imbrication of diaphragm for eventration, transthoracic or transabdominal, paralytic or nonparalytic

➔ *CPT Assistant* Nov 00:3

39560 Resection, diaphragm; with simple repair (eg, primary suture)

➔ *CPT Changes: An Insider's View* 2000

➔ *CPT Assistant* Nov 99:21, Nov 00:3

39561 with complex repair (eg, prosthetic material, local muscle flap)

➔ *CPT Changes: An Insider's View* 2000

➔ *CPT Assistant* Nov 99:21, Nov 00:3

Other Procedures

39599 Unlisted procedure, diaphragm

(For laparoscopic insertion or replacement of a permanent synchronized diaphragmatic stimulation system, see 0674T, 0675T, 0680T)

Surgery

Digestive System

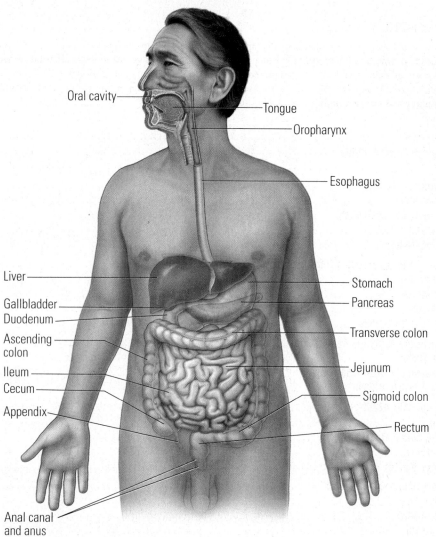

Oral cavity

Tongue

Oropharynx

Esophagus

Liver

Stomach

Gallbladder

Pancreas

Duodenum

Ascending colon

Transverse colon

Ileum

Jejunum

Cecum

Appendix

Sigmoid colon

Rectum

Anal canal and anus

Digestive System

Lips

(For procedures on skin of lips, see 10040 et seq)

Excision

40490   Biopsy of lip

40500   Vermilionectomy (lip shave), with mucosal advancement

40510   Excision of lip; transverse wedge excision with primary closure

40520   V-excision with primary direct linear closure

(For excision of mucous lesions, see 40810-40816)

40525   full thickness, reconstruction with local flap (eg, Estlander or fan)

40527   full thickness, reconstruction with cross lip flap (Abbe-Estlander)

40530   Resection of lip, more than one-fourth, without reconstruction

(For reconstruction, see 13131 et seq)

Repair (Cheiloplasty)

40650   Repair lip, full thickness; vermilion only
 ➔ *CPT Assistant* Jul 00:10, Nov 16:7

40652   up to half vertical height
 ➔ *CPT Assistant* Jul 00:10, Nov 16:7

40654   over one-half vertical height, or complex
 ➔ *CPT Assistant* Nov 16:7

40700   Plastic repair of cleft lip/nasal deformity; primary, partial or complete, unilateral
 ➔ *CPT Assistant* Dec 14:18

40701   primary bilateral, 1-stage procedure

40702   primary bilateral, 1 of 2 stages

40720   secondary, by recreation of defect and reclosure
 ➔ *CPT Assistant* Dec 14:18

(For bilateral procedure, report 40720 with modifier 50)

(To report rhinoplasty only for nasal deformity secondary to congenital cleft lip, see 30460, 30462)

(For repair of cleft lip, with cross lip pedicle flap (Abbe-Estlander type), use 40527)

40761   with cross lip pedicle flap (Abbe-Estlander type), including sectioning and inserting of pedicle

(For repair cleft palate, see 42200 et seq)

(For other reconstructive procedures, see 14060, 14061, 15120-15261, 15574, 15576, 15630)

Other Procedures

40799   Unlisted procedure, lips

Vestibule of Mouth

The vestibule is the part of the oral cavity outside the dentoalveolar structures; it includes the mucosal and submucosal tissue of lips and cheeks.

Incision

40800   Drainage of abscess, cyst, hematoma, vestibule of mouth; simple

40801   complicated

40804   Removal of embedded foreign body, vestibule of mouth; simple

40805   complicated

40806   Incision of labial frenum (frenotomy)

Excision, Destruction

40808   Biopsy, vestibule of mouth

40810   Excision of lesion of mucosa and submucosa, vestibule of mouth; without repair

40812   with simple repair

40814   with complex repair

40816   complex, with excision of underlying muscle

40818   Excision of mucosa of vestibule of mouth as donor graft

40819   Excision of frenum, labial or buccal (frenumectomy, frenulectomy, frenectomy)
 ➔ *CPT Assistant* Aug 20:14

40820   Destruction of lesion or scar of vestibule of mouth by physical methods (eg, laser, thermal, cryo, chemical)

Repair

40830   Closure of laceration, vestibule of mouth; 2.5 cm or less

40831   over 2.5 cm or complex

40840   Vestibuloplasty; anterior

40842   posterior, unilateral

40843   posterior, bilateral

40844   entire arch

40845   complex (including ridge extension, muscle repositioning)

(For skin grafts, see 15002 et seq)

Other Procedures

40899   Unlisted procedure, vestibule of mouth

Tongue and Floor of Mouth

Incision

41000   Intraoral incision and drainage of abscess, cyst, or hematoma of tongue or floor of mouth; lingual

41005   sublingual, superficial

41006   sublingual, deep, supramylohyoid

41007   submental space

41008   submandibular space

41009   masticator space

41010   Incision of lingual frenum (frenotomy)
➜ *CPT Assistant* Sep 17:14, Nov 17:10, Aug 20:14

41015   Extraoral incision and drainage of abscess, cyst, or hematoma of floor of mouth; sublingual

41016   submental

41017   submandibular

41018   masticator space

(For frenoplasty, use 41520)

41019   Placement of needles, catheters, or other device(s) into the head and/or neck region (percutaneous, transoral, or transnasal) for subsequent interstitial radioelement application
➜ *CPT Changes: An Insider's View* 2008

(For imaging guidance, see 76942, 77002, 77012, 77021)

(For stereotactic insertion of intracranial brachytherapy radiation sources, use 61770)

(For interstitial radioelement application, see 77770, 77771, 77772, 77778)

Excision

41100   Biopsy of tongue; anterior two-thirds

41105   posterior one-third

41108   Biopsy of floor of mouth

41110   Excision of lesion of tongue without closure

41112   Excision of lesion of tongue with closure; anterior two-thirds

41113   posterior one-third

41114   with local tongue flap

(Do not report 41114 in conjunction with 41112 or 41113)

41115   Excision of lingual frenum (frenectomy)
➜ *CPT Assistant* Sep 17:14, Nov 17:10

41116   Excision, lesion of floor of mouth

41120   Glossectomy; less than one-half tongue
➜ *CPT Assistant* Aug 10:10

41130   hemiglossectomy
➜ *CPT Assistant* Aug 10:5

41135   partial, with unilateral radical neck dissection
➜ *CPT Assistant* Aug 10:5

41140   complete or total, with or without tracheostomy, without radical neck dissection
➜ *CPT Assistant* Aug 10:5

41145   complete or total, with or without tracheostomy, with unilateral radical neck dissection
➜ *CPT Assistant* Aug 10:5

41150   composite procedure with resection floor of mouth and mandibular resection, without radical neck dissection
➜ *CPT Assistant* Aug 10:5

41153   composite procedure with resection floor of mouth, with suprahyoid neck dissection
➜ *CPT Assistant* Aug 10:3

41155   composite procedure with resection floor of mouth, mandibular resection, and radical neck dissection (Commando type)
➜ *CPT Assistant* Jan 01:13, Aug 10:3

Repair

41250   Repair of laceration 2.5 cm or less; floor of mouth and/or anterior two-thirds of tongue

41251   posterior one-third of tongue

41252   Repair of laceration of tongue, floor of mouth, over 2.6 cm or complex

Other Procedures

41510   Suture of tongue to lip for micrognathia (Douglas type procedure)
➜ *CPT Assistant* Aug 10:11

41512   Tongue base suspension, permanent suture technique
➜ *CPT Changes: An Insider's View* 2009
➜ *CPT Assistant* Aug 10:11, Aug 12:13

(For suture of tongue to lip for micrognathia, use 41510)

41520   Frenoplasty (surgical revision of frenum, eg, with Z-plasty)
➜ *CPT Assistant* Sep 17:14, Nov 17:10, Aug 20:14

(For frenotomy, see 40806, 41010)

41530   Submucosal ablation of the tongue base, radiofrequency, 1 or more sites, per session
→ *CPT Changes: An Insider's View* 2009
→ *CPT Assistant* Aug 10:10

41599   Unlisted procedure, tongue, floor of mouth
→ *CPT Assistant* Dec 00:14
→ *Clinical Examples in Radiology* Fall 09:11

Dentoalveolar Structures

Incision

41800   Drainage of abscess, cyst, hematoma from dentoalveolar structures

41805   Removal of embedded foreign body from dentoalveolar structures; soft tissues

41806   bone

Excision, Destruction

41820   Gingivectomy, excision gingiva, each quadrant

41821   Operculectomy, excision pericoronal tissues

41822   Excision of fibrous tuberosities, dentoalveolar structures

41823   Excision of osseous tuberosities, dentoalveolar structures

41825   Excision of lesion or tumor (except listed above), dentoalveolar structures; without repair

41826   with simple repair

41827   with complex repair

(For nonexcisional destruction, use 41850)

41828   Excision of hyperplastic alveolar mucosa, each quadrant (specify)

41830   Alveolectomy, including curettage of osteitis or sequestrectomy

41850   Destruction of lesion (except excision), dentoalveolar structures

Other Procedures

41870   Periodontal mucosal grafting

41872   Gingivoplasty, each quadrant (specify)

41874   Alveoloplasty, each quadrant (specify)

(For closure of lacerations, see 40830, 40831)

(For segmental osteotomy, use 21206)

(For reduction of fractures, see 21421-21490)

41899   Unlisted procedure, dentoalveolar structures

Palate and Uvula

Incision

42000   Drainage of abscess of palate, uvula

Excision, Destruction

42100   Biopsy of palate, uvula

42104   Excision, lesion of palate, uvula; without closure

42106   with simple primary closure

42107   with local flap closure

(For skin graft, see 14040-14302)

(For mucosal graft, use 40818)

42120   Resection of palate or extensive resection of lesion

(For reconstruction of palate with extraoral tissue, see 14040-14302, 15050, 15120, 15240, 15576)

42140   Uvulectomy, excision of uvula

42145   Palatopharyngoplasty (eg, uvulopalatopharyngoplasty, uvulopharyngoplasty)
→ *CPT Assistant* Dec 04:19

(For removal of exostosis of the bony palate, see 21031, 21032)

42160   Destruction of lesion, palate or uvula (thermal, cryo or chemical)
→ *CPT Assistant* Apr 10:10

Repair

42180   Repair, laceration of palate; up to 2 cm

42182   over 2 cm or complex

42200   Palatoplasty for cleft palate, soft and/or hard palate only
→ *CPT Assistant* Jul 14:8, Mar 15:9

42205   Palatoplasty for cleft palate, with closure of alveolar ridge; soft tissue only

42210   with bone graft to alveolar ridge (includes obtaining graft)

42215   Palatoplasty for cleft palate; major revision

42220   secondary lengthening procedure

42225   attachment pharyngeal flap

42226   Lengthening of palate, and pharyngeal flap

42227   Lengthening of palate, with island flap

42235   Repair of anterior palate, including vomer flap
➔ *CPT Assistant* Jul 14:8, Mar 15:9

(For repair of oronasal fistula, use 30600)

42260   Repair of nasolabial fistula

(For repair of cleft lip, see 40700 et seq)

42280   Maxillary impression for palatal prosthesis

42281   Insertion of pin-retained palatal prosthesis

Other Procedures

42299   Unlisted procedure, palate, uvula
➔ *CPT Assistant* Dec 04:19, Apr 10:10, Nov 10:9, Jul 14:8

Salivary Gland and Ducts

Incision

42300   Drainage of abscess; parotid, simple

42305   parotid, complicated

42310   Drainage of abscess; submaxillary or sublingual, intraoral
➔ *CPT Changes: An Insider's View* 2003

42320   submaxillary, external

42330   Sialolithotomy; submandibular (submaxillary), sublingual or parotid, uncomplicated, intraoral

42335   submandibular (submaxillary), complicated, intraoral

42340   parotid, extraoral or complicated intraoral

Excision

42400   Biopsy of salivary gland; needle
➔ *Clinical Examples in Radiology* Winter 17:5

(For fine needle aspiration biopsy, see 10004, 10005, 10006, 10007, 10008, 10009, 10010, 10011, 10012, 10021)

(For evaluation of fine needle aspirate, see 88172, 88173)

(If imaging guidance is performed, see 76942, 77002, 77012, 77021)

42405   incisional

(If imaging guidance is performed, see 76942, 77002, 77012, 77021)

42408   Excision of sublingual salivary cyst (ranula)

42409   Marsupialization of sublingual salivary cyst (ranula)

42410   Excision of parotid tumor or parotid gland; lateral lobe, without nerve dissection

42415   lateral lobe, with dissection and preservation of facial nerve

42420   total, with dissection and preservation of facial nerve
➔ *CPT Assistant* Aug 10:4

42425   total, en bloc removal with sacrifice of facial nerve

42426   total, with unilateral radical neck dissection

(For suture or grafting of facial nerve, see 64864, 64865, 69740, 69745)

42440   Excision of submandibular (submaxillary) gland

42450   Excision of sublingual gland

Repair

42500   Plastic repair of salivary duct, sialodochoplasty; primary or simple

42505   secondary or complicated

42507   Parotid duct diversion, bilateral (Wilke type procedure);

42509   with excision of both submandibular glands

42510   with ligation of both submandibular (Wharton's) ducts

Other Procedures

42550   Injection procedure for sialography
➔ *Clinical Examples in Radiology* Fall 09:9

(For radiological supervision and interpretation, use 70390)

42600   Closure salivary fistula

42650   Dilation salivary duct

42660   Dilation and catheterization of salivary duct, with or without injection

42665   Ligation salivary duct, intraoral

42699   Unlisted procedure, salivary glands or ducts

Pharynx, Adenoids, and Tonsils

Incision

42700   Incision and drainage abscess; peritonsillar
➔ *CPT Assistant* Apr 24:35

42720   retropharyngeal or parapharyngeal, intraoral approach

42725   retropharyngeal or parapharyngeal, external approach

Excision, Destruction

42800   Biopsy; oropharynx

42804   nasopharynx, visible lesion, simple

42806   nasopharynx, survey for unknown primary lesion

(For laryngoscopic biopsy, see 31510, 31535, 31536)

  ★=Telemedicine   ◀=Audio-only   +=Add-on code   ✗=FDA approval pending   #=Resequenced code   ⊘=Modifier 51 exempt   ➔➔➔=See p xxi for details

42808   Excision or destruction of lesion of pharynx, any method

42809   Removal of foreign body from pharynx

42810   Excision branchial cleft cyst or vestige, confined to skin and subcutaneous tissues

42815   Excision branchial cleft cyst, vestige, or fistula, extending beneath subcutaneous tissues and/or into pharynx

42820   Tonsillectomy and adenoidectomy; younger than age 12
➜ *CPT Assistant* Feb 98:11, Mar 08:15, May 08:14, Jun 21:14

42821   age 12 or over
➜ *CPT Assistant* Aug 97:18, Feb 98:11, Mar 08:15, May 08:14, Jun 21:14

42825   Tonsillectomy, primary or secondary; younger than age 12
➜ *CPT Assistant* Aug 97:18, Feb 98:11, Mar 08:15, Jun 21:14, Apr 24:35

42826   age 12 or over
➜ *CPT Assistant* Aug 97:18, Feb 98:11, Mar 08:15, Apr 10:10, Jun 21:14, Sep 21:14, Apr 24:35

42830   Adenoidectomy, primary; younger than age 12

42831   age 12 or over

42835   Adenoidectomy, secondary; younger than age 12

42836   age 12 or over
➜ *CPT Assistant* Feb 98:11, Nov 10:9

42842   Radical resection of tonsil, tonsillar pillars, and/or retromolar trigone; without closure
➜ *CPT Assistant* Aug 10:6

42844   closure with local flap (eg, tongue, buccal)
➜ *CPT Assistant* Aug 10:6

42845   closure with other flap
➜ *CPT Assistant* Aug 10:6

(For closure with other flap(s), use appropriate number for flap(s))

(When combined with radical neck dissection, use also 38720)

42860   Excision of tonsil tags

42870   Excision or destruction lingual tonsil, any method (separate procedure)

(For resection of the nasopharynx [eg, juvenile angiofibroma] by bicoronal and/or transzygomatic approach, see 61586 and 61600)

42890   Limited pharyngectomy

42892   Resection of lateral pharyngeal wall or pyriform sinus, direct closure by advancement of lateral and posterior pharyngeal walls
➜ *CPT Assistant* Aug 10:6

(When combined with radical neck dissection, use also 38720)

42894   Resection of pharyngeal wall requiring closure with myocutaneous or fasciocutaneous flap or free muscle, skin, or fascial flap with microvascular anastomosis
➜ *CPT Changes: An Insider's View* 2010
➜ *CPT Assistant* Nov 07:8, Aug 10:6

(When combined with radical neck dissection, use also 38720)

(For limited pharyngectomy with radical neck dissection, use 38720 with 42890)

(For flap used for reconstruction, see 15730, 15733, 15734, 15756, 15757, 15758)

Repair

42900   Suture pharynx for wound or injury

42950   Pharyngoplasty (plastic or reconstructive operation on pharynx)
➜ *CPT Assistant* Apr 16:8, Oct 19:10

(For pharyngeal flap, use 42225)

42953   Pharyngoesophageal repair

(For closure with myocutaneous or other flap, use appropriate number in addition)

Other Procedures

42955   Pharyngostomy (fistulization of pharynx, external for feeding)

42960   Control oropharyngeal hemorrhage, primary or secondary (eg, post-tonsillectomy); simple

42961   complicated, requiring hospitalization

42962   with secondary surgical intervention

42970   Control of nasopharyngeal hemorrhage, primary or secondary (eg, postadenoidectomy); simple, with posterior nasal packs, with or without anterior packs and/or cautery
➜ *CPT Changes: An Insider's View* 2002

42971   complicated, requiring hospitalization

42972   with secondary surgical intervention

42975   Drug-induced sleep endoscopy, with dynamic evaluation of velum, pharynx, tongue base, and larynx for evaluation of sleep-disordered breathing, flexible, diagnostic
➜ *CPT Changes: An Insider's View* 2022
➜ *CPT Assistant* Dec 21:20

(Do not report 42975 in conjunction with 31231, unless performed for a separate condition [ie, other than sleep-disordered breathing] and using a separate endoscope)

(Do not report 42975 in conjunction with 31575, 92511)

Digestive 40490-49999

Copying, photographing, or sharing this CPT® book violates AMA's copyright.

42999 Unlisted procedure, pharynx, adenoids, or tonsils

⊙ *CPT Assistant* Feb 14:11

Esophagus

Incision

(For esophageal intubation with laparotomy, use 43510)

43020 Esophagotomy, cervical approach, with removal of foreign body

43030 Cricopharyngeal myotomy

⊙ *CPT Assistant* Jul 20:13

43045 Esophagotomy, thoracic approach, with removal of foreign body

Excision

(For gastrointestinal reconstruction for previous esophagectomy, see 43360, 43361)

43100 Excision of lesion, esophagus, with primary repair; cervical approach

43101 thoracic or abdominal approach

⊙ *CPT Assistant* Aug 10:4

(For wide excision of malignant lesion of cervical esophagus, with total laryngectomy without radical neck dissection, see 43107, 43116, 43124, and 31360)

(For wide excision of malignant lesion of cervical esophagus, with total laryngectomy with radical neck dissection, see 43107, 43116, 43124, and 31365)

43107 Total or near total esophagectomy, without thoracotomy; with pharyngogastrostomy or cervical esophagogastrostomy, with or without pyloroplasty (transhiatal)

⊙ *CPT Assistant* Aug 10:4

43108 with colon interposition or small intestine reconstruction, including intestine mobilization, preparation and anastomosis(es)

⊙ *CPT Changes: An Insider's View* 2002

43112 Total or near total esophagectomy, with thoracotomy; with pharyngogastrostomy or cervical esophagogastrostomy, with or without pyloroplasty (ie, McKeown esophagectomy or tri-incisional esophagectomy)

⊙ *CPT Changes: An Insider's View* 2018
⊙ *CPT Assistant* Aug 13:14, Jul 18:7

43113 with colon interposition or small intestine reconstruction, including intestine mobilization, preparation, and anastomosis(es)

⊙ *CPT Changes: An Insider's View* 2002

43116 Partial esophagectomy, cervical, with free intestinal graft, including microvascular anastomosis, obtaining the graft and intestinal reconstruction

⊙ *CPT Assistant* Nov 97:17, Nov 98:16, Aug 10:4

(Do not report 43116 in conjunction with 69990)

(Report 43116 with the modifier 52 appended if intestinal or free jejunal graft with microvascular anastomosis is performed by another physician)

(For free jejunal graft with microvascular anastomosis performed by another physician, use 43496)

43117 Partial esophagectomy, distal two-thirds, with thoracotomy and separate abdominal incision, with or without proximal gastrectomy; with thoracic esophagogastrostomy, with or without pyloroplasty (Ivor Lewis)

43118 with colon interposition or small intestine reconstruction, including intestine mobilization, preparation, and anastomosis(es)

⊙ *CPT Changes: An Insider's View* 2002

(For total esophagectomy with gastropharyngostomy, see 43107, 43124)

(For esophagogastrectomy (lower third) and vagotomy, use 43122)

43121 Partial esophagectomy, distal two-thirds, with thoracotomy only, with or without proximal gastrectomy, with thoracic esophagogastrostomy, with or without pyloroplasty

43122 Partial esophagectomy, thoracoabdominal or abdominal approach, with or without proximal gastrectomy; with esophagogastrostomy, with or without pyloroplasty

43123 with colon interposition or small intestine reconstruction, including intestine mobilization, preparation, and anastomosis(es)

⊙ *CPT Changes: An Insider's View* 2002

43124 Total or partial esophagectomy, without reconstruction (any approach), with cervical esophagostomy

43130 Diverticulectomy of hypopharynx or esophagus, with or without myotomy; cervical approach

⊙ *CPT Assistant* Oct 10:12, Dec 10:12

43135 thoracic approach

⊙ *CPT Assistant* Oct 10:12, Dec 10:12

(For endoscopic diverticulectomy of hypopharynx or cervical esophagus, use 43180)

Endoscopy

When bleeding occurs as a result of an endoscopic procedure, control of bleeding is not reported separately during the same operative session.

★=Telemedicine ◀=Audio-only ✚=Add-on code ✗=FDA approval pending #=Resequenced code ⊘=Modifier 51 exempt ⊙⊙⊙=See p xxi for details

Esophagoscopy includes examination from the cricopharyngeus muscle (upper esophageal sphincter) to and including the gastroesophageal junction. It may also include examination of the proximal region of the stomach via retroflexion when performed.

Esophagoscopy

43180   Esophagoscopy, rigid, transoral with diverticulectomy of hypopharynx or cervical esophagus (eg, Zenker's diverticulum), with cricopharyngeal myotomy, includes use of telescope or operating microscope and repair, when performed

→ *CPT Changes: An Insider's View* 2015

→ *CPT Assistant* Nov 15:8

(Do not report 43180 in conjunction with 43210, 69990)

(For diverticulectomy of hypopharynx or esophagus [open], see 43130, 43135)

43191   Esophagoscopy, rigid, transoral; diagnostic, including collection of specimen(s) by brushing or washing when performed (separate procedure)

→ *CPT Changes: An Insider's View* 2014

→ *CPT Assistant* Dec 13:3, Feb 14:9, 11, Nov 15:8, Sep 22:13

►(Do not report 43191 in conjunction with 43192, 43193, 43194, 43195, 43196, 43197, 43198, 43210, 43497, 0884T)◄

(For diagnostic transnasal esophagoscopy, see 43197, 43198)

(For diagnostic flexible transoral esophagoscopy, use 43200)

43192   with directed submucosal injection(s), any substance

→ *CPT Changes: An Insider's View* 2014

→ *CPT Assistant* Dec 13:3, Sep 22:13

(Do not report 43192 in conjunction with 43191, 43197, 43198)

(For flexible transoral esophagoscopy with directed submucosal injection(s), use 43201)

(For flexible transoral esophagoscopy with injection sclerosis of esophageal varices, use 43204)

(For rigid transoral esophagoscopy with injection sclerosis of esophageal varices, use 43499)

43193   with biopsy, single or multiple

→ *CPT Changes: An Insider's View* 2014

→ *CPT Assistant* Dec 13:3, Sep 22:13

(Do not report 43193 in conjunction with 43191, 43197, 43198)

(For flexible transoral esophagoscopy with biopsy, use 43202)

43194   with removal of foreign body(s)

→ *CPT Changes: An Insider's View* 2014, 2015

→ *CPT Assistant* Dec 13:3, Sep 22:13

(Do not report 43194 in conjunction with 43191, 43197, 43198)

(If fluoroscopic guidance is performed, use 76000)

(For flexible transoral esophagoscopy with removal of foreign body(s), use 43215)

43195   with balloon dilation (less than 30 mm diameter)

→ *CPT Changes: An Insider's View* 2014

→ *CPT Assistant* Dec 13:3, Sep 22:13

►(Do not report 43195 in conjunction with 43191, 43197, 43198, 0884T)◄

(If fluoroscopic guidance is performed, use 74360)

(For esophageal dilation with balloon 30 mm diameter or larger, see 43214, 43233)

(For dilation without endoscopic visualization, see 43450, 43453)

(For flexible transoral esophagoscopy with balloon dilation [less than 30 mm diameter], use 43220)

43196   with insertion of guide wire followed by dilation over guide wire

→ *CPT Changes: An Insider's View* 2014

→ *CPT Assistant* Dec 13:3, Feb 14:9, Sep 22:13

►(Do not report 43196 in conjunction with 43191, 43197, 43198, 0884T)◄

(If fluoroscopic guidance is performed, use 74360)

(For flexible transoral esophagoscopy with insertion of guide wire followed by dilation over guide wire, use 43226)

43197   Esophagoscopy, flexible, transnasal; diagnostic, including collection of specimen(s) by brushing or washing, when performed (separate procedure)

→ *CPT Changes: An Insider's View* 2014, 2015

→ *CPT Assistant* Dec 13:3, Feb 14:9, Nov 15:8, Sep 22:13, Nov 22:12

(Do not report 43197 in conjunction with 31575, 43191, 43192, 43193, 43194, 43195, 43196, 43198, 43200-43232, 43235-43259, 43266, 43270, 43290, 43291, 43497, 92511, 0652T, 0653T, 0654T)

(Do not report 43197 in conjunction with 31231 unless separate type of endoscope [eg, rigid endoscope] is used)

(For transoral esophagoscopy, see 43191, 43200)

43198   with biopsy, single or multiple

→ *CPT Changes: An Insider's View* 2014

→ *CPT Assistant* Dec 13:3, Feb 14:9, Sep 22:13, Nov 22:12

(Do not report 43198 in conjunction with 31575, 43191, 43192, 43193, 43194, 43195, 43196, 43197, 43200-43232, 43235-43259, 43266, 43270, 43290, 43291, 92511, 0652T, 0653T, 0654T)

(Do not report 43198 in conjunction with 31231 unless separate type of endoscope [eg, rigid endoscope] is used)

(For transoral esophagoscopy with biopsy, see 43193, 43202)

43200 Esophagoscopy, flexible, transoral; diagnostic, including collection of specimen(s) by brushing or washing, when performed (separate procedure)

➲ *CPT Changes: An Insider's View* 2000, 2014, 2017

➲ *CPT Assistant* Spring 91:7, Spring 94:1, Jun 98:10, Nov 99:21, Sep 03:3, Oct 08:6, Jan 13:11, Feb 13:16, Dec 13:3, Feb 14:9, Nov 15:8, Sep 22:13

▶(Do not report 43200 in conjunction with 43197, 43198, 43201-43232, 43497, 0884T)◀

(For diagnostic rigid transoral esophagoscopy, use 43191)

(For diagnostic flexible transnasal esophagoscopy, use 43197)

(For diagnostic flexible esophagogastroduodenoscopy, use 43235)

43201 with directed submucosal injection(s), any substance

➲ *CPT Changes: An Insider's View* 2003, 2014, 2017

➲ *CPT Assistant* Jun 10:4, Jan 13:11, Dec 13:3

(Do not report 43201 in conjunction with 43204, 43211, 43227 for the same lesion)

(Do not report 43201 in conjunction with 43197, 43198, 43200)

(For rigid transoral esophagoscopy with directed submucosal injection[s], use 43192)

(For flexible transoral esophagoscopy with injection sclerosis of esophageal varices, use 43204)

(For rigid transoral esophagoscopy with injection sclerosis of esophageal varices, use 43499)

43202 with biopsy, single or multiple

➲ *CPT Changes: An Insider's View* 2014, 2017

➲ *CPT Assistant* Spring 94:1, Oct 08:6, Jan 13:11, Dec 13:3

(Do not report 43202 in conjunction with 43211 for the same lesion)

(Do not report 43202 in conjunction with 43197, 43198, 43200)

(For rigid transoral esophagoscopy with biopsy, use 43193)

(For flexible transnasal esophagoscopy with biopsy, use 43198)

43204 with injection sclerosis of esophageal varices

➲ *CPT Changes: An Insider's View* 2014, 2017

➲ *CPT Assistant* Spring 94:1, Oct 08:6, Jun 10:5, Jan 13:11, Dec 13:3

(Do not report 43204 in conjunction with 43201, 43227 for the same lesion)

(Do not report 43204 in conjunction with 43197, 43198, 43200)

(For rigid transoral esophagoscopy with injection sclerosis of esophageal varices, use 43499)

43205 with band ligation of esophageal varices

➲ *CPT Changes: An Insider's View* 2014, 2017

➲ *CPT Assistant* Spring 94:1, Oct 08:6, Jan 13:11, Dec 13:3

(Do not report 43205 in conjunction with 43227 for the same lesion)

(Do not report 43205 in conjunction with 43197, 43198, 43200)

(To report control of nonvariceal bleeding with band ligation, use 43227)

43206 with optical endomicroscopy

➲ *CPT Changes: An Insider's View* 2013, 2014, 2017

➲ *CPT Assistant* Jan 13:11, Aug 13:5, Dec 13:3, Nov 17:10

(Report supply of contrast agent separately)

(Do not report 43206 in conjunction with 43197, 43198, 43200, 88375)

43210 Code is out of numerical sequence. See 43254-43261

43211 Code is out of numerical sequence. See 43216-43227

43212 Code is out of numerical sequence. See 43216-43227

43213 Code is out of numerical sequence. See 43216-43227

43214 Code is out of numerical sequence. See 43216-43227

43215 with removal of foreign body(s)

➲ *CPT Changes: An Insider's View* 2014, 2015, 2017

➲ *CPT Assistant* Spring 94:1, Oct 08:6, Dec 13:3

(Do not report 43215 in conjunction with 43197, 43198, 43200)

(If fluoroscopic guidance is performed, use 76000)

(For rigid transoral esophagoscopy with removal of foreign body(s), use 43194)

43216 with removal of tumor(s), polyp(s), or other lesion(s) by hot biopsy forceps

➲ *CPT Changes: An Insider's View* 2014, 2015, 2017

➲ *CPT Assistant* Spring 94:1, Oct 08:6, Jan 13:11, Dec 13:3

(Do not report 43216 in conjunction with 43197, 43198, 43200)

43217 with removal of tumor(s), polyp(s), or other lesion(s) by snare technique

➲ *CPT Changes: An Insider's View* 2014, 2017

➲ *CPT Assistant* Spring 94:1, Oct 08:6, Jan 13:11, Dec 13:3, May 20:13

(Do not report 43217 in conjunction with 43211 for the same lesion)

(Do not report 43217 in conjunction with 43197, 43198, 43200)

(For esophagogastroduodenoscopy with removal of tumor[s], polyp[s], or other lesion[s] by snare technique, use 43251)

(For endoscopic mucosal resection, use 43211)

 # 43211   with endoscopic mucosal resection
➔ *CPT Changes: An Insider's View* 2014, 2017
➔ *CPT Assistant* Dec 13:3, Nov 17:10, Dec 19:14

(Do not report 43211 in conjunction with 43201, 43202, 43217 for the same lesion)

(Do not report 43211 in conjunction with 43197, 43198, 43200)

 # 43212   with placement of endoscopic stent (includes pre- and post-dilation and guide wire passage, when performed)
➔ *CPT Changes: An Insider's View* 2014, 2017
➔ *CPT Assistant* Dec 13:3

(Do not report 43212 in conjunction with 43197, 43198, 43200, 43220, 43226, 43241)

(If fluoroscopic guidance is performed, use 74360)

43220   with transendoscopic balloon dilation (less than 30 mm diameter)
➔ *CPT Changes: An Insider's View* 2014, 2017
➔ *CPT Assistant* Spring 94:2, Jan 97:10, May 05:3, Oct 08:6, Jan 13:11, Dec 13:3

►(Do not report 43220 in conjunction with 43197, 43198, 43200, 43212, 43226, 43229, 0884T)◄

(If fluoroscopic guidance is performed, use 74360)

(For rigid transoral esophagoscopy with balloon dilation [less than 30 mm diameter], use 43195)

(For esophageal dilation with balloon 30 mm diameter or larger, use 43214)

(For dilation without endoscopic visualization, see 43450, 43453)

►(For esophagoscopy with predilation followed by therapeutic drug delivery by drug-coated balloon catheter, use 0884T)◄

 # 43213   with dilation of esophagus, by balloon or dilator, retrograde (includes fluoroscopic guidance, when performed)
➔ *CPT Changes: An Insider's View* 2014, 2017
➔ *CPT Assistant* Dec 13:3

►(Do not report 43213 in conjunction with 43197, 43198, 43200, 74360, 76000, 0884T)◄

(For transendoscopic balloon dilation of multiple strictures during the same session, report 43213 with modifier 59 for each additional stricture dilated)

 # 43214   with dilation of esophagus with balloon (30 mm diameter or larger) (includes fluoroscopic guidance, when performed)
➔ *CPT Changes: An Insider's View* 2014, 2017
➔ *CPT Assistant* Dec 13:3

►(Do not report 43214 in conjunction with 43197, 43198, 43200, 74360, 76000, 0884T)◄

43226   with insertion of guide wire followed by passage of dilator(s) over guide wire
➔ *CPT Changes: An Insider's View* 2014, 2017
➔ *CPT Assistant* Spring 94:2, Jan 13:11, Dec 13:3

(Do not report 43226 in conjunction with 43229 for the same lesion)

►(Do not report 43226 in conjunction with 43197, 43198, 43200, 43212, 43220, 0884T)◄

(If fluoroscopic guidance is performed, use 74360)

(For rigid transoral esophagoscopy with insertion of guide wire followed by dilation over guide wire, use 43196)

►(For esophagoscopy with predilation followed by therapeutic drug delivery by drug-coated balloon catheter, use 0884T)◄

43227   with control of bleeding, any method
➔ *CPT Changes: An Insider's View* 2002, 2014, 2017
➔ *CPT Assistant* Spring 94:2, Oct 08:6, Jun 10:4, Jan 13:11, Dec 13:3, Feb 14:11

(Do not report 43227 in conjunction with 43201, 43204, 43205 for the same lesion)

(Do not report 43227 in conjunction with 43197, 43198, 43200)

43229   with ablation of tumor(s), polyp(s), or other lesion(s) (includes pre- and post-dilation and guide wire passage, when performed)
➔ *CPT Changes: An Insider's View* 2014, 2017
➔ *CPT Assistant* Dec 13:3

(Do not report 43229 in conjunction with 43220, 43226 for the same lesion)

(Do not report 43229 in conjunction with 43197, 43198, 43200)

(For esophagoscopic photodynamic therapy, report 43229 in conjunction with 96570, 96571 as appropriate)

43231   with endoscopic ultrasound examination
➔ *CPT Changes: An Insider's View* 2001, 2014, 2017
➔ *CPT Assistant* Oct 01:4, May 04:6, Oct 08:6, Mar 09:8, Jan 13:11, Dec 13:3

(Do not report 43231 in conjunction with 43197, 43198, 43200, 43232, 76975)

(Do not report 43231 more than once per session)

43232   with transendoscopic ultrasound-guided intramural or transmural fine needle aspiration/biopsy(s)

> *CPT Changes: An Insider's View* 2001, 2014, 2017

> *CPT Assistant* Oct 01:4, Mar 04:11, May 04:6, Oct 08:6, Mar 09:8, Jan 13:11, Dec 13:3, Feb 14:9, Sep 22:13

(Do not report 43232 in conjunction with 43197, 43198, 43200, 43231, 76942, 76975)

(Do not report 43232 more than once per session)

43233   Code is out of numerical sequence. See 43248-43251

Esophagogastroduodenoscopy

(For examination of the esophagus from the cricopharyngeus muscle [upper esophageal sphincter] to and including the gastroesophageal junction, including examination of the proximal region of the stomach via retroflexion when performed, see 43197, 43198, 43200, 43201, 43202, 43204, 43205, 43206, 43211, 43212, 43213, 43214, 43215, 43216, 43217, 43220, 43226, 43227, 43229, 43231, 43232)

(Use 43233, 43235-43259, 43266, 43270 for examination of a surgically altered stomach where the jejunum is examined distal to the anastomosis [eg, gastric bypass, gastroenterostomy {Billroth II}])

To report esophagogastroscopy where the duodenum is deliberately not examined (eg, judged clinically not pertinent), or because the clinical situation precludes such exam (eg, significant gastric retention precludes safe exam of duodenum), append modifier 52 if repeat examination is not planned, or modifier 53 if repeat examination is planned.

43235   Esophagogastroduodenoscopy, flexible, transoral; diagnostic, including collection of specimen(s) by brushing or washing, when performed (separate procedure)

> *CPT Changes: An Insider's View* 2014, 2017

> *CPT Assistant* Spring 94:4, Dec 97:11, Jun 03:11, Sep 03:3, Oct 08:6, May 09:8, Jan 13:11, Dec 13:3, Nov 15:8, Jul 17:10, Jul 18:14, Oct 19:10, Sep 22:13, Nov 22:12, May 23:27

(Do not report 43235 in conjunction with 43197, 43198, 43210, 43236-43259, 43266, 43270, 43290, 43291, 43497, 44360, 44361, 44363, 44364, 44365, 44366, 44369, 44370, 44372, 44373, 44376, 44377, 44378, 44379)

43236   with directed submucosal injection(s), any substance

> *CPT Changes: An Insider's View* 2003, 2014, 2017

> *CPT Assistant* Jun 10:4, Jan 13:11, Dec 13:3

(Do not report 43236 in conjunction with 43243, 43254, 43255 for the same lesion)

(Do not report 43236 in conjunction with 43197, 43198, 43235, 44360, 44361, 44363, 44364, 44365, 44366, 44369, 44370, 44372, 44373, 44376, 44377, 44378, 44379)

(For flexible, transoral esophagogastroduodenoscopy with injection sclerosis of esophageal and/or gastric varices, use 43243)

Esophagogastroduodenoscopy
43235

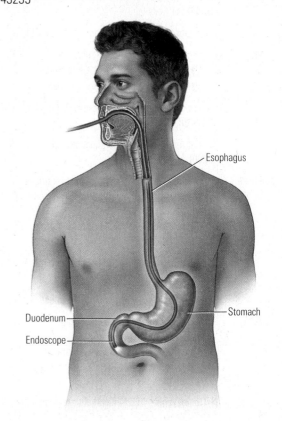

Esophagus

Stomach

Duodenum

Endoscope

43237   with endoscopic ultrasound examination limited to the esophagus, stomach or duodenum, and adjacent structures

> *CPT Changes: An Insider's View* 2004, 2014, 2017

> *CPT Assistant* Jan 13:11, Dec 13:3, Jan 16:11

(Do not report 43237 in conjunction with 43197, 43198, 43235, 43238, 43242, 43253, 43259, 44360, 44361, 44363, 44364, 44365, 44366, 44369, 44370, 44372, 44373, 44376, 44377, 44378, 44379, 76975)

(Do not report 43237 more than once per session)

43238   with transendoscopic ultrasound-guided intramural or transmural fine needle aspiration/biopsy(s), (includes endoscopic ultrasound examination limited to the esophagus, stomach or duodenum, and adjacent structures)

> *CPT Changes: An Insider's View* 2004, 2014, 2017

> *CPT Assistant* Jan 13:11, Dec 13:3

(Do not report 43238 in conjunction with 43197, 43198, 43235, 43237, 43242, 44360, 44361, 44363, 44364, 44365, 44366, 44369, 44370, 44372, 44373, 44376, 44377, 44378, 44379, 76942, 76975)

(Do not report 43238 more than once per session)

43239   with biopsy, single or multiple

➲ *CPT Changes: An Insider's View* 2014, 2017

➲ *CPT Assistant* Spring 94:4, Apr 98:14, Feb 99:11, Oct 01:4, Nov 07:9, Jan 13:11, Dec 13:3, Jul 18:14, Jan 20:12

(Do not report 43239 in conjunction with 43254 for the same lesion)

(Do not report 43239 in conjunction with 43197, 43198, 43235, 44360, 44361, 44363, 44364, 44365, 44366, 44369, 44370, 44372, 44373, 44376, 44377, 44378, 44379)

43240   with transmural drainage of pseudocyst (includes placement of transmural drainage catheter[s]/stent[s], when performed, and endoscopic ultrasound, when performed)

➲ *CPT Changes: An Insider's View* 2001, 2014, 2017

➲ *CPT Assistant* Oct 01:4, Jan 13:11, Dec 13:3

(Do not report 43240 in conjunction with 43253 for the same lesion)

(Do not report 43240 in conjunction with 43197, 43198, 43235, 43242, 43259, 43266, 44360, 44361, 44363, 44364, 44365, 44366, 44369, 44370, 44372, 44373, 44376, 44377, 44378, 44379)

(Do not report 43240 more than once per session)

(For endoscopic pancreatic necrosectomy, use 48999)

43241   with insertion of intraluminal tube or catheter

➲ *CPT Changes: An Insider's View* 2001, 2014, 2017

➲ *CPT Assistant* Spring 94:4, Nov 01:7, Apr 09:3, Jan 13:11, Dec 13:3, Oct 21:5-6, Nov 22:12

(Do not report 43241 in conjunction with 43197, 43198, 43212, 43235, 43266, 43290, 44360, 44361, 44363, 44364, 44365, 44366, 44369, 44370, 44372, 44373, 44376, 44377, 44378, 44379)

(For naso- or oro-gastric tube placement requiring physician's or other qualified health care professional's skill and fluoroscopic guidance, use 43752)

(For nonendoscopic enteric tube placement, see 44500, 74340)

43242   with transendoscopic ultrasound-guided intramural or transmural fine needle aspiration/biopsy(s) (includes endoscopic ultrasound examination of the esophagus, stomach, and either the duodenum or a surgically altered stomach where the jejunum is examined distal to the anastomosis)

➲ *CPT Changes: An Insider's View* 2001, 2004, 2014, 2017

➲ *CPT Assistant* Oct 01:4, Mar 09:8, Jan 13:11, Dec 13:3

(Do not report 43242 in conjunction with 43197, 43198, 43235, 43237, 43238, 43240, 43259, 44360, 44361, 44363, 44364, 44365, 44366, 44369, 44370, 44372, 44373, 44376, 44377, 44378, 44379, 76942, 76975)

(Do not report 43242 more than once per session)

(For transendoscopic ultrasound-guided transmural fine needle aspiration/biopsy limited to the esophagus, stomach, duodenum, or adjacent structure, use 43238)

43243   with injection sclerosis of esophageal/gastric varices

➲ *CPT Changes: An Insider's View* 2014, 2017

➲ *CPT Assistant* Spring 94:4, Jun 10:5, Jan 13:11, Dec 13:3

(Do not report 43243 in conjunction with 43236, 43255 for the same lesion)

(Do not report 43243 in conjunction with 43197, 43198, 43235, 44360, 44361, 44363, 44364, 44365, 44366, 44369, 44370, 44372, 44373, 44376, 44377, 44378, 44379)

43244   with band ligation of esophageal/gastric varices

➲ *CPT Changes: An Insider's View* 2014, 2017

➲ *CPT Assistant* Spring 94:4, Jun 11:13, Jan 13:11, Dec 13:3

(Do not report 43244 in conjunction with 43197, 43198, 43235, 43255, 44360, 44361, 44363, 44364, 44365, 44366, 44369, 44370, 44372, 44373, 44376, 44377, 44378, 44379)

(To report control of nonvariceal bleeding with band ligation, use 43255)

43245   with dilation of gastric/duodenal stricture(s) (eg, balloon, bougie)

➲ *CPT Changes: An Insider's View* 2002, 2003, 2014, 2017

➲ *CPT Assistant* Spring 94:4, Oct 01:4, Jan 04:26, Jan 13:11, Dec 13:3

(Do not report 43245 in conjunction with 43197, 43198, 43235, 43266, 44360, 44361, 44363, 44364, 44365, 44366, 44369, 44370, 44372, 44373, 44376, 44377, 44378, 44379)

(If fluoroscopic guidance is performed, use 74360)

43246   with directed placement of percutaneous gastrostomy tube

➲ *CPT Changes: An Insider's View* 2014, 2017

➲ *CPT Assistant* Spring 94:4, Feb 97:10, Mar 10:10, Jan 13:11, May 13:12, Dec 13:3, Feb 19:5, Oct 21:5, Jul 23:1

➲ *Clinical Examples in Radiology* Winter 19:12

(Do not report 43246 in conjunction with 43197, 43198, 43235, 44360, 44361, 44363, 44364, 44365, 44366, 44369, 44370, 44372, 44376, 44377, 44378, 44379)

(For percutaneous insertion of gastrostomy tube under fluoroscopic guidance, use 49440)

(For percutaneous replacement of gastrostomy tube without imaging or endoscopy, see 43762, 43763)

43247   with removal of foreign body(s)

➔ CPT Changes: An Insider's View 2014, 2015, 2017

➔ CPT Assistant Spring 94:4, Jan 13:11, Dec 13:3, Nov 22:12

(Do not report 43247 in conjunction with 43197, 43198, 43235, 43290, 43291, 44360, 44361, 44363, 44364, 44365, 44366, 44369, 44370, 44372, 44373, 44376, 44377, 44378, 44379)

(If fluoroscopic guidance is performed, use 76000)

 # 43290   with deployment of intragastric bariatric balloon

➔ CPT Changes: An Insider's View 2023

➔ CPT Assistant Nov 22:12, Dec 22:20

(Do not report 43290 in conjunction with 43197, 43198, 43235, 43241, 43247)

 # 43291   with removal of intragastric bariatric balloon(s)

➔ CPT Changes: An Insider's View 2023

➔ CPT Assistant Nov 22:12, Dec 22:20

(Do not report 43291 in conjunction with 43197, 43198, 43235, 43247)

43248   with insertion of guide wire followed by passage of dilator(s) through esophagus over guide wire

➔ CPT Changes: An Insider's View 2014, 2017

➔ CPT Assistant Spring 94:4, Dec 97:11, Oct 08:6, Jan 13:11, Dec 13:3, Jul 17:10

(Do not report 43248 in conjunction with 43197, 43198, 43235, 43266, 43270, 44360, 44361, 44363, 44364, 44365, 44366, 44369, 44370, 44372, 44373, 44376, 44377, 44378, 44379)

(If fluoroscopic guidance is performed, use 74360)

43249   with transendoscopic balloon dilation of esophagus (less than 30 mm diameter)

➔ CPT Changes: An Insider's View 2014, 2017

➔ CPT Assistant May 05:3, Jan 13:11, Dec 13:3, Jul 18:14

(Do not report 43249 in conjunction with 43197, 43198, 43235, 43266, 43270, 44360, 44361, 44363, 44364, 44365, 44366, 44369, 44370, 44372, 44373, 44376, 44377, 44378, 44379)

(If fluoroscopic guidance is performed, use 74360)

 # 43233   with dilation of esophagus with balloon (30 mm diameter or larger) (includes fluoroscopic guidance, when performed)

➔ CPT Changes: An Insider's View 2014, 2017

➔ CPT Assistant Dec 13:3, Oct 19:10, Sep 22:13

(Do not report 43233 in conjunction with 43197, 43198, 43235, 44360, 44361, 44363, 44364, 44365, 44366, 44369, 44370, 44372, 44373, 44376, 44377, 44378, 44379, 74360, 76000)

43250   with removal of tumor(s), polyp(s), or other lesion(s) by hot biopsy forceps

➔ CPT Changes: An Insider's View 2014, 2015, 2017

➔ CPT Assistant Spring 94:4, Feb 99:11, Nov 07:9, Jan 13:11, Dec 13:3

(Do not report 43250 in conjunction with 43197, 43198, 43235, 44360, 44361, 44363, 44364, 44365, 44366, 44369, 44370, 44372, 44373, 44376, 44377, 44378, 44379)

43251   with removal of tumor(s), polyp(s), or other lesion(s) by snare technique

➔ CPT Changes: An Insider's View 2014, 2017

➔ CPT Assistant Spring 94:4, Oct 04:12, Nov 07:9, Jun 11:13, Jan 13:11, Dec 13:3

(Do not report 43251 in conjunction with 43254 for the same lesion)

(Do not report 43251 in conjunction with 43197, 43198, 43235, 44360, 44361, 44363, 44364, 44365, 44366, 44369, 44370, 44372, 44373, 44376, 44377, 44378, 44379)

(For endoscopic mucosal resection, use 43254)

43252   with optical endomicroscopy

➔ CPT Changes: An Insider's View 2013, 2014, 2017

➔ CPT Assistant Jan 13:11, Aug 13:5, Dec 13:3

(Report supply of contrast agent separately)

(Do not report 43252 in conjunction with 43197, 43198, 43235, 44360, 44361, 44363, 44364, 44365, 44366, 44369, 44370, 44372, 44373, 44376, 44377, 44378, 44379, 88375)

43253   with transendoscopic ultrasound-guided transmural injection of diagnostic or therapeutic substance(s) (eg, anesthetic, neurolytic agent) or fiducial marker(s) (includes endoscopic ultrasound examination of the esophagus, stomach, and either the duodenum or a surgically altered stomach where the jejunum is examined distal to the anastomosis)

➔ CPT Changes: An Insider's View 2014, 2017

➔ CPT Assistant Dec 13:3, Apr 18:11

(Do not report 43253 in conjunction with 43240 for the same lesion)

(Do not report 43253 in conjunction with 43197, 43198, 43235, 43237, 43259, 44360, 44361, 44363, 44364, 44365, 44366, 44369, 44370, 44372, 44373, 44376, 44377, 44378, 44379, 76942, 76975)

(Do not report 43253 more than once per session)

(For transendoscopic ultrasound-guided transmural fine needle aspiration/biopsy, see 43238, 43242)

43254   with endoscopic mucosal resection

➔ CPT Changes: An Insider's View 2014, 2017

➔ CPT Assistant Dec 13:3, Dec 19:14

(Do not report 43254 in conjunction with 43236, 43239, 43251 for the same lesion)

(Do not report 43254 in conjunction with 43197, 43198, 43235, 44360, 44361, 44363, 44364, 44365, 44366, 44369, 44370, 44372, 44373, 44376, 44377, 44378, 44379)

43255   with control of bleeding, any method
> *CPT Changes: An Insider's View* 2014, 2017
> *CPT Assistant* Spring 94:4, Jun 10:4, Dec 13:3

(Do not report 43255 in conjunction with 43236, 43243, 43244 for the same lesion)

(Do not report 43255 in conjunction with 43197, 43198, 43235, 44360, 44361, 44363, 44364, 44365, 44366, 44369, 44370, 44372, 44373, 44376, 44377, 44378, 44379)

 # 43266   with placement of endoscopic stent (includes pre- and post-dilation and guide wire passage, when performed)
> *CPT Changes: An Insider's View* 2014, 2017
> *CPT Assistant* Dec 13:3, Oct 19:10, Sep 22:13

(Do not report 43266 in conjunction with 43197, 43198, 43235, 43240, 43241, 43245, 43248, 43249, 44360, 44361, 44363, 44364, 44365, 44366, 44369, 44370, 44372, 44373, 44376, 44377, 44378, 44379)

(If fluoroscopic guidance is performed, use 74360)

43257   with delivery of thermal energy to the muscle of lower esophageal sphincter and/or gastric cardia, for treatment of gastroesophageal reflux disease
> *CPT Changes: An Insider's View* 2005, 2014, 2017
> *CPT Assistant* May 05:3, Jan 13:11, Dec 13:3

(Do not report 43257 in conjunction with 43197, 43198, 43235, 44360, 44361, 44363, 44364, 44365, 44366, 44369, 44370, 44372, 44373, 44376, 44377, 44378, 44379)

(For ablation of metaplastic/dysplastic esophageal lesion [eg, Barrett's esophagus], see 43229, 43270)

 # 43270   with ablation of tumor(s), polyp(s), or other lesion(s) (includes pre- and post-dilation and guide wire passage, when performed)
> *CPT Changes: An Insider's View* 2014, 2017
> *CPT Assistant* Dec 13:3, Oct 19:10, Sep 22:13, May 23:27

(Do not report 43270 in conjunction with 43248, 43249 for the same lesion)

(Do not report 43270 in conjunction with 43197, 43198, 43235, 44360, 44361, 44363, 44364, 44365, 44366, 44369, 44370, 44372, 44373, 44376, 44377, 44378, 44379)

(For esophagoscopic photodynamic therapy, use 43270 in conjunction with 96570, 96571 as appropriate)

43259   with endoscopic ultrasound examination, including the esophagus, stomach, and either the duodenum or a surgically altered stomach where the jejunum is examined distal to the anastomosis
> *CPT Changes: An Insider's View* 2004, 2014, 2017
> *CPT Assistant* Spring 94:4, May 04:7, Mar 09:8, Jan 13:11, Dec 13:3, Jan 16:11, Oct 19:10, Sep 22:13

(Do not report 43259 in conjunction with 43197, 43198, 43235, 43237, 43240, 43242, 43253, 44360, 44361, 44363, 44364, 44365, 44366, 44369, 44370, 44372, 44373, 44376, 44377, 44378, 44379, 76975)

(Do not report 43259 more than once per session)

 # 43210   with esophagogastric fundoplasty, partial or complete, includes duodenoscopy when performed
> *CPT Changes: An Insider's View* 2016
> *CPT Assistant* Nov 15:8, Sep 22:13

(Do not report 43210 in conjunction with 43180, 43191, 43197, 43200, 43235)

Endoscopic Retrograde Cholangiopancreatography (ERCP)

Report the appropriate code(s) for each service performed. Therapeutic ERCP (43261, 43262, 43263, 43264, 43265, 43274, 43275, 43276, 43277, 43278) includes diagnostic ERCP (43260). ERCP includes guide wire passage when performed. An ERCP is considered complete if one or more of the ductal system(s), (pancreatic/biliary) is visualized. To report ERCP attempted but with unsuccessful cannulation of any ductal system, see 43235-43259, 43266, 43270.

(For percutaneous biliary catheter procedures, see 47490-47544)

Codes 43274, 43275, 43276, and 43277 describe ERCP with stent placement, removal or replacement (exchange) of stent(s), and balloon dilation within the pancreatico-biliary system. For reporting purposes, ducts that may be reported as stented or subject to stent replacement (exchange) or to balloon dilation include:

Pancreas: major and minor ducts

Biliary tree: common bile duct, right hepatic duct, left hepatic duct, cystic duct/gallbladder

ERCP with stent placement includes any balloon dilation performed in that duct. ERCP with more than one stent placement (eg, different ducts or side by side in the same duct) performed during the same day/session may be reported with 43274 more than once with modifier 59 appended to the subsequent procedure(s). For ERCP with more than one stent exchanged during the same day/session, 43276 may be reported for the initial stent exchange, and 43276 with modifier 59 for each additional stent exchange. ERCP with balloon dilation of more than one duct during the same day/session may be reported with modifier 59 appended to the subsequent procedure(s). Sphincteroplasty, which is balloon dilation of the ampulla (sphincter of Oddi), is reported with 43277, and includes sphincterotomy (43262) when performed.

To report ERCP via altered postoperative anatomy, see 43260, 43262, 43263, 43264, 43265, 43273, 43274, 43275, 43276, 43277, 43278, for Billroth II gastroenterostomy. See 47999 (Unlisted procedure, biliary tract) or 48999 (Unlisted procedure, pancreas) for ERCP via gastrostomy (laparoscopic or open) or via Roux-en-Y anatomy (eg, post-bariatric gastric bypass, post-total gastrectomy).

To report optical endomicroscopy of the biliary tract and pancreas, use 0397T. Do not report optical endomicroscopy more than once per session.

Stone destruction includes any stone removal in the same ductal system (biliary/pancreatic). Code 43277 may be separately reported if sphincteroplasty or dilation of a ductal stricture is required before proceeding to remove stones/debris from the duct during the same session. Dilation that is incidental to the passage of an instrument to clear stones or debris is not separately reported.

(Do not report 43277 for use of a balloon catheter to clear stones/debris from a duct. Any dilation of the duct that may occur during this maneuver is considered inherent to the work of 43264 and 43265)

(If imaging of the ductal systems is performed, including images saved to the permanent record and report of the imaging, see 74328, 74329, 74330)

43260 Endoscopic retrograde cholangiopancreatography (ERCP); diagnostic, including collection of specimen(s) by brushing or washing, when performed (separate procedure)

➡ CPT Changes: An Insider's View 2014, 2017

➡ CPT Assistant Spring 94:5, Oct 04:13, May 08:14, Aug 08:12, Jan 12:12, Jan 13:11, Dec 13:3

(Do not report 43260 in conjunction with 43261, 43262, 43263, 43264, 43265, 43274, 43275, 43276, 43277, 43278)

43261 with biopsy, single or multiple

➡ CPT Changes: An Insider's View 2017

➡ CPT Assistant Spring 94:5, Aug 08:12, Jun 11:13, Jan 13:11

(Do not report 43261 in conjunction with 43260)

(For percutaneous endoluminal biopsy of biliary tree, use 47543)

43262 with sphincterotomy/papillotomy

➡ CPT Changes: An Insider's View 2017

➡ CPT Assistant Spring 94:5, Oct 04:13, Jul 09:10, Jan 13:11

(43262 may be reported when sphincterotomy is performed in addition to 43261, 43263, 43264, 43265, 43275, 43278)

(Do not report 43262 in conjunction with 43274 for stent placement or with 43276 for stent replacement [exchange] in the same location)

(Do not report 43262 in conjunction with 43260, 43277)

(For percutaneous balloon dilation of biliary duct(s) or of ampulla, use 47542)

43263 with pressure measurement of sphincter of Oddi

➡ CPT Changes: An Insider's View 2014, 2017

➡ CPT Assistant Spring 94:5, Oct 04:13, Jan 13:11, Dec 13:3

(Do not report 43263 in conjunction with 43260)

(Do not report 43263 more than once per session)

43264 with removal of calculi/debris from biliary/pancreatic duct(s)

➡ CPT Changes: An Insider's View 2002, 2014, 2017

➡ CPT Assistant Spring 94:5, Jan 13:11, Dec 13:3

(Do not report 43264 if no calculi or debris are found, even if balloon catheter is deployed)

(Do not report 43264 in conjunction with 43260, 43265)

(For percutaneous removal of calculi/debris, use 47544)

Endoscopic Retrograde Cholangiopancreatography (ERCP)
43260

Examination of the hepatobiliary system (pancreatic ducts, hepatic ducts, common bile ducts, duodenal papilla [ampulla of Vater] and gallbladder [if present]) is performed through a side-viewing flexible fiberoptic endoscope.

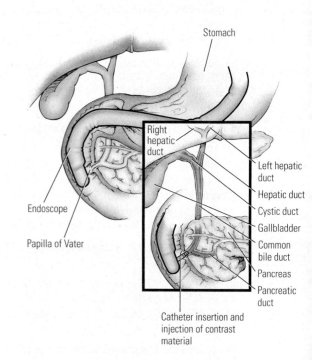

Stomach

Right hepatic duct

Left hepatic duct

Hepatic duct

Cystic duct

Gallbladder

Common bile duct

Pancreas

Pancreatic duct

Endoscope

Papilla of Vater

Catheter insertion and injection of contrast material

43265   with destruction of calculi, any method (eg,
                  mechanical, electrohydraulic, lithotripsy)
                  ➔ *CPT Changes: An Insider's View* 2002, 2014, 2017
                  ➔ *CPT Assistant* Spring 94:5, Jan 13:11, Dec 13:3

(Do not report 43265 in conjunction with 43260, 43264)

(For percutaneous removal of calculi/debris, use 47544)

43266   Code is out of numerical sequence. See 43254-43261

43270   Code is out of numerical sequence. See 43254-43261

 # 43274   with placement of endoscopic stent into biliary or
                  pancreatic duct, including pre- and post-dilation and
                  guide wire passage, when performed, including
                  sphincterotomy, when performed, each stent
                  ➔ *CPT Changes: An Insider's View* 2014, 2017
                  ➔ *CPT Assistant* Dec 13:3

(Do not report 43274 in conjunction with 43262, 43275,
43276, 43277 for stent placement or replacement
[exchange] in the same duct)

(For stent placement in both the pancreatic duct and the
common bile duct during the same operative session,
placement of separate stents in both the right and left
hepatic ducts, or placement of two side-by-side stents in
the same duct, 43274 may be reported for each
additional stent placed, using modifier 59 with the
subsequent procedure[s])

(To report naso-biliary or naso-pancreatic drainage tube
placement, use 43274)

(For percutaneous placement of biliary stent(s), see
47538, 47539, 47540)

 # 43275   with removal of foreign body(s) or stent(s) from
                  biliary/pancreatic duct(s)
                  ➔ *CPT Changes: An Insider's View* 2014, 2017
                  ➔ *CPT Assistant* Dec 13:3

(Do not report 43275 in conjunction with 43260, 43274,
43276)

(For removal of stent from biliary or pancreatic duct
without ERCP, use 43247)

(Report 43275 only once for removal of one or more
stents or foreign bodies from biliary/pancreatic duct[s]
during the same session)

(For percutaneous removal of calculi/debris, use 47544)

 # 43276   with removal and exchange of stent(s), biliary or
                  pancreatic duct, including pre- and post-dilation and
                  guide wire passage, when performed, including
                  sphincterotomy, when performed, each stent
                  exchanged
                  ➔ *CPT Changes: An Insider's View* 2014, 2017
                  ➔ *CPT Assistant* Dec 13:3

(43276 includes removal and replacement [exchange] of
one stent. For replacement [exchange] of additional
stent[s] during the same session, report 43276 with
modifier 59 for each additional replacement [exchange])

(Do not report 43276 in conjunction with 43260, 43275)

(Do not report 43276 in conjunction with 43262, 43274
for stent placement or exchange in the same duct)

 # 43277   with trans-endoscopic balloon dilation of biliary/
                  pancreatic duct(s) or of ampulla (sphincteroplasty),
                  including sphincterotomy, when performed, each duct
                  ➔ *CPT Changes: An Insider's View* 2014, 2017
                  ➔ *CPT Assistant* Dec 13:3

(Do not report 43277 in conjunction with 43278 for the
same lesion)

(Do not report 43277 in conjunction with 43260, 43262)

(Do not report 43277 for incidental dilation using balloon
for stone/debris removal performed with 43264, 43265)

(If sphincterotomy without sphincteroplasty is performed
on a separate pancreatic duct orifice during the same
session [ie, pancreas divisum], report 43262 with
modifier 59)

(Do not report 43277 in conjunction with 43274, 43276
for dilation and stent placement/replacement [exchange]
in the same duct)

(For transendoscopic balloon dilation of multiple
strictures during the same session, use 43277 with
modifier 59 for each additional stricture dilated)

(For bilateral balloon dilation [both right and left hepatic
ducts], 43277 may be reported twice with modifier 59
appended to the second procedure)

(For percutaneous balloon dilation of biliary duct(s) or of
ampulla (sphincteroplasty), use 47542)

 # 43278   with ablation of tumor(s), polyp(s), or other lesion(s),
                  including pre- and post-dilation and guide wire
                  passage, when performed
                  ➔ *CPT Changes: An Insider's View* 2014, 2017
                  ➔ *CPT Assistant* Dec 13:3

(Do not report 43278 in conjunction with 43277 for the
same lesion)

(Do not report 43278 in conjunction with 43260)

(For ampullectomy, use 43254)

+ 43273   Endoscopic cannulation of papilla with direct
               visualization of pancreatic/common bile duct(s) (List
               separately in addition to code(s) for primary procedure)
               ➔ *CPT Changes: An Insider's View* 2009, 2014, 2017
               ➔ *CPT Assistant* Jan 13:11, Dec 13:3

(Report 43273 once per procedure)

(Use 43273 in conjunction with 43260, 43261, 43262,
43263, 43264, 43265, 43274, 43275, 43276, 43277,
43278)

Digestive 40490-49999

Copying, photographing, or sharing this CPT® book violates AMA's copyright.

43274 Code is out of numerical sequence. See 43264-43279

43275 Code is out of numerical sequence. See 43264-43279

43276 Code is out of numerical sequence. See 43264-43279

43277 Code is out of numerical sequence. See 43264-43279

43278 Code is out of numerical sequence. See 43264-43279

Laparoscopy

Surgical laparoscopy always includes diagnostic laparoscopy. To report a diagnostic laparoscopy (peritoneoscopy) (separate procedure), use 49320.

43279 Laparoscopy, surgical, esophagomyotomy (Heller type), with fundoplasty, when performed

➜ *CPT Changes: An Insider's View* 2009

➜ *CPT Assistant* Feb 12:3

(For open approach, see 43330, 43331)

(Do not report 43279 in conjunction with 43280)

43280 Laparoscopy, surgical, esophagogastric fundoplasty (eg, Nissen, Toupet procedures)

➜ *CPT Changes: An Insider's View* 2000

➜ *CPT Assistant* Nov 99:22, Mar 00:8, Dec 02:2, Jun 11:8, Feb 12:3, Dec 14:16, Nov 15:8

(Do not report 43280 in conjunction with 43279, 43281, 43282)

(For open esophagogastric fundoplasty, see 43327, 43328)

(For laparoscopy, surgical, esophageal sphincter augmentation procedure, placement of sphincter augmentation device, see 43284, 43285)

(For esophagogastroduodenoscopy fundoplasty, partial or complete, transoral approach, use 43210)

43281 Laparoscopy, surgical, repair of paraesophageal hernia, includes fundoplasty, when performed; without implantation of mesh

➜ *CPT Changes: An Insider's View* 2010

➜ *CPT Assistant* Jun 11:9, Feb 12:3, Dec 14:16, Sep 18:14, Nov 18:11

43282 with implantation of mesh

➜ *CPT Changes: An Insider's View* 2010

➜ *CPT Assistant* Jun 11:9, Feb 12:3, Dec 14:16, Aug 16:9

(To report transabdominal paraesophageal hiatal hernia repair, see 43332, 43333)

(To report transthoracic diaphragmatic hernia repair, see 43334, 43335)

(Do not report 43281, 43282 in conjunction with 43280, 43450, 43453)

Laparoscopic Fundoplasty
43280

With the esophagus and fundus held aside, sutures are placed in both crus diaphragmatis muscles below the esophagus to bring them together to close the hiatal hernia, and the anterior and posterior walls of the fundus are wrapped and stitched around the esophagus to complete the laparoscopic fundoplasty.

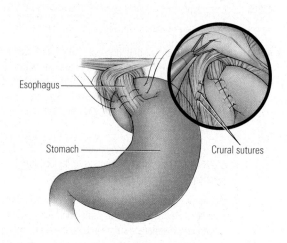

Esophagus

Stomach

Crural sutures

+ 43283 Laparoscopy, surgical, esophageal lengthening procedure (eg, Collis gastroplasty or wedge gastroplasty) (List separately in addition to code for primary procedure)

➜ *CPT Changes: An Insider's View* 2011

➜ *CPT Assistant* Jun 11:9, Feb 12:3

(Use 43283 in conjunction with 43280, 43281, 43282)

43284 Laparoscopy, surgical, esophageal sphincter augmentation procedure, placement of sphincter augmentation device (ie, magnetic band), including cruroplasty when performed

➜ *CPT Changes: An Insider's View* 2017

➜ *CPT Assistant* Aug 17:6, Sep 18:14, Apr 19:11

(Do not report 43284 in conjunction with 43279, 43280, 43281, 43282)

43285 Removal of esophageal sphincter augmentation device

➜ *CPT Changes: An Insider's View* 2017

➜ *CPT Assistant* Aug 17:6

43286 Esophagectomy, total or near total, with laparoscopic mobilization of the abdominal and mediastinal esophagus and proximal gastrectomy, with laparoscopic pyloric drainage procedure if performed, with open cervical pharyngogastrostomy or esophagogastrostomy (ie, laparoscopic transhiatal esophagectomy)

➜ *CPT Changes: An Insider's View* 2018

➜ *CPT Assistant* Jul 18:7

Laparoscopic Esophageal Sphincter Augmentation
43284

Ivor Lewis Esophagectomy
43287

Implanted magnetic sphincter augmentation device

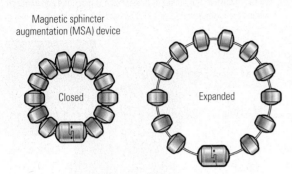

Magnetic sphincter augmentation (MSA) device

Closed

Expanded

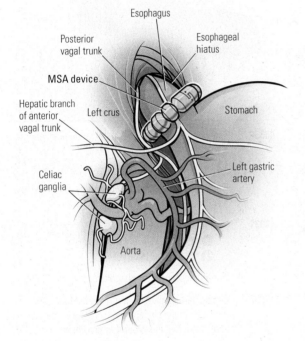

Esophagus

Posterior vagal trunk

Esophageal hiatus

MSA device

Hepatic branch of anterior vagal trunk

Left crus

Stomach

Celiac ganglia

Left gastric artery

Aorta

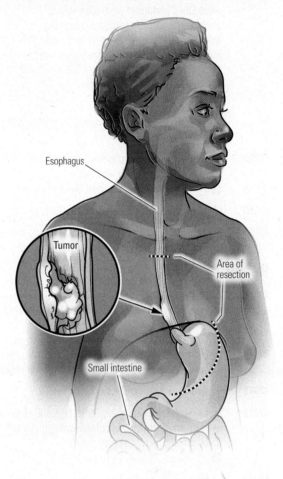

Esophagus

Tumor

Area of resection

Small intestine

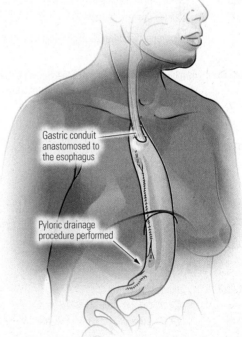

Gastric conduit anastomosed to the esophagus

Pyloric drainage procedure performed

43287   Esophagectomy, distal two-thirds, with laparoscopic mobilization of the abdominal and lower mediastinal esophagus and proximal gastrectomy, with laparoscopic pyloric drainage procedure if performed, with separate thoracoscopic mobilization of the middle and upper mediastinal esophagus and thoracic esophagogastrostomy (ie, laparoscopic thoracoscopic esophagectomy, Ivor Lewis esophagectomy)

➔ CPT Changes: An Insider's View 2018

➔ CPT Assistant Jul 18:7

(Do not report 43287 in conjunction with 32551 for right tube thoracostomy)

43288   Esophagectomy, total or near total, with thoracoscopic mobilization of the upper, middle, and lower mediastinal esophagus, with separate laparoscopic proximal gastrectomy, with laparoscopic pyloric drainage procedure if performed, with open cervical pharyngogastrostomy or esophagogastrostomy (ie, thoracoscopic, laparoscopic and cervical incision esophagectomy, McKeown esophagectomy, tri-incisional esophagectomy)

➲ *CPT Changes: An Insider's View* 2018

➲ *CPT Assistant* Jul 18:7

(Do not report 43288 in conjunction with 32551 for right tube thoracostomy)

43289   Unlisted laparoscopy procedure, esophagus

➲ *CPT Changes: An Insider's View* 2000

➲ *CPT Assistant* Nov 99:22, Mar 00:8, Dec 14:16, Jul 18:7

43290   Code is out of numerical sequence. See 43246-43249

43291   Code is out of numerical sequence. See 43246-43249

Repair

43300   Esophagoplasty (plastic repair or reconstruction), cervical approach; without repair of tracheoesophageal fistula

43305   with repair of tracheoesophageal fistula

43310   Esophagoplasty (plastic repair or reconstruction), thoracic approach; without repair of tracheoesophageal fistula

43312   with repair of tracheoesophageal fistula

43313   Esophagoplasty for congenital defect (plastic repair or reconstruction), thoracic approach; without repair of congenital tracheoesophageal fistula

➲ *CPT Changes: An Insider's View* 2002

43314   with repair of congenital tracheoesophageal fistula

➲ *CPT Changes: An Insider's View* 2002

(Do not report modifier 63 in conjunction with 43313, 43314)

43320   Esophagogastrostomy (cardioplasty), with or without vagotomy and pyloroplasty, transabdominal or transthoracic approach

(For laparoscopic procedure, use 43280)

43325   Esophagogastric fundoplasty, with fundic patch (Thal-Nissen procedure)

➲ *CPT Assistant* Winter 90:6

(For cricopharyngeal myotomy, use 43030)

43327   Esophagogastric fundoplasty partial or complete; laparotomy

➲ *CPT Changes: An Insider's View* 2011

➲ *CPT Assistant* Jun 11:8, Feb 12:3, Nov 15:8

43328   thoracotomy

➲ *CPT Changes: An Insider's View* 2011

➲ *CPT Assistant* Jun 11:8, Feb 12:3, Nov 15:8

(For esophagogastroduodenoscopy fundoplasty, partial or complete, transoral approach, use 43210)

Nissen Fundoplasty
43327, 43328

The lower esophagus is accessed through an upper abdominal or lower thoracic incision. The fundus of the stomach is mobilized and wrapped around the lower esophageal sphincter, and the wrap is sutured into place.

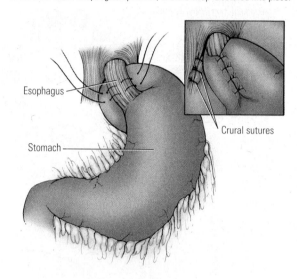

Esophagus

Crural sutures

Stomach

43330   Esophagomyotomy (Heller type); abdominal approach

➲ *CPT Changes: An Insider's View* 2000

➲ *CPT Assistant* Nov 99:22

(For laparoscopic esophagomyotomy procedure, use 43279)

43331   thoracic approach

➲ *CPT Changes: An Insider's View* 2000

➲ *CPT Assistant* Nov 99:22

(For thoracoscopic esophagomyotomy, use 32665)

43332   Repair, paraesophageal hiatal hernia (including fundoplication), via laparotomy, except neonatal; without implantation of mesh or other prosthesis

➲ *CPT Changes: An Insider's View* 2011

➲ *CPT Assistant* Feb 12:3

43333   with implantation of mesh or other prosthesis

➲ *CPT Changes: An Insider's View* 2011

➲ *CPT Assistant* Feb 12:3

(For neonatal diaphragmatic hernia repair, use 39503)

43334   Repair, paraesophageal hiatal hernia (including fundoplication), via thoracotomy, except neonatal; without implantation of mesh or other prosthesis

➲ *CPT Changes: An Insider's View* 2011

➲ *CPT Assistant* Feb 12:3

43335   with implantation of mesh or other prosthesis
➔ *CPT Changes: An Insider's View* 2011
➔ *CPT Assistant* Feb 12:3

(For neonatal diaphragmatic hernia repair, use 39503)

43336   Repair, paraesophageal hiatal hernia, (including fundoplication), via thoracoabdominal incision, except neonatal; without implantation of mesh or other prosthesis
➔ *CPT Changes: An Insider's View* 2011
➔ *CPT Assistant* Feb 12:3

43337   with implantation of mesh or other prosthesis
➔ *CPT Changes: An Insider's View* 2011
➔ *CPT Assistant* Feb 12:3

(For neonatal diaphragmatic hernia repair, use 39503)

+ 43338   Esophageal lengthening procedure (eg, Collis gastroplasty or wedge gastroplasty) (List separately in addition to code for primary procedure)
➔ *CPT Changes: An Insider's View* 2011
➔ *CPT Assistant* Jun 11:10, Feb 12:3

(Use 43338 in conjunction with 43280, 43327-43337)

43340   Esophagojejunostomy (without total gastrectomy); abdominal approach

43341   thoracic approach

43351   Esophagostomy, fistulization of esophagus, external; thoracic approach
➔ *CPT Changes: An Insider's View* 2015

43352   cervical approach
➔ *CPT Changes: An Insider's View* 2015

43360   Gastrointestinal reconstruction for previous esophagectomy, for obstructing esophageal lesion or fistula, or for previous esophageal exclusion; with stomach, with or without pyloroplasty

43361   with colon interposition or small intestine reconstruction, including intestine mobilization, preparation, and anastomosis(es)
➔ *CPT Changes: An Insider's View* 2002

43400   Ligation, direct, esophageal varices

43405   Ligation or stapling at gastroesophageal junction for pre-existing esophageal perforation

43410   Suture of esophageal wound or injury; cervical approach
➔ *CPT Assistant* Jun 96:7

43415   transthoracic or transabdominal approach

43420   Closure of esophagostomy or fistula; cervical approach

43425   transthoracic or transabdominal approach

(To report transabdominal paraesophageal hiatal hernia repair, see 43332, 43333. To report transthoracic diaphragmatic hernia repair, see 43334, 43335)

Manipulation

(For associated esophagogram, use 74220)

43450   Dilation of esophagus, by unguided sound or bougie, single or multiple passes
➔ *CPT Changes: An Insider's View* 2014
➔ *CPT Assistant* Spring 94:1, Jan 97:10, Apr 98:14, Jun 98:10, Dec 13:3, Jul 17:10

(For radiological supervision and interpretation, use 74360)

43453   Dilation of esophagus, over guide wire
➔ *CPT Changes: An Insider's View* 2017
➔ *CPT Assistant* Spring 94:1, Jan 97:10, Dec 97:11

(For dilation with endoscopic visualization, see 43195, 43226)

(For dilation of esophagus, by balloon or dilator, see 43214, 43220, 43233, 43249)

(For radiological supervision and interpretation, use 74360)

(For endoscopic dilation of esophagus with balloon less than 30 mm diameter, see 43195, 43220, 43249)

(For endoscopic dilation of esophagus with balloon 30 mm diameter or larger, see 43214, 43233)

43460   Esophagogastric tamponade, with balloon (Sengstaken type)
➔ *CPT Changes: An Insider's View* 2009

(For removal of esophageal foreign body by balloon catheter, see 43499, 74235)

Other Procedures

43496   Free jejunum transfer with microvascular anastomosis
➔ *CPT Assistant* Nov 96:8, Apr 97:4, Jun 97:10, Nov 97:17, Nov 98:16

(Do not report code 69990 in addition to code 43496)

43497   Lower esophageal myotomy, transoral (ie, peroral endoscopic myotomy [POEM])
➔ *CPT Changes: An Insider's View* 2022
➔ *CPT Assistant* Dec 21:20

(Do not report 43497 in conjunction with 32665, 43191, 43197, 43200, 43235)

43499   Unlisted procedure, esophagus
➔ *CPT Assistant* May 07:10, Oct 10:12, Dec 10:12, May 11:9, Dec 11:19, Mar 13:13, Nov 15:8, 11, Jul 18:7, Sep 22:13

Stomach

Incision

43500   Gastrotomy; with exploration or foreign body removal

43501   with suture repair of bleeding ulcer

43502   with suture repair of pre-existing esophagogastric laceration (eg, Mallory-Weiss)

43510   with esophageal dilation and insertion of permanent intraluminal tube (eg, Celestin or Mousseaux-Barbin)

43520   Pyloromyotomy, cutting of pyloric muscle (Fredet-Ramstedt type operation)

(Do not report modifier 63 in conjunction with 43520)

Excision

43605   Biopsy of stomach, by laparotomy
➔ *CPT Changes: An Insider's View* 2011

43610   Excision, local; ulcer or benign tumor of stomach

43611   malignant tumor of stomach

43620   Gastrectomy, total; with esophagoenterostomy

43621   with Roux-en-Y reconstruction

43622   with formation of intestinal pouch, any type

43631   Gastrectomy, partial, distal; with gastroduodenostomy

43632   with gastrojejunostomy

43633   with Roux-en-Y reconstruction

43634   with formation of intestinal pouch

+ 43635   Vagotomy when performed with partial distal gastrectomy (List separately in addition to code[s] for primary procedure)
➔ *CPT Assistant* Nov 97:17

(Use 43635 in conjunction with 43631, 43632, 43633, 43634)

43640   Vagotomy including pyloroplasty, with or without gastrostomy; truncal or selective

(For pyloroplasty, use 43800)

(For vagotomy, see 64755, 64760)

43641   parietal cell (highly selective)

(For upper gastrointestinal endoscopy, see 43235-43259)

Laparoscopy

Surgical laparoscopy always includes diagnostic laparoscopy. To report a diagnostic laparoscopy (peritoneoscopy) (separate procedure), use 49320.

(For upper gastrointestinal endoscopy including esophagus, stomach, and either the duodenum and/or jejunum, see 43235-43259)

43644   Laparoscopy, surgical, gastric restrictive procedure; with gastric bypass and Roux-en-Y gastroenterostomy (roux limb 150 cm or less)
➔ *CPT Changes: An Insider's View* 2005
➔ *CPT Assistant* May 05:3, Nov 22:12, Feb 24:33

(Do not report 43644 in conjunction with 43846, 49320)

(Esophagogastroduodenoscopy [EGD] performed for a separate condition should be reported with modifier 59)

(For greater than 150 cm, use 43645)

(For open procedure, use 43846)

43645   with gastric bypass and small intestine reconstruction to limit absorption
➔ *CPT Changes: An Insider's View* 2005
➔ *CPT Assistant* May 05:3, Nov 22:12, Feb 24:33

(Do not report 43645 in conjunction with 49320, 43847)

43647   Laparoscopy, surgical; implantation or replacement of gastric neurostimulator electrodes, antrum
➔ *CPT Changes: An Insider's View* 2007
➔ *CPT Assistant* Mar 07:4

43648   revision or removal of gastric neurostimulator electrodes, antrum
➔ *CPT Changes: An Insider's View* 2007
➔ *CPT Assistant* Mar 07:4

(For open approach, see 43881, 43882)

(For insertion of gastric neurostimulator pulse generator, use 64590)

(For revision or removal of gastric neurostimulator pulse generator, use 64595)

(For electronic analysis and programming of gastric neurostimulator pulse generator, see 95980, 95981, 95982)

(For laparoscopic implantation, revision, or removal of gastric neurostimulator electrodes, lesser curvature [morbid obesity], use 43659)

43651   Laparoscopy, surgical; transection of vagus nerves, truncal
➔ *CPT Changes: An Insider's View* 2000
➔ *CPT Assistant* Nov 99:22, Mar 00:8

43652   transection of vagus nerves, selective or highly selective
➔ *CPT Changes: An Insider's View* 2000
➔ *CPT Assistant* Nov 99:22, Mar 00:8

43653   gastrostomy, without construction of gastric tube (eg, Stamm procedure) (separate procedure)

➡ *CPT Changes: An Insider's View* 2000

➡ *CPT Assistant* Nov 99:22, Mar 00:8

43659   Unlisted laparoscopy procedure, stomach

➡ *CPT Changes: An Insider's View* 2000

➡ *CPT Assistant* Nov 99:22, Mar 00:8, Apr 06:19, Jun 06:16, Dec 07:12, Jun 11:8, Dec 11:19, Feb 13:13, Jun 13:13, Jul 18:7, Jun 23:27

Introduction

43752   Naso- or oro-gastric tube placement, requiring physician's skill and fluoroscopic guidance (includes fluoroscopy, image documentation and report)

➡ *CPT Changes: An Insider's View* 2001, 2004

➡ *CPT Assistant* Jan 02:11, Apr 03:7, Oct 03:2, Jul 06:4, Feb 07:10, Jul 07:1, Aug 08:7, Sep 11:4, May 14:4, Mar 18:11, Aug 19:8, Jan 22:3, Jun 22:19, Dec 22:10, Nov 23:26

➡ *Clinical Examples in Radiology* Fall 21:17

(Do not report 43752 in conjunction with critical care codes 99291-99292, neonatal critical care codes 99468, 99469, pediatric critical care codes 99471, 99472 or low birth weight intensive care service codes 99478, 99479)

(For percutaneous placement of gastrostomy tube, use 49440)

(For enteric tube placement, see 44500, 74340)

43753   Gastric intubation and aspiration(s) therapeutic, necessitating physician's skill (eg, for gastrointestinal hemorrhage), including lavage if performed

➡ *CPT Changes: An Insider's View* 2011

➡ *CPT Assistant* Sep 11:3, May 14:4, Aug 19:8, Jan 22:3, Jun 22:19, Dec 22:10

43754   Gastric intubation and aspiration, diagnostic; single specimen (eg, acid analysis)

➡ *CPT Changes: An Insider's View* 2011

➡ *CPT Assistant* Dec 10:10, Sep 11:3

43755   collection of multiple fractional specimens with gastric stimulation, single or double lumen tube (gastric secretory study) (eg, histamine, insulin, pentagastrin, calcium, secretin), includes drug administration

➡ *CPT Changes: An Insider's View* 2011

➡ *CPT Assistant* Dec 10:10, Sep 11:3

(For gastric acid analysis, use 82930)

(For naso- or oro-gastric tube placement by physician with fluoroscopic guidance, use 43752)

(Report the drug[s] or substance[s] administered. The fluid used to administer the drug[s] is not separately reported)

Gastric Intubation
43753

A large-bore gastric lavage tube is inserted orally through the esophagus into the stomach for expedient lavage and evacuation of stomach contents (eg, poisonings, hemorrhage).

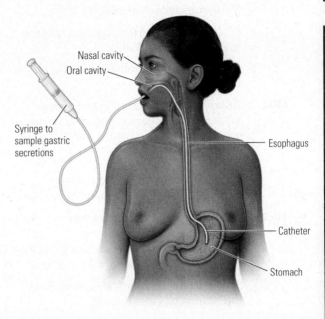

Nasal cavity

Oral cavity

Syringe to sample gastric secretions

Esophagus

Catheter

Stomach

43756   Duodenal intubation and aspiration, diagnostic, includes image guidance; single specimen (eg, bile study for crystals or afferent loop culture)

➡ *CPT Changes: An Insider's View* 2011

➡ *CPT Assistant* Dec 10:10, Sep 11:3

43757   collection of multiple fractional specimens with pancreatic or gallbladder stimulation, single or double lumen tube, includes drug administration

➡ *CPT Changes: An Insider's View* 2011

➡ *CPT Assistant* Dec 10:10, Sep 11:3

(For appropriate chemical analysis procedures, see 89049-89240)

(Report the substances[s] or drug[s] administered. The fluid used to administer the drug[s] is not separately reported)

(To report fluoroscopically guided replacement of gastrostomy tube, use 49450)

(For endoscopic placement of gastrostomy tube, use 43246)

Digestive 40490-49999

43761 Repositioning of a naso- or oro-gastric feeding tube, through the duodenum for enteric nutrition

➔ *CPT Changes: An Insider's View* 2000, 2008, 2010

➔ *CPT Assistant* Oct 96:9, Nov 99:22, Jun 08:8, Aug 08:7

(Do not report 43761 in conjunction with 44500, 49446)

(If imaging guidance is performed, use 76000)

(For endoscopic conversion of a gastrostomy tube to jejunostomy tube, use 44373)

(For placement of a long gastrointestinal tube into the duodenum, use 44500)

43762 Replacement of gastrostomy tube, percutaneous, includes removal, when performed, without imaging or endoscopic guidance; not requiring revision of gastrostomy tract

➔ *CPT Changes: An Insider's View* 2019

➔ *CPT Assistant* Feb 19:5, Oct 21:5-6, Jun 22:6-8

➔ *Clinical Examples in Radiology* Winter 19:12, Summer 22:15

43763 requiring revision of gastrostomy tract

➔ *CPT Changes: An Insider's View* 2019

➔ *CPT Assistant* Feb 19:5, Oct 19:10, Oct 21:5-6, Jun 22:6-8

➔ *Clinical Examples in Radiology* Winter 19:12, Summer 22:15

(For percutaneous replacement of gastrostomy tube under fluoroscopic guidance, use 49450)

(For endoscopically directed placement of gastrostomy tube, use 43246)

Bariatric Surgery

Bariatric surgical procedures may involve the stomach, duodenum, jejunum, and/or the ileum.

Laparoscopy

Surgical laparoscopy always includes diagnostic laparoscopy. To report a diagnostic laparoscopy (separate procedure), use 49320.

Typical postoperative follow-up care (see Surgery Guidelines, CPT Surgical Package Definition) after gastric restriction using the adjustable gastric restrictive device includes subsequent restrictive device adjustment(s) through the postoperative period for the typical patient. Adjustment consists of changing the gastric restrictive device component diameter by injection or aspiration of fluid through the subcutaneous port component.

43770 Laparoscopy, surgical, gastric restrictive procedure; placement of adjustable gastric restrictive device (eg, gastric band and subcutaneous port components)

➔ *CPT Changes: An Insider's View* 2006, 2008

➔ *CPT Assistant* Dec 10:13, Nov 22:12

(For individual component placement, report 43770 with modifier 52)

43771 revision of adjustable gastric restrictive device component only

➔ *CPT Changes: An Insider's View* 2006, 2008

➔ *CPT Assistant* Nov 22:12

43772 removal of adjustable gastric restrictive device component only

➔ *CPT Changes: An Insider's View* 2006, 2008

➔ *CPT Assistant* Nov 22:12

43773 removal and replacement of adjustable gastric restrictive device component only

➔ *CPT Changes: An Insider's View* 2006, 2008

➔ *CPT Assistant* Nov 22:12

(Do not report 43773 in conjunction with 43772)

43774 removal of adjustable gastric restrictive device and subcutaneous port components

➔ *CPT Changes: An Insider's View* 2006, 2008

➔ *CPT Assistant* Nov 22:12

(For removal and replacement of both gastric band and subcutaneous port components, use 43659)

43775 longitudinal gastrectomy (ie, sleeve gastrectomy)

➔ *CPT Changes: An Insider's View* 2010

➔ *CPT Assistant* Oct 19:10, Nov 22:12

(For open gastric restrictive procedure, without gastric bypass, for morbid obesity, other than vertical-banded gastroplasty, use 43843)

Other Procedures

43800 Pyloroplasty

(For pyloroplasty and vagotomy, use 43640)

43810 Gastroduodenostomy

43820 Gastrojejunostomy; without vagotomy

43825 with vagotomy, any type

43830 Gastrostomy, open; without construction of gastric tube (eg, Stamm procedure) (separate procedure)

➔ *CPT Changes: An Insider's View* 2000

➔ *CPT Assistant* Nov 99:22

43831 neonatal, for feeding

➔ *CPT Changes: An Insider's View* 2000

➔ *CPT Assistant* Nov 99:22, Feb 19:5

(For percutaneous replacement of gastrostomy tube with removal when performed without imaging or endoscopy, see 43762, 43763)

(For percutaneous replacement of gastrostomy tube under fluoroscopic guidance, use 49450)

(Do not report modifier 63 in conjunction with 43831)

43832   with construction of gastric tube (eg, Janeway
            procedure)
            ⟳ *CPT Changes: An Insider's View* 2000
            ⟳ *CPT Assistant* Nov 99:22

            (For percutaneous endoscopic gastrostomy, use 43246)

43840 Gastrorrhaphy, suture of perforated duodenal or gastric
            ulcer, wound, or injury

43842 Gastric restrictive procedure, without gastric bypass, for
            morbid obesity; vertical-banded gastroplasty
            ⟳ *CPT Assistant* May 98:5

43843   other than vertical-banded gastroplasty
            ⟳ *CPT Assistant* May 98:5

            (For laparoscopic longitudinal gastrectomy [ie, sleeve
            gastrectomy], use 43775)

43845 Gastric restrictive procedure with partial gastrectomy,
            pylorus-preserving duodenoileostomy and ileoileostomy
            (50 to 100 cm common channel) to limit absorption
            (biliopancreatic diversion with duodenal switch)
            ⟳ *CPT Changes: An Insider's View* 2005
            ⟳ *CPT Assistant* May 05:3, Nov 22:12

            (Do not report 43845 in conjunction with 43633, 43847,
            44130, 49000)

43846 Gastric restrictive procedure, with gastric bypass for
            morbid obesity; with short limb (150 cm or less) Roux-
            en-Y gastroenterostomy
            ⟳ *CPT Changes: An Insider's View* 2005
            ⟳ *CPT Assistant* May 98:5, May 05:3, Nov 22:12

            (For greater than 150 cm, use 43847)

            (For laparoscopic procedure, use 43644)

43847   with small intestine reconstruction to limit absorption
            ⟳ *CPT Changes: An Insider's View* 2015
            ⟳ *CPT Assistant* May 98:5, May 02:7

43848 Revision, open, of gastric restrictive procedure for morbid
            obesity, other than adjustable gastric restrictive device
            (separate procedure)
            ⟳ *CPT Changes: An Insider's View* 2006, 2008
            ⟳ *CPT Assistant* May 98:5, Apr 06:1

            (For laparoscopic adjustable gastric restrictive
            procedures, see 43770-43774)

            (For gastric restrictive port procedures, see 43886-43888)

43860 Revision of gastrojejunal anastomosis
            (gastrojejunostomy) with reconstruction, with or without
            partial gastrectomy or intestine resection; without
            vagotomy
            ⟳ *CPT Changes: An Insider's View* 2002

43865   with vagotomy

43870 Closure of gastrostomy, surgical
            ⟳ *CPT Assistant* Jul 18:14

43880 Closure of gastrocolic fistula

Gastric Bypass for Morbid Obesity
43846

The stomach is partitioned with a staple line on the lesser curvature (no
band, no gastric transection). A short limb of small bowel (less than 100 cm)
is divided and anastomosed to the small upper stomach pouch.

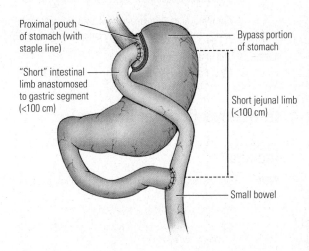

Proximal pouch of stomach (with staple line) — Bypass portion of stomach — "Short" intestinal limb anastomosed to gastric segment (<100 cm) — Short jejunal limb (<100 cm) — Small bowel

43881 Implantation or replacement of gastric neurostimulator
            electrodes, antrum, open
            ⟳ *CPT Changes: An Insider's View* 2007
            ⟳ *CPT Assistant* Mar 07:4

43882 Revision or removal of gastric neurostimulator
            electrodes, antrum, open
            ⟳ *CPT Changes: An Insider's View* 2007
            ⟳ *CPT Assistant* Mar 07:4

            (For laparoscopic approach, see 43647, 43648)

            (For insertion of gastric neurostimulator pulse generator,
            use 64590)

            (For revision or removal of gastric neurostimulator pulse
            generator, use 64595)

            (For electronic analysis and programming of gastric
            neurostimulator pulse generator, see 95980, 95981,
            95982)

            (For open implantation, revision, or removal of gastric
            neurostimulator electrodes, lesser curvature [morbid
            obesity] or vagal trunk [EGJ] neurostimulator electrodes,
            use 43999)

43886 Gastric restrictive procedure, open; revision of
            subcutaneous port component only
            ⟳ *CPT Changes: An Insider's View* 2006

43887   removal of subcutaneous port component only
            ⟳ *CPT Changes: An Insider's View* 2006

43888   removal and replacement of subcutaneous port component only

➔ *CPT Changes: An Insider's View* 2006

(Do not report 43888 in conjunction with 43774, 43887)

(For laparoscopic removal of both gastric restrictive device and subcutaneous port components, use 43774)

(For removal and replacement of both gastric restrictive device and subcutaneous port components, use 43659)

43999   Unlisted procedure, stomach

➔ *CPT Assistant* Mar 10:10, Jun 11:13, Feb 13:13, Jul 18:14, Dec 18:10, Dec 21:20, Sep 22:13

Intestines (Except Rectum)

Incision

44005   Enterolysis (freeing of intestinal adhesion) (separate procedure)

➔ *CPT Changes: An Insider's View* 2000

➔ *CPT Assistant* Winter 90:6, Nov 97:17, Nov 99:23, Jan 00:11, Apr 00:10, Feb 18:11

(Do not report 44005 in addition to 45136)

(For laparoscopic approach, use 44180)

44010   Duodenotomy, for exploration, biopsy(s), or foreign body removal

+ 44015   Tube or needle catheter jejunostomy for enteral alimentation, intraoperative, any method (List separately in addition to primary procedure)

➔ *CPT Assistant* Mar 02:10, Jul 10:10

44020   Enterotomy, small intestine, other than duodenum; for exploration, biopsy(s), or foreign body removal

➔ *CPT Changes: An Insider's View* 2002

44021   for decompression (eg, Baker tube)

44025   Colotomy, for exploration, biopsy(s), or foreign body removal

(For exteriorization of intestine (Mikulicz resection with crushing of spur), see 44602-44605)

44050   Reduction of volvulus, intussusception, internal hernia, by laparotomy

44055   Correction of malrotation by lysis of duodenal bands and/ or reduction of midgut volvulus (eg, Ladd procedure)

(Do not report modifier 63 in conjunction with 44055)

Excision

Intestinal allotransplantation involves three distinct components of physician work:

1. **Cadaver donor enterectomy,** which includes harvesting the intestine graft and cold preservation of the graft (perfusing with cold preservation solution and cold maintenance) (use 44132). **Living donor enterectomy,** which includes harvesting the intestine graft, cold preservation of the graft (perfusing with cold preservation solution and cold maintenance), and care of the donor (use 44133).

2. **Backbench work:**
Standard preparation of an intestine allograft prior to transplantation includes mobilization and fashioning of the superior mesenteric artery and vein (see 44715).

Additional reconstruction of an intestine allograft prior to transplantation may include venous and/or arterial anastomosis(es) (see 44720-44721).

3. **Recipient intestinal allotransplantation with or without recipient enterectomy,** which includes transplantation of allograft and care of the recipient (see 44135, 44136).

44100   Biopsy of intestine by capsule, tube, peroral (1 or more specimens)

44110   Excision of 1 or more lesions of small or large intestine not requiring anastomosis, exteriorization, or fistulization; single enterotomy

➔ *CPT Changes: An Insider's View* 2002

44111   multiple enterotomies

44120   Enterectomy, resection of small intestine; single resection and anastomosis

➔ *CPT Assistant* Mar 04:3, Aug 08:7, Nov 18:11, Nov 22:22

+ 44121   each additional resection and anastomosis (List separately in addition to code for primary procedure)

(Use 44121 in conjunction with 44120)

44125   with enterostomy

44126   Enterectomy, resection of small intestine for congenital atresia, single resection and anastomosis of proximal segment of intestine; without tapering

➔ *CPT Changes: An Insider's View* 2002

44127   with tapering

➔ *CPT Changes: An Insider's View* 2002

+ 44128   each additional resection and anastomosis (List separately in addition to code for primary procedure)

➔ *CPT Changes: An Insider's View* 2002

(Use 44128 in conjunction with 44126, 44127)

(Do not report modifier 63 in conjunction with 44126, 44127, 44128)

44130   Enteroenterostomy, anastomosis of intestine, with or without cutaneous enterostomy (separate procedure)

Enterectomy, Resection for Congenital Atresia
44127

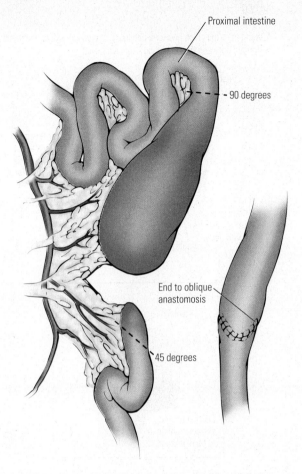

Proximal intestine

90 degrees

End to oblique
anastomosis

45 degrees

44132 Donor enterectomy (including cold preservation), open;
from cadaver donor

➲ *CPT Changes: An Insider's View* 2001, 2005

44133 partial, from living donor

➲ *CPT Changes: An Insider's View* 2001

(For backbench intestinal graft preparation or
reconstruction, see 44715, 44720, 44721)

44135 Intestinal allotransplantation; from cadaver donor

➲ *CPT Changes: An Insider's View* 2001

44136 from living donor

➲ *CPT Changes: An Insider's View* 2001

44137 Removal of transplanted intestinal allograft, complete

➲ *CPT Changes: An Insider's View* 2005

(For partial removal of transplant allograft, see 44120,
44121, 44140)

+ 44139 Mobilization (take-down) of splenic flexure performed in
conjunction with partial colectomy (List separately in
addition to primary procedure)

(Use 44139 in conjunction with 44140-44147)

44140 Colectomy, partial; with anastomosis

➲ *CPT Assistant* Fall 92:23, Aug 08:7, Nov 08:7, Sep 10:7,
Apr 20:10, Jul 23:1

(For laparoscopic procedure, use 44204)

Colectomy, Partial
44140

A segment of the colon is resected and an anastomosis is performed
between the remaining ends of the colon.

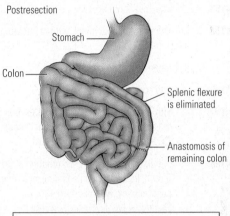

Postresection

Stomach

Colon

Splenic flexure
is eliminated

Anastomosis of
remaining colon

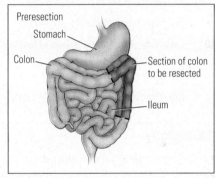

Preresection

Stomach

Colon

Section of colon
to be resected

Ileum

44141 with skin level cecostomy or colostomy

➲ *CPT Assistant* Fall 92:24, Nov 08:7

44143 with end colostomy and closure of distal segment
(Hartmann type procedure)

➲ *CPT Assistant* Fall 92:24, Nov 08:7

(For laparoscopic procedure, use 44206)

44144 with resection, with colostomy or ileostomy and
creation of mucofistula

➲ *CPT Assistant* Fall 92:24, Nov 08:7

44145 with coloproctostomy (low pelvic anastomosis)

➲ *CPT Assistant* Fall 92:24

(For laparoscopic procedure, use 44207)

44146 with coloproctostomy (low pelvic anastomosis), with colostomy
➔ *CPT Assistant* Fall 92:24, Nov 08:7, Jun 18:11

(For laparoscopic procedure, use 44208)

44147 abdominal and transanal approach
➔ *CPT Assistant* Fall 92:24, Nov 08:7

44150 Colectomy, total, abdominal, without proctectomy; with ileostomy or ileoproctostomy

(For laparoscopic procedure, use 44210)

44151 with continent ileostomy

44155 Colectomy, total, abdominal, with proctectomy; with ileostomy

(For laparoscopic procedure, use 44212)

44156 with continent ileostomy

44157 with ileoanal anastomosis, includes loop ileostomy, and rectal mucosectomy, when performed
➔ *CPT Changes: An Insider's View* 2007

44158 with ileoanal anastomosis, creation of ileal reservoir (S or J), includes loop ileostomy, and rectal mucosectomy, when performed
➔ *CPT Changes: An Insider's View* 2007

(For laparoscopic procedure, use 44211)

44160 Colectomy, partial, with removal of terminal ileum with ileocolostomy
➔ *CPT Changes: An Insider's View* 2002

(For laparoscopic procedure, use 44205)

Laparoscopy

Surgical laparoscopy always includes diagnostic laparoscopy. To report a diagnostic laparoscopy (peritoneoscopy) (separate procedure), use 49320.

Incision

44180 Laparoscopy, surgical, enterolysis (freeing of intestinal adhesion) (separate procedure)
➔ *CPT Changes: An Insider's View* 2006
➔ *CPT Assistant* Feb 18:11

(For laparoscopy with salpingolysis, ovariolysis, use 58660)

Enterostomy—External Fistulization of Intestines

44186 Laparoscopy, surgical; jejunostomy (eg, for decompression or feeding)
➔ *CPT Changes: An Insider's View* 2006

Colectomy With Removal of Terminal Ileum and Ileocolostomy
44160

A segment of the colon and terminal ileum is removed and an anastomosis is performed between the remaining ileum and colon.

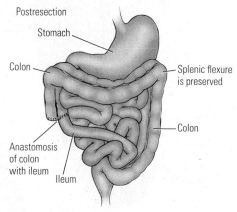

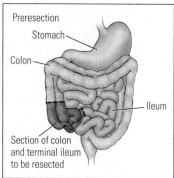

44187 ileostomy or jejunostomy, non-tube
➔ *CPT Changes: An Insider's View* 2006
➔ *CPT Assistant* Sep 19:11

(For open procedure, use 44310)

44188 Laparoscopy, surgical, colostomy or skin level cecostomy
➔ *CPT Changes: An Insider's View* 2006

(For open procedure, use 44320)

(Do not report 44188 in conjunction with 44970)

Excision

44202 Laparoscopy, surgical; enterectomy, resection of small intestine, single resection and anastomosis
➔ *CPT Changes: An Insider's View* 2000, 2002, 2006
➔ *CPT Assistant* Nov 99:23, Mar 00:9, May 03:2, Apr 06:1, Jul 20:14

+ 44203   each additional small intestine resection and anastomosis (List separately in addition to code for primary procedure)
> *CPT Changes: An Insider's View* 2002
> *CPT Assistant* May 03:2

(Use 44203 in conjunction with 44202)

(For open procedure, see 44120, 44121)

44204   colectomy, partial, with anastomosis
> *CPT Changes: An Insider's View* 2002
> *CPT Assistant* May 03:3, Apr 06:1, 19, Dec 17:14

(For open procedure, use 44140)

44205   colectomy, partial, with removal of terminal ileum with ileocolostomy
> *CPT Changes: An Insider's View* 2002
> *CPT Assistant* May 03:3, Apr 06:1

(For open procedure, use 44160)

44206   colectomy, partial, with end colostomy and closure of distal segment (Hartmann type procedure)
> *CPT Changes: An Insider's View* 2003
> *CPT Assistant* May 03:3, Apr 06:1

(For open procedure, use 44143)

44207   colectomy, partial, with anastomosis, with coloproctostomy (low pelvic anastomosis)
> *CPT Changes: An Insider's View* 2003
> *CPT Assistant* May 03:3, Apr 06:1

(For open procedure, use 44145)

44208   colectomy, partial, with anastomosis, with coloproctostomy (low pelvic anastomosis) with colostomy
> *CPT Changes: An Insider's View* 2003
> *CPT Assistant* May 03:3, Apr 06:1

(For open procedure, use 44146)

44210   colectomy, total, abdominal, without proctectomy, with ileostomy or ileoproctostomy
> *CPT Changes: An Insider's View* 2003
> *CPT Assistant* May 03:3

(For open procedure, use 44150)

44211   colectomy, total, abdominal, with proctectomy, with ileoanal anastomosis, creation of ileal reservoir (S or J), with loop ileostomy, includes rectal mucosectomy, when performed
> *CPT Changes: An Insider's View* 2003, 2007
> *CPT Assistant* May 03:3

(For open procedure, see 44157, 44158)

44212   colectomy, total, abdominal, with proctectomy, with ileostomy
> *CPT Changes: An Insider's View* 2003
> *CPT Assistant* May 03:3

(For open procedure, use 44155)

+ 44213   Laparoscopy, surgical, mobilization (take-down) of splenic flexure performed in conjunction with partial colectomy (List separately in addition to primary procedure)
> *CPT Changes: An Insider's View* 2006

(Use 44213 in conjunction with 44204-44208)

(For open procedure, use 44139)

Repair

44227   Laparoscopy, surgical, closure of enterostomy, large or small intestine, with resection and anastomosis
> *CPT Changes: An Insider's View* 2006

(For open procedure, see 44625, 44626)

Other Procedures

44238   Unlisted laparoscopy procedure, intestine (except rectum)
> *CPT Changes: An Insider's View* 2003
> *CPT Assistant* May 03:4, Jul 17:10, Oct 19:10, Jul 20:14

Enterostomy—External Fistulization of Intestines

44300   Placement, enterostomy or cecostomy, tube open (eg, for feeding or decompression) (separate procedure)
> *CPT Changes: An Insider's View* 2008
> *CPT Assistant* Mar 02:10, Aug 08:7

(Do not report 44300 in conjunction with 44701 for cannulation of the colon for intraoperative colonic lavage)

(For percutaneous placement of duodenostomy, jejunostomy, gastro-jejunostomy or cecostomy [or other colonic] tube including fluoroscopic imaging guidance, see 49441-49442)

44310   Ileostomy or jejunostomy, non-tube
> *CPT Changes: An Insider's View* 2006
> *CPT Assistant* Mar 02:10, Apr 06:1

(For laparoscopic procedure, use 44187)

(Do not report 44310 in conjunction with 44144, 44150-44151, 44155, 44156, 45113, 45119, 45136)

44312   Revision of ileostomy; simple (release of superficial scar) (separate procedure)
> *CPT Assistant* Spring 93:35

44314   complicated (reconstruction in-depth) (separate procedure)

44316   Continent ileostomy (Kock procedure) (separate procedure)

(For fiberoptic evaluation, use 44385)

44320 Colostomy or skin level cecostomy;

→ *CPT Changes: An Insider's View* 2006

(For laparoscopic procedure, use 44188)

(Do not report 44320 in conjunction with 44141, 44144, 44146, 44605, 45110, 45119, 45126, 45563, 45805, 45825, 50810, 51597, 57307, or 58240)

44322 with multiple biopsies (eg, for congenital megacolon) (separate procedure)

→ *CPT Changes: An Insider's View* 2002

44340 Revision of colostomy; simple (release of superficial scar) (separate procedure)

44345 complicated (reconstruction in-depth) (separate procedure)

44346 with repair of paracolostomy hernia (separate procedure)

Endoscopy, Small Intestine

When bleeding occurs as the result of an endoscopic procedure, control of bleeding is not reported separately during the same operative session.

Antegrade transoral small intestinal endoscopy (enteroscopy) is defined by the most distal segment of small intestine that is examined. Codes 44360, 44361, 44363, 44364, 44365, 44366, 44369, 44370, 44372, 44373 are endoscopic procedures to visualize the esophagus through the jejunum using an antegrade approach. Codes 44376, 44377, 44378, 44379 are endoscopic procedures to visualize the esophagus through the ileum using an antegrade approach. If an endoscope cannot be advanced at least 50 cm beyond the pylorus, see 43233, 43235-43259, 43266, 43270; if an endoscope can be passed at least 50 cm beyond pylorus but only into jejunum, see 44360, 44361, 44363, 44364, 44365, 44366, 44369, 44370, 44372, 44373.

To report retrograde examination of small intestine via anus or colon stoma, use 44799, unlisted procedure, intestine.

(Do not report 44360, 44361, 44363, 44364, 44365, 44366, 44369, 44370, 44372, 44373 in conjunction with 43233, 43235-43259, 43266, 43270, 44376, 44377, 44378, 44379)

(Do not report 44376, 44377, 44378, 44379 in conjunction with 43233, 43235-43259, 43266, 43270, 44360, 44361, 44363, 44364, 44365, 44366, 44369, 44370, 44372, 44373)

(For esophagogastroduodenoscopy, see 43233, 43235-43259, 43266, 43270)

44360 Small intestinal endoscopy, enteroscopy beyond second portion of duodenum, not including ileum; diagnostic, including collection of specimen(s) by brushing or washing, when performed (separate procedure)

→ *CPT Changes: An Insider's View* 2015, 2017

→ *CPT Assistant* Spring 94:7, Mar 11:10, Dec 13:3, Nov 14:3

44361 with biopsy, single or multiple

→ *CPT Changes: An Insider's View* 2017

44363 with removal of foreign body(s)

→ *CPT Changes: An Insider's View* 2015, 2017

→ *CPT Assistant* Oct 19:10

44364 with removal of tumor(s), polyp(s), or other lesion(s) by snare technique

→ *CPT Changes: An Insider's View* 2017

→ *CPT Assistant* Oct 19:10

44365 with removal of tumor(s), polyp(s), or other lesion(s) by hot biopsy forceps or bipolar cautery

→ *CPT Changes: An Insider's View* 2017

→ *CPT Assistant* Oct 19:10

44366 with control of bleeding (eg, injection, bipolar cautery, unipolar cautery, laser, heater probe, stapler, plasma coagulator)

→ *CPT Changes: An Insider's View* 2002, 2017

→ *CPT Assistant* Jun 10:4, Oct 19:10

44369 with ablation of tumor(s), polyp(s), or other lesion(s) not amenable to removal by hot biopsy forceps, bipolar cautery or snare technique

→ *CPT Changes: An Insider's View* 2017

→ *CPT Assistant* Oct 19:10

44370 with transendoscopic stent placement (includes predilation)

→ *CPT Changes: An Insider's View* 2001, 2017

→ *CPT Assistant* Nov 01:7, Oct 19:10

44372 with placement of percutaneous jejunostomy tube

→ *CPT Changes: An Insider's View* 2017

→ *CPT Assistant* Spring 94:7, Oct 19:10

44373 with conversion of percutaneous gastrostomy tube to percutaneous jejunostomy tube

→ *CPT Changes: An Insider's View* 2017

→ *CPT Assistant* Spring 94:7, Dec 13:3, Oct 19:10, Oct 21:5-6

(For fiberoptic jejunostomy through stoma, use 43235)

44376 Small intestinal endoscopy, enteroscopy beyond second portion of duodenum, including ileum; diagnostic, with or without collection of specimen(s) by brushing or washing (separate procedure)

→ *CPT Changes: An Insider's View* 2017

→ *CPT Assistant* Spring 94:7, Mar 11:10, Dec 13:3

(Do not report 44376 in conjunction with 44360, 44361, 44363, 44364, 44365, 44366, 44369, 44370, 44372, 44373)

44377 with biopsy, single or multiple

→ *CPT Changes: An Insider's View* 2017

→ *CPT Assistant* Spring 94:7

(Do not report 44377 in conjunction with 44360, 44361, 44363, 44364, 44365, 44366, 44369, 44370, 44372, 44373)

44378   with control of bleeding (eg, injection, bipolar cautery, unipolar cautery, laser, heater probe, stapler, plasma coagulator)

> ➔ *CPT Changes: An Insider's View* 2002, 2017

> ➔ *CPT Assistant* Spring 94:7, Jun 10:4, Apr 12:17, Dec 13:3

(Do not report 44378 in conjunction with 44360, 44361, 44363, 44364, 44365, 44366, 44369, 44370, 44372, 44373)

44379   with transendoscopic stent placement (includes predilation)

> ➔ *CPT Changes: An Insider's View* 2001, 2017

> ➔ *CPT Assistant* Nov 01:7, Nov 14:3

(Do not report 44379 in conjunction with 44360, 44361, 44363, 44364, 44365, 44366, 44369, 44370, 44372, 44373)

Endoscopy, Stomal

Definitions

Proctosigmoidoscopy is the examination of the rectum and may include examination of a portion of the sigmoid colon.

Sigmoidoscopy is the examination of the entire rectum, sigmoid colon and may include examination of a portion of the descending colon.

Colonoscopy is the examination of the entire colon, from the rectum to the cecum, and may include examination of the terminal ileum or small intestine proximal to an anastomosis.

Colonoscopy through stoma is the examination of the colon, from the colostomy stoma to the cecum or colon-small intestine anastomosis, and may include examination of the terminal ileum or small intestine proximal to an anastomosis.

When performing a diagnostic or screening endoscopic procedure on a patient who is scheduled and prepared for a total colonoscopy, if the physician is unable to advance the colonoscope to the cecum or colon-small intestine anastomosis due to unforeseen circumstances, report 45378 (colonoscopy) or 44388 (colonoscopy through stoma) with modifier 53 and provide appropriate documentation.

If a therapeutic colonoscopy (44389-44407, 45379, 45380, 45381, 45382, 45384, 45388, 45398) is performed and does not reach the cecum or colon-small intestine anastomosis, report the appropriate therapeutic colonoscopy code with modifier 52 and provide appropriate documentation.

Report ileoscopy through stoma (44380, 44381, 44382, 44384) for endoscopic examination of a patient who has an ileostomy.

Report colonoscopy through stoma (44388-44408) for endoscopic examination of a patient who has undergone segmental resection of the colon (eg, hemicolectomy, sigmoid colectomy, low anterior resection) and has a colostomy.

— *Coding Tip* —

For definitions of proctosigmoidoscopy, sigmoidoscopy, colonoscopy, and guidelines for colonoscopies that do not reach the cecum or colon-small intestine anastomosis, see Colon and Rectum/Endoscopy.

For colonoscopy per rectum, see 45378, 45390, 45392, 45393, 45398.

Report proctosigmoidoscopy (45300-45327), flexible sigmoidoscopy (45330-45347), or anoscopy (46600, 46604, 46606, 46608, 46610, 46611, 46612, 46614, 46615), as appropriate for endoscopic examination of the defunctionalized rectum or distal colon in a patient who has undergone colectomy, in addition to colonoscopy through stoma (44388-44408) or ileoscopy through stoma (44380, 44381, 44382, 44384) if appropriate.

When bleeding occurs as the result of an endoscopic procedure, control of bleeding is not reported separately during the same operative session.

For computed tomographic colonography, see 74261, 74262, 74263.

44380   Ileoscopy, through stoma; diagnostic, including collection of specimen(s) by brushing or washing, when performed (separate procedure)

> ➔ *CPT Changes: An Insider's View* 2015, 2017

> ➔ *CPT Assistant* Dec 13:3, Nov 14:3, Dec 14:3

(Do not report 44380 in conjunction with 44381, 44382, 44384)

44381   Code is out of numerical sequence. See 44380-44385

44382   with biopsy, single or multiple

> ➔ *CPT Changes: An Insider's View* 2017

> ➔ *CPT Assistant* Dec 13:3

(Do not report 44382 in conjunction with 44380)

 # 44381   with transendoscopic balloon dilation

> ➔ *CPT Changes: An Insider's View* 2015, 2017

> ➔ *CPT Assistant* Nov 14:3

(Do not report 44381 in conjunction with 44380, 44384)

(If fluoroscopic guidance is performed, use 74360)

(For transendoscopic balloon dilation of multiple strictures during the same session, report 44381 with modifier 59 for each additional stricture dilated)

44384 with placement of endoscopic stent (includes pre- and post-dilation and guide wire passage, when performed)
➔ *CPT Changes: An Insider's View* 2015, 2017
➔ *CPT Assistant* Nov 14:3

(Do not report 44384 in conjunction with 44380, 44381)

(If fluoroscopic guidance is performed, use 74360)

44385 Endoscopic evaluation of small intestinal pouch (eg, Kock pouch, ileal reservoir [S or J]); diagnostic, including collection of specimen(s) by brushing or washing, when performed (separate procedure)
➔ *CPT Changes: An Insider's View* 2015, 2017

(Do not report 44385 in conjunction with 44386)

44386 with biopsy, single or multiple
➔ *CPT Changes: An Insider's View* 2015, 2017
➔ *CPT Assistant* Dec 13:3

(Do not report 44386 in conjunction with 44385)

─── *Coding Tip* ───

Definition of Colonoscopy Through Stoma

Colonoscopy through stoma is the examination of the colon, from the stoma to the cecum, and may include the examination of the terminal ileum or small intestine proximal to an anastomosis. When performing an endoscopic procedure on a patient who is scheduled and prepared for a colonoscopy through stoma, if the physician is unable to advance the colonoscope to the cecum or colon-small intestine anastomosis due to unforeseen circumstances, report 44388 with modifier 53 and provide appropriate documentation.

44388 Colonoscopy through stoma; diagnostic, including collection of specimen(s) by brushing or washing, when performed (separate procedure)
➔ *CPT Changes: An Insider's View* 2015, 2017
➔ *CPT Assistant* Nov 07:8, Dec 13:3, Nov 14:3

(Do not report 44388 in conjunction with 44389-44408)

44389 with biopsy, single or multiple
➔ *CPT Changes: An Insider's View* 2017
➔ *CPT Assistant* Dec 14:3

(Do not report 44389 in conjunction with 44403 for the same lesion)

(Do not report 44389 in conjunction with 44388)

44390 with removal of foreign body(s)
➔ *CPT Changes: An Insider's View* 2015, 2017

(Do not report 44390 in conjunction with 44388)

(If fluoroscopic guidance is performed, use 76000)

44391 with control of bleeding, any method
➔ *CPT Changes: An Insider's View* 2002, 2015, 2017
➔ *CPT Assistant* Jun 10:4

(Do not report 44391 in conjunction with 44404 for the same lesion)

(Do not report 44391 in conjunction with 44388)

44392 with removal of tumor(s), polyp(s), or other lesion(s) by hot biopsy forceps
➔ *CPT Changes: An Insider's View* 2015, 2017

(Do not report 44392 in conjunction with 44388)

 # 44401 with ablation of tumor(s), polyp(s), or other lesion(s) (includes pre-and post-dilation and guide wire passage, when performed)
➔ *CPT Changes: An Insider's View* 2015, 2017
➔ *CPT Assistant* Nov 14:3

(Do not report 44401 in conjunction with 44405 for the same lesion)

(Do not report 44401 in conjunction with 44388)

44394 with removal of tumor(s), polyp(s), or other lesion(s) by snare technique
➔ *CPT Changes: An Insider's View* 2017

(Do not report 44394 in conjunction with 44403 for the same lesion)

(Do not report 44394 in conjunction with 44388)

(For endoscopic mucosal resection, use 44403)

44401 Code is out of numerical sequence. See 44391-44402

44402 with endoscopic stent placement (including pre- and post-dilation and guide wire passage, when performed)
➔ *CPT Changes: An Insider's View* 2015, 2017
➔ *CPT Assistant* Nov 14:3

(Do not report 44402 in conjunction with 44388, 44405)

(If fluoroscopic guidance is performed, use 74360)

44403 with endoscopic mucosal resection
➔ *CPT Changes: An Insider's View* 2015, 2017
➔ *CPT Assistant* Nov 14:3, Dec 19:14

(Do not report 44403 in conjunction with 44389, 44394, 44404 for the same lesion)

(Do not report 44403 in conjunction with 44388)

44404 with directed submucosal injection(s), any substance
➔ *CPT Changes: An Insider's View* 2015, 2017
➔ *CPT Assistant* Nov 14:3

(Do not report 44404 in conjunction with 44391, 44403 for the same lesion)

(Do not report 44404 in conjunction with 44388)

44405 with transendoscopic balloon dilation
➔ *CPT Changes: An Insider's View* 2015, 2017
➔ *CPT Assistant* Nov 14:3

(Do not report 44405 in conjunction with 44388, 44401, 44402)

(If fluoroscopic guidance is performed, use 74360)

(For transendoscopic balloon dilation of multiple strictures during the same session, report 44405 with modifier 59 for each additional stricture dilated)

44406   with endoscopic ultrasound examination, limited to the sigmoid, descending, transverse, or ascending colon and cecum and adjacent structures
➜ *CPT Changes: An Insider's View* 2015, 2017
➜ *CPT Assistant* Nov 14:3

(Do not report 44406 in conjunction with 44388, 44407, 76975)

(Do not report 44406 more than once per session)

44407   with transendoscopic ultrasound guided intramural or transmural fine needle aspiration/biopsy(s), includes endoscopic ultrasound examination limited to the sigmoid, descending, transverse, or ascending colon and cecum and adjacent structures
➜ *CPT Changes: An Insider's View* 2015, 2017
➜ *CPT Assistant* Nov 14:3, Dec 14:3

(Do not report 44407 in conjunction with 44388, 44406, 76942, 76975)

(Do not report 44407 more than once per session)

44408   with decompression (for pathologic distention) (eg, volvulus, megacolon), including placement of decompression tube, when performed
➜ *CPT Changes: An Insider's View* 2015, 2017
➜ *CPT Assistant* Nov 14:3, Dec 14:3

(Do not report 44408 in conjunction with 44388)

(Do not report 44408 more than once per session)

Introduction

⊘ **44500**   Introduction of long gastrointestinal tube (eg, Miller-Abbott) (separate procedure)
➜ *CPT Changes: An Insider's View* 2017
➜ *CPT Assistant* Sep 16:9

(For radiological supervision and interpretation, use 74340)

(For naso- or oro-gastric tube placement, use 43752)

Repair

44602   Suture of small intestine (enterorrhaphy) for perforated ulcer, diverticulum, wound, injury or rupture; single perforation
➜ *CPT Assistant* Feb 20:13

44603   multiple perforations

44604   Suture of large intestine (colorrhaphy) for perforated ulcer, diverticulum, wound, injury or rupture (single or multiple perforations); without colostomy
➜ *CPT Assistant* Jul 23:1

44605   with colostomy

44615   Intestinal strictureplasty (enterotomy and enterorrhaphy) with or without dilation, for intestinal obstruction

44620   Closure of enterostomy, large or small intestine;
➜ *CPT Assistant* Nov 97:17, May 02:7

44625   with resection and anastomosis other than colorectal
➜ *CPT Assistant* Nov 97:17

44626   with resection and colorectal anastomosis (eg, closure of Hartmann type procedure)
➜ *CPT Assistant* Nov 97:17

(For laparoscopic procedure, use 44227)

44640   Closure of intestinal cutaneous fistula

44650   Closure of enteroenteric or enterocolic fistula

44660   Closure of enterovesical fistula; without intestinal or bladder resection

44661   with intestine and/or bladder resection
➜ *CPT Changes: An Insider's View* 2002

(For closure of renocolic fistula, see 50525, 50526)

(For closure of gastrocolic fistula, use 43880)

(For closure of rectovesical fistula, see 45800, 45805)

44680   Intestinal plication (separate procedure)

Other Procedures

44700   Exclusion of small intestine from pelvis by mesh or other prosthesis, or native tissue (eg, bladder or omentum)
➜ *CPT Changes: An Insider's View* 2002
➜ *CPT Assistant* Nov 97:18

(For therapeutic radiation clinical treatment, see **Radiation Oncology** section)

+ **44701**   Intraoperative colonic lavage (List separately in addition to code for primary procedure)
➜ *CPT Changes: An Insider's View* 2003

(Use 44701 in conjunction with 44140, 44145, 44150, or 44604 as appropriate)

(Do not report 44701 in conjunction with 44950-44960)

44705   Preparation of fecal microbiota for instillation, including assessment of donor specimen
➜ *CPT Changes: An Insider's View* 2013
➜ *CPT Assistant* Jan 13:11, May 13:12

(Do not report 44705 in conjunction with 74283, 0780T)

(For fecal instillation by oro-nasogastric tube, use 44799)

(For instillation of fecal microbiota suspension via rectal enema, use 0780T)

44715 Backbench standard preparation of cadaver or living donor intestine allograft prior to transplantation, including mobilization and fashioning of the superior mesenteric artery and vein

➤ *CPT Changes: An Insider's View* 2005

44720 Backbench reconstruction of cadaver or living donor intestine allograft prior to transplantation; venous anastomosis, each

➤ *CPT Changes: An Insider's View* 2005

44721 arterial anastomosis, each

➤ *CPT Changes: An Insider's View* 2005

➤ *CPT Assistant* Apr 05:10-11

44799 Unlisted procedure, small intestine

➤ *CPT Changes: An Insider's View* 2015

➤ *CPT Assistant* Dec 00:14, May 08:15, Nov 08:11, Mar 10:10, Jul 10:10, Mar 11:10, May 11:9, May 13:12, Nov 14:3, Sep 22:13, Nov 23:26

(For unlisted laparoscopic procedure, intestine except rectum, use 44238)

(For unlisted procedure, colon, use 45399)

Meckel's Diverticulum and the Mesentery

Excision

44800 Excision of Meckel's diverticulum (diverticulectomy) or omphalomesenteric duct

44820 Excision of lesion of mesentery (separate procedure)

(With intestine resection, see 44120 or 44140 et seq)

Suture

44850 Suture of mesentery (separate procedure)

(For reduction and repair of internal hernia, use 44050)

Other Procedures

44899 Unlisted procedure, Meckel's diverticulum and the mesentery

➤ *CPT Assistant* Jul 20:14

Appendix

Incision

44900 Incision and drainage of appendiceal abscess, open

➤ *CPT Assistant* Nov 97:18

(For percutaneous image-guided drainage by catheter of appendiceal abscess, use 49406)

Excision

44950 Appendectomy;

➤ *CPT Assistant* Feb 92:22, Sep 96:4, Aug 02:2, Nov 08:7

(Incidental appendectomy during intra-abdominal surgery does not usually warrant a separate identification. If necessary to report, add modifier 52)

+ 44955 when done for indicated purpose at time of other major procedure (not as separate procedure) (List separately in addition to code for primary procedure)

➤ *CPT Assistant* Fall 92:22, Sep 96:4, Apr 97:3, Nov 08:7, Jan 12:13

44960 for ruptured appendix with abscess or generalized peritonitis

➤ *CPT Assistant* Fall 92:22, Nov 08:7, Dec 19:12

Laparoscopy

Surgical laparoscopy always includes diagnostic laparoscopy. To report a diagnostic laparoscopy (peritoneoscopy) (separate procedure), use 49320.

44970 Laparoscopy, surgical, appendectomy

➤ *CPT Changes: An Insider's View* 2000

➤ *CPT Assistant* Nov 99:23, Mar 00:9, Apr 06:1, 20, Mar 15:3, Dec 19:12, Jul 23:1

44979 Unlisted laparoscopy procedure, appendix

➤ *CPT Changes: An Insider's View* 2000

➤ *CPT Assistant* Nov 99:23, Mar 00:9, Jan 12:13

Colon and Rectum

Incision

45000 Transrectal drainage of pelvic abscess

(For transrectal image-guided fluid collection drainage by catheter of pelvic abscess, use 49407)

45005 Incision and drainage of submucosal abscess, rectum

45020 Incision and drainage of deep supralevator, pelvirectal, or retrorectal abscess

(See also 46050, 46060)

Excision

45100 Biopsy of anorectal wall, anal approach (eg, congenital megacolon)

(For endoscopic biopsy, use 45305)

45108 Anorectal myomectomy

45110   Proctectomy; complete, combined abdominoperineal, with colostomy

(For laparoscopic procedure, use 45395)

45111   partial resection of rectum, transabdominal approach

45112   Proctectomy, combined abdominoperineal, pull-through procedure (eg, colo-anal anastomosis)
➔ *CPT Assistant* Nov 97:18

(For colo-anal anastomosis with colonic reservoir or pouch, use 45119)

45113   Proctectomy, partial, with rectal mucosectomy, ileoanal anastomosis, creation of ileal reservoir (S or J), with or without loop ileostomy

45114   Proctectomy, partial, with anastomosis; abdominal and transsacral approach

45116   transsacral approach only (Kraske type)

45119   Proctectomy, combined abdominoperineal pull-through procedure (eg, colo-anal anastomosis), with creation of colonic reservoir (eg, J-pouch), with diverting enterostomy when performed
➔ *CPT Changes: An Insider's View* 2006
➔ *CPT Assistant* Nov 97:18, Apr 06:1

(For laparoscopic procedure, use 45397)

45120   Proctectomy, complete (for congenital megacolon), abdominal and perineal approach; with pull-through procedure and anastomosis (eg, Swenson, Duhamel, or Soave type operation)

45121   with subtotal or total colectomy, with multiple biopsies

45123   Proctectomy, partial, without anastomosis, perineal approach

45126   Pelvic exenteration for colorectal malignancy, with proctectomy (with or without colostomy), with removal of bladder and ureteral transplantations, and/or hysterectomy, or cervicectomy, with or without removal of tube(s), with or without removal of ovary(s), or any combination thereof
➔ *CPT Assistant* Nov 98:16

45130   Excision of rectal procidentia, with anastomosis; perineal approach

45135   abdominal and perineal approach

45136   Excision of ileoanal reservoir with ileostomy
➔ *CPT Changes: An Insider's View* 2002

(Do not report 45136 in conjunction with 44005, 44310)

45150   Division of stricture of rectum

45160   Excision of rectal tumor by proctotomy, transsacral or transcoccygeal approach

45171   Excision of rectal tumor, transanal approach; not including muscularis propria (ie, partial thickness)
➔ *CPT Changes: An Insider's View* 2010
➔ *CPT Assistant* Jun 10:3

45172   including muscularis propria (ie, full thickness)
➔ *CPT Changes: An Insider's View* 2010
➔ *CPT Assistant* Jun 10:3, Feb 18:11

(For destruction of rectal tumor, transanal approach, use 45190)

(For transanal endoscopic microsurgical [ie, TEMS] excision of rectal tumor, including muscularis propria [ie, full thickness], use 0184T)

Rectal Tumor Excision
45171-45172

A rectal tumor is excised via transanal approach.

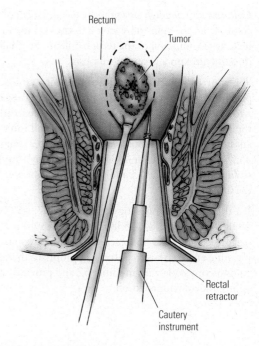

Rectum

Tumor

Rectal retractor

Cautery instrument

Destruction

45190   Destruction of rectal tumor (eg, electrodesiccation, electrosurgery, laser ablation, laser resection, cryosurgery) transanal approach
➔ *CPT Changes: An Insider's View* 2002
➔ *CPT Assistant* Jun 10:3

(For excision of rectal tumor, transanal approach, see 45171, 45172)

(For transanal endoscopic microsurgical [ie, TEMS] excision of rectal tumor, including muscularis propria [ie, full thickness], use 0184T)

Endoscopy

Definitions

Proctosigmoidoscopy is the examination of the rectum and may include examination of a portion of the sigmoid colon.

Sigmoidoscopy is the examination of the entire rectum, sigmoid colon and may include examination of a portion of the descending colon.

Colonoscopy is the examination of the entire colon, from the rectum to the cecum, and may include examination of the terminal ileum or small intestine proximal to an anastomosis.

Colonoscopy through stoma is the examination of the colon, from the colostomy stoma to the cecum, and may include examination of the terminal ileum or small intestine proximal to an anastomosis.

When performing a diagnostic or screening endoscopic procedure on a patient who is scheduled and prepared for a total colonoscopy, if the physician is unable to advance the colonoscope to the cecum or colon-small intestine anastomosis due to unforeseen circumstances, report 45378 (colonoscopy) or 44388 (colonoscopy through stoma) with modifier 53 and provide appropriate documentation.

If a therapeutic colonoscopy (44389-44407, 45379, 45380, 45381, 45382, 45384, 45388, 45398) is performed and does not reach the cecum or colon-small intestine anastomosis, report the appropriate therapeutic colonoscopy code with modifier 52 and provide appropriate documentation.

Report flexible sigmoidoscopy (45330-45347) for endoscopic examination during which the endoscope is not advanced beyond the splenic flexure.

Report flexible sigmoidoscopy (45330-45347) for endoscopic examination of a patient who has undergone resection of the colon proximal to the sigmoid (eg, subtotal colectomy) and has an ileo-sigmoid or ileo-rectal anastomosis. Report pouch endoscopy codes (44385, 44386) for endoscopic examination of a patient who has undergone resection of colon with ileo-anal anastomosis (eg, J-pouch).

Report colonoscopy (45378-45398) for endoscopic examination of a patient who has undergone segmental resection of the colon (eg, hemicolectomy, sigmoid colectomy, low anterior resection).

For colonoscopy through stoma, see 44388-44408.

Report proctosigmoidoscopy (45300-45327), flexible sigmoidoscopy (45330-45347), or anoscopy (46600, 46604, 46606, 46608, 46610, 46611, 46612, 46614, 46615), as appropriate for endoscopic examination of the defunctionalized rectum or distal colon in a patient who has undergone colectomy, in addition to colonoscopy through stoma (44388-44408) or ileoscopy through stoma (44380, 44381, 44382, 44384) if appropriate.

When bleeding occurs as a result of an endoscopic procedure, control of bleeding is not reported separately during the same operative session.

For computed tomographic colonography, see 74261-74263.

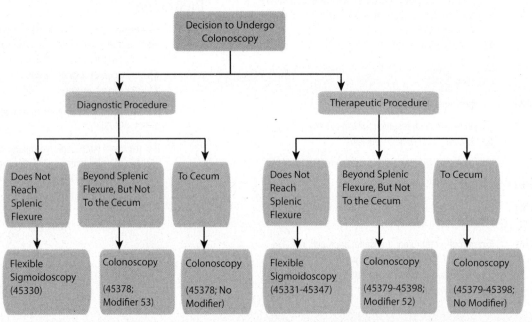

Colonoscopy Decision Tree

★ = Telemedicine ◀ = Audio-only ✛ = Add-on code ✗ = FDA approval pending # = Resequenced code ⊘ = Modifier 51 exempt ↻↻↻ = See p xxi for details

45300   Proctosigmoidoscopy, rigid; diagnostic, with or without collection of specimen(s) by brushing or washing (separate procedure)

→ *CPT Assistant* Spring 94:8, Oct 97:6, Apr 06:1

45303   with dilation (eg, balloon, guide wire, bougie)

→ *CPT Changes: An Insider's View* 2002, 2017

→ *CPT Assistant* Spring 94:8, Oct 97:6, Apr 06:1

▶(Do not report 45300, 45303 in conjunction with 0886T)◀

(For radiological supervision and interpretation, use 74360)

45305   with biopsy, single or multiple

→ *CPT Changes: An Insider's View* 2017

→ *CPT Assistant* Spring 94:8, Oct 97:6, Apr 06:1

45307   with removal of foreign body

→ *CPT Changes: An Insider's View* 2017

→ *CPT Assistant* Spring 94:8, Oct 97:6, Apr 06:1

45308   with removal of single tumor, polyp, or other lesion by hot biopsy forceps or bipolar cautery

→ *CPT Changes: An Insider's View* 2017

→ *CPT Assistant* Spring 94:8, Oct 97:6, Apr 06:1

45309   with removal of single tumor, polyp, or other lesion by snare technique

→ *CPT Changes: An Insider's View* 2017

→ *CPT Assistant* Spring 94:8, Oct 97:6, Apr 06:1

45315   with removal of multiple tumors, polyps, or other lesions by hot biopsy forceps, bipolar cautery or snare technique

→ *CPT Changes: An Insider's View* 2017

→ *CPT Assistant* Spring 94:8, Oct 97:6, Apr 06:1

45317   with control of bleeding (eg, injection, bipolar cautery, unipolar cautery, laser, heater probe, stapler, plasma coagulator)

→ *CPT Changes: An Insider's View* 2002, 2017

→ *CPT Assistant* Spring 94:8, Oct 97:6, Apr 06:1

45320   with ablation of tumor(s), polyp(s), or other lesion(s) not amenable to removal by hot biopsy forceps, bipolar cautery or snare technique (eg, laser)

→ *CPT Changes: An Insider's View* 2017

→ *CPT Assistant* Spring 94:8, Oct 97:6, Apr 06:1

45321   with decompression of volvulus

→ *CPT Changes: An Insider's View* 2017

→ *CPT Assistant* Spring 94:8, Oct 97:6, Apr 06:1

45327   with transendoscopic stent placement (includes predilation)

→ *CPT Changes: An Insider's View* 2001, 2017

→ *CPT Assistant* Nov 01:7, Apr 06:1

— *Coding Tip* —

Definition of Sigmoidoscopy

Sigmoidoscopy is the examination of the entire rectum, sigmoid colon and may include examination of a portion of the descending colon.

CPT Coding Guidelines, Endoscopy

45330   Sigmoidoscopy, flexible; diagnostic, including collection of specimen(s) by brushing or washing, when performed (separate procedure)

→ *CPT Changes: An Insider's View* 2015

→ *CPT Assistant* Spring 94:9, May 05:3, May 07:10, Nov 07:8, Dec 13:3, Dec 14:3, 19, Sep 15:12, Feb 16:13

▶(Do not report 45330 in conjunction with 45331-45342, 45346, 45347, 45349, 45350, 0886T)◀

45331   with biopsy, single or multiple

→ *CPT Assistant* Spring 94:9, Sep 96:6, Jan 07:28

(Do not report 45331 in conjunction with 45349 for the same lesion)

45332   with removal of foreign body(s)

→ *CPT Changes: An Insider's View* 2015, 2017

→ *CPT Assistant* Winter 90:3, Spring 94:9, Dec 14:3

(Do not report 45332 in conjunction with 45330)

(If fluoroscopic guidance is performed, use 76000)

45333   with removal of tumor(s), polyp(s), or other lesion(s) by hot biopsy forceps

→ *CPT Changes: An Insider's View* 2015, 2017

→ *CPT Assistant* Winter 90:3, Spring 94:9, Dec 14:3

(Do not report 45333 in conjunction with 45330)

45334   with control of bleeding, any method

→ *CPT Changes: An Insider's View* 2002, 2015, 2017

→ *CPT Assistant* Spring 94:9, Sep 96:6, Jan 07:28, Jun 10:5, Dec 14:3

(Do not report 45334 in conjunction with 45335, 45350 for the same lesion)

(Do not report 45334 in conjunction with 45330)

45335   with directed submucosal injection(s), any substance

→ *CPT Changes: An Insider's View* 2003, 2017

→ *CPT Assistant* Mar 03:22, Jun 10:5

(Do not report 45335 in conjunction with 45334, 45349 for the same lesion)

(Do not report 45335 in conjunction with 45330)

45337   with decompression (for pathologic distention) (eg, volvulus, megacolon), including placement of decompression tube, when performed

➔ *CPT Changes: An Insider's View* 2015, 2017

➔ *CPT Assistant* Spring 94:9, Dec 14:3

(Do not report 45337 in conjunction with 45330)

(Do not report 45337 more than once per session)

45338   with removal of tumor(s), polyp(s), or other lesion(s) by snare technique

➔ *CPT Changes: An Insider's View* 2017

➔ *CPT Assistant* Spring 94:9

(Do not report 45338 in conjunction with 45349 for the same lesion)

(Do not report 45338 in conjunction with 45330)

(For endoscopic mucosal resection, use 45349)

 # 45346   with ablation of tumor(s), polyp(s), or other lesion(s) (includes pre- and post-dilation and guide wire passage, when performed)

➔ *CPT Changes: An Insider's View* 2015, 2017

➔ *CPT Assistant* Dec 14:3

(Do not report 45346 in conjunction with 45330)

(Do not report 45346 in conjunction with 45340 for the same lesion)

45340   with transendoscopic balloon dilation

➔ *CPT Changes: An Insider's View* 2003, 2015, 2017

➔ *CPT Assistant* Dec 14:3

▶(Do not report 45340 in conjunction with 45330, 45346, 45347, 0886T)◀

(If fluoroscopic guidance is performed, use 74360)

▶(For sigmoidoscopy with predilation followed by therapeutic drug delivery by drug-coated balloon catheter, use 0886T)◀

(For transendoscopic balloon dilation of multiple strictures during the same session, use 45340 with modifier 59 for each additional stricture dilated)

45341   with endoscopic ultrasound examination

➔ *CPT Changes: An Insider's View* 2001, 2017

➔ *CPT Assistant* Oct 01:4, May 05:3, Dec 13:3

(Do not report 45341 in conjunction with 45330, 45342, 76872, 76975)

(Do not report 45341 more than once per session)

45342   with transendoscopic ultrasound guided intramural or transmural fine needle aspiration/biopsy(s)

➔ *CPT Changes: An Insider's View* 2001, 2017

➔ *CPT Assistant* Oct 01:4, May 05:3, Dec 13:3

(Do not report 45342 in conjunction with 45330, 45341, 76872, 76942, 76975)

(Do not report 45342 more than once per session)

45346   Code is out of numerical sequence. See 45337-45341

45347   with placement of endoscopic stent (includes pre- and post-dilation and guide wire passage, when performed)

➔ *CPT Changes: An Insider's View* 2015, 2017

➔ *CPT Assistant* Dec 14:3, Feb 16:13

(Do not report 45347 in conjunction with 45330, 45340)

(If fluoroscopic guidance is performed, use 74360)

45349   with endoscopic mucosal resection

➔ *CPT Changes: An Insider's View* 2015, 2017

➔ *CPT Assistant* Dec 14:3, Dec 19:14, May 20:13

(Do not report 45349 in conjunction with 45331, 45335, 45338, 45350 for the same lesion)

(Do not report 45349 in conjunction with 45330)

45350   with band ligation(s) (eg, hemorrhoids)

➔ *CPT Changes: An Insider's View* 2015, 2017

➔ *CPT Assistant* Dec 14:3

(Do not report 45350 in conjunction with 45334 for the same lesion)

(Do not report 45350 in conjunction with 45330, 45349, 46221)

(Do not report 45350 more than once per session)

(To report control of active bleeding with band ligation[s], use 45334)

Coding Tip

Definition of Colonoscopy

Colonoscopy is the examination of the entire colon, from the rectum to the cecum, and may include the examination of the terminal ileum or small intestine proximal to an anastomosis.

When performing a diagnostic or screening endoscopic procedure on a patient who is scheduled and prepared for a total colonoscopy, if the physician is unable to advance the colonoscope to the cecum or colon-small intestine anastomosis due to unforeseen circumstances, report 45378 (colonoscopy) or 44388 (colonoscopy through stoma) with modifier 53 and provide appropriate documentation.

CPT Coding Guidelines, Endoscopy

45378   Colonoscopy, flexible; diagnostic, including collection of specimen(s) by brushing or washing, when performed (separate procedure)

➔ *CPT Changes: An Insider's View* 2015, 2017

➔ *CPT Assistant* Spring 94:9, Aug 99:3, Jan 02:12, Jan 04:4, May 05:3, Dec 10:3, Apr 11:12, Jan 13:11, Nov 14:3, Dec 14:3, Sep 15:12, Sep 17:14, Jan 18:7, Aug 21:15

▶(Do not report 45378 in conjunction with 45379-45393, 45398, 0885T)◀

(For colonoscopy with decompression [pathologic distention], use 45393)

Colonoscopy
45378

A colonoscope is inserted in the anus and moved through the colon to the cecum in order to visualize the lumen of the rectum and colon.

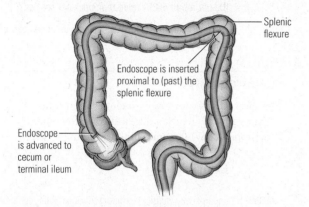

Splenic flexure

Endoscope is inserted proximal to (past) the splenic flexure

Endoscope is advanced to cecum or terminal ileum

45379   with removal of foreign body(s)
> *CPT Changes: An Insider's View* 2015, 2017
> *CPT Assistant* Spring 94:9, Aug 99:3, Dec 14:3, Aug 21:15

(Do not report 45379 in conjunction with 45378)

(If fluoroscopic guidance is performed, use 76000)

45380   with biopsy, single or multiple
> *CPT Changes: An Insider's View* 2015, 2017
> *CPT Assistant* Spring 94:9, Jan 96:7, Feb 99:11, Aug 99:3, Jan 04:7, Jul 04:15, Dec 14:3, Aug 21:15

(Do not report 45380 in conjunction with 45390 for the same lesion)

(Do not report 45380 in conjunction with 45378)

45381   with directed submucosal injection(s), any substance
> *CPT Changes: An Insider's View* 2003, 2015, 2017
> *CPT Assistant* Mar 03:22, Jan 04:7, Jun 10:5, Jan 17:6

(Do not report 45381 in conjunction with 45382, 45390 for the same lesion)

(Do not report 45381 in conjunction with 45378)

45382   with control of bleeding, any method
> *CPT Changes: An Insider's View* 2002, 2015, 2017
> *CPT Assistant* Spring 94:9, Aug 99:3, Jun 10:5, Dec 14:3

(Do not report 45382 in conjunction with 45381, 45398 for the same lesion)

(Do not report 45382 in conjunction with 45378)

 # 45388   with ablation of tumor(s), polyp(s), or other lesion(s) (includes pre- and post-dilation and guide wire passage, when performed)
> *CPT Changes: An Insider's View* 2015, 2017
> *CPT Assistant* Dec 14:3

(Do not report 45388 in conjunction with 45386 for the same lesion)

(Do not report 45388 in conjunction with 45378)

45384   with removal of tumor(s), polyp(s), or other lesion(s) by hot biopsy forceps
> *CPT Changes: An Insider's View* 2015, 2017
> *CPT Assistant* Spring 94:9, Jul 98:10, Feb 99:11, Aug 99:3, Jan 04:6, Jul 04:15, Apr 11:12, Dec 14:3, Jun 15:10

(Do not report 45384 in conjunction with 45378)

45385   with removal of tumor(s), polyp(s), or other lesion(s) by snare technique
> *CPT Changes: An Insider's View* 2015, 2017
> *CPT Assistant* Spring 94:9, Jan 96:7, Jul 98:10, Aug 99:3, Jan 04:5, Jul 04:15, Jun 10:5, Jan 17:6

(Do not report 45385 in conjunction with 45390 for the same lesion)

(Do not report 45385 in conjunction with 45378)

(For endoscopic mucosal resection, use 45390)

Colonoscopy With Lesion Ablation or Removal
45385, 45388

Insertion and advancement of a colonoscope through the colon and to the cecum for ablation (45388) or removal (45385) of tumors, polyps, or other lesions

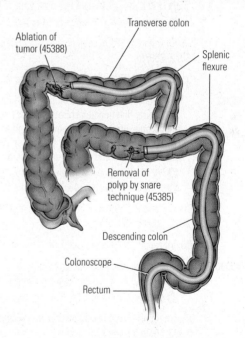

Transverse colon

Ablation of tumor (45388)

Splenic flexure

Removal of polyp by snare technique (45385)

Descending colon

Colonoscope

Rectum

45386   with transendoscopic balloon dilation
> *CPT Changes: An Insider's View* 2003, 2015, 2017
> *CPT Assistant* Dec 14:3

▶(Do not report 45386 in conjunction with 45378, 45388, 45389, 0885T)◀

(If fluoroscopic guidance is performed, use 74360)

▶(For colonoscopy with predilation followed by therapeutic drug delivery by drug-coated balloon catheter, use 0885T)◀

(For transendoscopic balloon dilation of multiple strictures during the same session, report 45386 with modifier 59 for each additional stricture dilated)

45388   Code is out of numerical sequence. See 45381-45385

45389   with endoscopic stent placement (includes pre- and post-dilation and guide wire passage, when performed)
> *CPT Changes: An Insider's View* 2015, 2017
> *CPT Assistant* Dec 14:3

(Do not report 45389 in conjunction with 45378, 45386)

(If fluoroscopic guidance is performed, use 74360)

45390   Code is out of numerical sequence. See 45391-45397

45391   with endoscopic ultrasound examination limited to the rectum, sigmoid, descending, transverse, or ascending colon and cecum, and adjacent structures
> *CPT Changes: An Insider's View* 2005, 2015, 2017
> *CPT Assistant* May 05:3, Dec 13:3, Dec 14:3

(Do not report 45391 in conjunction with 45378, 45392, 76872, 76975)

(Do not report 45391 more than once per session)

45392   with transendoscopic ultrasound guided intramural or transmural fine needle aspiration/biopsy(s), includes endoscopic ultrasound examination limited to the rectum, sigmoid, descending, transverse, or ascending colon and cecum, and adjacent structures
> *CPT Changes: An Insider's View* 2005, 2015, 2017
> *CPT Assistant* May 05:3, Dec 13:3, Dec 14:3

(Do not report 45392 in conjunction with 45378, 45391, 76872, 76942, 76975)

(Do not report 45392 more than once per session)

 # 45390   with endoscopic mucosal resection
> *CPT Changes: An Insider's View* 2015, 2017
> *CPT Assistant* Dec 14:3, Jan 17:6, Dec 19:14, May 20:13

(Do not report 45390 in conjunction with 45380, 45381, 45385, 45398 for the same lesion)

(Do not report 45390 in conjunction with 45378)

45393   with decompression (for pathologic distention) (eg, volvulus, megacolon), including placement of decompression tube, when performed
> *CPT Changes: An Insider's View* 2015, 2017
> *CPT Assistant* Dec 14:4

(Do not report 45393 in conjunction with 45378)

(Do not report 45393 more than once per session)

 # 45398   with band ligation(s) (eg, hemorrhoids)
> *CPT Changes: An Insider's View* 2015, 2017
> *CPT Assistant* Dec 14:3, Sep 17:14, Jan 18:7, Aug 21:15

(Do not report 45398 in conjunction with 45382 for the same lesion)

(Do not report 45398 in conjunction with 45378, 45390, 46221)

(Do not report 45398 more than once per session)

(To report control of active bleeding with band ligation[s], use 45382)

Laparoscopy

Surgical laparoscopy always includes diagnostic laparoscopy. To report a diagnostic laparoscopy (peritoneoscopy) (separate procedure), use 49320.

Excision

45395   Laparoscopy, surgical; proctectomy, complete, combined abdominoperineal, with colostomy
> *CPT Changes: An Insider's View* 2006

(For open procedure, use 45110)

45397   proctectomy, combined abdominoperineal pull-through procedure (eg, colo-anal anastomosis), with creation of colonic reservoir (eg, J-pouch), with diverting enterostomy, when performed
> *CPT Changes: An Insider's View* 2006

(For open procedure, use 45119)

45398   Code is out of numerical sequence. See 45391-45397

45399   Code is out of numerical sequence. See 45910-45999

Repair

45400   Laparoscopy, surgical; proctopexy (for prolapse)
> *CPT Changes: An Insider's View* 2006

(For open procedure, use 45540, 45541)

45402   proctopexy (for prolapse), with sigmoid resection
> *CPT Changes: An Insider's View* 2006

(For open procedure, use 45550)

45499   Unlisted laparoscopy procedure, rectum
> *CPT Changes: An Insider's View* 2006

Repair

45500   Proctoplasty; for stenosis

Digestive 40490-49999

45505   for prolapse of mucous membrane
> *CPT Assistant* Oct 13:19, Mar 15:10

45520   Perirectal injection of sclerosing solution for prolapse
> *CPT Assistant* Jul 01:11, Aug 01:10

45540   Proctopexy (eg, for prolapse); abdominal approach
> *CPT Changes: An Insider's View* 2006

(For laparoscopic procedure, use 45400)

45541   perineal approach

45550   with sigmoid resection, abdominal approach
> *CPT Changes: An Insider's View* 2006

(For laparoscopic procedure, use 45402)

45560   Repair of rectocele (separate procedure)

(For repair of rectocele with posterior colporrhaphy, use 57250)

45562   Exploration, repair, and presacral drainage for rectal injury;

45563   with colostomy

45800   Closure of rectovesical fistula;

45805   with colostomy

45820   Closure of rectourethral fistula;

45825   with colostomy

(For rectovaginal fistula closure, see 57300-57308)

Manipulation

45900   Reduction of procidentia (separate procedure) under anesthesia

45905   Dilation of anal sphincter (separate procedure) under anesthesia other than local

45910   Dilation of rectal stricture (separate procedure) under anesthesia other than local

45915   Removal of fecal impaction or foreign body (separate procedure) under anesthesia
> *CPT Changes: An Insider's View* 2003

Other Procedures

Surgical diagnostic anorectal exam (45990) includes the following elements: external perineal exam, digital rectal exam, pelvic exam (when performed), diagnostic anoscopy, and diagnostic rigid proctoscopy.

\# **45399**   Unlisted procedure, colon
> *CPT Changes: An Insider's View* 2015
> *CPT Assistant* Nov 14:3, Dec 14:4

45990   Anorectal exam, surgical, requiring anesthesia (general, spinal, or epidural), diagnostic
> *CPT Changes: An Insider's View* 2006

(Do not report 45990 in conjunction with 45300-45327, 46600, 57410, 99170)

45999   Unlisted procedure, rectum

(For unlisted laparoscopic procedure, rectum, use 45499)

Anus

For incision of thrombosed external hemorrhoid, use 46083. For ligation of internal hemorrhoid(s), see 46221, 46945, 46946. For excision of internal and/or external hemorrhoid(s), see 46250-46262, 46320. For injection of hemorrhoid(s), use 46500. For destruction of internal hemorrhoid(s) by thermal energy, use 46930. For destruction of hemorrhoid(s) by cryosurgery, use 46999. For transanal hemorrhoidal dearterialization, including ultrasound guidance, with mucopexy, when performed, use 46948. For hemorrhoidopexy, use 46947. Do not report 46600 in conjunction with 46020-46947, 0184T, during the same operative session.

Incision

(For subcutaneous fistulotomy, use 46270)

46020   Placement of seton
> *CPT Changes: An Insider's View* 2002

(Do not report 46020 in conjunction with 46060, 46280, 46600)

Placement of Seton
46020

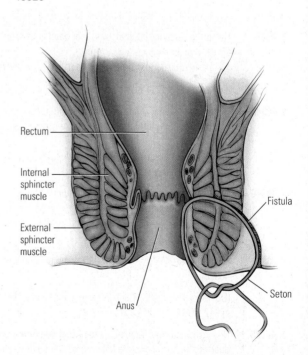

Rectum

Internal sphincter muscle

External sphincter muscle

Anus

Fistula

Seton

46030   Removal of anal seton, other marker

46040   Incision and drainage of ischiorectal and/or perirectal abscess (separate procedure)

46045   Incision and drainage of intramural, intramuscular, or submucosal abscess, transanal, under anesthesia

46050   Incision and drainage, perianal abscess, superficial

(See also 45020, 46060)

46060   Incision and drainage of ischiorectal or intramural abscess, with fistulectomy or fistulotomy, submuscular, with or without placement of seton

(Do not report 46060 in addition to 46020)

(See also 45020)

46070   Incision, anal septum (infant)

(For anoplasty, see 46700-46705)

(Do not report modifier 63 in conjunction with 46070)

46080   Sphincterotomy, anal, division of sphincter (separate procedure)

46083   Incision of thrombosed hemorrhoid, external
         ➔ CPT Assistant Jun 97:10

Excision

46200   Fissurectomy, including sphincterotomy, when performed
         ➔ CPT Changes: An Insider's View 2010

46220   Code is out of numerical sequence. See 46200-46255

46221   Hemorrhoidectomy, internal, by rubber band ligation(s)
         ➔ CPT Changes: An Insider's View 2010
         ➔ CPT Assistant Oct 97:8, Dec 14:3, Apr 15:10, Sep 17:14, Jan 18:7

(Do not report 46221 in conjunction with 45350, 45398)

46945 Hemorrhoidectomy, internal, by ligation other than rubber band; single hemorrhoid column/group, without imaging guidance
         ➔ CPT Changes: An Insider's View 2010, 2020
         ➔ CPT Assistant Apr 15:10, Feb 20:11

46946   2 or more hemorrhoid columns/groups, without imaging guidance
         ➔ CPT Changes: An Insider's View 2010, 2020
         ➔ CPT Assistant Apr 15:10, Feb 20:11

(Do not report 46221, 46945, 46946 in conjunction with 46948)

(Do not report 46945, 46946 in conjunction with 76872, 76942, 76998)

46948 Hemorrhoidectomy, internal, by transanal hemorrhoidal dearterialization, 2 or more hemorrhoid columns/groups, including ultrasound guidance, with mucopexy, when performed
         ➔ CPT Changes: An Insider's View 2020
         ➔ CPT Assistant Feb 20:11

(Do not report 46948 in conjunction with 76872, 76942, 76998)

(For transanal hemorrhoidal dearterialization, single hemorrhoid column/group, use 46999)

46220 Excision of single external papilla or tag, anus
         ➔ CPT Changes: An Insider's View 2010

46230   Excision of multiple external papillae or tags, anus
         ➔ CPT Changes: An Insider's View 2010

46320 Excision of thrombosed hemorrhoid, external
         ➔ CPT Changes: An Insider's View 2010

46250   Hemorrhoidectomy, external, 2 or more columns/groups
         ➔ CPT Changes: An Insider's View 2010
         ➔ CPT Assistant May 22:17

(For hemorrhoidectomy, external, single column/group, use 46999)

Hemorrhoidectomy of Internal Prolapsed Hemorrhoid Columns
46250-46262

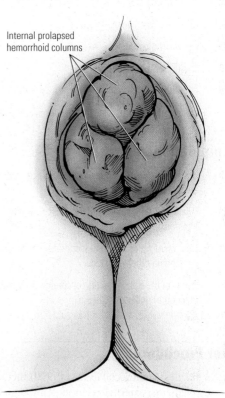

Internal prolapsed hemorrhoid columns

Anal column is considered to be an internal hemorrhoid with 3 major areas in the anal canal: right posterior (1 o'clock), right anterior (5 o'clock), and left lateral (9 o'clock) positions of the anus.

46255   Hemorrhoidectomy, internal and external, single column/
group;
➔ *CPT Changes: An Insider's View* 2010
➔ *CPT Assistant* Oct 14:15, May 22:17

46257   with fissurectomy

46258   with fistulectomy, including fissurectomy, when
performed
➔ *CPT Changes: An Insider's View* 2010

46260   Hemorrhoidectomy, internal and external, 2 or more
columns/groups;
➔ *CPT Changes: An Insider's View* 2010
➔ *CPT Assistant* Aug 21:15

46261   with fissurectomy

46262   with fistulectomy, including fissurectomy, when
performed
➔ *CPT Changes: An Insider's View* 2010
➔ *CPT Assistant* May 05:3

(Do not report 46250-46262 in conjunction with 46948)

46270   Surgical treatment of anal fistula (fistulectomy/
fistulotomy); subcutaneous

46275   intersphincteric
➔ *CPT Changes: An Insider's View* 2010

46280   transsphincteric, suprasphincteric, extrasphincteric or
multiple, including placement of seton, when
performed
➔ *CPT Changes: An Insider's View* 2010

(Do not report 46280 in conjunction with 46020)

46285   second stage

46288   Closure of anal fistula with rectal advancement flap

46320   Code is out of numerical sequence. See 46200-46255

Introduction

46500   Injection of sclerosing solution, hemorrhoids
➔ *CPT Assistant* May 05:3

46505   Chemodenervation of internal anal sphincter
➔ *CPT Changes: An Insider's View* 2006

(For chemodenervation of other muscles, see 64612,
64616, 64617, 64642, 64643, 64644, 64645, 64646,
64647. For destruction of nerve by neurolytic agent, use
64630)

(Report the specific service in conjunction with the
specific substance(s) or drug(s) provided)

Endoscopy

Surgical endoscopy always includes diagnostic endoscopy.

46600   Anoscopy; diagnostic, including collection of specimen(s)
by brushing or washing, when performed (separate
procedure)
➔ *CPT Changes: An Insider's View* 2015
➔ *CPT Assistant* Spring 94:9, Oct 97:6, Apr 06:1, Jun 10:3,
Aug 11:9, Jan 18:7

(Do not report 46600 in conjunction with 46020-46947,
0184T, during the same operative session)

(For diagnostic high-resolution anoscopy [HRA], use
46601)

46601   diagnostic, with high-resolution magnification (HRA)
(eg, colposcope, operating microscope) and chemical
agent enhancement, including collection of
specimen(s) by brushing or washing, when performed
➔ *CPT Changes: An Insider's View* 2015
➔ *CPT Assistant* Oct 18:11

(Do not report 46601 in conjunction with 69990)

46604   with dilation (eg, balloon, guide wire, bougie)
➔ *CPT Changes: An Insider's View* 2002
➔ *CPT Assistant* Spring 94:9, Oct 97:6

46606   with biopsy, single or multiple
➔ *CPT Assistant* Spring 94:9, Oct 97:6, Sep 19:11

(For high-resolution anoscopy [HRA] with biopsy, use
46607)

46607   with high-resolution magnification (HRA) (eg,
colposcope, operating microscope) and chemical
agent enhancement, with biopsy, single or multiple
➔ *CPT Changes: An Insider's View* 2015
➔ *CPT Assistant* Oct 18:11, Dec 19:12

(Do not report 46607 in conjunction with 69990)

46608   with removal of foreign body
➔ *CPT Assistant* Spring 94:9, Oct 97:6

46610   with removal of single tumor, polyp, or other lesion by
hot biopsy forceps or bipolar cautery
➔ *CPT Assistant* Spring 94:10, Oct 97:6

46611   with removal of single tumor, polyp, or other lesion by
snare technique
➔ *CPT Assistant* Spring 94:10, Oct 97:6

46612   with removal of multiple tumors, polyps, or other
lesions by hot biopsy forceps, bipolar cautery or snare
technique
➔ *CPT Assistant* Spring 94:10, Oct 97:6

Digestive 40490-49999

46614 with control of bleeding (eg, injection, bipolar cautery, unipolar cautery, laser, heater probe, stapler, plasma coagulator)
➔ *CPT Changes: An Insider's View* 2002
➔ *CPT Assistant* Spring 94:10, Oct 97:6

46615 with ablation of tumor(s), polyp(s), or other lesion(s) not amenable to removal by hot biopsy forceps, bipolar cautery or snare technique
➔ *CPT Assistant* Spring 94:10, Oct 97:6

Repair

46700 Anoplasty, plastic operation for stricture; adult

46705 infant

(Do not report modifier 63 in conjunction with 46705)

(For simple incision of anal septum, use 46070)

46706 Repair of anal fistula with fibrin glue
➔ *CPT Changes: An Insider's View* 2003

46707 Repair of anorectal fistula with plug (eg, porcine small intestine submucosa [SIS])
➔ *CPT Changes: An Insider's View* 2010
➔ *CPT Assistant* Jan 12:10, Oct 13:15

46710 Repair of ileoanal pouch fistula/sinus (eg, perineal or vaginal), pouch advancement; transperineal approach
➔ *CPT Changes: An Insider's View* 2006

46712 combined transperineal and transabdominal approach
➔ *CPT Changes: An Insider's View* 2006

46715 Repair of low imperforate anus; with anoperineal fistula (cut-back procedure)

46716 with transposition of anoperineal or anovestibular fistula

(Do not report modifier 63 in conjunction with 46715, 46716)

46730 Repair of high imperforate anus without fistula; perineal or sacroperineal approach

46735 combined transabdominal and sacroperineal approaches

(Do not report modifier 63 in conjunction with 46730, 46735)

46740 Repair of high imperforate anus with rectourethral or rectovaginal fistula; perineal or sacroperineal approach

46742 combined transabdominal and sacroperineal approaches

(Do not report modifier 63 in conjunction with 46740, 46742)

46744 Repair of cloacal anomaly by anorectovaginoplasty and urethroplasty, sacroperineal approach

(Do not report modifier 63 in conjunction with 46744)

46746 Repair of cloacal anomaly by anorectovaginoplasty and urethroplasty, combined abdominal and sacroperineal approach;

46748 with vaginal lengthening by intestinal graft or pedicle flaps

46750 Sphincteroplasty, anal, for incontinence or prolapse; adult

46751 child

46753 Graft (Thiersch operation) for rectal incontinence and/or prolapse

46754 Removal of Thiersch wire or suture, anal canal

46760 Sphincteroplasty, anal, for incontinence, adult; muscle transplant

46761 levator muscle imbrication (Park posterior anal repair)

 # 46947 Hemorrhoidopexy (eg, for prolapsing internal hemorrhoids) by stapling
➔ *CPT Changes: An Insider's View* 2005
➔ *CPT Assistant* May 05:3; 14

Destruction

46900 Destruction of lesion(s), anus (eg, condyloma, papilloma, molluscum contagiosum, herpetic vesicle), simple; chemical

46910 electrodesiccation
➔ *CPT Assistant* Dec 19:12

46916 cryosurgery

46917 laser surgery

46922 surgical excision

46924 Destruction of lesion(s), anus (eg, condyloma, papilloma, molluscum contagiosum, herpetic vesicle), extensive (eg, laser surgery, electrosurgery, cryosurgery, chemosurgery)
➔ *CPT Changes: An Insider's View* 2002

46930 Destruction of internal hemorrhoid(s) by thermal energy (eg, infrared coagulation, cautery, radiofrequency)
➔ *CPT Changes: An Insider's View* 2009
➔ *CPT Assistant* Apr 15:10, Jul 16:8, Dec 22:16

46940 Curettage or cautery of anal fissure, including dilation of anal sphincter (separate procedure); initial
➔ *CPT Changes: An Insider's View* 2002

46942 subsequent

46945 Code is out of numerical sequence. See 46200-46255

46946 Code is out of numerical sequence. See 46200-46255

46947 Code is out of numerical sequence. See 46760-46910

46948 Code is out of numerical sequence. See 46200-46255

Other Procedures

46999   Unlisted procedure, anus

➜ *CPT Assistant* Oct 97:8, Apr 15:10, Oct 18:11, May 22:17, Dec 22:16

Liver

Incision

47000   Biopsy of liver, needle; percutaneous

➜ *CPT Changes: An Insider's View* 2012, 2017

➜ *CPT Assistant* Fall 93:12, Nov 21:13

➜ *Clinical Examples in Radiology* Winter 17:4, Spring 22:5,6

(If imaging guidance is performed, see 76942, 77002, 77012, 77021)

+ 47001   when done for indicated purpose at time of other major procedure (List separately in addition to code for primary procedure)

➜ *CPT Assistant* Jun 07:10

(If imaging guidance is performed, see 76942, 77002)

(For fine needle aspiration biopsy in conjunction with 47000, 47001, see 10004, 10005, 10006, 10007, 10008, 10009, 10010, 10011, 10012, 10021)

(For evaluation of fine needle aspirate in conjunction with 47000, 47001, see 88172, 88173)

47010   Hepatotomy, for open drainage of abscess or cyst, 1 or 2 stages

➜ *CPT Assistant* Nov 97:18

(For percutaneous image-guided fluid collection drainage by catheter of hepatic abscess or cyst, use 49405)

47015   Laparotomy, with aspiration and/or injection of hepatic parasitic (eg, amoebic or echinococcal) cyst(s) or abscess(es)

Excision

47100   Biopsy of liver, wedge

47120   Hepatectomy, resection of liver; partial lobectomy

➜ *CPT Assistant* May 98:10, Sep 14:14, Oct 16:11

47122   trisegmentectomy

47125   total left lobectomy

47130   total right lobectomy

Liver Transplantation

Liver allotransplantation involves three distinct components of physician work:

1. ***Cadaver donor hepatectomy,*** which includes harvesting the graft and cold preservation of the graft (perfusing with cold preservation solution and cold maintenance) (use 47133). ***Living donor hepatectomy,*** which includes harvesting the graft, cold preservation of the graft (perfusing with cold preservation solution and cold maintenance), and care of the donor (see 47140-47142).

2. ***Backbench work:***

Standard preparation of the whole liver graft will include one of the following:

Preparation of whole liver graft (including cholecystectomy, if necessary, and dissection and removal of surrounding soft tissues to prepare vena cava, portal vein, hepatic artery, and common bile duct for implantation) (use 47143).

Preparation as described for whole liver graft, plus trisegment split into two partial grafts (use 47144).

Preparation as described for whole liver graft, plus lobe split into two partial grafts (use 47145).

Additional reconstruction of the liver graft may include venous and/or arterial anastomosis(es) (see 47146, 47147).

3. ***Recipient liver allotransplantation,*** which includes recipient hepatectomy (partial or whole), transplantation of the allograft (partial or whole), and care of the recipient (use 47135).

47133   Donor hepatectomy (including cold preservation), from cadaver donor

➜ *CPT Changes: An Insider's View* 2005

47135   Liver allotransplantation, orthotopic, partial or whole, from cadaver or living donor, any age

➜ *CPT Assistant* Dec 11:16

47140   Donor hepatectomy (including cold preservation), from living donor; left lateral segment only (segments II and III)

➜ *CPT Changes: An Insider's View* 2004, 2005

➜ *CPT Assistant* Aug 11:9

47141   total left lobectomy (segments II, III and IV)

➜ *CPT Changes: An Insider's View* 2004

47142   total right lobectomy (segments V, VI, VII and VIII)

➜ *CPT Changes: An Insider's View* 2004

47143   Backbench standard preparation of cadaver donor whole liver graft prior to allotransplantation, including cholecystectomy, if necessary, and dissection and removal of surrounding soft tissues to prepare the vena cava, portal vein, hepatic artery, and common bile duct for implantation; without trisegment or lobe split

➜ *CPT Changes: An Insider's View* 2005

➜ *CPT Assistant* Apr 05:10, 12

47144   with trisegment split of whole liver graft into 2 partial liver grafts (ie, left lateral segment [segments II and III] and right trisegment [segments I and IV through VIII])

➜ *CPT Changes: An Insider's View* 2005, 2009

47145   with lobe split of whole liver graft into 2 partial liver grafts (ie, left lobe [segments II, III, and IV] and right lobe [segments I and V through VIII])

➜ *CPT Changes: An Insider's View* 2005

47146   Backbench reconstruction of cadaver or living donor liver graft prior to allotransplantation; venous anastomosis, each

➜ *CPT Changes: An Insider's View* 2005

47147   arterial anastomosis, each

➜ *CPT Changes: An Insider's View* 2005

(Do not report 47143-47147 in conjunction with 47120-47125, 47600, 47610)

Repair

47300   Marsupialization of cyst or abscess of liver

47350   Management of liver hemorrhage; simple suture of liver wound or injury

➜ *CPT Assistant* Oct 20:14

47360   complex suture of liver wound or injury, with or without hepatic artery ligation

➜ *CPT Assistant* Oct 20:14

47361   exploration of hepatic wound, extensive debridement, coagulation and/or suture, with or without packing of liver

➜ *CPT Assistant* Oct 20:14

47362   re-exploration of hepatic wound for removal of packing

Laparoscopy

Surgical laparoscopy always includes diagnostic laparoscopy. To report a diagnostic laparoscopy (peritoneoscopy) (separate procedure), use 49320.

47370   Laparoscopy, surgical, ablation of 1 or more liver tumor(s); radiofrequency

➜ *CPT Changes: An Insider's View* 2002

➜ *CPT Assistant* Oct 02:2, Jan 21:13

(For imaging guidance, use 76940)

47371   cryosurgical

➜ *CPT Changes: An Insider's View* 2002

(For imaging guidance, use 76940)

47379   Unlisted laparoscopic procedure, liver

➜ *CPT Changes: An Insider's View* 2001

➜ *CPT Assistant* Aug 06:10, Dec 07:12, Dec 14:18, Aug 18:10

Other Procedures

47380   Ablation, open, of 1 or more liver tumor(s); radiofrequency

➜ *CPT Changes: An Insider's View* 2002

➜ *CPT Assistant* Oct 02:1

➜ *Clinical Examples in Radiology* Summer 08:3

(For imaging guidance, use 76940)

47381   cryosurgical

➜ *CPT Changes: An Insider's View* 2002

(For imaging guidance, use 76940)

47382   Ablation, 1 or more liver tumor(s), percutaneous, radiofrequency

➜ *CPT Changes: An Insider's View* 2002, 2010, 2017

➜ *CPT Assistant* Oct 02:1

➜ *Clinical Examples in Radiology* Spring 08:1-2, Summer 08:3, Summer 12:11

(For imaging guidance and monitoring, see 76940, 77013, 77022)

47383   Ablation, 1 or more liver tumor(s), percutaneous, cryoablation

➜ *CPT Changes: An Insider's View* 2015, 2017

➜ *CPT Assistant* Dec 14:18

(For imaging guidance and monitoring, see 76940, 77013, 77022)

47399   Unlisted procedure, liver

➜ *CPT Assistant* Dec 14:18, Mar 17:10

Biliary Tract

Incision

47400   Hepaticotomy or hepaticostomy with exploration, drainage, or removal of calculus

47420   Choledochotomy or choledochostomy with exploration, drainage, or removal of calculus, with or without cholecystotomy; without transduodenal sphincterotomy or sphincteroplasty

47425   with transduodenal sphincterotomy or sphincteroplasty

47460   Transduodenal sphincterotomy or sphincteroplasty, with or without transduodenal extraction of calculus (separate procedure)

47480   Cholecystotomy or cholecystostomy, open, with exploration, drainage, or removal of calculus (separate procedure)
> *CPT Changes: An Insider's View* 2011
> *CPT Assistant* Apr 11:12
> *Clinical Examples in Radiology* Summer 11:3

(For percutaneous cholecystostomy, use 47490)

Introduction

Percutaneous biliary procedures (eg, transhepatic, transcholecystic) are described by 47490 and 47531-47544, and are performed with imaging guidance. They are differentiated from endoscopic procedures that utilize an access to the biliary tree from a hollow viscus for diagnosis and therapy. Diagnostic cholangiography is typically performed with percutaneous biliary procedures, and is included in 47490, 47533, 47534, 47535, 47536, 47537, 47538, 47539, 47540, and 47541.

Codes 47531 and 47532 describe percutaneous diagnostic cholangiography that includes injection(s) of contrast material, all associated radiological supervision and interpretation, and procedural imaging guidance (eg, ultrasound and/or fluoroscopy). Code 47532 also includes accessing the biliary system with a needle or catheter. Codes 47531 and 47532 may not be reported with codes 47533, 47534, 47535, 47536, 47537, 47538, 47539, 47540, and 47541.

An external biliary drainage catheter is a catheter placed into a bile duct that does not terminate in bowel, and that drains bile externally only. An internal-external biliary drainage catheter is a single, externally accessible catheter that terminates in the small intestine, and may drain bile into the small intestine and/or externally. A "stent," as used in this code set, is a percutaneously placed device (eg, self-expanding metallic mesh stent, plastic tube) that is positioned within the biliary tree and is completely internal, with no portion extending outside the patient.

Codes 47533, 47534, 47535, 47536, 47537, 47538, 47539, and 47540 describe percutaneous therapeutic biliary procedures that include catheter or stent placement, catheter removal and replacement (exchange), and/or catheter removal. These codes include the elements of access, drainage catheter manipulations, diagnostic cholangiography, imaging guidance (eg, ultrasonography and/or fluoroscopy), and all associated radiological supervision and interpretation. Codes 47533, 47534, 47538, 47539, 47540 may be reported once for each catheter or stent placed (eg, bilobar placement, multi-segmental placement). Codes 47535, 47536, and 47537 may be reported once for each catheter conversion, exchange, or removal (eg, bilobar, bisegmental).

Codes 47538, 47539, 47540 may be reported only once per session to describe one or more overlapping or serial stent(s) placed within a single bile duct, or bridging more than one ductal segment (eg, left hepatic duct and

common bile duct) through a single percutaneous access. Codes 47538, 47539, 47540 may be reported more than once in the same session using modifier 59 for the additional procedures in the following circumstances: (i) placement of side-by-side (double-barrel) stents within a single bile duct; (ii) placement of two or more stents into separate bile ducts through a single percutaneous access; or (iii) placement of stents through two or more percutaneous access sites (eg, placement of one stent through the interstices of another stent). Code 47538 describes biliary stent placement through an existing access. Therefore, 47538 should not be reported together with 47536 if a biliary drainage catheter (eg, external or internal-external) is replaced after the biliary stent is placed. Code 47540 describes biliary stent placement with the additional service of placing a biliary drainage catheter (eg, external or internal-external). Therefore, 47540 should not be reported with 47533, 47534 for the same ductal system.

Code 47541 describes a procedure to assist with endoscopic procedures performed in conjunction with other physician specialists. Access placed may include wire and/or catheter. Code 47541 may not be reported if a wire is placed through existing percutaneous access.

Codes 47542, 47543, and 47544 describe procedures that may be performed in conjunction with other codes in this family, are add-on codes and do not include access, catheter placement, or diagnostic imaging. Do not report 47542 with 47538, 47539, 47540 because balloon dilation is included in 47538, 47539, and 47540. Code 47544 should not be reported with 47531-47543 for incidental removal of debris. Code 47542 should not be reported with 47544, if a balloon is used for removal of calculi or debris rather than for dilation.

47490   Cholecystostomy, percutaneous, complete procedure, including imaging guidance, catheter placement, cholecystogram when performed, and radiological supervision and interpretation
> *CPT Changes: An Insider's View* 2011
> *CPT Assistant* Apr 11:12, Dec 15:3, Feb 23:14
> *Clinical Examples in Radiology* Winter 11:10, Summer 11:1, 3

(Do not report 47490 in conjunction with 47531, 47532, 75989, 76942, 77002, 77012, 77021)

47531 Injection procedure for cholangiography, percutaneous, complete diagnostic procedure including imaging guidance (eg, ultrasound and/or fluoroscopy) and all associated radiological supervision and interpretation; existing access

➔ *CPT Changes: An Insider's View* 2016
➔ *CPT Assistant* Dec 15:3, Feb 23:14
➔ *Clinical Examples in Radiology* Fall 15:5

47532 new access (eg, percutaneous transhepatic cholangiogram)

➔ *CPT Changes: An Insider's View* 2016, 2017
➔ *CPT Assistant* Dec 15:3
➔ *Clinical Examples in Radiology* Fall 15:5

(Do not report 47531, 47532 in conjunction with 47490, 47533, 47534, 47535, 47536, 47537, 47538, 47539, 47540, 47541 for procedures performed through the same percutaneous access)

(For intraoperative cholangiography, see 74300, 74301)

47533 Placement of biliary drainage catheter, percutaneous, including diagnostic cholangiography when performed, imaging guidance (eg, ultrasound and/or fluoroscopy), and all associated radiological supervision and interpretation; external

➔ *CPT Changes: An Insider's View* 2016, 2017
➔ *CPT Assistant* Dec 15:3
➔ *Clinical Examples in Radiology* Fall 15:5, Spring 20:14

47534 internal-external

➔ *CPT Changes: An Insider's View* 2016, 2017
➔ *CPT Assistant* Dec 15:3
➔ *Clinical Examples in Radiology* Fall 15:4, Spring 20:14

47535 Conversion of external biliary drainage catheter to internal-external biliary drainage catheter, percutaneous, including diagnostic cholangiography when performed, imaging guidance (eg, fluoroscopy), and all associated radiological supervision and interpretation

➔ *CPT Changes: An Insider's View* 2016, 2017
➔ *CPT Assistant* Dec 15:3
➔ *Clinical Examples in Radiology* Fall 15:5, Spring 20:14

Percutaneous Biliary Stent(s) and Drain Placement
47533, 47534, 47538, 47539, 47540

Biliary catheters (eg, external 47533, internal-external 47534) and multiple stents (eg, 47538, 47539, 47540)

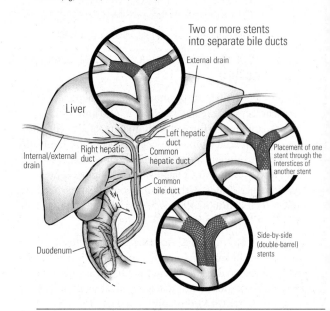

47536 Exchange of biliary drainage catheter (eg, external, internal-external, or conversion of internal-external to external only), percutaneous, including diagnostic cholangiography when performed, imaging guidance (eg, fluoroscopy), and all associated radiological supervision and interpretation

➔ *CPT Changes: An Insider's View* 2016, 2017
➔ *CPT Assistant* Dec 15:3
➔ *Clinical Examples in Radiology* Fall 15:5, Spring 20:14

(Do not report 47536 in conjunction with 47538 for the same access)

(47536 includes exchange of one catheter. For exchange of additional catheter[s] during the same session, report 47536 with modifier 59 for each additional exchange)

Exchanges/Conversions

(Existing Access)		To		
Do Not Report Exchange with Stent for Same Percutaneous Access		**Internal-External**	**External**	**Stent**
From	External Drain	47535 Conversion	47536 Exchange	47538 Stent
	Internal-External Drain	47536 Exchange	47536 Exchange	47538 Stent

47537   Removal of biliary drainage catheter, percutaneous, requiring fluoroscopic guidance (eg, with concurrent indwelling biliary stents), including diagnostic cholangiography when performed, imaging guidance (eg, fluoroscopy), and all associated radiological supervision and interpretation

     ➔ *CPT Changes: An Insider's View* 2016

     ➔ *CPT Assistant* Dec 15:3

     ➔ *Clinical Examples in Radiology* Fall 15:5

     (Do not report 47537 in conjunction with 47538 for the same access)

     (For removal of biliary drainage catheter not requiring fluoroscopic guidance, see E/M services and report the appropriate level of service provided [eg, 99202-99215, 99221, 99222, 99223, 99231, 99232, 99233])

47538   Placement of stent(s) into a bile duct, percutaneous, including diagnostic cholangiography, imaging guidance (eg, fluoroscopy and/or ultrasound), balloon dilation, catheter exchange(s) and catheter removal(s) when performed, and all associated radiological supervision and interpretation; existing access

     ➔ *CPT Changes: An Insider's View* 2016, 2017

     ➔ *CPT Assistant* Dec 15:3, Mar 16:10

     ➔ *Clinical Examples in Radiology* Fall 15:5

     (Do not report 47538 in conjunction with 47536, 47537 for the same percutaneous access)

47539   new access, without placement of separate biliary drainage catheter

     ➔ *CPT Changes: An Insider's View* 2016, 2017

     ➔ *CPT Assistant* Dec 15:3, Mar 16:10

     ➔ *Clinical Examples in Radiology* Fall 15:5

47540   new access, with placement of separate biliary drainage catheter (eg, external or internal-external)

     ➔ *CPT Changes: An Insider's View* 2016, 2017

     ➔ *CPT Assistant* Dec 15:3, Mar 16:10

     ➔ *Clinical Examples in Radiology* Fall 15:5

     (Do not report 47538, 47539, 47540 in conjunction with 43277, 47542, 47555, 47556 for the same lesion in the same session)

     (Do not report 47540 in conjunction with 47533, 47534 for the same percutaneous access)

     (47538, 47539, 47540 may be reported more than once per session, when specific conditions described in the **Introduction** within the **Biliary Tract** subsection guidelines are met)

47541   Placement of access through the biliary tree and into small bowel to assist with an endoscopic biliary procedure (eg, rendezvous procedure), percutaneous, including diagnostic cholangiography when performed, imaging guidance (eg, ultrasound and/or fluoroscopy), and all associated radiological supervision and interpretation, new access

     ➔ *CPT Changes: An Insider's View* 2016, 2017

     ➔ *CPT Assistant* Dec 15:3

     ➔ *Clinical Examples in Radiology* Fall 15:6

(Do not report 47541 in conjunction with 47531, 47532, 47533, 47534, 47535, 47536, 47537, 47538, 47539, 47540)

(Do not report 47541 when there is existing catheter access)

(For use of existing access through the biliary tree into small bowel to assist with an endoscopic biliary procedure, see 47535, 47536, 47537)

+ 47542   Balloon dilation of biliary duct(s) or of ampulla (sphincteroplasty), percutaneous, including imaging guidance (eg, fluoroscopy), and all associated radiological supervision and interpretation, each duct (List separately in addition to code for primary procedure)

     ➔ *CPT Changes: An Insider's View* 2016, 2017

     ➔ *CPT Assistant* Dec 15:3

     ➔ *Clinical Examples in Radiology* Fall 15:6

     (Use 47542 in conjunction with 47531, 47532, 47533, 47534, 47535, 47536, 47537, 47541)

     (Do not report 47542 in conjunction with 43262, 43277, 47538, 47539, 47540, 47555, 47556)

     (Do not report 47542 in conjunction with 47544 if a balloon is used for removal of calculi, debris, and/or sludge rather than for dilation)

     (For percutaneous balloon dilation of multiple ducts during the same session, report an additional dilation once with 47542 and modifier 59, regardless of the number of additional ducts dilated)

     (For endoscopic balloon dilation, see 43277, 47555, 47556)

+ 47543   Endoluminal biopsy(ies) of biliary tree, percutaneous, any method(s) (eg, brush, forceps, and/or needle), including imaging guidance (eg, fluoroscopy), and all associated radiological supervision and interpretation, single or multiple (List separately in addition to code for primary procedure)

     ➔ *CPT Changes: An Insider's View* 2016, 2017

     ➔ *CPT Assistant* Dec 15:3

     ➔ *Clinical Examples in Radiology* Fall 15:6

     (Use 47543 in conjunction with 47531, 47532, 47533, 47534, 47535, 47536, 47537, 47538, 47539, 47540)

     (Report 47543 once per session)

     (For endoscopic brushings, see 43260, 47552)

     (For endoscopic biopsy, see 43261, 47553)

+ 47544   Removal of calculi/debris from biliary duct(s) and/or gallbladder, percutaneous, including destruction of calculi by any method (eg, mechanical, electrohydraulic, lithotripsy) when performed, imaging guidance (eg, fluoroscopy), and all associated radiological supervision and interpretation (List separately in addition to code for primary procedure)
➔ *CPT Changes: An Insider's View* 2016, 2017
➔ *CPT Assistant* Dec 15:3, Feb 23:14
➔ *Clinical Examples in Radiology* Fall 15:6

(Use 47544 in conjunction with 47531, 47532, 47533, 47534, 47535, 47536, 47537, 47538, 47539, 47540)

(Do not report 47544 if no calculi or debris are found, even if removal device is deployed)

(Do not report 47544 in conjunction with 43264, 47554)

(Do not report 47544 in conjunction with 47531-47543 for incidental removal of debris)

(For endoscopic removal of calculi, see 43264, 47554)

(For endoscopic destruction of calculi, use 43265)

Endoscopy

Surgical endoscopy always includes diagnostic endoscopy.

+ 47550   Biliary endoscopy, intraoperative (choledochoscopy) (List separately in addition to code for primary procedure)

47552   Biliary endoscopy, percutaneous via T-tube or other tract; diagnostic, with collection of specimen(s) by brushing and/or washing, when performed (separate procedure)
➔ *CPT Changes: An Insider's View* 2014

47553   with biopsy, single or multiple

47554   with removal of calculus/calculi
➔ *CPT Changes: An Insider's View* 2002

47555   with dilation of biliary duct stricture(s) without stent

47556   with dilation of biliary duct stricture(s) with stent

(For ERCP, see 43260-43278, 74328, 74329, 74330, 74363)

(If imaging guidance is performed, use 74363)

Laparoscopy

Surgical laparoscopy always includes diagnostic laparoscopy. To report a diagnostic laparoscopy (peritoneoscopy) (separate procedure), use 49320.

(For percutaneous cholangiography, see 47531 or 47532)

47562   Laparoscopy, surgical; cholecystectomy
➔ *CPT Changes: An Insider's View* 2000
➔ *CPT Assistant* Nov 99:23, Mar 00:9, Sep 03:3, Dec 07:12, Aug 20:14, May 21:14, Jul 23:1, Dec 23:41

47563   cholecystectomy with cholangiography
➔ *CPT Changes: An Insider's View* 2000
➔ *CPT Assistant* Nov 99:23, Mar 00:9, Dec 00:14, Dec 07:12, Mar 19:10

(For intraoperative cholangiography radiological supervision and interpretation, see 74300, 74301)

(For percutaneous cholangiography, see 47531, 47532)

47564   cholecystectomy with exploration of common duct
➔ *CPT Changes: An Insider's View* 2000
➔ *CPT Assistant* Nov 99:23, Mar 00:9

47570   cholecystoenterostomy
➔ *CPT Changes: An Insider's View* 2000
➔ *CPT Assistant* Nov 99:23, Mar 00:9

47579   Unlisted laparoscopy procedure, biliary tract
➔ *CPT Changes: An Insider's View* 2000
➔ *CPT Assistant* Nov 99:23, Mar 00:9, Dec 23:41

Laparoscopic Cholecystectomy
47562

The gallbladder is dissected and removed from the liver bed under laparoscopic guidance.

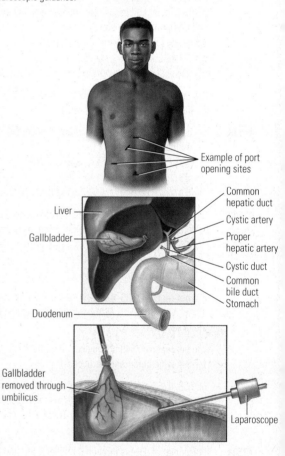

Example of port opening sites
Liver
Gallbladder
Duodenum
Common hepatic duct
Cystic artery
Proper hepatic artery
Cystic duct
Common bile duct
Stomach
Gallbladder removed through umbilicus
Laparoscope

Excision

47600   Cholecystectomy;
➔ *CPT Changes: An Insider's View* 2000
➔ *CPT Assistant* Fall 92:19, Nov 99:24

47605   with cholangiography
➔ *CPT Changes: An Insider's View* 2000
➔ *CPT Assistant* Nov 99:24, Apr 02:19

(For laparoscopic approach, see 47562-47564)

47610   Cholecystectomy with exploration of common duct;
➔ *CPT Assistant* Apr 02:19

(For cholecystectomy with exploration of common duct with biliary endoscopy, use 47610 with 47550)

47612   with choledochoenterostomy

47620   with transduodenal sphincterotomy or sphincteroplasty, with or without cholangiography

47700   Exploration for congenital atresia of bile ducts, without repair, with or without liver biopsy, with or without cholangiography

(Do not report modifier 63 in conjunction with 47700)

47701   Portoenterostomy (eg, Kasai procedure)

(Do not report modifier 63 in conjunction with 47701)

47711   Excision of bile duct tumor, with or without primary repair of bile duct; extrahepatic

47712   intrahepatic

(For anastomosis, see 47760-47800)

47715   Excision of choledochal cyst

Repair

47720   Cholecystoenterostomy; direct
➔ *CPT Changes: An Insider's View* 2000
➔ *CPT Assistant* Nov 99:24

(For laparoscopic approach, use 47570)

47721   with gastroenterostomy

47740   Roux-en-Y

47741   Roux-en-Y with gastroenterostomy

47760   Anastomosis, of extrahepatic biliary ducts and gastrointestinal tract

47765   Anastomosis, of intrahepatic ducts and gastrointestinal tract

47780   Anastomosis, Roux-en-Y, of extrahepatic biliary ducts and gastrointestinal tract

47785   Anastomosis, Roux-en-Y, of intrahepatic biliary ducts and gastrointestinal tract

47800   Reconstruction, plastic, of extrahepatic biliary ducts with end-to-end anastomosis

47801   Placement of choledochal stent
➔ *CPT Assistant* Dec 10:13

▶(47802 has been deleted)◀

47900   Suture of extrahepatic biliary duct for pre-existing injury (separate procedure)

Other Procedures

47999   Unlisted procedure, biliary tract
➔ *CPT Assistant* May 11:9
➔ *Clinical Examples in Radiology* Spring 20:15

Pancreas

(For peroral pancreatic endoscopic procedures, see 43260-43265, 43274-43278)

Incision

48000   Placement of drains, peripancreatic, for acute pancreatitis;

48001   with cholecystostomy, gastrostomy, and jejunostomy

48020   Removal of pancreatic calculus
➔ *CPT Assistant* Spring 91:7

Excision

48100   Biopsy of pancreas, open (eg, fine needle aspiration, needle core biopsy, wedge biopsy)
➔ *CPT Changes: An Insider's View* 2002

48102   Biopsy of pancreas, percutaneous needle
➔ *Clinical Examples in Radiology* Winter 17:5

(For radiological supervision and interpretation, see 76942, 77002, 77012, 77021)

(For fine needle aspiration biopsy, see 10005, 10006, 10007, 10008, 10009, 10010, 10011, 10012)

(For evaluation of fine needle aspirate, see 88172, 88173)

48105   Resection or debridement of pancreas and peripancreatic tissue for acute necrotizing pancreatitis
➔ *CPT Changes: An Insider's View* 2007

48120   Excision of lesion of pancreas (eg, cyst, adenoma)

48140   Pancreatectomy, distal subtotal, with or without splenectomy; without pancreaticojejunostomy
➔ *CPT Assistant* Jul 17:10

48145   with pancreaticojejunostomy

48146   Pancreatectomy, distal, near-total with preservation of duodenum (Child-type procedure)

48148   Excision of ampulla of Vater

48150 Pancreatectomy, proximal subtotal with total duodenectomy, partial gastrectomy, choledochoenterostomy and gastrojejunostomy (Whipple-type procedure); with pancreatojejunostomy
> *CPT Assistant* Dec 15:18

48152 without pancreatojejunostomy

48153 Pancreatectomy, proximal subtotal with near-total duodenectomy, choledochoenterostomy and duodenojejunostomy (pylorus-sparing, Whipple-type procedure); with pancreatojejunostomy

48154 without pancreatojejunostomy

48155 Pancreatectomy, total

48160 Pancreatectomy, total or subtotal, with autologous transplantation of pancreas or pancreatic islet cells
> *CPT Changes: An Insider's View* 2002
> *CPT Assistant* Aug 23:20

(To report pancreatic islet cell transplantation via portal vein catheterization and infusion, see 0584T, 0585T, 0586T)

Introduction

+ 48400 Injection procedure for intraoperative pancreatography (List separately in addition to code for primary procedure)
> *CPT Assistant* Dec 07:12

(For radiological supervision and interpretation, see 74300, 74301)

(For intraoperative pancreatography radiological supervision and interpretation, see 74300, 74301)

Repair

48500 Marsupialization of pancreatic cyst
> *CPT Changes: An Insider's View* 2002

48510 External drainage, pseudocyst of pancreas, open
> *CPT Assistant* Nov 97:18

(For percutaneous image-guided fluid collection drainage by catheter of pancreatic pseudocyst, use 49405)

48520 Internal anastomosis of pancreatic cyst to gastrointestinal tract; direct

48540 Roux-en-Y

48545 Pancreatorrhaphy for injury
> *CPT Changes: An Insider's View* 2002

48547 Duodenal exclusion with gastrojejunostomy for pancreatic injury
> *CPT Changes: An Insider's View* 2002

48548 Pancreaticojejunostomy, side-to-side anastomosis (Puestow-type operation)
> *CPT Changes: An Insider's View* 2007

Pancreas Transplantation

Pancreas allotransplantation involves three distinct components of physician work:

1. **Cadaver donor pancreatectomy,** which includes harvesting the pancreas graft, with or without duodenal segment, and cold preservation of the graft (perfusing with cold preservation solution and cold maintenance) (use 48550).

2. **Backbench work:**

   Standard preparation of a cadaver donor pancreas allograft prior to transplantation includes dissection of the allograft from surrounding soft tissues, splenectomy, duodenotomy, ligation of bile duct, ligation of mesenteric vessels, and Y-graft arterial anastomoses from the iliac artery to the superior mesenteric artery and to the splenic artery (use 48551).

   Additional reconstruction of a cadaver donor pancreas allograft prior to transplantation may include venous anastomosis(es) (use 48552).

3. **Recipient pancreas allotransplantation,** which includes transplantation of allograft, and care of the recipient (use 48554).

48550 Donor pancreatectomy (including cold preservation), with or without duodenal segment for transplantation
> *CPT Changes: An Insider's View* 2005
> *CPT Assistant* Apr 05:10, 12

48551 Backbench standard preparation of cadaver donor pancreas allograft prior to transplantation, including dissection of allograft from surrounding soft tissues, splenectomy, duodenotomy, ligation of bile duct, ligation of mesenteric vessels, and Y-graft arterial anastomoses from iliac artery to superior mesenteric artery and to splenic artery
> *CPT Changes: An Insider's View* 2005

48552 Backbench reconstruction of cadaver donor pancreas allograft prior to transplantation, venous anastomosis, each
> *CPT Changes: An Insider's View* 2005

(Do not report 48551 and 48552 in conjunction with 35531, 35563, 35685, 38100-38102, 44010, 44820, 44850, 47460, 47550-47556, 48100-48120, 48545)

48554 Transplantation of pancreatic allograft

48556 Removal of transplanted pancreatic allograft

Other Procedures

48999 Unlisted procedure, pancreas
↪ *CPT Assistant* Dec 07:12, May 11:9, Feb 13:13

Abdomen, Peritoneum, and Omentum

Incision

49000 Exploratory laparotomy, exploratory celiotomy with or without biopsy(s) (separate procedure)
↪ *CPT Assistant* Fall 92:23, Mar 01:10, Nov 08:7, Sep 12:11, Jan 20:6

(To report wound exploration due to penetrating trauma without laparotomy, use 20102)

49002 Reopening of recent laparotomy
↪ *CPT Assistant* Fall 92:23, Nov 08:7, Jan 20:6

(To report re-exploration of hepatic wound for removal of packing, use 47362)

(To report re-exploration of pelvic wound for removal, including repacking, when performed, use 49014)

49010 Exploration, retroperitoneal area with or without biopsy(s) (separate procedure)
↪ *CPT Assistant* Jan 20:6

(To report wound exploration due to penetrating trauma without laparotomy, use 20102)

49013 Preperitoneal pelvic packing for hemorrhage associated with pelvic trauma, including local exploration
↪ *CPT Changes: An Insider's View* 2020
↪ *CPT Assistant* Jan 20:6

49014 Re-exploration of pelvic wound with removal of preperitoneal pelvic packing, including repacking, when performed
↪ *CPT Changes: An Insider's View* 2020
↪ *CPT Assistant* Jan 20:6

49020 Drainage of peritoneal abscess or localized peritonitis, exclusive of appendiceal abscess, open

(For appendiceal abscess, use 44900)

(For percutaneous image-guided drainage of peritoneal abscess or localized peritonitis by catheter, use 49406)

(For transrectal or transvaginal image-guided drainage of peritoneal abscess by catheter, use 49407)

49040 Drainage of subdiaphragmatic or subphrenic abscess, open
↪ *CPT Assistant* Nov 97:18

(For percutaneous image-guided drainage of subdiaphragmatic or subphrenic abscess by catheter, use 49406)

49060 Drainage of retroperitoneal abscess, open
↪ *CPT Changes: An Insider's View* 2000
↪ *CPT Assistant* Nov 97:18, Nov 99:24, Jul 01:11, Aug 01:10

(For percutaneous image-guided drainage of retroperitoneal abscess by catheter, use 49406)

(For transrectal or transvaginal image-guided drainage of retroperitoneal abscess by catheter, use 49407)

49062 Drainage of extraperitoneal lymphocele to peritoneal cavity, open
↪ *CPT Assistant* Nov 97:19, Jul 01:11, Aug 01:10

(For laparoscopic drainage of lymphocele to peritoneal cavity, use 49323)

(For percutaneous image-guided drainage of peritoneal or retroperitoneal lymphocele by catheter, use 49406)

49082 Abdominal paracentesis (diagnostic or therapeutic); without imaging guidance
↪ *CPT Changes: An Insider's View* 2012
↪ *CPT Assistant* Dec 12:9
↪ *Clinical Examples in Radiology* Fall 11:11, Winter 12:9, Spring 12:10

49083 with imaging guidance
↪ *CPT Changes: An Insider's View* 2012
↪ *CPT Assistant* Dec 12:9, Mar 14:14, Feb 24:33
↪ *Clinical Examples in Radiology* Fall 11:11, Winter 12:9, Spring 12:10

(Do not report 49083 in conjunction with 76942, 77002, 77012, 77021)

(For percutaneous image-guided drainage of retroperitoneal abscess by catheter, use 49406)

49084 Peritoneal lavage, including imaging guidance, when performed
↪ *CPT Changes: An Insider's View* 2012
↪ *CPT Assistant* Dec 12:9
↪ *Clinical Examples in Radiology* Fall 11:11, Winter 12:9

(Do not report 49084 in conjunction with 76942, 77002, 77012, 77021)

(For percutaneous image-guided drainage of retroperitoneal abscess by catheter, use 49406)

Excision, Destruction

Code 49185 describes sclerotherapy of a fluid collection (eg, lymphocele, cyst, or seroma) through a percutaneous access. It includes contrast injection(s), sclerosant injection(s), sclerosant dwell time, diagnostic study, imaging guidance (eg, ultrasound, fluoroscopy), and radiological supervision and interpretation, when performed. Code 49185 may be reported once per day for each lesion treated through a separate catheter. Do not report 49185 more than once if treating multiple lesions through the same catheter. Codes for access to and drainage of the collection may be separately reportable according to location (eg, 10030, 10160, 49405, 49406, 49407, 50390).

▶Codes 49186, 49187, 49188, 49189, 49190 describe excision or destruction of intra-abdominal primary or secondary tumor(s) or cyst(s) via an open approach. Excision or destruction of intra-abdominal primary or secondary tumor(s) or cyst(s) via an open approach includes cytoreduction, debulking, or other methods of removal of the tumor(s) or cyst(s). Codes 49186, 49187, 49188, 49189, 49190 are reported based on the sum of the maximum length of each tumor or cyst excised or destroyed (eg, ultrasound desiccation). Only the tumor(s) and cyst(s) are measured, not the tissue (eg, mesentery) in which the tumor(s) and cyst(s) may be implanted. If only a portion of a tumor or cyst is excised or destroyed, then only the excised or destroyed portion is measured. The tumor(s) and cyst(s) should be measured in situ before excision or destruction and documented in the operative report. Measurement includes only the tumor(s) and cyst(s) and not the margins. Codes 49186, 49187, 49188, 49189, 49190 are reported when the resected or destroyed intra-abdominal tumor(s) and cyst(s) do not directly arise from a resected organ (eg, small bowel mass, renal mass, liver mass) or soft tissue that may be separately reportable. When the tumors arise directly from an organ or soft tissue, only the organ or soft tissue resection or destruction procedure code from which the tumors arise is reported. For example, if a partial ascending colon resection, including small tumor implants, is performed and a separate excision of multiple small tumor implants in the mesentery of the descending colon is also performed, the appropriate colectomy code (eg, 44140) would be reported for the partial ascending colon resection and the excision of the tumor implants in the mesentery of the descending colon would be separately reported with an appropriate tumor excision code (49186, 49187, 49188, 49189, 49190). The implants that were part of the ascending colon resection would not be included in the measurement for reporting the tumor excision code (49186, 49187, 49188, 49189, 49190).

Open resection of recurrent ovarian, endometrial, tubal, or primary peritoneal gynecological malignancies without lymphadenectomy should be reported with 49186, 49187, 49188, 49189, 49190. All other open resection of initial or recurrent ovarian, endometrial, tubal, or primary peritoneal gynecologic malignancies should be reported with 58943, 58950, 58951, 58952, 58953, 58954, 58956, 58958, 58960.◀

(For lysis of intestinal adhesions, use 44005)

49180 Biopsy, abdominal or retroperitoneal mass, percutaneous needle

➔ *CPT Assistant* Fall 93:11

➔ *Clinical Examples in Radiology* Fall 10:7, Winter 17:5, Summer 23:26, Fall 23:26

(If imaging guidance is performed, see 76942, 77002, 77012, 77021)

(For fine needle aspiration biopsy, see 10004, 10005, 10006, 10007, 10008, 10009, 10010, 10011, 10012, 10021)

(For evaluation of fine needle aspirate, see 88172, 88173)

49185 Sclerotherapy of a fluid collection (eg, lymphocele, cyst, or seroma), percutaneous, including contrast injection(s), sclerosant injection(s), diagnostic study, imaging guidance (eg, ultrasound, fluoroscopy) and radiological supervision and interpretation when performed

➔ *CPT Changes: An Insider's View* 2016

➔ *CPT Assistant* Mar 16:10

(Do not report 49185 in conjunction with 49424, 76080)

(For access/drainage with catheter, see 10030, 49405, 49406, 49407, 50390)

(For access/drainage with needle, see 10160, 50390)

(For pleurodesis, use 32560)

(For sclerosis of veins or endovenous ablation of incompetent extremity veins, see 36468, 36470, 36471, 36475, 36476, 36478, 36479)

(For sclerotherapy of a lymphatic/vascular malformation, use 37241)

(For treatment of multiple interconnected lesions treated through a single access, report 49185 once)

(For exchange of existing catheter, before or after injection of sclerosant, see 49423, 75984)

(For treatment of multiple lesions in a single day requiring separate access, use modifier 59 for each additional treated lesion)

● **49186** Excision or destruction, open, intra-abdominal (ie, peritoneal, mesenteric, retroperitoneal), primary or secondary tumor(s) or cyst(s), sum of the maximum length of tumor(s) or cyst(s); 5 cm or less

➔ *CPT Changes: An Insider's View* 2025

● **49187** 5.1 to 10 cm

➔ *CPT Changes: An Insider's View* 2025

● **49188** 10.1 to 20 cm

➔ *CPT Changes: An Insider's View* 2025

● **49189** 20.1 to 30 cm

➔ *CPT Changes: An Insider's View* 2025

● **49190** greater than 30 cm

➔ *CPT Changes: An Insider's View* 2025

▶(Do not report 49186, 49187, 49188, 49189, 49190 in conjunction with 49000, 49010, 49215, 58943, 58950, 58951, 58952, 58953, 58954, 58956, 58958, 58960)◀

★ = Telemedicine ◀ = Audio-only ✛ = Add-on code ✗ = FDA approval pending # = Resequenced code ⊘ = Modifier 51 exempt ➔➔➔ = See p xxi for details

►(For excision of perinephric cyst, use 50290)◄

►(49203, 49204, 49205 have been deleted. For open excision or destruction of intra-abdominal [ie, peritoneal, mesenteric, retroperitoneal] primary or secondary tumor[s] or cyst[s], see 49186, 49187, 49188, 49189, 49190)◄

►(For excision or destruction of endometriomas, open method, use 58999)◄

49215 Excision of presacral or sacrococcygeal tumor

(Do not report modifier 63 in conjunction with 49215)

49250 Umbilectomy, omphalectomy, excision of umbilicus (separate procedure)

49255 Omentectomy, epiploectomy, resection of omentum (separate procedure)

➲ *CPT Changes: An Insider's View* 2000

➲ *CPT Assistant* Nov 99:24, Mar 18:11

Laparoscopy

Surgical laparoscopy always includes diagnostic laparoscopy. To report a diagnostic laparoscopy (peritoneoscopy), (separate procedure), use 49320.

For laparoscopic fulguration or excision of lesions of the ovary, pelvic viscera, or peritoneal surface use 58662.

49320 Laparoscopy, abdomen, peritoneum, and omentum, diagnostic, with or without collection of specimen(s) by brushing or washing (separate procedure)

➲ *CPT Changes: An Insider's View* 2000, 2001

➲ *CPT Assistant* Nov 99:24, Mar 00:9, Apr 06:19, Mar 07:4, Nov 07:1, Dec 08:7, Jun 10:7, Dec 15:18, Apr 17:7

Laparoscopy
49320

The physician inserts a fiberoptic laparoscope to observe the necessary organs in these procedures.

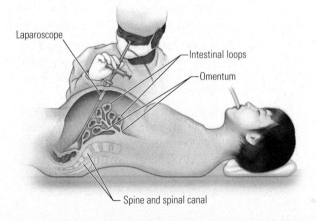

Laparoscope
Intestinal loops
Omentum
Spine and spinal canal

49321 Laparoscopy, surgical; with biopsy (single or multiple)

➲ *CPT Changes: An Insider's View* 2000, 2001

➲ *CPT Assistant* Nov 99:24, Mar 00:9, Aug 18:10

49322 with aspiration of cavity or cyst (eg, ovarian cyst) (single or multiple)

➲ *CPT Changes: An Insider's View* 2000

➲ *CPT Assistant* Nov 99:24, Mar 00:9, Jul 23:17

49323 with drainage of lymphocele to peritoneal cavity

➲ *CPT Changes: An Insider's View* 2000

➲ *CPT Assistant* Nov 99:24, Mar 00:9, May 00:4, Jul 01:11, Aug 01:10

(For open drainage of lymphocele to peritoneal cavity, use 49062)

49324 with insertion of tunneled intraperitoneal catheter

➲ *CPT Changes: An Insider's View* 2007, 2011

(For subcutaneous extension of intraperitoneal catheter with remote chest exit site, use 49435 in conjunction with 49324)

(For open insertion of tunneled intraperitoneal catheter, use 49421)

49325 with revision of previously placed intraperitoneal cannula or catheter, with removal of intraluminal obstructive material if performed

➲ *CPT Changes: An Insider's View* 2007

+ 49326 with omentopexy (omental tacking procedure) (List separately in addition to code for primary procedure)

➲ *CPT Changes: An Insider's View* 2007

(Use 49326 in conjunction with 49324, 49325)

+ 49327 with placement of interstitial device(s) for radiation therapy guidance (eg, fiducial markers, dosimeter), intra-abdominal, intrapelvic, and/or retroperitoneum, including imaging guidance, if performed, single or multiple (List separately in addition to code for primary procedure)

➲ *CPT Changes: An Insider's View* 2011

(Use 49327 in conjunction with laparoscopic abdominal, pelvic, or retroperitoneal procedure[s] performed concurrently)

(For placement of interstitial device[s] for intra-abdominal, intrapelvic, and/or retroperitoneal radiation therapy guidance concurrent with open procedure, use 49412)

(For percutaneous placement of interstitial device[s] for intra-abdominal, intrapelvic, and/or retroperitoneal radiation therapy guidance, use 49411)

49329 Unlisted laparoscopy procedure, abdomen, peritoneum and omentum

➲ *CPT Changes: An Insider's View* 2000

➲ *CPT Assistant* Nov 99:24, Mar 00:9, Feb 06:16, Dec 11:16, Oct 13:18, Mar 19:10, Feb 20:13

Introduction, Revision, Removal

49400   Injection of air or contrast into peritoneal cavity (separate procedure)

→ *CPT Assistant* Dec 10:13

→ *Clinical Examples in Radiology* Fall 07:1-2

(For radiological supervision and interpretation, use 74190)

49402   Removal of peritoneal foreign body from peritoneal cavity

→ *CPT Changes: An Insider's View* 2007

(For lysis of intestinal adhesions, use 44005)

(For open or percutaneous peritoneal drainage or lavage, see 49406, 49020, 49040, 49082-49084, as appropriate)

(For percutaneous insertion of a tunneled intraperitoneal catheter without subcutaneous port, use 49418)

49405   Image-guided fluid collection drainage by catheter (eg, abscess, hematoma, seroma, lymphocele, cyst); visceral (eg, kidney, liver, spleen, lung/mediastinum), percutaneous

→ *CPT Changes: An Insider's View* 2014, 2017

→ *CPT Assistant* May 14:9, Feb 20:13

→ *Clinical Examples in Radiology* Fall 13:6, Spring 15:8, Winter 16:10, Fall 18:15

(Do not report 49405 in conjunction with 75989, 76942, 77002, 77003, 77012, 77021)

(For percutaneous cholecystostomy, use 47490)

(For pneumonostomy, use 32200)

(For thoracentesis, see 32554, 32555)

(For percutaneous pleural drainage, see 32556, 32557)

(For open visceral drainage, see 32200 [lung abscess or cyst], 47010 [liver abscess or cyst], 48510 [pseudocyst of pancreas], 50020 [perirenal or renal abscess])

49406   peritoneal or retroperitoneal, percutaneous

→ *CPT Changes: An Insider's View* 2014, 2017

→ *CPT Assistant* May 14:9, Feb 20:13, Mar 24:26

→ *Clinical Examples in Radiology* Fall 13:6, Spring 15:8, Winter 16:10, Fall 18:15

(Do not report 49406 in conjunction with 75989, 76942, 77002, 77003, 77012, 77021)

(For abdominal paracentesis [diagnostic or therapeutic], see 49082, 49083)

(For transrectal or transvaginal image-guided peritoneal or retroperitoneal fluid collection drainage by catheter, use 49407)

(For open transrectal drainage of pelvic abscess, use 45000)

(For open peritoneal or retroperitoneal drainage, see 44900 [appendiceal abscess], 49020 [peritoneal abscess or localized peritonitis], 49040 [subdiaphragmatic or subphrenic abscess], 49060 [retroperitoneal abscess], 49062 [extraperitoneal lymphocele], 49084 [peritoneal lavage], 50020 [perirenal or renal abscess], 58805 [ovarian cyst], 58822 [ovarian abscess])

(For percutaneous paracentesis, see 49082, 49083)

(For percutaneous insertion of a tunneled intraperitoneal catheter without subcutaneous port, use 49418)

49407   peritoneal or retroperitoneal, transvaginal or transrectal

→ *CPT Changes: An Insider's View* 2014, 2017

→ *CPT Assistant* May 14:9

→ *Clinical Examples in Radiology* Fall 13:6, Spring 15:8, Winter 16:10, Fall 18:15

(Do not report 49407 in conjunction with 75989, 76942, 77002, 77003, 77012, 77021)

(Report 49405, 49406, 49407 separately for each individual collection drained with a separate catheter)

(For open transrectal or transvaginal drainage, see 45000 [pelvic abscess], 58800 [ovarian cyst], 58820 [ovarian abscess])

(For percutaneous image-guided fluid collection drainage by catheter [eg, abscess, hematoma, seroma, lymphocele, cyst] for soft tissue [eg, extremity, abdominal wall, neck], use 10030)

49411   Placement of interstitial device(s) for radiation therapy guidance (eg, fiducial markers, dosimeter), percutaneous, intra-abdominal, intra-pelvic (except prostate), and/or retroperitoneum, single or multiple

→ *CPT Changes: An Insider's View* 2010, 2017

→ *CPT Assistant* Feb 10:7, Jun 16:3

(Report supply of device separately)

(For imaging guidance, see 76942, 77002, 77012, 77021)

(For percutaneous placement of interstitial device[s] for intra-thoracic radiation therapy guidance, use 32553)

+ 49412   Placement of interstitial device(s) for radiation therapy guidance (eg, fiducial markers, dosimeter), open, intra-abdominal, intrapelvic, and/or retroperitoneum, including image guidance, if performed, single or multiple (List separately in addition to code for primary procedure)

→ *CPT Changes: An Insider's View* 2011

(Use 49412 in conjunction with open abdominal, pelvic, or retroperitoneal procedure[s] performed concurrently)

(For placement of interstitial device[s] for intra-abdominal, intrapelvic, and/or retroperitoneal radiation therapy guidance concurrent with laparoscopic procedure, use 49327)

(For percutaneous placement of interstitial device[s] for intra-abdominal, intrapelvic, and/or retroperitoneal radiation therapy guidance, use 49411)

49418   Insertion of tunneled intraperitoneal catheter (eg, dialysis, intraperitoneal chemotherapy instillation, management of ascites), complete procedure, including imaging guidance, catheter placement, contrast injection when performed, and radiological supervision and interpretation, percutaneous

➔ *CPT Changes: An Insider's View* 2011, 2017

49419   Insertion of tunneled intraperitoneal catheter, with subcutaneous port (ie, totally implantable)

➔ *CPT Changes: An Insider's View* 2003, 2011

(For removal, use 49422)

49421   Insertion of tunneled intraperitoneal catheter for dialysis, open

➔ *CPT Changes: An Insider's View* 2011

➔ *CPT Assistant* Fall 93:2, Jul 06:19

(For laparoscopic insertion of tunneled intraperitoneal catheter, use 49324)

(For subcutaneous extension of intraperitoneal catheter with remote chest exit site, use 49435 in conjunction with 49421)

49422   Removal of tunneled intraperitoneal catheter

➔ *CPT Changes: An Insider's View* 2011

(For removal of a non-tunneled catheter, use appropriate E/M code)

49423   Exchange of previously placed abscess or cyst drainage catheter under radiological guidance (separate procedure)

➔ *CPT Assistant* Nov 97:19, Mar 98:8

➔ *Clinical Examples in Radiology* Summer 13:6

(For radiological supervision and interpretation, use 75984)

49424   Contrast injection for assessment of abscess or cyst via previously placed drainage catheter or tube (separate procedure)

➔ *CPT Changes: An Insider's View* 2002

➔ *CPT Assistant* Nov 97:19, Mar 98:8, Nov 03:14

➔ *Clinical Examples in Radiology* Fall 09:9

(For radiological supervision and interpretation, use 76080)

49425   Insertion of peritoneal-venous shunt

49426   Revision of peritoneal-venous shunt

(For shunt patency test, use 78291)

49427   Injection procedure (eg, contrast media) for evaluation of previously placed peritoneal-venous shunt

(For radiological supervision and interpretation, see 75809, 78291)

49428   Ligation of peritoneal-venous shunt

49429   Removal of peritoneal-venous shunt

+ 49435   Insertion of subcutaneous extension to intraperitoneal cannula or catheter with remote chest exit site (List separately in addition to code for primary procedure)

➔ *CPT Changes: An Insider's View* 2007

(Use 49435 in conjunction with 49324, 49421)

49436   Delayed creation of exit site from embedded subcutaneous segment of intraperitoneal cannula or catheter

➔ *CPT Changes: An Insider's View* 2007

Initial Placement

Do not additionally report 43752 for placement of a nasogastric (NG) or orogastric (OG) tube to insufflate the stomach prior to percutaneous gastrointestinal tube placement. NG or OG tube placement is considered part of the procedure in this family of codes.

49440   Insertion of gastrostomy tube, percutaneous, under fluoroscopic guidance including contrast injection(s), image documentation and report

➔ *CPT Changes: An Insider's View* 2008, 2017

➔ *CPT Assistant* Jan 08:8, Jun 08:8, Aug 08:7, Sep 10:9, Sep 14:5, Dec 14:18, Oct 21:14, Oct 21:5

➔ *Clinical Examples in Radiology* Spring 20:6, Summer 22:15

(For conversion to a gastro-jejunostomy tube at the time of initial gastrostomy tube placement, use 49440 in conjunction with 49446)

49441   Insertion of duodenostomy or jejunostomy tube, percutaneous, under fluoroscopic guidance including contrast injection(s), image documentation and report

➔ *CPT Changes: An Insider's View* 2008, 2017

➔ *CPT Assistant* Jan 08:8, Jun 08:8, Aug 08:7, Dec 14:18

(For conversion of gastrostomy tube to gastro-jejunostomy tube, use 49446)

49442   Insertion of cecostomy or other colonic tube, percutaneous, under fluoroscopic guidance including contrast injection(s), image documentation and report

➔ *CPT Changes: An Insider's View* 2008, 2017

➔ *CPT Assistant* Jan 08:8, Jun 08:8, Aug 08:7, Dec 14:18

Conversion

49446   Conversion of gastrostomy tube to gastro-jejunostomy tube, percutaneous, under fluoroscopic guidance including contrast injection(s), image documentation and report

➔ *CPT Changes: An Insider's View* 2008, 2017

➔ *CPT Assistant* Oct 21:5

(For conversion to a gastro-jejunostomy tube at the time of initial gastrostomy tube placement, use 49446 in conjunction with 49440)

Replacement

If an existing gastrostomy, duodenostomy, jejunostomy, gastro-jejunostomy, or cecostomy (or other colonic) tube is removed and a new tube is placed via a separate percutaneous access site, the placement of the new tube is not considered a replacement and would be reported using the appropriate initial placement codes 49440-49442.

49450　Replacement of gastrostomy or cecostomy (or other colonic) tube, percutaneous, under fluoroscopic guidance including contrast injection(s), image documentation and report

➲ *CPT Changes: An Insider's View* 2008

➲ *CPT Assistant* Sep 10:9, Dec 13:17, Feb 19:5

➲ *Clinical Examples in Radiology* Winter 19:12, Summer 22:15

(For percutaneous replacement of gastrostomy tube with removal when performed without imaging or endoscopy, see 43762, 43763)

49451　Replacement of duodenostomy or jejunostomy tube, percutaneous, under fluoroscopic guidance including contrast injection(s), image documentation and report

➲ *CPT Changes: An Insider's View* 2008

➲ *CPT Assistant* Jan 08:8, Jun 08:8, Aug 08:7, Jul 10:10, Dec 14:18

49452　Replacement of gastro-jejunostomy tube, percutaneous, under fluoroscopic guidance including contrast injection(s), image documentation and report

➲ *CPT Changes: An Insider's View* 2008

➲ *CPT Assistant* Mar 10:10, Oct 21:6

Mechanical Removal of Obstructive Material

49460　Mechanical removal of obstructive material from gastrostomy, duodenostomy, jejunostomy, gastro-jejunostomy, or cecostomy (or other colonic) tube, any method, under fluoroscopic guidance including contrast injection(s), if performed, image documentation and report

➲ *CPT Changes: An Insider's View* 2008

(Do not report 49460 in conjunction with 49450-49452, 49465)

Other

49465　Contrast injection(s) for radiological evaluation of existing gastrostomy, duodenostomy, jejunostomy, gastro-jejunostomy, or cecostomy (or other colonic) tube, from a percutaneous approach including image documentation and report

➲ *CPT Changes: An Insider's View* 2008

➲ *CPT Assistant* Sep 14:5

(Do not report 49465 in conjunction with 49450-49460)

Repair

Hernioplasty, Herniorrhaphy, Herniotomy

The hernia repair codes in this section are categorized primarily by the type of hernia (inguinal, femoral, lumbar, omphalocele, anterior abdominal, parastomal).

Some types of hernias are further categorized as "initial" or "recurrent" based on whether or not the hernia has required previous repair(s).

Additional variables accounted for by some of the codes include patient age and clinical presentation (reducible vs. incarcerated or strangulated).

The excision/repair of strangulated organs or structures such as testicle(s), intestine, ovaries are reported by using the appropriate code for the excision/repair (eg, 44120, 54520, and 58940) in addition to the appropriate code for the repair of the strangulated hernia.

(For debridement of abdominal wall, see 11042, 11043)

(For reduction and repair of intra-abdominal hernia, use 44050)

(49491-49557, 49600, 49605, 49606, 49610, 49611, 49650, 49651 are unilateral procedures. For bilateral procedure, use modifier 50)

(Do not report modifier 50 in conjunction with 49591-49622)

49491　Repair, initial inguinal hernia, preterm infant (younger than 37 weeks gestation at birth), performed from birth up to 50 weeks postconception age, with or without hydrocelectomy; reducible

➲ *CPT Changes: An Insider's View* 2002

➲ *CPT Assistant* Mar 04:2, Jun 08:3, Sep 23:1

49492　incarcerated or strangulated

➲ *CPT Changes: An Insider's View* 2002

➲ *CPT Assistant* Mar 04:2, Jun 08:3, Sep 23:1

(Do not report modifier 63 in conjunction with 49491, 49492)

(Postconception age equals gestational age at birth plus age of infant in weeks at the time of the hernia repair. Initial inguinal hernia repairs that are performed on preterm infants who are older than 50 weeks postconception age and younger than age 6 months at the time of surgery, should be reported using codes 49495, 49496)

Digestive 40490-49999

49495   Repair, initial inguinal hernia, full term infant younger than age 6 months, or preterm infant older than 50 weeks postconception age and younger than age 6 months at the time of surgery, with or without hydrocelectomy; reducible

➔ *CPT Changes: An Insider's View* 2002

➔ *CPT Assistant* Winter 93:6, Winter 94:13, Jan 04:27, Mar 04:10, May 04:14, Nov 07:9, Jun 08:3, Sep 23:1

➔ *Clinical Examples in Radiology* Fall 18:15

49496   incarcerated or strangulated

➔ *CPT Assistant* Winter 93:6, Winter 94:13, Jan 04:27, Mar 04:10, May 04:14, Jun 08:3, Sep 23:1

(Do not report modifier 63 in conjunction with 49495, 49496)

(Postconception age equals gestational age at birth plus age in weeks at the time of the hernia repair. Initial inguinal hernia repairs that are performed on preterm infants who are younger than or up to 50 weeks postconception age but younger than 6 months of age since birth, should be reported using codes 49491, 49492. Inguinal hernia repairs on infants age 6 months to younger than 5 years should be reported using codes 49500-49501)

49500   Repair initial inguinal hernia, age 6 months to younger than 5 years, with or without hydrocelectomy; reducible

➔ *CPT Changes: An Insider's View* 2002

➔ *CPT Assistant* Winter 94:13, Jan 04:27, Mar 04:10, Nov 07:9, Jun 08:3, Nov 14:14, Sep 23:1

49501   incarcerated or strangulated

➔ *CPT Changes: An Insider's View* 2002

➔ *CPT Assistant* Winter 94:13, Jan 04:27, Mar 04:12, Jun 08:3, Sep 23:1

49505   Repair initial inguinal hernia, age 5 years or older; reducible

➔ *CPT Assistant* Winter 94:13, Sep 00:10, Jan 04:27, Mar 04:12, Jun 08:3, Sep 23:1

49507   incarcerated or strangulated

➔ *CPT Assistant* Winter 94:13, Jan 04:27, Mar 04:10, Jun 08:3, Sep 23:1

(For inguinal hernia repair, with simple orchiectomy, see 49505 or 49507 and 54520)

(For inguinal hernia repair, with excision of hydrocele or spermatocele, see 49505 or 49507 and 54840 or 55040)

49520   Repair recurrent inguinal hernia, any age; reducible

➔ *CPT Assistant* Winter 94:13, Sep 03:3, Jan 04:27, Mar 04:3, Jun 08:3, Sep 23:1

49521   incarcerated or strangulated

➔ *CPT Assistant* Winter 94:13, Jan 04:27, Mar 04:10, Jun 08:3, Sep 23:1

49525   Repair inguinal hernia, sliding, any age

➔ *CPT Assistant* Winter 94:14, Jan 04:27, Mar 04:10, Nov 07:9, Jun 08:3, Sep 23:1

(For incarcerated or strangulated inguinal hernia repair, see 49496, 49501, 49507, 49521)

49540   Repair lumbar hernia

➔ *CPT Assistant* Winter 94:14, Jun 08:3, Sep 23:1

49550   Repair initial femoral hernia, any age; reducible

➔ *CPT Assistant* Winter 94:14, Jun 08:3, Sep 23:1

49553   incarcerated or strangulated

➔ *CPT Assistant* Winter 94:14, Jun 08:3, Sep 23:1

49555   Repair recurrent femoral hernia; reducible

➔ *CPT Assistant* Winter 94:14, Jun 08:3, Sep 23:1

49557   incarcerated or strangulated

➔ *CPT Assistant* Winter 94:14, Jun 08:3, Sep 23:1

(49560, 49561 have been deleted. For repair of initial incisional or ventral hernia, see 49591, 49592, 49593, 49594, 49595, 49596)

(49565, 49566 have been deleted. For repair of recurrent incisional or ventral hernia, see 49613, 49614, 49615, 49616, 49617, 49618)

(49568 has been deleted. For implantation of mesh or other prosthesis for anterior abdominal hernia repair, see 49591-49618)

(49570, 49572 have been deleted. For epigastric hernia repair, see 49591-49618)

(49580, 49582 have been deleted. For umbilical hernia repair, younger than age 5 years, see 49591-49618)

(49585, 49587 have been deleted. For umbilical hernia repair, age 5 years and older, see 49591-49618)

(49590 has been deleted. For spigelian hernia repair, see 49591-49618)

Codes 49591-49618 describe repair of an anterior abdominal hernia(s) (ie, epigastric, incisional, ventral, umbilical, spigelian) by any approach (ie, open, laparoscopic, robotic). Codes 49591-49618 are reported only once, based on the total defect size for one or more anterior abdominal hernia(s), measured as the maximal craniocaudal or transverse distance between the outer margins of all defects repaired. For example, "Swiss cheese" defects (ie, multiple separate defects) would be measured from the superior most aspect of the upper defect to the inferior most aspect of the lowest defect. In addition, the hernia defect size should be measured prior to opening the hernia defect(s) (ie, during repair the fascia will typically retract creating a falsely elevated measurement).

When both reducible and incarcerated or strangulated anterior abdominal hernias are repaired at the same operative session, all hernias are reported as incarcerated or strangulated. For example, one 2-cm reducible initial incisional hernia and one 4-cm incarcerated initial incisional hernia separated by 2 cm would be reported as an initial incarcerated hernia repair with a maximum craniocaudal distance of 8 cm (49594).

Inguinal, femoral, lumbar, omphalocele, and/or parastomal hernia repair may be separately reported when performed at the same operative session as anterior abdominal hernia repair by appending modifier 59, as appropriate.

Codes 49621, 49622 describe repair of a parastomal hernia (initial or recurrent) by any approach (ie, open, laparoscopic, robotic). Code 49621 is reported for repair of a reducible parastomal hernia, and code 49622 is reported for an incarcerated or strangulated parastomal hernia.

Implantation of mesh or other prosthesis, when performed, is included in 49591-49622 and may not be separately reported. For total or near total removal of non-infected mesh when performed, use 49623 in conjunction with 49591-49622. For removal of infected mesh, use 11008.

49591 Repair of anterior abdominal hernia(s) (ie, epigastric, incisional, ventral, umbilical, spigelian), any approach (ie, open, laparoscopic, robotic), initial, including implantation of mesh or other prosthesis when performed, total length of defect(s); less than 3 cm, reducible
➔ *CPT Changes: An Insider's View* 2023
➔ *CPT Assistant* Apr 23:26, Sep 23:1

49592 less than 3 cm, incarcerated or strangulated
➔ *CPT Changes: An Insider's View* 2023
➔ *CPT Assistant* Sep 23:1

49593 3 cm to 10 cm, reducible
➔ *CPT Changes: An Insider's View* 2023
➔ *CPT Assistant* Apr 23:26, Sep 23:1

49594 3 cm to 10 cm, incarcerated or strangulated
➔ *CPT Changes: An Insider's View* 2023
➔ *CPT Assistant* Sep 23:1, Oct 23:22

49595 greater than 10 cm, reducible
➔ *CPT Changes: An Insider's View* 2023
➔ *CPT Assistant* Sep 23:1

49596 greater than 10 cm, incarcerated or strangulated
➔ *CPT Changes: An Insider's View* 2023
➔ *CPT Assistant* Sep 23:1, Oct 23:22

 # 49613 Repair of anterior abdominal hernia(s) (ie, epigastric, incisional, ventral, umbilical, spigelian), any approach (ie, open, laparoscopic, robotic), recurrent, including implantation of mesh or other prosthesis when performed, total length of defect(s); less than 3 cm, reducible
➔ *CPT Changes: An Insider's View* 2023
➔ *CPT Assistant* Sep 23:1

 # 49614 less than 3 cm, incarcerated or strangulated
➔ *CPT Changes: An Insider's View* 2023
➔ *CPT Assistant* Sep 23:1

 # 49615 3 cm to 10 cm, reducible
➔ *CPT Changes: An Insider's View* 2023
➔ *CPT Assistant* Sep 23:1

 # 49616 3 cm to 10 cm, incarcerated or strangulated
➔ *CPT Changes: An Insider's View* 2023
➔ *CPT Assistant* Sep 23:1

 # 49617 greater than 10 cm, reducible
➔ *CPT Changes: An Insider's View* 2023
➔ *CPT Assistant* Sep 23:1

 # 49618 greater than 10 cm, incarcerated or strangulated
➔ *CPT Changes: An Insider's View* 2023
➔ *CPT Assistant* Apr 23:26, Sep 23:1, Oct 23:22

 # 49621 Repair of parastomal hernia, any approach (ie, open, laparoscopic, robotic), initial or recurrent, including implantation of mesh or other prosthesis, when performed; reducible
➔ *CPT Changes: An Insider's View* 2023
➔ *CPT Assistant* Apr 23:26, Sep 23:1

 # 49622 incarcerated or strangulated
➔ *CPT Changes: An Insider's View* 2023
➔ *CPT Assistant* Apr 23:26, Sep 23:1

#+ 49623 Removal of total or near total non-infected mesh or other prosthesis at the time of initial or recurrent anterior abdominal hernia repair or parastomal hernia repair, any approach (ie, open, laparoscopic, robotic) (List separately in addition to code for primary procedure)
➔ *CPT Changes: An Insider's View* 2023
➔ *CPT Assistant* Sep 23:1

(Use 49623 in conjunction with 49591-49622)

(For removal of infected mesh, use 11008)

49600 Repair of small omphalocele, with primary closure
➔ *CPT Assistant* Winter 94:15, Sep 23:1

(Do not report modifier 63 in conjunction with 49600)

49605 Repair of large omphalocele or gastroschisis; with or without prosthesis
➔ *CPT Assistant* Winter 94:15, Sep 23:1

49606 with removal of prosthesis, final reduction and closure, in operating room
➔ *CPT Assistant* Winter 94:15, Sep 23:1

(Do not report modifier 63 in conjunction with 49605, 49606)

Measuring Total Length of Anterior Abdominal Hernia Defect(s)
49591-49618

Hernia measurements are performed either in the transverse or craniocaudal dimension. The total length of the defect(s) corresponds to the maximum width or height of an oval drawn to encircle the outer perimeter of all repaired defects. If the defects are not contiguous and are separated by greater than or equal to 10 cm of intact fascia, total defect size is the sum of each defect measured individually.

Codes 49591-49618 are reported only once, based on the total defect size for one or more anterior abdominal hernia(s), measured as the maximal craniocaudal or transverse distance between the outer margins of all defects repaired.

A. Single anterior abdominal hernia defect

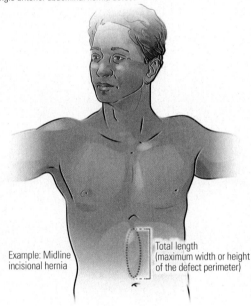

Example: Midline incisional hernia

Total length (maximum width or height of the defect perimeter)

B. Multiple anterior abdominal hernia defects

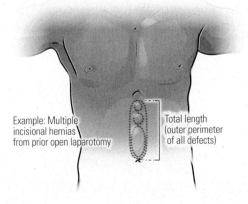

Example: Multiple incisional hernias from prior open laparotomy

Total length (outer perimeter of all defects)

C. Remote anterior abdominal hernia defects

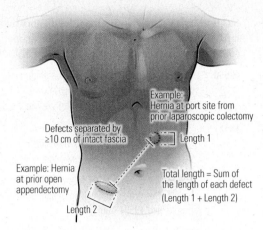

Example: Hernia at port site from prior laparoscopic colectomy

Defects separated by ≥10 cm of intact fascia

Length 1

Example: Hernia at prior open appendectomy

Length 2

Total length = Sum of the length of each defect (Length 1 + Length 2)

49610	Repair of omphalocele (Gross type operation); first stage

→ *CPT Assistant* Winter 94:15, Sep 23:1

49611	second stage

→ *CPT Assistant* Winter 94:15, Sep 23:1

(Do not report modifier 63 in conjunction with 49610, 49611)

(For diaphragmatic or hiatal hernia repair, see 39503, 43332)

(For surgical repair of omentum, use 49999)

49613	Code is out of numerical sequence. See 49595-49605
49614	Code is out of numerical sequence. See 49595-49605
49615	Code is out of numerical sequence. See 49595-49605
49616	Code is out of numerical sequence. See 49595-49605
49617	Code is out of numerical sequence. See 49595-49605
49618	Code is out of numerical sequence. See 49595-49605
49621	Code is out of numerical sequence. See 49595-49605
49622	Code is out of numerical sequence. See 49595-49605
49623	Code is out of numerical sequence. See 49595-49605

Laparoscopy

Surgical laparoscopy always includes diagnostic laparoscopy. To report a diagnostic laparoscopy (peritoneoscopy) (separate procedure), use 49320.

49650 Laparoscopy, surgical; repair initial inguinal hernia
➔ *CPT Changes: An Insider's View* 2000
➔ *CPT Assistant* Nov 99:24, Mar 00:9, Jul 14:5, Sep 23:1

49651 repair recurrent inguinal hernia
➔ *CPT Changes: An Insider's View* 2000
➔ *CPT Assistant* Nov 99:24, Mar 00:9, Sep 23:1

(49652, 49653 have been deleted. To report laparoscopic repair of ventral, umbilical, spigelian, or epigastric hernia, see 49591-49618)

(49654, 49655 have been deleted. To report laparoscopic repair of incisional hernia, see 49591-49618)

(49656, 49657 have been deleted. To report laparoscopic repair of recurrent incisional hernia, see 49613, 49614, 49615, 49616, 49617, 49618)

49659 Unlisted laparoscopy procedure, hernioplasty, herniorrhaphy, herniotomy
➔ *CPT Changes: An Insider's View* 2000
➔ *CPT Assistant* Nov 99:25, Mar 00:9, Sep 01:11, Nov 05:15, Feb 06:16, Jan 09:7, Jul 14:5, Dec 14:16, Jul 17:10, Jul 23:18

Suture

49900 Suture, secondary, of abdominal wall for evisceration or dehiscence
➔ *CPT Assistant* Sep 10:7

(For suture of ruptured diaphragm, see 39540, 39541)

(For debridement of abdominal wall, see 11042, 11043)

Other Procedures

49904 Omental flap, extra-abdominal (eg, for reconstruction of sternal and chest wall defects)
➔ *CPT Changes: An Insider's View* 2003

(Code 49904 includes harvest and transfer. If a second surgeon harvests the omental flap, then the 2 surgeons should code 49904 as co-surgeons, using modifier 62)

+ 49905 Omental flap, intra-abdominal (List separately in addition to code for primary procedure)
➔ *CPT Changes: An Insider's View* 2003
➔ *CPT Assistant* Nov 00:11, Feb 20:13

(Do not report 49905 in conjunction with 44700)

49906 Free omental flap with microvascular anastomosis
➔ *CPT Assistant* Nov 96:8, Apr 97:8, Nov 98:16

(Do not report code 69990 in addition to 49906)

49999 Unlisted procedure, abdomen, peritoneum and omentum
➔ *CPT Assistant* Jul 06:19, Sep 07:10, Nov 07:9, Aug 08:7, Apr 10:10, Dec 10:13, Jun 11:13, Jan 14:9, Nov 19:14, Jun 23:27
➔ *Clinical Examples in Radiology* Fall 07:1-2

★=Telemedicine ◀=Audio-only +=Add-on code ✗=FDA approval pending #=Resequenced code ⊘=Modifier 51 exempt ➔➔➔=See p xxi for details

Surgery

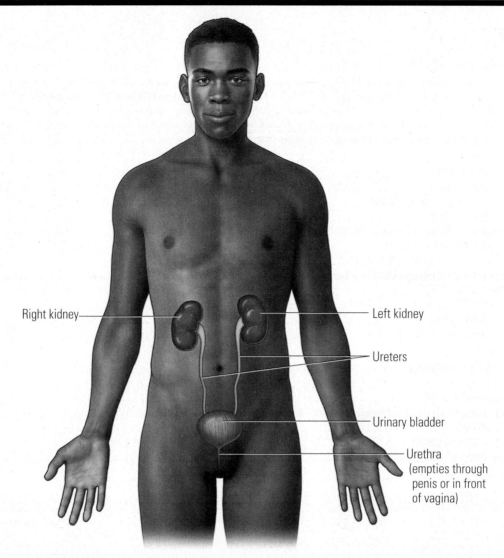

Right kidney

Left kidney

Ureters

Urinary bladder

Urethra
(empties through
penis or in front
of vagina)

Urinary System

Urinary System

(For provision of chemotherapeutic agents, report both the specific service in addition to code(s) for the specific substance(s) or drug(s) provided)

Kidney

Incision

Nephrolithotomy is the surgical removal of stones from the kidney, and pyelolithotomy is the surgical removal of stones from the renal pelvis. This section of the guidelines refers to the removal of stones from the kidney or renal pelvis using a percutaneous antegrade approach. Breaking and removing stones is separate from accessing the kidney (ie, 50040, 50432, 50433, 52334), accessing the kidney with dilation of the tract to accommodate an endoscope used in an endourologic procedure (ie, 50437), or dilation of a previously established tract to accommodate an endoscope used in an endourologic procedure (ie, 50436). These procedures include the antegrade removal of stones in the calyces, renal pelvis, and/or ureter with the antegrade placement of catheters, stents, and tubes, but do not include retrograde placement of catheters, stents, and tubes.

Code 50080 describes nephrolithotomy or pyelolithotomy using a percutaneous antegrade approach with endoscopic instruments to break and remove kidney stones of 2 cm or smaller.

Code 50081 includes the elements of 50080, but it is reported for stones larger than 2 cm, branching, stones in multiple locations, ureteral stones, or in patients with complicated anatomy.

Creation of percutaneous access or dilation of the tract to accommodate large endoscopic instruments used in stone removals (50436, 50437) is not included in 50080, 50081, and may be reported separately, if performed. Codes 50080, 50081 include placement of any stents or drainage catheters that remain indwelling after the procedure.

Report one unit of 50080 or 50081 per side (ie, per kidney), regardless of the number of stones broken and/or removed or locations of the stones. For bilateral procedure, report 50080, 50081 with modifier 50. When 50080 is performed on one side and 50081 is performed on the contralateral side, modifier 50 is not applicable. Placement of additional accesses, if needed, into the kidney, and removal of stones through other approaches (eg, open or retrograde) may be reported separately, if performed.

▶(For open retroperitoneal exploration, use 49010)◀

▶(For open drainage of retroperitoneal abscess, use 49060)◀

▶(For open excision or destruction of intra-abdominal [ie, peritoneal, mesenteric, retroperitoneal] primary or secondary tumor[s] or cyst[s], see 49186, 49187, 49188, 49189, 49190)◀

50010   Renal exploration, not necessitating other specific procedures

(For laparoscopic ablation of renal mass lesion(s), use 50542)

50020   Drainage of perirenal or renal abscess, open
➔ *CPT Assistant* Nov 97:19, Oct 01:8, May 14:9

Drainage of Renal Abscess
50020

An incision is made to the abscess cavity and the site is irrigated and drained.

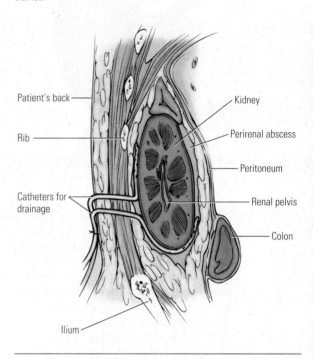

Patient's back —
Rib —
Catheters for drainage —
Ilium —
Kidney —
Perirenal abscess —
Peritoneum —
Renal pelvis —
Colon

(For percutaneous image-guided fluid collection drainage by catheter of perirenal/renal abscess, use 49405)

50040   Nephrostomy, nephrotomy with drainage
➔ *CPT Assistant* Spring 93:35, Oct 01:8

50045   Nephrotomy, with exploration
➔ *CPT Assistant* Oct 01:8

(For renal endoscopy performed in conjunction with this procedure, see 50570-50580)

50060   Nephrolithotomy; removal of calculus
➔ *CPT Assistant* Oct 01:8

50065 secondary surgical operation for calculus
➔ *CPT Assistant* Oct 01:8

50070 complicated by congenital kidney abnormality
➔ *CPT Assistant* Oct 01:8

50075 removal of large staghorn calculus filling renal pelvis and calyces (including anatrophic pyelolithotomy)
➔ *CPT Assistant* Oct 01:8

Nephrolithotomy With Calculus Removal
50060-50075

A kidney stone (calculus) is removed by an incision in the kidney. Use 50070 if complicated by a congenital kidney abnormality.

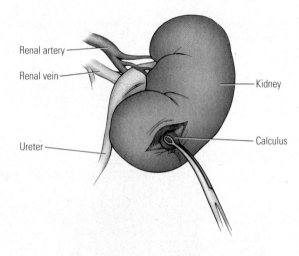

50080 Percutaneous nephrolithotomy or pyelolithotomy, lithotripsy, stone extraction, antegrade ureteroscopy, antegrade stent placement and nephrostomy tube placement, when performed, including imaging guidance; simple (eg, stone[s] up to 2 cm in single location of kidney or renal pelvis, nonbranching stones)
➔ *CPT Changes: An Insider's View* 2023
➔ *CPT Assistant* Oct 01:8, Dec 08:7, Jun 09:10, Sep 23:30

50081 complex (eg, stone[s] > 2 cm, branching stones, stones in multiple locations, ureter stones, complicated anatomy)
➔ *CPT Changes: An Insider's View* 2023
➔ *CPT Assistant* Oct 01:8, Dec 08:7, Jun 09:10, Sep 23:30

(50080, 50081 may only be reported once per side. For bilateral procedure, report 50080, 50081 with modifier 50)

(Do not report 50080, 50081 in conjunction with 50430, 50431, 50433, 50434, 50435, if performed on the same side)

(For establishment of nephrostomy without nephrolithotomy, see 50040, 50432, 50433, 52334)

(For dilation of an existing percutaneous access for an endourologic procedure, use 50436)

(For dilation of an existing percutaneous access for an endourologic procedure with new access into the collecting system, use 50437; for additional new access into the kidney, use 50437 for each new access that is dilated for an endourologic procedure)

(For removal of stone without lithotripsy, use 50561)

(For cystourethroscopy with insertion of ureteral guidewire through kidney to establish a percutaneous nephrostomy, retrograde, use 52334)

50100 Transection or repositioning of aberrant renal vessels (separate procedure)
➔ *CPT Assistant* Oct 01:8

50120 Pyelotomy; with exploration
➔ *CPT Assistant* Oct 01:8

(For renal endoscopy performed in conjunction with this procedure, see 50570-50580)

50125 with drainage, pyelostomy
➔ *CPT Assistant* Oct 01:8

50130 with removal of calculus (pyelolithotomy, pelviolithotomy, including coagulum pyelolithotomy)
➔ *CPT Assistant* Oct 01:8

▶(50135 has been deleted)◀

Excision

▶(For open excision or destruction of retroperitoneal tumor[s] or cyst[s] [other than endometriomas], see 49186, 49187, 49188, 49189, 49190)◀

(For laparoscopic ablation of renal mass lesion(s), use 50542)

▶(For excision or destruction of endometriomas, open method, use 58999)◀

50200 Renal biopsy; percutaneous, by trocar or needle
➔ *CPT Changes: An Insider's View* 2010, 2017
➔ *CPT Assistant* Fall 93:13, Oct 01:8, Feb 10:7
➔ *Clinical Examples in Radiology* Winter 17:5

(For radiological supervision and interpretation, see 76942, 77002, 77012, 77021)

(For fine needle aspiration biopsy, see 10005, 10006, 10007, 10008, 10009, 10010, 10011, 10012)

(For evaluation of fine needle aspirate, see 88172, 88173)

50205 by surgical exposure of kidney
➔ *CPT Assistant* Oct 01:8

50220   Nephrectomy, including partial ureterectomy, any open approach including rib resection;
➔ *CPT Changes: An Insider's View* 2002
➔ *CPT Assistant* Oct 01:8, Nov 02:3, Aug 08:7

50225   complicated because of previous surgery on same kidney
➔ *CPT Assistant* Oct 01:8, Nov 02:3

50230   radical, with regional lymphadenectomy and/or vena caval thrombectomy
➔ *CPT Assistant* Oct 01:8, Nov 02:3

(When vena caval resection with reconstruction is necessary, use 37799)

50234   Nephrectomy with total ureterectomy and bladder cuff; through same incision
➔ *CPT Assistant* Oct 01:8, Nov 02:3

50236   through separate incision
➔ *CPT Assistant* Oct 01:8, Nov 02:3

50240   Nephrectomy, partial
➔ *CPT Assistant* Oct 01:8, Nov 02:3, Jan 03:20, Apr 05:10, 12, Aug 08:7

(For laparoscopic partial nephrectomy, use 50543)

50250   Ablation, open, 1 or more renal mass lesion(s), cryosurgical, including intraoperative ultrasound guidance and monitoring, if performed
➔ *CPT Changes: An Insider's View* 2006, 2011
➔ *CPT Assistant* May 06:17

(For laparoscopic ablation of renal mass lesions, use 50542)

(For percutaneous ablation of renal tumors, see 50592, 50593)

50280   Excision or unroofing of cyst(s) of kidney
➔ *CPT Changes: An Insider's View* 2000
➔ *CPT Assistant* Nov 99:25, Oct 01:8

(For laparoscopic ablation of renal cysts, use 50541)

50290   Excision of perinephric cyst
➔ *CPT Assistant* Oct 01:8

Renal Transplantation

Renal *auto*transplantation includes reimplantation of the autograft as the primary procedure, along with secondary extra-corporeal procedure(s) (eg, partial nephrectomy, nephrolithotomy) reported with modifier 51 (see 50380 and applicable secondary procedure(s)).

Renal *allo*transplantation involves three distinct components of physician work:

1. ***Cadaver donor nephrectomy, unilateral or bilateral,*** which includes harvesting the graft(s) and cold preservation of the graft(s) (perfusing with cold preservation solution and cold maintenance) (use 50300). ***Living donor nephrectomy,*** which includes harvesting the graft, cold preservation of the graft (perfusing with cold preservation solution and cold

maintenance), and care of the donor (see 50320, 50547).

2. ***Backbench work:***
Standard preparation of a cadaver donor renal allograft prior to transplantation including dissection and removal of perinephric fat, diaphragmatic and retroperitoneal attachments; excision of adrenal gland; and preparation of ureter(s), renal vein(s), and renal artery(s), ligating branches, as necessary (use 50323).

Standard preparation of a living donor renal allograft (open or laparoscopic) prior to transplantation including dissection and removal of perinephric fat and preparation of ureter(s), renal vein(s), and renal artery(s), ligating branches, as necessary (use 50325).

Additional reconstruction of a cadaver or living donor renal allograft prior to transplantation may include venous, arterial, and/or ureteral anastomosis(es) necessary for implantation (see 50327-50329).

3. ***Recipient renal allotransplantation,*** which includes transplantation of the allograft (with or without recipient nephrectomy) and care of the recipient (see 50360, 50365).

(For dialysis, see 90935-90999)

(For laparoscopic donor nephrectomy, use 50547)

(For laparoscopic drainage of lymphocele to peritoneal cavity, use 49323)

50300   Donor nephrectomy (including cold preservation); from cadaver donor, unilateral or bilateral
➔ *CPT Changes: An Insider's View* 2000, 2005
➔ *CPT Assistant* Nov 99:25, Apr 05:10, 12

50320   open, from living donor
➔ *CPT Changes: An Insider's View* 2000, 2005
➔ *CPT Assistant* Nov 99:25, May 00:4

50323   Backbench standard preparation of cadaver donor renal allograft prior to transplantation, including dissection and removal of perinephric fat, diaphragmatic and retroperitoneal attachments, excision of adrenal gland, and preparation of ureter(s), renal vein(s), and renal artery(s), ligating branches, as necessary
➔ *CPT Changes: An Insider's View* 2005
➔ *CPT Assistant* Apr 05:10-11

(Do not report 50323 in conjunction with 60540, 60545)

50325   Backbench standard preparation of living donor renal allograft (open or laparoscopic) prior to transplantation, including dissection and removal of perinephric fat and preparation of ureter(s), renal vein(s), and renal artery(s), ligating branches, as necessary
➔ *CPT Changes: An Insider's View* 2005

50327 Backbench reconstruction of cadaver or living donor renal allograft prior to transplantation; venous anastomosis, each
➜ *CPT Changes: An Insider's View* 2005

50328 arterial anastomosis, each
➜ *CPT Changes: An Insider's View* 2005

50329 ureteral anastomosis, each
➜ *CPT Changes: An Insider's View* 2005

50340 Recipient nephrectomy (separate procedure)

(For bilateral procedure, report 50340 with modifier 50)

50360 Renal allotransplantation, implantation of graft; without recipient nephrectomy
➜ *CPT Changes: An Insider's View* 2005

50365 with recipient nephrectomy
➜ *CPT Assistant* Apr 05:10-11

(For bilateral procedure, report 50365 with modifier 50)

50370 Removal of transplanted renal allograft

50380 Renal autotransplantation, reimplantation of kidney
➜ *CPT Assistant* Apr 05:10, 12, Sep 19:11

(For renal autotransplantation extra-corporeal [bench] surgery, use autotransplantation as the primary procedure and report secondary procedure[s] [eg, partial nephrectomy, nephrolithotomy] with modifier 51)

Introduction

Renal Pelvis Catheter Procedures

Internally Dwelling

50382 Removal (via snare/capture) and replacement of internally dwelling ureteral stent via percutaneous approach, including radiological supervision and interpretation
➜ *CPT Changes: An Insider's View* 2006, 2017
➜ *CPT Assistant* Sep 06:1, 16, Oct 08:8, Dec 09:4, Jan 16:3
➜ *Clinical Examples in Radiology* Winter 06:15, Spring 08:5

(For bilateral procedure, use modifier 50)

(For removal and replacement of an internally dwelling ureteral stent via a transurethral approach, use 50385)

50384 Removal (via snare/capture) of internally dwelling ureteral stent via percutaneous approach, including radiological supervision and interpretation
➜ *CPT Changes: An Insider's View* 2006, 2017
➜ *CPT Assistant* Sep 06:2, 16, Oct 08:8, Jan 16:3
➜ *Clinical Examples in Radiology* Winter 06:16, Spring 08:5

(For bilateral procedure, use modifier 50)

(Do not report 50382, 50384 in conjunction with 50436, 50437)

(For removal of an internally dwelling ureteral stent via a transurethral approach, use 50386)

50385 Removal (via snare/capture) and replacement of internally dwelling ureteral stent via transurethral approach, without use of cystoscopy, including radiological supervision and interpretation
➜ *CPT Changes: An Insider's View* 2008, 2017
➜ *CPT Assistant* Oct 08:8, Dec 09:4, Jan 16:3, Jul 23:19
➜ *Clinical Examples in Radiology* Spring 08:5

50386 Removal (via snare/capture) of internally dwelling ureteral stent via transurethral approach, without use of cystoscopy, including radiological supervision and interpretation
➜ *CPT Changes: An Insider's View* 2008, 2017
➜ *CPT Assistant* Oct 08:8, Jan 16:3
➜ *Clinical Examples in Radiology* Spring 08:4

Externally Accessible

50387 Removal and replacement of externally accessible nephroureteral catheter (eg, external/internal stent) requiring fluoroscopic guidance, including radiological supervision and interpretation
➜ *CPT Changes: An Insider's View* 2006, 2016, 2017
➜ *CPT Assistant* Sep 06:2, 4, 16, Dec 09:4, Mar 12:3, Jan 16:3, Mar 16:10
➜ *Clinical Examples in Radiology* Winter 06:16, Spring 08:5, Fall 15:4

(For bilateral procedure, use modifier 50)

(For removal and replacement of externally accessible ureteral stent via ureterostomy or ileal conduit, use 50688)

(For removal without replacement of an externally accessible ureteral stent not requiring fluoroscopic guidance, see Evaluation and Management services codes)

50389 Removal of nephrostomy tube, requiring fluoroscopic guidance (eg, with concurrent indwelling ureteral stent)
➜ *CPT Changes: An Insider's View* 2006
➜ *CPT Assistant* Sep 06:1-2, 4, Jan 16:3
➜ *Clinical Examples in Radiology* Winter 06:16, Fall 21:8

(Removal of nephrostomy tube not requiring fluoroscopic guidance is considered inherent to E/M services. Report the appropriate level of E/M service provided)

Other Introduction (Injection/Change/Removal) Procedures

Percutaneous genitourinary procedures are performed with imaging guidance (eg, fluoroscopy and/or ultrasound). Diagnostic nephrostogram and/or ureterogram are typically performed with percutaneous genitourinary procedures and are included in 50432, 50433, 50434, 50435, 50436, 50437, 50693, 50694, 50695.

Code 50436 describes enlargement of an existing percutaneous tract to the renal collecting system to accommodate large instruments used in an endourologic procedure. Code 50436 includes predilation urinary tract imaging, postprocedure nephrostomy tube placement, when performed, and includes all radiological supervision and interpretation and imaging guidance (eg, ultrasound, fluoroscopy). Code 50436 may not be reported with 50432, 50433, 52334 for basic dilation of a percutaneous tract during initial placement of a catheter or device.

Code 50437 includes all elements of 50436, but also includes new access into the renal collecting system performed in the same session when a pre-existing tract is not present.

Codes 50430 and 50431 are diagnostic procedure codes that include injection(s) of contrast material, all associated radiological supervision and interpretation, and procedural imaging guidance (eg, ultrasound and/or fluoroscopy). Code 50430 also includes accessing the collecting system and/or associated ureter with a needle and/or catheter. Codes 50430 or 50431 may not be reported together with 50432, 50433, 50434, 50435, 50693, 50694, 50695.

Codes 50432, 50433, 50434, 50435 represent therapeutic procedures describing catheter placement or exchange, and include the elements of access, drainage catheter manipulations, and imaging guidance (eg, ultrasonography and/or fluoroscopy), as well as diagnostic imaging supervision and interpretation, when performed.

Code 50433 describes percutaneous nephrostomy with the additional accessing of the ureter/bladder to ultimately place a nephroureteral catheter (a single transnephric catheter with nephrostomy and ureteral components that allows drainage internally, externally, or both).

For codes 50430, 50431, 50432, 50433, 50434, 50435, 50606, 50693, 50694, 50695, 50705, and 50706, the renal pelvis and its associated ureter are considered a single entity for reporting purposes. Codes 50430, 50431, 50432, 50433, 50434, 50435, 50606, 50693, 50694, 50695, 50705, and 50706 may be reported once for each renal collecting system/ureter accessed (eg, two separate codes would be reported for bilateral nephrostomy tube placement or for unilateral duplicated collecting system/ureter requiring two separate procedures).

50390   Aspiration and/or injection of renal cyst or pelvis by needle, percutaneous
➔ *CPT Assistant* Fall 93:14, Dec 97:7, Oct 01:8, Oct 05:18, Oct 08:8

(For radiological supervision and interpretation, see 74425, 74470, 76942, 77002, 77012, 77021)

(For antegrade nephrostogram and/or antegrade pyelogram, see 50430, 50431)

50391   Instillation(s) of therapeutic agent into renal pelvis and/or ureter through established nephrostomy, pyelostomy or ureterostomy tube (eg, anticarcinogenic or antifungal agent)
➔ *CPT Changes: An Insider's View* 2005
➔ *CPT Assistant* Oct 05:18

 # 50436   Dilation of existing tract, percutaneous, for an endourologic procedure including imaging guidance (eg, ultrasound and/or fluoroscopy) and all associated radiological supervision and interpretation, with postprocedure tube placement, when performed;
➔ *CPT Changes: An Insider's View* 2019
➔ *CPT Assistant* Sep 23:30
➔ *Clinical Examples in Radiology* Winter 19:5

 # 50437   including new access into the renal collecting system
➔ *CPT Changes: An Insider's View* 2019
➔ *CPT Assistant* Sep 23:30
➔ *Clinical Examples in Radiology* Winter 19:4

(Do not report 50436, 50437 in conjunction with 50382, 50384, 50430, 50431, 50432, 50433, 52334, 74485)

(For nephrolithotomy, see 50080, 50081)

(For dilation of an existing percutaneous access for an endourologic procedure with a new access into the collecting system, use 50437; for additional new access into the kidney, use 50437 for each new access that is dilated for an endourologic procedure)

(For endoscopic surgery, see 50551-50561)

(For retrograde percutaneous nephrostomy, use 52334)

50396   Manometric studies through nephrostomy or pyelostomy tube, or indwelling ureteral catheter
➔ *CPT Assistant* Fall 93:16, Dec 97:7, Oct 01:8

(For radiological supervision and interpretation, use 74425)

50430 Injection procedure for antegrade nephrostogram and/or ureterogram, complete diagnostic procedure including imaging guidance (eg, ultrasound and fluoroscopy) and all associated radiological supervision and interpretation; new access

➔ *CPT Changes: An Insider's View* 2016, 2017

➔ *CPT Assistant* Oct 15:5, Jan 16:3, Sep 23:30

➔ *Clinical Examples in Radiology* Fall 15:3, Spring 16:12, Fall 20:12, Fall 21:7

50431 existing access

➔ *CPT Changes: An Insider's View* 2016

➔ *CPT Assistant* Oct 15:5, Jan 16:3, Sep 23:30

➔ *Clinical Examples in Radiology* Fall 15:3, Spring 16:12, Fall 20:12, Fall 21:7

(Do not report 50430, 50431 in conjunction with 50432, 50433, 50434, 50435, 50693, 50694, 50695, 74425 for the same renal collecting system and/or associated ureter)

50432 Placement of nephrostomy catheter, percutaneous, including diagnostic nephrostogram and/or ureterogram when performed, imaging guidance (eg, ultrasound and/or fluoroscopy) and all associated radiological supervision and interpretation

➔ *CPT Changes: An Insider's View* 2016, 2017

➔ *CPT Assistant* Oct 15:5, Jan 16:3, Mar 18:11

➔ *Clinical Examples in Radiology* Fall 15:2, Spring 16:12, Fall 20:12, Fall 21:7-8

(Do not report 50432 in conjunction with 50430, 50431, 50433, 50436, 50437, 50694, 50695, 74425, for the same renal collecting system and/or associated ureter)

(Do not report 50432 in conjunction with 50436, 50437, for dilation of the nephrostomy tube tract)

Introduction of Catheter Into Renal Pelvis
50432

The physician inserts a catheter into the renal pelvis in order to drain urine.

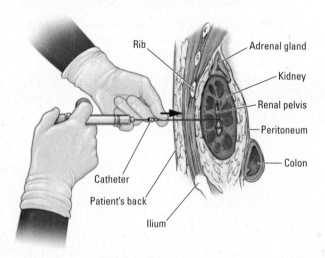

50433 Placement of nephroureteral catheter, percutaneous, including diagnostic nephrostogram and/or ureterogram when performed, imaging guidance (eg, ultrasound and/or fluoroscopy) and all associated radiological supervision and interpretation, new access

➔ *CPT Changes: An Insider's View* 2016, 2017

➔ *CPT Assistant* Oct 15:5, Jan 16:3, Mar 18:11, Sep 23:30

➔ *Clinical Examples in Radiology* Fall 15:3, Spring 16:12, Fall 20:12, Fall 21:7-8

(Do not report 50433 in conjunction with 50430, 50431, 50432, 50693, 50694, 50695, 74425 for the same renal collecting system and/or associated ureter)

(Do not report 50433 in conjunction with 50436, 50437, for dilation of the nephroureteral catheter tract)

(For nephroureteral catheter removal and replacement, use 50387)

50434 Convert nephrostomy catheter to nephroureteral catheter, percutaneous, including diagnostic nephrostogram and/or ureterogram when performed, imaging guidance (eg, ultrasound and/or fluoroscopy) and all associated radiological supervision and interpretation, via pre-existing nephrostomy tract

➔ *CPT Changes: An Insider's View* 2016, 2017

➔ *CPT Assistant* Oct 15:5, Jan 16:3, Sep 23:30

➔ *Clinical Examples in Radiology* Fall 15:3, Spring 16:12, Fall 20:12, Fall 21:7-8

(Do not report 50434 in conjunction with 50430, 50431, 50435, 50684, 50693, 74425 for the same renal collecting system and/or associated ureter)

50435 Exchange nephrostomy catheter, percutaneous, including diagnostic nephrostogram and/or ureterogram when performed, imaging guidance (eg, ultrasound and/or fluoroscopy) and all associated radiological supervision and interpretation

➔ *CPT Changes: An Insider's View* 2016

➔ *CPT Assistant* Oct 15:5, Jan 16:3, Mar 18:11, Dec 22:20, Sep 23:30

➔ *Clinical Examples in Radiology* Fall 15:3, Spring 16:12, Fall 20:12, Fall 21:7-8

(Do not report 50435 in conjunction with 50430, 50431, 50434, 50693, 74425 for the same renal collecting system and/or associated ureter)

(For removal of nephrostomy catheter requiring fluoroscopic guidance, use 50389)

Rib
Adrenal gland
Kidney
Renal pelvis
Peritoneum
Colon
Catheter
Patient's back
Ilium

★=Telemedicine ◀=Audio-only +=Add-on code ✔=FDA approval pending #=Resequenced code ⊘=Modifier 51 exempt ➔➔➔=See p xxi for details

Repair

50400 Pyeloplasty (Foley Y-pyeloplasty), plastic operation on renal pelvis, with or without plastic operation on ureter, nephropexy, nephrostomy, pyelostomy, or ureteral splinting; simple

➲ *CPT Changes: An Insider's View* 2000

➲ *CPT Assistant* Nov 99:25, May 00:4, Oct 01:8

50405 complicated (congenital kidney abnormality, secondary pyeloplasty, solitary kidney, calycoplasty)

➲ *CPT Changes: An Insider's View* 2000

➲ *CPT Assistant* Nov 99:25, May 00:4, Oct 01:8

(For laparoscopic approach, use 50544)

50430 Code is out of numerical sequence. See 50390-50405

50431 Code is out of numerical sequence. See 50390-50405

50432 Code is out of numerical sequence. See 50390-50405

50433 Code is out of numerical sequence. See 50390-50405

50434 Code is out of numerical sequence. See 50390-50405

50435 Code is out of numerical sequence. See 50390-50405

50436 Code is out of numerical sequence. See 50390-50405

50437 Code is out of numerical sequence. See 50390-50405

50500 Nephrorrhaphy, suture of kidney wound or injury

50520 Closure of nephrocutaneous or pyelocutaneous fistula

50525 Closure of nephrovisceral fistula (eg, renocolic), including visceral repair; abdominal approach

50526 thoracic approach

50540 Symphysiotomy for horseshoe kidney with or without pyeloplasty and/or other plastic procedure, unilateral or bilateral (1 operation)

Laparoscopy

Surgical laparoscopy always includes diagnostic laparoscopy. To report a diagnostic laparoscopy (peritoneoscopy) (separate procedure), use 49320.

50541 Laparoscopy, surgical; ablation of renal cysts

➲ *CPT Changes: An Insider's View* 2000

➲ *CPT Assistant* Nov 99:25, May 00:4, Oct 01:8, Nov 02:3, Jan 03:20

50542 ablation of renal mass lesion(s), including intraoperative ultrasound guidance and monitoring, when performed

➲ *CPT Changes: An Insider's View* 2003, 2011

➲ *CPT Assistant* Nov 02:3, Jan 03:21, Aug 04:12

(For open procedure, use 50250)

(For percutaneous ablation of renal tumors, see 50592, 50593)

50543 partial nephrectomy

➲ *CPT Changes: An Insider's View* 2003

➲ *CPT Assistant* Nov 02:3, Jan 03:21

(For open procedure, use 50240)

50544 pyeloplasty

➲ *CPT Changes: An Insider's View* 2000

➲ *CPT Assistant* Nov 99:25, May 00:4, Oct 01:8

50545 radical nephrectomy (includes removal of Gerota's fascia and surrounding fatty tissue, removal of regional lymph nodes, and adrenalectomy)

➲ *CPT Changes: An Insider's View* 2001

➲ *CPT Assistant* Oct 01:8

(For open procedure, use 50230)

Laparoscopic Radical Nephrectomy
50545

Radical nephrectomy (includes removal of Gerota's fascia and surrounding fatty tissue, removal of regional lymph nodes, and adrenalectomy)

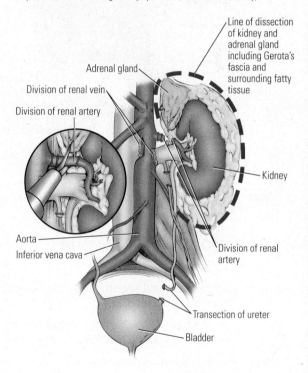

50546   nephrectomy, including partial ureterectomy
→ *CPT Changes: An Insider's View* 2000, 2001
→ *CPT Assistant* Nov 99:25, May 00:4, Oct 01:8

Laparoscopic Nephrectomy
50546

A kidney is dissected and removed under laparoscopic guidance.

Division of renal artery
Adrenal gland
Line of dissection of kidney from adrenal gland
Line of dissection of kidney from surrounding tissue
Tumor
Division of adrenal vein
Division of renal vein
Inferior vena cava
Aorta
Division of gonadal vein
Kidney
Division of renal artery
Transection of ureter

50547   donor nephrectomy (including cold preservation), from living donor
→ *CPT Changes: An Insider's View* 2000, 2005
→ *CPT Assistant* Nov 99:25, May 00:4, Oct 01:8

(For open procedure, use 50320)

(For backbench renal allograft standard preparation prior to transplantation, use 50325)

(For backbench renal allograft reconstruction prior to transplantation, see 50327-50329)

50548   nephrectomy with total ureterectomy
→ *CPT Changes: An Insider's View* 2000, 2001
→ *CPT Assistant* Nov 99:25, May 00:4, Oct 01:8

(For open procedure, see 50234, 50236)

50549   Unlisted laparoscopy procedure, renal
→ *CPT Changes: An Insider's View* 2000
→ *CPT Assistant* Nov 99:25, Mar 00:9, May 00:4, Feb 06:16

(For laparoscopic drainage of lymphocele to peritoneal cavity, use 49323)

Endoscopy

(For supplies and materials, use 99070)

50551   Renal endoscopy through established nephrostomy or pyelostomy, with or without irrigation, instillation, or ureteropyelography, exclusive of radiologic service;
→ *CPT Assistant* Oct 01:8, Jan 03:21

50553   with ureteral catheterization, with or without dilation of ureter
→ *CPT Assistant* Oct 01:8

(For image-guided dilation of ureter without endoscopic guidance, use 50706)

50555   with biopsy
→ *CPT Assistant* Oct 01:8

(For image-guided biopsy of ureter and/or renal pelvis without endoscopic guidance, use 50606)

50557   with fulguration and/or incision, with or without biopsy
→ *CPT Assistant* Oct 01:8

50561   with removal of foreign body or calculus
→ *CPT Assistant* Oct 01:8, Jan 03:21

50562   with resection of tumor
→ *CPT Changes: An Insider's View* 2003
→ *CPT Assistant* Jan 03:21

(When procedures 50570-50580 provide a significant identifiable service, they may be added to 50045 and 50120)

50570   Renal endoscopy through nephrotomy or pyelotomy, with or without irrigation, instillation, or ureteropyelography, exclusive of radiologic service;
→ *CPT Assistant* Oct 01:8

(For nephrotomy, use 50045)

(For pyelotomy, use 50120)

50572   with ureteral catheterization, with or without dilation of ureter
→ *CPT Assistant* Oct 01:8

(For image-guided dilation of ureter without endoscopic guidance, use 50706)

50574   with biopsy
→ *CPT Assistant* Oct 01:8

(For image-guided biopsy of ureter and/or renal pelvis without endoscopic guidance, use 50606)

50575   with endopyelotomy (includes cystoscopy, ureteroscopy, dilation of ureter and ureteral pelvic junction, incision of ureteral pelvic junction and insertion of endopyelotomy stent)
↪ *CPT Assistant* Oct 01:8, Aug 02:11

50576   with fulguration and/or incision, with or without biopsy
↪ *CPT Assistant* Oct 01:8

50580   with removal of foreign body or calculus
↪ *CPT Assistant* Oct 01:8

Other Procedures

50590   Lithotripsy, extracorporeal shock wave
↪ *CPT Assistant* Jul 01:11, Aug 01:10, Oct 01:8, Jul 03:16, Aug 03:14, Feb 22:14

Lithotripsy
50590

The physician breaks up a kidney stone (calculus) by directing shock waves through a liquid surrounding the patient.

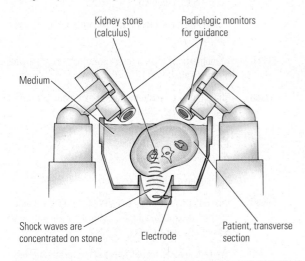

Kidney stone (calculus)   Radiologic monitors for guidance

Medium

Shock waves are concentrated on stone   Electrode   Patient, transverse section

50592   Ablation, 1 or more renal tumor(s), percutaneous, unilateral, radiofrequency
↪ *CPT Changes: An Insider's View* 2006, 2017
↪ *Clinical Examples in Radiology* Winter 06:16, Summer 12:11

(50592 is a unilateral procedure. For bilateral procedure, report 50592 with modifier 50)

(For imaging guidance and monitoring, see 76940, 77013, 77022)

50593   Ablation, renal tumor(s), unilateral, percutaneous, cryotherapy
↪ *CPT Changes: An Insider's View* 2008, 2017
↪ *CPT Assistant* May 17:3

(50593 is a unilateral procedure. For bilateral procedure, report 50593 with modifier 50)

(For imaging guidance and monitoring, see codes 76940, 77013, 77022)

Ureter

Incision/Biopsy

Code 50606 is an add-on code describing endoluminal biopsy (eg, brush) using non-endoscopic imaging guidance, which may be reported once per ureter per day. This code includes the work of the biopsy and the imaging guidance and radiological supervision and interpretation required to accomplish the biopsy. The biopsy may be performed through *de novo* transrenal access, an existing renal/ureteral access, transurethral access, an ileal conduit, or ureterostomy. The service of gaining access may be reported separately. Diagnostic pyelography/ureterography is not included in the work of 50606 and may be reported separately. Other interventions or catheter placements performed at the same setting as the biopsy may be reported separately.

For codes 50430, 50431, 50432, 50433, 50434, 50435, 50606, 50693, 50694, 50695, 50705, and 50706, the renal pelvis and its associated ureter are considered a single entity for reporting purposes. Codes 50430, 50431, 50432, 50433, 50434, 50435, 50606, 50693, 50694, 50695, 50705, and 50706 may be reported once for each renal collecting system/ureter accessed (eg, two separate codes would be reported for bilateral nephrostomy tube placement or for unilateral duplicated collecting system/ureter requiring two separate procedures).

50600   Ureterotomy with exploration or drainage (separate procedure)

(For ureteral endoscopy performed in conjunction with this procedure, see 50970-50980)

50605   Ureterotomy for insertion of indwelling stent, all types
↪ *CPT Assistant* Oct 01:8, Dec 09:4, Apr 12:18

+ 50606   Endoluminal biopsy of ureter and/or renal pelvis, non-endoscopic, including imaging guidance (eg, ultrasound and/or fluoroscopy) and all associated radiological supervision and interpretation (List separately in addition to code for primary procedure)
↪ *CPT Changes: An Insider's View* 2016, 2017
↪ *CPT Assistant* Jan 16:3
↪ *Clinical Examples in Radiology* Fall 15:3, Spring 16:12, Fall 21:7

(Use 50606 in conjunction with 50382, 50384, 50385, 50386, 50387, 50389, 50430, 50431, 50432, 50433, 50434, 50435, 50684, 50688, 50690, 50693, 50694, 50695, 51610)

(Do not report 50606 in conjunction with 50555, 50574, 50955, 50974, 52007, 74425 for the same renal collecting system and/or associated ureter)

Indwelling Ureteral Stent
50605

The physician makes an incision in the ureter (ureterotomy) and inserts a stent. For placement using cystourethroscopic technique, use 52332.

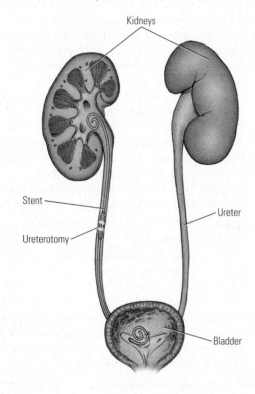

Kidneys

Stent

Ureterotomy

Ureter

Bladder

50610 Ureterolithotomy; upper one-third of ureter
> *CPT Changes: An Insider's View* 2000
> *CPT Assistant* Nov 99:26, Oct 01:8

50620 middle one-third of ureter
> *CPT Changes: An Insider's View* 2000
> *CPT Assistant* Nov 99:26, Oct 01:8

50630 lower one-third of ureter
> *CPT Changes: An Insider's View* 2000
> *CPT Assistant* Nov 99:26, Oct 01:8, May 14:3

(For laparoscopic approach, use 50945)

(For transvesical ureterolithotomy, use 51060)

(For cystotomy with stone basket extraction of ureteral calculus, use 51065)

(For endoscopic extraction or manipulation of ureteral calculus, see 50080, 50081, 50561, 50961, 50980, 52320-52330, 52352, 52353, 52356)

Excision

(For ureterocele, see 51535, 52300)

50650 Ureterectomy, with bladder cuff (separate procedure)

50660 Ureterectomy, total, ectopic ureter, combination abdominal, vaginal and/or perineal approach

Introduction

Other Introduction (Injection/Change/Removal) Procedures

Codes 50693, 50694, 50695 are therapeutic procedure codes describing percutaneous placement of ureteral stents. These codes include access, drainage, catheter manipulations, diagnostic nephrostogram and/or ureterogram, when performed, imaging guidance (eg, ultrasonography and/or fluoroscopy), and all associated radiological supervision and interpretation. When a separate ureteral stent and a nephrostomy catheter are placed into a ureter and its associated renal pelvis during the same session through a new percutaneous renal access, use 50695 to report the procedure.

50684 Injection procedure for ureterography or ureteropyelography through ureterostomy or indwelling ureteral catheter
> *CPT Assistant* Jan 16:3

(Do not report 50684 in conjunction with 50433, 50434, 50693, 50694, 50695)

(For radiological supervision and interpretation, use 74425)

50686 Manometric studies through ureterostomy or indwelling ureteral catheter

50688 Change of ureterostomy tube or externally accessible ureteral stent via ileal conduit
> *CPT Changes: An Insider's View* 2006
> *CPT Assistant* Jan 16:3, Jul 23:19
> *Clinical Examples in Radiology* Winter 06:20

(If imaging guidance is performed, use 75984)

50690 Injection procedure for visualization of ileal conduit and/or ureteropyelography, exclusive of radiologic service
> *CPT Assistant* Jan 16:3

(For radiological supervision and interpretation, see 74420 for retrograde or 74425 for antegrade injection)

50693 Placement of ureteral stent, percutaneous, including diagnostic nephrostogram and/or ureterogram when performed, imaging guidance (eg, ultrasound and/or fluoroscopy), and all associated radiological supervision and interpretation; pre-existing nephrostomy tract
> *CPT Changes: An Insider's View* 2016, 2017
> *CPT Assistant* Oct 15:5, Jan 16:3
> *Clinical Examples in Radiology* Fall 15:3, Spring 16:12, Fall 20:12, Fall 21:7

50694   new access, without separate nephrostomy catheter
⟳ *CPT Changes: An Insider's View* 2016, 2017
⟳ *CPT Assistant* Oct 15:5, Jan 16:3
⟳ *Clinical Examples in Radiology* Fall 15:3, Spring 16:12, Fall 20:12, Fall 21:7

50695   new access, with separate nephrostomy catheter
⟳ *CPT Changes: An Insider's View* 2016, 2017
⟳ *CPT Assistant* Oct 15:5, Jan 16:3
⟳ *Clinical Examples in Radiology* Fall 15:3, Spring 16:12, Fall 20:12, Fall 21:7

(Do not report 50693, 50694, 50695 in conjunction with 50430, 50431, 50432, 50433, 50434, 50435, 50684, 74425 for the same renal collecting system and/or associated ureter)

Repair

Codes 50705, 50706 are add-on codes describing embolization and balloon dilation of the ureter using non-endoscopic imaging guidance, and each may be reported once per ureter per day. These codes include embolization or dilation plus imaging guidance and radiological supervision and interpretation required to accomplish the embolization or dilation. These procedures may be performed through *de novo* transrenal access, an existing renal/ureteral access, transurethral access, an ileal conduit, or ureterostomy. The service of gaining access may be reported separately. Diagnostic pyelography/ureterography is not included in 50705 and 50706 and may be reported separately. Other interventions or catheter placements performed at the same setting as the embolization/dilation may be reported separately.

50700   Ureteroplasty, plastic operation on ureter (eg, stricture)

+ **50705**   Ureteral embolization or occlusion, including imaging guidance (eg, ultrasound and/or fluoroscopy) and all associated radiological supervision and interpretation (List separately in addition to code for primary procedure)
⟳ *CPT Changes: An Insider's View* 2016, 2017
⟳ *CPT Assistant* Jan 16:3
⟳ *Clinical Examples in Radiology* Fall 15:3, Spring 16:12, Fall 21:7

(Use 50705 in conjunction with 50382, 50384, 50385, 50386, 50387, 50389, 50430, 50431, 50432, 50433, 50434, 50435, 50684, 50688, 50690, 50693, 50694, 50695, 51610)

+ **50706**   Balloon dilation, ureteral stricture, including imaging guidance (eg, ultrasound and/or fluoroscopy) and all associated radiological supervision and interpretation (List separately in addition to code for primary procedure)
⟳ *CPT Changes: An Insider's View* 2016, 2017
⟳ *CPT Assistant* Jan 16:3
⟳ *Clinical Examples in Radiology* Fall 15:3, Spring 16:12, Fall 21:7

(Use 50706 in conjunction with 50382, 50384, 50385, 50386, 50387, 50389, 50430, 50431, 50432, 50433, 50434, 50435, 50684, 50688, 50690, 50693, 50694, 50695, 51610)

(Do not report 50706 in conjunction with 50553, 50572, 50953, 50972, 52341, 52344, 52345, 74485)

(For percutaneous nephrostomy, nephroureteral catheter, and/or ureteral catheter placement use 50385, 50387, 50432, 50433, 50434, 50435, 50693, 50694, 50695)

50715   Ureterolysis, with or without repositioning of ureter for retroperitoneal fibrosis

(For bilateral procedure, report 50715 with modifier 50)

50722   Ureterolysis for ovarian vein syndrome

50725   Ureterolysis for retrocaval ureter, with reanastomosis of upper urinary tract or vena cava

50727   Revision of urinary-cutaneous anastomosis (any type urostomy);

50728   with repair of fascial defect and hernia

50740   Ureteropyelostomy, anastomosis of ureter and renal pelvis
⟳ *CPT Assistant* Oct 01:8

50750   Ureterocalycostomy, anastomosis of ureter to renal calyx
⟳ *CPT Assistant* Oct 01:8

50760   Ureteroureterostomy
⟳ *CPT Assistant* Oct 01:8

50770   Transureteroureterostomy, anastomosis of ureter to contralateral ureter

(Codes 50780-50785 include minor procedures to prevent vesicoureteral reflux)

50780   Ureteroneocystostomy; anastomosis of single ureter to bladder
⟳ *CPT Assistant* Oct 01:8, Feb 18:11

(For bilateral procedure, report 50780 with modifier 50)

(When combined with cystourethroplasty or vesical neck revision, use 51820)

50782   anastomosis of duplicated ureter to bladder
⟳ *CPT Assistant* Oct 01:8

50783   with extensive ureteral tailoring
⟳ *CPT Assistant* Oct 01:8

50785   with vesico-psoas hitch or bladder flap
⟳ *CPT Assistant* Oct 01:8

(For bilateral procedure, report 50785 with modifier 50)

50800   Ureteroenterostomy, direct anastomosis of ureter to intestine
⟳ *CPT Assistant* Oct 01:8

(For bilateral procedure, report 50800 with modifier 50)

50810 Ureterosigmoidostomy, with creation of sigmoid bladder and establishment of abdominal or perineal colostomy, including intestine anastomosis
➲ *CPT Changes: An Insider's View* 2002
➲ *CPT Assistant* Oct 01:8

50815 Ureterocolon conduit, including intestine anastomosis
➲ *CPT Assistant* Oct 01:8

(For bilateral procedure, report 50815 with modifier 50)

50820 Ureteroileal conduit (ileal bladder), including intestine anastomosis (Bricker operation)
➲ *CPT Changes: An Insider's View* 2002
➲ *CPT Assistant* Oct 01:8, May 23:27

(For bilateral procedure, report 50820 with modifier 50)

(For combination of 50800-50820 with cystectomy, see 51580-51595)

Ureteroileal Conduit
50820

The ureters are connected to a segment of intestine to divert urine flow through an opening in the skin.

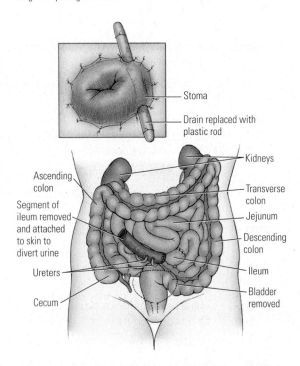

Stoma

Drain replaced with plastic rod

Kidneys

Ascending colon

Transverse colon

Segment of ileum removed and attached to skin to divert urine

Jejunum

Descending colon

Ureters

Ileum

Cecum

Bladder removed

50825 Continent diversion, including intestine anastomosis using any segment of small and/or large intestine (Kock pouch or Camey enterocystoplasty)
➲ *CPT Changes: An Insider's View* 2002
➲ *CPT Assistant* Oct 01:8

50830 Urinary undiversion (eg, taking down of ureteroileal conduit, ureterosigmoidostomy or ureteroenterostomy with ureteroureterostomy or ureteroneocystostomy)
➲ *CPT Assistant* Oct 01:8

50840 Replacement of all or part of ureter by intestine segment, including intestine anastomosis
➲ *CPT Changes: An Insider's View* 2002
➲ *CPT Assistant* Oct 01:8

(For bilateral procedure, report 50840 with modifier 50)

50845 Cutaneous appendico-vesicostomy

50860 Ureterostomy, transplantation of ureter to skin

(For bilateral procedure, report 50860 with modifier 50)

50900 Ureterorrhaphy, suture of ureter (separate procedure)

50920 Closure of ureterocutaneous fistula

50930 Closure of ureterovisceral fistula (including visceral repair)

50940 Deligation of ureter

(For ureteroplasty, ureterolysis, see 50700-50860)

Laparoscopy

Surgical laparoscopy always includes diagnostic laparoscopy. To report a diagnostic laparoscopy (peritoneoscopy) (separate procedure), use 49320.

50945 Laparoscopy, surgical; ureterolithotomy
➲ *CPT Changes: An Insider's View* 2000
➲ *CPT Assistant* Nov 99:26, May 00:4, Oct 01:8, Sep 06:13

50947 ureteroneocystostomy with cystoscopy and ureteral stent placement
➲ *CPT Changes: An Insider's View* 2001
➲ *CPT Assistant* Oct 01:8

50948 ureteroneocystostomy without cystoscopy and ureteral stent placement
➲ *CPT Changes: An Insider's View* 2001
➲ *CPT Assistant* Oct 01:8

(For open ureteroneocystostomy, see 50780-50785)

50949 Unlisted laparoscopy procedure, ureter
➲ *CPT Changes: An Insider's View* 2001
➲ *CPT Assistant* Oct 01:8

Endoscopy

50951 Ureteral endoscopy through established ureterostomy, with or without irrigation, instillation, or ureteropyelography, exclusive of radiologic service;
➲ *CPT Assistant* Oct 01:8

50953 with ureteral catheterization, with or without dilation of ureter
➲ *CPT Assistant* Oct 01:8

(For image-guided dilation of ureter without endoscopic guidance, use 50706)

Laparoscopic Ureteroneocystostomy
50947

Ureteroneocystostomy with cystoscopy and ureteral stent placement

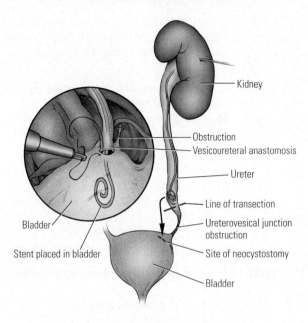

Kidney

Obstruction

Vesicoureteral anastomosis

Ureter

Line of transection

Ureterovesical junction obstruction

Bladder

Stent placed in bladder

Site of neocystostomy

Bladder

50955 with biopsy
➔ *CPT Assistant* Oct 01:8

(For image-guided biopsy of ureter and/or renal pelvis without endoscopic guidance, use 50606)

50957 with fulguration and/or incision, with or without biopsy
➔ *CPT Assistant* Oct 01:8

50961 with removal of foreign body or calculus
➔ *CPT Assistant* Oct 01:8, Mar 07:10, Apr 07:12

50970 Ureteral endoscopy through ureterotomy, with or without irrigation, instillation, or ureteropyelography, exclusive of radiologic service;
➔ *CPT Assistant* Oct 01:8

(For ureterotomy, use 50600)

50972 with ureteral catheterization, with or without dilation of ureter
➔ *CPT Assistant* Oct 01:8

(For image-guided dilation of ureter without endoscopic guidance, use 50706)

50974 with biopsy
➔ *CPT Assistant* Oct 01:8

(For image-guided biopsy of ureter and/or renal pelvis without endoscopic guidance, use 50606)

50976 with fulguration and/or incision, with or without biopsy
➔ *CPT Assistant* Oct 01:8

50980 with removal of foreign body or calculus
➔ *CPT Assistant* Oct 01:8

Bladder

Incision

▲ **51020** Cystotomy or cystostomy, with fulguration and/or insertion of radioactive material
➔ *CPT Changes: An Insider's View* 2025

►(51030 has been deleted)◄

51040 Cystostomy, cystotomy with drainage

51045 Cystotomy, with insertion of ureteral catheter or stent (separate procedure)

51050 Cystolithotomy, cystotomy with removal of calculus, without vesical neck resection

51060 Transvesical ureterolithotomy

51065 Cystotomy, with calculus basket extraction and/or ultrasonic or electrohydraulic fragmentation of ureteral calculus
➔ *CPT Changes: An Insider's View* 2002

51080 Drainage of perivesical or prevesical space abscess

(For percutaneous image-guided fluid collection drainage by catheter of perivesicular or prevesicular space abscess, use 49406)

Removal

51100 Aspiration of bladder; by needle
➔ *CPT Changes: An Insider's View* 2008
➔ *CPT Assistant* Jun 08:11

51101 by trocar or intracatheter
➔ *CPT Changes: An Insider's View* 2008
➔ *CPT Assistant* Jun 08:11

51102 with insertion of suprapubic catheter
➔ *CPT Changes: An Insider's View* 2008
➔ *CPT Assistant* Jun 08:11

(For imaging guidance, see 76942, 77002, 77012)

Excision

51500 Excision of urachal cyst or sinus, with or without umbilical hernia repair

51520 Cystotomy; for simple excision of vesical neck (separate procedure)

51525 for excision of bladder diverticulum, single or multiple (separate procedure)

51530 for excision of bladder tumor

(For transurethral resection, see 52234-52240, 52305)

51535 Cystotomy for excision, incision, or repair of ureterocele

(For bilateral procedure, report 51535 with modifier 50)

(For transurethral excision, use 52300)

51550 Cystectomy, partial; simple

51555 complicated (eg, postradiation, previous surgery, difficult location)

51565 Cystectomy, partial, with reimplantation of ureter(s) into bladder (ureteroneocystostomy)

51570 Cystectomy, complete; (separate procedure)
➔ *CPT Assistant* Spring 93:35

51575 with bilateral pelvic lymphadenectomy, including external iliac, hypogastric, and obturator nodes
➔ *CPT Assistant* Spring 93:35

51580 Cystectomy, complete, with ureterosigmoidostomy or ureterocutaneous transplantations;

51585 with bilateral pelvic lymphadenectomy, including external iliac, hypogastric, and obturator nodes

51590 Cystectomy, complete, with ureteroileal conduit or sigmoid bladder, including intestine anastomosis;
➔ *CPT Changes: An Insider's View* 2002
➔ *CPT Assistant* May 23:27

51595 with bilateral pelvic lymphadenectomy, including external iliac, hypogastric, and obturator nodes

51596 Cystectomy, complete, with continent diversion, any open technique, using any segment of small and/or large intestine to construct neobladder
➔ *CPT Changes: An Insider's View* 2002

51597 Pelvic exenteration, complete, for vesical, prostatic or urethral malignancy, with removal of bladder and ureteral transplantations, with or without hysterectomy and/or abdominoperineal resection of rectum and colon and colostomy, or any combination thereof

(For pelvic exenteration for gynecologic malignancy, use 58240)

Introduction

51600 Injection procedure for cystography or voiding urethrocystography
➔ *CPT Assistant* Oct 19:11
➔ *Clinical Examples in Radiology* Summer 19:11, Winter 21:3

(For radiological supervision and interpretation, see 74430, 74455)

51605 Injection procedure and placement of chain for contrast and/or chain urethrocystography

(For radiological supervision and interpretation, use 74430)

51610 Injection procedure for retrograde urethrocystography
➔ *CPT Assistant* Jan 16:3, Oct 19:11, Jan 21:11, Dec 23:41, Feb 24:21

(For radiological supervision and interpretation, use 74450)

51700 Bladder irrigation, simple, lavage and/or instillation
➔ *CPT Assistant* Jan 21:11

(Codes 51701-51702 are reported only when performed independently. Do not report 51701-51702 when catheter insertion is an inclusive component of another procedure.)

51701 Insertion of non-indwelling bladder catheter (eg, straight catheterization for residual urine)
➔ *CPT Changes: An Insider's View* 2003
➔ *CPT Assistant* Jul 06:4, Jan 07:31, Jul 07:1, Jan 21:11, Mar 23:1

51702 Insertion of temporary indwelling bladder catheter; simple (eg, Foley)
➔ *CPT Changes: An Insider's View* 2003
➔ *CPT Assistant* Oct 03:10, Jul 06:4, Jan 07:31, Jul 07:1, May 14:3, Jan 21:11
➔ *Clinical Examples in Radiology* Spring 12:1

(Do not report 51702 in conjunction with 0071T, 0072T)

51703 complicated (eg, altered anatomy, fractured catheter/balloon)
➔ *CPT Changes: An Insider's View* 2003
➔ *CPT Assistant* Jan 07:31, Jan 21:11

51705 Change of cystostomy tube; simple
➔ *CPT Assistant* Dec 07:13, Jan 21:11

51710 complicated
➔ *CPT Assistant* Dec 07:13

(If imaging guidance is performed, use 75984)

51715 Endoscopic injection of implant material into the submucosal tissues of the urethra and/or bladder neck

51720 Bladder instillation of anticarcinogenic agent (including retention time)
➔ *CPT Changes: An Insider's View* 2007
➔ *CPT Assistant* Nov 02:11

● **51721** Insertion of transurethral ablation transducer for delivery of thermal ultrasound for prostate tissue ablation, including suprapubic tube placement during the same session and placement of an endorectal cooling device, when performed
➔ *CPT Changes: An Insider's View* 2025

▶(Do not report 51721 in conjunction with 51701, 51702, 55881, 55882, 72195, 72196, 72197, 77022)◀

▶(For insertion of transurethral ultrasound transducer and ablation of prostate tissue using thermal ultrasound transducer performed by the same physician, use 55882)◀

Urodynamics

The following section (51725-51798) lists procedures that may be used separately or in many and varied combinations.

When multiple procedures are performed in the same investigative session, modifier 51 should be employed.

All procedures in this section imply that these services are performed by, or are under the direct supervision of, a physician or other qualified health care professional and that all instruments, equipment, fluids, gases, probes, catheters, technician's fees, medications, gloves, trays, tubing, and other sterile supplies be provided by that individual. When the individual only interprets the results and/or operates the equipment, a professional component, modifier 26, should be used to identify these services.

51725　Simple cystometrogram (CMG) (eg, spinal manometer)
➔ *CPT Assistant* Sep 02:6, Feb 10:7

51726　Complex cystometrogram (ie, calibrated electronic equipment);
➔ *CPT Changes: An Insider's View* 2010
➔ *CPT Assistant* Sep 02:6, Feb 10:7

51727　with urethral pressure profile studies (ie, urethral closure pressure profile), any technique
➔ *CPT Changes: An Insider's View* 2010
➔ *CPT Assistant* Feb 10:7

51728　with voiding pressure studies (ie, bladder voiding pressure), any technique
➔ *CPT Changes: An Insider's View* 2010
➔ *CPT Assistant* Feb 10:7

51729　with voiding pressure studies (ie, bladder voiding pressure) and urethral pressure profile studies (ie, urethral closure pressure profile), any technique
➔ *CPT Changes: An Insider's View* 2010
➔ *CPT Assistant* Feb 10:7

#+ 51797　Voiding pressure studies, intra-abdominal (ie, rectal, gastric, intraperitoneal) (List separately in addition to code for primary procedure)
➔ *CPT Changes: An Insider's View* 2008, 2010
➔ *CPT Assistant* Dec 01:7, Sep 02:6, Oct 09:7, Feb 10:7

(Use 51797 in conjunction with 51728, 51729)

51736　Simple uroflowmetry (UFR) (eg, stop-watch flow rate, mechanical uroflowmeter)
➔ *CPT Assistant* Sep 02:6, Feb 10:7, Nov 23:26, Feb 24:28

(Do not report 51736 in conjunction with 0811T, 0812T)

51741　Complex uroflowmetry (eg, calibrated electronic equipment)
➔ *CPT Assistant* Sep 02:6, Feb 10:7, Sep 14:14, Nov 23:26, Feb 24:28

(Do not report 51741 in conjunction with 0811T, 0812T)

51784　Electromyography studies (EMG) of anal or urethral sphincter, other than needle, any technique
➔ *CPT Assistant* Sep 02:6, Feb 10:7, Feb 14:11, Sep 14:14

(Do not report 51784 in conjunction with 51792)

51785　Needle electromyography studies (EMG) of anal or urethral sphincter, any technique
➔ *CPT Assistant* Apr 02:6, Sep 02:6, Jul 04:13, Feb 10:7

51792　Stimulus evoked response (eg, measurement of bulbocavernosus reflex latency time)
➔ *CPT Assistant* Apr 02:6, Sep 02:6, Feb 10:7, Feb 14:11

(Do not report 51792 in conjunction with 51784)

51797　Code is out of numerical sequence. See 51728-51741

51798　Measurement of post-voiding residual urine and/or bladder capacity by ultrasound, non-imaging
➔ *CPT Changes: An Insider's View* 2003
➔ *CPT Assistant* Dec 05:3, Feb 10:7, Jun 18:11

Measurement of Postvoiding
51798

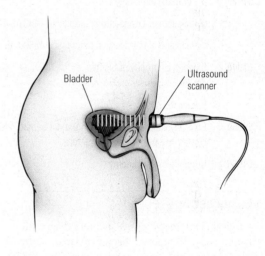

Bladder　　　　　Ultrasound scanner

Repair

51800　Cystoplasty or cystourethroplasty, plastic operation on bladder and/or vesical neck (anterior Y-plasty, vesical fundus resection), any procedure, with or without wedge resection of posterior vesical neck

51820　Cystourethroplasty with unilateral or bilateral ureteroneocystostomy

51840 Anterior vesicourethropexy, or urethropexy (eg, Marshall-Marchetti-Krantz, Burch); simple
→ *CPT Assistant* Jan 97:1, Nov 97:19, Apr 98:15, Jun 02:7, May 06:17, Jun 10:6, Aug 12:13

51841 complicated (eg, secondary repair)
→ *CPT Assistant* Jan 97:1, Jun 02:7, Jun 10:6, Aug 12:13

(For urethropexy (Pereyra type), use 57289)

51845 Abdomino-vaginal vesical neck suspension, with or without endoscopic control (eg, Stamey, Raz, modified Pereyra)
→ *CPT Assistant* Jan 97:3

51860 Cystorrhaphy, suture of bladder wound, injury or rupture; simple

51865 complicated

51880 Closure of cystostomy (separate procedure)

51900 Closure of vesicovaginal fistula, abdominal approach

(For vaginal approach, see 57320-57330)

51920 Closure of vesicouterine fistula;

51925 with hysterectomy

(For closure of vesicoenteric fistula, see 44660, 44661)

(For closure of rectovesical fistula, see 45800-45805)

51940 Closure, exstrophy of bladder
→ *CPT Changes: An Insider's View* 2002

(See also 54390)

51960 Enterocystoplasty, including intestinal anastomosis
→ *CPT Changes: An Insider's View* 2002

51980 Cutaneous vesicostomy

Laparoscopy

Surgical laparoscopy always includes diagnostic laparoscopy. To report a diagnostic laparoscopy (peritoneoscopy) (separate procedure), use 49320.

51990 Laparoscopy, surgical; urethral suspension for stress incontinence
→ *CPT Changes: An Insider's View* 2000
→ *CPT Assistant* Nov 99:26, May 00:4, Jun 10:6, Mar 12:10, Aug 12:13

51992 sling operation for stress incontinence (eg, fascia or synthetic)
→ *CPT Changes: An Insider's View* 2000
→ *CPT Assistant* Nov 99:26, May 00:4, Mar 12:10, Aug 12:13

(For open sling operation for stress incontinence, use 57288)

(For reversal or removal of sling operation for stress incontinence, use 57287)

51999 Unlisted laparoscopy procedure, bladder
→ *CPT Changes: An Insider's View* 2006
→ *CPT Assistant* Dec 17:14

Laparoscopic Sling Suspension Urinary Incontinence
51990

Nonabsorbable sutures are placed laparoscopically into the endopelvic fascia at the bladder neck region on each side and secured to the ipsilateral pectineal ligament. The sutures are tied using extra vaginal-urethral knots so as to create a hammock type suspension of the bladder neck, without urethral occlusion.

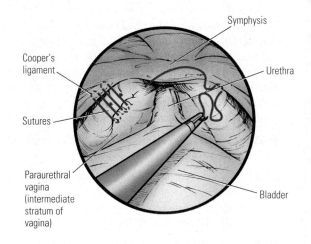

Endoscopy—Cystoscopy, Urethroscopy, Cystourethroscopy

Endoscopic descriptions are listed so that the main procedure can be identified without having to list all the minor related functions performed at the same time. For example: meatotomy, urethral calibration and/or dilation, urethroscopy, and cystoscopy prior to a transurethral resection of prostate; ureteral catheterization following extraction of ureteral calculus; internal urethrotomy and bladder neck fulguration when performing a cystourethroscopy for the female urethral syndrome. When the secondary procedure requires significant additional time and effort, it may be identified by the addition of modifier 22.

For example: urethrotomy performed for a documented pre-existing stricture or bladder neck contracture.

Because cutaneous urinary diversions utilizing ileum or colon serve as functional replacements of a native bladder, endoscopy of such bowel segments, as well as performance of secondary procedures can be captured by using the cystourethroscopy codes. For example, endoscopy of an ileal loop with removal of ureteral calculus would be coded as cystourethroscopy (including ureteral catheterization); with removal of ureteral calculus (52320).

52000   Cystourethroscopy (separate procedure)

➲ *CPT Assistant* Oct 00:7, May 01:5, Sep 04:11, Oct 05:23, Nov 07:9, Mar 13:14, May 14:3, Oct 17:9, Nov 18:10, Dec 23:41, Feb 24:21

▶(Do not report 52000 in conjunction with 52001, 52320, 52325, 52327, 52330, 52332, 52334, 52341, 52342, 52343, 52356, 57240, 57260, 57265, 0935T)◀

(Do not report 52000 in conjunction with 57240, 57260, 57265)

52001   Cystourethroscopy with irrigation and evacuation of multiple obstructing clots

➲ *CPT Changes: An Insider's View* 2002, 2003

(Do not report 52001 in conjunction with 52000)

— *Coding Tip* —

Restrictions for Reporting Temporary Catheter Insertion and Removal with Cystourethroscopy

The insertion and removal of a temporary ureteral catheter (52005) during diagnostic or therapeutic cystourethroscopy with ureteroscopy and/or pyeloscopy is included in 52320-52356 and should not be reported separately.

CPT Coding Guidelines, Urinary System, Bladder Transurethral Surgery, Ureter and Pelvis

52005   Cystourethroscopy, with ureteral catheterization, with or without irrigation, instillation, or ureteropyelography, exclusive of radiologic service;

➲ *CPT Assistant* Sep 00:11, Jan 01:13, May 01:5, Oct 01:8, Dec 10:15, Mar 19:11

▶(Do not report 52005 in conjunction with 0935T)◀

52007   with brush biopsy of ureter and/or renal pelvis

➲ *CPT Assistant* May 01:5, Oct 01:8

(For image-guided biopsy of ureter and/or renal pelvis without endoscopic guidance, use 50606)

52010   Cystourethroscopy, with ejaculatory duct catheterization, with or without irrigation, instillation, or duct radiography, exclusive of radiologic service

➲ *CPT Assistant* May 01:5

(For radiological supervision and interpretation, use 74440)

Transurethral Surgery

Urethra and Bladder

52204   Cystourethroscopy, with biopsy(s)

➲ *CPT Changes: An Insider's View* 2007

➲ *CPT Assistant* May 01:5, Sep 01:1, Sep 03:16, Aug 09:6, May 16:12

Cystourethroscopy With Ureteral Catheterization
52005

A cystourethroscope is passed through the urethra and bladder in order to view the urinary collecting system.

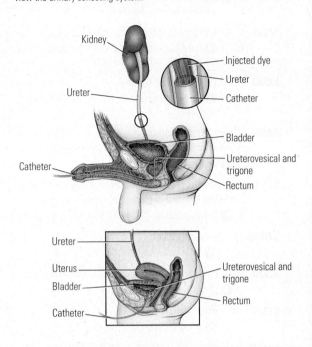

52214   Cystourethroscopy, with fulguration (including cryosurgery or laser surgery) of trigone, bladder neck, prostatic fossa, urethra, or periurethral glands

➲ *CPT Assistant* May 01:5, Sep 01:1, Aug 09:6, May 16:12

(For transurethral fulguration of prostate tissue performed within the postoperative period of 52601 or 52630 performed by the same physician, append modifier 78)

(For transurethral fulguration of prostate tissue performed within the postoperative period of a related procedure performed by the same physician, append modifier 78)

(For transurethral fulguration of prostate for postoperative bleeding performed by the same physician, append modifier 78)

52224   Cystourethroscopy, with fulguration (including cryosurgery or laser surgery) or treatment of MINOR (less than 0.5 cm) lesion(s) with or without biopsy

➲ *CPT Assistant* May 01:5, Sep 01:1, Dec 07:7, Jun 09:10, Aug 09:6, May 16:12

52234 Cystourethroscopy, with fulguration (including cryosurgery or laser surgery) and/or resection of; SMALL bladder tumor(s) (0.5 up to 2.0 cm)
→ *CPT Changes: An Insider's View* 2005
→ *CPT Assistant* May 01:5, Sep 01:1, Oct 02:12, Jan 03:21, Jun 09:10, Aug 09:6, May 16:12

52235 MEDIUM bladder tumor(s) (2.0 to 5.0 cm)
→ *CPT Assistant* May 01:5, Sep 01:1, Oct 02:12, Jan 03:21, Jun 09:10, Aug 09:6, May 16:12

52240 LARGE bladder tumor(s)
→ *CPT Assistant* May 01:5, Sep 01:1, Jun 09:10, Aug 09:6, May 16:12

52250 Cystourethroscopy with insertion of radioactive substance, with or without biopsy or fulguration
→ *CPT Assistant* May 01:5, Sep 01:1

52260 Cystourethroscopy, with dilation of bladder for interstitial cystitis; general or conduction (spinal) anesthesia
→ *CPT Assistant* May 01:5, Sep 01:1, Oct 05:23

52265 local anesthesia
→ *CPT Assistant* May 01:5, Sep 01:1

52270 Cystourethroscopy, with internal urethrotomy; female
→ *CPT Assistant* May 01:5, Sep 01:1

52275 male
→ *CPT Assistant* May 01:5, Sep 01:1

52276 Cystourethroscopy with direct vision internal urethrotomy
→ *CPT Assistant* May 01:5, Sep 01:1, May 09:8, Feb 10:7

52277 Cystourethroscopy, with resection of external sphincter (sphincterotomy)
→ *CPT Assistant* May 01:5, Sep 01:1

52281 Cystourethroscopy, with calibration and/or dilation of urethral stricture or stenosis, with or without meatotomy, with or without injection procedure for cystography, male or female
→ *CPT Assistant* Nov 97:20, May 01:5, Sep 01:1, Jun 07:10, Oct 17:9, Dec 23:41, Feb 24:21

(For cystourethroscopy with mechanical urethral dilation and urethral therapeutic drug delivery by drug-coated balloon catheter for urethral stricture or stenosis, including fluoroscopy, use 52284)

52282 Cystourethroscopy, with insertion of permanent urethral stent
→ *CPT Changes: An Insider's View* 2010
→ *CPT Assistant* Nov 97:20, May 01:5, Sep 01:1, Feb 10:7, Jun 15:5

(For placement of temporary prostatic urethral stent, use 53855)

►(For insertion of prostatic urethral scaffold, use 0941T)◄

52283 Cystourethroscopy, with steroid injection into stricture
→ *CPT Assistant* May 01:5, Sep 01:1, Mar 15:9, Dec 23:41, Feb 24:21

52284 Cystourethroscopy, with mechanical urethral dilation and urethral therapeutic drug delivery by drug-coated balloon catheter for urethral stricture or stenosis, male, including fluoroscopy, when performed
→ *CPT Changes: An Insider's View* 2024
→ *CPT Assistant* Dec 23:41, Feb 24:21

(Do not report 52284 in conjunction with 51610, 52000, 52281, 52283, 74450, 76000)

52285 Cystourethroscopy for treatment of the female urethral syndrome with any or all of the following: urethral meatotomy, urethral dilation, internal urethrotomy, lysis of urethrovaginal septal fibrosis, lateral incisions of the bladder neck, and fulguration of polyp(s) of urethra, bladder neck, and/or trigone
→ *CPT Assistant* May 01:5, Sep 01:1

52287 Cystourethroscopy, with injection(s) for chemodenervation of the bladder
→ *CPT Changes: An Insider's View* 2013

(The supply of the chemodenervation agent is reported separately)

52290 Cystourethroscopy; with ureteral meatotomy, unilateral or bilateral
→ *CPT Assistant* May 01:5, Sep 01:1

52300 with resection or fulguration of orthotopic ureterocele(s), unilateral or bilateral
→ *CPT Assistant* May 01:5, Sep 01:1

52301 with resection or fulguration of ectopic ureterocele(s), unilateral or bilateral
→ *CPT Assistant* May 01:5, Sep 01:1

52305 with incision or resection of orifice of bladder diverticulum, single or multiple
→ *CPT Assistant* May 01:5, Sep 01:1

—— *Coding Tip* ——

Instructions for Reporting Stent Removal

To report cystourethroscopic removal of a self-retaining, indwelling ureteral stent, see 52310, 52315, and append modifier 58, if appropriate.

CPT Coding Guidelines, Urinary System, Bladder Transurethral Surgery, Ureter and Pelvis

52310 Cystourethroscopy, with removal of foreign body, calculus, or ureteral stent from urethra or bladder (separate procedure); simple
→ *CPT Assistant* May 01:5, Sep 01:1

52315   complicated
   CPT Assistant May 01:5, Sep 01:1

   ►(For removal and replacement of prostatic urethral scaffold, use 0942T)◄

   ►(For removal of prostatic urethral scaffold, use 0943T)◄

52317   Litholapaxy: crushing or fragmentation of calculus by any means in bladder and removal of fragments; simple or small (less than 2.5 cm)
   CPT Assistant May 01:5, Sep 01:1, Feb 12:11

52318   complicated or large (over 2.5 cm)
   CPT Assistant May 01:5, Sep 01:1, Feb 12:11

Ureter and Pelvis

Therapeutic cystourethroscopy always includes diagnostic cystourethroscopy. To report a diagnostic cystourethroscopy, use 52000. Therapeutic cystourethroscopy with ureteroscopy and/or pyeloscopy always includes diagnostic cystourethroscopy with ureteroscopy and/or pyeloscopy. To report a diagnostic cystourethroscopy with ureteroscopy and/or pyeloscopy, use 52351.

Do not report 52000 in conjunction with 52320-52343, 52356.

Do not report 52351 in conjunction with 52344-52346, 52352-52356.

The insertion and removal of a temporary ureteral catheter (52005) during diagnostic or therapeutic cystourethroscopy with ureteroscopy and/or pyeloscopy is included in 52320-52356 and should not be reported separately.

To report insertion of a self-retaining, indwelling stent performed during diagnostic or therapeutic cystourethroscopy with ureteroscopy and/or pyeloscopy, report 52332, in addition to primary procedure(s) performed (52320-52330, 52334-52352, 52354, 52355), and append modifier 51. Code 52332 is used to report a unilateral procedure unless otherwise specified.

For bilateral insertion of self-retaining, indwelling ureteral stents, use code 52332, and append modifier 50.

To report cystourethroscopic removal of a self-retaining, indwelling ureteral stent, see 52310, 52315, and append modifier 58, if appropriate.

52320   Cystourethroscopy (including ureteral catheterization); with removal of ureteral calculus
   CPT Assistant Mar 96:1, May 96:11, Jan 01:13, May 01:5, Sep 01:1, Oct 01:8, May 14:3

52325   with fragmentation of ureteral calculus (eg, ultrasonic or electro-hydraulic technique)
   CPT Assistant Mar 96:1, May 96:11, May 01:5, Sep 01:1, Oct 01:8, Dec 07:13

52327   with subureteric injection of implant material
   CPT Assistant Mar 96:1, May 96:11, May 01:5, Sep 01:1, Oct 01:8

52330   with manipulation, without removal of ureteral calculus
   CPT Assistant Mar 96:1, May 96:11, Sep 00:11, May 01:5, Sep 01:1, Oct 01:8, May 14:3

(Do not report 52320, 52325, 52327, 52330 in conjunction with 52000)

52332   Cystourethroscopy, with insertion of indwelling ureteral stent (eg, Gibbons or double-J type)
   CPT Assistant Mar 96:1, May 96:11, Nov 96:8, Jan 01:13, May 01:5, Sep 01:1, Oct 01:8, Oct 05:18, Dec 09:4, 12, May 14:3, Jul 23:19

(Do not report 52332 in conjunction with 52000, 52353, 52356 when performed together on the same side)

52334   Cystourethroscopy with insertion of ureteral guide wire through kidney to establish a percutaneous nephrostomy, retrograde
   CPT Assistant Mar 96:11, May 96:11, May 01:5, Sep 01:1, Oct 01:8, May 14:3

(For percutaneous nephrolithotomy, see 50080, 50081; for establishment of percutaneous nephrostomy, see 50432, 50433)

(For cystourethroscopy, with ureteroscopy and/or pyeloscopy, see 52351-52356)

(For cystourethroscopy with incision, fulguration, or resection of congenital posterior urethral valves or obstructive hypertrophic mucosal folds, use 52400)

(Do not report 52334 in conjunction with 50437, 52000, 52351)

52341   Cystourethroscopy; with treatment of ureteral stricture (eg, balloon dilation, laser, electrocautery, and incision)
   CPT Changes: An Insider's View 2001
   CPT Assistant Nov 96:9, Apr 01:4, May 01:5, Sep 01:1, Oct 01:8

52342   with treatment of ureteropelvic junction stricture (eg, balloon dilation, laser, electrocautery, and incision)
   CPT Changes: An Insider's View 2001
   CPT Assistant Apr 01:4, May 01:5, Sep 01:1, Oct 01:8, Aug 02:11

52343   with treatment of intra-renal stricture (eg, balloon dilation, laser, electrocautery, and incision)
   CPT Changes: An Insider's View 2001
   CPT Assistant Apr 01:4, May 01:5, Sep 01:1, Oct 01:8, May 14:3

(Do not report 52341, 52342, 52343 in conjunction with 52000, 52351)

(For image-guided dilation of ureter, ureteropelvic junction stricture without endoscopic guidance, use 50706)

(For radiological supervision and interpretation, use 74485)

52344   Cystourethroscopy with ureteroscopy; with treatment of ureteral stricture (eg, balloon dilation, laser, electrocautery, and incision)

➜ *CPT Changes: An Insider's View* 2001

➜ *CPT Assistant* Apr 01:4, May 01:5, Sep 01:1, Oct 01:8

52345   with treatment of ureteropelvic junction stricture (eg, balloon dilation, laser, electrocautery, and incision)

➜ *CPT Changes: An Insider's View* 2001

➜ *CPT Assistant* Apr 01:4, May 01:5, Sep 01:1, Oct 01:8

52346   with treatment of intra-renal stricture (eg, balloon dilation, laser, electrocautery, and incision)

➜ *CPT Changes: An Insider's View* 2001

➜ *CPT Assistant* Apr 01:4, May 01:5, Sep 01:1, Oct 01:8, May 14:3

(For transurethral resection or incision of ejaculatory ducts, use 52402)

(Do not report 52344, 52345, 52346 in conjunction with 52351)

(For image-guided dilation of ureter, ureteropelvic junction stricture without endoscopic guidance, use 50706)

(For radiological supervision and interpretation, use 74485)

52351   Cystourethroscopy, with ureteroscopy and/or pyeloscopy; diagnostic

➜ *CPT Changes: An Insider's View* 2001

➜ *CPT Assistant* Apr 01:4, May 01:5, Sep 01:1, Oct 01:8, May 14:3

(Do not report 52351 in conjunction with 52341, 52342, 52343, 52344, 52345, 52346, 52352-52356)

52352   with removal or manipulation of calculus (ureteral catheterization is included)

➜ *CPT Changes: An Insider's View* 2001

➜ *CPT Assistant* Apr 01:4, May 01:5, Sep 01:1, Oct 01:8, Jun 07:10, Feb 10:13, May 14:3, Dec 19:12

52353   with lithotripsy (ureteral catheterization is included)

➜ *CPT Changes: An Insider's View* 2001

➜ *CPT Assistant* Apr 01:4, May 01:5, Sep 01:1, Oct 01:8, Dec 07:13, Apr 09:8, May 14:3, Dec 19:12

(Do not report 52353 in conjunction with 52332, 52356 when performed together on the same side)

 # 52356   with lithotripsy including insertion of indwelling ureteral stent (eg, Gibbons or double-J type)

➜ *CPT Changes: An Insider's View* 2014

➜ *CPT Assistant* May 14:3, Dec 19:12, Feb 22:14

(Do not report 52356 in conjunction with 52332, 52353 when performed together on the same side)

52354   with biopsy and/or fulguration of ureteral or renal pelvic lesion

➜ *CPT Changes: An Insider's View* 2001, 2003

➜ *CPT Assistant* Apr 01:4, May 01:5, Sep 01:1, Oct 01:8, May 14:3

(For image-guided biopsy of ureter and/or renal pelvis without endoscopic guidance, use 50606)

52355   with resection of ureteral or renal pelvic tumor

➜ *CPT Changes: An Insider's View* 2001, 2003

➜ *CPT Assistant* Apr 01:4, May 01:5, Sep 01:1, Oct 01:8, Jan 03:21, May 14:3

52356   Code is out of numerical sequence. See 52352-52355

Vesical Neck and Prostate

52400   Cystourethroscopy with incision, fulguration, or resection of congenital posterior urethral valves, or congenital obstructive hypertrophic mucosal folds

➜ *CPT Changes: An Insider's View* 2001

➜ *CPT Assistant* Apr 01:4

52402   Cystourethroscopy with transurethral resection or incision of ejaculatory ducts

➜ *CPT Changes: An Insider's View* 2005

52441   Cystourethroscopy, with insertion of permanent adjustable transprostatic implant; single implant

➜ *CPT Changes: An Insider's View* 2015

➜ *CPT Assistant* Jun 15:5

+ 52442   each additional permanent adjustable transprostatic implant (List separately in addition to code for primary procedure)

➜ *CPT Changes: An Insider's View* 2015

➜ *CPT Assistant* Jun 15:5

(Use 52442 in conjunction with 52441)

(To report removal of implant[s], use 52310)

▶(For insertion of a permanent urethral stent, use 52282. For insertion of a temporary prostatic urethral stent, use 53855. For insertion of prostatic urethral scaffold, use 0941T)◀

52450   Transurethral incision of prostate

➜ *CPT Assistant* Apr 01:4, Jul 05:15, Jun 15:5

52500   Transurethral resection of bladder neck (separate procedure)

➜ *CPT Assistant* Apr 01:4, Jan 04:27, Jul 05:15, May 09:8

52601   Transurethral electrosurgical resection of prostate, including control of postoperative bleeding, complete (vasectomy, meatotomy, cystourethroscopy, urethral calibration and/or dilation, and internal urethrotomy are included)

➜ *CPT Assistant* Nov 97:20, Apr 01:4, Jun 03:6, Oct 11:10, Jun 15:5, Jul 21:10

(For transurethral waterjet ablation of prostate, use 0421T)

(For other approaches, see 55801-55845)

Transurethral Resection of Prostate, Complete
52601

The physician removes the prostate gland using an electrocautery knife.

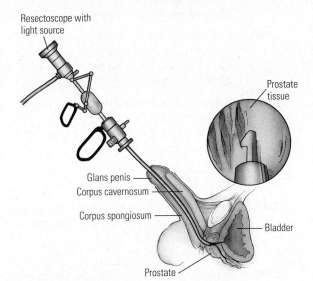

Resectoscope with light source

Prostate tissue

Glans penis
Corpus cavernosum
Corpus spongiosum

Bladder

Prostate

Contact Laser Vaporization of Prostate
52648

A laser is used to vaporize the prostate.

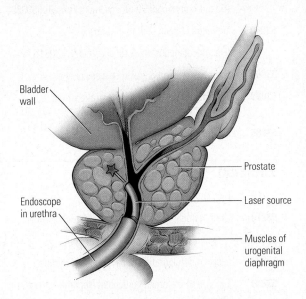

Bladder wall

Prostate

Laser source

Endoscope in urethra

Muscles of urogenital diaphragm

52630   Transurethral resection; residual or regrowth of obstructive prostate tissue including control of postoperative bleeding, complete (vasectomy, meatotomy, cystourethroscopy, urethral calibration and/or dilation, and internal urethrotomy are included)

➔ *CPT Changes: An Insider's View* 2009

➔ *CPT Assistant* Apr 01:4

(For resection of residual prostate tissue performed within the postoperative period of a related procedure performed by the same physician, append modifier 78)

(For transurethral waterjet ablation of prostate, use 0421T)

52640   of postoperative bladder neck contracture
➔ *CPT Assistant* Apr 01:4

52647   Laser coagulation of prostate, including control of postoperative bleeding, complete (vasectomy, meatotomy, cystourethroscopy, urethral calibration and/or dilation, and internal urethrotomy are included if performed)

➔ *CPT Changes: An Insider's View* 2006

➔ *CPT Assistant* Nov 97:20, Mar 98:11, Apr 01:4, Nov 06:21

52648   Laser vaporization of prostate, including control of postoperative bleeding, complete (vasectomy, meatotomy, cystourethroscopy, urethral calibration and/or dilation, internal urethrotomy and transurethral resection of prostate are included if performed)

➔ *CPT Changes: An Insider's View* 2006

➔ *CPT Assistant* Mar 98:11, Apr 01:5, Jul 05:15, Nov 06:21, Jun 15:5

52649   Laser enucleation of the prostate with morcellation, including control of postoperative bleeding, complete (vasectomy, meatotomy, cystourethroscopy, urethral calibration and/or dilation, internal urethrotomy and transurethral resection of prostate are included if performed)

➔ *CPT Changes: An Insider's View* 2008

➔ *CPT Assistant* Jun 15:5

(Do not report 52649 in conjunction with 52000, 52276, 52281, 52601, 52647, 52648, 53020, 55250)

52700   Transurethral drainage of prostatic abscess
➔ *CPT Assistant* Apr 01:4

(For litholapaxy, use 52317, 52318)

Urethra

(For endoscopy, see cystoscopy, urethroscopy, cystourethroscopy, 52000-52700)

(For injection procedure for urethrocystography, see 51600-51610)

Incision

53000   Urethrotomy or urethrostomy, external (separate procedure); pendulous urethra

53010   perineal urethra, external

53020   Meatotomy, cutting of meatus (separate procedure); except infant

53025   infant

(Do not report modifier 63 in conjunction with 53025)

53040   Drainage of deep periurethral abscess

(For subcutaneous abscess, see 10060, 10061)

53060   Drainage of Skene's gland abscess or cyst

53080   Drainage of perineal urinary extravasation; uncomplicated (separate procedure)

53085   complicated

Excision

53200   Biopsy of urethra

53210   Urethrectomy, total, including cystostomy; female

53215   male

53220   Excision or fulguration of carcinoma of urethra

53230   Excision of urethral diverticulum (separate procedure); female

53235   male

53240   Marsupialization of urethral diverticulum, male or female

53250   Excision of bulbourethral gland (Cowper's gland)

53260   Excision or fulguration; urethral polyp(s), distal urethra

(For endoscopic approach, see 52214, 52224)

53265   urethral caruncle

53270   Skene's glands

53275   urethral prolapse

Repair

(For hypospadias, see 54300-54352)

53400   Urethroplasty; first stage, for fistula, diverticulum, or stricture (eg, Johannsen type)

53405   second stage (formation of urethra), including urinary diversion

53410   Urethroplasty, 1-stage reconstruction of male anterior urethra

53415   Urethroplasty, transpubic or perineal, 1-stage, for reconstruction or repair of prostatic or membranous urethra

53420   Urethroplasty, 2-stage reconstruction or repair of prostatic or membranous urethra; first stage

53425   second stage

53430   Urethroplasty, reconstruction of female urethra

53431   Urethroplasty with tubularization of posterior urethra and/or lower bladder for incontinence (eg, Tenago, Leadbetter procedure)
➲ *CPT Changes: An Insider's View* 2002

53440   Sling operation for correction of male urinary incontinence (eg, fascia or synthetic)
➲ *CPT Changes: An Insider's View* 2003
➲ *CPT Assistant* Aug 20:6

53442   Removal or revision of sling for male urinary incontinence (eg, fascia or synthetic)
➲ *CPT Changes: An Insider's View* 2003
➲ *CPT Assistant* Aug 20:6

53444   Insertion of tandem cuff (dual cuff)
➲ *CPT Changes: An Insider's View* 2002

53445   Insertion of inflatable urethral/bladder neck sphincter, including placement of pump, reservoir, and cuff
➲ *CPT Changes: An Insider's View* 2002
➲ *CPT Assistant* Aug 20:6

53446   Removal of inflatable urethral/bladder neck sphincter, including pump, reservoir, and cuff
➲ *CPT Changes: An Insider's View* 2002
➲ *CPT Assistant* Aug 20:6

53447   Removal and replacement of inflatable urethral/bladder neck sphincter including pump, reservoir, and cuff at the same operative session
➲ *CPT Changes: An Insider's View* 2002
➲ *CPT Assistant* Aug 20:6

53448   Removal and replacement of inflatable urethral/bladder neck sphincter including pump, reservoir, and cuff through an infected field at the same operative session including irrigation and debridement of infected tissue
➲ *CPT Changes: An Insider's View* 2002
➲ *CPT Assistant* Aug 20:6

(Do not report 11042, 11043 in addition to 53448)

53449   Repair of inflatable urethral/bladder neck sphincter, including pump, reservoir, and cuff
➲ *CPT Changes: An Insider's View* 2002
➲ *CPT Assistant* Aug 20:6

53450   Urethromeatoplasty, with mucosal advancement
➲ *CPT Assistant* Sep 12:16

(For meatotomy, see 53020, 53025)

53451 Periurethral transperineal adjustable balloon continence device; bilateral insertion, including cystourethroscopy and imaging guidance
➲ *CPT Changes: An Insider's View* 2022
➲ *CPT Assistant* Dec 21:11, 21, Mar 22:12

(Do not report 53451 in conjunction with 52000, 53452, 53453, 53454, 76000)

53452 unilateral insertion, including cystourethroscopy and imaging guidance
➲ *CPT Changes: An Insider's View* 2022
➲ *CPT Assistant* Dec 21:11, Mar 22:12

(Do not report 53452 in conjunction with 52000, 53451, 53453, 53454, 76000)

53453 removal, each balloon
➲ *CPT Changes: An Insider's View* 2022
➲ *CPT Assistant* Dec 21:11, Mar 22:12

(Do not report 53453 in conjunction with 53451, 53452, 53454)

53454 percutaneous adjustment of balloon(s) fluid volume
➲ *CPT Changes: An Insider's View* 2022
➲ *CPT Assistant* Dec 21:11, Mar 22:12

(Do not report 53454 in conjunction with 53451, 53452, 53453)

(Report 53454 only once per patient encounter)

53460 Urethromeatoplasty, with partial excision of distal urethral segment (Richardson type procedure)

53500 Urethrolysis, transvaginal, secondary, open, including cystourethroscopy (eg, postsurgical obstruction, scarring)
➲ *CPT Changes: An Insider's View* 2004
➲ *CPT Assistant* Sep 04:11

(For urethrolysis by retropubic approach, use 53899)

(Do not report 53500 in conjunction with 52000)

53502 Urethrorrhaphy, suture of urethral wound or injury, female

53505 Urethrorrhaphy, suture of urethral wound or injury; penile

53510 perineal

53515 prostatomembranous

53520 Closure of urethrostomy or urethrocutaneous fistula, male (separate procedure)

(For closure of urethrovaginal fistula, use 57310)

(For closure of urethrorectal fistula, see 45820, 45825)

Manipulation

(For radiological supervision and interpretation, use 74485)

53600 Dilation of urethral stricture by passage of sound or urethral dilator, male; initial

53601 subsequent

53605 Dilation of urethral stricture or vesical neck by passage of sound or urethral dilator, male, general or conduction (spinal) anesthesia

(For dilation of urethral stricture, male, performed under local anesthesia, see 53600, 53601, 53620, 53621)

53620 Dilation of urethral stricture by passage of filiform and follower, male; initial

53621 subsequent

53660 Dilation of female urethra including suppository and/or instillation; initial

53661 subsequent

53665 Dilation of female urethra, general or conduction (spinal) anesthesia

(For urethral catheterization, see 51701-51703)

(For dilation of urethra performed under local anesthesia, female, see 53660, 53661)

Other Procedures

(For 2 or 3 glass urinalysis, use 81020)

53850 Transurethral destruction of prostate tissue; by microwave thermotherapy
➲ *CPT Assistant* Nov 97:20, Apr 01:6, Feb 10:7, Jun 15:5, Nov 18:10

53852 by radiofrequency thermotherapy
➲ *CPT Assistant* Nov 97:20, Apr 01:6, Jun 15:5, Nov 18:10

53854 by radiofrequency generated water vapor thermotherapy
➲ *CPT Changes: An Insider's View* 2019
➲ *CPT Assistant* Nov 18:10

(For transurethral ablation of malignant prostate tissue by high-energy water vapor thermotherapy, including intraoperative imaging and needle guidance, use 0582T)

53855 Insertion of a temporary prostatic urethral stent, including urethral measurement

➜ *CPT Changes: An Insider's View* 2010

➜ *CPT Assistant* Feb 10:7, Nov 18:10

(For insertion of permanent urethral stent, use 52282)

▶(For insertion of prostatic urethral scaffold, use 0941T)◀

Temporary Prostatic Urethral Stent Insertion
53855

A temporary prostatic urethral stent is inserted.

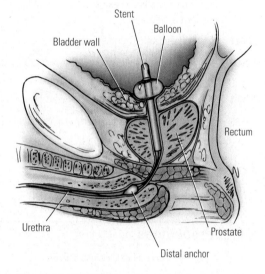

Stent

Balloon

Bladder wall

Rectum

Urethra

Prostate

Distal anchor

53860 Transurethral radiofrequency micro-remodeling of the female bladder neck and proximal urethra for stress urinary incontinence

➜ *CPT Changes: An Insider's View* 2011

● **53865** Cystourethroscopy with insertion of temporary device for ischemic remodeling (ie, pressure necrosis) of bladder neck and prostate

➜ *CPT Changes: An Insider's View* 2025

▶(For insertion of a permanent urethral stent, use 52282)◀

▶(For insertion of a temporary prostatic urethral stent without cystourethroscopy, including urethral measurement, use 53855)◀

▶(For catheterization with removal of temporary device for ischemic remodeling of bladder neck and prostate, use 53866)◀

● **53866** Catheterization with removal of temporary device for ischemic remodeling (ie, pressure necrosis) of bladder neck and prostate

➜ *CPT Changes: An Insider's View* 2025

▶(For cystourethroscopy with removal of temporary device for ischemic remodeling of bladder neck and prostate, use 52310)◀

▶(For insertion of temporary device for ischemic remodeling of bladder neck and prostate, use 53865)◀

53899 Unlisted procedure, urinary system

➜ *CPT Assistant* Aug 04:12, Sep 04:11, Oct 05:18, 23-24, Feb 06:14, May 10:10, Mar 15:9, Jun 15:5, Aug 19:10, Dec 23:41

➜ *Clinical Examples in Radiology* Summer 06:1, 3

Surgery

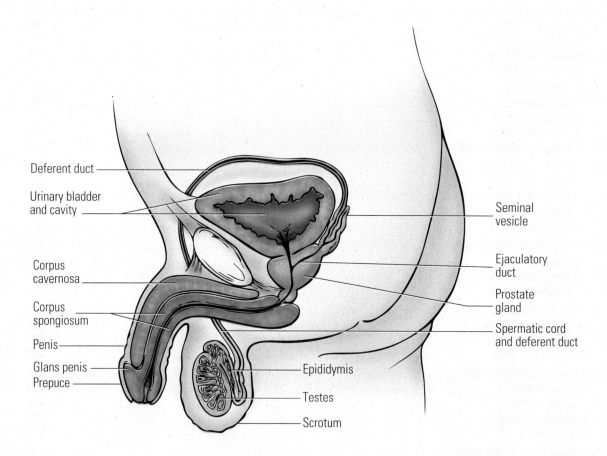

Male Genital System

Male Genital System

Penis

Incision

(For abdominal perineal gangrene debridement, see 11004-11006)

54000 Slitting of prepuce, dorsal or lateral (separate procedure); newborn

(Do not report modifier 63 in conjunction with 54000)

54001 except newborn

54015 Incision and drainage of penis, deep

(For skin and subcutaneous abscess, see 10060-10160)

Destruction

54050 Destruction of lesion(s), penis (eg, condyloma, papilloma, molluscum contagiosum, herpetic vesicle), simple; chemical

54055 electrodesiccation

54056 cryosurgery

54057 laser surgery

54060 surgical excision

54065 Destruction of lesion(s), penis (eg, condyloma, papilloma, molluscum contagiosum, herpetic vesicle), extensive (eg, laser surgery, electrosurgery, cryosurgery, chemosurgery)
➡ *CPT Changes: An Insider's View* 2002

(For destruction or excision of other lesions, see **Integumentary System**)

Excision

54100 Biopsy of penis; (separate procedure)
➡ *CPT Changes: An Insider's View* 2000
➡ *CPT Assistant* Nov 99:26

54105 deep structures

54110 Excision of penile plaque (Peyronie disease);

54111 with graft to 5 cm in length
➡ *CPT Assistant* Aug 99:5

54112 with graft greater than 5 cm in length

54115 Removal foreign body from deep penile tissue (eg, plastic implant)

54120 Amputation of penis; partial

54125 complete

54130 Amputation of penis, radical; with bilateral inguinofemoral lymphadenectomy

54135 in continuity with bilateral pelvic lymphadenectomy, including external iliac, hypogastric and obturator nodes

(For lymphadenectomy [separate procedure], see 38760-38770)

54150 Circumcision, using clamp or other device with regional dorsal penile or ring block
➡ *CPT Changes: An Insider's View* 2007
➡ *CPT Assistant* Sep 96:11, May 98:11, Apr 03:27, Aug 03:6, May 07:10, Jul 07:5

(Do not report modifier 63 in conjunction with 54150)

(Report 54150 with modifier 52 when performed without dorsal penile or ring block)

54160 Circumcision, surgical excision other than clamp, device, or dorsal slit; neonate (28 days of age or less)
➡ *CPT Changes: An Insider's View* 2007
➡ *CPT Assistant* Sep 96:11, May 98:11, May 07:10, Jul 07:5

(Do not report modifier 63 in conjunction with 54160)

54161 older than 28 days of age
➡ *CPT Changes: An Insider's View* 2007
➡ *CPT Assistant* Sep 96:11, Dec 96:10, May 98:11, Jul 07:5

54162 Lysis or excision of penile post-circumcision adhesions
➡ *CPT Changes: An Insider's View* 2002

54163 Repair incomplete circumcision
➡ *CPT Changes: An Insider's View* 2002

54164 Frenulotomy of penis
➡ *CPT Changes: An Insider's View* 2002

(Do not report 54164 with circumcision codes 54150-54161, 54162, 54163)

Introduction

54200 Injection procedure for Peyronie disease;

54205 with surgical exposure of plaque

54220 Irrigation of corpora cavernosa for priapism

54230 Injection procedure for corpora cavernosography

(For radiological supervision and interpretation, use 74445)

54231 Dynamic cavernosometry, including intracavernosal injection of vasoactive drugs (eg, papaverine, phentolamine)

54235 Injection of corpora cavernosa with pharmacologic agent(s) (eg, papaverine, phentolamine)
➡ *CPT Assistant* Sep 96:10

54240 Penile plethysmography

54250 Nocturnal penile tumescence and/or rigidity test

Repair

(For other urethroplasties, see 53400-53430)

(For penile revascularization, use 37788)

54300 Plastic operation of penis for straightening of chordee (eg, hypospadias), with or without mobilization of urethra
➔ *CPT Assistant* Dec 14:16

54304 Plastic operation on penis for correction of chordee or for first stage hypospadias repair with or without transplantation of prepuce and/or skin flaps

54308 Urethroplasty for second stage hypospadias repair (including urinary diversion); less than 3 cm

54312   greater than 3 cm

54316 Urethroplasty for second stage hypospadias repair (including urinary diversion) with free skin graft obtained from site other than genitalia

54318 Urethroplasty for third stage hypospadias repair to release penis from scrotum (eg, third stage Cecil repair)

54322 1-stage distal hypospadias repair (with or without chordee or circumcision); with simple meatal advancement (eg, Magpi, V-flap)

54324   with urethroplasty by local skin flaps (eg, flip-flap, prepucial flap)

54326   with urethroplasty by local skin flaps and mobilization of urethra

54328   with extensive dissection to correct chordee and urethroplasty with local skin flaps, skin graft patch, and/or island flap
➔ *CPT Assistant* Oct 04:15

(For urethroplasty and straightening of chordee, use 54308)

54332 1-stage proximal penile or penoscrotal hypospadias repair requiring extensive dissection to correct chordee and urethroplasty by use of skin graft tube and/or island flap
➔ *CPT Assistant* Mar 04:11, Sep 04:12

54336 1-stage perineal hypospadias repair requiring extensive dissection to correct chordee and urethroplasty by use of skin graft tube and/or island flap
➔ *CPT Assistant* Oct 04:15

54340 Repair of hypospadias complication(s) (ie, fistula, stricture, diverticula); by closure, incision, or excision, simple
➔ *CPT Changes: An Insider's View* 2022

54344   requiring mobilization of skin flaps and urethroplasty with flap or patch graft
➔ *CPT Changes: An Insider's View* 2022

54348   requiring extensive dissection, and urethroplasty with flap, patch or tubed graft (including urinary diversion, when performed)
➔ *CPT Changes: An Insider's View* 2022

54352 Revision of prior hypospadias repair requiring extensive dissection and excision of previously constructed structures including re-release of chordee and reconstruction of urethra and penis by use of local skin as grafts and island flaps and skin brought in as flaps or grafts
➔ *CPT Changes: An Insider's View* 2022

(Do not report 54352 in conjunction with 15275, 15574, 15740, 53235, 53410, 54300, 54336, 54340, 54344, 54348, 54360)

54360 Plastic operation on penis to correct angulation

54380 Plastic operation on penis for epispadias distal to external sphincter;

54385   with incontinence

54390   with exstrophy of bladder

54400 Insertion of penile prosthesis; non-inflatable (semi-rigid)

54401   inflatable (self-contained)

(For removal or replacement of penile prosthesis, see 54415, 54416)

54405 Insertion of multi-component, inflatable penile prosthesis, including placement of pump, cylinders, and reservoir
➔ *CPT Changes: An Insider's View* 2002

(For reduced services, report 54405 with modifier 52)

54406 Removal of all components of a multi-component, inflatable penile prosthesis without replacement of prosthesis
➔ *CPT Changes: An Insider's View* 2002

(For reduced services, report 54406 with modifier 52)

54408 Repair of component(s) of a multi-component, inflatable penile prosthesis
➔ *CPT Changes: An Insider's View* 2002

54410 Removal and replacement of all component(s) of a multi-component, inflatable penile prosthesis at the same operative session
➔ *CPT Changes: An Insider's View* 2002

54411 Removal and replacement of all components of a multi-component inflatable penile prosthesis through an infected field at the same operative session, including irrigation and debridement of infected tissue
➔ *CPT Changes: An Insider's View* 2002

(For reduced services, report 54411 with modifier 52)

(Do not report 11042, 11043 in addition to 54411)

54415   Removal of non-inflatable (semi-rigid) or inflatable (self-contained) penile prosthesis, without replacement of prosthesis

➔ *CPT Changes: An Insider's View* 2002

54416   Removal and replacement of non-inflatable (semi-rigid) or inflatable (self-contained) penile prosthesis at the same operative session

➔ *CPT Changes: An Insider's View* 2002

54417   Removal and replacement of non-inflatable (semi-rigid) or inflatable (self-contained) penile prosthesis through an infected field at the same operative session, including irrigation and debridement of infected tissue

➔ *CPT Changes: An Insider's View* 2002

(Do not report 11042, 11043 in addition to 54417)

54420   Corpora cavernosa-saphenous vein shunt (priapism operation), unilateral or bilateral

54430   Corpora cavernosa-corpus spongiosum shunt (priapism operation), unilateral or bilateral

54435   Corpora cavernosa-glans penis fistulization (eg, biopsy needle, Winter procedure, rongeur, or punch) for priapism

54437   Repair of traumatic corporeal tear(s)

➔ *CPT Changes: An Insider's View* 2016

(For repair of urethra, see 53410, 53415)

▶(54438 has been deleted)◀

54440   Plastic operation of penis for injury

Manipulation

54450   Foreskin manipulation including lysis of preputial adhesions and stretching

Testis

Excision

(For abdominal perineal gangrene debridement, see 11004-11006)

54500   Biopsy of testis, needle (separate procedure)

➔ *Clinical Examples in Radiology* Winter 17:5

(For fine needle aspiration biopsy, see 10004, 10005, 10006, 10007, 10008, 10009, 10010, 10011, 10012, 10021)

(For evaluation of fine needle aspirate, see 88172, 88173)

54505   Biopsy of testis, incisional (separate procedure)

➔ *CPT Assistant* Oct 01:8

(For bilateral procedure, report 54505 with modifier 50)

(When combined with vasogram, seminal vesiculogram, or epididymogram, use 55300)

54512   Excision of extraparenchymal lesion of testis

➔ *CPT Changes: An Insider's View* 2001

➔ *CPT Assistant* Oct 01:8, Aug 05:13

54520   Orchiectomy, simple (including subcapsular), with or without testicular prosthesis, scrotal or inguinal approach

➔ *CPT Assistant* Winter 94:13, Oct 01:8, Mar 04:3

(For bilateral procedure, report 54520 with modifier 50)

54522   Orchiectomy, partial

➔ *CPT Changes: An Insider's View* 2001
➔ *CPT Assistant* Oct 01:8

54530   Orchiectomy, radical, for tumor; inguinal approach

➔ *CPT Assistant* Oct 01:8

54535   with abdominal exploration

➔ *CPT Assistant* Oct 01:8

(For orchiectomy with repair of hernia, see 49505 or 49507 and 54520)

(For radical retroperitoneal lymphadenectomy, use 38780)

Exploration

54550   Exploration for undescended testis (inguinal or scrotal area)

➔ *CPT Assistant* Oct 01:8, Mar 17:10

(For bilateral procedure, report 54550 with modifier 50)

54560   Exploration for undescended testis with abdominal exploration

➔ *CPT Assistant* Oct 01:8

(For bilateral procedure, report 54560 with modifier 50)

Repair

54600   Reduction of torsion of testis, surgical, with or without fixation of contralateral testis

➔ *CPT Assistant* Aug 05:13

54620   Fixation of contralateral testis (separate procedure)

54640   Orchiopexy, inguinal or scrotal approach

➔ *CPT Changes: An Insider's View* 2020
➔ *CPT Assistant* Oct 01:8, Jan 04:27, Mar 04:10, Jun 08:4, Mar 17:11

(For bilateral procedure, report 54640 with modifier 50)

(For inguinal hernia repair performed in conjunction with inguinal orchiopexy, see 49495-49525)

54650   Orchiopexy, abdominal approach, for intra-abdominal testis (eg, Fowler-Stephens)

➔ *CPT Changes: An Insider's View* 2000
➔ *CPT Assistant* Nov 99:26, May 00:4, Oct 01:8

(For laparoscopic approach, use 54692)

54660	Insertion of testicular prosthesis (separate procedure)
	➔ *CPT Assistant* Oct 01:8

(For bilateral procedure, report 54660 with modifier 50)

54670	Suture or repair of testicular injury
	➔ *CPT Assistant* Oct 01:8

54680	Transplantation of testis(es) to thigh (because of scrotal destruction)
	➔ *CPT Assistant* Oct 01:8

Laparoscopy

Surgical laparoscopy always includes diagnostic laparoscopy. To report a diagnostic laparoscopy (peritoneoscopy) (separate procedure), use 49320.

54690	Laparoscopy, surgical; orchiectomy
	➔ *CPT Changes: An Insider's View* 2000
	➔ *CPT Assistant* Nov 99:26, Mar 00:5, Oct 01:8

54692	orchiopexy for intra-abdominal testis
	➔ *CPT Changes: An Insider's View* 2000
	➔ *CPT Assistant* Nov 99:27, May 00:4, Oct 01:8

Laparoscopic Orchiopexy
54692

Surgical fixation of an undescended testis in the scrotum under laparoscopic guidance

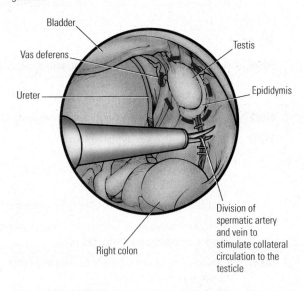

Bladder
Vas deferens
Ureter
Testis
Epididymis
Right colon
Division of spermatic artery and vein to stimulate collateral circulation to the testicle

54699	Unlisted laparoscopy procedure, testis
	➔ *CPT Changes: An Insider's View* 2000
	➔ *CPT Assistant* Nov 99:27, Mar 00:9

Epididymis

Incision

54700	Incision and drainage of epididymis, testis and/or scrotal space (eg, abscess or hematoma)
	➔ *CPT Assistant* Oct 01:8

(For debridement of necrotizing soft tissue infection of external genitalia, see 11004-11006)

Excision

54800	Biopsy of epididymis, needle
	➔ *CPT Assistant* Oct 01:8
	➔ *Clinical Examples in Radiology* Winter 17:5

(For fine needle aspiration biopsy, see 10004, 10005, 10006, 10007, 10008, 10009, 10010, 10011, 10012, 10021)

(For evaluation of fine needle aspirate, see 88172, 88173)

54830	Excision of local lesion of epididymis
	➔ *CPT Assistant* Oct 01:8

54840	Excision of spermatocele, with or without epididymectomy
	➔ *CPT Assistant* Oct 01:8

54860	Epididymectomy; unilateral
54861	bilateral

Exploration

54865	Exploration of epididymis, with or without biopsy
	➔ *CPT Changes: An Insider's View* 2007

Repair

54900	Epididymovasostomy, anastomosis of epididymis to vas deferens; unilateral
	➔ *CPT Assistant* Nov 98:16, Jun 04:11

54901	bilateral
	➔ *CPT Assistant* Nov 98:16, Jun 04:11

(For operating microscope, use 69990)

Tunica Vaginalis

Incision

55000	Puncture aspiration of hydrocele, tunica vaginalis, with or without injection of medication

Excision

55040   Excision of hydrocele; unilateral
➔ *CPT Assistant* Jun 08:4, Nov 17:10

55041   bilateral

(With hernia repair, see 49495-49501)

Repair

55060   Repair of tunica vaginalis hydrocele (Bottle type)
➔ *CPT Assistant* Nov 14:14

Scrotum

Incision

55100   Drainage of scrotal wall abscess

(See also 54700)

(For debridement of necrotizing soft tissue infection of external genitalia, see 11004-11006)

55110   Scrotal exploration

55120   Removal of foreign body in scrotum

Excision

(For excision of local lesion of skin of scrotum, see **Integumentary System**)

55150   Resection of scrotum

Repair

55175   Scrotoplasty; simple
➔ *CPT Assistant* Dec 14:16

55180   complicated

Vas Deferens

Incision

55200   Vasotomy, cannulization with or without incision of vas, unilateral or bilateral (separate procedure)

Excision

55250   Vasectomy, unilateral or bilateral (separate procedure), including postoperative semen examination(s)
➔ *CPT Assistant* Jun 98:10, Jul 98:10, Apr 21:13

Introduction

55300   Vasotomy for vasograms, seminal vesiculograms, or epididymograms, unilateral or bilateral

(For radiological supervision and interpretation, use 74440)

(When combined with biopsy of testis, see 54505 and use modifier 51)

Repair

55400   Vasovasostomy, vasovasorrhaphy
➔ *CPT Assistant* Nov 98:16, Oct 01:8, Jun 04:11

(For bilateral procedure, report 55400 with modifier 50)

(For operating microscope, use 69990)

Spermatic Cord

Excision

55500   Excision of hydrocele of spermatic cord, unilateral (separate procedure)
➔ *CPT Assistant* Oct 01:8

55520   Excision of lesion of spermatic cord (separate procedure)
➔ *CPT Assistant* Sep 00:10, Oct 01:8

55530   Excision of varicocele or ligation of spermatic veins for varicocele; (separate procedure)
➔ *CPT Assistant* Oct 01:8

55535   abdominal approach
➔ *CPT Assistant* Oct 01:8

55540   with hernia repair
➔ *CPT Assistant* Oct 01:8

Laparoscopy

Surgical laparoscopy always includes diagnostic laparoscopy. To report a diagnostic laparoscopy (peritoneoscopy) (separate procedure), use 49320.

55550   Laparoscopy, surgical, with ligation of spermatic veins for varicocele
➔ *CPT Changes: An Insider's View* 2000
➔ *CPT Assistant* Nov 99:27, Mar 00:9, Oct 01:8

55559   Unlisted laparoscopy procedure, spermatic cord
➔ *CPT Changes: An Insider's View* 2000
➔ *CPT Assistant* Nov 99:27, Mar 00:9

Seminal Vesicles

Incision

55600   Vesiculotomy;

(For bilateral procedure, report 55600 with modifier 50)

55605   complicated

Excision

55650 Vesiculectomy, any approach

(For bilateral procedure, report 55650 with modifier 50)

55680 Excision of Mullerian duct cyst

(For injection procedure, see 52010, 55300)

Prostate

Incision

55700 Biopsy, prostate; needle or punch, single or multiple, any approach
> *CPT Assistant* May 96:3, Nov 10:5, Jul 18:11, Jul 22:20
> *Clinical Examples in Radiology* Spring 15:10, Winter 17:5

(If imaging guidance is performed, see 76942, 77002, 77012, 77021)

(For fine needle aspiration biopsy, see 10004, 10005, 10006, 10007, 10008, 10009, 10010, 10011, 10012, 10021)

(For evaluation of fine needle aspirate, see 88172, 88173)

(For transperineal stereotactic template guided saturation prostate biopsies, use 55706)

55705 incisional, any approach

55706 Biopsies, prostate, needle, transperineal, stereotactic template guided saturation sampling, including imaging guidance
> *CPT Changes: An Insider's View* 2009
> *CPT Assistant* Nov 10:5

(Do not report 55706 in conjunction with 55700)

55720 Prostatotomy, external drainage of prostatic abscess, any approach; simple

55725 complicated

(For transurethral drainage, use 52700)

Excision

(For transurethral removal of prostate, see 52601-52640)

(For transurethral destruction of prostate, see 53850-53852)

(For limited pelvic lymphadenectomy for staging [separate procedure], use 38562)

(For independent node dissection, see 38770-38780)

55801 Prostatectomy, perineal, subtotal (including control of postoperative bleeding, vasectomy, meatotomy, urethral calibration and/or dilation, and internal urethrotomy)
> *CPT Assistant* Jun 03:6-7

55810 Prostatectomy, perineal radical;
> *CPT Assistant* Jun 03:7

55812 with lymph node biopsy(s) (limited pelvic lymphadenectomy)

55815 with bilateral pelvic lymphadenectomy, including external iliac, hypogastric and obturator nodes

(If 55815 is carried out on separate days, use 38770 with modifier 50 and 55810)

55821 Prostatectomy (including control of postoperative bleeding, vasectomy, meatotomy, urethral calibration and/or dilation, and internal urethrotomy); suprapubic, subtotal, 1 or 2 stages
> *CPT Assistant* Jun 03:6, Dec 22:8

55831 retropubic, subtotal
> *CPT Assistant* Jun 03:7, Dec 22:8

(For laparoscopy, surgical prostatectomy, simple subtotal, use 55867)

55840 Prostatectomy, retropubic radical, with or without nerve sparing;
> *CPT Assistant* Jun 03:8, Dec 22:8

55842 with lymph node biopsy(s) (limited pelvic lymphadenectomy)
> *CPT Assistant* Jun 03:8, Dec 22:8

55845 with bilateral pelvic lymphadenectomy, including external iliac, hypogastric, and obturator nodes
> *CPT Assistant* Jun 03:8, Dec 22:8

(If 55845 is carried out on separate days, use 38770 with modifier 50 and 55840)

(For laparoscopic retropubic radical prostatectomy, use 55866)

55860 Exposure of prostate, any approach, for insertion of radioactive substance;

(For application of interstitial radioelement, see 77770, 77771, 77772, 77778)

55862 with lymph node biopsy(s) (limited pelvic lymphadenectomy)

55865 with bilateral pelvic lymphadenectomy, including external iliac, hypogastric and obturator nodes

Laparoscopy

Surgical laparoscopy always includes diagnostic laparoscopy. To report a diagnostic laparoscopy (peritoneoscopy) (separate procedure), use 49320.

55866 Laparoscopy, surgical prostatectomy, retropubic radical, including nerve sparing, includes robotic assistance, when performed
> *CPT Changes: An Insider's View* 2003, 2011
> *CPT Assistant* Jun 03:8, Mar 12:10

(For open procedure, use 55840)

(For laparoscopy, surgical prostatectomy, simple subtotal, use 55867)

55867   Laparoscopy, surgical prostatectomy, simple subtotal (including control of postoperative bleeding, vasectomy, meatotomy, urethral calibration and/or dilation, and internal urethrotomy), includes robotic assistance, when performed

→ *CPT Changes: An Insider's View* 2023

→ *CPT Assistant* Dec 22:8

(For open subtotal prostatectomy, see 55821, 55831)

Other Procedures

(For artificial insemination, see 58321, 58322)

55870   Electroejaculation

55873   Cryosurgical ablation of the prostate (includes ultrasonic guidance and monitoring)

→ *CPT Changes: An Insider's View* 2001, 2010

→ *CPT Assistant* Apr 01:4, Sep 02:9, Jun 03:8, Feb 10:7, Sep 15:12, Sep 19:11

55874   Transperineal placement of biodegradable material, peri-prostatic, single or multiple injection(s), including image guidance, when performed

→ *CPT Changes: An Insider's View* 2018

(Do not report 55874 in conjunction with 76942)

55875   Transperineal placement of needles or catheters into prostate for interstitial radioelement application, with or without cystoscopy

→ *CPT Changes: An Insider's View* 2007

→ *CPT Assistant* May 07:1, Apr 09:3

(For placement of needles or catheters into pelvic organs and/or genitalia [except prostate] for interstitial radioelement application, use 55920)

(For interstitial radioelement application, see 77770, 77771, 77772, 77778)

(For ultrasonic guidance for interstitial radioelement application, use 76965)

55876   Placement of interstitial device(s) for radiation therapy guidance (eg, fiducial markers, dosimeter), prostate (via needle, any approach), single or multiple

→ *CPT Changes: An Insider's View* 2007, 2010, 2011

→ *CPT Assistant* May 07:1, Oct 07:1, Feb 10:7, 12, Jun 16:3

(Report supply of device separately)

(For imaging guidance, see 76942, 77002, 77012, 77021)

55880   Ablation of malignant prostate tissue, transrectal, with high intensity–focused ultrasound (HIFU), including ultrasound guidance

→ *CPT Changes: An Insider's View* 2021

→ *CPT Assistant* Sep 21:11

● **55881**   Ablation of prostate tissue, transurethral, using thermal ultrasound, including magnetic resonance imaging guidance for, and monitoring of, tissue ablation;

→ *CPT Changes: An Insider's View* 2025

►(Do not report 55881 in conjunction with 55882)◄

►(For insertion of transurethral ultrasound transducer and ablation of prostate tissue using thermal ultrasound transducer performed by the same physician, use 55882)◄

● **55882**   with insertion of transurethral ultrasound transducer for delivery of thermal ultrasound, including suprapubic tube placement and placement of an endorectal cooling device, when performed

→ *CPT Changes: An Insider's View* 2025

►(Do not report 55882 in conjunction with 55881)◄

►(Do not report 55881, 55882 in conjunction with 51701, 51702, 51721, 72195, 72196, 72197, 77022)◄

55899   Unlisted procedure, male genital system

→ *CPT Assistant* Jun 03:8, May 07:11, Jun 15:5, Jan 17:6, Jun 19:14, Dec 19:12, Aug 20:6

→ *Clinical Examples in Radiology* Spring 06:8-9

Reproductive System Procedures

55920   Placement of needles or catheters into pelvic organs and/or genitalia (except prostate) for subsequent interstitial radioelement application

→ *CPT Changes: An Insider's View* 2008

→ *CPT Assistant* Apr 09:10

(For placement of needles or catheters into prostate, use 55875)

(For insertion of uterine tandems and/or vaginal ovoids for clinical brachytherapy, use 57155)

(For insertion of Heyman capsules for clinical brachytherapy, use 58346)

Intersex Surgery

55970   Intersex surgery; male to female

55980   female to male

Notes

Surgery

The following is a listing of headings and subheadings that appear within the Female Genital System section of the CPT codebook. The subheadings or subsections denoted with asterisks (*) below have special instructions unique to that subsection. Where these are indicated, special notes or guidelines will be presented preceding those procedural terminology listings, referring to that subsection specifically. Note that all code ranges in each subsection are listed as they appear in the subsection, even if the code numbers are out of numerical sequence and/or repeated in the next subsection.

Female Genital System

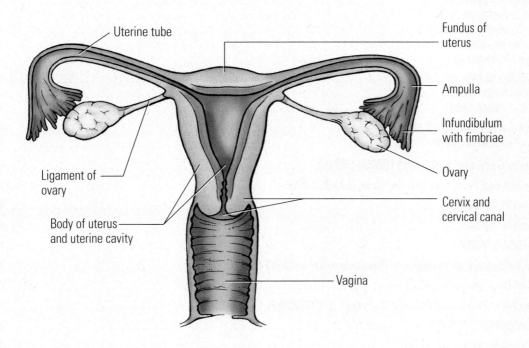

Female Genital System

(For pelvic laparotomy, use 49000)

(For paracentesis, see 49082, 49083, 49084)

(For secondary closure of abdominal wall evisceration or disruption, use 49900)

(For fulguration or excision of lesions, laparoscopic approach, use 58662)

▶(For excision or destruction of endometriomas, open method, use 58999)◀

(For chemotherapy, see 96401-96549)

Vulva, Perineum, and Introitus

Definitions

The following definitions apply to the vulvectomy codes (56620-56640):

A *simple* procedure is the removal of skin and superficial subcutaneous tissues.

A *radical* procedure is the removal of skin and deep subcutaneous tissue.

A *partial* procedure is the removal of less than 80% of the vulvar area.

A *complete* procedure is the removal of greater than 80% of the vulvar area.

Incision

(For incision and drainage of sebaceous cyst, furuncle, or abscess, see 10040, 10060, 10061)

56405 Incision and drainage of vulva or perineal abscess
➔ *CPT Assistant* Jul 19:6

56420 Incision and drainage of Bartholin's gland abscess

(For incision and drainage of Skene's gland abscess or cyst, use 53060)

56440 Marsupialization of Bartholin's gland cyst

56441 Lysis of labial adhesions
➔ *CPT Assistant* Winter 90:7

56442 Hymenotomy, simple incision
➔ *CPT Changes: An Insider's View* 2007

Destruction

56501 Destruction of lesion(s), vulva; simple (eg, laser surgery, electrosurgery, cryosurgery, chemosurgery)
➔ *CPT Changes: An Insider's View* 2002
➔ *CPT Assistant* Aug 19:10

56515 extensive (eg, laser surgery, electrosurgery, cryosurgery, chemosurgery)
➔ *CPT Changes: An Insider's View* 2002
➔ *CPT Assistant* Aug 19:10

(For destruction of Skene's gland cyst or abscess, use 53270)

(For cautery destruction of urethral caruncle, use 53265)

Excision

56605 Biopsy of vulva or perineum (separate procedure); 1 lesion
➔ *CPT Assistant* Sep 00:9, Jun 08:6

+ 56606   each separate additional lesion (List separately in addition to code for primary procedure)

(Use 56606 in conjunction with 56605)

(For excision of local lesion, see 11420-11426, 11620-11626)

56620 Vulvectomy simple; partial
➔ *CPT Assistant* Dec 13:14

56625   complete

(For skin graft, see 15002 et seq)

56630 Vulvectomy, radical, partial;

(For skin graft, if used, see 15004-15005, 15120, 15121, 15240, 15241)

56631   with unilateral inguinofemoral lymphadenectomy

56632   with bilateral inguinofemoral lymphadenectomy

(For partial radical vulvectomy with inguinofemoral lymph node biopsy without complete inguinofemoral lymphadenectomy, use 56630 in conjunction with 38531)

56633 Vulvectomy, radical, complete;

56634   with unilateral inguinofemoral lymphadenectomy

56637   with bilateral inguinofemoral lymphadenectomy

(For complete radical vulvectomy with inguinofemoral lymph node biopsy without complete inguinofemoral lymphadenectomy, use 56633 in conjunction with 38531)

56640 Vulvectomy, radical, complete, with inguinofemoral, iliac, and pelvic lymphadenectomy

(For bilateral procedure, report 56640 with modifier 50)

(For lymphadenectomy, see 38760-38780)

56700 Partial hymenectomy or revision of hymenal ring

56740 Excision of Bartholin's gland or cyst

(For excision of Skene's gland, use 53270)

(For excision of urethral caruncle, use 53265)

(For excision or fulguration of urethral carcinoma, use 53220)

(For excision or marsupialization of urethral diverticulum, see 53230, 53240)

Repair

(For repair of urethra for mucosal prolapse, use 53275)

56800 Plastic repair of introitus

56805 Clitoroplasty for intersex state

56810 Perineoplasty, repair of perineum, nonobstetrical (separate procedure)

(See also 56800)

(For repair of wounds to genitalia, see 12001-12007, 12041-12047, 13131-13133)

(For repair of recent injury of vagina and perineum, nonobstetrical, use 57210)

(For anal sphincteroplasty, see 46750, 46751)

(For episiorrhaphy, episioperineorrhaphy for recent injury of vulva and/or perineum, nonobstetrical, use 57210)

Endoscopy

56820 Colposcopy of the vulva;
➔ *CPT Changes: An Insider's View* 2003
➔ *CPT Assistant* Feb 03:5

56821 with biopsy(s)
➔ *CPT Changes: An Insider's View* 2003
➔ *CPT Assistant* Feb 03:5, Jun 03:11

(For colposcopic examinations/procedures involving the vagina, see 57420, 57421; cervix, see 57452-57461)

Vagina

Incision

57000 Colpotomy; with exploration
➔ *CPT Assistant* Nov 07:1

57010 with drainage of pelvic abscess

57020 Colpocentesis (separate procedure)

57022 Incision and drainage of vaginal hematoma; obstetrical/ postpartum
➔ *CPT Changes: An Insider's View* 2001, 2002

57023 non-obstetrical (eg, post-trauma, spontaneous bleeding)
➔ *CPT Changes: An Insider's View* 2001

Destruction

57061 Destruction of vaginal lesion(s); simple (eg, laser surgery, electrosurgery, cryosurgery, chemosurgery)
➔ *CPT Changes: An Insider's View* 2002
➔ *CPT Assistant* Apr 96:11

57065 extensive (eg, laser surgery, electrosurgery, cryosurgery, chemosurgery)
➔ *CPT Changes: An Insider's View* 2002
➔ *CPT Assistant* Apr 96:11

Excision

57100 Biopsy of vaginal mucosa; simple (separate procedure)

57105 extensive, requiring suture (including cysts)

57106 Vaginectomy, partial removal of vaginal wall;
➔ *CPT Assistant* Nov 98:17, Oct 99:5

57107 with removal of paravaginal tissue (radical vaginectomy)
➔ *CPT Assistant* Nov 98:17, Oct 99:5

57109 with removal of paravaginal tissue (radical vaginectomy) with bilateral total pelvic lymphadenectomy and para-aortic lymph node sampling (biopsy)
➔ *CPT Assistant* Nov 98:17, Oct 99:5

Vaginectomy, Partial Removal of Vaginal Wall
57106

A specific portion of the upper or lower vaginal wall is excised.

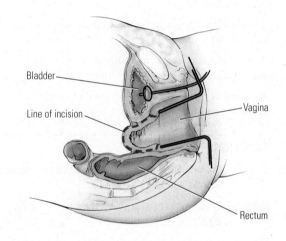

Bladder
Vagina
Line of incision
Rectum

57110 Vaginectomy, complete removal of vaginal wall;
➔ *CPT Assistant* Nov 98:17, Oct 99:5

57111 with removal of paravaginal tissue (radical vaginectomy)
➔ *CPT Assistant* Nov 98:17, Oct 99:5

57120 Colpocleisis (Le Fort type)

57130 Excision of vaginal septum

57135 Excision of vaginal cyst or tumor

Vaginectomy, Complete Removal of Vaginal Wall (Radical Vaginectomy)

57111

Removal of all of the vaginal wall and removal of paravaginal tissue (the highly vascular supporting connective tissue next to the vagina)

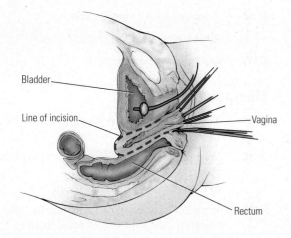

Bladder

Line of incision

Vagina

Rectum

Introduction

57150   Irrigation of vagina and/or application of medicament for treatment of bacterial, parasitic, or fungoid disease

57155   Insertion of uterine tandem and/or vaginal ovoids for clinical brachytherapy

➔ *CPT Changes: An Insider's View* 2002, 2011, 2017

➔ *CPT Assistant* Feb 02:8, Apr 09:3

(For placement of needles or catheters into pelvic organs and/or genitalia [except prostate] for interstitial radioelement application, use 55920)

(For insertion of radioelement sources or ribbons, see 77761-77763, 77770, 77771, 77772)

57156   Insertion of a vaginal radiation afterloading apparatus for clinical brachytherapy

➔ *CPT Changes: An Insider's View* 2011

57160   Fitting and insertion of pessary or other intravaginal support device

➔ *CPT Assistant* Nov 96:9, Oct 98:11, Jun 00:11, May 10:10

57170   Diaphragm or cervical cap fitting with instructions

57180   Introduction of any hemostatic agent or pack for spontaneous or traumatic nonobstetrical vaginal hemorrhage (separate procedure)

➔ *CPT Assistant* Nov 07:1

Repair

(For urethral suspension, Marshall-Marchetti-Krantz type, abdominal approach, see 51840, 51841)

(For laparoscopic suspension, use 51990)

57200   Colporrhaphy, suture of injury of vagina (nonobstetrical)

57210   Colpoperineorrhaphy, suture of injury of vagina and/or perineum (nonobstetrical)

57220   Plastic operation on urethral sphincter, vaginal approach (eg, Kelly urethral plication)

➔ *CPT Assistant* Winter 90:7

57230   Plastic repair of urethrocele

➔ *CPT Assistant* Winter 90:7

57240   Anterior colporrhaphy, repair of cystocele with or without repair of urethrocele, including cystourethroscopy, when performed

➔ *CPT Changes: An Insider's View* 2018

➔ *CPT Assistant* Winter 90:7, Jan 97:3, Jun 02:5, Jun 10:6

(Do not report 57240 in conjunction with 52000)

57250   Posterior colporrhaphy, repair of rectocele with or without perineorrhaphy

➔ *CPT Assistant* Winter 90:7, Jun 02:4, May 11:9

(For repair of rectocele [separate procedure] without posterior colporrhaphy, use 45560)

57260   Combined anteroposterior colporrhaphy, including cystourethroscopy, when performed;

➔ *CPT Changes: An Insider's View* 2018

➔ *CPT Assistant* Jun 02:5, Jun 10:6

(Do not report 57260 in conjunction with 52000)

57265   with enterocele repair

➔ *CPT Changes: An Insider's View* 2018

➔ *CPT Assistant* Jun 02:6, Jun 10:6

(Do not report 57265 in conjunction with 52000)

+ 57267   Insertion of mesh or other prosthesis for repair of pelvic floor defect, each site (anterior, posterior compartment), vaginal approach (List separately in addition to code for primary procedure)

➔ *CPT Changes: An Insider's View* 2005

➔ *CPT Assistant* Jul 05:16, May 11:9, Jan 12:10, Oct 13:15

(Use 57267 in conjunction with 45560, 57240-57265, 57285)

57268   Repair of enterocele, vaginal approach (separate procedure)

➔ *CPT Assistant* Jun 02:6

57270   Repair of enterocele, abdominal approach (separate procedure)

➔ *CPT Assistant* Jun 02:6

57280   Colpopexy, abdominal approach

➔ *CPT Assistant* Jan 97:3, Jun 02:6

57282 Colpopexy, vaginal; extra-peritoneal approach (sacrospinous, iliococcygeus)

➔ *CPT Changes: An Insider's View* 2005

➔ *CPT Assistant* Jan 97:3, Jun 02:6

57283 intra-peritoneal approach (uterosacral, levator myorrhaphy)

➔ *CPT Changes: An Insider's View* 2005

➔ *CPT Assistant* May 11:9

(Do not report 57283 in conjunction with 57556, 58263, 58270, 58280, 58292, 58294)

57284 Paravaginal defect repair (including repair of cystocele, if performed); open abdominal approach

➔ *CPT Changes: An Insider's View* 2008

➔ *CPT Assistant* Jan 97:1, Jun 02:7, Jul 05:16, Jun 10:6

(Do not report 57284 in conjunction with 51840, 51841, 51990, 57240, 57260, 57265, 58152, 58267)

57285 vaginal approach

➔ *CPT Changes: An Insider's View* 2008

➔ *CPT Assistant* Jun 10:6

(Do not report 57285 in conjunction with 51990, 57240, 57260, 57265, 58267)

57287 Removal or revision of sling for stress incontinence (eg, fascia or synthetic)

➔ *CPT Changes: An Insider's View* 2001

➔ *CPT Assistant* Jun 02:7, Nov 07:9

57288 Sling operation for stress incontinence (eg, fascia or synthetic)

➔ *CPT Changes: An Insider's View* 2000

➔ *CPT Assistant* Nov 99:28, May 00:4, Oct 00:7, Apr 02:18, Jun 02:7

(For laparoscopic approach, use 51992)

57289 Pereyra procedure, including anterior colporrhaphy

➔ *CPT Assistant* Jan 97:3, Jun 02:7

57291 Construction of artificial vagina; without graft

57292 with graft

57295 Revision (including removal) of prosthetic vaginal graft; vaginal approach

➔ *CPT Changes: An Insider's View* 2006

57296 open abdominal approach

➔ *CPT Changes: An Insider's View* 2007

(For laparoscopic approach, use 57426)

57300 Closure of rectovaginal fistula; vaginal or transanal approach

➔ *CPT Assistant* Nov 97:21

57305 abdominal approach

➔ *CPT Assistant* Nov 97:21

57307 abdominal approach, with concomitant colostomy

➔ *CPT Assistant* Nov 97:21

57308 transperineal approach, with perineal body reconstruction, with or without levator plication

➔ *CPT Assistant* Nov 97:21

57310 Closure of urethrovaginal fistula;

57311 with bulbocavernosus transplant

57320 Closure of vesicovaginal fistula; vaginal approach

(For concomitant cystostomy, see 51020-51040, 51101, 51102)

57330 transvesical and vaginal approach

(For abdominal approach, use 51900)

57335 Vaginoplasty for intersex state

Manipulation

57400 Dilation of vagina under anesthesia (other than local)

➔ *CPT Changes: An Insider's View* 2009

57410 Pelvic examination under anesthesia (other than local)

➔ *CPT Changes: An Insider's View* 2009

➔ *CPT Assistant* Spring 93:34, Apr 06:1, Nov 07:1

57415 Removal of impacted vaginal foreign body (separate procedure) under anesthesia (other than local)

➔ *CPT Changes: An Insider's View* 2009

(For removal without anesthesia of an impacted vaginal foreign body, use the appropriate E/M code)

Endoscopy/Laparoscopy

57420 Colposcopy of the entire vagina, with cervix if present;

➔ *CPT Changes: An Insider's View* 2003

➔ *CPT Assistant* Feb 03:5, Dec 20:10

57421 with biopsy(s) of vagina/cervix

➔ *CPT Changes: An Insider's View* 2003, 2006

➔ *CPT Assistant* Feb 03:5, Jun 03:11, Jun 06:16, Dec 20:10

(For colposcopic visualization of cervix and adjacent upper vagina, use 57452)

(When reporting colposcopies of multiple sites, use modifier 51 as appropriate. For colposcopic examinations/procedures involving the vulva, see 56820, 56821; cervix, see 57452-57461)

(For computer-aided mapping of cervix uteri during colposcopy, use 57465)

(For endometrial sampling [biopsy] performed in conjunction with colposcopy, use 58110)

57423 Paravaginal defect repair (including repair of cystocele, if performed), laparoscopic approach

➔ *CPT Changes: An Insider's View* 2008

➔ *CPT Assistant* Jun 10:6

(Do not report 57423 in conjunction with 49320, 51840, 51841, 51990, 57240, 57260, 58152, 58267)

★ = Telemedicine   ◀ = Audio-only   ✛ = Add-on code   ✗ = FDA approval pending   # = Resequenced code   ⊘ = Modifier 51 exempt   ➔➔➔ = See p xxi for details

57425 Laparoscopy, surgical, colpopexy (suspension of vaginal apex)

➔ *CPT Changes: An Insider's View* 2004

➔ *CPT Assistant* Jul 19:6

57426 Revision (including removal) of prosthetic vaginal graft, laparoscopic approach

➔ *CPT Changes: An Insider's View* 2010

(For vaginal approach, see 57295. For open abdominal approach, see 57296)

Laparoscopic Revision of Prosthetic Vaginal Graft
57426

Location of prosthetic vaginal graft

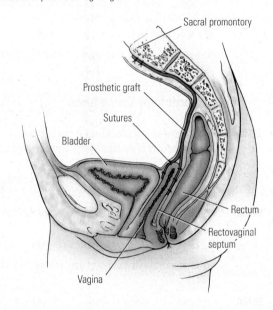

Sacral promontory

Prosthetic graft

Sutures

Bladder

Rectum

Rectovaginal septum

Vagina

Cervix Uteri

Endoscopy

(For colposcopic examinations/procedures involving the vulva, see 56820, 56821; vagina, see 57420, 57421)

57452 Colposcopy of the cervix including upper/adjacent vagina;

➔ *CPT Changes: An Insider's View* 2003

➔ *CPT Assistant* Apr 00:5, Feb 03:5, Jun 03:10, Jul 19:6, Dec 20:10

(Do not report 57452 in addition to 57454-57461)

57454 with biopsy(s) of the cervix and endocervical curettage

➔ *CPT Changes: An Insider's View* 2003

➔ *CPT Assistant* Apr 00:5, Feb 03:5, Jun 03:10, Aug 11:9, Jul 19:6, Dec 20:10

57455 with biopsy(s) of the cervix

➔ *CPT Changes: An Insider's View* 2003

➔ *CPT Assistant* Apr 00:5, Feb 03:5, Jun 03:10, Jul 19:6, Dec 20:10

57456 with endocervical curettage

➔ *CPT Changes: An Insider's View* 2003

➔ *CPT Assistant* Apr 00:5, Jan 03:23, Feb 03:5, Jun 03:10, Jul 19:6, Dec 20:10

57460 with loop electrode biopsy(s) of the cervix

➔ *CPT Changes: An Insider's View* 2003

➔ *CPT Assistant* Apr 00:5, Jan 03:23, Feb 03:5, Jun 03:10, Jul 05:15, Jul 19:6, Dec 20:10

57461 with loop electrode conization of the cervix

➔ *CPT Changes: An Insider's View* 2003

➔ *CPT Assistant* Jan 03:23, Feb 03:5, Jun 03:10, Dec 06:15, Jul 19:6, Dec 20:10

(Do not report 57461 in addition to 57456)

(For computer-aided mapping of cervix uteri during colposcopy, use 57465)

(For endometrial sampling [biopsy] performed in conjunction with colposcopy, use 58110)

+ 57465 Computer-aided mapping of cervix uteri during colposcopy, including optical dynamic spectral imaging and algorithmic quantification of the acetowhitening effect (List separately in addition to code for primary procedure)

➔ *CPT Changes: An Insider's View* 2021

(Use 57465 in conjunction with 57420, 57421, 57452, 57454, 57455, 57456, 57460, 57461)

Excision

(For radical surgical procedures, see 58200-58240)

57500 Biopsy of cervix, single or multiple, or local excision of lesion, with or without fulguration (separate procedure)

➔ *CPT Changes: An Insider's View* 2008

57505 Endocervical curettage (not done as part of a dilation and curettage)

➔ *CPT Assistant* Jul 05:15

57510 Cautery of cervix; electro or thermal

➔ *CPT Changes: An Insider's View* 2002

57511 cryocautery, initial or repeat

57513 laser ablation

57520 Conization of cervix, with or without fulguration, with or without dilation and curettage, with or without repair; cold knife or laser

➔ *CPT Assistant* Apr 00:5

(See also 58120)

57522 loop electrode excision

➔ *CPT Assistant* Apr 00:5, Mar 03:22, Jul 03:15

57530   Trachelectomy (cervicectomy), amputation of cervix (separate procedure)

57531   Radical trachelectomy, with bilateral total pelvic lymphadenectomy and para-aortic lymph node sampling biopsy, with or without removal of tube(s), with or without removal of ovary(s)
➔ *CPT Assistant* Nov 97:21

(For radical abdominal hysterectomy, use 58210)

57540   Excision of cervical stump, abdominal approach;

57545   with pelvic floor repair

57550   Excision of cervical stump, vaginal approach;

57555   with anterior and/or posterior repair

57556   with repair of enterocele

(For insertion of intrauterine device, use 58300)

(For insertion of any hemostatic agent or pack for control of spontaneous non-obstetrical hemorrhage, see 57180)

57558   Dilation and curettage of cervical stump
➔ *CPT Changes: An Insider's View* 2007

Repair

57700   Cerclage of uterine cervix, nonobstetrical

57720   Trachelorrhaphy, plastic repair of uterine cervix, vaginal approach

Manipulation

57800   Dilation of cervical canal, instrumental (separate procedure)

Corpus Uteri

Excision

58100   Endometrial sampling (biopsy) with or without endocervical sampling (biopsy), without cervical dilation, any method (separate procedure)
➔ *CPT Assistant* Oct 21:14

(For endocervical curettage only, use 57505)

(For endometrial sampling [biopsy] performed in conjunction with colposcopy [57420, 57421, 57452-57461], use 58110)

+ 58110   Endometrial sampling (biopsy) performed in conjunction with colposcopy (List separately in addition to code for primary procedure)
➔ *CPT Changes: An Insider's View* 2006
➔ *CPT Assistant* Jun 06:17

(Use 58110 in conjunction with 57420, 57421, 57452-57461)

58120   Dilation and curettage, diagnostic and/or therapeutic (nonobstetrical)
➔ *CPT Assistant* Fall 95:16, Nov 97:21, May 03:19, Oct 21:14, Dec 22:17

(For postpartum hemorrhage, use 59160)

58140   Myomectomy, excision of fibroid tumor(s) of uterus, 1 to 4 intramural myoma(s) with total weight of 250 g or less and/or removal of surface myomas; abdominal approach
➔ *CPT Changes: An Insider's View* 2002, 2003
➔ *CPT Assistant* Feb 03:15, Jun 03:5

58145   vaginal approach

58146   Myomectomy, excision of fibroid tumor(s) of uterus, 5 or more intramural myomas and/or intramural myomas with total weight greater than 250 g, abdominal approach
➔ *CPT Changes: An Insider's View* 2003
➔ *CPT Assistant* Feb 03:15, Jun 03:5

(Do not report 58146 in addition to 58140-58145, 58150-58240)

Hysterectomy Procedures

58150   Total abdominal hysterectomy (corpus and cervix), with or without removal of tube(s), with or without removal of ovary(s);
➔ *CPT Assistant* Dec 96:10, Apr 97:3, Nov 97:21, Sep 00:9, Aug 01:11

58152   with colpo-urethrocystopexy (eg, Marshall-Marchetti-Krantz, Burch)
➔ *CPT Assistant* Jan 97:1, Nov 97:22, Jun 10:6

(For urethrocystopexy without hysterectomy, see 51840, 51841)

58180   Supracervical abdominal hysterectomy (subtotal hysterectomy), with or without removal of tube(s), with or without removal of ovary(s)

58200   Total abdominal hysterectomy, including partial vaginectomy, with para-aortic and pelvic lymph node sampling, with or without removal of tube(s), with or without removal of ovary(s)
➔ *CPT Assistant* Nov 21:8

58210   Radical abdominal hysterectomy, with bilateral total pelvic lymphadenectomy and para-aortic lymph node sampling (biopsy), with or without removal of tube(s), with or without removal of ovary(s)
➔ *CPT Assistant* Fall 92:21, May 12:14, Nov 21:8

(For radical hysterectomy with ovarian transposition, use also 58825)

58240 Pelvic exenteration for gynecologic malignancy, with total abdominal hysterectomy or cervicectomy, with or without removal of tube(s), with or without removal of ovary(s), with removal of bladder and ureteral transplantations, and/or abdominoperineal resection of rectum and colon and colostomy, or any combination thereof
➜ *CPT Assistant* Nov 21:8

(For pelvic exenteration for lower urinary tract or male genital malignancy, use 51597)

58260 Vaginal hysterectomy, for uterus 250 g or less;
➜ *CPT Changes: An Insider's View* 2003
➜ *CPT Assistant* May 11:9

58262 with removal of tube(s), and/or ovary(s)

58263 with removal of tube(s), and/or ovary(s), with repair of enterocele

58267 with colpo-urethrocystopexy (Marshall-Marchetti-Krantz type, Pereyra type) with or without endoscopic control
➜ *CPT Assistant* Jun 10:6

58270 with repair of enterocele

(For repair of enterocele with removal of tubes and/or ovaries, use 58263)

58275 Vaginal hysterectomy, with total or partial vaginectomy;
➜ *CPT Changes: An Insider's View* 2002

58280 with repair of enterocele

58285 Vaginal hysterectomy, radical (Schauta type operation)
➜ *CPT Assistant* Nov 07:1

58290 Vaginal hysterectomy, for uterus greater than 250 g;
➜ *CPT Changes: An Insider's View* 2003

58291 with removal of tube(s) and/or ovary(s)
➜ *CPT Changes: An Insider's View* 2003

58292 with removal of tube(s) and/or ovary(s), with repair of enterocele
➜ *CPT Changes: An Insider's View* 2003

58294 with repair of enterocele
➜ *CPT Changes: An Insider's View* 2003

Introduction

(To report insertion of non-biodegradable drug delivery implant for contraception, use 11981. To report removal of implantable contraceptive capsules with subsequent insertion of non-biodegradable drug delivery implant, use 11976 and 11981)

58300 Insertion of intrauterine device (IUD)
➜ *CPT Assistant* Apr 98:14, Jan 23:31

58301 Removal of intrauterine device (IUD)
➜ *CPT Assistant* Apr 98:14

58321 Artificial insemination; intra-cervical

58322 intra-uterine

58323 Sperm washing for artificial insemination
➜ *CPT Assistant* Jan 98:6

58340 Catheterization and introduction of saline or contrast material for saline infusion sonohysterography (SIS) or hysterosalpingography
➜ *CPT Changes: An Insider's View* 2004
➜ *CPT Assistant* Nov 97:22, Jul 99:8, Mar 09:11
➜ *Clinical Examples in Radiology* Spring 23:32

(For radiological supervision and interpretation of saline infusion sonohysterography, use 76831)

(For radiological supervision and interpretation of hysterosalpingography, use 74740)

58345 Transcervical introduction of fallopian tube catheter for diagnosis and/or re-establishing patency (any method), with or without hysterosalpingography
➜ *CPT Assistant* Nov 97:22, Mar 09:11

(For radiological supervision and interpretation, use 74742)

58346 Insertion of Heyman capsules for clinical brachytherapy
➜ *CPT Changes: An Insider's View* 2002
➜ *CPT Assistant* Feb 02:8, Apr 09:3

(For placement of needles or catheters into pelvic organs and/or genitalia [except prostate] for interstitial radioelement application, use 55920)

(For insertion of radioelement sources or ribbons, see 77761-77763, 77770, 77771, 77772)

58350 Chromotubation of oviduct, including materials
➜ *CPT Assistant* May 02:19, Dec 08:7

(To report the supply of any materials, use 99070)

58353 Code is out of numerical sequence. See 58578-58600

58356 Code is out of numerical sequence. See 58578-58600

Repair

58400 Uterine suspension, with or without shortening of round ligaments, with or without shortening of sacrouterine ligaments; (separate procedure)

58410 with presacral sympathectomy
➜ *CPT Assistant* Mar 07:9

(For anastomosis of tubes to uterus, use 58752)

58520 Hysterorrhaphy, repair of ruptured uterus (nonobstetrical)

58540 Hysteroplasty, repair of uterine anomaly (Strassman type)

(For closure of vesicouterine fistula, use 51920)

Laparoscopy/Hysteroscopy

Surgical laparoscopy always includes diagnostic laparoscopy. To report a diagnostic laparoscopy (peritoneoscopy) (separate procedure), use 49320. To report a diagnostic hysteroscopy (separate procedure), use 58555.

\# **58674** Laparoscopy, surgical, ablation of uterine fibroid(s) including intraoperative ultrasound guidance and monitoring, radiofrequency

➡️ *CPT Changes: An Insider's View* 2017

➡️ *CPT Assistant* Feb 17:14, Apr 17:7, Dec 23:42, Feb 24:21

(Do not report 58674 in conjunction with 49320, 58541-58554, 58570, 58571, 58572, 58573, 58580, 76998)

(For transcervical radiofrequency ablation of uterine fibroid[s], including intraoperative ultrasound guidance and monitoring, use 58580)

58541 Laparoscopy, surgical, supracervical hysterectomy, for uterus 250 g or less;

➡️ *CPT Changes: An Insider's View* 2007

➡️ *CPT Assistant* Nov 07:1, Apr 17:7, Jul 19:6, Aug 21:8-9

58542 with removal of tube(s) and/or ovary(s)

➡️ *CPT Changes: An Insider's View* 2007

➡️ *CPT Assistant* Nov 07:1, Apr 17:7, Jul 19:6, Aug 21:8-9

(Do not report 58541, 58542 in conjunction with 49320, 57000, 57180, 57410, 58140-58146, 58545, 58546, 58561, 58661, 58670, 58671)

58543 Laparoscopy, surgical, supracervical hysterectomy, for uterus greater than 250 g;

➡️ *CPT Changes: An Insider's View* 2007

➡️ *CPT Assistant* Nov 07:1, Apr 17:7, Jul 19:6, Aug 21:8-9

58544 with removal of tube(s) and/or ovary(s)

➡️ *CPT Changes: An Insider's View* 2007

➡️ *CPT Assistant* Nov 07:1, Jul 19:6, Aug 21:8-9

(Do not report 58543-58544 in conjunction with 49320, 57000, 57180, 57410, 58140-58146, 58545, 58546, 58561, 58661, 58670, 58671)

58545 Laparoscopy, surgical, myomectomy, excision; 1 to 4 intramural myomas with total weight of 250 g or less and/or removal of surface myomas

➡️ *CPT Changes: An Insider's View* 2003

➡️ *CPT Assistant* Jun 03:5, 12, Jul 19:6

58546 5 or more intramural myomas and/or intramural myomas with total weight greater than 250 g

➡️ *CPT Changes: An Insider's View* 2003

➡️ *CPT Assistant* Jun 03:12, Jan 04:26, Apr 17:7, Jul 19:6

58548 Laparoscopy, surgical, with radical hysterectomy, with bilateral total pelvic lymphadenectomy and para-aortic lymph node sampling (biopsy), with removal of tube(s) and ovary(s), if performed

➡️ *CPT Changes: An Insider's View* 2007

➡️ *CPT Assistant* Nov 07:1, Sep 15:12, Apr 17:7, Mar 19:5, Jul 19:6, Aug 21:8-9, Dec 21:21, Dec 22:20

(Do not report 58548 in conjunction with 38570-38572, 58210, 58285, 58550-58554)

58550 Laparoscopy, surgical, with vaginal hysterectomy, for uterus 250 g or less;

➡️ *CPT Changes: An Insider's View* 2000, 2003

➡️ *CPT Assistant* Nov 99:28, Mar 00:9, Apr 17:7, Jul 19:6, Aug 21:8-9

Radical and Total Hysterectomy
58548, 58575

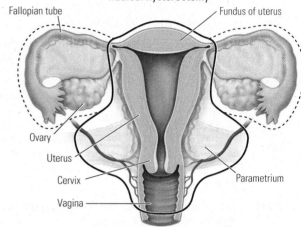

Radical hysterectomy

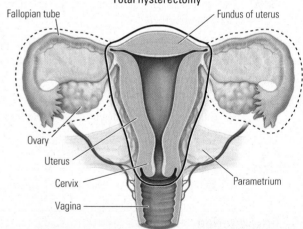

Total hysterectomy

- - - - - The dotted lines around the fallopian tube(s) and ovary(ies) indicate that both procedures may include the removal of tube(s) and ovary(ies), unilateral or bilateral.

——— The solid line indicates the organs or parts that are removed for the procedure.

58552   with removal of tube(s) and/or ovary(s)

➔ *CPT Changes: An Insider's View* 2003

➔ *CPT Assistant* Nov 07:1, Apr 17:7, Jul 19:6, Aug 21:8-9

(Do not report 58550-58552 in conjunction with 49320, 57000, 57180, 57410, 58140-58146, 58545, 58546, 58561, 58661, 58670, 58671)

58553   Laparoscopy, surgical, with vaginal hysterectomy, for uterus greater than 250 g;

➔ *CPT Changes: An Insider's View* 2003

➔ *CPT Assistant* Apr 17:7, Jul 19:6, Aug 21:8-9

58554   with removal of tube(s) and/or ovary(s)

➔ *CPT Changes: An Insider's View* 2003

➔ *CPT Assistant* Apr 17:7, Jul 19:6, Aug 21:8-9

(Do not report 58553-58554 in conjunction with 49320, 57000, 57180, 57410, 58140-58146, 58545, 58546, 58561, 58661, 58670, 58671)

58555   Hysteroscopy, diagnostic (separate procedure)

➔ *CPT Changes: An Insider's View* 2000

➔ *CPT Assistant* Nov 99:28, Mar 00:10

58558   Hysteroscopy, surgical; with sampling (biopsy) of endometrium and/or polypectomy, with or without D & C

➔ *CPT Changes: An Insider's View* 2000

➔ *CPT Assistant* Nov 99:28, Mar 00:10, Sep 02:10, Jan 03:7, May 03:19

58559   with lysis of intrauterine adhesions (any method)

➔ *CPT Changes: An Insider's View* 2000

➔ *CPT Assistant* Nov 99:28, Mar 00:10

58560   with division or resection of intrauterine septum (any method)

➔ *CPT Changes: An Insider's View* 2000

➔ *CPT Assistant* Nov 99:28, Mar 00:10

58561   with removal of leiomyomata

➔ *CPT Changes: An Insider's View* 2000

➔ *CPT Assistant* Nov 99:28, Mar 00:10, Jan 03:7, Dec 23:42

58562   with removal of impacted foreign body

➔ *CPT Changes: An Insider's View* 2000

➔ *CPT Assistant* Nov 99:28, Mar 00:10

58563   with endometrial ablation (eg, endometrial resection, electrosurgical ablation, thermoablation)

➔ *CPT Changes: An Insider's View* 2000, 2002

➔ *CPT Assistant* Nov 99:28, Mar 00:10, Mar 02:11, Apr 02:19, Jan 03:7, Feb 12:11, Jan 15:14

58565   with bilateral fallopian tube cannulation to induce occlusion by placement of permanent implants

➔ *CPT Changes: An Insider's View* 2005

➔ *CPT Assistant* Jan 11:9, Feb 12:11

(Do not report 58565 in conjunction with 58555 or 57800)

(For unilateral procedure, use modifier 52)

Hysteroscopy
58563

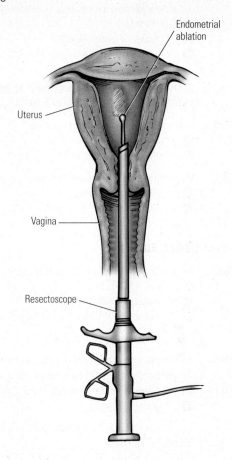

Endometrial ablation

Uterus

Vagina

Resectoscope

58570   Laparoscopy, surgical, with total hysterectomy, for uterus 250 g or less;

➔ *CPT Changes: An Insider's View* 2008

➔ *CPT Assistant* Apr 17:7, Jul 19:6, Aug 21:8-9

58571   with removal of tube(s) and/or ovary(s)

➔ *CPT Changes: An Insider's View* 2008

➔ *CPT Assistant* May 12:14, Aug 12:13, Apr 17:7, Feb 18:11, Jul 19:6, Mar 21:10, Aug 21:8-9

58572   Laparoscopy, surgical, with total hysterectomy, for uterus greater than 250 g;

➔ *CPT Changes: An Insider's View* 2008

➔ *CPT Assistant* Apr 17:7, Jul 19:6, Aug 21:8-9

58573   with removal of tube(s) and/or ovary(s)

➔ *CPT Changes: An Insider's View* 2008

➔ *CPT Assistant* May 12:14, Aug 12:13, Apr 17:7, Feb 18:11, Apr 18:11, Mar 19:5, Jul 19:6, Mar 21:10, Aug 21:8-9

(Do not report 58570-58573 in conjunction with 49320, 57000, 57180, 57410, 58140-58146, 58150, 58545, 58546, 58561, 58661, 58670, 58671)

58575　Laparoscopy, surgical, total hysterectomy for resection of malignancy (tumor debulking), with omentectomy including salpingo-oophorectomy, unilateral or bilateral, when performed

➲ *CPT Changes: An Insider's View* 2018

➲ *CPT Assistant* Mar 19:5, Jul 19:6, Mar 20:14, Mar 21:11, Aug 21:8-9, Dec 21:21

(Do not report 58575 in conjunction with 49255, 49320, 49321, 58570, 58571, 58572, 58573, 58661)

58578　Unlisted laparoscopy procedure, uterus

➲ *CPT Changes: An Insider's View* 2000

➲ *CPT Assistant* Nov 99:28, Mar 00:10, Mar 07:9

58579　Unlisted hysteroscopy procedure, uterus

➲ *CPT Changes: An Insider's View* 2000

➲ *CPT Assistant* Nov 99:28, Mar 00:10

Other Procedures

\# 58353　Endometrial ablation, thermal, without hysteroscopic guidance

➲ *CPT Changes: An Insider's View* 2001

➲ *CPT Assistant* Mar 02:11, Apr 02:19, Feb 24:21

(For hysteroscopic procedure, use 58563)

\# 58356　Endometrial cryoablation with ultrasonic guidance, including endometrial curettage, when performed

➲ *CPT Changes: An Insider's View* 2005

➲ *CPT Assistant* Feb 24:21

(Do not report 58356 in conjunction with 58100, 58120, 58340, 76700, 76856)

58580　Transcervical ablation of uterine fibroid(s), including intraoperative ultrasound guidance and monitoring, radiofrequency

➲ *CPT Changes: An Insider's View* 2024

➲ *CPT Assistant* Dec 23:42, Feb 24:21

(Do not report 58580 in conjunction with 58561, 58674, 76830, 76940, 76998)

(For laparoscopic radiofrequency ablation of uterine fibroid[s], including intraoperative ultrasound guidance and monitoring, use 58674)

Oviduct/Ovary

Incision

58600　Ligation or transection of fallopian tube(s), abdominal or vaginal approach, unilateral or bilateral

➲ *CPT Changes: An Insider's View* 2000

➲ *CPT Assistant* Nov 99:28

58605　Ligation or transection of fallopian tube(s), abdominal or vaginal approach, postpartum, unilateral or bilateral, during same hospitalization (separate procedure)

➲ *CPT Changes: An Insider's View* 2000

➲ *CPT Assistant* Nov 99:28

(For laparoscopic procedures, use 58670, 58671)

+ 58611　Ligation or transection of fallopian tube(s) when done at the time of cesarean delivery or intra-abdominal surgery (not a separate procedure) (List separately in addition to code for primary procedure)

➲ *CPT Changes: An Insider's View* 2002

58615　Occlusion of fallopian tube(s) by device (eg, band, clip, Falope ring) vaginal or suprapubic approach

➲ *CPT Changes: An Insider's View* 2000

➲ *CPT Assistant* Nov 99:28

(For laparoscopic approach, use 58671)

(For lysis of adnexal adhesions, use 58740)

Laparoscopy

Surgical laparoscopy always includes diagnostic laparoscopy. To report a diagnostic laparoscopy (peritoneoscopy) (separate procedure), use 49320.

58660　Laparoscopy, surgical; with lysis of adhesions (salpingolysis, ovariolysis) (separate procedure)

➲ *CPT Changes: An Insider's View* 2000

➲ *CPT Assistant* Nov 99:28, Mar 00:10, Mar 03:22, Dec 11:16, Jul 19:6

58661　with removal of adnexal structures (partial or total oophorectomy and/or salpingectomy)

➲ *CPT Changes: An Insider's View* 2000

➲ *CPT Assistant* Nov 99:28, Mar 00:10, Jan 02:11, Nov 07:1, May 10:10, Jul 19:6, Jan 20:12, Mar 22:12, Feb 24:34

(For bilateral procedure, report 58661 with modifier 50)

58662　with fulguration or excision of lesions of the ovary, pelvic viscera, or peritoneal surface by any method

➲ *CPT Changes: An Insider's View* 2000

➲ *CPT Assistant* Nov 99:28, Mar 00:10, Dec 17:14, Jul 19:6, Jul 23:17

58670　with fulguration of oviducts (with or without transection)

➲ *CPT Changes: An Insider's View* 2000

➲ *CPT Assistant* Nov 99:29, Mar 00:10, Nov 07:2, Jul 19:6, Mar 22:12

58671　with occlusion of oviducts by device (eg, band, clip, or Falope ring)

➲ *CPT Changes: An Insider's View* 2000

➲ *CPT Assistant* Nov 99:29, Mar 00:10, Jul 19:6

58672　with fimbrioplasty

➲ *CPT Changes: An Insider's View* 2000

➲ *CPT Assistant* Nov 99:29, Mar 00:10, Jul 19:6

58673　with salpingostomy (salpingoneostomy)

➲ *CPT Changes: An Insider's View* 2000

➲ *CPT Assistant* Nov 99:29, Mar 00:10, May 02:19, Jul 19:6

(Codes 58672 and 58673 are used to report unilateral procedures. For bilateral procedure, use modifier 50)

58674   Code is out of numerical sequence. See 58520-58542

58679   Unlisted laparoscopy procedure, oviduct, ovary
⮕ *CPT Changes: An Insider's View* 2000
⮕ *CPT Assistant* Nov 99:29, Mar 00:10, Jul 23:17

(For laparoscopic aspiration of ovarian cyst, use 49322)

(For laparoscopic biopsy of the ovary or fallopian tube, use 49321)

Excision

58700   Salpingectomy, complete or partial, unilateral or bilateral (separate procedure)
⮕ *CPT Assistant* Sep 18:14

58720   Salpingo-oophorectomy, complete or partial, unilateral or bilateral (separate procedure)
⮕ *CPT Assistant* Sep 00:9, Jul 06:19

Repair

58740   Lysis of adhesions (salpingolysis, ovariolysis)
⮕ *CPT Changes: An Insider's View* 2000
⮕ *CPT Assistant* Sep 96:9, Nov 99:29

(For laparoscopic approach, use 58660)

(For fulguration or excision of lesions, laparoscopic approach, use 58662)

►(For excision or destruction of endometriomas, open method, use 58999)◄

58750   Tubotubal anastomosis

58752   Tubouterine implantation

58760   Fimbrioplasty
⮕ *CPT Changes: An Insider's View* 2000
⮕ *CPT Assistant* Nov 99:29

(For laparoscopic approach, use 58672)

58770   Salpingostomy (salpingoneostomy)
⮕ *CPT Changes: An Insider's View* 2000
⮕ *CPT Assistant* Nov 99:29

(For laparoscopic approach, use 58673)

Ovary

Incision

58800   Drainage of ovarian cyst(s), unilateral or bilateral (separate procedure); vaginal approach

58805   abdominal approach
⮕ *CPT Assistant* Mar 24:26

58820   Drainage of ovarian abscess; vaginal approach, open
⮕ *CPT Assistant* Nov 97:22

58822   abdominal approach
⮕ *CPT Assistant* Nov 97:22

(For transrectal image-guided fluid collection drainage by catheter of pelvic abscess, use 49407)

58825   Transposition, ovary(s)

Excision

58900   Biopsy of ovary, unilateral or bilateral (separate procedure)
⮕ *CPT Changes: An Insider's View* 2000
⮕ *CPT Assistant* Nov 99:29

(For laparoscopic biopsy of the ovary or fallopian tube, use 49321)

58920   Wedge resection or bisection of ovary, unilateral or bilateral

58925   Ovarian cystectomy, unilateral or bilateral

58940   Oophorectomy, partial or total, unilateral or bilateral;
⮕ *CPT Assistant* Mar 04:3

(For oophorectomy with concomitant debulking for ovarian malignancy, use 58952)

58943   for ovarian, tubal or primary peritoneal malignancy, with para-aortic and pelvic lymph node biopsies, peritoneal washings, peritoneal biopsies, diaphragmatic assessments, with or without salpingectomy(s), with or without omentectomy
⮕ *CPT Changes: An Insider's View* 2001
⮕ *CPT Assistant* Oct 10:16, Dec 10:16

►(Do not report 58943 in conjunction with 49186, 49187, 49188, 49189, 49190)◄

58950   Resection (initial) of ovarian, tubal or primary peritoneal malignancy with bilateral salpingo-oophorectomy and omentectomy;
⮕ *CPT Changes: An Insider's View* 2001, 2007
⮕ *CPT Assistant* Oct 10:16, Dec 10:16, Nov 21:8

58951   with total abdominal hysterectomy, pelvic and limited para-aortic lymphadenectomy
⮕ *CPT Assistant* Aug 01:11, Oct 10:16, Dec 10:16, Nov 21:8

58952   with radical dissection for debulking (ie, radical excision or destruction, intra-abdominal or retroperitoneal tumors)
⮕ *CPT Changes: An Insider's View* 2001
⮕ *CPT Assistant* Dec 96:10, Aug 01:11, Oct 10:16, Dec 10:16, Nov 21:8

►(Do not report 58950, 58951, 58952 in conjunction with 49186, 49187, 49188, 49189, 49190)◄

►(For resection of recurrent ovarian, tubal, primary peritoneal, or uterine malignancy, use 58958)◄

58953 Bilateral salpingo-oophorectomy with omentectomy, total abdominal hysterectomy and radical dissection for debulking;

➡ *CPT Changes: An Insider's View* 2002

➡ *CPT Assistant* Feb 02:8, Oct 10:16, Dec 10:16, May 14:10, Nov 21:8

58954 with pelvic lymphadenectomy and limited para-aortic lymphadenectomy

➡ *CPT Changes: An Insider's View* 2002

➡ *CPT Assistant* Feb 02:9, Oct 10:16, Dec 10:16, Nov 21:8

▶(Do not report 58953, 58954 in conjunction with 49186, 49187, 49188, 49189, 49190)◀

58956 Bilateral salpingo-oophorectomy with total omentectomy, total abdominal hysterectomy for malignancy

➡ *CPT Changes: An Insider's View* 2005

➡ *CPT Assistant* May 14:10

▶(Do not report 58956 in conjunction with 49186, 49187, 49188, 49189, 49190, 49255, 58150, 58180, 58262, 58263, 58550, 58661, 58700, 58720, 58900, 58925, 58940, 58958)◀

▶(58957 has been deleted. For resection [tumor debulking] of recurrent ovarian, endometrial, tubal, or primary peritoneal gynecological malignancies, with omentectomy, if performed, without lymphadenectomy, see 49186, 49187, 49188, 49189, 49190)◀

▲ **58958** Resection (tumor debulking) of recurrent ovarian, tubal, primary peritoneal, uterine malignancy (intra-abdominal, retroperitoneal tumors), with omentectomy, if performed, with pelvic lymphadenectomy and limited para-aortic lymphadenectomy

➡ *CPT Changes: An Insider's View* 2007, 2025

▶(Do not report 58958 in conjunction with 38770, 38780, 44005, 49000, 49186, 49187, 49188, 49189, 49190, 49215, 49255, 58900-58960)◀

58960 Laparotomy, for staging or restaging of ovarian, tubal, or primary peritoneal malignancy (second look), with or without omentectomy, peritoneal washing, biopsy of abdominal and pelvic peritoneum, diaphragmatic assessment with pelvic and limited para-aortic lymphadenectomy

➡ *CPT Changes: An Insider's View* 2001

▶(Do not report 58960 in conjunction with 49186, 49187, 49188, 49189, 49190, 58958)◀

In Vitro Fertilization

58970 Follicle puncture for oocyte retrieval, any method

(For radiological supervision and interpretation, use 76948)

58974 Embryo transfer, intrauterine

58976 Gamete, zygote, or embryo intrafallopian transfer, any method

➡ *CPT Changes: An Insider's View* 2000

➡ *CPT Assistant* Nov 99:29

(For laparoscopic adnexal procedures, see 58660-58673)

Other Procedures

58999 Unlisted procedure, female genital system (nonobstetrical)

➡ *CPT Assistant* Apr 09:9-10, Jul 19:6, Aug 22:18, Mar 24:26

Maternity Care and Delivery

The services normally provided in uncomplicated maternity cases include antepartum care, delivery, and postpartum care. Pregnancy confirmation during a problem-oriented or preventive visit is not considered as part of antepartum care and should be reported using the appropriate E/M service codes 99202, 99203, 99204, 99205, 99211, 99212, 99213, 99214, 99215, 99242, 99243, 99244, 99245, 99281, 99282, 99283, 99284, 99285, 99384, 99385, 99386, 99394, 99395, 99396 for that visit.

Antepartum care includes the initial prenatal history and physical examination; subsequent prenatal history and physical examinations; recording of weight, blood pressures, fetal heart tones, routine chemical urinalysis, and monthly visits up to 28 weeks gestation; biweekly visits to 36 weeks gestation; and weekly visits until delivery. Any other visits or services within this time period should be coded separately.

Delivery services include admission to the hospital, the admission history and physical examination, management of uncomplicated labor, vaginal delivery (with or without episiotomy, with or without forceps), or cesarean delivery. When reporting delivery only services (59409, 59514, 59612, 59620), report inpatient postdelivery management and discharge services using E/M service codes (99238, 99239). Delivery and postpartum services (59410, 59515, 59614, 59622) include delivery services and all inpatient and outpatient postpartum services. Medical complications of pregnancy (eg, cardiac problems, neurological problems, diabetes, hypertension, toxemia, hyperemesis, preterm labor, premature rupture of membranes, trauma) and medical problems complicating labor and delivery management may require additional resources and may be reported separately.

Postpartum care only services (59430) include office or other outpatient visits following vaginal or cesarean section delivery.

For surgical complications of pregnancy (eg, appendectomy, hernia, ovarian cyst, Bartholin cyst), see services in the **Surgery** section.

If all or part of the antepartum and/or postpartum patient care is provided except delivery due to termination of pregnancy by abortion or referral to another physician or other qualified health care professional for delivery, see the antepartum and postpartum care codes 59425, 59426, and 59430.

(For circumcision of newborn, see 54150, 54160)

Antepartum and Fetal Invasive Services

(For fetal intrauterine transfusion, use 36460)

(For unlisted fetal invasive procedure, use 59897)

59000   Amniocentesis; diagnostic
> *CPT Changes: An Insider's View* 2002
> *CPT Assistant* Apr 97:2, Feb 02:7, Aug 02:2, May 04:2, Jul 19:6

(For radiological supervision and interpretation, use 76946)

59001   therapeutic amniotic fluid reduction (includes ultrasound guidance)
> *CPT Changes: An Insider's View* 2002
> *CPT Assistant* Feb 02:7, Aug 02:2

Amniocentesis, Therapeutic Amniotic Fluid Reduction
59001

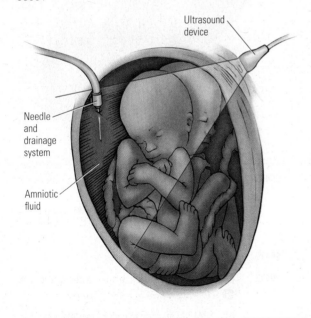

Ultrasound device

Needle and drainage system

Amniotic fluid

59012   Cordocentesis (intrauterine), any method
> *CPT Assistant* Aug 02:2

(For radiological supervision and interpretation, use 76941)

59015   Chorionic villus sampling, any method
> *CPT Assistant* Apr 97:2, Aug 02:2

(For radiological supervision and interpretation, use 76945)

59020   Fetal contraction stress test
> *CPT Assistant* Apr 97:2, Aug 02:2

59025   Fetal non-stress test
> *CPT Assistant* Apr 97:2, May 98:10, Oct 04:10, Dec 08:8

59030   Fetal scalp blood sampling
> *CPT Assistant* Aug 02:3

(For repeat fetal scalp blood sampling, use 59030 and see modifiers 76 and 77)

59050   Fetal monitoring during labor by consulting physician (ie, non-attending physician) with written report; supervision and interpretation
> *CPT Assistant* Nov 97:22

59051   interpretation only
> *CPT Assistant* Nov 97:22

59070   Transabdominal amnioinfusion, including ultrasound guidance
> *CPT Changes: An Insider's View* 2004
> *CPT Assistant* May 04:2, Jun 04:11

59072   Fetal umbilical cord occlusion, including ultrasound guidance
> *CPT Changes: An Insider's View* 2004
> *CPT Assistant* May 04:2, Jun 04:11

59074   Fetal fluid drainage (eg, vesicocentesis, thoracocentesis, paracentesis), including ultrasound guidance
> *CPT Changes: An Insider's View* 2004
> *CPT Assistant* May 04:2, 4, Jun 04:11, Dec 04:19

59076   Fetal shunt placement, including ultrasound guidance
> *CPT Changes: An Insider's View* 2004
> *CPT Assistant* May 04:2, 4, Jun 04:11, Dec 04:19

Excision

59100   Hysterotomy, abdominal (eg, for hydatidiform mole, abortion)

(When tubal ligation is performed at the same time as hysterotomy, use 58611 in addition to 59100)

59120   Surgical treatment of ectopic pregnancy; tubal or ovarian, requiring salpingectomy and/or oophorectomy, abdominal or vaginal approach

59121   tubal or ovarian, without salpingectomy and/or oophorectomy

59130   abdominal pregnancy

59136   interstitial, uterine pregnancy with partial resection of uterus

59140   cervical, with evacuation

59150   Laparoscopic treatment of ectopic pregnancy; without salpingectomy and/or oophorectomy
> *CPT Assistant* Sep 96:9

59151   with salpingectomy and/or oophorectomy

Laparoscopic Treatment of Ectopic Pregnancy
59150

The site of gestation is located with a laparoscope, and a small incision is made above the site. The ectopic pregnancy is then removed.

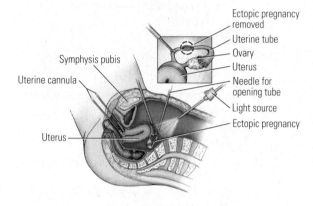

59160   Curettage, postpartum
> *CPT Assistant* Nov 97:22, Sep 02:11

Introduction

(For intrauterine fetal transfusion, use 36460)

(For introduction of hypertonic solution and/or prostaglandins to initiate labor, see 59850-59857)

59200   Insertion of cervical dilator (eg, laminaria, prostaglandin) (separate procedure)
> *CPT Assistant* Fall 93:9, Apr 97:3, Jul 05:15, Dec 17:14

Repair

(For tracheloplasty, use 57700)

59300   Episiotomy or vaginal repair, by other than attending
> *CPT Changes: An Insider's View* 2013
> *CPT Assistant* Dec 23:45

59320   Cerclage of cervix, during pregnancy; vaginal
> *CPT Assistant* Aug 02:2, Nov 06:21, Feb 07:10

59325   abdominal
> *CPT Assistant* Aug 02:2, Nov 06:21, Feb 07:10

59350   Hysterorrhaphy of ruptured uterus
> *CPT Assistant* Aug 02:2

Vaginal Delivery, Antepartum and Postpartum Care

—— *Coding Tip* ——

Instructions for Reporting Antepartum and Postpartum Care

The services normally provided in uncomplicated maternity cases include antepartum care, delivery, and postpartum care.

CPT Coding Guidelines, Maternity Care and Delivery

59400   Routine obstetric care including antepartum care, vaginal delivery (with or without episiotomy, and/or forceps) and postpartum care
> *CPT Assistant* Feb 96:1, Mar 96:11, Feb 97:11, Apr 97:3, Apr 98:15, Jun 98:10, Aug 02:3, Feb 03:15, Feb 22:14

Vaginal Delivery
59400-59410

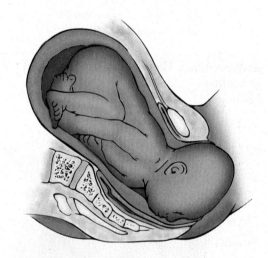

59409   Vaginal delivery only (with or without episiotomy and/or forceps);
> *CPT Assistant* Feb 96:1, Mar 96:11, Jul 96:11, Sep 96:4, Feb 97:11, Apr 97:1, Aug 02:3, Dec 07:13, Jun 09:10, Feb 22:15, Dec 23:45

59410   including postpartum care

59412   External cephalic version, with or without tocolysis
> *CPT Assistant* Fall 94:21, Feb 96:1, Aug 02:2-3

(Use 59412 in addition to code[s] for delivery)

59414   Delivery of placenta (separate procedure)
➔ *CPT Assistant* Jun 96:10, Jun 98:10, Aug 02:3, Dec 23:45

(For antepartum care only, see 59425, 59426 or appropriate E/M code[s])

(For 1-3 antepartum care visits, see appropriate E/M code[s])

59425   Antepartum care only; 4-6 visits
➔ *CPT Assistant* Fall 94:21, Apr 97:11, Aug 02:3

59426   7 or more visits
➔ *CPT Assistant* Fall 94:21, Apr 97:11, Aug 02:3

59430   Postpartum care only (separate procedure)
➔ *CPT Assistant* Jun 96:10, Aug 02:3

Cesarean Delivery

(For standby attendance for infant, use 99360)

(For low cervical cesarean section, see 59510, 59515, 59525)

─── *Coding Tip* ───

Instructions for Reporting Cesarean Delivery

Patients who have had a previous cesarean delivery and now present with the expectation of a vaginal delivery are coded using codes 59610-59622. If the patient has a successful vaginal delivery after a previous cesarean delivery (VBAC), use codes 59610-59614. If the attempt is unsuccessful and another cesarean delivery is carried out, use codes 59618-59622. To report elective cesarean deliveries, use code 59510, 59514 or 59515.

CPT Coding Guidelines, Maternity Care and Delivery, Delivery After Previous Cesarean Delivery

59510   Routine obstetric care including antepartum care, cesarean delivery, and postpartum care
➔ *CPT Assistant* Jul 96:11, Sep 96:4, Oct 96:10, Feb 97:11, Apr 97:2, Aug 02:3, Mar 13:13, Feb 22:14

59514   Cesarean delivery only;
➔ *CPT Assistant* Oct 96:10, Feb 97:11, Mar 13:13, Feb 22:15

59515   including postpartum care
➔ *CPT Assistant* Mar 13:13

(For classic cesarean section, see 59510, 59515, 59525)

+ 59525   Subtotal or total hysterectomy after cesarean delivery (List separately in addition to code for primary procedure)

(Use 59525 in conjunction with 59510, 59514, 59515, 59618, 59620, 59622)

(For extraperitoneal cesarean section, or cesarean section with subtotal or total hysterectomy, see 59510, 59515, 59525)

Cesarean Delivery
59510-59515

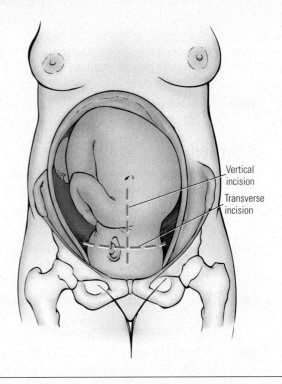

Vertical incision
Transverse incision

Delivery After Previous Cesarean Delivery

Patients who have had a previous cesarean delivery and now present with the expectation of a vaginal delivery are coded using codes 59610-59622. If the patient has a successful vaginal delivery after a previous cesarean delivery (VBAC), use codes 59610-59614. If the attempt is unsuccessful and another cesarean delivery is carried out, use codes 59618-59622. To report elective cesarean deliveries use code 59510, 59514 or 59515.

59610   Routine obstetric care including antepartum care, vaginal delivery (with or without episiotomy, and/or forceps) and postpartum care, after previous cesarean delivery
➔ *CPT Assistant* Feb 96:2, Apr 97:3, Aug 02:3

59612   Vaginal delivery only, after previous cesarean delivery (with or without episiotomy and/or forceps);
➔ *CPT Assistant* Feb 96:2, Aug 02:3

59614   including postpartum care
➔ *CPT Assistant* Feb 96:2

59618 Routine obstetric care including antepartum care, cesarean delivery, and postpartum care, following attempted vaginal delivery after previous cesarean delivery
→ *CPT Assistant* Feb 96:2, Aug 02:4

59620 Cesarean delivery only, following attempted vaginal delivery after previous cesarean delivery;
→ *CPT Assistant* Feb 96:2

59622 including postpartum care
→ *CPT Assistant* Feb 96:2

Abortion

(For medical treatment of spontaneous complete abortion, any trimester, use E/M codes 99202-99233)

(For surgical treatment of spontaneous abortion, use 59812)

59812 Treatment of incomplete abortion, any trimester, completed surgically
→ *CPT Assistant* Fall 93:9, Fall 95:16

59820 Treatment of missed abortion, completed surgically; first trimester
→ *CPT Assistant* Fall 93:9, Fall 95:16, Feb 99:10

59821 second trimester
→ *CPT Assistant* Fall 93:9, Fall 95:16

59830 Treatment of septic abortion, completed surgically
→ *CPT Assistant* Fall 93:9

59840 Induced abortion, by dilation and curettage
→ *CPT Assistant* Fall 93:9, Sep 03:16

59841 Induced abortion, by dilation and evacuation
→ *CPT Assistant* Fall 93:9

59850 Induced abortion, by 1 or more intra-amniotic injections (amniocentesis-injections), including hospital admission and visits, delivery of fetus and secundines;
→ *CPT Assistant* Fall 93:10

59851 with dilation and curettage and/or evacuation
→ *CPT Assistant* Fall 93:10

59852 with hysterotomy (failed intra-amniotic injection)
→ *CPT Assistant* Fall 93:10

(For insertion of cervical dilator, use 59200)

59855 Induced abortion, by 1 or more vaginal suppositories (eg, prostaglandin) with or without cervical dilation (eg, laminaria), including hospital admission and visits, delivery of fetus and secundines;

59856 with dilation and curettage and/or evacuation

59857 with hysterotomy (failed medical evacuation)

Other Procedures

59866 Multifetal pregnancy reduction(s) (MPR)

59870 Uterine evacuation and curettage for hydatidiform mole
→ *CPT Assistant* Feb 99:10

59871 Removal of cerclage suture under anesthesia (other than local)
→ *CPT Assistant* Nov 97:22, Nov 06:21, Feb 07:10

59897 Unlisted fetal invasive procedure, including ultrasound guidance, when performed
→ *CPT Changes: An Insider's View* 2004, 2010
→ *CPT Assistant* May 04:5

59898 Unlisted laparoscopy procedure, maternity care and delivery
→ *CPT Changes: An Insider's View* 2000
→ *CPT Assistant* Nov 99:29, Mar 00:10

59899 Unlisted procedure, maternity care and delivery
→ *CPT Assistant* Jun 97:10, May 04:2, Oct 13:3, Jul 19:6

Endocrine System

(For pituitary and pineal surgery, see **Nervous System**)

Thyroid Gland

Incision

60000 Incision and drainage of thyroglossal duct cyst, infected
→ *CPT Changes: An Insider's View* 2002

Excision

60100 Biopsy thyroid, percutaneous core needle
→ *CPT Assistant* Jun 97:5, Jun 07:10
→ *Clinical Examples in Radiology* Winter 17:5, Winter 19:3

(If imaging guidance is performed, see 76942, 77002, 77012, 77021)

(For fine needle aspiration biopsy, see 10004, 10005, 10006, 10007, 10008, 10009, 10010, 10011, 10012, 10021)

(For evaluation of fine needle aspirate, see 88172, 88173)

60200 Excision of cyst or adenoma of thyroid, or transection of isthmus
→ *CPT Assistant* Aug 11:10, Dec 12:3

60210 Partial thyroid lobectomy, unilateral; with or without isthmusectomy
→ *CPT Assistant* Winter 94:7, Aug 11:9, Dec 12:3

60212 with contralateral subtotal lobectomy, including isthmusectomy
→ *CPT Assistant* Dec 12:3

60220   Total thyroid lobectomy, unilateral; with or without isthmusectomy

➡ *CPT Assistant* Oct 10:13, Dec 10:13, Aug 11:10, Dec 12:3, Aug 20:14

60225   with contralateral subtotal lobectomy, including isthmusectomy

➡ *CPT Assistant* Dec 12:3

Thyroid Lobectomy
60220

The thyroid is exposed via a transverse cervical incision. The superior and inferior thyroid vessels serving the lobe are ligated, the isthmus is severed, and the entire thyroid lobe is resected.

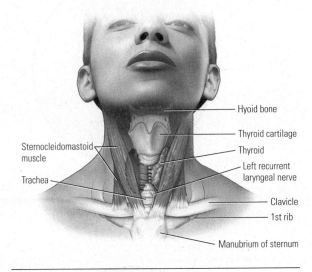

Hyoid bone
Thyroid cartilage
Sternocleidomastoid muscle
Thyroid
Left recurrent laryngeal nerve
Trachea
Clavicle
1st rib
Manubrium of sternum

60240   Thyroidectomy, total or complete

➡ *CPT Assistant* Dec 12:3

(For thyroidectomy, subtotal or partial, use 60271)

60252   Thyroidectomy, total or subtotal for malignancy; with limited neck dissection

➡ *CPT Assistant* Nov 00:10, Dec 12:3

60254   with radical neck dissection

➡ *CPT Assistant* Nov 00:10, Dec 12:3

60260   Thyroidectomy, removal of all remaining thyroid tissue following previous removal of a portion of thyroid

➡ *CPT Assistant* Oct 10:13, Dec 10:13, Dec 12:3

(For bilateral procedure, report 60260 with modifier 50)

60270   Thyroidectomy, including substernal thyroid; sternal split or transthoracic approach

➡ *CPT Changes: An Insider's View* 2002

➡ *CPT Assistant* Dec 12:3

60271   cervical approach

➡ *CPT Assistant* Dec 12:3, Aug 20:14

60280   Excision of thyroglossal duct cyst or sinus;

60281   recurrent

(For thyroid ultrasonography, use 76536)

Removal

60300   Aspiration and/or injection, thyroid cyst

➡ *CPT Changes: An Insider's View* 2008

➡ *CPT Assistant* May 21:14

(For fine needle aspiration biopsy, see 10004, 10005, 10006, 10007, 10008, 10009, 10010, 10011, 10012, 10021)

(If imaging guidance is performed, see 76942, 77012)

Parathyroid, Thymus, Adrenal Glands, Pancreas, and Carotid Body

Excision

(For pituitary and pineal surgery, see **Nervous System**)

60500   Parathyroidectomy or exploration of parathyroid(s);

➡ *CPT Assistant* Dec 12:3

60502   re-exploration

➡ *CPT Assistant* Dec 12:3

60505   with mediastinal exploration, sternal split or transthoracic approach

➡ *CPT Assistant* Dec 12:3

+ 60512   Parathyroid autotransplantation (List separately in addition to code for primary procedure)

➡ *CPT Assistant* Aug 11:9, Dec 12:3, Jan 17:7

(Use 60512 in conjunction with 60500, 60502, 60505, 60212, 60225, 60240, 60252, 60254, 60260, 60270, 60271)

60520   Thymectomy, partial or total; transcervical approach (separate procedure)

➡ *CPT Assistant* Mar 19:11

60521   sternal split or transthoracic approach, without radical mediastinal dissection (separate procedure)

➡ *CPT Assistant* Dec 07:12

60522   sternal split or transthoracic approach, with radical mediastinal dissection (separate procedure)

(For thoracoscopic [VATS] thymectomy, see 32673)

60540   Adrenalectomy, partial or complete, or exploration of adrenal gland with or without biopsy, transabdominal, lumbar or dorsal (separate procedure);

➡ *CPT Assistant* Nov 98:17

Posterior View of the Pharynx
60512

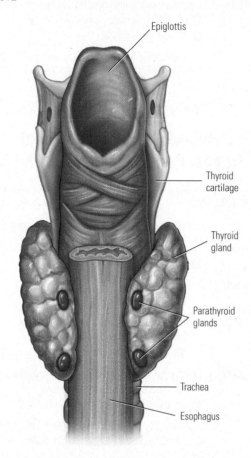

Epiglottis

Thyroid cartilage

Thyroid gland

Parathyroid glands

Trachea

Esophagus

60545   with excision of adjacent retroperitoneal tumor
> *CPT Assistant* Nov 98:17

(Do not report 60540, 60545 in conjunction with 50323)

▶(For open excision or destruction of remote or disseminated pheochromocytoma, see 49186, 49187, 49188, 49189, 49190)◀

(For laparoscopic approach, use 60650)

(For bilateral procedure, report 60540 with modifier 50)

60600   Excision of carotid body tumor; without excision of carotid artery

60605   with excision of carotid artery

Laparoscopy

Surgical laparoscopy always includes diagnostic laparoscopy. To report a diagnostic laparoscopy (peritoneoscopy) (separate procedure), use 49320.

60650   Laparoscopy, surgical, with adrenalectomy, partial or complete, or exploration of adrenal gland with or without biopsy, transabdominal, lumbar or dorsal
> *CPT Changes: An Insider's View* 2000
> *CPT Assistant* Nov 99:30, Mar 00:10, Nov 01:8

60659   Unlisted laparoscopy procedure, endocrine system
> *CPT Changes: An Insider's View* 2000
> *CPT Assistant* Nov 99:30, Mar 00:10

Laparoscopic Adrenalectomy
60650

An adrenal gland is dissected and removed under laparoscopic guidance. Multiple small blood vessels from the vena cava and the aorta do not follow standard anatomic pattern, requiring intricate dissection.

Left

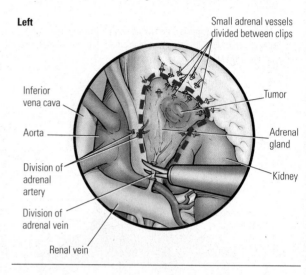

Small adrenal vessels divided between clips

Inferior vena cava

Tumor

Aorta

Adrenal gland

Division of adrenal artery

Kidney

Division of adrenal vein

Renal vein

Right

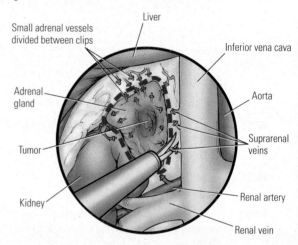

Liver

Small adrenal vessels divided between clips

Inferior vena cava

Adrenal gland

Aorta

Suprarenal veins

Tumor

Kidney

Renal artery

Renal vein

★=Telemedicine ◀=Audio-only +=Add-on code ✗=FDA approval pending #=Resequenced code ⊘=Modifier 51 exempt ➔➔➔=See p xxi for details

Other Procedures

● **60660** Ablation of 1 or more thyroid nodule(s), one lobe or the isthmus, percutaneous, including imaging guidance, radiofrequency

→ *CPT Changes: An Insider's View* 2025

▶(Do not report 60660 in conjunction with 76940, 76942, 77013, 77022)◀

▶(For laser ablation of benign thyroid nodule[s], use 0673T)◀

+● **60661** Ablation of 1 or more thyroid nodule(s), additional lobe, percutaneous, including imaging guidance, radiofrequency (List separately in addition to code for primary procedure)

→ *CPT Changes: An Insider's View* 2025

▶(Use 60661 in conjunction with 60660)◀

▶(Do not report 60661 in conjunction with 76940, 76942, 77013, 77022)◀

60699 Unlisted procedure, endocrine system

→ *CPT Assistant* Feb 06:16, Dec 07:12, Oct 22:18

Notes

Surgery

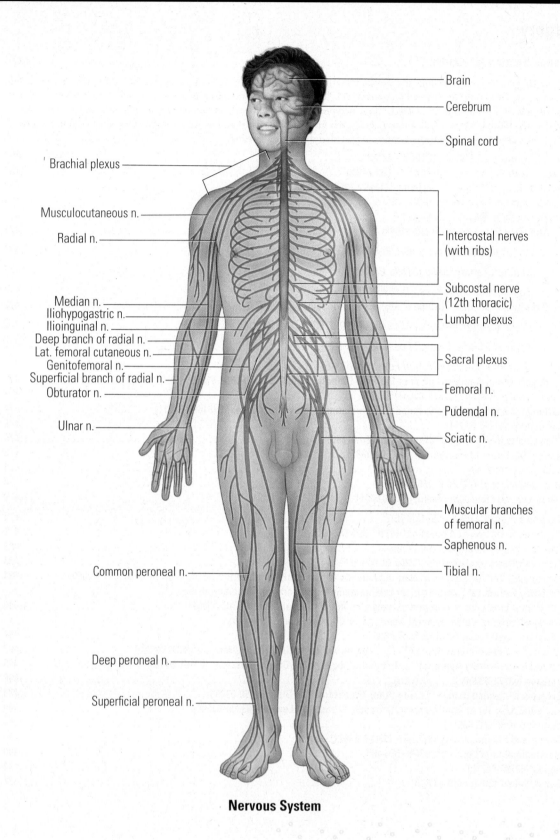

Brain

Cerebrum

Spinal cord

Brachial plexus

Musculocutaneous n.

Radial n.

Intercostal nerves
(with ribs)

Subcostal nerve
(12th thoracic)

Lumbar plexus

Median n.
Iliohypogastric n.
Ilioinguinal n.
Deep branch of radial n.
Lat. femoral cutaneous n.
Genitofemoral n.
Superficial branch of radial n.
Obturator n.

Sacral plexus

Femoral n.

Pudendal n.

Ulnar n.

Sciatic n.

Muscular branches
of femoral n.

Saphenous n.

Common peroneal n.

Tibial n.

Deep peroneal n.

Superficial peroneal n.

Nervous System

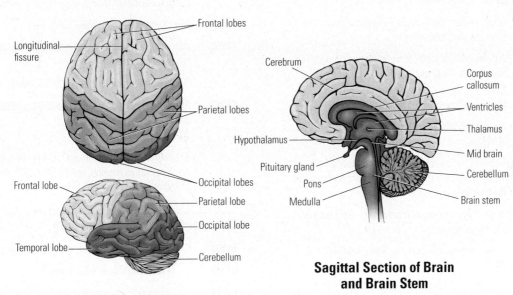

Brain Anatomy

**Sagittal Section of Brain
and Brain Stem**

Nervous System

Skull, Meninges, and Brain

(For injection procedure for cerebral angiography, see 36100-36218)

(For injection procedure for ventriculography, see 61026, 61120)

(For injection procedure for pneumoencephalography, use 61055)

Injection, Drainage, or Aspiration

61000 Subdural tap through fontanelle, or suture, infant, unilateral or bilateral; initial

61001 subsequent taps

61020 Ventricular puncture through previous burr hole, fontanelle, suture, or implanted ventricular catheter/reservoir; without injection

61026 with injection of medication or other substance for diagnosis or treatment
→ CPT Changes: An Insider's View 2002

61050 Cisternal or lateral cervical (C1-C2) puncture; without injection (separate procedure)

61055 with injection of medication or other substance for diagnosis or treatment
→ CPT Changes: An Insider's View 2002, 2015
→ Clinical Examples in Radiology Fall 14:7, Fall 15:10

(Do not report 61055 in conjunction with 62302, 62303, 62304, 62305)

(For radiological supervision and interpretation by a different physician or qualified health care professional, see **Radiology**)

61070 Puncture of shunt tubing or reservoir for aspiration or injection procedure

(For radiological supervision and interpretation, use 75809)

Twist Drill, Burr Hole(s), or Trephine

61105 Twist drill hole for subdural or ventricular puncture

⊘ **61107** Twist drill hole(s) for subdural, intracerebral, or ventricular puncture; for implanting ventricular catheter, pressure recording device, or other intracerebral monitoring device
→ CPT Changes: An Insider's View 2007

(For intracranial neuroendoscopic ventricular catheter placement, use 62160)

61108 for evacuation and/or drainage of subdural hematoma

61120 Burr hole(s) for ventricular puncture (including injection of gas, contrast media, dye, or radioactive material)

61140 Burr hole(s) or trephine; with biopsy of brain or intracranial lesion

61150 with drainage of brain abscess or cyst

61151 with subsequent tapping (aspiration) of intracranial abscess or cyst

61154 Burr hole(s) with evacuation and/or drainage of hematoma, extradural or subdural

(For bilateral procedure, report 61154 with modifier 50)

61156 Burr hole(s); with aspiration of hematoma or cyst, intracerebral

61210 for implanting ventricular catheter, reservoir, EEG electrode(s), pressure recording device, or other cerebral monitoring device (separate procedure)
→ CPT Changes: An Insider's View 2007, 2008

(For intracranial neuroendoscopic ventricular catheter placement, use 62160)

61215 Insertion of subcutaneous reservoir, pump or continuous infusion system for connection to ventricular catheter
→ CPT Assistant Spring 93:13

(For refilling and maintenance of an implantable infusion pump for spinal or brain drug therapy, use 95990)

(For chemotherapy, use 96450)

61250 Burr hole(s) or trephine, supratentorial, exploratory, not followed by other surgery

(For bilateral procedure, report 61250 with modifier 50)

61253 Burr hole(s) or trephine, infratentorial, unilateral or bilateral
→ CPT Assistant Sep 02:10

(If burr hole[s] or trephine are followed by craniotomy at same operative session, use 61304-61321; do not use 61250 or 61253)

Craniectomy or Craniotomy

61304 Craniectomy or craniotomy, exploratory; supratentorial

61305 infratentorial (posterior fossa)

61312 Craniectomy or craniotomy for evacuation of hematoma, supratentorial; extradural or subdural

61313 intracerebral

61314 Craniectomy or craniotomy for evacuation of hematoma, infratentorial; extradural or subdural

61315 intracerebellar

+ 61316   Incision and subcutaneous placement of cranial bone graft (List separately in addition to code for primary procedure)

> *CPT Changes: An Insider's View* 2003

(Use 61316 in conjunction with 61304, 61312, 61313, 61322, 61323, 61340, 61570, 61571, 61680-61705)

61320   Craniectomy or craniotomy, drainage of intracranial abscess; supratentorial

61321   infratentorial

61322   Craniectomy or craniotomy, decompressive, with or without duraplasty, for treatment of intracranial hypertension, without evacuation of associated intraparenchymal hematoma; without lobectomy

> *CPT Changes: An Insider's View* 2003
> *CPT Assistant* Aug 18:11, May 20:14

(Do not report 61313 in addition to 61322)

(For subtemporal decompression, use 61340)

61323   with lobectomy

> *CPT Changes: An Insider's View* 2003

(Do not report 61313 in addition to 61323)

(For subtemporal decompression, use 61340)

61330   Decompression of orbit only, transcranial approach

(For bilateral procedure, report 61330 with modifier 50)

61333   Exploration of orbit (transcranial approach), with removal of lesion

61340   Subtemporal cranial decompression (pseudotumor cerebri, slit ventricle syndrome)

> *CPT Changes: An Insider's View* 2003
> *CPT Assistant* May 20:14

(For bilateral procedure, report 61340 with modifier 50)

(For decompressive craniotomy or craniectomy for intracranial hypertension, without hematoma evacuation, see 61322, 61323)

61343   Craniectomy, suboccipital with cervical laminectomy for decompression of medulla and spinal cord, with or without dural graft (eg, Arnold-Chiari malformation)

61345   Other cranial decompression, posterior fossa

(For orbital decompression by lateral wall approach, Kroenlein type, use 67445)

61450   Craniectomy, subtemporal, for section, compression, or decompression of sensory root of gasserian ganglion

61458   Craniectomy, suboccipital; for exploration or decompression of cranial nerves

61460   for section of 1 or more cranial nerves

61500   Craniectomy; with excision of tumor or other bone lesion of skull

> *CPT Assistant* Jan 14:9

61501   for osteomyelitis

> *CPT Assistant* Jan 14:9

61510   Craniectomy, trephination, bone flap craniotomy; for excision of brain tumor, supratentorial, except meningioma

61512   for excision of meningioma, supratentorial

61514   for excision of brain abscess, supratentorial

61516   for excision or fenestration of cyst, supratentorial

(For excision of pituitary tumor or craniopharyngioma, see 61545, 61546, 61548)

+ 61517   Implantation of brain intracavitary chemotherapy agent (List separately in addition to code for primary procedure)

> *CPT Changes: An Insider's View* 2003

(Use 61517 only in conjunction with 61510 or 61518)

(Do not report 61517 for brachytherapy insertion. For intracavitary insertion of radioelement sources or ribbons, see 77770, 77771, 77772)

61518   Craniectomy for excision of brain tumor, infratentorial or posterior fossa; except meningioma, cerebellopontine angle tumor, or midline tumor at base of skull

61519   meningioma

61520   cerebellopontine angle tumor

61521   midline tumor at base of skull

61522   Craniectomy, infratentorial or posterior fossa; for excision of brain abscess

61524   for excision or fenestration of cyst

61526   Craniectomy, bone flap craniotomy, transtemporal (mastoid) for excision of cerebellopontine angle tumor;

> *CPT Assistant* Summer 91:8, Mar 18:11

61530   combined with middle/posterior fossa craniotomy/craniectomy

61531   Subdural implantation of strip electrodes through 1 or more burr or trephine hole(s) for long-term seizure monitoring

> *CPT Assistant* Jul 19:11

(For stereotactic implantation of electrodes, use 61760)

(For craniotomy for excision of intracranial arteriovenous malformation, see 61680-61692)

61533   Craniotomy with elevation of bone flap; for subdural implantation of an electrode array, for long-term seizure monitoring

(For continuous EEG monitoring, see 95700-95726)

61534   for excision of epileptogenic focus without electrocorticography during surgery

61535 for removal of epidural or subdural electrode array, without excision of cerebral tissue (separate procedure)
➔ *CPT Assistant* Jul 19:11

61536 for excision of cerebral epileptogenic focus, with electrocorticography during surgery (includes removal of electrode array)

61537 for lobectomy, temporal lobe, without electrocorticography during surgery
➔ *CPT Changes: An Insider's View* 2004

61538 for lobectomy, temporal lobe, with electrocorticography during surgery
➔ *CPT Changes: An Insider's View* 2004

61539 for lobectomy, other than temporal lobe, partial or total, with electrocorticography during surgery
➔ *CPT Changes: An Insider's View* 2004

61540 for lobectomy, other than temporal lobe, partial or total, without electrocorticography during surgery
➔ *CPT Changes: An Insider's View* 2004

61541 for transection of corpus callosum

61543 for partial or subtotal (functional) hemispherectomy
➔ *CPT Changes: An Insider's View* 2004

61544 for excision or coagulation of choroid plexus

61545 for excision of craniopharyngioma

(For craniotomy for selective amygdalohippocampectomy, use 61566)

(For craniotomy for multiple subpial transections during surgery, use 61567)

61546 Craniotomy for hypophysectomy or excision of pituitary tumor, intracranial approach

61548 Hypophysectomy or excision of pituitary tumor, transnasal or transseptal approach, nonstereotactic
➔ *CPT Assistant* Nov 98:17, Jul 11:13, Dec 19:12

(Do not report code 69990 in addition to code 61548)

61550 Craniectomy for craniosynostosis; single cranial suture
➔ *CPT Assistant* Feb 12:11, Oct 22:18

61552 multiple cranial sutures
➔ *CPT Assistant* Feb 12:11

(For cranial reconstruction for orbital hypertelorism, see 21260-21263)

(For reconstruction, see 21172-21180)

61556 Craniotomy for craniosynostosis; frontal or parietal bone flap

61557 bifrontal bone flap
➔ *CPT Assistant* Feb 12:11

61558 Extensive craniectomy for multiple cranial suture craniosynostosis (eg, cloverleaf skull); not requiring bone grafts
➔ *CPT Assistant* Feb 12:11

61559 recontouring with multiple osteotomies and bone autografts (eg, barrel-stave procedure) (includes obtaining grafts)
➔ *CPT Assistant* Feb 12:11, Oct 22:18

(For reconstruction, see 21172-21180)

61563 Excision, intra and extracranial, benign tumor of cranial bone (eg, fibrous dysplasia); without optic nerve decompression

61564 with optic nerve decompression

(For reconstruction, see 21181-21183)

61566 Craniotomy with elevation of bone flap; for selective amygdalohippocampectomy
➔ *CPT Changes: An Insider's View* 2004

61567 for multiple subpial transections, with electrocorticography during surgery
➔ *CPT Changes: An Insider's View* 2004

61570 Craniectomy or craniotomy; with excision of foreign body from brain

61571 with treatment of penetrating wound of brain

(For sequestrectomy for osteomyelitis, use 61501)

61575 Transoral approach to skull base, brain stem or upper spinal cord for biopsy, decompression or excision of lesion;

61576 requiring splitting of tongue and/or mandible (including tracheostomy)

(For arthrodesis, use 22548)

Surgery of Skull Base

The surgical management of lesions involving the skull base (base of anterior, middle, and posterior cranial fossae) often requires the skills of several surgeons of different surgical specialties working together or in tandem during the operative session. These operations are usually not staged because of the need for definitive closure of dura, subcutaneous tissues, and skin to avoid serious infections such as osteomyelitis and/or meningitis.

The procedures are categorized according to:

(1) **approach procedure** necessary to obtain adequate exposure to the lesion (pathologic entity), (2) **definitive procedure(s)** necessary to biopsy, excise or otherwise treat the lesion, and (3) **repair/reconstruction** of the defect present following the definitive procedure(s).

The ***approach procedure*** is described according to anatomical area involved, ie, anterior cranial fossa, middle cranial fossa, posterior cranial fossa, and brain stem or upper spinal cord.

The ***definitive procedure(s)*** describes the repair, biopsy, resection, or excision of various lesions of the skull base and, when appropriate, primary closure of the dura, mucous membranes, and skin.

The ***repair/reconstruction procedure(s)*** is reported separately if extensive dural grafting, cranioplasty, local or regional myocutaneous pedicle flaps, or extensive skin grafts are required.

For primary closure, see the appropriate codes (ie, 15730, 15733, 15756, 15757, 15758).

When one surgeon performs the approach procedure, another surgeon performs the definitive procedure, and another surgeon performs the repair/reconstruction procedure, each surgeon reports only the code for the specific procedure performed.

If one surgeon performs more than one procedure (ie, approach procedure and definitive procedure), then both codes are reported, adding modifier 51 to the secondary, additional procedure(s).

Approach Procedures

Anterior Cranial Fossa

61580   Craniofacial approach to anterior cranial fossa; extradural, including lateral rhinotomy, ethmoidectomy, sphenoidectomy, without maxillectomy or orbital exenteration
➔ *CPT Assistant* Winter 93:17, Spring 94:11

61581   extradural, including lateral rhinotomy, orbital exenteration, ethmoidectomy, sphenoidectomy and/or maxillectomy
➔ *CPT Assistant* Winter 93:17, Spring 94:11

61582   extradural, including unilateral or bifrontal craniotomy, elevation of frontal lobe(s), osteotomy of base of anterior cranial fossa
➔ *CPT Assistant* Winter 93:17, Spring 94:11

61583   intradural, including unilateral or bifrontal craniotomy, elevation or resection of frontal lobe, osteotomy of base of anterior cranial fossa
➔ *CPT Assistant* Winter 93:17, Spring 94:11, Dec 17:13

61584   Orbitocranial approach to anterior cranial fossa, extradural, including supraorbital ridge osteotomy and elevation of frontal and/or temporal lobe(s); without orbital exenteration
➔ *CPT Assistant* Winter 93:18

61585   with orbital exenteration
➔ *CPT Assistant* Winter 93:18

61586   Bicoronal, transzygomatic and/or LeFort I osteotomy approach to anterior cranial fossa with or without internal fixation, without bone graft
➔ *CPT Assistant* Winter 93:18, Nov 96:12

Middle Cranial Fossa

61590   Infratemporal pre-auricular approach to middle cranial fossa (parapharyngeal space, infratemporal and midline skull base, nasopharynx), with or without disarticulation of the mandible, including parotidectomy, craniotomy, decompression and/or mobilization of the facial nerve and/or petrous carotid artery
➔ *CPT Assistant* Winter 93:18, Apr 20:10

61591   Infratemporal post-auricular approach to middle cranial fossa (internal auditory meatus, petrous apex, tentorium, cavernous sinus, parasellar area, infratemporal fossa) including mastoidectomy, resection of sigmoid sinus, with or without decompression and/or mobilization of contents of auditory canal or petrous carotid artery
➔ *CPT Assistant* Winter 93:18

61592   Orbitocranial zygomatic approach to middle cranial fossa (cavernous sinus and carotid artery, clivus, basilar artery or petrous apex) including osteotomy of zygoma, craniotomy, extra- or intradural elevation of temporal lobe
➔ *CPT Assistant* Winter 93:18

Posterior Cranial Fossa

61595   Transtemporal approach to posterior cranial fossa, jugular foramen or midline skull base, including mastoidectomy, decompression of sigmoid sinus and/or facial nerve, with or without mobilization
➔ *CPT Assistant* Winter 93:18, Mar 18:11

61596   Transcochlear approach to posterior cranial fossa, jugular foramen or midline skull base, including labyrinthectomy, decompression, with or without mobilization of facial nerve and/or petrous carotid artery
➔ *CPT Assistant* Winter 93:18

61597   Transcondylar (far lateral) approach to posterior cranial fossa, jugular foramen or midline skull base, including occipital condylectomy, mastoidectomy, resection of C1-C3 vertebral body(s), decompression of vertebral artery, with or without mobilization
➔ *CPT Assistant* Winter 93:18

61598   Transpetrosal approach to posterior cranial fossa, clivus or foramen magnum, including ligation of superior petrosal sinus and/or sigmoid sinus
➔ *CPT Assistant* Winter 93:18

Definitive Procedures

Base of Anterior Cranial Fossa

61600 Resection or excision of neoplastic, vascular or infectious lesion of base of anterior cranial fossa; extradural
➔ *CPT Assistant* Winter 93:19, Spring 94:12, Nov 96:12

61601 intradural, including dural repair, with or without graft
➔ *CPT Assistant* Winter 93:19, Spring 94:12

Base of Middle Cranial Fossa

61605 Resection or excision of neoplastic, vascular or infectious lesion of infratemporal fossa, parapharyngeal space, petrous apex; extradural
➔ *CPT Assistant* Winter 93:19, Apr 20:10, Aug 21:15

61606 intradural, including dural repair, with or without graft
➔ *CPT Assistant* Winter 93:20

61607 Resection or excision of neoplastic, vascular or infectious lesion of parasellar area, cavernous sinus, clivus or midline skull base; extradural
➔ *CPT Assistant* Winter 93:20

61608 intradural, including dural repair, with or without graft
➔ *CPT Assistant* Winter 93:20

Code 61611 is reported in addition to code(s) for primary procedure(s) 61605-61608. Report only one transection or ligation of carotid artery code per operative session.

+ 61611 Transection or ligation, carotid artery in petrous canal; without repair (List separately in addition to code for primary procedure)
➔ *CPT Assistant* Winter 93:20

61613 Obliteration of carotid aneurysm, arteriovenous malformation, or carotid-cavernous fistula by dissection within cavernous sinus
➔ *CPT Assistant* Winter 93:20

Base of Posterior Cranial Fossa

61615 Resection or excision of neoplastic, vascular or infectious lesion of base of posterior cranial fossa, jugular foramen, foramen magnum, or C1-C3 vertebral bodies; extradural
➔ *CPT Assistant* Winter 93:20, Aug 21:15

61616 intradural, including dural repair, with or without graft
➔ *CPT Assistant* Mar 18:11

Repair and/or Reconstruction of Surgical Defects of Skull Base

61618 Secondary repair of dura for cerebrospinal fluid leak, anterior, middle or posterior cranial fossa following surgery of the skull base; by free tissue graft (eg, pericranium, fascia, tensor fascia lata, adipose tissue, homologous or synthetic grafts)
➔ *CPT Assistant* Winter 93:20, Spring 94:19, Mar 00:11

61619 by local or regionalized vascularized pedicle flap or myocutaneous flap (including galea, temporalis, frontalis or occipitalis muscle)
➔ *CPT Assistant* Winter 93:20, Spring 94:19, Mar 00:11

Endovascular Therapy

61623 Endovascular temporary balloon arterial occlusion, head or neck (extracranial/intracranial) including selective catheterization of vessel to be occluded, positioning and inflation of occlusion balloon, concomitant neurological monitoring, and radiologic supervision and interpretation of all angiography required for balloon occlusion and to exclude vascular injury post occlusion
➔ *CPT Changes: An Insider's View* 2003

(If selective catheterization and angiography of arteries other than artery to be occluded is performed, use appropriate catheterization and radiologic supervision and interpretation codes)

(If complete diagnostic angiography of the artery to be occluded is performed immediately prior to temporary occlusion, use appropriate radiologic supervision and interpretation codes only)

61624 Transcatheter permanent occlusion or embolization (eg, for tumor destruction, to achieve hemostasis, to occlude a vascular malformation), percutaneous, any method; central nervous system (intracranial, spinal cord)
➔ *CPT Changes: An Insider's View* 2003
➔ *CPT Assistant* Jun 99:10, Nov 06:8, Nov 13:6, Sep 19:6
➔ *Clinical Examples in Radiology* Summer 07:2, Summer 16:13, Winter 18:2, Spring 20:15

(For non-central nervous system and non-head or neck embolization, see 37241-37244)

(For radiological supervision and interpretation, use 75894)

61626 non-central nervous system, head or neck (extracranial, brachiocephalic branch)
➔ *CPT Assistant* Nov 13:6, Sep 19:6
➔ *Clinical Examples in Radiology* Spring 16:5, Spring 20:15

(For non-central nervous system and non-head or neck embolization, see 37241-37244)

(For radiological supervision and interpretation, use 75894)

61630 Balloon angioplasty, intracranial (eg, atherosclerotic stenosis), percutaneous
➔ *CPT Changes: An Insider's View* 2006
➔ *CPT Assistant* Apr 17:10
➔ *Clinical Examples in Radiology* Winter 06:16

61635 Transcatheter placement of intravascular stent(s), intracranial (eg, atherosclerotic stenosis), including balloon angioplasty, if performed

➲ *CPT Changes: An Insider's View* 2006
➲ *CPT Assistant* Mar 14:8
➲ *Clinical Examples in Radiology* Winter 06:16

(61630 and 61635 include all selective vascular catheterization of the target vascular territory, all diagnostic imaging for arteriography of the target vascular territory, and all related radiological supervision and interpretation. When diagnostic arteriogram (including imaging and selective catheterization) confirms the need for angioplasty or stent placement, 61630 and 61635 are inclusive of these services. If angioplasty or stenting are not indicated, then the appropriate codes for selective catheterization and imaging should be reported in lieu of 61630 and 61635)

(Do not report 61630 or 61635 in conjunction with 61645 for the same vascular territory)

(For definition of vascular territory, see the Nervous System Endovascular Therapy guidelines)

61640 Balloon dilatation of intracranial vasospasm, percutaneous; initial vessel

➲ *CPT Changes: An Insider's View* 2006
➲ *CPT Assistant* May 14:10
➲ *Clinical Examples in Radiology* Winter 06:16

+ 61641 each additional vessel in same vascular territory (List separately in addition to code for primary procedure)

➲ *CPT Changes: An Insider's View* 2006, 2019
➲ *CPT Assistant* May 14:10
➲ *Clinical Examples in Radiology* Winter 06:16

+ 61642 each additional vessel in different vascular territory (List separately in addition to code for primary procedure)

➲ *CPT Changes: An Insider's View* 2006, 2019
➲ *CPT Assistant* May 14:10
➲ *Clinical Examples in Radiology* Winter 06:16

(Use 61641 and 61642 in conjunction with 61640)

(61640, 61641, 61642 include all selective vascular catheterization of the target vessel, contrast injection[s], vessel measurement, roadmapping, postdilatation angiography, and fluoroscopic guidance for the balloon dilatation)

(Do not report 61640, 61642 in conjunction with 61650 or 61651 for the same vascular territory)

(For definition of vascular territory, see the Nervous System Endovascular Therapy guidelines)

Codes 61645, 61650, 61651 describe cerebral endovascular therapeutic interventions in any intracranial artery. They include selective catheterization, diagnostic angiography, and all subsequent angiography including associated radiological supervision and interpretation within the treated vascular territory, fluoroscopic guidance, neurologic and hemodynamic monitoring of the patient, and closure of the arteriotomy by manual pressure, an arterial closure device, or suture.

For purposes of reporting services described by 61645, 61650, 61651, the intracranial arteries are divided into three vascular territories: 1) right carotid circulation; 2) left carotid circulation; 3) vertebro-basilar circulation. Code 61645 may be reported once for each intracranial vascular territory treated. Code 61650 is reported once for the first intracranial vascular territory treated with intra-arterial prolonged administration of pharmacologic agent(s). If additional intracranial vascular territory(ies) is also treated with intra-arterial prolonged administration of pharmacologic agent(s) during the same session, the treatment of each additional vascular territory(ies) is reported using 61651 (may be reported maximally two times per day).

Code 61645 describes endovascular revascularization of thrombotic/embolic occlusion of intracranial arterial vessel(s) via any method, including mechanical thrombectomy (eg, mechanical retrieval device, aspiration catheter) and/or the administration of any agent(s) for the purpose of revascularization, such as thrombolytics or IIB/IIIA inhibitors.

Codes 61650, 61651 describe the cerebral endovascular continuous or intermittent therapeutic prolonged administration of any non-thrombolytic agent(s) (eg, spasmolytics or chemotherapy) into an artery to treat non-iatrogenic central nervous system diseases or sequelae thereof. These codes should not be used to report administration of agents (eg, heparin, nitroglycerin, saline) usually administered during endovascular interventions. These codes are used for prolonged administrations, ie, of at least 10 minutes continuous or intermittent duration.

Do not report 61645, 61650, or 61651 in conjunction with 36221, 36226, 36228, 37184, or 37186 for the treated vascular territory. Do not report 61645 in conjunction with 61650 or 61651 for the same vascular distribution. Diagnostic angiography of a non-treated vascular territory may be reported separately. For example, angiography of the left carotid and/or the vertebral circulations may be reported if the intervention is performed in the right carotid circulation.

61645 Percutaneous arterial transluminal mechanical thrombectomy and/or infusion for thrombolysis, intracranial, any method, including diagnostic angiography, fluoroscopic guidance, catheter placement, and intraprocedural pharmacological thrombolytic injection(s)

➲ *CPT Changes: An Insider's View* 2016
➲ *CPT Assistant* Nov 15:3, Dec 15:17, Mar 16:3, Sep 19:6
➲ *Clinical Examples in Radiology* Spring 16:2

(Do not report 61645 in conjunction with 36221, 36222, 36223, 36224, 36225, 36226, 37184, 61630, 61635, 61650, 61651 for the same vascular territory)

(To report venous mechanical thrombectomy and/or thrombolysis, see 37187, 37188, 37212, 37214)

61650 Endovascular intracranial prolonged administration of pharmacologic agent(s) other than for thrombolysis, arterial, including catheter placement, diagnostic angiography, and imaging guidance; initial vascular territory

➲ *CPT Changes: An Insider's View* 2016
➲ *CPT Assistant* Nov 15:3, Mar 16:3, Sep 19:6
➲ *Clinical Examples in Radiology* Spring 16:3

+ 61651 each additional vascular territory (List separately in addition to code for primary procedure)

➲ *CPT Changes: An Insider's View* 2016
➲ *CPT Assistant* Nov 15:3, Mar 16:3, Sep 19:6
➲ *Clinical Examples in Radiology* Spring 16:3

(Use 61651 in conjunction with 61650)

(Do not report 61650 or 61651 in conjunction with 36221, 36222, 36223, 36224, 36225, 36226, 61640, 61641, 61642, 61645 for the same vascular territory)

(Do not report 61650 or 61651 in conjunction with 96420, 96422, 96423, 96425 for the same vascular territory)

Surgery for Aneurysm, Arteriovenous Malformation, or Vascular Disease

Includes craniotomy when appropriate for procedure.

61680 Surgery of intracranial arteriovenous malformation; supratentorial, simple

61682 supratentorial, complex

➲ *CPT Assistant* Jun 13:14

61684 infratentorial, simple

61686 infratentorial, complex

➲ *CPT Assistant* Jun 13:14

61690 dural, simple

61692 dural, complex

➲ *CPT Assistant* Jun 13:14

61697 Surgery of complex intracranial aneurysm, intracranial approach; carotid circulation

➲ *CPT Changes: An Insider's View* 2001
➲ *CPT Assistant* Dec 17:13

61698 vertebrobasilar circulation

➲ *CPT Changes: An Insider's View* 2001

(61697, 61698 involve aneurysms that are larger than 15 mm or with calcification of the aneurysm neck, or with incorporation of normal vessels into the aneurysm neck, or a procedure requiring temporary vessel occlusion, trapping, or cardiopulmonary bypass to successfully treat the aneurysm)

61700 Surgery of simple intracranial aneurysm, intracranial approach; carotid circulation

➲ *CPT Changes: An Insider's View* 2001
➲ *CPT Assistant* Jun 99:11, Jul 99:10, Dec 17:13

61702 vertebrobasilar circulation

➲ *CPT Changes: An Insider's View* 2001

Intracranial Aneurysm, Intracranial Approach
61700

Placement of ligating clip across the neck of an intracranial aneurysm

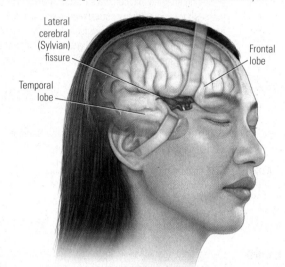

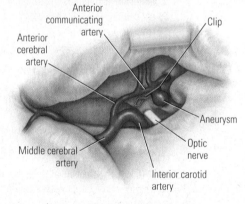

61703 Surgery of intracranial aneurysm, cervical approach by application of occluding clamp to cervical carotid artery (Selverstone-Crutchfield type)

(For cervical approach for direct ligation of carotid artery, see 37600-37606)

61705 Surgery of aneurysm, vascular malformation or carotid-cavernous fistula; by intracranial and cervical occlusion of carotid artery

61708 by intracranial electrothrombosis

(For ligation or gradual occlusion of internal/common carotid artery, see 37605, 37606)

61710 by intra-arterial embolization, injection procedure, or balloon catheter
➔ *CPT Assistant* Nov 13:6

61711 Anastomosis, arterial, extracranial-intracranial (eg, middle cerebral/cortical) arteries

(For carotid or vertebral thromboendarterectomy, use 35301)

(Use 69990 when the surgical microscope is employed for the microsurgical procedure. Do not use 69990 for visualization with magnifying loupes or corrected vision)

Stereotaxis

● **61715** Magnetic resonance image guided high intensity focused ultrasound (MRgFUS), stereotactic ablation of target, intracranial, including stereotactic navigation and frame placement, when performed
➔ *CPT Changes: An Insider's View* 2025

▶(Do not report 61715 in conjunction with 61781, 61800)◀

▶(Do not report 61715 in conjunction with 70540, 70542, 70543, 70544, 70545, 70546, 70551, 70552, 70553, when performed in the same session)◀

61720 Creation of lesion by stereotactic method, including burr hole(s) and localizing and recording techniques, single or multiple stages; globus pallidus or thalamus
➔ *CPT Assistant* Jul 11:12, Jul 14:9

61735 subcortical structure(s) other than globus pallidus or thalamus
➔ *CPT Assistant* Jul 11:12

61736 Laser interstitial thermal therapy (LITT) of lesion, intracranial, including burr hole(s), with magnetic resonance imaging guidance, when performed; single trajectory for 1 simple lesion
➔ *CPT Changes: An Insider's View* 2022
➔ *CPT Assistant* Dec 21:22

(Do not report 61736 in conjunction with 20660, 61737, 61781, 70551, 70552, 70553, 70557, 70558, 70559, 77021, 77022)

61737 multiple trajectories for multiple or complex lesion(s)
➔ *CPT Changes: An Insider's View* 2022
➔ *CPT Assistant* Dec 21:22

(Do not report 61737 in conjunction with 20660, 61736, 61781, 70551, 70552, 70553, 70557, 70558, 70559, 77021, 77022)

61750 Stereotactic biopsy, aspiration, or excision, including burr hole(s), for intracranial lesion;
➔ *CPT Changes: An Insider's View* 2000
➔ *CPT Assistant* Nov 99:30

61751 with computed tomography and/or magnetic resonance guidance
➔ *CPT Changes: An Insider's View* 2000, 2003
➔ *CPT Assistant* Jun 96:10, Nov 99:30, Dec 04:20, Jul 11:12

(For radiological supervision and interpretation of computerized tomography, see 70450, 70460, or 70470 as appropriate)

(For radiological supervision and interpretation of magnetic resonance imaging, see 70551, 70552, or 70553 as appropriate)

61760 Stereotactic implantation of depth electrodes into the cerebrum for long-term seizure monitoring
➔ *CPT Assistant* Jul 11:12

61770 Stereotactic localization, including burr hole(s), with insertion of catheter(s) or probe(s) for placement of radiation source
➔ *CPT Changes: An Insider's View* 2001
➔ *CPT Assistant* Jul 11:12

+ **61781** Stereotactic computer-assisted (navigational) procedure; cranial, intradural (List separately in addition to code for primary procedure)
➔ *CPT Changes: An Insider's View* 2011
➔ *CPT Assistant* Jul 11:12, Jul 14:9, Sep 14:14

(Do not report 61781 in conjunction with 61720-61791, 61796-61799, 61863-61868, 62201, 77371-77373, 77432)

+ **61782** cranial, extradural (List separately in addition to code for primary procedure)
➔ *CPT Changes: An Insider's View* 2011
➔ *CPT Assistant* Jul 11:12

(Do not report 61781, 61782 by the same individual during the same surgical session)

+ **61783** spinal (List separately in addition to code for primary procedure)
➔ *CPT Changes: An Insider's View* 2011
➔ *CPT Assistant* Jul 11:12

(Do not report 61783 in conjunction with 63620, 63621)

61790 Creation of lesion by stereotactic method, percutaneous, by neurolytic agent (eg, alcohol, thermal, electrical, radiofrequency); gasserian ganglion
➔ *CPT Assistant* Jul 11:12

61791 trigeminal medullary tract
➔ *CPT Assistant* Jul 11:12, Jul 14:9

Stereotactic Radiosurgery (Cranial)

Cranial stereotactic radiosurgery is a distinct procedure that utilizes externally generated ionizing radiation to inactivate or eradicate defined target(s) in the head without the need to make an incision. The target is defined by and the treatment is delivered using high-resolution stereotactic imaging. Stereotactic radiosurgery codes and headframe application procedures are reported by the neurosurgeon. The radiation oncologist reports the appropriate code(s) for clinical treatment planning, physics and dosimetry, treatment delivery, and management from the **Radiation Oncology** section (77261-77790). Any necessary planning, dosimetry, targeting, positioning, or blocking by the neurosurgeon is included in the stereotactic radiation surgery services. The same individual should not report stereotactic radiosurgery services with radiation treatment management codes (77427-77435).

Cranial stereotactic radiosurgery is typically performed in a single planning and treatment session, using a rigidly attached stereotactic guiding device, other immobilization technology and/or a stereotactic image-guidance system, but can be performed with more than one planning session and in a limited number of treatment sessions, up to a maximum of five sessions. Do not report stereotactic radiosurgery more than once per lesion per course of treatment when the treatment requires more than one session.

Codes 61796 and 61797 involve stereotactic radiosurgery for simple cranial lesions. Simple cranial lesions are lesions less than 3.5 cm in maximum dimension that do not meet the definition of a complex lesion provided below. Report code 61796 when all lesions are simple.

Codes 61798 and 61799 involve stereotactic radiosurgery for complex cranial lesions and procedures that create therapeutic lesions (eg, thalamotomy or pallidotomy). All lesions 3.5 cm in maximum dimension or greater are complex. When performing therapeutic lesion creation procedures, report code 61798 only once regardless of the number of lesions created. Schwannomas, arterio-venous malformations, pituitary tumors, glomus tumors, pineal region tumors and cavernous sinus/parasellar/petroclival tumors are complex. Any lesion that is adjacent (5 mm or less) to the optic nerve/optic chasm/optic tract or within the brainstem is complex. If treating multiple lesions, and any single lesion treated is complex, use 61798.

Do not report codes 61796-61800 in conjunction with code 20660.

Codes 61796-61799 include computer-assisted planning. Do not report codes 61796-61799 in conjunction with 61781-61783.

> (For intensity modulated beam delivery plan and treatment, see 77301, 77385, 77386. For stereotactic body radiation therapy, see 77373, 77435)

61796 Stereotactic radiosurgery (particle beam, gamma ray, or linear accelerator); 1 simple cranial lesion
➔ *CPT Changes: An Insider's View* 2009
➔ *CPT Assistant* Jul 11:12, Apr 12:11, Jul 14:9, Jun 15:6

(Do not report 61796 more than once per course of treatment)

(Do not report 61796 in conjunction with 61798)

+ 61797 each additional cranial lesion, simple (List separately in addition to code for primary procedure)
➔ *CPT Changes: An Insider's View* 2009
➔ *CPT Assistant* Jul 11:12, Apr 12:11, Jun 15:6

(Use 61797 in conjunction with 61796, 61798)

(For each course of treatment, 61797 and 61799 may be reported no more than once per lesion. Do not report any combination of 61797 and 61799 more than 4 times for entire course of treatment regardless of number of lesions treated)

61798 1 complex cranial lesion
➔ *CPT Changes: An Insider's View* 2009
➔ *CPT Assistant* Jul 11:12, Apr 12:11, Jun 15:6

(Do not report 61798 more than once per course of treatment)

(Do not report 61798 in conjunction with 61796)

+ 61799 each additional cranial lesion, complex (List separately in addition to code for primary procedure)
➔ *CPT Changes: An Insider's View* 2009
➔ *CPT Assistant* Jul 11:12, Apr 12:11, Jul 14:9, Jun 15:6

(Use 61799 in conjunction with 61798)

(For each course of treatment, 61797 and 61799 may be reported no more than once per lesion. Do not report any combination of 61797 and 61799 more than 4 times for entire course of treatment regardless of number of lesions treated)

+ 61800 Application of stereotactic headframe for stereotactic radiosurgery (List separately in addition to code for primary procedure)
➔ *CPT Changes: An Insider's View* 2009
➔ *CPT Assistant* Apr 12:11, Jun 15:6

(Use 61800 in conjunction with 61796, 61798)

Neurostimulators (Intracranial)

For electronic analysis with programming, when performed, of cranial nerve and brain neurostimulator pulse generator/transmitters, see codes 95970, 95976, 95977, 95983, 95984. Test stimulation to confirm correct target site placement of the electrode array(s) and/or to confirm the functional status of the system is inherent to placement and is not separately reported as electronic analysis or programming of the neurostimulator system. Electronic analysis (95970) at the time of implantation is not separately reported.

Microelectrode recording, when performed by the operating surgeon in association with implantation of neurostimulator electrode arrays, is an inclusive service and should not be reported separately. If another individual participates in neurophysiological mapping during a deep brain stimulator implantation procedure, this service may be reported by the second individual with codes 95961-95962.

61850   Twist drill or burr hole(s) for implantation of neurostimulator electrodes, cortical

➔ *CPT Changes: An Insider's View* 2000
➔ *CPT Assistant* Sep 99:5, Nov 99:30

61860   Craniectomy or craniotomy for implantation of neurostimulator electrodes, cerebral, cortical

➔ *CPT Changes: An Insider's View* 2000
➔ *CPT Assistant* Sep 99:5, Nov 99:30

61863   Twist drill, burr hole, craniotomy, or craniectomy with stereotactic implantation of neurostimulator electrode array in subcortical site (eg, thalamus, globus pallidus, subthalamic nucleus, periventricular, periaqueductal gray), without use of intraoperative microelectrode recording; first array

➔ *CPT Changes: An Insider's View* 2004
➔ *CPT Assistant* Sep 99:5, Oct 10:10, Jul 11:12, Jul 14:9, Oct 23:24

+ 61864   each additional array (List separately in addition to primary procedure)

➔ *CPT Changes: An Insider's View* 2004
➔ *CPT Assistant* Sep 99:5, Jul 11:12

(Use 61864 in conjunction with 61863)

61867   Twist drill, burr hole, craniotomy, or craniectomy with stereotactic implantation of neurostimulator electrode array in subcortical site (eg, thalamus, globus pallidus, subthalamic nucleus, periventricular, periaqueductal gray), with use of intraoperative microelectrode recording; first array

➔ *CPT Changes: An Insider's View* 2004
➔ *CPT Assistant* Jul 11:12

+ 61868   each additional array (List separately in addition to primary procedure)

➔ *CPT Changes: An Insider's View* 2004
➔ *CPT Assistant* Jul 11:12, Jul 14:9

(Use 61868 in conjunction with 61867)

Placement of Cranial Neurostimulator
61867-61868, 61885

Placement of subcortical (eg, thalamic) neurostimulator electrode via burr hole (61867-61868) with connection of the electrode to an implanted programmable pulse generator (61885) in the infraclavicular area

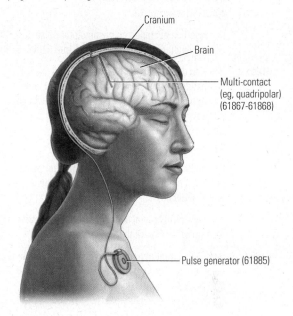

Cranium

Brain

Multi-contact (eg, quadripolar) (61867-61868)

Pulse generator (61885)

61880   Revision or removal of intracranial neurostimulator electrodes

61885   Insertion or replacement of cranial neurostimulator pulse generator or receiver, direct or inductive coupling; with connection to a single electrode array

➔ *CPT Changes: An Insider's View* 2000, 2005
➔ *CPT Assistant* Sep 99:5, Nov 99:30, Jun 00:3, Apr 01:8, Sep 03:3, Dec 10:14, Feb 11:5, Sep 11:8, Jul 21:10

61886   with connection to 2 or more electrode arrays

➔ *CPT Changes: An Insider's View* 2000
➔ *CPT Assistant* Nov 99:30, Jun 00:3, Apr 01:8, Feb 11:5, Sep 11:8, Jul 21:10

(For percutaneous placement of cranial nerve (eg, vagus, trigeminal) neurostimulator electrode(s), use 64553)

(For revision or removal of cranial nerve (eg, vagus, trigeminal) neurostimulator electrode array, use 64569)

61888   Revision or removal of cranial neurostimulator pulse generator or receiver

➔ *CPT Assistant* Sep 11:8, Mar 22:7

(Do not report 61888 in conjunction with 61885 or 61886 for the same pulse generator)

61889 Insertion of skull-mounted cranial neurostimulator pulse generator or receiver, including craniectomy or craniotomy, when performed, with direct or inductive coupling, with connection to depth and/or cortical strip electrode array(s)
  ➲ *CPT Changes: An Insider's View* 2024
  ➲ *CPT Assistant* Dec 23:1

(For insertion of cranial neurostimulator pulse generator or receiver other than skull mounted, see 61885, 61886)

61891 Revision or replacement of skull-mounted cranial neurostimulator pulse generator or receiver with connection to depth and/or cortical strip electrode array(s)
  ➲ *CPT Changes: An Insider's View* 2024
  ➲ *CPT Assistant* Dec 23:1

(For replacement of cranial neurostimulator pulse generator or receiver other than skull mounted, see 61885, 61886)

(For revision of cranial neurostimulator pulse generator or receiver other than skull mounted, use 61888)

61892 Removal of skull-mounted cranial neurostimulator pulse generator or receiver with cranioplasty, when performed
  ➲ *CPT Changes: An Insider's View* 2024
  ➲ *CPT Assistant* Dec 23:1

(Do not report 61892 in conjunction with 61891 for the same pulse generator)

(For removal of cranial neurostimulator pulse generator or receiver other than skull mounted, use 61888)

Repair

62000 Elevation of depressed skull fracture; simple, extradural

62005 compound or comminuted, extradural

62010 with repair of dura and/or debridement of brain

62100 Craniotomy for repair of dural/cerebrospinal fluid leak, including surgery for rhinorrhea/otorrhea
  ➲ *CPT Changes: An Insider's View* 2002

(For repair of spinal dural/CSF leak, see 63707, 63709)

62115 Reduction of craniomegalic skull (eg, treated hydrocephalus); not requiring bone grafts or cranioplasty

62117 requiring craniotomy and reconstruction with or without bone graft (includes obtaining grafts)

62120 Repair of encephalocele, skull vault, including cranioplasty

62121 Craniotomy for repair of encephalocele, skull base

62140 Cranioplasty for skull defect; up to 5 cm diameter
  ➲ *CPT Assistant* Jan 14:9

62141 larger than 5 cm diameter
  ➲ *CPT Assistant* Jan 14:9

62142 Removal of bone flap or prosthetic plate of skull
  ➲ *CPT Assistant* Jan 14:9

62143 Replacement of bone flap or prosthetic plate of skull
  ➲ *CPT Assistant* Jan 14:9

62145 Cranioplasty for skull defect with reparative brain surgery
  ➲ *CPT Assistant* Jan 14:9

62146 Cranioplasty with autograft (includes obtaining bone grafts); up to 5 cm diameter
  ➲ *CPT Assistant* Jan 14:9

62147 larger than 5 cm diameter
  ➲ *CPT Assistant* Jan 14:9

+ 62148 Incision and retrieval of subcutaneous cranial bone graft for cranioplasty (List separately in addition to code for primary procedure)
  ➲ *CPT Changes: An Insider's View* 2003

(Use 62148 in conjunction with 62140-62147)

Neuroendoscopy

Surgical endoscopy always includes diagnostic endoscopy.

+ 62160 Neuroendoscopy, intracranial, for placement or replacement of ventricular catheter and attachment to shunt system or external drainage (List separately in addition to code for primary procedure)
  ➲ *CPT Changes: An Insider's View* 2003
  ➲ *CPT Assistant* Jun 07:11, Dec 12:14

(Use 62160 only in conjunction with 61107, 61210, 62220-62230, 62258)

62161 Neuroendoscopy, intracranial; with dissection of adhesions, fenestration of septum pellucidum or intraventricular cysts (including placement, replacement, or removal of ventricular catheter)
  ➲ *CPT Changes: An Insider's View* 2003

62162 with fenestration or excision of colloid cyst, including placement of external ventricular catheter for drainage
  ➲ *CPT Changes: An Insider's View* 2003

62164 with excision of brain tumor, including placement of external ventricular catheter for drainage
  ➲ *CPT Changes: An Insider's View* 2003

62165 with excision of pituitary tumor, transnasal or trans-sphenoidal approach
  ➲ *CPT Changes: An Insider's View* 2003
  ➲ *CPT Assistant* Dec 17:14, Dec 19:12, Jul 22:18

Cerebrospinal Fluid (CSF) Shunt

62180   Ventriculocisternostomy (Torkildsen type operation)

62190   Creation of shunt; subarachnoid/subdural-atrial, -jugular, -auricular

62192   subarachnoid/subdural-peritoneal, -pleural, other terminus

62194   Replacement or irrigation, subarachnoid/subdural catheter

→ *CPT Assistant* Dec 11:6

62200   Ventriculocisternostomy, third ventricle;

→ *CPT Changes: An Insider's View* 2003

62201   stereotactic, neuroendoscopic method

→ *CPT Changes: An Insider's View* 2003

→ *CPT Assistant* Aug 07:15, Jul 11:12, Jul 14:9

(For intracranial neuroendoscopic procedures, see 62161-62165)

62220   Creation of shunt; ventriculo-atrial, -jugular, -auricular

→ *CPT Changes: An Insider's View* 2003

(For intracranial neuroendoscopic ventricular catheter placement, use 62160)

62223   ventriculo-peritoneal, -pleural, other terminus

→ *CPT Changes: An Insider's View* 2003

(For intracranial neuroendoscopic ventricular catheter placement, use 62160)

Cerebrospinal Fluid (CSF) Shunt (Ventricular Peritoneal)
62223

A ventriculostomy is performed to drain CSF into the peritoneal cavity.

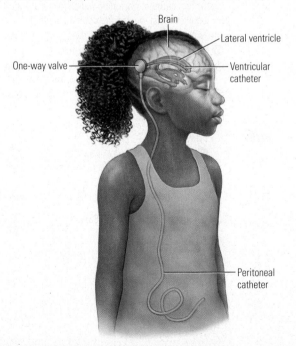

Brain

Lateral ventricle

One-way valve

Ventricular catheter

Peritoneal catheter

62225   Replacement or irrigation, ventricular catheter

→ *CPT Changes: An Insider's View* 2003

→ *CPT Assistant* Dec 11:6

(For intracranial neuroendoscopic ventricular catheter placement, use 62160)

62230   Replacement or revision of cerebrospinal fluid shunt, obstructed valve, or distal catheter in shunt system

→ *CPT Changes: An Insider's View* 2002, 2003

→ *CPT Assistant* Dec 11:6, Dec 12:14

(For intracranial neuroendoscopic ventricular catheter placement, use 62160)

(For replacement of **only** the valve and proximal catheter, use 62230 in conjunction with 62225)

62252   Reprogramming of programmable cerebrospinal shunt

→ *CPT Changes: An Insider's View* 2001, 2002

62256   Removal of complete cerebrospinal fluid shunt system; without replacement

→ *CPT Changes: An Insider's View* 2002

62258   with replacement by similar or other shunt at same operation

→ *CPT Assistant* Dec 11:6

(For percutaneous irrigation or aspiration of shunt reservoir, use 61070)

(For reprogramming of programmable CSF shunt, use 62252)

(For intracranial neuroendoscopic ventricular catheter placement, use 62160)

Spine and Spinal Cord

(For application of caliper or tongs, use 20660)

(For treatment of fracture or dislocation of spine, see 22310-22327)

Injection, Drainage, or Aspiration

Injection of contrast during fluoroscopic guidance and localization is an inclusive component of 62263, 62264, 62267, 62273, 62280, 62281, 62282, 62302, 62303, 62304, 62305, 62321, 62323, 62325, 62327, 62328, 62329. Fluoroscopic guidance and localization is reported with 77003, unless a formal contrast study (myelography or arthrography) is performed, in which case the use of fluoroscopy is included in the supervision and interpretation codes or the myelography via lumbar injection code. Image guidance and the injection of contrast are inclusive components and are required for the performance of myelography, as described by codes 62302, 62303, 62304, 62305.

Code 62263 describes a catheter-based treatment involving targeted injection of various substances (eg, hypertonic saline, steroid, anesthetic) via an indwelling epidural catheter. Code 62263 includes percutaneous insertion and removal of an epidural catheter (remaining in place over a several-day period), for the administration of multiple injections of a neurolytic agent(s) performed during serial treatment sessions (ie, spanning two or more treatment days). If required, adhesions or scarring may also be lysed by mechanical means. Code 62263 is **not** reported for each adhesiolysis treatment, but should be reported **once** to describe the entire series of injections/infusions spanning two or more treatment days.

Code 62264 describes multiple adhesiolysis treatment sessions performed on the same day. Adhesions or scarring may be lysed by injections of neurolytic agent(s). If required, adhesions or scarring may also be lysed mechanically using a percutaneously deployed catheter.

Codes 62263 and 62264 include fluoroscopic guidance and localization (77003) during initial or subsequent sessions.

Fluoroscopy or CT and any injection of contrast are inclusive components of 62321, 62323, 62325, 62327.

The placement and use of a catheter to administer one or more epidural or subarachnoid injections on a single calendar day should be reported in the same manner as if a needle had been used, ie, as a single injection using either 62320, 62321, 62322, or 62323. Such injections should not be reported with 62324, 62325, 62326, or 62327.

Threading a catheter into the epidural space, injecting substances at one or more levels and then removing the catheter should be treated as a single injection (62320, 62321, 62322, 62323). If the catheter is left in place to deliver substance(s) over a prolonged period (ie, more than a single calendar day) either continuously or via intermittent bolus, use 62324, 62325, 62326, 62327 as appropriate.

When reporting 62320, 62321, 62322, 62323, 62324, 62325, 62326, 62327 code choice is based on the region at which the needle or catheter entered the body (eg, lumbar). Codes 62320, 62321, 62322, 62323, 62324, 62325, 62326, 62327 should be reported only once, when the substance injected spreads or catheter tip insertion moves into another spinal region (eg, 62322 is reported only once for injection or catheter insertion at L3-4 with spread of the substance or placement of the catheter tip to the thoracic region).

Percutaneous spinal procedures are done with indirect visualization (eg, image guidance) (eg, 62287). Endoscopic assistance during an open procedure with continuous and direct visualization (light-based) is reported using excision codes (eg, 63020-63035).

(For transforaminal epidural injection, see 64479-64484)

(Report 01996 for daily hospital management of continuous epidural or subarachnoid drug administration performed in conjunction with 62324, 62325, 62326, 62327)

Definitions

For purposes of CPT coding, the following definitions of approach and visualization apply. The primary approach and visualization define the service, whether another method is incidentally applied. Surgical services are presumed open, unless otherwise specified.

Percutaneous: Image-guided procedures (eg, computer tomography [CT] or fluoroscopy) performed with indirect visualization of the spine without the use of any device that allows visualization through a surgical incision.

Endoscopic: Spinal procedures performed with continuous direct visualization of the spine through an endoscope.

Open: Spinal procedures performed with continuous direct visualization of the spine through a surgical opening.

Indirect visualization: Image-guided (eg, CT or fluoroscopy), not light-based visualization.

Direct visualization: Light-based visualization; can be performed by eye, or with surgical loupes, microscope, or endoscope.

(For the techniques of microsurgery and/or use of microscope, use 69990)

62263 Percutaneous lysis of epidural adhesions using solution injection (eg, hypertonic saline, enzyme) or mechanical means (eg, catheter) including radiologic localization (includes contrast when administered), multiple adhesiolysis sessions; 2 or more days
➡ *CPT Changes: An Insider's View* 2000, 2003
➡ *CPT Assistant* Nov 99:33, Dec 99:11, Mar 02:11, Dec 02:10, Nov 05:14, Jul 08:9, Oct 09:12, Nov 10:3, Jan 11:8, Jun 12:12
➡ *Clinical Examples in Radiology* Spring 11:10, Summer 16:4

(62263 includes code 77003)

62264 1 day
➡ *CPT Changes: An Insider's View* 2003
➡ *CPT Assistant* Nov 05:14, Jul 08:9, Oct 09:12, Nov 10:3, Jan 11:8, Jun 12:12
➡ *Clinical Examples in Radiology* Spring 11:10, Summer 16:4

(Do not report 62264 with 62263)

(62264 includes code 77003)

★ = Telemedicine ◀ = Audio-only ✛ = Add-on code � = FDA approval pending # = Resequenced code ⊘ = Modifier 51 exempt ➡➡➡ = See p xxi for details

62267   Percutaneous aspiration within the nucleus pulposus, intervertebral disc, or paravertebral tissue for diagnostic purposes

➔ *CPT Changes: An Insider's View* 2009

➔ *CPT Assistant* Nov 10:3, Jan 11:8, Jul 12:3

➔ *Clinical Examples in Radiology* Fall 10:8, Spring 11:10, Winter 14:10, Summer 16:4, Spring 22:10

(For imaging, use 77003)

(Do not report 62267 in conjunction with 10005, 10006, 10007, 10008, 10009, 10010, 10011, 10012, 20225, 62287, 62290, 62291)

62268   Percutaneous aspiration, spinal cord cyst or syrinx

➔ *CPT Assistant* Dec 17:13

(For radiological supervision and interpretation, see 76942, 77002, 77012)

62269   Biopsy of spinal cord, percutaneous needle

➔ *Clinical Examples in Radiology* Fall 10:7, Winter 17:5, Spring 22:9

(For radiological supervision and interpretation, see 76942, 77002, 77012)

(For fine needle aspiration biopsy, see 10004, 10005, 10006, 10007, 10008, 10009, 10010, 10011, 10012, 10021)

(For evaluation of fine needle aspirate, see 88172, 88173)

62270   Spinal puncture, lumbar, diagnostic;

➔ *CPT Changes: An Insider's View* 2000, 2002, 2020

➔ *CPT Assistant* Nov 99:32-33, Oct 03:2, Jul 06:4, Jul 07:1, Oct 09:12, Nov 10:3, Jan 11:8, Mar 12:3

➔ *Clinical Examples in Radiology* Spring 11:9, Winter 14:9-10, Summer 16:4, Summer 18:9, Fall 19:8, Winter 20:11

\# **62328**   with fluoroscopic or CT guidance

➔ *CPT Changes: An Insider's View* 2020

➔ *CPT Assistant* Jun 20:10

➔ *Clinical Examples in Radiology* Fall 19:9, Winter 20:11

(Do not report 62270, 62328 in conjunction with 77003, 77012)

(If ultrasound or MRI guidance is performed, see 76942, 77021)

62272   Spinal puncture, therapeutic, for drainage of cerebrospinal fluid (by needle or catheter);

➔ *CPT Changes: An Insider's View* 2000, 2020

➔ *CPT Assistant* Nov 99:32-33, Nov 10:3, Dec 13:14

➔ *Clinical Examples in Radiology* Spring 11:10, Winter 14:9-10, Summer 16:4, Fall 19:8

\# **62329**   with fluoroscopic or CT guidance

➔ *CPT Changes: An Insider's View* 2020

➔ *CPT Assistant* Jun 20:10

➔ *Clinical Examples in Radiology* Fall 19:9

(Do not report 62272, 62329 in conjunction with 77003, 77012)

(If ultrasound or MRI guidance is performed, see 76942, 77021)

62273   Injection, epidural, of blood or clot patch

➔ *CPT Changes: An Insider's View* 2000

➔ *CPT Assistant* Nov 99:32, 34, Oct 09:12, Nov 10:3

➔ *Clinical Examples in Radiology* Spring 11:10, Winter 14:10, Summer 16:4

(For injection of diagnostic or therapeutic substance[s], see 62320, 62321, 62322, 62323, 62324, 62325, 62326, 62327)

62280   Injection/infusion of neurolytic substance (eg, alcohol, phenol, iced saline solutions), with or without other therapeutic substance; subarachnoid

➔ *CPT Changes: An Insider's View* 2000

➔ *CPT Assistant* Nov 99:32, 34, Jan 00:2, Jul 08:9, Oct 09:12, Feb 10:11, Nov 10:3, Jan 11:8, Jun 12:12

➔ *Clinical Examples in Radiology* Spring 11:10, Winter 14:10, Summer 16:4

62281   epidural, cervical or thoracic

➔ *CPT Changes: An Insider's View* 2000

➔ *CPT Assistant* Apr 96:11, Nov 99:32, 34, Jan 00:2, Jul 08:9, Oct 09:12, Feb 10:11, May 10:10, Nov 10:3, Jan 11:8, Jun 12:12

➔ *Clinical Examples in Radiology* Spring 11:10, Winter 14:10, Summer 16:4

62282   epidural, lumbar, sacral (caudal)

➔ *CPT Changes: An Insider's View* 2000

➔ *CPT Assistant* Apr 96:11, Nov 99:32, 34, Jan 00:2, Jul 08:9, Oct 09:12, Feb 10:11, Nov 10:3, Jan 11:8, Jun 12:12

➔ *Clinical Examples in Radiology* Spring 11:10, Winter 14:10, Summer 16:4

62284   Injection procedure for myelography and/or computed tomography, lumbar

➔ *CPT Changes: An Insider's View* 2003, 2008, 2015

➔ *CPT Assistant* Fall 93:13, Sep 04:13

➔ *Clinical Examples in Radiology* Fall 06:5-6, 11-12, Spring 11:9, Fall 14:6-7, 11

(Do not report 62284 in conjunction with 62302, 62303, 62304, 62305, 72240, 72255, 72265, 72270)

(When both 62284 and 72240, 72255, 72265, 72270 are performed by the same physician or other qualified health care professional for myelography, see 62302, 62303, 62304, 62305)

(For injection procedure at C1-C2, use 61055)

(For radiological supervision and interpretation, see **Radiology**)

62287   Decompression procedure, percutaneous, of nucleus pulposus of intervertebral disc, any method utilizing needle based technique to remove disc material under fluoroscopic imaging or other form of indirect visualization, with discography and/or epidural injection(s) at the treated level(s), when performed, single or multiple levels, lumbar

➔ *CPT Changes: An Insider's View* 2000, 2009, 2012, 2017

➔ *CPT Assistant* Nov 99:34, Mar 02:11, Oct 10:9, Jul 12:3, Oct 12:14, Apr 14:11, Mar 15:10, Feb 17:12, Dec 19:12, Feb 21:13

(Do not report 62287 in conjunction with 62267, 62290, 62322, 77003, 77012, 72295, when performed at same level)

(For non-needle based technique for percutaneous decompression of nucleus pulposus of intervertebral disc, see 0274T, 0275T)

62290   Injection procedure for discography, each level; lumbar

➔ *CPT Changes: An Insider's View* 2000

➔ *CPT Assistant* Nov 99:35, Apr 03:27, Mar 11:7, Jul 12:3

➔ *Clinical Examples in Radiology* Fall 10:10

62291   cervical or thoracic

➔ *CPT Changes: An Insider's View* 2000

➔ *CPT Assistant* Nov 99:35, Mar 11:7

➔ *Clinical Examples in Radiology* Fall 10:10

(For radiological supervision and interpretation, see 72285, 72295)

62292   Injection procedure for chemonucleolysis, including discography, intervertebral disc, single or multiple levels, lumbar

➔ *CPT Assistant* Oct 99:10

62294   Injection procedure, arterial, for occlusion of arteriovenous malformation, spinal

62302   Myelography via lumbar injection, including radiological supervision and interpretation; cervical

➔ *CPT Changes: An Insider's View* 2015

➔ *Clinical Examples in Radiology* Fall 14:6, Fall 15:10, Summer 16:4

(Do not report 62302 in conjunction with 62284, 62303, 62304, 62305, 72240, 72255, 72265, 72270)

62303   thoracic

➔ *CPT Changes: An Insider's View* 2015

➔ *Clinical Examples in Radiology* Fall 14:6, Fall 15:10, Summer 16:4

(Do not report 62303 in conjunction with 62284, 62302, 62304, 62305, 72240, 72255, 72265, 72270)

62304   lumbosacral

➔ *CPT Changes: An Insider's View* 2015

➔ *Clinical Examples in Radiology* Fall 14:3, 6, Fall 15:10, Summer 16:4

(Do not report 62304 in conjunction with 62284, 62302, 62303, 62305, 72240, 72255, 72265, 72270)

62305   2 or more regions (eg, lumbar/thoracic, cervical/thoracic, lumbar/cervical, lumbar/thoracic/cervical)

➔ *CPT Changes: An Insider's View* 2015

➔ *Clinical Examples in Radiology* Fall 14:6-7, Fall 15:10, Summer 16:4

(Do not report 62305 in conjunction with 62284, 62302, 62303, 62304, 72240, 72255, 72265, 72270)

(For myelography lumbar injection and imaging performed by different physicians or other qualified health care professionals, see 62284 or 72240, 72255, 72265, 72270)

(For injection procedure at C1-C2, use 61055)

62320   Injection(s), of diagnostic or therapeutic substance(s) (eg, anesthetic, antispasmodic, opioid, steroid, other solution), not including neurolytic substances, including needle or catheter placement, interlaminar epidural or subarachnoid, cervical or thoracic; without imaging guidance

➔ *CPT Changes: An Insider's View* 2017

➔ *CPT Assistant* Sep 17:6

62321   with imaging guidance (ie, fluoroscopy or CT)

➔ *CPT Changes: An Insider's View* 2017

➔ *CPT Assistant* Sep 17:6, Sep 23:48

(Do not report 62321 in conjunction with 77003, 77012, 76942)

62322   Injection(s), of diagnostic or therapeutic substance(s) (eg, anesthetic, antispasmodic, opioid, steroid, other solution), not including neurolytic substances, including needle or catheter placement, interlaminar epidural or subarachnoid, lumbar or sacral (caudal); without imaging guidance

➔ *CPT Changes: An Insider's View* 2017

➔ *CPT Assistant* Sep 17:6, Mar 21:3

➔ *Clinical Examples in Radiology* Summer 18:9

62323   with imaging guidance (ie, fluoroscopy or CT)

➔ *CPT Changes: An Insider's View* 2017

➔ *CPT Assistant* Sep 17:6, Mar 21:3, Sep 23:48

➔ *Clinical Examples in Radiology* Summer 18:9

(Do not report 62323 in conjunction with 77003, 77012, 76942)

62324   Injection(s), including indwelling catheter placement, continuous infusion or intermittent bolus, of diagnostic or therapeutic substance(s) (eg, anesthetic, antispasmodic, opioid, steroid, other solution), not including neurolytic substances, interlaminar epidural or subarachnoid, cervical or thoracic; without imaging guidance

➔ *CPT Changes: An Insider's View* 2017

➔ *CPT Assistant* May 17:10, Sep 17:6

62325   with imaging guidance (ie, fluoroscopy or CT)

→ *CPT Changes: An Insider's View* 2017

→ *CPT Assistant* May 17:10, Sep 17:6

(Do not report 62325 in conjunction with 77003, 77012, 76942)

62326   Injection(s), including indwelling catheter placement, continuous infusion or intermittent bolus, of diagnostic or therapeutic substance(s) (eg, anesthetic, antispasmodic, opioid, steroid, other solution), not including neurolytic substances, interlaminar epidural or subarachnoid, lumbar or sacral (caudal); without imaging guidance

→ *CPT Changes: An Insider's View* 2017

→ *CPT Assistant* May 17:10, Sep 17:7

62327   with imaging guidance (ie, fluoroscopy or CT)

→ *CPT Changes: An Insider's View* 2017

→ *CPT Assistant* May 17:10, Sep 17:7

(Do not report 62327 in conjunction with 77003, 77012, 76942)

(Report 01996 for daily hospital management of continuous epidural or subarachnoid drug administration performed in conjunction with 62324, 62325, 62326, 62327)

62328   Code is out of numerical sequence. See 62269-62280

62329   Code is out of numerical sequence. See 62269-62280

Catheter Implantation

(For percutaneous placement of intrathecal or epidural catheter, see 62270, 62272, 62273, 62280, 62281, 62282, 62284, 62320, 62321, 62322, 62323, 62324, 62325, 62326, 62327, 62328, 62329)

62350   Implantation, revision or repositioning of tunneled intrathecal or epidural catheter, for long-term medication administration via an external pump or implantable reservoir/infusion pump; without laminectomy

→ *CPT Changes: An Insider's View* 2000, 2001

→ *CPT Assistant* Nov 99:36

62351   with laminectomy

→ *CPT Changes: An Insider's View* 2000

→ *CPT Assistant* Nov 99:36

(For refilling and maintenance of an implantable infusion pump for spinal or brain drug therapy, see 95990, 95991)

62355   Removal of previously implanted intrathecal or epidural catheter

Reservoir/Pump Implantation

62360   Implantation or replacement of device for intrathecal or epidural drug infusion; subcutaneous reservoir

62361   nonprogrammable pump

62362   programmable pump, including preparation of pump, with or without programming

→ *CPT Assistant* Mar 97:11

Intrathecal or Epidural Drug Infusion Pump Implantation
62362

The reservoir is placed in the subcutaneous tissues and attached to a previously placed catheter for intrathecal or epidural drug infusion.

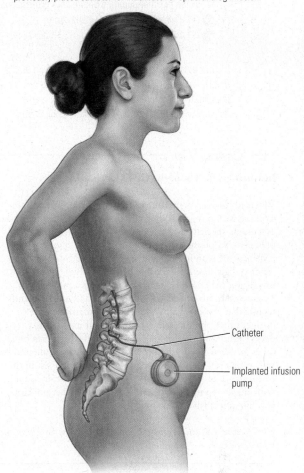

Catheter

Implanted infusion pump

62365   Removal of subcutaneous reservoir or pump, previously implanted for intrathecal or epidural infusion

62367   Electronic analysis of programmable, implanted pump for intrathecal or epidural drug infusion (includes evaluation of reservoir status, alarm status, drug prescription status); without reprogramming or refill

→ *CPT Changes: An Insider's View* 2012

→ *CPT Assistant* Jul 12:5-6, Aug 12:10-12, 15, May 22:18

62368   with reprogramming

→ *CPT Assistant* Nov 02:10, Jul 06:1, Jul 12:5-6, Aug 12:10-12, 15, May 22:18

(For refilling and maintenance of an implantable infusion pump for spinal or brain drug therapy, see 95990-95991)

62369   with reprogramming and refill
> *CPT Changes: An Insider's View* 2012
> *CPT Assistant* Jul 12:5-6, Aug 12:10-12, 15, May 22:18, Jul 22:18

62370   with reprogramming and refill (requiring skill of a physician or other qualified health care professional)
> *CPT Changes: An Insider's View* 2012, 2013
> *CPT Assistant* Jul 12:5-6, Aug 12:10-12, 15, Jun 21:14, May 22:18, Jul 22:18

(Do not report 62367-62370 in conjunction with 95990, 95991. For refilling and maintenance of a reservoir or an implantable infusion pump for spinal or brain drug delivery without reprogramming, see 95990, 95991)

—— *Coding Tip* ——

Instructions for Use of the CPT Codebook

When advanced practice nurses and physician assistants are working with physicians they are considered as working in the exact same specialty and exact same subspecialties as the physician. A "physician or other qualified health care professional" is an individual who is qualified by education, training, licensure/regulation (when applicable), and facility privileging (when applicable) who performs a professional service within his or her scope of practice and independently reports that professional service. These professionals are distinct from "clinical staff." A clinical staff member is a person who works under the supervision of a physician or other qualified health care professional, and who is allowed by law, regulation, and facility policy to perform or assist in the performance of a specific professional service, but does not individually report that professional service. Other policies may also affect who may report specific services.

CPT Coding Guidelines, Introduction, Instructions for Use of the CPT Codebook

Endoscopic Decompression of Neural Elements and/or Excision of Herniated Intervertebral Discs

Definitions

For purposes of CPT coding, the following definitions of approach and visualization apply. The primary approach and visualization define the service, whether another method is incidentally applied. Surgical services are presumed open, unless otherwise specified.

Percutaneous: Image-guided procedures (eg, computer tomography [CT] or fluoroscopy) performed with indirect visualization of the spine without the use of any device that allows visualization through a surgical incision.

Endoscopic: Spinal procedures performed with continuous direct visualization of the spine through an endoscope.

Open: Spinal procedures performed with continuous direct visualization of the spine through a surgical opening.

Indirect visualization: Image-guided (eg, CT or fluoroscopy), not light-based visualization.

Direct visualization: Light-based visualization; can be performed by eye, or with surgical loupes, microscope, or endoscope.

(For the techniques of microsurgery and/or use of microscope, use 69990)

(For percutaneous decompression, see 62287, 0274T, 0275T)

62380   Endoscopic decompression of spinal cord, nerve root(s), including laminotomy, partial facetectomy, foraminotomy, discectomy and/or excision of herniated intervertebral disc, 1 interspace, lumbar
> *CPT Changes: An Insider's View* 2017
> *CPT Assistant* Feb 17:12

(For open procedures, see 63030, 63056)

(For bilateral procedure, report 62380 with modifier 50)

Posterior Extradural Laminotomy or Laminectomy for Exploration/ Decompression of Neural Elements or Excision of Herniated Intervertebral Discs

Definitions

For purposes of CPT coding, the following definitions of approach and visualization apply. The primary approach and visualization define the service, whether another method is incidentally applied. Surgical services are presumed open, unless otherwise specified.

Percutaneous: Image-guided procedures (eg, computer tomography [CT] or fluoroscopy) performed with indirect visualization of the spine without the use of any device that allows visualization through a surgical incision.

Endoscopic: Spinal procedures performed with continuous direct visualization of the spine through an endoscope.

Open: Spinal procedures performed with continuous direct visualization of the spine through a surgical opening.

Indirect visualization: Image-guided (eg, CT or fluoroscopy), not light-based visualization.

Direct visualization: Light-based visualization; can be performed by eye, or with surgical loupes, microscope, or endoscope.

(When 63001-63048 are followed by arthrodesis, see 22590-22614)

(For the techniques of microsurgery and/or use of microscope, use 69990)

(For percutaneous decompression, see 62287, 0274T, 0275T)

63001   Laminectomy with exploration and/or decompression of spinal cord and/or cauda equina, without facetectomy, foraminotomy or discectomy (eg, spinal stenosis), 1 or 2 vertebral segments; cervical
→ *CPT Assistant* Jan 01:12, Jun 07:1, Jul 11:13, Jul 12:3, Jul 13:3

63003   thoracic
→ *CPT Assistant* Jan 01:12, Jul 12:3, Jul 13:3

63005   lumbar, except for spondylolisthesis
→ *CPT Assistant* Jan 01:12, Jul 12:3, Jul 13:3, Dec 13:17

63011   sacral
→ *CPT Assistant* Jan 01:12, Jul 13:3

Lumbar Laminectomy
63005

With the patient prone and under general anesthesia, the laminae and underlying ligamentum flavum are removed.

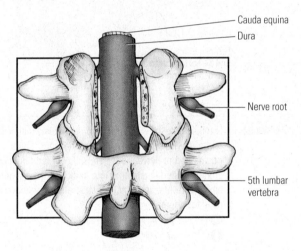

- Cauda equina
- Dura
- Nerve root
- 5th lumbar vertebra

63012   Laminectomy with removal of abnormal facets and/or pars inter-articularis with decompression of cauda equina and nerve roots for spondylolisthesis, lumbar (Gill type procedure)
→ *CPT Assistant* Jan 01:12, Jul 13:3, Dec 19:12

63015   Laminectomy with exploration and/or decompression of spinal cord and/or cauda equina, without facetectomy, foraminotomy or discectomy (eg, spinal stenosis), more than 2 vertebral segments; cervical
→ *CPT Assistant* Jan 01:12, Jul 13:3

63016   thoracic
→ *CPT Assistant* Jan 01:12, Jul 13:3

63017   lumbar
→ *CPT Assistant* Jan 01:12, Jul 13:3

63020   Laminotomy (hemilaminectomy), with decompression of nerve root(s), including partial facetectomy, foraminotomy and/or excision of herniated intervertebral disc; 1 interspace, cervical
→ *CPT Changes: An Insider's View* 2000, 2009, 2012
→ *CPT Assistant* Nov 99:36, Jan 01:12, Jul 12:4, Dec 12:13, Jul 13:3

(For bilateral procedure, report 63020 with modifier 50)

63030   1 interspace, lumbar
→ *CPT Changes: An Insider's View* 2000, 2009, 2012
→ *CPT Assistant* Mar 96:7, Nov 99:36, Jan 01:12, Feb 01:10, Sep 02:10, Oct 04:12, Oct 08:10, Oct 09:9, Nov 10:4, Mar 11:7, Jul 11:13, Jul 12:3-4, Dec 12:13, Jul 13:3, Dec 13:17, May 16:13, Feb 17:13, Nov 19:15, May 20:14

(For bilateral procedure, report 63030 with modifier 50)

+ 63035   each additional interspace, cervical or lumbar (List separately in addition to code for primary procedure)
→ *CPT Changes: An Insider's View* 2000, 2009, 2012
→ *CPT Assistant* Fall 91:8, Mar 96:7, Nov 99:36, Jan 01:12, Feb 01:10, Jul 12:4, Mar 22:5

(Use 63035 in conjunction with 63020-63030)

(Do not report 63030, 63035 in conjunction with 22630, 22632, 22633, 22634, for laminotomy performed to prepare the interspace for fusion on the same interspace[s] and vertebral segment[s])

(For decompression performed on the same interspace[s] and vertebral segment[s] as posterior interbody fusion that includes laminectomy, removal of facets, and/or opening/widening of the foramen for decompression of nerves or spinal components, such as spinal cord, cauda equina, or nerve roots, see 63052, 63053)

(For bilateral procedure, report 63035 twice. Do not report modifier 50 in conjunction with 63035)

(For percutaneous endoscopic approach, see 0274T, 0275T)

63040   Laminotomy (hemilaminectomy), with decompression of nerve root(s), including partial facetectomy, foraminotomy and/or excision of herniated intervertebral disc, reexploration, single interspace; cervical
→ *CPT Changes: An Insider's View* 2001
→ *CPT Assistant* Jan 99:11, Jan 01:12, Jul 13:3, May 20:14, Jul 21:7

(For bilateral procedure, report 63040 with modifier 50)

63042   lumbar
→ *CPT Assistant* Jan 99:11, Jan 01:12, Oct 08:10, Oct 09:9, Jul 11:13, Jul 13:3, May 20:14, Jul 21:7

(For bilateral procedure, report 63042 with modifier 50)

+ 63043   each additional cervical interspace (List separately in addition to code for primary procedure)

⮕ *CPT Changes: An Insider's View* 2001

⮕ *CPT Assistant* May 20:14, Jul 21:7

(Use 63043 in conjunction with 63040)

(For bilateral procedure, report 63043 twice. Do not report modifier 50 in conjunction with 63043)

+ 63044   each additional lumbar interspace (List separately in addition to code for primary procedure)

⮕ *CPT Changes: An Insider's View* 2001

⮕ *CPT Assistant* May 20:14, Jul 21:7, Mar 22:5

(Use 63044 in conjunction with 63042)

(Do not report 63040, 63042, 63043, 63044 in conjunction with 22630, 22632, 22633, 22634, for laminotomy to prepare the interspace for fusion on the same interspace[s] and vertebral segment[s])

(For decompression performed on the same interspace[s] and vertebral segment[s] as posterior interbody fusion that includes laminectomy, removal of facets, and/or opening/widening of the foramen for decompression of nerves or spinal components, such as spinal cord, cauda equina, or nerve roots, see 63052, 63053)

(For bilateral procedure, report 63044 twice. Do not report modifier 50 in conjunction with 63044)

Decompression performed on the same interspace[s] and vertebral segment(s) as posterior interbody fusion that includes laminectomy, facetectomy, or foraminotomy may be separately reported using 63052.

Codes 63052, 63053 may only be reported for decompression at the same anatomic site(s) when posterior interbody fusion (eg, 22630) requires decompression beyond preparation of the interspace(s) for fusion.

63045   Laminectomy, facetectomy and foraminotomy (unilateral or bilateral with decompression of spinal cord, cauda equina and/or nerve root[s], [eg, spinal or lateral recess stenosis]), single vertebral segment; cervical

⮕ *CPT Assistant* Jan 01:12, Dec 12:13, Jul 13:3, Jul 21:7, Mar 22:4-5, Mar 24:27

63046   thoracic

⮕ *CPT Assistant* Jan 99:11, Jan 01:12, Dec 12:13, Jul 13:3, Mar 22:4-5

63047   lumbar

⮕ *CPT Assistant* Jan 99:11, Jan 01:12, Feb 01:10, Nov 02:11, Apr 08:11, Jul 08:7, Oct 08:10, Oct 09:9, Nov 10:4, Jul 11:13, Dec 12:13, Jul 13:3, Dec 13:17, Dec 14:16, Oct 16:11, Feb 17:13, May 18:9, Dec 19:12, May 20:14, Jul 21:7, Dec 21:6, 22, Mar 22:4-5, Mar 24:27

+ 63048   each additional vertebral segment, cervical, thoracic, or lumbar (List separately in addition to code for primary procedure)

⮕ *CPT Changes: An Insider's View* 2022

⮕ *CPT Assistant* Fall 91:8, Jan 99:11, Jan 01:12, Dec 12:13, Jul 21:7, Dec 21:22, Mar 22:4-5, Mar 24:27

(Use 63048 in conjunction with 63045-63047)

(Do not report 63047, 63048 in conjunction with 22630, 22632, 22633, 22634, for laminectomy performed to prepare the interspace for fusion on the same interspace[s] and vertebral segment[s])

(For decompression performed on the same interspace[s] and vertebral segment[s] as posterior interbody fusion that includes laminectomy, removal of facets, and/or opening/widening of the foramen for decompression of nerves or spinal components, such as spinal cord, cauda equina, or nerve roots, see 63052, 63053)

Example of Laminectomy at Single Interspace
63047

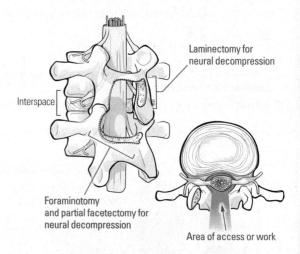

Laminectomy for neural decompression

Interspace

Foraminotomy and partial facetectomy for neural decompression

Area of access or work

#+ 63052   Laminectomy, facetectomy, or foraminotomy (unilateral or bilateral with decompression of spinal cord, cauda equina and/or nerve root[s] [eg, spinal or lateral recess stenosis]), during posterior interbody arthrodesis, lumbar; single vertebral segment (List separately in addition to code for primary procedure)

⮕ *CPT Changes: An Insider's View* 2022

⮕ *CPT Assistant* Mar 22:3-5

#+ 63053   each additional vertebral segment (List separately in addition to code for primary procedure)

⮕ *CPT Changes: An Insider's View* 2022

⮕ *CPT Assistant* Mar 22:3-5

(Use 63053 in conjunction with 63052)

(Use 63052, 63053 in conjunction with 22630, 22632, 22633, 22634)

63050   Laminoplasty, cervical, with decompression of the spinal cord, 2 or more vertebral segments;

⮕ *CPT Changes: An Insider's View* 2005, 2022

⮕ *CPT Assistant* Jul 13:3

63051	with reconstruction of the posterior bony elements (including the application of bridging bone graft and non-segmental fixation devices [eg, wire, suture, mini-plates], when performed)

➜ *CPT Changes: An Insider's View* 2005, 2022

➜ *CPT Assistant* Jul 11:13, Jul 13:3, Feb 23:14, Mar 24:27

(Do not report 63050 or 63051 in conjunction with 22600, 22614, 22840-22842, 63001, 63015, 63045, 63048, 63295 for the same vertebral segment(s))

63052   Code is out of numerical sequence. See 63047-63051

63053   Code is out of numerical sequence. See 63047-63051

Transpedicular or Costovertebral Approach for Posterolateral Extradural Exploration/Decompression

63055   Transpedicular approach with decompression of spinal cord, equina and/or nerve root(s) (eg, herniated intervertebral disc), single segment; thoracic

➜ *CPT Changes: An Insider's View* 2000

➜ *CPT Assistant* Nov 99:36, Jul 13:3

63056   lumbar (including transfacet, or lateral extraforaminal approach) (eg, far lateral herniated intervertebral disc)

➜ *CPT Changes: An Insider's View* 2000

➜ *CPT Assistant* Nov 99:36, Oct 09:9, Nov 11:10, Jul 12:3, Jul 13:3, Jan 14:9, Nov 19:15, May 21:14

+ 63057   each additional segment, thoracic or lumbar (List separately in addition to code for primary procedure)

➜ *CPT Changes: An Insider's View* 2000

➜ *CPT Assistant* Nov 99:36, Mar 22:5

(Use 63057 in conjunction with 63055, 63056)

(Do not report 63056, 63057 for a herniated disc in conjunction with 22630, 22632, 22633, 22634 for decompression to prepare the interspace on the same interspace[s] and vertebral segment[s])

(For decompression performed on the same interspace[s] and vertebral segment[s] as posterior interbody fusion that includes laminectomy, removal of facets, and/or opening/widening of the foramen for decompression of nerves or spinal components, such as spinal cord, cauda equina, or nerve roots, see 63052, 63053)

63064   Costovertebral approach with decompression of spinal cord or nerve root(s) (eg, herniated intervertebral disc), thoracic; single segment

➜ *CPT Assistant* Fall 92:19, Jul 13:3

+ 63066   each additional segment (List separately in addition to code for primary procedure)

(Use 63066 in conjunction with 63064)

(For excision of thoracic intraspinal lesions by laminectomy, see 63266, 63271, 63276, 63281, 63286)

Anterior or Anterolateral Approach for Extradural Exploration/Decompression

For the following codes, when two surgeons work together as primary surgeons performing distinct part(s) of spinal cord exploration/decompression operation, each surgeon should report his/her distinct operative work by appending modifier 62 to the procedure code (and any associated add-on codes for that procedure code as long as both surgeons continue to work together as primary surgeons). In this situation, modifier 62 may be appended to the definitive procedure code(s) 63075, 63077, 63081, 63085, 63087, 63090 and, as appropriate, to associated additional interspace add-on code(s) 63076, 63078 or additional segment add-on code(s) 63082, 63086, 63088, 63091 as long as both surgeons continue to work together as primary surgeons.

For vertebral corpectomy, the term **partial** is used to describe removal of a substantial portion of the body of the vertebra. In the cervical spine, the amount of bone removed is defined as at least one-half of the vertebral body. In the thoracic and lumbar spine, the amount of bone removed is defined as at least one-third of the vertebral body.

63075   Discectomy, anterior, with decompression of spinal cord and/or nerve root(s), including osteophytectomy; cervical, single interspace

➜ *CPT Changes: An Insider's View* 2002

➜ *CPT Assistant* Nov 98:18, Jan 01:12, Feb 02:4, Jul 13:3, Apr 15:7, Aug 23:11

(Do not report 63075 in conjunction with 22554, even if performed by separate individuals. To report anterior cervical discectomy and interbody fusion at the same level during the same session, use 22551)

+ 63076   cervical, each additional interspace (List separately in addition to code for primary procedure)

➜ *CPT Changes: An Insider's View* 2002

➜ *CPT Assistant* Nov 98:18, Jan 01:12, Feb 02:4

(Do not report 63076 in conjunction with 22554, even if performed by separate individuals. To report anterior cervical discectomy and interbody fusion at the same level during the same session, use 22552)

(Use 63076 in conjunction with 63075)

63077   thoracic, single interspace

➜ *CPT Changes: An Insider's View* 2002

➜ *CPT Assistant* Nov 98:18, Jan 01:12, Feb 02:4, Jul 13:3

+ 63078   thoracic, each additional interspace (List separately in addition to code for primary procedure)
➔ *CPT Changes: An Insider's View* 2002
➔ *CPT Assistant* Nov 98:18, Jan 01:12, Feb 02:4

(Use 63078 in conjunction with 63077)

(Do not report code 69990 in addition to codes 63075-63078)

63081   Vertebral corpectomy (vertebral body resection), partial or complete, anterior approach with decompression of spinal cord and/or nerve root(s); cervical, single segment
➔ *CPT Changes: An Insider's View* 2002
➔ *CPT Assistant* Spring 93:37, Feb 02:4, Jul 13:3, Jun 15:10, Apr 16:8, Aug 23:11

+ 63082   cervical, each additional segment (List separately in addition to code for primary procedure)
➔ *CPT Changes: An Insider's View* 2002
➔ *CPT Assistant* Spring 93:37, Feb 02:4, Apr 16:8, Aug 23:11

(Use 63082 in conjunction with 63081)

(For transoral approach, see 61575, 61576)

63085   Vertebral corpectomy (vertebral body resection), partial or complete, transthoracic approach with decompression of spinal cord and/or nerve root(s); thoracic, single segment
➔ *CPT Changes: An Insider's View* 2002
➔ *CPT Assistant* Spring 93:37, Feb 02:4, Jul 13:3, Apr 16:8

+ 63086   thoracic, each additional segment (List separately in addition to code for primary procedure)
➔ *CPT Changes: An Insider's View* 2002
➔ *CPT Assistant* Spring 93:37, Feb 02:4, Apr 16:8

(Use 63086 in conjunction with 63085)

63087   Vertebral corpectomy (vertebral body resection), partial or complete, combined thoracolumbar approach with decompression of spinal cord, cauda equina or nerve root(s), lower thoracic or lumbar; single segment
➔ *CPT Changes: An Insider's View* 2002
➔ *CPT Assistant* Spring 93:37, Feb 02:4, Jul 13:3, Apr 16:8

+ 63088   each additional segment (List separately in addition to code for primary procedure)
➔ *CPT Changes: An Insider's View* 2002
➔ *CPT Assistant* Spring 93:37, Feb 02:4, Apr 16:8

(Use 63088 in conjunction with 63087)

63090   Vertebral corpectomy (vertebral body resection), partial or complete, transperitoneal or retroperitoneal approach with decompression of spinal cord, cauda equina or nerve root(s), lower thoracic, lumbar, or sacral; single segment
➔ *CPT Changes: An Insider's View* 2002
➔ *CPT Assistant* Spring 93:37, Mar 96:6, Feb 02:4, Jul 13:3, Apr 16:8

+ 63091   each additional segment (List separately in addition to code for primary procedure)
➔ *CPT Changes: An Insider's View* 2002
➔ *CPT Assistant* Spring 93:37, Mar 96:6, Feb 02:4, Apr 16:8

(Use 63091 in conjunction with 63090)

(Procedures 63081-63091 include discectomy above and/or below vertebral segment)

(If followed by arthrodesis, see 22548-22812)

(For reconstruction of spine, use appropriate vertebral corpectomy codes 63081-63091, bone graft codes 20930-20938, arthrodesis codes 22548-22812, and spinal instrumentation codes 22840-22855, 22859)

Lateral Extracavitary Approach for Extradural Exploration/Decompression

For vertebral corpectomy, the term **partial** is used to describe removal of a substantial portion of the body of the vertebra. In the cervical spine, the amount of bone removed is defined as at least one-half of the vertebral body. In the thoracic and lumbar spine, the amount of bone removed is defined as at least one-third of the vertebral body.

63101   Vertebral corpectomy (vertebral body resection), partial or complete, lateral extracavitary approach with decompression of spinal cord and/or nerve root(s) (eg, for tumor or retropulsed bone fragments); thoracic, single segment
➔ *CPT Changes: An Insider's View* 2004
➔ *CPT Assistant* Jul 13:3

63102   lumbar, single segment
➔ *CPT Changes: An Insider's View* 2004
➔ *CPT Assistant* Jul 13:3

+ 63103   thoracic or lumbar, each additional segment (List separately in addition to code for primary procedure)
➔ *CPT Changes: An Insider's View* 2004

(Use 63103 in conjunction with 63101 and 63102)

Incision

63170   Laminectomy with myelotomy (eg, Bischof or DREZ type), cervical, thoracic, or thoracolumbar
➔ *CPT Assistant* Jul 13:3

63172   Laminectomy with drainage of intramedullary cyst/syrinx; to subarachnoid space
➔ *CPT Assistant* Jul 13:3

63173   to peritoneal or pleural space
➔ *CPT Changes: An Insider's View* 2004
➔ *CPT Assistant* Jul 13:3

63185   Laminectomy with rhizotomy; 1 or 2 segments
➔ *CPT Assistant* Jul 13:3, Mar 24:27

63190   more than 2 segments
➔ *CPT Assistant* Jul 13:3

★=Telemedicine   ◀=Audio-only   +=Add-on code   �=FDA approval pending   #=Resequenced code   ⊘=Modifier 51 exempt   ➔➔➔=See p xxi for details

63191 Laminectomy with section of spinal accessory nerve
➔ *CPT Assistant* Jul 13:3

(For bilateral procedure, report 63191 with modifier 50)

(For resection of sternocleidomastoid muscle, use 21720)

63197 Laminectomy with cordotomy, with section of both spinothalamic tracts, 1 stage, thoracic
➔ *CPT Changes: An Insider's View* 2022
➔ *CPT Assistant* Jul 13:3

63200 Laminectomy, with release of tethered spinal cord, lumbar
➔ *CPT Assistant* Jul 13:3

Excision by Laminectomy of Lesion Other Than Herniated Disc

63250 Laminectomy for excision or occlusion of arteriovenous malformation of spinal cord; cervical
➔ *CPT Assistant* Jul 13:3

63251 thoracic
➔ *CPT Assistant* Jul 13:3

63252 thoracolumbar
➔ *CPT Assistant* Jul 13:3

63265 Laminectomy for excision or evacuation of intraspinal lesion other than neoplasm, extradural; cervical
➔ *CPT Assistant* Jul 13:3

63266 thoracic

63267 lumbar
➔ *CPT Assistant* Jul 13:3

63268 sacral
➔ *CPT Assistant* Jul 13:3

63270 Laminectomy for excision of intraspinal lesion other than neoplasm, intradural; cervical
➔ *CPT Assistant* Jul 13:3

63271 thoracic
➔ *CPT Assistant* Jul 13:3

63272 lumbar
➔ *CPT Assistant* Jul 13:3

63273 sacral
➔ *CPT Assistant* Jul 13:3

63275 Laminectomy for biopsy/excision of intraspinal neoplasm; extradural, cervical
➔ *CPT Assistant* Jul 13:3

63276 extradural, thoracic
➔ *CPT Assistant* Jul 13:3

63277 extradural, lumbar
➔ *CPT Assistant* Jul 13:3

63278 extradural, sacral
➔ *CPT Assistant* Jul 13:3

63280 intradural, extramedullary, cervical
➔ *CPT Assistant* Jul 13:3

63281 intradural, extramedullary, thoracic
➔ *CPT Assistant* Jul 13:3

63282 intradural, extramedullary, lumbar
➔ *CPT Assistant* Jul 13:3

63283 intradural, sacral
➔ *CPT Assistant* Jul 13:3

63285 intradural, intramedullary, cervical
➔ *CPT Assistant* Jul 13:3

63286 intradural, intramedullary, thoracic
➔ *CPT Assistant* Jul 13:3

63287 intradural, intramedullary, thoracolumbar
➔ *CPT Assistant* Jul 13:3

63290 combined extradural-intradural lesion, any level
➔ *CPT Assistant* Jul 13:3

(For drainage of intramedullary cyst/syrinx, use 63172, 63173)

+ 63295 Osteoplastic reconstruction of dorsal spinal elements, following primary intraspinal procedure (List separately in addition to code for primary procedure)
➔ *CPT Changes: An Insider's View* 2005

(Use 63295 in conjunction with 63172, 63173, 63185, 63190, 63200-63290)

(Do not report 63295 in conjunction with 22590-22614, 22840-22844, 63050, 63051 for the same vertebral segment(s))

Excision, Anterior or Anterolateral Approach, Intraspinal Lesion

For the following codes, when two surgeons work together as primary surgeons performing distinct part(s) of an anterior approach for an intraspinal excision, each surgeon should report his/her distinct operative work by appending modifier 62 to the single definitive procedure code. In this situation, modifier 62 may be appended to the definitive procedure code(s) 63300-63307 and, as appropriate, to the associated additional segment add-on code 63308 as long as both surgeons continue to work together as primary surgeons.

For vertebral corpectomy, the term **partial** is used to describe removal of a substantial portion of the body of the vertebra. In the cervical spine, the amount of bone removed is defined as at least one-half of the vertebral body. In the thoracic and lumbar spine, the amount of bone removed is defined as at least one-third of the vertebral body.

(For arthrodesis, see 22548-22585)

(For reconstruction of spine, see 20930-20938)

63300   Vertebral corpectomy (vertebral body resection), partial or complete, for excision of intraspinal lesion, single segment; extradural, cervical

➜ *CPT Assistant* Feb 02:4, Jul 13:3

63301   extradural, thoracic by transthoracic approach

➜ *CPT Assistant* Feb 02:4, Jul 13:3

63302   extradural, thoracic by thoracolumbar approach

➜ *CPT Assistant* Feb 02:4, Jul 13:3

63303   extradural, lumbar or sacral by transperitoneal or retroperitoneal approach

➜ *CPT Assistant* Feb 02:4, Jul 13:3

63304   intradural, cervical

➜ *CPT Assistant* Feb 02:4, Jul 13:3

63305   intradural, thoracic by transthoracic approach

➜ *CPT Assistant* Feb 02:4, Jul 13:3

63306   intradural, thoracic by thoracolumbar approach

➜ *CPT Assistant* Feb 02:4, Jul 13:3

63307   intradural, lumbar or sacral by transperitoneal or retroperitoneal approach

➜ *CPT Assistant* Feb 02:4, Jul 13:3

+ 63308   each additional segment (List separately in addition to codes for single segment)

➜ *CPT Assistant* Feb 02:4

(Use 63308 in conjunction with 63300-63307)

Stereotaxis

63600   Creation of lesion of spinal cord by stereotactic method, percutaneous, any modality (including stimulation and/or recording)

63610   Stereotactic stimulation of spinal cord, percutaneous, separate procedure not followed by other surgery

Stereotactic Radiosurgery (Spinal)

Spinal stereotactic radiosurgery is a distinct procedure that utilizes externally generated ionizing radiation to inactivate or eradicate defined target(s) in the spine without the need to make an incision. The target is defined by and the treatment is delivered using high-resolution stereotactic imaging. These codes are reported by the surgeon. The radiation oncologist reports the appropriate code(s) for clinical treatment planning, physics and dosimetry, treatment delivery and management from the **Radiation Oncology** section (77261-77790). Any necessary planning, dosimetry, targeting, positioning, or blocking by the neurosurgeon is included in the stereotactic radiation surgery services. The same individual should not report stereotactic radiosurgery services with radiation treatment management codes (77427-77432).

Spinal stereotactic radiosurgery is typically performed in a single planning and treatment session using a stereotactic image-guidance system, but can be performed with a planning session and in a limited number of treatment sessions, up to a maximum of five sessions. Do not report stereotactic radiosurgery more than once per lesion per course of treatment when the treatment requires greater than one session.

Stereotactic spinal surgery is only used when the tumor being treated affects spinal neural tissue or abuts the dura mater. Arteriovenous malformations must be subdural. For other radiation services of the spine, see **Radiation Oncology** services.

Codes 63620, 63621 include computer-assisted planning. Do not report 63620, 63621 in conjunction with 61781-61783.

(For intensity modulated beam delivery plan and treatment, see 77301, 77385, 77386. For stereotactic body radiation therapy, see 77373, 77435)

63620   Stereotactic radiosurgery (particle beam, gamma ray, or linear accelerator); 1 spinal lesion

➜ *CPT Changes: An Insider's View* 2009

➜ *CPT Assistant* Oct 10:3, Jul 11:12, Jun 15:6

(Do not report 63620 more than once per course of treatment)

+ 63621   each additional spinal lesion (List separately in addition to code for primary procedure)

➜ *CPT Changes: An Insider's View* 2009

➜ *CPT Assistant* Oct 10:3, Jul 11:12, Jun 15:6

(Report 63621 in conjunction with 63620)

(For each course of treatment, 63621 may be reported no more than once per lesion. Do not report 63621 more than 2 times for entire course of treatment regardless of number of lesions treated)

Neurostimulators (Spinal)

For electronic analysis with programming, when performed, of spinal cord neurostimulator pulse generator or transmitters, see codes 95970, 95971, 95972. Test stimulation to confirm correct target site placement of the electrode array(s) and/or to confirm the functional status of the system is inherent to placement, and is not separately reported as electronic analysis or programming of the neurostimulator pulse generator or receiver system. Electronic analysis (95970) at the time of implantation is not separately reported.

Codes 63650, 63655, 63661, 63662, 63663, 63664 describe the operative placement, revision, replacement, or removal of the spinal neurostimulator system components to provide spinal electrical stimulation. A neurostimulator system includes an implanted pulse generator or implanted receiver with an external transmitter, a collection of contacts, electrodes (electrode array), an extension if applicable, an external controller, and an external charger, if applicable. The neurostimulator may be integrated with the electrode array (single-component implant, see 0784T, 0785T) or have a detachable connection to the electrode array (two or more component implant). Multiple contacts or electrodes (4 or more) provide the actual electrical stimulation in the epidural space.

For percutaneously placed neurostimulator systems (63650, 63661, 63663), the contacts are on a catheter-like lead. An array defines the collection of contacts that are on one catheter.

For systems placed via an open surgical exposure (63655, 63662, 63664), the contacts are on a plate or paddle-shaped surface.

Do not report 63661 or 63663 when removing or replacing a temporary percutaneously placed array for an external generator.

Codes 63650, 63661, 63663, 63685, 63688 describe insertion, replacement, revision, or removal of a percutaneous electrode array and neurostimulator requiring pocket creation and connection between electrode array and pulse generator or receiver. For insertion, replacement, revision, or removal of a percutaneous spinal cord or sacral electrode array and integrated neurostimulator, see 0784T, 0785T, 0786T, 0787T.

63650   Percutaneous implantation of neurostimulator electrode array, epidural
> *CPT Changes: An Insider's View* 2010
> *CPT Assistant* Jun 98:3-4, Nov 98:18, Mar 99:11, Apr 99:10, Sep 99:3, Dec 08:8, Feb 10:9, Aug 10:8, Dec 10:14, Apr 11:10, Oct 13:19, Dec 15:17, Jan 16:12, Dec 17:16, Oct 18:11

63655   Laminectomy for implantation of neurostimulator electrodes, plate/paddle, epidural
> *CPT Assistant* Jun 98:3-4, Nov 98:18, Sep 99:3-4, Dec 08:8, Aug 10:8, Dec 10:14, Apr 11:10, Dec 20:13

63661   Removal of spinal neurostimulator electrode percutaneous array(s), including fluoroscopy, when performed
> *CPT Changes: An Insider's View* 2010
> *CPT Assistant* Feb 10:9, Aug 10:8, Jan 11:8, Apr 11:10
> *Clinical Examples in Radiology* Spring 11:10

Percutaneous Implantation of Neurostimulator Electrodes
63650

Single catheter electrode array is inserted percutaneously into the epidural space. A simple or complex receiver is subcutaneously implanted.

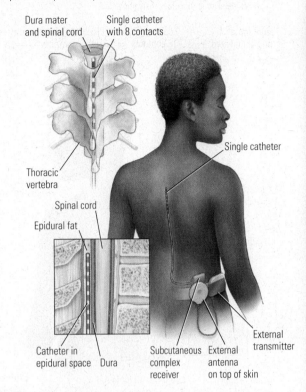

Dura mater and spinal cord
Single catheter with 8 contacts
Single catheter
Thoracic vertebra
Spinal cord
Epidural fat
Catheter in epidural space
Dura
Subcutaneous complex receiver
External antenna on top of skin
External transmitter

63662   Removal of spinal neurostimulator electrode plate/paddle(s) placed via laminotomy or laminectomy, including fluoroscopy, when performed
> *CPT Changes: An Insider's View* 2010
> *CPT Assistant* Feb 10:9, Aug 10:8, Apr 11:10, Dec 20:13
> *Clinical Examples in Radiology* Spring 11:10

63663   Revision including replacement, when performed, of spinal neurostimulator electrode percutaneous array(s), including fluoroscopy, when performed
> *CPT Changes: An Insider's View* 2010
> *CPT Assistant* Feb 10:9, Aug 10:8, Apr 11:10
> *Clinical Examples in Radiology* Spring 11:10

(Do not report 63663 in conjunction with 63661, 63662 for the same spinal level)

Placement of Neurostimulator Electrodes Through Laminectomy
63655

The electrode plate or paddle is placed in the epidural space via open exposure through large laminotomy or small laminectomy. The simple or complex receiver is subcutaneously implanted.

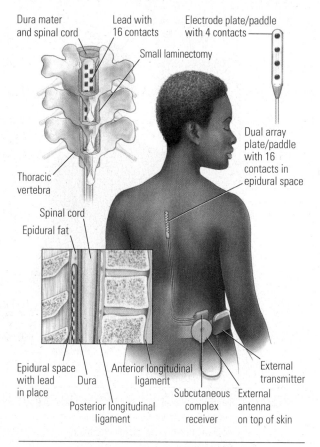

Dura mater and spinal cord
Lead with 16 contacts
Electrode plate/paddle with 4 contacts
Small laminectomy
Dual array plate/paddle with 16 contacts in epidural space
Thoracic vertebra
Spinal cord
Epidural fat
Epidural space with lead in place
Dura
Posterior longitudinal ligament
Anterior longitudinal ligament
Subcutaneous complex receiver
External antenna on top of skin
External transmitter

63664 Revision including replacement, when performed, of spinal neurostimulator electrode plate/paddle(s) placed via laminotomy or laminectomy, including fluoroscopy, when performed

➔ *CPT Changes: An Insider's View* 2010
➔ *CPT Assistant* Feb 10:9, Aug 10:8, Apr 11:10
➔ *Clinical Examples in Radiology* Spring 11:10

(Do not report 63664 in conjunction with 63661, 63662 for the same spinal level)

63685 Insertion or replacement of spinal neurostimulator pulse generator or receiver, requiring pocket creation and connection between electrode array and pulse generator or receiver

➔ *CPT Changes: An Insider's View* 2005, 2024
➔ *CPT Assistant* Jun 98:3-4, Sep 99:5, Feb 10:9, Oct 10:14, Dec 10:14, Apr 11:10, Dec 17:16, Dec 23:1

(Do not report 63685 in conjunction with 63688 for the same neurostimulator pulse generator or receiver)

(For insertion or replacement of spinal percutaneous electrode array with integrated neurostimulator, use 0784T)

63688 Revision or removal of implanted spinal neurostimulator pulse generator or receiver, with detachable connection to electrode array

➔ *CPT Changes: An Insider's View* 2024
➔ *CPT Assistant* Jun 98:3-4, Sep 99:5, Feb 10:9, Apr 11:11, Dec 23:1

(For electronic analysis with programming, when performed, of implanted spinal cord neurostimulator, see 95970, 95971, 95972)

(For revision or removal of spinal percutaneous electrode array and integrated neurostimulator, use 0785T)

(For revision or removal of sacral percutaneous electrode array and integrated neurostimulator, use 0787T)

Repair

63700 Repair of meningocele; less than 5 cm diameter

63702 larger than 5 cm diameter

(Do not use modifier 63 in conjunction with 63700, 63702)

63704 Repair of myelomeningocele; less than 5 cm diameter

63706 larger than 5 cm diameter

(Do not use modifier 63 in conjunction with 63704, 63706)

(For complex skin closure, see **Integumentary System**)

63707 Repair of dural/cerebrospinal fluid leak, not requiring laminectomy

➔ *CPT Changes: An Insider's View* 2002

63709 Repair of dural/cerebrospinal fluid leak or pseudomeningocele, with laminectomy

➔ *CPT Changes: An Insider's View* 2002

63710 Dural graft, spinal

Shunt, Spinal CSF

63740 Creation of shunt, lumbar, subarachnoid-peritoneal, -pleural, or other; including laminectomy

➔ *CPT Assistant* Winter 90:8

63741 percutaneous, not requiring laminectomy

➔ *CPT Assistant* Winter 90:8

63744 Replacement, irrigation or revision of lumbosubarachnoid shunt

63746 Removal of entire lumbosubarachnoid shunt system without replacement

★=Telemedicine ◀=Audio-only ✚=Add-on code ✗=FDA approval pending #=Resequenced code ⊘=Modifier 51 exempt ➔➔➔=See p xxi for details

(For insertion of subarachnoid catheter with reservoir and/or pump for intermittent or continuous infusion of drug including laminectomy, see 62351 and 62360, 62361 or 62362)

(For insertion or replacement of subarachnoid or epidural catheter, with reservoir and/or pump for drug infusion without laminectomy, see 62350 and 62360, 62361 or 62362)

Extracranial Nerves, Peripheral Nerves, and Autonomic Nervous System

(For intracranial surgery on cranial nerves, see 61450, 61460, 61790)

Introduction/Injection of Anesthetic Agent (Nerve Block), Diagnostic or Therapeutic

(For destruction by neurolytic agent or chemodenervation, see 62280-62282, 64600-64681)

(For epidural or subarachnoid injection, see 62320, 62321, 62322, 62323, 62324, 62325, 62326, 62327)

(64400-64455, 64461, 64462, 64463, 64479, 64480, 64483, 64484, 64490-64495 are unilateral procedures. For bilateral procedures, report 64400, 64405, 64408, 64415, 64416, 64417, 64418, 64420, 64425-64455, 64461, 64463, 64479, 64483, 64490, 64493 with modifier 50. Report add-on codes 64421, 64462, 64480, 64484, 64491, 64492, 64494, 64495 twice, when performed bilaterally. Do not report modifier 50 in conjunction with 64421, 64462, 64480, 64484, 64491, 64492, 64494, 64495)

Somatic Nerves

Codes 64400-64489 describe the introduction/injection of an anesthetic agent and/or steroid into the somatic nervous system for diagnostic or therapeutic purposes. For injection or destruction of genicular nerve branches, see 64454, 64624, respectively.

Codes 64400-64450, 64454 describe the injection of an anesthetic agent(s) and/or steroid into a nerve plexus, nerve, or branch. These codes are reported once per nerve plexus, nerve, or branch as described in the descriptor regardless of the number of injections performed along the nerve plexus, nerve, or branch described by the code.

Imaging guidance and localization may be reported separately for 64400, 64405, 64408, 64420, 64421, 64425, 64430, 64435, 64449, 64450. Imaging guidance and any injection of contrast are inclusive components of 64415, 64416, 64417, 64445, 64446, 64447, 64448, 64451, 64454.

Codes 64455, 64479, 64480, 64483, 64484 are reported for single or multiple injections on the same site. For 64479, 64480, 64483, 64484, imaging guidance (fluoroscopy or CT) and any injection of contrast are inclusive components and are not reported separately. For 64455, imaging guidance (ultrasound, fluoroscopy, CT) and localization may be reported separately.

▶Codes 64461, 64462, 64463 describe injection of a paravertebral block (PVB). Codes 64486, 64487, 64488, 64489 describe injection of an abdominal fascial plane block. Imaging guidance and any injection of contrast are inclusive components of 64461, 64462, 64463, 64486, 64487, 64488, 64489 and are not reported separately.◀

64400 Injection(s), anesthetic agent(s) and/or steroid; trigeminal nerve, each branch (ie, ophthalmic, maxillary, mandibular)
➔ *CPT Changes: An Insider's View* 2000, 2020
➔ *CPT Assistant* Jul 98:10, May 99:8, Nov 99:36, Apr 05:13, Feb 10:9, Jan 13:13, Feb 21:3, Jul 22:13,18, Dec 22:12, Jan 23:24
➔ *Clinical Examples in Radiology* Summer 14:6, Fall 20:14

64405 greater occipital nerve
➔ *CPT Changes: An Insider's View* 2020
➔ *CPT Assistant* Jul 98:10, Apr 05:13, Jan 13:13, Oct 16:11, Jan 23:24
➔ *Clinical Examples in Radiology* Fall 20:14

64408 vagus nerve
➔ *CPT Changes: An Insider's View* 2020
➔ *CPT Assistant* Jul 98:10, Apr 05:13, Jan 13:13, Jan 23:24

64415 brachial plexus, including imaging guidance, when performed
➔ *CPT Changes: An Insider's View* 2003, 2020, 2023
➔ *CPT Assistant* Fall 92:17, Jul 98:10, May 99:8, Oct 01:9, Feb 04:7, Apr 05:13, Nov 06:23, Jan 13:13, Jan 23:24

(Do not report 64415 in conjunction with 76942, 77002, 77003)

64416 brachial plexus, continuous infusion by catheter (including catheter placement), including imaging guidance, when performed
➔ *CPT Changes: An Insider's View* 2003, 2009, 2020, 2023
➔ *CPT Assistant* Feb 04:7, Apr 05:13, Jan 13:13, Jan 23:24

(Do not report 64416 in conjunction with 01996, 76942, 77002, 77003)

64417 axillary nerve, including imaging guidance, when performed
➔ *CPT Changes: An Insider's View* 2020, 2023
➔ *CPT Assistant* Jul 98:10, Apr 05:13, Jan 13:13, Jan 23:24

(Do not report 64417 in conjunction with 76942, 77002, 77003)

64418 suprascapular nerve
→ *CPT Changes: An Insider's View* 2020
→ *CPT Assistant* Jul 98:10, Apr 05:13, Aug 07:15, Jan 13:13

64420 intercostal nerve, single level
→ *CPT Changes: An Insider's View* 2020
→ *CPT Assistant* Jul 98:10, Apr 05:13, Aug 10:12, Nov 10:9, Jan 13:13, Jun 15:3, Jan 23:24

+ 64421 intercostal nerve, each additional level (List separately in addition to code for primary procedure)
→ *CPT Changes: An Insider's View* 2020
→ *CPT Assistant* Jul 98:10, Apr 05:13, Aug 10:12, Nov 10:9, Jan 13:13, Jun 15:3, May 18:10, Jan 23:24

(Use 64421 in conjunction with 64420)

64425 ilioinguinal, iliohypogastric nerves
→ *CPT Changes: An Insider's View* 2020
→ *CPT Assistant* Jul 98:10, Apr 05:13, Jan 13:13, Jun 15:3, Jan 23:24

64430 pudendal nerve
→ *CPT Changes: An Insider's View* 2020
→ *CPT Assistant* Jul 98:10, Apr 05:13, Jan 13:13, Jan 23:24

64435 paracervical (uterine) nerve
→ *CPT Changes: An Insider's View* 2020
→ *CPT Assistant* Jul 98:10, Mar 03:22, Jul 03:15, Apr 05:13, Feb 12:11, Jan 13:13, Jan 23:24

64445 sciatic nerve, including imaging guidance, when performed
→ *CPT Changes: An Insider's View* 2003, 2020, 2023
→ *CPT Assistant* Jul 98:10, May 99:8, Feb 04:8, Apr 05:13, Dec 11:8, Apr 12:19, Jan 13:13, Jan 23:24

(Do not report 64445 in conjunction with 76942, 77002, 77003)

64446 sciatic nerve, continuous infusion by catheter (including catheter placement), including imaging guidance, when performed
→ *CPT Changes: An Insider's View* 2003, 2009, 2020, 2023
→ *CPT Assistant* Feb 04:9, Apr 05:13, Jan 13:13, Jan 23:24

(Do not report 64446 in conjunction with 01996, 76942, 77002, 77003)

64447 femoral nerve, including imaging guidance, when performed
→ *CPT Changes: An Insider's View* 2003, 2020, 2023
→ *CPT Assistant* Feb 04:9, Apr 05:13, Jan 13:13, Nov 14:14, Dec 14:16, Sep 15:12, Mar 21:11, Jan 23:24, Feb 24:34

(Do not report 64447 in conjunction with 01996, 76942, 77002, 77003)

64448 femoral nerve, continuous infusion by catheter (including catheter placement), including imaging guidance, when performed
→ *CPT Changes: An Insider's View* 2003, 2009, 2020, 2023
→ *CPT Assistant* Feb 04:10, Apr 05:13, Jan 13:13, Nov 14:14, Dec 14:16, Sep 15:12, Jan 23:24, Feb 24:34

(Do not report 64448 in conjunction with 01996, 76942, 77002, 77003)

64449 lumbar plexus, posterior approach, continuous infusion by catheter (including catheter placement)
→ *CPT Changes: An Insider's View* 2004, 2009, 2020
→ *CPT Assistant* Apr 05:13, Jan 13:13, Jan 23:24

(Do not report 64449 in conjunction with 01996)

64450 other peripheral nerve or branch
→ *CPT Changes: An Insider's View* 2000, 2020
→ *CPT Assistant* Jul 98:10, Nov 99:37, Dec 99:7, Oct 01:9, Aug 03:6, Apr 05:13, Jan 09:6, Jan 13:13, Sep 15:12, Nov 15:11, Oct 16:11, May 18:10, Nov 18:10, Nov 19:15, Mar 21:11, May 22:17, Jul 22:13,18, Dec 22:12, Jan 23:24
→ *Clinical Examples in Radiology* Summer 14:6, Fall 20:14

(For injection, anesthetic agent, nerves innervating the sacroiliac joint, use 64451)

64451 nerves innervating the sacroiliac joint, with image guidance (ie, fluoroscopy or computed tomography)
→ *CPT Changes: An Insider's View* 2020
→ *CPT Assistant* Nov 19:15, Jul 20:14, May 22:17, Jan 23:24

(Do not report 64451 in conjunction with 64493, 64494, 64495, 77002, 77003, 77012, 95873, 95874)

(For injection, anesthetic agent, nerves innervating the sacroiliac joint, with ultrasound, use 76999)

(For bilateral procedure, report 64451 with modifier 50)

64454 genicular nerve branches, including imaging guidance, when performed
→ *CPT Changes: An Insider's View* 2020
→ *CPT Assistant* Dec 19:8, Dec 20:13, Jul 22:13,18, Jan 23:24

(Do not report 64454 in conjunction with 64624)

(64454 requires injecting all of the following genicular nerve branches: superolateral, superomedial, and inferomedial. If all 3 of these genicular nerve branches are not injected, report 64454 with modifier 52)

64455 plantar common digital nerve(s) (eg, Morton's neuroma)
→ *CPT Changes: An Insider's View* 2009, 2021
→ *CPT Assistant* Jan 13:13, Feb 21:3
→ *Clinical Examples in Radiology* Fall 20:15

(Do not report 64455 in conjunction with 64632)

64461 Code is out of numerical sequence. See 64483-64487

64462 Code is out of numerical sequence. See 64483-64487

64463 Code is out of numerical sequence. See 64483-64487

64466 Code is out of numerical sequence. See 64483-64487

64467 Code is out of numerical sequence. See 64483-64487

64468 Code is out of numerical sequence. See 64483-64487

64469   Code is out of numerical sequence. See 64483-64487

64473   Code is out of numerical sequence. See 64483-64487

64474   Code is out of numerical sequence. See 64483-64487

64479   transforaminal epidural, with imaging guidance
        (fluoroscopy or CT), cervical or thoracic, single level

➔ *CPT Changes: An Insider's View* 2000, 2011, 2021

➔ *CPT Assistant* Nov 99:33, 37, Feb 00:4, Jul 08:9, Nov 08:11,
  Feb 10:9, Jan 11:8, Feb 11:4, Jul 11:16, Jul 12:5, Jan 16:9,
  Feb 21:3

➔ *Clinical Examples in Radiology* Summer 08:9, Spring 11:10,
  Winter 18:7

+ **64480**   transforaminal epidural, with imaging guidance
              (fluoroscopy or CT), cervical or thoracic, each
              additional level (List separately in addition to code for
              primary procedure)

➔ *CPT Changes: An Insider's View* 2000, 2011, 2021

➔ *CPT Assistant* Nov 99:33, 37, Feb 00:4, Feb 05:14, Jul 08:9,
  Feb 10:9, Jan 11:8, Feb 11:4, Jul 11:16, Jul 12:5, Feb 21:3

➔ *Clinical Examples in Radiology* Summer 08:9, Spring 11:10,
  Winter 18:7

(Use 64480 in conjunction with 64479)

(For transforaminal epidural injection at the T12-L1 level,
use 64479)

Code(s)	Unit	Imaging Guidance Included	Imaging Guidance Separately Reported, When Performed
Extracranial Nerves, Peripheral Nerves, and Autonomic Nervous System			
Introduction/Injection of Anesthetic Agent (Nerve Block), Diagnostic or Therapeutic			
Somatic Nerve			
64400-64408	1 unit per plexus, nerve, or branch injected regardless of the number of injections		X
64415-64417	1 unit per plexus, nerve, or branch injected regardless of the number of injections	X	
64418-64435	1 unit per plexus, nerve, or branch injected regardless of the number of injections		X
64445-64448	1 unit per plexus, nerve, or branch injected regardless of the number of injections	X	
64449	1 unit per plexus, nerve, or branch injected regardless of the number of injections		X
64450	1 unit per plexus, nerve, or branch injected regardless of the number of injections		X
64451	1 unit for any number of nerves innervating the sacroiliac joint injected regardless of the number of injections	X	
64454	1 unit for any number of genicular nerve branches, with a required minimum of three nerve branches	X	
64455	1 or more injections per level		X
64479	1 or more injections per level	X	
+64480	1 or more additional injections per level (add-on)	X	
64483	1 or more injections per level	X	
+64484	1 or more additional injections per level (add-on)	X	
64461	1 injection site	X	
+64462	1 or more additional injections per code (add-on)	X	
64463	1 or more injections per code	X	
64486-64489	By injection site	X	
Destruction by Neurolytic Agent (Eg, Chemical, Thermal, Electrical, or Radiofrequency), Chemodenervation			
Code(s)	Unit	Imaging Guidance Included	Imaging Guidance Separately Reported, When Performed
Somatic Nerves			
64624	1 unit for any number of genicular nerve branches, with a required minimum of three nerve branches	X	

▲ = Revised code   ● = New code   ▶ ◀ = Contains new or revised text   ✋ = Duplicate PLA test   ↕ = Category I PLA   American Medical Association   **495**

64483   transforaminal epidural, with imaging guidance (fluoroscopy or CT), lumbar or sacral, single level

➔ *CPT Changes: An Insider's View* 2000, 2011, 2021

➔ *CPT Assistant* Nov 99:33, 37, Feb 00:4, Jul 08:9, Feb 10:9, Jan 11:8, Feb 11:4, Jul 11:16, May 12:14, Jul 12:5, Oct 16:11, Feb 21:3

➔ *Clinical Examples in Radiology* Spring 11:10, Winter 18:7

+ 64484   transforaminal epidural, with imaging guidance (fluoroscopy or CT), lumbar or sacral, each additional level (List separately in addition to code for primary procedure)

➔ *CPT Changes: An Insider's View* 2000, 2011, 2021

➔ *CPT Assistant* Nov 99:33, 37, Feb 00:4, Feb 05:14, Jul 08:9, Nov 08:11, Feb 10:9, Feb 11:4, Jul 11:16, Jul 12:5, Jan 16:9, Feb 21:3

➔ *Clinical Examples in Radiology* Spring 11:10, Winter 18:7

(Use 64484 in conjunction with 64483)

(64479-64484 are unilateral procedures. For bilateral procedures, report 64479, 64483 with modifier 50. Report add-on codes 64480, 64484 twice, when performed bilaterally. Do not report modifier 50 in conjunction with 64480, 64484)

(Imaging guidance [fluoroscopy or CT] and any injection of contrast are inclusive components of 64479-64484. Imaging guidance and localization are required for the performance of 64479-64484)

 # 64461   Paravertebral block (PVB) (paraspinous block), thoracic; single injection site (includes imaging guidance, when performed)

➔ *CPT Changes: An Insider's View* 2016

➔ *CPT Assistant* Jan 16:9, Dec 18:8, Jul 22:13, May 23:28

#+ 64462   second and any additional injection site(s) (includes imaging guidance, when performed) (List separately in addition to code for primary procedure)

➔ *CPT Changes: An Insider's View* 2016

➔ *CPT Assistant* Jan 16:9, Dec 18:8, May 23:28

(Use 64462 in conjunction with 64461)

(Do not report 64462 more than once per day)

 # 64463   continuous infusion by catheter (includes imaging guidance, when performed)

➔ *CPT Changes: An Insider's View* 2016

➔ *CPT Assistant* Jan 16:9, Dec 18:8

(Do not report 64461, 64462, 64463 in conjunction with 62320, 62324, 64420, 64421, 64479, 64480, 64490, 64491, 64492, 76942, 77002, 77003)

#● 64466   Thoracic fascial plane block, unilateral; by injection(s), including imaging guidance, when performed

➔ *CPT Changes: An Insider's View* 2025

#● 64467   by continuous infusion(s), including imaging guidance, when performed

➔ *CPT Changes: An Insider's View* 2025

▶(Do not report 64466, 64467 in conjunction with 76942, 77001, 77002, 77012, 77021)◀

#● 64468   Thoracic fascial plane block, bilateral; by injection(s), including imaging guidance, when performed

➔ *CPT Changes: An Insider's View* 2025

#● 64469   by continuous infusion(s), including imaging guidance, when performed

➔ *CPT Changes: An Insider's View* 2025

▶(Do not report 64468, 64469 in conjunction with 76942, 77001, 77002, 77012, 77021)◀

#● 64473   Lower extremity fascial plane block, unilateral; by injection(s), including imaging guidance, when performed

➔ *CPT Changes: An Insider's View* 2025

#● 64474   by continuous infusion(s), including imaging guidance, when performed

➔ *CPT Changes: An Insider's View* 2025

▶(Do not report 64473, 64474 in conjunction with 76942, 77001, 77002, 77012, 77021)◀

64486   Transversus abdominis plane (TAP) block (abdominal plane block, rectus sheath block) unilateral; by injection(s) (includes imaging guidance, when performed)

➔ *CPT Changes: An Insider's View* 2015

➔ *CPT Assistant* Jun 15:3, Jul 22:13, Dec 22:12, Mar 24:27

➔ *Clinical Examples in Radiology* Winter 18:8

64487   by continuous infusion(s) (includes imaging guidance, when performed)

➔ *CPT Changes: An Insider's View* 2015

➔ *CPT Assistant* Jun 15:3, Jul 22:13, Dec 22:12, Mar 24:27

➔ *Clinical Examples in Radiology* Winter 18:8

64488   Transversus abdominis plane (TAP) block (abdominal plane block, rectus sheath block) bilateral; by injections (includes imaging guidance, when performed)

➔ *CPT Changes: An Insider's View* 2015

➔ *CPT Assistant* Jun 15:3, Jul 22:13, Dec 22:12,17, Mar 24:27

➔ *Clinical Examples in Radiology* Winter 18:8

64489   by continuous infusions (includes imaging guidance, when performed)

➔ *CPT Changes: An Insider's View* 2015

➔ *CPT Assistant* Jun 15:3, Jul 22:13, Dec 22:12, Mar 24:27

➔ *Clinical Examples in Radiology* Winter 18:8

Paravertebral Spinal Nerves and Branches

Codes 64490, 64491, 64492, 64493, 64494, 64495 describe the introduction/injection of a diagnostic or therapeutic agent into the paravertebral facet joint or into the nerves that innervate that joint by level. Facet joints are paired joints with one pair at each vertebral level. Imaging guidance and localization are required for the performance of paravertebral facet joint injections described by 64490, 64491, 64492, 64493, 64494, 64495. If imaging is not used, report 20552, 20553. If ultrasound guidance is used, report 0213T, 0214T, 0215T, 0216T, 0217T, 0218T.

When determining a level, count the number of facet joints injected, not the number of nerves injected. Therefore, if multiple nerves of the same facet joint are injected, it would be considered as a single level. The add-on codes are reported when second, third, or additional levels are injected during the same session.

When the procedure is performed bilaterally at the same level, report one unit of the primary code with modifier 50.

When the procedure is performed on the left side at one level and the right side at a different level in the same region, report one unit of the primary procedure and one unit of the add-on code.

When the procedure is performed bilaterally at one level and unilaterally at a different level(s), report one unit of the primary procedure for each level and append modifier 50 for the bilateral procedure. If the procedure is performed unilaterally at different levels, report one unit of the primary procedure and the appropriate add-on code(s).

Procedure	Cervical/ Thoracic	Lumbar/Sacral
Multiple nerves injected at the same level	64490 X 1	64493 X 1
1 level injected unilaterally	64490 X 1	64493 X 1
1 level injected bilaterally	64490 50 X 1	64493 50 X 1
1 level injected bilaterally and 1 level injected unilaterally	64490 50 X 1 64491 X 1	64493 50 X 1 64494 X 1
2 levels injected unilaterally	64490 X 1 64491 X 1	64493 X 1 64494 X 1
2 levels injected bilaterally	64490 50 X 1 64491 X 2	64493 50 X 1 64494 X 2
3 or more levels injected unilaterally	64490 X 1 64491 X 1 64492 X 1	64493 X 1 64494 X 1 64495 X 1
3 or more levels injected bilaterally	64490 50 X 1 64491 X 2 64492 X 2	64493 50 X 1 64494 X 2 64495 X 2

(For bilateral paravertebral facet injection procedures, report 64490, 64493 with modifier 50. Report add-on codes 64491, 64492, 64494, 64495 twice, when performed bilaterally. Do not report modifier 50 in conjunction with 64491, 64492, 64494, 64495)

(For paravertebral facet injection of the T12-L1 joint, or nerves innervating that joint, use 64490)

(For unilateral paravertebral facet injection of the T12-L1 and L1-L2 levels or nerves innervating that joint, use 64490 and 64494 once)

(For bilateral paravertebral facet injection of the T12-L1 and L1-L2 levels or nerves innervating that joint, use 64490 with modifier 50 once and 64494 twice)

64490 Injection(s), diagnostic or therapeutic agent, paravertebral facet (zygapophyseal) joint (or nerves innervating that joint) with image guidance (fluoroscopy or CT), cervical or thoracic; single level
➔ *CPT Changes: An Insider's View* 2010
➔ *CPT Assistant* Feb 10:9, Aug 10:12, Dec 10:13, Jan 11:8, Feb 11:4, Jun 12:10, Oct 12:15
➔ *Clinical Examples in Radiology* Winter 10:15, Spring 11:10, Winter 18:8, Fall 23:31

+ 64491 second level (List separately in addition to code for primary procedure)
➔ *CPT Changes: An Insider's View* 2010
➔ *CPT Assistant* Aug 10:12, Jun 12:10, Oct 12:15
➔ *Clinical Examples in Radiology* Winter 10:15, Fall 23:32

(Use 64491 in conjunction with 64490)

+ 64492 third and any additional level(s) (List separately in addition to code for primary procedure)
➔ *CPT Changes: An Insider's View* 2010
➔ *CPT Assistant* Feb 10:9, Aug 10:12, Jan 11:8, Feb 11:4, Jun 12:10, Oct 12:15
➔ *Clinical Examples in Radiology* Winter 10:14, Spring 11:10, Winter 18:8, Fall 23:32

(Use 64492 in conjunction with 64490, 64491)

64493 Injection(s), diagnostic or therapeutic agent, paravertebral facet (zygapophyseal) joint (or nerves innervating that joint) with image guidance (fluoroscopy or CT), lumbar or sacral; single level
➔ *CPT Changes: An Insider's View* 2010
➔ *CPT Assistant* Feb 10:9, Aug 10:12, Jan 11:8, Feb 11:4, Jun 12:10, Oct 12:15, May 18:10, Jul 20:14
➔ *Clinical Examples in Radiology* Winter 10:14, Spring 11:10, Winter 18:8, Fall 23:32

(For injection, anesthetic agent, nerves innervating the sacroiliac joint, use 64451)

+ 64494 second level (List separately in addition to code for primary procedure)
➔ *CPT Changes: An Insider's View* 2010
➔ *CPT Assistant* Feb 10:9, Aug 10:12, Jan 11:8, Feb 11:4, Jun 12:10, May 18:10, Jul 20:14
➔ *Clinical Examples in Radiology* Winter 10:14, Spring 11:10, Winter 18:8, Fall 23:32

(Use 64494 in conjunction with 64490, 64493)

+ 64495   third and any additional level(s) (List separately in addition to code for primary procedure)

> *CPT Changes: An Insider's View* 2010

> *CPT Assistant* Feb 10:9, Aug 10:12, Jan 11:8, Feb 11:4, Jun 12:10, Oct 12:15, May 18:10

> *Clinical Examples in Radiology* Winter 10:14, Spring 11:10, Winter 18:8, Fall 23:32

(Use 64495 in conjunction with 64493, 64494)

Autonomic Nerves

64505   Injection, anesthetic agent; sphenopalatine ganglion

> *CPT Assistant* Jul 98:10, Apr 05:13, Jan 13:13, Jun 13:13, Jul 14:8, Jul 22:13

> *Clinical Examples in Radiology* Summer 14:6, Fall 20:14

64510   stellate ganglion (cervical sympathetic)

> *CPT Assistant* Jul 98:10, Apr 05:13, Jan 13:13

64517   superior hypogastric plexus

> *CPT Changes: An Insider's View* 2004

> *CPT Assistant* Oct 04:11, Apr 05:13, Jan 13:13, Jan 22:18

64520   lumbar or thoracic (paravertebral sympathetic)

> *CPT Assistant* Jul 98:10, Apr 05:13, Dec 10:14, Jan 13:13

64530   celiac plexus, with or without radiologic monitoring

> *CPT Assistant* Jul 98:10, Apr 05:13, Jan 13:13, Jul 22:13, Dec 22:21

> *Clinical Examples in Radiology* Summer 14:5-6, Fall 20:14

(For transendoscopic ultrasound-guided transmural injection, anesthetic, celiac plexus, use 43253)

Neurostimulators (Peripheral Nerve)

For electronic analysis with programming, when performed, of peripheral nerve neurostimulator pulse generator or transmitters, see codes 95970, 95971, 95972. An electrode array is a catheter or other device with more than one contact. The function of each contact may be capable of being adjusted during programming services. Test stimulation to confirm correct target site placement of the electrode array(s) and/or to confirm the functional status of the system is inherent to placement, and is not separately reported as electronic analysis or programming of the neurostimulator pulse generator or receiver system. Electronic analysis (95970) at the time of implantation is not separately reported.

A neurostimulator system includes an implanted pulse generator or implanted receiver with an external transmitter, a collection of contacts, electrodes (electrode array), an extension if applicable, an external controller, and an external charger, if applicable. The electrode array provides the actual electrical stimulation. The pulse generator or receiver may be integrated with the electrode array (single-component implant) or have a detachable connection to the electrode array (two or more component implant).

Codes 64553, 64555, and 64561 may be used to report both temporary and permanent placement of percutaneous electrode arrays.

Codes 64590, 64596 describe two different approaches to placing a neurostimulator pulse generator or receiver. Code 64590 is used in conjunction with 64555, 64561 for permanent placement. Codes 64555, 64561 are used to report electrode array placement for a trial and for the permanent placement of the electrode array. Code 64590 is used to report the insertion of a neurostimulator pulse generator or receiver that requires creation of a pocket and connection between the electrode array and the neurostimulator pulse generator or receiver. Code 64596 is used to report the permanent placement of an integrated system, including the electrode array and receiver.

(For transcutaneous nerve stimulation [TENS], use 97014 for electrical stimulation requiring supervision only or use 97032 for electrical stimulation requiring constant attendance)

64553   Percutaneous implantation of neurostimulator electrode array; cranial nerve

> *CPT Changes: An Insider's View* 2000, 2012

> *CPT Assistant* Nov 99:38, Apr 01:9, Oct 18:8, Oct 21:7

(For percutaneous electrical stimulation of a cranial nerve using needle[s] or needle electrode[s] [eg, PENS, PNT], use 64999)

(For open placement of cranial nerve (eg, vagus, trigeminal) neurostimulator pulse generator or receiver, see 61885, 61886, as appropriate)

▶(For open implantation of vagus nerve integrated neurostimulation system, see 0908T, 0909T)◀

64555   peripheral nerve (excludes sacral nerve)

> *CPT Changes: An Insider's View* 2002, 2012

> *CPT Assistant* Jan 15:14, Feb 16:13, Dec 17:16, Aug 18:10, Oct 18:8, Oct 21:7

(Do not report 64555 in conjunction with 64566)

(For percutaneous electrical stimulation of a peripheral nerve using needle[s] or needle electrode[s] [eg, PENS, PNT], use 64999)

64561   sacral nerve (transforaminal placement) including image guidance, if performed

> *CPT Changes: An Insider's View* 2002, 2012, 2013

> *CPT Assistant* Dec 12:14, Sep 14:5, Oct 18:8, Oct 21:7

(For percutaneous electrical neuromuscular stimulation or neuromodulation using needle[s] or needle electrode[s] [eg, PENS, PNT], use 64999)

Nervous 61000-64999

64566   Posterior tibial neurostimulation, percutaneous needle electrode, single treatment, includes programming

➔ *CPT Changes: An Insider's View* 2011

➔ *CPT Assistant* Feb 11:5, Sep 11:8

(Do not report 64566 in conjunction with 64555, 95970-95972)

(For peripheral nerve transcutaneous magnetic stimulation, see 0766T, 0767T)

64568   Open implantation of cranial nerve (eg, vagus nerve) neurostimulator electrode array and pulse generator

➔ *CPT Changes: An Insider's View* 2011, 2022

➔ *CPT Assistant* Feb 11:5, Sep 11:8, 10, 12, Nov 16:6, Mar 18:9, Mar 22:7-8

(Do not report 64568 in conjunction with 61885, 61886, 64570)

▶(For open implantation of vagus nerve integrated neurostimulation system, see 0908T, 0909T)◀

Open Implantation Neurostimulator Electrodes, Cranial Nerve (Vagus Nerve Stimulation)
64568-64570

Open implantation of a cranial nerve (eg, vagus nerve) neurostimulator electrode with connection of the electrode to an implanted programmable pulse generator in the infraclavicular area (64568). Revision or replacement of the cranial nerve electrode (64569). Replacement of the cranial nerve pulse generator (61885).

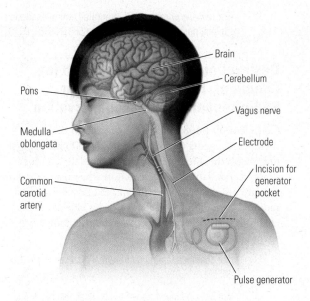

64569   Revision or replacement of cranial nerve (eg, vagus nerve) neurostimulator electrode array, including connection to existing pulse generator

➔ *CPT Changes: An Insider's View* 2011

➔ *CPT Assistant* Feb 11:5, Sep 11:8, Nov 16:6, Mar 18:9, Mar 22:7

(Do not report 64569 in conjunction with 64570 or 61888)

(For replacement of pulse generator, use 61885)

64570   Removal of cranial nerve (eg, vagus nerve) neurostimulator electrode array and pulse generator

➔ *CPT Changes: An Insider's View* 2011

➔ *CPT Assistant* Feb 11:5, Sep 11:10, Nov 16:6, Mar 18:9, Mar 22:7

(Do not report 64570 in conjunction with 61888)

▶(For removal of vagus nerve integrated neurostimulation system, use 0910T)◀

64575   Open implantation of neurostimulator electrode array; peripheral nerve (excludes sacral nerve)

➔ *CPT Changes: An Insider's View* 2002, 2011, 2012, 2022

➔ *CPT Assistant* Mar 22:7-8

64580   neuromuscular

➔ *CPT Changes: An Insider's View* 2012, 2022

➔ *CPT Assistant* Mar 22:7-8

64581   sacral nerve (transforaminal placement)

➔ *CPT Changes: An Insider's View* 2002, 2012, 2022

➔ *CPT Assistant* Dec 12:14, Sep 14:5, Oct 21:7, Mar 22:7-8

Open Implantation of Sacral Nerve Neurostimulator Electrode Array
64581

Posterior View

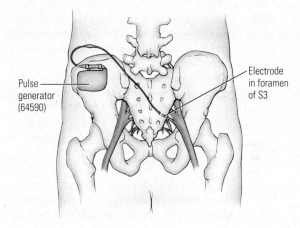

Pulse generator (64590)

Electrode in foramen of S3

64582   Open implantation of hypoglossal nerve neurostimulator array, pulse generator, and distal respiratory sensor electrode or electrode array

➔ *CPT Changes: An Insider's View* 2022

➔ *CPT Assistant* Mar 22:7-8

64583 Revision or replacement of hypoglossal nerve neurostimulator array and distal respiratory sensor electrode or electrode array, including connection to existing pulse generator

➔ *CPT Changes: An Insider's View* 2022

➔ *CPT Assistant* Mar 22:7-8

(Do not report 64583 in conjunction with 64582, 64584)

(For replacement of pulse generator, use 61886)

(For revision or replacement of either the hypoglossal nerve stimulator electrode array or distal respiratory sensor, use modifier 52)

64584 Removal of hypoglossal nerve neurostimulator array, pulse generator, and distal respiratory sensor electrode or electrode array

➔ *CPT Changes: An Insider's View* 2022

(Do not report 64584 in conjunction with 61888, 64582, 64583)

(For removal of one or two components of the hypoglossal nerve stimulator electrode array, pulse generator, or distal respiratory sensor, use modifier 52)

64585 Revision or removal of peripheral neurostimulator electrode array

➔ *CPT Changes: An Insider's View* 2012

64590 Insertion or replacement of peripheral, sacral, or gastric neurostimulator pulse generator or receiver, requiring pocket creation and connection between electrode array and pulse generator or receiver

➔ *CPT Changes: An Insider's View* 2002, 2005, 2007, 2024

➔ *CPT Assistant* Sep 99:4, Apr 01:8, Mar 07:4, Apr 07:7, Sep 11:9, Dec 12:14, Jan 15:14, Dec 17:16, Aug 18:10, Oct 21:7, Dec 23:1, 46, Mar 24:11

(Do not report 64590 in conjunction with 64595)

(Do not report 64590 in conjunction with 64596, 64597, 64598)

(For insertion or replacement of percutaneous electrode array with integrated neurostimulator, use 64596)

(For neurostimulators without a named target nerve [eg, field stimulation], use 64999)

64595 Revision or removal of peripheral, sacral, or gastric neurostimulator pulse generator or receiver, with detachable connection to electrode array

➔ *CPT Changes: An Insider's View* 2007, 2024

➔ *CPT Assistant* Sep 99:3, Mar 07:4, Jan 08:8, Dec 23:1, Mar 24:11

(For revision or removal of percutaneous electrode array with integrated neurostimulator, use 64598)

64596 Insertion or replacement of percutaneous electrode array, peripheral nerve, with integrated neurostimulator, including imaging guidance, when performed; initial electrode array

➔ *CPT Changes: An Insider's View* 2024

➔ *CPT Assistant* Dec 23:1

+ 64597 each additional electrode array (List separately in addition to code for primary procedure)

➔ *CPT Changes: An Insider's View* 2024

➔ *CPT Assistant* Dec 23:1

(Use 64597 in conjunction with 64596)

(Do not report 64596, 64597 in conjunction with 64555, 64561, 64590, 64595)

(For percutaneous implantation of electrode array only, peripheral nerve, use 64555)

(For implantation of trial or permanent electrode arrays or pulse generators for peripheral subcutaneous field stimulation, use 64999)

(For neurostimulators without a named target nerve [eg, field stimulation], use 64999)

(For percutaneous implantation or replacement of integrated neurostimulation system for bladder dysfunction, posterior tibial nerve, use 0587T)

(For open implantation or replacement of integrated neurostimulator system, posterior tibial nerve, see 0816T, 0817T)

64598 Revision or removal of neurostimulator electrode array, peripheral nerve, with integrated neurostimulator

➔ *CPT Changes: An Insider's View* 2024

➔ *CPT Assistant* Dec 23:1

(For revision or removal of electrode array only, use 64585)

(For revision or removal of integrated neurostimulation system, posterior tibial nerve, see 0588T, 0818T, 0819T)

Destruction by Neurolytic Agent (eg, Chemical, Thermal, Electrical or Radiofrequency), Chemodenervation

Codes 64600-64681 include the injection of other therapeutic agents (eg, corticosteroids). Do not report diagnostic/therapeutic injections separately. Do not report a code labeled as destruction when using therapies that are not destructive of the target nerve (eg, pulsed radiofrequency), use 64999. For codes labeled as chemodenervation, the supply of the chemodenervation agent is reported separately.

(For chemodenervation of internal anal sphincter, use 46505)

(For chemodenervation of the bladder, use 52287)

(For chemodenervation for strabismus involving the extraocular muscles, use 67345)

(For chemodenervation guided by needle electromyography or muscle electrical stimulation, see 95873, 95874)

Somatic Nerves

64600   Destruction by neurolytic agent, trigeminal nerve; supraorbital, infraorbital, mental, or inferior alveolar branch
➡ *CPT Assistant* Aug 05:13, Feb 10:9, Sep 12:14, Apr 19:9
➡ *Clinical Examples in Radiology* Winter 18:19

64605   second and third division branches at foramen ovale
➡ *CPT Assistant* Aug 05:13, Feb 10:9, Sep 12:14, Apr 19:9

64610   second and third division branches at foramen ovale under radiologic monitoring
➡ *CPT Assistant* Aug 05:13, Feb 10:9, Sep 12:14, Apr 17:10, Apr 19:9

 # 64624   Destruction by neurolytic agent, genicular nerve branches including imaging guidance, when performed
➡ *CPT Changes: An Insider's View* 2020
➡ *CPT Assistant* Dec 19:8

(Do not report 64624 in conjunction with 64454)

(64624 requires the destruction of each of the following genicular nerve branches: superolateral, superomedial, and inferomedial. If a neurolytic agent for the purposes of destruction is not applied to all of these nerve branches, report 64624 with modifier 52)

 # 64625   Radiofrequency ablation, nerves innervating the sacroiliac joint, with image guidance (ie, fluoroscopy or computed tomography)
➡ *CPT Changes: An Insider's View* 2020
➡ *CPT Assistant* Dec 19:8

(Do not report 64625 in conjunction with 64635, 77002, 77003, 77012, 95873, 95874)

(For radiofrequency ablation, nerves innervating the sacroiliac joint, with ultrasound, use 76999)

(For bilateral procedure, report 64625 with modifier 50)

 # 64628   Thermal destruction of intraosseous basivertebral nerve, including all imaging guidance; first 2 vertebral bodies, lumbar or sacral
➡ *CPT Changes: An Insider's View* 2022
➡ *CPT Assistant* Mar 22:10

#+ 64629   each additional vertebral body, lumbar or sacral (List separately in addition to code for primary procedure)
➡ *CPT Changes: An Insider's View* 2022
➡ *CPT Assistant* Mar 22:10

(Use 64629 in conjunction with 64628)

(Do not report 64628, 64629 in conjunction with 77003, 77012)

64611   Chemodenervation of parotid and submandibular salivary glands, bilateral
➡ *CPT Changes: An Insider's View* 2011
➡ *CPT Assistant* Feb 11:10, Sep 12:14, Apr 19:9, Dec 20:14, Aug 22:18

(Report 64611 with modifier 52 if fewer than four salivary glands are injected)

64612   Chemodenervation of muscle(s); muscle(s) innervated by facial nerve, unilateral (eg, for blepharospasm, hemifacial spasm)
➡ *CPT Changes: An Insider's View* 2000, 2001, 2013
➡ *CPT Assistant* Oct 98:10, Apr 01:2, Aug 05:13, Sep 06:5, Dec 08:9, Jan 09:8, Feb 10:9, 13, Dec 11:19, Sep 12:14, Apr 13:5, Dec 13:10, Jan 14:6, May 14:5, Apr 19:9, Aug 22:18

(For bilateral procedure, report 64612 with modifier 50)

64615   muscle(s) innervated by facial, trigeminal, cervical spinal and accessory nerves, bilateral (eg, for chronic migraine)
➡ *CPT Changes: An Insider's View* 2013
➡ *CPT Assistant* Apr 13:5, Jan 14:6, Apr 19:9, Aug 22:18

(Report 64615 only once per session)

(Do not report 64615 in conjunction with 64612, 64616, 64617, 64642, 64643, 64644, 64645, 64646, 64647)

(For guidance see 95873, 95874. Do not report more than one guidance code for 64615)

64616   neck muscle(s), excluding muscles of the larynx, unilateral (eg, for cervical dystonia, spasmodic torticollis)
➡ *CPT Changes: An Insider's View* 2014
➡ *CPT Assistant* Jan 14:6, May 14:5, Apr 19:9, Aug 22:18

(For bilateral procedure, report 64616 with modifier 50)

(For chemodenervation guided by needle electromyography or muscle electrical stimulation, see 95873, 95874. Do not report more than one guidance code for any unit of 64616)

64617   larynx, unilateral, percutaneous (eg, for spasmodic dysphonia), includes guidance by needle electromyography, when performed
➡ *CPT Changes: An Insider's View* 2014
➡ *CPT Assistant* Jan 14:6, Apr 19:9

(For bilateral procedure, report 64617 with modifier 50)

(Do not report 64617 in conjunction with 95873, 95874)

(For diagnostic needle electromyography of the larynx, use 95865)

(For chemodenervation of the larynx performed with direct laryngoscopy, see 31570, 31571)

Nervous 61000-64999

64620 Destruction by neurolytic agent, intercostal nerve
- ➔ *CPT Changes: An Insider's View* 2000
- ➔ *CPT Assistant* Nov 99:38, Aug 05:13, Sep 12:14, Jan 14:6, Apr 19:9, Nov 19:15

(Imaging guidance [fluoroscopy or CT] are inclusive components of 64633-64636)

(Image guidance [fluoroscopy or CT] and any injection of contrast are inclusive components of 64633-64636. Image guidance and localization are required for the performance of paravertebral facet joint nerve destruction by neurolytic agent described by 64633-64636. If CT or fluoroscopic imaging is not used, report 64999)

Report 64633, 64634, 64635, 64636 per joint, not per nerve. Although two nerves innervate each facet joint, only one code may be reported for each joint denervated, regardless of the number of nerves treated. Use 64634 or 64636 to report each additional facet joint at a different vertebral level in the same spinal region.

For neurolytic destruction of the nerves innervating the T12-L1 paravertebral facet joint, use 64633.

Do not report 64633, 64634, 64635, 64636 for non-thermal facet joint denervation including chemical, low-grade thermal energy (<80 degrees Celsius), or any form of pulsed radiofrequency. To appropriately report any of these modalities, use 64999.

64624 Code is out of numerical sequence. See 64605-64612

64625 Code is out of numerical sequence. See 64605-64612

64628 Code is out of numerical sequence. See 64610-64612

64629 Code is out of numerical sequence. See 64610-64612

 # 64633 Destruction by neurolytic agent, paravertebral facet joint nerve(s), with imaging guidance (fluoroscopy or CT); cervical or thoracic, single facet joint
- ➔ *CPT Changes: An Insider's View* 2012
- ➔ *CPT Assistant* Jun 12:10, Jul 12:6, Sep 12:14, Apr 13:10, Feb 15:9, Apr 19:9, Dec 20:13

(For bilateral procedure, report 64633 with modifier 50)

#+ 64634 cervical or thoracic, each additional facet joint (List separately in addition to code for primary procedure)
- ➔ *CPT Changes: An Insider's View* 2012
- ➔ *CPT Assistant* Jun 12:10, Jul 12:6, Sep 12:14, Apr 13:10, Feb 15:9, Apr 19:9, Dec 20:13

(Use 64634 in conjunction with 64633)

(For bilateral procedure, report 64634 twice. Do not report modifier 50 in conjunction with 64634)

 # 64635 lumbar or sacral, single facet joint
- ➔ *CPT Changes: An Insider's View* 2012
- ➔ *CPT Assistant* Jun 12:10, Jul 12:6, 14, Sep 12:14, Apr 13:10, Feb 15:9, Apr 19:9, Dec 19:8, May 20:14, Dec 20:13

(For bilateral procedure, report 64635 with modifier 50)

#+ 64636 lumbar or sacral, each additional facet joint (List separately in addition to code for primary procedure)
- ➔ *CPT Changes: An Insider's View* 2012
- ➔ *CPT Assistant* Jun 12:10, Jul 12:6, 14, Sep 12:14, Apr 13:10, Feb 15:9, Apr 19:9, May 20:14, Dec 20:13

(Use 64636 in conjunction with 64635)

(For bilateral procedure, report 64636 twice. Do not report modifier 50 in conjunction with 64636)

(Do not report 64633-64636 in conjunction with 77003, 77012)

(For radiofrequency ablation of nerves innervating the sacroiliac joint with image guidance, use 64625)

64630 Destruction by neurolytic agent; pudendal nerve
- ➔ *CPT Changes: An Insider's View* 2001
- ➔ *CPT Assistant* Aug 05:13, Feb 10:9, Sep 12:14, Oct 17:9, Apr 19:9

64632 plantar common digital nerve
- ➔ *CPT Changes: An Insider's View* 2009
- ➔ *CPT Assistant* Jan 09:6, Sep 12:14, Jan 13:13, Jul 15:11, Oct 17:9, Apr 19:9

(Do not report 64632 in conjunction with 64455)

64633 Code is out of numerical sequence. See 64617-64632

64634 Code is out of numerical sequence. See 64617-64632

64635 Code is out of numerical sequence. See 64617-64632

64636 Code is out of numerical sequence. See 64617-64632

64640 other peripheral nerve or branch
- ➔ *CPT Assistant* Aug 05:13, Dec 09:11, Feb 10:9, Jun 12:15, Sep 12:14, May 17:10, Oct 17:9, Jan 18:7, Apr 19:9, Dec 23:47

Report 64642, 64643, 64644, 64645 once per extremity. Codes 64642, 64643, 64644, 64645 can be reported together up to a combined total of four units of service per patient when all four extremities are injected. Report only one base code (64642 or 64644) per session. Report one unit of additional extremity code(s) (64643 or 64645) for each additional extremity injected.

Report 64646 or 64647 for chemodenervation of muscles of the trunk.

Trunk muscles include the erector spinae and paraspinal muscles, rectus abdominus and obliques. All other somatic muscles are extremity muscles, head muscles, or neck muscles.

(For chemodenervation guided by needle electromyography or muscle electrical stimulation, see 95873, 95874. Do not report more than one guidance code for each corresponding chemodenervation of extremity or trunk code)

(Do not report modifier 50 in conjunction with 64642, 64643, 64644, 64645, 64646, 64647)

64642   Chemodenervation of one extremity; 1-4 muscle(s)
→ *CPT Changes: An Insider's View* 2014
→ *CPT Assistant* Jan 14:6, Oct 14:15, Apr 19:9, Aug 19:10, Jul 22:17, Aug 22:18

+ 64643   each additional extremity, 1-4 muscle(s) (List separately in addition to code for primary procedure)
→ *CPT Changes: An Insider's View* 2014
→ *CPT Assistant* Jan 14:6, Oct 14:15, Apr 19:9, Aug 19:10, Jul 22:17, Aug 22:18

(Use 64643 in conjunction with 64642, 64644)

Chemodenervation of Extremity
64642

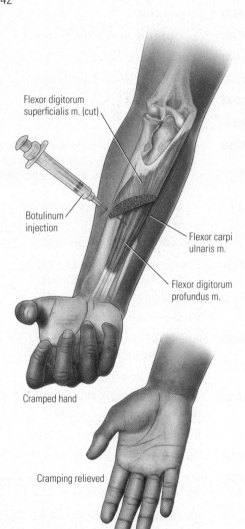

Flexor digitorum
superficialis m. (cut)

Botulinum
injection

Flexor carpi
ulnaris m.

Flexor digitorum
profundus m.

Cramped hand

Cramping relieved

64644   Chemodenervation of one extremity; 5 or more muscles
→ *CPT Changes: An Insider's View* 2014
→ *CPT Assistant* Jan 14:6, Oct 14:15, Apr 19:9, Aug 19:10, Jul 22:17, Aug 22:18

+ 64645   each additional extremity, 5 or more muscles (List separately in addition to code for primary procedure)
→ *CPT Changes: An Insider's View* 2014
→ *CPT Assistant* Jan 14:6, Oct 14:15, Apr 19:9, Aug 19:10, Jul 22:17, Aug 22:18

(Use 64645 in conjunction with 64644)

64646   Chemodenervation of trunk muscle(s); 1-5 muscle(s)
→ *CPT Changes: An Insider's View* 2014
→ *CPT Assistant* Jan 14:6, Apr 19:9, Oct 21:8, Aug 22:18

64647   6 or more muscles
→ *CPT Changes: An Insider's View* 2014
→ *CPT Assistant* Jan 14:6, Apr 19:9, Oct 21:8, Aug 22:18

(Report either 64646 or 64647 only once per session)

Sympathetic Nerves

64650   Chemodenervation of eccrine glands; both axillae
→ *CPT Changes: An Insider's View* 2006
→ *CPT Assistant* Jun 08:9, Feb 10:11, Sep 12:14, Apr 19:9

64653   other area(s) (eg, scalp, face, neck), per day
→ *CPT Changes: An Insider's View* 2006
→ *CPT Assistant* Jun 08:9, Sep 12:14, Apr 19:9

(Report the specific service in conjunction with code(s) for the specific substance(s) or drug(s) provided)

(For chemodenervation of extremities (eg, hands or feet), use 64999)

(For chemodenervation of bladder, use 52287)

64680   Destruction by neurolytic agent, with or without radiologic monitoring; celiac plexus
→ *CPT Changes: An Insider's View* 2004
→ *CPT Assistant* Feb 99:10, Aug 05:13, Jun 08:9, Sep 12:14, Apr 19:9
→ *Clinical Examples in Radiology* Winter 18:19

(For transendoscopic ultrasound-guided transmural injection, neurolytic agent, celiac plexus, use 43253)

64681   superior hypogastric plexus
→ *CPT Changes: An Insider's View* 2004
→ *CPT Assistant* Aug 05:13, Dec 07:13, Sep 12:14, Apr 19:9
→ *Clinical Examples in Radiology* Winter 18:19

Neuroplasty (Exploration, Neurolysis or Nerve Decompression)

Neuroplasty is the surgical decompression or freeing of intact nerve from scar tissue, including external neurolysis and/or transposition to repair or restore the nerve.

(For percutaneous neurolysis, see 62263, 62264, 62280-62282)

(For internal neurolysis requiring use of operating microscope, use 64727)

(For facial nerve decompression, use 69720)

(For neuroplasty with nerve wrapping, see 64702-64727, 64999)

64702 Neuroplasty; digital, 1 or both, same digit
➡ *CPT Assistant* Jun 01:11

64704 nerve of hand or foot
➡ *CPT Assistant* Jun 01:11

(Do not report 64702, 64704 in conjunction with 11960)

64708 Neuroplasty, major peripheral nerve, arm or leg, open; other than specified
➡ *CPT Changes: An Insider's View* 2011
➡ *CPT Assistant* Jun 01:11, Jun 12:12, Nov 17:10

64712 sciatic nerve
➡ *CPT Changes: An Insider's View* 2011
➡ *CPT Assistant* Jun 01:11, Jun 12:12

64713 brachial plexus
➡ *CPT Changes: An Insider's View* 2011
➡ *CPT Assistant* Jun 01:11, Jun 12:12, May 13:12, Aug 21:15

64714 lumbar plexus
➡ *CPT Changes: An Insider's View* 2011
➡ *CPT Assistant* Jun 97:11, Sep 98:16, Jun 01:11, Jun 12:12, Dec 13:17

(Do not report 64708, 64712, 64713, 64714 in conjunction with 11960)

64716 Neuroplasty and/or transposition; cranial nerve (specify)
➡ *CPT Assistant* Jun 01:11

64718 ulnar nerve at elbow
➡ *CPT Assistant* Jun 01:11, Mar 09:10

64719 ulnar nerve at wrist
➡ *CPT Assistant* Jun 01:11, Mar 09:10

64721 median nerve at carpal tunnel
➡ *CPT Assistant* Fall 92:17, Sep 97:10, Jun 01:11, Nov 06:23, Aug 09:11, Jun 12:15, Sep 12:16, Dec 13:14, Jul 15:10, Mar 21:9, Jul 22:18

(Do not report 64716, 64718, 64719, 64721 in conjunction with 11960)

(For endoscopic procedure, use 29848)

64722 Decompression; unspecified nerve(s) (specify)
➡ *CPT Assistant* Sep 98:16, May 99:11, Jun 01:11, Oct 04:12

64726 plantar digital nerve
➡ *CPT Assistant* Jun 01:11

(Do not report 64722, 64726 in conjunction with 11960)

+ 64727 Internal neurolysis, requiring use of operating microscope (List separately in addition to code for neuroplasty) (Neuroplasty includes external neurolysis)
➡ *CPT Assistant* Nov 98:19, Jun 01:11, Jun 12:13

(Do not report code 69990 in addition to code 64727)

Transection or Avulsion

(For stereotactic lesion of gasserian ganglion, use 61790)

64732 Transection or avulsion of; supraorbital nerve
➡ *CPT Changes: An Insider's View* 2000
➡ *CPT Assistant* Nov 99:39

64734 infraorbital nerve

64736 mental nerve

64738 inferior alveolar nerve by osteotomy

64740 lingual nerve

64742 facial nerve, differential or complete

64744 greater occipital nerve

64746 phrenic nerve

64755 vagus nerves limited to proximal stomach (selective proximal vagotomy, proximal gastric vagotomy, parietal cell vagotomy, supra- or highly selective vagotomy)
➡ *CPT Changes: An Insider's View* 2000, 2002
➡ *CPT Assistant* Nov 99:39

(For laparoscopic approach, use 43652)

64760 vagus nerve (vagotomy), abdominal
➡ *CPT Changes: An Insider's View* 2000
➡ *CPT Assistant* Nov 99:39

(For laparoscopic approach, use 43651)

64763 Transection or avulsion of obturator nerve, extrapelvic, with or without adductor tenotomy

(For bilateral procedure, report 64763 with modifier 50)

64766 Transection or avulsion of obturator nerve, intrapelvic, with or without adductor tenotomy

(For bilateral procedure, report 64766 with modifier 50)

64771 Transection or avulsion of other cranial nerve, extradural

64772 Transection or avulsion of other spinal nerve, extradural
➡ *CPT Assistant* Apr 15:10, Aug 21:15

(For excision of tender scar, skin and subcutaneous tissue, with or without tiny neuroma, see 11400-11446, 13100-13153)

Excision

Somatic Nerves

(For Morton neurectomy, use 28080)

64774 Excision of neuroma; cutaneous nerve, surgically identifiable

64776 digital nerve, 1 or both, same digit

+ 64778 digital nerve, each additional digit (List separately in addition to code for primary procedure)

(Use 64778 in conjunction with 64776)

64782 hand or foot, except digital nerve

+ 64783 hand or foot, each additional nerve, except same digit (List separately in addition to code for primary procedure)

(Use 64783 in conjunction with 64782)

64784 major peripheral nerve, except sciatic

64786 sciatic nerve

+ 64787 Implantation of nerve end into bone or muscle (List separately in addition to neuroma excision)

(Use 64787 in conjunction with 64774-64786)

64788 Excision of neurofibroma or neurolemmoma; cutaneous nerve
➡ *CPT Assistant* Apr 16:3

64790 major peripheral nerve
➡ *CPT Assistant* Apr 16:3

64792 extensive (including malignant type)
➡ *CPT Assistant* Apr 16:3

(For destruction of extensive cutaneous neurofibroma, see 0419T, 0420T)

64795 Biopsy of nerve

Sympathetic Nerves

64802 Sympathectomy, cervical
➡ *CPT Assistant* Apr 24:36

(For bilateral procedure, report 64802 with modifier 50)

64804 Sympathectomy, cervicothoracic
➡ *CPT Assistant* Apr 24:36

(For bilateral procedure, report 64804 with modifier 50)

64809 Sympathectomy, thoracolumbar

(For bilateral procedure, report 64809 with modifier 50)

64818 Sympathectomy, lumbar

(For bilateral procedure, report 64818 with modifier 50)

64820 Sympathectomy; digital arteries, each digit
➡ *CPT Changes: An Insider's View* 2002
➡ *CPT Assistant* Jan 04:27

(Do not report 69990 in addition to code 64820)

64821 radial artery
➡ *CPT Changes: An Insider's View* 2002

(Do not report 69990 in addition to code 64821)

64822 ulnar artery
➡ *CPT Changes: An Insider's View* 2002

(Do not report 69990 in addition to code 64822)

64823 superficial palmar arch
➡ *CPT Changes: An Insider's View* 2002

(Do not report 69990 in addition to code 64823)

Neurorrhaphy

64831 Suture of digital nerve, hand or foot; 1 nerve
➡ *CPT Assistant* Apr 00:6, Sep 14:13, Jan 21:13

+ 64832 each additional digital nerve (List separately in addition to code for primary procedure)
➡ *CPT Assistant* Apr 00:6, Jan 21:13

(Use 64832 in conjunction with 64831)

64834 Suture of 1 nerve; hand or foot, common sensory nerve
➡ *CPT Changes: An Insider's View* 2008
➡ *CPT Assistant* Jan 21:13

64835 median motor thenar
➡ *CPT Changes: An Insider's View* 2008

64836 ulnar motor
➡ *CPT Changes: An Insider's View* 2008

+ 64837 Suture of each additional nerve, hand or foot (List separately in addition to code for primary procedure)
➡ *CPT Assistant* Jan 21:13

(Use 64837 in conjunction with 64834-64836)

64840 Suture of posterior tibial nerve

64856 Suture of major peripheral nerve, arm or leg, except sciatic; including transposition

64857 without transposition

64858 Suture of sciatic nerve

+ 64859 Suture of each additional major peripheral nerve (List separately in addition to code for primary procedure)

(Use 64859 in conjunction with 64856, 64857)

64861 Suture of; brachial plexus

64862 lumbar plexus

64864 Suture of facial nerve; extracranial

64865 infratemporal, with or without grafting

64866 Anastomosis; facial-spinal accessory

64868   facial-hypoglossal

+ 64872 Suture of nerve; requiring secondary or delayed suture (List separately in addition to code for primary neurorrhaphy)

(Use 64872 in conjunction with 64831-64865)

+ 64874   requiring extensive mobilization, or transposition of nerve (List separately in addition to code for nerve suture)

(Use 64874 in conjunction with 64831-64865)

+ 64876   requiring shortening of bone of extremity (List separately in addition to code for nerve suture)

(Use 64876 in conjunction with 64831-64865)

Neurorrhaphy With Nerve Graft, Vein Graft, or Conduit

64885 Nerve graft (includes obtaining graft), head or neck; up to 4 cm in length
➔ *CPT Assistant* Nov 00:11, Dec 17:12

64886   more than 4 cm length
➔ *CPT Assistant* Nov 00:11, Dec 17:12

64890 Nerve graft (includes obtaining graft), single strand, hand or foot; up to 4 cm length
➔ *CPT Assistant* Apr 15:10, Aug 15:8, Dec 17:12, Apr 21:14

64891   more than 4 cm length
➔ *CPT Assistant* Dec 17:12, Apr 21:14

64892 Nerve graft (includes obtaining graft), single strand, arm or leg; up to 4 cm length
➔ *CPT Assistant* Dec 17:12

64893   more than 4 cm length
➔ *CPT Assistant* Dec 17:12

64895 Nerve graft (includes obtaining graft), multiple strands (cable), hand or foot; up to 4 cm length
➔ *CPT Assistant* Nov 00:11, Dec 17:12

64896   more than 4 cm length
➔ *CPT Assistant* Nov 00:11, Dec 17:12

64897 Nerve graft (includes obtaining graft), multiple strands (cable), arm or leg; up to 4 cm length
➔ *CPT Assistant* Nov 00:11, Dec 17:12

64898   more than 4 cm length
➔ *CPT Assistant* Nov 00:11, Dec 17:12

+ 64901 Nerve graft, each additional nerve; single strand (List separately in addition to code for primary procedure)
➔ *CPT Assistant* Nov 00:11, Dec 17:12, Apr 21:14

(Use 64901 in conjunction with 64885-64893)

+ 64902   multiple strands (cable) (List separately in addition to code for primary procedure)
➔ *CPT Assistant* Nov 00:11, Dec 17:12

(Use 64902 in conjunction with 64885, 64886, 64895-64898)

64905 Nerve pedicle transfer; first stage
➔ *CPT Assistant* Dec 17:12, Aug 21:15

64907   second stage
➔ *CPT Assistant* Dec 17:12

64910 Nerve repair; with synthetic conduit or vein allograft (eg, nerve tube), each nerve
➔ *CPT Changes: An Insider's View* 2007
➔ *CPT Assistant* Nov 07:4, Apr 15:10, Aug 15:8, Dec 17:12

64911   with autogenous vein graft (includes harvest of vein graft), each nerve
➔ *CPT Changes: An Insider's View* 2007
➔ *CPT Assistant* Nov 07:4, Dec 17:12

(Do not report 69990 in addition to 64910, 64911)

64912   with nerve allograft, each nerve, first strand (cable)
➔ *CPT Changes: An Insider's View* 2018
➔ *CPT Assistant* Dec 17:12

+ 64913   with nerve allograft, each additional strand (List separately in addition to code for primary procedure)
➔ *CPT Changes: An Insider's View* 2018
➔ *CPT Assistant* Dec 17:12

(Use 64913 in conjunction with 64912)

(Do not report 64912, 64913 in conjunction with 69990)

Other Procedures

64999 Unlisted procedure, nervous system
➔ *CPT Assistant* Apr 96:11, Sep 98:16, Oct 98:10, Jan 00:10, Aug 00:7, Sep 00:10, Feb 02:10, Nov 03:5, Oct 04:11, Apr 05:13, Aug 05:13, Sep 05:9, Sep 07:10, Nov 07:4, Dec 07:8, Jul 08:9, Sep 08:11, Aug 09:8, Dec 09:11, Jun 10:8, Sep 10:10, Nov 10:4, Apr 11:12, Jul 11:12, 16-17, Sep 11:12, Jan 12:14, Feb 12:11, May 12:14, Sep 12:16, Oct 12:14, Dec 12:13, Apr 13:5, 10, Jun 13:13, Nov 13:14, Dec 13:14, Jan 14:8-9, Feb 14:11, Jul 14:8, Feb 15:9, Apr 15:10, Jul 15:11, Aug 15:8, Oct 15:9, Feb 16:13, Oct 16:11, Nov 16:6, May 17:10, Dec 17:13, Jan 18:7, Mar 18:9, Aug 18:10, Oct 18:8, Dec 18:8, Apr 19:9, May 19:10, Jul 19:11, Dec 19:12, Jan 20:12, Feb 20:13, Dec 20:13, Jan 21:13, Aug 21:15, Oct 21:10, Dec 21:22, Jan 22:18, Jul 22:13, Dec 22:12,21, Jan 23:31, Apr 24:36
➔ *Clinical Examples in Radiology* Winter 17:3

★ =Telemedicine ◀ =Audio-only ✛ =Add-on code ✗ =FDA approval pending # =Resequenced code ⊘ =Modifier 51 exempt ➔➔➔ =See p xxi for details

Surgery

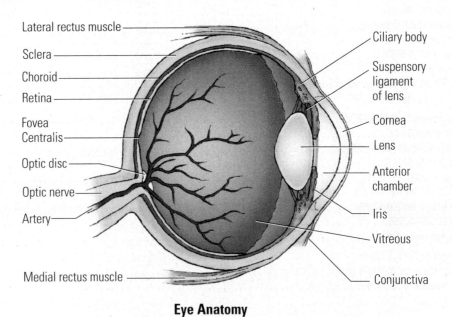

Eye Anatomy

Eye and Ocular Adnexa

(For diagnostic and treatment ophthalmological services, see **Medicine, Ophthalmology,** and 92002 et seq)

(Do not report code 69990 in addition to codes 65091-68850)

Eyeball

Removal of Eye

65091   Evisceration of ocular contents; without implant

65093   with implant

65101   Enucleation of eye; without implant

65103   with implant, muscles not attached to implant

65105   with implant, muscles attached to implant

(For conjunctivoplasty after enucleation, see 68320 et seq)

65110   Exenteration of orbit (does not include skin graft), removal of orbital contents; only

65112   with therapeutic removal of bone

65114   with muscle or myocutaneous flap

(For skin graft to orbit (split skin), see 15120, 15121; free, full thickness, see 15260, 15261)

(For eyelid repair involving more than skin, see 67930 et seq)

Secondary Implant(s) Procedures

An ocular implant is an implant inside muscular cone; an orbital implant is an implant outside muscular cone.

65125   Modification of ocular implant with placement or replacement of pegs (eg, drilling receptacle for prosthesis appendage) (separate procedure)

65130   Insertion of ocular implant secondary; after evisceration, in scleral shell

65135   after enucleation, muscles not attached to implant

65140   after enucleation, muscles attached to implant

65150   Reinsertion of ocular implant; with or without conjunctival graft

65155   with use of foreign material for reinforcement and/or attachment of muscles to implant

65175   Removal of ocular implant

(For orbital implant (implant outside muscle cone) insertion, use 67550; removal, use 67560)

Removal of Foreign Body

(For removal of implanted material: ocular implant, use 65175; anterior segment implant, use 65920; posterior segment implant, use 67120; orbital implant, use 67560)

(For diagnostic x-ray for foreign body, use 70030)

(For diagnostic echography for foreign body, use 76529)

(For removal of foreign body from orbit: frontal approach, use 67413; lateral approach, use 67430)

(For removal of foreign body from eyelid, embedded, use 67938)

(For removal of foreign body from lacrimal system, use 68530)

65205   Removal of foreign body, external eye; conjunctival superficial
> *CPT Assistant* Mar 05:17, Oct 13:19

65210   conjunctival embedded (includes concretions), subconjunctival, or scleral nonperforating

65220   corneal, without slit lamp

65222   corneal, with slit lamp

(For repair of corneal laceration with foreign body, use 65275)

65235   Removal of foreign body, intraocular; from anterior chamber of eye or lens
> *CPT Changes: An Insider's View* 2002

(For removal of implanted material from anterior segment, use 65920)

65260   from posterior segment, magnetic extraction, anterior or posterior route

65265   from posterior segment, nonmagnetic extraction

(For removal of implanted material from posterior segment, use 67120)

Repair of Laceration

(For fracture of orbit, see 21385 et seq)

(For repair of wound of eyelid, skin, linear, simple, see 12011-12018; intermediate, layered closure, see 12051-12057; linear, complex, see 13151-13160; other, see 67930, 67935)

(For repair of wound of lacrimal system, use 68700)

(For repair of operative wound, use 66250)

65270   Repair of laceration; conjunctiva, with or without nonperforating laceration sclera, direct closure
> *CPT Assistant* Aug 12:9

65272   conjunctiva, by mobilization and rearrangement, without hospitalization

65273   conjunctiva, by mobilization and rearrangement, with hospitalization

---

▲ = Revised code   ● = New code   ► ◄ = Contains new or revised text   ✖ = Duplicate PLA test   ↕ = Category I PLA   American Medical Association   **509**

65275	cornea, nonperforating, with or without removal foreign body
65280	cornea and/or sclera, perforating, not involving uveal tissue

> *CPT Assistant* Aug 12:9

65285	cornea and/or sclera, perforating, with reposition or resection of uveal tissue

> *CPT Assistant* Aug 12:9

(65280 and 65285 are not used for repair of a surgical wound)

65286	application of tissue glue, wounds of cornea and/or sclera

> *CPT Assistant* May 99:11, Apr 09:5

(Repair of laceration includes use of conjunctival flap and restoration of anterior chamber, by air or saline injection when indicated)

(For repair of iris or ciliary body, use 66680)

65290	Repair of wound, extraocular muscle, tendon and/or Tenon's capsule

Anterior Segment

Cornea

Excision

65400	Excision of lesion, cornea (keratectomy, lamellar, partial), except pterygium
65410	Biopsy of cornea
65420	Excision or transposition of pterygium; without graft

> *CPT Assistant* Dec 07:13

65426	with graft

> *CPT Assistant* May 18:11

Removal or Destruction

65430	Scraping of cornea, diagnostic, for smear and/or culture
65435	Removal of corneal epithelium; with or without chemocauterization (abrasion, curettage)

> *CPT Assistant* Feb 16:12

(Do not report 65435 in conjunction with 0402T)

65436	with application of chelating agent (eg, EDTA)
65450	Destruction of lesion of cornea by cryotherapy, photocoagulation or thermocauterization
65600	Multiple punctures of anterior cornea (eg, for corneal erosion, tattoo)

Anterior Segment of the Eye

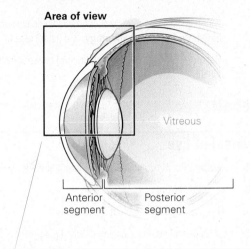

Anterior segment | **Posterior segment**

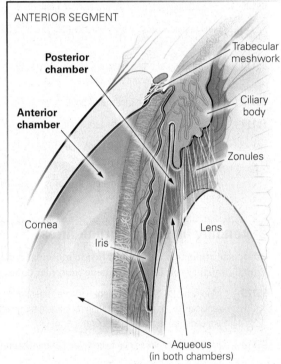

ANTERIOR SEGMENT

Posterior chamber

Anterior chamber

Cornea

Iris

Trabecular meshwork

Ciliary body

Zonules

Lens

Aqueous (in both chambers)

Cryotherapy of Lesion on Cornea
65450

A freezing probe is applied directly to the corneal defect to destroy it.

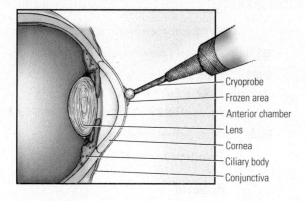

Cryoprobe
Frozen area
Anterior chamber
Lens
Cornea
Ciliary body
Conjunctiva

Keratoplasty

Corneal transplant includes use of fresh or preserved grafts. The preparation of donor material is included for penetrating or anterior lamellar keratoplasty, but reported separately for endothelial keratoplasty. Do not report 65710-65757 in conjunction with 92025.

(Keratoplasty excludes refractive keratoplasty procedures, 65760, 65765, and 65767)

65710 Keratoplasty (corneal transplant); anterior lamellar
➔ *CPT Changes: An Insider's View* 2009
➔ *CPT Assistant* Oct 02:8, Apr 09:5, Dec 09:13, Aug 12:15

65730 penetrating (except in aphakia or pseudophakia)
➔ *CPT Changes: An Insider's View* 2009
➔ *CPT Assistant* Oct 02:8, Feb 06:1, Apr 09:5, Dec 09:13, Aug 12:15

65750 penetrating (in aphakia)
➔ *CPT Assistant* Oct 02:8, Apr 09:5, Dec 09:13, Aug 12:15

65755 penetrating (in pseudophakia)
➔ *CPT Assistant* Winter 90:8, Oct 02:9, Apr 09:5, Dec 09:13, Aug 12:15

65756 endothelial
➔ *CPT Changes: An Insider's View* 2009

+ 65757 Backbench preparation of corneal endothelial allograft prior to transplantation (List separately in addition to code for primary procedure)
➔ *CPT Changes: An Insider's View* 2009
➔ *CPT Assistant* Aug 14:15

(Use 65757 in conjunction with 65756)

Other Procedures

Do not report 65760-65771 in conjunction with 92025.

65760 Keratomileusis
➔ *CPT Assistant* Oct 02:9

65765 Keratophakia
➔ *CPT Assistant* Oct 02:10

65767 Epikeratoplasty
➔ *CPT Assistant* Winter 90:8, Oct 02:10

65770 Keratoprosthesis
➔ *CPT Assistant* Oct 02:10

65771 Radial keratotomy
➔ *CPT Assistant* Winter 90:8, Oct 02:10

65772 Corneal relaxing incision for correction of surgically induced astigmatism
➔ *CPT Assistant* Oct 02:10, 12

65775 Corneal wedge resection for correction of surgically induced astigmatism
➔ *CPT Assistant* Oct 02:10, 12, Aug 12:9

(For fitting of contact lens for treatment of disease, see 92071, 92072)

(For unlisted procedures on cornea, use 66999)

65778 Placement of amniotic membrane on the ocular surface; without sutures
➔ *CPT Changes: An Insider's View* 2011, 2014
➔ *CPT Assistant* May 14:5, Feb 18:11

65779 single layer, sutured
➔ *CPT Changes: An Insider's View* 2011, 2014
➔ *CPT Assistant* May 14:5, Feb 18:11

(Do not report 65778, 65779 in conjunction with 65430, 65435, 65780)

(For placement of amniotic membrane using tissue glue, use 66999)

65780 Ocular surface reconstruction; amniotic membrane transplantation, multiple layers
➔ *CPT Changes: An Insider's View* 2004, 2011
➔ *CPT Assistant* May 04:10, Jun 09:9, May 14:5, Feb 18:11

(For placement of amniotic membrane without reconstruction using no sutures or single layer suture technique, see 65778, 65779)

65781 limbal stem cell allograft (eg, cadaveric or living donor)
➔ *CPT Changes: An Insider's View* 2004
➔ *CPT Assistant* May 04:10

65782 limbal conjunctival autograft (includes obtaining graft)
➔ *CPT Changes: An Insider's View* 2004
➔ *CPT Assistant* Feb 04:11, May 04:10, Feb 05:15-16

(For harvesting conjunctival allograft, living donor, use 68371)

65785 Implantation of intrastromal corneal ring segments
➔ *CPT Changes: An Insider's View* 2016

Eye / Ocular Adnexa   **65091-68899**

Anterior Chamber

Incision

65800 Paracentesis of anterior chamber of eye (separate procedure); with removal of aqueous
➔ *CPT Changes: An Insider's View* 2013
➔ *CPT Assistant* Nov 12:10

65810 with removal of vitreous and/or discission of anterior hyaloid membrane, with or without air injection
➔ *CPT Assistant* Nov 12:10

65815 with removal of blood, with or without irrigation and/or air injection
➔ *CPT Assistant* Nov 12:10

(For injection, see 66020-66030)

(For removal of blood clot, use 65930)

65820 Goniotomy
➔ *CPT Assistant* Sep 05:12, Jul 18:3, Dec 18:9, Sep 19:11, Sep 21:10, May 22:14, Aug 22:1, Nov 22:18

(Do not report modifier 63 in conjunction with 65820)

(For use of ophthalmic endoscope with 65820, use 66990)

Goniotomy
65820

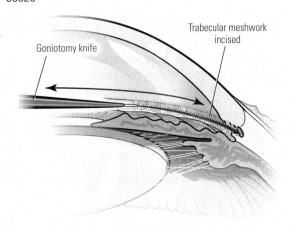

Goniotomy knife

Trabecular meshwork incised

65850 Trabeculotomy ab externo
➔ *CPT Assistant* Sep 23:42

(Do not report 65850 in conjunction with 0730T)

(For trabeculotomy by laser, including optical coherence tomography [OCT] image guidance, use 0730T)

65855 Trabeculoplasty by laser surgery
➔ *CPT Changes: An Insider's View* 2016
➔ *CPT Assistant* Mar 98:7, Mar 03:23, Sep 21:10, Sep 23:42

(Do not report 65855 in conjunction with 65860, 65865, 65870, 65875, 65880, 0730T)

(For trabeculectomy, use 66170)

(For trabeculotomy by laser, including optical coherence tomography [OCT] image guidance, use 0730T)

65860 Severing adhesions of anterior segment, laser technique (separate procedure)

65865 Severing adhesions of anterior segment of eye, incisional technique (with or without injection of air or liquid) (separate procedure); goniosynechiae

(For trabeculoplasty by laser surgery, use 65855)

65870 anterior synechiae, except goniosynechiae

65875 posterior synechiae
➔ *CPT Assistant* Sep 05:12

(For use of ophthalmic endoscope with 65875, use 66990)

65880 corneovitreal adhesions

(For laser surgery, use 66821)

Removal

65900 Removal of epithelial downgrowth, anterior chamber of eye
➔ *CPT Changes: An Insider's View* 2002

65920 Removal of implanted material, anterior segment of eye
➔ *CPT Changes: An Insider's View* 2002
➔ *CPT Assistant* Sep 05:12

(For use of ophthalmic endoscope with 65920, use 66990)

65930 Removal of blood clot, anterior segment of eye
➔ *CPT Changes: An Insider's View* 2002

Introduction

66020 Injection, anterior chamber of eye (separate procedure); air or liquid
➔ *CPT Changes: An Insider's View* 2002
➔ *CPT Assistant* Nov 12:10, Nov 21:14

66030 medication
➔ *CPT Assistant* Nov 12:10

(For unlisted procedures on anterior segment, use 66999)

Anterior Sclera

Excision

(For removal of intraocular foreign body, use 65235)

(For operations on posterior sclera, use 67250, 67255)

66130 Excision of lesion, sclera

66150 Fistulization of sclera for glaucoma; trephination with iridectomy
➔ *CPT Assistant* Jul 18:3

66155   thermocauterization with iridectomy
➥ *CPT Assistant* Jul 18:3

66160   sclerectomy with punch or scissors, with iridectomy
➥ *CPT Assistant* Jul 18:3

66170   trabeculectomy ab externo in absence of previous surgery
➥ *CPT Assistant* Jul 03:4, Nov 03:10, Dec 12:14, Jul 18:3, Dec 18:9

(For trabeculotomy ab externo, use 65850)

(For repair of operative wound, use 66250)

66172   trabeculectomy ab externo with scarring from previous ocular surgery or trauma (includes injection of antifibrotic agents)
➥ *CPT Assistant* Jul 03:4, Nov 03:10, Dec 12:14, Jul 18:3, Dec 18:10, Apr 19:7

66174   Transluminal dilation of aqueous outflow canal (eg, canaloplasty); without retention of device or stent
➥ *CPT Changes: An Insider's View* 2011, 2023
➥ *CPT Assistant* Dec 18:9, Sep 19:11, May 22:14,17

(Do not report 66174 in conjunction with 65820)

66175   with retention of device or stent
➥ *CPT Changes: An Insider's View* 2011, 2023
➥ *CPT Assistant* May 22:14

Minimally Invasive Glaucoma Surgery (External Approach)
66150, 66155, 66160, 66170, 66172, 66183

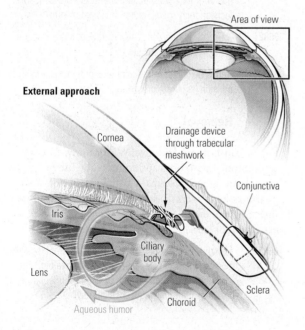

Area of view

External approach

Cornea

Drainage device through trabecular meshwork

Iris

Conjunctiva

Ciliary body

Lens

Sclera

Choroid

Aqueous humor

Aqueous Shunt

66179   Aqueous shunt to extraocular equatorial plate reservoir, external approach; without graft
➥ *CPT Changes: An Insider's View* 2015
➥ *CPT Assistant* Jan 15:10, Jul 18:3

66180   with graft
➥ *CPT Changes: An Insider's View* 2015
➥ *CPT Assistant* Winter 90:8, Aug 03:9, Sep 03:2, Jun 12:15, Jan 15:10, Jul 18:3

(Do not report 66180 in conjunction with 67255)

66183   Insertion of anterior segment aqueous drainage device, without extraocular reservoir, external approach
➥ *CPT Changes: An Insider's View* 2014
➥ *CPT Assistant* May 14:5, Jul 18:3

66184   Revision of aqueous shunt to extraocular equatorial plate reservoir; without graft
➥ *CPT Changes: An Insider's View* 2015
➥ *CPT Assistant* Jan 15:10

66185   with graft
➥ *CPT Changes: An Insider's View* 2015
➥ *CPT Assistant* Winter 90:8, Jan 15:10

(Do not report 66185 in conjunction with 67255)

(For removal of implanted shunt, use 67120)

Repair or Revision

(For scleral procedures in retinal surgery, see 67101 et seq)

66225   Repair of scleral staphyloma with graft

(For scleral reinforcement, see 67250, 67255)

66250   Revision or repair of operative wound of anterior segment, any type, early or late, major or minor procedure
➥ *CPT Assistant* Oct 10:15, Dec 10:15, Dec 18:9

(For unlisted procedures on anterior sclera, use 66999)

Iris, Ciliary Body

Incision

66500   Iridotomy by stab incision (separate procedure); except transfixion

66505   with transfixion as for iris bombe

(For iridotomy by photocoagulation, use 66761)

Excision

66600 Iridectomy, with corneoscleral or corneal section; for removal of lesion
➡ *CPT Assistant* Mar 21:7

66605 with cyclectomy

66625 peripheral for glaucoma (separate procedure)

66630 sector for glaucoma (separate procedure)

66635 optical (separate procedure)

(For coreoplasty by photocoagulation, use 66762)

Repair

66680 Repair of iris, ciliary body (as for iridodialysis)
➡ *CPT Assistant* Mar 21:7

(For reposition or resection of uveal tissue with perforating wound of cornea or sclera, use 65285)

66682 Suture of iris, ciliary body (separate procedure) with retrieval of suture through small incision (eg, McCannel suture)
➡ *CPT Assistant* Mar 21:7

● **66683** Implantation of iris prosthesis, including suture fixation and repair or removal of iris, when performed
➡ *CPT Changes: An Insider's View* 2025

▶(Use 66683 in conjunction with 66825, 66830, 66840, 66850, 66852, 66920, 66930, 66940, 66982, 66983, 66984, 66985, 66986, 66987, 66988, 66989, 66991, for lens or intraocular lens surgery[ies] performed concurrently)◀

▶(Do not report 66683 in conjunction with 65800, 65810, 65815, 65865, 65870, 65875, 66020, 66030, 66500, 66505, 66600, 66625, 66630, 66635, 66680, 66682, 66770, 67500, 67515, 69990, for the same eye, same surgeon, or same operative session)◀

▶(For severing adhesions of anterior segment, incisional technique, without concurrent iris prosthesis implantation, see 65865, 65870, 65875, 65880)◀

▶(For removal of iris tissue without concurrent iris prosthesis implantation, see 66600, 66605, 66625, 66630, 66635)◀

▶(For repair of iris without concurrent iris prosthesis implantation, see 66680, 66682)◀

Destruction

66700 Ciliary body destruction; diathermy

66710 cyclophotocoagulation, transscleral
➡ *CPT Changes: An Insider's View* 2005
➡ *CPT Assistant* Mar 05:20, Sep 05:5

66711 cyclophotocoagulation, endoscopic, without concomitant removal of crystalline lens
➡ *CPT Changes: An Insider's View* 2005, 2020
➡ *CPT Assistant* Mar 05:20, Sep 05:5, 12, Dec 19:6

(For endoscopic cyclophotocoagulation performed at same encounter as extracapsular cataract removal with intraocular lens insertion, see 66987, 66988)

(Do not report 66711 in conjunction with 66990)

66720 cryotherapy
➡ *CPT Changes: An Insider's View* 2017

66740 cyclodialysis

66761 Iridotomy/iridectomy by laser surgery (eg, for glaucoma) (per session)
➡ *CPT Changes: An Insider's View* 2011
➡ *CPT Assistant* Mar 98:7, Sep 21:10

66762 Iridoplasty by photocoagulation (1 or more sessions) (eg, for improvement of vision, for widening of anterior chamber angle)
➡ *CPT Assistant* Mar 98:7, Sep 21:10

66770 Destruction of cyst or lesion iris or ciliary body (nonexcisional procedure)

(For excision lesion iris, ciliary body, see 66600, 66605; for removal of epithelial downgrowth, use 65900)

(For unlisted procedures on iris, ciliary body, use 66999)

Lens

Incision

66820 Discission of secondary membranous cataract (opacified posterior lens capsule and/or anterior hyaloid); stab incision technique (Ziegler or Wheeler knife)

66821 laser surgery (eg, YAG laser) (1 or more stages)
➡ *CPT Assistant* Sep 21:10

66825 Repositioning of intraocular lens prosthesis, requiring an incision (separate procedure)

Removal

Lateral canthotomy, iridectomy, iridotomy, anterior capsulotomy, posterior capsulotomy, the use of viscoelastic agents, enzymatic zonulysis, use of other pharmacologic agents, and subconjunctival or sub-tenon injections are included as part of the code for the extraction of lens.

66830 Removal of secondary membranous cataract (opacified posterior lens capsule and/or anterior hyaloid) with corneo-scleral section, with or without iridectomy (iridocapsulotomy, iridocapsulectomy)

66840 Removal of lens material; aspiration technique, 1 or more stages
➡ *CPT Assistant* Fall 92:4, Jan 09:7, Apr 09:9, Sep 09:5, Apr 16:8, Jun 16:6, Sep 16:9

66850 phacofragmentation technique (mechanical or ultrasonic) (eg, phacoemulsification), with aspiration
➡ *CPT Assistant* Fall 92:6, Jan 09:7, Apr 09:9, Sep 09:5, Jun 16:6

66852 pars plana approach, with or without vitrectomy
➡ *CPT Assistant* Fall 92:8, Jan 09:7, Apr 09:9, Sep 09:5, Jun 16:6

66920 intracapsular
➡ *CPT Assistant* Fall 92:8, Sep 09:5

66930 intracapsular, for dislocated lens
➡ *CPT Assistant* Fall 92:8, Sep 09:5

66940 extracapsular (other than 66840, 66850, 66852)
➡ *CPT Assistant* Fall 92:4, Jan 09:7, Apr 09:9, Sep 09:5, Jun 16:6

(For removal of intralenticular foreign body without lens extraction, use 65235)

(For repair of operative wound, use 66250)

Intraocular Lens Procedures

66982 Extracapsular cataract removal with insertion of intraocular lens prosthesis (1-stage procedure), manual or mechanical technique (eg, irrigation and aspiration or phacoemulsification), complex, requiring devices or techniques not generally used in routine cataract surgery (eg, iris expansion device, suture support for intraocular lens, or primary posterior capsulorrhexis) or performed on patients in the amblyogenic developmental stage; without endoscopic cyclophotocoagulation
➡ *CPT Changes: An Insider's View* 2001, 2002, 2020
➡ *CPT Assistant* Feb 01:7, Nov 03:10, Sep 09:5, Mar 13:6, Mar 16:10, Dec 17:14, Dec 18:6, Dec 19:6, Mar 21:7, Jul 22:1

(For complex extracapsular cataract removal with concomitant endoscopic cyclophotocoagulation, use 66987)

(For complex extracapsular cataract removal with intraocular lens implant and concomitant intraocular aqueous drainage device by internal approach, use 66989)

(For insertion of ocular telescope prosthesis including removal of crystalline lens, use 0308T)

 # 66989 with insertion of intraocular (eg, trabecular meshwork, supraciliary, suprachoroidal) anterior segment aqueous drainage device, without extraocular reservoir, internal approach, one or more
➡ *CPT Changes: An Insider's View* 2022
➡ *CPT Assistant* Jun 22:2,5, Jul 22:1, Aug 22:1

(For complex extracapsular cataract removal with intraocular lens implant without concomitant aqueous drainage device, use 66982)

(For insertion of intraocular anterior segment drainage device into the trabecular meshwork without concomitant cataract removal with intraocular lens implant, use 0671T)

 # 66987 with endoscopic cyclophotocoagulation
➡ *CPT Changes: An Insider's View* 2020
➡ *CPT Assistant* Dec 19:6

(For complex extracapsular cataract removal without endoscopic cyclophotocoagulation, use 66982)

(For insertion of ocular telescope prosthesis including removal of crystalline lens, use 0308T)

66983 Intracapsular cataract extraction with insertion of intraocular lens prosthesis (1 stage procedure)
➡ *CPT Assistant* Fall 92:5, 8, Nov 03:10, Sep 09:5, Mar 13:6, Dec 19:6, Mar 21:7

(Do not report 66983 in conjunction with 0308T)

66984 Extracapsular cataract removal with insertion of intraocular lens prosthesis (1 stage procedure), manual or mechanical technique (eg, irrigation and aspiration or phacoemulsification); without endoscopic cyclophotocoagulation
➡ *CPT Changes: An Insider's View* 2020
➡ *CPT Assistant* Fall 92:5, 8, Feb 01:7, Nov 03:10, Mar 05:11, Sep 09:5, Mar 13:6, Dec 18:6, Dec 19:6, Dec 20:13, Mar 21:7, May 22:17, Jun 22:2,5

(For complex extracapsular cataract removal, use 66982)

(For extracapsular cataract removal with concomitant endoscopic cyclophotocoagulation, use 66988)

(For extracapsular cataract removal with concomitant intraocular aqueous drainage device by internal approach, use 66991)

(For insertion of ocular telescope prosthesis including removal of crystalline lens, use 0308T)

(For insertion of intraocular anterior segment drainage device into the trabecular meshwork without concomitant cataract removal with intraocular lens implant, use 0671T)

 # 66991 with insertion of intraocular (eg, trabecular meshwork, supraciliary, suprachoroidal) anterior segment aqueous drainage device, without extraocular reservoir, internal approach, one or more
➡ *CPT Changes: An Insider's View* 2022
➡ *CPT Assistant* May 22:17, Jun 22:2,5, Jul 22:1, Aug 22:1

(For extracapsular cataract removal with intraocular lens implant without concomitant aqueous drainage device, use 66984)

(For insertion of intraocular anterior segment drainage device into the trabecular meshwork without concomitant cataract removal with intraocular lens implant, use 0671T)

(For insertion of intraocular anterior segment drainage device into the trabecular meshwork without concomitant cataract removal with intraocular lens implant, use 0671T)

 # 66988 with endoscopic cyclophotocoagulation

➜ *CPT Changes: An Insider's View* 2020

➜ *CPT Assistant* Dec 19:6

(For extracapsular cataract removal without endoscopic cyclophotocoagulation, use 66984)

(For complex extracapsular cataract removal with endoscopic cyclophotocoagulation, use 66987)

(For insertion of ocular telescope prosthesis, including removal of crystalline lens, use 0308T)

66985 Insertion of intraocular lens prosthesis (secondary implant), not associated with concurrent cataract removal

➜ *CPT Assistant* Sep 05:12, Sep 09:5, Dec 11:16, Mar 13:6, Mar 21:7

(To code implant at time of concurrent cataract surgery, see 66982, 66983, 66984)

(To report supply of intraocular lens prosthesis, use 99070)

(For ultrasonic determination of intraocular lens power, use 76519)

(For removal of implanted material from anterior segment, use 65920)

(For secondary fixation (separate procedure), use 66682)

(For use of ophthalmic endoscope with 66985, use 66990)

66986 Exchange of intraocular lens

➜ *CPT Assistant* Sep 05:12, Mar 21:7

(For use of ophthalmic endoscope with 66986, use 66990)

66987 Code is out of numerical sequence. See 66940-66984

66988 Code is out of numerical sequence. See 66983-66986

66989 Code is out of numerical sequence. See 66940-66984

66991 Code is out of numerical sequence. See 66983-66986

Other Procedures

+ 66990 Use of ophthalmic endoscope (List separately in addition to code for primary procedure)

➜ *CPT Changes: An Insider's View* 2003

➜ *CPT Assistant* Sep 05:12, Oct 08:3

(66990 may be used only with codes 65820, 65875, 65920, 66985, 66986, 67036, 67039, 67040, 67041, 67042, 67043, 67113)

66999 Unlisted procedure, anterior segment of eye

➜ *CPT Assistant* Apr 16:8, Sep 21:10, Aug 22:1, Nov 22:18

Posterior Segment

Vitreous

67005 Removal of vitreous, anterior approach (open sky technique or limbal incision); partial removal

➜ *CPT Assistant* Fall 92:4

67010 subtotal removal with mechanical vitrectomy

➜ *CPT Assistant* Fall 92:4

(For removal of vitreous by paracentesis of anterior chamber, use 65810)

(For removal of corneovitreal adhesions, use 65880)

67015 Aspiration or release of vitreous, subretinal or choroidal fluid, pars plana approach (posterior sclerotomy)

➜ *CPT Assistant* Feb 24:35

67025 Injection of vitreous substitute, pars plana or limbal approach (fluid-gas exchange), with or without aspiration (separate procedure)

➜ *CPT Assistant* Feb 18:3, Aug 19:11

67027 Implantation of intravitreal drug delivery system (eg, ganciclovir implant), includes concomitant removal of vitreous

➜ *CPT Assistant* Nov 97:23, Nov 98:1, Feb 18:3

(For removal, use 67121)

Intravitreal Drug Delivery System
67027

A drug delivery system that releases medication into the vitreous is implanted into the vitreous by pars plana incision.

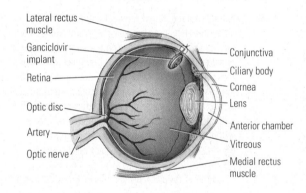

Lateral rectus muscle
Ganciclovir implant
Retina
Optic disc
Artery
Optic nerve
Conjunctiva
Ciliary body
Cornea
Lens
Anterior chamber
Vitreous
Medial rectus muscle

67028 Intravitreal injection of a pharmacologic agent (separate procedure)

➜ *CPT Assistant* Winter 90:9, Oct 12:15, Feb 18:3

67030 Discission of vitreous strands (without removal), pars plana approach

67031 Severing of vitreous strands, vitreous face adhesions, sheets, membranes or opacities, laser surgery (1 or more stages)

67036 Vitrectomy, mechanical, pars plana approach;

➜ *CPT Assistant* Fall 92:6, Oct 08:3

67039   with focal endolaser photocoagulation
      → *CPT Assistant* Winter 90:9, Sep 05:12

67040   with endolaser panretinal photocoagulation
      → *CPT Assistant* Winter 90:9, Sep 05:12, Jul 07:12

67041   with removal of preretinal cellular membrane (eg, macular pucker)
      → *CPT Changes: An Insider's View* 2008

67042   with removal of internal limiting membrane of retina (eg, for repair of macular hole, diabetic macular edema), includes, if performed, intraocular tamponade (ie, air, gas or silicone oil)
      → *CPT Changes: An Insider's View* 2008

67043   with removal of subretinal membrane (eg, choroidal neovascularization), includes, if performed, intraocular tamponade (ie, air, gas or silicone oil) and laser photocoagulation
      → *CPT Changes: An Insider's View* 2008

(For use of ophthalmic endoscope with 67036, 67039, 67040-67043, use 66990)

(For associated lensectomy, use 66850)

(For use of vitrectomy in retinal detachment surgery, see 67108, 67113)

(For associated removal of foreign body, see 65260, 65265)

(For unlisted procedures on vitreous, use 67299)

Retina or Choroid

Repair

(If diathermy, cryotherapy and/or photocoagulation are combined, report under principal modality used)

67101   Repair of retinal detachment, including drainage of subretinal fluid when performed; cryotherapy
      → *CPT Changes: An Insider's View* 2016, 2017
      → *CPT Assistant* Mar 98:7, Jun 16:6, Sep 16:5, Feb 17:14

67105   photocoagulation
      → *CPT Changes: An Insider's View* 2016, 2017
      → *CPT Assistant* Mar 98:7, Jun 16:6, Sep 16:5, Feb 17:14

67107   Repair of retinal detachment; scleral buckling (such as lamellar scleral dissection, imbrication or encircling procedure), including, when performed, implant, cryotherapy, photocoagulation, and drainage of subretinal fluid
      → *CPT Changes: An Insider's View* 2016
      → *CPT Assistant* Jun 16:6, Sep 16:5, Aug 19:11

67108   with vitrectomy, any method, including, when performed, air or gas tamponade, focal endolaser photocoagulation, cryotherapy, drainage of subretinal fluid, scleral buckling, and/or removal of lens by same technique
      → *CPT Changes: An Insider's View* 2016
      → *CPT Assistant* Winter 90:9, Mar 12:9, Jun 16:6, Sep 16:5

Repair of Retinal Detachment
67107

The retinal tear is treated externally by placing a hot or cold probe over the sclera and then depressing it. The burn seals the choroid to the retina at the site of the tear. The healing scar is supported by the encircling band, which buckles the eye.

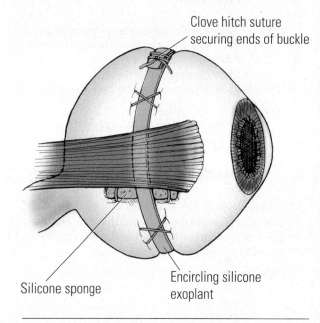

Clove hitch suture securing ends of buckle

Silicone sponge

Encircling silicone exoplant

67110   by injection of air or other gas (eg, pneumatic retinopexy)
      → *CPT Assistant* Winter 90:9, Sep 16:5

(For aspiration or drainage of subretinal or subchoroidal fluid, use 67015)

67113   Repair of complex retinal detachment (eg, proliferative vitreoretinopathy, stage C-1 or greater, diabetic traction retinal detachment, retinopathy of prematurity, retinal tear of greater than 90 degrees), with vitrectomy and membrane peeling, including, when performed, air, gas, or silicone oil tamponade, cryotherapy, endolaser photocoagulation, drainage of subretinal fluid, scleral buckling, and/or removal of lens
      → *CPT Changes: An Insider's View* 2008, 2016
      → *CPT Assistant* Jun 16:6, Sep 16:5

(To report vitrectomy, pars plana approach, other than in retinal detachment surgery, see 67036-67043)

(For use of ophthalmic endoscope with 67113, use 66990)

67115   Release of encircling material (posterior segment)

67120   Removal of implanted material, posterior segment; extraocular

Eye / Ocular Adnexa   65091-68899

67121   intraocular
→ *CPT Assistant* Nov 97:23, Nov 98:19

(For removal from anterior segment, use 65920)

(For removal of foreign body, see 65260, 65265)

Prophylaxis

67141   Prophylaxis of retinal detachment (eg, retinal break, lattice degeneration) without drainage; cryotherapy, diathermy
→ *CPT Changes: An Insider's View* 2022
→ *CPT Assistant* Mar 98:7, Oct 08:3, Sep 16:5, Nov 21:9

67145   photocoagulation
→ *CPT Changes: An Insider's View* 2022
→ *CPT Assistant* Fall 92:4, Mar 98:7, Sep 16:5, Nov 21:9

Destruction

Codes 67208, 67210, 67218, 67220, 67229 include treatment at one or more sessions that may occur at different encounters. These codes should be reported once during a defined treatment period.

67208   Destruction of localized lesion of retina (eg, macular edema, tumors), 1 or more sessions; cryotherapy, diathermy
→ *CPT Assistant* Mar 98:7, Nov 98:19, Oct 08:3

67210   photocoagulation
→ *CPT Assistant* Mar 98:7, Nov 98:19, Oct 08:3, Jan 12:3

67218   radiation by implantation of source (includes removal of source)
→ *CPT Assistant* Mar 98:7, Oct 08:3

67220   Destruction of localized lesion of choroid (eg, choroidal neovascularization); photocoagulation (eg, laser), 1 or more sessions
→ *CPT Changes: An Insider's View* 2000, 2001
→ *CPT Assistant* Nov 98:19, Nov 99:39, Feb 01:8, Oct 08:3, Jan 12:3

67221   photodynamic therapy (includes intravenous infusion)
→ *CPT Changes: An Insider's View* 2001
→ *CPT Assistant* Feb 01:8, Sep 01:10, Jun 02:10, Feb 18:10

+ 67225   photodynamic therapy, second eye, at single session (List separately in addition to code for primary eye treatment)
→ *CPT Changes: An Insider's View* 2002
→ *CPT Assistant* Jun 02:10

(Use 67225 in conjunction with 67221)

67227   Destruction of extensive or progressive retinopathy (eg, diabetic retinopathy), cryotherapy, diathermy
→ *CPT Changes: An Insider's View* 2008, 2016
→ *CPT Assistant* Mar 98:7, Oct 08:3

67228   Treatment of extensive or progressive retinopathy (eg, diabetic retinopathy), photocoagulation
→ *CPT Changes: An Insider's View* 2008, 2016
→ *CPT Assistant* Mar 98:7, Oct 08:3

67229   Treatment of extensive or progressive retinopathy, 1 or more sessions, preterm infant (less than 37 weeks gestation at birth), performed from birth up to 1 year of age (eg, retinopathy of prematurity), photocoagulation or cryotherapy
→ *CPT Changes: An Insider's View* 2008

(For bilateral procedure, use modifier 50 with 67208, 67210, 67218, 67220, 67227, 67228, 67229)

(For unlisted procedures on retina, use 67299)

▶(For photobiomodulation therapy of retina, single session, use 0936T)◀

Posterior Sclera

Repair

(For excision lesion sclera, use 66130)

67250   Scleral reinforcement (separate procedure); without graft

67255   with graft
→ *CPT Assistant* Jun 12:15, Jan 15:10

(Do not report 67255 in conjunction with 66180, 66185)

(For repair scleral staphyloma, use 66225)

Other Procedures

67299   Unlisted procedure, posterior segment

Ocular Adnexa

Extraocular Muscles

67311   Strabismus surgery, recession or resection procedure; 1 horizontal muscle
→ *CPT Assistant* Summer 93:20, Mar 97:5, Nov 98:19, Sep 02:10, Jan 17:7

67312   2 horizontal muscles
→ *CPT Assistant* Summer 93:20, Mar 97:5

67314   1 vertical muscle (excluding superior oblique)
→ *CPT Assistant* Summer 93:20, Mar 97:5

67316   2 or more vertical muscles (excluding superior oblique)
→ *CPT Assistant* Summer 93:20, Mar 97:5

(For adjustable sutures, use 67335 in addition to codes 67311-67334 for primary procedure reflecting number of muscles operated on)

Extraocular Muscles of Right Eye

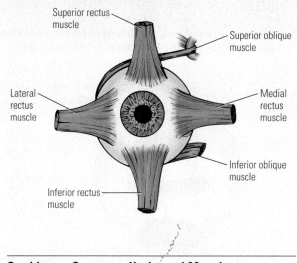

Superior rectus muscle
Superior oblique muscle
Lateral rectus muscle
Medial rectus muscle
Inferior oblique muscle
Inferior rectus muscle

Strabismus Surgery—Horizontal Muscles
67311-67312

In Figure A, the medial or lateral rectus muscle is made weaker by recession (retroplacement of the muscle attachment). In Figure B, it is made stronger by resection (removal of a segment). Use 67311 for one horizontal muscle and 67312 for two muscles of the same eye.

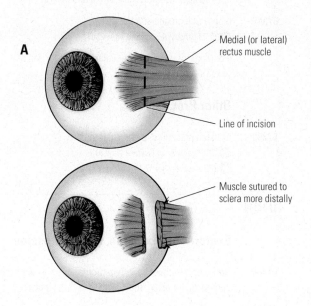

A
Medial (or lateral) rectus muscle
Line of incision
Muscle sutured to sclera more distally

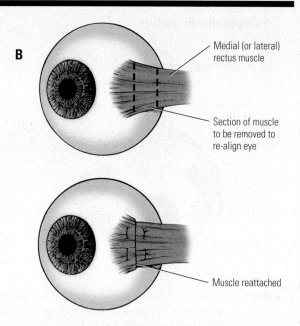

B
Medial (or lateral) rectus muscle
Section of muscle to be removed to re-align eye
Muscle reattached

Strabismus Surgery—Vertical Muscles
67314-67316

Either the superior or inferior rectus muscle is strengthened or weakened. Use 67316 for two muscles of the same eye.

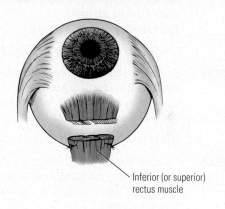

Inferior (or superior) rectus muscle

67318   Strabismus surgery, any procedure, superior oblique muscle
> *CPT Assistant* Summer 93:20, Mar 97:5, Nov 98:19

+ 67320   Transposition procedure (eg, for paretic extraocular muscle), any extraocular muscle (specify) (List separately in addition to code for primary procedure)
> *CPT Assistant* Summer 93:20, Mar 97:5

(Use 67320 in conjunction with 67311-67318)

Eye / Ocular Adnexa **65091-68899**

Transposition Procedure
67320

The extraocular muscles are transposed.

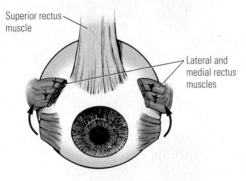

Superior rectus muscle

Lateral and medial rectus muscles

+ 67331   Strabismus surgery on patient with previous eye surgery or injury that did not involve the extraocular muscles (List separately in addition to code for primary procedure)
➔ *CPT Assistant* Summer 93:20, Mar 97:5

(Use 67331 in conjunction with 67311-67318)

+ 67332   Strabismus surgery on patient with scarring of extraocular muscles (eg, prior ocular injury, strabismus or retinal detachment surgery) or restrictive myopathy (eg, dysthyroid ophthalmopathy) (List separately in addition to code for primary procedure)
➔ *CPT Assistant* Summer 93:20, Mar 97:5

(Use 67332 in conjunction with 67311-67318)

+ 67334   Strabismus surgery by posterior fixation suture technique, with or without muscle recession (List separately in addition to code for primary procedure)
➔ *CPT Assistant* Summer 93:20, Mar 97:5

(Use 67334 in conjunction with 67311-67318)

+ 67335   Placement of adjustable suture(s) during strabismus surgery, including postoperative adjustment(s) of suture(s) (List separately in addition to code for specific strabismus surgery)
➔ *CPT Assistant* Summer 93:20, Mar 97:5

(Use 67335 in conjunction with 67311-67334)

+ 67340   Strabismus surgery involving exploration and/or repair of detached extraocular muscle(s) (List separately in addition to code for primary procedure)
➔ *CPT Assistant* Summer 93:20, Mar 97:5

(Use 67340 in conjunction with 67311-67334)

67343   Release of extensive scar tissue without detaching extraocular muscle (separate procedure)
➔ *CPT Assistant* Summer 93:20, Mar 97:5

(Use 67343 in conjunction with 67311-67340, when such procedures are performed other than on the affected muscle)

Strabismus Surgery—Adjustable Sutures
67335

Sutures are tied in such a way as to allow the tension on the muscle to be adjusted after the anesthetic is not affecting the position of the globe.

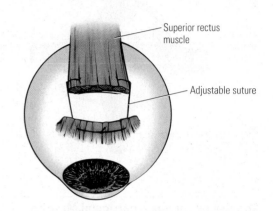

Superior rectus muscle

Adjustable suture

67345   Chemodenervation of extraocular muscle
➔ *CPT Assistant* Summer 93:20, Mar 97:5, Apr 00:2, Feb 10:13, Dec 13:10, May 14:5

(For chemodenervation for blepharospasm and other neurological disorders, see 64612 and 64616)

67346   Biopsy of extraocular muscle
➔ *CPT Changes: An Insider's View* 2007

(For repair of wound, extraocular muscle, tendon or Tenon's capsule, use 65290)

Other Procedures

67399   Unlisted procedure, extraocular muscle
➔ *CPT Changes: An Insider's View* 2015
➔ *CPT Assistant* Jul 17:10

Orbit

Exploration, Excision, Decompression

67400   Orbitotomy without bone flap (frontal or transconjunctival approach); for exploration, with or without biopsy
67405   with drainage only
67412   with removal of lesion
67413   with removal of foreign body
67414   with removal of bone for decompression
➔ *CPT Assistant* Jul 99:10

Eye / Ocular Adnexa 65091-68899

67415   Fine needle aspiration of orbital contents

(For exenteration, enucleation, and repair, see 65101 et seq; for optic nerve decompression, use 67570)

67420   Orbitotomy with bone flap or window, lateral approach (eg, Kroenlein); with removal of lesion

67430   with removal of foreign body

67440   with drainage

67445   with removal of bone for decompression
         ➔ *CPT Assistant* Dec 19:14

(For optic nerve sheath decompression, use 67570)

67450   for exploration, with or without biopsy

(For orbitotomy, transcranial approach, see 61330, 61333)

(For orbital implant, see 67550, 67560)

(For removal of eyeball or for repair after removal, see 65091-65175)

Other Procedures

67500   Retrobulbar injection; medication (separate procedure, does not include supply of medication)
         ➔ *CPT Assistant* Nov 12:10

67505   alcohol

67515   Injection of medication or other substance into Tenon's capsule
         ➔ *CPT Changes: An Insider's View* 2002
         ➔ *CPT Assistant* Nov 12:10

(For subconjunctival injection, use 68200)

67516   Suprachoroidal space injection of pharmacologic agent (separate procedure)
         ➔ *CPT Changes: An Insider's View* 2024
         ➔ *CPT Assistant* Nov 23:8

(Report medication separately)

67550   Orbital implant (implant outside muscle cone); insertion

67560   removal or revision

(For ocular implant (implant inside muscle cone), see 65093-65105, 65130-65175)

(For treatment of fractures of malar area, orbit, see 21355 et seq)

67570   Optic nerve decompression (eg, incision or fenestration of optic nerve sheath)

67599   Unlisted procedure, orbit

Eyelids

Incision

67700   Blepharotomy, drainage of abscess, eyelid
         ➔ *CPT Assistant* Mar 13:6

67710   Severing of tarsorrhaphy
         ➔ *CPT Assistant* Mar 13:6

67715   Canthotomy (separate procedure)
         ➔ *CPT Assistant* Mar 13:6

(For canthoplasty, use 67950)

(For division of symblepharon, use 68340)

 # 67810   Incisional biopsy of eyelid skin including lid margin
         ➔ *CPT Changes: An Insider's View* 2013
         ➔ *CPT Assistant* Dec 04:19, Feb 13:16, Mar 13:6

(For biopsy of skin of the eyelid, see 11102, 11103, 11104, 11105, 11106, 11107)

Excision, Destruction

Codes for removal of lesion include more than skin (ie, involving lid margin, tarsus, and/or palpebral conjunctiva).

(For removal of lesion, involving mainly skin of eyelid, see 11310-11313; 11440-11446, 11640-11646; 17000-17004)

(For repair of wounds, blepharoplasty, grafts, reconstructive surgery, see 67930-67975)

67800   Excision of chalazion; single
         ➔ *CPT Assistant* Sep 99:10

67801   multiple, same lid

67805   multiple, different lids
         ➔ *CPT Assistant* Sep 99:10

67808   under general anesthesia and/or requiring hospitalization, single or multiple

67810   Code is out of numerical sequence. See 67710-67801

67820   Correction of trichiasis; epilation, by forceps only
         ➔ *CPT Assistant* Jul 98:10

67825   epilation by other than forceps (eg, by electrosurgery, cryotherapy, laser surgery)
         ➔ *CPT Assistant* Jul 98:10

67830   incision of lid margin

67835   incision of lid margin, with free mucous membrane graft

Trichiasis
67820-67825

When the eyelashes are ingrown or misdirected (trichiasis), the physician uses a biomicroscope and forceps to remove the offending eyelashes. Report 67825 when cryosurgery or electrosurgery is used to destroy the follicles.

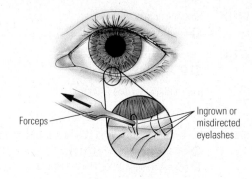

Forceps

Ingrown or misdirected eyelashes

67840 Excision of lesion of eyelid (except chalazion) without closure or with simple direct closure

(For excision and repair of eyelid by reconstructive surgery, see 67961, 67966)

67850 Destruction of lesion of lid margin (up to 1 cm)

(For Mohs micrographic surgery, see 17311-17315)

(For initiation or follow-up care of topical chemotherapy (eg, 5-FU or similar agents), see appropriate office visits)

Tarsorrhaphy

67875 Temporary closure of eyelids by suture (eg, Frost suture)
➔ *CPT Assistant* Winter 90:9

67880 Construction of intermarginal adhesions, median tarsorrhaphy, or canthorrhaphy;

67882 with transposition of tarsal plate

(For severing of tarsorrhaphy, use 67710)

(For canthoplasty, reconstruction canthus, use 67950)

(For canthotomy, use 67715)

Repair (Brow Ptosis, Blepharoptosis, Lid Retraction, Ectropion, Entropion)

67900 Repair of brow ptosis (supraciliary, mid-forehead or coronal approach)

(For forehead rhytidectomy, use 15824)

67901 Repair of blepharoptosis; frontalis muscle technique with suture or other material (eg, banked fascia)
➔ *CPT Changes: An Insider's View* 2006
➔ *CPT Assistant* Sep 00:7, Oct 06:11, Jul 17:10

67902 frontalis muscle technique with autologous fascial sling (includes obtaining fascia)
➔ *CPT Changes: An Insider's View* 2006
➔ *CPT Assistant* Sep 00:7, Oct 06:11

67903 (tarso) levator resection or advancement, internal approach
➔ *CPT Assistant* Sep 00:7, Oct 06:11

67904 (tarso) levator resection or advancement, external approach
➔ *CPT Assistant* Sep 00:7, Oct 06:11, Aug 11:8

67906 superior rectus technique with fascial sling (includes obtaining fascia)
➔ *CPT Assistant* Sep 00:7, Oct 06:11

67908 conjunctivo-tarso-Muller's muscle-levator resection (eg, Fasanella-Servat type)
➔ *CPT Assistant* Sep 00:7, Oct 06:11, Mar 21:11

67909 Reduction of overcorrection of ptosis

67911 Correction of lid retraction
➔ *CPT Assistant* Nov 21:13

(For obtaining autologous graft materials, see 15769, 20920, 20922)

(For correction of lid defects using fat harvested via liposuction technique, see 15773, 15774)

(For correction of trichiasis by mucous membrane graft, use 67835)

67912 Correction of lagophthalmos, with implantation of upper eyelid lid load (eg, gold weight)
➔ *CPT Changes: An Insider's View* 2004
➔ *CPT Assistant* May 04:12, Aug 04:10, Oct 06:11

67914 Repair of ectropion; suture

67915 thermocauterization

67916 excision tarsal wedge
➔ *CPT Changes: An Insider's View* 2004
➔ *CPT Assistant* Feb 04:11, May 04:12, Feb 05:16, Oct 06:11

67917 extensive (eg, tarsal strip operations)
➔ *CPT Changes: An Insider's View* 2004
➔ *CPT Assistant* Feb 04:11, May 04:12, Oct 06:11, Feb 20:13, Mar 20:14

(For correction of everted punctum, use 68705)

67921 Repair of entropion; suture

67922 thermocauterization

67923 excision tarsal wedge
➔ *CPT Changes: An Insider's View* 2004
➔ *CPT Assistant* May 04:12, Oct 06:11

67924 extensive (eg, tarsal strip or capsulopalpebral fascia repairs operation)
➔ *CPT Changes: An Insider's View* 2004
➔ *CPT Assistant* May 04:12, Oct 06:11

Eye / Ocular Adnexa 65091-68899

★=Telemedicine ◀=Audio-only +=Add-on code ✗=FDA approval pending #=Resequenced code ⊘=Modifier 51 exempt ➔➔➔=See p xxi for details

(For repair of cicatricial ectropion or entropion requiring scar excision or skin graft, see also 67961 et seq)

Reconstruction

Codes for blepharoplasty involve more than skin (ie, involving lid margin, tarsus, and/or palpebral conjunctiva).

67930 Suture of recent wound, eyelid, involving lid margin, tarsus, and/or palpebral conjunctiva direct closure; partial thickness

67935 full thickness

67938 Removal of embedded foreign body, eyelid
➲ *CPT Assistant* May 14:5

(For repair of skin of eyelid, see 12011-12018, 12051-12057, 13151-13153)

(For tarsorrhaphy, canthorrhaphy, see 67880, 67882)

(For repair of blepharoptosis and lid retraction, see 67901-67911)

(For blepharoplasty for entropion, ectropion, see 67916, 67917, 67923, 67924)

(For correction of blepharochalasis (blepharorhytidectomy), see 15820-15823)

(For repair of skin of eyelid, adjacent tissue transfer, see 14060, 14061; preparation for graft, use 15004; free graft, see 15120, 15121, 15260, 15261)

(For excision of lesion of eyelid, use 67800 et seq)

(For repair of lacrimal canaliculi, use 68700)

67950 Canthoplasty (reconstruction of canthus)

67961 Excision and repair of eyelid, involving lid margin, tarsus, conjunctiva, canthus, or full thickness, may include preparation for skin graft or pedicle flap with adjacent tissue transfer or rearrangement; up to one-fourth of lid margin

67966 over one-fourth of lid margin
➲ *CPT Assistant* Nov 12:13

(For canthoplasty, use 67950)

(For free skin grafts, see 15120, 15121, 15260, 15261)

(For tubed pedicle flap preparation, use 15576; for delay, use 15630; for attachment, use 15650)

67971 Reconstruction of eyelid, full thickness by transfer of tarsoconjunctival flap from opposing eyelid; up to two-thirds of eyelid, 1 stage or first stage

67973 total eyelid, lower, 1 stage or first stage

67974 total eyelid, upper, 1 stage or first stage

67975 second stage

Other Procedures

67999 Unlisted procedure, eyelids
➲ *CPT Assistant* Jul 17:10

Conjunctiva

(For removal of foreign body, see 65205 et seq)

Incision and Drainage

68020 Incision of conjunctiva, drainage of cyst

68040 Expression of conjunctival follicles (eg, for trachoma)
➲ *CPT Assistant* May 14:5

(To report automated evacuation of meibomian glands, use 0207T)

(For manual evacuation of meibomian glands, use 0563T)

Excision and/or Destruction

68100 Biopsy of conjunctiva

68110 Excision of lesion, conjunctiva; up to 1 cm
➲ *CPT Assistant* Jan 17:7, Feb 18:11

68115 over 1 cm
➲ *CPT Assistant* Feb 18:11

68130 with adjacent sclera

68135 Destruction of lesion, conjunctiva

Injection

(For injection into Tenon's capsule or retrobulbar injection, see 67500-67515)

68200 Subconjunctival injection
➲ *CPT Assistant* Aug 03:15, Nov 12:10

Conjunctivoplasty

(For wound repair, see 65270-65273)

68320 Conjunctivoplasty; with conjunctival graft or extensive rearrangement
➲ *CPT Assistant* Feb 04:11

68325 with buccal mucous membrane graft (includes obtaining graft)

68326 Conjunctivoplasty, reconstruction cul-de-sac; with conjunctival graft or extensive rearrangement

68328 with buccal mucous membrane graft (includes obtaining graft)

Eye / Ocular Adnexa   **65091-68899**

68330   Repair of symblepharon; conjunctivoplasty, without graft

68335   with free graft conjunctiva or buccal mucous membrane (includes obtaining graft)

68340   division of symblepharon, with or without insertion of conformer or contact lens

Other Procedures

68360   Conjunctival flap; bridge or partial (separate procedure)

68362   total (such as Gunderson thin flap or purse string flap)

(For conjunctival flap for perforating injury, see 65280, 65285)

(For repair of operative wound, use 66250)

(For removal of conjunctival foreign body, see 65205, 65210)

68371   Harvesting conjunctival allograft, living donor
➔ *CPT Changes: An Insider's View* 2004
➔ *CPT Assistant* May 04:10

68399   Unlisted procedure, conjunctiva

Lacrimal System

Incision

68400   Incision, drainage of lacrimal gland

68420   Incision, drainage of lacrimal sac (dacryocystotomy or dacryocystostomy)

68440   Snip incision of lacrimal punctum

Excision

68500   Excision of lacrimal gland (dacryoadenectomy), except for tumor; total

68505   partial

68510   Biopsy of lacrimal gland

68520   Excision of lacrimal sac (dacryocystectomy)

68525   Biopsy of lacrimal sac

68530   Removal of foreign body or dacryolith, lacrimal passages

68540   Excision of lacrimal gland tumor; frontal approach

68550   involving osteotomy

Repair

68700   Plastic repair of canaliculi

68705   Correction of everted punctum, cautery
➔ *CPT Assistant* Feb 20:13

68720   Dacryocystorhinostomy (fistulization of lacrimal sac to nasal cavity)
➔ *CPT Assistant* Sep 01:10, Jul 03:15, Aug 03:14, Aug 09:11

68745   Conjunctivorhinostomy (fistulization of conjunctiva to nasal cavity); without tube

68750   with insertion of tube or stent

68760   Closure of the lacrimal punctum; by thermocauterization, ligation, or laser surgery

68761   by plug, each
➔ *CPT Assistant* Jun 96:10, Jan 07:28

(For insertion and removal of drug-eluting implant into lacrimal canaliculus for intraocular pressure, use 68841)

(For placement of drug-eluting insert under the eyelid[s], see 0444T, 0445T)

68770   Closure of lacrimal fistula (separate procedure)

Closure of Lacrimal Punctum by Plug
68761

The physician inserts a lacrimal duct implant into a lacrimal punctum.

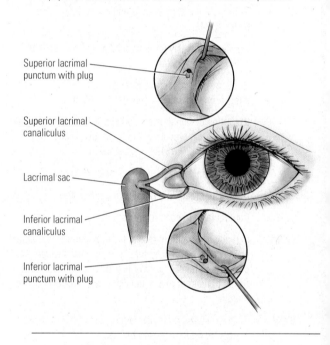

Superior lacrimal punctum with plug

Superior lacrimal canaliculus

Lacrimal sac

Inferior lacrimal canaliculus

Inferior lacrimal punctum with plug

Probing and/or Related Procedures

68801   Dilation of lacrimal punctum, with or without irrigation

(To report a bilateral procedure, use 68801 with modifier 50)

68810   Probing of nasolacrimal duct, with or without irrigation;
➔ *CPT Assistant* Nov 02:11, Oct 08:3

(For bilateral procedure, report 68810 with modifier 50)

68811   requiring general anesthesia
　　　→ *CPT Assistant* Nov 02:11, Oct 08:3

　　(For bilateral procedure, report 68811 with modifier 50)

68815   with insertion of tube or stent
　　　→ *CPT Assistant* Nov 02:11, Oct 08:3, Aug 09:11, Nov 10:9

　　(See also 92018)

　　(For bilateral procedure, report 68815 with modifier 50)

　　(For insertion and removal of drug-eluting implant into lacrimal canaliculus for intraocular pressure, use 68841)

　　(For placement of drug-eluting insert under the eyelid[s], see 0444T, 0445T)

68816   with transluminal balloon catheter dilation
　　　→ *CPT Changes: An Insider's View* 2008

　　(Do not report 68816 in conjunction with 68810, 68811, 68815)

　　(For bilateral procedure, report 68816 with modifier 50)

Probing of Nasolacrimal Duct
68816

A balloon catheter is in the nasolacrimal duct.

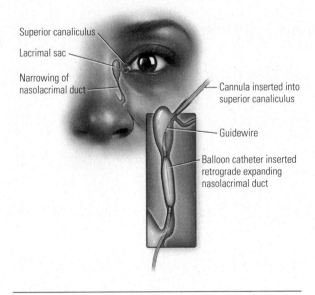

68840   Probing of lacrimal canaliculi, with or without irrigation

68841   Insertion of drug-eluting implant, including punctal dilation when performed, into lacrimal canaliculus, each
　　　→ *CPT Changes: An Insider's View* 2022

　　(For placement of drug-eluting ocular insert under the eyelid[s], see 0444T, 0445T)

　　(Report drug-eluting implant separately with 99070 or appropriate supply code)

68850   Injection of contrast medium for dacryocystography
　　　→ *CPT Assistant* Feb 01:9

　　(For radiological supervision and interpretation, see 70170, 78660)

Other Procedures

68899   Unlisted procedure, lacrimal system

Notes

Surgery

The following is a listing of headings and subheadings that appear within the Auditory System and Operating Microscope sections of the CPT codebook. The subheadings or subsections denoted with asterisks (*) below have special instructions unique to that subsection. Where these are indicated, special notes or guidelines will be presented preceding those procedural terminology listings, referring to that subsection specifically. Note that all code ranges in each subsection are listed as they appear in the subsection, even if the code numbers are out of numerical sequence and/or repeated in the next subsection.

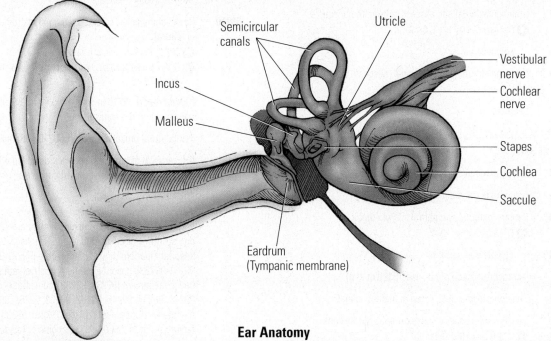

Semicircular canals — Utricle — Vestibular nerve — Cochlear nerve — Incus — Malleus — Stapes — Cochlea — Saccule — Eardrum (Tympanic membrane)

Ear Anatomy

Auditory System

(For diagnostic services (eg, audiometry, vestibular tests), see 92502 et seq)

External Ear

Incision

69000   Drainage external ear, abscess or hematoma; simple
➜ *CPT Assistant* Oct 97:11, Oct 99:10

69005   complicated

69020   Drainage external auditory canal, abscess
➜ *CPT Assistant* Oct 97:11

69090   Ear piercing

Excision

69100   Biopsy external ear

69105   Biopsy external auditory canal

69110   Excision external ear; partial, simple repair
➜ *CPT Assistant* Dec 23:42

69120   complete amputation

(For reconstruction of ear, see 15120 et seq)

69140   Excision exostosis(es), external auditory canal

69145   Excision soft tissue lesion, external auditory canal
➜ *CPT Assistant* Dec 19:14

69150   Radical excision external auditory canal lesion; without neck dissection

69155   with neck dissection

(For resection of temporal bone, use 69535)

(For skin grafting, see 15004-15261)

Removal

69200   Removal foreign body from external auditory canal; without general anesthesia

69205   with general anesthesia
➜ *CPT Assistant* Apr 13:10

69209   Removal impacted cerumen using irrigation/lavage, unilateral
➜ *CPT Changes: An Insider's View* 2016
➜ *CPT Assistant* Jan 16:7, Feb 16:14, Mar 16:11

(Do not report 69209 in conjunction with 69210 when performed on the same ear)

(For bilateral procedure, report 69209 with modifier 50)

(For removal of impacted cerumen requiring instrumentation, use 69210)

(For cerumen removal that is not impacted, see E/M service code, which may include new or established patient office or other outpatient services [99202-99215], hospital inpatient or observation care [99221-99223, 99231-99233], hospital inpatient or observation discharge day management [99238, 99239], consultations [99242, 99243, 99244, 99245, 99252, 99253, 99254, 99255], emergency department services [99281-99285], nursing facility services [99304-99316], home or residence services [99341-99350])

69210   Removal impacted cerumen requiring instrumentation, unilateral
➜ *CPT Changes: An Insider's View* 2014
➜ *CPT Assistant* Apr 03:9, Jul 05:14, Oct 13:14, Nov 14:14, Jan 16:7, Feb 16:14, Mar 16:11

(Do not report 69210 in conjunction with 69209 when performed on the same ear)

(For bilateral procedure, report 69210 with modifier 50)

(For removal of impacted cerumen achieved with irrigation and/or lavage but without instrumentation, use 69209)

(For cerumen removal that is not impacted, see E/M service code, which may include new or established patient office or other outpatient services [99202-99215], hospital inpatient or observation care [99221-99223, 99231-99233], hospital inpatient or observation discharge day management [99238, 99239], consultations [99242, 99243, 99244, 99245, 99252, 99253, 99254, 99255], emergency department services [99281-99285], nursing facility services [99304-99316], home or residence services [99341-99350])

69220   Debridement, mastoidectomy cavity, simple (eg, routine cleaning)

(For bilateral procedure, report 69220 with modifier 50)

69222   Debridement, mastoidectomy cavity, complex (eg, with anesthesia or more than routine cleaning)

(For bilateral procedure, report 69222 with modifier 50)

Repair

(For suture of wound or injury of external ear, see 12011-14302)

69300   Otoplasty, protruding ear, with or without size reduction
➜ *CPT Changes: An Insider's View* 2017

(For bilateral procedure, report 69300 with modifier 50)

★ = Telemedicine   ◀ = Audio-only   ✛ = Add-on code   ✗ = FDA approval pending   # = Resequenced code   ⊘ = Modifier 51 exempt   ➜➜➜ = See p xxi for details

69310 Reconstruction of external auditory canal (meatoplasty) (eg, for stenosis due to injury, infection) (separate procedure)

➔ *CPT Changes: An Insider's View* 2002

➔ *CPT Assistant* Jan 14:9, Jul 14:9

69320 Reconstruction external auditory canal for congenital atresia, single stage

(For combination with middle ear reconstruction, see 69631, 69641)

(For other reconstructive procedures with grafts (eg, skin, cartilage, bone), see 13151-15760, 21230-21235)

Other Procedures

(For otoscopy under general anesthesia, use 92502)

69399 Unlisted procedure, external ear

Middle Ear

Incision

69420 Myringotomy including aspiration and/or eustachian tube inflation

➔ *CPT Assistant* May 11:8, Apr 21:12

69421 Myringotomy including aspiration and/or eustachian tube inflation requiring general anesthesia

➔ *CPT Assistant* May 11:8, Apr 21:12

69424 Ventilating tube removal requiring general anesthesia

➔ *CPT Changes: An Insider's View* 2003

➔ *CPT Assistant* Mar 05:17, Jun 10:11, Nov 10:9

(For bilateral procedure, report 69424 with modifier 50)

(Do not report code 69424 in conjunction with 69205, 69210, 69420, 69421, 69433-69676, 69710-69745, 69801-69930)

69433 Tympanostomy (requiring insertion of ventilating tube), local or topical anesthesia

➔ *CPT Assistant* May 11:8, Feb 18:11, Apr 21:14

(For bilateral procedure, report 69433 with modifier 50)

(For tympanostomy requiring insertion of ventilating tube, with iontophoresis, using an automated tube delivery system, use 0583T)

69436 Tympanostomy (requiring insertion of ventilating tube), general anesthesia

➔ *CPT Assistant* May 11:8, May 12:14, Feb 18:11, Apr 21:14

(For bilateral procedure, report 69436 with modifier 50)

69440 Middle ear exploration through postauricular or ear canal incision

(For atticotomy, see 69601 et seq)

69450 Tympanolysis, transcanal

➔ *CPT Assistant* May 21:14

Tympanostomy
69433-69436

A ventilating tube is inserted into the opening of the tympanum.

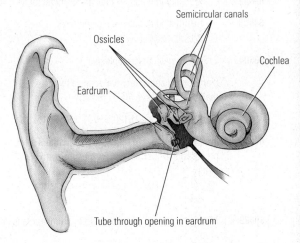

Semicircular canals

Ossicles

Cochlea

Eardrum

Tube through opening in eardrum

Excision

69501 Transmastoid antrotomy (simple mastoidectomy)

➔ *CPT Assistant* Apr 23:7

69502 Mastoidectomy; complete

69505 modified radical

69511 radical

(For skin graft, see 15004 et seq)

(For mastoidectomy cavity debridement, see 69220, 69222)

69530 Petrous apicectomy including radical mastoidectomy

69535 Resection temporal bone, external approach

(For middle fossa approach, see 69950-69970)

69540 Excision aural polyp

69550 Excision aural glomus tumor; transcanal

69552 transmastoid

69554 extended (extratemporal)

Auditory 69000-69979

Repair

69601 Revision mastoidectomy; resulting in complete mastoidectomy

69602 resulting in modified radical mastoidectomy

69603 resulting in radical mastoidectomy
→ *CPT Assistant* Dec 22:21

69604 resulting in tympanoplasty

(For planned secondary tympanoplasty after mastoidectomy, see 69631, 69632)

(For skin graft, see 15120, 15121, 15260, 15261)

69610 Tympanic membrane repair, with or without site preparation of perforation for closure, with or without patch
→ *CPT Assistant* Mar 01:10, Mar 03:21, Aug 08:4, Apr 15:11, May 15:11

69620 Myringoplasty (surgery confined to drumhead and donor area)
→ *CPT Assistant* Mar 01:10, Aug 08:4, Apr 15:11, May 15:11

69631 Tympanoplasty without mastoidectomy (including canalplasty, atticotomy and/or middle ear surgery), initial or revision; without ossicular chain reconstruction
→ *CPT Assistant* Jul 98:11, Mar 01:10, Mar 07:9, Aug 08:4, Dec 12:11

69632 with ossicular chain reconstruction (eg, postfenestration)
→ *CPT Assistant* May 21:14

69633 with ossicular chain reconstruction and synthetic prosthesis (eg, partial ossicular replacement prosthesis [PORP], total ossicular replacement prosthesis [TORP])
→ *CPT Assistant* May 21:14

69635 Tympanoplasty with antrotomy or mastoidotomy (including canalplasty, atticotomy, middle ear surgery, and/or tympanic membrane repair); without ossicular chain reconstruction

69636 with ossicular chain reconstruction

69637 with ossicular chain reconstruction and synthetic prosthesis (eg, partial ossicular replacement prosthesis [PORP], total ossicular replacement prosthesis [TORP])

69641 Tympanoplasty with mastoidectomy (including canalplasty, middle ear surgery, tympanic membrane repair); without ossicular chain reconstruction

69642 with ossicular chain reconstruction

69643 with intact or reconstructed wall, without ossicular chain reconstruction

69644 with intact or reconstructed canal wall, with ossicular chain reconstruction

Tympanoplasty
69635-69646

A graft is used to repair the tympanic membrane perforation.

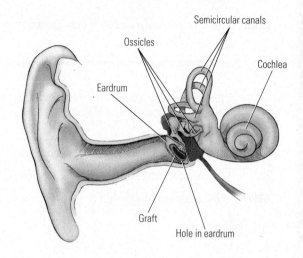

69645 radical or complete, without ossicular chain reconstruction
→ *CPT Assistant* May 21:14

69646 radical or complete, with ossicular chain reconstruction

69650 Stapes mobilization

69660 Stapedectomy or stapedotomy with reestablishment of ossicular continuity, with or without use of foreign material;
→ *CPT Assistant* May 21:14

69661 with footplate drill out
→ *CPT Assistant* May 21:14

69662 Revision of stapedectomy or stapedotomy
→ *CPT Assistant* May 21:14

69666 Repair oval window fistula
→ *CPT Assistant* May 21:14

69667 Repair round window fistula
→ *CPT Assistant* May 21:14

69670 Mastoid obliteration (separate procedure)

69676 Tympanic neurectomy
→ *CPT Assistant* Apr 23:7

(For bilateral procedure, report 69676 with modifier 50)

Osseointegrated Implants

The following codes are for implantation of an osseointegrated implant into the skull. These devices treat hearing loss through surgical placement of an abutment or device into the skull that facilitates transduction of acoustic energy to be received by the better-hearing inner ear or both inner ears when the implant is coupled to a speech processor and vibratory element. This coupling may occur in a percutaneous or a transcutaneous fashion. Other middle ear and mastoid procedures (69501-69676) may be performed for different indications and may be reported separately, when performed.

 # 69714 Implantation, osseointegrated implant, skull; with percutaneous attachment to external speech processor

➜ *CPT Changes: An Insider's View* 2001, 2022

➜ *CPT Assistant* Oct 13:19, Nov 21:5-6, Apr 23:7

(69715 has been deleted. To report mastoidectomy performed at the same operative session as osseointegrated implant placement, revision, replacement, or removal, see 69501-69676)

 # 69716   with magnetic transcutaneous attachment to external speech processor, within the mastoid and/or resulting in removal of less than 100 sq mm surface area of bone deep to the outer cranial cortex

➜ *CPT Changes: An Insider's View* 2022, 2023

➜ *CPT Assistant* Nov 21:5-6, Apr 23:7

 # 69729   with magnetic transcutaneous attachment to external speech processor, outside of the mastoid and resulting in removal of greater than or equal to 100 sq mm surface area of bone deep to the outer cranial cortex

➜ *CPT Changes: An Insider's View* 2023

➜ *CPT Assistant* Apr 23:7

(For diagnostic analysis, programming, and verification of an auditory osseointegrated sound processor, use 92622)

 # 69717 Replacement (including removal of existing device), osseointegrated implant, skull; with percutaneous attachment to external speech processor

➜ *CPT Changes: An Insider's View* 2001, 2022, 2023

➜ *CPT Assistant* Nov 21:5, Apr 23:7

(69718 has been deleted. To report mastoidectomy performed at the same operative session as osseointegrated implant placement, revision, replacement, or removal, see 69501-69676)

 # 69719   with magnetic transcutaneous attachment to external speech processor, within the mastoid and/or involving a bony defect less than 100 sq mm surface area of bone deep to the outer cranial cortex

➜ *CPT Changes: An Insider's View* 2022, 2023

➜ *CPT Assistant* Nov 21:5-6, Apr 23:7

 # 69730   with magnetic transcutaneous attachment to external speech processor, outside the mastoid and involving a bony defect greater than or equal to 100 sq mm surface area of bone deep to the outer cranial cortex

➜ *CPT Changes: An Insider's View* 2023

➜ *CPT Assistant* Apr 23:7

 # 69726 Removal, entire osseointegrated implant, skull; with percutaneous attachment to external speech processor

➜ *CPT Changes: An Insider's View* 2022, 2023

➜ *CPT Assistant* Nov 21:5-6, Apr 23:7

(To report partial removal of the device [ie, abutment only], use appropriate evaluation and management code)

 # 69727   with magnetic transcutaneous attachment to external speech processor, within the mastoid and/or involving a bony defect less than 100 sq mm surface area of bone deep to the outer cranial cortex

➜ *CPT Changes: An Insider's View* 2022, 2023

➜ *CPT Assistant* Nov 21:5-6, Apr 23:7

 # 69728   with magnetic transcutaneous attachment to external speech processor, outside the mastoid and involving a bony defect greater than or equal to 100 sq mm surface area of bone deep to the outer cranial cortex

➜ *CPT Changes: An Insider's View* 2023

➜ *CPT Assistant* Apr 23:7

Other Procedures

69700 Closure postauricular fistula, mastoid (separate procedure)

69705 Nasopharyngoscopy, surgical, with dilation of eustachian tube (ie, balloon dilation); unilateral

➜ *CPT Changes: An Insider's View* 2021

➜ *CPT Assistant* Apr 21:12

69706   bilateral

➜ *CPT Changes: An Insider's View* 2021

➜ *CPT Assistant* Apr 21:12

(Do not report 69705, 69706 in conjunction with 31231, 92511)

69710 Implantation or replacement of electromagnetic bone conduction hearing device in temporal bone

(Replacement procedure includes removal of old device)

69711 Removal or repair of electromagnetic bone conduction hearing device in temporal bone

69714 Code is out of numerical sequence. See 69670-69705

69716 Code is out of numerical sequence. See 69670-69705

69717 Code is out of numerical sequence. See 69670-69705

69719 Code is out of numerical sequence. See 69670-69705

69720 Decompression facial nerve, intratemporal; lateral to geniculate ganglion

69725 including medial to geniculate ganglion

69726 Code is out of numerical sequence. See 69670-69705

69727 Code is out of numerical sequence. See 69670-69705

69728 Code is out of numerical sequence. See 69670-69705

69729 Code is out of numerical sequence. See 69670-69705

69730 Code is out of numerical sequence. See 69670-69705

69740 Suture facial nerve, intratemporal, with or without graft or decompression; lateral to geniculate ganglion

69745 including medial to geniculate ganglion

(For extracranial suture of facial nerve, use 64864)

69799 Unlisted procedure, middle ear
> *CPT Assistant* Oct 99:10, Jan 19:14, Apr 21:12

Inner Ear

Incision and/or Destruction

69801 Labyrinthotomy, with perfusion of vestibuloactive drug(s), transcanal
> *CPT Changes: An Insider's View* 2011
> *CPT Assistant* Nov 96:12, May 11:8

(Do not report 69801 more than once per day)

(Do not report 69801 in conjunction with 69420, 69421, 69433, 69436 when performed on the same ear)

69805 Endolymphatic sac operation; without shunt

69806 with shunt
> *CPT Assistant* Nov 96:12

Excision

69905 Labyrinthectomy; transcanal

69910 with mastoidectomy

69915 Vestibular nerve section, translabyrinthine approach

(For transcranial approach, use 69950)

Introduction

69930 Cochlear device implantation, with or without mastoidectomy
> *CPT Assistant* Jan 23:32, Dec 23:32

(For implantation of vestibular device, use 0725T)

Cochlear Device Implantation
69930

An internal coil is attached to the temporal bone and the ground wire attached to the internal coil is connected to the temporalis muscle.

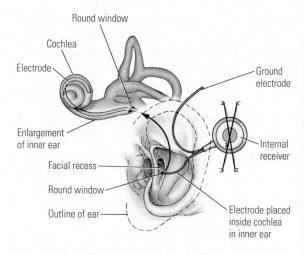

Other Procedures

69949 Unlisted procedure, inner ear
> *CPT Assistant* Dec 23:32

Temporal Bone, Middle Fossa Approach

(For external approach, use 69535)

69950 Vestibular nerve section, transcranial approach

69955 Total facial nerve decompression and/or repair (may include graft)

69960 Decompression internal auditory canal

69970 Removal of tumor, temporal bone

Other Procedures

69979 Unlisted procedure, temporal bone, middle fossa approach
> *CPT Assistant* Jan 07:30, Sep 14:14

Operating Microscope

The surgical microscope is employed when the surgical services are performed using the techniques of microsurgery. Code 69990 should be reported (without modifier 51 appended) in addition to the code for the primary procedure performed. Do not use 69990 for visualization with magnifying loupes or corrected vision. Do not report 69990 in addition to procedures where use of the operating microscope is an inclusive component (15756-15758, 15842, 19364, 19368, 20955-20962, 20969-20973, 22551, 22552, 22856-22861, 26551-26554, 26556, 31526, 31531, 31536, 31541, 31545, 31546, 31561, 31571, 43116, 43180, 43496, 46601, 46607, 49906, 61548, 63075-63078, 64727, 64820-64823, 64912, 64913, 65091-68850, 0184T, 0308T, 0402T, 0583T).

+ **69990**   Microsurgical techniques, requiring use of operating microscope (List separately in addition to code for primary procedure)

⮕ *CPT Changes: An Insider's View* 2002

⮕ *CPT Assistant* Nov 98:20, Apr 99:11, Jun 99:11, Jul 99:10, Oct 99:10, Oct 00:3, Oct 02:8, Jan 04:28, Mar 05:11, Jul 05:14, Aug 05:1, Nov 07:4, Sep 08:10, Mar 09:10, Dec 11:14, Mar 12:9, Jun 12:17, Dec 12:13, Oct 13:14, Jan 14:8, Apr 14:10, Sep 14:13-14, Feb 16:12, Dec 17:13, Feb 18:11, Aug 21:15

Operating Microscope
69990

A surgical operating microscope is used to obtain good visualization of the fine structures in the operating field. The lens system may be operated by hand or foot controls to adjust to working distance, with interchangeable oculars providing magnification as needed.

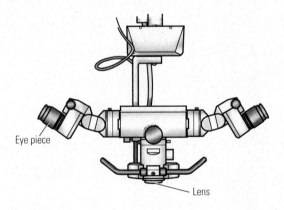

Eye piece

Lens

Notes

Radiology Guidelines (Including Nuclear Medicine and Diagnostic Ultrasound)

Radiology

The following is a listing of headings and subheadings that appear within the Radiology section of the CPT codebook. The subheadings or subsections denoted with asterisks (*) below have special instructions unique to that subsection. Where these are indicated, special notes or guidelines will be presented preceding those procedural terminology listings, referring to that subsection specifically. Note that all code ranges in each subsection are listed as they appear in the subsection, even if the code numbers are out of numerical sequence and/or repeated in the next subsection.

Radiology 70010-79999

Radiology 70010-79999

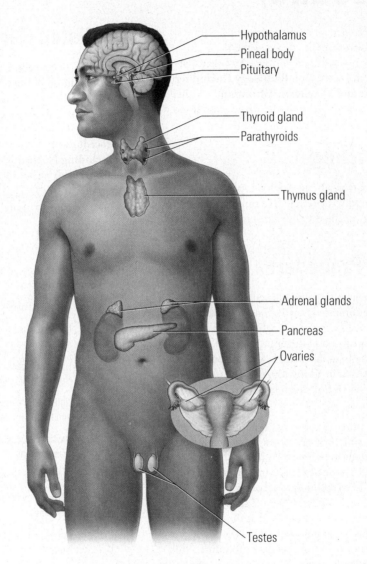

Hypothalamus
Pineal body
Pituitary

Thyroid gland
Parathyroids

Thymus gland

Adrenal glands

Pancreas

Ovaries

Testes

Endocrine System

Radiology 70010-79999

Radiology Guidelines (Including Nuclear Medicine and Diagnostic Ultrasound)

Guidelines to direct general reporting of services are presented in the **Introduction.** Some of the commonalities are repeated here for the convenience of those referring to this section on **Radiology (Including Nuclear Medicine and Diagnostic Ultrasound).** Other definitions and items unique to Radiology are also listed.

Subject Listings

Subject listings apply when radiological services are performed by or under the responsible supervision of a physician or other qualified health care professional.

Separate Procedures

Some of the procedures or services listed in the CPT codebook that are commonly carried out as an integral component of a total service or procedure have been identified by the inclusion of the term "separate procedure." The codes designated as "separate procedure" should not be reported in addition to the code for the total procedure or service of which it is considered an integral component.

However, when a procedure or service that is designated as a "separate procedure" is carried out independently or considered to be unrelated or distinct from other procedures/services provided at that time, it may be reported by itself, or in addition to other procedures/services by appending modifier 59 to the specific "separate procedure" code to indicate that the procedure is not considered to be a component of another procedure, but is a distinct, independent procedure. This may represent a different session or patient encounter, different procedure or surgery, different site or organ system, separate incision/excision, separate lesion, separate injury, or area of injury in extensive injuries.

Unlisted Service or Procedure

A service or procedure may be provided that is not listed in this edition of the CPT codebook. When reporting such a service, the appropriate "Unlisted Procedure" code may be used to indicate the service, identifying it by "Special Report" as discussed below. The "Unlisted Procedures" and accompanying codes for **Radiology (Including Nuclear Medicine and Diagnostic Ultrasound)** are as follows:

76496	Unlisted fluoroscopic procedure (eg, diagnostic, interventional)
76497	Unlisted computed tomography procedure (eg, diagnostic, interventional)
76498	Unlisted magnetic resonance procedure (eg, diagnostic, interventional)
76499	Unlisted diagnostic radiographic procedure
76999	Unlisted ultrasound procedure (eg, diagnostic, interventional)
77299	Unlisted procedure, therapeutic radiology clinical treatment planning
77399	Unlisted procedure, medical radiation physics, dosimetry and treatment devices, and special services
77499	Unlisted procedure, therapeutic radiology treatment management
77799	Unlisted procedure, clinical brachytherapy
78099	Unlisted endocrine procedure, diagnostic nuclear medicine
78199	Unlisted hematopoietic, reticuloendothelial and lymphatic procedure, diagnostic nuclear medicine
78299	Unlisted gastrointestinal procedure, diagnostic nuclear medicine
78399	Unlisted musculoskeletal procedure, diagnostic nuclear medicine
78499	Unlisted cardiovascular procedure, diagnostic nuclear medicine
78599	Unlisted respiratory procedure, diagnostic nuclear medicine
78699	Unlisted nervous system procedure, diagnostic nuclear medicine

★=Telemedicine ◀=Audio-only ✚=Add-on code ✔=FDA approval pending #=Resequenced code ⊘=Modifier 51 exempt ➲➲➲=See p xxi for details

78799   Unlisted genitourinary procedure, diagnostic nuclear medicine

78999   Unlisted miscellaneous procedure, diagnostic nuclear medicine

79999   Radiopharmaceutical therapy, unlisted procedure

Special Report

A service that is rarely provided, unusual, variable, or new may require a special report. Pertinent information should include an adequate definition or description of the nature, extent, and need for the procedure; and the time, effort, and equipment necessary to provide the service.

Supervision and Interpretation, Imaging Guidance

Imaging may be required during the performance of certain procedures or certain imaging procedures may require surgical procedures to access the imaged area. Many services include image guidance, and imaging guidance is not separately reportable when it is included in the base service. The CPT code set typically defines in descriptors and/or guidelines when imaging guidance is included. When imaging is not included in a surgical procedure or procedure from the **Medicine** section, image guidance codes or codes labeled "radiological supervision and interpretation" (RS&I) may be reported for the portion of the service that requires imaging. All imaging guidance codes require: (1) image documentation in the patient record and (2) description of imaging guidance in the procedure report. All RS&I codes require: (1) image documentation in the patient's permanent record and (2) a procedure report or separate imaging report that includes written documentation of interpretive findings of information contained in the images and radiologic supervision of the service.

(The RS&I codes are not applicable to the Radiation Oncology subsection.)

Administration of Contrast Material(s)

The phrase "with contrast" used in the codes for procedures performed using contrast for imaging enhancement represents contrast material administered intravascularly, intra-articularly, or intrathecally.

For intra-articular injection, use the appropriate joint injection code. If radiographic arthrography is performed, also use the arthrography supervision and interpretation code for the appropriate joint (which includes fluoroscopy). If computed tomography (CT) or magnetic resonance (MR) arthrography are performed without radiographic arthrography, use the appropriate joint injection code, the appropriate CT or MR code ("with contrast" or "without followed by contrast"), and the appropriate imaging guidance code for needle placement for contrast injection.

For spine examinations using computed tomography, magnetic resonance imaging, magnetic resonance angiography, "with contrast" includes intrathecal or intravascular injection. For intrathecal injection, use also 61055 or 62284.

Injection of intravascular contrast material is part of the "with contrast" CT, computed tomographic angiography (CTA), magnetic resonance imaging (MRI), and magnetic resonance angiography (MRA) procedures.

Oral and/or rectal contrast administration alone does not qualify as a study "with contrast."

Written Report(s)

A written report (eg, handwritten or electronic) signed by the interpreting individual should be considered an integral part of a radiologic procedure or interpretation.

With regard to CPT descriptors for imaging services, "images" must contain anatomic information unique to the patient for which the imaging service is provided. "Images" refer to those acquired in either an analog (ie, film) or digital (ie, electronic) manner.

Foreign Body/Implant Definition

An object intentionally placed by a physician or other qualified health care professional for any purpose (eg, diagnostic or therapeutic) is considered an implant. An object that is unintentionally placed (eg, trauma or ingestion) is considered a foreign body. If an implant (or part thereof) has moved from its original position or is structurally broken and no longer serves its intended purpose or presents a hazard to the patient, it qualifies as a foreign body for coding purposes, unless CPT coding instructions direct otherwise or a specific CPT code exists to describe the removal of that broken/moved implant.

Radiology

Diagnostic Radiology (Diagnostic Imaging)

Head and Neck

70010 Myelography, posterior fossa, radiological supervision and interpretation
> *CPT Assistant* Mar 05:11, Dec 07:16

70015 Cisternography, positive contrast, radiological supervision and interpretation

70030 Radiologic examination, eye, for detection of foreign body

70100 Radiologic examination, mandible; partial, less than 4 views

70110   complete, minimum of 4 views

70120 Radiologic examination, mastoids; less than 3 views per side

70130   complete, minimum of 3 views per side

70134 Radiologic examination, internal auditory meati, complete

70140 Radiologic examination, facial bones; less than 3 views

70150   complete, minimum of 3 views

70160 Radiologic examination, nasal bones, complete, minimum of 3 views

70170 Dacryocystography, nasolacrimal duct, radiological supervision and interpretation

70190 Radiologic examination; optic foramina

70200   orbits, complete, minimum of 4 views

70210 Radiologic examination, sinuses, paranasal, less than 3 views

70220 Radiologic examination, sinuses, paranasal, complete, minimum of 3 views

70240 Radiologic examination, sella turcica

70250 Radiologic examination, skull; less than 4 views
> *CPT Changes: An Insider's View* 2004

70260   complete, minimum of 4 views
> *CPT Changes: An Insider's View* 2004

70300 Radiologic examination, teeth; single view

70310   partial examination, less than full mouth

70320   complete, full mouth

70328 Radiologic examination, temporomandibular joint, open and closed mouth; unilateral

70330   bilateral
> *CPT Assistant* May 11:10

70332 Temporomandibular joint arthrography, radiological supervision and interpretation
> *CPT Assistant* Feb 07:11

(Do not report 70332 in conjunction with 77002)

70336 Magnetic resonance (eg, proton) imaging, temporomandibular joint(s)
> *CPT Changes: An Insider's View* 2001
> *CPT Assistant* Jul 99:11, Jul 01:7, Aug 15:6, Jul 22:19

70350 Cephalogram, orthodontic
> *CPT Assistant* Aug 12:14

70355 Orthopantogram (eg, panoramic x-ray)
> *CPT Changes: An Insider's View* 2012
> *Clinical Examples in Radiology* Fall 11:11

70360 Radiologic examination; neck, soft tissue

70370   pharynx or larynx, including fluoroscopy and/or magnification technique

70371 Complex dynamic pharyngeal and speech evaluation by cine or video recording
> *CPT Assistant* Dec 04:17, Jul 14:5
> *Clinical Examples in Radiology* Spring 18:15

(For laryngeal computed tomography, see 70490, 70491, 70492)

70380 Radiologic examination, salivary gland for calculus

70390 Sialography, radiological supervision and interpretation
> *Clinical Examples in Radiology* Fall 09:9

70450 Computed tomography, head or brain; without contrast material
> *CPT Changes: An Insider's View* 2003
> *CPT Assistant* Apr 96:11
> *Clinical Examples in Radiology* Winter 08:6, Fall 14:8, Summer 20:13, Winter 22:15

70460   with contrast material(s)
> *CPT Assistant* Apr 96:11
> *Clinical Examples in Radiology* Winter 10:11, Fall 14:8, Summer 23:24

70470   without contrast material, followed by contrast material(s) and further sections
> *CPT Assistant* Apr 96:11
> *Clinical Examples in Radiology* Fall 14:8

(To report 3D rendering, see 76376, 76377)

Radiology 70010-79999

70480   Computed tomography, orbit, sella, or posterior fossa or outer, middle, or inner ear; without contrast material
➲ *CPT Changes: An Insider's View* 2003

70481   with contrast material(s)
➲ *CPT Assistant* Apr 08:11

70482   without contrast material, followed by contrast material(s) and further sections

(To report 3D rendering, see 76376, 76377)

70486   Computed tomography, maxillofacial area; without contrast material
➲ *CPT Changes: An Insider's View* 2003
➲ *CPT Assistant* Mar 02:11
➲ *Clinical Examples in Radiology* Winter 07:4-5, Spring 07:4, Fall 09:9

70487   with contrast material(s)

70488   without contrast material, followed by contrast material(s) and further sections

(To report 3D rendering, see 76376, 76377)

70490   Computed tomography, soft tissue neck; without contrast material
➲ *CPT Changes: An Insider's View* 2003

70491   with contrast material(s)
➲ *Clinical Examples in Radiology* Summer 22:3

70492   without contrast material followed by contrast material(s) and further sections

(To report 3D rendering, see 76376, 76377)

(For cervical spine, see 72125, 72126)

70496   Computed tomographic angiography, head, with contrast material(s), including noncontrast images, if performed, and image postprocessing
➲ *CPT Changes: An Insider's View* 2001, 2008
➲ *CPT Assistant* Jul 01:4, Dec 05:7, Jan 07:31
➲ *Clinical Examples in Radiology* Summer 20:12

(For noninvasive arterial plaque analysis using software processing of data from computerized tomography angiography to quantify structure and composition of the vessel wall, including assessment for lipid-rich necrotic core plaque, see 0710T, 0711T, 0712T, 0713T)

70498   Computed tomographic angiography, neck, with contrast material(s), including noncontrast images, if performed, and image postprocessing
➲ *CPT Changes: An Insider's View* 2001, 2008
➲ *CPT Assistant* Jul 01:4, Dec 05:7, Jan 07:31
➲ *Clinical Examples in Radiology* Winter 09:2, Summer 19:11, Summer 22:2

(For noninvasive arterial plaque analysis using software processing of data from computerized tomography angiography to quantify structure and composition of the vessel wall, including assessment for lipid-rich necrotic core plaque, see 0710T, 0711T, 0712T, 0713T)

70540   Magnetic resonance (eg, proton) imaging, orbit, face, and/or neck; without contrast material(s)
➲ *CPT Changes: An Insider's View* 2001, 2007
➲ *CPT Assistant* Jul 01:6, Mar 07:7, Sep 10:10
➲ *Clinical Examples in Radiology* Spring 05:3, Summer 07:7, Summer 13:9

(For head or neck magnetic resonance angiography studies, see 70544-70546, 70547-70549)

70542   with contrast material(s)
➲ *CPT Changes: An Insider's View* 2001
➲ *CPT Assistant* Jul 01:6, Sep 10:10, Jul 22:19
➲ *Clinical Examples in Radiology* Spring 05:3, Summer 07:7, Summer 13:9

70543   without contrast material(s), followed by contrast material(s) and further sequences
➲ *CPT Changes: An Insider's View* 2001
➲ *CPT Assistant* Jul 01:6, Sep 10:10
➲ *Clinical Examples in Radiology* Spring 05:2-3, Winter 07:7, 11, Summer 07:7, Summer 13:9

(Report 70540-70543 once per imaging session)

70544   Magnetic resonance angiography, head; without contrast material(s)
➲ *CPT Changes: An Insider's View* 2001
➲ *CPT Assistant* Sep 01:5, Dec 05:7, Jan 07:31
➲ *Clinical Examples in Radiology* Summer 23:16

70545   with contrast material(s)
➲ *CPT Changes: An Insider's View* 2001
➲ *CPT Assistant* Jul 01:5, Dec 05:7
➲ *Clinical Examples in Radiology* Summer 23:16

70546   without contrast material(s), followed by contrast material(s) and further sequences
➲ *CPT Changes: An Insider's View* 2001
➲ *CPT Assistant* Jul 01:5, Dec 05:7, Jan 07:31
➲ *Clinical Examples in Radiology* Summer 23:16

70547   Magnetic resonance angiography, neck; without contrast material(s)
➲ *CPT Changes: An Insider's View* 2001
➲ *CPT Assistant* Sep 01:5, Dec 05:7, Jan 07:31
➲ *Clinical Examples in Radiology* Winter 09:2

70548   with contrast material(s)
➲ *CPT Changes: An Insider's View* 2001
➲ *CPT Assistant* Sep 01:6, Dec 05:7, Jan 07:31
➲ *Clinical Examples in Radiology* Winter 09:2

70549   without contrast material(s), followed by contrast material(s) and further sequences
➲ *CPT Changes: An Insider's View* 2001
➲ *CPT Assistant* Sep 01:6, Dec 05:7, Jan 07:31
➲ *Clinical Examples in Radiology* Winter 09:2

Radiology 70010-79999

Radiology 70010-79999

70551 Magnetic resonance (eg, proton) imaging, brain (including brain stem); without contrast material

➔ *CPT Assistant* May 98:10, Mar 05:20, Feb 07:6

➔ *Clinical Examples in Radiology* Spring 15:9, Summer 23:16, Fall 23:14, Winter 24:11

70552 with contrast material(s)

➔ *CPT Assistant* Jul 01:6, Mar 05:20, Feb 07:6

➔ *Clinical Examples in Radiology* Spring 15:9, Summer 23:16, Fall 23:14, Winter 24:11

70553 without contrast material, followed by contrast material(s) and further sequences

➔ *CPT Assistant* Nov 97:24, Jul 01:6, Mar 05:20, Feb 07:6

➔ *Clinical Examples in Radiology* Spring 05:2, Spring 06:4-5, Spring 15:9, Summer 15:13, Summer 23:16, Fall 23:14, Winter 24:10

(For magnetic spectroscopy, use 76390)

▶Functional MRI involves identification and mapping of stimulation of brain function. When neurofunctional tests are administered by a technologist or other non-physician or non-psychologist, use 70554. When neurofunctional tests are entirely administered by a physician or other qualified health care professional or psychologist, use 70555.◀

70554 Magnetic resonance imaging, brain, functional MRI; including test selection and administration of repetitive body part movement and/or visual stimulation, not requiring physician or psychologist administration

➔ *CPT Changes: An Insider's View* 2007

➔ *CPT Assistant* Feb 07:6, Mar 07:7, Aug 08:13

➔ *Clinical Examples in Radiology* Fall 23:14

(Do not report 70554 in conjunction with 96020)

70555 requiring physician or psychologist administration of entire neurofunctional testing

➔ *CPT Changes: An Insider's View* 2007

➔ *CPT Assistant* Feb 07:6, Mar 07:7

➔ *Clinical Examples in Radiology* Fall 23:13

(Do not report 70555 unless 96020 is performed)

(Do not report 70554, 70555 in conjunction with 70551-70553 unless a separate diagnostic MRI is performed)

70557 Magnetic resonance (eg, proton) imaging, brain (including brain stem and skull base), during open intracranial procedure (eg, to assess for residual tumor or residual vascular malformation); without contrast material

➔ *CPT Changes: An Insider's View* 2004

70558 with contrast material(s)

➔ *CPT Changes: An Insider's View* 2004

70559 without contrast material(s), followed by contrast material(s) and further sequences

➔ *CPT Changes: An Insider's View* 2004

(For stereotactic biopsy of intracranial lesion with magnetic resonance guidance, use 61751, 70557, 70558, or 70559 may be reported only if a separate report is generated. Report only 1 of the above codes once per operative session. Do not use these codes in conjunction with 61751, 77021, 77022)

Chest

(For fluoroscopic or ultrasonic guidance for needle placement procedures (eg, biopsy, aspiration, injection, localization device) of the thorax, see 76942, 77002)

71045 Radiologic examination, chest; single view

➔ *CPT Changes: An Insider's View* 2018

➔ *CPT Assistant* Apr 18:7, Mar 19:10, May 19:10, Aug 19:8, Jan 22:3, Jun 22:19, Dec 22:10

➔ *Clinical Examples in Radiology* Fall 18:9, Summer 19:14

71046 2 views

➔ *CPT Changes: An Insider's View* 2018

➔ *CPT Assistant* Apr 18:7, Mar 19:10, Aug 19:8, Jan 22:3, Jun 22:19, Dec 22:10

➔ *Clinical Examples in Radiology* Fall 18:9, Summer 19:14

71047 3 views

➔ *CPT Changes: An Insider's View* 2018

➔ *CPT Assistant* Apr 18:7, Mar 19:10

➔ *Clinical Examples in Radiology* Fall 18:9, Summer 19:14

71048 4 or more views

➔ *CPT Changes: An Insider's View* 2018

➔ *CPT Assistant* Apr 18:7, Mar 19:10

➔ *Clinical Examples in Radiology* Fall 18:9, Summer 19:14

(For complete acute abdomen series that includes 2 or more views of the abdomen [eg, supine, erect, decubitus], and a single view chest, use 74022)

(For concurrent computer-aided detection [CAD] performed in addition to 71045, 71046, 71047, 71048, use 0174T)

(Do not report 71045, 71046, 71047, 71048 in conjunction with 0175T for computer-aided detection [CAD] performed remotely from the primary interpretation)

71100 Radiologic examination, ribs, unilateral; 2 views

➔ *Clinical Examples in Radiology* Spring 14:6

71101 including posteroanterior chest, minimum of 3 views

➔ *CPT Assistant* Dec 22:22

71110 Radiologic examination, ribs, bilateral; 3 views

➔ *Clinical Examples in Radiology* Spring 14:6

71111 including posteroanterior chest, minimum of 4 views

➔ *CPT Assistant* Dec 22:22

➔ *Clinical Examples in Radiology* Spring 14:6

71120 Radiologic examination; sternum, minimum of 2 views

71130 sternoclavicular joint or joints, minimum of 3 views

71250   Computed tomography, thorax, diagnostic; without contrast material
>   *CPT Changes: An Insider's View* 2003, 2021
>   *CPT Assistant* Jul 07:13, Aug 11:10, Feb 21:9
>   *Clinical Examples in Radiology* Fall 08:7, Fall 13:9-10, Winter 18:17, Summer 19:10, Winter 20:9, Spring 20:13, Fall 20:13, Summer 21:3, Winter 23:17

71260   with contrast material(s)
>   *CPT Changes: An Insider's View* 2021
>   *CPT Assistant* Jul 01:4, Jun 09:9, Feb 21:9
>   *Clinical Examples in Radiology* Summer 05:4, Fall 08:7, 11-12, Fall 13:9-10, Fall 20:13

71270   without contrast material, followed by contrast material(s) and further sections
>   *CPT Changes: An Insider's View* 2021
>   *CPT Assistant* Jun 01:10, Jul 07:13, Feb 21:9
>   *Clinical Examples in Radiology* Fall 08:7, Fall 13:9-10, Fall 20:13

(Do not report 71270 in conjunction with 71250, 71260, 71271)

(Do not report 71250, 71260, 71270 for breast CT procedures)

(For cardiac computed tomography of the heart, see 75571-75574)

(To report 3D rendering, see 76376, 76377)

71271   Computed tomography, thorax, low dose for lung cancer screening, without contrast material(s)
>   *CPT Changes: An Insider's View* 2021
>   *CPT Assistant* Feb 21:9
>   *Clinical Examples in Radiology* Fall 20:13, Spring 21:10, Winter 23:17, Spring 23:25

(Do not report 71271 in conjunction with 71250, 71260, 71270)

(Do not report 71271 for breast CT procedures)

(For cardiac computed tomography of the heart, see 75571, 75572, 75573, 75574)

71275   Computed tomographic angiography, chest (noncoronary), with contrast material(s), including noncontrast images, if performed, and image postprocessing
>   *CPT Changes: An Insider's View* 2001, 2007, 2008
>   *CPT Assistant* Jul 01:4, Jun 05:11, Dec 05:7, Jan 07:31, Mar 07:7, Jun 09:9, Aug 11:10
>   *Clinical Examples in Radiology* Spring 05:7, Fall 08:11-12, Spring 09:11, Fall 09:10, Winter 10:2, Fall 13:9-10, Spring 16:13, Winter 20:8, Summer 20:12, Summer 21:3

(For coronary artery computed tomographic angiography including calcification score and/or cardiac morphology, use 75574)

71550   Magnetic resonance (eg, proton) imaging, chest (eg, for evaluation of hilar and mediastinal lymphadenopathy); without contrast material(s)
>   *CPT Changes: An Insider's View* 2001
>   *CPT Assistant* Jul 01:7, Apr 10:10, Sep 10:10
>   *Clinical Examples in Radiology* Summer 13:9, Winter 20:14, Winter 21:12

71551   with contrast material(s)
>   *CPT Changes: An Insider's View* 2001
>   *CPT Assistant* Jul 01:7, Sep 10:10
>   *Clinical Examples in Radiology* Summer 13:9, Winter 20:14, Winter 21:12, Winter 23:19

71552   without contrast material(s), followed by contrast material(s) and further sequences
>   *CPT Changes: An Insider's View* 2001
>   *CPT Assistant* Jul 01:7, Apr 10:10, Sep 10:10, Apr 21:14
>   *Clinical Examples in Radiology* Summer 13:9, Winter 20:14, Winter 21:12, Winter 23:18

(For breast MRI, see 77046, 77047, 77048, 77049)

71555   Magnetic resonance angiography, chest (excluding myocardium), with or without contrast material(s)
>   *CPT Assistant* Fall 95:2, Dec 05:7, Jan 07:31
>   *Clinical Examples in Radiology* Spring 16:13, Spring 17:14

Spine and Pelvis

72020   Radiologic examination, spine, single view, specify level
>   *CPT Assistant* Jul 13:10, Oct 15:9
>   *Clinical Examples in Radiology* Spring 13:8-9, Winter 18:15

(For a single view that includes the entire thoracic and lumbar spine, use 72081)

72040   Radiologic examination, spine, cervical; 2 or 3 views
>   *CPT Changes: An Insider's View* 2001, 2013, 2014
>   *CPT Assistant* Sep 01:7, Jul 13:10, Aug 18:11
>   *Clinical Examples in Radiology* Fall 09:10, Summer 11:8, Fall 11:9, Spring 13:8-9, Winter 18:15

72050   4 or 5 views
>   *CPT Changes: An Insider's View* 2013
>   *Clinical Examples in Radiology* Summer 11:8, Fall 11:9, Spring 13:9, Winter 18:15

72052   6 or more views
>   *CPT Changes: An Insider's View* 2013
>   *Clinical Examples in Radiology* Summer 11:8, Fall 11:9, Spring 13:9, Winter 18:15

72070   Radiologic examination, spine; thoracic, 2 views
>   *CPT Changes: An Insider's View* 2001
>   *CPT Assistant* Sep 01:7
>   *Clinical Examples in Radiology* Fall 11:9, Spring 13:9, Winter 18:15

72072   thoracic, 3 views
>   *CPT Changes: An Insider's View* 2001
>   *CPT Assistant* Sep 01:7
>   *Clinical Examples in Radiology* Fall 11:9, Spring 13:9, Winter 18:15

72074 thoracic, minimum of 4 views

➔ *CPT Changes: An Insider's View* 2001

➔ *CPT Assistant* Sep 01:7

➔ *Clinical Examples in Radiology* Fall 11:9, Spring 13:9, Winter 18:15

72080 thoracolumbar junction, minimum of 2 views

➔ *CPT Changes: An Insider's View* 2001, 2016

➔ *CPT Assistant* Sep 01:7, Oct 15:9, Sep 16:4

➔ *Clinical Examples in Radiology* Fall 11:9, Spring 13:8-9, Fall 15:7, Winter 18:15

(For a single view examination of the thoracolumbar junction, use 72020)

72081 Radiologic examination, spine, entire thoracic and lumbar, including skull, cervical and sacral spine if performed (eg, scoliosis evaluation); one view

➔ *CPT Changes: An Insider's View* 2016

➔ *CPT Assistant* Sep 16:4

➔ *Clinical Examples in Radiology* Fall 15:7, Winter 18:15

72082 2 or 3 views

➔ *CPT Changes: An Insider's View* 2016

➔ *CPT Assistant* Sep 16:4

➔ *Clinical Examples in Radiology* Fall 15:7, Winter 18:15

72083 4 or 5 views

➔ *CPT Changes: An Insider's View* 2016

➔ *CPT Assistant* Sep 16:4

➔ *Clinical Examples in Radiology* Fall 15:7, Winter 18:15

72084 minimum of 6 views

➔ *CPT Changes: An Insider's View* 2016

➔ *CPT Assistant* Sep 16:4

➔ *Clinical Examples in Radiology* Fall 15:7, Winter 18:15

72100 Radiologic examination, spine, lumbosacral; 2 or 3 views

➔ *CPT Changes: An Insider's View* 2001

➔ *CPT Assistant* Sep 01:7

➔ *Clinical Examples in Radiology* Fall 11:9-10, Spring 13:8-9, Spring 14:10, Winter 18:15

72110 minimum of 4 views

➔ *CPT Changes: An Insider's View* 2001

➔ *CPT Assistant* Sep 01:7

➔ *Clinical Examples in Radiology* Fall 11:10, Spring 13:9, Winter 18:15

72114 complete, including bending views, minimum of 6 views

➔ *CPT Changes: An Insider's View* 2012

➔ *Clinical Examples in Radiology* Summer 12:11, Spring 13:9, Winter 18:15

72120 bending views only, 2 or 3 views

➔ *CPT Changes: An Insider's View* 2012

➔ *CPT Assistant* Aug 16:7

➔ *Clinical Examples in Radiology* Fall 11:9-10, Spring 13:8-9, Spring 14:10, Winter 18:15

(Contrast material in CT of spine is either by intrathecal or intravenous injection. For intrathecal injection, use also 61055 or 62284. IV injection of contrast material is part of the CT procedure)

72125 Computed tomography, cervical spine; without contrast material

➔ *CPT Changes: An Insider's View* 2003

➔ *Clinical Examples in Radiology* Fall 14:7, 11

72126 with contrast material

➔ *CPT Assistant* Sep 14:3

➔ *Clinical Examples in Radiology* Fall 15:10, Summer 19:11, Summer 22:3

72127 without contrast material, followed by contrast material(s) and further sections

(For intrathecal injection procedure, see 61055, 62284)

72128 Computed tomography, thoracic spine; without contrast material

➔ *CPT Changes: An Insider's View* 2003

72129 with contrast material

➔ *CPT Assistant* Sep 14:3, Jan 19:15

➔ *Clinical Examples in Radiology* Fall 15:10

(For intrathecal injection procedure, see 61055, 62284)

72130 without contrast material, followed by contrast material(s) and further sections

(For intrathecal injection procedure, see 61055, 62284)

72131 Computed tomography, lumbar spine; without contrast material

➔ *CPT Changes: An Insider's View* 2003

➔ *Clinical Examples in Radiology* Summer 07:11, Spring 12:10

72132 with contrast material

➔ *CPT Assistant* Fall 93:13, Sep 14:3, Jan 19:15

➔ *Clinical Examples in Radiology* Fall 06:5-6, 11-12, Fall 14:6, Fall 15:10

72133 without contrast material, followed by contrast material(s) and further sections

➔ *Clinical Examples in Radiology* Fall 14:7, 11

(For intrathecal injection procedure, see 61055, 62284)

(To report 3D rendering, see 76376, 76377)

72141 Magnetic resonance (eg, proton) imaging, spinal canal and contents, cervical; without contrast material

➔ *CPT Assistant* Apr 10:10, Jun 14:14

➔ *Clinical Examples in Radiology* Winter 21:6, 12

72142 with contrast material(s)

➔ *CPT Assistant* Apr 10:10, Jul 21:6

➔ *Clinical Examples in Radiology* Winter 21:6

(For cervical spinal canal imaging without contrast material followed by contrast material, use 72156)

(For magnetic resonance spectroscopy, determination and localization of discogenic pain, see 0609T, 0610T)

72146 Magnetic resonance (eg, proton) imaging, spinal canal and contents, thoracic; without contrast material
➔ *CPT Assistant* May 99:10, Apr 10:10, Jun 14:14
➔ *Clinical Examples in Radiology* Winter 21:6

72147   with contrast material(s)
➔ *CPT Assistant* May 99:10, Apr 10:10, Jul 21:6
➔ *Clinical Examples in Radiology* Winter 21:6, 12

(For thoracic spinal canal imaging without contrast material followed by contrast material, use 72157)

(For magnetic resonance spectroscopy, determination and localization of discogenic pain, see 0609T, 0610T)

72148 Magnetic resonance (eg, proton) imaging, spinal canal and contents, lumbar; without contrast material
➔ *CPT Assistant* Nov 05:15, Jun 14:14
➔ *Clinical Examples in Radiology* Spring 06:6, 11, Winter 21:6

72149   with contrast material(s)
➔ *CPT Assistant* Jul 21:6
➔ *Clinical Examples in Radiology* Winter 21:6

(For lumbar spinal canal imaging without contrast material followed by contrast material, use 72158)

(For magnetic resonance spectroscopy, determination and localization of discogenic pain, see 0609T, 0610T)

72156 Magnetic resonance (eg, proton) imaging, spinal canal and contents, without contrast material, followed by contrast material(s) and further sequences; cervical
➔ *Clinical Examples in Radiology* Winter 21:6

72157   thoracic
➔ *Clinical Examples in Radiology* Winter 21:6

72158   lumbar
➔ *CPT Assistant* Jul 21:6
➔ *Clinical Examples in Radiology* Winter 21:6

(For magnetic resonance spectroscopy, determination and localization of discogenic pain, see 0609T, 0610T)

72159 Magnetic resonance angiography, spinal canal and contents, with or without contrast material(s)
➔ *CPT Assistant* Dec 05:7, Jan 07:31
➔ *Clinical Examples in Radiology* Winter 21:6

72170 Radiologic examination, pelvis; 1 or 2 views
➔ *CPT Changes: An Insider's View* 2001
➔ *CPT Assistant* Sep 01:7, Mar 03:23, Aug 16:7
➔ *Clinical Examples in Radiology* Spring 05:12, Fall 15:8, Winter 16:13, Summer 16:8

72190   complete, minimum of 3 views
➔ *Clinical Examples in Radiology* Fall 15:9, Winter 16:13, Summer 16:8

(For a combined computed tomography [CT] or computed tomographic angiography abdomen and pelvis study, see 74174, 74176-74178)

72191 Computed tomographic angiography, pelvis, with contrast material(s), including noncontrast images, if performed, and image postprocessing
➔ *CPT Changes: An Insider's View* 2001, 2008
➔ *CPT Assistant* Jul 01:4, 6, Dec 05:7, Jan 07:31
➔ *Clinical Examples in Radiology* Summer 08:8, Fall 09:10, Fall 11:9

(Do not report 72191 in conjunction with 73706 or 75635. For CTA aorto-iliofemoral runoff, use 75635)

(Do not report 72191 in conjunction with 74175. For a combined computed tomographic angiography abdomen and pelvis study, use 74174)

(For noninvasive arterial plaque analysis using software processing of data from computerized tomography angiography to quantify structure and composition of the vessel wall, including assessment for lipid-rich necrotic core plaque, see 0710T, 0711T, 0712T, 0713T)

72192 Computed tomography, pelvis; without contrast material
➔ *CPT Changes: An Insider's View* 2003
➔ *CPT Assistant* Mar 05:1, 4, Mar 07:10, Apr 10:9, Nov 11:6, Oct 12:12
➔ *Clinical Examples in Radiology* Winter 06:11, Spring 07:3, 11, Summer 07:11, Fall 09:9, Winter 11:8, 10, Fall 11:8, Spring 16:9, Summer 20:7, Winter 21:3

72193   with contrast material(s)
➔ *CPT Assistant* Mar 05:1, 4, Mar 07:10, Apr 10:9, Nov 11:6, Oct 12:12
➔ *Clinical Examples in Radiology* Winter 05:1, 7, Spring 07:3, 11, Winter 11:8, 10, Fall 11:8, Spring 16:9, Summer 20:7

72194   without contrast material, followed by contrast material(s) and further sections
➔ *CPT Assistant* Mar 05:1, 4, Mar 07:10, Apr 10:9, Nov 11:6, Oct 12:12
➔ *Clinical Examples in Radiology* Spring 07:3, 11, Winter 11:8, 10, Fall 11:8, Spring 16:9, Summer 20:7

(For a combined CT abdomen and pelvis study, see 74176-74178)

(To report 3D rendering, see 76376, 76377)

(For computed tomographic colonography, diagnostic, see 74261-74262. For computed tomographic colonography, screening, use 74263)

(Do not report 72192-72194 in conjunction with 74261-74263)

Radiology 70010-79999

72195　Magnetic resonance (eg, proton) imaging, pelvis; without contrast material(s)

➔ *CPT Changes: An Insider's View* 2001

➔ *CPT Assistant* Jul 01:7, Jun 06:17, Jun 14:14, Jun 16:5, Jul 18:11, Jun 22:20-21

➔ *Clinical Examples in Radiology* Spring 06:8-9, Fall 06:7-8, Summer 07:4-5, Winter 16:12, Spring 18:12, Spring 19:12, Summer 22:10

72196　with contrast material(s)

➔ *CPT Changes: An Insider's View* 2001

➔ *CPT Assistant* Jul 01:7, Jun 06:17, Jun 16:5, Jul 18:11

➔ *Clinical Examples in Radiology* Spring 06:8-9, Fall 06:7-8, Winter 16:12, Spring 18:12, Spring 19:12, Winter 21:12, Summer 22:10, Winter 23:19

72197　without contrast material(s), followed by contrast material(s) and further sequences

➔ *CPT Changes: An Insider's View* 2001

➔ *CPT Assistant* Jul 01:7, Jun 16:5, Jul 18:11, Apr 21:14, Jun 22:20-21

➔ *Clinical Examples in Radiology* Spring 06:8-9, Fall 06:2-3, 7-8, Spring 15:10, Winter 16:12, Spring 18:12, Spring 19:12, Winter 21:12, Summer 21:6, Summer 22:10, Winter 23:19

(Do not report 72195, 72196, 72197 in conjunction with 74712, 74713)

(For magnetic resonance imaging of a fetus[es], see 74712, 74713)

72198　Magnetic resonance angiography, pelvis, with or without contrast material(s)

➔ *CPT Assistant* Dec 05:7, Jan 07:31

72200　Radiologic examination, sacroiliac joints; less than 3 views

72202　　3 or more views

72220　Radiologic examination, sacrum and coccyx, minimum of 2 views

72240　Myelography, cervical, radiological supervision and interpretation

➔ *CPT Assistant* Fall 93:13, Sep 14:3

➔ *Clinical Examples in Radiology* Fall 06:5-6, 11-12, Fall 14:6-7, 11, Fall 15:10

(Do not report 72240 in conjunction with 62284, 62302, 62303, 62304, 62305)

(When both 62284 and 72240 are performed by the same physician or other qualified health care professional for cervical myelography, use 62302)

(For complete cervical myelography via injection procedure at C1-C2, see 61055, 72240)

72255　Myelography, thoracic, radiological supervision and interpretation

➔ *CPT Assistant* Sep 14:3

➔ *Clinical Examples in Radiology* Fall 14:7, 11, Fall 15:10

(Do not report 72255 in conjunction with 62284, 62302, 62303, 62304, 62305)

(When both 62284 and 72255 are performed by the same physician or other qualified health care professional for thoracic myelography, use 62303)

(For complete thoracic myelography via injection procedure at C1-C2, see 61055, 72255)

72265　Myelography, lumbosacral, radiological supervision and interpretation

➔ *CPT Assistant* Fall 93:13, Aug 00:7, Sep 14:3

➔ *Clinical Examples in Radiology* Fall 14:7, 11, Fall 15:10

(Do not report 72265 in conjunction with 62284, 62302, 62303, 62304, 62305)

(When both 62284 and 72265 are performed by the same physician or other qualified health care professional for lumbosacral myelography, use 62304)

(For complete lumbosacral myelography via injection procedure at C1-C2, see 61055, 72265)

72270　Myelography, 2 or more regions (eg, lumbar/thoracic, cervical/thoracic, lumbar/cervical, lumbar/thoracic/cervical), radiological supervision and interpretation

➔ *CPT Changes: An Insider's View* 2004

➔ *CPT Assistant* Sep 14:3

➔ *Clinical Examples in Radiology* Fall 14:6-7, 11, Fall 15:10

(Do not report 72270 in conjunction with 62284, 62302, 62303, 62304, 62305)

(When both 62284 and 72270 are performed by the same physician or other qualified health care professional for myelography of 2 or more regions, use 62305)

(For complete myelography of 2 or more regions via injection procedure at C1-C2, see 61055, 72270)

72285　Discography, cervical or thoracic, radiological supervision and interpretation

➔ *CPT Changes: An Insider's View* 2000

➔ *CPT Assistant* Nov 99:35, 40, Mar 11:7, Dec 23:46

➔ *Clinical Examples in Radiology* Fall 10:10

72295　Discography, lumbar, radiological supervision and interpretation

➔ *CPT Assistant* Apr 03:27, Mar 11:7, Jul 12:3, Dec 23:46

➔ *Clinical Examples in Radiology* Fall 10:10

Upper Extremities

(For stress views, any joint, use 77071)

73000　Radiologic examination; clavicle, complete

73010　　scapula, complete

73020   Radiologic examination, shoulder; 1 view

73030   complete, minimum of 2 views

73040   Radiologic examination, shoulder, arthrography, radiological supervision and interpretation

→ *CPT Assistant* Jul 01:7, Feb 07:11

→ *Clinical Examples in Radiology* Spring 05:6, Spring 09:6-7, Summer 18:14

(Do not report 77002 in conjunction with 73040)

73050   Radiologic examination; acromioclavicular joints, bilateral, with or without weighted distraction

73060   humerus, minimum of 2 views

73070   Radiologic examination, elbow; 2 views

→ *CPT Changes: An Insider's View* 2001

→ *CPT Assistant* Winter 90:9, Sep 01:8

73080   complete, minimum of 3 views

73085   Radiologic examination, elbow, arthrography, radiological supervision and interpretation

→ *CPT Assistant* Feb 07:11

→ *Clinical Examples in Radiology* Spring 05:6

(Do not report 77002 in conjunction with 73085)

73090   Radiologic examination; forearm, 2 views

→ *CPT Changes: An Insider's View* 2001

→ *CPT Assistant* Sep 01:8, Apr 02:14

73092   upper extremity, infant, minimum of 2 views

73100   Radiologic examination, wrist; 2 views

→ *CPT Changes: An Insider's View* 2001

→ *CPT Assistant* Winter 90:9, Sep 01:8, Oct 18:11

73110   complete, minimum of 3 views

→ *CPT Assistant* Mar 97:10, Nov 06:22, Oct 18:11

73115   Radiologic examination, wrist, arthrography, radiological supervision and interpretation

→ *CPT Assistant* Feb 07:11

→ *Clinical Examples in Radiology* Spring 05:6

(Do not report 77002 in conjunction with 73115)

73120   Radiologic examination, hand; 2 views

→ *CPT Assistant* Winter 90:9, Oct 18:11

73130   minimum of 3 views

→ *Clinical Examples in Radiology* Winter 05:9, Spring 11:8, Summer 21:8

73140   Radiologic examination, finger(s), minimum of 2 views

→ *CPT Assistant* Jan 07:29

→ *Clinical Examples in Radiology* Spring 11:8

73200   Computed tomography, upper extremity; without contrast material

→ *CPT Changes: An Insider's View* 2003

→ *CPT Assistant* Jul 11:17

→ *Clinical Examples in Radiology* Spring 22:13, 14

73201   with contrast material(s)

→ *CPT Assistant* Jul 11:17, Aug 15:6

→ *Clinical Examples in Radiology* Spring 09:6-7, Summer 18:14, Spring 22:13, 14

73202   without contrast material, followed by contrast material(s) and further sections

→ *Clinical Examples in Radiology* Spring 22:13, 14

(To report 3D rendering, see 76376, 76377)

73206   Computed tomographic angiography, upper extremity, with contrast material(s), including noncontrast images, if performed, and image postprocessing

→ *CPT Changes: An Insider's View* 2001, 2008

→ *CPT Assistant* Jul 01:5, Dec 05:7, Jan 07:31

73218   Magnetic resonance (eg, proton) imaging, upper extremity, other than joint; without contrast material(s)

→ *CPT Changes: An Insider's View* 2001

→ *CPT Assistant* Jul 01:7, Sep 10:10, Feb 11:9

→ *Clinical Examples in Radiology* Summer 13:9

73219   with contrast material(s)

→ *CPT Changes: An Insider's View* 2001

→ *CPT Assistant* Jul 01:7, Sep 10:10

→ *Clinical Examples in Radiology* Summer 13:9

73220   without contrast material(s), followed by contrast material(s) and further sequences

→ *CPT Changes: An Insider's View* 2001

→ *CPT Assistant* Jul 01:7, Sep 10:10

→ *Clinical Examples in Radiology* Summer 13:9

73221   Magnetic resonance (eg, proton) imaging, any joint of upper extremity; without contrast material(s)

→ *CPT Changes: An Insider's View* 2001

→ *CPT Assistant* Jul 01:7, Sep 10:10, Feb 11:9

→ *Clinical Examples in Radiology* Summer 13:9

73222   with contrast material(s)

→ *CPT Changes: An Insider's View* 2001

→ *CPT Assistant* Jul 01:7, Sep 10:10, Aug 15:6

→ *Clinical Examples in Radiology* Spring 05:5, Summer 13:9

73223   without contrast material(s), followed by contrast material(s) and further sequences

→ *CPT Changes: An Insider's View* 2001

→ *CPT Assistant* Jul 01:7, Sep 10:10

→ *Clinical Examples in Radiology* Spring 09:6, Summer 13:9

73225   Magnetic resonance angiography, upper extremity, with or without contrast material(s)

→ *CPT Assistant* Dec 05:7, Jan 07:31

→ *Clinical Examples in Radiology* Summer 13:9-10

Radiology 70010-79999

Lower Extremities

(For stress views, any joint, use 77071)

73501 Radiologic examination, hip, unilateral, with pelvis when performed; 1 view
- ➡ *CPT Changes: An Insider's View* 2016
- ➡ *CPT Assistant* Oct 15:9, Jun 16:9, Aug 16:7, Nov 16:10
- ➡ *Clinical Examples in Radiology* Fall 15:9, Spring 16:14, Summer 16:9, 13

73502 2-3 views
- ➡ *CPT Changes: An Insider's View* 2016
- ➡ *CPT Assistant* Oct 15:9, Jun 16:9, Aug 16:7, Nov 16:10
- ➡ *Clinical Examples in Radiology* Fall 15:9, Spring 16:14, Summer 16:8, 13

73503 minimum of 4 views
- ➡ *CPT Changes: An Insider's View* 2016
- ➡ *CPT Assistant* Oct 15:9, Jun 16:9, Aug 16:7, Nov 16:10
- ➡ *Clinical Examples in Radiology* Fall 15:9, Summer 16:9, 13

73521 Radiologic examination, hips, bilateral, with pelvis when performed; 2 views
- ➡ *CPT Changes: An Insider's View* 2016
- ➡ *CPT Assistant* Oct 15:9, Jun 16:9, Aug 16:7, Nov 16:10
- ➡ *Clinical Examples in Radiology* Fall 15:9, Winter 16:13, Summer 16:9, 13

73522 3-4 views
- ➡ *CPT Changes: An Insider's View* 2016
- ➡ *CPT Assistant* Oct 15:9, Jun 16:9, Aug 16:7, Nov 16:10
- ➡ *Clinical Examples in Radiology* Fall 15:8, Winter 16:13, Summer 16:9, 13

73523 minimum of 5 views
- ➡ *CPT Changes: An Insider's View* 2016
- ➡ *CPT Assistant* Oct 15:9, Jun 16:9, Aug 16:7, Nov 16:10
- ➡ *Clinical Examples in Radiology* Fall 15:9, Winter 16:13, Summer 16:9, 13

73525 Radiologic examination, hip, arthrography, radiological supervision and interpretation
- ➡ *CPT Assistant* Feb 07:11, Jun 12:14, Nov 16:10
- ➡ *Clinical Examples in Radiology* Spring 05:6, Spring 21:7

(Do not report 73525 in conjunction with 77002)

73551 Radiologic examination, femur; 1 view
- ➡ *CPT Changes: An Insider's View* 2016
- ➡ *CPT Assistant* Aug 16:7, Nov 16:10
- ➡ *Clinical Examples in Radiology* Fall 15:9, Summer 16:8

73552 minimum 2 views
- ➡ *CPT Changes: An Insider's View* 2016
- ➡ *CPT Assistant* Aug 16:7, Nov 16:10, Nov 17:10
- ➡ *Clinical Examples in Radiology* Fall 15:9

73560 Radiologic examination, knee; 1 or 2 views
- ➡ *CPT Assistant* Feb 15:10, May 15:10
- ➡ *Clinical Examples in Radiology* Winter 15:11, Fall 22:16

73562 3 views
- ➡ *CPT Assistant* Apr 02:15, Sep 21:14-15, Feb 22:15
- ➡ *Clinical Examples in Radiology* Fall 06:4, Fall 22:15

73564 complete, 4 or more views
- ➡ *CPT Assistant* Jun 98:11, Nov 98:21, Feb 15:10, May 15:10
- ➡ *Clinical Examples in Radiology* Fall 06:4, Winter 15:11, Fall 22:16

73565 both knees, standing, anteroposterior
- ➡ *CPT Assistant* Winter 90:9, Feb 15:10, May 15:10
- ➡ *Clinical Examples in Radiology* Fall 06:4, Winter 15:11

73580 Radiologic examination, knee, arthrography, radiological supervision and interpretation
- ➡ *CPT Assistant* Feb 07:11, Aug 15:6, Aug 19:7
- ➡ *Clinical Examples in Radiology* Spring 05:6, Winter 19:15

(Do not report 73580 in conjunction with 77002)

73590 Radiologic examination; tibia and fibula, 2 views
- ➡ *CPT Changes: An Insider's View* 2001
- ➡ *CPT Assistant* Sep 01:8, Nov 17:10

73592 lower extremity, infant, minimum of 2 views
- ➡ *CPT Assistant* Nov 17:10

73600 Radiologic examination, ankle; 2 views
- ➡ *CPT Changes: An Insider's View* 2001
- ➡ *CPT Assistant* Sep 01:8, Apr 02:15, Mar 03:9
- ➡ *Clinical Examples in Radiology* Winter 13:11

73610 complete, minimum of 3 views
- ➡ *CPT Assistant* Apr 02:15, Mar 03:9

73615 Radiologic examination, ankle, arthrography, radiological supervision and interpretation
- ➡ *CPT Assistant* Feb 07:11

(Do not report 73615 in conjunction with 77002)

73620 Radiologic examination, foot; 2 views
- ➡ *CPT Changes: An Insider's View* 2001
- ➡ *CPT Assistant* Sep 01:8, Apr 02:15, Mar 03:9
- ➡ *Clinical Examples in Radiology* Summer 18:6

73630 complete, minimum of 3 views
- ➡ *Clinical Examples in Radiology* Summer 07:12, Summer 18:6, Summer 21:8

73650 Radiologic examination; calcaneus, minimum of 2 views
- ➡ *Clinical Examples in Radiology* Summer 18:6, Summer 21:8

73660 toe(s), minimum of 2 views
- ➡ *Clinical Examples in Radiology* Summer 18:6

73700 Computed tomography, lower extremity; without contrast material
- ➡ *CPT Changes: An Insider's View* 2003
- ➡ *CPT Assistant* Mar 07:10, Jul 11:17
- ➡ *Clinical Examples in Radiology* Fall 08:10, Fall 10:6, Fall 19:11, Spring 22:13, 14

Radiology 70010-79999

548   ★=Telemedicine   ◀=Audio-only   ✚=Add-on code   ✗=FDA approval pending   #=Resequenced code   ⊘=Modifier 51 exempt   ➡➡➡=See p xxi for details

73701   with contrast material(s)

➜ *CPT Assistant* Mar 07:10, Jul 11:17, Aug 19:7

➜ *Clinical Examples in Radiology* Summer 10:10, Summer 18:12, Winter 19:14, Spring 22:13, 14

73702   without contrast material, followed by contrast material(s) and further sections

➜ *CPT Assistant* Mar 07:10, Jul 11:17, Aug 19:7

➜ *Clinical Examples in Radiology* Winter 19:14, Spring 22:13, 14

(To report 3D rendering, see 76376, 76377)

73706   Computed tomographic angiography, lower extremity, with contrast material(s), including noncontrast images, if performed, and image postprocessing

➜ *CPT Changes: An Insider's View* 2001, 2008

➜ *CPT Assistant* Jul 01:5-6, Dec 05:7, Jan 07:31, Apr 08:11, Apr 11:13

➜ *Clinical Examples in Radiology* Summer 08:8

(For CTA aorto-iliofemoral runoff, use 75635)

(For noninvasive arterial plaque analysis using software processing of data from computerized tomography angiography to quantify structure and composition of the vessel wall, including assessment for lipid-rich necrotic core plaque, see 0710T, 0711T, 0712T, 0713T)

73718   Magnetic resonance (eg, proton) imaging, lower extremity other than joint; without contrast material(s)

➜ *CPT Changes: An Insider's View* 2001

➜ *CPT Assistant* Jul 01:3

➜ *Clinical Examples in Radiology* Spring 07:7, 9, 12, Summer 07:4-5

73719   with contrast material(s)

➜ *CPT Changes: An Insider's View* 2001

➜ *CPT Assistant* Jul 01:3, Aug 19:7

➜ *Clinical Examples in Radiology* Spring 07:7, 9, 12, Summer 07:4-5

73720   without contrast material(s), followed by contrast material(s) and further sequences

➜ *CPT Changes: An Insider's View* 2001

➜ *CPT Assistant* Jul 01:3, Aug 19:7

➜ *Clinical Examples in Radiology* Spring 07:7, 9, 12, Summer 07:4-5

73721   Magnetic resonance (eg, proton) imaging, any joint of lower extremity; without contrast material

➜ *CPT Changes: An Insider's View* 2001

➜ *CPT Assistant* Jul 01:3, Jun 06:17

➜ *Clinical Examples in Radiology* Spring 07:7, 9, 12, Summer 07:4-5, Fall 18:11

73722   with contrast material(s)

➜ *CPT Changes: An Insider's View* 2001

➜ *CPT Assistant* Jul 01:3, Jun 06:17, Aug 15:6

➜ *Clinical Examples in Radiology* Spring 07:7, 9, 12, Summer 07:4-5, Spring 13:11, Winter 19:15, Spring 21:7

73723   without contrast material(s), followed by contrast material(s) and further sequences

➜ *CPT Changes: An Insider's View* 2001

➜ *CPT Assistant* Jul 01:3

➜ *Clinical Examples in Radiology* Spring 07:7, 9, 12, Summer 07:4-5, Winter 19:14, Spring 21:7

73725   Magnetic resonance angiography, lower extremity, with or without contrast material(s)

➜ *CPT Assistant* Dec 05:7, Jan 07:31

➜ *Clinical Examples in Radiology* Spring 06:1, 3

Abdomen

74018   Radiologic examination, abdomen; 1 view

➜ *CPT Changes: An Insider's View* 2018

➜ *CPT Assistant* Apr 18:7, May 19:10, Apr 20:11, Feb 21:13

➜ *Clinical Examples in Radiology* Summer 18:13, Spring 19:12, Summer 19:14, Summer 20:14, Winter 22:16

74019   2 views

➜ *CPT Changes: An Insider's View* 2018

➜ *CPT Assistant* Apr 18:7

➜ *Clinical Examples in Radiology* Summer 18:13, Spring 19:12, Summer 19:14, Summer 20:14, Winter 22:16

74021   3 or more views

➜ *CPT Changes: An Insider's View* 2018

➜ *CPT Assistant* Apr 18:7

➜ *Clinical Examples in Radiology* Summer 18:13, Summer 19:14, Summer 20:14

74022   Radiologic examination, complete acute abdomen series, including 2 or more views of the abdomen (eg, supine, erect, decubitus), and a single view chest

➜ *CPT Changes: An Insider's View* 2003, 2020

➜ *CPT Assistant* May 19:10

➜ *Clinical Examples in Radiology* Summer 19:14

74150   Computed tomography, abdomen; without contrast material

➜ *CPT Changes: An Insider's View* 2003

➜ *CPT Assistant* Oct 02:12, Mar 05:1, 4, Apr 10:9, Nov 11:6, Oct 12:12

➜ *Clinical Examples in Radiology* Spring 07:3, 11, Fall 08:7, Fall 09:9, Winter 11:8-9, Fall 11:8, Spring 16:9, Summer 20:7

74160   with contrast material(s)

➜ *CPT Assistant* Mar 05:1, 4, Apr 10:9, Nov 11:6, Oct 12:12

➜ *Clinical Examples in Radiology* Spring 07:3, 11, Fall 08:7, Summer 10:10, Winter 11:8-9, Fall 11:8, Spring 16:9, Summer 20:7

74170   without contrast material, followed by contrast material(s) and further sections

➜ *CPT Assistant* Mar 05:4, Apr 10:9, Nov 11:6, Oct 12:12

➜ *Clinical Examples in Radiology* Winter 05:1, 7-8, 12, Spring 07:3, 11, Fall 08:7, Winter 11:8-9, Fall 11:8, Spring 16:10, Summer 20:7

(For a combined CT abdomen and pelvis study, see 74176-74178)

(To report 3D rendering, see 76376, 76377)

Radiology 70010-79999

(For computed tomographic colonography, diagnostic, see 74261-74262. For computed tomographic colonography, screening, use 74263)

(Do not report 74150-74170 in conjunction with 74261-74263)

74174 Computed tomographic angiography, abdomen and pelvis, with contrast material(s), including noncontrast images, if performed, and image postprocessing

→ *CPT Changes: An Insider's View* 2012

→ *Clinical Examples in Radiology* Fall 11:8, Spring 17:7, Spring 20:13

(Do not report 74174 in conjunction with 72191, 73706, 74175, 75635, 76376, 76377)

(For CTA aorto-iliofemoral runoff, use 75635)

74175 Computed tomographic angiography, abdomen, with contrast material(s), including noncontrast images, if performed, and image postprocessing

→ *CPT Changes: An Insider's View* 2001, 2008

→ *CPT Assistant* Jul 01:6, Dec 05:7, Jan 07:31, Apr 11:13

→ *Clinical Examples in Radiology* Summer 08:8, Fall 09:10, Fall 11:8

(Do not report 74175 in conjunction with 73706 or 75635. For CTA aorto-iliofemoral runoff, use 75635)

(Do not report 74175 in conjunction with 72191. For a combined computed tomographic angiography abdomen and pelvis study, use 74174)

(For noninvasive arterial plaque analysis using software processing of data from computerized tomography angiography to quantify structure and composition of the vessel wall, including assessment for lipid-rich necrotic core plaque, see 0710T, 0711T, 0712T, 0713T)

For combinations of CT of the abdomen with CT of the pelvis performed at the same session, use the following table. Do not report more than one CT of the abdomen or CT of the pelvis for any session.

Stand Alone Code	74150 CT Abdomen WO Contrast	74160 CT Abdomen W Contrast	74170 CT Abdomen WO/W Contrast
72192 CT Pelvis WO Contrast	74176	74178	74178
72193 CT Pelvis W Contrast	74178	74177	74178
72194 CT Pelvis WO/W Contrast	74178	74178	74178

74176 Computed tomography, abdomen and pelvis; without contrast material

→ *CPT Changes: An Insider's View* 2011

→ *CPT Assistant* Nov 11:6

→ *Clinical Examples in Radiology* Winter 11:9, Fall 11:8, Spring 16:10, Spring 17:7, Spring 20:13

74177 with contrast material(s)

→ *CPT Changes: An Insider's View* 2011

→ *CPT Assistant* Nov 11:6

→ *Clinical Examples in Radiology* Winter 11:9, Fall 11:8, Spring 16:10, Spring 17:7

74178 without contrast material in one or both body regions, followed by contrast material(s) and further sections in one or both body regions

→ *CPT Changes: An Insider's View* 2011

→ *CPT Assistant* Nov 11:6

→ *Clinical Examples in Radiology* Winter 11:8, Fall 11:8, Spring 16:10, Spring 17:7, Summer 20:7

(Do not report 74176-74178 in conjunction with 72192-72194, 74150-74170)

(Report 74176, 74177, or 74178 only once per CT abdomen and pelvis examination)

74181 Magnetic resonance (eg, proton) imaging, abdomen; without contrast material(s)

→ *CPT Changes: An Insider's View* 2001

→ *CPT Assistant* Jul 01:3, Nov 07:9, May 09:9, Jul 09:10, Mar 18:11

→ *Clinical Examples in Radiology* Fall 07:3, Spring 09:4, Summer 22:7, Fall 22:17

74182 with contrast material(s)

→ *CPT Changes: An Insider's View* 2001

→ *CPT Assistant* Jul 01:3, May 09:9, Jul 09:10, Mar 18:11

→ *Clinical Examples in Radiology* Winter 21:12, Summer 22:7, Winter 23:19

74183 without contrast material(s), followed by with contrast material(s) and further sequences

→ *CPT Changes: An Insider's View* 2001

→ *CPT Assistant* Jul 01:3, May 09:9, Jul 09:10, Mar 18:11, Apr 21:14

→ *Clinical Examples in Radiology* Winter 21:12, Summer 21:6, Winter 22:6, Summer 22:7, Winter 23:19

74185 Magnetic resonance angiography, abdomen, with or without contrast material(s)

→ *CPT Assistant* Dec 05:7, Jan 07:31

→ *Clinical Examples in Radiology* Spring 06:1, 3

74190 Peritoneogram (eg, after injection of air or contrast), radiological supervision and interpretation

→ *CPT Assistant* Dec 10:13

→ *Clinical Examples in Radiology* Fall 07:1-2

(For procedure, use 49400)

(For computed tomography, see 72192 or 74150)

Radiology 70010-79999

550 ★=Telemedicine ◀=Audio-only ✚=Add-on code ✔=FDA approval pending #=Resequenced code ⊘=Modifier 51 exempt ➲➲➲=See p xxi for details

Gastrointestinal Tract

(For percutaneous placement of gastrostomy tube, use 43246)

74210 Radiologic examination, pharynx and/or cervical esophagus, including scout neck radiograph(s) and delayed image(s), when performed, contrast (eg, barium) study
➜ *CPT Changes: An Insider's View* 2020
➜ *CPT Assistant* Aug 20:9
➜ *Clinical Examples in Radiology* Fall 19:4, Summer 20:4

74220 Radiologic examination, esophagus, including scout chest radiograph(s) and delayed image(s), when performed; single-contrast (eg, barium) study
➜ *CPT Changes: An Insider's View* 2020
➜ *CPT Assistant* Aug 20:9
➜ *Clinical Examples in Radiology* Spring 18:15, Fall 19:4, Summer 20:4

(Do not report 74220 in conjunction with 74221, 74240, 74246, 74248)

74221 double-contrast (eg, high-density barium and effervescent agent) study
➜ *CPT Changes: An Insider's View* 2020
➜ *Clinical Examples in Radiology* Fall 19:4, Summer 20:4

(Do not report 74221 in conjunction with 74220, 74240, 74246, 74248)

74230 Radiologic examination, swallowing function, with cineradiography/videoradiography, including scout neck radiograph(s) and delayed image(s), when performed, contrast (eg, barium) study
➜ *CPT Changes: An Insider's View* 2002, 2020
➜ *CPT Assistant* Dec 04:17, Jul 14:5, Aug 20:9
➜ *Clinical Examples in Radiology* Summer 06:4-5, Spring 18:14, Fall 19:4, Summer 20:4

(For otorhinolaryngologic services fluoroscopic evaluation of swallowing function, use 92611)

74235 Removal of foreign body(s), esophageal, with use of balloon catheter, radiological supervision and interpretation

(For procedure, use 43499)

74240 Radiologic examination, upper gastrointestinal tract, including scout abdominal radiograph(s) and delayed image(s), when performed; single-contrast (eg, barium) study
➜ *CPT Changes: An Insider's View* 2016, 2020
➜ *CPT Assistant* Sep 16:7, Aug 20:9
➜ *Clinical Examples in Radiology* Fall 19:3, Summer 20:4

(Do not report 74240 in conjunction with 74220, 74221, 74246)

74246 double-contrast (eg, high-density barium and effervescent agent) study, including glucagon, when administered
➜ *CPT Changes: An Insider's View* 2016, 2020
➜ *CPT Assistant* Sep 16:7, Aug 20:9
➜ *Clinical Examples in Radiology* Fall 19:4, Summer 20:4

(Do not report 74246 in conjunction with 74220, 74221, 74240)

+ 74248 Radiologic small intestine follow-through study, including multiple serial images (List separately in addition to code for primary procedure for upper GI radiologic examination)
➜ *CPT Changes: An Insider's View* 2020
➜ *Clinical Examples in Radiology* Fall 19:4, Summer 20:4

(Use 74248 in conjunction with 74240, 74246)

(Do not report 74248 in conjunction with 74250, 74251)

74250 Radiologic examination, small intestine, including multiple serial images and scout abdominal radiograph(s), when performed; single-contrast (eg, barium) study
➜ *CPT Changes: An Insider's View* 2002, 2016, 2020
➜ *CPT Assistant* Sep 16:7, Aug 20:9, Feb 21:13
➜ *Clinical Examples in Radiology* Fall 19:4, Summer 20:4

(Do not report 74250 in conjunction with 74248, 74251)

74251 double-contrast (eg, high-density barium and air via enteroclysis tube) study, including glucagon, when administered
➜ *CPT Changes: An Insider's View* 2016, 2020
➜ *CPT Assistant* Sep 16:7, Aug 20:9
➜ *Clinical Examples in Radiology* Fall 19:4, Summer 20:4

(For placement of enteroclysis tube, see 44500, 74340)

(Do not report 74251 in conjunction with 74248, 74250)

74261 Computed tomographic (CT) colonography, diagnostic, including image postprocessing; without contrast material
➜ *CPT Changes: An Insider's View* 2010
➜ *CPT Assistant* Apr 10:9, Feb 20:13
➜ *Clinical Examples in Radiology* Winter 10:6, Spring 20:12, Spring 23:4

74262 with contrast material(s) including non-contrast images, if performed
➜ *CPT Changes: An Insider's View* 2010
➜ *CPT Assistant* Apr 10:9, Feb 20:13
➜ *Clinical Examples in Radiology* Winter 10:4, 6, Spring 20:12, Spring 23:4

(Do not report 74261, 74262 in conjunction with 72192-72194, 74150-74170, 74263, 76376, 76377)

74263 Computed tomographic (CT) colonography, screening, including image postprocessing
➜ *CPT Changes: An Insider's View* 2010
➜ *CPT Assistant* Apr 10:9, Feb 20:13
➜ *Clinical Examples in Radiology* Winter 10:6, Spring 20:12, Spring 23:4

(Do not report 74263 in conjunction with 72192-72194, 74150-74170, 74261, 74262, 76376, 76377)

Radiology 70010-79999

74270 Radiologic examination, colon, including scout abdominal radiograph(s) and delayed image(s), when performed; single-contrast (eg, barium) study

➔ *CPT Changes: An Insider's View* 2009, 2020

➔ *CPT Assistant* May 03:19, Aug 20:9

➔ *Clinical Examples in Radiology* Fall 19:4, Summer 20:4

(Do not report 74270 in conjunction with 74280)

74280 double-contrast (eg, high density barium and air) study, including glucagon, when administered

➔ *CPT Changes: An Insider's View* 2020

➔ *CPT Assistant* Aug 20:9

➔ *Clinical Examples in Radiology* Fall 19:4, Summer 20:4

(Do not report 74280 in conjunction with 74270)

74283 Therapeutic enema, contrast or air, for reduction of intussusception or other intraluminal obstruction (eg, meconium ileus)

➔ *CPT Assistant* Nov 97:24

➔ *Clinical Examples in Radiology* Spring 13:9

74290 Cholecystography, oral contrast

74300 Cholangiography and/or pancreatography; intraoperative, radiological supervision and interpretation

➔ *CPT Changes: An Insider's View* 2000

➔ *CPT Assistant* Nov 99:41, Dec 00:14

+ 74301 additional set intraoperative, radiological supervision and interpretation (List separately in addition to code for primary procedure)

(Use 74301 in conjunction with 74300)

74328 Endoscopic catheterization of the biliary ductal system, radiological supervision and interpretation

(For procedure, see 43260-43278 as appropriate)

74329 Endoscopic catheterization of the pancreatic ductal system, radiological supervision and interpretation

(For procedure, see 43260-43278 as appropriate)

74330 Combined endoscopic catheterization of the biliary and pancreatic ductal systems, radiological supervision and interpretation

(For procedure, see 43260-43278 as appropriate)

74340 Introduction of long gastrointestinal tube (eg, Miller-Abbott), including multiple fluoroscopies and images, radiological supervision and interpretation

➔ *CPT Changes: An Insider's View* 2016

➔ *CPT Assistant* Sep 16:9

(For tube placement, use 44500)

74355 Percutaneous placement of enteroclysis tube, radiological supervision and interpretation

➔ *CPT Assistant* Feb 07:11, Nov 10:3, Jan 11:8

74360 Intraluminal dilation of strictures and/or obstructions (eg, esophagus), radiological supervision and interpretation

➔ *CPT Assistant* Spring 94:3, Oct 08:6

(Do not report 74360 in conjunction with 43213, 43214, 43233)

74363 Percutaneous transhepatic dilation of biliary duct stricture with or without placement of stent, radiological supervision and interpretation

➔ *CPT Changes: An Insider's View* 2002

(For procedure, see 47555, 47556)

Urinary Tract

74400 Urography (pyelography), intravenous, with or without KUB, with or without tomography

74410 Urography, infusion, drip technique and/or bolus technique;

74415 with nephrotomography

74420 Urography, retrograde, with or without KUB

➔ *CPT Assistant* Sep 00:11, Dec 10:15

74425 Urography, antegrade, radiological supervision and interpretation

➔ *CPT Changes: An Insider's View* 2021

➔ *CPT Assistant* Fall 93:14, Dec 97:7, Oct 05:18

➔ *Clinical Examples in Radiology* Summer 06:1, 3, Fall 15:2, Spring 16:12, Fall 20:12

(Use 74425 in conjunction with 50390, 50396, 50684, 50690)

(Do not report 74425 in conjunction with 50430, 50431, 50432, 50433, 50434, 50435, 50693, 50694, 50695)

74430 Cystography, minimum of 3 views, radiological supervision and interpretation

➔ *Clinical Examples in Radiology* Summer 19:11, Winter 21:3

74440 Vasography, vesiculography, or epididymography, radiological supervision and interpretation

74445 Corpora cavernosography, radiological supervision and interpretation

➔ *CPT Assistant* Feb 07:11, Nov 10:3, Jan 11:8

74450 Urethrocystography, retrograde, radiological supervision and interpretation

➔ *CPT Assistant* Oct 19:11, Dec 23:41, Feb 24:21

74455 Urethrocystography, voiding, radiological supervision and interpretation

➔ *CPT Assistant* Oct 19:11

➔ *Clinical Examples in Radiology* Summer 19:11

74470 Radiologic examination, renal cyst study, translumbar, contrast visualization, radiological supervision and interpretation

➔ *CPT Assistant* Oct 05:18, Feb 07:11, Nov 10:3, Jan 11:8

★ = Telemedicine ◀ = Audio-only + = Add-on code ⊁ = FDA approval pending # = Resequenced code ⦸ = Modifier 51 exempt ➔➔➔ = See p xxi for details

74485 Dilation of ureter(s) or urethra, radiological supervision and interpretation

➜ *CPT Changes: An Insider's View* 2019
➜ *CPT Assistant* Oct 05:18, Dec 08:7, Jan 09:7, Oct 15:5
➜ *Clinical Examples in Radiology* Summer 06:1, 3, Winter 19:6

(Do not report 74485 in conjunction with 50436, 50437)

(For dilation of ureter without radiologic guidance, use 52341, 52344)

(For change of nephrostomy or pyelostomy tube, use 50435)

(For dilation of a nephrostomy tract for endourologic procedure, see 50436, 50437)

Gynecological and Obstetrical

(For abdomen and pelvis, see 72170-72190, 74018, 74019, 74021, 74022, 74150, 74160, 74170)

(74710 has been deleted)

74712 Magnetic resonance (eg, proton) imaging, fetal, including placental and maternal pelvic imaging when performed; single or first gestation

➜ *CPT Changes: An Insider's View* 2016
➜ *CPT Assistant* Jun 16:5
➜ *Clinical Examples in Radiology* Winter 16:12

+ 74713 each additional gestation (List separately in addition to code for primary procedure)

➜ *CPT Changes: An Insider's View* 2016
➜ *CPT Assistant* Jun 16:5
➜ *Clinical Examples in Radiology* Winter 16:12

(Use 74713 in conjunction with 74712)

(Do not report 74712, 74713 in conjunction with 72195, 72196, 72197)

(If only placenta or maternal pelvis is imaged without fetal imaging, see 72195, 72196, 72197)

74740 Hysterosalpingography, radiological supervision and interpretation

➜ *CPT Assistant* Nov 97:24, Jul 99:8, Mar 09:11
➜ *Clinical Examples in Radiology* Spring 23:32

(For introduction of saline or contrast for hysterosalpingography, see 58340)

74742 Transcervical catheterization of fallopian tube, radiological supervision and interpretation

(For procedure, use 58345)

74775 Perineogram (eg, vaginogram, for sex determination or extent of anomalies)

Heart

Cardiac magnetic imaging differs from traditional magnetic resonance imaging (MRI) in its ability to provide a physiologic evaluation of cardiac function. Traditional MRI relies on static images to obtain clinical diagnoses based upon anatomic information.

Improvement in spatial and temporal resolution has expanded the application from an anatomic test and includes physiologic evaluation of cardiac function. Flow and velocity assessment for valves and intracardiac shunts is performed in addition to a function and morphologic evaluation. Use 75559 with 75565 to report flow with pharmacologic wall motion stress evaluation without contrast. Use 75563 with 75565 to report flow with pharmacologic perfusion stress with contrast.

Cardiac MRI for velocity flow mapping can be reported in conjunction with 75557, 75559, 75561, or 75563.

▶Listed procedures may be performed independently or in the course of overall medical care. If the individual providing these services is also responsible for diagnostic workup and/or follow-up care of the patient, also see appropriate sections. Only one procedure in the series 75557-75563 is appropriately reported per session.

To report absolute quantitation of myocardial blood flow (AQMBF), cardiac magnetic resonance (CMR), see 0899T, 0900T. Report 0899T, 0900T in conjunction with code for primary procedure.◀

Cardiac MRI studies may be performed at rest and/or during pharmacologic stress. Therefore, the appropriate stress testing code from the 93015-93018 series should be reported in addition to 75559 or 75563.

Cardiac computed tomography (CT) and coronary computed tomographic angiography (CTA) include the axial source images of the pre-contrast, arterial phase sequence, and venous phase sequence (if performed), as well as the two-dimensional and three-dimensional reformatted images resulting from the study, including cine review. Each of the contrast enhanced cardiac CT and coronary CTA codes (75572, 75573, 75574) includes conventional quantitative assessment(s) intrinsic to the service listed in the code descriptor (ie, quantification of coronary percentage stenosis, ventricular volume[s], ejection fraction[s], and stroke volume[s]), when performed. Report only one computed tomography heart service per encounter (75571, 75572, 75573, 75574).

(For separate injection procedures for vascular radiology, see **Surgery** section, 36000-36299)

(For cardiac catheterization procedures, see 93451-93572)

75557 Cardiac magnetic resonance imaging for morphology and function without contrast material;

➜ *CPT Changes: An Insider's View* 2008
➜ *CPT Assistant* Jul 10:7
➜ *Clinical Examples in Radiology* Spring 09:2, Fall 22:17, Winter 24:32

75559   with stress imaging
→ *CPT Changes: An Insider's View* 2008
→ *CPT Assistant* Jul 10:7
→ *Clinical Examples in Radiology* Spring 09:2, Winter 24:32

75561   Cardiac magnetic resonance imaging for morphology and function without contrast material(s), followed by contrast material(s) and further sequences;
→ *CPT Changes: An Insider's View* 2008
→ *CPT Assistant* Jul 10:7
→ *Clinical Examples in Radiology* Spring 09:2, Spring 16:13, Spring 17:14, Summer 23:4, Winter 24:32

75563   with stress imaging
→ *CPT Changes: An Insider's View* 2008
→ *CPT Assistant* Jul 10:7
→ *Clinical Examples in Radiology* Spring 09:2, Winter 24:32

▶(Use 75563 in conjunction with 0899T, 0900T for absolute quantification of myocardial blood flow [AQMBF] with cardiac magnetic resonance [CMR])◀

+ 75565   Cardiac magnetic resonance imaging for velocity flow mapping (List separately in addition to code for primary procedure)
→ *CPT Changes: An Insider's View* 2010
→ *CPT Assistant* Jul 10:7
→ *Clinical Examples in Radiology* Summer 23:4, Winter 24:32

(Use 75565 in conjunction with 75557, 75559, 75561, 75563)

(Do not report 75557, 75559, 75561, 75563, 75565 in conjunction with 76376, 76377)

75571   Computed tomography, heart, without contrast material, with quantitative evaluation of coronary calcium
→ *CPT Changes: An Insider's View* 2010
→ *CPT Assistant* Jul 10:7, Jul 20:5
→ *Clinical Examples in Radiology* Winter 10:2-3

75572   Computed tomography, heart, with contrast material, for evaluation of cardiac structure and morphology (including 3D image postprocessing, assessment of cardiac function, and evaluation of venous structures, if performed)
→ *CPT Changes: An Insider's View* 2010
→ *CPT Assistant* Jul 10:7, Oct 21:3
→ *Clinical Examples in Radiology* Winter 10:2-3, Spring 16:13

75573   Computed tomography, heart, with contrast material, for evaluation of cardiac structure and morphology in the setting of congenital heart disease (including 3D image postprocessing, assessment of left ventricular [LV] cardiac function, right ventricular [RV] structure and function and evaluation of vascular structures, if performed)
→ *CPT Changes: An Insider's View* 2010, 2022
→ *CPT Assistant* Jul 10:7, Oct 21:3
→ *Clinical Examples in Radiology* Winter 10:2-3

75574   Computed tomographic angiography, heart, coronary arteries and bypass grafts (when present), with contrast material, including 3D image postprocessing (including

evaluation of cardiac structure and morphology, assessment of cardiac function, and evaluation of venous structures, if performed)
→ *CPT Changes: An Insider's View* 2010
→ *CPT Assistant* Jul 10:7, Oct 21:3, Mar 24:14
→ *Clinical Examples in Radiology* Winter 10:1, 3, Spring 21:11, Winter 22:10-12

(For noninvasive estimate of coronary fractional flow reserve [FFR] derived from augmentative software analysis of the data set from a coronary computed tomography angiography with interpretation and report by a physician or other qualified health care professional, use 75580)

(For automated quantification and characterization of coronary atherosclerotic plaque, see 0623T, 0624T, 0625T, 0626T)

75580   Noninvasive estimate of coronary fractional flow reserve (FFR) derived from augmentative software analysis of the data set from a coronary computed tomography angiography, with interpretation and report by a physician or other qualified health care professional
→ *CPT Changes: An Insider's View* 2024
→ *CPT Assistant* Mar 24:14

(Use 75580 only once per coronary computed tomography angiogram)

(When noninvasive estimate of coronary FFR derived from augmentative software analysis of the data set from a coronary computed tomography angiography with interpretation and report by a physician or other qualified health care professional is performed on the same day as the coronary computed tomography angiography, use 75580 in conjunction with 75574)

Vascular Procedures

Aorta and Arteries

Selective vascular catheterizations should be coded to include introduction and all lesser order selective catheterizations used in the approach (eg, the description for a selective right middle cerebral artery catheterization includes the introduction and placement catheterization of the right common and internal carotid arteries).

Additional second and/or third order arterial catheterizations within the same family of arteries supplied by a single first order artery should be expressed by 36218 or 36248. Additional first order or higher catheterizations in vascular families supplied by a first order vessel different from a previously selected and coded family should be separately coded using the conventions described above.

Radiology 70010-79999

554   ★=Telemedicine   ◀=Audio-only   +=Add-on code   ✔=FDA approval pending   #=Resequenced code   ⊘=Modifier 51 exempt   →→→=See p xxi for details

The lower extremity endovascular revascularization codes describing services performed for occlusive disease (37220-37235) include catheterization (36200, 36140, 36245-36248) in the work described by the codes. Catheterization codes are not additionally reported for diagnostic lower extremity angiography when performed through the same access site as the therapy (37220-37235) performed in the same session. However, catheterization for the diagnostic lower extremity angiogram may be reported separately if a different arterial puncture site is necessary.

For angiography performed in conjunction with therapeutic transcatheter radiological supervision and interpretation services, see the radiology **Transcatheter Procedures** guidelines.

Diagnostic angiography (radiological supervision and interpretation) codes should NOT be used with interventional procedures for:

1. Contrast injections, angiography, roadmapping, and/or fluoroscopic guidance for the intervention,

2. Vessel measurement, and

3. Post-angioplasty/stent/atherectomy angiography, as this work is captured in the radiological supervision and interpretation code(s). In those therapeutic codes that include radiological supervision and interpretation, this work is captured in the therapeutic code.

Diagnostic angiography performed at the time of an interventional procedure is separately reportable if:

1. No prior catheter-based angiographic study is available and a full diagnostic study is performed, and the decision to intervene is based on the diagnostic study, OR

2. A prior study is available, but as documented in the medical record:

   a. The patient's condition with respect to the clinical indication has changed since the prior study, OR

   b. There is inadequate visualization of the anatomy and/or pathology, OR

   c. There is a clinical change during the procedure that requires new evaluation outside the target area of intervention.

►Diagnostic angiography performed at a separate session from an interventional procedure is separately reported.◄

If diagnostic angiography is necessary, is performed at the same session as the interventional procedure and meets the above criteria, modifier 59 must be appended to the diagnostic radiological supervision and interpretation code(s) to denote that diagnostic work has been done following these guidelines.

Diagnostic angiography performed at the time of an interventional procedure is NOT separately reportable if it is specifically included in the interventional code descriptor.

►Add-on code 75774 may be used with both arteries and veins for each additional vessel.◄

(For intravenous procedure, see 36000, 36005-36015, and for intra-arterial procedure, see 36100-36248)

(For radiological supervision and interpretation, see 75600-75893)

75600   Aortography, thoracic, without serialography, radiological supervision and interpretation

(For supravalvular aortography performed at the time of cardiac catheterization, use 93567, which includes imaging supervision, interpretation, and report)

75605   Aortography, thoracic, by serialography, radiological supervision and interpretation
➜ *CPT Assistant* Spring 94:29, Dec 98:9, Jan 13:6
➜ *Clinical Examples in Radiology* Spring 13:4-6

(For supravalvular aortography performed at the time of cardiac catheterization, use 93567, which includes imaging supervision, interpretation, and report)

75625   Aortography, abdominal, by serialography, radiological supervision and interpretation
➜ *CPT Assistant* Fall 93:16, Jan 01:14, Dec 07:14, Apr 08:11, Dec 09:13, Jan 13:6, Feb 13:16, Sep 20:14
➜ *Clinical Examples in Radiology* Winter 08:1-2, 4-5, 9, Spring 13:11

75630   Aortography, abdominal plus bilateral iliofemoral lower extremity, catheter, by serialography, radiological supervision and interpretation
➜ *CPT Assistant* Fall 93:16, Jan 01:14, Apr 08:11, Dec 09:13, Sep 20:14
➜ *Clinical Examples in Radiology* Winter 14:5, 7

75635   Computed tomographic angiography, abdominal aorta and bilateral iliofemoral lower extremity runoff, with contrast material(s), including noncontrast images, if performed, and image postprocessing
➜ *CPT Changes: An Insider's View* 2001, 2008
➜ *CPT Assistant* Jul 01:4-5, Dec 05:7, Jan 07:31, Apr 11:13
➜ *Clinical Examples in Radiology* Spring 06:1, 3, Summer 08:7-8, Summer 10:10, Summer 18:12

(Do not report 75635 in conjunction with 72191, 73706, 74174 or 74175)

(For noninvasive arterial plaque analysis using software processing of data from computerized tomography angiography to quantify structure and composition of the vessel wall, including assessment for lipid-rich necrotic core plaque, see 0710T, 0711T, 0712T, 0713T)

Aortography
75600-75630

A radiographic contrast study is performed on the abdominal or thoracic aorta.

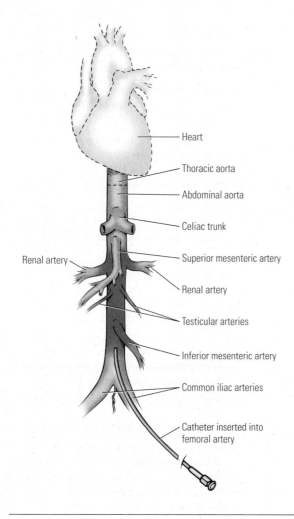

Heart

Thoracic aorta

Abdominal aorta

Celiac trunk

Superior mesenteric artery

Renal artery

Renal artery

Testicular arteries

Inferior mesenteric artery

Common iliac arteries

Catheter inserted into femoral artery

75705 Angiography, spinal, selective, radiological supervision and interpretation

➔ *Clinical Examples in Radiology* Winter 18:2

75710 Angiography, extremity, unilateral, radiological supervision and interpretation

➔ *CPT Assistant* Apr 99:11, Jan 01:14, Mar 17:4, Jul 21:4

➔ *Clinical Examples in Radiology* Winter 11:1, Spring 11:1, Spring 12:4

(Do not report 75710 in conjunction with 36836, 36837)

75716 Angiography, extremity, bilateral, radiological supervision and interpretation

➔ *CPT Assistant* Fall 93:16, Jan 01:14, Dec 07:14, Apr 08:11, Dec 09:13, Sep 20:14

➔ *Clinical Examples in Radiology* Winter 08:1-2, 4-5, 9, Winter 13:1-3, Spring 13:5-6

(Do not report 75716 in conjunction with 36836, 36837)

75726 Angiography, visceral, selective or supraselective (with or without flush aortogram), radiological supervision and interpretation

➔ *Clinical Examples in Radiology* Summer 08:1-3, Fall 13:2-3, 5, Summer 15:2, Winter 18:11, Summer 18:2, Spring 19:2

(For selective angiography, each additional visceral vessel studied after basic examination, use 75774)

75731 Angiography, adrenal, unilateral, selective, radiological supervision and interpretation

➔ *Clinical Examples in Radiology* Spring 19:2

75733 Angiography, adrenal, bilateral, selective, radiological supervision and interpretation

75736 Angiography, pelvic, selective or supraselective, radiological supervision and interpretation

➔ *Clinical Examples in Radiology* Spring 05:14, Winter 08:4-5, Winter 14:1, 3, Summer 19:4

75741 Angiography, pulmonary, unilateral, selective, radiological supervision and interpretation

➔ *CPT Assistant* Mar 12:10, Jan 13:6, Jun 19:3

➔ *Clinical Examples in Radiology* Spring 13:1-2

75743 Angiography, pulmonary, bilateral, selective, radiological supervision and interpretation

➔ *CPT Assistant* Spring 94:29, Apr 98:7, Jan 13:6, Jun 19:3, May 23:1

➔ *Clinical Examples in Radiology* Summer 12:1-2, Winter 23:8

(For selective pulmonary arterial angiography during cardiac catheterization, see 93569, 93573)

(For selective pulmonary venous angiography during cardiac catheterization, each distinct vein, use 93574)

(For selective pulmonary angiography of major aortopulmonary collateral arteries [MAPCAs] arising off the aorta or its systemic branches, use 93575)

75746 Angiography, pulmonary, by nonselective catheter or venous injection, radiological supervision and interpretation

➔ *CPT Assistant* Jun 19:3, May 23:1

(For nonselective pulmonary arterial angiography by catheter injection performed at the time of cardiac catheterization, use 93568, which includes imaging supervision, interpretation, and report)

75756 Angiography, internal mammary, radiological supervision and interpretation

(For internal mammary angiography performed at the time of cardiac catheterization, see 93455, 93457, 93459, 93461, 93564, which include imaging supervision, interpretation, and report)

+ 75774   Angiography, selective, each additional vessel studied after basic examination, radiological supervision and interpretation (List separately in addition to code for primary procedure)

➔ *CPT Assistant* Fall 93:17, Spring 94:29, Apr 11:13, Feb 13:17, Jun 13:12, Oct 13:18, May 17:3, Sep 20:14, Sep 22:20, May 23:1

➔ *Clinical Examples in Radiology* Winter 08:1-2, 4-5, Summer 08:1, 3, Winter 13:1, 3, Spring 13:6, Fall 13:2-3, 5, Winter 15:4, 6, Winter 18:2, Summer 18:2, Summer 19:4, Winter 23:8

(Use 75774 in addition to code for specific initial vessel studied)

(Do not report 75774 as part of diagnostic angiography of the extracranial and intracranial cervicocerebral vessels. It may be appropriate to report 75774 for diagnostic angiography of upper extremities and other vascular beds performed in the same session)

(For cardiac catheterization procedures, see 93452-93462, 93563, 93564, 93565, 93566, 93567, 93568, 93569, 93573, 93574, 93575, 93593, 93594, 93595, 93596, 93597)

(For radiological supervision and interpretation of dialysis circuit angiography performed through existing access[es] or catheter-based arterial access, use 36901 with modifier 52)

Veins and Lymphatics

For venography performed in conjunction with therapeutic transcatheter radiological supervision and interpretation services, see the radiology **Transcatheter Procedures** guidelines.

Diagnostic venography (radiological supervision and interpretation) codes should NOT be used with interventional procedures for:

1. Contrast injections, venography, roadmapping, and/or fluoroscopic guidance for the intervention,

2. Vessel measurement, and

3. Post-angioplasty/stent venography, as this work is captured in the radiological supervision and interpretation code(s).

Diagnostic venography performed at the time of an interventional procedure is separately reportable if:

1. No prior catheter-based venographic study is available and a full diagnostic study is performed, and decision to intervene is based on the diagnostic study, OR

2. A prior study is available, but as documented in the medical record:

   a. The patient's condition with respect to the clinical indication has changed since the prior study, OR

   b. There is inadequate visualization of the anatomy and/or pathology, OR

   c. There is a clinical change during the procedure that requires new evaluation outside the target area of intervention.

Diagnostic venography performed at a separate setting from an interventional procedure is separately reported.

Diagnostic venography performed at the time of an interventional procedure is NOT separately reportable if it is specifically included in the interventional code descriptor.

(For injection procedure for venous system, see 36000-36015, 36400-36510)

(For injection procedure for lymphatic system, use 38790)

75801   Lymphangiography, extremity only, unilateral, radiological supervision and interpretation

➔ *Clinical Examples in Radiology* Summer 15:8, Winter 23:19

75803   Lymphangiography, extremity only, bilateral, radiological supervision and interpretation

➔ *Clinical Examples in Radiology* Summer 15:8, Winter 21:12, Winter 23:19

75805   Lymphangiography, pelvic/abdominal, unilateral, radiological supervision and interpretation

➔ *Clinical Examples in Radiology* Summer 15:8, Winter 23:19

75807   Lymphangiography, pelvic/abdominal, bilateral, radiological supervision and interpretation

➔ *Clinical Examples in Radiology* Summer 15:8, Winter 23:19

75809   Shuntogram for investigation of previously placed indwelling nonvascular shunt (eg, LeVeen shunt, ventriculoperitoneal shunt, indwelling infusion pump), radiological supervision and interpretation

➔ *CPT Changes: An Insider's View* 2001

➔ *CPT Assistant* Feb 07:11, Jul 08:13, Aug 08:13, Sep 08:10, Nov 10:3, Jan 11:8

(For procedure, see 49427 or 61070)

75810   Splenoportography, radiological supervision and interpretation

➔ *CPT Assistant* Feb 07:11, Nov 10:3, Jan 11:8

75820   Venography, extremity, unilateral, radiological supervision and interpretation

➔ *CPT Assistant* Oct 97:10, May 08:14, May 15:3, May 16:5

➔ *Clinical Examples in Radiology* Summer 06:8-9, Spring 08:12, Spring 14:7, Winter 16:2

(Do not report 75820 in conjunction with 36836, 36837)

Radiology 70010-79999

Venography
75820-75822

A radiographic contrast study is performed on the veins of the lower extremities.

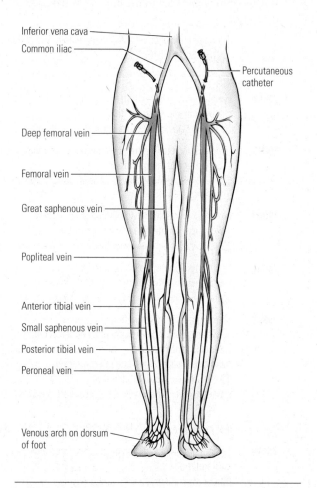

Inferior vena cava
Common iliac
Percutaneous catheter
Deep femoral vein
Femoral vein
Great saphenous vein
Popliteal vein
Anterior tibial vein
Small saphenous vein
Posterior tibial vein
Peroneal vein
Venous arch on dorsum of foot

75822 Venography, extremity, bilateral, radiological supervision and interpretation

(Do not report 75822 in conjunction with 36836, 36837)

75825 Venography, caval, inferior, with serialography, radiological supervision and interpretation
➔ *CPT Assistant* Feb 17:14, Apr 24:1
➔ *Clinical Examples in Radiology* Winter 05:5-6, Winter 12:3, Winter 16:2

75827 Venography, caval, superior, with serialography, radiological supervision and interpretation
➔ *CPT Assistant* Apr 98:12, Apr 24:1
➔ *Clinical Examples in Radiology* Winter 12:3

75831 Venography, renal, unilateral, selective, radiological supervision and interpretation
➔ *CPT Assistant* Sep 98:7
➔ *Clinical Examples in Radiology* Winter 12:3

75833 Venography, renal, bilateral, selective, radiological supervision and interpretation
➔ *CPT Assistant* Sep 98:7
➔ *Clinical Examples in Radiology* Winter 12:3

75840 Venography, adrenal, unilateral, selective, radiological supervision and interpretation

75842 Venography, adrenal, bilateral, selective, radiological supervision and interpretation

75860 Venography, venous sinus (eg, petrosal and inferior sagittal) or jugular, catheter, radiological supervision and interpretation
➔ *CPT Changes: An Insider's View* 2004
➔ *Clinical Examples in Radiology* Summer 16:3

75870 Venography, superior sagittal sinus, radiological supervision and interpretation
➔ *Clinical Examples in Radiology* Summer 16:3

75872 Venography, epidural, radiological supervision and interpretation

75880 Venography, orbital, radiological supervision and interpretation

75885 Percutaneous transhepatic portography with hemodynamic evaluation, radiological supervision and interpretation
➔ *CPT Assistant* Oct 96:4, Mar 02:10, Dec 03:2, Feb 07:11, Nov 10:3, Jan 11:8
➔ *Clinical Examples in Radiology* Winter 18:11

75887 Percutaneous transhepatic portography without hemodynamic evaluation, radiological supervision and interpretation
➔ *CPT Assistant* Mar 02:10, Dec 03:2, Feb 07:11, Jan 11:8
➔ *Clinical Examples in Radiology* Winter 18:11

75889 Hepatic venography, wedged or free, with hemodynamic evaluation, radiological supervision and interpretation

75891 Hepatic venography, wedged or free, without hemodynamic evaluation, radiological supervision and interpretation

75893 Venous sampling through catheter, with or without angiography (eg, for parathyroid hormone, renin), radiological supervision and interpretation
➔ *Clinical Examples in Radiology* Summer 16:2

(For procedure, use 36500)

★ =Telemedicine ◀ =Audio-only +=Add-on code ✗ =FDA approval pending #=Resequenced code ⊘=Modifier 51 exempt ➔➔➔=See p xxi for details

Transcatheter Procedures

Therapeutic transcatheter radiological supervision and interpretation code(s) include the following services associated with that intervention:

1. Contrast injections, angiography/venography, roadmapping, and fluoroscopic guidance for the intervention,

2. Vessel measurement, and

3. Completion angiography/venography (except for those uses permitted by 75898).

Unless specifically included in the code descriptor, diagnostic angiography/venography performed at the time of transcatheter therapeutic radiological and interpretation service(s) is separately reportable (eg, no prior catheter-based diagnostic angiography/venography study of the target vessel is available, prior diagnostic study is inadequate, patient's condition with respect to the clinical indication has changed since the prior study or during the intervention). See 75600-75893.

Codes 75956 and 75957 include all angiography of the thoracic aorta and its branches for diagnostic imaging prior to deployment of the primary endovascular devices (including all routine components of modular devices), fluoroscopic guidance in the delivery of the endovascular components, and intraprocedural arterial angiography (eg, confirm position, detect endoleak, evaluate runoff).

Code 75958 includes the analogous services for placement of each proximal thoracic endovascular extension. Code 75959 includes the analogous services for placement of a distal thoracic endovascular extension(s) placed during a procedure after the primary repair.

75894   Transcatheter therapy, embolization, any method, radiological supervision and interpretation

➔ *CPT Assistant* Sep 98:7, Feb 08:5, Apr 12:5, Nov 13:6-7, 15, Oct 14:6

➔ *Clinical Examples in Radiology* Winter 07:1, 3, Summer 07:2, Winter 08:4-5, Summer 08:1-3, Fall 11:3, Fall 13:2-4, Spring 14:8, Spring 16:5, Summer 16:13, Winter 18:2

(Do not report 75894 in conjunction with 36475, 36476, 36478, 36479, 36836, 36837, 37241, 37242, 37243, 37244)

75898   Angiography through existing catheter for follow-up study for transcatheter therapy, embolization or infusion, other than for thrombolysis

➔ *CPT Changes: An Insider's View* 2002, 2013

➔ *CPT Assistant* Dec 07:11, Nov 11:11, Nov 13:6, 15, Oct 14:6, Nov 15:3, Sep 19:6

➔ *Clinical Examples in Radiology* Summer 07:2, Winter 08:4-5, Summer 08:1-3, Summer 12:3, Fall 13:2-4, Spring 16:4, Winter 18:2

(Do not report 75898 in conjunction with 36836, 36837, 37211, 37212, 37213, 37214, 37241, 37242, 37243, 37244, 61645, 61650, 61651)

(For thrombolysis infusion management other than coronary, see 37211-37214, 61645)

(For non-thrombolysis infusion management other than coronary, see 61650, 61651)

75901   Mechanical removal of pericatheter obstructive material (eg, fibrin sheath) from central venous device via separate venous access, radiologic supervision and interpretation

➔ *CPT Changes: An Insider's View* 2003

➔ *CPT Assistant* Jul 03:13, Dec 04:12

(For procedure, use 36595)

(For venous catheterization, see 36010-36012)

75902   Mechanical removal of intraluminal (intracatheter) obstructive material from central venous device through device lumen, radiologic supervision and interpretation

➔ *CPT Changes: An Insider's View* 2003

➔ *CPT Assistant* Jul 03:13, Dec 04:12

(For procedure, use 36596)

(For venous catheterization, see 36010-36012)

75956   Endovascular repair of descending thoracic aorta (eg, aneurysm, pseudoaneurysm, dissection, penetrating ulcer, intramural hematoma, or traumatic disruption); involving coverage of left subclavian artery origin, initial endoprosthesis plus descending thoracic aortic extension(s), if required, to level of celiac artery origin, radiological supervision and interpretation

➔ *CPT Changes: An Insider's View* 2006

➔ *Clinical Examples in Radiology* Winter 06:17

(For implantation of endovascular graft, use 33880)

75957   not involving coverage of left subclavian artery origin, initial endoprosthesis plus descending thoracic aortic extension(s), if required, to level of celiac artery origin, radiological supervision and interpretation

➔ *CPT Changes: An Insider's View* 2006

➔ *Clinical Examples in Radiology* Winter 06:17

(For implantation of endovascular graft, use 33881)

75958   Placement of proximal extension prosthesis for endovascular repair of descending thoracic aorta (eg, aneurysm, pseudoaneurysm, dissection, penetrating ulcer, intramural hematoma, or traumatic disruption), radiological supervision and interpretation

➔ *CPT Changes: An Insider's View* 2006

➔ *Clinical Examples in Radiology* Winter 06:17

(Report 75958 for each proximal extension)

(For implantation of proximal endovascular extension, see 33883, 33884)

75959 Placement of distal extension prosthesis(s) (delayed) after endovascular repair of descending thoracic aorta, as needed, to level of celiac origin, radiological supervision and interpretation

➔ *CPT Changes: An Insider's View* 2006

➔ *Clinical Examples in Radiology* Winter 06:17

(Do not report 75959 in conjunction with 75956, 75957)

(Report 75959 once, regardless of number of modules deployed)

(For implantation of distal endovascular extension, use 33886)

(Radiologic supervision for transcatheter placement of stent[s] is included in the therapeutic service codes)

(For removal of a vena cava filter, use 37193)

75970 Transcatheter biopsy, radiological supervision and interpretation

➔ *CPT Assistant* May 17:3

(For injection procedure only for transcatheter therapy or biopsy, see 36100-36299)

(For transcatheter renal and ureteral biopsy, use 52007)

(For percutaneous needle biopsy of pancreas, use 48102; of retroperitoneal lymph node or mass, use 49180)

(For radiological supervision and interpretation of transluminal balloon angioplasty within the peripheral and/or central segments of a dialysis circuit performed through the dialysis circuit, see 36902, 36905, 36907)

75984 Change of percutaneous tube or drainage catheter with contrast monitoring (eg, genitourinary system, abscess), radiological supervision and interpretation

➔ *CPT Changes: An Insider's View* 2008

➔ *CPT Assistant* Nov 97:24

➔ *Clinical Examples in Radiology* Summer 10:11, Fall 15:2, Spring 16:12

(For percutaneous replacement of gastrostomy, duodenostomy, jejunostomy, gastro-jejunostomy, or cecostomy [or other colonic] tube including fluoroscopic imaging guidance, see 49450-49452)

(To report exchange of a percutaneous nephrostomy catheter, use 50435)

(For percutaneous cholecystostomy, use 47490)

(For percutaneous biliary procedures, including radiological supervision and interpretation, see 47531-47544)

(For percutaneous nephrolithotomy or pyelolithotomy, see 50080, 50081)

(For removal and/or replacement of an internally dwelling ureteral stent via a transurethral approach, see 50385-50386)

75989 Radiological guidance (ie, fluoroscopy, ultrasound, or computed tomography), for percutaneous drainage (eg, abscess, specimen collection), with placement of catheter, radiological supervision and interpretation

➔ *CPT Changes: An Insider's View* 2001, 2002

➔ *CPT Assistant* Nov 97:24, Mar 98:8, Feb 07:11, Nov 10:3, Apr 11:12, Nov 12:3, Nov 13:9, May 14:9

➔ *Clinical Examples in Radiology* Summer 10:3, Winter 11:10, Summer 11:3, Winter 13:5, Fall 13:5-6, Spring 14:10, Spring 15:8, Winter 16:10

(Do not report 75989 in conjunction with 10030, 32554, 32555, 32556, 32557, 33017, 33018, 33019, 47490, 49405, 49406, 49407)

► Magnetic Resonance Safety Implant/Foreign Body Procedures ◄

►Implanted medical devices or foreign bodies can increase the risk of injury or death for a patient entering the magnetic resonance (MR) environment, either for diagnostic MR procedures or for procedures performed under MR imaging guidance.

Implants may have FDA-approved labeling specifying conditions under which an MR examination could be safely performed. These conditions can specify the type of MR equipment to use, preparation of the implant before the MR procedure, anatomical regions that should be excluded from MR examination, limitations on MR scan time and energy deposition, and/or implant components that may contraindicate MR examination.

Codes 76014, 76015, 76016 describe MR safety-planning services performed in advance of the date of the MR procedure. For 76014, implant-safety conditions and additional procedures required to safely perform the requested MR examination are documented for inclusion in the medical record by a technologist or other MR safety-trained clinical staff. Contraindications to MR are also documented. For patients with complex, multiple, or incompletely documented implants, use 76015 to report prolonged MR safety implant/foreign body assessment by clinical staff. For an implant and/or foreign body that lacks MR conditional labeling, is contraindicated for MR, or may result in a limited MR examination, use 76016 to report the performance of an MR safety determination by a physician or other qualified health care professional (QHP) responsible for the safe performance of the MR procedure, with a written report.

Codes 76017, 76018, 76019 describe MR safety services performed on the day of the MR examination under supervision of the physician or other QHP responsible

★ = Telemedicine   ◀ = Audio-only   ✦ = Add-on code   ✗ = FDA approval pending   # = Resequenced code   ⊘ = Modifier 51 exempt   ➔➔➔ = See p xxi for details

for the safe performance of the MR procedure. The need for these services depends on the design of the medical implant, and the MR conditional labeling of the implant, if available. Use 76017 to report medical physics services provided during the MR examination, with a written report. Use 76018 to report the preparation and documentation of an electronic implant into an MR-protective mode. Use 76019 to report specified positioning and/or immobilization of an implant during the MR examination, with documentation for inclusion in the medical record.

Cardiac devices (eg, pacemakers and defibrillators) may require interrogation or programming services before or after the performance of the MR examination to put them in a mode safe for the MR scan. For cardiac device interrogation or programming, see the appropriate cardiac device evaluation code. Similarly, neurostimulation devices may require analysis-programming before being placed into an MR-protective mode, or after the performance of the MR examination. For electronic analysis-programming of neurostimulation devices, see the appropriate analysis-programming code. If cardiac device evaluation or neurostimulator analysis-programming is performed on the same day, report 76018 only if a separate individual performs additional preparation of the electronic implant into an MR-protective mode immediately before patient entry to the MR environment. For reprogramming of programmable cerebrospinal shunt after the performance of the MR examination, use 62252.◀

#● **76014**   MR safety implant and/or foreign body assessment by trained clinical staff, including identification and verification of implant components from appropriate sources (eg, surgical reports, imaging reports, medical device databases, device vendors, review of prior imaging), analyzing current MR conditional status of individual components and systems, and consulting published professional guidance with written report; initial 15 minutes

⮕ *CPT Changes: An Insider's View* 2025

#+● **76015**   each additional 30 minutes (List separately in addition to code for primary procedure)

⮕ *CPT Changes: An Insider's View* 2025

▶(Use 76015 in conjunction with 76014)◀

▶(Do not report 76015 more than three times per encounter)◀

#● **76016**   MR safety determination by a physician or other qualified health care professional responsible for the safety of the MR procedure, including review of implant MR conditions for indicated MR examination, analysis of risk vs clinical benefit of performing MR examination, and determination of MR equipment, accessory equipment, and expertise required to perform examination, with written report

⮕ *CPT Changes: An Insider's View* 2025

#⊘● **76017**   MR safety medical physics examination customization, planning and performance monitoring by medical physicist or MR safety expert, with review and analysis by physician or other qualified health care professional to prioritize and select views and imaging sequences, to tailor MR acquisition specific to restrictive requirements or artifacts associated with MR conditional implants or to mitigate risk of non-conditional implants or foreign bodies, with written report

⮕ *CPT Changes: An Insider's View* 2025

▶(Use 76017 in conjunction with 76018, 76019, when implant requires electronics preparation or positioning and/or immobilization before MR)◀

#⊘● **76018**   MR safety implant electronics preparation under supervision of physician or other qualified health care professional, including MR-specific programming of pulse generator and/or transmitter to verify device integrity, protection of device internal circuitry from MR electromagnetic fields, and protection of patient from risks of unintended stimulation or heating while in the MR room, with written report

⮕ *CPT Changes: An Insider's View* 2025

▶(Use 76018 in conjunction with 76017, when implant also requires medical physics examination customization)◀

#⊘● **76019**   MR safety implant positioning and/or immobilization under supervision of physician or other qualified health care professional, including application of physical protections to secure implanted medical device from MR-induced translational or vibrational forces, magnetically induced functional changes, and/or prevention of radiofrequency burns from inadvertent tissue contact while in the MR room, with written report

⮕ *CPT Changes: An Insider's View* 2025

▶(Use 76019 in conjunction with 76017, when implant also requires medical physics examination customization)◀

Other Procedures

(For computed tomography cerebral perfusion analysis, see Category III code 0042T)

(For arthrography of shoulder, use 73040; elbow, use 73085; wrist, use 73115; hip, use 73525; knee, use 73580; ankle, use 73615)

76000 Fluoroscopy (separate procedure), up to 1 hour physician or other qualified health care professional time

➡ *CPT Changes: An Insider's View* 2000, 2013, 2018

➡ *CPT Assistant* Apr 96:11, Nov 99:32, Dec 00:14, Apr 03:7, Jul 03:16, Aug 03:14, Jul 08:9, Aug 08:7, Dec 08:7, 9, Aug 10:8, Oct 10:14, Nov 10:3, Dec 10:14, Jul 11:5, Nov 11:11, Feb 13:3, Mar 13:10, Sep 13:17, Sep 14:5, Oct 14:6, May 15:3, Sep 15:3, Jan 16:12, Mar 16:5, May 16:5, Aug 16:5, Mar 19:6, Jun 19:3, Sep 19:11, Dec 23:41, Feb 24:21, Mar 24:1

➡ *Clinical Examples in Radiology* Spring 18:14, Spring 20:6, Summer 21:13, Summer 22:15

(Do not report 76000 in conjunction with 33274, 33275, 33957, 33958, 33959, 33962, 33963, 33964, 0515T, 0516T, 0517T, 0518T, 0519T, 0520T, 0795T, 0796T, 0797T, 0798T, 0799T, 0800T, 0801T, 0802T, 0803T, 0823T, 0824T, 0825T, 0861T, 0862T, 0863T)

76010 Radiologic examination from nose to rectum for foreign body, single view, child

➡ *CPT Changes: An Insider's View* 2001

➡ *CPT Assistant* Feb 10:12

➡ *Clinical Examples in Radiology* Summer 09:11

76014 Code is out of numerical sequence. See 75984-76010

76015 Code is out of numerical sequence. See 75984-76010

76016 Code is out of numerical sequence. See 75984-76010

76017 Code is out of numerical sequence. See 75984-76010

76018 Code is out of numerical sequence. See 75984-76010

76019 Code is out of numerical sequence. See 75984-76010

76080 Radiologic examination, abscess, fistula or sinus tract study, radiological supervision and interpretation

➡ *CPT Assistant* Nov 97:24, Mar 98:8, Nov 03:14, Dec 06:10, Jan 09:8

➡ *Clinical Examples in Radiology* Fall 09:9, Summer 15:8

(For contrast injection[s] and radiological assessment of gastrostomy, duodenostomy, jejunostomy, gastro-jejunostomy, or cecostomy [or other colonic] tube including fluoroscopic imaging guidance, use 49465)

76098 Radiological examination, surgical specimen

➡ *Clinical Examples in Radiology* Fall 10:1, Summer 12:10, Fall 13:10-11, Spring 14:10

(Do not report 76098 in conjunction with 19081-19086, 0694T)

(For 3-dimensional volumetric specimen imaging, use 0694T)

76100 Radiologic examination, single plane body section (eg, tomography), other than with urography

(For nephrotomography, use 74415)

(For panoramic X-ray, use 70355)

76120 Cineradiography/videoradiography, except where specifically included

➡ *CPT Changes: An Insider's View* 2002

➡ *CPT Assistant* Sep 00:4, Apr 04:15, Apr 11:13

+ 76125 Cineradiography/videoradiography to complement routine examination (List separately in addition to code for primary procedure)

➡ *CPT Changes: An Insider's View* 2002

➡ *CPT Assistant* Oct 97:1, Sep 00:4

76140 Consultation on X-ray examination made elsewhere, written report

➡ *CPT Assistant* Summer 91:13, Oct 97:1, Mar 21:11

➡ *Clinical Examples in Radiology* Summer 21:11

(2D reformatting is no longer separately reported. To report 3D rendering, see 76376, 76377)

76145 Medical physics dose evaluation for radiation exposure that exceeds institutional review threshold, including report

➡ *CPT Changes: An Insider's View* 2021

➡ *CPT Assistant* Mar 22:13

➡ *Clinical Examples in Radiology* Fall 20:10-11

76376 3D rendering with interpretation and reporting of computed tomography, magnetic resonance imaging, ultrasound, or other tomographic modality with image postprocessing under concurrent supervision; not requiring image postprocessing on an independent workstation

➡ *CPT Changes: An Insider's View* 2006, 2013

➡ *CPT Assistant* Dec 05:1, 7, Jan 07:31, Jul 08:3, May 09:9, Jun 09:9, Jul 09:10, Apr 10:5, Jul 10:7, May 13:3, Jun 13:12, Apr 16:9, May 17:11, Jul 18:11, Aug 19:5, Sep 19:11, Oct 19:11, Oct 21:3

➡ *Clinical Examples in Radiology* Winter 06:17, Spring 06:8-9, Fall 06:9-10, Winter 07:4-5, Summer 08:8, Fall 08:12, Spring 09:4, Summer 09:14, Fall 09:9, Winter 10:6, Spring 10:2, Summer 10:10, Fall 10:6, Winter 13:10, Fall 14:8, 11, Winter 17:14, Spring 17:7, Spring 19:7, Winter 20:8, Spring 20:13, Spring 21:6, 11, Summer 22:2, 3, 7, 11, 17, 18, Winter 23:1, Spring 23:5, Summer 23:4, Winter 24:33

(Use 76376 in conjunction with code[s] for base imaging procedure[s])

▶(Do not report 76376 in conjunction with 31627, 34839, 70496, 70498, 70544, 70545, 70546, 70547, 70548, 70549, 71275, 71555, 72159, 72191, 72198, 73206, 73225, 73706, 73725, 74174, 74175, 74185, 74261, 74262, 74263, 75557, 75559, 75561, 75563, 75565, 75571, 75572, 75573, 75574, 75635, 76377, 77046, 77047, 77048, 77049, 77061, 77062, 77063, 78012-78999, 93319, 93355, 0523T, 0559T, 0560T, 0561T, 0562T, 0623T, 0624T, 0625T, 0626T, 0633T, 0634T, 0635T, 0636T, 0637T, 0638T, 0710T, 0711T, 0712T, 0713T, 0876T)◀

★=Telemedicine ◀=Audio-only +=Add-on code ✚=FDA approval pending #=Resequenced code ⊘=Modifier 51 exempt ➡➡➡=See p xxi for details

(For noninvasive arterial plaque analysis using software processing of data from computerized tomography angiography to quantify structure and composition of the vessel wall, including assessment for lipid-rich necrotic core plaque, see 0710T, 0711T, 0712T, 0713T)

76377   requiring image postprocessing on an independent workstation

➔ *CPT Changes: An Insider's View* 2006, 2013

➔ *CPT Assistant* Dec 05:1, Jan 07:31, Jul 08:3, May 09:9, Jun 09:9, Jul 09:10, Dec 09:13, Feb 10:6, Apr 10:5, 9, Jul 10:7, May 13:3, Jun 13:12, Apr 16:9, May 17:11, Jul 18:11, Aug 19:5, Sep 19:11, Oct 19:11, Oct 21:3, Jun 22:20-21

➔ *Clinical Examples in Radiology* Winter 06:17, Spring 06:8-9, Fall 06:9-10, Winter 07:4-5, Summer 07:1-2, Summer 08:8, Fall 08:12, Spring 09:5, Summer 09:14, Fall 09:9, Winter 10:6, Spring 10:2, Summer 10:10, Fall 10:6, Winter 13:10, Winter 17:14, Spring 17:7, Summer 18:13, Spring 19:7, Winter 20:8, Spring 20:13, Spring 21:6, 11, Summer 22:2, 3, 7, 10, 11, 17, 18, Winter 23:1, Spring 23:5, Summer 23:4, Fall 23:14, Winter 24:33

(Use 76377 in conjunction with code[s] for base imaging procedure[s])

▶(Do not report 76377 in conjunction with 34839, 70496, 70498, 70544, 70545, 70546, 70547, 70548, 70549, 71275, 71555, 72159, 72191, 72198, 73206, 73225, 73706, 73725, 74174, 74175, 74185, 74261, 74262, 74263, 75557, 75559, 75561, 75563, 75565, 75571, 75572, 75573, 75574, 75635, 76376, 77046, 77047, 77048, 77049, 77061, 77062, 77063, 78012-78999, 93319, 93355, 0523T, 0559T, 0560T, 0561T, 0562T, 0623T, 0624T, 0625T, 0626T, 0633T, 0634T, 0635T, 0636T, 0637T, 0638T, 0710T, 0711T, 0712T, 0713T, 0876T)◀

(76376, 76377 require concurrent supervision of image postprocessing 3D manipulation of volumetric data set and image rendering)

(For noninvasive arterial plaque analysis using software processing of data from computerized tomography angiography to quantify structure and composition of the vessel wall, including assessment for lipid-rich necrotic core plaque, see 0710T, 0711T, 0712T, 0713T)

76380   Computed tomography, limited or localized follow-up study

➔ *CPT Changes: An Insider's View* 2002, 2003

➔ *CPT Assistant* Jul 07:13, Mar 19:11

➔ *Clinical Examples in Radiology* Summer 16:4, Spring 22:10, Spring 23:27

76390   Magnetic resonance spectroscopy

➔ *CPT Assistant* Nov 97:25, Jul 21:6

➔ *Clinical Examples in Radiology* Winter 21:5-6

(For magnetic resonance imaging, use appropriate MRI body site code)

(For magnetic resonance spectroscopy, determination and localization of discogenic pain, see 0609T, 0610T)

76391   Magnetic resonance (eg, vibration) elastography

➔ *CPT Changes: An Insider's View* 2019

➔ *CPT Assistant* Aug 19:3

➔ *Clinical Examples in Radiology* Fall 18:5

76496   Unlisted fluoroscopic procedure (eg, diagnostic, interventional)

➔ *CPT Changes: An Insider's View* 2003

➔ *CPT Assistant* Sep 22:20

➔ *Clinical Examples in Radiology* Fall 07:3

76497   Unlisted computed tomography procedure (eg, diagnostic, interventional)

➔ *CPT Changes: An Insider's View* 2003

➔ *CPT Assistant* Jun 05:11, Sep 18:10

➔ *Clinical Examples in Radiology* Spring 05:1, 7, Summer 18:13, Fall 19:11

76498   Unlisted magnetic resonance procedure (eg, diagnostic, interventional)

➔ *CPT Changes: An Insider's View* 2003

➔ *CPT Assistant* Dec 11:17, Jul 22:20

➔ *Clinical Examples in Radiology* Fall 08:11, Spring 09:11, Winter 13:11, Spring 18:12, Fall 18:6, Spring 19:12, Summer 19:11, Winter 20:14, Winter 22:6, Summer 22:10, 11, Fall 22:16

76499   Unlisted diagnostic radiographic procedure

➔ *CPT Changes: An Insider's View* 2003

➔ *CPT Assistant* Jul 99:10, Sep 00:4, Apr 04:15, Nov 06:22, Mar 08:15, Dec 11:17, Dec 13:17, Jul 16:8, Apr 24:34

➔ *Clinical Examples in Radiology* Spring 11:8, Fall 14:10, Summer 15:8, Fall 18:5, Fall 21:4

Diagnostic Ultrasound

All diagnostic ultrasound examinations require permanently recorded images with measurements, when such measurements are clinically indicated. For those codes whose sole diagnostic goal is a biometric measure (ie, 76514, 76516, and 76519), permanently recorded images are not required. A final, written report should be issued for inclusion in the patient's medical record. The prescription form for the intraocular lens satisfies the written report requirement for 76519. For those anatomic regions that have "complete" and "limited" ultrasound codes, note the elements that comprise a "complete" exam. The report should contain a description of these elements or the reason that an element could not be visualized (eg, obscured by bowel gas, surgically absent).

If less than the required elements for a "complete" exam are reported (eg, limited number of organs or limited portion of region evaluated), the "limited" code for that anatomic region should be used once per patient exam session. A "limited" exam of an anatomic region should not be reported for the same exam session as a "complete" exam of that same region.

Evaluation of vascular structures using both color and spectral Doppler is separately reportable. To report, see **Noninvasive Vascular Diagnostic Studies** (93880-93990). However, color Doppler alone, when performed for anatomic structure identification in conjunction with a real-time ultrasound examination, is not reported separately.

Ultrasound guidance procedures also require permanently recorded images of the site to be localized, as well as a documented description of the localization process, either separately or within the report of the procedure for which the guidance is utilized.

Use of ultrasound, without thorough evaluation of organ(s) or anatomic region, image documentation, and final, written report, is not separately reportable.

Definitions

A-mode implies a one-dimensional ultrasonic measurement procedure.

M-mode implies a one-dimensional ultrasonic measurement procedure with movement of the trace to record amplitude and velocity of moving echo-producing structures.

B-scan implies a two-dimensional ultrasonic scanning procedure with a two-dimensional display.

Real-time scan implies a two-dimensional ultrasonic scanning procedure with display of both two-dimensional structure and motion with time.

> (To report diagnostic vascular ultrasound studies, see 93880-93990)

> (For focused ultrasound ablation treatment of uterine leiomyomata, see Category III codes 0071T, 0072T)

Head and Neck

76506   Echoencephalography, real time with image documentation (gray scale) (for determination of ventricular size, delineation of cerebral contents, and detection of fluid masses or other intracranial abnormalities), including A-mode encephalography as secondary component where indicated
→ *CPT Changes: An Insider's View* 2007, 2008
→ *CPT Assistant* Mar 07:7

76510   Ophthalmic ultrasound, diagnostic; B-scan and quantitative A-scan performed during the same patient encounter
→ *CPT Changes: An Insider's View* 2005
→ *CPT Assistant* Dec 05:3

76511   quantitative A-scan only
→ *CPT Changes: An Insider's View* 2005
→ *CPT Assistant* Winter 93:12, Oct 96:9, Nov 99:42, Jul 04:12, Dec 05:3

76512   B-scan (with or without superimposed non-quantitative A-scan)
→ *CPT Changes: An Insider's View* 2005
→ *CPT Assistant* Winter 93:12, Oct 96:9, Dec 05:3

76513   anterior segment ultrasound, immersion (water bath) B-scan or high resolution biomicroscopy, unilateral or bilateral
→ *CPT Changes: An Insider's View* 2000, 2021
→ *CPT Assistant* Winter 93:12, Nov 99:42, Nov 09:9, Apr 13:7

> ▶(For computerized ophthalmic diagnostic imaging of the anterior and posterior segments using technology other than ultrasound, see 92132, 92133, 92134, 92137)◀

76514   corneal pachymetry, unilateral or bilateral (determination of corneal thickness)
→ *CPT Changes: An Insider's View* 2004
→ *CPT Assistant* Jul 04:12, 15, Feb 05:13, Jun 05:11, Dec 05:3, Feb 16:12

> (Do not report 76514 in conjunction with 0402T)

76516   Ophthalmic biometry by ultrasound echography, A-scan;
→ *CPT Assistant* Oct 03:10, Dec 05:3

76519   with intraocular lens power calculation
→ *CPT Assistant* Winter 93:12, Oct 03:10, Dec 05:3, Sep 09:5

> (For partial coherence interferometry, use 92136)

76529   Ophthalmic ultrasonic foreign body localization
→ *CPT Assistant* Winter 93:12

76536   Ultrasound, soft tissues of head and neck (eg, thyroid, parathyroid, parotid), real time with image documentation
→ *CPT Changes: An Insider's View* 2002, 2007
→ *CPT Assistant* Mar 07:7, May 09:7, Oct 17:10, Dec 22:17
→ *Clinical Examples in Radiology* Winter 13:8, Spring 15:4, Spring 18:13, Fall 18:4, Winter 22:3, Summer 22:15, 19-21

Chest

Code 76641 represents a complete ultrasound examination of the breast. Code 76641 consists of an ultrasound examination of all four quadrants of the breast and the retroareolar region. It also includes ultrasound examination of the axilla, if performed.

Code 76642 consists of a focused ultrasound examination of the breast limited to the assessment of one or more, but not all of the elements listed in code 76641. It also includes ultrasound examination of the axilla, if performed.

Use of ultrasound, without thorough evaluation of organ(s) or anatomic region, image documentation, and final written report, is not separately reportable.

76604 Ultrasound, chest (includes mediastinum), real time with image documentation
- ➔ *CPT Changes: An Insider's View* 2002, 2007
- ➔ *CPT Assistant* Nov 12:3, Oct 17:10, Dec 22:17
- ➔ *Clinical Examples in Radiology* Spring 15:4, Summer 15:14, Winter 16:13, Fall 18:4, Spring 19:12, Winter 22:3, Summer 22:19, 20, Winter 24:16

76641 Ultrasound, breast, unilateral, real time with image documentation, including axilla when performed; complete
- ➔ *CPT Changes: An Insider's View* 2015
- ➔ *CPT Assistant* Aug 15:11, Oct 17:10, Dec 22:17
- ➔ *Clinical Examples in Radiology* Winter 15:10, Spring 15:4, Fall 18:4, Winter 22:3, Summer 22:19, 20, Winter 24:18

76642 limited
- ➔ *CPT Changes: An Insider's View* 2015
- ➔ *CPT Assistant* Oct 17:10, Dec 22:17
- ➔ *Clinical Examples in Radiology* Winter 15:10, Spring 15:4, Winter 16:13, Spring 18:13, Fall 18:4, Winter 22:2, Summer 22:19, 20, Winter 24:17

(Report 76641, 76642 only once per breast, per session)

(For axillary ultrasound only, use 76882)

Abdomen and Retroperitoneum

A complete ultrasound examination of the abdomen (76700) consists of real time scans of the liver, gall bladder, common bile duct, pancreas, spleen, kidneys, and the upper abdominal aorta and inferior vena cava including any demonstrated abdominal abnormality.

A complete ultrasound examination of the retroperitoneum (76770) consists of real time scans of the kidneys, abdominal aorta, common iliac artery origins, and inferior vena cava, including any demonstrated retroperitoneal abnormality. Alternatively, if clinical history suggests urinary tract pathology, complete evaluation of the kidneys and urinary bladder also comprises a complete retroperitoneal ultrasound.

Use of ultrasound, without thorough evaluation of organ(s) or anatomic region, image documentation and final, written report, is not separately reportable.

76700 Ultrasound, abdominal, real time with image documentation; complete
- ➔ *CPT Changes: An Insider's View* 2002, 2007
- ➔ *CPT Assistant* Fall 93:13, Oct 01:3, Dec 05:3, Mar 07:7, Oct 17:10, Dec 22:17
- ➔ *Clinical Examples in Radiology* Winter 05:9, 11, Fall 07:4, Spring 08:10, Summer 14:9, Spring 15:4, Winter 17:14, Fall 18:4, Fall 21:17, Summer 22:19, 20

76705 limited (eg, single organ, quadrant, follow-up)
- ➔ *CPT Assistant* Fall 93:13, Oct 01:3, Apr 03:27, Dec 05:3, Feb 09:22, May 09:7, Mar 12:10, Dec 12:9, Oct 17:10, Dec 22:17, Feb 23:14, Feb 24:35
- ➔ *Clinical Examples in Radiology* Winter 05:9, 11, Fall 07:4, Summer 11:11, Winter 12:10, Spring 12:10, Summer 14:8-9, Spring 15:4, Summer 15:13, Summer 16:10, Winter 17:14, Spring 18:13, Fall 18:2, Winter 22:3, Summer 22:19, 20

76706 Ultrasound, abdominal aorta, real time with image documentation, screening study for abdominal aortic aneurysm (AAA)
- ➔ *CPT Changes: An Insider's View* 2017
- ➔ *CPT Assistant* May 17:3, Sep 17:12
- ➔ *Clinical Examples in Radiology* Spring 17:5, Fall 18:4, Fall 22:15, Spring 23:18

(For ultrasound or duplex ultrasound of the abdominal aorta other than screening, see 76770, 76775, 93978, 93979)

76770 Ultrasound, retroperitoneal (eg, renal, aorta, nodes), real time with image documentation; complete
- ➔ *CPT Changes: An Insider's View* 2002, 2007
- ➔ *CPT Assistant* May 99:10, Jun 99:10, Mar 15:10, May 17:8, Oct 17:10, Dec 22:17
- ➔ *Clinical Examples in Radiology* Winter 05:9, 11, Fall 07:4, Winter 08:12, Summer 09:12, Summer 12:10, Summer 13:10, Spring 15:4, Spring 17:5, Fall 18:4, Summer 21:5, Winter 22:3, Summer 22:19, 20, Fall 22:15, Spring 23:18, Fall 23:20

76775 limited
- ➔ *CPT Assistant* May 99:10, Jun 99:10, Dec 05:3, Feb 09:22, Mar 15:10, May 17:8, Oct 17:10, Dec 22:17
- ➔ *Clinical Examples in Radiology* Winter 05:9, 11, Winter 07:8, 10, Spring 07:5-6, Fall 07:4, Summer 09:12, Summer 12:10, Summer 13:10, Spring 15:4, Summer 16:11, Spring 17:5, Fall 18:4, Summer 21:5, Winter 22:3, Summer 22:19, 20, Fall 22:15, Spring 23:18, Fall 23:20

76776 Ultrasound, transplanted kidney, real time and duplex Doppler with image documentation
- ➔ *CPT Changes: An Insider's View* 2007
- ➔ *CPT Assistant* Mar 07:7
- ➔ *Clinical Examples in Radiology* Summer 12:10, Fall 23:19

(For ultrasound of transplanted kidney without duplex Doppler, use 76775)

(For ultrasound and duplex Doppler of a transplanted kidney, do not report 76776 in conjunction with 93975, 93976)

Spinal Canal

76800 Ultrasound, spinal canal and contents
- ➔ *CPT Changes: An Insider's View* 2002
- ➔ *CPT Assistant* Apr 98:15

Pelvis

Obstetrical

Codes 76801 and 76802 include determination of the number of gestational sacs and fetuses, gestational sac/fetal measurements appropriate for gestation (younger than 14 weeks 0 days), survey of visible fetal and placental anatomic structure, qualitative assessment of amniotic fluid volume/gestational sac shape and examination of the maternal uterus and adnexa.

Codes 76805 and 76810 include determination of number of fetuses and amniotic/chorionic sacs, measurements appropriate for gestational age (older than or equal to 14 weeks 0 days), survey of intracranial/spinal/abdominal anatomy, 4 chambered heart, umbilical cord insertion site, placenta location and amniotic fluid assessment and, when visible, examination of maternal adnexa.

Codes 76811 and 76812 include all elements of codes 76805 and 76810 plus detailed anatomic evaluation of the fetal brain/ventricles, face, heart/outflow tracts and chest anatomy, abdominal organ specific anatomy, number/length/architecture of limbs and detailed evaluation of the umbilical cord and placenta and other fetal anatomy as clinically indicated.

Report should document the results of the evaluation of each element described above or the reason for non-visualization.

Code 76815 represents a focused "quick look" exam limited to the assessment of one or more of the elements listed in code 76815.

Code 76816 describes an examination designed to reassess fetal size and interval growth or reevaluate one or more anatomic abnormalities of a fetus previously demonstrated on ultrasound, and should be coded once for each fetus requiring reevaluation using modifier 59 for each fetus after the first.

Code 76817 describes a transvaginal obstetric ultrasound performed separately or in addition to one of the transabdominal examinations described above. For transvaginal examinations performed for non-obstetrical purposes, use code 76830.

76801 Ultrasound, pregnant uterus, real time with image documentation, fetal and maternal evaluation, first trimester (< 14 weeks 0 days), transabdominal approach; single or first gestation
➜ *CPT Changes: An Insider's View* 2003
➜ *CPT Assistant* Mar 03:7, Nov 05:15
➜ *Clinical Examples in Radiology* Winter 07:6-7, Summer 10:8, Winter 19:7, Spring 19:9, Winter 20:12, Fall 21:16, Winter 22:16

(To report first trimester fetal nuchal translucency measurement, use 76813)

+ **76802** each additional gestation (List separately in addition to code for primary procedure)
➜ *CPT Changes: An Insider's View* 2003
➜ *CPT Assistant* Mar 03:7, Nov 05:15
➜ *Clinical Examples in Radiology* Winter 07:6-7, Summer 11:10, Spring 19:10, Winter 20:12, Fall 21:16, Winter 22:16

(Use 76802 in conjunction with 76801)

(To report first trimester fetal nuchal translucency measurement, use 76814)

76805 Ultrasound, pregnant uterus, real time with image documentation, fetal and maternal evaluation, after first trimester (> or = 14 weeks 0 days), transabdominal approach; single or first gestation
➜ *CPT Changes: An Insider's View* 2002, 2003
➜ *CPT Assistant* Apr 97:2, Nov 97:25, Oct 01:3, Aug 02:2, Mar 03:7, Jun 22:21-22
➜ *Clinical Examples in Radiology* Winter 05:3-4, Summer 12:11, Winter 14:11, Spring 19:9, Summer 20:10, Fall 21:12-13, 16

+ **76810** each additional gestation (List separately in addition to code for primary procedure)
➜ *CPT Changes: An Insider's View* 2003
➜ *CPT Assistant* Apr 97:2, Oct 01:3, Aug 02:2, Mar 03:7, Jun 22:21-22
➜ *Clinical Examples in Radiology* Winter 05:4, Summer 11:10, Winter 14:11, Fall 21:12-13, 16

(Use 76810 in conjunction with 76805)

76811 Ultrasound, pregnant uterus, real time with image documentation, fetal and maternal evaluation plus detailed fetal anatomic examination, transabdominal approach; single or first gestation
➜ *CPT Changes: An Insider's View* 2003
➜ *CPT Assistant* Mar 03:7
➜ *Clinical Examples in Radiology* Winter 05:4, Winter 14:11, Fall 21:13, 16

+ **76812** each additional gestation (List separately in addition to code for primary procedure)
➜ *CPT Changes: An Insider's View* 2003
➜ *CPT Assistant* Mar 03:7
➜ *Clinical Examples in Radiology* Summer 11:10, Winter 14:11, Fall 21:13

(Use 76812 in conjunction with 76811)

76813 Ultrasound, pregnant uterus, real time with image documentation, first trimester fetal nuchal translucency measurement, transabdominal or transvaginal approach; single or first gestation
➜ *CPT Changes: An Insider's View* 2007
➜ *CPT Assistant* Mar 07:7
➜ *Clinical Examples in Radiology* Winter 07:6

Radiology 70010-79999

+ 76814   each additional gestation (List separately in addition
                to code for primary procedure)

> *CPT Changes: An Insider's View* 2007

> *CPT Assistant* Mar 07:7

> *Clinical Examples in Radiology* Winter 07:6, Summer 11:10

(Use 76814 in conjunction with 76813)

76815   Ultrasound, pregnant uterus, real time with image
             documentation, limited (eg, fetal heart beat, placental
             location, fetal position and/or qualitative amniotic fluid
             volume), 1 or more fetuses

> *CPT Changes: An Insider's View* 2003

> *CPT Assistant* Apr 97:2, Nov 97:25, Oct 01:3, Dec 01:6, Aug 02:2,
> Mar 03:7, Nov 03:14, May 10:9

> *Clinical Examples in Radiology* Winter 07:6-7, Summer 10:8-9,
> Summer 12:11, Summer 14:7-8, Summer 16:12, Spring 19:9,
> Winter 20:12, Spring 20:13, Summer 20:10, Fall 21:13

(Use 76815 only once per exam and not per element)

(To report first trimester fetal nuchal translucency
measurement, see 76813, 76814)

76816   Ultrasound, pregnant uterus, real time with image
             documentation, follow-up (eg, re-evaluation of fetal size
             by measuring standard growth parameters and amniotic
             fluid volume, re-evaluation of organ system(s) suspected
             or confirmed to be abnormal on a previous scan),
             transabdominal approach, per fetus

> *CPT Changes: An Insider's View* 2003

> *CPT Assistant* Apr 97:2, Oct 01:3, Aug 02:2, Mar 03:7, May 10:9,
> Nov 11:10

> *Clinical Examples in Radiology* Summer 10:9, Summer 12:11,
> Summer 14:7-8, Spring 16:13, Spring 19:9, Winter 20:12,
> Fall 21:14

(Report 76816 with modifier 59 for each additional fetus
examined in a multiple pregnancy)

76817   Ultrasound, pregnant uterus, real time with image
             documentation, transvaginal

> *CPT Changes: An Insider's View* 2003

> *CPT Assistant* Mar 03:7, Nov 11:10

> *Clinical Examples in Radiology* Summer 10:8, Summer 11:10,
> Winter 14:11, Winter 16:13, Spring 19:9, Winter 20:12,
> Spring 20:13, Fall 21:14

(For non-obstetrical transvaginal ultrasound, use 76830)

(If transvaginal examination is done in addition to
transabdominal obstetrical ultrasound exam, use 76817
in addition to appropriate transabdominal exam code)

76818   Fetal biophysical profile; with non-stress testing

> *CPT Changes: An Insider's View* 2001

> *CPT Assistant* Apr 97:2, May 98:10, Sep 01:4, Oct 01:3, Dec 01:6,
> Nov 04:10

> *Clinical Examples in Radiology* Summer 14:7-8

76819   without non-stress testing

> *CPT Changes: An Insider's View* 2001, 2002

> *CPT Assistant* Sep 01:8, Dec 01:6

> *Clinical Examples in Radiology* Summer 14:7-8

(Fetal biophysical profile assessments for the second and
any additional fetuses, should be reported separately by
code 76818 or 76819 with the modifier 59 appended)

(For amniotic fluid index without non-stress test, use
76815)

76820   Doppler velocimetry, fetal; umbilical artery

> *CPT Changes: An Insider's View* 2005

> *CPT Assistant* Dec 05:3, Jul 16:9

76821   middle cerebral artery

> *CPT Changes: An Insider's View* 2005

> *CPT Assistant* Dec 05:3

76825   Echocardiography, fetal, cardiovascular system, real time
             with image documentation (2D), with or without M-mode
             recording;

> *CPT Assistant* Apr 97:2, Aug 02:2, Sep 17:15

> *Clinical Examples in Radiology* Fall 21:16, Spring 22:15

76826   follow-up or repeat study

> *CPT Assistant* Apr 97:2, Aug 02:2, Sep 17:15

> *Clinical Examples in Radiology* Spring 22:15

76827   Doppler echocardiography, fetal, pulsed wave and/or
             continuous wave with spectral display; complete

> *CPT Changes: An Insider's View* 2005

> *CPT Assistant* Apr 97:2, Aug 02:2, Dec 05:3, Sep 22:20

> *Clinical Examples in Radiology* Spring 22:15

76828   follow-up or repeat study

> *CPT Assistant* Apr 97:2, Aug 02:2, Dec 05:3, Sep 22:20

> *Clinical Examples in Radiology* Spring 22:15

(To report the use of color mapping, use 93325)

Nonobstetrical

Code 76856 includes the complete evaluation of the
female pelvic anatomy. Elements of this examination
include a description and measurements of the uterus and
adnexal structures, measurement of the endometrium,
measurement of the bladder (when applicable), and a
description of any pelvic pathology (eg, ovarian cysts,
uterine leiomyomata, free pelvic fluid).

Code 76856 is also applicable to a complete evaluation of
the male pelvis. Elements of the examination include
evaluation and measurement (when applicable) of the
urinary bladder, evaluation of the prostate and seminal
vesicles to the extent that they are visualized
transabdominally, and any pelvic pathology (eg, bladder
tumor, enlarged prostate, free pelvic fluid, pelvic abscess).

Code 76857 represents a focused examination limited to
the assessment of one or more elements listed in code
76856 and/or the reevaluation of one or more pelvic
abnormalities previously demonstrated on ultrasound.
Code 76857, rather than 76770, should be utilized if the

Radiology 70010-79999

urinary bladder alone (ie, not including the kidneys) is imaged, whereas code 51798 should be utilized if a bladder volume or post-void residual measurement is obtained without imaging the bladder.

Use of ultrasound, without thorough evaluation of organ(s) or anatomic region, image documentation, and final, written report, is not separately reportable.

76830 Ultrasound, transvaginal

➔ *CPT Changes: An Insider's View* 2002

➔ *CPT Assistant* Aug 96:10, Jul 99:8, Aug 02:2, Mar 03:7, Dec 05:3, Feb 09:22, Nov 11:10, Oct 17:10, Dec 22:17, Mar 23:35, May 23:28, Nov 23:27, Dec 23:42

➔ *Clinical Examples in Radiology* Inaugural 04:6-7, Spring 08:9, Summer 10:8-9, Summer 12:7, Spring 15:4, Summer 15:10, Winter 16:13, Fall 18:4, Spring 20:9, Winter 22:3, 17, Summer 22:20, Fall 22:9-12, Spring 23:33

(For obstetrical transvaginal ultrasound, use 76817)

(If transvaginal examination is done in addition to transabdominal non-obstetrical ultrasound exam, use 76830 in addition to appropriate transabdominal exam code)

76831 Saline infusion sonohysterography (SIS), including color flow Doppler, when performed

➔ *CPT Changes: An Insider's View* 2004

➔ *CPT Assistant* Nov 97:25, Jul 99:8, Dec 05:3, Mar 09:11

➔ *Clinical Examples in Radiology* Spring 23:32

(For introduction of saline for saline infusion sonohysterography, use 58340)

76856 Ultrasound, pelvic (nonobstetric), real time with image documentation; complete

➔ *CPT Changes: An Insider's View* 2002, 2007

➔ *CPT Assistant* Oct 01:3, Dec 05:3, Jan 06:47, Mar 07:7, Feb 09:22, Aug 16:10, Oct 17:10, Dec 22:17, Nov 23:27

➔ *Clinical Examples in Radiology* Inaugural 04:6-7, Spring 08:9, Summer 10:8, Summer 12:7, Summer 14:9, Spring 15:4, Summer 15:10, Winter 18:15, Fall 18:4, Spring 20:9, Winter 21:13, Winter 22:3, 16, Summer 22:20, Fall 22:9-12, Spring 23:28

76857 limited or follow-up (eg, for follicles)

➔ *CPT Assistant* Jun 97:10, Oct 01:3, Dec 05:3, Sep 07:10, May 09:7, Oct 17:10, Dec 22:17, Nov 23:27

➔ *Clinical Examples in Radiology* Spring 08:9, Summer 10:8, Summer 12:7, Summer 13:11, Summer 14:8-9, Spring 15:4, Summer 15:10, Winter 18:15, Spring 18:13, Fall 18:4, Spring 20:9, Winter 21:13, Winter 22:3, 16, Summer 22:20, Fall 22:9-12

Genitalia

76870 Ultrasound, scrotum and contents

➔ *CPT Changes: An Insider's View* 2002

➔ *CPT Assistant* May 05:3, Oct 17:10, Dec 22:17

➔ *Clinical Examples in Radiology* Spring 15:4, Winter 18:15, Fall 18:4, Winter 22:3, Summer 22:20

76872 Ultrasound, transrectal;

➔ *CPT Changes: An Insider's View* 2000, 2004

➔ *CPT Assistant* May 96:3, Nov 99:42, Oct 17:10, Jul 18:11, Nov 18:10, Jul 22:20, Dec 22:17

➔ *Clinical Examples in Radiology* Spring 15:4, Fall 18:4, Winter 22:3, Summer 22:20

(Do not report 76872 in conjunction with 45341, 45342, 45391, 45392, 46948, 0421T, 0619T)

76873 prostate volume study for brachytherapy treatment planning (separate procedure)

➔ *CPT Changes: An Insider's View* 2000

➔ *CPT Assistant* Nov 99:42

Extremities

Code 76881 represents a complete evaluation of a specific joint in an extremity. Code 76881 requires ultrasound examination of all of the following joint elements: joint space (eg, effusion), peri-articular soft-tissue structures that surround the joint (ie, muscles, tendons, other soft-tissue structures), and any identifiable abnormality. In some circumstances, additional evaluations such as dynamic imaging or stress maneuvers may be performed as part of the complete evaluation. Code 76881 also requires permanently recorded images and a written report containing a description of each of the required elements or reason that an element(s) could not be visualized (eg, absent secondary to surgery or trauma).

When fewer than all of the required elements for a "complete" exam (76881) are performed, report the "limited" code (76882).

Code 76882 represents a limited evaluation of a joint or focal evaluation of a structure(s) in an extremity other than a joint (eg, soft-tissue mass, fluid collection, or nerve[s]). Limited evaluation of a joint includes assessment of a specific anatomic structure(s) (eg, joint space only [effusion] or tendon, muscle, and/or other soft-tissue structure[s] that surround the joint) that does not assess all of the required elements included in 76881. Code 76882 also requires permanently recorded images and a written report containing a description of each of the elements evaluated.

Comprehensive evaluation of a nerve is defined as evaluation of the nerve throughout its course in an extremity. Documentation of the entire course of a nerve throughout an extremity includes the acquisition and permanent archive of cine clips and static images to demonstrate the anatomy.

For spectral and color Doppler evaluation of the extremities, use 93925, 93926, 93930, 93931, 93970, or 93971 as appropriate.

76881   Ultrasound, complete joint (ie, joint space and peri-articular soft-tissue structures), real-time with image documentation

➔ *CPT Changes: An Insider's View* 2011, 2018

➔ *CPT Assistant* Sep 16:9, Oct 17:10, Nov 22:8, Dec 22:17

➔ *Clinical Examples in Radiology* Winter 11:7, 11, Summer 14:8, Winter 15:8-9, Spring 15:4, Spring 17:12, Spring 18:12, Fall 18:4, Winter 19:13, Summer 19:8, Winter 21:8, Winter 22:3, Summer 22:20, Summer 23:11

76882   Ultrasound, limited, joint or focal evaluation of other nonvascular extremity structure(s) (eg, joint space, peri-articular tendon[s], muscle[s], nerve[s], other soft-tissue structure[s], or soft-tissue mass[es]), real-time with image documentation

➔ *CPT Changes: An Insider's View* 2011, 2018, 2023

➔ *CPT Assistant* Sep 16:9, Oct 17:10, Nov 22:8, Dec 22:17

➔ *Clinical Examples in Radiology* Winter 11:7, Summer 11:11, Summer 14:8-9, Winter 15:8, 10, Spring 15:4, Summer 15:13, Spring 17:12, Fall 18:4, Winter 19:7, Summer 19:8, Winter 21:8, Summer 22:20, Summer 23:10

(Do not report 76882 in conjunction with 76883)

76883   Ultrasound, nerve(s) and accompanying structures throughout their entire anatomic course in one extremity, comprehensive, including real-time cine imaging with image documentation, per extremity

➔ *CPT Changes: An Insider's View* 2023

➔ *CPT Assistant* Nov 22:8

➔ *Clinical Examples in Radiology* Summer 23:10

76885   Ultrasound, infant hips, real time with imaging documentation; dynamic (requiring physician or other qualified health care professional manipulation)

➔ *CPT Changes: An Insider's View* 2002, 2013

➔ *CPT Assistant* Nov 97:25

➔ *Clinical Examples in Radiology* Summer 19:8

76886   limited, static (not requiring physician or other qualified health care professional manipulation)

➔ *CPT Changes: An Insider's View* 2002, 2013

➔ *CPT Assistant* Nov 97:25

➔ *Clinical Examples in Radiology* Summer 19:8

Ultrasonic Guidance Procedures

76932   Ultrasonic guidance for endomyocardial biopsy, imaging supervision and interpretation

➔ *CPT Changes: An Insider's View* 2001

76936   Ultrasound guided compression repair of arterial pseudoaneurysm or arteriovenous fistulae (includes diagnostic ultrasound evaluation, compression of lesion and imaging)

+ 76937   Ultrasound guidance for vascular access requiring ultrasound evaluation of potential access sites, documentation of selected vessel patency, concurrent

realtime ultrasound visualization of vascular needle entry, with permanent recording and reporting (List separately in addition to code for primary procedure)

➔ *CPT Changes: An Insider's View* 2004

➔ *CPT Assistant* Dec 04:13, Jan 09:7, Jul 10:6, Nov 10:3, Jan 11:8, Apr 12:6, Feb 13:3, May 13:3, Jun 13:12, Sep 13:18, Oct 14:6, Jul 15:10, Mar 17:4, Jul 17:5, Jan 23:32, Mar 24:1

➔ *Clinical Examples in Radiology* Inaugural 04:1-2, Winter 05:5-6, Summer 06:8-9, Spring 08:7-8, Fall 08:5-6, Winter 09:8-9, Spring 09:10, Summer 10:1, 3-4, Winter 12:3, Spring 12:4, Summer 12:3, Winter 13:1-3, Summer 13:4, Fall 13:1-4, Winter 14:1, 5, 7, Summer 14:10, Winter 15:2-6, Summer 15:2, Winter 16:2, Winter 17:8, Spring 18:8, Summer 18:4, Fall 18:8, Spring 19:2, Summer 19:4, Winter 23:9

(Do not report 76937 in conjunction with 33274, 33275, 36568, 36569, 36572, 36573, 36584, 36836, 36837, 37191, 37192, 37193, 37760, 37761, 76942, 0795T, 0796T, 0797T, 0798T, 0799T, 0800T, 0801T, 0802T, 0803T, 0823T, 0824T, 0825T)

(Do not report 76937 in conjunction with 0505T, 0620T for ultrasound guidance for vascular access)

(If extremity venous non-invasive vascular diagnostic study is performed separate from venous access guidance, see 93970, 93971)

76940   Ultrasound guidance for, and monitoring of, parenchymal tissue ablation

➔ *CPT Changes: An Insider's View* 2004, 2007

➔ *CPT Assistant* Oct 02:2, Mar 07:7, Jul 15:8, May 17:3, Nov 17:8, Mar 21:5, Dec 23:42

➔ *Clinical Examples in Radiology* Spring 08:1-2, Summer 12:11, Spring 15:3, Fall 17:3

(Do not report 76940 in conjunction with 20982, 20983, 32994, 32998, 50250, 50542, 76942, 76998, 0582T, 0600T, 0601T)

(For ablation, see 47370-47382, 47383, 50592, 50593)

76941   Ultrasonic guidance for intrauterine fetal transfusion or cordocentesis, imaging supervision and interpretation

➔ *CPT Changes: An Insider's View* 2001

(For procedure, see 36460, 59012)

Radiology 70010-79999

76942 Ultrasonic guidance for needle placement (eg, biopsy, aspiration, injection, localization device), imaging supervision and interpretation

➔ *CPT Changes: An Insider's View* 2001

➔ *CPT Assistant* Fall 93:12, Fall 94:2, May 96:3, Jun 97:5, Oct 01:2, May 04:7, Dec 04:12, Apr 05:15-16, Aug 08:7, Mar 09:8, Feb 10:6, Mar 10:9, Jul 10:6, Feb 11:4, Mar 11:10, Apr 11:12, Nov 12:3, Dec 12:9, Nov 13:9, Oct 14:6, Feb 15:6, Aug 15:8, Nov 15:10, Jan 16:9, Jun 16:3, Jun 17:10, Dec 17:16, Mar 18:3, Jul 18:11, Aug 19:10, Jan 21:13, Apr 21:10, May 21:14, Aug 21:14, Nov 21:13, Jul 22:20, Dec 22:1, Jan 23:24, Dec 23:47

➔ *Clinical Examples in Radiology* Summer 05:1-2, 6, Fall 05:1, Summer 08:5-6, Fall 08:2-3, Winter 09:9, Fall 09:8, Summer 10:1, 3-4, Fall 10:3, Summer 11:3, Spring 14:2, 4, 7, Summer 14:9, Spring 15:10, Summer 15:7, Winter 16:6, Winter 17:3, Winter 18:8, Spring 18:3, Winter 19:2, Fall 19:9, Winter 20:5, Fall 20:4, 14-15, Winter 21:12, Spring 21:12, 13, Spring 22:5, 6, Winter 23:12, Summer 23:23

▶(Do not report 76942 in conjunction with 10004, 10005, 10006, 10021, 10030, 19083, 19285, 20604, 20606, 20611, 27096, 32408, 32554, 32555, 32556, 32557, 37760, 37761, 43232, 43237, 43242, 45341, 45342, 46948, 55874, 64415, 64416, 64417, 64445, 64446, 64447, 64448, 64466, 64467, 64468, 64469, 64473, 64474, 64479, 64480, 64483, 64484, 64490, 64491, 64493, 64494, 64495, 76975, 0213T, 0214T, 0215T, 0216T, 0217T, 0218T, 0232T, 0481T, 0582T)◀

(For harvesting, preparation, and injection[s] of platelet rich plasma, use 0232T)

76945 Ultrasonic guidance for chorionic villus sampling, imaging supervision and interpretation

➔ *CPT Changes: An Insider's View* 2001

(For procedure, use 59015)

76946 Ultrasonic guidance for amniocentesis, imaging supervision and interpretation

➔ *CPT Changes: An Insider's View* 2001

76948 Ultrasonic guidance for aspiration of ova, imaging supervision and interpretation

➔ *CPT Changes: An Insider's View* 2001

(For placement of interstitial device[s] for radiation therapy guidance, see 31627, 32553, 49411, 55876)

76965 Ultrasonic guidance for interstitial radioelement application

Other Procedures

76975 Gastrointestinal endoscopic ultrasound, supervision and interpretation

➔ *CPT Changes: An Insider's View* 2001

➔ *CPT Assistant* Spring 94:5, May 04:7, Mar 09:8

(Do not report 76975 in conjunction with 43231, 43232, 43237, 43238, 43240, 43242, 43259, 44406, 44407, 45341, 45342, 45391, 45392, 76942)

76977 Ultrasound bone density measurement and interpretation, peripheral site(s), any method

➔ *CPT Assistant* Nov 98:21

➔ *Clinical Examples in Radiology* Winter 19:7

76978 Ultrasound, targeted dynamic microbubble sonographic contrast characterization (non-cardiac); initial lesion

➔ *CPT Changes: An Insider's View* 2019

➔ *CPT Assistant* Jun 19:9, Nov 21:13, Aug 23:21

➔ *Clinical Examples in Radiology* Fall 18:14, Spring 22:5, Fall 23:25

+ 76979 each additional lesion with separate injection (List separately in addition to code for primary procedure)

➔ *CPT Changes: An Insider's View* 2019

➔ *CPT Assistant* Jun 19:9, Nov 21:13, Aug 23:21

➔ *Clinical Examples in Radiology* Fall 18:14, Spring 22:5, Fall 23:25

(Use 76979 in conjunction with 76978)

(Do not report 76978, 76979 in conjunction with 96374)

76981 Ultrasound, elastography; parenchyma (eg, organ)

➔ *CPT Changes: An Insider's View* 2019

➔ *CPT Assistant* Aug 19:3, Dec 22:17

➔ *Clinical Examples in Radiology* Fall 18:3, Fall 21:17, Winter 22:3, Summer 22:20

76982 first target lesion

➔ *CPT Changes: An Insider's View* 2019

➔ *CPT Assistant* Aug 19:3, Dec 22:17

➔ *Clinical Examples in Radiology* Fall 18:3, Winter 22:3, Summer 22:20

+ 76983 each additional target lesion (List separately in addition to code for primary procedure)

➔ *CPT Changes: An Insider's View* 2019

➔ *CPT Assistant* Aug 19:3, Dec 22:17

➔ *Clinical Examples in Radiology* Fall 18:3, Winter 22:3, Summer 22:20

(Use 76983 in conjunction with 76982)

(Report 76981 only once per session for evaluation of the same parenchymal organ)

(To report shear wave liver elastography without imaging, use 91200)

(For evaluation of a parenchymal organ and lesion[s] in the same parenchymal organ at the same session, report only 76981)

(Do not report 76981, 76982, 76983 in conjunction with 0689T)

(Do not report 76983 more than two times per organ)

76984 Ultrasound, intraoperative thoracic aorta (eg, epiaortic), diagnostic

➔ *CPT Changes: An Insider's View* 2024

(For diagnostic intraoperative epicardial cardiac ultrasound [ie, echocardiography], see 76987, 76988, 76989)

Radiology 70010-79999

76987 Intraoperative epicardial cardiac ultrasound (ie, echocardiography) for congenital heart disease, diagnostic; including placement and manipulation of transducer, image acquisition, interpretation and report

➔ *CPT Changes: An Insider's View* 2024

76988   placement, manipulation of transducer, and image acquisition only

➔ *CPT Changes: An Insider's View* 2024

76989   interpretation and report only

➔ *CPT Changes: An Insider's View* 2024

(For diagnostic intraoperative thoracic aorta (eg, epiaortic) ultrasound, use 76984)

76998 Ultrasonic guidance, intraoperative

➔ *CPT Changes: An Insider's View* 2007

➔ *CPT Assistant* Mar 07:7, Jul 10:6, Jan 13:6, Jan 14:5, Oct 14:6, Aug 15:8, Apr 17:7, Dec 23:42

➔ *Clinical Examples in Radiology* Winter 12:11

(Do not report 76998 in conjunction with 36475, 36479, 37760, 37761, 46948, 47370, 47371, 47380, 47381, 47382, 76984, 76987, 76988, 76989, 0515T, 0516T, 0517T, 0518T, 0519T, 0520T, 0861T, 0862T, 0863T)

(For ultrasound guidance for open and laparoscopic radiofrequency tissue ablation, use 76940)

76999 Unlisted ultrasound procedure (eg, diagnostic, interventional)

➔ *CPT Changes: An Insider's View* 2003

➔ *CPT Assistant* Dec 19:8, Sep 22:20, Dec 22:17

➔ *Clinical Examples in Radiology* Summer 12:10, Winter 15:8-9, Spring 15:10, Winter 19:7, Winter 22:3, Summer 22:20

Radiologic Guidance

Fluoroscopic Guidance

(Do not report guidance codes 77001, 77002, 77003 for services in which fluoroscopic guidance is included in the descriptor)

+ 77001 Fluoroscopic guidance for central venous access device placement, replacement (catheter only or complete), or removal (includes fluoroscopic guidance for vascular access and catheter manipulation, any necessary contrast injections through access site or catheter with related venography radiologic supervision and interpretation, and radiographic documentation of final catheter position) (List separately in addition to code for primary procedure)

➔ *CPT Changes: An Insider's View* 2007

➔ *CPT Assistant* Mar 07:7, Jul 08:9, Nov 10:3, Jan 11:8, Jul 23:17

➔ *Clinical Examples in Radiology* Spring 08:7-8, Fall 08:5-6, Winter 09:8-9, Summer 10:11, Winter 17:8, Fall 18:7, Fall 23:28

▶(Do not report 77001 in conjunction with 33957, 33958, 33959, 33962, 33963, 33964, 36568, 36569, 36572, 36573, 36584, 36836, 36837, 64466, 64467, 64468, 64469, 64473, 64474, 77002)◀

(If formal extremity venography is performed from separate venous access and separately interpreted, use 36005 and 75820, 75822, 75825, or 75827)

+ 77002 Fluoroscopic guidance for needle placement (eg, biopsy, aspiration, injection, localization device) (List separately in addition to code for primary procedure)

➔ *CPT Changes: An Insider's View* 2007, 2017

➔ *CPT Assistant* Feb 07:11; Mar 07:7, May 07:1, Jun 07:10, Jul 08:9, Aug 08:7, Dec 08:9, Dec 09:12, Feb 10:6, Nov 10:3, Jan 11:8, Apr 11:12, Feb 12:11, Apr 12:19, Jun 12:14, Nov 12:3, Dec 12:9, Nov 13:9, Jul 15:8, Aug 15:6, Jan 16:9, Jun 16:3, Sep 16:10, May 17:3, Jun 17:10, Nov 17:8, Dec 18:11, Dec 19:8, Mar 21:5, Apr 21:10, Jun 21:14, Dec 22:1, Jan 23:24, Mar 24:1

➔ *Clinical Examples in Radiology* Summer 08:5-6, Winter 09:9, Spring 09:6-7, Fall 09:7, Fall 10:10, Summer 11:3, Spring 13:11, Winter 14:9-10, Spring 14:4, 10, Spring 15:3, Winter 16:6, Winter 17:5, Spring 18:3, Summer 18:9, Fall 18:12, Winter 19:3, Winter 20:5, Spring 20:6, Fall 20:4, 15, Spring 21:7, 13, Spring 22:9, Summer 22:15, Winter 23:12, Summer 23:27

(Use 77002 in conjunction with 10160, 20206, 20220, 20225, 20520, 20525, 20526, 20550, 20551, 20552, 20553, 20555, 20600, 20605, 20610, 20612, 20615, 21116, 21550, 23350, 24220, 25246, 27093, 27095, 27369, 27648, 32400, 32553, 36002, 38220, 38221, 38222, 38505, 38794, 41019, 42400, 42405, 47000, 47001, 48102, 49180, 49411, 50200, 50390, 51100, 51101, 51102, 55700, 55876, 60100, 62268, 62269, 64400, 64405, 64408, 64418, 64420, 64421, 64425, 64430, 64435, 64450, 64455, 64505, 64600, 64605)

(77002 is included in all arthrography radiological supervision and interpretation codes. See **Administration of Contrast Material[s]** introductory guidelines for reporting of arthrography procedures)

+ 77003 Fluoroscopic guidance and localization of needle or catheter tip for spine or paraspinous diagnostic or therapeutic injection procedures (epidural or subarachnoid) (List separately in addition to code for primary procedure)

➔ *CPT Changes: An Insider's View* 2007, 2010, 2011, 2012, 2017

➔ *CPT Assistant* Mar 07:7, Jul 08:9, Feb 10:12, May 10:10, Aug 10:8, Oct 10:14, Nov 10:3, Dec 10:14, Jan 11:8, Feb 11:4, Mar 11:7, Jul 11:17, Jun 12:12, Jul 12:3, 5-6, Sep 12:14, Nov 13:9, Dec 13:14, Jan 16:9, 12, May 17:3, Dec 17:13, Dec 19:8, Mar 21:3, Oct 21:10, Jan 23:24

➔ *Clinical Examples in Radiology* Summer 08:9, 13, Winter 09:9, Spring 11:9, Winter 14:9-10, Spring 14:4, Fall 15:10, Summer 16:4, Winter 18:8, Summer 18:9, Fall 19:8, Fall 20:15, Winter 22:18, Spring 22:10

(Use 77003 in conjunction with 61050, 61055, 62267, 62273, 62280, 62281, 62282, 62284, 64449, 64510, 64517, 64520, 64610, 96450)

Radiology 70010-79999

(Do not report 77003 in conjunction with 62270, 62272, 62320, 62321, 62322, 62323, 62324, 62325, 62326, 62327, 62328, 62329, 64415, 64416, 64417, 64445, 64446, 64447, 64448, 0627T, 0628T)

Computed Tomography Guidance

77011 Computed tomography guidance for stereotactic localization

➲ *CPT Changes: An Insider's View* 2007

➲ *CPT Assistant* Mar 07:7

77012 Computed tomography guidance for needle placement (eg, biopsy, aspiration, injection, localization device), radiological supervision and interpretation

➲ *CPT Changes: An Insider's View* 2007

➲ *CPT Assistant* Mar 07:7, May 07:1, Jun 07:10, Aug 08:7, Feb 10:6, Feb 11:4, Apr 11:12, Jul 12:3, 6, Sep 12:14, Nov 12:3, Dec 12:9, Nov 13:9, Feb 15:6, Jun 16:3, Dec 19:8, Apr 21:10, May 21:14, Oct 21:10, Mar 24:26

➲ *Clinical Examples in Radiology* Summer 08:5-6, Fall 08:3, Fall 09:6, Fall 10:3, Summer 11:3, Spring 14:4, Spring 15:7, Winter 16:6, Summer 16:4, Winter 17:5, Winter 18:8, Spring 18:3, Winter 19:3, Fall 19:9, Winter 20:5, Fall 20:3-4, Spring 21:13, Winter 22:19, Spring 22:9, 10, Winter 23:12, Summer 23:26

(Do not report 77011, 77012 in conjunction with 22586)

▶(Do not report 77012 in conjunction with 10009, 10010, 10030, 27096, 32408, 32554, 32555, 32556, 32557, 62270, 62272, 62328, 62329, 64466, 64467, 64468, 64469, 64473, 64474, 64479, 64480, 64483, 64484, 64490, 64491, 64492, 64493, 64494, 64495, 64633, 64634, 64635, 64636, 0232T, 0481T, 0629T, 0630T)◀

(For harvesting, preparation, and injection[s] of platelet-rich plasma, use 0232T)

77013 Computed tomography guidance for, and monitoring of, parenchymal tissue ablation

➲ *CPT Changes: An Insider's View* 2007

➲ *CPT Assistant* Mar 07:7, Jul 15:8, May 17:3, Nov 17:8, Mar 21:5

➲ *Clinical Examples in Radiology* Summer 12:11, Spring 15:3, Fall 17:3

(Do not report 77013 in conjunction with 20982, 20983, 32994, 32998, 0600T)

(For percutaneous ablation, see 47382, 47383, 50592, 50593)

77014 Computed tomography guidance for placement of radiation therapy fields

➲ *CPT Changes: An Insider's View* 2007

➲ *CPT Assistant* Mar 07:7, Apr 15:11, Feb 16:3

➲ *Clinical Examples in Radiology* Summer 09:2, 4, Spring 12:10, Winter 13:11, Fall 20:12

(For placement of interstitial device[s] for radiation therapy guidance, see 31627, 32553, 49411, 55876)

Magnetic Resonance Imaging Guidance

77021 Magnetic resonance imaging guidance for needle placement (eg, for biopsy, needle aspiration, injection, or placement of localization device) radiological supervision and interpretation

➲ *CPT Changes: An Insider's View* 2007, 2019

➲ *CPT Assistant* Mar 07:7, May 07:1, Jun 07:10, Aug 08:7, Feb 10:6, Apr 11:12, Nov 12:3, Dec 12:9, Nov 13:9, Feb 15:6, Jun 16:3, Jun 17:10, Jul 18:11, Apr 21:10

➲ *Clinical Examples in Radiology* Summer 08:5-6, 13, Fall 08:3, Fall 10:3, Summer 11:3, Spring 14:4, Spring 15:7, Winter 16:6, Winter 17:5, Spring 18:3, Winter 19:3, Fall 19:9, Winter 20:5, Fall 20:4, Spring 21:13, Spring 22:9, Winter 23:12, Summer 23:27

(For procedure, see appropriate organ or site)

▶(Do not report 77021 in conjunction with 10011, 10012, 10030, 19085, 19287, 32408, 32554, 32555, 32556, 32557, 64466, 64467, 64468, 64469, 64473, 64474, 0232T, 0481T)◀

(For harvesting, preparation, and injection[s] of platelet-rich plasma, use 0232T)

77022 Magnetic resonance imaging guidance for, and monitoring of, parenchymal tissue ablation

➲ *CPT Changes: An Insider's View* 2007, 2019

➲ *CPT Assistant* Mar 07:7, Oct 14:6, Jul 15:8, May 17:3, Sep 19:11, Mar 21:5

➲ *Clinical Examples in Radiology* Summer 12:11, Spring 15:3, Fall 17:3

(Do not report 77022 in conjunction with 20982, 20983, 32994, 32998, 0071T, 0072T, 0600T)

(For percutaneous ablation, see 47382, 47383, 50592, 50593)

(For focused ultrasound ablation treatment of uterine leiomyomata, see Category III codes 0071T, 0072T)

(To report stereotactic localization guidance for breast biopsy or for placement of breast localization device[s], see 19081, 19283)

(To report mammographic guidance for placement of breast localization device[s], use 19281)

Breast, Mammography

77046 Magnetic resonance imaging, breast, without contrast material; unilateral

➲ *CPT Changes: An Insider's View* 2019

➲ *CPT Assistant* Aug 19:5

➲ *Clinical Examples in Radiology* Summer 19:11, Winter 20:14

77047   bilateral

          ➔ *CPT Changes: An Insider's View* 2019

          ➔ *CPT Assistant* Aug 19:5

          ➔ *Clinical Examples in Radiology* Summer 19:11, Winter 20:14

77048   Magnetic resonance imaging, breast, without and with contrast material(s), including computer-aided detection (CAD real-time lesion detection, characterization and pharmacokinetic analysis), when performed; unilateral

    ➔ *CPT Changes: An Insider's View* 2019

    ➔ *CPT Assistant* Aug 19:5, Dec 19:15, Sep 21:5

    ➔ *Clinical Examples in Radiology* Summer 19:11, Winter 20:11

77049   bilateral

          ➔ *CPT Changes: An Insider's View* 2019

          ➔ *CPT Assistant* Aug 19:5, Dec 19:15, Sep 21:5

          ➔ *Clinical Examples in Radiology* Summer 19:11, Winter 20:11

77053   Mammary ductogram or galactogram, single duct, radiological supervision and interpretation

    ➔ *CPT Changes: An Insider's View* 2007

    ➔ *CPT Assistant* Mar 07:7

    ➔ *Clinical Examples in Radiology* Fall 22:6

    (For mammary ductogram or galactogram injection, use 19030)

77054   Mammary ductogram or galactogram, multiple ducts, radiological supervision and interpretation

    ➔ *CPT Changes: An Insider's View* 2007

    ➔ *CPT Assistant* Mar 07:7

    ➔ *Clinical Examples in Radiology* Fall 22:6

77061   Diagnostic digital breast tomosynthesis; unilateral

    ➔ *CPT Changes: An Insider's View* 2015, 2019

    ➔ *CPT Assistant* May 17:3, Sep 20:15

    ➔ *Clinical Examples in Radiology* Fall 14:10, Fall 20:12, Summer 21:11

77062   bilateral

          ➔ *CPT Changes: An Insider's View* 2015, 2019

          ➔ *CPT Assistant* Dec 16:15, May 17:3, Sep 20:15

          ➔ *Clinical Examples in Radiology* Fall 14:10, Fall 20:12, Summer 21:11

    (Do not report 77061, 77062 in conjunction with 76376, 76377, 77067)

+ 77063   Screening digital breast tomosynthesis, bilateral (List separately in addition to code for primary procedure)

    ➔ *CPT Changes: An Insider's View* 2015

    ➔ *CPT Assistant* Dec 16:15, May 17:3, Sep 20:15

    ➔ *Clinical Examples in Radiology* Fall 14:10, Fall 20:12

    (Do not report 77063 in conjunction with 76376, 76377, 77065, 77066)

    (Use 77063 in conjunction with 77067)

77065   Diagnostic mammography, including computer-aided detection (CAD) when performed; unilateral

    ➔ *CPT Changes: An Insider's View* 2017

    ➔ *CPT Assistant* Dec 16:15, May 17:3, Sep 20:15, Sep 21:5

    ➔ *Clinical Examples in Radiology* Winter 17:15, Spring 18:3, Fall 20:12, Summer 21:11, Spring 23:11

77066   bilateral

          ➔ *CPT Changes: An Insider's View* 2017

          ➔ *CPT Assistant* Dec 16:15, May 17:3, Sep 20:15, Sep 21:5

          ➔ *Clinical Examples in Radiology* Winter 17:15, Spring 18:12, Fall 20:12, Summer 21:11, Spring 23:11

77067   Screening mammography, bilateral (2-view study of each breast), including computer-aided detection (CAD) when performed

    ➔ *CPT Changes: An Insider's View* 2017

    ➔ *CPT Assistant* Dec 16:15, May 17:3, Sep 20:15, Sep 21:5

    ➔ *Clinical Examples in Radiology* Winter 17:15, Spring 18:12, Fall 20:12

    (For electrical impedance breast scan, use 76499)

Screening Mammography
77067

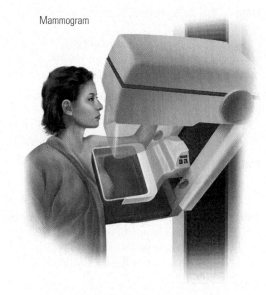

Mammogram

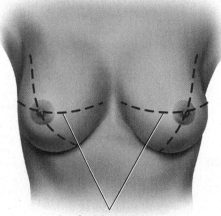

Medial lateral oblique view

Cranial caudal view

Radiology 70010-79999

Bone/Joint Studies

77071 Manual application of stress performed by physician or other qualified health care professional for joint radiography, including contralateral joint if indicated

➔ *CPT Changes: An Insider's View* 2007, 2013

➔ *CPT Assistant* Mar 07:7, Oct 18:11

(For radiographic interpretation of stressed images, see appropriate anatomic site and number of views)

77072 Bone age studies

➔ *CPT Changes: An Insider's View* 2007

➔ *CPT Assistant* Mar 07:7

77073 Bone length studies (orthoroentgenogram, scanogram)

➔ *CPT Changes: An Insider's View* 2007

➔ *CPT Assistant* Mar 07:7, Sep 21:14-15, Feb 22:15

➔ *Clinical Examples in Radiology* Summer 07:12, Fall 08:10, Fall 10:6, Fall 22:15

77074 Radiologic examination, osseous survey; limited (eg, for metastases)

➔ *CPT Changes: An Insider's View* 2007

➔ *CPT Assistant* Mar 07:7

➔ *Clinical Examples in Radiology* Summer 21:8

77075 complete (axial and appendicular skeleton)

➔ *CPT Changes: An Insider's View* 2007

➔ *CPT Assistant* Mar 07:7

➔ *Clinical Examples in Radiology* Summer 21:8-9

77076 Radiologic examination, osseous survey, infant

➔ *CPT Changes: An Insider's View* 2007

➔ *CPT Assistant* Mar 07:7

77077 Joint survey, single view, 2 or more joints (specify)

➔ *CPT Changes: An Insider's View* 2007

➔ *CPT Assistant* Mar 07:7

➔ *Clinical Examples in Radiology* Summer 21:9

77078 Computed tomography, bone mineral density study, 1 or more sites, axial skeleton (eg, hips, pelvis, spine)

➔ *CPT Changes: An Insider's View* 2007

➔ *CPT Assistant* Mar 07:7

77080 Dual-energy X-ray absorptiometry (DXA), bone density study, 1 or more sites; axial skeleton (eg, hips, pelvis, spine)

➔ *CPT Changes: An Insider's View* 2007

➔ *CPT Assistant* Mar 07:7

➔ *Clinical Examples in Radiology* Fall 07:11, Summer 10:6, Summer 15:12, Spring 19:14,15

(Do not report 77080 in conjunction with 77085, 77086)

77081 appendicular skeleton (peripheral) (eg, radius, wrist, heel)

➔ *CPT Changes: An Insider's View* 2007

➔ *CPT Assistant* Mar 07:7

➔ *Clinical Examples in Radiology* Spring 19:14,15

(For dual energy x-ray absorptiometry [DXA] body composition study, use 76499)

 # 77085 axial skeleton (eg, hips, pelvis, spine), including vertebral fracture assessment

➔ *CPT Changes: An Insider's View* 2015

➔ *Clinical Examples in Radiology* Summer 15:12

(Do not report 77085 in conjunction with 77080, 77086)

 # 77086 Vertebral fracture assessment via dual-energy X-ray absorptiometry (DXA)

➔ *CPT Changes: An Insider's View* 2015

➔ *Clinical Examples in Radiology* Summer 15:12

(Do not report 77086 in conjunction with 77080, 77085)

77084 Magnetic resonance (eg, proton) imaging, bone marrow blood supply

➔ *CPT Changes: An Insider's View* 2007

➔ *CPT Assistant* Mar 07:7

➔ *Clinical Examples in Radiology* Spring 22:17

77085 Code is out of numerical sequence. See 77080-77261

77086 Code is out of numerical sequence. See 77080-77261

77089 Trabecular bone score (TBS), structural condition of the bone microarchitecture; using dual X-ray absorptiometry (DXA) or other imaging data on gray-scale variogram, calculation, with interpretation and report on fracture-risk

➔ *CPT Changes: An Insider's View* 2022

➔ *CPT Assistant* Dec 21:16

➔ *Clinical Examples in Radiology* Fall 21:4

(Do not report 77089 in conjunction with 77090, 77091, 77092)

77090 technical preparation and transmission of data for analysis to be performed elsewhere

➔ *CPT Changes: An Insider's View* 2022

➔ *CPT Assistant* Dec 21:16

➔ *Clinical Examples in Radiology* Fall 21:4

77091 technical calculation only

➔ *CPT Changes: An Insider's View* 2022

➔ *CPT Assistant* Dec 21:16

➔ *Clinical Examples in Radiology* Fall 21:4

77092 interpretation and report on fracture-risk only by other qualified health care professional

➔ *CPT Changes: An Insider's View* 2022

➔ *CPT Assistant* Dec 21:16

➔ *Clinical Examples in Radiology* Fall 21:4

(Do not report 77090, 77091, 77092 in conjunction with 77089)

Radiation Oncology

Listings for Radiation Oncology provide for teletherapy and brachytherapy to include initial consultation, clinical treatment planning, simulation, medical radiation physics, dosimetry, treatment devices, special services, and clinical treatment management procedures. They include normal follow-up care during course of treatment and for three months following its completion.

When a service or procedure is provided that is not listed in this edition of the CPT codebook it should be identified by a Special Report (see page 539) and one of the following unlisted procedure codes:

77299   Unlisted procedure, therapeutic radiology clinical treatment planning

77399   Unlisted procedure, medical radiation physics, dosimetry and treatment devices, and special services

77499   Unlisted procedure, therapeutic radiology treatment management

77799   Unlisted procedure, clinical brachytherapy

For treatment by injectable or ingestible isotopes, see subsection Nuclear Medicine.

Consultation: Clinical Management

Preliminary consultation, evaluation of patient prior to decision to treat, or full medical care (in addition to treatment management) when provided by the therapeutic radiologist may be identified by the appropriate procedure codes from **Evaluation and Management, Medicine,** or **Surgery** sections.

Clinical Treatment Planning (External and Internal Sources)

The clinical treatment planning process is a complex service including interpretation of special testing, tumor localization, treatment volume determination, treatment time/dosage determination, choice of treatment modality, determination of number and size of treatment ports, selection of appropriate treatment devices, and other procedures.

Definitions

Simple planning requires a single treatment area of interest encompassed in a single port or simple parallel opposed ports with simple or no blocking.

Intermediate planning requires 3 or more converging ports, 2 separate treatment areas, multiple blocks, or special time dose constraints.

Complex planning requires highly complex blocking, custom shielding blocks, tangential ports, special wedges or compensators, three or more separate treatment areas, rotational or special beam considerations, combination of therapeutic modalities.

77261   Therapeutic radiology treatment planning; simple
➔ *CPT Assistant* Fall 91:12, 15, Oct 97:2, Oct 10:3, Feb 16:3
➔ *Clinical Examples in Radiology* Summer 09:2, 4, Fall 23:4

77262   intermediate
➔ *CPT Assistant* Fall 91:12, 15, Oct 97:2, Apr 09:3, Nov 09:6, Oct 10:3, Feb 16:3
➔ *Clinical Examples in Radiology* Summer 09:2, 4, Fall 23:5

77263   complex
➔ *CPT Assistant* Fall 91:15, Oct 97:2, Apr 09:3, Nov 09:6, Oct 10:3, Feb 16:3
➔ *Clinical Examples in Radiology* Summer 09:2, 4, Summer 15:5, Fall 23:5

Simulation is the process of defining relevant normal and abnormal target anatomy, and acquiring the images and data necessary to develop the optimal radiation treatment process for the patient. A simulation is defined as complex if any of these criteria are met: particle, rotation or arc therapy, complex or custom blocking, brachytherapy simulation, hyperthermia probe verification, or any use of contrast material. If a simulation does not meet any of these criteria, the complexity is defined by the number of treatment areas: one treatment area is simple, two treatment areas are intermediate, and three or more treatment areas are complex.

A treatment area is a contiguous anatomic location that will be treated with radiation therapy. Generally, this includes the primary tumor organ or the resection bed and the draining lymph node chains, if indicated. An example is a breast cancer patient for whom a single treatment area could be the breast alone or the breast, adjacent supraclavicular fossa, and internal mammary nodes. In some cases, a patient might receive radiation therapy to more than one discontinuous anatomic location. An example would be a patient with multiple bone metastases in separate sites (eg, femur and cervical spine); in this case, each distinct and separate anatomic site to be irradiated is a separate treatment area.

Definitions

Simple: simulation of a single treatment area.

Intermediate: two separate treatment areas.

Complex: three or more treatment areas, or any number of treatment areas if any of the following are involved: particle, rotation or arc therapy, complex blocking, custom shielding blocks, brachytherapy simulation, hyperthermia probe verification, any use of contrast materials.

Radiology 70010-79999

77280 Therapeutic radiology simulation-aided field setting; simple

➔ *CPT Assistant* Fall 91:15, Oct 97:2, Nov 97:26, Apr 09:10, Nov 09:6, Oct 10:3, Nov 13:11, Apr 15:11

➔ *Clinical Examples in Radiology* Summer 08:12, Summer 09:2, 4-5, Fall 20:12-13, Fall 23:4

77285 intermediate

➔ *CPT Assistant* Fall 91:15, Oct 97:3, Nov 09:6, Oct 10:3, Apr 15:11

➔ *Clinical Examples in Radiology* Summer 08:12, Summer 09:4, Fall 20:12-13, Fall 23:5

77290 complex

➔ *CPT Assistant* Fall 91:12, 15, Oct 97:3, Apr 09:3, 10, Nov 09:6, Oct 10:3, Nov 13:11, Apr 15:11, Sep 16:10

➔ *Clinical Examples in Radiology* Summer 08:12, Summer 09:4, Fall 20:12-13, Fall 23:5

+ 77293 Respiratory motion management simulation (List separately in addition to code for primary procedure)

➔ *CPT Changes: An Insider's View* 2014

➔ *CPT Assistant* Nov 13:11, Dec 15:16

(Use 77293 in conjunction with 77295, 77301)

77295 Code is out of numerical sequence. See 77293-77301

77299 Unlisted procedure, therapeutic radiology clinical treatment planning

➔ *CPT Assistant* Oct 10:3

Medical Radiation Physics, Dosimetry, Treatment Devices, and Special Services

 # 77295 3-dimensional radiotherapy plan, including dose-volume histograms

➔ *CPT Changes: An Insider's View* 2014

➔ *CPT Assistant* Fall 91:15, Oct 97:3, Nov 97:26, May 05:7, Oct 07:1, Nov 09:3, Oct 10:3, Nov 13:11, Jun 15:6, Dec 15:16, Jun 21:14

➔ *Clinical Examples in Radiology* Summer 08:12, Summer 09:2, 5, Fall 20:12

77300 Basic radiation dosimetry calculation, central axis depth dose calculation, TDF, NSD, gap calculation, off axis factor, tissue inhomogeneity factors, calculation of non-ionizing radiation surface and depth dose, as required during course of treatment, only when prescribed by the treating physician

➔ *CPT Changes: An Insider's View* 2002

➔ *CPT Assistant* Fall 91:14, Oct 97:3, Dec 08:9, Nov 09:3, Oct 10:3

➔ *Clinical Examples in Radiology* Summer 08:12, Summer 09:2, 5-6, Summer 15:5, Fall 20:10-11

(Do not report 77300 in conjunction with 77306, 77307, 77316, 77317, 77318, 77321, 77767, 77768, 77770, 77771, 77772, 0394T, 0395T)

77301 Intensity modulated radiotherapy plan, including dose-volume histograms for target and critical structure partial tolerance specifications

➔ *CPT Changes: An Insider's View* 2002

➔ *CPT Assistant* Mar 05:1, 6, May 05:7, Oct 07:1, Nov 09:3, Oct 10:3, Nov 13:11

➔ *Clinical Examples in Radiology* Fall 20:12-13

(Dose plan is optimized using inverse or forward planning technique for modulated beam delivery [eg, binary, dynamic MLC] to create highly conformal dose distribution. Computer plan distribution must be verified for positional accuracy based on dosimetric verification of the intensity map with verification of treatment set-up and interpretation of verification methodology)

77306 Teletherapy isodose plan; simple (1 or 2 unmodified ports directed to a single area of interest), includes basic dosimetry calculation(s)

➔ *CPT Changes: An Insider's View* 2015

➔ *CPT Assistant* Feb 16:3

➔ *Clinical Examples in Radiology* Fall 20:12, Fall 23:7

77307 complex (multiple treatment areas, tangential ports, the use of wedges, blocking, rotational beam, or special beam considerations), includes basic dosimetry calculation(s)

➔ *CPT Changes: An Insider's View* 2015

➔ *CPT Assistant* Feb 16:3

➔ *Clinical Examples in Radiology* Fall 23:4

(Only 1 teletherapy isodose plan may be reported for a given course of therapy to a specific treatment area)

(Do not report 77306, 77307 in conjunction with 77300)

77316 Brachytherapy isodose plan; simple (calculation[s] made from 1 to 4 sources, or remote afterloading brachytherapy, 1 channel), includes basic dosimetry calculation(s)

➔ *CPT Changes: An Insider's View* 2015

➔ *CPT Assistant* Feb 16:3

(For definition of source, see clinical brachytherapy introductory guidelines)

77317 intermediate (calculation[s] made from 5 to 10 sources, or remote afterloading brachytherapy, 2-12 channels), includes basic dosimetry calculation(s)

➔ *CPT Changes: An Insider's View* 2015

➔ *CPT Assistant* Feb 16:3

77318 complex (calculation[s] made from over 10 sources, or remote afterloading brachytherapy, over 12 channels), includes basic dosimetry calculation(s)

➔ *CPT Changes: An Insider's View* 2015

➔ *CPT Assistant* Feb 16:3

(Do not report 77316, 77317, 77318 in conjunction with 77300)

77321 Special teletherapy port plan, particles, hemibody, total body
> *CPT Assistant* Fall 91:14, Oct 97:4, Oct 10:3
> *Clinical Examples in Radiology* Summer 09:5-6, Fall 20:12

77331 Special dosimetry (eg, TLD, microdosimetry) (specify), only when prescribed by the treating physician
> *CPT Assistant* Fall 91:13, Oct 97:4, Jun 15:6
> *Clinical Examples in Radiology* Summer 09:5-6, Fall 20:10-12

77332 Treatment devices, design and construction; simple (simple block, simple bolus)
> *CPT Assistant* Oct 97:4, Oct 10:3, Feb 16:3
> *Clinical Examples in Radiology* Summer 07:10, Summer 08:12, Summer 09:6, Fall 23:6

77333 intermediate (multiple blocks, stents, bite blocks, special bolus)
> *CPT Assistant* Oct 97:3, Oct 10:3, Feb 16:3
> *Clinical Examples in Radiology* Summer 07:10, Summer 08:12, Summer 09:6, Fall 23:6

77334 complex (irregular blocks, special shields, compensators, wedges, molds or casts)
> *CPT Assistant* Fall 91:14, Oct 97:4, Dec 08:9, Nov 09:3, Oct 10:3, Dec 10:15, Dec 15:16, Feb 16:3, Sep 16:10
> *Clinical Examples in Radiology* Summer 07:9-10, Summer 08:12, Summer 09:2, 6, Fall 23:4

77336 Continuing medical physics consultation, including assessment of treatment parameters, quality assurance of dose delivery, and review of patient treatment documentation in support of the radiation oncologist, reported per week of therapy
> *CPT Assistant* Fall 91:15, Oct 97:4, Nov 98:21, Oct 10:3, Feb 16:3, Mar 22:13
> *Clinical Examples in Radiology* Summer 08:12, Summer 09:2, 6, Fall 20:10-11

77338 Multi-leaf collimator (MLC) device(s) for intensity modulated radiation therapy (IMRT), design and construction per IMRT plan
> *CPT Changes: An Insider's View* 2010
> *CPT Assistant* Oct 10:3, Dec 10:15

(Do not report 77338 in conjunction with 77385 for compensator based IMRT)

(Do not report 77338 more than once per IMRT plan)

(For immobilization in IMRT treatment, see 77332-77334)

77370 Special medical radiation physics consultation
> *CPT Assistant* Fall 91:14, Oct 97:4, May 09:8, Oct 10:3, Jun 15:6, Feb 16:3, Mar 22:13
> *Clinical Examples in Radiology* Summer 08:12, Summer 09:6, 9, Fall 20:12

Stereotactic Radiation Treatment Delivery

77371 Radiation treatment delivery, stereotactic radiosurgery (SRS), complete course of treatment of cranial lesion(s) consisting of 1 session; multi-source Cobalt 60 based
> *CPT Changes: An Insider's View* 2007, 2008, 2010, 2017
> *CPT Assistant* Mar 07:7, Oct 07:1, Oct 10:3, Jul 11:12, Jul 14:9
> *Clinical Examples in Radiology* Summer 09:7

77372 linear accelerator based
> *CPT Changes: An Insider's View* 2007, 2008
> *CPT Assistant* Mar 07:7, Oct 07:1, Oct 10:3, Jul 11:12
> *Clinical Examples in Radiology* Summer 09:7

(For radiation treatment management, use 77432)

77373 Stereotactic body radiation therapy, treatment delivery, per fraction to 1 or more lesions, including image guidance, entire course not to exceed 5 fractions
> *CPT Changes: An Insider's View* 2007
> *CPT Assistant* Mar 07:7, Oct 07:1, Oct 10:3, Jul 11:12, Jul 14:9, Jun 15:6
> *Clinical Examples in Radiology* Summer 09:7

(Do not report 77373 in conjunction with 77385, 77386, 77401, 77402, 77407, 77412)

(For single fraction cranial lesion[s], see 77371, 77372)

77385 Code is out of numerical sequence. See 77412-77427

77386 Code is out of numerical sequence. See 77412-77427

77387 Code is out of numerical sequence. See 77412-77427

Other Procedures

77399 Unlisted procedure, medical radiation physics, dosimetry and treatment devices, and special services
> *CPT Assistant* Nov 98:21, Oct 10:3
> *Clinical Examples in Radiology* Fall 20:10-11

Radiation Treatment Delivery

Following dosimetry calculations, there are a number of alternative methods to deliver external radiation treatments, which are described with specific CPT codes:

- X-ray (photon), including conventional and intensity modulated radiation therapy (IMRT) beams;
- Electron beams;
- Neutron beams;
- Proton beams.

Radiology 70010-79999

All treatment delivery codes are reported once per treatment session. The treatment delivery codes recognize technical-only services and contain no physician work (the professional component). In contrast, the treatment management codes contain only the professional component.

Radiation treatment delivery with conventional X-ray or electron beams is assigned levels of complexity based on the number of treatment sites and complexity of the treatment fields, blocking, wedges, and physical or virtual tissue compensators. A simple block is straight-edged or an approximation of a straight edge created by a multileaf collimator (MLC). Energy of the megavoltage (≥ 1 MeV) beam does not contribute to complexity. Techniques such as treating a field-in-field to ensure dose homogeneity reflect added complexity.

Energies below the megavoltage range may be used in the treatment of skin lesions. Superficial radiation energies (up to 200 kV) may be generated by a variety of technologies and should not be reported with megavoltage (77402, 77407, 77412) for surface application. Do not report clinical treatment planning (77261, 77262, 77263), treatment devices (77332, 77333, 77334), isodose planning (77306, 77307, 77316, 77317, 77318), physics consultation (77336), or radiation treatment management (77427, 77431, 77432, 77435, 77469, 77470, 77499) with 77401, 0394T, or 0395T. When reporting 77401 alone, evaluation and management, when performed, may be reported with the appropriate E/M codes.

Intensity modulated radiation therapy (IMRT) uses computer-based optimization techniques with non-uniform radiation beam intensities to create highly conformal dose distributions that can be delivered by a radiotherapy treatment machine. A number of technologies, including spatially and temporally modulated beams, cylindrical beamlets, dynamic MLC, single or multiple fields or arcs, or compensators, may be used to generate IMRT. The complexity of IMRT may vary depending on the area being treated or the technique being used.

Image guided radiation therapy (IGRT) may be used to direct the radiation beam and to reflect motion during treatment. A variety of techniques may be used to perform this guidance including imaging (eg, ultrasound, CT, MRI, stereoscopic imaging) and non-imaging (eg, electromagnetic or infrared) techniques. Guidance may be used with any radiation treatment delivery technique and is typically used with IMRT delivery. IMRT delivery codes include the technical component of guidance or tracking, if performed. Because only the technical portion of IGRT is bundled into IMRT, the physician involvement in guidance or tracking may be reported separately. When guidance is required with conventional radiation treatment delivery, both the professional and technical components are reported because neither component of guidance is bundled into conventional radiation treatment delivery services.

The technical and professional components of guidance are handled differently with each radiation delivery code depending on the type of radiation being administered. The **Radiation Management and Treatment Table** is provided for clarity.

Definitions

Radiation Treatment Delivery, megavoltage (≥ 1 MeV), any energy

Simple: All of the following criteria are met (and none of the complex or intermediate criteria are met): single treatment area, one or two ports, and two or fewer simple blocks.

Intermediate: Any of the following criteria are met (and none of the complex criteria are met): 2 separate treatment areas, 3 or more ports on a single treatment area, or 3 or more simple blocks.

Complex: Any of the following criteria are met: 3 or more separate treatment areas, custom blocking, tangential ports, wedges, rotational beam, field-in-field or other tissue compensation that does not meet IMRT guidelines, or electron beam.

IMRT, any energy, includes the technical services for guidance.

Simple: Any of the following: prostate, breast, and all sites using physical compensator based IMRT.

Complex: Includes all other sites if not using physical compensator based IMRT.

77401 Radiation treatment delivery, superficial and/or ortho voltage, per day

> *CPT Changes: An Insider's View* 2015
> *CPT Assistant* Apr 03:14, Aug 03:10, Oct 07:1, Oct 10:3, Dec 15:14, Feb 16:3
> *Clinical Examples in Radiology* Summer 08:12, Summer 09:7

(Do not report 77401 in conjunction with 77373)

77402 Radiation treatment delivery, ≥1 MeV; simple

> *CPT Changes: An Insider's View* 2015
> *CPT Assistant* Apr 03:14, Aug 03:10, Oct 07:1, Oct 10:3, Dec 15:14, Feb 16:3, Mar 16:7
> *Clinical Examples in Radiology* Spring 07:7, 9, 12, Summer 08:12, Summer 09:7

(Do not report 77402 in conjunction with 77373)

Radiology 70010-79999

578 ★=Telemedicine ◀=Audio-only ╋=Add-on code ✗=FDA approval pending #=Resequenced code ⊘=Modifier 51 exempt ⟳⟳⟳=See p xxi for details

77407   intermediate

➜ *CPT Changes: An Insider's View* 2015

➜ *CPT Assistant* Apr 03:14, Aug 03:10, Oct 07:1, Dec 15:14, Feb 16:3, Mar 16:7

➜ *Clinical Examples in Radiology* Spring 07:7, 9, 12, Summer 08:12, Summer 09:7

(Do not report 77407 in conjunction with 77373)

77412   complex

➜ *CPT Changes: An Insider's View* 2006, 2015

➜ *CPT Assistant* Apr 03:14, Aug 03:10, Oct 07:1, Dec 15:14, Feb 16:3, Mar 16:7

➜ *Clinical Examples in Radiology* Winter 06:20, Spring 07:7, 9, 12, Summer 08:12, Summer 09:7

(Do not report 77412 in conjunction with 77373)

77417   Therapeutic radiology port image(s)

➜ *CPT Changes: An Insider's View* 2016

➜ *CPT Assistant* Fall 91:14, Dec 97:11, Feb 06:14, Oct 07:1, Dec 15:14, Dec 17:15

➜ *Clinical Examples in Radiology* Summer 09:2, 7

(For intensity modulated treatment planning, use 77301)

 # 77385   Intensity modulated radiation treatment delivery (IMRT), includes guidance and tracking, when performed; simple

➜ *CPT Changes: An Insider's View* 2015

➜ *CPT Assistant* Feb 16:3

(To report professional component [PC] of guidance and tracking, use 77387 with modifier 26)

 # 77386   complex

➜ *CPT Changes: An Insider's View* 2015

➜ *CPT Assistant* Feb 16:3

(To report professional component [PC] of guidance and tracking, use 77387 with modifier 26)

(Do not report 77385, 77386 in conjunction with 77371, 77372, 77373)

 # 77387   Guidance for localization of target volume for delivery of radiation treatment, includes intrafraction tracking, when performed

➜ *CPT Changes: An Insider's View* 2015, 2019

➜ *CPT Assistant* Dec 15:14, 17, Feb 16:3

(Do not report technical component [TC] with 77385, 77386, 77371, 77372, 77373)

(For placement of interstitial device[s] for radiation therapy guidance, see 31627, 32553, 49411, 55876)

 # 77424   Intraoperative radiation treatment delivery, x-ray, single treatment session

➜ *CPT Changes: An Insider's View* 2012

➜ *CPT Assistant* Dec 15:14

➜ *Clinical Examples in Radiology* Fall 11:11

 # 77425   Intraoperative radiation treatment delivery, electrons, single treatment session

➜ *CPT Changes: An Insider's View* 2012

➜ *CPT Assistant* Dec 15:14

➜ *Clinical Examples in Radiology* Fall 11:11

Neutron Beam Treatment Delivery

77423   High energy neutron radiation treatment delivery, 1 or more isocenter(s) with coplanar or non-coplanar geometry with blocking and/or wedge, and/or compensator(s)

➜ *CPT Changes: An Insider's View* 2006, 2018

➜ *CPT Assistant* Dec 15:14

➜ *Clinical Examples in Radiology* Winter 06:18

77424   Code is out of numerical sequence. See 77412-77427

77425   Code is out of numerical sequence. See 77412-77427

Radiation Treatment Management

Radiation treatment management is reported in units of five fractions or treatment sessions, regardless of the actual time period in which the services are furnished. The services need not be furnished on consecutive days. Multiple fractions representing two or more treatment sessions furnished on the same day may be counted separately as long as there has been a distinct break in therapy sessions, and the fractions are of the character usually furnished on different days. Code 77427 is also reported if there are three or four fractions beyond a multiple of five at the end of a course of treatment; one or two fractions beyond a multiple of five at the end of a course of treatment are not reported separately.

Radiation treatment management requires **and includes** a minimum of one examination of the patient by the physician for medical evaluation and management (eg, assessment of the patient's response to treatment, coordination of care and treatment, review of imaging and/or lab test results with documentation) for each reporting of the radiation treatment management service. Code 77469 represents only the intraoperative session management and does not include medical evaluation and management outside of that session. The professional services furnished during treatment management typically include:

- Review of port images;
- Review of dosimetry, dose delivery, and treatment parameters;
- Review of patient treatment set-up.

Stereotactic radiosurgery (SRS-[77432]) and stereotactic body radiation treatment (SBRT-[77435]) management also include the professional component of guidance for localization of target volume for the delivery of radiation therapy (77387). *See also the Radiation Management and Treatment Table.*

Radiation Management and Treatment Table

Category	Code	Descriptor	IGRT TC (77387-TC) Bundled into Code?	IGRT PC (77387-PC) Bundled into Code?	Code Type (Technical/ Professional)
SRS: Stereotactic radiosurgery IMRT: Intensity modulated radiation therapy TC: Technical component		SBRT: Stereotactic body radiation therapy IGRT: Image guided radiation therapy PC: Professional component (modifier 26)			
Radiation Treatment Management	77427	Treatment Management, 1-5 Treatments	N	N	Professional
	77431	Treatment Management, 1-2 Fractions	N	N	Professional
	77432	SRS Management, Cranial Lesion(s)	N	Y	Professional
	77435	SBRT Management	N	Y	Professional
SRS Treatment Delivery	77371	SRS Multisource 60 Based	Y	N	Technical
	77372	SRS Linear Based	Y	N	Technical
SBRT Treatment Delivery	77373	SBRT, 1 or More Lesions, 1-5 Fractions	Y	N	Technical
Radiation Treatment Delivery	77401	Superficial and/or Ortho Voltage	N	N	Technical
	77402	Radiation Treatment Delivery, Simple	N	N	Technical
	77407	Radiation Treatment Delivery, Intermediate	N	N	Technical
	77412	Radiation Treatment Delivery, Complex	N	N	Technical
IMRT Treatment Delivery	77385	IMRT Treatment Delivery, Simple	Y	N	Technical
	77386	IMRT Treatment Delivery, Complex	Y	N	Technical
Neutron Beam Treatment Delivery	77423	Neutron Beam Treatment, Complex	N	N	Technical
Proton Treatment Delivery	77520	Proton Treatment, Simple	N	N	Technical
	77522	Proton Treatment, Simple	N	N	Technical
	77523	Proton Treatment, Intermediate	N	N	Technical
	77525	Proton Treatment, Complex	N	N	Technical

77427 Radiation treatment management, 5 treatments

➜ *CPT Changes: An Insider's View* 2000

➜ *CPT Assistant* Nov 99:42, Feb 00:7, Oct 07:1, Nov 09:6, Jun 15:6, Feb 16:3

➜ *Clinical Examples in Radiology* Summer 08:12, Summer 09:2, 7-8

77431 Radiation therapy management with complete course of therapy consisting of 1 or 2 fractions only

➜ *CPT Assistant* Winter 90:10, Oct 97:4, Nov 09:6, Feb 16:3

➜ *Clinical Examples in Radiology* Summer 08:12, Summer 09:7-8

(77431 is not to be used to fill in the last week of a long course of therapy)

77432   Stereotactic radiation treatment management of cranial lesion(s) (complete course of treatment consisting of 1 session)
> *CPT Changes: An Insider's View* 2008
> *CPT Assistant* Oct 97:4, Nov 09:6, Jul 11:12, Jul 14:9, Dec 15:14, 17, Feb 16:3
> *Clinical Examples in Radiology* Summer 09:7-8

(The same physician should not report both stereotactic radiosurgery services [61796-61800] and radiation treatment management [77432 or 77435] for cranial lesions)

(For stereotactic body radiation therapy treatment, use 77435)

(To report the technical component of guidance for localization of target volume, use 77387 with a technical component modifier [TC])

77435   Stereotactic body radiation therapy, treatment management, per treatment course, to 1 or more lesions, including image guidance, entire course not to exceed 5 fractions
> *CPT Changes: An Insider's View* 2007
> *CPT Assistant* Mar 07:7, Oct 07:1, Nov 09:6, Jun 15:6, Dec 15:14, Feb 16:3
> *Clinical Examples in Radiology* Summer 09:7-8

(Do not report 77435 in conjunction with 77427-77432)

(The same physician should not report both stereotactic radiosurgery services [32701, 63620, 63621] and radiation treatment management [77435])

(To report the technical component of guidance for localization of target volume, use 77387 with a technical component modifier [TC])

77469   Intraoperative radiation treatment management
> *CPT Changes: An Insider's View* 2012
> *CPT Assistant* Feb 16:3
> *Clinical Examples in Radiology* Summer 09:7, Fall 11:11

77470   Special treatment procedure (eg, total body irradiation, hemibody radiation, per oral or endocavitary irradiation)
> *CPT Changes: An Insider's View* 2001, 2012
> *CPT Assistant* Winter 91:22, Oct 97:1, Apr 09:3, Feb 16:3
> *Clinical Examples in Radiology* Summer 08:12, Summer 09:7-8, Spring 12:11

(77470 assumes that the procedure is performed 1 or more times during the course of therapy, in addition to daily or weekly patient management)

(For intraoperative radiation treatment delivery and management, see 77424, 77425, 77469)

77499   Unlisted procedure, therapeutic radiology treatment management
> *CPT Changes: An Insider's View* 2000
> *CPT Assistant* Nov 99:42, Feb 00:7, Nov 09:6, Jun 15:6, Feb 16:3
> *Clinical Examples in Radiology* Summer 09:7-8

Proton Beam Treatment Delivery

Definitions

Simple proton treatment delivery to a single treatment area utilizing a single non-tangential/oblique port, custom block with compensation (77522) and without compensation (77520).

Intermediate proton treatment delivery to one or more treatment areas utilizing two or more ports or one or more tangential/oblique ports, with custom blocks and compensators.

Complex proton treatment delivery to one or more treatment areas utilizing two or more ports per treatment area with matching or patching fields and/or multiple isocenters, with custom blocks and compensators.

77520   Proton treatment delivery; simple, without compensation
> *CPT Changes: An Insider's View* 2000, 2001
> *CPT Assistant* Nov 99:43

77522   simple, with compensation
> *CPT Changes: An Insider's View* 2001

77523   intermediate
> *CPT Changes: An Insider's View* 2000, 2001
> *CPT Assistant* Nov 99:43

77525   complex
> *CPT Changes: An Insider's View* 2001

Hyperthermia

Hyperthermia treatments as listed in this section include external (superficial and deep), interstitial, and intracavitary.

Radiation therapy when given concurrently is listed separately.

Hyperthermia is used only as an adjunct to radiation therapy or chemotherapy. It may be induced by a variety of sources (eg, microwave, ultrasound, low energy radio-frequency conduction, or by probes).

The listed treatments include management during the course of therapy and follow-up care for three months after completion.

Preliminary consultation is not included (see **evaluation and management** services).

Physics planning and interstitial insertion of temperature sensors, and use of external or interstitial heat generating sources are included.

The following descriptors are included in the treatment schedule:

Radiology 70010-79999

77600   Hyperthermia, externally generated; superficial (ie, heating to a depth of 4 cm or less)
  ➲ *CPT Changes: An Insider's View* 2017
  ➲ *CPT Assistant* Winter 91:22, Dec 13:17

77605   deep (ie, heating to depths greater than 4 cm)
  ➲ *CPT Changes: An Insider's View* 2017
  ➲ *CPT Assistant* Winter 91:22, Dec 13:17, Dec 23:27

(For intraoperative hyperthermic intraperitoneal chemotherapy [HIPEC], see 96547, 96548)

77610   Hyperthermia generated by interstitial probe(s); 5 or fewer interstitial applicators
  ➲ *CPT Changes: An Insider's View* 2017
  ➲ *CPT Assistant* Winter 91:22
  ➲ *Clinical Examples in Radiology* Spring 14:11

77615   more than 5 interstitial applicators
  ➲ *CPT Changes: An Insider's View* 2017
  ➲ *CPT Assistant* Winter 91:22

Clinical Intracavitary Hyperthermia

77620   Hyperthermia generated by intracavitary probe(s)
  ➲ *CPT Assistant* Winter 91:22, Dec 13:17

Clinical Brachytherapy

Clinical brachytherapy requires the use of either natural or man-made radioelements applied into or around a treatment field of interest. The supervision of radioelements and dose interpretation are performed solely by the therapeutic radiologist.

Services 77750-77799 include admission to the hospital and daily visits.

For insertion of ovoids and tandems, use 57155.

For insertion of Heyman capsules, use 58346.

Definitions

(Sources refer to intracavitary placement or permanent interstitial placement; ribbons refer to temporary interstitial placement)

A simple application has one to four sources/ribbons.

An intermediate application has five to 10 sources/ribbons.

A complex application has greater than 10 sources/ribbons.

High dose-rate brachytherapy involves treatment with radiation sources that cannot safely be handled manually. These systems are remotely controlled and place a radionuclide source (radioelement or radioisotope) within an applicator placed in or near the target. These applicators may be placed in the body or on the skin surface.

Small electronic X-ray sources placed into an applicator within or close to the target may also be used to generate radiation at high-dose rates. This is referred to as high dose-rate electronic brachytherapy.

To report high dose-rate electronic brachytherapy, see 0394T, 0395T.

77750   Infusion or instillation of radioelement solution (includes 3-month follow-up care)
  ➲ *CPT Changes: An Insider's View* 2005
  ➲ *CPT Assistant* Sep 05:1

(For administration of radiolabeled monoclonal antibodies, use 79403)

(For non-antibody radiopharmaceutical therapy by intravenous administration only, not including 3-month follow-up care, use 79101)

77761   Intracavitary radiation source application; simple
  ➲ *CPT Changes: An Insider's View* 2001
  ➲ *CPT Assistant* Winter 91:23, Jan 96:7, Mar 99:3, Feb 02:7, Sep 05:1

77762   intermediate
  ➲ *CPT Assistant* Winter 91:23, Feb 02:7, Sep 05:1

77763   complex
  ➲ *CPT Assistant* Winter 91:23, Mar 99:3, Feb 02:7, Sep 05:1

(Do not report 77761-77763 in conjunction with Category III code 0394T, 0395T)

77767   Remote afterloading high dose rate radionuclide skin surface brachytherapy, includes basic dosimetry, when performed; lesion diameter up to 2.0 cm or 1 channel
  ➲ *CPT Changes: An Insider's View* 2016

77768   lesion diameter over 2.0 cm and 2 or more channels, or multiple lesions
  ➲ *CPT Changes: An Insider's View* 2016

77770   Remote afterloading high dose rate radionuclide interstitial or intracavitary brachytherapy, includes basic dosimetry, when performed; 1 channel
  ➲ *CPT Changes: An Insider's View* 2016

77771   2-12 channels
  ➲ *CPT Changes: An Insider's View* 2016

77772   over 12 channels
  ➲ *CPT Changes: An Insider's View* 2016

(Do not report 77767, 77768, 77770, 77771, 77772 in conjunction with 77300, 0394T, 0395T)

(For non-brachytherapy superficial [eg, ≤200 kV] radiation treatment delivery, use 77401)

77778   Interstitial radiation source application, complex, includes supervision, handling, loading of radiation source, when performed
  ➲ *CPT Changes: An Insider's View* 2016
  ➲ *CPT Assistant* Winter 91:23, Apr 04:6, Sep 05:1, May 07:1
  ➲ *Clinical Examples in Radiology* Summer 15:5

Radiology 70010-79999

(Do not report 77778 in conjunction with Category III codes 0394T, 0395T)

(Do not report 77778 in conjunction with 77790)

77789   Surface application of low dose rate radionuclide source
➔ *CPT Changes: An Insider's View* 2001, 2016
➔ *CPT Assistant* Sep 05:1

(Do not report 77789 in conjunction with 77401, 77767, 77768, 0394T, 0395T)

77790   Supervision, handling, loading of radiation source
➔ *CPT Changes: An Insider's View* 2001
➔ *CPT Assistant* Sep 05:1
➔ *Clinical Examples in Radiology* Summer 15:5

(Do not report 77790 in conjunction with 77778)

77799   Unlisted procedure, clinical brachytherapy
➔ *CPT Assistant* Sep 05:1

Nuclear Medicine

Listed procedures may be performed independently or in the course of overall medical care. If the individual providing these services is also responsible for diagnostic workup and/or follow-up care of patient, see appropriate sections also.

Radioimmunoassay tests are found in the **Clinical Pathology** section (codes 82009-84999). These codes can be appropriately used by any specialist performing such tests in a laboratory licensed and/or certified for radioimmunoassays. The reporting of these tests is not confined to clinical pathology laboratories alone.

The services listed do not include the radiopharmaceutical or drug. To separately report supply of diagnostic and therapeutic radiopharmaceuticals and drugs, use the appropriate supply code(s), in addition to the procedure code.

Diagnostic

Endocrine System

78012   Thyroid uptake, single or multiple quantitative measurement(s) (including stimulation, suppression, or discharge, when performed)
➔ *CPT Changes: An Insider's View* 2013
➔ *CPT Assistant* Jun 13:9
➔ *Clinical Examples in Radiology* Winter 13:9

78013   Thyroid imaging (including vascular flow, when performed);
➔ *CPT Changes: An Insider's View* 2013
➔ *CPT Assistant* Jun 13:9
➔ *Clinical Examples in Radiology* Winter 13:9

78014   with single or multiple uptake(s) quantitative measurement(s) (including stimulation, suppression, or discharge, when performed)
➔ *CPT Changes: An Insider's View* 2013
➔ *CPT Assistant* Jun 13:9
➔ *Clinical Examples in Radiology* Winter 13:9

78015   Thyroid carcinoma metastases imaging; limited area (eg, neck and chest only)
➔ *CPT Assistant* Nov 98:21, Jan 07:31

78016   with additional studies (eg, urinary recovery)
➔ *CPT Assistant* Jan 07:31

78018   whole body
➔ *CPT Assistant* Apr 99:4, Jan 07:31
➔ *Clinical Examples in Radiology* Fall 09:3, 5, Fall 19:14

+ 78020   Thyroid carcinoma metastases uptake (List separately in addition to code for primary procedure)
➔ *CPT Assistant* Nov 98:21, Apr 99:4, Jan 07:31
➔ *Clinical Examples in Radiology* Fall 09:3, 5, Fall 19:14

(Use 78020 in conjunction with 78018 only)

78070   Parathyroid planar imaging (including subtraction, when performed);
➔ *CPT Changes: An Insider's View* 2013
➔ *CPT Assistant* Jan 07:31, Dec 16:10
➔ *Clinical Examples in Radiology* Summer 11:4-5

78071   with tomographic (SPECT)
➔ *CPT Changes: An Insider's View* 2013
➔ *CPT Assistant* Dec 16:10, Oct 20:3

78072   with tomographic (SPECT), and concurrently acquired computed tomography (CT) for anatomical localization
➔ *CPT Changes: An Insider's View* 2013
➔ *CPT Assistant* Dec 16:10, Oct 20:3

(Do not report 78070, 78071, 78072 in conjunction with 78800, 78801, 78802, 78803, 78804, 78830, 78831, 78832, 78835)

78075   Adrenal imaging, cortex and/or medulla
➔ *CPT Assistant* Jan 07:31, Feb 12:9
➔ *Clinical Examples in Radiology* Summer 12:9

78099   Unlisted endocrine procedure, diagnostic nuclear medicine
➔ *CPT Assistant* Dec 05:7, Jan 07:31, Dec 16:10
➔ *Clinical Examples in Radiology* Fall 19:14

(For chemical analysis, see **Chemistry** section)

Radiology 70010-79999

Hematopoietic, Reticuloendothelial and Lymphatic System

78102 Bone marrow imaging; limited area
➔ *CPT Assistant* Dec 05:7, Feb 12:9

78103 multiple areas

78104 whole body

78110 Plasma volume, radiopharmaceutical volume-dilution technique (separate procedure); single sampling

78111 multiple samplings

78120 Red cell volume determination (separate procedure); single sampling

78121 multiple samplings

78122 Whole blood volume determination, including separate measurement of plasma volume and red cell volume (radiopharmaceutical volume-dilution technique)

78130 Red cell survival study
➔ *CPT Changes: An Insider's View* 2021

78140 Labeled red cell sequestration, differential organ/tissue (eg, splenic and/or hepatic)

78185 Spleen imaging only, with or without vascular flow

(If combined with liver study, use procedures 78215 and 78216)

78191 Platelet survival study

78195 Lymphatics and lymph nodes imaging
➔ *CPT Changes: An Insider's View* 2000, 2002
➔ *CPT Assistant* Nov 98:22, Jul 99:6, Nov 99:43, Dec 99:8, Sep 08:5, Feb 12:9

(For sentinel node identification without scintigraphy imaging, use 38792)

(For sentinel node excision, see 38500-38542)

78199 Unlisted hematopoietic, reticuloendothelial and lymphatic procedure, diagnostic nuclear medicine
➔ *CPT Assistant* Dec 05:7

(For chemical analysis, see **Chemistry** section)

Gastrointestinal System

78201 Liver imaging; static only
➔ *CPT Assistant* Dec 05:7, Feb 12:9

78202 with vascular flow
➔ *CPT Assistant* Feb 12:9

(For spleen imaging only, use 78185)

78215 Liver and spleen imaging; static only

78216 with vascular flow

78226 Hepatobiliary system imaging, including gallbladder when present;
➔ *CPT Changes: An Insider's View* 2012
➔ *Clinical Examples in Radiology* Winter 12:6, Summer 22:16, 17

78227 with pharmacologic intervention, including quantitative measurement(s) when performed
➔ *CPT Changes: An Insider's View* 2012
➔ *Clinical Examples in Radiology* Winter 12:5, Summer 22:16, 17

78230 Salivary gland imaging;

78231 with serial images

78232 Salivary gland function study

78258 Esophageal motility

78261 Gastric mucosa imaging

78262 Gastroesophageal reflux study
➔ *CPT Assistant* Dec 15:10

78264 Gastric emptying imaging study (eg, solid, liquid, or both);
➔ *CPT Changes: An Insider's View* 2016
➔ *CPT Assistant* Dec 15:10

78265 with small bowel transit
➔ *CPT Changes: An Insider's View* 2016
➔ *CPT Assistant* Dec 15:10
➔ *Clinical Examples in Radiology* Winter 17:12

78266 with small bowel and colon transit, multiple days
➔ *CPT Changes: An Insider's View* 2016
➔ *CPT Assistant* Dec 15:10
➔ *Clinical Examples in Radiology* Winter 17:6

(Report 78264, 78265, 78266 only once per imaging study)

78267 Urea breath test, C-14 (isotopic); acquisition for analysis
➔ *CPT Changes: An Insider's View* 2000, 2005
➔ *CPT Assistant* Nov 99:43
➔ *Clinical Examples in Radiology* Fall 07:9

78268 analysis
➔ *CPT Changes: An Insider's View* 2000
➔ *CPT Assistant* Nov 99:43
➔ *Clinical Examples in Radiology* Fall 07:9

(For breath hydrogen or methane testing and analysis, use 91065)

78278 Acute gastrointestinal blood loss imaging
➔ *Clinical Examples in Radiology* Summer 19:2

78282 Gastrointestinal protein loss
➔ *CPT Assistant* Jul 18:15

78290 Intestine imaging (eg, ectopic gastric mucosa, Meckel's localization, volvulus)
➔ *CPT Changes: An Insider's View* 2002

78291 Peritoneal-venous shunt patency test (eg, for LeVeen, Denver shunt)
➔ *CPT Assistant* Feb 12:9

(For injection procedure, use 49427)

★=Telemedicine ◀=Audio-only ✚=Add-on code ✗=FDA approval pending #=Resequenced code ⊘=Modifier 51 exempt ➔➔➔=See p xxi for details

78299   Unlisted gastrointestinal procedure, diagnostic nuclear medicine
➔ *CPT Assistant* Dec 05:7
➔ *Clinical Examples in Radiology* Summer 19:2

Musculoskeletal System

Bone and joint imaging can be used in the diagnosis of a variety of inflammatory processes (eg, osteomyelitis), as well as for localization of primary and/or metastatic neoplasms.

78300   Bone and/or joint imaging; limited area
➔ *CPT Assistant* Mar 97:11, Dec 05:7, Feb 12:9
➔ *Clinical Examples in Radiology* Winter 09:5, Spring 10:9

78305   multiple areas
➔ *CPT Assistant* Mar 97:11
➔ *Clinical Examples in Radiology* Winter 09:5, Spring 10:9

78306   whole body
➔ *CPT Assistant* Mar 97:11, Jan 02:10, Jun 03:11, Feb 12:10
➔ *Clinical Examples in Radiology* Summer 06:7, 12, Winter 09:3-5, Spring 10:9, Spring 13:10, Spring 21:3

78315   3 phase study
➔ *CPT Assistant* Jan 02:10
➔ *Clinical Examples in Radiology* Summer 06:7, 12, Winter 09:4-5, Spring 10:9

78350   Bone density (bone mineral content) study, 1 or more sites; single photon absorptiometry
➔ *CPT Assistant* Nov 97:26

78351   dual photon absorptiometry, 1 or more sites
➔ *CPT Assistant* Nov 97:26, Feb 12:9

78399   Unlisted musculoskeletal procedure, diagnostic nuclear medicine
➔ *CPT Assistant* Dec 05:7

Cardiovascular System

Myocardial perfusion (SPECT and PET) and cardiac blood pool imaging studies may be performed at rest and/ or during stress. When performed during exercise and/or pharmacologic stress, the appropriate stress testing code from the 93015-93018 series may be reported in addition to 78430, 78431, 78432, 78433, 78451-78454, 78472, 78491, 78492. PET can be performed on either a dedicated PET machine (which uses a PET source for attenuation correction) or a combination PET/CT camera (78429, 78430, 78431, 78433). A cardiac PET study performed on a PET/CT camera includes examination of the CT transmission images for review of anatomy in the field of view.

78414   Determination of central c-v hemodynamics (non-imaging) (eg, ejection fraction with probe technique) with or without pharmacologic intervention or exercise, single or multiple determinations
➔ *CPT Assistant* Dec 05:7, May 10:6, Feb 12:9

78428   Cardiac shunt detection
➔ *CPT Assistant* May 10:6

78429   Code is out of numerical sequence. See 78458-78468

78430   Code is out of numerical sequence. See 78483-78496

78431   Code is out of numerical sequence. See 78483-78496

78432   Code is out of numerical sequence. See 78483-78496

78433   Code is out of numerical sequence. See 78483-78496

78434   Code is out of numerical sequence. See 78483-78496

78445   Non-cardiac vascular flow imaging (ie, angiography, venography)
➔ *CPT Assistant* May 10:6
➔ *Clinical Examples in Radiology* Spring 10:9

78451   Myocardial perfusion imaging, tomographic (SPECT) (including attenuation correction, qualitative or quantitative wall motion, ejection fraction by first pass or gated technique, additional quantification, when performed); single study, at rest or stress (exercise or pharmacologic)
➔ *CPT Changes: An Insider's View* 2010
➔ *CPT Assistant* May 10:5, Feb 11:9, Feb 12:10, Jul 20:5, Oct 20:3
➔ *Clinical Examples in Radiology* Winter 10:11, Spring 10:9

(Do not report 78451 in conjunction with 78800, 78801, 78802, 78803, 78804, 78830, 78831, 78832, 78835)

(For absolute quantification of myocardial blood flow [AQMBF] with single-photon emission computed tomography [SPECT], use 0742T)

78452   multiple studies, at rest and/or stress (exercise or pharmacologic) and/or redistribution and/or rest reinjection
➔ *CPT Changes: An Insider's View* 2010
➔ *CPT Assistant* May 10:5, Feb 11:9, Feb 12:9, Jul 20:5, Oct 20:3
➔ *Clinical Examples in Radiology* Winter 10:10-11, Spring 10:9

(Do not report 78452 in conjunction with 78800, 78801, 78802, 78803, 78804, 78830, 78831, 78832, 78835)

(For absolute quantification of myocardial blood flow [AQMBF] with single-photon emission computed tomography [SPECT], use 0742T)

78453   Myocardial perfusion imaging, planar (including qualitative or quantitative wall motion, ejection fraction by first pass or gated technique, additional quantification, when performed); single study, at rest or stress (exercise or pharmacologic)
➔ *CPT Changes: An Insider's View* 2010
➔ *CPT Assistant* May 10:5, Jul 20:5
➔ *Clinical Examples in Radiology* Winter 10:11

Radiology 70010-79999

78454   multiple studies, at rest and/or stress (exercise or pharmacologic) and/or redistribution and/or rest reinjection
> *CPT Changes: An Insider's View* 2010
> *CPT Assistant* May 10:5, Jul 20:5
> *Clinical Examples in Radiology* Winter 10:11

78456   Acute venous thrombosis imaging, peptide
> *CPT Changes: An Insider's View* 2000
> *CPT Assistant* Nov 99:43, May 10:6

78457   Venous thrombosis imaging, venogram; unilateral
> *CPT Changes: An Insider's View* 2000
> *CPT Assistant* Nov 99:43

78458   bilateral
> *CPT Changes: An Insider's View* 2000
> *CPT Assistant* Nov 99:43, May 10:6

78459   Myocardial imaging, positron emission tomography (PET), metabolic evaluation study (including ventricular wall motion[s] and/or ejection fraction[s], when performed), single study;
> *CPT Changes: An Insider's View* 2020
> *CPT Assistant* Jun 96:5, Nov 97:26, May 10:6, Jul 20:5
> *Clinical Examples in Radiology* Summer 10:11

 # 78429   with concurrently acquired computed tomography transmission scan
> *CPT Changes: An Insider's View* 2020
> *CPT Assistant* Jul 20:5
> *Clinical Examples in Radiology* Spring 20:3

(For CT coronary calcium scoring, use 75571)

(CT performed for other than attenuation correction and anatomical localization is reported using the appropriate site specific CT code with modifier 59)

78466   Myocardial imaging, infarct avid, planar; qualitative or quantitative
> *CPT Assistant* May 10:6

78468   with ejection fraction by first pass technique
> *CPT Assistant* May 10:6

78469   tomographic SPECT with or without quantification
> *CPT Assistant* May 10:6, Nov 18:11

(For myocardial sympathetic innervation imaging, see 0331T, 0332T)

(Do not report 78469 in conjunction with 78800, 78801, 78802, 78803, 78804, 78830, 78831, 78832, 78835)

78472   Cardiac blood pool imaging, gated equilibrium; planar, single study at rest or stress (exercise and/or pharmacologic), wall motion study plus ejection fraction, with or without additional quantitative processing
> *CPT Changes: An Insider's View* 2000
> *CPT Assistant* Nov 98:22, Nov 99:44, May 10:6
> *Clinical Examples in Radiology* Summer 20:2

(For assessment of right ventricular ejection fraction by first pass technique, use 78496)

78473   multiple studies, wall motion study plus ejection fraction, at rest and stress (exercise and/or pharmacologic), with or without additional quantification
> *CPT Assistant* May 10:6

(Do not report 78472, 78473 in conjunction with 78451-78454, 78481, 78483, 78494)

78481   Cardiac blood pool imaging (planar), first pass technique; single study, at rest or with stress (exercise and/or pharmacologic), wall motion study plus ejection fraction, with or without quantification
> *CPT Assistant* May 10:6

78483   multiple studies, at rest and with stress (exercise and/or pharmacologic), wall motion study plus ejection fraction, with or without quantification
> *CPT Assistant* May 10:6

(For cerebral blood flow study, use 78610)

(Do not report 78481-78483 in conjunction with 78451-78454)

78491   Myocardial imaging, positron emission tomography (PET), perfusion study (including ventricular wall motion[s] and/or ejection fraction[s], when performed); single study, at rest or stress (exercise or pharmacologic)
> *CPT Changes: An Insider's View* 2020
> *CPT Assistant* Nov 97:27, May 10:6, Jul 20:5
> *Clinical Examples in Radiology* Summer 10:11

 # 78430   single study, at rest or stress (exercise or pharmacologic), with concurrently acquired computed tomography transmission scan
> *CPT Changes: An Insider's View* 2020
> *CPT Assistant* Jul 20:5

78492   multiple studies at rest and stress (exercise or pharmacologic)
> *CPT Changes: An Insider's View* 2020
> *CPT Assistant* Nov 97:27, May 10:6, Jul 20:5
> *Clinical Examples in Radiology* Summer 10:11

 # 78431   multiple studies at rest and stress (exercise or pharmacologic), with concurrently acquired computed tomography transmission scan
> *CPT Changes: An Insider's View* 2020
> *CPT Assistant* Jul 20:5
> *Clinical Examples in Radiology* Fall 22:3

78432 Myocardial imaging, positron emission tomography (PET), combined perfusion with metabolic evaluation study (including ventricular wall motion[s] and/or ejection fraction[s], when performed), dual radiotracer (eg, myocardial viability);
➔ *CPT Changes: An Insider's View* 2020
➔ *CPT Assistant* Jul 20:5

78433 with concurrently acquired computed tomography transmission scan
➔ *CPT Changes: An Insider's View* 2020
➔ *CPT Assistant* Jul 20:5

(CT performed for other than attenuation correction and anatomical localization is reported using the appropriate site specific CT code with modifier 59)

#+ 78434 Absolute quantitation of myocardial blood flow (AQMBF), positron emission tomography (PET), rest and pharmacologic stress (List separately in addition to code for primary procedure)
➔ *CPT Changes: An Insider's View* 2020
➔ *CPT Assistant* Jul 20:5
➔ *Clinical Examples in Radiology* Fall 22:3

(Use 78434 in conjunction with 78431, 78492)

(For CT coronary calcium scoring, use 75571)

(For myocardial imaging by planar or SPECT, see 78451, 78452, 78453, 78454)

(For absolute quantification of myocardial blood flow [AQMBF] with single-photon emission computed tomography [SPECT], use 0742T)

78494 Cardiac blood pool imaging, gated equilibrium, SPECT, at rest, wall motion study plus ejection fraction, with or without quantitative processing
➔ *CPT Assistant* Nov 98:22, Jun 99:3, May 10:6
➔ *Clinical Examples in Radiology* Summer 20:2

(Do not report 78494 in conjunction with 78800, 78801, 78802, 78803, 78804, 78830, 78831, 78832, 78835)

+ 78496 Cardiac blood pool imaging, gated equilibrium, single study, at rest, with right ventricular ejection fraction by first pass technique (List separately in addition to code for primary procedure)
➔ *CPT Assistant* Nov 98:22, Jun 99:3, 11, May 10:6, Feb 12:9
➔ *Clinical Examples in Radiology* Summer 20:3

(Use 78496 in conjunction with 78472)

78499 Unlisted cardiovascular procedure, diagnostic nuclear medicine
➔ *CPT Assistant* Dec 05:7, May 10:6
➔ *Clinical Examples in Radiology* Summer 08:12

Respiratory System

78579 Pulmonary ventilation imaging (eg, aerosol or gas)
➔ *CPT Changes: An Insider's View* 2012
➔ *CPT Assistant* Feb 12:9
➔ *Clinical Examples in Radiology* Fall 11:5

78580 Pulmonary perfusion imaging (eg, particulate)
➔ *CPT Changes: An Insider's View* 2012
➔ *CPT Assistant* Mar 99:4, Dec 05:7, May 10:6

78582 Pulmonary ventilation (eg, aerosol or gas) and perfusion imaging
➔ *CPT Changes: An Insider's View* 2012
➔ *Clinical Examples in Radiology* Fall 11:4-5

78597 Quantitative differential pulmonary perfusion, including imaging when performed
➔ *CPT Changes: An Insider's View* 2012
➔ *Clinical Examples in Radiology* Fall 11:5-6

78598 Quantitative differential pulmonary perfusion and ventilation (eg, aerosol or gas), including imaging when performed
➔ *CPT Changes: An Insider's View* 2012
➔ *CPT Assistant* Feb 12:9
➔ *Clinical Examples in Radiology* Fall 11:5

(Report 78579, 78580, 78582-78598 only once per imaging session)

(Do not report 78580, 78582-78598 in conjunction with 78451-78454)

78599 Unlisted respiratory procedure, diagnostic nuclear medicine
➔ *CPT Assistant* Dec 05:7

Nervous System

78600 Brain imaging, less than 4 static views;
➔ *CPT Changes: An Insider's View* 2008
➔ *CPT Assistant* Dec 05:7, Feb 12:9

78601 with vascular flow
➔ *CPT Changes: An Insider's View* 2008

78605 Brain imaging, minimum 4 static views;
➔ *CPT Changes: An Insider's View* 2008

78606 with vascular flow
➔ *CPT Changes: An Insider's View* 2008

78608 Brain imaging, positron emission tomography (PET); metabolic evaluation
➔ *Clinical Examples in Radiology* Spring 10:1-2, Spring 22:16

78609 perfusion evaluation

78610 Brain imaging, vascular flow only

78630 Cerebrospinal fluid flow, imaging (not including introduction of material); cisternography
➔ *CPT Assistant* May 17:3

(For injection procedure, see 61000-61070, 62270-62327)

78635 ventriculography

(For injection procedure, see 61000-61070, 62270-62294)

78645 shunt evaluation

(For injection procedure, see 61000-61070, 62270-62294)

78650 Cerebrospinal fluid leakage detection and localization
➔ *CPT Changes: An Insider's View* 2002

(For injection procedure, see 61000-61070, 62270-62294)

78660 Radiopharmaceutical dacryocystography
➔ *CPT Assistant* Feb 12:9

78699 Unlisted nervous system procedure, diagnostic nuclear medicine
➔ *CPT Assistant* Dec 05:7

Genitourinary System

78700 Kidney imaging morphology;
➔ *CPT Changes: An Insider's View* 2007
➔ *CPT Assistant* Dec 05:7, Mar 07:7, Feb 12:9
➔ *Clinical Examples in Radiology* Fall 09:2

78701 with vascular flow
➔ *Clinical Examples in Radiology* Fall 09:2

78707 with vascular flow and function, single study without pharmacological intervention
➔ *CPT Changes: An Insider's View* 2007
➔ *CPT Assistant* Nov 97:27, Mar 07:7

78708 with vascular flow and function, single study, with pharmacological intervention (eg, angiotensin converting enzyme inhibitor and/or diuretic)
➔ *CPT Changes: An Insider's View* 2007
➔ *CPT Assistant* Nov 97:27, Mar 07:7
➔ *Clinical Examples in Radiology* Fall 09:2

78709 with vascular flow and function, multiple studies, with and without pharmacological intervention (eg, angiotensin converting enzyme inhibitor and/or diuretic)
➔ *CPT Changes: An Insider's View* 2007
➔ *CPT Assistant* Nov 97:27, Mar 07:7
➔ *Clinical Examples in Radiology* Fall 09:2

(For introduction of radioactive substance in association with renal endoscopy, use 77778)

78725 Kidney function study, non-imaging radioisotopic study
➔ *CPT Assistant* Nov 98:22
➔ *Clinical Examples in Radiology* Fall 09:2

+ 78730 Urinary bladder residual study (List separately in addition to code for primary procedure)
➔ *CPT Changes: An Insider's View* 2007
➔ *CPT Assistant* Mar 07:7
➔ *Clinical Examples in Radiology* Spring 12:2

(Use 78730 in conjunction with 78740)

(For measurement of postvoid residual urine and/or bladder capacity by ultrasound, nonimaging, use 51798)

(For ultrasound imaging of the bladder only, with measurement of postvoid residual urine when performed, use 76857)

78740 Ureteral reflux study (radiopharmaceutical voiding cystogram)
➔ *Clinical Examples in Radiology* Spring 12:1

(Use 78740 in conjunction with 78730 for urinary bladder residual study)

(For catheterization, see 51701, 51702, 51703)

78761 Testicular imaging with vascular flow
➔ *CPT Changes: An Insider's View* 2007
➔ *CPT Assistant* Mar 07:7, Feb 12:9

78799 Unlisted genitourinary procedure, diagnostic nuclear medicine
➔ *CPT Assistant* Dec 05:7

(For chemical analysis, see **Chemistry** section)

Other Procedures

(For specific organ, see appropriate heading)

78800 Radiopharmaceutical localization of tumor, inflammatory process or distribution of radiopharmaceutical agent(s) (includes vascular flow and blood pool imaging, when performed); planar, single area (eg, head, neck, chest, pelvis), single day imaging
➔ *CPT Changes: An Insider's View* 2004, 2020
➔ *CPT Assistant* Dec 05:7, Dec 11:17, Feb 12:9, Nov 18:11, Oct 20:3
➔ *Clinical Examples in Radiology* Summer 06:6, 10-11, Spring 10:4, 8, Fall 10:11, Fall 19:6

(For specific organ, see appropriate heading)

78801 planar, 2 or more areas (eg, abdomen and pelvis, head and chest), 1 or more days imaging or single area imaging over 2 or more days
➔ *CPT Changes: An Insider's View* 2020
➔ *CPT Assistant* Dec 11:17, Feb 12:9, Oct 20:3
➔ *Clinical Examples in Radiology* Fall 19:6, Fall 20:7

78802 planar, whole body, single day imaging
➔ *CPT Changes: An Insider's View* 2004, 2020
➔ *CPT Assistant* Jun 03:11, Feb 12:9, Oct 20:3
➔ *Clinical Examples in Radiology* Summer 06:6, 10-11, Fall 19:6, Fall 20:6-7

 # 78804 planar, whole body, requiring 2 or more days imaging
➔ *CPT Changes: An Insider's View* 2004, 2020
➔ *CPT Assistant* Feb 12:9, Oct 20:3
➔ *Clinical Examples in Radiology* Summer 12:8, Fall 19:6

★=Telemedicine   ◀=Audio-only   +=Add-on code   ✘=FDA approval pending   #=Resequenced code   ⊘=Modifier 51 exempt   ➔➔➔=See p xxi for details

78803   tomographic (SPECT), single area (eg, head, neck, chest, pelvis) or acquisition, single day imaging

> ➔ *CPT Changes: An Insider's View* 2020, 2023
> ➔ *CPT Assistant* Jun 03:11, Feb 12:9, Oct 15:9, Dec 16:10, Nov 18:11, Oct 20:14, Sep 23:38
> ➔ *Clinical Examples in Radiology* Summer 06:6, 10-11, Summer 12:8, Spring 15:10, Fall 19:6, Winter 21:12

78804   Code is out of numerical sequence. See 78801-78811

(For imaging bone infectious or inflammatory disease with a bone imaging radiopharmaceutical, see 78300, 78305, 78306, 78315)

 # 78830   tomographic (SPECT) with concurrently acquired computed tomography (CT) transmission scan for anatomical review, localization and determination/detection of pathology, single area (eg, head, neck, chest, pelvis) or acquisition, single day imaging

> ➔ *CPT Changes: An Insider's View* 2020, 2023
> ➔ *CPT Assistant* Oct 20:3, Sep 23:38
> ➔ *Clinical Examples in Radiology* Fall 19:6, Fall 20:6-7, Spring 21:3

 # 78831   tomographic (SPECT), minimum 2 areas (eg, pelvis and knees, chest and abdomen) or separate acquisitions (eg, lung ventilation and perfusion), single day imaging, or single area or acquisition over 2 or more days

> ➔ *CPT Changes: An Insider's View* 2020, 2023
> ➔ *CPT Assistant* Oct 20:3, Sep 23:38
> ➔ *Clinical Examples in Radiology* Fall 19:6, Winter 21:12

 # 78832   tomographic (SPECT) with concurrently acquired computed tomography (CT) transmission scan for anatomical review, localization and determination/detection of pathology, minimum 2 areas (eg, pelvis and knees, chest and abdomen) or separate acquisitions (eg, lung ventilation and perfusion), single day imaging, or single area or acquisition over 2 or more days

> ➔ *CPT Changes: An Insider's View* 2020, 2023
> ➔ *CPT Assistant* Oct 20:3, Sep 23:38
> ➔ *Clinical Examples in Radiology* Fall 19:6, Spring 21:3

(For cerebrospinal fluid studies that require injection procedure, see 61055, 61070, 62320, 62321, 62322, 62323)

#+ 78835   Radiopharmaceutical quantification measurement(s) single area (List separately in addition to code for primary procedure)

> ➔ *CPT Changes: An Insider's View* 2020
> ➔ *CPT Assistant* Oct 20:3
> ➔ *Clinical Examples in Radiology* Fall 19:6

(Use 78835 in conjunction with 78830, 78832)

(Report multiple units of 78835 if quantitation is more than 1 area or more than 1 day imaging)

(Report myocardial SPECT imaging with 78451, 78452, 78469, 78494)

(For all nuclear medicine codes, select the organ/system-specific code[s] first; if there is no organ/system-specific code[s], see 78800, 78801, 78802, 78803, 78830, 78831, 78832)

(For parathyroid imaging, see 78070, 78071, 78072)

78808   Injection procedure for radiopharmaceutical localization by non-imaging probe study, intravenous (eg, parathyroid adenoma)

> ➔ *CPT Changes: An Insider's View* 2009
> ➔ *CPT Assistant* Feb 12:9, Dec 16:10

(For sentinel lymph node identification, use 38792)

(For PET of brain, see 78608, 78609)

(For PET myocardial imaging, see 78459, 78491, 78492)

78811   Positron emission tomography (PET) imaging; limited area (eg, chest, head/neck)

> ➔ *CPT Changes: An Insider's View* 2005, 2008
> ➔ *CPT Assistant* Dec 05:7, Feb 12:9
> ➔ *Clinical Examples in Radiology* Spring 05:13, 15, Spring 10:2, 7, Spring 13:10, Winter 23:1

78812   skull base to mid-thigh

> ➔ *CPT Changes: An Insider's View* 2005, 2008
> ➔ *CPT Assistant* Dec 05:7, Feb 12:9, Feb 13:16
> ➔ *Clinical Examples in Radiology* Spring 05:13, 15, Spring 10:1-2

78813   whole body

> ➔ *CPT Changes: An Insider's View* 2005, 2008
> ➔ *CPT Assistant* Dec 05:7, Feb 12:9, Feb 13:16
> ➔ *Clinical Examples in Radiology* Spring 05:13, 15, Spring 10:2

78814   Positron emission tomography (PET) with concurrently acquired computed tomography (CT) for attenuation correction and anatomical localization imaging; limited area (eg, chest, head/neck)

> ➔ *CPT Changes: An Insider's View* 2005, 2008
> ➔ *CPT Assistant* Feb 05:13, Jun 05:10, Dec 05:7, Feb 12:9, Feb 13:16
> ➔ *Clinical Examples in Radiology* Spring 05:13, 15, Spring 10:2, 4, Spring 13:10, Spring 22:15, 16, Winter 23:1, Fall 23:26

78815   skull base to mid-thigh

> ➔ *CPT Changes: An Insider's View* 2005, 2008
> ➔ *CPT Assistant* Feb 05:13, Jun 05:10, Dec 05:7, Feb 12:9, Feb 13:16
> ➔ *Clinical Examples in Radiology* Spring 05:13, 15, Spring 10:2, 4, Spring 13:10

Radiology 70010-79999

78816 whole body
→ *CPT Changes: An Insider's View* 2005, 2008
→ *CPT Assistant* Feb 05:13, Jun 05:10, Dec 05:7, Feb 12:9, Feb 13:16
→ *Clinical Examples in Radiology* Spring 05:13, 15, Spring 10:2, Spring 13:10

(Report 78811-78816 only once per imaging session)

(Computed tomography [CT] performed for other than attenuation correction and anatomical localization is reported using the appropriate site specific CT code with modifier 59)

78830 Code is out of numerical sequence. See 78801-78811

78831 Code is out of numerical sequence. See 78801-78811

78832 Code is out of numerical sequence. See 78801-78811

78835 Code is out of numerical sequence. See 78801-78811

78999 Unlisted miscellaneous procedure, diagnostic nuclear medicine
→ *CPT Assistant* Dec 05:7, Feb 12:9, Oct 15:9, Dec 16:16
→ *Clinical Examples in Radiology* Summer 08:12, Spring 10:2, 11, Spring 15:9

Therapeutic

The oral and intravenous administration codes in this section are inclusive of the mode of administration. For intra-arterial, intra-cavitary, and intra-articular administration, also use the appropriate injection and/or procedure codes, as well as imaging guidance and radiological supervision and interpretation codes, when appropriate.

79005 Radiopharmaceutical therapy, by oral administration
→ *CPT Changes: An Insider's View* 2005
→ *CPT Assistant* Sep 05:1, Feb 12:9
→ *Clinical Examples in Radiology* Spring 05:14, Fall 09:5, Winter 12:8

(For monoclonal antibody therapy, use 79403)

79101 Radiopharmaceutical therapy, by intravenous administration
→ *CPT Changes: An Insider's View* 2005
→ *CPT Assistant* Sep 05:1, Feb 12:9
→ *Clinical Examples in Radiology* Spring 10:8, Winter 12:8, Winter 24:3

(Do not report 79101 in conjunction with 36400, 36410, 79403, 96360, 96374 or 96375, 96409)

(For radiolabeled monoclonal antibody by intravenous infusion, use 79403)

(For infusion or instillation of non-antibody radioelement solution that includes 3 months follow-up care, use 77750)

79200 Radiopharmaceutical therapy, by intracavitary administration
→ *CPT Changes: An Insider's View* 2005
→ *CPT Assistant* Sep 05:1, Feb 12:9

79300 Radiopharmaceutical therapy, by interstitial radioactive colloid administration
→ *CPT Changes: An Insider's View* 2005
→ *CPT Assistant* Sep 05:1, Feb 12:9

79403 Radiopharmaceutical therapy, radiolabeled monoclonal antibody by intravenous infusion
→ *CPT Changes: An Insider's View* 2004
→ *CPT Assistant* Sep 05:1, Feb 12:9

(For pre-treatment imaging, see 78802, 78804)

(Do not report 79403 in conjunction with 79101)

79440 Radiopharmaceutical therapy, by intra-articular administration
→ *CPT Changes: An Insider's View* 2005
→ *CPT Assistant* Sep 05:1, Feb 12:9

79445 Radiopharmaceutical therapy, by intra-arterial particulate administration
→ *CPT Changes: An Insider's View* 2005
→ *CPT Assistant* Sep 05:1, Dec 06:10, Feb 12:9, Nov 13:6
→ *Clinical Examples in Radiology* Summer 15:3, Winter 18:12

(Do not report 79445 in conjunction with 96373, 96420)

(Use appropriate procedural and radiological supervision and interpretation codes for the angiographic and interventional procedures provided prerequisite to intra-arterial radiopharmaceutical therapy)

79999 Radiopharmaceutical therapy, unlisted procedure
→ *CPT Changes: An Insider's View* 2005
→ *CPT Assistant* Mar 05:11, Sep 05:1, Jan 07:30, Feb 12:9
→ *Clinical Examples in Radiology* Winter 12:8

Radiology 70010-79999

Pathology and Laboratory Guidelines

Pathology and Laboratory

The following is a listing of headings and subheadings that appear within the Pathology and Laboratory section of the CPT code set. The subheadings or subsections denoted with asterisks (*) below have special instructions unique to that subsection. Where these are indicated, special notes or guidelines will be presented preceding those procedural terminology listings, referring to that subsection specifically. Note that all code ranges in each subsection are listed as they appear in the subsection, even if the code numbers are out of numerical sequence and/or repeated in the next subsection.

Molecular Pathology Gene Table

Claim Designation	Abbreviated Gene Name	Full Gene Name	Commonly Associated Proteins/Diseases (Not a complete list)	CPT Code(s)
ABCA4	ABCA4	ATP-binding cassette, sub-family A (ABC1), member 4	Stargardt disease, age-related macular degeneration, hereditary retinal disorders	81408, 81434
ABCC8	ABCC8	ATP-binding cassette, sub-family C (CFTR/MRP), member 8	Familial hyperinsulinism	81401, 81407
ABCD1	ABCD1	ATP-binding cassette, sub-family D (ALD), member 1	Adrenoleukodystrophy	81405
ABL1	ABL1	ABL proto-oncogene 1 non-receptor tyrosine kinase	Acquired imatinib resistance	81401
	ABL1	ABL proto-oncogene 1, non-receptor tyrosine kinase	Acquired imatinib tyrosine kinase inhibitor resistance	81170
ACADM	ACADM	Acyl-coa dehydrogenase, C-4 to C-12 straight chain, MCAD	Medium chain acyl dehydrogenase deficiency, severe inherited conditions	81400, 81401, 81443
ACADS	ACADS	Acyl-coa dehydrogenase, C-2 to C-3 short chain	Short chain acyl-CoA dehydrogenase deficiency	81404, 81405
ACADVL	ACADVL	Acyl-coa dehydrogenase, very long chain	Very long chain acyl-coenzyme A dehydrogenase deficiency	81406
ACE	ACE	Angiotensin converting enzyme	Hereditary blood pressure regulation	81400
ACTA2	ACTA2	Actin, alpha 2, smooth muscle, aorta	Thoracic aortic aneurysms and aortic dissections, aortic dysfunction or dilation	81405, 81410
ACTC1	ACTC1	Actin, alpha, cardiac muscle 1	Familial hypertrophic cardiomyopathy	81405
ACTN4	ACTN4	Actinin, alpha 4	Focal segmental glomerulosclerosis	81406
ADRB2	ADRB2	Adrenergic beta-2 receptor surface	Drug metabolism	81401
AFF2	AFF2	ALF transcription elongation factor 2	Fragile X intellectual disability 2 (FRAXE)	81171, 81172
AFG3L2	AFG3L2	AFG3 atpase family gene 3-like 2 (S. Cerevisiae)	Spinocerebellar ataxia	81406
AGL	AGL	Amylo-alpha-1, 6-glucosidase, 4-alpha-glucanotransferase	Glycogen storage disease type III	81407
AGTR1	AGTR1	Angiotensin II receptor, type 1	Essential hypertension	81400
AHI1	AHI1	Abelson helper integration site 1	Joubert syndrome	81407
AIRE	AIRE	Autoimmune regulator	Autoimmune polyendocrinopathy syndrome type 1	81406
ALDH7A1	ALDH7A1	Aldehyde dehydrogenase 7 family, member A1	Pyridoxine-dependent epilepsy, epilepsy	81406, 81419
ANG	ANG	Angiogenin, ribonuclease, rnase A family, 5	Amyotrophic lateral sclerosis	81403
ANK2	ANK2	Ankyrin-2	Cardiac ion channelopathies	81413
ANKRD1	ANKRD1	Ankyrin repeat domain 1	Dilated cardiomyopathy	81405
ANO5	ANO5	Anoctamin 5	Limb-girdle muscular dystrophy	81406
ANOS1	ANOS1	Anosmin- 1	Kallmann syndrome 1	81406
	APC	Adenomatous polyposis coli	Familial adenomatosis polyposis (FAP), attenuated FAP, hereditary colon cancer disorders	81201, 81202, 81203
APOB	APOB	Apolipoprotein B	Familial hypercholesterolemia type B	81401, 81407
APOE	APOE	Apolipoprotein E	Hyperlipoproteinemia type III, cardiovascular disease, Alzheimer disease	81401
APP	APP	Amyloid beta (A4) precursor protein	Alzheimer disease	81406
APTX	APTX	Aprataxin	Ataxia with oculomotor apraxia 1	81405
AQP2	AQP2	Aquaporin 2 (collecting duct)	Nephrogenic diabetes insipidus	81404
AR	AR	Androgen receptor	Spinal and bulbar muscular atrophy, Kennedy disease, X chromosome inactivation, androgen insensitivity syndrome	81173, 81174, 81204
ARSA	ARSA	Arylsulfatase A	Arylsulfatase A deficiency, severe inherited conditions	81405, 81443
ARX	ARX	Aristaless related homeobox	X-linked lissencephaly with ambiguous genitalia, X-linked intellectual disability (XLID)	81403, 81404, 81470, 81471
	ASPA	Aspartoacylase	Canavan disease, Ashkenazi Jewish-associated disorders, severe inherited conditions	81200, 81412, 81443
ASPM	ASPM	Asp (abnormal spindle) homolog, microcephaly associated (Drosophila)	Primary microcephaly	81407

Pathology and Laboratory 80047-89398, 0001U-0520U

Molecular Pathology Gene Table, *continued*

Claim Designation	Abbreviated Gene Name	Full Gene Name	Commonly Associated Proteins/Diseases (Not a complete list)	CPT Code(s)
ASS1	ASS1	Argininosuccinate synthase 1	Citrullinemia type I	81406
ASXL1	ASXL1	Additional sex combs like 1, transcriptional regulator	Myelodysplastic syndrome, myeloproliferative neoplasms, chronic myelomonocytic leukemia	81175, 81176
ATL1	ATL1	Atlastin gtpase 1	Spastic paraplegia	81406
ATM	ATM	Ataxia telangiectasia mutated	Ataxia telangiectasia	81408
ATN1	ATN1	Atrophin 1	Dentatorubral-pallidoluysian atrophy	81177
ATP1A2	ATP1A2	Atpase, Na+/K+ transporting, alpha 2 polypeptide	Familial hemiplegic migraine	81406
ATP7B	ATP7B	Atpase, Cu++ transporting, beta polypeptide	Wilson disease, severe inherited conditions	81406, 81443
ATRX	ATRX	ATRX chromatin remodeler	X-linked intellectual disability (XLID)	81470, 81471
ATXN1	ATXN1	Ataxin 1	Spinocerebellar ataxia	81178
ATXN2	ATXN2	Ataxin 2	Spinocerebellar ataxia	81179
ATXN3	ATXN3	Ataxin 3	Spinocerebellar ataxia, Machado-Joseph disease	81180
ATXN7	ATXN7	Ataxin 7	Spinocerebellar ataxia	81181
ATXN8OS	ATXN8OS	ATXN8 opposite strand (non-protein coding)	Spinocerebellar ataxia	81182
ATXN10	ATXN10	Ataxin 10	Spinocerebellar ataxia	81183
AVPR2	AVPR2	Arginine vasopressin receptor 2	Nephrogenic diabetes insipidus	81404
BBS1	BBS1	Bardet-Biedl syndrome 1	Bardet-Biedl syndrome	81406
BBS2	BBS2	Bardet-Biedl syndrome 2	Bardet-Biedl syndrome	81406
BBS10	BBS10	Bardet-Biedl syndrome 10	Bardet-Biedl syndrome	81404
BCKDHA	BCKDHA	Branched-chain keto acid dehydrogenase E1, alpha polypeptide	Maple syrup urine disease type 1A, severe inherited conditions	81400, 81405, 81443
BCKDHB	BCKDHB	Branched-chain keto acid dehydrogenase E1, beta polypeptide	Maple syrup urine disease, maple syrup urine disease type 1B, severe inherited conditions	81205, 81406, 81443
	BCR/ABL1	t(9;22)	Chronic myelogenous leukemia	81206, 81207, 81208
BCS1L	BCS1L	BCS1-like (S. Cerevisiae)	Leigh syndrome, mitochondrial complex III deficiency, GRACILE syndrome, mitochondrial disorders	81405, 81440
BEST1	BEST1	Bestrophin 1	Vitelliform macular dystrophy	81406
	BLM	Bloom syndrome, recq helicase-like	Bloom syndrome, Ashkenazi Jewish-associated disorders, severe inherited conditions	81209, 81412, 81443
BMPR2	BMPR2	Bone morphogenetic protein receptor, type II (serine/threonine kinase)	Heritable pulmonary arterial hypertension	81405, 81406
	BRAF	V-raf murine sarcoma viral oncogene homolog B1	Colon cancer	81210
BRAF	BRAF	B-Raf proto-oncogene, serine/threonine kinase	Noonan syndrome, Noonan spectrum disorders, solid organ neoplasm, hematolymphoid neoplasm or disorder	81406, 81442
	BRCA1	BRCA1, DNA repair associated	Hereditary breast and ovarian cancer, hereditary breast cancer-related disorders	81165, 81166, 81215
	BRCA2	BRCA2, DNA repair associated	Hereditary breast and ovarian cancer, hereditary breast cancer-related disorders, inherited bone marrow failure syndromes (IBMFS)	81167, 81216, 81217, 81441
	BRCA1 and BRCA2	BRCA1, DNA repair associated BRCA2, DNA repair associated	Hereditary breast and ovarian cancer	81162, 81163, 81164, 81212
	BRIP1	BRCA1 interacting helicase 1	Inherited bone marrow failure syndromes (IBMFS)	81441
BSCL2	BSCL2	Berardinelli-Seip congenital lipodystrophy 2 (seipin)	Berardinelli-Seip congenital lipodystrophy, hereditary peripheral neuropathies	81406, 81448
BTD	BTD	Biotinidase	Biotinidase deficiency	81404
BTK	BTK	Bruton agammaglobulinemia tyrosine kinase	X-linked agammaglobulinemia, chronic lymphocytic leukemia	81406, 81233

Molecular Pathology Gene Table, *continued*

Claim Designation	Abbreviated Gene Name	Full Gene Name	Commonly Associated Proteins/Diseases (Not a complete list)	CPT Code(s)
C10ORF2	C10orf2	Chromosome 10 open reading frame 2	Mitochondrial DNA depletion syndrome, mitochondrial disorders	81404, 81440
C1P19Q	Chromosome 1p-/19q- deletion analysis	N/A	Glial tumors	81402
CACNA1A	CACNA1A	Calcium channel, voltage-dependent, P/Q type, alpha 1A subunit	Spinocerebellar ataxia, epilepsy	81184, 81185, 81186, 81419
CACNB2	CACNB2	Calcium channel, voltage-dependent, beta 2 subunit	Brugada syndrome	81406
	CALR	Calreticulin	Myeloproliferative disorders	81219
CAPN3	CAPN3	Calpain 3	Limb-girdle muscular dystrophy (LGMD) type 2A, calpainopathy	81406
CASQ2	CASQ2	Calsequestrin 2 (cardiac muscle)	Catecholaminergic polymorphic ventricular tachycardia, cardiac ion channelopathies	81405, 81413
CASR	CASR	Calcium-sensing receptor	Hypocalcemia	81405
CAV3	CAV3	Caveolin 3	CAV3-related distal myopathy, limb-girdle muscular dystrophy type 1C, cardiac ion channelopathies	81404, 81413
CBFBMYH11	CBFB/MYH11	Inv(16)	Acute myeloid leukemia	81401
CBL	CBL	Cbl proto-oncogene, E3 ubiquitin protein ligase	Noonan spectrum disorders	81442
CBS	CBS	Cystathionine-beta-synthase	Homocystinuria, cystathionine beta-synthase deficiency	81401, 81406
CCND1IGH	CCND1/IGH	t(11;14)	Mantle cell lymphoma	81168
CCR5	CCR5	Chemokine C-C motif receptor 5	HIV resistance	81400
CD40LG	CD40LG	CD40 ligand	X-linked hyper IgM syndrome	81404
CDH1	CDH1	Cadherin 1, type 1, E-cadherin (epithelial)	Hereditary diffuse gastric cancer, hereditary breast cancer-related disorders, hereditary colon cancer disorders	81406
CDH23	CDH23	Cadherin-related 23	Usher syndrome, type 1, hearing loss	81408, 81430
CDKL5	CDKL5	Cyclin-dependent kinase-like 5	Early infantile epileptic encephalopathy, X-linked intellectual disability (XLID), epilepsy	81405, 81406, 81419, 81470, 81471
CDKN2A	CDKN2A	Cyclin-dependent kinase inhibitor 2A	CDKN2A-related cutaneous malignant melanoma, solid organ neoplasm or hematolymphoid neoplasm	81404
	CEBPA	CCAAT/enhancer binding protein (C/EBP), alpha	Acute myeloid leukemia, hematolymphoid neoplasm or disorder, solid organ neoplasm	81218
CEL	CEL	Carboxyl ester lipase (bile salt-stimulated lipase)	Maturity-onset diabetes of the young (MODY)	81403
CEP290	CEP290	Centrosomal protein 290kda	Joubert syndrome	81408
CFHARMS2	CFH/ARMS2	Complement factor H/age-related maculopathy susceptibility 2	Macular degeneration	81401
	CFTR	Cystic fibrosis transmembrane conductance regulator	Cystic fibrosis, Ashkenazi Jewish-associated disorders, severe inherited conditions	81220, 81221, 81222, 81223, 81224, 81412, 81443
Ch22Q13	Cytogenomic constitutional targeted microarray analysis of chromosome 22q13 by interrogation of genomic regions for copy number and single nucleotide polymorphism variants	N/A	N/A	81405

Molecular Pathology Gene Table, *continued*

Claim Designation	Abbreviated Gene Name	Full Gene Name	Commonly Associated Proteins/Diseases (Not a complete list)	CPT Code(s)
	CHD2	Chromodomain helicase DNA binding protein 2	Epilepsy	81419
CHD7	CHD7	Chromodomain helicase DNA binding protein 7	CHARGE syndrome	81407
	Chimerism engraftment analysis	N/A	Post transplantation specimen (eg, hematopoietic stem cell)	81267, 81268
CHRNA4	CHRNA4	Cholinergic receptor, nicotinic, alpha 4	Nocturnal frontal lobe epilepsy	81405
CHRNB2	CHRNB2	Cholinergic receptor, nicotinic, beta 2 (neuronal)	Nocturnal frontal lobe epilepsy	81405
CHROM18Q	Chromosome 18q-		Colon cancer	81402
CLCN1	CLCN1	Chloride channel 1, skeletal muscle	Myotonia congenita	81406
CLCNKB	CLCNKB	Chloride channel, voltage-sensitive Kb	Bartter syndrome 3 and 4b	81406
CLRN1	CLRN1	Clarin 1	Usher syndrome, type 3, hearing loss	81400, 81404, 81430
CNBP	CNBP	CCHC-type zinc finger, nucleic acid binding protein	Myotonic dystrophy type 2	81187
CNGA1	CNGA1	Cyclic nucleotide gated channel alpha 1	Hereditary retinal disorders	81434
CNTNAP2	CNTNAP2	Contactin associated protein-like 2	Pitt-Hopkins-like syndrome 1	81406
COL1A1	COL1A1	Collagen, type I, alpha 1	Osteogenesis imperfecta, type I	81408
COL1A1PDGFB	COL1A1/PDGFB	t(17;22)	Dermatofibrosarcoma protuberans	81402
COL1A2	COL1A2	Collagen, type I, alpha 2	Osteogenesis imperfecta, type I	81408
COL3A1	COL3A1	Collagen, type III, alpha 1	Aortic dysfunction or dilation	81410, 81411
COL4A1	COL4A1	Collagen, type IV, alpha 1	Brain small-vessel disease with hemorrhage	81408
COL4A3	COL4A3	Collagen, type IV, alpha 3 (Goodpasture antigen)	Alport syndrome	81408
COL4A4	COL4A4	Collagen, type IV, alpha 4	Alport syndrome	81407
COL4A5	COL4A5	Collagen, type IV, alpha 5	Alport syndrome	81407, 81408
COL6A1	COL6A1	Collagen, type VI, alpha 1	Collagen type VI-related disorders	81407
COL6A2	COL6A2	Collagen, type VI, alpha 2	Collagen type VI-related disorders	81406, 81407
COL6A3	COL6A3	Collagen, type VI, alpha 3	Collagen type VI-related disorders	81407
COQ2	COQ2	Coenzyme Q2, polyprenyltransferase	Mitochondrial disorders	81440
COX10	COX10	COX10 homolog, cytochrome c oxidase assembly protein	Mitochondrial respiratory chain complex IV deficiency, mitochondrial disorders	81405, 81440
COX15	COX15	COX15 homolog, cytochrome c oxidase assembly protein	Mitochondrial respiratory chain complex IV deficiency	81405
COX6B1	COX6B1	Cytochrome c oxidase subunit vib polypeptide 1	Mitochondrial respiratory chain complex IV deficiency	81404
CPOX	CPOX	Coproporphyrinogen oxidase	Hereditary coproporphyria	81405
CPT1A	CPT1A	Carnitine palmitoyltransferase 1A (liver)	Carnitine palmitoyltransferase 1A (CPT1A) deficiency	81406
CPT2	CPT2	Carnitine palmitoyltransferase 2	Carnitine palmitoyltransferase II deficiency	81404
CRB1	CRB1	Crumbs homolog 1 (Drosophila)	Leber congenital amaurosis, hereditary retinal disorders	81406, 81434
CREBBP	CREBBP	CREB binding protein	Rubinstein-Taybi syndrome	81406, 81407
CRX	CRX	Cone-rod homeobox	Cone-rod dystrophy 2, Leber congenital amaurosis	81404
CSTB	CSTB	Cystatin B (stefin B)	Unverricht-Lundborg disease	81188, 81189, 81190
CTNNB1	CTNNB1	Catenin (cadherin-associated protein), beta 1, 88kda	Desmoid tumors	81403
CTRC	CTRC	Chymotrypsin C	Hereditary pancreatitis	81405
CYP11B1	CYP11B1	Cytochrome P450, family 11, subfamily B, polypeptide 1	Congenital adrenal hyperplasia	81405

Molecular Pathology Gene Table, *continued*

Claim Designation	Abbreviated Gene Name	Full Gene Name	Commonly Associated Proteins/Diseases (Not a complete list)	CPT Code(s)
CYP17A1	CYP17A1	Cytochrome P450, family 17, subfamily A, polypeptide 1	Congenital adrenal hyperplasia	81405
CYP1B1	CYP1B1	Cytochrome P450, family 1, subfamily B, polypeptide 1	Primary congenital glaucoma	81404
CYP21A2	CYP21A2	Cytochrome P450, family 21, subfamily A, polypeptide 2	Congenital adrenal hyperplasia, 21-hydroxylase deficiency, steroid 21-hydroxylase isoform	81402, 81405
	CYP2C9	Cytochrome P450, family 2, subfamily C, polypeptide 9	Drug metabolism	81227
	CYP2C19	Cytochrome P450, family 2, subfamily C, polypeptide 19	Drug metabolism	81225, 81418
	CYP2D6	Cytochrome P450, family 2, subfamily D, polypeptide 6	Drug metabolism	81226, 81418
CYP3A4	CYP3A4	Cytochrome P450 family 3 subfamily A member 4	Drug metabolism	81230
CYP3A5	CYP3A5	Cytochrome P450 family 3 subfamily A member 5	Drug metabolism	81231
	Cytogenomic (genome-wide) analysis for constitutional chromosomal abnormalities	N/A	N/A	81228, 81229, 81349
	Cytogenomic (genome-wide) analysis, hematologic malignancy, structural variants and copy number variants, optical genome mapping (OGM)	N/A	N/A	81195
	Cytogenomic neoplasia (genome-wide) microarray analysis	N/A	N/A	81277
DAZSRY	DAZ/SRY	Deleted in azoospermia and sex determining region Y	Male infertility	81403
DBT	DBT	Dihydrolipoamide branched chain transacylase E2	Maple syrup urine disease, type 2	81405, 81406
DCX	DCX	Doublecortin	X-linked lissencephaly	81405
DEKNUP214	DEK/NUP214	t(6;9)	Acute myeloid leukemia	81401
DES	DES	Desmin	Myofibrillar myopathy	81405
DFNB1	DFNB1	N/A	Hearing loss	81431
DFNB59	DFNB59	Deafness, autosomal recessive 59	Autosomal recessive nonsyndromic hearing impairment	81405
DGUOK	DGUOK	Deoxyguanosine kinase	Hepatocerebral mitochondrial DNA depletion syndrome, mitochondrial disorders	81405, 81440
DHCR7	DHCR7	7-dehydrocholesterol reductase	Smith-Lemli-Opitz syndrome, severe inherited conditions	81405, 81443
	DKC1	Dyskerin pseudouridine synthase 1	Inherited bone marrow failure syndromes (IBMFS)	81441
DLAT	DLAT	Dihydrolipoamide S-acetyltransferase	Pyruvate dehydrogenase E2 deficiency	81406
DLD	DLD	Dihydrolipoamide dehydrogenase	Maple syrup urine disease, type III	81406
	DMD	Dystrophin	Duchenne/Becker muscular dystrophy	81161
DMD	DMD	Dystrophin	Duchenne/Becker muscular dystrophy	81408
DMPK	DMPK	Dystrophia myotonica-protein kinase	Myotonic dystrophy, type 1	81234, 81239
DNMT3A	DNMT3A	DNA (cytosine-5-)-methyltransferase 3 alpha	Acute myeloid leukemia, hematolymphoid neoplasm or disorder, solid organ neoplasm	81403
DPYD	DPYD	Dihydropyrimidine dehydrogenase	5-fluorouracil/5-FU and capecitabine drug metabolism	81232

Molecular Pathology Gene Table, *continued*

Claim Designation	Abbreviated Gene Name	Full Gene Name	Commonly Associated Proteins/Diseases (Not a complete list)	CPT Code(s)
DSC2	DSC2	Desmocollin	Arrhythmogenic right ventricular dysplasia/cardiomyopathy 11	81406
DSG2	DSG2	Desmoglein 2	Arrhythmogenic right ventricular dysplasia/cardiomyopathy 10, hereditary cardiomyopathy	81406, 81439
DSP	DSP	Desmoplakin	Arrhythmogenic right ventricular dysplasia/cardiomyopathy 8	81406
DYSF	DYSF	Dysferlin, limb-girdle muscular dystrophy 2B (autosomal recessive)	Limb-girdle muscular dystrophy	81408
E2APBX1	E2A/PBX1	t(1;19)	Acute lymphocytic leukemia	81401
EFHC1	EFHC1	EF-hand domain (C-terminal) containing 1	Juvenile myoclonic epilepsy	81406
	EGFR	Epidermal growth factor receptor	Non-small cell lung cancer, solid organ neoplasm or hematolymphoid neoplasm	81235
EGR2	EGR2	Early growth response 2	Charcot-Marie-Tooth disease	81404
EIF2B2	EIF2B2	Eukaryotic translation initiation factor 2B, subunit 2 beta, 39kda	Leukoencephalopathy with vanishing white matter	81405
EIF2B3	EIF2B3	Eukaryotic translation initiation factor 2B, subunit 3 gamma, 58kda	Leukoencephalopathy with vanishing white matter	81406
EIF2B4	EIF2B4	Eukaryotic translation initiation factor 2B, subunit 4 delta, 67kda	Leukoencephalopathy with vanishing white matter	81406
EIF2B5	EIF2B5	Eukaryotic translation initiation factor 2B, subunit 5 epsilon, 82kda	Childhood ataxia with central nervous system hypomyelination/vanishing white matter	81406
EMD	EMD	Emerin	Emery-Dreifuss muscular dystrophy	81404, 81405
EML4ALK	EML4/ALK	Inv(2)	Non-small cell lung cancer	81401
ENG	ENG	Endoglin	Hereditary hemorrhagic telangiectasia, type 1	81405, 81406
EPCAM	EPCAM	Epithelial cell adhesion molecule	Lynch syndrome, hereditary colon cancer disorders	81403
EPM2A	EPM2A	Epilepsy, progressive myoclonus type 2A, Lafora disease (laforin)	Progressive myoclonus epilepsy	81404
ESR1PGR	ESR1/PGR	Receptor 1/progesterone receptor	Breast cancer	81402
ETV6RUNX1	ETV6/RUNX1	t(12;21)	Acute lymphocytic leukemia	81401
EWSR1ATF1	EWSR1/ATF1	t(12;22)	Clear cell sarcoma	81401
EWSR1ERG	EWSR1/ERG	t(21;22)	Ewing sarcoma/peripheral neuroectodermal tumor	81401
EWSR1FLI1	EWSR1/FLI1	t(11;22)	Ewing sarcoma/peripheral neuroectodermal tumor	81401
EWSR1WT1	EWSR1/WT1	t(11;22)	Desmoplastic small round cell tumor	81401
EYA1	EYA1	Eyes absent homolog 1 (Drosophila)	Branchio-oto-renal (BOR) spectrum disorders	81405, 81406
EYS	EYS	Eyes shut homolog (Drosophila)	Hereditary retinal disorders	81434
EZH2	EZH2	Enhancer of zeste 2 polycomb repressive complex 2 subunit	Myelodysplastic syndrome, myeloproliferative neoplasms, diffuse large B-cell lymphoma, solid organ or hematolymphoid neoplasm or disorder	81236, 81237
	F2	Prothrombin, coagulation factor II	Hereditary hypercoagulability	81240
F2	F2	Prothrombin, coagulation factor II	Hereditary hypercoagulability	81400
	F5	Coagulation factor V	Hereditary hypercoagulability	81241
F5	F5	Coagulation factor V	Hereditary hypercoagulability	81400
F7	F7	Coagulation factor VII (serum prothrombin conversion accelerator)	Hereditary hypercoagulability	81400
F8	F8	Coagulation factor VIII	Hemophilia A	81403, 81406, 81407
F9	F9	Coagulation factor IX	Hemophilia B	81238

Molecular Pathology Gene Table, *continued*

Claim Designation	Abbreviated Gene Name	Full Gene Name	Commonly Associated Proteins/Diseases (Not a complete list)	CPT Code(s)
F11	F11	Coagulation factor XI	Coagulation disorder	81401
F12	F12	Coagulation factor XII (Hageman factor)	Angioedema, hereditary, type III; factor XII deficiency	81403
F13B	F13B	Coagulation factor XIII, B polypeptide	Hereditary hypercoagulability	81400
FAH	FAH	Fumarylacetoacetate hydrolase (fumarylacetoacetase)	Tyrosinemia, type 1	81406
	FANCA	FA complementation group A	Inherited bone marrow failure syndromes (IBMFS)	81441
	FANCB	FA complementation group B	Inherited bone marrow failure syndromes (IBMFS)	81441
	FANCC	Fanconi anemia, complementation group C	Fanconi anemia, type C, Ashkenazi Jewish-associated disorders, severe inherited conditions, inherited bone marrow failure syndromes (IBMFS)	81242, 81412, 81441, 81443
	FANCD2	FA complementation group D2	Inherited bone marrow failure syndromes (IBMFS)	81441
	FANCE2	FA complementation group E	Inherited bone marrow failure syndromes (IBMFS)	81441
	FANCF	FA complementation group F	Inherited bone marrow failure syndromes (IBMFS)	81441
	FANCG	FA complementation group G	Inherited bone marrow failure syndromes (IBMFS)	81441
	FANCI	FA complementation group I	Inherited bone marrow failure syndromes (IBMFS)	81441
	FANCL	FA complementation group L	Inherited bone marrow failure syndromes (IBMFS)	81441
FASTKD2	FASTKD2	FAST kinase domains 2	Mitochondrial respiratory chain complex IV deficiency	81406
FBN1	FBN1	Fibrillin 1	Marfan syndrome, aortic dysfunction or dilation	81408, 81410
FGB	FGB	Fibrinogen beta chain	Hereditary ischemic heart disease	81400
FGD1	FGD1	FYVE, rhogef and PH domain containing 1	X-linked intellectual disability (XLID)	81470, 81471
FGF23	FGF23	Fibroblast growth factor 23	Hypophosphatemic rickets	81404
FGFR1	FGFR1	Fibroblast growth factor receptor 1	Pfeiffer syndrome type 1, craniosynostosis, Kallmann syndrome	81400, 81405
FGFR2	FGFR2	Fibroblast growth factor receptor 2	Craniosynostosis, Apert syndrome, Crouzon syndrome	81404
FGFR3	FGFR3	Fibroblast growth factor receptor 3	Muenke syndrome, achondroplasia, hypochondroplasia, isolated craniosynostosis	81400, 81401, 81403, 81404
FH	FH	Fumarate hydratase	Fumarate hydratase deficiency, hereditary leiomyomatosis with renal cell cancer	81405
FHL1	FHL1	Four and a half LIM domains 1	Emery-Dreifuss muscular dystrophy	81404
FIG4	FIG4	FIG4 homolog, SAC1 lipid phosphatase domain containing (S. Cerevisiae)	Charcot-Marie-Tooth disease	81406
FIP1L1PDGFRA	FIP1L1/PDGFRA	Del(4q12)	Imatinib-sensitive chronic eosinophilic leukemia	81401
FKRP	FKRP	Fukutin related protein	Congenital muscular dystrophy type 1C (MDC1C), limb-girdle muscular dystrophy (LGMD) type 2I	81404
FKTN	FKTN	Fukutin	Fukuyama congenital muscular dystrophy, limb-girdle muscular dystrophy (LGMD) type 2M or 2L	81400, 81405
FLG	FLG	Filaggrin	Ichthyosis vulgaris	81401
	FLT3	Fms-related tyrosine kinase 3	Acute myeloid leukemia, hematolymphoid neoplasm or disorder, solid organ neoplasm	81245, 81246
	FMR1	Fragile X messenger ribonucleoprotein 1	X-linked intellectual disability (XLID)	81243, 81244, 81470, 81471
FOXG1	FOXG1	Forkhead box G1	Rett syndrome	81404
FOXO1PAX3	FOXO1/PAX3	t(2;13)	Ewing sarcoma/peripheral neuroectodermal tumor, alveolar rhabdomyosarcoma	81401
FOXO1PAX7	FOXO1/PAX7	t(1;13)	Ewing sarcoma/peripheral neuroectodermal tumor, alveolar rhabdomyosarcoma	81401

Molecular Pathology Gene Table, *continued*

Claim Designation	Abbreviated Gene Name	Full Gene Name	Commonly Associated Proteins/Diseases (Not a complete list)	CPT Code(s)
FSHMD1A	FSHMD1A	Facioscapulohumeral muscular dystrophy 1A	Facioscapulohumeral muscular dystrophy	81404
FTSJ1	FTSJ1	FtsJ RNA 2'-O-methyltransferase 1	X-linked intellectual disability 9	81405, 81406
FUS	FUS	Fused in sarcoma	Amyotrophic lateral sclerosis	81406
FUSDDIT3	FUS/DDIT3	t(12;16)	Myxoid liposarcoma	81401
FXN	FXN	Frataxin	Friedreich ataxia	81284, 81285, 81286, 81289
G6PC	G6PC	Glucose-6-phosphatase, catalytic subunit	Glycogen storage disease, type 1a, von Gierke disease, severe inherited conditions	81250, 81443
G6PD	G6PD	Glucose-6-phosphate dehydrogenase	Hemolytic anemia, jaundice	81247, 81248, 81249
GAA	GAA	Glucosidase, alpha; acid	Glycogen storage disease type II (Pompe disease), severe inherited conditions	81406, 81443
GABRG2	GABRG2	Gamma-aminobutyric acid (GABA) A receptor, gamma 2	Generalized epilepsy with febrile seizures, epilepsy	81405, 81419
GALC	GALC	Galactosylceramidase	Krabbe disease	81401, 81406
GALT	GALT	Galactose-1-phosphate uridylyltransferase	Galactosemia, severe inherited conditions	81401, 81406, 81443
GARS	GARS	Glycyl-trna synthetase	Charcot-Marie-Tooth disease	81406
	GATA1	GATA binding protein 1	Inherited bone marrow failure syndromes (IBMFS)	81441
	GATA2	GATA binding protein 2	Inherited bone marrow failure syndromes (IBMFS)	81441
	GBA	Glucosidase, beta, acid	Gaucher disease, Ashkenazi Jewish-associated disorders, severe inherited conditions	81251, 81412, 81443
GBE1		1,4-alpha-glucan branching enzyme 1	Severe inherited conditions	81443
GCDH	GCDH	Glutaryl-coa dehydrogenase	Glutaricacidemia type 1	81406
GCH1	GCH1	GTP cyclohydrolase 1	Autosomal dominant dopa-responsive dystonia	81405
GCK	GCK	Glucokinase (hexokinase 4)	Maturity-onset diabetes of the young (MODY)	81406
GDAP1	GDAP1	Ganglioside-induced differentiation-associated protein 1	Charcot-Marie-Tooth disease	81405
GFAP	GFAP	Glial fibrillary acidic protein	Alexander disease	81405
GH1	GH1	Growth hormone 1	Growth hormone deficiency	81404
GHR	GHR	Growth hormone receptor	Laron syndrome	81405
GHRHR	GHRHR	Growth hormone releasing hormone receptor	Growth hormone deficiency	81405
GJB1	GJB1	Gap junction protein, beta 1	Charcot-Marie-Tooth X-linked, hereditary peripheral neuropathies	81403, 81448
	GJB2	Gap junction protein, beta 2, 26kda, connexin 26	Nonsyndromic hearing loss	81252, 81253, 81430, 81431
	GJB6	Gap junction protein, beta 6, 30kda, connexin 30	Nonsyndromic hearing loss	81254, 81431
GLA	GLA	Galactosidase, alpha	Fabry disease	81405
GLUD1	GLUD1	Glutamate dehydrogenase 1	Familial hyperinsulinism	81406
GNAQ	GNAQ	Guanine nucleotide-binding protein G(q) subunit alpha	Uveal melanoma	81403
GNE	GNE	Glucosamine (UDP-N-acetyl)-2-epimerase/N-acetylmannosamine kinase	Inclusion body myopathy 2 (IBM2), Nonaka myopathy	81400, 81406
GP1BB	GP1BB	Glycoprotein Ib (platelet), beta polypeptide	Bernard-Soulier syndrome type B	81404
GPR98	GPR98	G-protein coupled receptor 98	Hearing loss	81430

Molecular Pathology Gene Table, *continued*

Claim Designation	Abbreviated Gene Name	Full Gene Name	Commonly Associated Proteins/Diseases (Not a complete list)	CPT Code(s)
	GRIN2A	Glutamate ionotropic receptor NMDA type subunit 2A	Epilepsy	81419
GRN	GRN	Granulin	Frontotemporal dementia	81406
H19	H19	Imprinted maternally expressed transcript (non-protein coding)	Beckwith-Wiedemann syndrome	81401
HADHA	HADHA	Hydroxyacyl-coa dehydrogenase/3-ketoacyl-coa thiolase/enoyl-coa hydratase (trifunctional protein) alpha subunit	Long chain acyl-coenzyme A dehydrogenase deficiency	81406
HADHB	HADHB	Hydroxyacyl-coa dehydrogenase/3-ketoacyl-coa thiolase/enoyl-coa hydratase (trifunctional protein), beta subunit	Trifunctional protein deficiency	81406
HBA1/HBA2	HBA1/HBA2	Alpha globin 1 and alpha globin 2	Alpha thalassemia, thalassemia, Hb Bart hydrops fetalis syndrome, HbH disease	81257, 81258, 81259, 81269
HBB	HBB	Hemoglobin, subunit beta	Sickle cell anemia, beta thalassemia, hemoglobinopathy, severe inherited conditions	81361, 81362, 81363, 81364, 81443
HEA	HEA	Human erythrocyte antigen	Sickle-cell disease, thalassemia, hemolytic transfusion reactions, hemolytic disease of the fetus or newborn	81403
	HEXA	Hexosaminidase A (alpha polypeptide)	Tay-Sachs disease, Ashkenazi Jewish-associated disorders, severe inherited conditions	81255, 81406, 81412, 81443
	HFE	Hemochromatosis	Hereditary hemochromatosis	81256
	HLA	Human leukocyte antigen genes	Pretransplant and drug therapy testing	81370-81383
HLCS	HLCS	HLCS holocarboxylase synthetase	Holocarboxylase synthetase deficiency	81406
HMBS	HMBS	Hydroxymethylbilane synthase	Acute intermittent porphyria	81406
HNF1A	HNF1A	HNF1 homeobox A	Maturity-onset diabetes of the young (MODY)	81405
HNF1B	HNF1B	HNF1 homeobox B	Maturity-onset diabetes of the young (MODY)	81404, 81405
HNF4A	HNF4A	Hepatocyte nuclear factor 4, alpha	Maturity-onset diabetes of the young (MODY)	81406
HPA1	Human Platelet Antigen 1 genotyping (HPA-1), ITGB3	Integrin, beta 3 (platelet glycoprotein iiia), antigen CD61 (gpiiia)	Neonatal alloimmune thrombocytopenia (NAIT), post-transfusion purpura	81105
HPA2	Human Platelet Antigen 2 genotyping (HPA-2), GP1BA	Glycoprotein Ib (platelet), alpha polypeptide (gpiba)	Neonatal alloimmune thrombocytopenia (NAIT), post-transfusion purpura	81106
HPA3	Human Platelet Antigen 3 genotyping (HPA-3), ITGA2B	Integrin, alpha 2b (platelet glycoprotein iib of iib/iiia complex), antigen CD41 (gpiib)	Neonatal alloimmune thrombocytopenia (NAIT), post-transfusion purpura	81107
HPA4	Human Platelet Antigen 4 genotyping (HPA-4), ITGB3	Integrin, beta 3 (platelet glycoprotein iiia), antigen CD61 (gpiiia)	Neonatal alloimmune thrombocytopenia (NAIT), post-transfusion purpura	81108
HPA5	Human Platelet Antigen 5 genotyping (HPA-5), ITGA2	Integrin, alpha 2 (CD49B, alpha 2 subunit of VLA-2 receptor) (gpia)	Neonatal alloimmune thrombocytopenia (NAIT), post-transfusion purpura	81109
HPA6	Human Platelet Antigen 6 genotyping (HPA-6w), ITGB3	Integrin, beta 3 (platelet glycoprotein iiia, antigen CD61) (gpiiia)	Neonatal alloimmune thrombocytopenia (NAIT), post-transfusion purpura	81110

Molecular Pathology Gene Table, *continued*

Claim Designation	Abbreviated Gene Name	Full Gene Name	Commonly Associated Proteins/Diseases (Not a complete list)	CPT Code(s)
HPA9	Human Platelet Antigen 9 genotyping (HPA-9w), ITGA2B	Integrin, alpha 2b (platelet glycoprotein iib of iib/iiia complex, antigen CD41) (gpiib)	Neonatal alloimmune thrombocytopenia (NAIT), post-transfusion purpura	81111
HPA15	Human Platelet Antigen 15 genotyping (HPA-15), CD109	CD109 molecule	Neonatal alloimmune thrombocytopenia (NAIT), post-transfusion purpura	81112
HRAS	HRAS	V-Ha-ras Harvey rat sarcoma viral oncogene homolog	Costello syndrome, Noonan spectrum disorders	81403, 81404, 81442
HSD3B2	HSD3B2	Hydroxy-delta-5-steroid dehydrogenase, 3 beta- and steroid delta-isomerase 2	3-beta-hydroxysteroid dehydrogenase type II deficiency	81404
HSD11B2	HSD11B2	Hydroxysteroid (11-beta) dehydrogenase 2	Mineralocorticoid excess syndrome	81404
HSPB1	HSPB1	Heat shock 27kda protein 1	Charcot-Marie-Tooth disease	81404
HTRA1	HTRA1	Htra serine peptidase 1	Macular degeneration	81405
HTT	HTT	Huntingtin	Huntington disease	81271, 81274
HUWE1	HUWE1	HECT, UBA and WWE domain containing 1, E3 ubiquitin protein ligase	X-linked intellectual disability (XLID)	81470, 81471
IDH1	IDH1	Isocitrate dehydrogenase 1 (NADP+), soluble	Glioma, hematolymphoid neoplasm or disorder, solid organ neoplasm	81120
IDH2	IDH2	Isocitrate dehydrogenase 2 (NADP+), mitochondrial	Glioma, hematolymphoid neoplasm or disorder, solid organ neoplasm	81121
IDS	IDS	Iduronate 2-sulfatase	Mucopolysacchridosis, type II	81405
IDUA	IDUA	Iduronidase, alpha-L-	Mucopolysaccharidosis type I	81406
IFNL3	IFNL3	Interferon, lambda 3	Drug response	81283
	IGH@	Immunoglobulin heavy chain locus	Leukemias and lymphomas, B-cell	81261, 81262, 81263
IGHBCL2	IGH@/BCL2	t(14;18)	Follicular lymphoma	81278, 81401
	IGK@	Immunoglobulin kappa light chain locus	Leukemia and lymphoma, B-cell	81264
	IKBKAP	Inhibitor of kappa light polypeptide geneenhancer in B-cells, kinase complex-associated protein	Familial dysautonomia, Ashkenazi Jewish-associated disorders, severe inherited conditions	81260, 81412, 81443
IL1RAPL	IL1RAPL	Interleukin 1 receptor accessory protein	X-linked intellectual disability (XLID)	81470, 81471
IL2RG	IL2RG	Interleukin 2 receptor, gamma	X-linked severe combined immunodeficiency	81405
INF2	INF2	Inverted formin, FH2 and WH2 domain containing	Focal segmental glomerulosclerosis	81406
INS	INS	Insulin	Diabetes mellitus	81404
ISPD	ISPD	Isoprenoid synthase domain containing	Muscle-eye-brain disease, Walker-Warburg syndrome	81405
ITPR1	ITPR1	Inositol 1,4,5-trisphosphate receptor, type 1	Spinocerebellar ataxia	81408
IVD	IVD	Isovaleryl-coa dehydrogenase	Isovaleric acidemia	81400, 81406
JAG1	JAG1	Jagged 1	Alagille syndrome	81406, 81407
	JAK2	Janus kinase 2	Myeloproliferative disorder, hematolymphoid neoplasm or disorder, solid organ neoplasm	81270, 81279
JUP	JUP	Junction plakoglobin	Arrhythmogenic right ventricular dysplasia/cardiomyopathy 11	81406
KCNC3	KCNC3	Potassium voltage-gated channel, Shaw-related subfamily, member 3	Spinocerebellar ataxia	81403
KCNE1	KCNE1	Potassium voltage-gated channel, subfamily E, member 1	Cardiac ion channelopathies	81413

Molecular Pathology Gene Table, *continued*

Claim Designation	Abbreviated Gene Name	Full Gene Name	Commonly Associated Proteins/Diseases (Not a complete list)	CPT Code(s)
KCNE2	KCNE2	Potassium voltage-gated channel, subfamily E, member 2	Cardiac ion channelopathies	81413
KCNH2	KCNH2	Potassium voltage-gated channel, subfamily H (eag-related), member 2	Short QT syndrome, long QT syndrome, cardiac ion channelopathies	81406, 81413, 81414
KCNJ1	KCNJ1	Potassium inwardly-rectifying channel, subfamily J, member 1	Bartter syndrome	81404
KCNJ2	KCNJ2	Potassium inwardly-rectifying channel, subfamily J, member 2	Andersen-Tawil syndrome, cardiac ion channelopathies	81403, 81413
KCNJ10	KCNJ10	Potassium inwardly-rectifying channel, subfamily J, member 10	SeSAME syndrome, EAST syndrome, sensorineural hearing loss	81404
KCNJ11	KCNJ11	Potassium inwardly-rectifying channel, subfamily J, member 11	Familial hyperinsulinism	81403
KCNQ1	KCNQ1	Potassium voltage-gated channel, KQT-like subfamily, member 1	Short QT syndrome, long QT syndrome, cardiac ion channelopathies	81406, 81413, 81414
KCNQ1OT1	KCNQ1OT1	KCNQ1 overlapping transcript 1 (non-protein coding)	Beckwith-Wiedemann syndrome	81401
KCNQ2	KCNQ2	Potassium voltage-gated channel, KQT-like subfamily, member 2	Epileptic encephalopathy, epilepsy	81406, 81419
KDM5C	KDM5C	Lysine demethylase 5C	X-linked intellectual disability (XLID)	81407, 81470, 81471
KIAA0196	KIAA0196	Kiaa0196	Spastic paraplegia	81407
KIR	KIR	Killer cell immunoglobulin-like receptor	Hematopoietic stem cell transplantation	81403
	KIT	V-kit Hardy-Zuckerman 4 feline sarcoma viral oncogene homolog	Gastrointestinal stromal tumor, acute myeloid leukemia, melanoma, solid organ neoplasm, hematolymphoid neoplasm or disorder	81272, 81273
	KRAS	V-Ki-ras2 Kirsten rat sarcoma viral oncogene homolog	Carcinoma, Noonan syndrome	81275, 81276
KRAS	KRAS	Kirsten rat sarcoma viral oncogene homolog	Noonan syndrome, Noonan spectrum disorders, solid organ neoplasm, hematolymphoid neoplasm or disorder	81405, 81442
L1CAM	L1CAM	L1 cell adhesion molecule	MASA syndrome, X-linked hydrocephaly, X-linked intellectual disability (XLID)	81407, 81470, 81471
LAMA2	LAMA2	Laminin, alpha 2	Congenital muscular dystrophy	81408
LAMB2	LAMB2	Laminin, beta 2 (laminin S)	Pierson syndrome	81407
LAMP2	LAMP2	Lysosomal-associated membrane protein 2	Danon disease	81405
LCT	LCT	Lactase-phlorizin hydrolase	Lactose intolerance	81400
LDB3	LDB3	LIM domain binding 3	Familial dilated cardiomyopathy, myofibrillar myopathy	81406
LDLR	LDLR	Low density lipoprotein receptor	Familial hypercholesterolemia	81405, 81406
LEPR	LEPR	Leptin receptor	Obesity with hypogonadism	81406
LHCGR	LHCGR	Luteinizing hormone/choriogonadotropin receptor	Precocious male puberty	81406
LINC00518	LINC00518	Long intergenic non-protein coding RNA 518	Melanoma	81401
LITAF	LITAF	Lipopolysaccharide-induced TNF factor	Charcot-Marie-Tooth disease	81404
LMNA	LMNA	Lamin A/C	Emery-Dreifuss muscular dystrophy (EDMD1, 2, and 3), limb-girdle muscular dystrophy (LGMD) type 1B, dilated cardiomyopathy (CMD1A), familial partial lipodystrophy (FPLD2)	81406
LRP5	LRP5	Low density lipoprotein receptor-related protein 5	Osteopetrosis	81406
LRRK2	LRRK2	Leucine-rich repeat kinase 2	Parkinson disease	81401, 81408
MAP2K1	MAP2K1	Mitogen-activated protein kinase 1	Cardiofaciocutaneous syndrome, Noonan spectrum disorders	81406, 81442

Molecular Pathology Gene Table, *continued*

Claim Designation	Abbreviated Gene Name	Full Gene Name	Commonly Associated Proteins/Diseases (Not a complete list)	CPT Code(s)
MAP2K2	MAP2K2	Mitogen-activated protein kinase 2	Cardiofaciocutaneous syndrome, Noonan spectrum disorders	81406, 81442
MAPT	MAPT	Microtubule-associated protein tau	Frontotemporal dementia	81406
MC4R	MC4R	Melanocortin 4 receptor	Obesity	81403
MCCC1	MCCC1	Methylcrotonoyl-coa carboxylase 1 (alpha)	3-methylcrotonyl-CoA carboxylase deficiency	81406
MCCC2	MCCC2	Methylcrotonoyl-coa carboxylase 2 (beta)	3-methylcrotonyl carboxylase deficiency	81406
	MCOLN1	Mucolipin 1	Mucolipidosis, type IV, Ashkenazi Jewish-associated disorders, severe inherited conditions	81290, 81412, 81443
	MECP2	Methyl cpg binding protein 2	Rett syndrome, X-linked intellectual disability (XLID), epilepsy	81302, 81303, 81304, 81419, 81470, 81471
MED12	MED12	Mediator complex subunit 12	FG syndrome type 1, Lujan syndrome, X-linked intellectual disability (XLID)	81401, 81470, 81471
MEFV	MEFV	Mediterranean fever	Familial Mediterranean fever	81402, 81404
MEG3DLK1	MEG3/DLK1	Maternally expressed 3 (non-protein coding)/delta-like 1 homolog (Drosophila)	Intrauterine growth retardation	81401
MEN1	MEN1	Multiple endocrine neoplasia 1	Multiple endocrine neoplasia type 1, Wermer syndrome	81404, 81405
MFN2	MFN2	Mitofusin 2	Charcot-Marie-Tooth disease, hereditary peripheral neuropathies	81406, 81448
	MGMT	O-6-methylguanine-DNA methyltransferase	Glioblastoma multiforme	81287
MICA	MICA	MHC class I polypeptide-related sequence A	Solid organ transplantation	81403
	Microsatellite instability analysis	N/A	Hereditary nonpolyposis colorectal cancer, Lynch syndrome	81301
MID1	MID1	Midline 1	X-linked intellectual disability (XLID)	81470, 81471
	MLH1	Mutl homolog 1, colon cancer, nonpolyposis type 2	Hereditary nonpolyposis colorectal cancer, Lynch syndrome, hereditary breast cancer-related disorders, hereditary colon cancer disorders	81288, 81292, 81293, 81294
MLLAFF1	MLL/AFF1	t(4;11)	Acute lymphoblastic leukemia	81401
MLLMLLT3	MLL/MLLT3	t(9;11)	Acute myeloid leukemia	81401
MMAA	MMAA	Methylmalonic aciduria (cobalamine deficiency) type A	MMAA-related methylmalonic acidemia	81405
MMAB	MMAB	Methylmalonic aciduria (cobalamine deficiency) type B	MMAA-related methylmalonic acidemia	81405
MMACHC	MMACHC	Methylmalonic aciduria (cobalamin deficiency) cblc type, with homocystinuria	Methylmalonic acidemia and homocystinuria	81404
MPI	MPI	Mannose phosphate isomerase	Congenital disorder of glycosylation 1b	81405
MPL	MPL	MPL proto-oncogene, thrombopoietin receptor	Myeloproliferative disorder, inherited bone marrow failure syndromes (IBMFS)	81338, 81339, 81441
MPV17	MPV17	Mpv17 mitochondrial inner membrane protein	Mitochondrial DNA depletion syndrome, mitochondrial disorders	81404, 81405, 81440
MPZ	MPZ	Myelin protein zero	Charcot-Marie-Tooth disease, hereditary peripheral neuropathies	81405, 81448
	MSH2	Muts homolog 2, colon cancer, nonpolyposis type 1	Hereditary nonpolyposis colorectal cancer, Lynch syndrome, hereditary breast cancer-related disorders, hereditary colon cancer disorders	81295, 81296, 81297
	MSH6	Muts homolog 6 (E. Coli)	Hereditary nonpolyposis colorectal cancer, Lynch syndrome, hereditary breast cancer-related disorders, hereditary colon cancer disorders	81298, 81299, 81300
MTATP6	MT-ATP6	Mitochondrially encoded ATP synthase 6	Neuropathy with ataxia and retinitis pigmentosa (NARP), Leigh syndrome	81401

Molecular Pathology Gene Table, *continued*

Claim Designation	Abbreviated Gene Name	Full Gene Name	Commonly Associated Proteins/Diseases (Not a complete list)	CPT Code(s)
	MTHFR	5,10-methylenetetrahydrofolate reductase	Hereditary hypercoagulability	81291
MTM1	MTM1	Myotubularin 1	X-linked centronuclear myopathy	81405, 81406
MTND4ND6	MT-ND4, MT-ND6	Mitochondrially encoded NADH dehydrogenase 4, mitochondrially encoded NADH dehydrogenase 6	Leber hereditary optic neuropathy (LHON)	81401
MTND5	MT-ND5	Mitochondrially encoded trna leucine 1 (UUA/G), mitochondrially encoded NADH dehydrogenase 5	Mitochondrial encephalopathy with lactic acidosis and stroke-like episodes (MELAS)	81401
MTRNR1	MT-RNR1	Mitochondrially encoded 12S RNA	Nonsyndromic hearing loss	81401, 81403, 81430
MTTK	MT-TK	Mitochondrially encoded trna lysine	Myoclonic epilepsy with ragged-red fibers (MERRF)	81401
MTTL1	MT-TL1	Mitochondrially encoded trna leucine 1 (UUA/G)	Diabetes and hearing loss	81401
MTTS1	MT-TS1	Mitochondrially encoded trna serine 1	Nonsyndromic hearing loss	81403
MTTS1RNR1	MT-TS1, MT-RNR1	Mitochondrially encoded trna serine 1 (UCN), mitochondrially encoded 12S RNA	Nonsyndromic sensorineural deafness (including aminoglycoside-induced nonsyndromic deafness)	81401
MUT	MUT	Methylmalonyl coa mutase	Methylmalonic acidemia	81406
MUTYH	MUTYH	Muty homolog (E. Coli)	MYH-associated polyposis, hereditary colon cancer disorders	81401, 81406
MYBPC3	MYBPC3	Myosin binding protein C, cardiac	Familial hypertrophic cardiomyopathy, hereditary cardiomyopathy	81407, 81439
MYD88	MYD88	Myeloid differentiation primary response 88	Waldenstrom's macroglobulinemia, lymphoplasmacytic leukemia	81305
MYH6	MYH6	Myosin, heavy chain 6, cardiac muscle, alpha	Familial dilated cardiomyopathy	81407
MYH7	MYH7	Myosin, heavy chain 7, cardiac muscle, beta	Familial hypertrophic cardiomyopathy, Laing distal myopathy, hereditary cardiomyopathy	81407, 81439
MYH11	MYH11	Myosin, heavy chain 11, smooth muscle	Thoracic aortic aneurysms and aortic dissections, aortic dysfunction or dilation	81408, 81410, 81411
MYL2	MYL2	Myosin, light chain 2, regulatory, cardiac, slow	Familial hypertrophic cardiomyopathy	81405
MYL3	MYL3	Myosin, light chain 3, alkali, ventricular, skeletal, slow	Familial hypertrophic cardiomyopathy	81405
MYLK	MYLK	Myosin light chain kinase	Aortic dysfunction or dilation	81410
MYO7A	MYO7A	Myosin VIIA	Usher syndrome, type 1, hearing loss	81407, 81430
MYO15A	MYO15A	Myosin XVA	Hearing loss	81430
MYOT	MYOT	Myotilin	Limb-girdle muscular dystrophy	81405
NDP	NDP	Norrie disease (pseudoglioma)	Norrie disease	81403, 81404
NDUFA1	NDUFA1	NADH dehydrogenase (ubiquinone) 1 alpha subcomplex, 1, 7.5kda	Leigh syndrome, mitochondrial complex I deficiency	81404
NDUFAF2	NDUFAF2	NADH dehydrogenase (ubiquinone) 1 alpha subcomplex, assembly factor 2	Leigh syndrome, mitochondrial complex I deficiency	81404
NDUFS1	NDUFS1	NADH dehydrogenase (ubiquinone) Fe-S protein 1, 75kda (NADH-coenzyme Q reductase)	Leigh syndrome, mitochondrial complex I deficiency	81406
NDUFS4	NDUFS4	NADH dehydrogenase (ubiquinone) Fe-S protein 4, 18kda (NADH-coenzyme Q reductase)	Leigh syndrome, mitochondrial complex I deficiency	81404
NDUFS7	NDUFS7	NADH dehydrogenase (ubiquinone) Fe-S protein 7, 20kda (NADH-coenzyme Q reductase)	Leigh syndrome, mitochondrial complex I deficiency	81405
NDUFS8	NDUFS8	NADH dehydrogenase (ubiquinone) Fe-S protein 8, 23kda (NADH-coenzyme Q reductase)	Leigh syndrome, mitochondrial complex I deficiency	81405

Molecular Pathology Gene Table, *continued*

Claim Designation	Abbreviated Gene Name	Full Gene Name	Commonly Associated Proteins/Diseases (Not a complete list)	CPT Code(s)
NDUFV1	NDUFV1	NADH dehydrogenase (ubiquinone) flavoprotein 1, 51kda	Leigh syndrome, mitochondrial complex I deficiency	81405
NEB	NEB	Nebulin	Nemaline myopathy 2	81400, 81408
NEFL	NEFL	Neurofilament, light polypeptide	Charcot-Marie-Tooth disease	81405
NF1	NF1	Neurofibromin 1	Neurofibromatosis, type 1	81408
NF2	NF2	Neurofibromin 2 (merlin)	Neurofibromatosis, type 2	81405, 81406
NHLRC1	NHLRC1	NHL repeat containing 1	Progressive myoclonus epilepsy	81403
	NHP2	NHP2 ribonucleoprotein	Inherited bone marrow failure syndromes (IBMFS)	81441
NIPA1	NIPA1	Non-imprinted in Prader-Willi/Angelman syndrome 1	Spastic paraplegia	81404
NLGN3	NLGN3	Neuroligin 3	Autism spectrum disorders	81405
NLGN4X	NLGN4X	Neuroligin 4, X-linked	Autism spectrum disorders	81404, 81405
NOD2	NOD2	Nucleotide-binding oligomerization domain containing 2	Crohn's disease, Blau syndrome	81401
	NOP10	NOP10 ribonucleoprotein	Inherited bone marrow failure syndromes (IBMFS)	81441
NOS	Known familial variant NOS	N/A	N/A	81403
NOTCH1	NOTCH1	Notch 1	Aortic valve disease, hematolymphoid neoplasm or disorder or solid organ neoplasm	81407
NOTCH3	NOTCH3	Notch 3	Cerebral autosomal dominant arteriopathy with subcortical infarcts and leukoencephalopathy (CADASIL)	81406
NPC1	NPC1	Niemann-Pick disease, type C1	Niemann-Pick disease	81406
NPC2	NPC2	Niemann-Pick disease, type C2 (epididymal secretory protein E1)	Niemann-Pick disease type C2	81404
NPHP1	NPHP1	Nephronophthisis 1 (juvenile)	Joubert syndrome	81405, 81406
NPHS1	NPHS1	Nephrosis 1, congenital, Finnish type (nephrin)	Congenital Finnish nephrosis	81407
NPHS2	NPHS2	Nephrosis 2, idiopathic, steroid-resistant (podocin)	Steroid-resistant nephrotic syndrome	81405
	NPM1	Nucleophosmin	Acute myeloid leukemia, hematolymphoid neoplasm or disorder or solid organ neoplasm	81310
NPM1ALK	NPM1/ALK	t(2;5)	Anaplastic large cell lymphoma	81401
NR0B1	NR0B1	Nuclear receptor subfamily 0, group B, member 1	Congenital adrenal hypoplasia	81404
	NRAS	Neuroblastoma RAS viral (v-ras) oncogene homolog	Colorectal carcinoma, Noonan spectrum disorders, solid organ neoplasm, hematolymphoid neoplasm or disorder	81311, 81442
NSD1	NSD1	Nuclear receptor binding SET domain protein 1	Sotos syndrome	81405, 81406
	NTRK	Neurotrophic-tropomyosin receptor tyrosine kinase 1, 2, and 3	Solid tumors	81194
	NTRK1	Neurotrophic receptor tyrosine kinase 1	Solid tumors	81191
	NTRK2	Neurotrophic receptor tyrosine kinase 2	Solid tumors	81192
	NTRK3	Neurotrophic receptor tyrosine kinase 3	Solid tumors	01193
	NUDT15	Nudix hydrolase 15	Drug metabolism	81306
OCRL	OCRL	Oculocerebrorenal syndrome of Lowe	X-linked intellectual disability (XLID)	81470, 81471
OPA1	OPA1	Optic atrophy 1	Optic atrophy, mitochondrial disorders	81406, 81407, 81440
OPTN	OPTN	Optineurin	Amyotrophic lateral sclerosis	81406
OTC	OTC	Ornithine carbamoyltransferase	Ornithine transcarbamylase deficiency	81405

Molecular Pathology Gene Table, *continued*

Claim Designation	Abbreviated Gene Name	Full Gene Name	Commonly Associated Proteins/Diseases (Not a complete list)	CPT Code(s)
OTOF	OTOF	Otoferlin	Hearing loss	81430
PABPN1	PABPN1	Poly(A) binding protein, nuclear 1	Oculopharyngeal muscular dystrophy	81312
PAFAH1B1	PAFAH1B1	Platelet-activating factor acetylhydrolase 1b, regulatory subunit 1 (45kda)	Lissencephaly, Miller-Dieker syndrome	81405, 81406
PAH	PAH	Phenylalanine hydroxylase	Phenylketonuria, severe inherited conditions	81406, 81443
PALB2	PALB2	Partner and localizer of BRCA2	Breast and pancreatic cancer, hereditary breast cancer-related disorders, inherited bone marrow failure syndromes (IBMFS)	81307, 81308, 81441
PARK2	PARK2	Parkinson protein 2, E3 ubiquitin protein ligase (parkin)	Parkinson disease	81405, 81406
PAX2	PAX2	Paired box 2	Renal coloboma syndrome	81406
PAX8PPARG	PAX8/PPARG	t(2;3) (q13;p25)	Follicular thyroid carcinoma	81401
PC	PC	Pyruvate carboxylase	Pyruvate carboxylase deficiency	81406
	PCA3/KLK3	Prostate cancer antigen 3/kallikrein-related peptidase 3	Prostate cancer	81313
PCCA	PCCA	Propionyl coa carboxylase, alpha polypeptide	Propionic acidemia, type 1	81405, 81406
PCCB	PCCB	Propionyl coa carboxylase, beta polypeptide	Propionic acidemia	81406
PCDH15	PCDH15	Protocadherin-related 15	Usher syndrome type 1F, Usher syndrome type 1, hearing loss	81400, 81406, 81407, 81430
PCDH19	PCDH19	Protocadherin 19	Epileptic encephalopathy, epilepsy	81405, 81419
PCSK9	PCSK9	Proprotein convertase subtilisin/kexin type 9	Familial hypercholesterolemia	81406
PDE6A	PDE6A	Phosphodiesterase 6A, CGMP-specific, rod, alpha	Hereditary retinal disorders	81434
PDE6B	PDE6B	Phosphodiesterase 6B, CGMP-specific, rod, beta	Hereditary retinal disorders	81434
	PDGFRA	Platelet-derived growth factor receptor, alpha polypeptide	Gastrointestinal stromal tumor, solid organ neoplasm or hematolymphoid neoplasm	81314
PDHA1	PDHA1	Pyruvate dehydrogenase (lipoamide) alpha 1	Lactic acidosis	81405, 81406
PDHB	PDHB	Pyruvate dehydrogenase (lipoamide) beta	Lactic acidosis	81405
PDHX	PDHX	Pyruvate dehydrogenase complex, component X	Lactic acidosis	81406
PDSS2	PDSS2	Decaprenyl diphosphate synthase subunit 2	Mitochondrial disorders	81440
PDX1	PDX1	Pancreatic and duodenal homeobox 1	Maturity-onset diabetes of the young (MODY)	81404
PHEX	PHEX	Phosphate regulating endopeptidase homolog, X-linked	Hypophosphatemic rickets	81406
PHOX2B	PHOX2B	Paired-like homeobox 2b	Congenital central hypoventilation syndrome	81403, 81404
PIK3CA	PIK3CA	Phosphatidylinositol-4,5-bisphosphate 3-kinase, catalytic subunit alpha	Colorectal cancer, breast cancer, solid organ neoplasm or hematolymphoid neoplasm	81309
PINK1	PINK1	PTEN induced putative kinase 1	Parkinson disease	81405
PKD1	PKD1	Polycystic kidney disease 1 (autosomal dominant)	Polycystic kidney disease	81407
PKD2	PKD2	Polycystic kidney disease 2 (autosomal dominant)	Polycystic kidney disease	81406
PKHD1	PKHD1	Polycystic kidney and hepatic disease 1	Autosomal recessive polycystic kidney disease	81408
PKLR	PKLR	Pyruvate kinase, liver and RBC	Pyruvate kinase deficiency	81405
PKP2	PKP2	Plakophilin 2	Arrhythmogenic right ventricular dysplasia/cardiomyopathy 9, hereditary cardiomyopathy	81406, 81439
PLCE1	PLCE1	Phospholipase C, epsilon 1	Nephrotic syndrome type 3	81407
	PLCG2	Phospholipase C gamma 2	Chronic lymphocytic leukemia	81320

Molecular Pathology Gene Table, *continued*

Claim Designation	Abbreviated Gene Name	Full Gene Name	Commonly Associated Proteins/Diseases (Not a complete list)	CPT Code(s)
PLN	PLN	Phospholamban	Dilated cardiomyopathy, hypertrophic cardiomyopathy	81403
PLP1	PLP1	Proteolipid protein 1	Pelizaeus-Merzbacher disease, spastic paraplegia	81404, 81405
	PML/RARalpha	t(15;17) promyelocytic leukemia/retinoic acid receptor alpha	Promyelocytic leukemia	81315, 81316
	PMP22	Peripheral myelin protein 22	Charcot-Marie-Tooth disease, hereditary neuropathy with liability to pressure palsies	81324, 81325, 81326
	PMS2	Postmeiotic segregation increased 2 (S. Cerevisiae)	Hereditary nonpolyposis colorectal cancer, Lynch syndrome	81317, 81318, 81319
PNKD	PNKD	Paroxysmal nonkinesigenic dyskinesia	Paroxysmal nonkinesigenic dyskinesia	81406
POLG	POLG	Polymerase (DNA directed), gamma	Alpers-Huttenlocher syndrome, autosomal dominant progressive external ophthalmoplegia, mitochondrial disorders, epilepsy	81406, 81419, 81440
POLG2	POLG2	Polymerase (DNA directed), gamma 2	Mitochondrial disorders	81440
POMGNT1	POMGNT1	Protein O-linked mannose beta1,2-N acetylglucosaminyltransferase	Muscle-eye-brain disease, Walker-Warburg syndrome	81406
POMT1	POMT1	Protein-O-mannosyltransferase 1	Limb-girdle muscular dystrophy (LGMD) type 2K, Walker-Warburg syndrome	81406
POMT2	POMT2	Protein-O-mannosyltransferase 2	Limb-girdle muscular dystrophy (LGMD) type 2N, Walker-Warburg syndrome	81406
POU1F1	POU1F1	POU class 1 homeobox 1	Combined pituitary hormone deficiency	81405
PPOX	PPOX	Protoporphyrinogen oxidase	Variegate porphyria	81406
PPP2R2B	PPP2R2B	Protein phosphatase 2, regulatory subunit B, beta	Spinocerebellar ataxia	81343
PQBP1	PQBP1	Polyglutamine binding protein 1	Renpenning syndrome	81404, 81405
PRAME	PRAME	Preferentially expressed antigen in melanoma	Melanoma	81401
PRKAG2	PRKAG2	Protein kinase, AMP-activated, gamma 2 non-catalytic subunit	Familial hypertrophic cardiomyopathy with Wolff-Parkinson-White syndrome, lethal congenital glycogen storage disease of heart	81406
PRKCG	PRKCG	Protein kinase C, gamma; (sodium channel, voltage-gated, type IV, alpha subunit)	Spinocerebellar ataxia; hyperkalemic periodic paralysis	81406
PRNP	PRNP	Srion protein	Genetic prion disease	81404
PROP1	PROP1	PROP paired-like homeobox 1	Combined pituitary hormone deficiency	81404
PRPF31	PRPF31	Pre-MRNA processing factor 31	Hereditary retinal disorders	81434
PRPH2	PRPH2	Peripherin 2 (retinal degeneration, slow)	Retinitis pigmentosa, hereditary retinal disorders	81404, 81434
	PRRT2	Proline rich transmembrane protein 2	Epilepsy	81419
PRSS1	PRSS1	Protease, serine, 1 (trypsin 1)	Hereditary pancreatitis	81401, 81404
PRX	PRX	Periaxin	Charcot-Marie-Tooth disease	81405
PSEN1	PSEN1	Presenilin 1	Alzheimer disease	81405
PSEN2	PSEN2	Presenilin 2 (Alzheimer disease 4)	Alzheimer disease	81406
	PTEN	Phosphatase and tensin homolog	Cowden syndrome, PTEN hamartoma tumor syndrome, hereditary breast cancer-related disorders, hereditary colon cancer disorders, solid organ neoplasm or hematolymphoid neoplasm	81321, 81322, 81323
PTPN11	PTPN11	Protein tyrosine phosphatase, non-receptor type 11	Noonan syndrome, LEOPARD syndrome, Noonan spectrum disorders	81406, 81442
PYGM	PYGM	Phosphorylase, glycogen, muscle	Glycogen storage disease type V, McArdle disease	81401, 81406

Molecular Pathology Gene Table, *continued*

Claim Designation	Abbreviated Gene Name	Full Gene Name	Commonly Associated Proteins/Diseases (Not a complete list)	CPT Code(s)
RAB7A	RAB7A	RAB7A, member RAS oncogene family	Charcot-Marie-Tooth disease	81405
	RAD51C	RAD51 paralog C	Inherited bone marrow failure syndromes (IBMFS)	81441
RAF1	RAF1	V-raf-1 murine leukemia viral oncogene homolog 1	LEOPARD syndrome, Noonan spectrum disorder	81404, 81406, 81442
RAI1	RAI1	Retinoic acid induced 1	Smith-Magenis syndrome	81405
RDH12	RDH12	Retinol dehydrogenase 12 (All-Trans/9-Cis/11-Cis)	Hereditary retinal disorders	81434
REEP1	REEP1	Receptor accessory protein 1	Spastic paraplegia, hereditary peripheral neuropathies	81405, 81448
RET	RET	Ret proto-oncogene	Multiple endocrine neoplasia, type 2A and familial medullary thyroid carcinoma, Hirschsprung disease, solid organ neoplasm or hematolymphoid neoplasm	81404, 81405, 81406
RHDDA	RHD, deletion analysis	Rh blood group, D antigen	Hemolytic disease of the fetus and newborn, Rh maternal/fetal compatibility	81403
RHDDAMB	RHD, deletion analysis, cell-free fetal DNA in maternal blood	Rh blood group, D antigen	Hemolytic disease of the fetus and newborn, Rh maternal/fetal compatibility	81403
RHO	RHO	Rhodopsin	Retinitis pigmentosa, hereditary retinal disorders	81404, 81434
RIT1	RIT1	Ras-like without CAAX 1	Noonan spectrum disorders	81442
RP1	RP1	Retinitis pigmentosa 1	Retinitis pigmentosa, hereditary retinal disorders	81404, 81434
RP2	RP2	Retinitis pigmentosa 2	Hereditary retinal disorders	81434
RPE65	RPE65	Retinal pigment epithelium-specific protein 65kda	Retinitis pigmentosa, Leber congenital amaurosis, hereditary retinal disorders	81406, 81434
RPGR	RPGR	Retinitis pigmentosa gtpase regulator	Hereditary retinal disorders	81434
	RPL11	Ribosomal protein L11	Inherited bone marrow failure syndromes (IBMFS)	81441
	RPL35A	Ribosomal protein l35a	Inherited bone marrow failure syndromes (IBMFS)	81441
	RPL5	Ribosomal protein L5	Inherited bone marrow failure syndromes (IBMFS)	81441
	RPS10	Ribosomal protein S10	Inherited bone marrow failure syndromes (IBMFS)	81441
RPS19	RPS19	Ribosomal protein S19	Diamond-Blackfan anemia, inherited bone marrow failure syndromes (IBMFS)	81405, 81441
	RPS24	Ribosomal protein S24	Inherited bone marrow failure syndromes (IBMFS)	81441
	RPS26	Ribosomal protein S26	Inherited bone marrow failure syndromes (IBMFS)	81441
RPS6KA3	RPS6KA3	Ribosomal protein S6 kinase, 90kda, polypeptide 3	X-linked intellectual disability (XLID)	81470, 81471
	RPS7	Ribosomal protein S7	Inherited bone marrow failure syndromes (IBMFS)	81441
RRM2B	RRM2B	Ribonucleotide reductase M2 B (TP53 inducible)	Mitochondrial DNA depletion, mitochondrial disorders	81405, 81440
RUNX1	RUNX1	Runt related transcription factor 1	Acute myeloid leukemia, familial platelet disorder with associated myeloid malignancy	81334
RUNX1RUNX1T1	RUNX1/RUNX1T1	t(8;21)	Acute myeloid leukemia	81401
RYR1	RYR1	Ryanodine receptor 1, skeletal	Malignant hyperthermia	81406, 81408
RYR2	RYR2	Ryanodine receptor 2 (cardiac)	Catecholaminergic polymorphic ventricular tachycardia, arrhythmogenic right ventricular dysplasia, cardiac ion channelopathies	81408, 81413
	SBDS	Ribosome maturation factor	Inherited bone marrow failure syndromes (IBMFS)	81441
SCN1A	SCN1A	Sodium channel, voltage-gated, type 1, alpha subunit	Generalized epilepsy with febrile seizures, epilepsy	81407, 81419
SCN1B	SCN1B	Sodium channel, voltage-gated, type I, beta	Brugada syndrome, epilepsy	81404, 81419
	SCN2A	Sodium voltage-gated channel alpha subunit 2	Epilepsy	81419

Molecular Pathology Gene Table, *continued*

Claim Designation	Abbreviated Gene Name	Full Gene Name	Commonly Associated Proteins/Diseases (Not a complete list)	CPT Code(s)
SCN4A	SCN4A	Sodium channel, voltage-gated, type IV, alpha subunit	Hyperkalemic periodic paralysis	81406
	SCN8A	Sodium voltage-gated channel alpha subunit 8	Epilepsy	81419
SCN5A	SCN5A	Sodium channel, voltage-gated, type V, alpha subunit	Familial dilated cardiomyopathy, cardiac ion channelopathies	81407, 81413
SCNN1A	SCNN1A	Sodium channel, nonvoltage-gated 1 alpha	Pseudohypoaldosteronism	81406
SCNN1B	SCNN1B	Sodium channel, nonvoltage-gated 1, beta	Liddle syndrome, pseudohypoaldosteronism	81406
SCNN1G	SCNN1G	Sodium channel, nonvoltage-gated 1, gamma	Liddle syndrome, pseudohypoaldosteronism	81406
SCO1	SCO1	SCO cytochrome oxidase deficient homolog 1	Mitochondrial respiratory chain complex IV deficiency, mitochondrial disorders	81405, 81440
SCO2	SCO2	SCO cytochrome oxidase deficient homolog 2 (SCO1L)	Mitochondrial respiratory chain complex IV deficiency, mitochondrial disorders	81404, 81440
SDHA	SDHA	Succinate dehydrogenase complex, subunit A, flavoprotein (Fp)	Leigh syndrome, mitochondrial complex II deficiency	81406
SDHB	SDHB	Succinate dehydrogenase complex, subunit B, iron sulfur	Hereditary paraganglioma, hereditary neuroendocrine tumor disorders	81405
SDHC	SDHC	Succinate dehydrogenase complex, subunit C, integral membrane protein, 15kda	Hereditary paraganglioma-pheochromocytoma syndrome, hereditary neuroendocrine tumor disorders	81404, 81405
SDHD	SDHD	Succinate dehydrogenase complex, subunit D, integral membrane protein	Hereditary paraganglioma, hereditary neuroendocrine tumor disorders	81404
SEPT9	SEPT9	Septin 9	Colorectal cancer	81327
	SERPINA1	Serpin peptidase inhibitor, clade A, alpha-1 antiproteinase, antitrypsin, member 1	Alpha-1-antitrypsin deficiency	81332
SERPINE1	SERPINE1	Serpine peptidase inhibitor clade E, member 1, plasminogen activator inhibitor -1, PAI-1	Thrombophilia	81400
SETX	SETX	Senataxin	Ataxia	81406
	SF3B1	Splicing factor [3b] subunit B1	Myelodysplastic syndrome/acute myeloid leukemia	81347
SGCA	SGCA	Sarcoglycan, alpha (50kda dystrophin-associated glycoprotein)	Limb-girdle muscular dystrophy	81405
SGCB	SGCB	Sarcoglycan, beta (43kda dystrophin-associated glycoprotein)	Limb-girdle muscular dystrophy	81405
SGCD	SGCD	Sarcoglycan, delta (35kda dystrophin-associated glycoprotein)	Limb-girdle muscular dystrophy	81405
SGCE	SGCE	Sarcoglycan, epsilon	Myoclonic dystonia	81405, 81406
SGCG	SGCG	Sarcoglycan, gamma (35kda dystrophin-associated glycoprotein)	Limb-girdle muscular dystrophy	81404, 81405
SH2D1A	SH2D1A	SH2 domain containing 1A	X-linked lymphoproliferative syndrome	81403, 81404
SH3TC2	SH3TC2	SH3 domain and tetratricopeptide repeats 2	Charcot-Marie-Tooth disease	81406
SHOC2	SHOC2	Soc-2 suppressor of clear homolog	Noonan-like syndrome with loose anagen hair, Noonan spectrum disorders	81400, 81405, 81442
	Short Tandem Repeat (STR)	N/A	Pre-transplant recipient, donor germline testing, post-transplant recipient	81265, 81266
SHOX	SHOX	Short stature homeobox	Langer mesomelic dysplasia	81405
SIL1	SIL1	SIL1 homolog, endoplasmic reticulum chaperone (S. Cerevisiae)	Ataxia	81405
SLC2A1	SLC2A1	Solute carrier family 2 (facilitated glucose transporter), member 1	Glucose transporter type 1 (GLUT 1) deficiency syndrome, epilepsy	81405, 81419

Molecular Pathology Gene Table, *continued*

Claim Designation	Abbreviated Gene Name	Full Gene Name	Commonly Associated Proteins/Diseases (Not a complete list)	CPT Code(s)
SLC2A10	SLC2A10	Solute carrier family 2 (facilitated glucose transporter), member 10	Aortic dysfunction or dilation	81410
SLC9A6	SLC9A6	Solute carrier family 9 (sodium/hydrogen exchanger), member 6	Christianson syndrome, epilepsy	81406, 81419
SLC12A1	SLC12A1	Solute carrier family 12 (sodium/potassium/chloride transporters), member 1	Bartter syndrome	81407
SLC12A3	SLC12A3	Solute carrier family 12 (sodium/chloride transporters), member 3	Gitelman syndrome	81407
SLC16A2	SLC16A2	Solute carrier family 16, member 2 (thyroid hormone transporter)	Specific thyroid hormone cell transporter deficiency, Allan-Herndon-Dudley syndrome, X-linked intellectual disability (XLID)	81404, 81405, 81470, 81471
SLC22A5	SLC22A5	Solute carrier family 22 (organic cation/carnitine transporter), member 5	Systemic primary carnitine deficiency	81405
SLC25A4	SLC25A4	Solute carrier family 25 (mitochondrial carrier; adenine nucleotide translocator), member 4	Progressive external ophthalmoplegia, mitochondrial disorders	81404, 81440
SLC25A20	SLC25A20	Solute carrier family 25 (carnitine/acylcarnitine translocase), member 20	Carnitine-acylcarnitine translocase deficiency	81404, 81405
SLC26A4	SLC26A4	Solute carrier family 26, member 4	Pendred syndrome, hearing loss	81406, 81430
SLC37A4	SLC37A4	Solute carrier family 37 (glucose-6-phosphate transporter), member 4	Glycogen storage disease type Ib	81406
SLCO1B1	SLCO1B1	Solute carrier organic anion transporter family, member 1B1	Adverse drug reaction	81328
SMAD3	SMAD3	SMAD family member 3	Aortic dysfunction or dilation	81410
SMAD4	SMAD4	SMAD family member 4	Hemorrhagic telangiectasia syndrome, juvenile polyposis, hereditary colon cancer disorders	81405, 81406
SMN1	SMN1	Survival of motor neuron 1, telomeric	Spinal muscular atrophy	81329, 81336, 81337
SMN1SMN2	SMN1/SMN2	Survival of motor neuron 1, telomeric/survival of motor neuron 2, centromeric	Spinal muscular atrophy	81329
	SMPD1	Sphingomyelin phosphodiesterase 1, acid lysosomal	Niemann-Pick disease, type A, Ashkenazi Jewish-associated disorders	81330, 81412
	SNRPN/UBE3A	Small nuclear ribonucleoprotein polypeptide N and ubiquitin protein ligase E3A	Prader-Willi syndrome and/or Angelman syndrome	81331
SOD1	SOD1	Superoxide dismutase 1, soluble	Amyotrophic lateral sclerosis	81404
SOS1	SOS1	Son of sevenless homolog 1	Noonan syndrome, gingival fibromatosis, Noonan spectrum disorders	81406, 81442
SPAST	SPAST	Spastin	Spastic paraplegia, hereditary peripheral neuropathies	81405, 81406, 81448
SPG11	SPG11	Spastic paraplegia 11 (autosomal recessive)	Spastic paraplegia, hereditary peripheral neuropathies	81407, 81448
SPG7	SPG7	Spastic paraplegia 7 (pure and complicated autosomal recessive)	Spastic paraplegia	81405, 81406
SPINK1	SPINK1	Serine peptidase inhibitor, Kazal type 1	Hereditary pancreatitis	81404
SPRED1	SPRED1	Sprouty-related, EVH1 domain containing 1	Legius syndrome	81405
SPTBN2	SPTBN2	Spectrin, beta, non-erythrocytic 2	Spinocerebellar ataxia	81407
SPTLC1	SPTLC1	Serine palmitoyltransferase, long chain base subunit 1	Hereditary peripheral neuropathies	81448
	SRSF2	Serine and arginine-rich splicing factor 2	Myelodysplastic syndrome, acute myeloid leukemia	81348
SRY	SRY	Sex determining region Y	46, XX testicular disorder of sex development, gonadal dysgenesis	81400

Molecular Pathology Gene Table, *continued*

Claim Designation	Abbreviated Gene Name	Full Gene Name	Commonly Associated Proteins/Diseases (Not a complete list)	CPT Code(s)
SS18SSX1	SS18/SSX1	t(x;18)	Synovial sarcoma	81401
SS18SSX2	SS18/SSX2	t(x;18)	Synovial sarcoma	81401
STAT3	STAT3	Signal transducer and activator of transcription 3 (acute-phase response factor)	Autosomal dominant hyper-IgE syndrome	81405
STK11	STK11	Serine/threonine kinase 11	Peutz-Jeghers syndrome, hereditary breast cancer-related disorders, hereditary colon cancer disorders	81404, 81405
STRC	STRC	Stereocilin	Hearing loss	81431
STXBP1	STXBP1	Syntaxin binding protein 1	Epileptic encephalopathy, epilepsy	81406, 81419
SUCLA2	SUCLA2	Succinate-coa ligase ADP-forming beta subunit	Mitochondrial disorders	81440
SUCLG1	SUCLG1	Succinate-coa ligase alpha subunit	Mitochondrial disorders	81440
SURF1	SURF1	Surfeit 1	Mitochondrial respiratory chain complex IV deficiency	81405
	SYNGAP1	Synaptic Ras gtpase activating protein 1	Epilepsy	81419
TACO1	TACO1	Translational activator of mitochondrial encoded cytochrome c oxidase I	Mitochondrial respiratory chain complex IV deficiency	81404
TARDBP	TARDBP	TAR DNA binding protein	Amyotrophic lateral sclerosis	81405
TAZ	TAZ	Tafazzin	Methylglutaconic aciduria type 2, Barth syndrome, mitochondrial disorders	81406, 81440
TBP	TBP	TATA box binding protein	Spinocerebellar ataxia	81344
TBX5	TBX5	T-box 5	Holt-Oram syndrome	81405
TCF4	TCF4	Transcription factor 4	Pitt-Hopkins syndrome, epilepsy	81405, 81406, 81419
	TERT	Telomerase reverse transcriptase	Thyroid carcinoma, glioblastoma multiforme, inherited bone marrow failure syndromes (IBMFS)	81345, 81441
	TGFBI	Transforming growth factor beta-induced	Corneal dystrophy	81333
TGFBR1	TGFBR1	Transforming growth factor, beta receptor 1	Marfan syndrome, aortic dysfunction or dilation	81405, 81410, 81411
TGFBR2	TGFBR2	Transforming growth factor, beta receptor 2	Marfan syndrome, aortic dysfunction or dilation	81405, 81410, 81411
TH	TH	Tyrosine hydroxylase	Segawa syndrome	81406
THAP1	THAP1	THAP domain containing, apoptosis associated protein 1	Torsion dystonia	81404
THRB	THRB	Thyroid hormone receptor, beta	Thyroid hormone resistance, thyroid hormone beta receptor deficiency	81405
	TINF2	TERF1 interacting nuclear factor 2	Inherited bone marrow failure syndromes (IBMFS)	81441
TK2	TK2	Thymidine kinase 2, mitochondrial	Mitochondrial DNA depletion syndrome, mitochondrial disorders	81405, 81440
TMC1	TMC1	Transmembrane channel-like 1	Hearing loss	81430
TMEM43	TMEM43	Transmembrane protein 43	Arrhythmogenic right ventricular cardiomyopathy	81406
TMEM67	TMEM67	Transmembrane protein 67	Joubert syndrome	81407
TMPRSS3	TMPRSS3	Transmembrane protease, serine 3	Hearing loss	81430
TNNC1	TNNC1	Troponin C type 1 (slow)	Hypertrophic cardiomyopathy or dilated cardiomyopathy	81405
TNNI3	TNNI3	Troponin I, type 3 (cardiac)	Familial hypertrophic cardiomyopathy	81405
TNNT2	TNNT2	Troponin T, type 2 (cardiac)	Familial hypertrophic cardiomyopathy	81406
TOR1A	TOR1A	Torsin family 1, member A (torsin A)	Early-onset primary dystonia (DYT1), torsion dystonia	81400, 81404

Molecular Pathology Gene Table, *continued*

Claim Designation	Abbreviated Gene Name	Full Gene Name	Commonly Associated Proteins/Diseases (Not a complete list)	CPT Code(s)
TP53	TP53	Tumor protein 53	Li-Fraumeni syndrome, hereditary breast cancer–related disorders	81351, 81352, 81353
TPM1	TPM1	Tropomyosin 1 (alpha)	Familial hypertrophic cardiomyopathy	81405
TPMT	TPMT	Thiopurine S-methyltransferase	Drug metabolism	81335
	TPP1	Tripeptidyl peptidase 1	Epilepsy	81419
	TRB@	T cell antigen receptor, beta	Leukemia and lymphoma	81340, 81341
TRD	TRD@	T cell antigen receptor, delta	Leukemia and lymphoma	81402
	TRG@	T cell antigen receptor, gamma	Leukemia and lymphoma	81342
TRPC6	TRPC6	Transient receptor potential cation channel, subfamily C, member 6	Focal segmental glomerulosclerosis	81406
TSC1	TSC1	Tuberous sclerosis 1	Tuberous sclerosis, epilepsy	81405, 81406, 81419
TSC2	TSC2	Tuberous sclerosis 2	Tuberous sclerosis, epilepsy	81406, 81407, 81419
TTN	TTN	Titin	Hereditary cardiomyopathy	81439
TTPA	TTPA	Tocopherol (alpha) transfer protein	Ataxia	81404
TTR	TTR	Transthyretin	Familial transthyretin amyloidosis	81404
TWIST1	TWIST1	Twist homolog 1 (Drosophila)	Saethre-Chotzen syndrome	81403, 81404
TYMP	TYMP	Thymidine phosphorylase	Mitochondrial DNA depletion syndrome, mitochondrial disorders	81405, 81440
TYMS	TYMS	Thymidylate synthetase	5-fluorouracil/5-FU drug metabolism	81346
TYR	TYR	Tyrosinase (oculocutaneous albinism IA)	Oculocutaneous albinism IA	81404
	U2AF1	U2 small nuclear RNA auxiliary factor 1	Myelodysplastic syndrome, acute myeloid leukemia	81357
UBA1	UBA1	Ubiquitin-like modifier activating enzyme 1	Spinal muscular atrophy, X-linked	81403
UBE3A	UBE3A	Ubiquitin protein ligase E3A	Angelman syndrome	81406
UGT1A1	UGT1A1	UDP glucuronosyltransferase 1 family, polypeptide A1	Drug metabolism, Gilbert syndrome, Crigler-Najjar syndrome	81350, 81404
UMOD	UMOD	Uromodulin	Glomerulocystic kidney disease with hyperuricemia and isosthenuria	81406
UPD	UPD	Uniparental disomy	Russell-Silver syndrome, Prader-Willi/Angelman syndrome	81402
USH1C	USH1C	Usher syndrome 1C (autosomal recessive, severe)	Usher syndrome, type 1, hearing loss	81407, 81430
USH1G	USH1G	Usher syndrome 1G (autosomal recessive)	Usher syndrome, type 1, hearing loss	81404, 81430
USH2A	USH2A	Usher syndrome 2A (autosomal recessive, mild)	Usher syndrome, type 2, hearing loss, hereditary retinal disorders	81408, 81430, 81434
VHL	VHL	Von Hippel-Lindau tumor suppressor	Von Hippel-Lindau familial cancer syndrome, hereditary neuroendocrine tumor disorders	81403, 81404
	VKORC1	Vitamin K epoxide reductase complex, subunit 1	Warfarin metabolism	81355
VPS13B	VPS13B	Vacuolar protein sorting 13 homolog B (yeast)	Cohen syndrome	81407, 81408
VWF	VWF	Von Willebrand factor	Von Willebrand disease types 1, 1C, 2A, 2B, 2M, 2N, 3	81401, 81403, 81404, 81405, 81406, 81408
WAS	WAS	Wiskott-Aldrich syndrome (eczema-thrombocytopenia)	Wiskott-Aldrich syndrome	81406
WDR62	WDR62	WD repeat domain 62	Primary autosomal recessive microcephaly	81407
WFS1	WFS1	Wolfram syndrome 1	Hearing loss	81430

Molecular Pathology Gene Table, *continued*

Claim Designation	Abbreviated Gene Name	Full Gene Name	Commonly Associated Proteins/Diseases (Not a complete list)	CPT Code(s)
WT1	WT1	Wilms tumor 1	Denys-Drash syndrome, familial Wilms tumor	81405
ZEB2	ZEB2	Zinc finger E-box binding homeobox 2	Mowat-Wilson syndrome, epilepsy	81404, 81405, 81419
ZNF41	ZNF41	Zinc finger protein 41	X-linked intellectual disability 89	81404
	ZRSR2	Zinc finger CCCH-type, RNA binding motif and serine/arginine rich 2	Myelodysplastic syndrome, acute myeloid leukemia	81360

Pathology and Laboratory Guidelines

Guidelines to direct general reporting of services are presented in the **Introduction.** Some of the commonalities are repeated here for the convenience of those referring to this section on **Pathology and Laboratory.** Other definitions and items unique to Pathology and Laboratory are also listed.

Services in Pathology and Laboratory

Services in Pathology and Laboratory are provided by a physician or by technologists under responsible supervision of a physician.

Separate or Multiple Procedures

It is appropriate to designate multiple procedures that are rendered on the same date by separate entries.

Unlisted Service or Procedure

A service or procedure may be provided that is not listed in this edition of the CPT codebook. When reporting such a service, the appropriate "Unlisted Procedure" code may be used to indicate the service, identifying it by "Special Report" as discussed below. The "Unlisted Procedures" and accompanying codes for **Pathology and Laboratory** are as follows:

81099	Unlisted urinalysis procedure
81479	Unlisted molecular pathology procedure
81599	Unlisted multianalyte assay with algorithmic analysis
84999	Unlisted chemistry procedure
85999	Unlisted hematology and coagulation procedure
86486	unlisted antigen, each
86849	Unlisted immunology procedure
86999	Unlisted transfusion medicine procedure
87999	Unlisted microbiology procedure
88099	Unlisted necropsy (autopsy) procedure

88199	Unlisted cytopathology procedure
88299	Unlisted cytogenetic study
88399	Unlisted surgical pathology procedure
88749	Unlisted in vivo (eg, transcutaneous) laboratory service
89240	Unlisted miscellaneous pathology test
89398	Unlisted reproductive medicine laboratory procedure

Special Report

A service that is rarely provided, unusual, variable, or new may require a special report. Pertinent information should include an adequate definition or description of the nature, extent, and need for the procedure; and the time, effort, and equipment necessary to provide the service.

Pathology and Laboratory

Organ or Disease-Oriented Panels

These panels were developed for coding purposes only and should not be interpreted as clinical parameters. The tests listed with each panel identify the defined components of that panel.

These panel components are not intended to limit the performance of other tests. If one performs tests in addition to those specifically indicated for a particular panel, those tests should be reported separately in addition to the panel code.

Do not report two or more panel codes that include any of the same constituent tests performed from the same patient collection. If a group of tests overlaps two or more panels, report the panel that incorporates the greater number of tests to fulfill the code definition and report the remaining tests using individual test codes (eg, do not report 80047 in conjunction with 80053).

80047   Basic metabolic panel (Calcium, ionized)

This panel must include the following:

Calcium, ionized (82330)

Carbon dioxide (bicarbonate) (82374)

Chloride (82435)

Creatinine (82565)

Glucose (82947)

Potassium (84132)

Sodium (84295)

Urea Nitrogen (BUN) (84520)

➔ CPT Changes: An Insider's View 2008

➔ CPT Assistant Apr 08:5, Apr 13:10, Dec 20:3, Jan 21:12, May 21:8, Jul 22:20

80048   Basic metabolic panel (Calcium, total)

This panel must include the following:

Calcium, total (82310)

Carbon dioxide (bicarbonate) (82374)

Chloride (82435)

Creatinine (82565)

Glucose (82947)

Potassium (84132)

Sodium (84295)

Urea nitrogen (BUN) (84520)

➔ CPT Changes: An Insider's View 2000, 2008, 2009

➔ CPT Assistant Jan 98:6, Sep 99:11, Nov 99:44, Jan 00:7, Aug 05:9

80050   General health panel

This panel must include the following:

Comprehensive metabolic panel (80053)

Blood count, complete (CBC), automated and automated differential WBC count (85025 or 85027 and 85004)

OR

Blood count, complete (CBC), automated (85027) and appropriate manual differential WBC count (85007 or 85009)

Thyroid stimulating hormone (TSH) (84443)

➔ CPT Changes: An Insider's View 2001, 2004

➔ CPT Assistant Winter 92:14, Summer 93:14, Jun 97:10, Nov 97:28, Jan 98:6, Sep 99:11

80051   Electrolyte panel

This panel must include the following:

Carbon dioxide (bicarbonate) (82374)

Chloride (82435)

Potassium (84132)

Sodium (84295)

➔ CPT Assistant Nov 97:28, Jan 98:7, Sep 99:11

80053   Comprehensive metabolic panel

This panel must include the following:

Albumin (82040)

Bilirubin, total (82247)

Calcium, total (82310)

Carbon dioxide (bicarbonate) (82374)

Chloride (82435)

Creatinine (82565)

Glucose (82947)

Phosphatase, alkaline (84075)

Potassium (84132)

Protein, total (84155)

Sodium (84295)

Transferase, alanine amino (ALT) (SGPT) (84460)

Transferase, aspartate amino (AST) (SGOT) (84450)

Urea nitrogen (BUN) (84520)

➔ CPT Changes: An Insider's View 2000, 2009

➔ CPT Assistant Jan 98:6, Nov 98:23, Sep 99:11, Nov 99:44, May 00:11, Jan 05:46, Apr 08:5, Apr 10:11, Apr 13:10, May 21:9, Jul 22:20

80055   Obstetric panel

This panel must include the following:

Blood count, complete (CBC), automated and automated differential WBC count (85025 or 85027 and 85004)

OR

Blood count, complete (CBC), automated (85027) and appropriate manual differential WBC count (85007 or 85009)

Hepatitis B surface antigen (HBsAg) (87340)

Antibody, rubella (86762)

Syphilis test, non-treponemal antibody; qualitative (eg, VDRL, RPR, ART) (86592)

Antibody screen, RBC, each serum technique (86850)

Blood typing, ABO (86900) AND

Blood typing, Rh (D) (86901)

➥ *CPT Changes: An Insider's View* 2004

➥ *CPT Assistant* Winter 92:14, Summer 93:14, Jun 97:10, Apr 99:6, Sep 99:11

(When syphilis screening is performed using a treponemal antibody approach [86780], do not use 80055. Use the individual codes for the tests performed in the obstetric panel)

\# **80081**   Obstetric panel (includes HIV testing)

This panel must include the following:

Blood count, complete (CBC), and automated differential WBC count (85025 or 85027 and 85004)

OR

Blood count, complete (CBC), automated (85027) and appropriate manual differential WBC count (85007 or 85009)

Hepatitis B surface antigen (HBsAg) (87340)

HIV-1 antigen(s), with HIV-1 and HIV-2 antibodies, single result (87389)

Antibody, rubella (86762)

Syphilis test, non-treponemal antibody; qualitative (eg, VDRL, RPR, ART) (86592)

Antibody screen, RBC, each serum technique (86850)

Blood typing, ABO (86900) AND

Blood typing, Rh (D) (86901)

➥ *CPT Changes: An Insider's View* 2016

(When syphilis screening is performed using a treponemal antibody approach [86780], do not use 80081. Use the individual codes for the tests performed in the Obstetric panel)

80061   Lipid panel

This panel must include the following:

Cholesterol, serum, total (82465)

Lipoprotein, direct measurement, high density cholesterol (HDL cholesterol) (83718)

Triglycerides (84478)

➥ *CPT Assistant* Winter 92:14, Summer 93:14, Jun 97:10, Sep 99:11, Mar 00:11, Feb 05:9, Sep 17:12

80069   Renal function panel

This panel must include the following:

Albumin (82040)

Calcium, total (82310)

Carbon dioxide (bicarbonate) (82374)

Chloride (82435)

Creatinine (82565)

Glucose (82947)

Phosphorus inorganic (phosphate) (84100)

Potassium (84132)

Sodium (84295)

Urea nitrogen (BUN) (84520)

➥ *CPT Changes: An Insider's View* 2000, 2009

➥ *CPT Assistant* Sep 99:11, Nov 99:44

80074   Acute hepatitis panel

This panel must include the following:

Hepatitis A antibody (HAAb), IgM antibody (86709)

Hepatitis B core antibody (HBcAb), IgM antibody (86705)

Hepatitis B surface antigen (HBsAg) (87340)

Hepatitis C antibody (86803)

➥ *CPT Changes: An Insider's View* 2000

➥ *CPT Assistant* Sep 99:11, Nov 99:45

80076   Hepatic function panel

This panel must include the following:

Albumin (82040)

Bilirubin, total (82247)

Bilirubin, direct (82248)

Phosphatase, alkaline (84075)

Protein, total (84155)

Transferase, alanine amino (ALT) (SGPT) (84460)

Transferase, aspartate amino (AST) (SGOT) (84450)

➥ *CPT Changes: An Insider's View* 2000

➥ *CPT Assistant* Winter 92:14, Summer 93:14, Jun 97:10, Jan 98:6, Apr 99:6, Sep 99:11, Nov 99:45, Jan 00:7, Aug 05:9

80081   Code is out of numerical sequence. See 80053-80069

Pathology and Laboratory 80047-89398, 0001U-0520U

Drug Assay

Drug procedures are divided into three subsections:

Therapeutic Drug Assay, **Drug Assay**, and **Chemistry**—with code selection dependent on the purpose and type of patient results obtained. Therapeutic Drug Assays are performed to monitor clinical response to a known, prescribed medication. The two major categories for drug testing in the Drug Assay subsection are:

1. **Presumptive Drug Class** procedures are used to identify possible use or non-use of a drug or drug class. A presumptive test may be followed by a definitive test in order to specifically identify drugs or metabolites.

2. **Definitive Drug Class** procedures are qualitative or quantitative test to identify possible use or non-use of a drug. These test identify specific drugs and associated metabolites, if performed. A presumptive test is not required prior to a definitive drug test.

The material for drug class procedures may be any specimen type unless otherwise specified in the code descriptor (eg, urine, blood, oral fluid, meconium, hair). Procedures can be qualitative (eg, positive/negative or present/absent), semi-quantitative, or quantitative (measured) depending on the purpose of the testing. Therapeutic drug assay (TDA) procedures are typically quantitative tests and the specimen type is whole blood, serum, plasma, or cerebrospinal fluid.

When the same procedure(s) is performed on more than one specimen type (eg, blood and urine), the appropriate code is reported separately for each specimen type using modifier 59.

Drugs or classes of drugs may be commonly assayed first by a presumptive screening method followed by a definitive drug identification method. Presumptive

(continued on page 621)

DEFINITIONS AND ACRONYM CONVERSION LISTING

Drug Testing Term/Acronym	Definition
6-MAM	Acronym for the heroin drug metabolite 6-monacetylmorphine
Acid	Descriptor for classifying drug/drug metabolite molecules based upon chemical ionization properties. Laboratory procedures for drug isolation and identification may include acid, base, or neutral groupings.
AM	A category of synthetic marijuana drugs discovered by and named after Alexandros Makriyannis at Northeastern University
Analog	A structural derivative of a parent chemical compound that often differs from it by a single element
Analyte	The substance or chemical constituent that is of interest in an analytical procedure
Base	Descriptor for classifying drug/drug metabolite molecules based upon chemical ionization properties. Laboratory procedures for drug isolation and identification may include acid, base, or neutral groupings.
Card(s)	Multiplexed presumptive drug class(es) immunoassay product that is read by visual observation, including instrumented when performed
Cassette(s)	Multiplexed presumptive drug class immunoassay product(s) that is read by visual observation, including instrumented when performed
CEDIA	Acronym for Cloned-Enzyme-Donor-Immuno-Assay. CEDIA immunoassay is a competitive antibody binding procedure that utilizes enzyme donor fragment-labeled antigens (drugs) to compete for antigens (drugs) contained in the patient sample. Recombination of enzyme donor fragment and enzyme acceptor fragment produces a functional enzyme. CEDIA immunoassay enzyme activity is proportional to concentration of drug(s) detected.
Chromatography	An analytical technique used to separate components of a mixture. See thin layer chromatography, gas chromatography, and high performance chromatography.
Confirmatory	Term used to describe definitive identification/quantitation procedures that are secondary to presumptive screening methods
DART	Acronym for Direct-Analysis-in-Real-Time. DART is an atmospheric pressure ionization method for mass spectrometry analysis

DEFINITIONS AND ACRONYM CONVERSION LISTING

Drug Testing Term/Acronym	Definition
Definitive Drug Procedure	A procedure that provides specific identification of individual drugs and drug metabolites
DESI	Acronym for Desorption-ElectroSpray-Ionization. DESI is a combination of electrospray ionization and desorption ionization methods for mass spectrometry analysis.
Dipstick	A multiplexed presumptive drug class immunoassay product that is read by visual observation, including instrumented when performed
Drug test cup	A multiplexed presumptive drug class immunoassay product that is read by visual observation, including instrumented when performed
EDDP	Acronym for the methadone drug metabolite 2-ethylidene-1,5-dimethyl-3,3-diphenylpyrrolidine
EIA	Acronym for Enzyme Immuno-Assay. Enzyme immunoassay is a competitive antibody binding procedure that utilizes enzyme-labeled antigens (drugs) to compete for antigens (drugs) contained in the patient sample. Enzyme immunoassay enzyme activity is proportional to concentration of drug(s) detected
ELISA	Acronym for Enzyme-Linked Immunosorbent Assay. ELISA is a competitive binding immunoassay that is designed to measure antigens (drugs) or antibodies. ELISA immunoassay results are proportional to concentration of drug(s) detected.
EMIT	Acronym for Enzyme-Multiplied-Immunoassay-Test. EMIT is a trade name for a type of enzyme immunoassay (EIA).
FPIA	Acronym for Fluorescence Polarization Immuno-Assay. FPIA is a competitive binding immunoassay that utilizes fluorescein-labeled antigens (drugs) to compete for antigens (drugs) contained in the patient sample. The measure of polarized light emission is inversely proportional to the concentration of drug(s) detected.
Gas chromatography	Gas chromatography is a chromatography technique in which patient sample preparations are vaporized into a gas (mobile phase) which flows through a tubular column (containing a stationary phase) and into a detector. The retention time of a drug on the column is determined by partitioning characteristics of the drug into the mobile and stationary phases. Chromatography column detectors may be non-specific (eg, flame ionization) or specific (eg, mass spectrometry). The combination of column retention time and specific detector response provides a definitive identification of the drug or drug metabolite.
GC	Acronym for gas chromatography
GC-MS	Acronym for gas chromatography mass spectrometry
GC-MS/MS	Acronym for gas chromatography mass spectrometry/mass spectrometry
High performance liquid chromatography	High performance liquid chromatography is a chromatography technique in which patient sample preparations are injected into a liquid (mobile phase) which flows through a tubular column (containing a stationary phase) and into a detector. The retention time of a drug on the column is determined by partitioning characteristics of the drug into the mobile and stationary phases. Chromatography column detectors may be non-specific (eg, ultra-violet spectrophotometry) or specific (eg, mass spectrometry). The combination of column retention time and specific detector response provides a definitive identification of the drug or drug metabolite. High performance liquid chromatography is also called high pressure liquid chromatography.
HPLC	Acronym for high performance liquid chromatography
HU	A category of synthetic marijuana drugs discovered by and named after Raphael Mechoulam at Hebrew University
IA	Acronym for immunoassay
Immunoassay	Antigen-antibody binding procedures utilized to detect antigens (eg, drugs and/or drug metabolites) in patient samples. Immunoassay designs include competitive or non-competitive with various mechanisms for detection.

(continued on page 620)

Pathology and Laboratory 80047-89398, 0001U-0520U

DEFINITIONS AND ACRONYM CONVERSION LISTING

Drug Testing Term/Acronym	Definition
Isobaric	In mass spectrometry, ions with the same mass
Isomers	Compounds that have the same molecular formula but differ in structural formula
JWH	A category of synthetic marijuana drugs discovered by and named after John W. Huffman at Clemson University.
KIMS	Acronym for kinetic interaction of microparticles in solution. KIMS immunoassay is a competitive antibody binding procedure that utilizes microparticle-labeled antigens (drugs) to compete for antigens (drugs) contained in the patient sample. Microparticle immunoassay absorbance increase is inversely proportional to concentration of drug(s) detected.
LC-MS	Acronym for liquid chromatography mass spectrometry
LC-MS/MS	Acronym for liquid chromatography mass spectrometry/mass spectrometry
LDTD	Acronym for laser diode thermal desorption. LDTD is a combination of atmospheric pressure chemical ionization and laser diode thermal desorption methods for mass spectrometry analysis.
MALDI	Acronym for matrix assisted laser desorption/ionization mass spectrometry. MALDI is a soft ionization technique that reduces molecular fragmentation.
MDA	Acronym for the drug 3,4-methylenedioxyamphetamine. MDA is also a drug metabolite of MDMA.
MDEA	Acronym for the drug 3,4-methylenedioxy-N-ethylamphetamine
MDMA	Acronym for the drug 3,4-methylenedioxy-N-methylamphetamine
MDPV	Acronym for the drug methylenedioxypyrovalerone
MS	Acronym for mass spectrometry. MS is an identification technique that measures the charge-to-mass ratio of charged particles. There are several types of mass spectrometry instruments, such as magnetic sectoring, time of flight, quadrupole mass filter, ion traps, and Fourier transformation. Mass spectrometry is used as part of the process to assign definitive identification of drugs and drug metabolites.
MS/MS	Acronym for mass spectrometry/mass spectrometry. MS/MS instruments combine multiple units of mass spectrometry filters into a single instrument. MS/MS is also called tandem mass spectrometry.
MS-TOF	Acronym for mass spectrometry time of flight. Time of flight is a mass spectrometry identification technique that utilizes ion velocity to determine the mass-to-charge ratio.
Multiplexed	Descriptor for a multiple component test device that simultaneously measures multiple analytes (drug classes) in a single analysis.
Neutral	Descriptor for classifying drug/drug metabolite molecules based upon chemical ionization properties. Laboratory procedures for drug isolation and identification may include acid, base, or neutral groupings.
ng/mL	Unit of measure for weight per volume calculated as nanograms per milliliter. The ng/mL unit of measure is equivalent to the µ/L unit of measure.
Optical observation	Optical observation refers to procedure results that are interpreted visually with or without instrumentation assistance.
Opiate	Medicinal category of narcotic alkaloid drugs that are natural products in the opium poppy plant Papaver somniferum. This immunoassay class of drugs typically includes detection of codeine, dihydrocodeine, hydrocodone, hydromorphone, and morphine.
Opioids	A category of medicinal synthetic or semi-synthetic narcotic alkaloid opioid receptor stimulating drugs including butorphanol, desomorphine, dextromethorphan, dextrorphan, levorphanol, meperidine, naloxone, naltrexone, normeperidine, and pentazocine.
Presumptive	Drug test results that indicate possible, but not definitive, presence of drugs and/or drug metabolites

DEFINITIONS AND ACRONYM CONVERSION LISTING

Drug Testing Term/Acronym	Definition
QTOF	Acronym for quadrupole-time of flight mass spectrometry. QTOF is a hybrid mass spectrometry identification technique that combines ion velocity with tandem quadrupole mass spectrometry (MS or MS/MS) to determine the mass-to-charge ratio.
RCS	A category of synthetic marijuana drugs that are analogs of JHW compounds. See JWH.
RIA	Acronym for radio-immuno-assay. Radioimmunoassay is a competitive antibody binding procedure that utilizes radioactive-labeled antigens (drugs) to compete for antigens (drugs) contained in the patient sample. The measure of radioactivity is inversely proportional to concentration of drug(s) detected.
Stereoisomers	Isomeric molecules that have the same molecular formula and sequence of bonded atoms (constitution), but that differ only in the three-dimensional orientations of their atoms in space
Substance	A substance is a drug that does not have an established therapeutic use as distinguished from other analytes listed in the Chemistry section (82009-84999).
TDM	Acronym for therapeutic drug monitoring
THC	Acronym for marijuana active drug ingredient tetrahydrocannabinol
Therapeutic Drug Monitoring	Analysis of blood (serum, plasma) drug concentration to monitor clinical response to therapy
Time of flight	Time of flight is a mass spectrometry technique that utilizes ion velocity to determine the mass-to-charge ratio
TLC	Acronym for thin layer chromatography
TOF	Acronym for time of flight
μ/L	Unit of measure for mass per volume calculated as micrograms per liter. The μ/L unit of measure is equivalent to the ng/mL unit of measure.

(continued from page 618)

methods include, but are not limited to, immunoassays (IA, EIA, ELISA, RIA, EMIT, FPIA, etc), enzymatic methods (alcohol dehydrogenase, etc), chromatographic methods without mass spectrometry (TLC, HPLC, GC, etc), or mass spectrometry without adequate drug resolution by chromatography (MS-TOF, DART, DESI, LDTD, MALDI). LC-MS, LCMS/MS, or mass spectrometry without adequate drug resolution by chromatography may also be used for presumptive testing if the chromatographic phase is not adequate to identify individual drugs and distinguish between structural isomers or isobaric compounds. All drug class immunoassays are considered presumptive, whether qualitative, semi-quantitative, or quantitative. Methods that cannot distinguish between structural isomers (such as morphine and hydromorphone or methamphetamine and phentermine) are also considered presumptive.

Definitive drug identification methods are able to identify individual drugs and distinguish between structural isomers but not necessarily stereoisomers. Definitive methods include, but are not limited to, gas chromatography with mass spectrometry (any type, single or tandem) and liquid chromatography mass spectrometry (any type, single or tandem) and excludes immunoassays (eg, IA, EIA, ELISA, RIA, EMIT, FPIA), and enzymatic methods (eg, alcohol dehydrogenase).

For chromatography, each combination of stationary and mobile phase is to be counted as one procedure.

Presumptive Drug Class Screening

Drugs or classes of drugs may be commonly assayed first by a presumptive screening method followed by a definitive drug identification method. The methodology is considered when coding presumptive procedures. Each code (80305, 80306, 80307) represents all drugs and drug classes performed by the respective methodology per date of service. Each code also includes all sample validation procedures performed. Examples of sample validation procedures may include, but are not limited to, pH, specific gravity, and nitrite. The codes (80305, 80306, 80307) represent three different method categories:

1. Code 80305 is used to report procedures in which the results are read by direct optical observation. The results are visually read. Examples of these procedures are dipsticks, cups, cards, and cartridges. Report

80305 once, irrespective of the number of direct observation drug class procedures performed or results on any date of service.

2. Code 80306 is used to report procedures when an instrument is used to assist in determining the result of a direct optical observation methodology. Examples of these procedures are dipsticks, cards, and cartridges inserted into an instrument that determines the final result of an optical observation methodology. Report 80306 once, irrespective of the number of drug class procedures or results on any date of service.

3. Code 80307 is used to report any number of devices or procedures by instrumented chemistry analyzers. There are many different instrumented methodologies available to perform presumptive drug assays. Examples include immunoassay (eg, EIA, ELISA, EMIT, FPIA, IA, KIMS, RIA), chromatography (eg, GC, HPLC), and mass spectrometry, either with or without chromatography (eg, DART, DESI, GC-MS, GC-MS/MS, LC-MS, LC-MS/MS, LDTD, MALDI, TOF). Some of these methodologies may be used for definitive drug testing also, but, for the purpose of presumptive drug testing, the presumptive method is insufficient to provide definitive drug identification. Report 80307 once, irrespective of the number of drug class procedures or results on any date of service.

 # 80305 Drug test(s), presumptive, any number of drug classes, any number of devices or procedures; capable of being read by direct optical observation only (eg, utilizing immunoassay [eg, dipsticks, cups, cards, or cartridges]), includes sample validation when performed, per date of service

➲ *CPT Changes: An Insider's View* 2017, 2018

➲ *CPT Assistant* Mar 17:6, Jul 18:15

 # 80306 read by instrument assisted direct optical observation (eg, utilizing immunoassay [eg, dipsticks, cups, cards, or cartridges]), includes sample validation when performed, per date of service

➲ *CPT Changes: An Insider's View* 2017, 2018

➲ *CPT Assistant* Mar 17:6

 # 80307 by instrument chemistry analyzers (eg, utilizing immunoassay [eg, EIA, ELISA, EMIT, FPIA, IA, KIMS, RIA]), chromatography (eg, GC, HPLC), and mass spectrometry either with or without chromatography, (eg, DART, DESI, GC-MS, GC-MS/MS, LC-MS, LC-MS/MS, LDTD, MALDI, TOF) includes sample validation when performed, per date of service

➲ *CPT Changes: An Insider's View* 2017, 2018

➲ *CPT Assistant* Mar 17:6

Definitive Drug Testing

Definitive drug identification methods are able to identify individual drugs and distinguish between structural isomers but not necessarily stereoisomers. Definitive methods include, but are not limited to, gas chromatography with mass spectrometry (any type, single or tandem) and liquid chromatography mass spectrometry (any type, single or tandem) and exclude immunoassays (eg, IA, EIA, ELISA, RIA, EMIT, FPIA) and enzymatic methods (eg, alcohol dehydrogenase).

Use 80320-80377 to report definitive drug class procedures. Definitive testing may be qualitative, quantitative, or a combination of qualitative and quantitative for the same patient on the same date of service.

The **Definitive Drug Classes Listing** provides the drug classes, their associated CPT codes, and the drugs included in each class. Each category of a drug class, including metabolite(s) if performed (except stereoisomers), is reported once per date of service. Metabolites not listed in the table may be reported using the code for the parent drug. Drug class metabolite(s) is not reported separately unless the metabolite(s) is listed as a separate category in **Definitive Drug Classes Listing** (eg, heroin metabolite).

Drug classes may contain one or more codes based on the number of analytes. For example, an analysis in which five or more amphetamines and/or amphetamine metabolites would be reported with 80326. The code is based on the number of reported analytes and not the capacity of the analysis.

Definitive drug procedures that are not specified in 80320-80373 should be reported using the unlisted definitive procedure codes 80375, 80376, 80377, unless the specific analyte is listed in the **Therapeutic Drug Assays** (80143-80203) or **Chemistry** (82009-84830) sections.

See the **Definitive Drug Classes Listing** table for a listing of the more common analytes within each drug class.

 # 80320 Alcohols

➲ *CPT Changes: An Insider's View* 2015

➲ *CPT Assistant* Apr 15:3

(For alcohol [ethanol] by immunoassay and enzymatic methods, use 82077)

 # 80321 Alcohol biomarkers; 1 or 2

➲ *CPT Changes: An Insider's View* 2015

 # 80322 3 or more

➲ *CPT Changes: An Insider's View* 2015

 # 80323 Alkaloids, not otherwise specified

➲ *CPT Changes: An Insider's View* 2015

 # 80324 Amphetamines; 1 or 2

➲ *CPT Changes: An Insider's View* 2015

 # 80325 3 or 4

➲ *CPT Changes: An Insider's View* 2015

\# **80326**   5 or more
➔ *CPT Changes: An Insider's View* 2015

\# **80327**   Anabolic steroids; 1 or 2
➔ *CPT Changes: An Insider's View* 2015
➔ *CPT Assistant* Apr 15:5

\# **80328**   3 or more
➔ *CPT Changes: An Insider's View* 2015
➔ *CPT Assistant* Apr 15:5

(For dihydrotestosterone analysis for endogenous hormone levels or therapeutic monitoring, use 82642)

\# **80329**   Analgesics, non-opioid; 1 or 2
➔ *CPT Changes: An Insider's View* 2015
➔ *CPT Assistant* Jan 21:8

\# **80330**   3-5
➔ *CPT Changes: An Insider's View* 2015
➔ *CPT Assistant* Jan 21:8

\# **80331**   6 or more
➔ *CPT Changes: An Insider's View* 2015
➔ *CPT Assistant* Jan 21:8

(For acetaminophen by immunoassay or enzymatic methods, use 80143)

(For salicylate by immunoassay or enzymatic methods, use 80179)

\# **80332**   Antidepressants, serotonergic class; 1 or 2
➔ *CPT Changes: An Insider's View* 2015

\# **80333**   3-5
➔ *CPT Changes: An Insider's View* 2015

\# **80334**   6 or more
➔ *CPT Changes: An Insider's View* 2015

\# **80335**   Antidepressants, tricyclic and other cyclicals; 1 or 2
➔ *CPT Changes: An Insider's View* 2015

\# **80336**   3-5
➔ *CPT Changes: An Insider's View* 2015

\# **80337**   6 or more
➔ *CPT Changes: An Insider's View* 2015

\# **80338**   Antidepressants, not otherwise specified
➔ *CPT Changes: An Insider's View* 2015

\# **80339**   Antiepileptics, not otherwise specified; 1-3
➔ *CPT Changes: An Insider's View* 2015

\# **80340**   4-6
➔ *CPT Changes: An Insider's View* 2015

\# **80341**   7 or more
➔ *CPT Changes: An Insider's View* 2015

(To report definitive drug testing for antihistamines, see 80375, 80376, 80377)

(To report therapeutic drug assay for carbamazepine, see 80156, 80157, 80161)

\# **80342**   Antipsychotics, not otherwise specified; 1-3
➔ *CPT Changes: An Insider's View* 2015

\# **80343**   4-6
➔ *CPT Changes: An Insider's View* 2015

\# **80344**   7 or more
➔ *CPT Changes: An Insider's View* 2015

\# **80345**   Barbiturates
➔ *CPT Changes: An Insider's View* 2015

\# **80346**   Benzodiazepines; 1-12
➔ *CPT Changes: An Insider's View* 2015

\# **80347**   13 or more
➔ *CPT Changes: An Insider's View* 2015

\# **80348**   Buprenorphine
➔ *CPT Changes: An Insider's View* 2015

\# **80349**   Cannabinoids, natural
➔ *CPT Changes: An Insider's View* 2015

\# **80350**   Cannabinoids, synthetic; 1-3
➔ *CPT Changes: An Insider's View* 2015

\# **80351**   4-6
➔ *CPT Changes: An Insider's View* 2015

\# **80352**   7 or more
➔ *CPT Changes: An Insider's View* 2015

\# **80353**   Cocaine
➔ *CPT Changes: An Insider's View* 2015

\# **80354**   Fentanyl
➔ *CPT Changes: An Insider's View* 2015

\# **80355**   Gabapentin, non-blood
➔ *CPT Changes: An Insider's View* 2015
➔ *CPT Assistant* Apr 15:3

(For therapeutic drug assay, use 80171)

\# **80356**   Heroin metabolite
➔ *CPT Changes: An Insider's View* 2015

\# **80357**   Ketamine and norketamine
➔ *CPT Changes: An Insider's View* 2015

\# **80358**   Methadone
➔ *CPT Changes: An Insider's View* 2015

\# **80359**   Methylenedioxyamphetamines (MDA, MDEA, MDMA)
➔ *CPT Changes: An Insider's View* 2015

\# **80360**   Methylphenidate
➔ *CPT Changes: An Insider's View* 2015

\# **80361**   Opiates, 1 or more
➔ *CPT Changes: An Insider's View* 2015

\# **80362**   Opioids and opiate analogs; 1 or 2
➔ *CPT Changes: An Insider's View* 2015

Pathology and Laboratory 80047-89398, 0001U-0520U

80363   3 or 4
➔ CPT Changes: An Insider's View 2015

80364   5 or more
➔ CPT Changes: An Insider's View 2015

80365   Oxycodone
➔ CPT Changes: An Insider's View 2015

83992   Phencyclidine (PCP)
➔ CPT Assistant Apr 15:3

(Phenobarbital, use 80345)

80366   Pregabalin
➔ CPT Changes: An Insider's View 2015

80367   Propoxyphene
➔ CPT Changes: An Insider's View 2015

80368   Sedative hypnotics (non-benzodiazepines)
➔ CPT Changes: An Insider's View 2015

80369   Skeletal muscle relaxants; 1 or 2
➔ CPT Changes: An Insider's View 2015

80370   3 or more
➔ CPT Changes: An Insider's View 2015

80371   Stimulants, synthetic
➔ CPT Changes: An Insider's View 2015

80372   Tapentadol
➔ CPT Changes: An Insider's View 2015

80373   Tramadol
➔ CPT Changes: An Insider's View 2015

80374   Stereoisomer (enantiomer) analysis, single drug class
➔ CPT Changes: An Insider's View 2015

(Use 80374 in conjunction with an index drug analysis, when performed)

80375   Drug(s) or substance(s), definitive, qualitative or quantitative, not otherwise specified; 1-3
➔ CPT Changes: An Insider's View 2015
➔ CPT Assistant Apr 15:3

80376   4-6
➔ CPT Changes: An Insider's View 2015
➔ CPT Assistant Apr 15:3

80377   7 or more
➔ CPT Changes: An Insider's View 2015
➔ CPT Assistant Apr 15:3

(To report definitive drug testing for antihistamines, see 80375, 80376, 80377)

For Example:

To report amphetamine and methamphetamine using any number of definitive procedures, report 80324 once per facility per date of service.

To report codeine, hydrocodone, hydromorphone, morphine using any number of definitive procedures, report 80361 once per facility per date of service.

To report codeine, hydrocodone, hydromorphone, morphine, oxycodone, oxymorphone, naloxone, naltrexone performed using any number of definitive procedures report 80361 X 1, 80362 X 1, and 80365 X 1 per facility per date of service.

To report benzoylecgonine, cocaine, carboxy-THC, meperidine, normeperidine using any number of definitive procedures, report 80349 X 1, 80353 X 1, and 80362 X 1 per facility per date of service.

Definitive Drug Classes Listing

Drugs and metabolites included in each definitive drug class are listed in the Definitive Drug Classes Listing table. This is not a comprehensive list. FDA classification of drugs not listed should be used where possible within the defined drug classes. Any metabolites that are not listed should be categorized with the parent drug. Drugs and metabolites not listed may be reported using codes from the Therapeutic Drug Assay (80143-80299) or Chemistry (82009-84999) sections.

DEFINITIVE DRUG CLASSES LISTING

Codes	Classes	Drugs
80320	Alcohol(s)	Acetone, ethanol, ethchlorvynol, ethylene glycol, isopropanol, isopropyl alcohol, methanol
80321-80322	Alcohol Biomarkers	Ethanol conjugates (ethyl glucuronide [ETG], ethyl sulfate [ETS], fatty acid ethyl esters, phosphatidylethanol)
80323	Alkaloids, not otherwise specified	7-Hydroxymitragynine, atropine, cotinine, lysergic acid diethylamide (LSD), mescaline, mitragynine, nicotine, psilocin, psilocybin, scopolamine
80324-80326	Amphetamines	Amphetamine, ephedrine, lisdexamphetamine, methamphetamine, phentermine, phenylpropanolamine, pseudoephedrine

DEFINITIVE DRUG CLASSES LISTING

Codes	Classes	Drugs
80327-80328	Anabolic steroids	1-Androstenediol, 1-androstenedione, 1-testosterone, 4-hydroxy-testosterone, 6-oxo, 19-norandrostenedione, androstenedione, androstanolone, bolandiol, bolasterone, boldenone, boldione, calusterone, clostebol, danazol, dehydrochlormethyltestosterone, dihydrotestosterone, drostanolone, epiandrosterone, epitestosterone, fluoxymesterone, furazabol, mestanolone, mesterolone, methandienone, methandriol, methenolone, methydienolone, methyl-1-testosterone, methylnortestosterone, methyltestosterone, mibolerone, nandrolone, norbolethone, norclostebol, norethandrolone, norethindrone, oxabolone, oxandrolone, oxymesterone, oxymetholone, stanozolol, stenbolone, tibolone, trenbolone, zeranol
80329-80331	Analgesics, non-opioid	Acetaminophen, diclofenac ibuprofen, ketoprofen, naproxen, oxaprozin, salicylate
80332-80334	Antidepressants, serotonergic class	Citalopram, duloxetine, escitalopram, fluoxetine, fluvoxamine, paroxetine, sertraline
80335-80337	Antidepressants, tricyclic and other cyclicals	Amitriptyline, amoxapine, clomipramine, demexiptiline, desipramine, doxepin, imipramine, maprotiline, mirtazpine, nortriptyline, protriptyline
80338	Antidepressants, not otherwise specified	Bupropion, desyenlafaxine, isocarboxazid, nefazodone, phenelzine, selegiline, tranylcypromine, trazodone, venlafaxine
80339-80341	Antiepileptics not otherwise specified	Carbamazepine, clobazam, diamethadione, ethosuximide, ezogabine, lamotrigine, levetiracetam, methsuximide, oxcarbazepine, phenytoin, primidone, rufinamide, tiagabine, topiramate, trimethadione, valproic acid, zonisamide
80342-80344	Antipsychotics not otherwise specified	Aripiprazole, chlorpromazine, clozapine, fluphenazine, haloperidol, loxapine, mesoridazine, molindone, olanzapine, paliperidone, perphenazine, phenothiazine, pimozide, prochlorperazine, quetiapine, risperidone, trifluoperazine, thiothixene, thoridazine, ziprasidone
80345	Barbiturates	Amobarbital, aprobarbital, butalbital, cyclobarbital, mephobarbital, pentobarbital, phenobarbital, secobarbital, talbutal, thiopental
80346, 80347	Benzodiazepines	Alprazolam, chlordiazepoxide, clonazepam, clorazepate, diazepam, estazolam, flunitrazepam, flurazepam, halazepam, lorazepam, midazolam, nitrazepam, nordazepam, oxazepam, prazepam, quazepam, temazepam
80348	Buprenorphine	Buprenorphine
80349	Cannabinoids, natural	Marijuana, dronabinol carboxy-THC
80350-80352	Cannabinoids, synthetic	CP-47,497, CP497 C8-homolog, JWH-018 and AM678, JWH-073, JWH-019, JWH-200, JWH-210, JWH-250, JWH-081, JWH-122, HWH-398, AM-2201, AM-694, SR-19 and RCS-4, SR-18 and RCS-8, JWH-203, UR-144, XLR-11, MAM-2201, AKB-48
80353	Cocaine	Benzoylecgonine, cocaethylene, cocaine, ecgonine methyl ester, norcocaine
80354	Fentanyls	Acetylfentanyl, alfentanil, fentanyl, remifentanil, sufentanil
80355	Gabapentin, non-blood	Gabapentin
80356	Heroin metabolite	6-acetylmorphine, acetylcodeine, diacetylmorphine
80368	Hypnotics, sedative (non-benzodiazepines)	See Sedative Hypnotics
80357	Ketamine and Norketamine	Ketamine, norketamine
80358	Methadone	Methadone and EDDP

(continued on page 626)

DEFINITIVE DRUG CLASSES LISTING

Codes	Classes	Drugs
80359	Methylenedioxyamphetamines	MDA, MDEA, MDMA
80360	Methylphenidate	Methylphenidate, ritalinic acid
80357	Norketamine	See Ketamine
80368	Non-Benzodiazepines	See Hypnotics, sedative
80361	Opiates	Codeine, dihydrocodeine, hydrocodone, hydromorphone, morphine
80362-80364	Opioids and opiate analogs	Butorphanol, desomorphine, dextromethorphan, dextrorphan, levorphanol, meperidine, naloxone, naltrexone, normeperidine, pentazocine
80365	Oxycodone	Oxycodone, oxymorphone
83992	Phencyclidine	Phencyclidine
80366	Pregabalin	Pregabalin
80367	Propoxyphene	Norpropoxyphene, propoxyphene
80368	Sedative hypnotics (non-benzodiazepines)	Eszopiclone, zaleplon, zolpidem
80369, 80370	Skeletal muscle relaxants	Baclofen, carisoprodol, cyclobenzaprine, meprobamate, metaxalone, methocarbamol, orphenadrine, tizanidide
80371	Stimulants, synthetic	2C-B, 2C-E, 2C-I, 2C-H, 3TFMPP, 4-methylethcathinone, alpha-PVP, benzylpiperazine, bromodragonfly, cathinone, m-CPP, MDPBP, MDPPP, MDPV, mephedrone, methcathinone, methylone, phenethylamines, salvinorin, tryptamines
80372	Tapentadol	Tapentadol
80373	Tramadol	Tramadol

Therapeutic Drug Assays

Therapeutic drug assays are performed to monitor levels of a known, prescribed, or over-the-counter medication.

The material for examination is whole blood, serum, plasma, or cerebrospinal fluid. Examination is quantitative. Coding is by parent drug; measured metabolites of the drug are included in the code, if performed.

80143 Acetaminophen
➤ *CPT Changes: An Insider's View* 2021
➤ *CPT Assistant* Jan 21:8

(For definitive drug testing for acetaminophen, see 80329, 80330, 80331)

80145 Adalimumab
➤ *CPT Changes: An Insider's View* 2020

80150 Amikacin
➤ *CPT Changes: An Insider's View* 2015
➤ *CPT Assistant* Aug 05:9, Oct 10:7, Dec 10:7, Mar 11:10, Apr 15:3

80151 Amiodarone
➤ *CPT Changes: An Insider's View* 2021
➤ *CPT Assistant* Jan 21:8

80155 Caffeine
➤ *CPT Changes: An Insider's View* 2014

80156 Carbamazepine; total
➤ *CPT Changes: An Insider's View* 2001
➤ *CPT Assistant* Oct 10:7, Mar 11:10, Jan 21:8

80157 free
➤ *CPT Changes: An Insider's View* 2001
➤ *CPT Assistant* Oct 10:7, Mar 11:10, Jan 21:8

 # 80161 -10,11-epoxide
➤ *CPT Changes: An Insider's View* 2021
➤ *CPT Assistant* Jan 21:8

80158 Cyclosporine
➤ *CPT Assistant* Oct 10:7, Mar 11:10

80159 Clozapine
➤ *CPT Changes: An Insider's View* 2014

80161 Code is out of numerical sequence. See 80156-80159

80162 Digoxin; total
➤ *CPT Changes: An Insider's View* 2015
➤ *CPT Assistant* Oct 10:7, Mar 11:10, Apr 15:3

80163	free
	➲ *CPT Changes: An Insider's View* 2015
	➲ *CPT Assistant* Apr 15:3

80164   Code is out of numerical sequence. See 80200-80203

80165   Code is out of numerical sequence. See 80200-80203

80167   Code is out of numerical sequence. See 80168-80173

| 80168 | Ethosuximide |
| | ➲ *CPT Assistant* Oct 10:7, Mar 11:10 |

| 80169 | Everolimus |
| | ➲ *CPT Changes: An Insider's View* 2014 |

# 80167	Felbamate
	➲ *CPT Changes: An Insider's View* 2021
	➲ *CPT Assistant* Jan 21:8

# 80181	Flecainide
	➲ *CPT Changes: An Insider's View* 2021
	➲ *CPT Assistant* Jan 21:8

# 80171	Gabapentin, whole blood, serum, or plasma
	➲ *CPT Changes: An Insider's View* 2014, 2015
	➲ *CPT Assistant* Apr 15:3

| 80170 | Gentamicin |
| | ➲ *CPT Assistant* Oct 10:7, Mar 11:10 |

80171   Code is out of numerical sequence. See 80168-80173

80173	Haloperidol
	➲ *CPT Changes: An Insider's View* 2001
	➲ *CPT Assistant* Oct 10:7, Mar 11:10

| # 80220 | Hydroxychloroquine |
| | ➲ *CPT Changes: An Insider's View* 2022 |

| # 80230 | Infliximab |
| | ➲ *CPT Changes: An Insider's View* 2020 |

# 80189	Itraconazole
	➲ *CPT Changes: An Insider's View* 2021
	➲ *CPT Assistant* Jan 21:8

| # 80235 | Lacosamide |
| | ➲ *CPT Changes: An Insider's View* 2020 |

| 80175 | Lamotrigine |
| | ➲ *CPT Changes: An Insider's View* 2014 |

80176   Code is out of numerical sequence. See 80170-80183

# 80193	Leflunomide
	➲ *CPT Changes: An Insider's View* 2021
	➲ *CPT Assistant* Jan 21:8

| 80177 | Levetiracetam |
| | ➲ *CPT Changes: An Insider's View* 2014 |

| # 80176 | Lidocaine |
| | ➲ *CPT Assistant* Oct 10:7, Mar 11:10 |

| 80178 | Lithium |
| | ➲ *CPT Assistant* Oct 10:7, Mar 11:10 |

80179   Code is out of numerical sequence. See 80192-80197

# 80204	Methotrexate
	➲ *CPT Changes: An Insider's View* 2021
	➲ *CPT Assistant* Jan 21:8

| 80180 | Mycophenolate (mycophenolic acid) |
| | ➲ *CPT Changes: An Insider's View* 2014 |

80181   Code is out of numerical sequence. See 80168-80173

| 80183 | Oxcarbazepine |
| | ➲ *CPT Changes: An Insider's View* 2014 |

| 80184 | Phenobarbital |
| | ➲ *CPT Assistant* Oct 10:7, Mar 11:10 |

| 80185 | Phenytoin; total |
| | ➲ *CPT Assistant* Oct 10:7, Mar 11:10 |

| 80186 | free |
| | ➲ *CPT Assistant* Oct 10:7, Mar 11:10 |

| 80187 | Posaconazole |
| | ➲ *CPT Changes: An Insider's View* 2020 |

| 80188 | Primidone |
| | ➲ *CPT Assistant* Oct 10:7, Mar 11:10 |

80189   Code is out of numerical sequence. See 80173-80175

| 80190 | Procainamide; |
| | ➲ *CPT Assistant* Oct 10:7, Mar 11:10 |

| 80192 | with metabolites (eg, n-acetyl procainamide) |
| | ➲ *CPT Assistant* Oct 10:7, Mar 11:10 |

80193   Code is out of numerical sequence. See 80170-80183

| 80194 | Quinidine |
| | ➲ *CPT Assistant* Oct 10:7, Mar 11:10 |

# 80210	Rufinamide
	➲ *CPT Changes: An Insider's View* 2021
	➲ *CPT Assistant* Jan 21:8

# 80179	Salicylate
	➲ *CPT Changes: An Insider's View* 2021
	➲ *CPT Assistant* Jan 21:8

(For definitive drug testing for salicylate, see 80329, 80330, 80331)

80195	Sirolimus
	➲ *CPT Changes: An Insider's View* 2006
	➲ *CPT Assistant* Mar 06:6, Oct 10:7, Mar 11:10

| 80197 | Tacrolimus |
| | ➲ *CPT Assistant* Oct 10:7, Mar 11:10 |

| 80198 | Theophylline |
| | ➲ *CPT Assistant* Oct 10:7, Mar 11:10 |

| 80199 | Tiagabine |
| | ➲ *CPT Changes: An Insider's View* 2014 |

Pathology and Laboratory 80047-89398, 0001U-0520U

80200 Tobramycin

➔ *CPT Assistant* Oct 10:7, Mar 11:10

80201 Topiramate

➔ *CPT Assistant* Nov 97:28, Oct 10:7, Mar 11:10

 # 80164 Valproic acid (dipropylacetic acid); total

➔ *CPT Changes: An Insider's View* 2015

➔ *CPT Assistant* Oct 10:7, Mar 11:10, Apr 15:3

 # 80165 free

➔ *CPT Changes: An Insider's View* 2015

➔ *CPT Assistant* Apr 15:3

80202 Vancomycin

➔ *CPT Assistant* Oct 10:7, Mar 11:10, Apr 15:3

 # 80280 Vedolizumab

➔ *CPT Changes: An Insider's View* 2020

 # 80285 Voriconazole

➔ *CPT Changes: An Insider's View* 2020

80203 Zonisamide

➔ *CPT Changes: An Insider's View* 2014

80204 Code is out of numerical sequence. See 80170-80183

80210 Code is out of numerical sequence. See 80192-80195

80220 Code is out of numerical sequence. See 80170-80175

80230 Code is out of numerical sequence. See 80170-80183

80235 Code is out of numerical sequence. See 80170-80183

80280 Code is out of numerical sequence. See 80201-80299

80285 Code is out of numerical sequence. See 80201-80299

80299 Quantitation of therapeutic drug, not elsewhere specified

➔ *CPT Changes: An Insider's View* 2015

➔ *CPT Assistant* Mar 00:3, Oct 04:14, Aug 05:9, Oct 10:7, Dec 10:3, Mar 11:10, Apr 15:3

80305 Code is out of numerical sequence. See Presumptive Drug Class Screening subsection

80306 Code is out of numerical sequence. See Presumptive Drug Class Screening subsection

80307 Code is out of numerical sequence. See Presumptive Drug Class Screening subsection

80320 Code is out of numerical sequence. See Definitive Drug Testing subsection

80321 Code is out of numerical sequence. See Definitive Drug Testing subsection

80322 Code is out of numerical sequence. See Definitive Drug Testing subsection

80323 Code is out of numerical sequence. See Definitive Drug Testing subsection

80324 Code is out of numerical sequence. See Definitive Drug Testing subsection

80325 Code is out of numerical sequence. See Definitive Drug Testing subsection

80326 Code is out of numerical sequence. See Definitive Drug Testing subsection

80327 Code is out of numerical sequence. See Definitive Drug Testing subsection

80328 Code is out of numerical sequence. See Definitive Drug Testing subsection

80329 Code is out of numerical sequence. See Definitive Drug Testing subsection

80330 Code is out of numerical sequence. See Definitive Drug Testing subsection

80331 Code is out of numerical sequence. See Definitive Drug Testing subsection

80332 Code is out of numerical sequence. See Definitive Drug Testing subsection

80333 Code is out of numerical sequence. See Definitive Drug Testing subsection

80334 Code is out of numerical sequence. See Definitive Drug Testing subsection

80335 Code is out of numerical sequence. See Definitive Drug Testing subsection

80336 Code is out of numerical sequence. See Definitive Drug Testing subsection

80337 Code is out of numerical sequence. See Definitive Drug Testing subsection

80338 Code is out of numerical sequence. See Definitive Drug Testing subsection

80339 Code is out of numerical sequence. See Definitive Drug Testing subsection

80340 Code is out of numerical sequence. See Definitive Drug Testing subsection

80341 Code is out of numerical sequence. See Definitive Drug Testing subsection

80342 Code is out of numerical sequence. See Definitive Drug Testing subsection

80343 Code is out of numerical sequence. See Definitive Drug Testing subsection

80344 Code is out of numerical sequence. See Definitive Drug Testing subsection

80345 Code is out of numerical sequence. See Definitive Drug Testing subsection

80346 Code is out of numerical sequence. See Definitive Drug Testing subsection

80347 Code is out of numerical sequence. See Definitive Drug Testing subsection

80348 Code is out of numerical sequence. See Definitive Drug Testing subsection

★ = Telemedicine ◀ = Audio-only ✚ = Add-on code ✗ = FDA approval pending # = Resequenced code ⊘ = Modifier 51 exempt ➔➔➔ = See p xxi for details

80349   Code is out of numerical sequence. See Definitive Drug Testing subsection

80350   Code is out of numerical sequence. See Definitive Drug Testing subsection

80351   Code is out of numerical sequence. See Definitive Drug Testing subsection

80352   Code is out of numerical sequence. See Definitive Drug Testing subsection

80353   Code is out of numerical sequence. See Definitive Drug Testing subsection

80354   Code is out of numerical sequence. See Definitive Drug Testing subsection

80355   Code is out of numerical sequence. See Definitive Drug Testing subsection

80356   Code is out of numerical sequence. See Definitive Drug Testing subsection

80357   Code is out of numerical sequence. See Definitive Drug Testing subsection

80358   Code is out of numerical sequence. See Definitive Drug Testing subsection

80359   Code is out of numerical sequence. See Definitive Drug Testing subsection

80360   Code is out of numerical sequence. See Definitive Drug Testing subsection

80361   Code is out of numerical sequence. See Definitive Drug Testing subsection

80362   Code is out of numerical sequence. See Definitive Drug Testing subsection

80363   Code is out of numerical sequence. See Definitive Drug Testing subsection

80364   Code is out of numerical sequence. See Definitive Drug Testing subsection

80365   Code is out of numerical sequence. See Definitive Drug Testing subsection

80366   Code is out of numerical sequence. See Definitive Drug Testing subsection

80367   Code is out of numerical sequence. See Definitive Drug Testing subsection

80368   Code is out of numerical sequence. See Definitive Drug Testing subsection

80369   Code is out of numerical sequence. See Definitive Drug Testing subsection

80370   Code is out of numerical sequence. See Definitive Drug Testing subsection

80371   Code is out of numerical sequence. See Definitive Drug Testing subsection

80372   Code is out of numerical sequence. See Definitive Drug Testing subsection

80373   Code is out of numerical sequence. See Definitive Drug Testing subsection

80374   Code is out of numerical sequence. See Definitive Drug Testing subsection

80375   Code is out of numerical sequence. See Definitive Drug Testing subsection

80376   Code is out of numerical sequence. See Definitive Drug Testing subsection

80377   Code is out of numerical sequence. See Definitive Drug Testing subsection

Evocative/Suppression Testing

The following test panels involve the administration of evocative or suppressive agents and the baseline and subsequent measurement of their effects on chemical constituents. These codes are to be used for the reporting of the laboratory component of the overall testing protocol. For the administration of the evocative or suppressive agents, see Hydration, Therapeutic, Prophylactic, Diagnostic Injections and Infusions, and Chemotherapy and Other Highly Complex Drug or Highly Complex Biologic Agent Administration (eg, 96365, 96366, 96367, 96368, 96372, 96374, 96375, 96376). In the code descriptors where reference is made to a particular analyte (eg, Cortisol: 82533 x 2) the "x 2" refers to the number of times the test for that particular analyte is performed.

80400   ACTH stimulation panel; for adrenal insufficiency

This panel must include the following:

Cortisol (82533 x 2)

➔ *CPT Assistant* Summer 94:1, Fall 94:10, Aug 05:9

80402   for 21 hydroxylase deficiency

This panel must include the following:

Cortisol (82533 x 2)

17 hydroxyprogesterone (83498 x 2)

➔ *CPT Assistant* Summer 94:1, Fall 94:10

80406   for 3 beta-hydroxydehydrogenase deficiency

This panel must include the following:

Cortisol (82533 x 2)

17 hydroxypregnenolone (84143 x 2)

➔ *CPT Assistant* Summer 94:1, Fall 94:10

80408   Aldosterone suppression evaluation panel (eg, saline infusion)

This panel must include the following:

Aldosterone (82088 x 2)

Renin (84244 x 2)

➔ *CPT Assistant* Summer 94:1, Fall 94:10

Pathology and Laboratory   80047-89398, 0001U-0520U

80410   Calcitonin stimulation panel (eg, calcium, pentagastrin)

This panel must include the following:

Calcitonin (82308 x 3)

➔ *CPT Assistant* Summer 94:1, Fall 94:11

80412   Corticotropic releasing hormone (CRH) stimulation panel

This panel must include the following:

Cortisol (82533 x 6)

Adrenocorticotropic hormone (ACTH) (82024 x 6)

➔ *CPT Assistant* Summer 94:1, Fall 94:11

80414   Chorionic gonadotropin stimulation panel; testosterone response

This panel must include the following:

Testosterone (84403 x 2 on 3 pooled blood samples)

➔ *CPT Changes: An Insider's View* 2009

➔ *CPT Assistant* Summer 94:1, Fall 94:11

80415   estradiol response

This panel must include the following:

Estradiol, total (82670 x 2 on 3 pooled blood samples)

➔ *CPT Changes: An Insider's View* 2009, 2021

➔ *CPT Assistant* Summer 94:1, Fall 94:11

80416   Renal vein renin stimulation panel (eg, captopril)

This panel must include the following:

Renin (84244 x 6)

➔ *CPT Assistant* Summer 94:1

80417   Peripheral vein renin stimulation panel (eg, captopril)

This panel must include the following:

Renin (84244 x 2)

80418   Combined rapid anterior pituitary evaluation panel

This panel must include the following:

Adrenocorticotropic hormone (ACTH) (82024 x 4)

Luteinizing hormone (LH) (83002 x 4)

Follicle stimulating hormone (FSH) (83001 x 4)

Prolactin (84146 x 4)

Human growth hormone (HGH) (83003 x 4)

Cortisol (82533 x 4)

Thyroid stimulating hormone (TSH) (84443 x 4)

➔ *CPT Assistant* Summer 94:1, Fall 94:13

80420   Dexamethasone suppression panel, 48 hour

This panel must include the following:

Free cortisol, urine (82530 x 2)

Cortisol (82533 x 2)

Volume measurement for timed collection (81050 x 2)

➔ *CPT Assistant* Fall 94:13

(For single dose dexamethasone, use 82533)

80422   Glucagon tolerance panel; for insulinoma

This panel must include the following:

Glucose (82947 x 3)

Insulin (83525 x 3)

➔ *CPT Assistant* Summer 94:1, Fall 94:13

80424   for pheochromocytoma

This panel must include the following:

Catecholamines, fractionated (82384 x 2)

➔ *CPT Assistant* Summer 94:1, Fall 94:14

80426   Gonadotropin releasing hormone stimulation panel

This panel must include the following:

Follicle stimulating hormone (FSH) (83001 x 4)

Luteinizing hormone (LH) (83002 x 4)

➔ *CPT Assistant* Summer 94:1, Fall 94:14

80428   Growth hormone stimulation panel (eg, arginine infusion, l-dopa administration)

This panel must include the following:

Human growth hormone (HGH) (83003 x 4)

➔ *CPT Assistant* Summer 94:1, Fall 94:14

80430   Growth hormone suppression panel (glucose administration)

This panel must include the following:

Glucose (82947 x 3)

Human growth hormone (HGH) (83003 x 4)

➔ *CPT Assistant* Summer 94:1, Fall 94:14

80432   Insulin-induced C-peptide suppression panel

This panel must include the following:

Insulin (83525)

C-peptide (84681 x 5)

Glucose (82947 x 5)

➔ *CPT Assistant* Summer 94:1, Fall 94:15

80434   Insulin tolerance panel; for ACTH insufficiency

This panel must include the following:

Cortisol (82533 x 5)

Glucose (82947 x 5)

➔ *CPT Assistant* Summer 94:1, Fall 94:15

80435   for growth hormone deficiency

This panel must include the following:

Glucose (82947 x 5)

Human growth hormone (HGH) (83003 x 5)

➔ *CPT Assistant* Summer 94:1, Fall 94:15, Oct 21:14

★ = Telemedicine   ◀ = Audio-only   + = Add-on code   ✗ = FDA approval pending   # = Resequenced code   ⊘ = Modifier 51 exempt   ➔➔➔ = See p xxi for details

80436   Metyrapone panel

This panel must include the following:

Cortisol (82533 x 2)

11 deoxycortisol (82634 x 2)

➔ *CPT Assistant* Summer 94:1, Fall 94:16

80438   Thyrotropin releasing hormone (TRH) stimulation panel; 1 hour

This panel must include the following:

Thyroid stimulating hormone (TSH) (84443 x 3)

➔ *CPT Assistant* Summer 94:1, Fall 94:16

80439   2 hour

This panel must include the following:

Thyroid stimulating hormone (TSH) (84443 x 4)

➔ *CPT Assistant* Summer 94:1, Fall 94:16

Pathology Clinical Consultations

Physician review of pathology and laboratory findings is frequently performed in the course of providing care to patients. Review of pathology and laboratory test results occurs in conjunction with the provision of an evaluation and management (E/M) service. Considered part of the non-face-to-face time activities associated with the overall E/M service, reviewing pathology and laboratory results is not a separately reportable service. Communicating results to the patient, family, or caregiver of independent interpretation of results (not separately reported) may constitute an E/M service.

Pathology clinical consultation services codes (80503, 80504, 80505, 80506) describe physician pathology clinical consultation services provided at the request of another physician or other qualified health care professional at the same or another facility or institution.

A pathology clinical consultation is a service, including a written report, rendered by the pathologist in response to a request (eg, written request, electronic request, phone request, or face-to-face request) from a physician or other qualified health care professional that is related to clinical assessment, evaluation of pathology and laboratory findings, or other relevant clinical or diagnostic information that requires additional medical interpretive judgment. Reporting pathology and laboratory findings or other relevant clinical or diagnostic information without medical interpretive judgment is not considered a pathology clinical consultation.

The pathology clinical consultation services (80503, 80504, 80505, 80506) may be reported when the following criteria have been met:

- The pathologist renders a pathology clinical consultation at the request of a physician or other qualified health care professional at the same or another institution.

- The pathology clinical consultation request is related to pathology and laboratory findings or other relevant clinical or diagnostic information (eg, radiology findings or operative/procedural notes) that require additional medical interpretive judgment.

A pathologist may also render a pathology clinical consultation when mandated by federal or state regulation (eg, Clinical Laboratory Improvement Amendments [CLIA]).

Instructions for Selecting a Level of Pathology Clinical Consultation Services

Selection of the appropriate level of pathology clinical consultation services may be based on either the total time for pathology clinical consultation services performed on the date of consultation **or** the level of medical decision making as defined for each service.

Medical Decision Making

See Medical Decision Making table on page 632.

Pathology and Laboratory 80047-89398, 0001U-0520U

Elements of Medical Decision Making

Code	Level of MDM (Based on 2 out of 3 Elements of MDM)	Number and Complexity of Problems Addressed	Amount and/or Complexity of Data to Be Reviewed and Analyzed *Each unique test, order, or document contributes to the combination of 2 or combination of 3 in Category 1 below.*	Risk of Complications and/or Morbidity or Mortality of Patient Management
80503	Straightforward	**Low** ■ **1** to **2** laboratory or pathology findings; **or** ■ **2** or more self-limited problems	**Limited** *(Must meet the requirements of at least 1 of the 2 categories)* **Category 1: Tests and documents** ■ **Any combination of 2 from the following:** • Review of prior note(s) from each unique source*; • Review of the result(s) of each unique test*; • Ordering or recommending additional or follow-up testing* **or** **Category 2: Assessment requiring an independent historian(s)** *(For the categories of independent interpretation of tests and discussion of management or test interpretation, see moderate or high)*	**Low risk of morbidity from additional diagnostic testing or treatment**
80504	Moderate	**Moderate** ■ **3** to **4** laboratory or pathology findings; **or** ■ **1** or more chronic illnesses with exacerbation, progression, or side effects of treatment; **or** ■ **2** or more stable chronic illnesses; **or** ■ **1** undiagnosed new problem with uncertain prognosis; **or** ■ **1** acute illness with systemic symptoms	**Moderate** *(Must meet the requirements of at least 1 out of 3 categories)* **Category 1: Tests, documents, or independent historian(s)** ■ **Any combination of 3 from the following:** • Review of prior note(s) from each unique source*; • Review of the result(s) of each unique test*; • Ordering or recommending additional or follow-up testing*; • Assessment requiring an independent historian(s) **or** **Category 2: Independent interpretation of tests** ■ Independent interpretation of a test performed by another physician/other qualified health care professional (not separately reported); **or** **Category 3: Discussion of management or test interpretation** ■ Discussion of management or test interpretation with external physician/other qualified health care professional/appropriate source (not separately reported)	**Moderate risk of morbidity from additional diagnostic testing or treatment** *Examples only:* Prescription drug management ■ Decision regarding minor surgery with identified patient or procedure risk factors ■ Decision regarding elective major surgery without identified patient or procedure risk factors ■ Diagnosis or treatment significantly limited by social determinants of health

Elements of Medical Decision Making

Code	Level of MDM (Based on 2 out of 3 Elements of MDM)	Number and Complexity of Problems Addressed	Amount and/or Complexity of Data to Be Reviewed and Analyzed *Each unique test, order, or document contributes to the combination of 2 or combination of 3 in Category 1 below.*	Risk of Complications and/or Morbidity or Mortality of Patient Management
80505	High	**High** ■ **5** or more laboratory or pathology findings; **or** ■ **1** or more chronic illnesses with severe exacerbation, progression, or side effects of treatment; **or** ■ **1** acute or chronic illness or injury that poses a threat to life or bodily function	**Extensive** *(Must meet the requirements of at least 2 out of 3 categories)* **Category 1: Tests, documents, or independent historian(s)** ■ **Any combination of 3 from the following:** ● Review of prior note(s) from each unique source*; ● Review of the result(s) of each unique test*; ● Ordering or recommending additional or follow-up testing*; ● Assessment requiring an independent historian(s) **or** **Category 2: Independent interpretation of tests** ■ Independent interpretation of a test performed by another physician/other qualified health care professional (not separately reported); **or** ■ **Category 3: Discussion of management or test interpretation** Discussion of management or test interpretation with external physician/other qualified health care professional/appropriate source (not separately reported)	**High risk of morbidity from additional diagnostic testing or treatment** *Examples only:* ■ Drug therapy requiring intensive monitoring for toxicity ■ Decision regarding elective major surgery with identified patient or procedure risk factors ■ Decision regarding emergency major surgery ■ Decision regarding hospitalization

Time

Time alone may be used to select the appropriate code level for the pathology clinical consultation services codes (ie, 80503, 80504, 80505). When time is used to select the appropriate level for pathology clinical consultation codes, time is defined by the service descriptions. When prolonged service time occurs, add-on code 80506 may be reported. The appropriate time should be documented in the medical record when it is used as the basis for code selection.

Total time on the date of the consultation (pathology clinical consultation services): For coding purposes, time for these services is the total time on the date of the consultation. It includes time personally spent by the consultant on the day of the consultation (includes time in activities that require the consultant and does not include time in activities normally performed by clinical staff).

Consultant time includes the following activities, when performed:

■ Review of available medical history, including presenting complaint, signs and symptoms, personal and family history
■ Review of test results

■ Review of all relevant past and current laboratory, pathology, and clinical findings
■ Arriving at a tentative conclusion/differential diagnosis
■ Comparing against previous study reports, including radiographic reports, images as applicable, and results of other clinical testing
■ Ordering or recommending additional or follow-up testing
■ Referring and communicating with other health care professionals (not separately reported)
■ Counseling and educating the clinician or other qualified health care professional
■ Documenting the clinical consultation report in the electronic or other health record

80503   Pathology clinical consultation; for a clinical problem, with limited review of patient's history and medical records and straightforward medical decision making

When using time for code selection, 5-20 minutes of total time is spent on the date of the consultation.
➜ *CPT Changes: An Insider's View* 2022
➜ *CPT Assistant* Feb 22:3, Mar 22:13

(For consultations involving the examination and evaluation of the patient, see evaluation and management services)

80504   for a moderately complex clinical problem, with review of patient's history and medical records and moderate level of medical decision making

When using time for code selection, 21-40 minutes of total time is spent on the date of the consultation.
➜ *CPT Changes: An Insider's View* 2022
➜ *CPT Assistant* Feb 22:3, Mar 22:13

80505   for a highly complex clinical problem, with comprehensive review of patient's history and medical records and high level of medical decision making

When using time for code selection, 41-60 minutes of total time is spent on the date of the consultation.
➜ *CPT Changes: An Insider's View* 2022
➜ *CPT Assistant* Feb 22:3, Mar 22:13

+ 80506   prolonged service, each additional 30 minutes (List separately in addition to code for primary procedure)
➜ *CPT Changes: An Insider's View* 2022
➜ *CPT Assistant* Feb 22:3, Mar 22:13

(Use 80506 in conjunction with 80505)

(Do not report 80503, 80504, 80505, 80506 in conjunction with 88321, 88323, 88325)

(Prolonged pathology clinical consultation service of less than 15 additional minutes is not reported separately)

(For consultations involving the examination and evaluation of the patient, see evaluation and management services)

Urinalysis

Urinalysis procedures that are not specified in 81000, 81001, 81002, 81003, 81005, 81007, 81015, 81020, 81025, 81050 may be reported using either the appropriate analyte-specific code in the Chemistry (82009-84830) subsection or the unlisted urinalysis procedure code 81099, if an analyte-specific code is not available.

81000   Urinalysis, by dip stick or tablet reagent for bilirubin, glucose, hemoglobin, ketones, leukocytes, nitrite, pH, protein, specific gravity, urobilinogen, any number of these constituents; non-automated, with microscopy
➜ *CPT Assistant* Winter 90:4, Winter 91:10, Fall 93:25, Aug 05:9, Jul 18:15, Jan 24:17

81001   automated, with microscopy

81002   non-automated, without microscopy
➜ *CPT Assistant* Mar 98:3, Apr 07:1

81003   automated, without microscopy
➜ *CPT Assistant* Apr 07:1

81005   Urinalysis; qualitative or semiquantitative, except immunoassays
➜ *CPT Assistant* Winter 90:4, Winter 91:10, Fall 93:25

(For non-immunoassay reagent strip urinalysis, see 81000, 81002)

(For immunoassay, qualitative or semiquantitative, use 83518)

(For microalbumin, see 82043, 82044)

81007   bacteriuria screen, except by culture or dipstick
➜ *CPT Changes: An Insider's View* 2001

(For culture, see 87086-87088)

(For dipstick, use 81000 or 81002)

81015   microscopic only
➜ *CPT Assistant* Nov 17:11

(For sperm evaluation for retrograde ejaculation, use 89331)

81020   2 or 3 glass test
➜ *CPT Assistant* Winter 90:4, Winter 91:10

81025   Urine pregnancy test, by visual color comparison methods
➜ *CPT Assistant* Mar 98:3

81050   Volume measurement for timed collection, each
➜ *CPT Assistant* Jan 24:17

81099   Unlisted urinalysis procedure
➜ *CPT Assistant* Aug 05:9, Jan 24:17

Molecular Pathology

Molecular pathology procedures are medical laboratory procedures involving the analyses of nucleic acid (ie, DNA, RNA) to detect variants in genes that may be indicative of germline (eg, constitutional disorders) or somatic (eg, neoplasia) conditions, or to test for histocompatibility antigens (eg, HLA). Code selection is typically based on the specific gene(s) that is being analyzed. Genes are described using Human Genome Organization (HUGO) approved gene names and are italicized in the code descriptors. Gene names were taken from tables of the HUGO Gene Nomenclature Committee (HGNC) at the time the CPT codes were developed. For the most part, Human Genome Variation

Society (HGVS) recommendations were followed for the names of specific molecular variants. The familiar name is used for some variants because defined criteria were not in place when the variant was first described or because HGVS recommendations were changed over time (eg, intronic variants, processed proteins). When the gene name is represented by an abbreviation, the abbreviation is listed first, followed by the full gene name italicized in parentheses (eg, "F5 *[coagulation Factor V]*"), except for the HLA series of codes. Proteins or diseases commonly associated with the genes are listed as examples in the code descriptors. The examples do not represent all conditions in which testing of the gene may be indicated.

Codes that describe tests to assess for the presence of gene variants (see definitions) use common gene variant names. Typically, all of the listed variants would be tested. However, these lists are not exclusive. If other variants are also tested in the analysis, they would be included in the procedure and not reported separately. Full gene sequencing should not be reported using codes that assess for the presence of gene variants unless specifically stated in the code descriptor.

The molecular pathology codes include all analytical services performed in the test (eg, cell lysis, nucleic acid stabilization, extraction, digestion, amplification, and detection). Any procedures required prior to cell lysis (eg, microdissection, codes 88380 and 88381) should be reported separately.

The results of the procedure may require interpretation by a physician or other qualified health care professional. When only the interpretation and report are performed, modifier 26 may be appended to the specific molecular pathology code.

All analyses are qualitative unless otherwise noted.

For microbial identification, see 87149-87153 and 87471-87801, and 87900-87904. For in situ hybridization analyses, see 88271-88275 and 88365-88368.

Molecular pathology procedures that are not specified in 81161, 81200-81383 should be reported using either the appropriate Tier 2 code (81400-81408) or the unlisted molecular pathology procedure code, 81479.

Definitions

For purposes of CPT reporting, the following definitions apply:

Abnormal allele: an alternative form of a gene that contains a disease-related variation from the normal sequence.

Breakpoint: the region at which a chromosome breaks during a translocation (defined elsewhere). These regions are often consistent for a given translocation.

Codon: a discrete unit of three nucleotides of a DNA or mRNA sequence that encodes a specific amino acid within, or signals the termination of, a polypeptide.

Common variants: variants (as defined elsewhere) that are associated with compromised gene function and are interrogated in a single round of laboratory testing (in a single, typically multiplex, assay format or using more than one assay to encompass all variants to be tested). These variants typically fit the definition of a "mutation," and are usually the predominant ones causing disease. Testing for additional uncommon variants may provide additional limited value in assessment of a patient. Often there are professional society recommendations or guidelines for which variants are most appropriate to test (eg, American College of Medical Genetics/American College of Obstetrics and Gynecology guidelines for variants used in population screening for cystic fibrosis).

Constitutional: synonymous with germline, often used in reference to the genetic code that is present at birth.

Copy number variants (CNVs): structural changes in the genome composed of large deletions or duplications. CNVs can be found in the germline, but can also occur in somatic cells. See also Duplication/Deletion (Dup/Del).

▶***Cytogenomic:*** a comprehensive genome-wide analysis of chromosomal and genetic abnormalities using molecular-based technologies.◀

DNA methylation: the process of adding methyl groups to a DNA sequence, specifically adenine and cytosine nucleotides, thereby affecting transcription of that sequence. DNA hyper-methylation in a gene promoter typically represses gene transcription. DNA methylation serves as a regulatory mechanism in numerous scenarios including development, chromosome inactivation, and carcinogenesis.

DNA methylation analysis: analytical protocols are designed to evaluate the degree of DNA methylation related to specific disease processes. This analysis has various applications, qualitative or quantitative, and could be gene specific or encompass global degrees of methylation. All assays employ specific maneuvers (eg, chemical, enzymatic) that allow for distinguishable evaluation of methylated and non-methylated sequences.

Duplication/Deletion (Dup/Del): terms that are usually used together with the "/" to refer to molecular testing, which assesses the dosage of a particular genomic region. The region tested is typically of modest to substantial size—from several dozen to several million or more nucleotides. Normal gene dosage is two copies per cell, except for the sex chromosomes (X and Y). Thus, zero or one copy represents a deletion, and three (or more) copies represent a duplication.

Dynamic mutation: polynucleotide (eg, trinucleotide) repeats that are in or associated with genes that can undergo disease-producing increases or decreases in the numbers of repeats within tissues and across generations.

Exome: DNA sequences within the human genome that code for proteins (coding regions).

Exon: typically, one of multiple nucleic acid sequences used to encode information for a gene product (polypeptide or protein). Exons are separated from each other by non-protein-coding sequences known as introns. Exons at the respective ends of a gene also contain nucleic acid sequence that does not code for the gene's protein product.

Gene: a nucleic acid sequence that typically contains information for coding a protein as well as for the regulated expression of that protein. Human genes usually contain multiple protein coding regions (exons) separated by non-protein coding regions (introns). See also *exon*, *intron*, and *polypeptide*.

Gene expression: the sequence of events that results in the production and assembly of a protein product corresponding to the information encoded in a specific gene. The process begins with the transcription of gene sequences to produce an mRNA intermediary, which is subsequently translated to produce a specific protein product.

Genome: the total (nuclear) human genetic content.

Heteroplasmy: the copy number of a variant within a cell; it is expressed as a percent. It reflects the varied distribution and dosage of mutant mitochondria in tissues and organs (mitotic segregation).

Intron: a nucleic acid sequence found between exons in human genes. An intron contains essential sequences for its proper removal (by a process known as *splicing*) to join exons together and thus facilitate production of a functional protein from a gene. An intron is sometimes referred to as an intervening sequence (IVS).

Inversion: a defect in a chromosome in which a segment breaks and reinserts in the same place but in the opposite orientation.

Loss of heterozygosity (LOH, allelic imbalance): an event that can occur in dividing cells that are heterozygous for one or more alleles, in which a daughter cell becomes hemizygous or homozygous for the allele(s) through mitotic recombination, deletion, or other chromosomal event.

Low-pass sequencing: a method of genome sequencing intended for cytogenomic analysis of chromosomal abnormalities, such as that performed for trait mapping or copy number variation, typically performed to an average depth of sequencing ranging from 0.1 to 5X.

Microarray: surface(s) on which multiple specific nucleic acid sequences are attached in a known arrangement. Sometimes referred to as a "gene chip." Examples of uses of microarrays include evaluation of a patient specimen for gains or losses of DNA sequences (copy number variants, CNVs), identification of the presence of specific nucleotide sequence variants (also known as single nucleotide polymorphisms, SNPs), mRNA expression levels, or DNA sequence analysis.

Mitochondrial DNA (mtDNA): DNA located in the mitochondria, which are cytoplasmic organelles involved with energy production. MtDNA contains 37 genes coding for oxidative phosphorylation enzymes, transfer RNAs (tRNAs) and ribosomal RNAs (rRNAs).

Mutations: typically are variants associated with altered gene function that lead to functional deficits or disease (pathogenic).

Mutation scanning: a technique (eg, single strand conformation polymorphism, temperature gradient gel electrophoresis, etc.) typically employed on multiple PCR amplicons to indicate the presence of DNA sequence variants by differences in physical properties compared to normal. Variants are then further characterized by DNA sequence analysis only in amplicons which demonstrate differences.

Nuclear DNA: DNA located in the nucleus of a cell, generally packaged in chromosomes.

Polymorphisms: typically are variants that do not compromise gene function or produce disease (benign).

Polypeptide: a sequence of amino acids covalently linked in a specified order. Polypeptides alone or in combination with other polypeptide subunits are the building blocks of proteins.

Promoter: a region of DNA associated with a gene (on the same strand) which regulates gene expression. Promoter regions can affect gene transcription through the binding of specific transcription factors.

Short tandem repeat (STR): a region of DNA where a pattern of two or more nucleotides are repeated. The number of repeating segments can be used as genetic markers for human identity testing.

Single-nucleotide polymorphism (SNP): a DNA sequence variation existing at a significant frequency in the population, in which a single nucleotide (A, T, C, or G) differs between individuals and/or within an individual's paired chromosomes.

Somatic: synonymous with acquired, referring to genetic code alterations that develop after birth (eg, occurring in neoplastic cells).

Translocation: an abnormality resulting from the breakage of a chromosome and the relocation of a portion of that chromosome's DNA sequence to the same or another chromosome. Most common translocations involve a reciprocal exchange of DNA sequences between two differently numbered (ie, non-homologous) chromosomes, with or without a clinically significant loss of DNA.

Uniparental disomy (UPD): abnormal inheritance of both members of a chromosome pair from one parent, with absence of the other parent's chromosome for the pair.

Variant: a nucleotide sequence difference from the "normal" (predominant) sequence for a given region. Variants are typically of two types: substitutions of one nucleotide for another, and deletions or insertions of nucleotides. Occasionally, variants reflect several nucleotide sequence changes in reasonably close proximity on the same chromosomal strand of DNA (a haplotype). These nucleotide sequence variants often result in amino acid changes in the protein made by the gene. The term *variant* does not itself carry a functional implication for those protein changes.

Variants in introns are typically described in one of two ways. The altered nucleotide(s) within a defined intervening sequence (eg, IVS3-2A>G) of a gene is listed with a "+" or "-" sign, which indicates the position relative to the first or last nucleotide of the intron. Or, the variant position is indicated relative to the last nucleotide of the preceding exon or first nucleotide of the following exon (eg, c.171+1G>A c.172-1G>T are single nucleotide changes at the first and last nucleotide of a given intron for a specific gene).

The majority of the variants described here are listed by the amino acid change using the single letter amino acid code for the original amino acid followed by the numerical position in the protein product and the amino acid substitution, eg, for *ASPA* E285A, Glutamic acid (E) at position 285 is replaced with an alanine (A). A few of the variants are described by the DNA change using the numerical position followed by the original nucleotide, a greater than sign (>) and the new nucleotide, eg, *MTHFR.* 677C>T.

A known familial variant is a specific mutation that has previously been identified within a patient's family.

Tier 1 Molecular Pathology Procedures

The following codes represent gene-specific and genomic procedures:

81105   Code is out of numerical sequence. See 81255-81270

81106   Code is out of numerical sequence. See 81255-81270

81107   Code is out of numerical sequence. See 81255-81270

81108   Code is out of numerical sequence. See 81255-81270

81109   Code is out of numerical sequence. See 81255-81270

81110   Code is out of numerical sequence. See 81255-81270

81111   Code is out of numerical sequence. See 81255-81270

81112   Code is out of numerical sequence. See 81255-81270

81120   Code is out of numerical sequence. See 81255-81270

81121   Code is out of numerical sequence. See 81255-81270

81161   Code is out of numerical sequence. See 81228-81235

81162   Code is out of numerical sequence. See 81182-81216

81163   Code is out of numerical sequence. See 81182-81216

81164   Code is out of numerical sequence. See 81182-81216

81165   Code is out of numerical sequence. See 81182-81216

81166   Code is out of numerical sequence. See 81182-81216

81167   Code is out of numerical sequence. See 81215-81220

81168   Code is out of numerical sequence. See 81215-81220

81170   *ABL1 (ABL proto-oncogene 1, non-receptor tyrosine kinase)* (eg, acquired imatinib tyrosine kinase inhibitor resistance), gene analysis, variants in the kinase domain
➔ *CPT Changes: An Insider's View* 2016
➔ *CPT Assistant* Aug 16:10

81171   *AFF2 (ALF transcription elongation factor 2 [FMR2])* (eg, fragile X intellectual disability 2 [FRAXE]) gene analysis; evaluation to detect abnormal (eg, expanded) alleles
➔ *CPT Changes: An Insider's View* 2019, 2024

81172   characterization of alleles (eg, expanded size and methylation status)
➔ *CPT Changes: An Insider's View* 2019, 2024

81173   Code is out of numerical sequence. See 81171-81176

81174   Code is out of numerical sequence. See 81171-81176

 # 81201   *APC (adenomatous polyposis coli)* (eg, familial adenomatosis polyposis [FAP], attenuated FAP) gene analysis; full gene sequence
➔ *CPT Changes: An Insider's View* 2013
➔ *CPT Assistant* May 12:4, Sep 13:3, Aug 16:10, Nov 18:9

 # 81202   known familial variants
➔ *CPT Changes: An Insider's View* 2013
➔ *CPT Assistant* May 12:4, Sep 13:3, Aug 16:10, Nov 18:9

 # 81203   duplication/deletion variants
➔ *CPT Changes: An Insider's View* 2013
➔ *CPT Assistant* May 12:4, Sep 13:3, Aug 16:10, Nov 18:9

 # 81204 *AR (androgen receptor)* (eg, spinal and bulbar muscular atrophy, Kennedy disease, X chromosome inactivation) gene analysis; characterization of alleles (eg, expanded size or methylation status)

➲ *CPT Changes: An Insider's View* 2019

➲ *CPT Assistant* Nov 18:9

 # 81173 full gene sequence

➲ *CPT Changes: An Insider's View* 2019

 # 81174 known familial variant

➲ *CPT Changes: An Insider's View* 2019

 # 81200 *ASPA (aspartoacylase)* (eg, Canavan disease) gene analysis, common variants (eg, E285A, Y231X)

➲ *CPT Changes: An Insider's View* 2012

➲ *CPT Assistant* May 12:4, Aug 16:10, Nov 18:9

81175 *ASXL1 (additional sex combs like 1, transcriptional regulator)* (eg, myelodysplastic syndrome, myeloproliferative neoplasms, chronic myelomonocytic leukemia), gene analysis; full gene sequence

➲ *CPT Changes: An Insider's View* 2018

81176 targeted sequence analysis (eg, exon 12)

➲ *CPT Changes: An Insider's View* 2018

81177 *ATN1 (atrophin 1)* (eg, dentatorubral-pallidoluysian atrophy) gene analysis, evaluation to detect abnormal (eg, expanded) alleles

➲ *CPT Changes: An Insider's View* 2019

81178 *ATXN1 (ataxin 1)* (eg, spinocerebellar ataxia) gene analysis, evaluation to detect abnormal (eg, expanded) alleles

➲ *CPT Changes: An Insider's View* 2019

➲ *CPT Assistant* Sep 19:7

81179 *ATXN2 (ataxin 2)* (eg, spinocerebellar ataxia) gene analysis, evaluation to detect abnormal (eg, expanded) alleles

➲ *CPT Changes: An Insider's View* 2019

➲ *CPT Assistant* Sep 19:7

81180 *ATXN3 (ataxin 3)* (eg, spinocerebellar ataxia, Machado-Joseph disease) gene analysis, evaluation to detect abnormal (eg, expanded) alleles

➲ *CPT Changes: An Insider's View* 2019

➲ *CPT Assistant* Sep 19:7

81181 *ATXN7 (ataxin 7)* (eg, spinocerebellar ataxia) gene analysis, evaluation to detect abnormal (eg, expanded) alleles

➲ *CPT Changes: An Insider's View* 2019

➲ *CPT Assistant* Sep 19:7

81182 *ATXN8OS (ATXN8 opposite strand [non-protein coding])* (eg, spinocerebellar ataxia) gene analysis, evaluation to detect abnormal (eg, expanded) alleles

➲ *CPT Changes: An Insider's View* 2019

➲ *CPT Assistant* Sep 19:7

81183 *ATXN10 (ataxin 10)* (eg, spinocerebellar ataxia) gene analysis, evaluation to detect abnormal (eg, expanded) alleles

➲ *CPT Changes: An Insider's View* 2019

➲ *CPT Assistant* Sep 19:7

81184 Code is out of numerical sequence. See 81215-81220

81185 Code is out of numerical sequence. See 81215-81220

81186 Code is out of numerical sequence. See 81215-81220

81187 Code is out of numerical sequence. See 81223-81226

81188 Code is out of numerical sequence. See 81223-81226

81189 Code is out of numerical sequence. See 81223-81226

81190 Code is out of numerical sequence. See 81223-81226

81191 Code is out of numerical sequence. See 81310-81314

81192 Code is out of numerical sequence. See 81310-81314

81193 Code is out of numerical sequence. See 81310-81314

81194 Code is out of numerical sequence. See 81310-81314

81195 Code is out of numerical sequence. See 81228-81235

81200 Code is out of numerical sequence. See 81171-81176

81201 Code is out of numerical sequence. See 81171-81176

81202 Code is out of numerical sequence. See 81171-81176

81203 Code is out of numerical sequence. See 81171-81176

81204 Code is out of numerical sequence. See 81171-81176

81205 Code is out of numerical sequence. See 81182-81216

81206 Code is out of numerical sequence. See 81182-81216

81207 Code is out of numerical sequence. See 81182-81216

81208 Code is out of numerical sequence. See 81182-81216

81209 Code is out of numerical sequence. See 81182-81216

81210 Code is out of numerical sequence. See 81182-81216

 # 81205 *BCKDHB (branched-chain keto acid dehydrogenase E1, beta polypeptide)* (eg, maple syrup urine disease) gene analysis, common variants (eg, R183P, G278S, E422X)

➲ *CPT Changes: An Insider's View* 2012

➲ *CPT Assistant* May 12:4, Aug 16:10, Nov 18:9

 # 81206 *BCR/ABL1 (t(9;22))* (eg, chronic myelogenous leukemia) translocation analysis; major breakpoint, qualitative or quantitative

➲ *CPT Changes: An Insider's View* 2012

➲ *CPT Assistant* May 12:4, Aug 16:10, Nov 18:9

 # 81207 minor breakpoint, qualitative or quantitative

➲ *CPT Changes: An Insider's View* 2012

➲ *CPT Assistant* May 12:4, Aug 16:10, Nov 18:9

81208   other breakpoint, qualitative or quantitative
→ *CPT Changes: An Insider's View* 2012
→ *CPT Assistant* May 12:4, Aug 16:10, Nov 18:9

81209   *BLM (Bloom syndrome, RecQ helicase-like)* (eg, Bloom syndrome) gene analysis, 2281del6ins7 variant
→ *CPT Changes: An Insider's View* 2012
→ *CPT Assistant* May 12:4, Aug 16:10, Nov 18:9

81210   *BRAF (B-Raf proto-oncogene, serine/threonine kinase)* (eg, colon cancer, melanoma), gene analysis, V600 variant(s)
→ *CPT Changes: An Insider's View* 2012, 2016
→ *CPT Assistant* May 12:4, Aug 16:10, Nov 18:9

81162   *BRCA1 (BRCA1, DNA repair associated), BRCA2 (BRCA2, DNA repair associated)* (eg, hereditary breast and ovarian cancer) gene analysis; full sequence analysis and full duplication/deletion analysis (ie, detection of large gene rearrangements)
→ *CPT Changes: An Insider's View* 2016, 2019
→ *CPT Assistant* Aug 16:10, May 19:5

(Do not report 81162 in conjunction with 81163, 81164, 81165, 81166, 81167, 81215, 81216, 81217, 81432)

81163   full sequence analysis
→ *CPT Changes: An Insider's View* 2019
→ *CPT Assistant* May 19:5

81164   full duplication/deletion analysis (ie, detection of large gene rearrangements)
→ *CPT Changes: An Insider's View* 2019
→ *CPT Assistant* May 19:5

(To report *BRCA1, BRCA2* full sequence analysis and full duplication/deletion analysis on the same date of service, use 81162)

(For analysis of common duplication/deletion variant(s) in *BRCA1* [ie, exon 13 del 3.835kb, exon 13 dup 6kb, exon 14-20 del 26kb, exon 22 del 510bp, exon 8-9 del 7.1kb], use 81479)

(Do not report 81163 in conjunction with 81162, 81164, 81165, 81216, 81432)

(Do not report 81164 in conjunction with 81162, 81163, 81166, 81167, 81217)

81212   185delAG, 5385insC, 6174delT variants
→ *CPT Changes: An Insider's View* 2012, 2019
→ *CPT Assistant* May 12:4, Aug 16:10, Nov 18:9, May 19:5

81165   *BRCA1 (BRCA1, DNA repair associated)* (eg, hereditary breast and ovarian cancer) gene analysis; full sequence analysis
→ *CPT Changes: An Insider's View* 2019
→ *CPT Assistant* May 19:5

81166   full duplication/deletion analysis (ie, detection of large gene rearrangements)
→ *CPT Changes: An Insider's View* 2019
→ *CPT Assistant* May 19:5

81215   known familial variant
→ *CPT Changes: An Insider's View* 2012, 2019
→ *CPT Assistant* May 12:4, Aug 16:10, Nov 18:9, May 19:5

(For analysis of common duplication/deletion variant(s) in *BRCA1* [ie, exon 13 del 3.835kb, exon 13 dup 6kb, exon 14-20 del 26kb, exon 22 del 510bp, exon 8-9 del 7.1kb], use 81479)

(Do not report 81165 in conjunction with 81162, 81163, 81432)

(Do not report 81166 in conjunction with 81162, 81164)

81216   *BRCA2 (BRCA2, DNA repair associated)* (eg, hereditary breast and ovarian cancer) gene analysis; full sequence analysis
→ *CPT Changes: An Insider's View* 2012, 2019
→ *CPT Assistant* May 12:4, Aug 16:10, Nov 18:9, May 19:5

81167   full duplication/deletion analysis (ie, detection of large gene rearrangements)
→ *CPT Changes: An Insider's View* 2019
→ *CPT Assistant* May 19:5

81217   known familial variant
→ *CPT Changes: An Insider's View* 2012, 2019
→ *CPT Assistant* May 12:4, Aug 16:10, Nov 18:9, May 19:5

(Do not report 81216 in conjunction with 81162, 81163, 81432)

(Do not report 81167 in conjunction with 81162, 81164, 81217)

(Do not report 81217 in conjunction with 81162, 81164, 81167)

81233   *BTK (Bruton's tyrosine kinase)* (eg, chronic lymphocytic leukemia) gene analysis, common variants (eg, C481S, C481R, C481F)
→ *CPT Changes: An Insider's View* 2019
→ *CPT Assistant* Nov 18:9

81184   *CACNA1A (calcium voltage-gated channel subunit alpha1 A)* (eg, spinocerebellar ataxia) gene analysis; evaluation to detect abnormal (eg, expanded) alleles
→ *CPT Changes: An Insider's View* 2019

81185   full gene sequence
→ *CPT Changes: An Insider's View* 2019

81186   known familial variant
→ *CPT Changes: An Insider's View* 2019

81219   *CALR (calreticulin)* (eg, myeloproliferative disorders), gene analysis, common variants in exon 9
→ *CPT Changes: An Insider's View* 2016
→ *CPT Assistant* Aug 16:10, Nov 18:9

81168 *CCND1/IGH (t(11;14))* (eg, mantle cell lymphoma) translocation analysis, major breakpoint, qualitative and quantitative, if performed

➔ *CPT Changes: An Insider's View* 2021

81218 *CEBPA (CCAAT/enhancer binding protein [C/EBP], alpha)* (eg, acute myeloid leukemia), gene analysis, full gene sequence

➔ *CPT Changes: An Insider's View* 2016

➔ *CPT Assistant* Aug 16:10

81219 Code is out of numerical sequence. See 81215-81220

81220 *CFTR (cystic fibrosis transmembrane conductance regulator)* (eg, cystic fibrosis) gene analysis; common variants (eg, ACMG/ACOG guidelines)

➔ *CPT Changes: An Insider's View* 2012

➔ *CPT Assistant* May 12:4, Aug 16:10, Nov 18:9

(When Intron 8 poly-T analysis is performed in conjunction with 81220 in a R117H positive patient, do not report 81224)

81221 known familial variants

➔ *CPT Changes: An Insider's View* 2012

➔ *CPT Assistant* May 12:4, Aug 16:10, Nov 18:9

81222 duplication/deletion variants

➔ *CPT Changes: An Insider's View* 2012

➔ *CPT Assistant* May 12:4, Aug 16:10, Nov 18:9

81223 full gene sequence

➔ *CPT Changes: An Insider's View* 2012

➔ *CPT Assistant* May 12:4, Aug 16:10, Nov 18:9

81224 intron 8 poly-T analysis (eg, male infertility)

➔ *CPT Changes: An Insider's View* 2012

➔ *CPT Assistant* May 12:4, Aug 16:10, Nov 18:9

81267 Chimerism (engraftment) analysis, post transplantation specimen (eg, hematopoietic stem cell), includes comparison to previously performed baseline analyses; without cell selection

➔ *CPT Changes: An Insider's View* 2012

➔ *CPT Assistant* May 12:4, Aug 16:10, Nov 18:9

81268 with cell selection (eg, CD3, CD33), each cell type

➔ *CPT Changes: An Insider's View* 2012

➔ *CPT Assistant* May 12:4, Aug 16:10, Nov 18:9

(If comparative STR analysis of recipient [using buccal swab or other germline tissue sample] and donor are performed after hematopoietic stem cell transplantation, report 81265, 81266 in conjunction with 81267, 81268 for chimerism testing)

81187 *CNBP (CCHC-type zinc finger nucleic acid binding protein)* (eg, myotonic dystrophy type 2) gene analysis, evaluation to detect abnormal (eg, expanded) alleles

➔ *CPT Changes: An Insider's View* 2019

81265 Comparative analysis using Short Tandem Repeat (STR) markers; patient and comparative specimen (eg, pre-transplant recipient and donor germline testing, post-transplant non-hematopoietic recipient germline [eg, buccal swab or other germline tissue sample] and donor testing, twin zygosity testing, or maternal cell contamination of fetal cells)

➔ *CPT Changes: An Insider's View* 2012

➔ *CPT Assistant* May 12:4, Aug 16:10, Nov 18:9

#+ 81266 each additional specimen (eg, additional cord blood donor, additional fetal samples from different cultures, or additional zygosity in multiple birth pregnancies) (List separately in addition to code for primary procedure)

➔ *CPT Changes: An Insider's View* 2012

➔ *CPT Assistant* May 12:4, Aug 16:10, Nov 18:9

(Use 81266 in conjunction with 81265)

81188 *CSTB (cystatin B)* (eg, Unverricht-Lundborg disease) gene analysis; evaluation to detect abnormal (eg, expanded) alleles

➔ *CPT Changes: An Insider's View* 2019

81189 full gene sequence

➔ *CPT Changes: An Insider's View* 2019

81190 known familial variant(s)

➔ *CPT Changes: An Insider's View* 2019

81227 *CYP2C9 (cytochrome P450, family 2, subfamily C, polypeptide 9)* (eg, drug metabolism), gene analysis, common variants (eg, *2, *3, *5, *6)

➔ *CPT Changes: An Insider's View* 2012

➔ *CPT Assistant* May 12:4, Aug 16:10, Nov 18:9

81225 *CYP2C19 (cytochrome P450, family 2, subfamily C, polypeptide 19)* (eg, drug metabolism), gene analysis, common variants (eg, *2, *3, *4, *8, *17)

➔ *CPT Changes: An Insider's View* 2012

➔ *CPT Assistant* May 12:4, Aug 16:10, Nov 18:9

81226 *CYP2D6 (cytochrome P450, family 2, subfamily D, polypeptide 6)* (eg, drug metabolism), gene analysis, common variants (eg, *2, *3, *4, *5, *6, *9, *10, *17, *19, *29, *35, *41, *1XN, *2XN, *4XN)

➔ *CPT Changes: An Insider's View* 2012

➔ *CPT Assistant* May 12:4, Aug 16:10, Nov 18:9

81227 Code is out of numerical sequence. See 81223-81226

81230 *CYP3A4 (cytochrome P450 family 3 subfamily A member 4)* (eg, drug metabolism), gene analysis, common variant(s) (eg, *2, *22)

➔ *CPT Changes: An Insider's View* 2018

➔ *CPT Assistant* Nov 18:9

81231   *CYP3A5 (cytochrome P450 family 3 subfamily A member 5)* (eg, drug metabolism), gene analysis, common variants (eg, *2, *3, *4, *5, *6, *7)
➔ *CPT Changes: An Insider's View* 2018
➔ *CPT Assistant* Nov 18:9

81228   Cytogenomic (genome-wide) analysis for constitutional chromosomal abnormalities; interrogation of genomic regions for copy number variants, comparative genomic hybridization [CGH] microarray analysis
➔ *CPT Changes: An Insider's View* 2012, 2022
➔ *CPT Assistant* May 12:4, Sep 13:4, 6, Aug 16:10, Nov 18:9

(Do not report 81228 in conjunction with 81229, 81349)

81229   interrogation of genomic regions for copy number and single nucleotide polymorphism (SNP) variants, comparative genomic hybridization (CGH) microarray analysis
➔ *CPT Changes: An Insider's View* 2012, 2022
➔ *CPT Assistant* May 12:4, Sep 13:4, Aug 16:10, Nov 18:9, Apr 24:36

(Do not report 81229 in conjunction with 81228, 81349)

(Do not report 88271 when performing cytogenomic [genome-wide] analysis for constitutional chromosomal abnormalities)

(For genomic sequencing procedures or other molecular multianalyte assays for copy number analysis using circulating cell-free fetal DNA in maternal blood, see 81420, 81422, 81479)

81349   interrogation of genomic regions for copy number and loss-of-heterozygosity variants, low-pass sequencing analysis
➔ *CPT Changes: An Insider's View* 2022

(When performing cytogenomic [genome-wide] analysis for constitutional chromosomal abnormalities that is not genome-wide [ie, regionally targeted], report the specific code for the targeted analysis if available [eg, 81405], or the unlisted molecular pathology code [81479])

(Do not report 81349 in conjunction with 81228, 81229)

(Do not report 81349 when analysis for chromosomal abnormalities is performed by sequence analysis included in 81425, 81426)

(Do not report analyte-specific molecular pathology procedures separately in conjunction with 81228, 81229, 81349, when the specific analytes are included as part of the cytogenomic [genome-wide] analysis for constitutional chromosomal abnormalities)

81277   Cytogenomic neoplasia (genome-wide) microarray analysis, interrogation of genomic regions for copy number and loss-of-heterozygosity variants for chromosomal abnormalities
➔ *CPT Changes: An Insider's View* 2020
➔ *CPT Assistant* Feb 20:10

(Do not report analyte-specific molecular pathology procedures separately when the specific analytes are included as part of the cytogenomic microarray analysis for neoplasia)

(Do not report 88271 when performing cytogenomic microarray analysis)

#● 81195   Cytogenomic (genome-wide) analysis, hematologic malignancy, structural variants and copy number variants, optical genome mapping (OGM)
➔ *CPT Changes: An Insider's View* 2025

81230   Code is out of numerical sequence. See 81225-81229

81231   Code is out of numerical sequence. See 81225-81229

81161   *DMD (dystrophin)* (eg, Duchenne/Becker muscular dystrophy) deletion analysis, and duplication analysis, if performed
➔ *CPT Changes: An Insider's View* 2013
➔ *CPT Assistant* Aug 16:10, Nov 18:9

81234   *DMPK (DM1 protein kinase)* (eg, myotonic dystrophy type 1) gene analysis; evaluation to detect abnormal (expanded) alleles
➔ *CPT Changes: An Insider's View* 2019
➔ *CPT Assistant* Nov 18:9

81239   characterization of alleles (eg, expanded size)
➔ *CPT Changes: An Insider's View* 2019
➔ *CPT Assistant* Nov 18:9

81232   *DPYD (dihydropyrimidine dehydrogenase)* (eg, 5-fluorouracil/5-FU and capecitabine drug metabolism), gene analysis, common variant(s) (eg, *2A, *4, *5, *6)
➔ *CPT Changes: An Insider's View* 2018
➔ *CPT Assistant* Nov 18:9

81233   Code is out of numerical sequence. See 81215-81220

81234   Code is out of numerical sequence. See 81228-81235

81235   *EGFR (epidermal growth factor receptor)* (eg, non-small cell lung cancer) gene analysis, common variants (eg, exon 19 LREA deletion, L858R, T790M, G719A, G719S, L861Q)
➔ *CPT Changes: An Insider's View* 2013
➔ *CPT Assistant* Sep 13:3, Aug 16:10, Nov 18:9

81236   *EZH2 (enhancer of zeste 2 polycomb repressive complex 2 subunit)* (eg, myelodysplastic syndrome, myeloproliferative neoplasms) gene analysis, full gene sequence
➔ *CPT Changes: An Insider's View* 2019
➔ *CPT Assistant* Nov 18:9, Jul 19:3

81237   *EZH2 (enhancer of zeste 2 polycomb repressive complex 2 subunit)* (eg, diffuse large B-cell lymphoma) gene analysis, common variant(s) (eg, codon 646)
➔ *CPT Changes: An Insider's View* 2019
➔ *CPT Assistant* Nov 18:9, Jul 19:3

81238   Code is out of numerical sequence. See 81240-81248

81239   Code is out of numerical sequence. See 81228-81235

81240   *F2 (prothrombin, coagulation factor II)* (eg, hereditary hypercoagulability) gene analysis, 20210G>A variant
> *CPT Changes: An Insider's View* 2012
> *CPT Assistant* May 12:4, Aug 16:10, Nov 18:9

81241   *F5 (coagulation factor V)* (eg, hereditary hypercoagulability) gene analysis, Leiden variant
> *CPT Changes: An Insider's View* 2012
> *CPT Assistant* May 12:4, Aug 16:10, Nov 18:9

 # 81238   *F9 (coagulation factor IX)* (eg, hemophilia B), full gene sequence
> *CPT Changes: An Insider's View* 2018
> *CPT Assistant* Nov 18:9

81242   *FANCC (Fanconi anemia, complementation group C)* (eg, Fanconi anemia, type C) gene analysis, common variant (eg, IVS4+4A>T)
> *CPT Changes: An Insider's View* 2012
> *CPT Assistant* May 12:4, Aug 16:10, Nov 18:9

 # 81245   *FLT3 (fms-related tyrosine kinase 3)* (eg, acute myeloid leukemia), gene analysis; internal tandem duplication (ITD) variants (ie, exons 14, 15)
> *CPT Changes: An Insider's View* 2012, 2015
> *CPT Assistant* May 12:4, Jan 15:3, Aug 16:10, Nov 18:9

 # 81246   tyrosine kinase domain (TKD) variants (eg, D835, I836)
> *CPT Changes: An Insider's View* 2015
> *CPT Assistant* Jan 15:3, Aug 16:10, Nov 18:9

81243   *FMR1 (fragile X messenger ribonucleoprotein 1)* (eg, fragile X syndrome, X-linked intellectual disability [XLID]) gene analysis; evaluation to detect abnormal (eg, expanded) alleles
> *CPT Changes: An Insider's View* 2012, 2024
> *CPT Assistant* May 12:4, Aug 16:10, Nov 18:9

(For evaluation to detect and characterize abnormal alleles, see 81243, 81244)

(For evaluation to detect and characterize abnormal alleles using a single assay [eg, PCR], use 81243)

81244   characterization of alleles (eg, expanded size and promoter methylation status)
> *CPT Changes: An Insider's View* 2012, 2019, 2024
> *CPT Assistant* May 12:4, Aug 16:10, Nov 18:9, Jul 19:3

81245   Code is out of numerical sequence. See 81240-81248

81246   Code is out of numerical sequence. See 81240-81248

 # 81284   *FXN (frataxin)* (eg, Friedreich ataxia) gene analysis; evaluation to detect abnormal (expanded) alleles
> *CPT Changes: An Insider's View* 2019
> *CPT Assistant* Nov 18:9

 # 81285   characterization of alleles (eg, expanded size)
> *CPT Changes: An Insider's View* 2019
> *CPT Assistant* Nov 18:9

 # 81286   full gene sequence
> *CPT Changes: An Insider's View* 2019
> *CPT Assistant* Nov 18:9

 # 81289   known familial variant(s)
> *CPT Changes: An Insider's View* 2019
> *CPT Assistant* Nov 18:9

 # 81250   *G6PC (glucose-6-phosphatase, catalytic subunit)* (eg, Glycogen storage disease, type 1a, von Gierke disease) gene analysis, common variants (eg, R83C, Q347X)
> *CPT Changes: An Insider's View* 2012
> *CPT Assistant* May 12:4, Aug 16:10, Nov 18:9

81247   *G6PD (glucose-6-phosphate dehydrogenase)* (eg, hemolytic anemia, jaundice), gene analysis; common variant(s) (eg, A, A-)
> *CPT Changes: An Insider's View* 2018
> *CPT Assistant* Nov 18:9

81248   known familial variant(s)
> *CPT Changes: An Insider's View* 2018

81249   full gene sequence
> *CPT Changes: An Insider's View* 2018
> *CPT Assistant* Nov 18:9

81250   Code is out of numerical sequence. See 81243-81248

81251   *GBA (glucosidase, beta, acid)* (eg, Gaucher disease) gene analysis, common variants (eg, N370S, 84GG, L444P, IVS2+1G>A)
> *CPT Changes: An Insider's View* 2012
> *CPT Assistant* May 12:4, Aug 16:10, Nov 18:9

81252   *GJB2 (gap junction protein, beta 2, 26kDa, connexin 26)* (eg, nonsyndromic hearing loss) gene analysis; full gene sequence
> *CPT Changes: An Insider's View* 2013
> *CPT Assistant* Sep 13:3, Aug 16:10, Nov 18:9

81253   known familial variants
> *CPT Changes: An Insider's View* 2013
> *CPT Assistant* Sep 13:3, Aug 16:10, Nov 18:9

81254   *GJB6 (gap junction protein, beta 6, 30kDa, connexin 30)* (eg, nonsyndromic hearing loss) gene analysis, common variants (eg, 309kb [del(GJB6-D13S1830)] and 232kb [del(GJB6-D13S1854)])
> *CPT Changes: An Insider's View* 2013
> *CPT Assistant* Sep 13:3, Aug 16:10, Nov 18:9

 # 81257   *HBA1/HBA2 (alpha globin 1 and alpha globin 2)* (eg, alpha thalassemia, Hb Bart hydrops fetalis syndrome, HbH disease), gene analysis; common deletions or variant (eg, Southeast Asian, Thai, Filipino, Mediterranean, alpha3.7, alpha4.2, alpha20.5, Constant Spring)
> *CPT Changes: An Insider's View* 2012, 2018
> *CPT Assistant* May 12:4, Aug 16:10, Nov 18:9

 # 81258   known familial variant
> *CPT Changes: An Insider's View* 2018
> *CPT Assistant* Nov 18:9

 # 81259   full gene sequence
> *CPT Changes: An Insider's View* 2018
> *CPT Assistant* Nov 18:9

 # 81269   duplication/deletion variants
> *CPT Changes: An Insider's View* 2018
> *CPT Assistant* Nov 18:9

 # 81361   *HBB (hemoglobin, subunit beta)* (eg, sickle cell anemia, beta thalassemia, hemoglobinopathy); common variant(s) (eg, HbS, HbC, HbE)
> *CPT Changes: An Insider's View* 2018
> *CPT Assistant* Nov 18:9

 # 81362   known familial variant(s)
> *CPT Changes: An Insider's View* 2018
> *CPT Assistant* Nov 18:9

 # 81363   duplication/deletion variant(s)
> *CPT Changes: An Insider's View* 2018
> *CPT Assistant* Sep 18:14, Nov 18:9

 # 81364   full gene sequence
> *CPT Changes: An Insider's View* 2018
> *CPT Assistant* Sep 18:14, Nov 18:9

81255   *HEXA (hexosaminidase A [alpha polypeptide])* (eg, Tay-Sachs disease) gene analysis, common variants (eg, 1278insTATC, 1421+1G>C, G269S)
> *CPT Changes: An Insider's View* 2012
> *CPT Assistant* May 12:4, Aug 16:10, Nov 18:9

81256   *HFE (hemochromatosis)* (eg, hereditary hemochromatosis) gene analysis, common variants (eg, C282Y, H63D)
> *CPT Changes: An Insider's View* 2012
> *CPT Assistant* May 12:4, Aug 16:10, Nov 18:9

81257   Code is out of numerical sequence. See 81253-81256

81258   Code is out of numerical sequence. See 81253-81256

81259   Code is out of numerical sequence. See 81253-81256

 # 81271   *HTT (huntingtin)* (eg, Huntington disease) gene analysis; evaluation to detect abnormal (eg, expanded) alleles
> *CPT Changes: An Insider's View* 2019
> *CPT Assistant* Nov 18:9

 # 81274   characterization of alleles (eg, expanded size)
> *CPT Changes: An Insider's View* 2019
> *CPT Assistant* Nov 18:9

 # 81105   *Human Platelet Antigen 1 genotyping (HPA-1), ITGB3 (integrin, beta 3 [platelet glycoprotein IIIa], antigen CD61 [GPIIIa])* (eg, neonatal alloimmune thrombocytopenia [NAIT], post-transfusion purpura), gene analysis, common variant, HPA-1a/b (L33P)
> *CPT Changes: An Insider's View* 2018

 # 81106   *Human Platelet Antigen 2 genotyping (HPA-2), GP1BA (glycoprotein Ib [platelet], alpha polypeptide [GPIba])* (eg, neonatal alloimmune thrombocytopenia [NAIT], post-transfusion purpura), gene analysis, common variant, HPA-2a/b (T145M)
> *CPT Changes: An Insider's View* 2018

 # 81107   *Human Platelet Antigen 3 genotyping (HPA-3), ITGA2B (integrin, alpha 2b [platelet glycoprotein IIb of IIb/IIIa complex], antigen CD41 [GPIIb])* (eg, neonatal alloimmune thrombocytopenia [NAIT], post-transfusion purpura), gene analysis, common variant, HPA-3a/b (I843S)
> *CPT Changes: An Insider's View* 2018

 # 81108   *Human Platelet Antigen 4 genotyping (HPA-4), ITGB3 (integrin, beta 3 [platelet glycoprotein IIIa], antigen CD61 [GPIIIa])* (eg, neonatal alloimmune thrombocytopenia [NAIT], post-transfusion purpura), gene analysis, common variant, HPA-4a/b (R143Q)
> *CPT Changes: An Insider's View* 2018

 # 81109   *Human Platelet Antigen 5 genotyping (HPA-5), ITGA2 (integrin, alpha 2 [CD49B, alpha 2 subunit of VLA-2 receptor] [GPIa])* (eg, neonatal alloimmune thrombocytopenia [NAIT], post-transfusion purpura), gene analysis, common variant (eg, HPA-5a/b [K505E])
> *CPT Changes: An Insider's View* 2018

 # 81110   *Human Platelet Antigen 6 genotyping (HPA-6w), ITGB3 (integrin, beta 3 [platelet glycoprotein IIIa, antigen CD61] [GPIIIa])* (eg, neonatal alloimmune thrombocytopenia [NAIT], post-transfusion purpura), gene analysis, common variant, HPA-6a/b (R489Q)
> *CPT Changes: An Insider's View* 2018

 # 81111   *Human Platelet Antigen 9 genotyping (HPA-9w), ITGA2B (integrin, alpha 2b [platelet glycoprotein IIb of IIb/IIIa complex, antigen CD41] [GPIIb])* (eg, neonatal alloimmune thrombocytopenia [NAIT], post-transfusion purpura), gene analysis, common variant, HPA-9a/b (V837M)
> *CPT Changes: An Insider's View* 2018

 # 81112   *Human Platelet Antigen 15 genotyping (HPA-15), CD109 (CD109 molecule)* (eg, neonatal alloimmune thrombocytopenia [NAIT], post-transfusion purpura), gene analysis, common variant, HPA-15a/b (S682Y)
> *CPT Changes: An Insider's View* 2018

 # 81120   *IDH1 (isocitrate dehydrogenase 1 [NADP+], soluble)* (eg, glioma), common variants (eg, R132H, R132C)
> *CPT Changes: An Insider's View* 2018

 # 81121   *IDH2 (isocitrate dehydrogenase 2 [NADP+], mitochondrial)* (eg, glioma), common variants (eg, R140W, R172M)
> *CPT Changes: An Insider's View* 2018

81283   IFNL3 (interferon, lambda 3) (eg, drug response), gene analysis, rs12979860 variant
➔ CPT Changes: An Insider's View 2018
➔ CPT Assistant Nov 18:9

81261   IGH@ (Immunoglobulin heavy chain locus) (eg, leukemias and lymphomas, B-cell), gene rearrangement analysis to detect abnormal clonal population(s); amplified methodology (eg, polymerase chain reaction)
➔ CPT Changes: An Insider's View 2012
➔ CPT Assistant May 12:4, Sep 13:7, Aug 16:10, Nov 18:9

81262   direct probe methodology (eg, Southern blot)
➔ CPT Changes: An Insider's View 2012
➔ CPT Assistant May 12:4, Aug 16:10, Nov 18:9

81263   IGH@ (Immunoglobulin heavy chain locus) (eg, leukemia and lymphoma, B-cell), variable region somatic mutation analysis
➔ CPT Changes: An Insider's View 2012
➔ CPT Assistant May 12:4, Aug 16:10, Nov 18:9

81278   IGH@/BCL2 (t(14;18)) (eg, follicular lymphoma) translocation analysis, major breakpoint region (MBR) and minor cluster region (mcr) breakpoints, qualitative or quantitative
➔ CPT Changes: An Insider's View 2021
➔ CPT Assistant Aug 21:10

81264   IGK@ (Immunoglobulin kappa light chain locus) (eg, leukemia and lymphoma, B-cell), gene rearrangement analysis, evaluation to detect abnormal clonal population(s)
➔ CPT Changes: An Insider's View 2012
➔ CPT Assistant May 12:4, Aug 16:10, Nov 18:9

(For immunoglobulin lambda gene [IGL@] rearrangement or immunoglobulin kappa deleting element, [IGKDEL] analysis, use 81479)

81260   IKBKAP (inhibitor of kappa light polypeptide gene enhancer in B-cells, kinase complex-associated protein) (eg, familial dysautonomia) gene analysis, common variants (eg, 2507+6T>C, R696P)
➔ CPT Changes: An Insider's View 2012
➔ CPT Assistant May 12:4, Aug 16:10, Nov 18:9

81261   Code is out of numerical sequence. See 81255-81270

81262   Code is out of numerical sequence. See 81255-81270

81263   Code is out of numerical sequence. See 81255-81270

81264   Code is out of numerical sequence. See 81255-81270

81265   Code is out of numerical sequence. See 81223-81226

81266   Code is out of numerical sequence. See 81223-81226

81267   Code is out of numerical sequence. See 81223-81226

81268   Code is out of numerical sequence. See 81223-81226

81269   Code is out of numerical sequence. See 81253-81256

81270   JAK2 (Janus kinase 2) (eg, myeloproliferative disorder) gene analysis, p.Val617Phe (V617F) variant
➔ CPT Changes: An Insider's View 2012
➔ CPT Assistant May 12:4, Aug 16:10, Nov 18:9

81279   JAK2 (Janus kinase 2) (eg, myeloproliferative disorder) targeted sequence analysis (eg, exons 12 and 13)
➔ CPT Changes: An Insider's View 2021
➔ CPT Assistant Aug 21:10

81271   Code is out of numerical sequence. See 81255-81270

81272   KIT (v-kit Hardy-Zuckerman 4 feline sarcoma viral oncogene homolog) (eg, gastrointestinal stromal tumor [GIST], acute myeloid leukemia, melanoma), gene analysis, targeted sequence analysis (eg, exons 8, 11, 13, 17, 18)
➔ CPT Changes: An Insider's View 2016
➔ CPT Assistant Aug 16:10, Nov 18:9

81273   KIT (v-kit Hardy-Zuckerman 4 feline sarcoma viral oncogene homolog) (eg, mastocytosis), gene analysis, D816 variant(s)
➔ CPT Changes: An Insider's View 2016
➔ CPT Assistant Aug 16:10, Nov 18:9

81274   Code is out of numerical sequence. See 81255-81270

81275   KRAS (Kirsten rat sarcoma viral oncogene homolog) (eg, carcinoma) gene analysis; variants in exon 2 (eg, codons 12 and 13)
➔ CPT Changes: An Insider's View 2012, 2016
➔ CPT Assistant May 12:4, Sep 13:6, Aug 16:10, Nov 18:9

81276   additional variant(s) (eg, codon 61, codon 146)
➔ CPT Changes: An Insider's View 2016
➔ CPT Assistant Aug 16:10, Nov 18:9

81277   Code is out of numerical sequence. See 81228-81235

81278   Code is out of numerical sequence. See 81255-81260

81279   Code is out of numerical sequence. See 81260-81273

81283   Code is out of numerical sequence. See 81255-81270

81284   Code is out of numerical sequence. See 81243-81248

81285   Code is out of numerical sequence. See 81243-81248

81286   Code is out of numerical sequence. See 81243-81248

81287   Code is out of numerical sequence. See 81276-81297

81288   Code is out of numerical sequence. See 81276-81297

81289   Code is out of numerical sequence. See 81243-81248

81290   MCOLN1 (mucolipin 1) (eg, Mucolipidosis, type IV) gene analysis, common variants (eg, IVS3-2A>G, del6.4kb)
➔ CPT Changes: An Insider's View 2012
➔ CPT Assistant May 12:4, Aug 16:10, Nov 18:9

81302   MECP2 (methyl CpG binding protein 2) (eg, Rett syndrome) gene analysis; full sequence analysis
➔ CPT Changes: An Insider's View 2012
➔ CPT Assistant May 12:4, Aug 16:10, Nov 18:9

Pathology and Laboratory   80047-89398, 0001U-0520U

644   ★=Telemedicine   ◀=Audio-only   +=Add-on code   ✒=FDA approval pending   #=Resequenced code   ⊘=Modifier 51 exempt   ➔➔➔=See p xxi for details

81303   known familial variant
- *CPT Changes: An Insider's View* 2012
- *CPT Assistant* May 12:4, Aug 16:10, Nov 18:9

81304   duplication/deletion variants
- *CPT Changes: An Insider's View* 2012
- *CPT Assistant* May 12:4, Aug 16:10, Nov 18:9

81287   *MGMT (O-6-methylguanine-DNA methyltransferase)* (eg, glioblastoma multiforme) promoter methylation analysis
- *CPT Changes: An Insider's View* 2014, 2019
- *CPT Assistant* Aug 16:10, Nov 18:9, Dec 18:10, Jul 19:3

81301   Microsatellite instability analysis (eg, hereditary non-polyposis colorectal cancer, Lynch syndrome) of markers for mismatch repair deficiency (eg, BAT25, BAT26), includes comparison of neoplastic and normal tissue, if performed
- *CPT Changes: An Insider's View* 2012
- *CPT Assistant* May 12:4, Aug 16:10, Nov 18:9

81292   *MLH1 (mutL homolog 1, colon cancer, nonpolyposis type 2)* (eg, hereditary non-polyposis colorectal cancer, Lynch syndrome) gene analysis; full sequence analysis
- *CPT Changes: An Insider's View* 2012
- *CPT Assistant* May 12:4, Jan 15:3, Aug 16:10, Nov 18:9

81288   promoter methylation analysis
- *CPT Changes: An Insider's View* 2015
- *CPT Assistant* Jan 15:3, Aug 16:10, Nov 18:9

81293   known familial variants
- *CPT Changes: An Insider's View* 2012
- *CPT Assistant* May 12:4, Aug 16:10, Nov 18:9

81294   duplication/deletion variants
- *CPT Changes: An Insider's View* 2012
- *CPT Assistant* May 12:4, Aug 16:10, Nov 18:9

81338   *MPL (MPL proto-oncogene, thrombopoietin receptor)* (eg, myeloproliferative disorder) gene analysis; common variants (eg, W515A, W515K, W515L, W515R)
- *CPT Changes: An Insider's View* 2021
- *CPT Assistant* Aug 21:10

81339   sequence analysis, exon 10
- *CPT Changes: An Insider's View* 2021
- *CPT Assistant* Aug 21:10

81295   *MSH2 (mutS homolog 2, colon cancer, nonpolyposis type 1)* (eg, hereditary non-polyposis colorectal cancer, Lynch syndrome) gene analysis; full sequence analysis
- *CPT Changes: An Insider's View* 2012
- *CPT Assistant* May 12:4, Aug 16:10, Nov 18:9

81291   Code is out of numerical sequence. See 81299-81310

81292   Code is out of numerical sequence. See 81276-81297

81293   Code is out of numerical sequence. See 81276-81297

81294   Code is out of numerical sequence. See 81276-81297

81295   Code is out of numerical sequence. See 81276-81297

81296   known familial variants
- *CPT Changes: An Insider's View* 2012
- *CPT Assistant* May 12:3, Aug 16:10, Nov 18:9

81297   duplication/deletion variants
- *CPT Changes: An Insider's View* 2012
- *CPT Assistant* May 12:4, Aug 16:10, Nov 18:9

81298   *MSH6 (mutS homolog 6 [E. coli])* (eg, hereditary non-polyposis colorectal cancer, Lynch syndrome) gene analysis; full sequence analysis
- *CPT Changes: An Insider's View* 2012
- *CPT Assistant* May 12:4, Aug 16:10, Nov 18:9

81299   known familial variants
- *CPT Changes: An Insider's View* 2012
- *CPT Assistant* May 12:4, Aug 16:10, Nov 18:9

81300   duplication/deletion variants
- *CPT Changes: An Insider's View* 2012
- *CPT Assistant* May 12:4, Aug 16:10, Nov 18:9

81301   Code is out of numerical sequence. See 81276-81297

81302   Code is out of numerical sequence. See 81276-81297

81303   Code is out of numerical sequence. See 81276-81297

81304   Code is out of numerical sequence. See 81276-81297

81291   *MTHFR (5,10-methylenetetrahydrofolate reductase)* (eg, hereditary hypercoagulability) gene analysis, common variants (eg, 677T, 1298C)
- *CPT Changes: An Insider's View* 2012
- *CPT Assistant* May 12:4, Aug 16:10, Nov 18:9

81305   *MYD88 (myeloid differentiation primary response 88)* (eg, Waldenstrom's macroglobulinemia, lymphoplasmacytic leukemia) gene analysis, p.Leu265Pro (L265P) variant
- *CPT Changes: An Insider's View* 2019
- *CPT Assistant* Nov 18:9, Jul 19:3

81306   Code is out of numerical sequence. See 81310-81316

81307   Code is out of numerical sequence. See 81310-81316

81308   Code is out of numerical sequence. See 81310-81316

81309   Code is out of numerical sequence. See 81310-81316

81310   *NPM1 (nucleophosmin)* (eg, acute myeloid leukemia) gene analysis, exon 12 variants
- *CPT Changes: An Insider's View* 2012
- *CPT Assistant* May 12:4, Aug 16:10, Nov 18:9

81311   *NRAS (neuroblastoma RAS viral [v-ras] oncogene homolog)* (eg, colorectal carcinoma), gene analysis, variants in exon 2 (eg, codons 12 and 13) and exon 3 (eg, codon 61)
- *CPT Changes: An Insider's View* 2016
- *CPT Assistant* Aug 16:10

81312   Code is out of numerical sequence. See 81310-81316

▲ = Revised code   ● = New code   ▶ ◀ = Contains new or revised text   ✕ = Duplicate PLA test   ↕ = Category I PLA   American Medical Association   **645**

Pathology and Laboratory 80047-89398, 0001U-0520U

 # 81191   *NTRK1 (neurotrophic receptor tyrosine kinase 1)* (eg, solid tumors) translocation analysis
➔ *CPT Changes: An Insider's View* 2021

 # 81192   *NTRK2 (neurotrophic receptor tyrosine kinase 2)* (eg, solid tumors) translocation analysis
➔ *CPT Changes: An Insider's View* 2021

 # 81193   *NTRK3 (neurotrophic receptor tyrosine kinase 3)* (eg, solid tumors) translocation analysis
➔ *CPT Changes: An Insider's View* 2021

 # 81194   *NTRK (neurotrophic receptor tyrosine kinase 1, 2, and 3)* (eg, solid tumors) translocation analysis
➔ *CPT Changes: An Insider's View* 2021, 2022

(For translocation analysis *NTRK1, NTRK2,* and *NTRK3* using a single assay, use 81194)

 # 81306   *NUDT15 (nudix hydrolase 15)* (eg, drug metabolism) gene analysis, common variant(s) (eg, *2, *3, *4, *5, *6)
➔ *CPT Changes: An Insider's View* 2019
➔ *CPT Assistant* Nov 18:9, Jul 19:3

 # 81312   *PABPN1 (poly[A] binding protein nuclear 1)* (eg, oculopharyngeal muscular dystrophy) gene analysis, evaluation to detect abnormal (eg, expanded) alleles
➔ *CPT Changes: An Insider's View* 2019

 # 81307   *PALB2 (partner and localizer of BRCA2)* (eg, breast and pancreatic cancer) gene analysis; full gene sequence
➔ *CPT Changes: An Insider's View* 2020
➔ *CPT Assistant* Mar 20:13

 # 81308   known familial variant
➔ *CPT Changes: An Insider's View* 2020
➔ *CPT Assistant* Mar 20:13

81313   *PCA3/KLK3 (prostate cancer antigen 3 [non-protein coding]/kallikrein-related peptidase 3 [prostate specific antigen])* ratio (eg, prostate cancer)
➔ *CPT Changes: An Insider's View* 2015
➔ *CPT Assistant* Jan 15:3, Aug 16:10

81314   *PDGFRA (platelet-derived growth factor receptor, alpha polypeptide)* (eg, gastrointestinal stromal tumor [GIST]), gene analysis, targeted sequence analysis (eg, exons 12, 18)
➔ *CPT Changes: An Insider's View* 2016
➔ *CPT Assistant* Aug 16:10

 # 81309   *PIK3CA (phosphatidylinositol-4, 5-biphosphate 3-kinase, catalytic subunit alpha)* (eg, colorectal and breast cancer) gene analysis, targeted sequence analysis (eg, exons 7, 9, 20)
➔ *CPT Changes: An Insider's View* 2020
➔ *CPT Assistant* Apr 20:11

 # 81320   *PLCG2 (phospholipase C gamma 2)* (eg, chronic lymphocytic leukemia) gene analysis, common variants (eg, R665W, S707F, L845F)
➔ *CPT Changes: An Insider's View* 2019
➔ *CPT Assistant* Jul 19:3

81315   *PML/RARalpha, (t(15;17)), (promyelocytic leukemia/ retinoic acid receptor alpha)* (eg, promyelocytic leukemia) translocation analysis; common breakpoints (eg, intron 3 and intron 6), qualitative or quantitative
➔ *CPT Changes: An Insider's View* 2012
➔ *CPT Assistant* May 12:4, Aug 16:10

81316   single breakpoint (eg, intron 3, intron 6 or exon 6), qualitative or quantitative
➔ *CPT Changes: An Insider's View* 2012
➔ *CPT Assistant* May 12:4, Aug 16:10

(For intron 3 and intron 6 [including exon 6 if performed] analysis, use 81315)

(If both intron 6 and exon 6 are analyzed, without intron 3, use one unit of 81316)

 # 81324   *PMP22 (peripheral myelin protein 22)* (eg, Charcot-Marie-Tooth, hereditary neuropathy with liability to pressure palsies) gene analysis; duplication/deletion analysis
➔ *CPT Changes: An Insider's View* 2013
➔ *CPT Assistant* Sep 13:3, Aug 16:10, Nov 18:9

 # 81325   full sequence analysis
➔ *CPT Changes: An Insider's View* 2013
➔ *CPT Assistant* Sep 13:3, Aug 16:10, May 18:6, Nov 18:9

 # 81326   known familial variant
➔ *CPT Changes: An Insider's View* 2013
➔ *CPT Assistant* Sep 13:3, Aug 16:10, Nov 18:9

81317   *PMS2 (postmeiotic segregation increased 2 [S. cerevisiae])* (eg, hereditary non-polyposis colorectal cancer, Lynch syndrome) gene analysis; full sequence analysis
➔ *CPT Changes: An Insider's View* 2012
➔ *CPT Assistant* May 12:4, Aug 16:10, Nov 18:9

81318   known familial variants
➔ *CPT Changes: An Insider's View* 2012
➔ *CPT Assistant* May 12:4, Aug 16:10, Nov 18:9

81319   duplication/deletion variants
➔ *CPT Changes: An Insider's View* 2012
➔ *CPT Assistant* May 12:4, Aug 16:10, Nov 18:9

81320   Code is out of numerical sequence. See 81310-81316

 # 81343   *PPP2R2B (protein phosphatase 2 regulatory subunit Bbeta)* (eg, spinocerebellar ataxia) gene analysis, evaluation to detect abnormal (eg, expanded) alleles
➔ *CPT Changes: An Insider's View* 2019
➔ *CPT Assistant* Nov 18:9

81321   PTEN (phosphatase and tensin homolog) (eg, Cowden syndrome, PTEN hamartoma tumor syndrome) gene analysis; full sequence analysis

➔ CPT Changes: An Insider's View 2013

➔ CPT Assistant Sep 13:3, Aug 16:10, Nov 18:9

81322   known familial variant

➔ CPT Changes: An Insider's View 2013

➔ CPT Assistant Sep 13:3, Aug 16:10, Nov 18:9

81323   duplication/deletion variant

➔ CPT Changes: An Insider's View 2013

➔ CPT Assistant Sep 13:3, Aug 16:10, Nov 18:9

81324   Code is out of numerical sequence. See 81310-81318

81325   Code is out of numerical sequence. See 81310-81318

81326   Code is out of numerical sequence. See 81310-81318

 # 81334   RUNX1 (runt related transcription factor 1) (eg, acute myeloid leukemia, familial platelet disorder with associated myeloid malignancy) gene analysis, targeted sequence analysis (eg, exons 3-8)

➔ CPT Changes: An Insider's View 2018

➔ CPT Assistant Nov 18:9

81327   SEPT9 (Septin9) (eg, colorectal cancer) promoter methylation analysis

➔ CPT Changes: An Insider's View 2017, 2019

➔ CPT Assistant Nov 18:9, Jul 19:3

 # 81332   SERPINA1 (serpin peptidase inhibitor, clade A, alpha-1 antiproteinase, antitrypsin, member 1) (eg, alpha-1-antitrypsin deficiency), gene analysis, common variants (eg, *S and *Z)

➔ CPT Changes: An Insider's View 2012

➔ CPT Assistant May 12:4, Aug 16:10, Nov 18:9

 # 81347   SF3B1 (splicing factor [3b] subunit B1) (eg, myelodysplastic syndrome/acute myeloid leukemia) gene analysis, common variants (eg, A672T, E622D, L833F, R625C, R625L)

➔ CPT Changes: An Insider's View 2021

➔ CPT Assistant Jun 21:9

81328   SLCO1B1 (solute carrier organic anion transporter family, member 1B1) (eg, adverse drug reaction), gene analysis, common variant(s) (eg, *5)

➔ CPT Changes: An Insider's View 2018

➔ CPT Assistant Nov 18:9

81329   SMN1 (survival of motor neuron 1, telomeric) (eg, spinal muscular atrophy) gene analysis; dosage/deletion analysis (eg, carrier testing), includes SMN2 (survival of motor neuron 2, centromeric) analysis, if performed

➔ CPT Changes: An Insider's View 2019

➔ CPT Assistant Nov 18:9, Jul 19:3

 # 81336   full gene sequence

➔ CPT Changes: An Insider's View 2019

➔ CPT Assistant Nov 18:9, Jul 19:3

 # 81337   known familial sequence variant(s)

➔ CPT Changes: An Insider's View 2019

➔ CPT Assistant Nov 18:9, Jul 19:3

81330   SMPD1 (sphingomyelin phosphodiesterase 1, acid lysosomal) (eg, Niemann-Pick disease, Type A) gene analysis, common variants (eg, R496L, L302P, fsP330)

➔ CPT Changes: An Insider's View 2012

➔ CPT Assistant May 12:4, Aug 16:10, Nov 18:9

81331   SNRPN/UBE3A (small nuclear ribonucleoprotein polypeptide N and ubiquitin protein ligase E3A) (eg, Prader-Willi syndrome and/or Angelman syndrome), methylation analysis

➔ CPT Changes: An Insider's View 2012

➔ CPT Assistant May 12:4, Aug 16:10, Nov 18:9

81332   Code is out of numerical sequence. See 81318-81335

 # 81348   SRSF2 (serine and arginine-rich splicing factor 2) (eg, myelodysplastic syndrome, acute myeloid leukemia) gene analysis, common variants (eg, P95H, P95L)

➔ CPT Changes: An Insider's View 2021

➔ CPT Assistant Jun 21:9

 # 81344   TBP (TATA box binding protein) (eg, spinocerebellar ataxia) gene analysis, evaluation to detect abnormal (eg, expanded) alleles

➔ CPT Changes: An Insider's View 2019

➔ CPT Assistant Nov 18:9

 # 81345   TERT (telomerase reverse transcriptase) (eg, thyroid carcinoma, glioblastoma multiforme) gene analysis, targeted sequence analysis (eg, promoter region)

➔ CPT Changes: An Insider's View 2019

➔ CPT Assistant Nov 18:9, Jul 19:3

81333   TGFBI (transforming growth factor beta-induced) (eg, corneal dystrophy) gene analysis, common variants (eg, R124H, R124C, R124L, R555W, R555Q)

➔ CPT Changes: An Insider's View 2019

➔ CPT Assistant Nov 18:9, Jul 19:3

81334   Code is out of numerical sequence. See 81318-81335

 # 81351   TP53 (tumor protein 53) (eg, Li-Fraumeni syndrome) gene analysis; full gene sequence

➔ CPT Changes: An Insider's View 2021

 # 81352   targeted sequence analysis (eg, 4 oncology)

➔ CPT Changes: An Insider's View 2021

 # 81353   known familial variant

➔ CPT Changes: An Insider's View 2021

81335   TPMT (thiopurine S-methyltransferase) (eg, drug metabolism), gene analysis, common variants (eg, *2, *3)

➔ CPT Changes: An Insider's View 2018

➔ CPT Assistant Nov 18:9, Apr 23:18

81336   Code is out of numerical sequence. See 81318-81335

81337   Code is out of numerical sequence. See 81318-81335

Pathology and Laboratory 80047-89398, 0001U-0520U

81338 Code is out of numerical sequence. See 81276-81297

81339 Code is out of numerical sequence. See 81276-81297

81340 *TRB@ (T cell antigen receptor, beta)* (eg, leukemia and lymphoma), gene rearrangement analysis to detect abnormal clonal population(s); using amplification methodology (eg, polymerase chain reaction)

➔ *CPT Changes: An Insider's View* 2012

➔ *CPT Assistant* May 12:4, Aug 16:10, Nov 18:9

81341 using direct probe methodology (eg, Southern blot)

➔ *CPT Changes: An Insider's View* 2012

➔ *CPT Assistant* May 12:4, Aug 16:10, Nov 18:9

81342 *TRG@ (T cell antigen receptor, gamma)* (eg, leukemia and lymphoma), gene rearrangement analysis, evaluation to detect abnormal clonal population(s)

➔ *CPT Changes: An Insider's View* 2012

➔ *CPT Assistant* May 12:4, Aug 16:10, Nov 18:9

(For T cell antigen alpha *[TRA@]* gene rearrangement analysis, use 81479)

(For T cell antigen delta *[TRD@]* gene rearrangement analysis, use 81402)

81343 Code is out of numerical sequence. See 81318-81335

81344 Code is out of numerical sequence. See 81318-81335

81345 Code is out of numerical sequence. See 81318-81335

81346 *TYMS (thymidylate synthetase)* (eg, 5-fluorouracil/5-FU drug metabolism), gene analysis, common variant(s) (eg, tandem repeat variant)

➔ *CPT Changes: An Insider's View* 2018

➔ *CPT Assistant* Nov 18:9

81347 Code is out of numerical sequence. See 81327-81329

81348 Code is out of numerical sequence. See 81330-81340

81349 Code is out of numerical sequence. See 81228-81235

 # 81357 *U2AF1 (U2 small nuclear RNA auxiliary factor 1)* (eg, myelodysplastic syndrome, acute myeloid leukemia) gene analysis, common variants (eg, S34F, S34Y, Q157R, Q157P)

➔ *CPT Changes: An Insider's View* 2021

➔ *CPT Assistant* Jun 21:9

81350 *UGT1A1 (UDP glucuronosyltransferase 1 family, polypeptide A1)* (eg, drug metabolism, hereditary unconjugated hyperbilirubinemia [Gilbert syndrome]) gene analysis, common variants (eg, *28, *36, *37)

➔ *CPT Changes: An Insider's View* 2012, 2020

➔ *CPT Assistant* May 12:4, Aug 16:10, Nov 18:9, Apr 20:9

81351 Code is out of numerical sequence. See 81330-81340

81352 Code is out of numerical sequence. See 81330-81340

81353 Code is out of numerical sequence. See 81330-81340

81355 *VKORC1 (vitamin K epoxide reductase complex, subunit 1)* (eg, warfarin metabolism), gene analysis, common variant(s) (eg, -1639G>A, c.173+1000C>T)

➔ *CPT Changes: An Insider's View* 2012, 2016

➔ *CPT Assistant* May 12:4, Aug 16:10, Nov 18:9

81357 Code is out of numerical sequence. See 81342-81355

81360 *ZRSR2 (zinc finger CCCH-type, RNA binding motif and serine/arginine-rich 2)* (eg, myelodysplastic syndrome, acute myeloid leukemia) gene analysis, common variant(s) (eg, E65fs, E122fs, R448fs)

➔ *CPT Changes: An Insider's View* 2021

➔ *CPT Assistant* Jun 21:9

81361 Code is out of numerical sequence. See 81253-81256

81362 Code is out of numerical sequence. See 81253-81256

81363 Code is out of numerical sequence. See 81253-81256

81364 Code is out of numerical sequence. See 81253-81256

Human leukocyte antigen (HLA) typing is performed to assess compatibility of recipients and potential donors as a part of solid organ and hematopoietic stem cell pretransplant testing. HLA testing is also performed to identify HLA alleles and allele groups (antigen equivalents) associated with specific diseases and individualized responses to drug therapy (eg, HLA-B*27 and ankylosing spondylitis and HLA-B*57:01 and abacavir hypersensitivity), as well as other clinical uses. One or more HLA genes may be tested in specific clinical situations (eg, HLA-DQB1 for narcolepsy and HLA-A, -B, -C, -DRB1, and -DQB1 for kidney transplantation). Each HLA gene typically has multiple variant alleles or allele groups that can be identified by typing. For HLA result reporting, a low resolution HLA type is denoted by a two digit HLA name (eg, A*02) and intermediate resolution typing by a string of alleles or an NMDP (National Marrow Donor Program) code (eg, B*14:01/07N/08/12/14, B*39CKGN). Both low and intermediate resolutions are considered low resolution for code assignment. High resolution typing resolves the common well defined (CWD) alleles and is usually denoted by at least 4 digits (eg, A*02:02, *03:01:01:01, A*26:01:01G, and C*03:04P), however, high resolution typing may include some ambiguities for rare alleles, which may be reported as a string of alleles or an NMDP code.

If additional testing is required to resolve ambiguous allele combinations for high resolution typing, this is included in the base HLA typing codes below. The gene names have been italicized similar to the other molecular pathology codes.

(For HLA antigen typing by non-molecular pathology techniques, see 86812, 86813, 86816, 86817, 86821)

81370   HLA Class I and II typing, low resolution (eg, antigen equivalents); *HLA-A, -B, -C, -DRB1/3/4/5,* and *-DQB1*
➔ *CPT Changes: An Insider's View* 2012
➔ *CPT Assistant* May 12:4, Aug 16:10, Nov 18:9

81371   *HLA-A, -B, and -DRB1* (eg, verification typing)
➔ *CPT Changes: An Insider's View* 2012, 2014
➔ *CPT Assistant* May 12:4, Aug 16:10, Nov 18:9

(When HLA typing includes a determination of the presence or absence of the DRB3/4/5 genes, that service is included in the typing and is not separately reported)

81372   HLA Class I typing, low resolution (eg, antigen equivalents); complete *(ie, HLA-A, -B,* and *-C)*
➔ *CPT Changes: An Insider's View* 2012
➔ *CPT Assistant* May 12:4, Aug 16:10, Nov 18:9

(When performing both Class I and II low resolution *HLA typing for HLA-A,-B,-C, -DRB1/3/4/5,* and *-DQB1,* use 81370)

81373   one locus *(eg, HLA-A, -B,* or *-C),* each
➔ *CPT Changes: An Insider's View* 2012
➔ *CPT Assistant* May 12:4, Jun 12:16, Aug 16:10, Nov 18:9

(When performing a complete Class I *[HLA-A,-B,* and*-C]* low resolution HLA typing, use 81372)

(When the presence or absence of a single antigen equivalent is reported using low resolution testing, use 81374)

81374   one antigen equivalent (eg, *B*27*), each
➔ *CPT Changes: An Insider's View* 2012
➔ *CPT Assistant* May 12:4, Jun 12:16, Aug 16:10, Nov 18:9

(When testing for presence or absence of more than 2 antigen equivalents at a locus, use 81373 for each locus tested)

81375   HLA Class II typing, low resolution (eg, antigen equivalents); *HLA-DRB1/3/4/5* and *-DQB1*
➔ *CPT Changes: An Insider's View* 2012
➔ *CPT Assistant* May 12:4, Aug 16:10, Nov 18:9

(When performing both Class I and II low resolution HLA typing *for HLA-A,-B,-C, -DRB1/3/4/5,* and*-DQB1,* use 81370)

81376   one locus *(eg, HLA-DRB1, -DRB3/4/5, -DQB1, -DQA1, -DPB1,* or *-DPA1),* each
➔ *CPT Changes: An Insider's View* 2012, 2014
➔ *CPT Assistant* May 12:4, Jun 12:16, Aug 16:10, Nov 18:9

(When low resolution typing is performed for *HLA-DRB1/3/4/5* and*-DQB1,* use 81375)

(When HLA typing includes a determination of the presence or absence of the DRB3/4/5 genes, that service is included in the typing and is not separately reported. When low or intermediate resolution typing of any or all of the DRB3/4/5 genes is performed, treat as one locus)

81377   one antigen equivalent, each
➔ *CPT Changes: An Insider's View* 2012
➔ *CPT Assistant* May 12:4, Jun 12:16, Aug 16:10, Nov 18:9

(When testing for presence or absence of more than 2 antigen equivalents at a locus, use 81376 for each locus)

81378   HLA Class I and II typing, high resolution (ie, alleles or allele groups), *HLA-A, -B, -C,* and *-DRB1*
➔ *CPT Changes: An Insider's View* 2012
➔ *CPT Assistant* May 12:4, Jun 12:16, Aug 16:10, Nov 18:9

81379   HLA Class I typing, high resolution (ie, alleles or allele groups); complete (ie, *HLA-A, -B,* and *-C)*
➔ *CPT Changes: An Insider's View* 2012
➔ *CPT Assistant* May 12:4, Aug 16:10, Nov 18:9, Jan 24:17

81380   one locus (eg, *HLA-A, -B,* or *-C),* each
➔ *CPT Changes: An Insider's View* 2012
➔ *CPT Assistant* May 12:4, Jun 12:16, Aug 16:10, Nov 18:9

(When a complete Class I high resolution typing for *HLA-A,-B,* and*-C* is performed, use 81379)

(When the presence or absence of a single allele or allele group is reported using high resolution testing, use 81381)

81381   one allele or allele group (eg, *B*57:01P),* each
➔ *CPT Changes: An Insider's View* 2012
➔ *CPT Assistant* May 12:4, Jun 12:16, Aug 16:10, Nov 18:9

(When testing for the presence or absence of more than 2 alleles or allele groups at a locus, use 81380 for each locus)

81382   HLA Class II typing, high resolution (ie, alleles or allele groups); one locus (eg, *HLA-DRB1, -DRB3/4/5, -DQB1, -DQA1, -DPB1,* or *-DPA1),* each
➔ *CPT Changes: An Insider's View* 2012, 2014
➔ *CPT Assistant* May 12:4, Jun 12:16, Nov 18:9

(When only the presence or absence of a single allele or allele group is reported using high resolution testing, use 81383)

(When high resolution typing of any or all of the DRB3/4/5 genes is performed, treat as one locus)

81383   one allele or allele group (eg, *HLA-DQB1*06:02P),* each
➔ *CPT Changes: An Insider's View* 2012
➔ *CPT Assistant* May 12:4, Jun 12:16, Nov 18:9

(When testing for the presence or absence of more than 2 alleles or allele groups at a locus, use 81382 for each locus)

Pathology and Laboratory   80047-89398, 0001U-0520U

Tier 2 Molecular Pathology Procedures

The following molecular pathology procedure (Tier 2) codes are used to report procedures not listed in the Tier 1 molecular pathology codes (81161, 81200-81383). They represent medically useful procedures that are generally performed in lower volumes than Tier 1 procedures (eg, the incidence of the disease being tested is rare). They are arranged by level of technical resources and interpretive work by the physician or other qualified health care professional. The individual analyses listed under each code (ie, level of procedure) utilize the definitions and coding principles as described in the introduction preceding the Tier 1 molecular pathology codes. The parenthetical examples of methodologies presented near the beginning of each code provide general guidelines used to group procedures for a given level and are not all-inclusive.

Use the appropriate molecular pathology procedure level code that includes the specific analyte listed after the code descriptor. If the analyte tested is not listed under one of the Tier 2 codes or is not represented by a Tier 1 code, use the unlisted molecular pathology procedure code, 81479. See the Introduction section of the CPT code set for a complete list of the dates of release and implementation.

81400 Molecular pathology procedure, Level 1 (eg, identification of single germline variant [eg, SNP] by techniques such as restriction enzyme digestion or melt curve analysis)

ACADM (acyl-CoA dehydrogenase, C-4 to C-12 straight chain, MCAD) (eg, medium chain acyl dehydrogenase deficiency), K304E variant

ACE (angiotensin converting enzyme) (eg, hereditary blood pressure regulation), insertion/deletion variant

AGTR1 (angiotensin II receptor, type 1) (eg, essential hypertension), 1166A>C variant

BCKDHA (branched chain keto acid dehydrogenase E1, alpha polypeptide) (eg, maple syrup urine disease, type 1A), Y438N variant

CCR5 (chemokine C-C motif receptor 5) (eg, HIV resistance), 32-bp deletion mutation/794 825del32 deletion

CLRN1 (clarin 1) (eg, Usher syndrome, type 3), N48K variant

F2 (coagulation factor 2) (eg, hereditary hypercoagulability), 1199G>A variant

F5 (coagulation factor V) (eg, hereditary hypercoagulability), HR2 variant

F7 (coagulation factor VII [serum prothrombin conversion accelerator]) (eg, hereditary hypercoagulability), R353Q variant

F13B (coagulation factor XIII, B polypeptide) (eg, hereditary hypercoagulability), V34L variant

FGB (fibrinogen beta chain) (eg, hereditary ischemic heart disease), -455G>A variant

FGFR1 (fibroblast growth factor receptor 1) (eg, Pfeiffer syndrome type 1, craniosynostosis), P252R variant

FGFR3 (fibroblast growth factor receptor 3) (eg, Muenke syndrome), P250R variant

FKTN (fukutin) (eg, Fukuyama congenital muscular dystrophy), retrotransposon insertion variant

GNE (glucosamine [UDP-N-acetyl]-2-epimerase/N-acetylmannosamine kinase) (eg, inclusion body myopathy 2 [IBM2], Nonaka myopathy), M712T variant

IVD (isovaleryl-CoA dehydrogenase) (eg, isovaleric acidemia), A282V variant

LCT (lactase-phlorizin hydrolase) (eg, lactose intolerance), 13910 C>T variant

NEB (nebulin) (eg, nemaline myopathy 2), exon 55 deletion variant

PCDH15 (protocadherin-related 15) (eg, Usher syndrome type 1F), R245X variant

SERPINE1 (serpine peptidase inhibitor clade E, member 1, plasminogen activator inhibitor -1, PAI-1) (eg, thrombophilia), 4G variant

SHOC2 (soc-2 suppressor of clear homolog) (eg, Noonan-like syndrome with loose anagen hair), S2G variant

SRY (sex determining region Y) (eg, 46,XX testicular disorder of sex development, gonadal dysgenesis), gene analysis

TOR1A (torsin family 1, member A [torsin A]) (eg, early-onset primary dystonia [DYT1]), 907_909delGAG (904_906delGAG) variant

➔ *CPT Changes: An Insider's View* 2012, 2013, 2014, 2018, 2019

➔ *CPT Assistant* May 12:4, Jul 13:12, Sep 13:4-5, 8, Jan 15:3, Aug 16:10, Nov 18:9, Jul 19:3

81401 Molecular pathology procedure, Level 2 (eg, 2-10 SNPs, 1 methylated variant, or 1 somatic variant [typically using nonsequencing target variant analysis], or detection of a dynamic mutation disorder/triplet repeat)

ABCC8 (ATP-binding cassette, sub-family C [CFTR/MRP], member 8) (eg, familial hyperinsulinism), common variants (eg, c.3898-9G>A [c.3992-9G>A], F1388del)

ABL1 (ABL proto-oncogene 1, non-receptor tyrosine kinase) (eg, acquired imatinib resistance), T315I variant

ACADM (acyl-CoA dehydrogenase, C-4 to C-12 straight chain, MCAD) (eg, medium chain acyl dehydrogenase deficiency), commons variants (eg, K304E, Y42H)

ADRB2 (adrenergic beta-2 receptor surface) (eg, drug metabolism), common variants (eg, G16R, Q27E)

APOB (apolipoprotein B) (eg, familial hypercholesterolemia type B), common variants (eg, R3500Q, R3500W)

APOE (apolipoprotein E) (eg, hyperlipoproteinemia type III, cardiovascular disease, Alzheimer disease), common variants (eg, *2, *3, *4)

CBFB/MYH11 (inv(16)) (eg, acute myeloid leukemia), qualitative, and quantitative, if performed

CBS (cystathionine-beta-synthase) (eg, homocystinuria, cystathionine beta-synthase deficiency), common variants (eg, I278T, G307S)

CFH/ARMS2 (complement factor H/age-related maculopathy susceptibility 2) (eg, macular degeneration), common variants (eg, Y402H [CFH], A69S [ARMS2])

DEK/NUP214 (t(6;9)) (eg, acute myeloid leukemia), translocation analysis, qualitative, and quantitative, if performed

E2A/PBX1 (t(1;19)) (eg, acute lymphocytic leukemia), translocation analysis, qualitative, and quantitative, if performed

EML4/ALK (inv(2)) (eg, non-small cell lung cancer), translocation or inversion analysis

ETV6/RUNX1 (t(12;21)) (eg, acute lymphocytic leukemia), translocation analysis, qualitative, and quantitative, if performed

EWSR1/ATF1 (t(12;22)) (eg, clear cell sarcoma), translocation analysis, qualitative, and quantitative, if performed

EWSR1/ERG (t(21;22)) (eg, Ewing sarcoma/peripheral neuroectodermal tumor), translocation analysis, qualitative, and quantitative, if performed

EWSR1/FLI1 (t(11;22)) (eg, Ewing sarcoma/peripheral neuroectodermal tumor), translocation analysis, qualitative, and quantitative, if performed

EWSR1/WT1 (t(11;22)) (eg, desmoplastic small round cell tumor), translocation analysis, qualitative, and quantitative, if performed

F11 (coagulation factor XI) (eg, coagulation disorder), common variants (eg, E117X [Type II], F283L [Type III], IVS14del14, and IVS14+1G>A [Type I])

FGFR3 (fibroblast growth factor receptor 3) (eg, achondroplasia, hypochondroplasia), common variants (eg, 1138G>A, 1138G>C, 1620C>A, 1620C>G)

FIP1L1/PDGFRA (del[4q12]) (eg, imatinib-sensitive chronic eosinophilic leukemia), qualitative, and quantitative, if performed

FLG (filaggrin) (eg, ichthyosis vulgaris), common variants (eg, R501X, 2282del4, R2447X, S3247X, 3702delG)

FOXO1/PAX3 (t(2;13)) (eg, alveolar rhabdomyosarcoma), translocation analysis, qualitative, and quantitative, if performed

FOXO1/PAX7 (t(1;13)) (eg, alveolar rhabdomyosarcoma), translocation analysis, qualitative, and quantitative, if performed

FUS/DDIT3 (t(12;16)) (eg, myxoid liposarcoma), translocation analysis, qualitative, and quantitative, if performed

GALC (galactosylceramidase) (eg, Krabbe disease), common variants (eg, c.857G>A, 30-kb deletion)

GALT (galactose-1-phosphate uridylyltransferase) (eg, galactosemia), common variants (eg, Q188R, S135L, K285N, T138M, L195P, Y209C, IVS2-2A>G, P171S, del5kb, N314D, L218L/N314D)

H19 (imprinted maternally expressed transcript [non-protein coding]) (eg, Beckwith-Wiedemann syndrome), methylation analysis

IGH@/BCL2 (t(14;18)) (eg, follicular lymphoma), translocation analysis; single breakpoint (eg, major breakpoint region [MBR] or minor cluster region [mcr]), qualitative or quantitative

(When both MBR and mcr breakpoints are performed, use 81278)

KCNQ1OT1 (KCNQ1 overlapping transcript 1 [non-protein coding]) (eg, Beckwith-Wiedemann syndrome), methylation analysis

LINC00518 (long intergenic non-protein coding RNA 518) (eg, melanoma), expression analysis

LRRK2 (leucine-rich repeat kinase 2) (eg, Parkinson disease), common variants (eg, R1441G, G2019S, I2020T)

MED12 (mediator complex subunit 12) (eg, FG syndrome type 1, Lujan syndrome), common variants (eg, R961W, N1007S)

MEG3/DLK1 (maternally expressed 3 [non-protein coding]/delta-like 1 homolog [Drosophila]) (eg, intrauterine growth retardation), methylation analysis

MLL/AFF1 (t(4;11)) (eg, acute lymphoblastic leukemia), translocation analysis, qualitative, and quantitative, if performed

MLL/MLLT3 (t(9;11)) (eg, acute myeloid leukemia), translocation analysis, qualitative, and quantitative, if performed

MT-ATP6 (mitochondrially encoded ATP synthase 6) (eg, neuropathy with ataxia and retinitis pigmentosa [NARP], Leigh syndrome), common variants (eg, m.8993T>G, m.8993T>C)

Pathology and Laboratory 80047-89398, 0001U-0520U

MT-ND4, MT-ND6 (mitochondrially encoded NADH dehydrogenase 4, mitochondrially encoded NADH dehydrogenase 6) (eg, Leber hereditary optic neuropathy [LHON]), common variants (eg, m.11778G>A, m.3460G>A, m.14484T>C)

MT-ND5 (mitochondrially encoded tRNA leucine 1 [UUA/G], mitochondrially encoded NADH dehydrogenase 5) (eg, mitochondrial encephalopathy with lactic acidosis and stroke-like episodes [MELAS]), common variants (eg, m.3243A>G, m.3271T>C, m.3252A>G, m.13513G>A)

MT-RNR1 (mitochondrially encoded 12S RNA) (eg, nonsyndromic hearing loss), common variants (eg, m.1555A>G, m.1494C>T)

MT-TK (mitochondrially encoded tRNA lysine) (eg, myoclonic epilepsy with ragged-red fibers [MERRF]), common variants (eg, m.8344A>G, m.8356T>C)

MT-TL1 (mitochondrially encoded tRNA leucine 1 [UUA/G]) (eg, diabetes and hearing loss), common variants (eg, m.3243A>G, m.14709 T>C) MT-TL1

MT-TS1, MT-RNR1 (mitochondrially encoded tRNA serine 1 [UCN], mitochondrially encoded 12S RNA) (eg, nonsyndromic sensorineural deafness [including aminoglycoside-induced nonsyndromic deafness]), common variants (eg, m.7445A>G, m.1555A>G)

MUTYH (mutY homolog [E. coli]) (eg, MYH-associated polyposis), common variants (eg, Y165C, G382D)

NOD2 (nucleotide-binding oligomerization domain containing 2) (eg, Crohn's disease, Blau syndrome), common variants (eg, SNP 8, SNP 12, SNP 13)

NPM1/ALK (t(2;5)) (eg, anaplastic large cell lymphoma), translocation analysis

PAX8/PPARG (t(2;3) (q13;p25)) (eg, follicular thyroid carcinoma), translocation analysis

PRAME (preferentially expressed antigen in melanoma) (eg, melanoma), expression analysis

PRSS1 (protease, serine, 1 [trypsin 1]) (eg, hereditary pancreatitis), common variants (eg, N29I, A16V, R122H)

PYGM (phosphorylase, glycogen, muscle) (eg, glycogen storage disease type V, McArdle disease), common variants (eg, R50X, G205S)

RUNX1/RUNX1T1 (t(8;21)) (eg, acute myeloid leukemia) translocation analysis, qualitative, and quantitative, if performed

SS18/SSX1 (t(X;18)) (eg, synovial sarcoma), translocation analysis, qualitative, and quantitative, if performed

SS18/SSX2 (t(X;18)) (eg, synovial sarcoma), translocation analysis, qualitative, and quantitative, if performed

VWF (von Willebrand factor) (eg, von Willebrand disease type 2N), common variants (eg, T791M, R816W, R854Q)

➔ *CPT Changes: An Insider's View* 2012, 2013, 2014, 2016, 2017, 2018, 2019, 2021

➔ *CPT Assistant* May 12:4, Jul 13:12, Sep 13:5, Jan 15:3, Aug 16:10, Nov 18:9, Jul 19:3

81402 Molecular pathology procedure, Level 3 (eg, >10 SNPs, 2-10 methylated variants, or 2-10 somatic variants [typically using non-sequencing target variant analysis], immunoglobulin and T-cell receptor gene rearrangements, duplication/deletion variants of 1 exon, loss of heterozygosity [LOH], uniparental disomy [UPD])

Chromosome 1p-/19q- (eg, glial tumors), deletion analysis

Chromosome 18q- (eg, D18S55, D18S58, D18S61, D18S64, and D18S69) (eg, colon cancer), allelic imbalance assessment (ie, loss of heterozygosity)

COL1A1/PDGFB (t(17;22)) (eg, dermatofibrosarcoma protuberans), translocation analysis, multiple breakpoints, qualitative, and quantitative, if performed

CYP21A2 (cytochrome P450, family 21, subfamily A, polypeptide 2) (eg, congenital adrenal hyperplasia, 21-hydroxylase deficiency), common variants (eg, IVS2-13G, P30L, I172N, exon 6 mutation cluster [I235N, V236E, M238K], V281L, L307FfsX6, Q318X, R356W, P453S, G110VfsX21, 30-kb deletion variant)

ESR1/PGR (receptor 1/progesterone receptor) ratio (eg, breast cancer)

MEFV (Mediterranean fever) (eg, familial Mediterranean fever), common variants (eg, E148Q, P369S, F479L, M680I, I692del, M694V, M694I, K695R, V726A, A744S, R761H)

TRD@ (T cell antigen receptor, delta) (eg, leukemia and lymphoma), gene rearrangement analysis, evaluation to detect abnormal clonal population

Uniparental disomy (UPD) (eg, Russell-Silver syndrome, Prader-Willi/Angelman syndrome), short tandem repeat (STR) analysis

➔ *CPT Changes: An Insider's View* 2012, 2013, 2014, 2015, 2016, 2021

➔ *CPT Assistant* May 12:4, Jul 13:12, Sep 13:5, 9, Jan 15:3, Aug 16:10, Nov 18:9, Aug 21:10

81403 Molecular pathology procedure, Level 4 (eg, analysis of single exon by DNA sequence analysis, analysis of >10 amplicons using multiplex PCR in 2 or more independent reactions, mutation scanning or duplication/deletion variants of 2-5 exons)

ANG (angiogenin, ribonuclease, RNase A family, 5) (eg, amyotrophic lateral sclerosis), full gene sequence

ARX (aristaless related homeobox) (eg, X-linked lissencephaly with ambiguous genitalia, X-linked intellectual disability), duplication/deletion analysis

CEL (carboxyl ester lipase [bile salt-stimulated lipase]) (eg, maturity-onset diabetes of the young [MODY]), targeted sequence analysis of exon 11 (eg, c.1785delC, c.1686delT)

CTNNB1 (catenin [cadherin-associated protein], beta 1, 88kDa) (eg, desmoid tumors), targeted sequence analysis (eg, exon 3)

DAZ/SRY (deleted in azoospermia and sex determining region Y) (eg, male infertility), common deletions (eg, AZFa, AZFb, AZFc, AZFd)

DNMT3A (DNA [cytosine-5-]-methyltransferase 3 alpha) (eg, acute myeloid leukemia), targeted sequence analysis (eg, exon 23)

EPCAM (epithelial cell adhesion molecule) (eg, Lynch syndrome), duplication/deletion analysis

F8 (coagulation factor VIII) (eg, hemophilia A), inversion analysis, intron 1 and intron 22A

F12 (coagulation factor XII [Hageman factor]) (eg, angioedema, hereditary, type III; factor XII deficiency), targeted sequence analysis of exon 9

FGFR3 (fibroblast growth factor receptor 3) (eg, isolated craniosynostosis), targeted sequence analysis (eg, exon 7)

(For targeted sequence analysis of multiple FGFR3 exons, use 81404)

GJB1 (gap junction protein, beta 1) (eg, Charcot-Marie-Tooth X-linked), full gene sequence

GNAQ (guanine nucleotide-binding protein G[q] subunit alpha) (eg, uveal melanoma), common variants (eg, R183, Q209)

Human erythrocyte antigen gene analyses (eg, SLC14A1 [Kidd blood group], BCAM [Lutheran blood group], ICAM4 [Landsteiner-Wiener blood group], SLC4A1 [Diego blood group], AQP1 [Colton blood group], ERMAP [Scianna blood group], RHCE [Rh blood group, CcEe antigens], KEL [Kell blood group], DARC [Duffy blood group], GYPA, GYPB, GYPE [MNS blood group], ART4 [Dombrock blood group]) (eg, sickle-cell disease, thalassemia, hemolytic transfusion reactions, hemolytic disease of the fetus or newborn), common variants

HRAS (v-Ha-ras Harvey rat sarcoma viral oncogene homolog) (eg, Costello syndrome), exon 2 sequence

KCNC3 (potassium voltage-gated channel, Shaw-related subfamily, member 3) (eg, spinocerebellar ataxia), targeted sequence analysis (eg, exon 2)

KCNJ2 (potassium inwardly-rectifying channel, subfamily J, member 2) (eg, Andersen-Tawil syndrome), full gene sequence

KCNJ11 (potassium inwardly-rectifying channel, subfamily J, member 11) (eg, familial hyperinsulinism), full gene sequence

Killer cell immunoglobulin-like receptor (KIR) gene family (eg, hematopoietic stem cell transplantation), genotyping of KIR family genes

Known familial variant not otherwise specified, for gene listed in Tier 1 or Tier 2, or identified during a genomic sequencing procedure, DNA sequence analysis, each variant exon

(For a known familial variant that is considered a common variant, use specific common variant Tier 1 or Tier 2 code)

MC4R (melanocortin 4 receptor) (eg, obesity), full gene sequence

MICA (MHC class I polypeptide-related sequence A) (eg, solid organ transplantation), common variants (eg, *001, *002)

MT-RNR1 (mitochondrially encoded 12S RNA) (eg, nonsyndromic hearing loss), full gene sequence

MT-TS1 (mitochondrially encoded tRNA serine 1) (eg, nonsyndromic hearing loss), full gene sequence

NDP (Norrie disease [pseudoglioma]) (eg, Norrie disease), duplication/deletion analysis

NHLRC1 (NHL repeat containing 1) (eg, progressive myoclonus epilepsy), full gene sequence

PHOX2B (paired-like homeobox 2b) (eg, congenital central hypoventilation syndrome), duplication/deletion analysis

PLN (phospholamban) (eg, dilated cardiomyopathy, hypertrophic cardiomyopathy), full gene sequence

RHD (Rh blood group, D antigen) (eg, hemolytic disease of the fetus and newborn, Rh maternal/fetal compatibility), deletion analysis (eg, exons 4, 5, and 7, pseudogene)

RHD (Rh blood group, D antigen) (eg, hemolytic disease of the fetus and newborn, Rh maternal/fetal compatibility), deletion analysis (eg, exons 4, 5, and 7, pseudogene), performed on cell-free fetal DNA in maternal blood

(For human erythrocyte gene analysis of RHD, use a separate unit of 81403)

SH2D1A (SH2 domain containing 1A) (eg, X-linked lymphoproliferative syndrome), duplication/deletion analysis

TWIST1 (twist homolog 1 [Drosophila]) (eg, Saethre-Chotzen syndrome), duplication/deletion analysis

UBA1 (ubiquitin-like modifier activating enzyme 1) (eg, spinal muscular atrophy, X-linked), targeted sequence analysis (eg, exon 15)

VHL (von Hippel-Lindau tumor suppressor) (eg, von Hippel-Lindau familial cancer syndrome), deletion/duplication analysis

VWF (von Willebrand factor) (eg, von Willebrand disease types 2A, 2B, 2M), targeted sequence analysis (eg, exon 28)

➡ *CPT Changes: An Insider's View* 2012, 2013, 2014, 2015, 2016, 2017, 2018, 2019, 2021, 2024

➡ *CPT Assistant* May 12:4, Jul 13:12, Sep 13:3, Jan 15:3, Aug 16:10, May 18:6, Nov 18:9, Jul 19:3, Aug 21:10

81404 Molecular pathology procedure, Level 5 (eg, analysis of 2-5 exons by DNA sequence analysis, mutation scanning or duplication/deletion variants of 6-10 exons, or characterization of a dynamic mutation disorder/triplet repeat by Southern blot analysis)

ACADS (acyl-CoA dehydrogenase, C-2 to C-3 short chain) (eg, short chain acyl-CoA dehydrogenase deficiency), targeted sequence analysis (eg, exons 5 and 6)

AQP2 (aquaporin 2 [collecting duct]) (eg, nephrogenic diabetes insipidus), full gene sequence

ARX (aristaless related homeobox) (eg, X-linked lissencephaly with ambiguous genitalia, X-linked intellectual disability), full gene sequence

AVPR2 (arginine vasopressin receptor 2) (eg, nephrogenic diabetes insipidus), full gene sequence

BBS10 (Bardet-Biedl syndrome 10) (eg, Bardet-Biedl syndrome), full gene sequence

BTD (biotinidase) (eg, biotinidase deficiency), full gene sequence

C10orf2 (chromosome 10 open reading frame 2) (eg, mitochondrial DNA depletion syndrome), full gene sequence

CAV3 (caveolin 3) (eg, CAV3-related distal myopathy, limb-girdle muscular dystrophy type 1C), full gene sequence

CD40LG (CD40 ligand) (eg, X-linked hyper IgM syndrome), full gene sequence

CDKN2A (cyclin-dependent kinase inhibitor 2A) (eg, CDKN2A-related cutaneous malignant melanoma, familial atypical mole-malignant melanoma syndrome), full gene sequence

CLRN1 (clarin 1) (eg, Usher syndrome, type 3), full gene sequence

COX6B1 (cytochrome c oxidase subunit VIb polypeptide 1) (eg, mitochondrial respiratory chain complex IV deficiency), full gene sequence

CPT2 (carnitine palmitoyltransferase 2) (eg, carnitine palmitoyltransferase II deficiency), full gene sequence

CRX (cone-rod homeobox) (eg, cone-rod dystrophy 2, Leber congenital amaurosis), full gene sequence

CYP1B1 (cytochrome P450, family 1, subfamily B, polypeptide 1) (eg, primary congenital glaucoma), full gene sequence

EGR2 (early growth response 2) (eg, Charcot-Marie-Tooth), full gene sequence

EMD (emerin) (eg, Emery-Dreifuss muscular dystrophy), duplication/deletion analysis

EPM2A (epilepsy, progressive myoclonus type 2A, Lafora disease [laforin]) (eg, progressive myoclonus epilepsy), full gene sequence

FGF23 (fibroblast growth factor 23) (eg, hypophosphatemic rickets), full gene sequence

FGFR2 (fibroblast growth factor receptor 2) (eg, craniosynostosis, Apert syndrome, Crouzon syndrome), targeted sequence analysis (eg, exons 8, 10)

FGFR3 (fibroblast growth factor receptor 3) (eg, achondroplasia, hypochondroplasia), targeted sequence analysis (eg, exons 8, 11, 12, 13)

FHL1 (four and a half LIM domains 1) (eg, Emery-Dreifuss muscular dystrophy), full gene sequence

FKRP (fukutin related protein) (eg, congenital muscular dystrophy type 1C [MDC1C], limb-girdle muscular dystrophy [LGMD] type 2I), full gene sequence

FOXG1 (forkhead box G1) (eg, Rett syndrome), full gene sequence

FSHMD1A (facioscapulohumeral muscular dystrophy 1A) (eg, facioscapulohumeral muscular dystrophy), evaluation to detect abnormal (eg, deleted) alleles

FSHMD1A (facioscapulohumeral muscular dystrophy 1A) (eg, facioscapulohumeral muscular dystrophy), characterization of haplotype(s) (ie, chromosome 4A and 4B haplotypes)

GH1 (growth hormone 1) (eg, growth hormone deficiency), full gene sequence

GP1BB (glycoprotein Ib [platelet], beta polypeptide) (eg, Bernard-Soulier syndrome type B), full gene sequence

(For common deletion variants of alpha globin 1 and alpha globin 2 genes, use 81257)

HNF1B (HNF1 homeobox B) (eg, maturity-onset diabetes of the young [MODY]), duplication/deletion analysis

HRAS (v-Ha-ras Harvey rat sarcoma viral oncogene homolog) (eg, Costello syndrome), full gene sequence

HSD3B2 (hydroxy-delta-5-steroid dehydrogenase, 3 beta- and steroid delta-isomerase 2) (eg, 3-beta-hydroxysteroid dehydrogenase type II deficiency), full gene sequence

HSD11B2 (hydroxysteroid [11-beta] dehydrogenase 2) (eg, mineralocorticoid excess syndrome), full gene sequence

HSPB1 (heat shock 27kDa protein 1) (eg, Charcot-Marie-Tooth disease), full gene sequence

INS (insulin) (eg, diabetes mellitus), full gene sequence

KCNJ1 (potassium inwardly-rectifying channel, subfamily J, member 1) (eg, Bartter syndrome), full gene sequence

KCNJ10 (potassium inwardly-rectifying channel, subfamily J, member 10) (eg, SeSAME syndrome, EAST syndrome, sensorineural hearing loss), full gene sequence

LITAF (lipopolysaccharide-induced TNF factor) (eg, Charcot-Marie-Tooth), full gene sequence

MEFV (Mediterranean fever) (eg, familial Mediterranean fever), full gene sequence

MEN1 (multiple endocrine neoplasia I) (eg, multiple endocrine neoplasia type 1, Wermer syndrome), duplication/deletion analysis

MMACHC (methylmalonic aciduria [cobalamin deficiency] cblC type, with homocystinuria) (eg, methylmalonic acidemia and homocystinuria), full gene sequence

MPV17 (MpV17 mitochondrial inner membrane protein) (eg, mitochondrial DNA depletion syndrome), duplication/deletion analysis

NDP (Norrie disease [pseudoglioma]) (eg, Norrie disease), full gene sequence

NDUFA1 (NADH dehydrogenase [ubiquinone] 1 alpha subcomplex, 1, 7.5kDa) (eg, Leigh syndrome, mitochondrial complex I deficiency), full gene sequence

NDUFAF2 (NADH dehydrogenase [ubiquinone] 1 alpha subcomplex, assembly factor 2) (eg, Leigh syndrome, mitochondrial complex I deficiency), full gene sequence

NDUFS4 (NADH dehydrogenase [ubiquinone] Fe-S protein 4, 18kDa [NADH-coenzyme Q reductase]) (eg, Leigh syndrome, mitochondrial complex I deficiency), full gene sequence

NIPA1 (non-imprinted in Prader-Willi/Angelman syndrome 1) (eg, spastic paraplegia), full gene sequence

NLGN4X (neuroligin 4, X-linked) (eg, autism spectrum disorders), duplication/deletion analysis

NPC2 (Niemann-Pick disease, type C2 [epididymal secretory protein E1]) (eg, Niemann-Pick disease type C2), full gene sequence

NR0B1 (nuclear receptor subfamily 0, group B, member 1) (eg, congenital adrenal hypoplasia), full gene sequence

PDX1 (pancreatic and duodenal homeobox 1) (eg, maturity-onset diabetes of the young [MODY]), full gene sequence

PHOX2B (paired-like homeobox 2b) (eg, congenital central hypoventilation syndrome), full gene sequence

PLP1 (proteolipid protein 1) (eg, Pelizaeus-Merzbacher disease, spastic paraplegia), duplication/deletion analysis

PQBP1 (polyglutamine binding protein 1) (eg, Renpenning syndrome), duplication/deletion analysis

PRNP (prion protein) (eg, genetic prion disease), full gene sequence

PROP1 (PROP paired-like homeobox 1) (eg, combined pituitary hormone deficiency), full gene sequence

PRPH2 (peripherin 2 [retinal degeneration, slow]) (eg, retinitis pigmentosa), full gene sequence

PRSS1 (protease, serine, 1 [trypsin 1]) (eg, hereditary pancreatitis), full gene sequence

RAF1 (v-raf-1 murine leukemia viral oncogene homolog 1) (eg, LEOPARD syndrome), targeted sequence analysis (eg, exons 7, 12, 14, 17)

RET (ret proto-oncogene) (eg, multiple endocrine neoplasia, type 2B and familial medullary thyroid carcinoma), common variants (eg, M918T, 2647_2648delinsTT, A883F)

RHO (rhodopsin) (eg, retinitis pigmentosa), full gene sequence

RP1 (retinitis pigmentosa 1) (eg, retinitis pigmentosa), full gene sequence

SCN1B (sodium channel, voltage-gated, type I, beta) (eg, Brugada syndrome), full gene sequence

SCO2 (SCO cytochrome oxidase deficient homolog 2 [SCO1L]) (eg, mitochondrial respiratory chain complex IV deficiency), full gene sequence

SDHC (succinate dehydrogenase complex, subunit C, integral membrane protein, 15kDa) (eg, hereditary paraganglioma-pheochromocytoma syndrome), duplication/deletion analysis

SDHD (succinate dehydrogenase complex, subunit D, integral membrane protein) (eg, hereditary paraganglioma), full gene sequence

SGCG (sarcoglycan, gamma [35kDa dystrophin-associated glycoprotein]) (eg, limb-girdle muscular dystrophy), duplication/deletion analysis

SH2D1A (SH2 domain containing 1A) (eg, X-linked lymphoproliferative syndrome), full gene sequence

SLC16A2 (solute carrier family 16, member 2 [thyroid hormone transporter]) (eg, specific thyroid hormone cell transporter deficiency, Allan-Herndon-Dudley syndrome), duplication/deletion analysis

SLC25A20 (solute carrier family 25 [carnitine/acylcarnitine translocase], member 20) (eg, carnitine-acylcarnitine translocase deficiency), duplication/deletion analysis

---

▲=Revised code   ●=New code   ▶◀=Contains new or revised text   ✦=Duplicate PLA test   ↕=Category I PLA   American Medical Association   **655**

SLC25A4 (solute carrier family 25 [mitochondrial carrier; adenine nucleotide translocator], member 4) (eg, progressive external ophthalmoplegia), full gene sequence

SOD1 (superoxide dismutase 1, soluble) (eg, amyotrophic lateral sclerosis), full gene sequence

SPINK1 (serine peptidase inhibitor, Kazal type 1) (eg, hereditary pancreatitis), full gene sequence

STK11 (serine/threonine kinase 11) (eg, Peutz-Jeghers syndrome), duplication/deletion analysis

TACO1 (translational activator of mitochondrial encoded cytochrome c oxidase I) (eg, mitochondrial respiratory chain complex IV deficiency), full gene sequence

THAP1 (THAP domain containing, apoptosis associated protein 1) (eg, torsion dystonia), full gene sequence

TOR1A (torsin family 1, member A [torsin A]) (eg, torsion dystonia), full gene sequence

TTPA (tocopherol [alpha] transfer protein) (eg, ataxia), full gene sequence

TTR (transthyretin) (eg, familial transthyretin amyloidosis), full gene sequence

TWIST1 (twist homolog 1 [Drosophila]) (eg, Saethre-Chotzen syndrome), full gene sequence

TYR (tyrosinase [oculocutaneous albinism IA]) (eg, oculocutaneous albinism IA), full gene sequence

UGT1A1 (UDP glucuronosyltransferase 1 family, polypeptide A1) (eg, hereditary unconjugated hyperbilirubinemia [Crigler-Najjar syndrome]) full gene sequence

USH1G (Usher syndrome 1G [autosomal recessive]) (eg, Usher syndrome, type 1), full gene sequence

VHL (von Hippel-Lindau tumor suppressor) (eg, von Hippel-Lindau familial cancer syndrome), full gene sequence

VWF (von Willebrand factor) (eg, von Willebrand disease type 1C), targeted sequence analysis (eg, exons 26, 27, 37)

ZEB2 (zinc finger E-box binding homeobox 2) (eg, Mowat-Wilson syndrome), duplication/deletion analysis

ZNF41 (zinc finger protein 41) (eg, X-linked intellectual disability 89), full gene sequence

➲ CPT Changes: An Insider's View 2012, 2013, 2014, 2015, 2016, 2018, 2019, 2020, 2021, 2024

➲ CPT Assistant May 12:4, Jul 13:12, Sep 13:6-7, 9, Jan 15:3, Aug 16:10, May 18:6, Nov 18:9, Jul 19:3, Apr 20:9

81405   Molecular pathology procedure, Level 6 (eg, analysis of 6-10 exons by DNA sequence analysis, mutation scanning or duplication/deletion variants of 11-25 exons, regionally targeted cytogenomic array analysis)

ABCD1 (ATP-binding cassette, sub-family D [ALD], member 1) (eg, adrenoleukodystrophy), full gene sequence

ACADS (acyl-CoA dehydrogenase, C-2 to C-3 short chain) (eg, short chain acyl-CoA dehydrogenase deficiency), full gene sequence

ACTA2 (actin, alpha 2, smooth muscle, aorta) (eg, thoracic aortic aneurysms and aortic dissections), full gene sequence

ACTC1 (actin, alpha, cardiac muscle 1) (eg, familial hypertrophic cardiomyopathy), full gene sequence

ANKRD1 (ankyrin repeat domain 1) (eg, dilated cardiomyopathy), full gene sequence

APTX (aprataxin) (eg, ataxia with oculomotor apraxia 1), full gene sequence

ARSA (arylsulfatase A) (eg, arylsulfatase A deficiency), full gene sequence

BCKDHA (branched chain keto acid dehydrogenase E1, alpha polypeptide) (eg, maple syrup urine disease, type 1A), full gene sequence

BCS1L (BCS1-like [S. cerevisiae]) (eg, Leigh syndrome, mitochondrial complex III deficiency, GRACILE syndrome), full gene sequence

BMPR2 (bone morphogenetic protein receptor, type II [serine/threonine kinase]) (eg, heritable pulmonary arterial hypertension), duplication/deletion analysis

CASQ2 (calsequestrin 2 [cardiac muscle]) (eg, catecholaminergic polymorphic ventricular tachycardia), full gene sequence

CASR (calcium-sensing receptor) (eg, hypocalcemia), full gene sequence

CDKL5 (cyclin-dependent kinase-like 5) (eg, early infantile epileptic encephalopathy), duplication/deletion analysis

CHRNA4 (cholinergic receptor, nicotinic, alpha 4) (eg, nocturnal frontal lobe epilepsy), full gene sequence

CHRNB2 (cholinergic receptor, nicotinic, beta 2 [neuronal]) (eg, nocturnal frontal lobe epilepsy), full gene sequence

COX10 (COX10 homolog, cytochrome c oxidase assembly protein) (eg, mitochondrial respiratory chain complex IV deficiency), full gene sequence

COX15 (COX15 homolog, cytochrome c oxidase assembly protein) (eg, mitochondrial respiratory chain complex IV deficiency), full gene sequence

CPOX (coproporphyrinogen oxidase) (eg, hereditary coproporphyria), full gene sequence

CTRC (chymotrypsin C) (eg, hereditary pancreatitis), full gene sequence

Pathology and Laboratory 80047-89398, 0001U-0520U

CYP11B1 (cytochrome P450, family 11, subfamily B, polypeptide 1) (eg, congenital adrenal hyperplasia), full gene sequence

CYP17A1 (cytochrome P450, family 17, subfamily A, polypeptide 1) (eg, congenital adrenal hyperplasia), full gene sequence

CYP21A2 (cytochrome P450, family 21, subfamily A, polypeptide2) (eg, steroid 21-hydroxylase isoform, congenital adrenal hyperplasia), full gene sequence

Cytogenomic constitutional targeted microarray analysis of chromosome 22q13 by interrogation of genomic regions for copy number and single nucleotide polymorphism (SNP) variants for chromosomal abnormalities

(When performing cytogenomic [genome-wide] analysis for constitutional chromosomal abnormalities, see 81228, 81229, 81349)

(Do not report analyte-specific molecular pathology procedures separately when the specific analytes are included as part of the microarray analysis of chromosome 22q13)

(Do not report 88271 when performing cytogenomic microarray analysis)

DBT (dihydrolipoamide branched chain transacylase E2) (eg, maple syrup urine disease, type 2), duplication/deletion analysis

DCX (doublecortin) (eg, X-linked lissencephaly), full gene sequence

DES (desmin) (eg, myofibrillar myopathy), full gene sequence

DFNB59 (deafness, autosomal recessive 59) (eg, autosomal recessive nonsyndromic hearing impairment), full gene sequence

DGUOK (deoxyguanosine kinase) (eg, hepatocerebral mitochondrial DNA depletion syndrome), full gene sequence

DHCR7 (7-dehydrocholesterol reductase) (eg, Smith-Lemli-Opitz syndrome), full gene sequence

EIF2B2 (eukaryotic translation initiation factor 2B, subunit 2 beta, 39kDa) (eg, leukoencephalopathy with vanishing white matter), full gene sequence

EMD (emerin) (eg, Emery-Dreifuss muscular dystrophy), full gene sequence

ENG (endoglin) (eg, hereditary hemorrhagic telangiectasia, type 1), duplication/deletion analysis

EYA1 (eyes absent homolog 1 [Drosophila]) (eg, branchio-oto-renal [BOR] spectrum disorders), duplication/deletion analysis

FGFR1 (fibroblast growth factor receptor 1) (eg, Kallmann syndrome 2), full gene sequence

FH (fumarate hydratase) (eg, fumarate hydratase deficiency, hereditary leiomyomatosis with renal cell cancer), full gene sequence

FKTN (fukutin) (eg, limb-girdle muscular dystrophy [LGMD] type 2M or 2L), full gene sequence

FTSJ1 (FtsJ RNA 2'-O-methyltransferase 1) (eg, X-linked intellectual disability 9), duplication/deletion analysis

GABRG2 (gamma-aminobutyric acid [GABA] A receptor, gamma 2) (eg, generalized epilepsy with febrile seizures), full gene sequence

GCH1 (GTP cyclohydrolase 1) (eg, autosomal dominant dopa-responsive dystonia), full gene sequence

GDAP1 (ganglioside-induced differentiation-associated protein 1) (eg, Charcot-Marie-Tooth disease), full gene sequence

GFAP (glial fibrillary acidic protein) (eg, Alexander disease), full gene sequence

GHR (growth hormone receptor) (eg, Laron syndrome), full gene sequence

GHRHR (growth hormone releasing hormone receptor) (eg, growth hormone deficiency), full gene sequence

GLA (galactosidase, alpha) (eg, Fabry disease), full gene sequence

HNF1A (HNF1 homeobox A) (eg, maturity-onset diabetes of the young [MODY]), full gene sequence

HNF1B (HNF1 homeobox B) (eg, maturity-onset diabetes of the young [MODY]), full gene sequence

HTRA1 (HtrA serine peptidase 1) (eg, macular degeneration), full gene sequence

IDS (iduronate 2-sulfatase) (eg, mucopolysacchridosis, type II), full gene sequence

IL2RG (interleukin 2 receptor, gamma) (eg, X-linked severe combined immunodeficiency), full gene sequence

ISPD (isoprenoid synthase domain containing) (eg, muscle-eye-brain disease, Walker-Warburg syndrome), full gene sequence

KRAS (Kirsten rat sarcoma viral oncogene homolog) (eg, Noonan syndrome), full gene sequence

LAMP2 (lysosomal-associated membrane protein 2) (eg, Danon disease), full gene sequence

LDLR (low density lipoprotein receptor) (eg, familial hypercholesterolemia), duplication/deletion analysis

MEN1 (multiple endocrine neoplasia I) (eg, multiple endocrine neoplasia type 1, Wermer syndrome), full gene sequence

▲ = Revised code　● = New code　▶ ◀ = Contains new or revised text　✦ = Duplicate PLA test　↕ = Category I PLA　　American Medical Association　**657**

Pathology and Laboratory　80047-89398, 0001U-0520U

MMAA (methylmalonic aciduria [cobalamine deficiency] type A) (eg, MMAA-related methylmalonic acidemia), full gene sequence

MMAB (methylmalonic aciduria [cobalamine deficiency] type B) (eg, MMAA-related methylmalonic acidemia), full gene sequence

MPI (mannose phosphate isomerase) (eg, congenital disorder of glycosylation 1b), full gene sequence

MPV17 (MpV17 mitochondrial inner membrane protein) (eg, mitochondrial DNA depletion syndrome), full gene sequence

MPZ (myelin protein zero) (eg, Charcot-Marie-Tooth), full gene sequence

MTM1 (myotubularin 1) (eg, X-linked centronuclear myopathy), duplication/deletion analysis

MYL2 (myosin, light chain 2, regulatory, cardiac, slow) (eg, familial hypertrophic cardiomyopathy), full gene sequence

MYL3 (myosin, light chain 3, alkali, ventricular, skeletal, slow) (eg, familial hypertrophic cardiomyopathy), full gene sequence

MYOT (myotilin) (eg, limb-girdle muscular dystrophy), full gene sequence

NDUFS7 (NADH dehydrogenase [ubiquinone] Fe-S protein 7, 20kDa [NADH-coenzyme Q reductase]) (eg, Leigh syndrome, mitochondrial complex I deficiency), full gene sequence

NDUFS8 (NADH dehydrogenase [ubiquinone] Fe-S protein 8, 23kDa [NADH-coenzyme Q reductase]) (eg, Leigh syndrome, mitochondrial complex I deficiency), full gene sequence

NDUFV1 (NADH dehydrogenase [ubiquinone] flavoprotein 1, 51kDa) (eg, Leigh syndrome, mitochondrial complex I deficiency), full gene sequence

NEFL (neurofilament, light polypeptide) (eg, Charcot-Marie-Tooth), full gene sequence

NF2 (neurofibromin 2 [merlin]) (eg, neurofibromatosis, type 2), duplication/deletion analysis

NLGN3 (neuroligin 3) (eg, autism spectrum disorders), full gene sequence

NLGN4X (neuroligin 4, X-linked) (eg, autism spectrum disorders), full gene sequence

NPHP1 (nephronophthisis 1 [juvenile]) (eg, Joubert syndrome), deletion analysis, and duplication analysis, if performed

NPHS2 (nephrosis 2, idiopathic, steroid-resistant [podocin]) (eg, steroid-resistant nephrotic syndrome), full gene sequence

NSD1 (nuclear receptor binding SET domain protein 1) (eg, Sotos syndrome), duplication/deletion analysis

OTC (ornithine carbamoyltransferase) (eg, ornithine transcarbamylase deficiency), full gene sequence

PAFAH1B1 (platelet-activating factor acetylhydrolase 1b, regulatory subunit 1 [45kDa]) (eg, lissencephaly, Miller-Dieker syndrome), duplication/deletion analysis

PARK2 (Parkinson protein 2, E3 ubiquitin protein ligase [parkin]) (eg, Parkinson disease), duplication/deletion analysis

PCCA (propionyl CoA carboxylase, alpha polypeptide) (eg, propionic acidemia, type 1), duplication/deletion analysis

PCDH19 (protocadherin 19) (eg, epileptic encephalopathy), full gene sequence

PDHA1 (pyruvate dehydrogenase [lipoamide] alpha 1) (eg, lactic acidosis), duplication/deletion analysis

PDHB (pyruvate dehydrogenase [lipoamide] beta) (eg, lactic acidosis), full gene sequence

PINK1 (PTEN induced putative kinase 1) (eg, Parkinson disease), full gene sequence

PKLR (pyruvate kinase, liver and RBC) (eg, pyruvate kinase deficiency), full gene sequence

PLP1 (proteolipid protein 1) (eg, Pelizaeus-Merzbacher disease, spastic paraplegia), full gene sequence

POU1F1 (POU class 1 homeobox 1) (eg, combined pituitary hormone deficiency), full gene sequence

PRX (periaxin) (eg, Charcot-Marie-Tooth disease), full gene sequence

PQBP1 (polyglutamine binding protein 1) (eg, Renpenning syndrome), full gene sequence

PSEN1 (presenilin 1) (eg, Alzheimer disease), full gene sequence

RAB7A (RAB7A, member RAS oncogene family) (eg, Charcot-Marie-Tooth disease), full gene sequence

RAI1 (retinoic acid induced 1) (eg, Smith-Magenis syndrome), full gene sequence

REEP1 (receptor accessory protein 1) (eg, spastic paraplegia), full gene sequence

RET (ret proto-oncogene) (eg, multiple endocrine neoplasia, type 2A and familial medullary thyroid carcinoma), targeted sequence analysis (eg, exons 10, 11, 13-16)

RPS19 (ribosomal protein S19) (eg, Diamond-Blackfan anemia), full gene sequence

RRM2B (ribonucleotide reductase M2 B [TP53 inducible]) (eg, mitochondrial DNA depletion), full gene sequence

SCO1 (SCO cytochrome oxidase deficient homolog 1) (eg, mitochondrial respiratory chain complex IV deficiency), full gene sequence

SDHB (succinate dehydrogenase complex, subunit B, iron sulfur) (eg, hereditary paraganglioma), full gene sequence

SDHC (succinate dehydrogenase complex, subunit C, integral membrane protein, 15kDa) (eg, hereditary paraganglioma-pheochromocytoma syndrome), full gene sequence

SGCA (sarcoglycan, alpha [50kDa dystrophin-associated glycoprotein]) (eg, limb-girdle muscular dystrophy), full gene sequence

SGCB (sarcoglycan, beta [43kDa dystrophin-associated glycoprotein]) (eg, limb-girdle muscular dystrophy), full gene sequence

SGCD (sarcoglycan, delta [35kDa dystrophin-associated glycoprotein]) (eg, limb-girdle muscular dystrophy), full gene sequence

SGCE (sarcoglycan, epsilon) (eg, myoclonic dystonia), duplication/deletion analysis

SGCG (sarcoglycan, gamma [35kDa dystrophin-associated glycoprotein]) (eg, limb-girdle muscular dystrophy), full gene sequence

SHOC2 (soc-2 suppressor of clear homolog) (eg, Noonan-like syndrome with loose anagen hair), full gene sequence

SHOX (short stature homeobox) (eg, Langer mesomelic dysplasia), full gene sequence

SIL1 (SIL1 homolog, endoplasmic reticulum chaperone [S. cerevisiae]) (eg, ataxia), full gene sequence

SLC2A1 (solute carrier family 2 [facilitated glucose transporter], member 1) (eg, glucose transporter type 1 [GLUT 1] deficiency syndrome), full gene sequence

SLC16A2 (solute carrier family 16, member 2 [thyroid hormone transporter]) (eg, specific thyroid hormone cell transporter deficiency, Allan-Herndon-Dudley syndrome), full gene sequence

SLC22A5 (solute carrier family 22 [organic cation/ carnitine transporter], member 5) (eg, systemic primary carnitine deficiency), full gene sequence

SLC25A20 (solute carrier family 25 [carnitine/ acylcarnitine translocase], member 20) (eg, carnitine-acylcarnitine translocase deficiency), full gene sequence

SMAD4 (SMAD family member 4) (eg, hemorrhagic telangiectasia syndrome, juvenile polyposis), duplication/ deletion analysis

SPAST (spastin) (eg, spastic paraplegia), duplication/ deletion analysis

SPG7 (spastic paraplegia 7 [pure and complicated autosomal recessive]) (eg, spastic paraplegia), duplication/deletion analysis

SPRED1 (sprouty-related, EVH1 domain containing 1) (eg, Legius syndrome), full gene sequence

STAT3 (signal transducer and activator of transcription 3 [acute-phase response factor]) (eg, autosomal dominant hyper-IgE syndrome), targeted sequence analysis (eg, exons 12, 13, 14, 16, 17, 20, 21)

STK11 (serine/threonine kinase 11) (eg, Peutz-Jeghers syndrome), full gene sequence

SURF1 (surfeit 1) (eg, mitochondrial respiratory chain complex IV deficiency), full gene sequence

TARDBP (TAR DNA binding protein) (eg, amyotrophic lateral sclerosis), full gene sequence

TBX5 (T-box 5) (eg, Holt-Oram syndrome), full gene sequence

TCF4 (transcription factor 4) (eg, Pitt-Hopkins syndrome), duplication/deletion analysis

TGFBR1 (transforming growth factor, beta receptor 1) (eg, Marfan syndrome), full gene sequence

TGFBR2 (transforming growth factor, beta receptor 2) (eg, Marfan syndrome), full gene sequence

THRB (thyroid hormone receptor, beta) (eg, thyroid hormone resistance, thyroid hormone beta receptor deficiency), full gene sequence or targeted sequence analysis of >5 exons

TK2 (thymidine kinase 2, mitochondrial) (eg, mitochondrial DNA depletion syndrome), full gene sequence

TNNC1 (troponin C type 1 [slow]) (eg, hypertrophic cardiomyopathy or dilated cardiomyopathy), full gene sequence

TNNI3 (troponin I, type 3 [cardiac]) (eg, familial hypertrophic cardiomyopathy), full gene sequence

TPM1 (tropomyosin 1 [alpha]) (eg, familial hypertrophic cardiomyopathy), full gene sequence

TSC1 (tuberous sclerosis 1) (eg, tuberous sclerosis), duplication/deletion analysis

TYMP (thymidine phosphorylase) (eg, mitochondrial DNA depletion syndrome), full gene sequence

VWF (von Willebrand factor) (eg, von Willebrand disease type 2N), targeted sequence analysis (eg, exons 18-20, 23-25)

WT1 (Wilms tumor 1) (eg, Denys-Drash syndrome, familial Wilms tumor), full gene sequence

ZEB2 (zinc finger E-box binding homeobox 2) (eg, Mowat-Wilson syndrome), full gene sequence

➲ *CPT Changes: An Insider's View* 2012, 2013, 2014, 2015, 2024

➲ *CPT Assistant* May 12:4, Jul 13:12, Sep 13:8, 10, Jan 15:3, Aug 16:10, May 18:6, Sep 18:15, Nov 18:9, Jul 19:3

Pathology and Laboratory   80047-89398, 0001U-0520U

81406 Molecular pathology procedure, Level 7 (eg, analysis of 11-25 exons by DNA sequence analysis, mutation scanning or duplication/deletion variants of 26-50 exons)

ACADVL (acyl-CoA dehydrogenase, very long chain) (eg, very long chain acyl-coenzyme A dehydrogenase deficiency), full gene sequence

ACTN4 (actinin, alpha 4) (eg, focal segmental glomerulosclerosis), full gene sequence

AFG3L2 (AFG3 ATPase family gene 3-like 2 [S. cerevisiae]) (eg, spinocerebellar ataxia), full gene sequence

AIRE (autoimmune regulator) (eg, autoimmune polyendocrinopathy syndrome type 1), full gene sequence

ALDH7A1 (aldehyde dehydrogenase 7 family, member A1) (eg, pyridoxine-dependent epilepsy), full gene sequence

ANO5 (anoctamin 5) (eg, limb-girdle muscular dystrophy), full gene sequence

ANOS1 (anosmin-1) (eg, Kallmann syndrome 1), full gene sequence

APP (amyloid beta [A4] precursor protein) (eg, Alzheimer disease), full gene sequence

ASS1 (argininosuccinate synthase 1) (eg, citrullinemia type I), full gene sequence

ATL1 (atlastin GTPase 1) (eg, spastic paraplegia), full gene sequence

ATP1A2 (ATPase, Na+/K+ transporting, alpha 2 polypeptide) (eg, familial hemiplegic migraine), full gene sequence

ATP7B (ATPase, Cu++ transporting, beta polypeptide) (eg, Wilson disease), full gene sequence

BBS1 (Bardet-Biedl syndrome 1) (eg, Bardet-Biedl syndrome), full gene sequence

BBS2 (Bardet-Biedl syndrome 2) (eg, Bardet-Biedl syndrome), full gene sequence

BCKDHB (branched-chain keto acid dehydrogenase E1, beta polypeptide) (eg, maple syrup urine disease, type 1B), full gene sequence

BEST1 (bestrophin 1) (eg, vitelliform macular dystrophy), full gene sequence

BMPR2 (bone morphogenetic protein receptor, type II [serine/threonine kinase]) (eg, heritable pulmonary arterial hypertension), full gene sequence

BRAF (B-Raf proto-oncogene, serine/threonine kinase) (eg, Noonan syndrome), full gene sequence

BSCL2 (Berardinelli-Seip congenital lipodystrophy 2 [seipin]) (eg, Berardinelli-Seip congenital lipodystrophy), full gene sequence

BTK (Bruton agammaglobulinemia tyrosine kinase) (eg, X-linked agammaglobulinemia), full gene sequence

CACNB2 (calcium channel, voltage-dependent, beta 2 subunit) (eg, Brugada syndrome), full gene sequence

CAPN3 (calpain 3) (eg, limb-girdle muscular dystrophy [LGMD] type 2A, calpainopathy), full gene sequence

CBS (cystathionine-beta-synthase) (eg, homocystinuria, cystathionine beta-synthase deficiency), full gene sequence

CDH1 (cadherin 1, type 1, E-cadherin [epithelial]) (eg, hereditary diffuse gastric cancer), full gene sequence

CDKL5 (cyclin-dependent kinase-like 5) (eg, early infantile epileptic encephalopathy), full gene sequence

CLCN1 (chloride channel 1, skeletal muscle) (eg, myotonia congenita), full gene sequence

CLCNKB (chloride channel, voltage-sensitive Kb) (eg, Bartter syndrome 3 and 4b), full gene sequence

CNTNAP2 (contactin-associated protein-like 2) (eg, Pitt-Hopkins-like syndrome 1), full gene sequence

COL6A2 (collagen, type VI, alpha 2) (eg, collagen type VI-related disorders), duplication/deletion analysis

CPT1A (carnitine palmitoyltransferase 1A [liver]) (eg, carnitine palmitoyltransferase 1A [CPT1A] deficiency), full gene sequence

CRB1 (crumbs homolog 1 [Drosophila]) (eg, Leber congenital amaurosis), full gene sequence

CREBBP (CREB binding protein) (eg, Rubinstein-Taybi syndrome), duplication/deletion analysis

DBT (dihydrolipoamide branched chain transacylase E2) (eg, maple syrup urine disease, type 2), full gene sequence

DLAT (dihydrolipoamide S-acetyltransferase) (eg, pyruvate dehydrogenase E2 deficiency), full gene sequence

DLD (dihydrolipoamide dehydrogenase) (eg, maple syrup urine disease, type III), full gene sequence

DSC2 (desmocollin) (eg, arrhythmogenic right ventricular dysplasia/cardiomyopathy 11), full gene sequence

DSG2 (desmoglein 2) (eg, arrhythmogenic right ventricular dysplasia/cardiomyopathy 10), full gene sequence

DSP (desmoplakin) (eg, arrhythmogenic right ventricular dysplasia/cardiomyopathy 8), full gene sequence

EFHC1 (EF-hand domain [C-terminal] containing 1) (eg, juvenile myoclonic epilepsy), full gene sequence

EIF2B3 (eukaryotic translation initiation factor 2B, subunit 3 gamma, 58kDa) (eg, leukoencephalopathy with vanishing white matter), full gene sequence

EIF2B4 (eukaryotic translation initiation factor 2B, subunit 4 delta, 67kDa) (eg, leukoencephalopathy with vanishing white matter), full gene sequence

EIF2B5 (eukaryotic translation initiation factor 2B, subunit 5 epsilon, 82kDa) (eg, childhood ataxia with central nervous system hypomyelination/vanishing white matter), full gene sequence

ENG (endoglin) (eg, hereditary hemorrhagic telangiectasia, type 1), full gene sequence

EYA1 (eyes absent homolog 1 [Drosophila]) (eg, branchio-oto-renal [BOR] spectrum disorders), full gene sequence

F8 (coagulation factor VIII) (eg, hemophilia A), duplication/deletion analysis

FAH (fumarylacetoacetate hydrolase [fumarylacetoacetase]) (eg, tyrosinemia, type 1), full gene sequence

FASTKD2 (FAST kinase domains 2) (eg, mitochondrial respiratory chain complex IV deficiency), full gene sequence

FIG4 (FIG4 homolog, SAC1 lipid phosphatase domain containing [S. cerevisiae]) (eg, Charcot-Marie-Tooth disease), full gene sequence

FTSJ1 (FtsJ RNA 2'-O-methyltransferase 1) (eg, X-linked intellectual disability 9), full gene sequence

FUS (fused in sarcoma) (eg, amyotrophic lateral sclerosis), full gene sequence

GAA (glucosidase, alpha; acid) (eg, glycogen storage disease type II [Pompe disease]), full gene sequence

GALC (galactosylceramidase) (eg, Krabbe disease), full gene sequence

GALT (galactose-1-phosphate uridylyltransferase) (eg, galactosemia), full gene sequence

GARS (glycyl-tRNA synthetase) (eg, Charcot-Marie-Tooth disease), full gene sequence

GCDH (glutaryl-CoA dehydrogenase) (eg, glutaricacidemia type 1), full gene sequence

GCK (glucokinase [hexokinase 4]) (eg, maturity-onset diabetes of the young [MODY]), full gene sequence

GLUD1 (glutamate dehydrogenase 1) (eg, familial hyperinsulinism), full gene sequence

GNE (glucosamine [UDP-N-acetyl]-2-epimerase/N-acetylmannosamine kinase) (eg, inclusion body myopathy 2 [IBM2], Nonaka myopathy), full gene sequence

GRN (granulin) (eg, frontotemporal dementia), full gene sequence

HADHA (hydroxyacyl-CoA dehydrogenase/3-ketoacyl-CoA thiolase/enoyl-CoA hydratase [trifunctional protein] alpha subunit) (eg, long chain acyl-coenzyme A dehydrogenase deficiency), full gene sequence

HADHB (hydroxyacyl-CoA dehydrogenase/3-ketoacyl-CoA thiolase/enoyl-CoA hydratase [trifunctional protein], beta subunit) (eg, trifunctional protein deficiency), full gene sequence

HEXA (hexosaminidase A, alpha polypeptide) (eg, Tay-Sachs disease), full gene sequence

HLCS (HLCS holocarboxylase synthetase) (eg, holocarboxylase synthetase deficiency), full gene sequence

HMBS (hydroxymethylbilane synthase) (eg, acute intermittent porphyria), full gene sequence

HNF4A (hepatocyte nuclear factor 4, alpha) (eg, maturity-onset diabetes of the young [MODY]), full gene sequence

IDUA (iduronidase, alpha-L-) (eg, mucopolysaccharidosis type I), full gene sequence

INF2 (inverted formin, FH2 and WH2 domain containing) (eg, focal segmental glomerulosclerosis), full gene sequence

IVD (isovaleryl-CoA dehydrogenase) (eg, isovaleric acidemia), full gene sequence

JAG1 (jagged 1) (eg, Alagille syndrome), duplication/deletion analysis

JUP (junction plakoglobin) (eg, arrhythmogenic right ventricular dysplasia/cardiomyopathy 11), full gene sequence

KCNH2 (potassium voltage-gated channel, subfamily H [eag-related], member 2) (eg, short QT syndrome, long QT syndrome), full gene sequence

KCNQ1 (potassium voltage-gated channel, KQT-like subfamily, member 1) (eg, short QT syndrome, long QT syndrome), full gene sequence

KCNQ2 (potassium voltage-gated channel, KQT-like subfamily, member 2) (eg, epileptic encephalopathy), full gene sequence

LDB3 (LIM domain binding 3) (eg, familial dilated cardiomyopathy, myofibrillar myopathy), full gene sequence

LDLR (low density lipoprotein receptor) (eg, familial hypercholesterolemia), full gene sequence

LEPR (leptin receptor) (eg, obesity with hypogonadism), full gene sequence

LHCGR (luteinizing hormone/choriogonadotropin receptor) (eg, precocious male puberty), full gene sequence

Pathology and Laboratory 80047-89398, 0001U-0520U

LMNA (lamin A/C) (eg, Emery-Dreifuss muscular dystrophy [EDMD1, 2 and 3] limb-girdle muscular dystrophy [LGMD] type 1B, dilated cardiomyopathy [CMD1A], familial partial lipodystrophy [FPLD2]), full gene sequence

LRP5 (low density lipoprotein receptor-related protein 5) (eg, osteopetrosis), full gene sequence

MAP2K1 (mitogen-activated protein kinase 1) (eg, cardiofaciocutaneous syndrome), full gene sequence

MAP2K2 (mitogen-activated protein kinase 2) (eg, cardiofaciocutaneous syndrome), full gene sequence

MAPT (microtubule-associated protein tau) (eg, frontotemporal dementia), full gene sequence

MCCC1 (methylcrotonoyl-CoA carboxylase 1 [alpha]) (eg, 3-methylcrotonyl-CoA carboxylase deficiency), full gene sequence

MCCC2 (methylcrotonoyl-CoA carboxylase 2 [beta]) (eg, 3-methylcrotonyl carboxylase deficiency), full gene sequence

MFN2 (mitofusin 2) (eg, Charcot-Marie-Tooth disease), full gene sequence

MTM1 (myotubularin 1) (eg, X-linked centronuclear myopathy), full gene sequence

MUT (methylmalonyl CoA mutase) (eg, methylmalonic acidemia), full gene sequence

MUTYH (mutY homolog [E. coli]) (eg, MYH-associated polyposis), full gene sequence

NDUFS1 (NADH dehydrogenase [ubiquinone] Fe-S protein 1, 75kDa [NADH-coenzyme Q reductase]) (eg, Leigh syndrome, mitochondrial complex I deficiency), full gene sequence

NF2 (neurofibromin 2 [merlin]) (eg, neurofibromatosis, type 2), full gene sequence

NOTCH3 (notch 3) (eg, cerebral autosomal dominant arteriopathy with subcortical infarcts and leukoencephalopathy [CADASIL]), targeted sequence analysis (eg, exons 1-23)

NPC1 (Niemann-Pick disease, type C1) (eg, Niemann-Pick disease), full gene sequence

NPHP1 (nephronophthisis 1 [juvenile]) (eg, Joubert syndrome), full gene sequence

NSD1 (nuclear receptor binding SET domain protein 1) (eg, Sotos syndrome), full gene sequence

OPA1 (optic atrophy 1) (eg, optic atrophy), duplication/deletion analysis

OPTN (optineurin) (eg, amyotrophic lateral sclerosis), full gene sequence

PAFAH1B1 (platelet-activating factor acetylhydrolase 1b, regulatory subunit 1 [45kDa]) (eg, lissencephaly, Miller-Dieker syndrome), full gene sequence

PAH (phenylalanine hydroxylase) (eg, phenylketonuria), full gene sequence

PARK2 (Parkinson protein 2, E3 ubiquitin protein ligase [parkin]) (eg, Parkinson disease), full gene sequence

PAX2 (paired box 2) (eg, renal coloboma syndrome), full gene sequence

PC (pyruvate carboxylase) (eg, pyruvate carboxylase deficiency), full gene sequence

PCCA (propionyl CoA carboxylase, alpha polypeptide) (eg, propionic acidemia, type 1), full gene sequence

PCCB (propionyl CoA carboxylase, beta polypeptide) (eg, propionic acidemia), full gene sequence

PCDH15 (protocadherin-related 15) (eg, Usher syndrome type 1F), duplication/deletion analysis

PCSK9 (proprotein convertase subtilisin/kexin type 9) (eg, familial hypercholesterolemia), full gene sequence

PDHA1 (pyruvate dehydrogenase [lipoamide] alpha 1) (eg, lactic acidosis), full gene sequence

PDHX (pyruvate dehydrogenase complex, component X) (eg, lactic acidosis), full gene sequence

PHEX (phosphate-regulating endopeptidase homolog, X-linked) (eg, hypophosphatemic rickets), full gene sequence

PKD2 (polycystic kidney disease 2 [autosomal dominant]) (eg, polycystic kidney disease), full gene sequence

PKP2 (plakophilin 2) (eg, arrhythmogenic right ventricular dysplasia/cardiomyopathy 9), full gene sequence

PNKD (paroxysmal nonkinesigenic dyskinesia) (eg, paroxysmal nonkinesigenic dyskinesia), full gene sequence

POLG (polymerase [DNA directed], gamma) (eg, Alpers-Huttenlocher syndrome, autosomal dominant progressive external ophthalmoplegia), full gene sequence

POMGNT1 (protein O-linked mannose beta1,2-N acetylglucosaminyltransferase) (eg, muscle-eye-brain disease, Walker-Warburg syndrome), full gene sequence

POMT1 (protein-O-mannosyltransferase 1) (eg, limb-girdle muscular dystrophy [LGMD] type 2K, Walker-Warburg syndrome), full gene sequence

POMT2 (protein-O-mannosyltransferase 2) (eg, limb-girdle muscular dystrophy [LGMD] type 2N, Walker-Warburg syndrome), full gene sequence

PPOX (protoporphyrinogen oxidase) (eg, variegate porphyria), full gene sequence

PRKAG2 (protein kinase, AMP-activated, gamma 2 non-catalytic subunit) (eg, familial hypertrophic cardiomyopathy with Wolff-Parkinson-White syndrome, lethal congenital glycogen storage disease of heart), full gene sequence

PRKCG (protein kinase C, gamma) (eg, spinocerebellar ataxia), full gene sequence

PSEN2 (presenilin 2 [Alzheimer disease 4]) (eg, Alzheimer disease), full gene sequence

PTPN11 (protein tyrosine phosphatase, non-receptor type 11) (eg, Noonan syndrome, LEOPARD syndrome), full gene sequence

PYGM (phosphorylase, glycogen, muscle) (eg, glycogen storage disease type V, McArdle disease), full gene sequence

RAF1 (v-raf-1 murine leukemia viral oncogene homolog 1) (eg, LEOPARD syndrome), full gene sequence

RET (ret proto-oncogene) (eg, Hirschsprung disease), full gene sequence

RPE65 (retinal pigment epithelium-specific protein 65kDa) (eg, retinitis pigmentosa, Leber congenital amaurosis), full gene sequence

RYR1 (ryanodine receptor 1, skeletal) (eg, malignant hyperthermia), targeted sequence analysis of exons with functionally-confirmed mutations

SCN4A (sodium channel, voltage-gated, type IV, alpha subunit) (eg, hyperkalemic periodic paralysis), full gene sequence

SCNN1A (sodium channel, nonvoltage-gated 1 alpha) (eg, pseudohypoaldosteronism), full gene sequence

SCNN1B (sodium channel, nonvoltage-gated 1, beta) (eg, Liddle syndrome, pseudohypoaldosteronism), full gene sequence

SCNN1G (sodium channel, nonvoltage-gated 1, gamma) (eg, Liddle syndrome, pseudohypoaldosteronism), full gene sequence

SDHA (succinate dehydrogenase complex, subunit A, flavoprotein [Fp]) (eg, Leigh syndrome, mitochondrial complex II deficiency), full gene sequence

SETX (senataxin) (eg, ataxia), full gene sequence

SGCE (sarcoglycan, epsilon) (eg, myoclonic dystonia), full gene sequence

SH3TC2 (SH3 domain and tetratricopeptide repeats 2) (eg, Charcot-Marie-Tooth disease), full gene sequence

SLC9A6 (solute carrier family 9 [sodium/hydrogen exchanger], member 6) (eg, Christianson syndrome), full gene sequence

SLC26A4 (solute carrier family 26, member 4) (eg, Pendred syndrome), full gene sequence

SLC37A4 (solute carrier family 37 [glucose-6-phosphate transporter], member 4) (eg, glycogen storage disease type Ih), full gene sequence

SMAD4 (SMAD family member 4) (eg, hemorrhagic telangiectasia syndrome, juvenile polyposis), full gene sequence

SOS1 (son of sevenless homolog 1) (eg, Noonan syndrome, gingival fibromatosis), full gene sequence

SPAST (spastin) (eg, spastic paraplegia), full gene sequence

SPG7 (spastic paraplegia 7 [pure and complicated autosomal recessive]) (eg, spastic paraplegia), full gene sequence

STXBP1 (syntaxin-binding protein 1) (eg, epileptic encephalopathy), full gene sequence

TAZ (tafazzin) (eg, methylglutaconic aciduria type 2, Barth syndrome), full gene sequence

TCF4 (transcription factor 4) (eg, Pitt-Hopkins syndrome), full gene sequence

TH (tyrosine hydroxylase) (eg, Segawa syndrome), full gene sequence

TMEM43 (transmembrane protein 43) (eg, arrhythmogenic right ventricular cardiomyopathy), full gene sequence

TNNT2 (troponin T, type 2 [cardiac]) (eg, familial hypertrophic cardiomyopathy), full gene sequence

TRPC6 (transient receptor potential cation channel, subfamily C, member 6) (eg, focal segmental glomerulosclerosis), full gene sequence

TSC1 (tuberous sclerosis 1) (eg, tuberous sclerosis), full gene sequence

TSC2 (tuberous sclerosis 2) (eg, tuberous sclerosis), duplication/deletion analysis

UBE3A (ubiquitin protein ligase E3A) (eg, Angelman syndrome), full gene sequence

UMOD (uromodulin) (eg, glomerulocystic kidney disease with hyperuricemia and isosthenuria), full gene sequence

VWF (von Willebrand factor) (von Willebrand disease type 2A), extended targeted sequence analysis (eg, exons 11-16, 24-26, 51, 52)

WAS (Wiskott-Aldrich syndrome [eczema-thrombocytopenia]) (eg, Wiskott-Aldrich syndrome), full gene sequence

➔ *CPT Changes: An Insider's View* 2012, 2013, 2014, 2016, 2017, 2018, 2020, 2024

➔ *CPT Assistant* May 12:4, Jul 13:12, Sep 13:5-6, 8, 11, Jan 15:3, Aug 16:10, Apr 17:10, May 18:6, Nov 18:9, Feb 20:10, Mar 20:13, Mar 23:36

81407   Molecular pathology procedure, Level 8 (eg, analysis of 26-50 exons by DNA sequence analysis, mutation scanning or duplication/deletion variants of >50 exons, sequence analysis of multiple genes on one platform)

ABCC8 (ATP-binding cassette, sub-family C [CFTR/MRP], member 8) (eg, familial hyperinsulinism), full gene sequence

AGL (amylo-alpha-1, 6-glucosidase, 4-alpha-glucanotransferase) (eg, glycogen storage disease type III), full gene sequence

AHI1 (Abelson helper integration site 1) (eg, Joubert syndrome), full gene sequence

APOB (apolipoprotein B) (eg, familial hypercholesterolemia type B) full gene sequence

ASPM (asp [abnormal spindle] homolog, microcephaly associated [Drosophila]) (eg, primary microcephaly), full gene sequence

CHD7 (chromodomain helicase DNA binding protein 7) (eg, CHARGE syndrome), full gene sequence

COL4A4 (collagen, type IV, alpha 4) (eg, Alport syndrome), full gene sequence

COL4A5 (collagen, type IV, alpha 5) (eg, Alport syndrome), duplication/deletion analysis

COL6A1 (collagen, type VI, alpha 1) (eg, collagen type VI-related disorders), full gene sequence

COL6A2 (collagen, type VI, alpha 2) (eg, collagen type VI-related disorders), full gene sequence

COL6A3 (collagen, type VI, alpha 3) (eg, collagen type VI-related disorders), full gene sequence

CREBBP (CREB binding protein) (eg, Rubinstein-Taybi syndrome), full gene sequence

F8 (coagulation factor VIII) (eg, hemophilia A), full gene sequence

JAG1 (jagged 1) (eg, Alagille syndrome), full gene sequence

KDM5C (lysine demethylase 5C) (eg, X-linked intellectual disability), full gene sequence

KIAA0196 (KIAA0196) (eg, spastic paraplegia), full gene sequence

L1CAM (L1 cell adhesion molecule) (eg, MASA syndrome, X-linked hydrocephaly), full gene sequence

LAMB2 (laminin, beta 2 [laminin S]) (eg, Pierson syndrome), full gene sequence

MYBPC3 (myosin binding protein C, cardiac) (eg, familial hypertrophic cardiomyopathy), full gene sequence

MYH6 (myosin, heavy chain 6, cardiac muscle, alpha) (eg, familial dilated cardiomyopathy), full gene sequence

MYH7 (myosin, heavy chain 7, cardiac muscle, beta) (eg, familial hypertrophic cardiomyopathy, Liang distal myopathy), full gene sequence

MYO7A (myosin VIIA) (eg, Usher syndrome, type 1), full gene sequence

NOTCH1 (notch 1) (eg, aortic valve disease), full gene sequence

NPHS1 (nephrosis 1, congenital, Finnish type [nephrin]) (eg, congenital Finnish nephrosis), full gene sequence

OPA1 (optic atrophy 1) (eg, optic atrophy), full gene sequence

PCDH15 (protocadherin-related 15) (eg, Usher syndrome, type 1), full gene sequence

PKD1 (polycystic kidney disease 1 [autosomal dominant]) (eg, polycystic kidney disease), full gene sequence

PLCE1 (phospholipase C, epsilon 1) (eg, nephrotic syndrome type 3), full gene sequence

SCN1A (sodium channel, voltage-gated, type 1, alpha subunit) (eg, generalized epilepsy with febrile seizures), full gene sequence

SCN5A (sodium channel, voltage-gated, type V, alpha subunit) (eg, familial dilated cardiomyopathy), full gene sequence

SLC12A1 (solute carrier family 12 [sodium/potassium/chloride transporters], member 1) (eg, Bartter syndrome), full gene sequence

SLC12A3 (solute carrier family 12 [sodium/chloride transporters], member 3) (eg, Gitelman syndrome), full gene sequence

SPG11 (spastic paraplegia 11 [autosomal recessive]) (eg, spastic paraplegia), full gene sequence

SPTBN2 (spectrin, beta, non-erythrocytic 2) (eg, spinocerebellar ataxia), full gene sequence

TMEM67 (transmembrane protein 67) (eg, Joubert syndrome), full gene sequence

TSC2 (tuberous sclerosis 2) (eg, tuberous sclerosis), full gene sequence

USH1C (Usher syndrome 1C [autosomal recessive, severe]) (eg, Usher syndrome, type 1), full gene sequence

VPS13B (vacuolar protein sorting 13 homolog B [yeast]) (eg, Cohen syndrome), duplication/deletion analysis

WDR62 (WD repeat domain 62) (eg, primary autosomal recessive microcephaly), full gene sequence

➲ *CPT Changes: An Insider's View* 2012, 2013, 2014, 2019, 2020, 2024

➲ *CPT Assistant* May 12:4, Jul 13:12, Sep 13:14, Jan 15:3, Aug 16:10, May 18:6, Nov 18:9, Jul 19:3

Pathology and Laboratory 80047-89398, 0001U-0520U

664   ★ = Telemedicine   ◀ = Audio-only   ✚ = Add-on code   ✒ = FDA approval pending   # = Resequenced code   ⊘ = Modifier 51 exempt   ➲➲➲ = See p xxi for details

81408   Molecular pathology procedure, Level 9 (eg, analysis of >50 exons in a single gene by DNA sequence analysis)

ABCA4 (ATP-binding cassette, sub-family A [ABC1], member 4) (eg, Stargardt disease, age-related macular degeneration), full gene sequence

ATM (ataxia telangiectasia mutated) (eg, ataxia telangiectasia), full gene sequence

CDH23 (cadherin-related 23) (eg, Usher syndrome, type 1), full gene sequence

CEP290 (centrosomal protein 290kDa) (eg, Joubert syndrome), full gene sequence

COL1A1 (collagen, type I, alpha 1) (eg, osteogenesis imperfecta, type I), full gene sequence

COL1A2 (collagen, type I, alpha 2) (eg, osteogenesis imperfecta, type I), full gene sequence

COL4A1 (collagen, type IV, alpha 1) (eg, brain small-vessel disease with hemorrhage), full gene sequence

COL4A3 (collagen, type IV, alpha 3 [Goodpasture antigen]) (eg, Alport syndrome), full gene sequence

COL4A5 (collagen, type IV, alpha 5) (eg, Alport syndrome), full gene sequence

DMD (dystrophin) (eg, Duchenne/Becker muscular dystrophy), full gene sequence

DYSF (dysferlin, limb girdle muscular dystrophy 2B [autosomal recessive]) (eg, limb-girdle muscular dystrophy), full gene sequence

FBN1 (fibrillin 1) (eg, Marfan syndrome), full gene sequence

ITPR1 (inositol 1,4,5-trisphosphate receptor, type 1) (eg, spinocerebellar ataxia), full gene sequence

LAMA2 (laminin, alpha 2) (eg, congenital muscular dystrophy), full gene sequence

LRRK2 (leucine-rich repeat kinase 2) (eg, Parkinson disease), full gene sequence

MYH11 (myosin, heavy chain 11, smooth muscle) (eg, thoracic aortic aneurysms and aortic dissections), full gene sequence

NEB (nebulin) (eg, nemaline myopathy 2), full gene sequence

NF1 (neurofibromin 1) (eg, neurofibromatosis, type 1), full gene sequence

PKHD1 (polycystic kidney and hepatic disease 1) (eg, autosomal recessive polycystic kidney disease), full gene sequence

RYR1 (ryanodine receptor 1, skeletal) (eg, malignant hyperthermia), full gene sequence

RYR2 (ryanodine receptor 2 [cardiac]) (eg, catecholaminergic polymorphic ventricular tachycardia, arrhythmogenic right ventricular dysplasia), full gene sequence or targeted sequence analysis of > 50 exons

USH2A (Usher syndrome 2A [autosomal recessive, mild]) (eg, Usher syndrome, type 2), full gene sequence

VPS13B (vacuolar protein sorting 13 homolog B [yeast]) (eg, Cohen syndrome), full gene sequence

VWF (von Willebrand factor) (eg, von Willebrand disease types 1 and 3), full gene sequence

➡ *CPT Changes: An Insider's View* 2012, 2013, 2014

➡ *CPT Assistant* May 12:4, Jul 13:12, Sep 13:4-5, 14, Jan 15:3, Aug 16:10, May 18:6, Nov 18:9

 # 81479   Unlisted molecular pathology procedure

➡ *CPT Changes: An Insider's View* 2013

➡ *CPT Assistant* Jul 13:12, Sep 13:4, 8, Jan 15:3, Apr 16:4, Aug 16:10, Sep 16:10, Apr 17:10, Jun 18:8, Sep 18:15, Nov 18:9, Dec 18:10, May 19:5, Jun 19:11, Oct 20:8, Dec 20:14, Feb 21:14, Mar 23:36

Genomic Sequencing Procedures and Other Molecular Multianalyte Assays

Genomic sequencing procedures (GSPs) and other molecular multianalyte assays are DNA and/or RNA sequence analysis methods that simultaneously assay multiple genes or genetic regions relevant to a clinical situation. They may target specific combinations of genes or genetic material, or they may assay the exome or genome. The technology typically used for genomic sequencing is massively parallel sequencing (MPS) (eg, next-generation sequencing [NGS]) although other technologies may be employed. GSPs are performed on nucleic acids from germline or neoplastic samples. Examples of applications include aneuploidy analysis of cell-free circulating fetal DNA, gene panels for somatic alterations in neoplasms, and sequence analysis of the exome or genome to determine the cause of developmental delay. Exome and genome procedures are designed to evaluate the genetic material in totality or near totality. Although commonly used to identify sequence (base) changes, they can also be used to identify copy number, structural changes, and abnormal zygosity patterns, and these analyses may be performed in combination or as separate and distinct studies. Another unique feature of GSPs is the ability to "re-query" or re-evaluate the sequence data (eg, complex phenotype such as developmental delay is reassessed when new genetic knowledge is attained, or for a separate unrelated clinical indication). The analyses below are often performed using NGS/MPS technology; however, they

Pathology and Laboratory 80047-89398, 0001U-0520U

may also be performed using molecular techniques (eg, polymerase chain reaction [PCR] methods and microarrays). These codes should be used when the components of the descriptor(s) are fulfilled regardless of the technique used for analysis, unless specifically noted in the code descriptor. When a GSP assay includes gene(s) that is listed in more than one code descriptor, the code for the most specific test for the primary disorder sought should be reported, rather than reporting multiple codes for the same gene(s). When all of the components of the descriptor are not performed, use individual Tier 1 codes, Tier 2 codes, or 81479 (Unlisted molecular pathology procedure).

Testing for somatic alterations in neoplasms may be reported differently depending on whether combined or separate methods and analyses are used for both DNA and RNA analytes. Procedures for somatic alterations in neoplasms which include DNA analysis or DNA and RNA analysis using a single combined method are reported with 81445, 81450, 81455, 81457, 81458, 81459, 81462, 81463, 81464. RNA analysis performed using a separate method is reported with 81449, 81451, 81456. When evaluation for tumor mutation burden (TMB) and/or microsatellite instability (MSI) is performed as part of the same test for somatic alterations in neoplasms, report 81457, 81458, 81459. When a genomic sequencing procedure (GSP) is performed on cell-free nucleic acid (eg, plasma), sometimes referred to as a liquid biopsy, report 81462, 81463, 81464.

Definitions

Cell-free nucleic acid: DNA or RNA released into the blood and other body fluids. Cell-free nucleic acid released from fetal cells can be sampled for non-invasive prenatal testing (NIPT) while that released from tumor cells can be sampled for cancer, sometimes referred to as tumor liquid biopsy.

Copy number variants (CNVs): structural changes in the genome which are composed of large deletions or duplications. CNVs can be found in the germline but can also occur in somatic cells. See also Duplication/Deletion (Dup/Del). Duplications may also be referred to as amplifications.

Duplication/Deletion (Dup/Del): terms that are usually used together with the "/" to refer to molecular testing, which assesses the dosage of a particular genomic region. The region tested is typically of modest to substantial size, from several dozen to several million or more nucleotides. Normal gene dosage is two copies per cell, except for the sex chromosomes (X and Y). Thus, zero or one copy represents a deletion and three (or more) copies represent a duplication.

Low-pass sequencing: a method of genome sequencing intended for cytogenomic analysis of chromosomal abnormalities, such as that performed for trait mapping or copy number variation, typically performed to an average depth of sequencing ranging from 0.1 to 5X.

Massively parallel sequencing (MPS): high-throughput method used to determine a portion of the nucleotide sequences in an individual patient's genome, utilizing advanced (non-Sanger) sequencing technologies that are capable of processing multiple DNA and/or RNA sequences in parallel. While other technologies exist, next-generation sequencing (NGS) is a common technique used to achieve MPS.

Microsatellite instability (MSI): a type of DNA hypermutation or predisposition to mutation in which replication errors are not corrected due to defective DNA mismatch repair (dMMR) mechanism. MSI manifests as insertions or deletions in short tandem repeat (STR) (defined in the molecular pathology guidelines) alleles and can be identified by changes in the DNA repeat sequence length.

Rearrangements: structural chromosomal variations such as deletions, insertions, inversions (defined in the molecular pathology guidelines), or translocations (defined in the molecular pathology guidelines) that bring together genetic material that is not normally adjacent in the unmodified genome. It can manifest as abnormal gene expression or as an abnormal fusion product at the RNA and/or protein level. Rearrangement can also refer to the process by which immunoglobulin and T cell receptor genes are normally modified.

Tumor mutational burden (TMB): the number of somatic mutations detected per million bases (Mb) of genomic sequence investigated from a cancer specimen. It is usually obtained from analysis using a next generation sequencing method. It is considered a biomarker to guide immunotherapy decisions for patients with cancer.

The assays in this section represent discrete genetic values, properties, or characteristics in which the measurement or analysis of each analyte is potentially of independent medical significance or useful in medical management. In contrast to multianalyte assays with algorithmic analyses (MAAAs), the assays in this section do not represent algorithmically combined results to obtain a risk score or other value, which in itself represents a new and distinct medical property that is of independent medical significance relative to the individual, component test results.

(For cytogenomic [genome-wide] analysis for constitutional chromosomal abnormalities, see 81228, 81229, 81349, 81405, 81406)

Code	Specimen Source			Nucleic Acid	Sequence Variants	Copy Number Variants	Microsatellite Instability	Tumor Mutation Burden	Rearrangements
	Solid Organ	**Hematolymphoid**	**Cell-Free**						
81445	X		No	DNA or DNA/RNA	X	X			X
81449	X		No	RNA	X				X
81450		X	No	DNA or DNA/RNA	X	X			X
81451		X	No	RNA	X				X
81455	X	X	No	DNA or DNA/RNA	X	X			X
81456	X	X	No	RNA	X				X
81457	X		No	DNA	X		X		
81458	X		No	DNA	X	X	X		
81459	X		No	DNA or DNA/RNA	X	X	X	X	X
81462	X		Yes	DNA or DNA/RNA	X	X			X
81463	X		Yes	DNA	X	X	X		
81464	X		Yes	DNA or DNA/RNA	X	X	X	X	X

81410 Aortic dysfunction or dilation (eg, Marfan syndrome, Loeys Dietz syndrome, Ehler Danlos syndrome type IV, arterial tortuosity syndrome); genomic sequence analysis panel, must include sequencing of at least 9 genes, including *FBN1, TGFBR1, TGFBR2, COL3A1, MYH11, ACTA2, SLC2A10, SMAD3,* and *MYLK*

➔ *CPT Changes: An Insider's View* 2015

➔ *CPT Assistant* Jan 15:3

81411 duplication/deletion analysis panel, must include analyses for *TGFBR1, TGFBR2, MYH11,* and *COL3A1*

➔ *CPT Changes: An Insider's View* 2015

➔ *CPT Assistant* Jan 15:3

81412 Ashkenazi Jewish associated disorders (eg, Bloom syndrome, Canavan disease, cystic fibrosis, familial dysautonomia, Fanconi anemia group C, Gaucher disease, Tay-Sachs disease), genomic sequence analysis panel, must include sequencing of at least 9 genes, including *ASPA, BLM, CFTR, FANCC, GBA, HEXA, IKBKAP, MCOLN1,* and *SMPD1*

➔ *CPT Changes: An Insider's View* 2016

➔ *CPT Assistant* Apr 16:4, Nov 18:9

81413 Cardiac ion channelopathies (eg, Brugada syndrome, long QT syndrome, short QT syndrome, catecholaminergic polymorphic ventricular tachycardia); genomic sequence analysis panel, must include sequencing of at least 10 genes, including *ANK2, CASQ2, CAV3, KCNE1, KCNE2, KCNH2, KCNJ2, KCNQ1, RYR2,* and *SCN5A*

➔ *CPT Changes: An Insider's View* 2017

➔ *CPT Assistant* Apr 17:3

81414 duplication/deletion gene analysis panel, must include analysis of at least 2 genes, including *KCNH2* and *KCNQ1*

➔ *CPT Changes: An Insider's View* 2017

➔ *CPT Assistant* Apr 17:3

(For genomic sequencing panel testing for cardiomyopathies, use 81439)

(Do not report 81413, 81414 in conjunction with 81439 when performed on the same date of service)

Pathology and Laboratory 80047-89398, 0001U-0520U

81418   Drug metabolism (eg, pharmacogenomics) genomic sequence analysis panel, must include testing of at least 6 genes, including *CYP2C19*, *CYP2D6*, and *CYP2D6* duplication/deletion analysis

➔ *CPT Changes: An Insider's View* 2023

81419   Epilepsy genomic sequence analysis panel, must include analyses for *ALDH7A1*, *CACNA1A*, *CDKL5*, *CHD2*, *GABRG2*, *GRIN2A*, *KCNQ2*, *MECP2*, *PCDH19*, *POLG*, *PRRT2*, *SCN1A*, *SCN1B*, *SCN2A*, *SCN8A*, *SLC2A1*, *SLC9A6*, *STXBP1*, *SYNGAP1*, *TCF4*, *TPP1*, *TSC1*, *TSC2*, and *ZEB2*

➔ *CPT Changes: An Insider's View* 2021

81415   Exome (eg, unexplained constitutional or heritable disorder or syndrome); sequence analysis

➔ *CPT Changes: An Insider's View* 2015

➔ *CPT Assistant* Jan 15:3

+ 81416   sequence analysis, each comparator exome (eg, parents, siblings) (List separately in addition to code for primary procedure)

➔ *CPT Changes: An Insider's View* 2015

➔ *CPT Assistant* Jan 15:3

(Use 81416 in conjunction with 81415)

81417   re-evaluation of previously obtained exome sequence (eg, updated knowledge or unrelated condition/syndrome)

➔ *CPT Changes: An Insider's View* 2015

➔ *CPT Assistant* Jan 15:3

(Do not report 81417 for incidental findings)

(Do not report 81349 when analysis for chromosomal abnormalities is performed by sequence analysis included in 81415, 81416)

(For cytogenomic [genome-wide] copy number assessment, see 81228, 81229)

81418   Code is out of numerical sequence. See 81414-81416

81419   Code is out of numerical sequence. See 81413-81416

81420   Fetal chromosomal aneuploidy (eg, trisomy 21, monosomy X) genomic sequence analysis panel, circulating cell-free fetal DNA in maternal blood, must include analysis of chromosomes 13, 18, and 21

➔ *CPT Changes: An Insider's View* 2015

➔ *CPT Assistant* Jan 15:3, Dec 15:17, Apr 18:11

(Do not report 81228, 81229, 88271 when performing genomic sequencing procedures or other molecular multianalyte assays for copy number analysis)

(Do not report 81349 when analysis for chromosomal abnormalities is performed by sequence analysis included in 81425, 81426)

81422   Fetal chromosomal microdeletion(s) genomic sequence analysis (eg, DiGeorge syndrome, Cri-du-chat syndrome), circulating cell-free fetal DNA in maternal blood

➔ *CPT Changes: An Insider's View* 2017

➔ *CPT Assistant* Apr 17:3

(Do not report 81228, 81229, 88271 when performing genomic sequencing procedures or other molecular multianalyte assays for copy number analysis)

(Do not report 81349 when analysis for chromosomal abnormalities is performed by sequence analysis included in 81425, 81426)

81443   Genetic testing for severe inherited conditions (eg, cystic fibrosis, Ashkenazi Jewish-associated disorders [eg, Bloom syndrome, Canavan disease, Fanconi anemia type C, mucolipidosis type VI, Gaucher disease, Tay-Sachs disease], beta hemoglobinopathies, phenylketonuria, galactosemia), genomic sequence analysis panel, must include sequencing of at least 15 genes (eg, *ACADM*, *ARSA*, *ASPA*, *ATP7B*, *BCKDHA*, *BCKDHB*, *BLM*, *CFTR*, *DHCR7*, *FANCC*, *G6PC*, *GAA*, *GALT*, *GBA*, *GBE1*, *HBB*, *HEXA*, *IKBKAP*, *MCOLN1*, *PAH*)

➔ *CPT Changes: An Insider's View* 2019

➔ *CPT Assistant* Nov 18:9, Jul 19:3

(If spinal muscular atrophy testing is performed separately, use 81329)

(If testing is performed only for Ashkenazi Jewish-associated disorders, use 81412)

(If *FMR1* [expanded allele] testing is performed separately, use 81243)

(If hemoglobin A testing is performed separately, use 81257)

(Do not report 81443 in conjunction with 81412)

81425   Genome (eg, unexplained constitutional or heritable disorder or syndrome); sequence analysis

➔ *CPT Changes: An Insider's View* 2015

➔ *CPT Assistant* Jan 15:3, Apr 24:36

+ 81426   sequence analysis, each comparator genome (eg, parents, siblings) (List separately in addition to code for primary procedure)

➔ *CPT Changes: An Insider's View* 2015

➔ *CPT Assistant* Jan 15:3, Apr 24:36

(Use 81426 in conjunction with 81425)

81427   re-evaluation of previously obtained genome sequence (eg, updated knowledge or unrelated condition/syndrome)

➔ *CPT Changes: An Insider's View* 2015

➔ *CPT Assistant* Jan 15:3, Apr 24:36

(Do not report 81427 for incidental findings)

(Do not report 81349 when analysis for chromosomal abnormalities is performed by sequence analysis included in 81425, 81426)

(For copy number assessment by cytogenomic [genome-wide] analysis for constitutional chromosomal abnormalities, see 81228, 81229)

(For cytogenomic [genome-wide] analysis for constitutional chromosomal abnormalities interrogation of genomic regions for copy number and loss-of-heterozygosity variants, low-pass sequencing analysis, use 81349)

81430   Hearing loss (eg, nonsyndromic hearing loss, Usher syndrome, Pendred syndrome); genomic sequence analysis panel, must include sequencing of at least 60 genes, including *CDH23, CLRN1, GJB2, GPR98, MTRNR1, MYO7A, MYO15A, PCDH15, OTOF, SLC26A4, TMC1, TMPRSS3, USH1C, USH1G, USH2A,* and *WFS1*

→ *CPT Changes: An Insider's View* 2015
→ *CPT Assistant* Jan 15:3

81431   duplication/deletion analysis panel, must include copy number analyses for *STRC* and *DFNB1* deletions in *GJB2* and *GJB6* genes

→ *CPT Changes: An Insider's View* 2015
→ *CPT Assistant* Jan 15:3

▲ **81432**   Hereditary breast cancer-related disorders (eg, hereditary breast cancer, hereditary ovarian cancer, hereditary endometrial cancer, hereditary pancreatic cancer, hereditary prostate cancer), genomic sequence analysis panel, 5 or more genes, interrogation for sequence variants and copy number variants

→ *CPT Changes: An Insider's View* 2016, 2018, 2025
→ *CPT Assistant* Apr 16:4, May 19:5, Feb 21:14

►(Do not report 81432 in conjunction with 81435, 81437)◄

►(81433 has been deleted. To report only a duplication/deletion analysis panel for hereditary breast cancer-related disorders, use 81479)◄

81434   Hereditary retinal disorders (eg, retinitis pigmentosa, Leber congenital amaurosis, cone-rod dystrophy), genomic sequence analysis panel, must include sequencing of at least 15 genes, including *ABCA4, CNGA1, CRB1, EYS, PDE6A, PDE6B, PRPF31, PRPH2, RDH12, RHO, RP1, RP2, RPE65, RPGR,* and *USH2A*

→ *CPT Changes: An Insider's View* 2016
→ *CPT Assistant* Apr 16:4

▲ **81435**   Hereditary colon cancer-related disorders (eg, Lynch syndrome, PTEN hamartoma syndrome, Cowden syndrome, familial adenomatosis polyposis), genomic sequence analysis panel, 5 or more genes, interrogation for sequence variants and copy number variants

→ *CPT Changes: An Insider's View* 2015, 2016, 2025
→ *CPT Assistant* Apr 15:3, April 16:4, Feb 21:14

►(Do not report 81435 in conjunction with 81432, 81437)◄

►(81436 has been deleted. To report only a duplication/deletion analysis panel for hereditary colon cancer-related disorders, use 81479)◄

▲ **81437**   Hereditary neuroendocrine tumor-related disorders (eg, medullary thyroid carcinoma, parathyroid carcinoma, malignant pheochromocytoma or paraganglioma), genomic sequence analysis panel, 5 or more genes, interrogation for sequence variants and copy number variants

→ *CPT Changes: An Insider's View* 2016, 2025
→ *CPT Assistant* Apr 16:4

►(Do not report 81437 in conjunction with 81432, 81435)◄

►(81438 has been deleted. To report only a duplication/deletion analysis panel for hereditary neuroendocrine tumor-related disorders, use 81479)◄

81448   Hereditary peripheral neuropathies (eg, Charcot-Marie-Tooth, spastic paraplegia), genomic sequence analysis panel, must include sequencing of at least 5 peripheral neuropathy-related genes (eg, *BSCL2, GJB1, MFN2, MPZ, REEP1, SPAST, SPG11, SPTLC1*)

→ *CPT Changes: An Insider's View* 2018
→ *CPT Assistant* May 18:6

81439   Hereditary cardiomyopathy (eg, hypertrophic cardiomyopathy, dilated cardiomyopathy, arrhythmogenic right ventricular cardiomyopathy), genomic sequence analysis panel, must include sequencing of at least 5 cardiomyopathy-related genes (eg, *DSG2, MYBPC3, MYH7, PKP2, TTN*)

→ *CPT Changes: An Insider's View* 2017, 2018
→ *CPT Assistant* Apr 17:3, Sep 18:15, Dec 20:14

(Do not report 81439 in conjunction with 81413, 81414 when performed on the same date of service)

(For genomic sequencing panel testing for cardiac ion channelopathies, see 81413, 81414)

81441   Inherited bone marrow failure syndromes (IBMFS) (eg, Fanconi anemia, dyskeratosis congenita, Diamond-Blackfan anemia, Shwachman-Diamond syndrome, GATA2 deficiency syndrome, congenital amegakaryocytic thrombocytopenia) sequence analysis panel, must include sequencing of at least 30 genes, including *BRCA2, BRIP1, DKC1, FANCA, FANCB, FANCC, FANCD2, FANCE, FANCF, FANCG, FANCI, FANCL, GATA1, GATA2, MPL, NHP2, NOP10, PALB2, RAD51C, RPL11, RPL35A, RPL5, RPS10, RPS19, RPS24, RPS26, RPS7, SBDS, TERT,* and *TINF2*

→ *CPT Changes: An Insider's View* 2023

81440   Nuclear encoded mitochondrial genes (eg, neurologic or myopathic phenotypes), genomic sequence panel, must include analysis of at least 100 genes, including *BCS1L, C10orf2, COQ2, COX10, DGUOK, MPV17, OPA1, PDSS2, POLG, POLG2, RRM2B, SCO1, SCO2, SLC25A4, SUCLA2, SUCLG1, TAZ, TK2,* and *TYMP*

→ *CPT Changes: An Insider's View* 2015
→ *CPT Assistant* Jan 15:3

▲ = Revised code   ● = New code   ►◄ = Contains new or revised text   ✄ = Duplicate PLA test   ↕ = Category I PLA   American Medical Association   **669**

Pathology and Laboratory   80047-89398, 0001U-0520U

81441 Code is out of numerical sequence. See 81437-81442

81442 Noonan spectrum disorders (eg, Noonan syndrome, cardio-facio-cutaneous syndrome, Costello syndrome, LEOPARD syndrome, Noonan-like syndrome), genomic sequence analysis panel, must include sequencing of at least 12 genes, including *BRAF, CBL, HRAS, KRAS, MAP2K1, MAP2K2, NRAS, PTPN11, RAF1, RIT1, SHOC2,* and *SOS1*

➔ *CPT Changes: An Insider's View* 2016

➔ *CPT Assistant* Apr 16:4

81443 Code is out of numerical sequence. See 81420-81426

81445 Solid organ neoplasm, genomic sequence analysis panel, 5-50 genes, interrogation for sequence variants and copy number variants or rearrangements, if performed; DNA analysis or combined DNA and RNA analysis

➔ *CPT Changes: An Insider's View* 2015, 2016, 2023, 2024

➔ *CPT Assistant* Jan 15:3, Apr 16:4, May 23:11, Feb 24:8

81448 Code is out of numerical sequence. See 81437-81442

81449 RNA analysis

➔ *CPT Changes: An Insider's View* 2023, 2024

➔ *CPT Assistant* May 23:11, Feb 24:8

(For copy number assessment by microarray, use 81277)

81450 Hematolymphoid neoplasm or disorder, genomic sequence analysis panel, 5-50 genes, interrogation for sequence variants, and copy number variants or rearrangements, or isoform expression or mRNA expression levels, if performed; DNA analysis or combined DNA and RNA analysis

➔ *CPT Changes: An Insider's View* 2015, 2016, 2023, 2024

➔ *CPT Assistant* Jan 15:3, Apr 16:4, Feb 21:14, May 23:11, Feb 24:8

81451 RNA analysis

➔ *CPT Changes: An Insider's View* 2023, 2024

➔ *CPT Assistant* May 23:11, Feb 24:8

(For copy number assessment by microarray, use 81406)

81455 Solid organ or hematolymphoid neoplasm or disorder, 51 or greater genes, genomic sequence analysis panel, interrogation for sequence variants and copy number variants or rearrangements, or isoform expression or mRNA expression levels, if performed; DNA analysis or combined DNA and RNA analysis

➔ *CPT Changes: An Insider's View* 2015, 2016, 2023, 2024

➔ *CPT Assistant* Jan 15:3, Apr 16:4, Feb 21:14, May 23:11, Feb 24:8

81456 RNA analysis

➔ *CPT Changes: An Insider's View* 2023, 2024

➔ *CPT Assistant* May 23:11, Feb 24:8

(For copy number assessment by microarray, use 81406)

(For genomic sequence DNA analysis and RNA analysis performed separately rather than via a combined method, report 81445, 81450, 81455, 81457, 81458, 81459 for the DNA analysis and report 81449, 81451, 81456 for the RNA analysis)

(For genomic sequence RNA analysis using a separate method, see 81449, 81451, 81456)

81457 Solid organ neoplasm, genomic sequence analysis panel, interrogation for sequence variants; DNA analysis, microsatellite instability

➔ *CPT Changes: An Insider's View* 2024

➔ *CPT Assistant* Feb 24:8

81458 DNA analysis, copy number variants and microsatellite instability

➔ *CPT Changes: An Insider's View* 2024

➔ *CPT Assistant* Feb 24:8

81459 DNA analysis or combined DNA and RNA analysis, copy number variants, microsatellite instability, tumor mutation burden, and rearrangements

➔ *CPT Changes: An Insider's View* 2024

➔ *CPT Assistant* Feb 24:8

(For solid organ genomic sequence DNA analysis or combined DNA and RNA analysis from cell-free nucleic acid, see 81462, 81463, 81464)

81462 Solid organ neoplasm, genomic sequence analysis panel, cell-free nucleic acid (eg, plasma), interrogation for sequence variants; DNA analysis or combined DNA and RNA analysis, copy number variants and rearrangements

➔ *CPT Changes: An Insider's View* 2024

➔ *CPT Assistant* Feb 24:8

81463 DNA analysis, copy number variants, and microsatellite instability

➔ *CPT Changes: An Insider's View* 2024

➔ *CPT Assistant* Feb 24:8

81464 DNA analysis or combined DNA and RNA analysis, copy number variants, microsatellite instability, tumor mutation burden, and rearrangements

➔ *CPT Changes: An Insider's View* 2024

➔ *CPT Assistant* Feb 24:8

81460 Whole mitochondrial genome (eg, Leigh syndrome, mitochondrial encephalomyopathy, lactic acidosis, and stroke-like episodes [MELAS], myoclonic epilepsy with ragged-red fibers [MERFF], neuropathy, ataxia, and retinitis pigmentosa [NARP], Leber hereditary optic neuropathy [LHON]), genomic sequence, must include sequence analysis of entire mitochondrial genome with heteroplasmy detection

➔ *CPT Changes: An Insider's View* 2015

➔ *CPT Assistant* Jan 15:3

81462 Code is out of numerical sequence. See 81458-81465

81463 Code is out of numerical sequence. See 81458-81465

81464 Code is out of numerical sequence. See 81458-81465

81465   Whole mitochondrial genome large deletion analysis panel (eg, Kearns-Sayre syndrome, chronic progressive external ophthalmoplegia), including heteroplasmy detection, if performed
➔ *CPT Changes: An Insider's View* 2015
➔ *CPT Assistant* Jan 15:3

81470   X-linked intellectual disability (XLID) (eg, syndromic and non-syndromic XLID); genomic sequence analysis panel, must include sequencing of at least 60 genes, including *ARX, ATRX, CDKL5, FGD1, FMR1, HUWE1, IL1RAPL, KDM5C, L1CAM, MECP2, MED12, MID1, OCRL, RPS6KA3,* and *SLC16A2*
➔ *CPT Changes: An Insider's View* 2015
➔ *CPT Assistant* Jan 15:3

81471   duplication/deletion gene analysis, must include analysis of at least 60 genes, including *ARX, ATRX, CDKL5, FGD1, FMR1, HUWE1, IL1RAPL, KDM5C, L1CAM, MECP2, MED12, MID1, OCRL, RPS6KA3,* and *SLC16A2*
➔ *CPT Changes: An Insider's View* 2015
➔ *CPT Assistant* Jan 15:3

81479   Code is out of numerical sequence. See 81407-81411

Multianalyte Assays with Algorithmic Analyses

Multianalyte Assays with Algorithmic Analyses (MAAAs) are procedures that utilize multiple results derived from panels of analyses of various types, including molecular pathology assays, fluorescent in situ hybridization assays, and non-nucleic acid based assays (eg, proteins, polypeptides, lipids, carbohydrates). Algorithmic analysis using the results of these assays as well as other patient information (if used) is then performed and typically reported as a numeric score(s) or as a probability. MAAAs are typically unique to a single clinical laboratory or manufacturer. The results of individual component procedure(s) that are inputs to the MAAAs may be provided on the associated laboratory report; however, these assays are not separately reported using additional codes.

The format for the code descriptors of MAAAs usually include (in order):

- Disease type (eg, oncology, autoimmune, tissue rejection),

- Material(s) analyzed (eg, DNA, RNA, protein, antibody),

- Number of markers (eg, number of genes, number of proteins),

- Methodology(ies) (eg, microarray, real-time [RT]-PCR, in situ hybridization [ISH], enzyme linked immunosorbent assays [ELISA]),

- Number of functional domains (if indicated),

- Specimen type (eg, blood, fresh tissue, formalin-fixed paraffin-embedded),

- Algorithm result type (eg, prognostic, diagnostic),

- Report (eg, probability index, risk score)

In contrast to GSPs and other molecular multianalyte assays, the assays in this section represent algorithmically combined results of analyses of multiple analytes to obtain a risk score or other value which in itself represents a new and distinct medical property that is of independent medical significance relative to the individual component test results in clinical context in which the assay is performed.

MAAAs, including those that do not have a Category I code, may be found in Appendix O. MAAAs that do not have a Category I code are identified in Appendix O by a four-digit number followed by the letter "M." The Category I MAAA codes that are included in this subsection are also included in Appendix O. All MAAA codes are listed in Appendix O along with the procedure's proprietary name. In order to report a MAAA code, the analysis performed must fulfill the code descriptor **and**, if proprietary, must be the test represented by the proprietary name listed in Appendix O.

When a specific MAAA procedure is not listed below or in Appendix O, the procedure must be reported using the Category I MAAA unlisted code (81599).

These codes encompass all analytical services required (eg, cell lysis, nucleic acid stabilization, extraction, digestion, amplification, hybridization, and detection) in addition to the algorithmic analysis itself. Procedures that are required prior to cell lysis (eg, microdissection, codes 88380 and 88381) should be reported separately.

81490   Autoimmune (rheumatoid arthritis), analysis of 12 biomarkers using immunoassays, utilizing serum, prognostic algorithm reported as a disease activity score
➔ *CPT Changes: An Insider's View* 2016

(Do not report 81490 in conjunction with 86140)

 # 81595   Cardiology (heart transplant), mRNA, gene expression profiling by real-time quantitative PCR of 20 genes (11 content and 9 housekeeping), utilizing subfraction of peripheral blood, algorithm reported as a rejection risk score
➔ *CPT Changes: An Insider's View* 2016

81493   Coronary artery disease, mRNA, gene expression profiling by real-time RT-PCR of 23 genes, utilizing whole peripheral blood, algorithm reported as a risk score
➔ *CPT Changes: An Insider's View* 2016

Pathology and Laboratory 80047-89398, 0001U-0520U

81500 Code is out of numerical sequence. See 81536-81541

81503 Code is out of numerical sequence. See 81536-81541

81504 Code is out of numerical sequence. See 81542-81554

81506 Endocrinology (type 2 diabetes), biochemical assays of seven analytes (glucose, HbA1c, insulin, hs-CRP, adiponectin, ferritin, interleukin 2-receptor alpha), utilizing serum or plasma, algorithm reporting a risk score

➔ *CPT Changes: An Insider's View* 2013

(Do not report 81506 in conjunction with constituent components [ie, 82728, 82947, 83036, 83525, 86141], 84999 [for adopectin], and 83520 [for interleukin 2-receptor alpha])

81507 Fetal aneuploidy (trisomy 21, 18, and 13) DNA sequence analysis of selected regions using maternal plasma, algorithm reported as a risk score for each trisomy

➔ *CPT Changes: An Insider's View* 2014

➔ *CPT Assistant* Apr 18:11

(Do not report 81228, 81229, 88271 when performing genomic sequencing procedures or other molecular multianalyte assays for copy number analysis)

(For cytogenomic [genome-wide] analysis for constitutional chromosomal abnormalities interrogation of genomic regions for copy number and loss-of-heterozygosity variants, low-pass sequencing analysis, use 81349)

81508 Fetal congenital abnormalities, biochemical assays of two proteins (PAPP-A, hCG [any form]), utilizing maternal serum, algorithm reported as a risk score

➔ *CPT Changes: An Insider's View* 2013

(Do not report 81508 in conjunction with 84163, 84702)

81509 Fetal congenital abnormalities, biochemical assays of three proteins (PAPP-A, hCG [any form], DIA), utilizing maternal serum, algorithm reported as a risk score

➔ *CPT Changes: An Insider's View* 2013

(Do not report 81509 in conjunction with 84163, 84702, 86336)

81510 Fetal congenital abnormalities, biochemical assays of three analytes (AFP, uE3, hCG [any form]), utilizing maternal serum, algorithm reported as a risk score

➔ *CPT Changes: An Insider's View* 2013

(Do not report 81510 in conjunction with 82105, 82677, 84702)

81511 Fetal congenital abnormalities, biochemical assays of four analytes (AFP, uE3, hCG [any form], DIA) utilizing maternal serum, algorithm reported as a risk score (may include additional results from previous biochemical testing)

➔ *CPT Changes: An Insider's View* 2013

(Do not report 81511 in conjunction with 82105, 82677, 84702, 86336)

81512 Fetal congenital abnormalities, biochemical assays of five analytes (AFP, uE3, total hCG, hyperglycosylated hCG, DIA) utilizing maternal serum, algorithm reported as a risk score

➔ *CPT Changes: An Insider's View* 2013

(Do not report 81512 in conjunction with 82105, 82677, 84702, 86336)

81513 Infectious disease, bacterial vaginosis, quantitative real-time amplification of RNA markers for Atopobium vaginae, Gardnerella vaginalis, and Lactobacillus species, utilizing vaginal-fluid specimens, algorithm reported as a positive or negative result for bacterial vaginosis

➔ *CPT Changes: An Insider's View* 2021

➔ *CPT Assistant* Mar 21:8

81514 Infectious disease, bacterial vaginosis and vaginitis, quantitative real-time amplification of DNA markers for Gardnerella vaginalis, Atopobium vaginae, Megasphaera type 1, Bacterial Vaginosis Associated Bacteria-2 (BVAB-2), and Lactobacillus species (L. crispatus and L. jensenii), utilizing vaginal-fluid specimens, algorithm reported as a positive or negative for high likelihood of bacterial vaginosis, includes separate detection of Trichomonas vaginalis and/or Candida species (C. albicans, C. tropicalis, C. parapsilosis, C. dubliniensis), Candida glabrata, Candida krusei, when reported

➔ *CPT Changes: An Insider's View* 2021

➔ *CPT Assistant* Mar 21:8

(Do not report 81514 in conjunction with 87480, 87481, 87482, 87510, 87511, 87512, 87660, 87661)

● **81515** Infectious disease, bacterial vaginosis and vaginitis, real-time PCR amplification of DNA markers for Atopobium vaginae, Atopobium species, Megasphaera type 1, and Bacterial Vaginosis Associated Bacteria-2 (BVAB-2), utilizing vaginal-fluid specimens, algorithm reported as positive or negative for high likelihood of bacterial vaginosis, includes separate detection of Trichomonas vaginalis and Candida species (C. albicans, C. tropicalis, C. parapsilosis, C. dubliniensis), Candida glabrata/Candida krusei, when reported

➔ *CPT Changes: An Insider's View* 2025

\# **81596** Infectious disease, chronic hepatitis C virus (HCV) infection, six biochemical assays (ALT, A2-macroglobulin, apolipoprotein A-1, total bilirubin, GGT, and haptoglobin) utilizing serum, prognostic algorithm reported as scores for fibrosis and necroinflammatory activity in liver

➔ *CPT Changes: An Insider's View* 2019

➔ *CPT Assistant* Jul 19:3

81517   Liver disease, analysis of 3 biomarkers (hyaluronic acid [HA], procollagen III amino terminal peptide [PIIINP], tissue inhibitor of metalloproteinase 1 [TIMP-1]), using immunoassays, utilizing serum, prognostic algorithm reported as a risk score and risk of liver fibrosis and liver-related clinical events within 5 years

➔ *CPT Changes: An Insider's View* 2024

(Do not report 81517 in conjunction with 83520 for identification of biomarkers included for liver disease analysis)

81518   Oncology (breast), mRNA, gene expression profiling by real-time RT-PCR of 11 genes (7 content and 4 housekeeping), utilizing formalin-fixed paraffin-embedded tissue, algorithms reported as percentage risk for metastatic recurrence and likelihood of benefit from extended endocrine therapy

➔ *CPT Changes: An Insider's View* 2019

➔ *CPT Assistant* Jul 19:3

 # 81522   Oncology (breast), mRNA, gene expression profiling by RT-PCR of 12 genes (8 content and 4 housekeeping), utilizing formalin-fixed paraffin-embedded tissue, algorithm reported as recurrence risk score

➔ *CPT Changes: An Insider's View* 2020

81519   Oncology (breast), mRNA, gene expression profiling by real-time RT-PCR of 21 genes, utilizing formalin-fixed paraffin-embedded tissue, algorithm reported as recurrence score

➔ *CPT Changes: An Insider's View* 2015

➔ *CPT Assistant* Jan 15:3

81520   Oncology (breast), mRNA gene expression profiling by hybrid capture of 58 genes (50 content and 8 housekeeping), utilizing formalin-fixed paraffin-embedded tissue, algorithm reported as a recurrence risk score

➔ *CPT Changes: An Insider's View* 2018

➔ *CPT Assistant* Jun 18:8

81521   Oncology (breast), mRNA, microarray gene expression profiling of 70 content genes and 465 housekeeping genes, utilizing fresh frozen or formalin-fixed paraffin-embedded tissue, algorithm reported as index related to risk of distant metastasis

➔ *CPT Changes: An Insider's View* 2018

➔ *CPT Assistant* Jun 18:8

(Do not report 81521 in conjunction with 81523 for the same specimen)

81522   Code is out of numerical sequence. See 81513-81520

81523   Oncology (breast), mRNA, next-generation sequencing gene expression profiling of 70 content genes and 31 housekeeping genes, utilizing formalin-fixed paraffin-embedded tissue, algorithm reported as index related to risk to distant metastasis

➔ *CPT Changes: An Insider's View* 2022

(Do not report 81523 in conjunction with 81521 for the same specimen)

81525   Oncology (colon), mRNA, gene expression profiling by real-time RT-PCR of 12 genes (7 content and 5 housekeeping), utilizing formalin-fixed paraffin-embedded tissue, algorithm reported as a recurrence score

81528   Oncology (colorectal) screening, quantitative real-time target and signal amplification of 10 DNA markers (*KRAS* mutations, promoter methylation of *NDRG4* and *BMP3*) and fecal hemoglobin, utilizing stool, algorithm reported as a positive or negative result

➔ *CPT Changes: An Insider's View* 2016

(Do not report 81528 in conjunction with 81275, 82274)

81529   Oncology (cutaneous melanoma), mRNA, gene expression profiling by real-time RT-PCR of 31 genes (28 content and 3 housekeeping), utilizing formalin-fixed paraffin-embedded tissue, algorithm reported as recurrence risk, including likelihood of sentinel lymph node metastasis

➔ *CPT Changes: An Insider's View* 2021

81535   Oncology (gynecologic), live tumor cell culture and chemotherapeutic response by DAPI stain and morphology, predictive algorithm reported as a drug response score; first single drug or drug combination

➔ *CPT Changes: An Insider's View* 2016

+ 81536   each additional single drug or drug combination (List separately in addition to code for primary procedure)

➔ *CPT Changes: An Insider's View* 2016

(Use 81536 in conjunction with 81535)

81538   Oncology (lung), mass spectrometric 8-protein signature, including amyloid A, utilizing serum, prognostic and predictive algorithm reported as good versus poor overall survival

➔ *CPT Changes: An Insider's View* 2016

 # 81500   Oncology (ovarian), biochemical assays of two proteins (CA-125 and HE4), utilizing serum, with menopausal status, algorithm reported as a risk score

➔ *CPT Changes: An Insider's View* 2013

➔ *CPT Assistant* Jun 19:11

(Do not report 81500 in conjunction with 86304, 86305)

 # 81503   Oncology (ovarian), biochemical assays of five proteins (CA-125, apolipoprotein A1, beta-2 microglobulin, transferrin, and pre-albumin), utilizing serum, algorithm reported as a risk score

➔ *CPT Changes: An Insider's View* 2013

(Do not report 81503 in conjunction with 82172, 82232, 84134, 84466, 86304)

Pathology and Laboratory 80047-89398, 0001U-0520U

81539 Oncology (high-grade prostate cancer), biochemical assay of four proteins (Total PSA, Free PSA, Intact PSA, and human kallikrein-2 [hK2]), utilizing plasma or serum, prognostic algorithm reported as a probability score

➔ CPT Changes: An Insider's View 2017

➔ CPT Assistant Apr 17:4

81540 Code is out of numerical sequence. See 81542-81554

81541 Oncology (prostate), mRNA gene expression profiling by real-time RT-PCR of 46 genes (31 content and 15 housekeeping), utilizing formalin-fixed paraffin-embedded tissue, algorithm reported as a disease-specific mortality risk score

➔ CPT Changes: An Insider's View 2018

➔ CPT Assistant Aug 18:8

81542 Oncology (prostate), mRNA, microarray gene expression profiling of 22 content genes, utilizing formalin-fixed paraffin-embedded tissue, algorithm reported as metastasis risk score

➔ CPT Changes: An Insider's View 2020

➔ CPT Assistant Oct 20:8

81546 Code is out of numerical sequence. See 81542-81554

81551 Oncology (prostate), promoter methylation profiling by real-time PCR of 3 genes (*GSTP1, APC, RASSF1*), utilizing formalin-fixed paraffin-embedded tissue, algorithm reported as a likelihood of prostate cancer detection on repeat biopsy

➔ CPT Changes: An Insider's View 2018

➔ CPT Assistant Aug 18:8

 # 81546 Oncology (thyroid), mRNA, gene expression analysis of 10,196 genes, utilizing fine needle aspirate, algorithm reported as a categorical result (eg, benign or suspicious)

➔ CPT Changes: An Insider's View 2021

 # 81504 Oncology (tissue of origin), microarray gene expression profiling of > 2000 genes, utilizing formalin-fixed paraffin-embedded tissue, algorithm reported as tissue similarity scores

➔ CPT Changes: An Insider's View 2014

 # 81540 Oncology (tumor of unknown origin), mRNA, gene expression profiling by real-time RT-PCR of 92 genes (87 content and 5 housekeeping) to classify tumor into main cancer type and subtype, utilizing formalin-fixed paraffin-embedded tissue, algorithm reported as a probability of a predicted main cancer type and subtype

➔ CPT Changes: An Insider's View 2016

81552 Oncology (uveal melanoma), mRNA, gene expression profiling by real-time RT-PCR of 15 genes (12 content and 3 housekeeping), utilizing fine needle aspirate or formalin-fixed paraffin-embedded tissue, algorithm reported as risk of metastasis

➔ CPT Changes: An Insider's View 2020

➔ CPT Assistant Jan 20:10

81554 Pulmonary disease (idiopathic pulmonary fibrosis [IPF]), mRNA, gene expression analysis of 190 genes, utilizing transbronchial biopsies, diagnostic algorithm reported as categorical result (eg, positive or negative for high probability of usual interstitial pneumonia [UIP])

➔ CPT Changes: An Insider's View 2021

➔ CPT Assistant Mar 21:6

● 81558 Transplantation medicine (allograft rejection, kidney), mRNA, gene expression profiling by quantitative polymerase chain reaction (qPCR) of 139 genes, utilizing whole blood, algorithm reported as a binary categorization as transplant excellence, which indicates immune quiescence, or not transplant excellence, indicating subclinical rejection

➔ CPT Changes: An Insider's View 2025

81560 Transplantation medicine (allograft rejection, pediatric liver and small bowel), measurement of donor and third-party-induced CD154+T-cytotoxic memory cells, utilizing whole peripheral blood, algorithm reported as a rejection risk score

➔ CPT Changes: An Insider's View 2022

(Do not report 81560 in conjunction with 85032, 86353, 86821, 88184, 88185, 88187, 88230, 88240, 88241, 0018M)

81595 Code is out of numerical sequence. See 81490-81506

81596 Code is out of numerical sequence. See 81513-81520

81599 Unlisted multianalyte assay with algorithmic analysis

➔ CPT Changes: An Insider's View 2013

➔ CPT Assistant Apr 18:11, Jun 18:8, Jun 19:11

(Do not use 81599 for multianalyte assays with algorithmic analyses listed in Appendix O)

Chemistry

The material for examination may be from any source unless otherwise specified in the code descriptor. When an analyte is measured in multiple specimens from different sources, or in specimens that are obtained at different times, the analyte is reported separately for each source and for each specimen. The examination is quantitative unless specified. To report an organ or disease oriented panel, see codes 80048-80076.

Clinical information or mathematically calculated values, which are not specifically requested by the ordering physician and are derived from the results of other ordered or performed laboratory tests, are considered part of the ordered test procedure(s) and therefore are not separately reportable service(s).

When the requested analyte result is derived using a calculation that requires values from nonrequested laboratory analyses, only the requested analyte code should be reported.

When the calculated analyte determination requires values derived from other requested and nonrequested laboratory analyses, the requested analyte codes (including those calculated) should be reported.

An exception to the above is when an analyte (eg, urinary creatinine) is performed to compensate for variations in urine concentration (eg, microalbumin, thromboxane metabolites) in random urine samples; the appropriate CPT code is reported for both the ordered analyte and the additional required analyte. When the calculated result(s) represent an algorithmically derived numeric score or probability, see the appropriate multianalyte assay with algorithmic analyses (MAAA) code or the MAAA unlisted code (81599).

Analytes that are not specified by either an analyte-specific or method-specific code in the Chemistry (82009-84830) subsection may be reported using the unlisted chemistry procedure code 84999.

82009 Ketone body(s) (eg, acetone, acetoacetic acid, beta-hydroxybutyrate); qualitative
➔ *CPT Changes: An Insider's View* 2013
➔ *CPT Assistant* Oct 11:11, Jun 15:10, Jan 24:17

82010 quantitative
➔ *CPT Changes: An Insider's View* 2013
➔ *CPT Assistant* Oct 11:11

82013 Acetylcholinesterase

(For gastric acid analysis, use 82930)

(Acid phosphatase, see 84060-84066)

82016 Acylcarnitines; qualitative, each specimen
➔ *CPT Assistant* Nov 98:23

82017 quantitative, each specimen
➔ *CPT Changes: An Insider's View* 2000
➔ *CPT Assistant* Nov 98:23

(For carnitine, use 82379)

82024 Adrenocorticotropic hormone (ACTH)

82030 Adenosine, 5-monophosphate, cyclic (cyclic AMP)

82040 Albumin; serum, plasma or whole blood
➔ *CPT Changes: An Insider's View* 2009
➔ *CPT Assistant* Dec 99:2

82042 Code is out of numerical sequence. See 82044-82077

82043 urine (eg, microalbumin), quantitative
➔ *CPT Changes: An Insider's View* 2018
➔ *CPT Assistant* Summer 94:2

82044 urine (eg, microalbumin), semiquantitative (eg, reagent strip assay)
➔ *CPT Changes: An Insider's View* 2018
➔ *CPT Assistant* Summer 94:2, Mar 98:3, Sep 02:10

(For prealbumin, use 84134)

82045 ischemia modified
➔ *CPT Changes: An Insider's View* 2005

 # 82042 other source, quantitative, each specimen
➔ *CPT Changes: An Insider's View* 2001, 2018

(For total protein, see 84155, 84156, 84157, 84160)

82075 Alcohol (ethanol); breath
➔ *CPT Changes: An Insider's View* 2015, 2021

82077 any specimen except urine and breath, immunoassay (eg, IA, EIA, ELISA, RIA, EMIT, FPIA) and enzymatic methods (eg, alcohol dehydrogenase)
➔ *CPT Changes: An Insider's View* 2021

(For definitive drug testing for alcohol [ethanol], use 80320)

82085 Aldolase

82088 Aldosterone
➔ *CPT Assistant* Oct 10:7

(Alkaline phosphatase, see 84075, 84080)

(Alphaketoglutarate, see 82009, 82010)

(Alpha tocopherol [Vitamin E], use 84446)

82103 Alpha-1-antitrypsin; total

82104 phenotype

82105 Alpha-fetoprotein (AFP); serum

82106 amniotic fluid

82107 AFP-L3 fraction isoform and total AFP (including ratio)
➔ *CPT Changes: An Insider's View* 2007

82108 Aluminum

82120 Amines, vaginal fluid, qualitative
➔ *CPT Changes: An Insider's View* 2000
➔ *CPT Assistant* Nov 99:45

(For combined pH and amines test for vaginitis, use 82120 and 83986)

82127 Amino acids; single, qualitative, each specimen
➔ *CPT Assistant* Nov 98:24

82128 multiple, qualitative, each specimen
➔ *CPT Assistant* Nov 98:24

82131 single, quantitative, each specimen
➔ *CPT Assistant* May 98:11, Nov 98:24

82135 Aminolevulinic acid, delta (ALA)

82136 Amino acids, 2 to 5 amino acids, quantitative, each specimen
➔ *CPT Assistant* Nov 98:24

82139 Amino acids, 6 or more amino acids, quantitative, each specimen
↪ *CPT Assistant* Nov 98:24

82140 Ammonia

82143 Amniotic fluid scan (spectrophotometric)

(For L/S ratio, use 83661)

(Amobarbital, use 80345)

82150 Amylase

▶(For amyloid, beta, see 82233, 82234)◀

82154 Androstanediol glucuronide
↪ *CPT Assistant* Summer 94:5

82157 Androstenedione

82160 Androsterone

82163 Angiotensin II

82164 Angiotensin I - converting enzyme (ACE)

(Antidiuretic hormone (ADH), use 84588)

(Antimony, use 83015)

(Antitrypsin, alpha-1-, see 82103, 82104)

82166 Anti-mullerian hormone (AMH)
↪ *CPT Changes: An Insider's View* 2024

82172 Apolipoprotein, each

82175 Arsenic

(For heavy metal screening, use 83015)

82180 Ascorbic acid (Vitamin C), blood

(Aspirin, see acetylsalicylic acid, 80329, 80330, 80331)

(For salicylate by immunoassay or enzymatic methods, use 80179)

(Atherogenic index, blood, ultracentrifugation, quantitative, use 83701)

82190 Atomic absorption spectroscopy, each analyte
↪ *CPT Assistant* Oct 10:7

82232 Beta-2 microglobulin

(Bicarbonate, use 82374)

● **82233** Beta-amyloid; 1-40 (Abeta 40)
↪ *CPT Changes: An Insider's View* 2025

● **82234** 1-42 (Abeta 42)
↪ *CPT Changes: An Insider's View* 2025

82239 Bile acids; total

82240 cholylglycine

(For bile pigments, urine, see 81000-81005)

82247 Bilirubin; total
↪ *CPT Assistant* Nov 98:24, Apr 99:6, Dec 99:1, Jan 00:7, Dec 08:5, Apr 10:11

82248 direct
↪ *CPT Assistant* Nov 98:24, Apr 99:6, Dec 99:1, Apr 10:11

82252 feces, qualitative

82261 Biotinidase, each specimen
↪ *CPT Assistant* Nov 98:24

82270 Blood, occult, by peroxidase activity (eg, guaiac), qualitative; feces, consecutive collected specimens with single determination, for colorectal neoplasm screening (ie, patient was provided 3 cards or single triple card for consecutive collection)
↪ *CPT Changes: An Insider's View* 2002, 2006
↪ *CPT Assistant* Sep 03:15, Feb 06:7, Apr 08:5

82271 other sources
↪ *CPT Changes: An Insider's View* 2006
↪ *CPT Assistant* Feb 06:7

82272 Blood, occult, by peroxidase activity (eg, guaiac), qualitative, feces, 1-3 simultaneous determinations, performed for other than colorectal neoplasm screening
↪ *CPT Changes: An Insider's View* 2006, 2008
↪ *CPT Assistant* Feb 06:7, Apr 08:5, Jun 09:10

(Blood urea nitrogen [BUN], see 84520, 84525)

82274 Blood, occult, by fecal hemoglobin determination by immunoassay, qualitative, feces, 1-3 simultaneous determinations
↪ *CPT Changes: An Insider's View* 2002

82286 Bradykinin
↪ *CPT Assistant* Oct 10:7

82300 Cadmium
↪ *CPT Assistant* Aug 05:9, Oct 10:7

82306 Vitamin D; 25 hydroxy, includes fraction(s), if performed
↪ *CPT Changes: An Insider's View* 2010

\# **82652** 1, 25 dihydroxy, includes fraction(s), if performed
↪ *CPT Changes: An Insider's View* 2010

82308 Calcitonin

82310 Calcium; total
↪ *CPT Assistant* Dec 99:2

82330 ionized
↪ *CPT Assistant* Apr 13:10, Jul 22:20

82331 after calcium infusion test

82340 urine quantitative, timed specimen

82355 Calculus; qualitative analysis
↪ *CPT Changes: An Insider's View* 2002

82360 quantitative analysis, chemical

82365 infrared spectroscopy

82370 X-ray diffraction
↪ *CPT Changes: An Insider's View* 2001

★=Telemedicine ◀=Audio-only ✚=Add-on code ✗=FDA approval pending #=Resequenced code ⊘=Modifier 51 exempt =See p xxi for details

(Carbamates, see individual listings)

82373 Carbohydrate deficient transferrin

➔ *CPT Changes: An Insider's View* 2001

82374 Carbon dioxide (bicarbonate)

➔ *CPT Assistant* Dec 99:2, Apr 13:10, Jul 22:20

(See also 82803)

82375 Carboxyhemoglobin; quantitative

➔ *CPT Changes: An Insider's View* 2009

82376 qualitative

➔ *CPT Changes: An Insider's View* 2009

(For transcutaneous measurement of carboxyhemoglobin, use 88740)

82378 Carcinoembryonic antigen (CEA)

➔ *CPT Assistant* Fall 93:25, Aug 96:11

82379 Carnitine (total and free), quantitative, each specimen

➔ *CPT Assistant* Nov 98:24

(For acylcarnitine, see 82016, 82017)

82380 Carotene

82382 Catecholamines; total urine

82383 blood

82384 fractionated

(For urine metabolites, see 83835, 84585)

82387 Cathepsin-D

82390 Ceruloplasmin

82397 Chemiluminescent assay

➔ *CPT Assistant* Fall 93:25, Oct 10:7

82415 Chloramphenicol

➔ *CPT Assistant* Aug 05:9, Oct 10:7

82435 Chloride; blood

➔ *CPT Assistant* Dec 99:2, Apr 13:10, Jul 22:20

82436 urine

82438 other source

➔ *CPT Assistant* Jul 03:7

(For sweat collection by iontophoresis, use 89230)

82441 Chlorinated hydrocarbons, screen

(Cholecalciferol [Vitamin D], use 82306)

82465 Cholesterol, serum or whole blood, total

➔ *CPT Changes: An Insider's View* 2001

➔ *CPT Assistant* Dec 99:2, Mar 00:11, Feb 05:9

(For high density lipoprotein [HDL], use 83718)

82480 Cholinesterase; serum

82482 RBC

82485 Chondroitin B sulfate, quantitative

(Chorionic gonadotropin, see gonadotropin, 84702, 84703)

82495 Chromium

➔ *CPT Assistant* Oct 10:7

82507 Citrate

➔ *CPT Assistant* Aug 05:9, Oct 10:7

(Cocaine, qualitative analysis, use 80353)

(Codeine, qualitative analysis, use 80361)

(Complement, see 86160-86162)

82523 Collagen cross links, any method

82525 Copper

(Coproporphyrin, see 84119, 84120)

(Corticosteroids, use 83491)

82528 Corticosterone

82530 Cortisol; free

➔ *CPT Assistant* Summer 94:3

82533 total

➔ *CPT Assistant* Summer 94:3

(C-peptide, use 84681)

82540 Creatine

82542 Column chromatography, includes mass spectrometry, if performed (eg, HPLC, LC, LC/MS, LC/MS-MS, GC, GC/MS-MS, GC/MS, HPLC/MS), non-drug analyte(s) not elsewhere specified, qualitative or quantitative, each specimen

➔ *CPT Changes: An Insider's View* 2015, 2016

➔ *CPT Assistant* Nov 98:24-25, Apr 15:3

(Do not report more than one unit of 82542 for each specimen)

(For column chromatography/mass spectrometry of drugs or substances, see 80305, 80306, 80307, 80320-80377, or specific analyte code[s] in the **Chemistry** section)

82550 Creatine kinase (CK), (CPK); total

➔ *CPT Assistant* Feb 98:1, Dec 99:2

82552 isoenzymes

➔ *CPT Assistant* Feb 98:1

82553 MB fraction only

➔ *CPT Assistant* Feb 98:1, Oct 21:14

82554 isoforms

➔ *CPT Assistant* Feb 98:1

82565 Creatinine; blood

➔ *CPT Assistant* Dec 99:2, Apr 13:10, Jul 22:20

82570 other source

82575 clearance

Pathology and Laboratory 80047-89398, 0001U-0520U

82585   Cryofibrinogen

82595   Cryoglobulin, qualitative or semi-quantitative (eg, cryocrit)
→ *CPT Changes: An Insider's View* 2001
→ *CPT Assistant* Oct 10:7

(For quantitative, cryoglobulin, see 82784, 82785)

(Crystals, pyrophosphate vs urate, use 89060)

82600   Cyanide
→ *CPT Assistant* Aug 05:9, Oct 10:7

82607   Cyanocobalamin (Vitamin B-12);
→ *CPT Assistant* Oct 21:14

82608   unsaturated binding capacity

(Cyclic AMP, use 82030)

(Cyclosporine, use 80158)

82610   Cystatin C
→ *CPT Changes: An Insider's View* 2008
→ *CPT Assistant* Apr 08:5, Aug 08:13

82615   Cystine and homocystine, urine, qualitative

82626   Dehydroepiandrosterone (DHEA)
→ *CPT Assistant* Summer 94:4

(Do not report 82626 in conjunction with 80327, 80328 to identify anabolic steroid testing for testosterone)

82627   Dehydroepiandrosterone-sulfate (DHEA-S)
→ *CPT Assistant* Summer 94:4

(Delta-aminolevulinic acid (ALA), use 82135)

82633   Desoxycorticosterone, 11-

82634   Deoxycortisol, 11-

(Dexamethasone suppression test, use 80420)

(Diastase, urine, use 82150)

82638   Dibucaine number

(Dichloroethane, use 82441)

(Dichloromethane, use 82441)

(Diethylether, use 84600)

82642   Dihydrotestosterone (DHT)
→ *CPT Changes: An Insider's View* 2019

(For dihydrotestosterone analysis for anabolic drug testing, see 80327, 80328)

(Dipropylacetic acid, use 80164)

(Dopamine, see 82382-82384)

(Duodenal contents, see individual enzymes; for intubation and collection, see 43756, 43757)

82652   Code is out of numerical sequence. See 82300-82310

82653   Code is out of numerical sequence. See 82642-82658

82656   Elastase, pancreatic (EL-1), fecal; qualitative or semi-quantitative
→ *CPT Changes: An Insider's View* 2005, 2022
→ *CPT Assistant* Sep 05:9

82653   quantitative
→ *CPT Changes: An Insider's View* 2022

82657   Enzyme activity in blood cells, cultured cells, or tissue, not elsewhere specified; nonradioactive substrate, each specimen
→ *CPT Assistant* Nov 98:25, Apr 23:18

82658   radioactive substrate, each specimen
→ *CPT Assistant* Nov 98:25

82664   Electrophoretic technique, not elsewhere specified

(Endocrine receptor assays, see 84233-84235)

82668   Erythropoietin

82670   Estradiol; total
→ *CPT Changes: An Insider's View* 2021

82681   free, direct measurement (eg, equilibrium dialysis)
→ *CPT Changes: An Insider's View* 2021

82671   Estrogens; fractionated

82672   total

(Estrogen receptor assay, use 84233)

82677   Estriol

82679   Estrone

(For definitive drug testing for alcohol [ethanol], use 80320)

(For alcohol [ethanol] by immunoassay or enzymatic methods, use 82077)

82681   Code is out of numerical sequence. See 82668-82672

82693   Ethylene glycol

82696   Etiocholanolone
→ *CPT Assistant* Oct 10:7

(For fractionation of ketosteroids, use 83593)

82705   Fat or lipids, feces; qualitative
→ *CPT Assistant* Aug 05:9, Oct 10:7

82710   quantitative

82715   Fat differential, feces, quantitative

82725   Fatty acids, nonesterified

82726   Very long chain fatty acids
→ *CPT Assistant* Nov 98:25

82728   Ferritin

(Fetal hemoglobin, see hemoglobin 83030, 83033, and 85460)

(Fetoprotein, alpha-1, see 82105, 82106)

★=Telemedicine   ◀=Audio-only   +=Add-on code   ✗=FDA approval pending   #=Resequenced code   ⊘=Modifier 51 exempt   →→→=See p xxi for details

82731   Fetal fibronectin, cervicovaginal secretions, semi-quantitative
  ➔ *CPT Assistant* Nov 98:25

82735   Fluoride

(Foam stability test, use 83662)

82746   Folic acid; serum

82747   RBC

(Follicle stimulating hormone [FSH], use 83001)

82757   Fructose, semen

(Fructosamine, use 82985)

(Fructose, TLC screen, use 84375)

82759   Galactokinase, RBC

82760   Galactose

82775   Galactose-1-phosphate uridyl transferase; quantitative

82776   screen

82777   Galectin-3
  ➔ *CPT Changes: An Insider's View* 2013

82784   Gammaglobulin (immunoglobulin); IgA, IgD, IgG, IgM, each
  ➔ *CPT Changes: An Insider's View* 2010
  ➔ *CPT Assistant* Spring 94:31, Aug 00:11

82785   IgE
  ➔ *CPT Changes: An Insider's View* 2010
  ➔ *CPT Assistant* Spring 94:31

(For allergen specific IgE, see 86003, 86005)

82787   immunoglobulin subclasses (eg, IgG1, 2, 3, or 4), each
  ➔ *CPT Changes: An Insider's View* 2001, 2010
  ➔ *CPT Assistant* Oct 10:7

(Gamma-glutamyltransferase [GGT], use 82977)

82800   Gases, blood, pH only
  ➔ *CPT Assistant* Aug 05:9, Oct 10:7

82803   Gases, blood, any combination of pH, pCO_2, pO_2, CO_2, HCO_3 (including calculated O_2 saturation);

(Use 82803 for 2 or more of the above listed analytes)

82805   with O_2 saturation, by direct measurement, except pulse oximetry

82810   Gases, blood, O_2 saturation only, by direct measurement, except pulse oximetry

(For pulse oximetry, use 94760)

82820   Hemoglobin-oxygen affinity (pO_2 for 50% hemoglobin saturation with oxygen)
  ➔ *CPT Assistant* Oct 10:7

(For gastric acid analysis, use 82930)

82930   Gastric acid analysis, includes pH if performed, each specimen
  ➔ *CPT Changes: An Insider's View* 2011
  ➔ *CPT Assistant* Oct 10:7, Dec 10:7, Sep 11:3

82938   Gastrin after secretin stimulation

82941   Gastrin
  ➔ *CPT Assistant* Aug 05:9

(Gentamicin, use 80170)

(GGT, use 82977)

(For a qualitative column chromatography procedure [eg, gas liquid chromatography], use the appropriate specific analyte code, if available, or 82542)

82943   Glucagon

82945   Glucose, body fluid, other than blood
  ➔ *CPT Changes: An Insider's View* 2001

82946   Glucagon tolerance test

82947   Glucose; quantitative, blood (except reagent strip)
  ➔ *CPT Changes: An Insider's View* 2001
  ➔ *CPT Assistant* Summer 93:14, Summer 94:5, Sep 99:10, Dec 99:2, Jun 02:3, Feb 05:9, Apr 13:10, May 21:8, Oct 21:14, Jul 22:20

82948   blood, reagent strip
  ➔ *CPT Assistant* Summer 94:5, Jan 99:10, Nov 10:10, Oct 11:8

82950   post glucose dose (includes glucose)
  ➔ *CPT Assistant* Sep 99:10, Jun 02:3, Feb 05:9

82951   tolerance test (GTT), 3 specimens (includes glucose)
  ➔ *CPT Assistant* Feb 01:10, Feb 05:9, Oct 10:7

+ 82952   tolerance test, each additional beyond 3 specimens (List separately in addition to code for primary procedure)
  ➔ *CPT Changes: An Insider's View* 2011
  ➔ *CPT Assistant* Feb 01:10, Oct 10:7, Dec 10:7

(Use 82952 in conjunction with 82951)

(For insulin tolerance test, see 80434, 80435)

(For leucine tolerance test, use 80428)

(For semiquantitative urine glucose, see 81000, 81002, 81005, 81099)

82955   Glucose-6-phosphate dehydrogenase (G6PD); quantitative

82960   screen

(For glucose tolerance test with medication, use 96374 in addition)

82962   Glucose, blood by glucose monitoring device(s) cleared by the FDA specifically for home use
  ➔ *CPT Assistant* Summer 94:4, Jan 99:10, Nov 10:10, Oct 11:8

82963   Glucosidase, beta

82965   Glutamate dehydrogenase

82977 Glutamyltransferase, gamma (GGT)
> *CPT Assistant* Dec 99:1

82978 Glutathione

82979 Glutathione reductase, RBC

(Glycohemoglobin, use 83036)

82985 Glycated protein
> *CPT Assistant* Summer 94:2

(Gonadotropin, chorionic, see 84702, 84703)

83001 Gonadotropin; follicle stimulating hormone (FSH)
> *CPT Assistant* Aug 05:9, Oct 10:7

83002 luteinizing hormone (LH)

(For luteinizing releasing factor [LRH], use 83727)

83003 Growth hormone, human (HGH) (somatotropin)
> *CPT Assistant* Oct 21:14

(For antibody to human growth hormone, use 86277)

83006 Growth stimulation expressed gene 2 (ST2, Interleukin 1 receptor like-1)
> *CPT Changes: An Insider's View* 2015

83009 Helicobacter pylori, blood test analysis for urease activity, non-radioactive isotope (eg, C-13)
> *CPT Changes: An Insider's View* 2005

(For H. pylori, breath test analysis for urease activity, see 83013, 83014)

83010 Haptoglobin; quantitative

83012 phenotypes

83013 Helicobacter pylori; breath test analysis for urease activity, non-radioactive isotope (eg, C-13)
> *CPT Changes: An Insider's View* 2001, 2002, 2005
> *CPT Assistant* Nov 98:25, Feb 99:8, Nov 99:45

83014 drug administration
> *CPT Changes: An Insider's View* 2005
> *CPT Assistant* Nov 98:25, Feb 99:8, Nov 99:45

(For H. pylori, stool, use 87338. For H. pylori, liquid scintillation counter, see 78267, 78268. For H. pylori, immunoassay, use 87339)

(For H. pylori, blood test analysis for urease activity, use 83009)

83015 Heavy metal (eg, arsenic, barium, beryllium, bismuth, antimony, mercury); qualitative, any number of analytes
> *CPT Changes: An Insider's View* 2017
> *CPT Assistant* Apr 22:14

83018 quantitative, each, not elsewhere specified
> *CPT Changes: An Insider's View* 2017
> *CPT Assistant* Apr 22:14

(Use an analyte-specific heavy metal quantitative code, instead of 83018, when available)

83020 Hemoglobin fractionation and quantitation; electrophoresis (eg, A2, S, C, and/or F)
> *CPT Assistant* Nov 98:25

83021 chromatography (eg, A2, S, C, and/or F)
> *CPT Assistant* Nov 98:25, Dec 99:7

(For glycosylated [A1c] hemoglobin analysis, by electrophoresis or chromatography, in the absence of an identified hemoglobin variant, use 83036)

83026 Hemoglobin; by copper sulfate method, non-automated

83030 F (fetal), chemical

83033 F (fetal), qualitative
> *CPT Changes: An Insider's View* 2001

83036 glycosylated (A1C)
> *CPT Changes: An Insider's View* 2006
> *CPT Assistant* Summer 94:2, Feb 06:7, Oct 06:15

(For glycosylated [A1C] hemoglobin analysis, by electrophoresis or chromatography, in the setting of an identified hemoglobin variant, see 83020, 83021)

(For fecal hemoglobin detection by immunoassay, use 82274)

83037 glycosylated (A1C) by device cleared by FDA for home use
> *CPT Changes: An Insider's View* 2006
> *CPT Assistant* Feb 06:7, Oct 06:15

83045 methemoglobin, qualitative

83050 methemoglobin, quantitative

(For transcutaneous quantitative methemoglobin determination, use 88741)

83051 plasma

83060 sulfhemoglobin, quantitative

83065 thermolabile

83068 unstable, screen

83069 urine

83070 Hemosiderin, qualitative

(HIAA, use 83497)

(For a qualitative column chromatography procedure [eg, high performance liquid chromatography], use the appropriate specific analyte code, if available, or 82542)

83080 b-Hexosaminidase, each assay
> *CPT Assistant* Nov 98:25

83088 Histamine

(Hollander test, see 43754, 43755)

83090 Homocysteine
> *CPT Changes: An Insider's View* 2001
> *CPT Assistant* Jan 01:13, Oct 10:7

★=Telemedicine ◀=Audio-only +=Add-on code ⊿=FDA approval pending #=Resequenced code ⊘=Modifier 51 exempt =See p xxi for details

83150   Homovanillic acid (HVA)
  CPT Assistant Aug 05:9, Oct 10:7

  (Hormones, see individual alphabetic listings in **Chemistry** section)

  (For hydrogen/methane breath test, use 91065)

83491   Hydroxycorticosteroids, 17- (17-OHCS)
  CPT Assistant Aug 05:9, Oct 10:7

  (For cortisol, see 82530, 82533. For deoxycortisol, use 82634)

83497   Hydroxyindolacetic acid, 5-(HIAA)

  (For urine qualitative test, use 81005)

  (5-Hydroxytryptamine, use 84260)

83498   Hydroxyprogesterone, 17-d

83500   Hydroxyproline; free
  CPT Assistant Aug 05:9, Oct 10:7

83505   total

83516   Immunoassay for analyte other than infectious agent antibody or infectious agent antigen; qualitative or semiquantitative, multiple step method
  CPT Changes: An Insider's View 2010
  CPT Assistant Nov 98:25, Mar 22:11

83518   qualitative or semiquantitative, single step method (eg, reagent strip)
  CPT Changes: An Insider's View 2010
  CPT Assistant Fall 93:26

83519   quantitative, by radioimmunoassay (eg, RIA)
  CPT Changes: An Insider's View 2010
  CPT Assistant Fall 93:26, Summer 94:2

83520   quantitative, not otherwise specified
  CPT Changes: An Insider's View 2010
  CPT Assistant Fall 93:26

  (For multianalyte assay with algorithmic analysis [MAAA] for liver disease using analysis of 3 biomarkers, use 81517)

  (Immunoglobulins, see 82784, 82785)

  (For immunoassay of tumor antigen not elsewhere specified, use 86316)

  (For immunoassays for antibodies to infectious agent antigens, see analyte and method specific codes in the **Immunology** section)

83521   Immunoglobulin light chains (ie, kappa, lambda), free, each
  CPT Changes: An Insider's View 2022

83525   Insulin; total

  (For proinsulin, use 84206)

83527   free
  CPT Assistant Summer 94:5

83529   Interleukin-6 (IL-6)
  CPT Changes: An Insider's View 2022

83528   Intrinsic factor

  (For intrinsic factor antibodies, use 86340)

83529   Code is out of numerical sequence. See 83525-83540

83540   Iron
  CPT Assistant Fall 93:25

83550   Iron binding capacity

83570   Isocitric dehydrogenase (IDH)

  (Isonicotinic acid hydrazide, INH, see code for specific method)

  (Isopropyl alcohol, use 80320)

83582   Ketogenic steroids, fractionation

  (Ketone bodies, for serum, see 82009, 82010; for urine, see 81000-81003)

83586   Ketosteroids, 17- (17-KS); total

83593   fractionation
  CPT Assistant Oct 10:7

83605   Lactate (lactic acid)
  CPT Assistant Aug 05:9, Oct 10:7

83615   Lactate dehydrogenase (LD), (LDH);
  CPT Assistant Fall 93:25, Feb 98:1, Dec 99:2

83625   isoenzymes, separation and quantitation
  CPT Assistant Fall 93:25, Feb 98:1

83630   Lactoferrin, fecal; qualitative
  CPT Changes: An Insider's View 2005, 2006
  CPT Assistant Feb 06:7

83631   quantitative
  CPT Changes: An Insider's View 2006
  CPT Assistant Feb 06:7, Jan 07:29

83632   Lactogen, human placental (HPL) human chorionic somatomammotropin

83633   Lactose, urine, qualitative

  (For tolerance, see 82951, 82952)

  (For breath hydrogen/methane test for lactase deficiency, use 91065)

83655   Lead

83661   Fetal lung maturity assessment; lecithin sphingomyelin (L/S) ratio
  CPT Changes: An Insider's View 2001

83662   foam stability test

83663   fluorescence polarization
  CPT Changes: An Insider's View 2001

83664   lamellar body density
  CPT Changes: An Insider's View 2001

  (For phosphatidylglycerol, use 84081)

83670 Leucine aminopeptidase (LAP)

83690 Lipase

83695 Lipoprotein (a)
> *CPT Changes: An Insider's View* 2006
> *CPT Assistant* Feb 06:7

83698 Lipoprotein-associated phospholipase A$_2$ (Lp-PLA$_2$)
> *CPT Changes: An Insider's View* 2007
> *CPT Assistant* Oct 10:7

83700 Lipoprotein, blood; electrophoretic separation and quantitation
> *CPT Changes: An Insider's View* 2006
> *CPT Assistant* Feb 06:7, Oct 10:7

83701 high resolution fractionation and quantitation of lipoproteins including lipoprotein subclasses when performed (eg, electrophoresis, ultracentrifugation)
> *CPT Changes: An Insider's View* 2006
> *CPT Assistant* Feb 06:7

83704 quantitation of lipoprotein particle number(s) (eg, by nuclear magnetic resonance spectroscopy), includes lipoprotein particle subclass(es), when performed
> *CPT Changes: An Insider's View* 2006, 2017
> *CPT Assistant* Feb 06:7

83718 Lipoprotein, direct measurement; high density cholesterol (HDL cholesterol)
> *CPT Assistant* Oct 99:11, Mar 00:11, Feb 05:9

83719 VLDL cholesterol
> *CPT Assistant* Oct 99:11

83721 LDL cholesterol
> *CPT Assistant* Nov 98:25, Oct 99:11

83722 small dense LDL cholesterol
> *CPT Changes: An Insider's View* 2019

(For fractionation by high resolution electrophoresis or ultracentrifugation, use 83701)

(For lipoprotein particle numbers and subclasses analysis by nuclear magnetic resonance spectroscopy, use 83704)

83727 Luteinizing releasing factor (LRH)

(Luteinizing hormone [LH], use 83002)

(Macroglobulins, alpha-2, use 86329)

83735 Magnesium

83775 Malate dehydrogenase

(Maltose tolerance, see 82951, 82952)

(Mammotropin, use 84146)

83785 Manganese

83789 Mass spectrometry and tandem mass spectrometry (eg, MS, MS/MS, MALDI, MS-TOF, QTOF), non-drug analyte(s) not elsewhere specified, qualitative or quantitative, each specimen
> *CPT Changes: An Insider's View* 2016
> *CPT Assistant* Nov 98:26, Oct 10:7

(Do not report more than one unit of 83789 for each specimen)

(For column chromatography/mass spectrometry of drugs or substances, see 80305, 80306, 80307, 80320-80377, or specific analyte code[s] in the **Chemistry** section)

83825 Mercury, quantitative

(Mercury screen, use 83015)

83835 Metanephrines

(For catecholamines, see 82382-82384)

(Methamphetamine, see 80324, 80325, 80326)

(Methane breath test, use 91065)

83857 Methemalbumin

(Methemoglobin, see hemoglobin 83045, 83050)

(Methyl alcohol, use 80320)

(Microalbumin, see 82043 for quantitative, see 82044 for semiquantitative)

83861 Microfluidic analysis utilizing an integrated collection and analysis device, tear osmolarity
> *CPT Changes: An Insider's View* 2011
> *CPT Assistant* Dec 10:7

(Microglobulin, beta-2, use 82232)

(For microfluidic tear osmolarity of both eyes, report 83861 twice)

83864 Mucopolysaccharides, acid, quantitative

83872 Mucin, synovial fluid (Ropes test)

83873 Myelin basic protein, cerebrospinal fluid
> *CPT Changes: An Insider's View* 2002

(For oligoclonal bands, use 83916)

83874 Myoglobin
> *CPT Assistant* Feb 98:1

83876 Myeloperoxidase (MPO)
> *CPT Changes: An Insider's View* 2009

83880 Natriuretic peptide
> *CPT Changes: An Insider's View* 2003
> *CPT Assistant* Jul 03:7

83883 Nephelometry, each analyte not elsewhere specified

● **83884** Neurofilament light chain (NfL)
> *CPT Changes: An Insider's View* 2025

83885 Nickel

83915 Nucleotidase 5'-

83916   Oligoclonal immune (oligoclonal bands)
➔ *CPT Changes: An Insider's View* 2002

83918   Organic acids; total, quantitative, each specimen
➔ *CPT Changes: An Insider's View* 2001
➔ *CPT Assistant* Mar 96:11, Nov 98:26

83919   qualitative, each specimen
➔ *CPT Assistant* Nov 98:26

83921   Organic acid, single, quantitative
➔ *CPT Changes: An Insider's View* 2001

83930   Osmolality; blood

83935   urine

(For tear osmolarity using microfluidic analysis, use 83861)

83937   Osteocalcin (bone g1a protein)
➔ *CPT Assistant* Summer 94:5

83945   Oxalate

83950   Oncoprotein; HER-2/neu
➔ *CPT Changes: An Insider's View* 2002, 2009

(For tissue, see 88342, 88365)

83951   des-gamma-carboxy-prothrombin (DCP)
➔ *CPT Changes: An Insider's View* 2009

83970   Parathormone (parathyroid hormone)

(Pesticide, quantitative, see code for specific method. For screen for chlorinated hydrocarbons, use 82441)

83986   pH; body fluid, not otherwise specified
➔ *CPT Changes: An Insider's View* 2010
➔ *CPT Assistant* Sep 13:13, May 16:14

83987   exhaled breath condensate
➔ *CPT Changes: An Insider's View* 2010

(For blood pH, see 82800, 82803)

(Phenobarbital, use 80345)

83992   Code is out of numerical sequence. See Definitive Drug Testing subsection

83993   Calprotectin, fecal
➔ *CPT Changes: An Insider's View* 2008
➔ *CPT Assistant* Apr 08:5, Oct 10:7

84030   Phenylalanine (PKU), blood

(Phenylalanine-tyrosine ratio, see 84030, 84510)

84035   Phenylketones, qualitative

84060   Phosphatase, acid; total

84066   prostatic

84075   Phosphatase, alkaline;
➔ *CPT Assistant* Dec 99:2

84078   heat stable (total not included)

84080   isoenzymes

84081   Phosphatidylglycerol

(Phosphates inorganic, use 84100)

(Phosphates, organic, see code for specific method. For cholinesterase, see 82480, 82482)

84085   Phosphogluconate, 6-, dehydrogenase, RBC

84087   Phosphohexose isomerase
➔ *CPT Assistant* Oct 10:7

84100   Phosphorus inorganic (phosphate);
➔ *CPT Assistant* Dec 99:2, Aug 05:9, Oct 10:7

84105   urine

(Pituitary gonadotropins, see 83001-83002)

(PKU, see 84030, 84035)

84106   Porphobilinogen, urine; qualitative

84110   quantitative

84112   Evaluation of cervicovaginal fluid for specific amniotic fluid protein(s) (eg, placental alpha microglobulin-1 [PAMG-1], placental protein 12 [PP12], alpha-fetoprotein), qualitative, each specimen
➔ *CPT Changes: An Insider's View* 2011, 2014
➔ *CPT Assistant* Oct 10:8, Dec 10:8

84119   Porphyrins, urine; qualitative

84120   quantitation and fractionation

84126   Porphyrins, feces, quantitative

(Porphyrin precursors, see 82135, 84106, 84110)

(For protoporphyrin, RBC, see 84202, 84203)

84132   Potassium; serum, plasma or whole blood
➔ *CPT Changes: An Insider's View* 2009
➔ *CPT Assistant* Dec 99:2, Jun 02:3, Apr 13:10, Jul 22:20

84133   urine

84134   Prealbumin

(For microalbumin, see 82043, 82044)

84135   Pregnanediol

84138   Pregnanetriol

84140   Pregnenolone
➔ *CPT Assistant* Summer 94:6

84143   17-hydroxypregnenolone
➔ *CPT Assistant* Summer 94:6

84144   Progesterone

(Progesterone receptor assay, use 84234)

(For proinsulin, use 84206)

84145   Procalcitonin (PCT)
➔ *CPT Changes: An Insider's View* 2010

84146   Prolactin

84150   Prostaglandin, each

84152   Prostate specific antigen (PSA); complexed (direct measurement)
> *CPT Changes: An Insider's View* 2001

84153   total
> *CPT Assistant* Fall 93:26, May 96:10, Aug 96:10, Jan 97:10, Nov 98:26, Aug 99:5, Dec 99:10

84154   free
> *CPT Assistant* Nov 98:26, Aug 99:5, Dec 99:10

84155   Protein, total, except by refractometry; serum, plasma or whole blood
> *CPT Changes: An Insider's View* 2004, 2009
> *CPT Assistant* Dec 99:2, Jan 00:7

84156   urine
> *CPT Changes: An Insider's View* 2004

84157   other source (eg, synovial fluid, cerebrospinal fluid)
> *CPT Changes: An Insider's View* 2004

84160   Protein, total, by refractometry, any source
> *CPT Changes: An Insider's View* 2004

(For urine total protein by dipstick method, use 81000-81003)

84163   Pregnancy-associated plasma protein-A (PAPP-A)
> *CPT Changes: An Insider's View* 2005

84165   Protein; electrophoretic fractionation and quantitation, serum
> *CPT Changes: An Insider's View* 2004, 2005

84166   electrophoretic fractionation and quantitation, other fluids with concentration (eg, urine, CSF)
> *CPT Changes: An Insider's View* 2005

84181   Western Blot, with interpretation and report, blood or other body fluid

84182   Western Blot, with interpretation and report, blood or other body fluid, immunological probe for band identification, each
> *CPT Assistant* Oct 10:7

(For Western Blot tissue analysis, use 88371)

84202   Protoporphyrin, RBC; quantitative
> *CPT Assistant* Aug 05:9, Oct 10:7

84203   screen

84206   Proinsulin

(Pseudocholinesterase, use 82480)

84207   Pyridoxal phosphate (Vitamin B-6)

84210   Pyruvate

84220   Pyruvate kinase

84228   Quinine
> *CPT Assistant* Apr 15:3

84233   Receptor assay; estrogen

84234   progesterone

84235   endocrine, other than estrogen or progesterone (specify hormone)

84238   non-endocrine (specify receptor)
> *CPT Changes: An Insider's View* 2006
> *CPT Assistant* Nov 05:14

84244   Renin

84252   Riboflavin (Vitamin B-2)

(Salicylates, see 80329, 80330, 80331)

(For salicylate by immunoassay or enzymatic methods, use 80179)

(Secretin test, see 99070, 43756, 43757 and appropriate analyses)

84255   Selenium

84260   Serotonin

(For urine metabolites (HIAA), use 83497)

84270   Sex hormone binding globulin (SHBG)
> *CPT Assistant* Summer 94:4

84275   Sialic acid

(Sickle hemoglobin, use 85660)

84285   Silica

84295   Sodium; serum, plasma or whole blood
> *CPT Changes: An Insider's View* 2009
> *CPT Assistant* Dec 99:2, Oct 10:7, Apr 13:10, Jul 22:20

84300   urine
> *CPT Assistant* Aug 05:9, Oct 10:7

84302   other source
> *CPT Changes: An Insider's View* 2003
> *CPT Assistant* Jul 03:7

(Somatomammotropin, use 83632)

(Somatotropin, use 83003)

84305   Somatomedin
> *CPT Assistant* Summer 94:4

84307   Somatostatin
> *CPT Assistant* Summer 94:4

84311   Spectrophotometry, analyte not elsewhere specified

84315   Specific gravity (except urine)

(For specific gravity, urine, see 81000-81003)

(Stone analysis, see 82355-82370)

(For suppression of growth stimulation expressed gene 2 [ST2] testing, use 83006)

84375 Sugars, chromatographic, TLC or paper chromatography

84376 Sugars (mono-, di-, and oligosaccharides); single qualitative, each specimen
➡ *CPT Assistant* Nov 98:26-27, Dec 99:7

84377 multiple qualitative, each specimen
➡ *CPT Assistant* Nov 98:26-27, Jul 03:7

84378 single quantitative, each specimen
➡ *CPT Assistant* Nov 98:26-27

84379 multiple quantitative, each specimen
➡ *CPT Assistant* Nov 98:26-27, Dec 99:7, Jul 03:7

84392 Sulfate, urine
➡ *CPT Assistant* Oct 10:7

(Sulfhemoglobin, use hemoglobin, 83060)

(T-3, see 84479-84481)

(T-4, see 84436-84439)

● **84393** Tau, phosphorylated (eg, pTau 181, pTau 217), each
➡ *CPT Changes: An Insider's View* 2025

● **84394** Tau, total (tTau)
➡ *CPT Changes: An Insider's View* 2025

84402 Testosterone; free
➡ *CPT Assistant* Aug 05:9, Oct 10:7

84403 total

84410 bioavailable, direct measurement (eg, differential precipitation)
➡ *CPT Changes: An Insider's View* 2017

(Do not report 84402, 84403 in conjunction with 80327, 80328 to identify anabolic steroid testing for testosterone)

84425 Thiamine (Vitamin B-1)

84430 Thiocyanate

84433 Thiopurine S-methyltransferase (TPMT)
➡ *CPT Changes: An Insider's View* 2023
➡ *CPT Assistant* Apr 23:18

84431 Thromboxane metabolite(s), including thromboxane if performed, urine
➡ *CPT Changes: An Insider's View* 2010

(For concurrent urine creatinine determination, use 84431 in conjunction with 82570)

84432 Thyroglobulin
➡ *CPT Assistant* Summer 94:2

(Thyroglobulin, antibody, use 86800)

(Thyrotropin releasing hormone [TRH] test, see 80438, 80439)

84433 Code is out of numerical sequence. See 84425-84432

84436 Thyroxine; total
➡ *CPT Assistant* Fall 93:25, Summer 94:3

84437 requiring elution (eg, neonatal)

84439 free

84442 Thyroxine binding globulin (TBG)

84443 Thyroid stimulating hormone (TSH)
➡ *CPT Assistant* Summer 94:3, Jul 22:20

84445 Thyroid stimulating immune globulins (TSI)
➡ *CPT Changes: An Insider's View* 2002
➡ *CPT Assistant* Summer 94:3

(Tobramycin, use 80200)

84446 Tocopherol alpha (Vitamin E)

84449 Transcortin (cortisol binding globulin)
➡ *CPT Assistant* Summer 94:6

84450 Transferase; aspartate amino (AST) (SGOT)
➡ *CPT Assistant* Dec 99:2

84460 alanine amino (ALT) (SGPT)
➡ *CPT Assistant* Dec 99:2

84466 Transferrin
➡ *CPT Assistant* Summer 94:4

(Iron binding capacity, use 83550)

84478 Triglycerides
➡ *CPT Assistant* Dec 99:2, Mar 00:11, Feb 05:9

84479 Thyroid hormone (T3 or T4) uptake or thyroid hormone binding ratio (THBR)
➡ *CPT Assistant* Fall 93:25, Summer 94:3

84480 Triiodothyronine T3; total (TT-3)

84481 free

84482 reverse
➡ *CPT Assistant* Summer 94:2

84484 Troponin, quantitative
➡ *CPT Assistant* Nov 97:29, Jan 98:6, Feb 98:1

(For troponin, qualitative assay, use 84512)

84485 Trypsin; duodenal fluid

84488 feces, qualitative

84490 feces, quantitative, 24-hour collection
➡ *CPT Assistant* Oct 10:7

84510 Tyrosine
➡ *CPT Assistant* Oct 10:7

(Urate crystal identification, use 89060)

84512 Troponin, qualitative
➡ *CPT Assistant* Nov 97:29, Jan 98:6, Feb 98:1

(For troponin, quantitative assay, use 84484)

84520 Urea nitrogen; quantitative
➡ *CPT Assistant* Dec 99:2, Apr 13:10, Jul 22:20

84525 semiquantitative (eg, reagent strip test)
➔ *CPT Assistant* Mar 98:3

84540 Urea nitrogen, urine

84545 Urea nitrogen, clearance

84550 Uric acid; blood
➔ *CPT Assistant* Dec 99:2

84560 other source

84577 Urobilinogen, feces, quantitative

84578 Urobilinogen, urine; qualitative

84580 quantitative, timed specimen

84583 semiquantitative

(Uroporphyrins, use 84120)

(Valproic acid [dipropylacetic acid], use 80164)

84585 Vanillylmandelic acid (VMA), urine

84586 Vasoactive intestinal peptide (VIP)
➔ *CPT Assistant* Summer 94:6

84588 Vasopressin (antidiuretic hormone, ADH)
➔ *CPT Assistant* Jan 18:7

84590 Vitamin A
➔ *CPT Assistant* Aug 05:9

(Vitamin B-1, use 84425)

(Vitamin B-2, use 84252)

(Vitamin B-6, use 84207)

(Vitamin B-12, use 82607)

(Vitamin C, use 82180)

(Vitamin D, see 82306, 82652)

(Vitamin E, use 84446)

84591 Vitamin, not otherwise specified
➔ *CPT Changes: An Insider's View* 2001
➔ *CPT Assistant* Oct 21:14

84597 Vitamin K
➔ *CPT Assistant* Oct 10:7

(VMA, use 84585)

84600 Volatiles (eg, acetic anhydride, diethylether)
➔ *CPT Changes: An Insider's View* 2015
➔ *CPT Assistant* Aug 05:9, Oct 10:7

(For carbon tetrachloride, dichloroethane, dichloromethane, use 82441)

(For isopropyl alcohol and methanol, use 80320)

(Volume, blood, RISA or Cr-51, see 78110, 78111)

84620 Xylose absorption test, blood and/or urine

(For administration, use 99070)

84630 Zinc

84681 C-peptide
➔ *CPT Assistant* Oct 10:7

84702 Gonadotropin, chorionic (hCG); quantitative
➔ *CPT Assistant* Oct 10:7

84703 qualitative

(For urine pregnancy test by visual color comparison, use 81025)

84704 free beta chain
➔ *CPT Changes: An Insider's View* 2008
➔ *CPT Assistant* Apr 08:5, Aug 08:13, Oct 10:7

84830 Ovulation tests, by visual color comparison methods for human luteinizing hormone
➔ *CPT Assistant* Oct 10:7, Jun 15:10, Jan 24:17

84999 Unlisted chemistry procedure
➔ *CPT Assistant* Oct 00:24, Aug 05:9, Oct 10:7, Dec 10:7, Apr 15:3, Oct 21:14, Jan 24:17

(For definitive testing of a drug, not otherwise specified, see 80299, 80375, 80376, 80377)

Hematology and Coagulation

Hematology and coagulation analytes/procedures that are not specified in 85002-85810 and are not in the Chemistry (82009-84830), Immunology (86015-86835), or Transfusion Medicine (86850-86985) subsections may be reported using the unlisted hematology and coagulation procedure code 85999.

(For blood banking procedures, see **Transfusion Medicine**)

(Agglutinins, see **Immunology**)

(Antiplasmin, use 85410)

(Antithrombin III, see 85300, 85301)

85002 Bleeding time
➔ *CPT Assistant* Aug 05:9

85004 Blood count; automated differential WBC count
➔ *CPT Changes: An Insider's View* 2003
➔ *CPT Assistant* Jan 04:26

85007 blood smear, microscopic examination with manual differential WBC count
➔ *CPT Changes: An Insider's View* 2003
➔ *CPT Assistant* Jul 03:7, Jan 04:26

85008 blood smear, microscopic examination without manual differential WBC count
➔ *CPT Changes: An Insider's View* 2003
➔ *CPT Assistant* Jul 03:8, Jan 04:26

(For other fluids [eg, CSF], see 89050, 89051)

85009   manual differential WBC count, buffy coat

→ *CPT Changes: An Insider's View* 2003

→ *CPT Assistant* Jul 03:7, Jan 04:26

(Eosinophils, nasal smear, use 89190)

85013   spun microhematocrit

85014   hematocrit (Hct)

→ *CPT Changes: An Insider's View* 2003

→ *CPT Assistant* Jul 03:7

85018   hemoglobin (Hgb)

→ *CPT Changes: An Insider's View* 2003

→ *CPT Assistant* Jul 03:8

(For other hemoglobin determination, see 83020-83069)

(For immunoassay, hemoglobin, fecal, use 82274)

(For transcutaneous hemoglobin measurement, use 88738)

85025   complete (CBC), automated (Hgb, Hct, RBC, WBC and platelet count) and automated differential WBC count

→ *CPT Changes: An Insider's View* 2003

→ *CPT Assistant* Jul 00:11, Jul 03:7, Jan 04:26, Jul 11:16, Jul 22:20

85027   complete (CBC), automated (Hgb, Hct, RBC, WBC and platelet count)

→ *CPT Changes: An Insider's View* 2003

→ *CPT Assistant* Jul 03:8, Jan 04:26, May 21:9

85032   manual cell count (erythrocyte, leukocyte, or platelet) each

→ *CPT Changes: An Insider's View* 2003

→ *CPT Assistant* Jul 03:8, Nov 03:15

85041   red blood cell (RBC), automated

→ *CPT Changes: An Insider's View* 2003

→ *CPT Assistant* Jul 03:8

(Do not report code 85041 in conjunction with 85025 or 85027)

85044   reticulocyte, manual

→ *CPT Changes: An Insider's View* 2003

→ *CPT Assistant* Jul 03:8

85045   reticulocyte, automated

→ *CPT Changes: An Insider's View* 2003

→ *CPT Assistant* Jul 03:8

85046   reticulocytes, automated, including 1 or more cellular parameters (eg, reticulocyte hemoglobin content [CHr], immature reticulocyte fraction [IRF], reticulocyte volume [MRV], RNA content), direct measurement

→ *CPT Changes: An Insider's View* 2005

→ *CPT Assistant* Nov 98:27

85048   leukocyte (WBC), automated

→ *CPT Changes: An Insider's View* 2003

→ *CPT Assistant* Jul 03:8

85049   platelet, automated

→ *CPT Changes: An Insider's View* 2003

85055   Reticulated platelet assay

→ *CPT Changes: An Insider's View* 2004

85060   Blood smear, peripheral, interpretation by physician with written report

(Use 0854T in conjunction with 85060, when the digitization of glass microscope slides is performed)

85097   Bone marrow, smear interpretation

→ *CPT Changes: An Insider's View* 2002

→ *CPT Assistant* Winter 92:17, Jul 98:4, Mar 03:22

(Use 0855T in conjunction with 85097, when the digitization of glass microscope slides is performed)

(For special stains, see 88312, 88313)

(For bone biopsy, see 20220, 20225, 20240, 20245, 20250, 20251)

85130   Chromogenic substrate assay

→ *CPT Assistant* Aug 05:9

(Circulating anti-coagulant screen [mixing studies], see 85611, 85732)

85170   Clot retraction

85175   Clot lysis time, whole blood dilution

(Clotting factor I [fibrinogen], see 85384, 85385)

85210   Clotting; factor II, prothrombin, specific

→ *CPT Assistant* Aug 05:9

(See also 85610-85613)

85220   factor V (AcG or proaccelerin), labile factor

85230   factor VII (proconvertin, stable factor)

85240   factor VIII (AHG), 1-stage

85244   factor VIII related antigen

85245   factor VIII, VW factor, ristocetin cofactor

85246   factor VIII, VW factor antigen

85247   factor VIII, von Willebrand factor, multimetric analysis

85250   factor IX (PTC or Christmas)

85260   factor X (Stuart-Prower)

85270   factor XI (PTA)

85280   factor XII (Hageman)

85290   factor XIII (fibrin stabilizing)

85291   factor XIII (fibrin stabilizing), screen solubility

85292   prekallikrein assay (Fletcher factor assay)

85293   high molecular weight kininogen assay (Fitzgerald factor assay)

85300   Clotting inhibitors or anticoagulants; antithrombin III, activity
⟳ *CPT Assistant* Aug 05:9

85301   antithrombin III, antigen assay

85302   protein C, antigen

85303   protein C, activity

85305   protein S, total

85306   protein S, free

85307   Activated Protein C (APC) resistance assay
⟳ *CPT Changes: An Insider's View* 2001

85335   Factor inhibitor test

85337   Thrombomodulin

(For mixing studies for inhibitors, use 85732)

85345   Coagulation time; Lee and White

85347   activated
⟳ *CPT Assistant* Apr 19:11

85348   other methods

(Differential count, see 85007 et seq)

(Duke bleeding time, use 85002)

(Eosinophils, nasal smear, use 89190)

85360   Euglobulin lysis

(Fetal hemoglobin, see 83030, 83033, 85460)

85362   Fibrin(ogen) degradation (split) products (FDP) (FSP); agglutination slide, semiquantitative

(Immunoelectrophoresis, use 86320)

85366   paracoagulation

85370   quantitative

85378   Fibrin degradation products, D-dimer; qualitative or semiquantitative
⟳ *CPT Changes: An Insider's View* 2003
⟳ *CPT Assistant* Jul 03:8

85379   quantitative

(For ultrasensitive and standard sensitivity quantitative D-dimer, use 85379)

85380   ultrasensitive (eg, for evaluation for venous thromboembolism), qualitative or semiquantitative
⟳ *CPT Changes: An Insider's View* 2003
⟳ *CPT Assistant* Jul 03:8

85384   Fibrinogen; activity
⟳ *CPT Assistant* Apr 19:11

85385   antigen

85390   Fibrinolysins or coagulopathy screen, interpretation and report
⟳ *CPT Assistant* Apr 19:11

85396   Coagulation/fibrinolysis assay, whole blood (eg, viscoelastic clot assessment), including use of any pharmacologic additive(s), as indicated, including interpretation and written report, per day
⟳ *CPT Changes: An Insider's View* 2004
⟳ *CPT Assistant* Apr 19:11

85397   Coagulation and fibrinolysis, functional activity, not otherwise specified (eg, ADAMTS-13), each analyte
⟳ *CPT Changes: An Insider's View* 2009

85400   Fibrinolytic factors and inhibitors; plasmin
⟳ *CPT Assistant* Aug 05:9

85410   alpha-2 antiplasmin

85415   plasminogen activator

85420   plasminogen, except antigenic assay

85421   plasminogen, antigenic assay

(Fragility, red blood cell, see 85547, 85555-85557)

85441   Heinz bodies; direct

85445   induced, acetyl phenylhydrazine

(Hematocrit [PCV], see 85014, 85025, 85027)

(Hemoglobin, see 83020-83068, 85018, 85025, 85027)

85460   Hemoglobin or RBCs, fetal, for fetomaternal hemorrhage; differential lysis (Kleihauer-Betke)
⟳ *CPT Assistant* Fall 93:25

(See also 83030, 83033)

(Hemolysins, see 86940, 86941)

85461   rosette

85475   Hemolysin, acid

(See also 86940, 86941)

85520   Heparin assay
⟳ *CPT Assistant* Aug 05:9

85525   Heparin neutralization
⟳ *CPT Assistant* Aug 17:10

85530   Heparin-protamine tolerance test

85536   Iron stain, peripheral blood
⟳ *CPT Changes: An Insider's View* 2001

(For iron stains on bone marrow or other tissues with physician evaluation, use 88313)

85540   Leukocyte alkaline phosphatase with count

85547   Mechanical fragility, RBC

85549   Muramidase

(Nitroblue tetrazolium dye test, use 86384)

85555 Osmotic fragility, RBC; unincubated

85557   incubated

(Packed cell volume, use 85013)

(Partial thromboplastin time, see 85730, 85732)

(Parasites, blood [eg, malaria smears], use 87207)

(Plasmin, use 85400)

(Plasminogen, use 85420)

(Plasminogen activator, use 85415)

85576 Platelet, aggregation (in vitro), each agent
➜ *CPT Changes: An Insider's View* 2003
➜ *CPT Assistant* Jul 96:10, Apr 19:11

(For thromboxane metabolite[s], including thromboxane, if performed, measurement[s] in urine, use 84431)

85597 Phospholipid neutralization; platelet
➜ *CPT Changes: An Insider's View* 2011
➜ *CPT Assistant* Oct 10:8, Dec 10:8, Apr 11:9

85598   hexagonal phospholipid
➜ *CPT Changes: An Insider's View* 2011
➜ *CPT Assistant* Oct 10:8, Dec 10:8, Apr 11:9

85610 Prothrombin time;
➜ *CPT Assistant* Aug 05:9

85611   substitution, plasma fractions, each

85612 Russell viper venom time (includes venom); undiluted

85613   diluted

(Red blood cell count, see 85025, 85027, 85041)

85635 Reptilase test

(Reticulocyte count, see 85044, 85045)

85651 Sedimentation rate, erythrocyte; non-automated

85652   automated

85660 Sickling of RBC, reduction

(Hemoglobin electrophoresis, use 83020)

(Smears [eg, for parasites, malaria], use 87207)

85670 Thrombin time; plasma

85675   titer

85705 Thromboplastin inhibition, tissue
➜ *CPT Assistant* Aug 05:9

(For individual clotting factors, see 85245-85247)

85730 Thromboplastin time, partial (PTT); plasma or whole blood

85732   substitution, plasma fractions, each
➜ *CPT Assistant* Apr 11:9

85810 Viscosity

(von Willebrand factor assay, see 85245-85247)

(WBC count, see 85025, 85027, 85048, 89050)

85999 Unlisted hematology and coagulation procedure
➜ *CPT Assistant* Aug 05:9, Oct 09:12, Aug 17:10

Immunology

Immunology analytes/procedures that are not specified in 86015-86835 and are not in the Chemistry subsection (82009-84830) may be reported using the unlisted immunology procedure code 86849.

\# **86041** Acetylcholine receptor (AChR); binding antibody
➜ *CPT Changes: An Insider's View* 2024

\# **86042**   blocking antibody
➜ *CPT Changes: An Insider's View* 2024

\# **86043**   modulating antibody
➜ *CPT Changes: An Insider's View* 2024

\# **86015** Actin (smooth muscle) antibody (ASMA), each
➜ *CPT Changes: An Insider's View* 2022
➜ *CPT Assistant* Sep 22:3, Jan 24:17

(Actinomyces, antibodies to, use 86602)

(Adrenal cortex antibodies, see 86255, 86256)

86000 Agglutinins, febrile (eg, Brucella, Francisella, Murine typhus, Q fever, Rocky Mountain spotted fever, scrub typhus), each antigen
➜ *CPT Assistant* Aug 05:9

(For antibodies to infectious agents, see 86602-86804)

86001 Allergen specific IgG quantitative or semiquantitative, each allergen
➜ *CPT Changes: An Insider's View* 2001

(Agglutinins and autohemolysins, see 86940, 86941)

86003 Allergen specific IgE; quantitative or semiquantitative, crude allergen extract, each
➜ *CPT Changes: An Insider's View* 2018
➜ *CPT Assistant* Spring 94:31

(For total quantitative IgE, use 82785)

86005   qualitative, multiallergen screen (eg, disk, sponge, card)
➜ *CPT Changes: An Insider's View* 2018
➜ *CPT Assistant* Spring 94:31

86008   quantitative or semiquantitative, recombinant or purified component, each
➜ *CPT Changes: An Insider's View* 2018

▶(For amyloid, beta, see 82233, 82234)◀

(For total qualitative IgE, use 83518)

(Alpha-1 antitrypsin, see 82103, 82104)

(Alpha-1 feto-protein, see 82105, 82106)

(Anti-AChR [acetylcholine receptor] antibody, see 86041, 86042, 86043)

(Anticardiolipin antibody, use 86147)

(Anti-DNA, use 86225)

(Anti-deoxyribonuclease titer, use 86215)

86015 Code is out of numerical sequence. See 85810-86001

86021 Antibody identification; leukocyte antibodies

86022 platelet antibodies

86023 platelet associated immunoglobulin assay

86036 Antineutrophil cytoplasmic antibody (ANCA); screen, each antibody
➔ *CPT Changes: An Insider's View* 2022
➔ *CPT Assistant* Sep 22:3

86037 titer, each antibody
➔ *CPT Changes: An Insider's View* 2022
➔ *CPT Assistant* Sep 22:3

86038 Antinuclear antibodies (ANA);
➔ *CPT Assistant* Feb 22:15

86039 titer
➔ *CPT Assistant* Feb 22:15

(Antistreptococcal antibody, ie, anti-DNAse, use 86215)

(Antistreptokinase titer, use 86590)

86041 Code is out of numerical sequence. See 85810-86001

86042 Code is out of numerical sequence. See 85810-86001

86043 Code is out of numerical sequence. See 85810-86001

86051 Code is out of numerical sequence. See 86060-86078

86052 Code is out of numerical sequence. See 86060-86078

86053 Code is out of numerical sequence. See 86060-86078

86060 Antistreptolysin O; titer

(For antibodies to infectious agents, see 86602-86804)

86063 screen

(For antibodies to infectious agents, see 86602-86804)

(Blastomyces, antibodies to, use 86612)

 # 86051 Aquaporin-4 (neuromyelitis optica [NMO]) antibody; enzyme-linked immunosorbent immunoassay (ELISA)
➔ *CPT Changes: An Insider's View* 2022
➔ *CPT Assistant* Apr 22:3

 # 86052 cell-based immunofluorescence assay (CBA), each
➔ *CPT Changes: An Insider's View* 2022
➔ *CPT Assistant* Apr 22:3

 # 86053 flow cytometry (ie, fluorescence-activated cell sorting [FACS]), each
➔ *CPT Changes: An Insider's View* 2022
➔ *CPT Assistant* Apr 22:3

86077 Blood bank physician services; difficult cross match and/or evaluation of irregular antibody(s), interpretation and written report

86078 investigation of transfusion reaction including suspicion of transmissible disease, interpretation and written report

86079 authorization for deviation from standard blood banking procedures (eg, use of outdated blood, transfusion of Rh incompatible units), with written report

(Brucella, antibodies to, use 86622)

(Candida, antibodies to, use 86628. For skin testing, use 86485)

86140 C-reactive protein;
➔ *CPT Changes: An Insider's View* 2002
➔ *CPT Assistant* Aug 05:9

(Candidiasis, use 86628)

86141 high sensitivity (hsCRP)
➔ *CPT Changes: An Insider's View* 2002

86146 Beta 2 Glycoprotein I antibody, each
➔ *CPT Changes: An Insider's View* 2001

86147 Cardiolipin (phospholipid) antibody, each Ig class
➔ *CPT Changes: An Insider's View* 2001

 # 86152 Cell enumeration using immunologic selection and identification in fluid specimen (eg, circulating tumor cells in blood);
➔ *CPT Changes: An Insider's View* 2013

(For physician interpretation and report, use 86153. For cell enumeration with interpretation and report, use 86152 and 86153)

 # 86153 physician interpretation and report, when required
➔ *CPT Changes: An Insider's View* 2013

(For cell enumeration, use 86152. For cell enumeration with interpretation and report, use 86152 and 86153)

(For flow cytometric immunophenotyping, see 88184-88189)

(For flow cytometric quantitation, see 86355, 86356, 86357, 86359, 86360, 86361, 86367)

86148 Anti-phosphatidylserine (phospholipid) antibody
➔ *CPT Assistant* Nov 97:30, Jul 03:8, Nov 03:5

(To report antiprothrombin [phospholipid cofactor] antibody, use 86849)

86152 Code is out of numerical sequence. See 86146-86155

86153 Code is out of numerical sequence. See 86146-86155

86155 Chemotaxis assay, specify method

(Clostridium difficile toxin, use 87230)

►(Coccidioides, antibodies to, use 86635)◄

86156 Cold agglutinin; screen

86157 titer

★ = Telemedicine   ◀ = Audio-only   + = Add-on code   ✔ = FDA approval pending   # = Resequenced code   ⊘ = Modifier 51 exempt   ➔➔➔ = See p xxi for details

86160	Complement; antigen, each component
86161	functional activity, each component
86162	total hemolytic (CH50)
86171	Complement fixation tests, each antigen

(Coombs test, see 86880-86886)

86200 Cyclic citrullinated peptide (CCP), antibody
➜ *CPT Changes: An Insider's View* 2006
➜ *CPT Assistant* Mar 06:6

86215 Deoxyribonuclease, antibody
➜ *CPT Assistant* Aug 05:9

86225 Deoxyribonucleic acid (DNA) antibody; native or double stranded

(Echinococcus, antibodies to, see code for specific method)

(For HIV antibody tests, see 86701-86703)

86226   single stranded
➜ *CPT Assistant* Feb 22:15

(Anti D.S., DNA, IFA, eg, using C.Lucilae, see 86255 and 86256)

86231 Endomysial antibody (EMA), each immunoglobulin (Ig) class
➜ *CPT Changes: An Insider's View* 2022
➜ *CPT Assistant* Mar 22:11

86235 Extractable nuclear antigen, antibody to, any method (eg, nRNP, SS-A, SS-B, Sm, RNP, Sc170, J01), each antibody

86255 Fluorescent noninfectious agent antibody; screen, each antibody
➜ *CPT Assistant* Nov 98:27, Feb 22:15, Mar 22:11, Sep 22:3

86256   titer, each antibody
➜ *CPT Assistant* Feb 22:15, Sep 22:3

(Fluorescent technique for antigen identification in tissue, use 88346; for indirect fluorescence, see 88346, 88350)

(FTA, use 86780)

(Gel [agar] diffusion tests, use 86331)

86258 Gliadin (deamidated) (DGP) antibody, each immunoglobulin (Ig) class
➜ *CPT Changes: An Insider's View* 2022
➜ *CPT Assistant* Mar 22:11

86277 Growth hormone, human (HGH), antibody

86280 Hemagglutination inhibition test (HAI)

(For rubella, use 86762)

(For antibodies to infectious agents, see 86602-86804)

86294 Immunoassay for tumor antigen, qualitative or semiquantitative (eg, bladder tumor antigen)
➜ *CPT Changes: An Insider's View* 2001

(For qualitative NMP22 protein, use 86386)

86300 Immunoassay for tumor antigen, quantitative; CA 15-3 (27.29)
➜ *CPT Changes: An Insider's View* 2001
➜ *CPT Assistant* Aug 05:9

86301   CA 19-9
➜ *CPT Changes: An Insider's View* 2001

86304   CA 125
➜ *CPT Changes: An Insider's View* 2001

(For measurement of serum HER-2/neu oncoprotein, see 83950)

(For hepatitis delta agent, antibody, use 86692)

(For hepatitis delta agent, antigen, use 87380)

(For hepatitis D [delta], quantification, use 87523)

86305 Human epididymis protein 4 (HE4)
➜ *CPT Changes: An Insider's View* 2010

86308 Heterophile antibodies; screening

(For antibodies to infectious agents, see 86602-86804)

86309   titer

(For antibodies to infectious agents, see 86602-86804)

86310   titers after absorption with beef cells and guinea pig kidney

(Histoplasma, antibodies to, use 86698. For skin testing, use 86510)

(For antibodies to infectious agents, see 86602-86804)

(Human growth hormone antibody, use 86277)

86316 Immunoassay for tumor antigen, other antigen, quantitative (eg, CA 50, 72-4, 549), each
➜ *CPT Changes: An Insider's View* 2001
➜ *CPT Assistant* May 96:11, Aug 96:11, Apr 98:15, Aug 99:5, Dec 99:10

86317 Immunoassay for infectious agent antibody, quantitative, not otherwise specified
➜ *CPT Assistant* Nov 97:30-31

(For immunoassay techniques for non-infectious agent antigens, see 83516, 83518, 83519, 83520)

(For particle agglutination procedures, use 86403)

(For infectious agent antigen detection by immunoassay technique, see 87301-87451. For infectious agent antigen detection by immunoassay technique with direct optical [ie, visual] observation, see 87802-87899)

Pathology and Laboratory **80047-89398, 0001U-0520U**

86318   Immunoassay for infectious agent antibody(ies), qualitative or semiquantitative, single-step method (eg, reagent strip);
➡ *CPT Changes: An Insider's View* 2021
➡ *CPT Assistant* Mar 07:10

 # 86328   severe acute respiratory syndrome coronavirus 2 (SARS-CoV-2) (coronavirus disease [COVID-19])
➡ *CPT Changes: An Insider's View* 2021

(For severe acute respiratory syndrome coronavirus 2 [SARS-CoV-2] [coronavirus disease {COVID-19}] antibody testing using multiple-step method, use 86769)

86320   Immunoelectrophoresis; serum

86325   other fluids (eg, urine, cerebrospinal fluid) with concentration
➡ *CPT Changes: An Insider's View* 2002

►(86327 has been deleted)◄

86328   Code is out of numerical sequence. See 86317-86325

86329   Immunodiffusion; not elsewhere specified
➡ *CPT Assistant* Aug 00:11

86331   gel diffusion, qualitative (Ouchterlony), each antigen or antibody

86332   Immune complex assay

86334   Immunofixation electrophoresis; serum
➡ *CPT Changes: An Insider's View* 2005

86335   other fluids with concentration (eg, urine, CSF)
➡ *CPT Changes: An Insider's View* 2005

86336   Inhibin A
➡ *CPT Changes: An Insider's View* 2002

86337   Insulin antibodies

86340   Intrinsic factor antibodies

(Leptospira, antibodies to, use 86720)

(Leukoagglutinins, use 86021)

86341   Islet cell antibody
➡ *CPT Assistant* Summer 94:6

86343   Leukocyte histamine release test (LHR)

86344   Leukocyte phagocytosis

86352   Cellular function assay involving stimulation (eg, mitogen or antigen) and detection of biomarker (eg, ATP)
➡ *CPT Changes: An Insider's View* 2010

86353   Lymphocyte transformation, mitogen (phytomitogen) or antigen induced blastogenesis

(Malaria antibodies, use 86750)

(For cellular function assay involving stimulation and detection of biomarker, use 86352)

86355   B cells, total count
➡ *CPT Changes: An Insider's View* 2006
➡ *CPT Assistant* Mar 06:6, Apr 08:5

86356   Mononuclear cell antigen, quantitative (eg, flow cytometry), not otherwise specified, each antigen
➡ *CPT Changes: An Insider's View* 2008
➡ *CPT Assistant* Apr 08:5

(Do not report 88187-88189 for interpretation of 86355, 86356, 86357, 86359, 86360, 86361, 86367)

 # 86366   Muscle-specific kinase (MuSK) antibody
➡ *CPT Changes: An Insider's View* 2024

 # 86362   Myelin oligodendrocyte glycoprotein (MOG-IgG1) antibody; cell-based immunofluorescence assay (CBA), each
➡ *CPT Changes: An Insider's View* 2022
➡ *CPT Assistant* Apr 22:3

 # 86363   flow cytometry (ie, fluorescence-activated cell sorting [FACS]), each
➡ *CPT Changes: An Insider's View* 2022
➡ *CPT Assistant* Apr 22:3

86357   Natural killer (NK) cells, total count
➡ *CPT Changes: An Insider's View* 2006
➡ *CPT Assistant* Mar 06:6, Apr 08:5

 # 86364   Tissue transglutaminase, each immunoglobulin (Ig) class
➡ *CPT Changes: An Insider's View* 2022
➡ *CPT Assistant* Mar 22:11

86359   T cells; total count
➡ *CPT Assistant* Nov 97:30, Apr 08:5

86360   absolute CD4 and CD8 count, including ratio
➡ *CPT Assistant* Nov 97:30, Jan 07:29, Apr 08:5

86361   absolute CD4 count
➡ *CPT Assistant* Nov 97:30, Apr 08:5

86362   Code is out of numerical sequence. See 86355-86360

86363   Code is out of numerical sequence. See 86355-86360

86364   Code is out of numerical sequence. See 86355-86360

86366   Code is out of numerical sequence. See 86355-86360

86367   Stem cells (ie, CD34), total count
➡ *CPT Changes: An Insider's View* 2006
➡ *CPT Assistant* Mar 06:6, Apr 08:5, Oct 13:3

(For flow cytometric immunophenotyping for the assessment of potential hematolymphoid neoplasia, see 88184-88189)

86376   Microsomal antibodies (eg, thyroid or liver-kidney), each

86381   Mitochondrial antibody (eg, M2), each
➡ *CPT Changes: An Insider's View* 2022
➡ *CPT Assistant* Sep 22:3

86382   Neutralization test, viral

\# **86408**   Neutralizing antibody, severe acute respiratory syndrome coronavirus 2 (SARS-CoV-2) (coronavirus disease [COVID-19]); screen
➔ *CPT Changes: An Insider's View* 2022

\# **86409**   titer
➔ *CPT Changes: An Insider's View* 2022

\# **86413**   Severe acute respiratory syndrome coronavirus 2 (SARS-CoV-2) (coronavirus disease [COVID-19]) antibody, quantitative
➔ *CPT Changes: An Insider's View* 2022

86384   Nitroblue tetrazolium dye test (NTD)

86386   Nuclear Matrix Protein 22 (NMP22), qualitative
➔ *CPT Changes: An Insider's View* 2012

(Ouchterlony diffusion, use 86331)

(Platelet antibodies, see 86022, 86023)

86403   Particle agglutination; screen, each antibody
➔ *CPT Assistant* Aug 05:9

86406   titer, each antibody

(Pregnancy test, see 84702, 84703)

(Rapid plasma reagin test (RPR), see 86592, 86593)

86408   Code is out of numerical sequence. See 86376-86386

86409   Code is out of numerical sequence. See 86376-86386

86413   Code is out of numerical sequence. See 86376-86386

86430   Rheumatoid factor; qualitative

86431   quantitative

(Serologic test for syphilis, see 86592, 86593)

86480   Tuberculosis test, cell mediated immunity antigen response measurement; gamma interferon
➔ *CPT Changes: An Insider's View* 2006, 2011
➔ *CPT Assistant* Mar 06:6, Oct 10:7, Dec 10:8, Dec 19:13

86481   enumeration of gamma interferon-producing T-cells in cell suspension
➔ *CPT Changes: An Insider's View* 2011
➔ *CPT Assistant* Oct 10:8, Dec 10:8, Dec 19:13

86485   Skin test; candida

(For antibody, candida, use 86628)

86486   unlisted antigen, each
➔ *CPT Changes: An Insider's View* 2008

▶(86490 has been deleted)◀

86510   histoplasmosis
➔ *CPT Assistant* Aug 05:9

(For histoplasma, antibody, use 86698)

86580   tuberculosis, intradermal

(For tuberculosis test, cell mediated immunity measurement of gamma interferon antigen response, use 86480)

(For skin tests for allergy, see 95012-95199)

(Smooth muscle antibody, use 86015)

(Sporothrix, antibodies to, see code for specific method)

● **86581**   Streptococcus pneumoniae antibody (IgG), serotypes, multiplex immunoassay, quantitative
➔ *CPT Changes: An Insider's View* 2025

86590   Streptokinase, antibody

(For antibodies to infectious agents, see 86602-86804)

(Streptolysin O antibody, see antistreptolysin O, 86060, 86063)

86592   Syphilis test, non-treponemal antibody; qualitative (eg, VDRL, RPR, ART)
➔ *CPT Changes: An Insider's View* 2010

(For antibodies to infectious agents, see 86602-86804)

86593   quantitative
➔ *CPT Changes: An Insider's View* 2010

(For antibodies to infectious agents, see 86602-86804)

(Tetanus antibody, use 86774)

(Thyroglobulin antibody, use 86800)

(Thyroglobulin, use 84432)

(Thyroid microsomal antibody, use 86376)

(For toxoplasma antibody, see 86777-86778)

86596   Voltage-gated calcium channel antibody, each
➔ *CPT Changes: An Insider's View* 2022
➔ *CPT Assistant* Sep 22:3

The following codes (86602-86804) are qualitative or semiquantitative immunoassays performed by multiple-step methods for the detection of antibodies to infectious agents. For immunoassays by single-step method (eg, reagent strips), see codes 86318, 86328. Procedures for the identification of antibodies should be coded as precisely as possible. For example, an antibody to a virus could be coded with increasing specificity for virus, family, genus, species, or type. In some cases, further precision may be added to codes by specifying the class of immunoglobulin being detected. When multiple tests are done to detect antibodies to organisms classified more precisely than the specificity allowed by available codes, it is appropriate to code each as a separate service. For example, a test for antibody to an enterovirus is coded as 86658. Coxsackie viruses are enteroviruses, but there are no codes for the individual species of enterovirus. If assays are performed for antibodies to coxsackie A and B species, each assay should be separately coded. Similarly, if multiple assays are performed for antibodies of different immunoglobulin classes, each assay should be coded separately. When a coding option exists for reporting IgM specific antibodies (eg, 86632), the corresponding nonspecific code (eg, 86631) may be reported for performance of either an antibody analysis not specific for a particular immunoglobulin class or for an IgG analysis.

(For the detection of antibodies other than those to infectious agents, see specific antibody [eg, 86015, 86021-86023, 86376, 86800, 86850-86870] or specific method [eg, 83516, 86255, 86256])

(For infectious agent/antigen detection, see 87260-87899)

86602   Antibody; actinomyces
➔ *CPT Assistant* Aug 05:9

86603   adenovirus

86606   Aspergillus

86609   bacterium, not elsewhere specified

86611   Bartonella
➔ *CPT Changes: An Insider's View* 2001

86612   Blastomyces

86615   Bordetella

86617   Borrelia burgdorferi (Lyme disease) confirmatory test (eg, Western Blot or immunoblot)

86618   Borrelia burgdorferi (Lyme disease)

86619   Borrelia (relapsing fever)

86622   Brucella

86625   Campylobacter

86628   Candida

(For skin test, candida, use 86485)

86631   Chlamydia

86632   Chlamydia, IgM
➔ *CPT Assistant* Nov 97:31

(For chlamydia antigen, see 87270, 87320. For fluorescent antibody technique, see 86255, 86256)

86635   Coccidioides

(For severe acute respiratory syndrome coronavirus 2 [SARS-CoV-2] [coronavirus disease {COVID-19}] antibody testing, see 86328, 86769)

86638   Coxiella burnetii (Q fever)

86641   Cryptococcus

86644   cytomegalovirus (CMV)

86645   cytomegalovirus (CMV), IgM
➔ *CPT Assistant* Jul 03:7

86648   Diphtheria

86651   encephalitis, California (La Crosse)

86652   encephalitis, Eastern equine

86653   encephalitis, St. Louis

86654   encephalitis, Western equine

86658   enterovirus (eg, coxsackie, echo, polio)

(Trichinella, antibodies to, use 86784)

(Trypanosoma, antibodies to, see code for specific method)

(Tuberculosis, use 86580 for skin testing)

(Viral antibodies, see code for specific method)

86663   Epstein-Barr (EB) virus, early antigen (EA)

86664   Epstein-Barr (EB) virus, nuclear antigen (EBNA)

86665   Epstein-Barr (EB) virus, viral capsid (VCA)

86666   Ehrlichia
➔ *CPT Changes: An Insider's View* 2001

86668   Francisella tularensis

86671   fungus, not elsewhere specified

86674   Giardia lamblia

86677   Helicobacter pylori
➔ *CPT Assistant* Jan 98:6

86682   helminth, not elsewhere specified

86684   Haemophilus influenza

86687   HTLV-I

86688   HTLV-II

86689   HTLV or HIV antibody, confirmatory test (eg, Western Blot)
➔ *CPT Assistant* Mar 08:3

86692   hepatitis, delta agent
➔ *CPT Assistant* Nov 97:31

(For hepatitis delta agent, antigen, use 87380)

(For hepatitis D [delta], quantification, use 87523)

86694   herpes simplex, non-specific type test

86695   herpes simplex, type 1

86696   herpes simplex, type 2
➔ *CPT Changes: An Insider's View* 2001

86698   histoplasma

86701   HIV-1
➔ *CPT Assistant* Aug 05:9, Mar 08:3, Apr 08:5

86702   HIV-2
➔ *CPT Assistant* Mar 08:3, Apr 08:5

86703   HIV-1 and HIV-2, single result
➔ *CPT Changes: An Insider's View* 2012
➔ *CPT Assistant* Nov 97:31, Mar 08:3, Apr 08:5

(For HIV-1 antigen(s) with HIV-1 and HIV-2 antibodies, single result, use 87389)

(When HIV immunoassay [HIV testing 86701-86703 or 87389] is performed using a kit or transportable instrument that wholly or in part consists of a single use, disposable analytical chamber, the service may be identified by adding modifier 92 to the usual code)

(For HIV-1 antigen, use 87390)

(For HIV-2 antigen, use 87391)

(For confirmatory test for HIV antibody (eg, Western Blot), use 86689)

86704 Hepatitis B core antibody (HBcAb); total
➔ *CPT Changes: An Insider's View* 2001
➔ *CPT Assistant* Nov 97:31-32

86705 IgM antibody
➔ *CPT Assistant* Nov 97:31-32

86706 Hepatitis B surface antibody (HBsAb)
➔ *CPT Assistant* Nov 97:31-32

86707 Hepatitis Be antibody (HBeAb)
➔ *CPT Assistant* Nov 97:31-32

86708 Hepatitis A antibody (HAAb)
➔ *CPT Changes: An Insider's View* 2001, 2016
➔ *CPT Assistant* Nov 97:31-32, Jun 00:11

86709 Hepatitis A antibody (HAAb), IgM antibody
➔ *CPT Changes: An Insider's View* 2016
➔ *CPT Assistant* Nov 97:31-32, Jun 00:11

86710 Antibody; influenza virus

86711 JC (John Cunningham) virus
➔ *CPT Changes: An Insider's View* 2013

86713 Legionella

86717 Leishmania

86720 Leptospira

86723 Listeria monocytogenes

86727 lymphocytic choriomeningitis

86732 mucormycosis

86735 mumps

86738 mycoplasma

86741 Neisseria meningitidis

86744 Nocardia

86747 parvovirus

86750 Plasmodium (malaria)

86753 protozoa, not elsewhere specified

86756 respiratory syncytial virus

86757 Rickettsia
➔ *CPT Changes: An Insider's View* 2001

86759 rotavirus

86762 rubella

86765 rubeola

86768 Salmonella

86769 severe acute respiratory syndrome coronavirus 2 (SARS-CoV-2) (coronavirus disease [COVID-19])
➔ *CPT Changes: An Insider's View* 2021

(For severe acute respiratory syndrome coronavirus 2 [SARS-CoV-2] [coronavirus disease {COVID-19}] antibody testing using single-step method, use 86328)

86771 Shigella

86774 tetanus

86777 Toxoplasma

86778 Toxoplasma, IgM

86780 Treponema pallidum
➔ *CPT Changes: An Insider's View* 2010

(For syphilis testing by non-treponemal antibody analysis, see 86592-86593)

86784 Trichinella

86787 varicella-zoster

86788 West Nile virus, IgM
➔ *CPT Changes: An Insider's View* 2007

86789 West Nile virus
➔ *CPT Changes: An Insider's View* 2007

86790 virus, not elsewhere specified

86793 Yersinia

86794 Zika virus, IgM
➔ *CPT Changes: An Insider's View* 2018

86800 Thyroglobulin antibody
➔ *CPT Assistant* Aug 05:9

(For thyroglobulin, use 84432)

86803 Hepatitis C antibody;
➔ *CPT Assistant* Nov 97:31-32

86804 confirmatory test (eg, immunoblot)
➔ *CPT Assistant* Nov 97:31-32

Tissue Typing

86805 Lymphocytotoxicity assay, visual crossmatch; with titration

86806 without titration

86807 Serum screening for cytotoxic percent reactive antibody (PRA); standard method
➔ *CPT Assistant* Jun 01:11

86808 quick method
➔ *CPT Assistant* Jun 01:11

86812 HLA typing; A, B, or C (eg, A10, B7, B27), single antigen
➔ *CPT Assistant* Mar 03:23, Jun 06:17

86813 A, B, or C, multiple antigens
➔ *CPT Assistant* Mar 03:23, Jun 06:17

86816 DR/DQ, single antigen
➔ *CPT Assistant* Mar 03:23

86817 DR/DQ, multiple antigens
➔ *CPT Assistant* Mar 03:23

86821 lymphocyte culture, mixed (MLC)
➔ *CPT Assistant* Mar 03:23

86825 Human leukocyte antigen (HLA) crossmatch, non-cytotoxic (eg, using flow cytometry); first serum sample or dilution
➔ *CPT Changes: An Insider's View* 2010
➔ *CPT Assistant* Aug 20:14

+ 86826 each additional serum sample or sample dilution (List separately in addition to primary procedure)
➔ *CPT Changes: An Insider's View* 2010
➔ *CPT Assistant* Aug 20:14

(Use 86826 in conjunction with 86825)

(Do not report 86825, 86826 in conjunction with 86355, 86359, 88184-88189 for antibody surface markers integral to crossmatch testing)

(For autologous HLA crossmatch, see 86825, 86826)

(For lymphocytotoxicity visual crossmatch, see 86805, 86806)

86828 Antibody to human leukocyte antigens (HLA), solid phase assays (eg, microspheres or beads, ELISA, flow cytometry); qualitative assessment of the presence or absence of antibody(ies) to HLA Class I and Class II HLA antigens
➔ *CPT Changes: An Insider's View* 2013

86829 qualitative assessment of the presence or absence of antibody(ies) to HLA Class I or Class II HLA antigens
➔ *CPT Changes: An Insider's View* 2013

(If solid phase testing is performed to assess presence or absence of antibody to both HLA classes, use 86828)

86830 antibody identification by qualitative panel using complete HLA phenotypes, HLA Class I
➔ *CPT Changes: An Insider's View* 2013

86831 antibody identification by qualitative panel using complete HLA phenotypes, HLA Class II
➔ *CPT Changes: An Insider's View* 2013

86832 high definition qualitative panel for identification of antibody specificities (eg, individual antigen per bead methodology), HLA Class I
➔ *CPT Changes: An Insider's View* 2013

86833 high definition qualitative panel for identification of antibody specificities (eg, individual antigen per bead methodology), HLA Class II
➔ *CPT Changes: An Insider's View* 2013

(If solid phase testing is performed to test for HLA Class I or II antibody after treatment [eg, to remove IgM antibodies or other interfering substances], report 86828-86833 once for each panel with the untreated serum and once for each panel with the treated serum)

86834 semi-quantitative panel (eg, titer), HLA Class I
➔ *CPT Changes: An Insider's View* 2013

86835 semi-quantitative panel (eg, titer), HLA Class II
➔ *CPT Changes: An Insider's View* 2013
➔ *CPT Assistant* Jan 24:17

86849 Unlisted immunology procedure
➔ *CPT Assistant* Mar 98:10, Dec 19:13, Jan 24:17

Transfusion Medicine

Transfusion medicine analytes/procedures that are not specified in 86850-86985 and are not in the Chemistry (82009-84830) or Immunology (86015-86835) subsections may be reported using the unlisted transfusion medicine procedure code 86999.

(For apheresis, use 36511, 36512)

(For therapeutic phlebotomy, use 99195)

86850 Antibody screen, RBC, each serum technique
➔ *CPT Assistant* Fall 93:25, Aug 05:9, Apr 08:5, Jan 24:17

86860 Antibody elution (RBC), each elution

86870 Antibody identification, RBC antibodies, each panel for each serum technique
➔ *CPT Assistant* Fall 93:25, Mar 01:10

86880 Antihuman globulin test (Coombs test); direct, each antiserum

86885 indirect, qualitative, each reagent red cell
➔ *CPT Changes: An Insider's View* 2008
➔ *CPT Assistant* Apr 08:5

86886 indirect, each antibody titer
➔ *CPT Changes: An Insider's View* 2008
➔ *CPT Assistant* Apr 08:5

(For indirect antihuman globulin [Coombs] test for RBC antibody screening, use 86850)

(For indirect antihuman globulin [Coombs] test for RBC antibody identification using reagent red cell panels, use 86870)

86890 Autologous blood or component, collection processing and storage; predeposited
➔ *CPT Assistant* Apr 96:2

86891 intra- or postoperative salvage

Pathology and Laboratory 80047-89398, 0001U-0520U

86900	Blood typing, serologic; ABO
	➔ *CPT Changes: An Insider's View* 2015
	➔ *CPT Assistant* Aug 05:9
86901	Rh (D)
	➔ *CPT Changes: An Insider's View* 2015
	➔ *CPT Assistant* Fall 93:25
86902	antigen testing of donor blood using reagent serum, each antigen test
	➔ *CPT Changes: An Insider's View* 2011, 2015
	➔ *CPT Assistant* Oct 10:8, Dec 10:8

(If multiple blood units are tested for the same antigen, 86902 should be reported once for each antigen for each unit tested)

86904	antigen screening for compatible unit using patient serum, per unit screened
	➔ *CPT Changes: An Insider's View* 2015
86905	RBC antigens, other than ABO or Rh (D), each
	➔ *CPT Changes: An Insider's View* 2015
86906	Rh phenotyping, complete
	➔ *CPT Changes: An Insider's View* 2015

(For human erythrocyte antigen typing by molecular pathology techniques, use 81403)

86910	Blood typing, for paternity testing, per individual; ABO, Rh and MN
86911	each additional antigen system
86920	Compatibility test each unit; immediate spin technique
	➔ *CPT Assistant* Mar 06:6
86921	incubation technique
	➔ *CPT Assistant* Mar 06:6
86922	antiglobulin technique
	➔ *CPT Assistant* Mar 06:6
86923	electronic
	➔ *CPT Changes: An Insider's View* 2006
	➔ *CPT Assistant* Mar 06:6

(Do not use 86923 in conjunction with 86920-86922 for same unit crossmatch)

86927	Fresh frozen plasma, thawing, each unit
86930	Frozen blood, each unit; freezing (includes preparation)
	➔ *CPT Changes: An Insider's View* 2003
	➔ *CPT Assistant* Apr 96:2, Jul 03:8
86931	thawing
	➔ *CPT Changes: An Insider's View* 2003
	➔ *CPT Assistant* Jul 03:8
86932	freezing (includes preparation) and thawing
	➔ *CPT Changes: An Insider's View* 2003
	➔ *CPT Assistant* Jul 03:8
86940	Hemolysins and agglutinins; auto, screen, each
86941	incubated
86945	Irradiation of blood product, each unit
	➔ *CPT Assistant* Dec 07:14

86950	Leukocyte transfusion
	➔ *CPT Assistant* Oct 13:3

(For allogeneic lymphocyte infusion, use 38242)

(For leukapheresis, use 36511)

86960	Volume reduction of blood or blood product (eg, red blood cells or platelets), each unit
	➔ *CPT Changes: An Insider's View* 2006
	➔ *CPT Assistant* Mar 06:6
86965	Pooling of platelets or other blood products
	➔ *CPT Assistant* Oct 10:8, Dec 10:8

(For harvesting, preparation, and injection[s] of platelet rich plasma, use 0232T)

(For harvesting, preparation, and injection[s] of autologous white blood cell/autologous protein solution, use 0481T)

86970	Pretreatment of RBCs for use in RBC antibody detection, identification, and/or compatibility testing; incubation with chemical agents or drugs, each
86971	incubation with enzymes, each
86972	by density gradient separation
86975	Pretreatment of serum for use in RBC antibody identification; incubation with drugs, each
86976	by dilution
86977	incubation with inhibitors, each
86978	by differential red cell absorption using patient RBCs or RBCs of known phenotype, each absorption
86985	Splitting of blood or blood products, each unit
	➔ *CPT Assistant* Apr 96:2, May 12:11, Jan 24:17
86999	Unlisted transfusion medicine procedure
	➔ *CPT Assistant* Aug 05:9, Nov 05:14, Mar 09:10, Apr 09:9, May 12:11, Jan 24:17

Microbiology

Includes bacteriology, mycology, parasitology, and virology.

Presumptive identification of microorganisms is defined as identification by colony morphology, growth on selective media, Gram stains, or up to three tests (eg, catalase, oxidase, indole, urease). Definitive identification of microorganisms is defined as an identification to the genus or species level that requires additional tests (eg, biochemical panels, slide cultures). If additional studies involve molecular probes, nucleic acid sequencing, chromatography, or immunologic techniques, these should be separately coded using 87140-87158, in addition to definitive identification codes. The molecular diagnostic codes (eg, 81161, 81200-81408) are not to be used in combination with or instead of the procedures represented by 87140-87158. For multiple specimens/sites use modifier 59. For repeat laboratory tests performed on the same day, use modifier 91.

Microbiology analytes/procedures that are not specified in 87003-87912 and are not in the Chemistry (82009-84830) or Immunology (86015-86835) subsections may be reported using the unlisted microbiology procedure code 87999.

87003 Animal inoculation, small animal, with observation and dissection
➔ *CPT Assistant* Jan 24:17

87015 Concentration (any type), for infectious agents
➔ *CPT Changes: An Insider's View* 2001

(Do not report 87015 in conjunction with 87177)

87040 Culture, bacterial; blood, aerobic, with isolation and presumptive identification of isolates (includes anaerobic culture, if appropriate)
➔ *CPT Changes: An Insider's View* 2001, 2004
➔ *CPT Assistant* Aug 97:18, Jun 02:2, Oct 10:17, Dec 10:17

87045 stool, aerobic, with isolation and preliminary examination (eg, KIA, LIA), Salmonella and Shigella species
➔ *CPT Changes: An Insider's View* 2001, 2002, 2004

87046 stool, aerobic, additional pathogens, isolation and presumptive identification of isolates, each plate
➔ *CPT Changes: An Insider's View* 2001, 2002, 2004, 2005

87070 any other source except urine, blood or stool, aerobic, with isolation and presumptive identification of isolates
➔ *CPT Changes: An Insider's View* 2001, 2004
➔ *CPT Assistant* Aug 97:18, Nov 01:10, Oct 03:10, Nov 11:11

(For urine, use 87088)

87071 quantitative, aerobic with isolation and presumptive identification of isolates, any source except urine, blood or stool
➔ *CPT Changes: An Insider's View* 2001
➔ *CPT Assistant* Jun 02:3, Sep 03:3

(For urine, use 87088)

87073 quantitative, anaerobic with isolation and presumptive identification of isolates, any source except urine, blood or stool
➔ *CPT Changes: An Insider's View* 2001
➔ *CPT Assistant* Jun 02:3

(For definitive identification of isolates, use 87076 or 87077. For typing of isolates see 87140-87158)

87075 any source, except blood, anaerobic with isolation and presumptive identification of isolates
➔ *CPT Changes: An Insider's View* 2001, 2004

87076 anaerobic isolate, additional methods required for definitive identification, each isolate
➔ *CPT Changes: An Insider's View* 2001

87077 aerobic isolate, additional methods required for definitive identification, each isolate
➔ *CPT Changes: An Insider's View* 2001
➔ *CPT Assistant* Nov 01:10, Nov 11:10

87081 Culture, presumptive, pathogenic organisms, screening only;
➔ *CPT Changes: An Insider's View* 2001
➔ *CPT Assistant* Nov 01:10

87084 with colony estimation from density chart

87086 Culture, bacterial; quantitative colony count, urine
➔ *CPT Changes: An Insider's View* 2001
➔ *CPT Assistant* Nov 11:10

87088 with isolation and presumptive identification of each isolate, urine
➔ *CPT Changes: An Insider's View* 2001, 2007
➔ *CPT Assistant* Nov 11:10

87101 Culture, fungi (mold or yeast) isolation, with presumptive identification of isolates; skin, hair, or nail
➔ *CPT Changes: An Insider's View* 2001
➔ *CPT Assistant* Sep 99:10, Aug 05:9

87102 other source (except blood)

87103 blood

87106 Culture, fungi, definitive identification, each organism; yeast
➔ *CPT Changes: An Insider's View* 2001

87107 mold
➔ *CPT Changes: An Insider's View* 2001

87109 Culture, mycoplasma, any source

87110 Culture, chlamydia, any source
➔ *CPT Changes: An Insider's View* 2001

(For immunofluorescence staining of shell vials, use 87140)

87116 Culture, tubercle or other acid-fast bacilli (eg, TB, AFB, mycobacteria) any source, with isolation and presumptive identification of isolates
➔ *CPT Changes: An Insider's View* 2001

(For concentration, use 87015)

87118 Culture, mycobacterial, definitive identification, each isolate
➔ *CPT Changes: An Insider's View* 2001

87140   Culture, typing; immunofluorescent method, each antiserum
> *CPT Changes: An Insider's View* 2001
> *CPT Assistant* Nov 01:10, Sep 03:3

87143   gas liquid chromatography (GLC) or high pressure liquid chromatography (HPLC) method
> *CPT Changes: An Insider's View* 2001

87147   immunologic method, other than immunofluorescence (eg, agglutination grouping), per antiserum
> *CPT Changes: An Insider's View* 2001
> *CPT Assistant* Apr 02:18, Oct 03:10

87149   identification by nucleic acid (DNA or RNA) probe, direct probe technique, per culture or isolate, each organism probed
> *CPT Changes: An Insider's View* 2001, 2010
> *CPT Assistant* Nov 01:10, May 12:5, Sep 13:3

(Do not report 87149 in conjunction with 81161, 81200-81408)

87150   identification by nucleic acid (DNA or RNA) probe, amplified probe technique, per culture or isolate, each organism probed
> *CPT Changes: An Insider's View* 2010
> *CPT Assistant* May 12:5, Sep 13:3

(Do not report 87150 in conjunction with 81161, 81200-81408)

 # 87154   identification of blood pathogen and resistance typing, when performed, by nucleic acid (DNA or RNA) probe, multiplexed amplified probe technique including multiplex reverse transcription, when performed, per culture or isolate, 6 or more targets
> *CPT Changes: An Insider's View* 2022

87152   identification by pulse field gel typing
> *CPT Changes: An Insider's View* 2001
> *CPT Assistant* May 12:5, Sep 13:3

(Do not report 87152 in conjunction with 81161, 81200-81408)

87153   identification by nucleic acid sequencing method, each isolate (eg, sequencing of the 16S rRNA gene)
> *CPT Changes: An Insider's View* 2010
> *CPT Assistant* May 12:5, Sep 13:3

87154   Code is out of numerical sequence. See 87149-87153

87158   other methods
> *CPT Assistant* Nov 01:10, Sep 03:3

87164   Dark field examination, any source (eg, penile, vaginal, oral, skin); includes specimen collection

87166   without collection

87168   Macroscopic examination; arthropod
> *CPT Changes: An Insider's View* 2001

87169   parasite
> *CPT Changes: An Insider's View* 2001

87172   Pinworm exam (eg, cellophane tape prep)
> *CPT Changes: An Insider's View* 2001

87176   Homogenization, tissue, for culture
> *CPT Changes: An Insider's View* 2001

87177   Ova and parasites, direct smears, concentration and identification
> *CPT Assistant* Jul 03:8, Nov 03:15, Mar 06:6

(Do not report 87177 in conjunction with 87015)

(For direct smears from a primary source, use 87207)

(For coccidia or microsporidia exam, use 87207)

(For complex special stain (trichrome, iron hematoxylin), use 87209)

(For nucleic acid probes in cytologic material, use 88365)

87181   Susceptibility studies, antimicrobial agent; agar dilution method, per agent (eg, antibiotic gradient strip)
> *CPT Changes: An Insider's View* 2001
> *CPT Assistant* Nov 01:10

87184   disk method, per plate (12 or fewer agents)
> *CPT Changes: An Insider's View* 2001
> *CPT Assistant* Nov 01:10

87185   enzyme detection (eg, beta lactamase), per enzyme
> *CPT Changes: An Insider's View* 2001
> *CPT Assistant* Nov 01:10

87186   microdilution or agar dilution (minimum inhibitory concentration [MIC] or breakpoint), each multi-antimicrobial, per plate
> *CPT Changes: An Insider's View* 2001
> *CPT Assistant* Nov 01:10

+ 87187   microdilution or agar dilution, minimum lethal concentration (MLC), each plate (List separately in addition to code for primary procedure)
> *CPT Changes: An Insider's View* 2001
> *CPT Assistant* Nov 01:10

(Use 87187 in conjunction with 87186 or 87188)

87188   macrobroth dilution method, each agent
> *CPT Changes: An Insider's View* 2001
> *CPT Assistant* Nov 01:10

87190   mycobacteria, proportion method, each agent
> *CPT Changes: An Insider's View* 2001

(For other mycobacterial susceptibility studies, see 87181, 87184, 87186, or 87188)

87197   Serum bactericidal titer (Schlichter test)

87205   Smear, primary source with interpretation; Gram or Giemsa stain for bacteria, fungi, or cell types
> *CPT Changes: An Insider's View* 2001
> *CPT Assistant* Aug 05:9, Oct 09:12

Pathology and Laboratory 80047-89398, 0001U-0520U

87206   fluorescent and/or acid fast stain for bacteria, fungi, parasites, viruses or cell types

➔ *CPT Changes: An Insider's View* 2001

87207   special stain for inclusion bodies or parasites (eg, malaria, coccidia, microsporidia, trypanosomes, herpes viruses)

➔ *CPT Changes: An Insider's View* 2001, 2003

➔ *CPT Assistant* Jul 03:8, Mar 06:6

(For direct smears with concentration and identification, use 87177)

(For thick smear preparation, use 87015)

(For fat, meat, fibers, nasal eosinophils, and starch, see miscellaneous section)

87209   complex special stain (eg, trichrome, iron hemotoxylin) for ova and parasites

➔ *CPT Changes: An Insider's View* 2006

➔ *CPT Assistant* Mar 06:6

87210   wet mount for infectious agents (eg, saline, India ink, KOH preps)

➔ *CPT Changes: An Insider's View* 2001

➔ *CPT Assistant* May 16:14

(For KOH examination of skin, hair or nails, see 87220)

87220   Tissue examination by KOH slide of samples from skin, hair, or nails for fungi or ectoparasite ova or mites (eg, scabies)

➔ *CPT Changes: An Insider's View* 2001

87230   Toxin or antitoxin assay, tissue culture (eg, Clostridium difficile toxin)

87250   Virus isolation; inoculation of embryonated eggs, or small animal, includes observation and dissection

➔ *CPT Changes: An Insider's View* 2001

87252   tissue culture inoculation, observation, and presumptive identification by cytopathic effect

➔ *CPT Changes: An Insider's View* 2001

87253   tissue culture, additional studies or definitive identification (eg, hemabsorption, neutralization, immunofluorescence stain), each isolate

➔ *CPT Changes: An Insider's View* 2001

(Electron microscopy, use 88348)

(Inclusion bodies in tissue sections, see 88304-88309; in smears, see 87207-87210; in fluids, use 88106)

87254   centrifuge enhanced (shell vial) technique, includes identification with immunofluorescence stain, each virus

➔ *CPT Changes: An Insider's View* 2001, 2003

➔ *CPT Assistant* Jul 03:8

(Report 87254 in addition to 87252 as appropriate)

87255   including identification by non-immunologic method, other than by cytopathic effect (eg, virus specific enzymatic activity)

➔ *CPT Changes: An Insider's View* 2003

➔ *CPT Assistant* Jul 03:9

These codes are intended for primary source only. For similar studies on culture material, refer to codes 87140-87158. Infectious agents by antigen detection, immunofluorescence microscopy, or nucleic acid probe techniques should be reported as precisely as possible. The molecular pathology procedures codes (81161, 81200-81408) are not to be used in combination with or instead of the procedures represented by 87471-87801. The most specific code possible should be reported. If there is no specific agent code, the general methodology code (eg, 87299, 87449, 87797, 87798, 87799, 87899) should be used. For identification of antibodies to many of the listed infectious agents, see 86602-86804. When separate results are reported for different species or strain of organisms, each result should be coded separately. Use modifier 59 when separate results are reported for different species or strains that are described by the same code.

When identifying infectious agents on primary-source specimens (eg, tissue, smear) microscopically by direct/indirect immunofluorescent assay [IFA] techniques, see 87260-87300. When identifying infectious agents on primary-source specimens or derivatives via non-microscopic immunochemical techniques with fluorescence detection (ie, fluorescence immunoassay [FIA]), see 87301-87451, 87802-87899. When identifying infectious agents on primary-source specimens using antigen detection by immunoassay with direct optical (ie, visual) observation, see 87802-87899.

87260   Infectious agent antigen detection by immunofluorescent technique; adenovirus

➔ *CPT Changes: An Insider's View* 2001

➔ *CPT Assistant* Nov 97:32

87265   Bordetella pertussis/parapertussis

➔ *CPT Assistant* Nov 97:32

87267   Enterovirus, direct fluorescent antibody (DFA)

➔ *CPT Assistant* Jul 03:8

87269   giardia

➔ *CPT Changes: An Insider's View* 2004

87270   Chlamydia trachomatis

➔ *CPT Assistant* Nov 97:32

87271   Cytomegalovirus, direct fluorescent antibody (DFA)

➔ *CPT Assistant* Jul 03:7

87272   cryptosporidium

➔ *CPT Changes: An Insider's View* 2004

➔ *CPT Assistant* Nov 97:32

87273   Herpes simplex virus type 2

➔ *CPT Changes: An Insider's View* 2001

Pathology and Laboratory 80047-89398, 0001U-0520U

87274   Herpes simplex virus type 1
➜ *CPT Changes: An Insider's View* 2001
➜ *CPT Assistant* Nov 97:32

87275   influenza B virus
➜ *CPT Changes: An Insider's View* 2001

87276   influenza A virus
➜ *CPT Assistant* Nov 97:32, May 09:6

87278   Legionella pneumophila
➜ *CPT Assistant* Nov 97:32

87279   Parainfluenza virus, each type
➜ *CPT Changes: An Insider's View* 2001

87280   respiratory syncytial virus
➜ *CPT Assistant* Nov 97:32

87281   Pneumocystis carinii
➜ *CPT Changes: An Insider's View* 2001

87283   Rubeola
➜ *CPT Changes: An Insider's View* 2001

87285   Treponema pallidum
➜ *CPT Assistant* Nov 97:32

87290   Varicella zoster virus
➜ *CPT Assistant* Nov 97:32

87299   not otherwise specified, each organism
➜ *CPT Changes: An Insider's View* 2001
➜ *CPT Assistant* Nov 97:32, Nov 01:10

87300   Infectious agent antigen detection by immunofluorescent technique, polyvalent for multiple organisms, each polyvalent antiserum
➜ *CPT Changes: An Insider's View* 2001
➜ *CPT Assistant* Aug 05:9

(For physician evaluation of infectious disease agents by immunofluorescence, use 88346)

87301   Infectious agent antigen detection by immunoassay technique (eg, enzyme immunoassay [EIA], enzyme-linked immunosorbent assay [ELISA], fluorescence immunoassay [FIA], immunochemiluminometric assay [IMCA]), qualitative or semiquantitative; adenovirus enteric types 40/41
➜ *CPT Changes: An Insider's View* 2016, 2022
➜ *CPT Assistant* Nov 97:32, Nov 99:46

87305   Aspergillus
➜ *CPT Changes: An Insider's View* 2007, 2016, 2022

87320   Chlamydia trachomatis
➜ *CPT Changes: An Insider's View* 2016, 2022
➜ *CPT Assistant* Nov 97:32

87324   Clostridium difficile toxin(s)
➜ *CPT Changes: An Insider's View* 2001, 2016, 2022
➜ *CPT Assistant* Nov 97:32

87327   Cryptococcus neoformans
➜ *CPT Changes: An Insider's View* 2001, 2016, 2022

(For Cryptococcus latex agglutination, use 86403)

87328   cryptosporidium
➜ *CPT Changes: An Insider's View* 2004, 2016, 2022
➜ *CPT Assistant* Nov 97:32

87329   giardia
➜ *CPT Changes: An Insider's View* 2004, 2016, 2022

87332   cytomegalovirus
➜ *CPT Changes: An Insider's View* 2016, 2022
➜ *CPT Assistant* Nov 97:32

87335   Escherichia coli O157
➜ *CPT Changes: An Insider's View* 2016, 2022
➜ *CPT Assistant* Nov 97:32

(For giardia antigen, use 87329)

87336   Entamoeba histolytica dispar group
➜ *CPT Changes: An Insider's View* 2001, 2016, 2022

87337   Entamoeba histolytica group
➜ *CPT Changes: An Insider's View* 2001, 2016, 2022

87338   Helicobacter pylori, stool
➜ *CPT Changes: An Insider's View* 2000, 2016, 2022
➜ *CPT Assistant* Nov 99:46

87339   Helicobacter pylori
➜ *CPT Changes: An Insider's View* 2001, 2016, 2022

(For H. pylori, stool, use 87338. For H. pylori, breath and blood by mass spectrometry, see 83013, 83014. For H. pylori, liquid scintillation counter, see 78267, 78268)

87340   hepatitis B surface antigen (HBsAg)
➜ *CPT Changes: An Insider's View* 2016, 2022
➜ *CPT Assistant* Nov 97:32, Jan 00:11

(For quantitative hepatitis B surface antigen [HBsAg], use 87467)

87341   hepatitis B surface antigen (HBsAg) neutralization
➜ *CPT Changes: An Insider's View* 2001, 2016, 2022

87350   hepatitis Be antigen (HBeAg)
➜ *CPT Changes: An Insider's View* 2016, 2022
➜ *CPT Assistant* Nov 97:32

87380   hepatitis, delta agent
➜ *CPT Changes: An Insider's View* 2016, 2022
➜ *CPT Assistant* Nov 97:32

(For hepatitis delta agent, antibody, use 86692)

(For hepatitis D [delta], quantification, use 87523)

87385   Histoplasma capsulatum
➜ *CPT Changes: An Insider's View* 2016, 2022
➜ *CPT Assistant* Nov 97:32

87389 HIV-1 antigen(s), with HIV-1 and HIV-2 antibodies, single result
➜ *CPT Changes: An Insider's View* 2012, 2016, 2022

87390 HIV-1
➜ *CPT Changes: An Insider's View* 2016, 2022
➜ *CPT Assistant* Nov 97:32

87391 HIV-2
➜ *CPT Changes: An Insider's View* 2016, 2022
➜ *CPT Assistant* Nov 97:32

87400 Influenza, A or B, each
➜ *CPT Changes: An Insider's View* 2001, 2016, 2022
➜ *CPT Assistant* Jun 01:11, Dec 01:6, Aug 05:9, May 09:6

87420 respiratory syncytial virus
➜ *CPT Changes: An Insider's View* 2016, 2022
➜ *CPT Assistant* Nov 97:32

87425 rotavirus
➜ *CPT Changes: An Insider's View* 2016, 2022
➜ *CPT Assistant* Nov 97:32

87426 severe acute respiratory syndrome coronavirus (eg, SARS-CoV, SARS-CoV-2 [COVID-19])
➜ *CPT Changes: An Insider's View* 2021, 2022

87428 severe acute respiratory syndrome coronavirus (eg, SARS-CoV, SARS-CoV-2 [COVID-19]) and influenza virus types A and B
➜ *CPT Changes: An Insider's View* 2022

87427 Shiga-like toxin
➜ *CPT Changes: An Insider's View* 2001, 2016, 2022

87428 Code is out of numerical sequence. See 87425-87430

87430 Streptococcus, group A
➜ *CPT Changes: An Insider's View* 2016, 2022
➜ *CPT Assistant* Nov 97:32

87449 not otherwise specified, each organism
➜ *CPT Changes: An Insider's View* 2001, 2016, 2022
➜ *CPT Assistant* Nov 97:32, Jan 00:11, Nov 01:10

87451 polyvalent for multiple organisms, each polyvalent antiserum
➜ *CPT Changes: An Insider's View* 2001, 2016, 2022

87467 hepatitis B surface antigen (HBsAg), quantitative
➜ *CPT Changes: An Insider's View* 2023

(For qualitative hepatitis B surface antigen [HBsAg], use 87340)

87468 Infectious agent detection by nucleic acid (DNA or RNA); Anaplasma phagocytophilum, amplified probe technique
➜ *CPT Changes: An Insider's View* 2023
➜ *CPT Assistant* Feb 23:9

87469 Babesia microti, amplified probe technique
➜ *CPT Changes: An Insider's View* 2023
➜ *CPT Assistant* Feb 23:9

87471 Bartonella henselae and Bartonella quintana, amplified probe technique
➜ *CPT Assistant* May 12:5, Sep 13:3, Oct 20:11, Feb 23:9

87472 Bartonella henselae and Bartonella quintana, quantification
➜ *CPT Assistant* Sep 13:3

87475 Borrelia burgdorferi, direct probe technique
➜ *CPT Assistant* May 12:5, Sep 13:3

87476 Borrelia burgdorferi, amplified probe technique
➜ *CPT Assistant* Sep 13:3

87478 Borrelia miyamotoi, amplified probe technique
➜ *CPT Changes: An Insider's View* 2023
➜ *CPT Assistant* Feb 23:9

87480 Candida species, direct probe technique
➜ *CPT Assistant* May 12:5, Sep 13:3, Mar 21:8

87481 Candida species, amplified probe technique
➜ *CPT Assistant* Sep 13:3, Mar 21:8

87482 Candida species, quantification
➜ *CPT Assistant* Sep 13:3, Mar 21:8

87483 central nervous system pathogen (eg, Neisseria meningitidis, Streptococcus pneumoniae, Listeria, Haemophilus influenzae, E. coli, Streptococcus agalactiae, enterovirus, human parechovirus, herpes simplex virus type 1 and 2, human herpesvirus 6, cytomegalovirus, varicella zoster virus, Cryptococcus), includes multiplex reverse transcription, when performed, and multiplex amplified probe technique, multiple types or subtypes, 12-25 targets
➜ *CPT Changes: An Insider's View* 2017

87484 Code is out of numerical sequence. See 87496-87500

87485 Chlamydia pneumoniae, direct probe technique
➜ *CPT Assistant* May 12:5, Sep 13:3

87486 Chlamydia pneumoniae, amplified probe technique
➜ *CPT Assistant* Sep 13:3

87487 Chlamydia pneumoniae, quantification
➜ *CPT Assistant* Sep 13:3

87490 Chlamydia trachomatis, direct probe technique
➜ *CPT Assistant* Sep 13:3

87491 Chlamydia trachomatis, amplified probe technique
➜ *CPT Assistant* Jun 13:14, Sep 13:3

87492 Chlamydia trachomatis, quantification
➜ *CPT Assistant* Sep 13:3

87493 Clostridium difficile, toxin gene(s), amplified probe technique
➜ *CPT Changes: An Insider's View* 2010
➜ *CPT Assistant* Sep 10:8, May 12:5, Sep 13:3

87495 cytomegalovirus, direct probe technique
➜ *CPT Assistant* May 12:5, Sep 13:3

87496	cytomegalovirus, amplified probe technique	

→ *CPT Assistant* Sep 13:3

87497   cytomegalovirus, quantification

→ *CPT Assistant* Sep 13:3

 # 87484   Ehrlichia chaffeensis, amplified probe technique

→ *CPT Changes: An Insider's View* 2023

→ *CPT Assistant* Feb 23:9

87498   enterovirus, amplified probe technique, includes reverse transcription when performed

→ *CPT Changes: An Insider's View* 2007, 2013, 2014

→ *CPT Assistant* May 12:5, Sep 13:3

87500   vancomycin resistance (eg, enterococcus species van A, van B), amplified probe technique

→ *CPT Changes: An Insider's View* 2008

→ *CPT Assistant* Apr 08:5, May 12:5, Sep 13:3

87501   influenza virus, includes reverse transcription, when performed, and amplified probe technique, each type or subtype

→ *CPT Changes: An Insider's View* 2011, 2015

→ *CPT Assistant* Oct 10:8, Dec 10:8, May 12:5, Sep 13:3

87502   influenza virus, for multiple types or sub-types, includes multiplex reverse transcription, when performed, and multiplex amplified probe technique, first 2 types or sub-types

→ *CPT Changes: An Insider's View* 2011, 2012, 2015, 2016

→ *CPT Assistant* Oct 10:8, Dec 10:8, Sep 13:3

+ 87503   influenza virus, for multiple types or sub-types, includes multiplex reverse transcription, when performed, and multiplex amplified probe technique, each additional influenza virus type or sub-type beyond 2 (List separately in addition to code for primary procedure)

→ *CPT Changes: An Insider's View* 2011, 2015, 2016

→ *CPT Assistant* Oct 10:8, Dec 10:8, Sep 13:3

(Use 87503 in conjunction with 87502)

87505   gastrointestinal pathogen (eg, Clostridium difficile, E. coli, Salmonella, Shigella, norovirus, Giardia), includes multiplex reverse transcription, when performed, and multiplex amplified probe technique, multiple types or subtypes, 3-5 targets

→ *CPT Changes: An Insider's View* 2015

87506   gastrointestinal pathogen (eg, Clostridium difficile, E. coli, Salmonella, Shigella, norovirus, Giardia), includes multiplex reverse transcription, when performed, and multiplex amplified probe technique, multiple types or subtypes, 6-11 targets

→ *CPT Changes: An Insider's View* 2015

87507   gastrointestinal pathogen (eg, Clostridium difficile, E. coli, Salmonella, Shigella, norovirus, Giardia), includes multiplex reverse transcription, when performed, and multiplex amplified probe technique, multiple types or subtypes, 12-25 targets

→ *CPT Changes: An Insider's View* 2015, 2018

87510   Gardnerella vaginalis, direct probe technique

→ *CPT Assistant* Aug 05:9, May 12:5, Sep 13:3, Mar 21:8

87511   Gardnerella vaginalis, amplified probe technique

→ *CPT Assistant* May 12:5, Sep 13:3, Mar 21:8

87512   Gardnerella vaginalis, quantification

→ *CPT Assistant* Sep 13:3, Mar 21:8

● 87513   Helicobacter pylori (H. pylori), clarithromycin resistance, amplified probe technique

→ *CPT Changes: An Insider's View* 2025

►(For H. pylori, stool, use 87338)◄

►(For H. pylori, immunoassay, use 87339)◄

►(For assays that detect clarithromycin resistance and identify H. pylori using a single procedure, use 87513)◄

►(For H. pylori, without clarithromycin resistance by amplified probe nucleic acid testing, use 87798)◄

87516   hepatitis B virus, amplified probe technique

→ *CPT Assistant* Sep 13:3

87517   hepatitis B virus, quantification

→ *CPT Assistant* Sep 13:3

87520   hepatitis C, direct probe technique

→ *CPT Assistant* Sep 13:3

87521   hepatitis C, amplified probe technique, includes reverse transcription when performed

→ *CPT Changes: An Insider's View* 2013, 2014

→ *CPT Assistant* Sep 13:3

87522   hepatitis C, quantification, includes reverse transcription when performed

→ *CPT Changes: An Insider's View* 2013, 2014

→ *CPT Assistant* Sep 13:3

87523   hepatitis D (delta), quantification, including reverse transcription, when performed

→ *CPT Changes: An Insider's View* 2024

87525   hepatitis G, direct probe technique

→ *CPT Assistant* Sep 13:3

87526   hepatitis G, amplified probe technique

→ *CPT Assistant* Sep 13:3

87527   hepatitis G, quantification

→ *CPT Assistant* Sep 13:3

87528   Herpes simplex virus, direct probe technique

→ *CPT Assistant* May 12:5, Sep 13:3

87529   Herpes simplex virus, amplified probe technique

→ *CPT Assistant* Sep 13:3

87530   Herpes simplex virus, quantification

→ *CPT Assistant* Sep 13:3

Pathology and Laboratory   80047-89398, 0001U-0520U

87531 Herpes virus-6, direct probe technique
→ *CPT Assistant* Sep 13:3

87532 Herpes virus-6, amplified probe technique
→ *CPT Assistant* Sep 13:3

87533 Herpes virus-6, quantification
→ *CPT Assistant* Sep 13:3

87534 HIV-1, direct probe technique
→ *CPT Assistant* May 12:5, Sep 13:3

87535 HIV-1, amplified probe technique, includes reverse transcription when performed
→ *CPT Changes: An Insider's View* 2013, 2014
→ *CPT Assistant* Mar 08:3, Sep 13:3

87536 HIV-1, quantification, includes reverse transcription when performed
→ *CPT Changes: An Insider's View* 2013, 2014
→ *CPT Assistant* Sep 13:3

87537 HIV-2, direct probe technique
→ *CPT Assistant* Sep 13:3

87538 HIV-2, amplified probe technique, includes reverse transcription when performed
→ *CPT Changes: An Insider's View* 2013, 2014
→ *CPT Assistant* Sep 13:3

87539 HIV-2, quantification, includes reverse transcription when performed
→ *CPT Changes: An Insider's View* 2013, 2014
→ *CPT Assistant* Sep 13:3

 # 87623 Human Papillomavirus (HPV), low-risk types (eg, 6, 11, 42, 43, 44)
→ *CPT Changes: An Insider's View* 2015

#▲ 87624 Human Papillomavirus (HPV), high-risk types (eg, 16, 18, 31, 33, 35, 39, 45, 51, 52, 56, 58, 59, 68), pooled result
→ *CPT Changes: An Insider's View* 2015, 2025
→ *CPT Assistant* Oct 15:10

(When both low-risk and high-risk HPV types are performed in a single assay, use only 87624)

#● 87626 Human Papillomavirus (HPV), separately reported high-risk types (eg, 16, 18, 31, 45, 51, 52) and high-risk pooled result(s)
→ *CPT Changes: An Insider's View* 2025

▶(Do not report 87626 in conjunction with 87624, 87625, for the same procedure)◀

▶(For singular pooled result of high-risk HPV types [eg, 16, 18, 31, 33, 35, 39, 45, 51, 52, 58, 59, 68], use 87624)◀

▶(For separately reported high-risk HPV types 16 and 18 only, including type 45, if performed, use 87625)◀

 # 87625 Human Papillomavirus (HPV), types 16 and 18 only, includes type 45, if performed
→ *CPT Changes: An Insider's View* 2015
→ *CPT Assistant* Jun 15:10, Oct 15:10

▶ (For Human Papillomavirus [HPV] detection of five or greater separately reported high-risk HPV types [ie, genotyping], use 87626)◀

87540 Legionella pneumophila, direct probe technique
→ *CPT Assistant* May 12:5, Sep 13:3

87541 Legionella pneumophila, amplified probe technique
→ *CPT Assistant* Sep 13:3

87542 Legionella pneumophila, quantification
→ *CPT Assistant* Sep 13:3

87550 Mycobacteria species, direct probe technique
→ *CPT Assistant* May 12:5, Sep 13:3

87551 Mycobacteria species, amplified probe technique
→ *CPT Assistant* Sep 13:3

87552 Mycobacteria species, quantification
→ *CPT Assistant* Sep 13:3

87555 Mycobacteria tuberculosis, direct probe technique
→ *CPT Assistant* Sep 13:3

87556 Mycobacteria tuberculosis, amplified probe technique
→ *CPT Assistant* Sep 13:3

87557 Mycobacteria tuberculosis, quantification
→ *CPT Assistant* Sep 13:3

87560 Mycobacteria avium-intracellulare, direct probe technique
→ *CPT Assistant* Sep 13:3

87561 Mycobacteria avium-intracellulare, amplified probe technique
→ *CPT Assistant* Sep 13:3

87562 Mycobacteria avium-intracellulare, quantification
→ *CPT Assistant* Sep 13:3

#● 87564 Mycobacterium tuberculosis, rifampin resistance, amplified probe technique
→ *CPT Changes: An Insider's View* 2025

▶(For assays that detect rifampin resistance and identify Mycobacterium tuberculosis using a single procedure, use 87564)◀

87563 Mycoplasma genitalium, amplified probe technique
→ *CPT Changes: An Insider's View* 2020
→ *CPT Assistant* Oct 20:11

87564 Code is out of numerical sequence. See 87561-87580

87580 Mycoplasma pneumoniae, direct probe technique
→ *CPT Assistant* Sep 13:3

87581 Mycoplasma pneumoniae, amplified probe technique
→ *CPT Assistant* Sep 13:3

Pathology and Laboratory   80047-89398, 0001U-0520U

87582   Mycoplasma pneumoniae, quantification
➲ *CPT Assistant* Sep 13:3

87590   Neisseria gonorrhoeae, direct probe technique
➲ *CPT Assistant* May 12:5, Sep 13:3

87591   Neisseria gonorrhoeae, amplified probe technique
➲ *CPT Assistant* Jun 13:14, Sep 13:3

87592   Neisseria gonorrhoeae, quantification
➲ *CPT Assistant* Sep 13:3

87593   Orthopoxvirus (eg, monkeypox virus, cowpox virus, vaccinia virus), amplified probe technique, each
➲ *CPT Changes: An Insider's View* 2024

● **87594**   Pneumocystis jirovecii, amplified probe technique
➲ *CPT Changes: An Insider's View* 2025

87623   Code is out of numerical sequence. See 87538-87541

87624   Code is out of numerical sequence. See 87538-87541

87625   Code is out of numerical sequence. See 87538-87541

87626   Code is out of numerical sequence. See 87538-87541

87631   respiratory virus (eg, adenovirus, influenza virus, coronavirus, metapneumovirus, parainfluenza virus, respiratory syncytial virus, rhinovirus), includes multiplex reverse transcription, when performed, and multiplex amplified probe technique, multiple types or subtypes, 3-5 targets
➲ *CPT Changes: An Insider's View* 2013, 2015
➲ *CPT Assistant* Sep 13:3, Apr 20:3

87632   respiratory virus (eg, adenovirus, influenza virus, coronavirus, metapneumovirus, parainfluenza virus, respiratory syncytial virus, rhinovirus), includes multiplex reverse transcription, when performed, and multiplex amplified probe technique, multiple types or subtypes, 6-11 targets
➲ *CPT Changes: An Insider's View* 2013, 2015
➲ *CPT Assistant* Sep 13:3, Apr 20:3

87633   respiratory virus (eg, adenovirus, influenza virus, coronavirus, metapneumovirus, parainfluenza virus, respiratory syncytial virus, rhinovirus), includes multiplex reverse transcription, when performed, and multiplex amplified probe technique, multiple types or subtypes, 12-25 targets
➲ *CPT Changes: An Insider's View* 2013, 2015
➲ *CPT Assistant* Sep 13:3, Apr 20:3

(Use 87631-87633 for nucleic acid assays which detect multiple respiratory viruses in a multiplex reaction [ie, single procedure with multiple results])

(For assays that are used to type or subtype influenza viruses only, see 87501-87503)

(For assays that include influenza viruses with additional respiratory viruses, see 87631-87633)

(For detection of multiple infectious agents not otherwise specified which report a single result, see 87800, 87801)

87634   respiratory syncytial virus, amplified probe technique
➲ *CPT Changes: An Insider's View* 2018

(For assays that include respiratory syncytial virus with additional respiratory viruses, see 87631, 87632, 87633)

87635   severe acute respiratory syndrome coronavirus 2 (SARS-CoV-2) (coronavirus disease [COVID-19]), amplified probe technique
➲ *CPT Changes: An Insider's View* 2021
➲ *CPT Assistant* Apr 20:3, Oct 23:10

87636   severe acute respiratory syndrome coronavirus 2 (SARS-CoV-2) (coronavirus disease [COVID-19]) and influenza virus types A and B, multiplex amplified probe technique
➲ *CPT Changes: An Insider's View* 2022
➲ *CPT Assistant* Oct 23:10

87637   severe acute respiratory syndrome coronavirus 2 (SARS-CoV-2) (coronavirus disease [COVID-19]), influenza virus types A and B, and respiratory syncytial virus, multiplex amplified probe technique
➲ *CPT Changes: An Insider's View* 2022
➲ *CPT Assistant* Oct 23:10

(For nucleic acid detection of multiple respiratory infectious agents, not including severe acute respiratory syndrome coronavirus 2 [SARS-CoV-2] [coronavirus disease {COVID-19}], see 87631, 87632, 87633)

(For nucleic acid detection of multiple respiratory infectious agents, including severe acute respiratory syndrome coronavirus 2 [SARS-CoV-2] [coronavirus disease {COVID-19}] in conjunction with additional target[s] beyond influenza virus types A and B and respiratory syncytial virus, see 87631, 87632, 87633)

(For infectious agent genotype analysis by nucleic acid [DNA or RNA] for severe acute respiratory syndrome coronavirus 2 [SARS-CoV-2] [coronavirus disease {COVID-19}], mutation identification in targeted region[s], use 87913)

(For SARS-CoV-2 variant analysis, use 87913)

87640   Staphylococcus aureus, amplified probe technique
➲ *CPT Changes: An Insider's View* 2007
➲ *CPT Assistant* Aug 07:7, May 12:5, Sep 13:3

87641   Staphylococcus aureus, methicillin resistant, amplified probe technique
➲ *CPT Changes: An Insider's View* 2007
➲ *CPT Assistant* Aug 07:7, Sep 13:3

(For assays that detect methicillin resistance and identify Staphylococcus aureus using a single nucleic acid sequence, use 87641)

87650   Streptococcus, group A, direct probe technique
➲ *CPT Assistant* Sep 13:4

Pathology and Laboratory   80047-89398, 0001U-0520U

87651 Streptococcus, group A, amplified probe technique
➲ CPT Assistant Sep 13:4

87652 Streptococcus, group A, quantification
➲ CPT Assistant Sep 13:4

87653 Streptococcus, group B, amplified probe technique
➲ CPT Changes: An Insider's View 2007
➲ CPT Assistant Aug 07:7, Sep 13:3

87660 Trichomonas vaginalis, direct probe technique
➲ CPT Changes: An Insider's View 2004
➲ CPT Assistant May 12:5, Sep 13:3, Mar 21:8

87661 Trichomonas vaginalis, amplified probe technique
➲ CPT Changes: An Insider's View 2014
➲ CPT Assistant Mar 21:8

87662 Zika virus, amplified probe technique
➲ CPT Changes: An Insider's View 2018

87797 Infectious agent detection by nucleic acid (DNA or RNA), not otherwise specified; direct probe technique, each organism
➲ CPT Changes: An Insider's View 2001
➲ CPT Assistant Nov 97:34, Nov 01:10, Aug 05:9, May 12:5, Sep 13:3, Aug 16:10

87798 amplified probe technique, each organism
➲ CPT Changes: An Insider's View 2001
➲ CPT Assistant Nov 97:34, Nov 01:10, Aug 07:7, Sep 13:3, Oct 20:11, Feb 23:9

87799 quantification, each organism
➲ CPT Changes: An Insider's View 2001
➲ CPT Assistant Nov 97:34, Sep 13:3

87800 Infectious agent detection by nucleic acid (DNA or RNA), multiple organisms; direct probe(s) technique
➲ CPT Changes: An Insider's View 2001
➲ CPT Assistant Aug 05:9, May 12:5, Sep 13:3, Aug 16:10

87801 amplified probe(s) technique
➲ CPT Changes: An Insider's View 2001
➲ CPT Assistant May 12:5, Jun 13:14, Sep 13:3, Mar 21:8

(For each specific organism nucleic acid detection from a primary source, see 87471-87660. For detection of specific infectious agents not otherwise specified, see 87797, 87798, or 87799 1 time for each agent)

(For detection of multiple infectious agents not otherwise specified which report a single result, see 87800, 87801)

(Do not use 87801 for nucleic acid assays that detect multiple respiratory viruses in a multiplex reaction [ie, single procedure with multiple results], see 87631-87633)

87802 Infectious agent antigen detection by immunoassay with direct optical (ie, visual) observation; Streptococcus, group B
➲ CPT Changes: An Insider's View 2002, 2022
➲ CPT Assistant Jun 03:12

87803 Clostridium difficile toxin A
➲ CPT Changes: An Insider's View 2002, 2022
➲ CPT Assistant Jun 03:12

 # 87806 HIV-1 antigen(s), with HIV-1 and HIV-2 antibodies
➲ CPT Changes: An Insider's View 2015, 2022

87804 Influenza
➲ CPT Changes: An Insider's View 2002, 2022
➲ CPT Assistant Jun 03:11-12, May 09:6

87806 Code is out of numerical sequence. See 87802-87903

87807 respiratory syncytial virus
➲ CPT Changes: An Insider's View 2005, 2022

 # 87811 severe acute respiratory syndrome coronavirus 2 (SARS-CoV-2) (coronavirus disease [COVID-19])
➲ CPT Changes: An Insider's View 2022

87808 Trichomonas vaginalis
➲ CPT Changes: An Insider's View 2007, 2022

87809 adenovirus
➲ CPT Changes: An Insider's View 2008, 2022
➲ CPT Assistant Apr 08:5

87810 Chlamydia trachomatis
➲ CPT Changes: An Insider's View 2009, 2022
➲ CPT Assistant Nov 97:34, Jan 98:6

87811 Code is out of numerical sequence. See 87804-87809

87850 Neisseria gonorrhoeae
➲ CPT Changes: An Insider's View 2022
➲ CPT Assistant Nov 97:34, Jan 98:6

87880 Streptococcus, group A
➲ CPT Changes: An Insider's View 2022
➲ CPT Assistant Nov 97:34, Jan 98:6, Dec 98:8

87899 not otherwise specified
➲ CPT Changes: An Insider's View 2022
➲ CPT Assistant Jan 98:6, Jun 01:11

87900 Infectious agent drug susceptibility phenotype prediction using regularly updated genotypic bioinformatics
➲ CPT Changes: An Insider's View 2006
➲ CPT Assistant Mar 06:6, May 12:5, Sep 13:3, Dec 15:17

 # 87910 Infectious agent genotype analysis by nucleic acid (DNA or RNA); cytomegalovirus
➲ CPT Changes: An Insider's View 2013
➲ CPT Assistant Sep 13:3

(For infectious agent drug susceptibility phenotype prediction for HIV-1, use 87900)

▶(For Human Papillomavirus [HPV] for high-risk types [ie, genotyping] of five or greater separately reported HPV types, use 87626)◀

★ = Telemedicine ◀ = Audio-only + = Add-on code ✗ = FDA approval pending # = Resequenced code ⊘ = Modifier 51 exempt ➲➲➲ = See p xxi for details

87901   HIV-1, reverse transcriptase and protease regions

➔ *CPT Changes: An Insider's View* 2001, 2002, 2011, 2013

➔ *CPT Assistant* Aug 05:9, Mar 06:6, Oct 10:9, Dec 10:9, May 12:5, Sep 13:3

87906   HIV-1, other region (eg, integrase, fusion)

➔ *CPT Changes: An Insider's View* 2011

➔ *CPT Assistant* Oct 10:8, Dec 10:8, Sep 13:3

(For infectious agent drug susceptibility phenotype prediction for HIV-1, use 87900)

87912   Hepatitis B virus

➔ *CPT Changes: An Insider's View* 2013

➔ *CPT Assistant* Sep 13:3, Jan 24:17

87902   Hepatitis C virus

➔ *CPT Changes: An Insider's View* 2002

➔ *CPT Assistant* May 12:5, Sep 13:3, Nov 15:11, Dec 15:17

87913   severe acute respiratory syndrome coronavirus 2 (SARS-CoV-2) (coronavirus disease [COVID-19]), mutation identification in targeted region(s)

➔ *CPT Changes: An Insider's View* 2023

➔ *CPT Assistant* Oct 23:10

(For infectious agent detection by nucleic acid [DNA or RNA] for severe acute respiratory syndrome coronavirus 2 [SARS-CoV-2] [coronavirus disease {COVID-19}], see 87635, 87636, 87637)

(For SARS-CoV-2 variant analysis, use 87913)

87903   Infectious agent phenotype analysis by nucleic acid (DNA or RNA) with drug resistance tissue culture analysis, HIV 1; first through 10 drugs tested

➔ *CPT Changes: An Insider's View* 2001, 2002

➔ *CPT Assistant* Apr 04:15, Mar 06:6, May 12:3, Sep 13:3

+ **87904**   each additional drug tested (List separately in addition to code for primary procedure)

➔ *CPT Changes: An Insider's View* 2001, 2002, 2006

➔ *CPT Assistant* Apr 04:15, Mar 06:6, May 12:3, Sep 13:3

(Use 87904 in conjunction with 87903)

87905   Infectious agent enzymatic activity other than virus (eg, sialidase activity in vaginal fluid)

➔ *CPT Changes: An Insider's View* 2009

(For virus isolation including identification by non-immunologic method, other than by cytopathic effect, use 87255)

87906   Code is out of numerical sequence. See 87802-87903

87910   Code is out of numerical sequence. See 87802-87903

87912   Code is out of numerical sequence. See 87802-87903

87913   Code is out of numerical sequence. See 87899-87904

87999   Unlisted microbiology procedure

➔ *CPT Assistant* Aug 05:9, Jan 24:17

Anatomic Pathology

Postmortem Examination

Procedures 88000 through 88099 represent physician services only. Use modifier 90 for outside laboratory services.

Postmortem examination procedures that are not specified in 88000-88045 may be reported using the unlisted necropsy (autopsy) procedure code 88099.

88000   Necropsy (autopsy), gross examination only; without CNS

➔ *CPT Assistant* Aug 05:9, Jan 24:17

88005   with brain

88007   with brain and spinal cord

88012   infant with brain

88014   stillborn or newborn with brain

88016   macerated stillborn

88020   Necropsy (autopsy), gross and microscopic; without CNS

88025   with brain

88027   with brain and spinal cord

88028   infant with brain

88029   stillborn or newborn with brain

88036   Necropsy (autopsy), limited, gross and/or microscopic; regional

88037   single organ

88040   Necropsy (autopsy); forensic examination

88045   coroner's call

➔ *CPT Assistant* Jan 24:17

88099   Unlisted necropsy (autopsy) procedure

➔ *CPT Assistant* Jan 24:17

Cytopathology

Cytopathology procedures that are not specified in 88104-88189 may be reported using the unlisted cytopathology procedure code 88199.

88104   Cytopathology, fluids, washings or brushings, except cervical or vaginal; smears with interpretation

➔ *CPT Assistant* Spring 91:6, Fall 94:3, Aug 05:9, Jan 24:17

(Use 0827T in conjunction with 88104, when the digitization of glass microscope slides is performed)

Pathology and Laboratory   80047-89398, 0001U-0520U

88106   simple filter method with interpretation

→ *CPT Changes: An Insider's View* 2007

→ *CPT Assistant* Fall 94:3

(Use 0828T in conjunction with 88106, when the digitization of glass microscope slides is performed)

(Do not report 88106 in conjunction with 88104)

(For nongynecological selective cellular enhancement including filter transfer techniques, use 88112)

88108 Cytopathology, concentration technique, smears and interpretation (eg, Saccomanno technique)

→ *CPT Assistant* Fall 94:3, Nov 97:34, Jan 98:6

(Use 0829T in conjunction with 88108, when the digitization of glass microscope slides is performed)

(For cervical or vaginal smears, see 88150-88155)

(For gastric intubation with lavage, see 43754, 43755)

(For x-ray localization, use 74340)

88112 Cytopathology, selective cellular enhancement technique with interpretation (eg, liquid based slide preparation method), except cervical or vaginal

→ *CPT Changes: An Insider's View* 2004

(Use 0830T in conjunction with 88112, when the digitization of glass microscope slides is performed)

(Do not report 88112 with 88108)

88120 Cytopathology, in situ hybridization (eg, FISH), urinary tract specimen with morphometric analysis, 3-5 molecular probes, each specimen; manual

→ *CPT Changes: An Insider's View* 2011

→ *CPT Assistant* Oct 10:9, Dec 10:9

88121   using computer-assisted technology

→ *CPT Changes: An Insider's View* 2011

→ *CPT Assistant* Oct 10:9, Dec 10:9

(For morphometric in situ hybridization on cytologic specimens other than urinary tract, see 88367, 88368)

(For more than 5 probes, use 88399)

88125 Cytopathology, forensic (eg, sperm)

88130 Sex chromatin identification; Barr bodies

88140   peripheral blood smear, polymorphonuclear drumsticks

→ *CPT Assistant* Nov 98:27-28, Mar 06:6

(For Guard stain, use 88313)

Codes 88141-88155, 88164-88167, 88174-88175 are used to report cervical or vaginal screening by various methods and to report physician interpretation services. Use codes 88150, 88152, 88153 to report conventional Pap smears that are examined using non-Bethesda reporting. Use codes 88164-88167 to report conventional Pap smears that are examined using the Bethesda System of reporting. Use codes 88142-88143 to report liquid-based specimens processed as thin-layer preparations that are examined using any system of reporting (Bethesda or non-Bethesda). Use codes 88174-88175 to report

automated screening of liquid-based specimens that are examined using any system of reporting (Bethesda or non-Bethesda). Within each of these three code families choose the one code that describes the screening method(s) used. Codes 88141 and 88155 should be reported in addition to the screening code chosen when the additional services are provided. Manual rescreening requires a complete visual reassessment of the entire slide initially screened by either an automated or manual process. Manual review represents an assessment of selected cells or regions of a slide identified by initial automated review.

88141 Cytopathology, cervical or vaginal (any reporting system), requiring interpretation by physician

→ *CPT Assistant* Nov 97:35, Jan 98:6, Jan 99:11, May 99:6, Nov 99:46, Mar 04:6, Mar 05:16, May 11:10, Dec 11:17

(Use 88141 in conjunction with 88142, 88143, 88147, 88148, 88150, 88152, 88153, 88164-88167, 88174-88175)

(Use 0831T in conjunction with 88141, when the digitization of glass microscope slides is performed)

88142 Cytopathology, cervical or vaginal (any reporting system), collected in preservative fluid, automated thin layer preparation; manual screening under physician supervision

→ *CPT Assistant* Nov 97:34-35, Jan 98:6, Nov 98:28, May 99:6, Jul 03:7, Mar 04:4

88143   with manual screening and rescreening under physician supervision

→ *CPT Assistant* Nov 97:34-35, Nov 98:28, May 99:6, Jul 03:7, Mar 04:4, Mar 05:16

(For automated screening of automated thin layer preparation, see 88174, 88175)

88147 Cytopathology smears, cervical or vaginal; screening by automated system under physician supervision

→ *CPT Assistant* Nov 97:35, Nov 98:28, Jan 99:11, May 99:6, Nov 99:46, Mar 04:6

88148   screening by automated system with manual rescreening under physician supervision

→ *CPT Changes: An Insider's View* 2000

→ *CPT Assistant* Jan 99:1, May 99:6, Nov 99:46, Mar 04:6

88150 Cytopathology, slides, cervical or vaginal; manual screening under physician supervision

→ *CPT Assistant* Winter 91:19, Nov 97:34-35, Nov 98:28, May 99:6, Mar 04:5

88152   with manual screening and computer-assisted rescreening under physician supervision

→ *CPT Assistant* Nov 97:35, Jan 98:6, May 99:6, Mar 04:5

★ = Telemedicine   ◀ = Audio-only   + = Add-on code   ✔ = FDA approval pending   # = Resequenced code   ⊘ = Modifier 51 exempt   →→→ = See p xxi for details

88153   with manual screening and rescreening under
physician supervision
➔ *CPT Assistant* Nov 97:34-35, Nov 98:28, May 99:6, Mar 04:5,
Mar 05:16

+ 88155   Cytopathology, slides, cervical or vaginal, definitive
hormonal evaluation (eg, maturation index, karyopyknotic
index, estrogenic index) (List separately in addition to
code[s] for other technical and interpretation services)
➔ *CPT Assistant* Nov 97:35, Nov 98:28, May 99:6, Nov 99:46,
Mar 04:5, May 11:10

(Use 88155 in conjunction with 88142, 88143, 88147,
88148, 88150, 88152, 88153, 88164-88167, 88174-88175)

88160   Cytopathology, smears, any other source; screening and
interpretation
➔ *CPT Assistant* Jan 98:6

(Use 0832T in conjunction with 88160, when the
digitization of glass microscope slides is performed)

88161   preparation, screening and interpretation
➔ *CPT Assistant* Aug 97:18, Jan 98:6

(Use 0833T in conjunction with 88161, when the
digitization of glass microscope slides is performed)

88162   extended study involving over 5 slides and/or multiple
stains

(Use 0834T in conjunction with 88162, when the
digitization of glass microscope slides is performed)

(For aerosol collection of sputum, use 89220)

(For special stains, see 88312-88314)

88164   Cytopathology, slides, cervical or vaginal (the Bethesda
System); manual screening under physician supervision
➔ *CPT Assistant* Nov 98:28, May 99:6, Mar 04:5

88165   with manual screening and rescreening under
physician supervision
➔ *CPT Assistant* Nov 98:28, May 99:6, Mar 04:5, Mar 05:16

88166   with manual screening and computer-assisted
rescreening under physician supervision
➔ *CPT Assistant* Nov 98:28, May 99:6, Mar 04:5

88167   with manual screening and computer-assisted
rescreening using cell selection and review under
physician supervision
➔ *CPT Assistant* Nov 98:28, May 99:6, Jul 03:7, Mar 04:5

(For collection of specimen via fine needle aspiration
biopsy, see 10004, 10005, 10006, 10007, 10008, 10009,
10010, 10011, 10012, 10021)

88172   Cytopathology, evaluation of fine needle aspirate;
immediate cytohistologic study to determine adequacy
for diagnosis, first evaluation episode, each site
➔ *CPT Changes: An Insider's View* 2001, 2011
➔ *CPT Assistant* Fall 93:26, Fall 94:2, Dec 98:8, Aug 07:15,
Oct 10:9, Dec 10:9, Jan 16:12, Apr 19:4

(Use 0835T in conjunction with 88172, when the
digitization of glass microscope slides is performed)

(The evaluation episode represents a complete set of
cytologic material submitted for evaluation and is
independent of the number of needle passes or slides
prepared. A separate evaluation episode occurs if the
proceduralist provider obtains additional material from
the same site, based on the prior immediate adequacy
assessment, or a separate lesion is aspirated)

88173   interpretation and report
➔ *CPT Assistant* Fall 93:26, Fall 94:2, Dec 98:8, Oct 10:9,
Dec 10:9, Apr 19:4

(Use 0837T in conjunction with 88173, when the
digitization of glass microscope slides is performed)

(Report one unit of 88173 for the interpretation and
report from each anatomic site, regardless of the number
of passes or evaluation episodes performed during the
aspiration procedure)

(For fine needle aspirate biopsy, see 10004, 10005,
10006, 10007, 10008, 10009, 10010, 10011, 10012,
10021)

(Do not report 88172, 88173 in conjunction with 88333
and 88334 for the same specimen)

#+ 88177   immediate cytohistologic study to determine
adequacy for diagnosis, each separate additional
evaluation episode, same site (List separately in
addition to code for primary procedure)
➔ *CPT Changes: An Insider's View* 2011
➔ *CPT Assistant* Oct 10:9, Dec 10:9, Jan 16:12, Apr 19:4

(Use 88177 in conjunction with 88172)

(Use 0836T in conjunction with 88177, when the
digitization of glass microscope slides is performed)

(When repeat immediate evaluation episode(s) is
required on subsequent cytologic material from the same
site, eg, following determination the prior sampling that
was not adequate for diagnosis, use 1 unit of 88177 for
each additional evaluation episode)

88174   Cytopathology, cervical or vaginal (any reporting system),
collected in preservative fluid, automated thin layer
preparation; screening by automated system, under
physician supervision
➔ *CPT Changes: An Insider's View* 2003
➔ *CPT Assistant* Jul 03:9, Mar 04:4

88175   with screening by automated system and manual
rescreening or review, under physician supervision
➔ *CPT Changes: An Insider's View* 2003, 2006
➔ *CPT Assistant* Jul 03:9, Mar 04:4, Mar 06:6, May 11:10

(For manual screening, see 88142, 88143)

88177   Code is out of numerical sequence. See 88172-88175

88182   Flow cytometry, cell cycle or DNA analysis

➡ *CPT Assistant* Oct 13:3

(For DNA ploidy analysis by morphometric technique, use 88358)

88184   Flow cytometry, cell surface, cytoplasmic, or nuclear marker, technical component only; first marker

➡ *CPT Changes: An Insider's View* 2005

➡ *CPT Assistant* Dec 07:14, Oct 13:3

+ 88185   each additional marker (List separately in addition to code for first marker)

➡ *CPT Changes: An Insider's View* 2005

➡ *CPT Assistant* Dec 07:14, Oct 13:3

(Report 88185 in conjunction with 88184)

88187   Flow cytometry, interpretation; 2 to 8 markers

➡ *CPT Changes: An Insider's View* 2005

➡ *CPT Assistant* Apr 05:14, Oct 13:3

88188   9 to 15 markers

➡ *CPT Changes: An Insider's View* 2005

➡ *CPT Assistant* Apr 05:14, Oct 13:3

88189   16 or more markers

➡ *CPT Changes: An Insider's View* 2005

➡ *CPT Assistant* Apr 05:14, Oct 13:3, Jan 24:17

(Do not report 88187-88189 for interpretation of 86355, 86356, 86357, 86359, 86360, 86361, 86367)

(For assessment of circulating antibodies by flow cytometric techniques, see analyte and method-specific codes in the Chemistry section [83516-83520] or Immunology section [86000-86849])

(For cell enumeration using immunologic selection and identification in fluid specimen [eg, circulating tumor cells in blood], see 86152, 86153)

88199   Unlisted cytopathology procedure

➡ *CPT Assistant* Jan 24:17

(For electron microscopy, use 88348)

Cytogenetic Studies

▶Cytogenetic study procedures that are not specified in 88230-88291 and are not in the Surgical Pathology (88300-88387) subsection may be reported using the unlisted cytogenetic study code 88299.◀

Molecular pathology procedures should be reported using the appropriate code from Tier 1 (81161, 81200-81383), Tier 2 (81400-81408), Genomic Sequencing Procedures and Other Molecular Multianalyte Assays (81410-81471), or Multianalyte Assays with Algorithmic Analyses (81500-81512) sections. If no specific code exists, one of the unlisted codes (81479 or 81599) should be used.

(For acetylcholinesterase, use 82013)

(For alpha-fetoprotein, serum or amniotic fluid, see 82105, 82106)

(For laser microdissection of cells from tissue sample, see 88380)

88230   Tissue culture for non-neoplastic disorders; lymphocyte

➡ *CPT Assistant* Nov 98:29, Oct 99:2, Aug 05:9, May 08:5, Jan 24:17

88233   skin or other solid tissue biopsy

➡ *CPT Assistant* Nov 98:29, Oct 99:2, May 08:5

88235   amniotic fluid or chorionic villus cells

➡ *CPT Assistant* Nov 98:29, Oct 99:2, May 08:5

88237   Tissue culture for neoplastic disorders; bone marrow, blood cells

➡ *CPT Assistant* Nov 98:29, Oct 99:2, May 08:5

88239   solid tumor

➡ *CPT Assistant* Nov 98:29, Oct 99:2, May 08:5

88240   Cryopreservation, freezing and storage of cells, each cell line

➡ *CPT Assistant* Nov 98:29, Oct 99:2, Jul 03:9, May 08:5, Oct 13:3

(For therapeutic cryopreservation and storage, use 38207)

88241   Thawing and expansion of frozen cells, each aliquot

➡ *CPT Assistant* Nov 98:29, Oct 99:2, Jul 03:9, May 08:5, Oct 13:3

(For therapeutic thawing of previous harvest, use 38208)

88245   Chromosome analysis for breakage syndromes; baseline Sister Chromatid Exchange (SCE), 20-25 cells

➡ *CPT Assistant* Nov 98:29, Oct 99:2, Jul 05:1, May 08:5

88248   baseline breakage, score 50-100 cells, count 20 cells, 2 karyotypes (eg, for ataxia telangiectasia, Fanconi anemia, fragile X)

➡ *CPT Assistant* Nov 98:29, Oct 99:2, Jul 05:1, May 08:5

88249   score 100 cells, clastogen stress (eg, diepoxybutane, mitomycin C, ionizing radiation, UV radiation)

➡ *CPT Assistant* Nov 98:29, Oct 99:2, Jul 05:1, May 08:5

88261   Chromosome analysis; count 5 cells, 1 karyotype, with banding

➡ *CPT Assistant* Nov 98:29, Oct 99:2, Jul 05:1, May 08:5

88262   count 15-20 cells, 2 karyotypes, with banding

➡ *CPT Assistant* Nov 98:29, Oct 99:2, May 08:5, May 11:10, Aug 19:11

88263   count 45 cells for mosaicism, 2 karyotypes, with banding

➡ *CPT Assistant* Nov 98:29, Oct 99:2, Jul 05:1, May 08:5

88264   analyze 20-25 cells

➡ *CPT Assistant* Nov 98:29, Oct 99:2, Jul 05:1, May 08:5, Aug 19:11

710   ★ = Telemedicine   ◀ = Audio-only   + = Add-on code   ✗ = FDA approval pending   # = Resequenced code   ⊘ = Modifier 51 exempt   ➡➡➡ = See p xxi for details

Pathology and Laboratory 80047-89398, 0001U-0520U

88267   Chromosome analysis, amniotic fluid or chorionic villus, count 15 cells, 1 karyotype, with banding
⮕ *CPT Assistant* Jul 05:1

88269   Chromosome analysis, in situ for amniotic fluid cells, count cells from 6-12 colonies, 1 karyotype, with banding
⮕ *CPT Assistant* Jul 05:1

88271   Molecular cytogenetics; DNA probe, each (eg, FISH)
⮕ *CPT Assistant* Nov 98:29, Mar 99:10, Oct 99:3, Jun 02:11, Jul 05:1, May 08:5, May 12:5, Sep 13:3, Feb 20:10

(For cytogenomic [genome-wide] analysis for constitutional chromosomal abnormalities, see 81228, 81229, 81349, 81405, 81406, 81479)

(For genomic sequencing procedures or other molecular multianalyte assays for copy number analysis using circulating cell-free fetal DNA in maternal blood, see 81420, 81422, 81479)

88272   chromosomal in situ hybridization, analyze 3-5 cells (eg, for derivatives and markers)
⮕ *CPT Assistant* Nov 98:29, Mar 99:10, Oct 99:3, Jun 02:11, Jul 05:1, May 08:5, May 12:5, Sep 13:3

88273   chromosomal in situ hybridization, analyze 10-30 cells (eg, for microdeletions)
⮕ *CPT Assistant* Nov 98:29, Mar 99:10, Oct 99:3, Jun 02:11, Jul 05:1, May 08:5, May 12:5, Sep 13:3

88274   interphase in situ hybridization, analyze 25-99 cells
⮕ *CPT Assistant* Nov 98:29, Mar 99:10, Oct 99:3, Jun 02:11, Jul 05:1, May 08:5, May 12:5, Sep 13:3

88275   interphase in situ hybridization, analyze 100-300 cells
⮕ *CPT Assistant* Nov 98:29, Mar 99:10, Oct 99:3, Jun 02:11, Jul 05:1, May 08:5, May 12:5, Sep 13:3

88280   Chromosome analysis; additional karyotypes, each study
⮕ *CPT Assistant* Jul 05:1, May 08:5

88283   additional specialized banding technique (eg, NOR, C-banding)
⮕ *CPT Assistant* Jul 05:1, May 08:5

88285   additional cells counted, each study
⮕ *CPT Assistant* Jul 05:1, Dec 07:14, May 08:5, May 11:10

88289   additional high resolution study
⮕ *CPT Assistant* Oct 99:3, Jul 05:1

88291   Cytogenetics and molecular cytogenetics, interpretation and report
⮕ *CPT Assistant* Nov 98:29, Oct 99:3, Jul 05:1, May 08:5, Jan 24:17

88299   Unlisted cytogenetic study
⮕ *CPT Assistant* Oct 99:3, Jan 24:17

Surgical Pathology

▶Services 88300 through 88309 include accession, examination, and reporting. They do not include the services designated in codes 88311 through 88387 and 88399, which are coded in addition when provided.◄

The unit of service for codes 88300 through 88309 is the specimen.

A specimen is defined as tissue or tissues that is (are) submitted for individual and separate attention, requiring individual examination and pathologic diagnosis. Two or more such specimens from the same patient (eg, separately identified endoscopic biopsies, skin lesions) are each appropriately assigned an individual code reflective of its proper level of service.

Service code 88300 is used for any specimen that in the opinion of the examining pathologist can be accurately diagnosed without microscopic examination. Service code 88302 is used when gross and microscopic examination is performed on a specimen to confirm identification and the absence of disease. Service codes 88304 through 88309 describe all other specimens requiring gross and microscopic examination, and represent additional ascending levels of physician work. Levels 88302 through 88309 are specifically defined by the assigned specimens.

Any unlisted specimen should be assigned to the code which most closely reflects the physician work involved when compared to other specimens assigned to that code.

▶Surgical pathology procedures that are not specified in 88300-88387 may be reported using the unlisted surgical pathology procedure code 88399.◄

(Do not report 88302-88309 on the same specimen as part of Mohs surgery)

88300   **Level I** - Surgical pathology, gross examination only
⮕ *CPT Assistant* Winter 91:18, Sep 00:10, Aug 05:9, Jun 21:6, Aug 21:3, 6-7, Jan 24:17

88302   **Level II** - Surgical pathology, gross and microscopic examination

Appendix, incidental

Fallopian tube, sterilization

Fingers/toes, amputation, traumatic

Foreskin, newborn

Hernia sac, any location

Hydrocele sac

Nerve

Skin, plastic repair

Sympathetic ganglion

Testis, castration

Vaginal mucosa, incidental

Vas deferens, sterilization
⮕ *CPT Assistant* Winter 91:18, Sep 00:10, Nov 06:1, Jan 07:29, Dec 11:17, Feb 14:10, Jun 21:6, Aug 21:3, 6-7

(Use 0751T in conjunction with 88302 when the digitization of glass microscope slides is performed)

88304 **Level III** - Surgical pathology, gross and microscopic examination

Abortion, induced

Abscess

Aneurysm - arterial/ventricular

Anus, tag

Appendix, other than incidental

Artery, atheromatous plaque

Bartholin's gland cyst

Bone fragment(s), other than pathologic fracture

Bursa/synovial cyst

Carpal tunnel tissue

Cartilage, shavings

Cholesteatoma

Colon, colostomy stoma

Conjunctiva - biopsy/pterygium

Cornea

Diverticulum - esophagus/small intestine

Dupuytren's contracture tissue

Femoral head, other than fracture

Fissure/fistula

Foreskin, other than newborn

Gallbladder

Ganglion cyst

Hematoma

Hemorrhoids

Hydatid of Morgagni

Intervertebral disc

Joint, loose body

Meniscus

Mucocele, salivary

Neuroma - Morton's/traumatic

Pilonidal cyst/sinus

Polyps, inflammatory - nasal/sinusoidal

Skin - cyst/tag/debridement

Soft tissue, debridement

Soft tissue, lipoma

Spermatocele

Tendon/tendon sheath

Testicular appendage

Thrombus or embolus

Tonsil and/or adenoids

Varicocele

Vas deferens, other than sterilization

Vein, varicosity

➲ *CPT Changes: An Insider's View* 2002

➲ *CPT Assistant* Winter 91:18, Spring 91:2, Aug 97:18, Sep 00:10, Jan 07:29, Dec 11:17, Jun 21:6, Aug 21:3, 6-7, Jul 23:20

(Use 0752T in conjunction with 88304 when the digitization of glass microscope slides is performed)

88305 **Level IV** - Surgical pathology, gross and microscopic examination

Abortion - spontaneous/missed

Artery, biopsy

Bone marrow, biopsy

Bone exostosis

Brain/meninges, other than for tumor resection

Breast, biopsy, not requiring microscopic evaluation of surgical margins

Breast, reduction mammoplasty

Bronchus, biopsy

Cell block, any source

Cervix, biopsy

Colon, biopsy

Duodenum, biopsy

Endocervix, curettings/biopsy

Endometrium, curettings/biopsy

Esophagus, biopsy

Extremity, amputation, traumatic

Fallopian tube, biopsy

Fallopian tube, ectopic pregnancy

Femoral head, fracture

Fingers/toes, amputation, non-traumatic

Gingiva/oral mucosa, biopsy

Heart valve

Joint, resection

Kidney, biopsy

Larynx, biopsy

★ = Telemedicine   ◀ = Audio-only   ✛ = Add-on code   ✗ = FDA approval pending   # = Resequenced code   ⊘ = Modifier 51 exempt   ➲➲➲ = See p xxi for details

Leiomyoma(s), uterine myomectomy - without uterus

Lip, biopsy/wedge resection

Lung, transbronchial biopsy

Lymph node, biopsy

Muscle, biopsy

Nasal mucosa, biopsy

Nasopharynx/oropharynx, biopsy

Nerve, biopsy

Odontogenic/dental cyst

Omentum, biopsy

Ovary with or without tube, non-neoplastic

Ovary, biopsy/wedge resection

Parathyroid gland

Peritoneum, biopsy

Pituitary tumor

Placenta, other than third trimester

Pleura/pericardium - biopsy/tissue

Polyp, cervical/endometrial

Polyp, colorectal

Polyp, stomach/small intestine

Prostate, needle biopsy

Prostate, TUR

Salivary gland, biopsy

Sinus, paranasal biopsy

Skin, other than cyst/tag/debridement/plastic repair

Small intestine, biopsy

Soft tissue, other than tumor/mass/lipoma/debridement

Spleen

Stomach, biopsy

Synovium

Testis, other than tumor/biopsy/castration

Thyroglossal duct/brachial cleft cyst

Tongue, biopsy

Tonsil, biopsy

Trachea, biopsy

Ureter, biopsy

Urethra, biopsy

Urinary bladder, biopsy

Uterus, with or without tubes and ovaries, for prolapse

Vagina, biopsy

Vulva/labia, biopsy

➲ *CPT Changes: An Insider's View* 2002

➲ *CPT Assistant* Winter 90:2, Winter 91:18, Spring 91:6, Winter 92:17, Aug 97:18, Jul 98:4, Nov 98:29-30, Jul 00:4, Sep 00:10, Dec 00:15, Jul 05:13, Nov 06:1, Jan 07:29, Dec 11:17, Jun 21:6, Aug 21:3, 6-7, Jun 23:31, Jul 23:20

(Use 0753T in conjunction with 88305 when the digitization of glass microscope slides is performed)

88307　**Level V** - Surgical pathology, gross and microscopic examination

Adrenal, resection

Bone - biopsy/curettings

Bone fragment(s), pathologic fracture

Brain, biopsy

Brain/meninges, tumor resection

Breast, excision of lesion, requiring microscopic evaluation of surgical margins

Breast, mastectomy - partial/simple

Cervix, conization

Colon, segmental resection, other than for tumor

Extremity, amputation, non-traumatic

Eye, enucleation

Kidney, partial/total nephrectomy

Larynx, partial/total resection

Liver, biopsy - needle/wedge

Liver, partial resection

Lung, wedge biopsy

Lymph nodes, regional resection

Mediastinum, mass

Myocardium, biopsy

Odontogenic tumor

Ovary with or without tube, neoplastic

Pancreas, biopsy

Placenta, third trimester

Prostate, except radical resection

Salivary gland

Sentinel lymph node

Small intestine, resection, other than for tumor

Soft tissue mass (except lipoma) - biopsy/simple excision

Stomach - subtotal/total resection, other than for tumor

Testis, biopsy

Thymus, tumor

Thyroid, total/lobe

Ureter, resection

Urinary bladder, TUR

Uterus, with or without tubes and ovaries, other than neoplastic/prolapse

➡ *CPT Changes: An Insider's View* 2001

➡ *CPT Assistant* Winter 91:18, Winter 92:18, Jul 98:4, Nov 98:29-30, Jul 99:10, Jul 00:4, Sep 00:10, Dec 00:15, Dec 03:11, Nov 06:1, Jan 07:29, Dec 11:17, Jun 21:6, Aug 21:3, 6

(Use 0754T in conjunction with 88307 when the digitization of glass microscope slides is performed)

88309 Level VI - Surgical pathology, gross and microscopic examination

Bone resection

Breast, mastectomy - with regional lymph nodes

Colon, segmental resection for tumor

Colon, total resection

Esophagus, partial/total resection

Extremity, disarticulation

Fetus, with dissection

Larynx, partial/total resection - with regional lymph nodes

Lung - total/lobe/segment resection

Pancreas, total/subtotal resection

Prostate, radical resection

Small intestine, resection for tumor

Soft tissue tumor, extensive resection

Stomach - subtotal/total resection for tumor

Testis, tumor

Tongue/tonsil - resection for tumor

Urinary bladder, partial/total resection

Uterus, with or without tubes and ovaries, neoplastic

Vulva, total/subtotal resection

➡ *CPT Assistant* Winter 91:18, Spring 91:2, Fall 93:2, 26, Jul 00:4, Sep 00:10, Dec 03:11, Nov 06:1, Jan 07:29, Dec 11:18, Feb 14:10, Jun 21:6, Aug 21:3, 6

(Use 0755T in conjunction with 88309 when the digitization of glass microscope slides is performed)

(Do not report 88302-88309 on the same specimen as part of Mohs surgery)

(For fine needle aspiration biopsy, see 10004, 10005, 10006, 10007, 10008, 10009, 10010, 10011, 10012, 10021)

(For evaluation of fine needle aspirate, see 88172-88173)

+ 88311 Decalcification procedure (List separately in addition to code for surgical pathology examination)

➡ *CPT Assistant* Winter 92:18, Jul 98:4, Jun 02:11, Nov 02:7, Nov 06:1, Dec 11:18, Jun 21:6, Aug 21:3, 6

88312 Special stain including interpretation and report; Group I for microorganisms (eg, acid fast, methenamine silver)

➡ *CPT Changes: An Insider's View* 2004, 2010, 2012

➡ *CPT Assistant* Winter 91:19, Jun 02:11, Nov 02:7, Nov 06:1, Dec 11:18

(Use 0756T in conjunction with 88312 when the digitization of glass microscope slides is performed)

(Report one unit of 88312 for each special stain, on each surgical pathology block, cytologic specimen, or hematologic smear)

88313 Group II, all other (eg, iron, trichrome), except stain for microorganisms, stains for enzyme constituents, or immunocytochemistry and immunohistochemistry

➡ *CPT Changes: An Insider's View* 2010, 2012

➡ *CPT Assistant* Jun 02:11, Nov 02:7, Mar 03:22, Nov 03:15, Jun 06:17, Nov 06:1, Dec 11:18

(Use 0757T in conjunction with 88313 when the digitization of glass microscope slides is performed)

(Report one unit of 88313 for each special stain, on each surgical pathology block, cytologic specimen, or hematologic smear)

(For immunocytochemistry and immunohistochemistry, use 88342)

+ 88314 histochemical stain on frozen tissue block (List separately in addition to code for primary procedure)

➡ *CPT Changes: An Insider's View* 2010, 2012

➡ *CPT Assistant* Nov 02:7, Nov 06:1, Dec 11:18

(Use 88314 in conjunction with 17311-17315, 88302-88309, 88331, 88332)

(Use 0758T in conjunction with 88314 when the digitization of glass microscope slides is performed)

(Do not report 88314 with 17311-17315 for routine frozen section stain [eg, hematoxylin and eosin, toluidine blue], performed during Mohs surgery. When a nonroutine histochemical stain on frozen tissue during Mohs surgery is utilized, report 88314 with modifier 59)

(Report one unit of 88314 for each special stain on each frozen surgical pathology block)

(For a special stain performed on frozen tissue section material to identify enzyme constituents, use 88319)

(For determinative histochemistry to identify chemical components, use 88313)

88319   Group III, for enzyme constituents
> *CPT Changes: An Insider's View* 2012
> *CPT Assistant* Dec 11:18

(Use 0759T in conjunction with 88319 when the digitization of glass microscope slides is performed)

(For each stain on each surgical pathology block, cytologic specimen, or hematologic smear, use one unit of 88319)

(For detection of enzyme constituents by immunohistochemical or immunocytochemical technique, use 88342)

88321   Consultation and report on referred slides prepared elsewhere
> *CPT Assistant* Winter 91:19, Apr 97:9, Oct 00:7, Dec 02:10, Jan 10:11, Dec 11:18, Jun 13:15, Feb 22:6

(Use 0838T in conjunction with 88321, when the digitization of glass microscope slides is performed)

88323   Consultation and report on referred material requiring preparation of slides
> *CPT Assistant* Winter 91:19, Apr 97:9, Oct 00:7, Dec 02:10, Dec 11:18, Jun 13:15, Feb 22:6

(Use 0839T in conjunction with 88323, when the digitization of glass microscope slides is performed)

88325   Consultation, comprehensive, with review of records and specimens, with report on referred material
> *CPT Assistant* Winter 91:19, Apr 97:9, Dec 02:10, Dec 11:18, Jun 13:15, Feb 22:6

(Use 0840T in conjunction with 88325, when the digitization of glass microscope slides is performed)

88329   Pathology consultation during surgery;
> *CPT Assistant* Winter 91:19, Apr 97:12, Aug 97:18, Jan 07:29, Dec 11:18

88331   first tissue block, with frozen section(s), single specimen
> *CPT Changes: An Insider's View* 2001
> *CPT Assistant* Winter 91:19, Spring 91:2, Apr 97:12, Aug 97:18, Jul 00:4, Nov 02:7, Mar 06:6, Nov 06:1, Jan 07:29, Oct 10:9, Dec 10:9, Dec 11:18

(Use 0841T in conjunction with 88331, when the digitization of glass microscope slides is performed)

+ 88332   each additional tissue block with frozen section(s) (List separately in addition to code for primary procedure)
> *CPT Changes: An Insider's View* 2011
> *CPT Assistant* Winter 91:19, Apr 97:12, Aug 97:18, Jul 00:4, Mar 06:6, Jan 07:29, Oct 10:9, Dec 10:9, Dec 11:18

(Use 88332 in conjunction with 88331)

(Use 0842T in conjunction with 88332, when the digitization of glass microscope slides is performed)

88333   cytologic examination (eg, touch prep, squash prep), initial site
> *CPT Changes: An Insider's View* 2006
> *CPT Assistant* Mar 06:6, Jan 07:29, Jun 08:15, Dec 10:9, Dec 11:18

(Use 0843T in conjunction with 88333, when the digitization of glass microscope slides is performed)

+ 88334   cytologic examination (eg, touch prep, squash prep), each additional site (List separately in addition to code for primary procedure)
> *CPT Changes: An Insider's View* 2006, 2011
> *CPT Assistant* Mar 06:6, Jan 07:29, Oct 10:9, Dec 11:18

(Use 88334 in conjunction with 88331, 88333)

(Use 0844T in conjunction with 88334, when the digitization of glass microscope slides is performed)

(For intraoperative consultation on a specimen requiring both frozen section and cytologic evaluation, use 88331 and 88334)

(For percutaneous needle biopsy requiring intraprocedural cytologic examination, use 88333)

(Do not report 88333 and 88334 for non-intraoperative cytologic examination, see 88160-88162)

(Do not report 88333 and 88334 for intraprocedural cytologic evaluation of fine needle aspirate, see 88172)

88341   Code is out of numerical sequence. See 88334-88372

88342   Immunohistochemistry or immunocytochemistry, per specimen; initial single antibody stain procedure
> *CPT Changes: An Insider's View* 2004, 2014, 2015
> *CPT Assistant* Winter 91:17, Jul 00:10, Nov 02:6-7, Nov 06:1, Dec 11:18, Jun 14:15, Jun 15:11

(Use 0760T in conjunction with 88342 when the digitization of glass microscope slides is performed)

(For quantitative or semiquantitative immunohistochemistry, see 88360, 88361)

#+ 88341   each additional single antibody stain procedure (List separately in addition to code for primary procedure)
> *CPT Changes: An Insider's View* 2015
> *CPT Assistant* Jun 15:11

(Use 88341 in conjunction with 88342)

(Use 0761T in conjunction with 88341 when the digitization of glass microscope slides is performed)

(For multiplex antibody stain procedure, use 88344)

88344   each multiplex antibody stain procedure
> *CPT Changes: An Insider's View* 2015
> *CPT Assistant* Jun 15:11

(Use 0762T in conjunction with 88344 when the digitization of glass microscope slides is performed)

(Do not use more than one unit of 88341, 88342, or 88344 for the same separately identifiable antibody per specimen)

(Do not report 88341, 88342, 88344 in conjunction with 88360, 88361 unless each procedure is for a different antibody)

(When multiple separately identifiable antibodies are applied to the same specimen [ie, multiplex antibody stain procedure], use one unit of 88344)

(When multiple antibodies are applied to the same slide that are not separately identifiable, [eg, antibody cocktails], use 88342, unless an additional separately identifiable antibody is also used, then use 88344)

88346 Immunofluorescence, per specimen; initial single antibody stain procedure

➔ *CPT Changes: An Insider's View* 2016

➔ *CPT Assistant* Dec 11:18

(Use 0845T in conjunction with 88346, when the digitization of glass microscope slides is performed)

#+ 88350 each additional single antibody stain procedure (List separately in addition to code for primary procedure)

➔ *CPT Changes: An Insider's View* 2016

(Use 0846T in conjunction with 88350, when the digitization of glass microscope slides is performed)

(Report 88350 in conjunction with 88346)

(Do not report 88346 and 88350 for fluorescent in situ hybridization studies, see 88364, 88365, 88366, 88367, 88368, 88369, 88373, 88374, and 88377)

(Do not report 88346 and 88350 for multiplex immunofluorescence analysis, use 88399)

88348 Electron microscopy, diagnostic

➔ *CPT Assistant* Dec 11:18

(Use 0856T in conjunction with 88348, when the digitization of glass microscope slides is performed)

88350 Code is out of numerical sequence. See 88334-88372

88355 Morphometric analysis; skeletal muscle

➔ *CPT Assistant* Dec 11:18

88356 nerve

➔ *CPT Assistant* Dec 11:18, Jun 14:15

88358 tumor (eg, DNA ploidy)

➔ *CPT Changes: An Insider's View* 2004

➔ *CPT Assistant* Jul 98:4, Jul 99:11, Jun 02:11, Jun 06:17, Dec 11:18

(Do not report 88358 with 88313 unless each procedure is for a different special stain)

88360 Morphometric analysis, tumor immunohistochemistry (eg, Her-2/neu, estrogen receptor/progesterone receptor), quantitative or semiquantitative, per specimen, each single antibody stain procedure; manual

➔ *CPT Changes: An Insider's View* 2005, 2015

➔ *CPT Assistant* Dec 11:18, Jun 14:15

(Use 0763T in conjunction with 88360 when the digitization of glass microscope slides is performed)

88361 using computer-assisted technology

➔ *CPT Changes: An Insider's View* 2004, 2005, 2015

➔ *CPT Assistant* Dec 11:18, Jun 14:15

(Do not report 88360, 88361 in conjunction with 88341, 88342, or 88344 unless each procedure is for a different antibody)

(Morphometric analysis of a multiplex antibody stain should be reported with one unit of 88360 or 88361, per specimen)

(For morphometric analysis using in situ hybridization techniques, see 88367, 88368)

(When semi-thin plastic-embedded sections are performed in conjunction with morphometric analysis, only the morphometric analysis should be reported; if performed as an independent procedure, see codes 88300-88309 for surgical pathology.)

88362 Nerve teasing preparations

➔ *CPT Assistant* Dec 11:18

88363 Examination and selection of retrieved archival (ie, previously diagnosed) tissue(s) for molecular analysis (eg, *KRAS* mutational analysis)

➔ *CPT Changes: An Insider's View* 2011

➔ *CPT Assistant* Oct 10:10, Dec 10:10, Dec 11:18

(Use 0847T in conjunction with 88363, when the digitization of glass microscope slides is performed)

88364 Code is out of numerical sequence. See 88334-88372

88365 In situ hybridization (eg, FISH), per specimen; initial single probe stain procedure

➔ *CPT Changes: An Insider's View* 2005, 2015

➔ *CPT Assistant* Jun 02:11, Mar 05:16, Dec 11:18, May 12:3, Sep 13:3, Nov 18:11, Jun 21:6, Aug 21:3, 6

(Use 0848T in conjunction with 88365, when the digitization of glass microscope slides is performed)

#+ 88364 each additional single probe stain procedure (List separately in addition to code for primary procedure)

➔ *CPT Changes: An Insider's View* 2015

(Use 88364 in conjunction with 88365)

(Use 0849T in conjunction with 88364, when the digitization of glass microscope slides is performed)

88366 each multiplex probe stain procedure

➔ *CPT Changes: An Insider's View* 2015

(Use 0850T in conjunction with 88366, when the digitization of glass microscope slides is performed)

(Do not report 88365, 88366 in conjunction with 88367, 88368, 88374, 88377 for the same probe)

88367   Morphometric analysis, in situ hybridization (quantitative or semi-quantitative), using computer-assisted technology, per specimen; initial single probe stain procedure
➜ *CPT Changes: An Insider's View* 2005, 2015
➜ *CPT Assistant* Mar 05:16, Oct 10:9, Dec 11:18, May 12:5, Sep 13:3

#+ 88373   each additional single probe stain procedure (List separately in addition to code for primary procedure)
➜ *CPT Changes: An Insider's View* 2015

(Use 88373 in conjunction with 88367)

 # 88374   each multiplex probe stain procedure
➜ *CPT Changes: An Insider's View* 2015

(Do not report 88367, 88374 in conjunction with 88365, 88366, 88368, 88377 for the same probe)

88368   Morphometric analysis, in situ hybridization (quantitative or semi-quantitative), manual, per specimen; initial single probe stain procedure
➜ *CPT Changes: An Insider's View* 2005, 2015
➜ *CPT Assistant* Mar 05:16, Oct 10:9, Dec 11:18, May 12:5, Sep 13:3

(Use 0851T in conjunction with 88368, when the digitization of glass microscope slides is performed)

+ 88369   each additional single probe stain procedure (List separately in addition to code for primary procedure)
➜ *CPT Changes: An Insider's View* 2015

(Use 88369 in conjunction with 88368)

(Use 0852T in conjunction with 88369, when the digitization of glass microscope slides is performed)

 # 88377   each multiplex probe stain procedure
➜ *CPT Changes: An Insider's View* 2015

(Use 0853T in conjunction with 88377, when the digitization of glass microscope slides is performed)

(Do not report 88368 or 88377 in conjunction with 88365, 88366, 88367, 88374 for the same probe)

(For morphometric in situ hybridization evaluation of urinary tract cytologic specimens, see 88120, 88121)

88371   Protein analysis of tissue by Western Blot, with interpretation and report;
➜ *CPT Assistant* Dec 11:18, Dec 15:17

88372   immunological probe for band identification, each
➜ *CPT Assistant* Dec 11:8

88373   Code is out of numerical sequence. See 88334-88372

88374   Code is out of numerical sequence. See 88334-88372

88375   Optical endomicroscopic image(s), interpretation and report, real-time or referred, each endoscopic session
➜ *CPT Changes: An Insider's View* 2013
➜ *CPT Assistant* Aug 13:5

(Do not report 88375 in conjunction with 43206, 43252, 0397T)

88377   Code is out of numerical sequence. See 88334-88372

88380   Microdissection (ie, sample preparation of microscopically identified target); laser capture
➜ *CPT Changes: An Insider's View* 2002, 2008
➜ *CPT Assistant* Apr 02:17, Apr 08:5, Dec 11:18, May 12:8, 10, Sep 13:3

88381   manual
➜ *CPT Changes: An Insider's View* 2008
➜ *CPT Assistant* Apr 08:5, Dec 11:18, May 12:8, 10, Sep 13:3

(Do not report 88380 in conjunction with 88381)

▲ 88387   Macroscopic examination, dissection, and preparation of tissue for non-microscopic analytical studies (eg, nucleic acid-based molecular studies), each tissue preparation (eg, a single lymph node)
➜ *CPT Changes: An Insider's View* 2010, 2025
➜ *CPT Assistant* Dec 11:18

(Do not report 88387 for tissue preparation for microbiologic cultures or flow cytometric studies)

▶(Do not report 88387 in conjunction with 88329-88334)◀

▶(88388 has been deleted)◀

88399   Unlisted surgical pathology procedure
➜ *CPT Assistant* Jun 14:15, Jun 21:6, Aug 21:3, 6, Jan 24:17

In Vivo (eg, Transcutaneous) Laboratory Procedures

In vivo measurement procedures that are not specified in 88720, 88738, 88740, 88741 may be reported using the unlisted in vivo pathology procedure code 88749.

(For wavelength fluorescent spectroscopy of advanced glycation end products [skin], use 88749)

88720   Bilirubin, total, transcutaneous
➜ *CPT Changes: An Insider's View* 2009
➜ *CPT Assistant* Dec 10:10, May 20:14, Jan 24:17

(For transdermal oxygen saturation, see 94760-94762)

88738   Hemoglobin (Hgb), quantitative, transcutaneous
➜ *CPT Changes: An Insider's View* 2010

(For in vitro hemoglobin measurement, use 85018)

88740   Hemoglobin, quantitative, transcutaneous, per day; carboxyhemoglobin
➜ *CPT Changes: An Insider's View* 2009

(For in vitro carboxyhemoglobin measurement, use 82375)

88741 methemoglobin
⊙ *CPT Changes: An Insider's View* 2009
⊙ *CPT Assistant* Jan 24:17

(For in vitro quantitative methemoglobin determination, use 83050)

88749 Unlisted in vivo (eg, transcutaneous) laboratory service
⊙ *CPT Changes: An Insider's View* 2011
⊙ *CPT Assistant* Oct 10:10, Dec 10:10, Jan 24:17

Other Procedures

Other procedures that are not specified in 89049-89230 or in other subsections (Chemistry, Hematology and Coagulation, Immunology, Transfusion Medicine, Microbiology, Cytopathology) may be reported using the unlisted miscellaneous pathology test code 89240.

89049 Caffeine halothane contracture test (CHCT) for malignant hyperthermia susceptibility, including interpretation and report
⊙ *CPT Changes: An Insider's View* 2006
⊙ *CPT Assistant* Mar 06:6, May 06:19, Sep 11:4, Jan 24:17

89050 Cell count, miscellaneous body fluids (eg, cerebrospinal fluid, joint fluid), except blood;
⊙ *CPT Changes: An Insider's View* 2002
⊙ *CPT Assistant* Aug 05:9, Sep 11:4

89051 with differential count
⊙ *CPT Assistant* Sep 11:4

89055 Leukocyte assessment, fecal, qualitative or semiquantitative
⊙ *CPT Changes: An Insider's View* 2003, 2004
⊙ *CPT Assistant* Jul 03:9, Sep 11:4

89060 Crystal identification by light microscopy with or without polarizing lens analysis, tissue or any body fluid (except urine)
⊙ *CPT Changes: An Insider's View* 2007
⊙ *CPT Assistant* Sep 11:4

(Do not report 89060 for crystal identification on paraffin-embedded tissue)

89125 Fat stain, feces, urine, or respiratory secretions
⊙ *CPT Changes: An Insider's View* 2001
⊙ *CPT Assistant* Sep 11:4

89160 Meat fibers, feces
⊙ *CPT Assistant* Sep 11:4

89190 Nasal smear for eosinophils
⊙ *CPT Assistant* Sep 11:4

(Occult blood, feces, use 82270)

(Paternity tests, use 86910)

89220 Sputum, obtaining specimen, aerosol induced technique (separate procedure)
⊙ *CPT Changes: An Insider's View* 2004
⊙ *CPT Assistant* Aug 05:9, Sep 11:4

89230 Sweat collection by iontophoresis
⊙ *CPT Changes: An Insider's View* 2004
⊙ *CPT Assistant* Sep 11:4, Jan 24:17

89240 Unlisted miscellaneous pathology test
⊙ *CPT Changes: An Insider's View* 2004
⊙ *CPT Assistant* Nov 05:14, Jan 07:30, Sep 11:4, Jan 24:17

Reproductive Medicine Procedures

Reproductive medicine procedures that are not specified in 89250-89356 may be reported using the unlisted reproductive medicine laboratory procedure code 89398.

89250 Culture of oocyte(s)/embryo(s), less than 4 days;
⊙ *CPT Changes: An Insider's View* 2004
⊙ *CPT Assistant* Nov 97:35-36, Jan 98:6, Oct 98:1, Apr 04:2, May 04:16, Jun 04:9, Sep 11:4, Jan 24:17

89251 with co-culture of oocyte(s)/embryos
⊙ *CPT Changes: An Insider's View* 2004
⊙ *CPT Assistant* Nov 97:35-36, Jan 98:6, Oct 98:1, Apr 04:2

(For extended culture of oocyte[s]/embryo[s], see 89272)

89253 Assisted embryo hatching, microtechniques (any method)
⊙ *CPT Assistant* Nov 97:35-36, Jan 98:6, Oct 98:1, Apr 04:2, May 04:16, Jun 04:9

89254 Oocyte identification from follicular fluid
⊙ *CPT Assistant* Nov 97:35-36, Jan 98:6, Oct 98:1, Apr 04:2, May 04:16, Jun 04:9

89255 Preparation of embryo for transfer (any method)
⊙ *CPT Assistant* Nov 97:35-36, Jan 98:6, Oct 98:1, Apr 04:2, May 04:16, Jun 04:9

89257 Sperm identification from aspiration (other than seminal fluid)
⊙ *CPT Assistant* Nov 97:35-36, Jan 98:6, Oct 98:1, Nov 98:30, Apr 04:2

(For semen analysis, see 89300-89320)

(For sperm identification from testis tissue, use 89264)

89258 Cryopreservation; embryo(s)
⊙ *CPT Changes: An Insider's View* 2004
⊙ *CPT Assistant* Nov 97:36, Jan 98:6, Oct 98:1, Apr 04:2, 4

89259 sperm
⊙ *CPT Assistant* Nov 97:36, Jan 98:6, Oct 98:1, Apr 04:2, 4

(For cryopreservation of reproductive tissue, testicular, use 89335)

Pathology and Laboratory 80047-89398, 0001U-0520U

89260 Sperm isolation; simple prep (eg, sperm wash and swim-up) for insemination or diagnosis with semen analysis

➜ *CPT Assistant* Nov 97:36, Jan 98:6, Oct 98:1, Apr 04:3-4

89261 complex prep (eg, Percoll gradient, albumin gradient) for insemination or diagnosis with semen analysis

➜ *CPT Assistant* Nov 97:36, Jan 98:6, Oct 98:1, Apr 04:3-4

(For semen analysis without sperm wash or swim-up, use 89320)

89264 Sperm identification from testis tissue, fresh or cryopreserved

➜ *CPT Assistant* Nov 98:30, Apr 04:3-4

(For biopsy of testis, see 54500, 54505)

(For sperm identification from aspiration, use 89257)

(For semen analysis, see 89300-89320)

89268 Insemination of oocytes

➜ *CPT Changes: An Insider's View* 2004

➜ *CPT Assistant* Apr 04:3-4

89272 Extended culture of oocyte(s)/embryo(s), 4-7 days

➜ *CPT Changes: An Insider's View* 2004

➜ *CPT Assistant* Apr 04:3-4

89280 Assisted oocyte fertilization, microtechnique; less than or equal to 10 oocytes

➜ *CPT Changes: An Insider's View* 2004

➜ *CPT Assistant* Apr 04:3-4

89281 greater than 10 oocytes

➜ *CPT Changes: An Insider's View* 2004

➜ *CPT Assistant* Apr 04:3-4

89290 Biopsy, oocyte polar body or embryo blastomere, microtechnique (for pre-implantation genetic diagnosis); less than or equal to 5 embryos

➜ *CPT Changes: An Insider's View* 2004

➜ *CPT Assistant* Apr 04:5

89291 greater than 5 embryos

➜ *CPT Changes: An Insider's View* 2004

➜ *CPT Assistant* Apr 04:3, 5

89300 Semen analysis; presence and/or motility of sperm including Huhner test (post coital)

➜ *CPT Assistant* Nov 97:36, Jul 98:10, Oct 98:4, Apr 04:3, Aug 05:9

89310 motility and count (not including Huhner test)

➜ *CPT Changes: An Insider's View* 2003

➜ *CPT Assistant* Jul 03:9, Apr 04:3

89320 volume, count, motility, and differential

➜ *CPT Changes: An Insider's View* 2008

➜ *CPT Assistant* Apr 04:3, Apr 08:5

(Skin tests, see 86485-86580 and 95012-95199)

89321 sperm presence and motility of sperm, if performed

➜ *CPT Changes: An Insider's View* 2001, 2008

(To report Hyaluronan binding assay [HBA], use 89398)

89322 volume, count, motility, and differential using strict morphologic criteria (eg, Kruger)

➜ *CPT Changes: An Insider's View* 2008

➜ *CPT Assistant* Apr 08:5

89325 Sperm antibodies

(For medicolegal identification of sperm, use 88125)

89329 Sperm evaluation; hamster penetration test

89330 cervical mucus penetration test, with or without spinnbarkeit test

➜ *CPT Assistant* Nov 05:14

89331 Sperm evaluation, for retrograde ejaculation, urine (sperm concentration, motility, and morphology, as indicated)

➜ *CPT Changes: An Insider's View* 2008

➜ *CPT Assistant* Apr 08:5

(For semen analysis on concurrent semen specimen, see 89300-89322 in conjunction with 89331)

(For detection of sperm in urine, use 81015)

89335 Cryopreservation, reproductive tissue, testicular

➜ *CPT Changes: An Insider's View* 2004

➜ *CPT Assistant* Apr 04:5

(For cryopreservation of embryo[s], use 89258. For cryopreservation of sperm, use 89259; for mature oocytes, use 89337)

89337 Cryopreservation, mature oocyte(s)

➜ *CPT Changes: An Insider's View* 2015

89342 Storage (per year); embryo(s)

➜ *CPT Changes: An Insider's View* 2004

➜ *CPT Assistant* Apr 04:5

89343 sperm/semen

➜ *CPT Changes: An Insider's View* 2004

➜ *CPT Assistant* Apr 04:5

89344 reproductive tissue, testicular/ovarian

➜ *CPT Changes: An Insider's View* 2004

➜ *CPT Assistant* Apr 04:5

89346 oocyte(s)

➜ *CPT Changes: An Insider's View* 2004, 2005

➜ *CPT Assistant* Apr 04:5

89352 Thawing of cryopreserved; embryo(s)

➜ *CPT Changes: An Insider's View* 2004

➜ *CPT Assistant* Apr 04:5

89353 sperm/semen, each aliquot

➜ *CPT Changes: An Insider's View* 2004

➜ *CPT Assistant* Apr 04:5

Pathology and Laboratory   80047-89398, 0001U-0520U

89354   reproductive tissue, testicular/ovarian
➲ *CPT Changes: An Insider's View* 2004
➲ *CPT Assistant* Apr 04:5

89356   oocytes, each aliquot
➲ *CPT Changes: An Insider's View* 2004
➲ *CPT Assistant* Apr 04:5, Aug 05:9, Jan 24:17

89398   Unlisted reproductive medicine laboratory procedure
➲ *CPT Changes: An Insider's View* 2010
➲ *CPT Assistant* Dec 20:3, Jan 24:17

Proprietary Laboratory Analyses

Proprietary laboratory analyses (PLA) codes describe proprietary clinical laboratory analyses and can be either provided by a single ("sole-source") laboratory or licensed or marketed to multiple providing laboratories (eg, cleared or approved by the Food and Drug Administration [FDA]).

This subsection includes advanced diagnostic laboratory tests (ADLTs) and clinical diagnostic laboratory tests (CDLTs), as defined under the Protecting Access to Medicare Act (PAMA) of 2014. These analyses may include a range of medical laboratory tests including, but not limited to, multianalyte assays with algorithmic analyses (MAAA) and genomic sequencing procedures (GSP). The descriptor nomenclature follows, where possible, existing code conventions (eg, MAAA, GSP).

Unless specifically noted, even though the Proprietary Laboratory Analyses section of the code set is located at the end of the Pathology and Laboratory section of the code set, a PLA code does not fulfill Category I code criteria. PLA codes are not required to fulfill the Category I criteria. The standards for inclusion in the PLA section are:

■ The test must be commercially available in the United States for use on human specimens and

■ The clinical laboratory or manufacturer that offers the test must request the code.

For similar laboratory analyses that fulfill Category I criteria, see codes listed in the numeric 80000 series.

When a PLA code is available to report a given proprietary laboratory service, that PLA code takes precedence. The service should not be reported with any other CPT code(s) and other CPT code(s) should not be used to report services that may be reported with that specific PLA code. These codes encompass all analytical services required for the analysis (eg, cell lysis, nucleic acid stabilization, extraction, digestion, amplification, hybridization and detection). For molecular analyses, additional procedures that are required prior to cell lysis (eg, microdissection [codes 88380 and 88381]) may be reported separately.

Codes in this subsection are released on a quarterly basis to expedite dissemination for reporting. PLA codes will be published electronically on the AMA CPT website (ama-assn.org/cpt-pla-codes), distributed via CPT data files on a quarterly basis, and, at a minimum, made available in print annually in the CPT codebook. See the Introduction section of the CPT code set for a complete list of the dates of release and implementation.

All codes that are included in this section are also included in Appendix O, with the procedure's proprietary name. In order to report a PLA code, the analysis performed must fulfill the code descriptor and must be the test represented by the proprietary name listed in Appendix O. In some instances, the descriptor language of PLA codes may be identical and the code may only be differentiated by the listed proprietary name in Appendix O. When more than one PLA has an identical descriptor, the codes will be denoted by the symbol "⌧."

All PLA tests will have assigned codes in the PLA section of the code set. Any PLA coded test(s) that satisfies Category I criteria and has been accepted by the CPT Editorial Panel will be designated by the addition of the symbol "↕" to the existing PLA code and will remain in the PLA section of the code set.

If a proprietary test has already been accepted for a Category I code and a code has not been published, subsequent application for a PLA code will take precedence. The code will only be placed in the PLA section.

The accuracy of a PLA code is to be maintained by the original applicant, or the current owner of the test kit or laboratory performing the proprietary test.

A new PLA code is required when:

1. Additional nucleic acid (DNA or RNA) and/or protein analysis(es) are added to the current PLA test, or

2. The name of the PLA test has changed in association with changes in test performance or test characteristics.

The addition or modification of the therapeutic applications of the test require submission of a code change application, but it may not require a new code number.

0001U   Red blood cell antigen typing, DNA, human erythrocyte antigen gene analysis of 35 antigens from 11 blood groups, utilizing whole blood, common RBC alleles reported
➲ *CPT Changes: An Insider's View* 2018

Pathology and Laboratory 80047-89398, 0001U-0520U

0002U   Oncology (colorectal), quantitative assessment of three urine metabolites (ascorbic acid, succinic acid and carnitine) by liquid chromatography with tandem mass spectrometry (LC-MS/MS) using multiple reaction monitoring acquisition, algorithm reported as likelihood of adenomatous polyps

➔ *CPT Changes: An Insider's View* 2018

➔ *CPT Assistant* Aug 18:4

0003U   Oncology (ovarian) biochemical assays of five proteins (apolipoprotein A-1, CA 125 II, follicle stimulating hormone, human epididymis protein 4, transferrin), utilizing serum, algorithm reported as a likelihood score

➔ *CPT Changes: An Insider's View* 2018

0005U   Oncology (prostate) gene expression profile by real-time RT-PCR of 3 genes *(ERG, PCA3,* and *SPDEF),* urine, algorithm reported as risk score

➔ *CPT Changes: An Insider's View* 2018

0007U   Drug test(s), presumptive, with definitive confirmation of positive results, any number of drug classes, urine, includes specimen verification including DNA authentication in comparison to buccal DNA, per date of service

➔ *CPT Changes: An Insider's View* 2018, 2020

0008U   Helicobacter pylori detection and antibiotic resistance, DNA, 16S and 23S rRNA, gyrA, pbp1, rdxA and rpoB, next generation sequencing, formalin-fixed paraffin-embedded or fresh tissue or fecal sample, predictive, reported as positive or negative for resistance to clarithromycin, fluoroquinolones, metronidazole, amoxicillin, tetracycline, and rifabutin

➔ *CPT Changes: An Insider's View* 2018, 2020

0009U   Oncology (breast cancer), *ERBB2* (HER2) copy number by FISH, tumor cells from formalin-fixed paraffin-embedded tissue isolated using image-based dielectrophoresis (DEP) sorting, reported as *ERBB2* gene amplified or non-amplified

➔ *CPT Changes: An Insider's View* 2018

0010U   Infectious disease (bacterial), strain typing by whole genome sequencing, phylogenetic-based report of strain relatedness, per submitted isolate

➔ *CPT Changes: An Insider's View* 2018

0011U   Prescription drug monitoring, evaluation of drugs present by LC-MS/MS, using oral fluid, reported as a comparison to an estimated steady-state range, per date of service including all drug compounds and metabolites

➔ *CPT Changes: An Insider's View* 2018

(0012U has been deleted)

(0013U has been deleted)

(0014U has been deleted)

0016U   Oncology (hematolymphoid neoplasia), RNA, *BCR/ABL1* major and minor breakpoint fusion transcripts, quantitative PCR amplification, blood or bone marrow, report of fusion not detected or detected with quantitation

➔ *CPT Changes: An Insider's View* 2018

0017U   Oncology (hematolymphoid neoplasia), *JAK2* mutation, DNA, PCR amplification of exons 12-14 and sequence analysis, blood or bone marrow, report of *JAK2* mutation not detected or detected

➔ *CPT Changes: An Insider's View* 2018

0018U   Oncology (thyroid), microRNA profiling by RT-PCR of 10 microRNA sequences, utilizing fine needle aspirate, algorithm reported as a positive or negative result for moderate to high risk of malignancy

➔ *CPT Changes: An Insider's View* 2019

0019U   Oncology, RNA, gene expression by whole transcriptome sequencing, formalin-fixed paraffin-embedded tissue or fresh frozen tissue, predictive algorithm reported as potential targets for therapeutic agents

➔ *CPT Changes: An Insider's View* 2019

0021U   Oncology (prostate), detection of 8 autoantibodies (ARF 6, NKX3-1, 5'-UTR-BMI1, CEP 164, 3'-UTR-Ropporin, Desmocollin, AURKAIP-1, CSNK2A2), multiplexed immunoassay and flow cytometry serum, algorithm reported as risk score

➔ *CPT Changes: An Insider's View* 2019

0022U   Targeted genomic sequence analysis panel, non-small cell lung neoplasia, DNA and RNA analysis, 23 genes, interrogation for sequence variants and rearrangements, reported as presence or absence of variants and associated therapy(ies) to consider

➔ *CPT Changes: An Insider's View* 2019, 2023, 2024

0023U   Oncology (acute myelogenous leukemia), DNA, genotyping of internal tandem duplication, p.D835, p. I836, using mononuclear cells, reported as detection or non-detection of *FLT3* mutation and indication for or against the use of midostaurin

➔ *CPT Changes: An Insider's View* 2019

0024U   Glycosylated acute phase proteins (GlycA), nuclear magnetic resonance spectroscopy, quantitative

➔ *CPT Changes: An Insider's View* 2019

0025U   Tenofovir, by liquid chromatography with tandem mass spectrometry (LC-MS/MS), urine, quantitative

➔ *CPT Changes: An Insider's View* 2019

0026U   Oncology (thyroid), DNA and mRNA of 112 genes, next-generation sequencing, fine needle aspirate of thyroid nodule, algorithmic analysis reported as a categorical result ("Positive, high probability of malignancy" or "Negative, low probability of malignancy")

➔ *CPT Changes: An Insider's View* 2019

0027U   *JAK2 (Janus kinase 2)* (eg, myeloproliferative disorder) gene analysis, targeted sequence analysis exons 12-15

➔ *CPT Changes: An Insider's View* 2019

Pathology and Laboratory   80047-89398, 0001U-0520U

0029U   Drug metabolism (adverse drug reactions and drug response), targeted sequence analysis (ie, *CYP1A2, CYP2C19, CYP2C9, CYP2D6, CYP3A4, CYP3A5, CYP4F2, SLCO1B1, VKORC1* and rs12777823)

➔ *CPT Changes: An Insider's View* 2019

0030U   Drug metabolism (warfarin drug response), targeted sequence analysis (ie, *CYP2C9, CYP4F2, VKORC1,* rs12777823)

➔ *CPT Changes: An Insider's View* 2019

0031U   *CYP1A2 (cytochrome P450 family 1, subfamily A, member 2)* (eg, drug metabolism) gene analysis, common variants (ie, *1F, *1K, *6, *7)

➔ *CPT Changes: An Insider's View* 2019

0032U   *COMT (catechol-O-methyltransferase)* (eg, drug metabolism) gene analysis, c.472G>A (rs4680) variant

➔ *CPT Changes: An Insider's View* 2019

0033U   *HTR2A (5-hydroxytryptamine receptor 2A), HTR2C (5-hydroxytryptamine receptor 2C)* (eg, citalopram metabolism) gene analysis, common variants (ie, *HTR2A* rs7997012 [c.614-2211T>C], *HTR2C* rs3813929 [c.-759C>T] and rs1414334 [c.551-3008C>G])

➔ *CPT Changes: An Insider's View* 2019

0034U   *TPMT (thiopurine S-methyltransferase), NUDT15 (nudix hydroxylase 15)* (eg, thiopurine metabolism) gene analysis, common variants (ie, *TPMT* *2, *3A, *3B, *3C, *4, *5, *6, *8, *12; *NUDT15* *3, *4, *5)

➔ *CPT Changes: An Insider's View* 2019

0035U   Neurology (prion disease), cerebrospinal fluid, detection of prion protein by quaking-induced conformational conversion, qualitative

➔ *CPT Changes: An Insider's View* 2019

0036U   Exome (ie, somatic mutations), paired formalin-fixed paraffin-embedded tumor tissue and normal specimen, sequence analyses

➔ *CPT Changes: An Insider's View* 2019

0037U   Targeted genomic sequence analysis, solid organ neoplasm, DNA analysis of 324 genes, interrogation for sequence variants, gene copy number amplifications, gene rearrangements, microsatellite instability and tumor mutational burden

➔ *CPT Changes: An Insider's View* 2019

0038U   Vitamin D, 25 hydroxy D2 and D3, by LC-MS/MS, serum microsample, quantitative

➔ *CPT Changes: An Insider's View* 2019

0039U   Deoxyribonucleic acid (DNA) antibody, double stranded, high avidity

➔ *CPT Changes: An Insider's View* 2019

0040U   *BCR/ABL1 (t(9;22))* (eg, chronic myelogenous leukemia) translocation analysis, major breakpoint, quantitative

➔ *CPT Changes: An Insider's View* 2019

0041U   Borrelia burgdorferi, antibody detection of 5 recombinant protein groups, by immunoblot, IgM

➔ *CPT Changes: An Insider's View* 2019

0042U   Borrelia burgdorferi, antibody detection of 12 recombinant protein groups, by immunoblot, IgG

➔ *CPT Changes: An Insider's View* 2019

0043U   Tick-borne relapsing fever Borrelia group, antibody detection to 4 recombinant protein groups, by immunoblot, IgM

➔ *CPT Changes: An Insider's View* 2019

0044U   Tick-borne relapsing fever Borrelia group, antibody detection to 4 recombinant protein groups, by immunoblot, IgG

➔ *CPT Changes: An Insider's View* 2019

0045U   Oncology (breast ductal carcinoma in situ), mRNA, gene expression profiling by real-time RT-PCR of 12 genes (7 content and 5 housekeeping), utilizing formalin-fixed paraffin-embedded tissue, algorithm reported as recurrence score

➔ *CPT Changes: An Insider's View* 2019

0046U   *FLT3 (fms-related tyrosine kinase 3)* (eg, acute myeloid leukemia) internal tandem duplication (ITD) variants, quantitative

➔ *CPT Changes: An Insider's View* 2019

0047U   Oncology (prostate), mRNA, gene expression profiling by real-time RT-PCR of 17 genes (12 content and 5 housekeeping), utilizing formalin-fixed paraffin-embedded tissue, algorithm reported as a risk score

➔ *CPT Changes: An Insider's View* 2019

0048U   Oncology (solid organ neoplasia), DNA, targeted sequencing of protein-coding exons of 468 cancer-associated genes, including interrogation for somatic mutations and microsatellite instability, matched with normal specimens, utilizing formalin-fixed paraffin-embedded tumor tissue, report of clinically significant mutation(s)

➔ *CPT Changes: An Insider's View* 2019

0049U   *NPM1 (nucleophosmin)* (eg, acute myeloid leukemia) gene analysis, quantitative

➔ *CPT Changes: An Insider's View* 2019

0050U   Targeted genomic sequence analysis panel, acute myelogenous leukemia, DNA analysis, 194 genes, interrogation for sequence variants, copy number variants or rearrangements

➔ *CPT Changes: An Insider's View* 2019

0051U   Prescription drug monitoring, evaluation of drugs present by liquid chromatography tandem mass spectrometry (LC-MS/MS), urine or blood, 31 drug panel, reported as quantitative results, detected or not detected, per date of service

➔ *CPT Changes: An Insider's View* 2019, 2022

0052U   Lipoprotein, blood, high resolution fractionation and quantitation of lipoproteins, including all five major lipoprotein classes and subclasses of HDL, LDL, and VLDL by vertical auto profile ultracentrifugation

→ *CPT Changes: An Insider's View* 2019

(0053U has been deleted)

0054U   Prescription drug monitoring, 14 or more classes of drugs and substances, definitive tandem mass spectrometry with chromatography, capillary blood, quantitative report with therapeutic and toxic ranges, including steady-state range for the prescribed dose when detected, per date of service

→ *CPT Changes: An Insider's View* 2019

0055U   Cardiology (heart transplant), cell-free DNA, PCR assay of 96 DNA target sequences (94 single nucleotide polymorphism targets and two control targets), plasma

→ *CPT Changes: An Insider's View* 2019

(0056U has been deleted)

0058U   Oncology (Merkel cell carcinoma), detection of antibodies to the Merkel cell polyoma virus oncoprotein (small T antigen), serum, quantitative

→ *CPT Changes: An Insider's View* 2019

0059U   Oncology (Merkel cell carcinoma), detection of antibodies to the Merkel cell polyoma virus capsid protein (VP1), serum, reported as positive or negative

→ *CPT Changes: An Insider's View* 2019

0060U   Twin zygosity, genomic-targeted sequence analysis of chromosome 2, using circulating cell-free fetal DNA in maternal blood

→ *CPT Changes: An Insider's View* 2019

0061U   Transcutaneous measurement of five biomarkers (tissue oxygenation [StO_2], oxyhemoglobin [$ctHbO_2$], deoxyhemoglobin [ctHbR], papillary and reticular dermal hemoglobin concentrations [ctHb1 and ctHb2]), using spatial frequency domain imaging (SFDI) and multi-spectral analysis

→ *CPT Changes: An Insider's View* 2019

0062U   Autoimmune (systemic lupus erythematosus), IgG and IgM analysis of 80 biomarkers, utilizing serum, algorithm reported with a risk score

→ *CPT Changes: An Insider's View* 2020

0063U   Neurology (autism), 32 amines by LC-MS/MS, using plasma, algorithm reported as metabolic signature associated with autism spectrum disorder

→ *CPT Changes: An Insider's View* 2020

0064U   Antibody, Treponema pallidum, total and rapid plasma reagin (RPR), immunoassay, qualitative

→ *CPT Changes: An Insider's View* 2020

0065U   Syphilis test, non-treponemal antibody, immunoassay, qualitative (RPR)

→ *CPT Changes: An Insider's View* 2020

(0066U has been deleted)

0067U   Oncology (breast), immunohistochemistry, protein expression profiling of 4 biomarkers (matrix metalloproteinase-1 [MMP-1], carcinoembryonic antigen-related cell adhesion molecule 6 [CEACAM6], hyaluronoglucosaminidase [HYAL1], highly expressed in cancer protein [HEC1]), formalin-fixed paraffin-embedded precancerous breast tissue, algorithm reported as carcinoma risk score

→ *CPT Changes: An Insider's View* 2020

0068U   Candida species panel *(C. albicans, C. parapsilosis, C. kruseii, C. tropicalis,* and *C. auris),* amplified probe technique with qualitative report of the presence or absence of each species

→ *CPT Changes: An Insider's View* 2020

0069U   Oncology (colorectal), microRNA, RT-PCR expression profiling of miR-31-3p, formalin-fixed paraffin-embedded tissue, algorithm reported as an expression score

→ *CPT Changes: An Insider's View* 2020

0070U   *CYP2D6 (cytochrome P450, family 2, subfamily D, polypeptide 6)* (eg, drug metabolism) gene analysis, common and select rare variants (ie, *2, *3, *4, *4N, *5, *6, *7, *8, *9, *10, *11, *12, *13, *14A, *14B, *15, *17, *29, *35, *36, *41, *57, *61, *63, *68, *83, *xN)

→ *CPT Changes: An Insider's View* 2020

+ 0071U   *CYP2D6 (cytochrome P450, family 2, subfamily D, polypeptide 6)* (eg, drug metabolism) gene analysis, full gene sequence (List separately in addition to code for primary procedure)

→ *CPT Changes: An Insider's View* 2020

(Use 0071U in conjunction with 0070U)

+ 0072U   *CYP2D6 (cytochrome P450, family 2, subfamily D, polypeptide 6)* (eg, drug metabolism) gene analysis, targeted sequence analysis (ie, *CYP2D6-2D7* hybrid gene) (List separately in addition to code for primary procedure)

→ *CPT Changes: An Insider's View* 2020

(Use 0072U in conjunction with 0070U)

+ 0073U   *CYP2D6 (cytochrome P450, family 2, subfamily D, polypeptide 6)* (eg, drug metabolism) gene analysis, targeted sequence analysis (ie, *CYP2D7-2D6* hybrid gene) (List separately in addition to code for primary procedure)

→ *CPT Changes: An Insider's View* 2020

(Use 0073U in conjunction with 0070U)

+ 0074U   *CYP2D6 (cytochrome P450, family 2, subfamily D, polypeptide 6)* (eg, drug metabolism) gene analysis, targeted sequence analysis (ie, non-duplicated gene when duplication/multiplication is trans) (List separately in addition to code for primary procedure)

→ *CPT Changes: An Insider's View* 2020

(Use 0074U in conjunction with 0070U)

Pathology and Laboratory **80047-89398, 0001U-0520U**

+ 0075U CYP2D6 (cytochrome P450, family 2, subfamily D, polypeptide 6) (eg, drug metabolism) gene analysis, targeted sequence analysis (ie, 5' gene duplication/multiplication) (List separately in addition to code for primary procedure)

→ CPT Changes: An Insider's View 2020

(Use 0075U in conjunction with 0070U)

+ 0076U CYP2D6 (cytochrome P450, family 2, subfamily D, polypeptide 6) (eg, drug metabolism) gene analysis, targeted sequence analysis (ie, 3' gene duplication/multiplication) (List separately in addition to code for primary procedure)

→ CPT Changes: An Insider's View 2020

(Use 0076U in conjunction with 0070U)

0077U Immunoglobulin paraprotein (M-protein), qualitative, immunoprecipitation and mass spectrometry, blood or urine, including isotype

→ CPT Changes: An Insider's View 2020

▶(0078U has been deleted)◀

0079U Comparative DNA analysis using multiple selected single-nucleotide polymorphisms (SNPs), urine and buccal DNA, for specimen identity verification

→ CPT Changes: An Insider's View 2020

0080U Oncology (lung), mass spectrometric analysis of galectin-3-binding protein and scavenger receptor cysteine-rich type 1 protein M130, with five clinical risk factors (age, smoking status, nodule diameter, nodule-spiculation status and nodule location), utilizing plasma, algorithm reported as a categorical probability of malignancy

→ CPT Changes: An Insider's View 2020

0082U Drug test(s), definitive, 90 or more drugs or substances, definitive chromatography with mass spectrometry, and presumptive, any number of drug classes, by instrument chemistry analyzer (utilizing immunoassay), urine, report of presence or absence of each drug, drug metabolite or substance with description and severity of significant interactions per date of service

→ CPT Changes: An Insider's View 2020

0083U Oncology, response to chemotherapy drugs using motility contrast tomography, fresh or frozen tissue, reported as likelihood of sensitivity or resistance to drugs or drug combinations

→ CPT Changes: An Insider's View 2020

0084U Red blood cell antigen typing, DNA, genotyping of 10 blood groups with phenotype prediction of 37 red blood cell antigens

→ CPT Changes: An Insider's View 2020

0086U Infectious disease (bacterial and fungal), organism identification, blood culture, using rRNA FISH, 6 or more organism targets, reported as positive or negative with phenotypic minimum inhibitory concentration (MIC)-based antimicrobial susceptibility

→ CPT Changes: An Insider's View 2020

0087U Cardiology (heart transplant), mRNA gene expression profiling by microarray of 1283 genes, transplant biopsy tissue, allograft rejection and injury algorithm reported as a probability score

→ CPT Changes: An Insider's View 2020

0088U Transplantation medicine (kidney allograft rejection), microarray gene expression profiling of 1494 genes, utilizing transplant biopsy tissue, algorithm reported as a probability score for rejection

→ CPT Changes: An Insider's View 2020

0089U Oncology (melanoma), gene expression profiling by RTqPCR, PRAME and LINC00518, superficial collection using adhesive patch(es)

→ CPT Changes: An Insider's View 2020

0090U Oncology (cutaneous melanoma), mRNA gene expression profiling by RT-PCR of 23 genes (14 content and 9 housekeeping), utilizing formalin-fixed paraffin-embedded (FFPE) tissue, algorithm reported as a categorical result (ie, benign, intermediate, malignant)

→ CPT Changes: An Insider's View 2020, 2023

0091U Oncology (colorectal) screening, cell enumeration of circulating tumor cells, utilizing whole blood, algorithm, for the presence of adenoma or cancer, reported as a positive or negative result

→ CPT Changes: An Insider's View 2020

0092U Oncology (lung), three protein biomarkers, immunoassay using magnetic nanosensor technology, plasma, algorithm reported as risk score for likelihood of malignancy

→ CPT Changes: An Insider's View 2020

0093U Prescription drug monitoring, evaluation of 65 common drugs by LC-MS/MS, urine, each drug reported detected or not detected

→ CPT Changes: An Insider's View 2020

0094U Genome (eg, unexplained constitutional or heritable disorder or syndrome), rapid sequence analysis

→ CPT Changes: An Insider's View 2020

0095U Eosinophilic esophagitis (Eotaxin-3 [CCL26 {C-C motif chemokine ligand 26}] and major basic protein [PRG2 {proteoglycan 2, pro eosinophil major basic protein}]), enzyme-linked immunosorbent assays (ELISA), specimen obtained by esophageal string test device, algorithm reported as probability of active or inactive eosinophilic esophagitis

→ CPT Changes: An Insider's View 2020, 2024

0096U Human papillomavirus (HPV), high-risk types (ie, 16, 18, 31, 33, 35, 39, 45, 51, 52, 56, 58, 59, 66, 68), male urine

→ CPT Changes: An Insider's View 2020

(0097U has been deleted)

0101U   Hereditary colon cancer disorders (eg, Lynch syndrome, *PTEN* hamartoma syndrome, Cowden syndrome, familial adenomatosis polyposis), genomic sequence analysis panel utilizing a combination of NGS, Sanger, MLPA, and array CGH, with mRNA analytics to resolve variants of unknown significance when indicated (15 genes [sequencing and deletion/duplication], *EPCAM* and *GREM1* [deletion/duplication only])

➔ *CPT Changes: An Insider's View* 2020

0102U   Hereditary breast cancer-related disorders (eg, hereditary breast cancer, hereditary ovarian cancer, hereditary endometrial cancer), genomic sequence analysis panel utilizing a combination of NGS, Sanger, MLPA, and array CGH, with mRNA analytics to resolve variants of unknown significance when indicated (17 genes [sequencing and deletion/duplication])

➔ *CPT Changes: An Insider's View* 2020

0103U   Hereditary ovarian cancer (eg, hereditary ovarian cancer, hereditary endometrial cancer), genomic sequence analysis panel utilizing a combination of NGS, Sanger, MLPA, and array CGH, with mRNA analytics to resolve variants of unknown significance when indicated (24 genes [sequencing and deletion/duplication], *EPCAM* [deletion/duplication only])

➔ *CPT Changes: An Insider's View* 2020

0105U   Nephrology (chronic kidney disease), multiplex electrochemiluminescent immunoassay (ECLIA) of tumor necrosis factor receptor 1A, receptor superfamily 2 *(TNFR1, TNFR2),* and kidney injury molecule-1 (KIM-1) combined with longitudinal clinical data, including *APOL1* genotype if available, and plasma (isolated fresh or frozen), algorithm reported as probability score for rapid kidney function decline (RKFD)

➔ *CPT Changes: An Insider's View* 2020

0106U   Gastric emptying, serial collection of 7 timed breath specimens, non-radioisotope carbon-13 (^{13}C) spirulina substrate, analysis of each specimen by gas isotope ratio mass spectrometry, reported as rate of $^{13}CO_2$ excretion

➔ *CPT Changes: An Insider's View* 2020

0107U   Clostridium difficile toxin(s) antigen detection by immunoassay technique, stool, qualitative, multiple-step method

➔ *CPT Changes: An Insider's View* 2020

0108U   Gastroenterology (Barrett's esophagus), whole slide–digital imaging, including morphometric analysis, computer-assisted quantitative immunolabeling of 9 protein biomarkers (p16, AMACR, p53, CD68, COX-2, CD45RO, HIF1a, HER-2, K20) and morphology, formalin-fixed paraffin-embedded tissue, algorithm reported as risk of progression to high-grade dysplasia or cancer

➔ *CPT Changes: An Insider's View* 2020

0109U   Infectious disease (Aspergillus species), real-time PCR for detection of DNA from 4 species *(A. fumigatus, A. terreus, A. niger,* and *A. flavus),* blood, lavage fluid, or tissue, qualitative reporting of presence or absence of each species

➔ *CPT Changes: An Insider's View* 2020

0110U   Prescription drug monitoring, one or more oral oncology drug(s) and substances, definitive tandem mass spectrometry with chromatography, serum or plasma from capillary blood or venous blood, quantitative report with steady-state range for the prescribed drug(s) when detected

➔ *CPT Changes: An Insider's View* 2020

0111U   Oncology (colon cancer), targeted *KRAS* (codons 12, 13, and 61) and *NRAS* (codons 12, 13, and 61) gene analysis, utilizing formalin-fixed paraffin-embedded tissue

➔ *CPT Changes: An Insider's View* 2020

0112U   Infectious agent detection and identification, targeted sequence analysis (16S and 18S rRNA genes) with drug-resistance gene

➔ *CPT Changes: An Insider's View* 2020

0113U   Oncology (prostate), measurement of *PCA3* and *TMPRSS2-ERG* in urine and PSA in serum following prostatic massage, by RNA amplification and fluorescence-based detection, algorithm reported as risk score

➔ *CPT Changes: An Insider's View* 2020

0114U   Gastroenterology (Barrett's esophagus), *VIM* and *CCNA1* methylation analysis, esophageal cells, algorithm reported as likelihood for Barrett's esophagus

➔ *CPT Changes: An Insider's View* 2020

0115U   Respiratory infectious agent detection by nucleic acid (DNA and RNA), 18 viral types and subtypes and 2 bacterial targets, amplified probe technique, including multiplex reverse transcription for RNA targets, each analyte reported as detected or not detected

➔ *CPT Changes: An Insider's View* 2020

0116U   Prescription drug monitoring, enzyme immunoassay of 35 or more drugs confirmed with LC-MS/MS, oral fluid, algorithm results reported as a patient-compliance measurement with risk of drug to drug interactions for prescribed medications

➔ *CPT Changes: An Insider's View* 2020

0117U   Pain management, analysis of 11 endogenous analytes (methylmalonic acid, xanthurenic acid, homocysteine, pyroglutamic acid, vanilmandelate, 5-hydroxyindoleacetic acid, hydroxymethylglutarate, ethylmalonate, 3-hydroxypropyl mercapturic acid (3-HPMA), quinolinic acid, kynurenic acid), LC-MS/MS, urine, algorithm reported as a pain-index score with likelihood of atypical biochemical function associated with pain

➔ *CPT Changes: An Insider's View* 2020

0118U Transplantation medicine, quantification of donor-derived cell-free DNA using whole genome next-generation sequencing, plasma, reported as percentage of donor-derived cell-free DNA in the total cell-free DNA

➔ *CPT Changes: An Insider's View* 2020

0119U Cardiology, ceramides by liquid chromatography–tandem mass spectrometry, plasma, quantitative report with risk score for major cardiovascular events

➔ *CPT Changes: An Insider's View* 2020

0120U Oncology (B-cell lymphoma classification), mRNA, gene expression profiling by fluorescent probe hybridization of 58 genes (45 content and 13 housekeeping genes), formalin-fixed paraffin-embedded tissue, algorithm reported as likelihood for primary mediastinal B-cell lymphoma (PMBCL) and diffuse large B-cell lymphoma (DLBCL) with cell of origin subtyping in the latter

➔ *CPT Changes: An Insider's View* 2020

(Do not report 0120U in conjunction with 0017M)

0121U Sickle cell disease, microfluidic flow adhesion (VCAM-1), whole blood

➔ *CPT Changes: An Insider's View* 2020

0122U Sickle cell disease, microfluidic flow adhesion (P-Selectin), whole blood

➔ *CPT Changes: An Insider's View* 2020

0123U Mechanical fragility, RBC, shear stress and spectral analysis profiling

➔ *CPT Changes: An Insider's View* 2020

0129U Hereditary breast cancer–related disorders (eg, hereditary breast cancer, hereditary ovarian cancer, hereditary endometrial cancer), genomic sequence analysis and deletion/duplication analysis panel *(ATM, BRCA1, BRCA2, CDH1, CHEK2, PALB2, PTEN, and TP53)*

➔ *CPT Changes: An Insider's View* 2020

+ 0130U Hereditary colon cancer disorders (eg, Lynch syndrome, PTEN hamartoma syndrome, Cowden syndrome, familial adenomatosis polyposis), targeted mRNA sequence analysis panel *(APC, CDH1, CHEK2, MLH1, MSH2, MSH6, MUTYH, PMS2, PTEN,* and *TP53)* (List separately in addition to code for primary procedure)

➔ *CPT Changes: An Insider's View* 2020

(Use 0130U in conjunction with 81435, 0101U)

+ 0131U Hereditary breast cancer–related disorders (eg, hereditary breast cancer, hereditary ovarian cancer, hereditary endometrial cancer), targeted mRNA sequence analysis panel (13 genes) (List separately in addition to code for primary procedure)

➔ *CPT Changes: An Insider's View* 2020

(Use 0131U in conjunction with 81162, 81432, 0102U)

+ 0132U Hereditary ovarian cancer–related disorders (eg, hereditary breast cancer, hereditary ovarian cancer, hereditary endometrial cancer), targeted mRNA sequence analysis panel (17 genes) (List separately in addition to code for primary procedure)

➔ *CPT Changes: An Insider's View* 2020

(Use 0132U in conjunction with 81162, 81432, 0103U)

+ 0133U Hereditary prostate cancer–related disorders, targeted mRNA sequence analysis panel (11 genes) (List separately in addition to code for primary procedure)

➔ *CPT Changes: An Insider's View* 2020

(Use 0133U in conjunction with 81162)

+ 0134U Hereditary pan cancer (eg, hereditary breast and ovarian cancer, hereditary endometrial cancer, hereditary colorectal cancer), targeted mRNA sequence analysis panel (18 genes) (List separately in addition to code for primary procedure)

➔ *CPT Changes: An Insider's View* 2020

(Use 0134U in conjunction with 81162, 81432, 81435)

+ 0135U Hereditary gynecological cancer (eg, hereditary breast and ovarian cancer, hereditary endometrial cancer, hereditary colorectal cancer), targeted mRNA sequence analysis panel (12 genes) (List separately in addition to code for primary procedure)

➔ *CPT Changes: An Insider's View* 2020

(Use 0135U in conjunction with 81162)

+ 0136U *ATM (ataxia telangiectasia mutated)* (eg, ataxia telangiectasia) mRNA sequence analysis (List separately in addition to code for primary procedure)

➔ *CPT Changes: An Insider's View* 2020

(Use 0136U in conjunction with 81408)

+ 0137U *PALB2 (partner and localizer of BRCA2)* (eg, breast and pancreatic cancer) mRNA sequence analysis (List separately in addition to code for primary procedure)

➔ *CPT Changes: An Insider's View* 2020

(Use 0137U in conjunction with 81307)

+ 0138U *BRCA1 (BRCA1, DNA repair associated), BRCA2 (BRCA2, DNA repair associated)* (eg, hereditary breast and ovarian cancer) mRNA sequence analysis (List separately in addition to code for primary procedure)

➔ *CPT Changes: An Insider's View* 2020

(Use 0138U in conjunction with 81162)

0140U Infectious disease (fungi), fungal pathogen identification, DNA (15 fungal targets), blood culture, amplified probe technique, each target reported as detected or not detected

➔ *CPT Changes: An Insider's View* 2021

0141U Infectious disease (bacteria and fungi), gram-positive organism identification and drug resistance element detection, DNA (20 gram-positive bacterial targets, 4 resistance genes, 1 pan gram-negative bacterial target, 1 pan Candida target), blood culture, amplified probe technique, each target reported as detected or not detected

➔ *CPT Changes: An Insider's View* 2021

Pathology and Laboratory 80047-89398, 0001U-0520U

0142U   Infectious disease (bacteria and fungi), gram-negative bacterial identification and drug resistance element detection, DNA (21 gram-negative bacterial targets, 6 resistance genes, 1 pan gram-positive bacterial target, 1 pan Candida target), amplified probe technique, each target reported as detected or not detected

➔ *CPT Changes: An Insider's View* 2021

(0143U has been deleted)

(0144U has been deleted)

(0145U has been deleted)

(0146U has been deleted)

(0147U has been deleted)

(0148U has been deleted)

(0149U has been deleted)

(0150U has been deleted)

(0151U has been deleted)

0152U   Infectious disease (bacteria, fungi, parasites, and DNA viruses), microbial cell-free DNA, plasma, untargeted next-generation sequencing, report for significant positive pathogens

➔ *CPT Changes: An Insider's View* 2021, 2022

0153U   Oncology (breast), mRNA, gene expression profiling by next-generation sequencing of 101 genes, utilizing formalin-fixed paraffin-embedded tissue, algorithm reported as a triple negative breast cancer clinical subtype(s) with information on immune cell involvement

➔ *CPT Changes: An Insider's View* 2021

0154U   Oncology (urothelial cancer), RNA, analysis by real-time RT-PCR of the *FGFR3 (fibroblast growth factor receptor 3)* gene analysis (ie, p.R248C [c.742C>T], p.S249C [c.746C>G], p.G370C [c.1108G>T], p.Y373C [c.1118A>G], FGFR3-TACC3v1, and FGFR3-TACC3v3), utilizing formalin-fixed paraffin-embedded urothelial cancer tumor tissue, reported as *FGFR* gene alteration status

➔ *CPT Changes: An Insider's View* 2021
➔ *CPT Assistant* Jun 20:11

0155U   Oncology (breast cancer), DNA, *PIK3CA (phosphatidylinositol-4,5-bisphosphate 3-kinase, catalytic subunit alpha)* (eg, breast cancer) gene analysis (ie, p. C420R, p.E542K, p.E545A, p.E545D [g.1635G>T only], p. E545G, p.E545K, p.Q546E, p.Q546R, p.H1047L, p.H1047R, p.H1047Y), utilizing formalin-fixed paraffin-embedded breast tumor tissue, reported as *PIK3CA* gene mutation status

➔ *CPT Changes: An Insider's View* 2021
➔ *CPT Assistant* Jun 20:11

0156U   Copy number (eg, intellectual disability, dysmorphology), sequence analysis

➔ *CPT Changes: An Insider's View* 2021

+ 0157U   *APC (APC regulator of WNT signaling pathway)* (eg, familial adenomatosis polyposis [FAP]) mRNA sequence analysis (List separately in addition to code for primary procedure)

➔ *CPT Changes: An Insider's View* 2021

(Use 0157U in conjunction with 81201)

+ 0158U   *MLH1 (mutL homolog 1)* (eg, hereditary non-polyposis colorectal cancer, Lynch syndrome) mRNA sequence analysis (List separately in addition to code for primary procedure)

➔ *CPT Changes: An Insider's View* 2021

(Use 0158U in conjunction with 81292)

+ 0159U   *MSH2 (mutS homolog 2)* (eg, hereditary colon cancer, Lynch syndrome) mRNA sequence analysis (List separately in addition to code for primary procedure)

➔ *CPT Changes: An Insider's View* 2021

(Use 0159U in conjunction with 81295)

+ 0160U   *MSH6 (mutS homolog 6)* (eg, hereditary colon cancer, Lynch syndrome) mRNA sequence analysis (List separately in addition to code for primary procedure)

➔ *CPT Changes: An Insider's View* 2021

(Use 0160U in conjunction with 81298)

+ 0161U   *PMS2 (PMS1 homolog 2, mismatch repair system component)* (eg, hereditary non-polyposis colorectal cancer, Lynch syndrome) mRNA sequence analysis (List separately in addition to code for primary procedure)

➔ *CPT Changes: An Insider's View* 2021

(Use 0161U in conjunction with 81317)

+ 0162U   Hereditary colon cancer (Lynch syndrome), targeted mRNA sequence analysis panel *(MLH1, MSH2, MSH6, PMS2)* (List separately in addition to code for primary procedure)

➔ *CPT Changes: An Insider's View* 2021

(Use 0162U in conjunction with 81292, 81295, 81298, 81317, 81435)

0163U   Oncology (colorectal) screening, biochemical enzyme-linked immunosorbent assay (ELISA) of 3 plasma or serum proteins (teratocarcinoma derived growth factor-1 [TDGF-1, Cripto-1], carcinoembryonic antigen [CEA], extracellular matrix protein [ECM]), with demographic data (age, gender, CRC-screening compliance) using a proprietary algorithm and reported as likelihood of CRC or advanced adenomas

➔ *CPT Changes: An Insider's View* 2021
➔ *CPT Assistant* Jun 20:11

Pathology and Laboratory 80047-89398, 0001U-0520U

0164U Gastroenterology (irritable bowel syndrome [IBS]), immunoassay for anti-CdtB and anti-vinculin antibodies, utilizing plasma, algorithm for elevated or not elevated qualitative results

➥ *CPT Changes: An Insider's View* 2021
➥ *CPT Assistant* Jun 20:12

0165U Peanut allergen-specific quantitative assessment of multiple epitopes using enzyme-linked immunosorbent assay (ELISA), blood, individual epitope results and probability of peanut allergy

➥ *CPT Changes: An Insider's View* 2021
➥ *CPT Assistant* Jun 20:12

0166U Liver disease, 10 biochemical assays (α2-macroglobulin, haptoglobin, apolipoprotein A1, bilirubin, GGT, ALT, AST, triglycerides, cholesterol, fasting glucose) and biometric and demographic data, utilizing serum, algorithm reported as scores for fibrosis, necroinflammatory activity, and steatosis with a summary interpretation

➥ *CPT Changes: An Insider's View* 2021
➥ *CPT Assistant* Jun 20:12

▶(0167U has been deleted)◀

0169U *NUDT15 (nudix hydrolase 15)* and *TPMT (thiopurine S-methyltransferase)* (eg, drug metabolism) gene analysis, common variants

➥ *CPT Changes: An Insider's View* 2021
➥ *CPT Assistant* Jun 20:12

0170U Neurology (autism spectrum disorder [ASD]), RNA, next-generation sequencing, saliva, algorithmic analysis, and results reported as predictive probability of ASD diagnosis

➥ *CPT Changes: An Insider's View* 2021
➥ *CPT Assistant* Jun 20:12

0171U Targeted genomic sequence analysis panel, acute myeloid leukemia, myelodysplastic syndrome, and myeloproliferative neoplasms, DNA analysis, 23 genes, interrogation for sequence variants, rearrangements and minimal residual disease, reported as presence/absence

➥ *CPT Changes: An Insider's View* 2021
➥ *CPT Assistant* Jun 20:12

0172U Oncology (solid tumor as indicated by the label), somatic mutation analysis of *BRCA1 (BRCA1, DNA repair associated), BRCA2 (BRCA2, DNA repair associated)* and analysis of homologous recombination deficiency pathways, DNA, formalin-fixed paraffin-embedded tissue, algorithm quantifying tumor genomic instability score

➥ *CPT Changes: An Insider's View* 2021

0173U Psychiatry (ie, depression, anxiety), genomic analysis panel, includes variant analysis of 14 genes

➥ *CPT Changes: An Insider's View* 2021

0174U Oncology (solid tumor), mass spectrometric 30 protein targets, formalin-fixed paraffin-embedded tissue, prognostic and predictive algorithm reported as likely, unlikely, or uncertain benefit of 39 chemotherapy and targeted therapeutic oncology agents

➥ *CPT Changes: An Insider's View* 2021

0175U Psychiatry (eg, depression, anxiety), genomic analysis panel, variant analysis of 15 genes

➥ *CPT Changes: An Insider's View* 2021

0176U Cytolethal distending toxin B (CdtB) and vinculin IgG antibodies by immunoassay (ie, ELISA)

➥ *CPT Changes: An Insider's View* 2021

0177U Oncology (breast cancer), DNA, *PIK3CA (phosphatidylinositol-4,5-bisphosphate 3-kinase catalytic subunit alpha)* gene analysis of 11 gene variants utilizing plasma, reported as *PIK3CA* gene mutation status

➥ *CPT Changes: An Insider's View* 2021

0178U Peanut allergen-specific quantitative assessment of multiple epitopes using enzyme-linked immunosorbent assay (ELISA), blood, report of minimum eliciting exposure for a clinical reaction

➥ *CPT Changes: An Insider's View* 2021

0179U Oncology (non-small cell lung cancer), cell-free DNA, targeted sequence analysis of 23 genes (single nucleotide variations, insertions and deletions, fusions without prior knowledge of partner/breakpoint, copy number variations), with report of significant mutation(s)

➥ *CPT Changes: An Insider's View* 2021

0180U Red cell antigen (ABO blood group) genotyping (ABO), gene analysis Sanger/chain termination/conventional sequencing, *ABO (ABO, alpha 1-3-N-acetylgalactosaminyltransferase and alpha 1-3-galactosyltransferase)* gene, including subtyping, 7 exons

➥ *CPT Changes: An Insider's View* 2021

0181U Red cell antigen (Colton blood group) genotyping (CO), gene analysis, *AQP1 (aquaporin 1 [Colton blood group])* exon 1

➥ *CPT Changes: An Insider's View* 2021

0182U Red cell antigen (Cromer blood group) genotyping (CROM), gene analysis, *CD55 (CD55 molecule [Cromer blood group])* exons 1-10

➥ *CPT Changes: An Insider's View* 2021

0183U Red cell antigen (Diego blood group) genotyping (DI), gene analysis, *SLC4A1 (solute carrier family 4 member 1 [Diego blood group])* exon 19

➥ *CPT Changes: An Insider's View* 2021

0184U Red cell antigen (Dombrock blood group) genotyping (DO), gene analysis, *ART4 (ADP-ribosyltransferase 4 [Dombrock blood group])* exon 2

➥ *CPT Changes: An Insider's View* 2021

0185U Red cell antigen (H blood group) genotyping (FUT1), gene analysis, *FUT1 (fucosyltransferase 1 [H blood group])* exon 4

➥ *CPT Changes: An Insider's View* 2021

0186U   Red cell antigen (H blood group) genotyping (FUT2), gene analysis, *FUT2 (fucosyltransferase 2)* exon 2
➔ *CPT Changes: An Insider's View* 2021

0187U   Red cell antigen (Duffy blood group) genotyping (FY), gene analysis, *ACKR1 (atypical chemokine receptor 1 [Duffy blood group])* exons 1-2
➔ *CPT Changes: An Insider's View* 2021

0188U   Red cell antigen (Gerbich blood group) genotyping (GE), gene analysis, *GYPC (glycophorin C [Gerbich blood group])* exons 1-4
➔ *CPT Changes: An Insider's View* 2021

0189U   Red cell antigen (MNS blood group) genotyping (GYPA), gene analysis, *GYPA (glycophorin A [MNS blood group])* introns 1, 5, exon 2
➔ *CPT Changes: An Insider's View* 2021

0190U   Red cell antigen (MNS blood group) genotyping (GYPB), gene analysis, *GYPB (glycophorin B [MNS blood group])* introns 1, 5, pseudoexon 3
➔ *CPT Changes: An Insider's View* 2021

0191U   Red cell antigen (Indian blood group) genotyping (IN), gene analysis, *CD44 (CD44 molecule [Indian blood group])* exons 2, 3, 6
➔ *CPT Changes: An Insider's View* 2021

0192U   Red cell antigen (Kidd blood group) genotyping (JK), gene analysis, *SLC14A1 (solute carrier family 14 member 1 [Kidd blood group])* gene promoter, exon 9
➔ *CPT Changes: An Insider's View* 2021

0193U   Red cell antigen (JR blood group) genotyping (JR), gene analysis, *ABCG2 (ATP binding cassette subfamily G member 2 [Junior blood group])* exons 2-26
➔ *CPT Changes: An Insider's View* 2021

0194U   Red cell antigen (Kell blood group) genotyping (KEL), gene analysis, *KEL (Kell metallo-endopeptidase [Kell blood group])* exon 8
➔ *CPT Changes: An Insider's View* 2021

0195U   *KLF1 (Kruppel-like factor 1)*, targeted sequencing (ie, exon 13)
➔ *CPT Changes: An Insider's View* 2021

0196U   Red cell antigen (Lutheran blood group) genotyping (LU), gene analysis, *BCAM (basal cell adhesion molecule [Lutheran blood group])* exon 3
➔ *CPT Changes: An Insider's View* 2021

0197U   Red cell antigen (Landsteiner-Wiener blood group) genotyping (LW), gene analysis, *ICAM4 (intercellular adhesion molecule 4 [Landsteiner-Wiener blood group])* exon 1
➔ *CPT Changes: An Insider's View* 2021

0198U   Red cell antigen (RH blood group) genotyping (RHD and RHCE), gene analysis Sanger/chain termination/conventional sequencing, *RHD (Rh blood group D antigen)* exons 1-10 and *RHCE (Rh blood group CcEe antigens)* exon 5

0199U   Red cell antigen (Scianna blood group) genotyping (SC), gene analysis, *ERMAP (erythroblast membrane associated protein [Scianna blood group])* exons 4, 12
➔ *CPT Changes: An Insider's View* 2021

0200U   Red cell antigen (Kx blood group) genotyping (XK), gene analysis, *XK (X-linked Kx blood group)* exons 1-3
➔ *CPT Changes: An Insider's View* 2021

0201U   Red cell antigen (Yt blood group) genotyping (YT), gene analysis, *ACHE (acetylcholinesterase [Cartwright blood group])* exon 2
➔ *CPT Changes: An Insider's View* 2021

✘ **0202U**   Infectious disease (bacterial or viral respiratory tract infection), pathogen-specific nucleic acid (DNA or RNA), 22 targets including severe acute respiratory syndrome coronavirus 2 (SARS-CoV-2), qualitative RT-PCR, nasopharyngeal swab, each pathogen reported as detected or not detected
➔ *CPT Changes: An Insider's View* 2021

(For additional PLA code with identical clinical descriptor, see 0223U. See Appendix O or the most current listing on the AMA CPT website to determine appropriate code assignment)

0203U   Autoimmune (inflammatory bowel disease), mRNA, gene expression profiling by quantitative RT-PCR, 17 genes (15 target and 2 reference genes), whole blood, reported as a continuous risk score and classification of inflammatory bowel disease aggressiveness
➔ *CPT Changes: An Insider's View* 2021

▶(0204U has been deleted)◀

0205U   Ophthalmology (age-related macular degeneration), analysis of 3 gene variants (2 *CFH* gene, 1 *ARMS2* gene), using PCR and MALDI-TOF, buccal swab, reported as positive or negative for neovascular age-related macular-degeneration risk associated with zinc supplements
➔ *CPT Changes: An Insider's View* 2021

0206U   Neurology (Alzheimer disease); cell aggregation using morphometric imaging and protein kinase C-epsilon (PKCe) concentration in response to amylospheroid treatment by ELISA, cultured skin fibroblasts, each reported as positive or negative for Alzheimer disease
➔ *CPT Changes: An Insider's View* 2021

+ **0207U**   quantitative imaging of phosphorylated *ERK1* and *ERK2* in response to bradykinin treatment by in situ immunofluorescence, using cultured skin fibroblasts, reported as a probability index for Alzheimer disease (List separately in addition to code for primary procedure)
➔ *CPT Changes: An Insider's View* 2021

(Use 0207U in conjunction with 0206U)

▲=Revised code   ●=New code   ▶◀=Contains new or revised text   ✘=Duplicate PLA test   ↕=Category I PLA

(0208U has been deleted)

0209U   Cytogenomic constitutional (genome-wide) analysis, interrogation of genomic regions for copy number, structural changes and areas of homozygosity for chromosomal abnormalities

➔ *CPT Changes: An Insider's View* 2021

0210U   Syphilis test, non-treponemal antibody, immunoassay, quantitative (RPR)

➔ *CPT Changes: An Insider's View* 2021

0211U   Oncology (pan-tumor), DNA and RNA by next-generation sequencing, utilizing formalin-fixed paraffin-embedded tissue, interpretative report for single nucleotide variants, copy number alterations, tumor mutational burden, and microsatellite instability, with therapy association

➔ *CPT Changes: An Insider's View* 2021

0212U   Rare diseases (constitutional/heritable disorders), whole genome and mitochondrial DNA sequence analysis, including small sequence changes, deletions, duplications, short tandem repeat gene expansions, and variants in non-uniquely mappable regions, blood or saliva, identification and categorization of genetic variants, proband

➔ *CPT Changes: An Insider's View* 2021

(Do not report 0212U in conjunction with 81425)

0213U   Rare diseases (constitutional/heritable disorders), whole genome and mitochondrial DNA sequence analysis, including small sequence changes, deletions, duplications, short tandem repeat gene expansions, and variants in non-uniquely mappable regions, blood or saliva, identification and categorization of genetic variants, each comparator genome (eg, parent, sibling)

➔ *CPT Changes: An Insider's View* 2021

(Do not report 0213U in conjunction with 81426)

0214U   Rare diseases (constitutional/heritable disorders), whole exome and mitochondrial DNA sequence analysis, including small sequence changes, deletions, duplications, short tandem repeat gene expansions, and variants in non-uniquely mappable regions, blood or saliva, identification and categorization of genetic variants, proband

➔ *CPT Changes: An Insider's View* 2021

(Do not report 0214U in conjunction with 81415)

0215U   Rare diseases (constitutional/heritable disorders), whole exome and mitochondrial DNA sequence analysis, including small sequence changes, deletions, duplications, short tandem repeat gene expansions, and variants in non-uniquely mappable regions, blood or saliva, identification and categorization of genetic variants, each comparator exome (eg, parent, sibling)

➔ *CPT Changes: An Insider's View* 2021

(Do not report 0215U in conjunction with 81416)

0216U   Neurology (inherited ataxias), genomic DNA sequence analysis of 12 common genes including small sequence changes, deletions, duplications, short tandem repeat

gene expansions, and variants in non-uniquely mappable regions, blood or saliva, identification and categorization of genetic variants

➔ *CPT Changes: An Insider's View* 2021

0217U   Neurology (inherited ataxias), genomic DNA sequence analysis of 51 genes including small sequence changes, deletions, duplications, short tandem repeat gene expansions, and variants in non-uniquely mappable regions, blood or saliva, identification and categorization of genetic variants

➔ *CPT Changes: An Insider's View* 2021

0218U   Neurology (muscular dystrophy), *DMD* gene sequence analysis, including small sequence changes, deletions, duplications, and variants in non-uniquely mappable regions, blood or saliva, identification and characterization of genetic variants

➔ *CPT Changes: An Insider's View* 2021

0219U   Infectious agent (human immunodeficiency virus), targeted viral next-generation sequence analysis (ie, protease [PR], reverse transcriptase [RT], integrase [INT]), algorithm reported as prediction of antiviral drug susceptibility

➔ *CPT Changes: An Insider's View* 2021

0220U   Oncology (breast cancer), image analysis with artificial intelligence assessment of 12 histologic and immunohistochemical features, reported as a recurrence score

➔ *CPT Changes: An Insider's View* 2021

0221U   Red cell antigen (ABO blood group) genotyping (ABO), gene analysis, next-generation sequencing, *ABO (ABO, alpha 1-3-N-acetylgalactosaminyltransferase and alpha 1-3-galactosyltransferase)* gene

➔ *CPT Changes: An Insider's View* 2021

0222U   Red cell antigen (RH blood group) genotyping (RHD and RHCE), gene analysis, next-generation sequencing, RH proximal promoter, exons 1-10, portions of introns 2-3

➔ *CPT Changes: An Insider's View* 2021

⋇ **0223U**   Infectious disease (bacterial or viral respiratory tract infection), pathogen-specific nucleic acid (DNA or RNA), 22 targets including severe acute respiratory syndrome coronavirus 2 (SARS-CoV-2), qualitative RT-PCR, nasopharyngeal swab, each pathogen reported as detected or not detected

➔ *CPT Changes: An Insider's View* 2022

(For additional PLA code with identical clinical descriptor, see 0202U. See Appendix O or the most current listing on the AMA CPT website to determine appropriate code assignment)

0224U Antibody, severe acute respiratory syndrome coronavirus 2 (SARS-CoV-2) (coronavirus disease [COVID-19]), includes titer(s), when performed
➲ *CPT Changes: An Insider's View* 2022

(Do not report 0224U in conjunction with 86769)

0225U Infectious disease (bacterial or viral respiratory tract infection) pathogen-specific DNA and RNA, 21 targets, including severe acute respiratory syndrome coronavirus 2 (SARS-CoV-2), amplified probe technique, including multiplex reverse transcription for RNA targets, each analyte reported as detected or not detected
➲ *CPT Changes: An Insider's View* 2022

0226U Surrogate viral neutralization test (sVNT), severe acute respiratory syndrome coronavirus 2 (SARS-CoV-2) (coronavirus disease [COVID-19]), ELISA, plasma, serum
➲ *CPT Changes: An Insider's View* 2022

0227U Drug assay, presumptive, 30 or more drugs or metabolites, urine, liquid chromatography with tandem mass spectrometry (LC-MS/MS) using multiple reaction monitoring (MRM), with drug or metabolite description, includes sample validation
➲ *CPT Changes: An Insider's View* 2022

0228U Oncology (prostate), multianalyte molecular profile by photometric detection of macromolecules adsorbed on nanosponge array slides with machine learning, utilizing first morning voided urine, algorithm reported as likelihood of prostate cancer
➲ *CPT Changes: An Insider's View* 2022

0229U *BCAT1 (Branched chain amino acid transaminase 1)* and *IKZF1 (IKAROS family zinc finger 1)* (eg, colorectal cancer) promoter methylation analysis
➲ *CPT Changes: An Insider's View* 2022, 2023
➲ *CPT Assistant* Aug 22:8-10

0230U *AR (androgen receptor)* (eg, spinal and bulbar muscular atrophy, Kennedy disease, X chromosome inactivation), full sequence analysis, including small sequence changes in exonic and intronic regions, deletions, duplications, short tandem repeat (STR) expansions, mobile element insertions, and variants in non-uniquely mappable regions
➲ *CPT Changes: An Insider's View* 2022

0231U *CACNA1A (calcium voltage-gated channel subunit alpha 1A)* (eg, spinocerebellar ataxia), full gene analysis, including small sequence changes in exonic and intronic regions, deletions, duplications, short tandem repeat (STR) gene expansions, mobile element insertions, and variants in non-uniquely mappable regions
➲ *CPT Changes: An Insider's View* 2022

0232U *CSTB (cystatin B)* (eg, progressive myoclonic epilepsy type 1A, Unverricht-Lundborg disease), full gene analysis, including small sequence changes in exonic and intronic regions, deletions, duplications, short tandem repeat (STR) expansions, mobile element insertions, and variants in non-uniquely mappable regions
➲ *CPT Changes: An Insider's View* 2022

0233U *FXN (frataxin)* (eg, Friedreich ataxia), gene analysis, including small sequence changes in exonic and intronic regions, deletions, duplications, short tandem repeat (STR) expansions, mobile element insertions, and variants in non-uniquely mappable regions
➲ *CPT Changes: An Insider's View* 2022

0234U *MECP2 (methyl CpG binding protein 2)* (eg, Rett syndrome), full gene analysis, including small sequence changes in exonic and intronic regions, deletions, duplications, mobile element insertions, and variants in non-uniquely mappable regions
➲ *CPT Changes: An Insider's View* 2022

0235U *PTEN (phosphatase and tensin homolog)* (eg, Cowden syndrome, PTEN hamartoma tumor syndrome), full gene analysis, including small sequence changes in exonic and intronic regions, deletions, duplications, mobile element insertions, and variants in non-uniquely mappable regions
➲ *CPT Changes: An Insider's View* 2022

0236U *SMN1 (survival of motor neuron 1, telomeric)* and *SMN2 (survival of motor neuron 2, centromeric)* (eg, spinal muscular atrophy) full gene analysis, including small sequence changes in exonic and intronic regions, duplications, deletions, and mobile element insertions
➲ *CPT Changes: An Insider's View* 2022

0237U Cardiac ion channelopathies (eg, Brugada syndrome, long QT syndrome, short QT syndrome, catecholaminergic polymorphic ventricular tachycardia), genomic sequence analysis panel including *ANK2, CASQ2, CAV3, KCNE1, KCNE2, KCNH2, KCNJ2, KCNQ1, RYR2,* and *SCN5A,* including small sequence changes in exonic and intronic regions, deletions, duplications, mobile element insertions, and variants in non-uniquely mappable regions
➲ *CPT Changes: An Insider's View* 2022

0238U Oncology (Lynch syndrome), genomic DNA sequence analysis of *MLH1, MSH2, MSH6, PMS2,* and *EPCAM,* including small sequence changes in exonic and intronic regions, deletions, duplications, mobile element insertions, and variants in non-uniquely mappable regions
➲ *CPT Changes: An Insider's View* 2022

0239U Targeted genomic sequence analysis panel, solid organ neoplasm, cell-free DNA, analysis of 311 or more genes, interrogation for sequence variants, including substitutions, insertions, deletions, select rearrangements, and copy number variations
➲ *CPT Changes: An Insider's View* 2022

0240U Infectious disease (viral respiratory tract infection), pathogen-specific RNA, 3 targets (severe acute respiratory syndrome coronavirus 2 [SARS-CoV-2], influenza A, influenza B), upper respiratory specimen, each pathogen reported as detected or not detected
➡ *CPT Changes: An Insider's View 2022*

0241U Infectious disease (viral respiratory tract infection), pathogen-specific RNA, 4 targets (severe acute respiratory syndrome coronavirus 2 [SARS-CoV-2], influenza A, influenza B, respiratory syncytial virus [RSV]), upper respiratory specimen, each pathogen reported as detected or not detected
➡ *CPT Changes: An Insider's View 2022*

0242U Targeted genomic sequence analysis panel, solid organ neoplasm, cell-free circulating DNA analysis of 55-74 genes, interrogation for sequence variants, gene copy number amplifications, and gene rearrangements
➡ *CPT Changes: An Insider's View 2022*

0243U Obstetrics (preeclampsia), biochemical assay of placental-growth factor, time-resolved fluorescence immunoassay, maternal serum, predictive algorithm reported as a risk score for preeclampsia
➡ *CPT Changes: An Insider's View 2022*

0244U Oncology (solid organ), DNA, comprehensive genomic profiling, 257 genes, interrogation for single-nucleotide variants, insertions/deletions, copy number alterations, gene rearrangements, tumor-mutational burden and microsatellite instability, utilizing formalin-fixed paraffin-embedded tumor tissue
➡ *CPT Changes: An Insider's View 2022*

0245U Oncology (thyroid), mutation analysis of 10 genes and 37 RNA fusions and expression of 4 mRNA markers using next-generation sequencing, fine needle aspirate, report includes associated risk of malignancy expressed as a percentage
➡ *CPT Changes: An Insider's View 2022*

0246U Red blood cell antigen typing, DNA, genotyping of at least 16 blood groups with phenotype prediction of at least 51 red blood cell antigens
➡ *CPT Changes: An Insider's View 2022*

0247U Obstetrics (preterm birth), insulin-like growth factor–binding protein 4 (IBP4), sex hormone–binding globulin (SHBG), quantitative measurement by LC-MS/MS, utilizing maternal serum, combined with clinical data, reported as predictive-risk stratification for spontaneous preterm birth
➡ *CPT Changes: An Insider's View 2022*

▲ **0248U** Oncology, spheroid cell culture in 3D microenvironment, 12-drug panel, brain- or brain metastasis–response prediction for each drug
➡ *CPT Changes: An Insider's View 2022, 2025*

0249U Oncology (breast), semiquantitative analysis of 32 phosphoproteins and protein analytes, includes laser capture microdissection, with algorithmic analysis and interpretative report
➡ *CPT Changes: An Insider's View 2022*

0250U Oncology (solid organ neoplasm), targeted genomic sequence DNA analysis of 505 genes, interrogation for somatic alterations (SNVs [single nucleotide variant], small insertions and deletions, one amplification, and four translocations), microsatellite instability and tumor-mutation burden
➡ *CPT Changes: An Insider's View 2022*

0251U Hepcidin-25, enzyme-linked immunosorbent assay (ELISA), serum or plasma
➡ *CPT Changes: An Insider's View 2022*

0252U Fetal aneuploidy short tandem–repeat comparative analysis, fetal DNA from products of conception, reported as normal (euploidy), monosomy, trisomy, or partial deletion/duplication, mosaicism, and segmental aneuploidy
➡ *CPT Changes: An Insider's View 2022*

0253U Reproductive medicine (endometrial receptivity analysis), RNA gene expression profile, 238 genes by next-generation sequencing, endometrial tissue, predictive algorithm reported as endometrial window of implantation (eg, pre-receptive, receptive, post-receptive)
➡ *CPT Changes: An Insider's View 2022*

0254U Reproductive medicine (preimplantation genetic assessment), analysis of 24 chromosomes using embryonic DNA genomic sequence analysis for aneuploidy, and a mitochondrial DNA score in euploid embryos, results reported as normal (euploidy), monosomy, trisomy, or partial deletion/duplication, mosaicism, and segmental aneuploidy, per embryo tested
➡ *CPT Changes: An Insider's View 2022*

0255U Andrology (infertility), sperm-capacitation assessment of ganglioside GM1 distribution patterns, fluorescence microscopy, fresh or frozen specimen, reported as percentage of capacitated sperm and probability of generating a pregnancy score
➡ *CPT Changes: An Insider's View 2022*

0256U Trimethylamine/trimethylamine N-oxide (TMA/TMAO) profile, tandem mass spectrometry (MS/MS), urine, with algorithmic analysis and interpretive report
➡ *CPT Changes: An Insider's View 2022*

0257U Very long chain acyl-coenzyme A (CoA) dehydrogenase (VLCAD), leukocyte enzyme activity, whole blood
➡ *CPT Changes: An Insider's View 2022*

0258U   Autoimmune (psoriasis), mRNA, next-generation sequencing, gene expression profiling of 50-100 genes, skin-surface collection using adhesive patch, algorithm reported as likelihood of response to psoriasis biologics

➜ *CPT Changes: An Insider's View* 2022

0259U   Nephrology (chronic kidney disease), nuclear magnetic resonance spectroscopy measurement of myo-inositol, valine, and creatinine, algorithmically combined with cystatin C (by immunoassay) and demographic data to determine estimated glomerular filtration rate (GFR), serum, quantitative

➜ *CPT Changes: An Insider's View* 2022

✱ **0260U**   Rare diseases (constitutional/heritable disorders), identification of copy number variations, inversions, insertions, translocations, and other structural variants by optical genome mapping

➜ *CPT Changes: An Insider's View* 2022

▶(For additional PLA codes with identical clinical descriptor, see 0264U, 0454U. See Appendix O or the most current listing on the AMA CPT website to determine appropriate code assignment)◀

0261U   Oncology (colorectal cancer), image analysis with artificial intelligence assessment of 4 histologic and immunohistochemical features (CD3 and CD8 within tumor-stroma border and tumor core), tissue, reported as immune response and recurrence-risk score

➜ *CPT Changes: An Insider's View* 2022

0262U   Oncology (solid tumor), gene expression profiling by real-time RT-PCR of 7 gene pathways (*ER, AR, PI3K, MAPK, HH, TGFB,* Notch), formalin-fixed paraffin-embedded (FFPE), algorithm reported as gene pathway activity score

➜ *CPT Changes: An Insider's View* 2022

0263U   Neurology (autism spectrum disorder [ASD]), quantitative measurements of 16 central carbon metabolites (ie, α-ketoglutarate, alanine, lactate, phenylalanine, pyruvate, succinate, carnitine, citrate, fumarate, hypoxanthine, inosine, malate, S-sulfocysteine, taurine, urate, and xanthine), liquid chromatography tandem mass spectrometry (LC-MS/MS), plasma, algorithmic analysis with result reported as negative or positive (with metabolic subtypes of ASD)

➜ *CPT Changes: An Insider's View* 2022

✱ **0264U**   Rare diseases (constitutional/heritable disorders), identification of copy number variations, inversions, insertions, translocations, and other structural variants by optical genome mapping

➜ *CPT Changes: An Insider's View* 2022

▶(For additional PLA codes with identical clinical descriptor, see 0260U, 0454U. See Appendix O or the most current listing on the AMA CPT website to determine appropriate code assignment)◀

0265U   Rare constitutional and other heritable disorders, whole genome and mitochondrial DNA sequence analysis, blood, frozen and formalin-fixed paraffin-embedded (FFPE) tissue, saliva, buccal swabs or cell lines, identification of single nucleotide and copy number variants

➜ *CPT Changes: An Insider's View* 2022

0266U   Unexplained constitutional or other heritable disorders or syndromes, tissue-specific gene expression by whole-transcriptome and next-generation sequencing, blood, formalin-fixed paraffin-embedded (FFPE) tissue or fresh frozen tissue, reported as presence or absence of splicing or expression changes

➜ *CPT Changes: An Insider's View* 2022

0267U   Rare constitutional and other heritable disorders, identification of copy number variations, inversions, insertions, translocations, and other structural variants by optical genome mapping and whole genome sequencing

➜ *CPT Changes: An Insider's View* 2022

0268U   Hematology (atypical hemolytic uremic syndrome [aHUS]), genomic sequence analysis of 15 genes, blood, buccal swab, or amniotic fluid

➜ *CPT Changes: An Insider's View* 2022

0269U   Hematology (autosomal dominant congenital thrombocytopenia), genomic sequence analysis of 22 genes, blood, buccal swab, or amniotic fluid

➜ *CPT Changes: An Insider's View* 2022, 2024

0270U   Hematology (congenital coagulation disorders), genomic sequence analysis of 20 genes, blood, buccal swab, or amniotic fluid

➜ *CPT Changes: An Insider's View* 2022

0271U   Hematology (congenital neutropenia), genomic sequence analysis of 24 genes, blood, buccal swab, or amniotic fluid

➜ *CPT Changes: An Insider's View* 2022, 2024

0272U   Hematology (genetic bleeding disorders), genomic sequence analysis of 60 genes and duplication/deletion of *PLAU*, blood, buccal swab, or amniotic fluid, comprehensive

➜ *CPT Changes: An Insider's View* 2022, 2024

0273U   Hematology (genetic hyperfibrinolysis, delayed bleeding), analysis of 9 genes (*F13A1, F13B, FGA, FGB, FGG, SERPINA1, SERPINE1, SERPINF2* by next-generation sequencing, and *PLAU* by array comparative genomic hybridization), blood, buccal swab, or amniotic fluid

➜ *CPT Changes: An Insider's View* 2022

Pathology and Laboratory   80047-89398, 0001U-0520U

0274U   Hematology (genetic platelet disorders), genomic sequence analysis of 62 genes and duplication/deletion of *PLAU,* blood, buccal swab, or amniotic fluid
➔ *CPT Changes: An Insider's View 2022, 2024*

0275U   Hematology (heparin-induced thrombocytopenia), platelet antibody reactivity by flow cytometry, serum
➔ *CPT Changes: An Insider's View 2022*

0276U   Hematology (inherited thrombocytopenia), genomic sequence analysis of 42 genes, blood, buccal swab, or amniotic fluid
➔ *CPT Changes: An Insider's View 2022, 2023*

0277U   Hematology (genetic platelet function disorder), genomic sequence analysis of 40 genes and duplication/deletion of *PLAU,* blood, buccal swab, or amniotic fluid
➔ *CPT Changes: An Insider's View 2022, 2024*

0278U   Hematology (genetic thrombosis), genomic sequence analysis of 14 genes, blood, buccal swab, or amniotic fluid
➔ *CPT Changes: An Insider's View 2022, 2024*

0279U   Hematology (von Willebrand disease [VWD]), von Willebrand factor (VWF) and collagen III binding by enzyme-linked immunosorbent assays (ELISA), plasma, report of collagen III binding
➔ *CPT Changes: An Insider's View 2022*

0280U   Hematology (von Willebrand disease [VWD]), von Willebrand factor (VWF) and collagen IV binding by enzyme-linked immunosorbent assays (ELISA), plasma, report of collagen IV binding
➔ *CPT Changes: An Insider's View 2022*

0281U   Hematology (von Willebrand disease [VWD]), von Willebrand propeptide, enzyme-linked immunosorbent assays (ELISA), plasma, diagnostic report of von Willebrand factor (VWF) propeptide antigen level
➔ *CPT Changes: An Insider's View 2022*

0282U   Red blood cell antigen typing, DNA, genotyping of 12 blood group system genes to predict 44 red blood cell antigen phenotypes
➔ *CPT Changes: An Insider's View 2022*

0283U   von Willebrand factor (VWF), type 2B, platelet-binding evaluation, radioimmunoassay, plasma
➔ *CPT Changes: An Insider's View 2022*

0284U   von Willebrand factor (VWF), type 2N, factor VIII and VWF binding evaluation, enzyme-linked immunosorbent assays (ELISA), plasma
➔ *CPT Changes: An Insider's View 2022*

0285U   Oncology, response to radiation, cell-free DNA, quantitative branched chain DNA amplification, plasma, reported as a radiation toxicity score
➔ *CPT Changes: An Insider's View 2023*

0286U   *CEP72 (centrosomal protein, 72-KDa), NUDT15 (nudix hydrolase 15)* and *TPMT (thiopurine S-methyltransferase)* (eg, drug metabolism) gene analysis, common variants
➔ *CPT Changes: An Insider's View 2023*

0287U   Oncology (thyroid), DNA and mRNA, next-generation sequencing analysis of 112 genes, fine needle aspirate or formalin-fixed paraffin-embedded (FFPE) tissue, algorithmic prediction of cancer recurrence, reported as a categorical risk result (low, intermediate, high)
➔ *CPT Changes: An Insider's View 2023*

0288U   Oncology (lung), mRNA, quantitative PCR analysis of 11 genes *(BAG1, BRCA1, CDC6, CDK2AP1, ERBB3, FUT3, IL11, LCK, RND3, SH3BGR, WNT3A)* and 3 reference genes *(ESD, TBP, YAP1),* formalin-fixed paraffin-embedded (FFPE) tumor tissue, algorithmic interpretation reported as a recurrence risk score
➔ *CPT Changes: An Insider's View 2023*

0289U   Neurology (Alzheimer disease), mRNA, gene expression profiling by RNA sequencing of 24 genes, whole blood, algorithm reported as predictive risk score
➔ *CPT Changes: An Insider's View 2023*

0290U   Pain management, mRNA, gene expression profiling by RNA sequencing of 36 genes, whole blood, algorithm reported as predictive risk score
➔ *CPT Changes: An Insider's View 2023*

0291U   Psychiatry (mood disorders), mRNA, gene expression profiling by RNA sequencing of 144 genes, whole blood, algorithm reported as predictive risk score
➔ *CPT Changes: An Insider's View 2023*

0292U   Psychiatry (stress disorders), mRNA, gene expression profiling by RNA sequencing of 72 genes, whole blood, algorithm reported as predictive risk score
➔ *CPT Changes: An Insider's View 2023*

0293U   Psychiatry (suicidal ideation), mRNA, gene expression profiling by RNA sequencing of 54 genes, whole blood, algorithm reported as predictive risk score
➔ *CPT Changes: An Insider's View 2023*

0294U   Longevity and mortality risk, mRNA, gene expression profiling by RNA sequencing of 18 genes, whole blood, algorithm reported as predictive risk score
➔ *CPT Changes: An Insider's View 2023*

0295U   Oncology (breast ductal carcinoma in situ), protein expression profiling by immunohistochemistry of 7 proteins (COX2, FOXA1, HER2, Ki-67, p16, PR, SIAH2), with 4 clinicopathologic factors (size, age, margin status, palpability), utilizing formalin-fixed paraffin-embedded (FFPE) tissue, algorithm reported as a recurrence risk score
➔ *CPT Changes: An Insider's View 2023*

0296U Oncology (oral and/or oropharyngeal cancer), gene expression profiling by RNA sequencing of at least 20 molecular features (eg, human and/or microbial mRNA), saliva, algorithm reported as positive or negative for signature associated with malignancy

➲ *CPT Changes: An Insider's View* 2023

0297U Oncology (pan tumor), whole genome sequencing of paired malignant and normal DNA specimens, fresh or formalin-fixed paraffin-embedded (FFPE) tissue, blood or bone marrow, comparative sequence analyses and variant identification

➲ *CPT Changes: An Insider's View* 2023

0298U Oncology (pan tumor), whole transcriptome sequencing of paired malignant and normal RNA specimens, fresh or formalin-fixed paraffin-embedded (FFPE) tissue, blood or bone marrow, comparative sequence analyses and expression level and chimeric transcript identification

➲ *CPT Changes: An Insider's View* 2023

0299U Oncology (pan tumor), whole genome optical genome mapping of paired malignant and normal DNA specimens, fresh frozen tissue, blood, or bone marrow, comparative structural variant identification

➲ *CPT Changes: An Insider's View* 2023

0300U Oncology (pan tumor), whole genome sequencing and optical genome mapping of paired malignant and normal DNA specimens, fresh tissue, blood, or bone marrow, comparative sequence analyses and variant identification

➲ *CPT Changes: An Insider's View* 2023

0301U Infectious agent detection by nucleic acid (DNA or RNA), Bartonella henselae and Bartonella quintana, droplet digital PCR (ddPCR);

➲ *CPT Changes: An Insider's View* 2023

0302U following liquid enrichment

➲ *CPT Changes: An Insider's View* 2023

0303U Hematology, red blood cell (RBC) adhesion to endothelial/ subendothelial adhesion molecules, functional assessment, whole blood, with algorithmic analysis and result reported as an RBC adhesion index; hypoxic

➲ *CPT Changes: An Insider's View* 2023

0304U normoxic

➲ *CPT Changes: An Insider's View* 2023

0305U Hematology, red blood cell (RBC) functionality and deformity as a function of shear stress, whole blood, reported as a maximum elongation index

➲ *CPT Changes: An Insider's View* 2023

0306U Oncology (minimal residual disease [MRD]), next-generation targeted sequencing analysis, cell-free DNA, initial (baseline) assessment to determine a patient-specific panel for future comparisons to evaluate for MRD

➲ *CPT Changes: An Insider's View* 2023

(Do not report 0306U in conjunction with 0307U)

0307U Oncology (minimal residual disease [MRD]), next-generation targeted sequencing analysis of a patient-specific panel, cell-free DNA, subsequent assessment with comparison to previously analyzed patient specimens to evaluate for MRD

➲ *CPT Changes: An Insider's View* 2023

(Do not report 0307U in conjunction with 0306U)

0308U Cardiology (coronary artery disease [CAD]), analysis of 3 proteins (high sensitivity [hs] troponin, adiponectin, and kidney injury molecule-1 [KIM-1]) with 3 clinical parameters (age, sex, history of cardiac intervention), plasma, algorithm reported as a risk score for obstructive CAD

➲ *CPT Changes: An Insider's View* 2023, 2024

0309U Cardiology (cardiovascular disease), analysis of 4 proteins (NT-proBNP, osteopontin, tissue inhibitor of metalloproteinase-1 [TIMP-1], and kidney injury molecule-1 [KIM-1]), plasma, algorithm reported as a risk score for major adverse cardiac event

➲ *CPT Changes: An Insider's View* 2023

0310U Pediatrics (vasculitis, Kawasaki disease [KD]), analysis of 3 biomarkers (NT-proBNP, C-reactive protein, and T-uptake), plasma, algorithm reported as a risk score for KD

➲ *CPT Changes: An Insider's View* 2023

0311U Infectious disease (bacterial), quantitative antimicrobial susceptibility reported as phenotypic minimum inhibitory concentration (MIC)–based antimicrobial susceptibility for each organism identified

➲ *CPT Changes: An Insider's View* 2023

(Do not report 0311U in conjunction with 87076, 87077, 0086U)

0312U Autoimmune diseases (eg, systemic lupus erythematosus [SLE]), analysis of 8 IgG autoantibodies and 2 cell-bound complement activation products using enzyme-linked immunosorbent immunoassay (ELISA), flow cytometry and indirect immunofluorescence, serum, or plasma and whole blood, individual components reported along with an algorithmic SLE-likelihood assessment

➲ *CPT Changes: An Insider's View* 2023

0313U Oncology (pancreas), DNA and mRNA next-generation sequencing analysis of 74 genes and analysis of CEA (CEACAM5) gene expression, pancreatic cyst fluid, algorithm reported as a categorical result (ie, negative, low probability of neoplasia or positive, high probability of neoplasia)

➲ *CPT Changes: An Insider's View* 2023

0314U Oncology (cutaneous melanoma), mRNA gene expression profiling by RT-PCR of 35 genes (32 content and 3 housekeeping), utilizing formalin-fixed paraffin-embedded (FFPE) tissue, algorithm reported as a categorical result (ie, benign, intermediate, malignant)

➡ *CPT Changes: An Insider's View* 2023

0315U Oncology (cutaneous squamous cell carcinoma), mRNA gene expression profiling by RT-PCR of 40 genes (34 content and 6 housekeeping), utilizing formalin-fixed paraffin-embedded (FFPE) tissue, algorithm reported as a categorical risk result (ie, Class 1, Class 2A, Class 2B)

➡ *CPT Changes: An Insider's View* 2023

0316U Borrelia burgdorferi (Lyme disease), OspA protein evaluation, urine

➡ *CPT Changes: An Insider's View* 2023

0317U Oncology (lung cancer), four-probe FISH (3q29, 3p22.1, 10q22.3, 10cen) assay, whole blood, predictive algorithm-generated evaluation reported as decreased or increased risk for lung cancer

➡ *CPT Changes: An Insider's View* 2023

0318U Pediatrics (congenital epigenetic disorders), whole genome methylation analysis by microarray for 50 or more genes, blood

➡ *CPT Changes: An Insider's View* 2023

0319U Nephrology (renal transplant), RNA expression by select transcriptome sequencing, using pretransplant peripheral blood, algorithm reported as a risk score for early acute rejection

➡ *CPT Changes: An Insider's View* 2023

0320U Nephrology (renal transplant), RNA expression by select transcriptome sequencing, using posttransplant peripheral blood, algorithm reported as a risk score for acute cellular rejection

➡ *CPT Changes: An Insider's View* 2023

0321U Infectious agent detection by nucleic acid (DNA or RNA), genitourinary pathogens, identification of 20 bacterial and fungal organisms and identification of 16 associated antibiotic-resistance genes, multiplex amplified probe technique

➡ *CPT Changes: An Insider's View* 2023

0322U Neurology (autism spectrum disorder [ASD]), quantitative measurements of 14 acyl carnitines and microbiome-derived metabolites, liquid chromatography with tandem mass spectrometry (LC-MS/MS), plasma, results reported as negative or positive for risk of metabolic subtypes associated with ASD

➡ *CPT Changes: An Insider's View* 2023

0323U Infectious agent detection by nucleic acid (DNA and RNA), central nervous system pathogen, metagenomic next-generation sequencing, cerebrospinal fluid (CSF), identification of pathogenic bacteria, viruses, parasites, or fungi

➡ *CPT Changes: An Insider's View* 2023
➡ *CPT Assistant* Aug 22:8-10

(0324U has been deleted)

(0325U has been deleted)

0326U Targeted genomic sequence analysis panel, solid organ neoplasm, cell-free circulating DNA analysis of 83 or more genes, interrogation for sequence variants, gene copy number amplifications, gene rearrangements, microsatellite instability and tumor mutational burden

➡ *CPT Changes: An Insider's View* 2023
➡ *CPT Assistant* Aug 22:8-10

0327U Fetal aneuploidy (trisomy 13, 18, and 21), DNA sequence analysis of selected regions using maternal plasma, algorithm reported as a risk score for each trisomy, includes sex reporting, if performed

➡ *CPT Changes: An Insider's View* 2023
➡ *CPT Assistant* Aug 22:8-10

0328U Drug assay, definitive, 120 or more drugs and metabolites, urine, quantitative liquid chromatography with tandem mass spectrometry (LC-MS/MS), includes specimen validity and algorithmic analysis describing drug or metabolite and presence or absence of risks for a significant patient-adverse event, per date of service

➡ *CPT Changes: An Insider's View* 2023
➡ *CPT Assistant* Aug 22:8-10

0329U Oncology (neoplasia), exome and transcriptome sequence analysis for sequence variants, gene copy number amplifications and deletions, gene rearrangements, microsatellite instability and tumor mutational burden utilizing DNA and RNA from tumor with DNA from normal blood or saliva for subtraction, report of clinically significant mutation(s) with therapy associations

➡ *CPT Changes: An Insider's View* 2023
➡ *CPT Assistant* Aug 22:8-10

0330U Infectious agent detection by nucleic acid (DNA or RNA), vaginal pathogen panel, identification of 27 organisms, amplified probe technique, vaginal swab

➡ *CPT Changes: An Insider's View* 2023
➡ *CPT Assistant* Aug 22:8-10

0331U Oncology (hematolymphoid neoplasia), optical genome mapping for copy number alterations and gene rearrangements utilizing DNA from blood or bone marrow, report of clinically significant alterations

➡ *CPT Changes: An Insider's View* 2023
➡ *CPT Assistant* Aug 22:8-10

0332U   Oncology (pan-tumor), genetic profiling of 8 DNA-regulatory (epigenetic) markers by quantitative polymerase chain reaction (qPCR), whole blood, reported as a high or low probability of responding to immune checkpoint–inhibitor therapy
➜ *CPT Changes: An Insider's View* 2023

0333U   Oncology (liver), surveillance for hepatocellular carcinoma (HCC) in high-risk patients, analysis of methylation patterns on circulating cell-free DNA (cfDNA) plus measurement of serum of AFP/AFP-L3 and oncoprotein des-gamma-carboxy-prothrombin (DCP), algorithm reported as normal or abnormal result
➜ *CPT Changes: An Insider's View* 2023

0334U   Oncology (solid organ), targeted genomic sequence analysis, formalin-fixed paraffin-embedded (FFPE) tumor tissue, DNA analysis, 84 or more genes, interrogation for sequence variants, gene copy number amplifications, gene rearrangements, microsatellite instability and tumor mutational burden
➜ *CPT Changes: An Insider's View* 2023

0335U   Rare diseases (constitutional/heritable disorders), whole genome sequence analysis, including small sequence changes, copy number variants, deletions, duplications, mobile element insertions, uniparental disomy (UPD), inversions, aneuploidy, mitochondrial genome sequence analysis with heteroplasmy and large deletions, short tandem repeat (STR) gene expansions, fetal sample, identification and categorization of genetic variants
➜ *CPT Changes: An Insider's View* 2023

(Do not report 0335U in conjunction with 81425, 0212U)

0336U   Rare diseases (constitutional/heritable disorders), whole genome sequence analysis, including small sequence changes, copy number variants, deletions, duplications, mobile element insertions, uniparental disomy (UPD), inversions, aneuploidy, mitochondrial genome sequence analysis with heteroplasmy and large deletions, short tandem repeat (STR) gene expansions, blood or saliva, identification and categorization of genetic variants, each comparator genome (eg, parent)
➜ *CPT Changes: An Insider's View* 2023

(Do not report 0336U in conjunction with 81426, 0213U)

0337U   Oncology (plasma cell disorders and myeloma), circulating plasma cell immunologic selection, identification, morphological characterization, and enumeration of plasma cells based on differential CD138, CD38, CD19, and CD45 protein biomarker expression, peripheral blood
➜ *CPT Changes: An Insider's View* 2023

0338U   Oncology (solid tumor), circulating tumor cell selection, identification, morphological characterization, detection and enumeration based on differential EpCAM, cytokeratins 8, 18, and 19, and CD45 protein biomarkers, and quantification of HER2 protein biomarker–expressing cells, peripheral blood
➜ *CPT Changes: An Insider's View* 2023

0339U   Oncology (prostate), mRNA expression profiling of *HOXC6* and *DLX1*, reverse transcription polymerase chain reaction (RT-PCR), first-void urine following digital rectal examination, algorithm reported as probability of high-grade cancer
➜ *CPT Changes: An Insider's View* 2023

0340U   Oncology (pan-cancer), analysis of minimal residual disease (MRD) from plasma, with assays personalized to each patient based on prior next-generation sequencing of the patient's tumor and germline DNA, reported as absence or presence of MRD, with disease-burden correlation, if appropriate
➜ *CPT Changes: An Insider's View* 2023

0341U   Fetal aneuploidy DNA sequencing comparative analysis, fetal DNA from products of conception, reported as normal (euploidy), monosomy, trisomy, or partial deletion/duplication, mosaicism, and segmental aneuploid
➜ *CPT Changes: An Insider's View* 2023

0342U   Oncology (pancreatic cancer), multiplex immunoassay of C5, C4, cystatin C, factor B, osteoprotegerin (OPG), gelsolin, IGFBP3, CA125 and multiplex electrochemiluminescent immunoassay (ECLIA) for CA19-9, serum, diagnostic algorithm reported qualitatively as positive, negative, or borderline
➜ *CPT Changes: An Insider's View* 2023

0343U   Oncology (prostate), exosome-based analysis of 442 small noncoding RNAs (sncRNAs) by quantitative reverse transcription polymerase chain reaction (RT-qPCR), urine, reported as molecular evidence of no-, low-, intermediate- or high-risk of prostate cancer
➜ *CPT Changes: An Insider's View* 2023

0344U   Hepatology (nonalcoholic fatty liver disease [NAFLD]), semiquantitative evaluation of 28 lipid markers by liquid chromatography with tandem mass spectrometry (LC-MS/MS), serum, reported as at-risk for nonalcoholic steatohepatitis (NASH) or not NASH
➜ *CPT Changes: An Insider's View* 2023

✷ **0345U**   Psychiatry (eg, depression, anxiety, attention deficit hyperactivity disorder [ADHD]), genomic analysis panel, variant analysis of 15 genes, including deletion/duplication analysis of *CYP2D6*
➜ *CPT Changes: An Insider's View* 2023

(For additional PLA code with identical clinical descriptor, see 0411U. See Appendix O to determine appropriate code assignment)

0346U   Beta amyloid, Aß40 and Aß42 by liquid chromatography with tandem mass spectrometry (LC-MS/MS), ratio, plasma
➜ *CPT Changes: An Insider's View* 2023

Pathology and Laboratory   **80047-89398, 0001U-0520U**

0347U Drug metabolism or processing (multiple conditions), whole blood or buccal specimen, DNA analysis, 16 gene report, with variant analysis and reported phenotypes

➔ *CPT Changes: An Insider's View* 2023

0348U Drug metabolism or processing (multiple conditions), whole blood or buccal specimen, DNA analysis, 25 gene report, with variant analysis and reported phenotypes

➔ *CPT Changes: An Insider's View* 2023

0349U Drug metabolism or processing (multiple conditions), whole blood or buccal specimen, DNA analysis, 27 gene report, with variant analysis, including reported phenotypes and impacted gene-drug interactions

➔ *CPT Changes: An Insider's View* 2023

0350U Drug metabolism or processing (multiple conditions), whole blood or buccal specimen, DNA analysis, 27 gene report, with variant analysis and reported phenotypes

➔ *CPT Changes: An Insider's View* 2023

▲ **0351U** Infectious disease (bacterial or viral), biochemical assays, tumor necrosis factor-related apoptosis-inducing ligand (TRAIL), interferon gamma-induced protein-10 (IP-10), and C-reactive protein, serum, or venous whole blood, algorithm reported as likelihood of bacterial infection

➔ *CPT Changes: An Insider's View* 2023, 2025

▶(0352U has been deleted. To report infectious disease, bacterial vaginosis and vaginitis, real-time PCR amplification of DNA markers for algorithm reported as high likelihood of bacterial vaginosis, use 81515)◀

▶(0353U has been deleted)◀

▶(0354U has been deleted)◀

0355U *APOL1 (apolipoprotein L1)* (eg, chronic kidney disease), risk variants (G1, G2)

➔ *CPT Changes: An Insider's View* 2024

▲ **0356U** Oncology (oropharyngeal or anal), evaluation of 17 DNA biomarkers using droplet digital PCR (ddPCR), cell-free DNA, algorithm reported as a prognostic risk score for cancer recurrence

➔ *CPT Changes: An Insider's View* 2024, 2025

(0357U has been deleted)

0358U Neurology (mild cognitive impairment), analysis of ß-amyloid 1-42 and 1-40, chemiluminescence enzyme immunoassay, cerebral spinal fluid, reported as positive, likely positive, or negative

➔ *CPT Changes: An Insider's View* 2024

0359U Oncology (prostate cancer), analysis of all prostate-specific antigen (PSA) structural isoforms by phase separation and immunoassay, plasma, algorithm reports risk of cancer

➔ *CPT Changes: An Insider's View* 2024

0360U Oncology (lung), enzyme-linked immunosorbent assay (ELISA) of 7 autoantibodies (p53, NY-ESO-1, CAGE, GBU4-5, SOX2, MAGE A4, and HuD), plasma, algorithm reported as a categorical result for risk of malignancy

➔ *CPT Changes: An Insider's View* 2024

0361U Neurofilament light chain, digital immunoassay, plasma, quantitative

➔ *CPT Changes: An Insider's View* 2024

0362U Oncology (papillary thyroid cancer), gene-expression profiling via targeted hybrid capture–enrichment RNA sequencing of 82 content genes and 10 housekeeping genes, fine needle aspirate or formalin-fixed paraffin-embedded (FFPE) tissue, algorithm reported as one of three molecular subtypes

➔ *CPT Changes: An Insider's View* 2024

0363U Oncology (urothelial), mRNA, gene-expression profiling by real-time quantitative PCR of 5 genes (*MDK, HOXA13, CDC2 [CDK1], IGFBP5,* and *CXCR2*), utilizing urine, algorithm incorporates age, sex, smoking history, and macrohematuria frequency, reported as a risk score for having urothelial carcinoma

➔ *CPT Changes: An Insider's View* 2024

0364U Oncology (hematolymphoid neoplasm), genomic sequence analysis using multiplex (PCR) and next-generation sequencing with algorithm, quantification of dominant clonal sequence(s), reported as presence or absence of minimal residual disease (MRD) with quantitation of disease burden, when appropriate

➔ *CPT Changes: An Insider's View* 2024

0365U Oncology (bladder), analysis of 10 protein biomarkers (A1AT, ANG, APOE, CA9, IL8, MMP9, MMP10, PAI1, SDC1, and VEGFA) by immunoassays, urine, algorithm reported as a probability of bladder cancer

➔ *CPT Changes: An Insider's View* 2024

0366U Oncology (bladder), analysis of 10 protein biomarkers (A1AT, ANG, APOE, CA9, IL8, MMP9, MMP10, PAI1, SDC1, and VEGFA) by immunoassays, urine, algorithm reported as a probability of recurrent bladder cancer

➔ *CPT Changes: An Insider's View* 2024

0367U Oncology (bladder), analysis of 10 protein biomarkers (A1AT, ANG, APOE, CA9, IL8, MMP9, MMP10, PAI1, SDC1, and VEGFA) by immunoassays, urine, diagnostic algorithm reported as a risk score for probability of rapid recurrence of recurrent or persistent cancer following transurethral resection

➔ *CPT Changes: An Insider's View* 2024

0368U Oncology (colorectal cancer), evaluation for mutations of *APC, BRAF, CTNNB1, KRAS, NRAS, PIK3CA, SMAD4,* and *TP53,* and methylation markers (MYO1G, KCNQ5, C9ORF50, FLI1, CLIP4, ZNF132, and TWIST1), multiplex quantitative polymerase chain reaction (qPCR), circulating cell-free DNA (cfDNA), plasma, report of risk score for advanced adenoma or colorectal cancer

➔ *CPT Changes: An Insider's View* 2024

Pathology and Laboratory 80047-89398, 0001U-0520U

0369U Infectious agent detection by nucleic acid (DNA and RNA), gastrointestinal pathogens, 31 bacterial, viral, and parasitic organisms and identification of 21 associated antibiotic-resistance genes, multiplex amplified probe technique

➔ *CPT Changes: An Insider's View* 2024

0370U Infectious agent detection by nucleic acid (DNA and RNA), surgical wound pathogens, 34 microorganisms and identification of 21 associated antibiotic-resistance genes, multiplex amplified probe technique, wound swab

➔ *CPT Changes: An Insider's View* 2024

0371U Infectious agent detection by nucleic acid (DNA or RNA), genitourinary pathogen, semiquantitative identification, DNA from 16 bacterial organisms and 1 fungal organism, multiplex amplified probe technique via quantitative polymerase chain reaction (qPCR), urine

➔ *CPT Changes: An Insider's View* 2024

0372U Infectious disease (genitourinary pathogens), antibiotic-resistance gene detection, multiplex amplified probe technique, urine, reported as an antimicrobial stewardship risk score

➔ *CPT Changes: An Insider's View* 2024

0373U Infectious agent detection by nucleic acid (DNA and RNA), respiratory tract infection, 17 bacteria, 8 fungus, 13 virus, and 16 antibiotic-resistance genes, multiplex amplified probe technique, upper or lower respiratory specimen

➔ *CPT Changes: An Insider's View* 2024

0374U Infectious agent detection by nucleic acid (DNA or RNA), genitourinary pathogens, identification of 21 bacterial and fungal organisms and identification of 21 associated antibiotic-resistance genes, multiplex amplified probe technique, urine

➔ *CPT Changes: An Insider's View* 2024

0375U Oncology (ovarian), biochemical assays of 7 proteins (follicle stimulating hormone, human epididymis protein 4, apolipoprotein A-1, transferrin, beta-2 macroglobulin, prealbumin [ie, transthyretin], and cancer antigen 125), algorithm reported as ovarian cancer risk score

➔ *CPT Changes: An Insider's View* 2024

0376U Oncology (prostate cancer), image analysis of at least 128 histologic features and clinical factors, prognostic algorithm determining the risk of distant metastases, and prostate cancer-specific mortality, includes predictive algorithm to androgen deprivation-therapy response, if appropriate

➔ *CPT Changes: An Insider's View* 2024

0377U Cardiovascular disease, quantification of advanced serum or plasma lipoprotein profile, by nuclear magnetic resonance (NMR) spectrometry with report of a lipoprotein profile (including 23 variables)

➔ *CPT Changes: An Insider's View* 2024

0378U *RFC1 (replication factor C subunit 1)*, repeat expansion variant analysis by traditional and repeat-primed PCR, blood, saliva, or buccal swab

➔ *CPT Changes: An Insider's View* 2024

0379U Targeted genomic sequence analysis panel, solid organ neoplasm, DNA (523 genes) and RNA (55 genes) by next-generation sequencing, interrogation for sequence variants, gene copy number amplifications, gene rearrangements, microsatellite instability, and tumor mutational burden

➔ *CPT Changes: An Insider's View* 2024

0380U Drug metabolism (adverse drug reactions and drug response), targeted sequence analysis, 20 gene variants and *CYP2D6* deletion or duplication analysis with reported genotype and phenotype

➔ *CPT Changes: An Insider's View* 2024

0381U Maple syrup urine disease monitoring by patient-collected blood card sample, quantitative measurement of allo-isoleucine, leucine, isoleucine, and valine, liquid chromatography with tandem mass spectrometry (LC-MS/MS)

➔ *CPT Changes: An Insider's View* 2024

0382U Hyperphenylalaninemia monitoring by patient-collected blood card sample, quantitative measurement of phenylalanine and tyrosine, liquid chromatography with tandem mass spectrometry (LC-MS/MS)

➔ *CPT Changes: An Insider's View* 2024

0383U Tyrosinemia type I monitoring by patient-collected blood card sample, quantitative measurement of tyrosine, phenylalanine, methionine, succinylacetone, nitisinone, liquid chromatography with tandem mass spectrometry (LC-MS/MS)

➔ *CPT Changes: An Insider's View* 2024

0384U Nephrology (chronic kidney disease), carboxymethyllysine, methylglyoxal hydroimidazolone, and carboxyethyl lysine by liquid chromatography with tandem mass spectrometry (LC-MS/MS) and HbA1c and estimated glomerular filtration rate (GFR), with risk score reported for predictive progression to high-stage kidney disease

➔ *CPT Changes: An Insider's View* 2024

0385U Nephrology (chronic kidney disease), apolipoprotein A4 (ApoA4), CD5 antigen-like (CD5L), and insulin-like growth factor binding protein 3 (IGFBP3) by enzyme-linked immunoassay (ELISA), plasma, algorithm combining results with HDL, estimated glomerular filtration rate (GFR) and clinical data reported as a risk score for developing diabetic kidney disease

➔ *CPT Changes: An Insider's View* 2024

(0386U has been deleted)

0387U Oncology (melanoma), autophagy and beclin 1 regulator 1 (AMBRA1) and loricrin (AMLo) by immunohistochemistry, formalin-fixed paraffin-embedded (FFPE) tissue, report for risk of progression

➔ *CPT Changes: An Insider's View* 2024

(Do not report 0387U in conjunction with 88341, 88342)

0388U Oncology (non-small cell lung cancer), next-generation sequencing with identification of single nucleotide variants, copy number variants, insertions and deletions, and structural variants in 37 cancer-related genes, plasma, with report for alteration detection

➔ *CPT Changes: An Insider's View* 2024

0389U Pediatric febrile illness (Kawasaki disease [KD]), interferon alpha-inducible protein 27 (IFI27) and mast cell-expressed membrane protein 1 (MCEMP1), RNA, using quantitative reverse transcription polymerase chain reaction (RT-qPCR), blood, reported as a risk score for KD

➔ *CPT Changes: An Insider's View* 2024

0390U Obstetrics (preeclampsia), kinase insert domain receptor (KDR), Endoglin (ENG), and retinol-binding protein 4 (RBP4), by immunoassay, serum, algorithm reported as a risk score

➔ *CPT Changes: An Insider's View* 2024

0391U Oncology (solid tumor), DNA and RNA by next-generation sequencing, utilizing formalin-fixed paraffin-embedded (FFPE) tissue, 437 genes, interpretive report for single nucleotide variants, splice-site variants, insertions/ deletions, copy number alterations, gene fusions, tumor mutational burden, and microsatellite instability, with algorithm quantifying immunotherapy response score

➔ *CPT Changes: An Insider's View* 2024

0392U Drug metabolism (depression, anxiety, attention deficit hyperactivity disorder [ADHD]), gene-drug interactions, variant analysis of 16 genes, including deletion/ duplication analysis of *CYP2D6*, reported as impact of gene-drug interaction for each drug

➔ *CPT Changes: An Insider's View* 2024

0393U Neurology (eg, Parkinson disease, dementia with Lewy bodies), cerebrospinal fluid (CSF), detection of misfolded α-synuclein protein by seed amplification assay, qualitative

➔ *CPT Changes: An Insider's View* 2024

0394U Perfluoroalkyl substances (PFAS) (eg, perfluorooctanoic acid, perfluorooctane sulfonic acid), 16 PFAS compounds by liquid chromatography with tandem mass spectrometry (LC-MS/MS), plasma or serum, quantitative

➔ *CPT Changes: An Insider's View* 2024

0395U Oncology (lung), multi-omics (microbial DNA by shotgun next-generation sequencing and carcinoembryonic antigen and osteopontin by immunoassay), plasma, algorithm reported as malignancy risk for lung nodules in early-stage disease

➔ *CPT Changes: An Insider's View* 2024

▶(0396U has been deleted)◀

(0397U has been deleted)

0398U Gastroenterology (Barrett's esophagus), *P16*, *RUNX3*, *HPP1*, and *FBN1* DNA methylation analysis using PCR, formalin-fixed paraffin-embedded (FFPE) tissue, algorithm reported as risk score for progression to high-grade dysplasia or cancer

➔ *CPT Changes: An Insider's View* 2024

0399U Neurology (cerebral folate deficiency), serum, detection of anti-human folate receptor IgG-binding antibody and blocking autoantibodies by enzyme-linked immunoassay (ELISA), qualitative, and blocking autoantibodies, using a functional blocking assay for IgG or IgM, quantitative, reported as positive or not detected

➔ *CPT Changes: An Insider's View* 2024

0400U Obstetrics (expanded carrier screening), 145 genes by next-generation sequencing, fragment analysis and multiplex ligation-dependent probe amplification, DNA, reported as carrier positive or negative

➔ *CPT Changes: An Insider's View* 2024

0401U Cardiology (coronary heart disease [CHD]), 9 genes (12 variants), targeted variant genotyping, blood, saliva, or buccal swab, algorithm reported as a genetic risk score for a coronary event

➔ *CPT Changes: An Insider's View* 2024

0402U Infectious agent (sexually transmitted infection), Chlamydia trachomatis, Neisseria gonorrhoeae, Trichomonas vaginalis, Mycoplasma genitalium, multiplex amplified probe technique, vaginal, endocervical, or male urine, each pathogen reported as detected or not detected

➔ *CPT Changes: An Insider's View* 2024

▲ **0403U** Oncology (prostate), mRNA, gene expression profiling of 18 genes, first-catch urine, algorithm reported as percentage of likelihood of detecting clinically significant prostate cancer

➔ *CPT Changes: An Insider's View* 2024, 2025

0404U Oncology (breast), semiquantitative measurement of thymidine kinase activity by immunoassay, serum, results reported as risk of disease progression

➔ *CPT Changes: An Insider's View* 2024

0405U Oncology (pancreatic), 59 methylation haplotype block markers, next-generation sequencing, plasma, reported as cancer signal detected or not detected

➔ *CPT Changes: An Insider's View* 2024

0406U Oncology (lung), flow cytometry, sputum, 5 markers (meso-tetra [4-carboxyphenyl] porphyrin [TCPP], CD206, CD66b, CD3, CD19), algorithm reported as likelihood of lung cancer

➔ *CPT Changes: An Insider's View* 2024

Pathology and Laboratory 80047-89398, 0001U-0520U

0407U Nephrology (diabetic chronic kidney disease [CKD]), multiplex electrochemiluminescent immunoassay (ECLIA) of soluble tumor necrosis factor receptor 1 (sTNFR1), soluble tumor necrosis receptor 2 (sTNFR2), and kidney injury molecule 1 (KIM-1) combined with clinical data, plasma, algorithm reported as risk for progressive decline in kidney function
➔ *CPT Changes: An Insider's View* 2024

0408U Infectious agent antigen detection by bulk acoustic wave biosensor immunoassay, severe acute respiratory syndrome coronavirus 2 (SARS-CoV-2) (coronavirus disease [COVID-19])
➔ *CPT Changes: An Insider's View* 2024

0409U Oncology (solid tumor), DNA (80 genes) and RNA (36 genes), by next-generation sequencing from plasma, including single nucleotide variants, insertions/deletions, copy number alterations, microsatellite instability, and fusions, report showing identified mutations with clinical actionability
➔ *CPT Changes: An Insider's View* 2024

0410U Oncology (pancreatic), DNA, whole genome sequencing with 5-hydroxymethylcytosine enrichment, whole blood or plasma, algorithm reported as cancer detected or not detected
➔ *CPT Changes: An Insider's View* 2024

✳ **0411U** Psychiatry (eg, depression, anxiety, attention deficit hyperactivity disorder [ADHD]), genomic analysis panel, variant analysis of 15 genes, including deletion/duplication analysis of *CYP2D6*
➔ *CPT Changes: An Insider's View* 2024

(For additional PLA code with identical clinical descriptor, see 0345U. See Appendix O to determine appropriate code assignment)

0412U Beta amyloid, Aβ42/40 ratio, immunoprecipitation with quantitation by liquid chromatography with tandem mass spectrometry (LC-MS/MS) and qualitative ApoE isoform-specific proteotyping, plasma combined with age, algorithm reported as presence or absence of brain amyloid pathology
➔ *CPT Changes: An Insider's View* 2024

0413U Oncology (hematolymphoid neoplasm), optical genome mapping for copy number alterations, aneuploidy, and balanced/complex structural rearrangements, DNA from blood or bone marrow, report of clinically significant alterations
➔ *CPT Changes: An Insider's View* 2024

0414U Oncology (lung), augmentative algorithmic analysis of digitized whole slide imaging for 8 genes *(ALK, BRAF, EGFR, ERBB2, MET, NTRK1-3, RET, ROS1),* and *KRAS* G12C and PD-L1, if performed, formalin-fixed paraffin-embedded (FFPE) tissue, reported as positive or negative for each biomarker
➔ *CPT Changes: An Insider's View* 2024

0415U Cardiovascular disease (acute coronary syndrome [ACS]), IL-16, FAS, FASLigand, HGF, CTACK, EOTAXIN, and MCP-3 by immunoassay combined with age, sex, family history, and personal history of diabetes, blood, algorithm reported as a 5-year (deleted risk) score for ACS
➔ *CPT Changes: An Insider's View* 2024

▶(0416U has been deleted)◀

0417U Rare diseases (constitutional/heritable disorders), whole mitochondrial genome sequence with heteroplasmy detection and deletion analysis, nuclear-encoded mitochondrial gene analysis of 335 nuclear genes, including sequence changes, deletions, insertions, and copy number variants analysis, blood or saliva, identification and categorization of mitochondrial disorder—associated genetic variants
➔ *CPT Changes: An Insider's View* 2024

0418U Oncology (breast), augmentative algorithmic analysis of digitized whole slide imaging of 8 histologic and immunohistochemical features, reported as a recurrence score
➔ *CPT Changes: An Insider's View* 2024

0419U Neuropsychiatry (eg, depression, anxiety), genomic sequence analysis panel, variant analysis of 13 genes, saliva or buccal swab, report of each gene phenotype
➔ *CPT Changes: An Insider's View* 2024

● **0420U** Oncology (urothelial), mRNA expression profiling by real-time quantitative PCR of *MDK, HOXA13, CDC2, IGFBP5,* and *CXCR2* in combination with droplet digital PCR (ddPCR) analysis of 6 single-nucleotide polymorphisms (SNPs) of genes *TERT* and *FGFR3,* urine, algorithm reported as a risk score for urothelial carcinoma
➔ *CPT Changes: An Insider's View* 2025

● **0421U** Oncology (colorectal) screening, quantitative real-time target and signal amplification of 8 RNA markers *(GAPDH, SMAD4, ACY1, AREG, CDH1, KRAS, TNFRSF10B, EGLN2)* and fecal hemoglobin, algorithm reported as a positive or negative for colorectal cancer risk
➔ *CPT Changes: An Insider's View* 2025

● **0422U** Oncology (pan-solid tumor), analysis of DNA biomarker response to anti-cancer therapy using cell-free circulating DNA, biomarker comparison to a previous baseline pre-treatment cell-free circulating DNA analysis using next-generation sequencing, algorithm reported as a quantitative change from baseline, including specific alterations, if appropriate
➔ *CPT Changes: An Insider's View* 2025

Pathology and Laboratory 80047-89398, 0001U-0520U

● **0423U**   Psychiatry (eg, depression, anxiety), genomic analysis panel, including variant analysis of 26 genes, buccal swab, report including metabolizer status and risk of drug toxicity by condition
→ *CPT Changes: An Insider's View* 2025

● **0424U**   Oncology (prostate), exosome-based analysis of 53 small noncoding RNAs (sncRNAs) by quantitative reverse transcription polymerase chain reaction (RT-qPCR), urine, reported as no molecular evidence, low-, moderate-, or elevated-risk of prostate cancer
→ *CPT Changes: An Insider's View* 2025

● **0425U**   Genome (eg, unexplained constitutional or heritable disorder or syndrome), rapid sequence analysis, each comparator genome (eg, parents, siblings)
→ *CPT Changes: An Insider's View* 2025

● **0426U**   Genome (eg, unexplained constitutional or heritable disorder or syndrome), ultra-rapid sequence analysis
→ *CPT Changes: An Insider's View* 2025

+● **0427U**   Monocyte distribution width, whole blood (List separately in addition to code for primary procedure)
→ *CPT Changes: An Insider's View* 2025

▶(Use 0427U in conjunction with 85004, 85025)◀

● **0428U**   Oncology (breast), targeted hybrid-capture genomic sequence analysis panel, circulating tumor DNA (ctDNA) analysis of 56 or more genes, interrogation for sequence variants, gene copy number amplifications, gene rearrangements, microsatellite instability, and tumor mutation burden
→ *CPT Changes: An Insider's View* 2025

● **0429U**   Human papillomavirus (HPV), oropharyngeal swab, 14 high-risk types (ie, 16, 18, 31, 33, 35, 39, 45, 51, 52, 56, 58, 59, 66, and 68)
→ *CPT Changes: An Insider's View* 2025

● **0430U**   Gastroenterology, malabsorption evaluation of alpha-1-antitrypsin, calprotectin, pancreatic elastase and reducing substances, feces, quantitative
→ *CPT Changes: An Insider's View* 2025

● **0431U**   Glycine receptor alpha1 IgG, serum or cerebrospinal fluid (CSF), live cell-binding assay (LCBA), qualitative
→ *CPT Changes: An Insider's View* 2025

● **0432U**   Kelch-like protein 11 (KLHL11) antibody, serum or cerebrospinal fluid (CSF), cell-binding assay, qualitative
→ *CPT Changes: An Insider's View* 2025

● **0433U**   Oncology (prostate), 5 DNA regulatory markers by quantitative PCR, whole blood, algorithm, including prostate-specific antigen, reported as likelihood of cancer
→ *CPT Changes: An Insider's View* 2025

● **0434U**   Drug metabolism (adverse drug reactions and drug response), genomic analysis panel, variant analysis of 25 genes with reported phenotypes
→ *CPT Changes: An Insider's View* 2025

● **0435U**   Oncology, chemotherapeutic drug cytotoxicity assay of cancer stem cells (CSCs), from cultured CSCs and primary tumor cells, categorical drug response reported based on cytotoxicity percentage observed, minimum of 14 drugs or drug combinations
→ *CPT Changes: An Insider's View* 2025

● **0436U**   Oncology (lung), plasma analysis of 388 proteins, using aptamer-based proteomics technology, predictive algorithm reported as clinical benefit from immune checkpoint inhibitor therapy
→ *CPT Changes: An Insider's View* 2025

● **0437U**   Psychiatry (anxiety disorders), mRNA, gene expression profiling by RNA sequencing of 15 biomarkers, whole blood, algorithm reported as predictive risk score
→ *CPT Changes: An Insider's View* 2025

● **0438U**   Drug metabolism (adverse drug reactions and drug response), buccal specimen, gene-drug interactions, variant analysis of 33 genes, including deletion/duplication analysis of *CYP2D6*, including reported phenotypes and impacted gene-drug interactions
→ *CPT Changes: An Insider's View* 2025

● **0439U**   Cardiology (coronary heart disease [CHD]), DNA, analysis of 5 single-nucleotide polymorphisms (SNPs) (rs11716050 [LOC105376934], rs6560711 [WDR37], rs3735222 [SCIN/LOC107986769], rs6820447 [intergenic], and rs9638144 [ESYT2]) and 3 DNA methylation markers (cg00300879 [transcription start site {TSS200} of CNKSR1], cg09552548 [intergenic], and cg14789911 [body of SPATC1L]), qPCR and digital PCR, whole blood, algorithm reported as a 4-tiered risk score for a 3-year risk of symptomatic CHD
→ *CPT Changes: An Insider's View* 2025

● **0440U**   Cardiology (coronary heart disease [CHD]), DNA, analysis of 10 single-nucleotide polymorphisms (SNPs) (rs710987 [LINC010019], rs1333048 [CDKN2B-AS1], rs12129789 [KCND3], rs942317 [KTN1-AS1], rs1441433 [PPP3CA], rs2869675 [PREX1], rs4639796 [ZBTB41], rs4376434 [LINC00972], rs12714414 [TMEM18], and rs7585056 [TMEM18]) and 6 DNA methylation markers (cg03725309 [SARS1], cg12586707 [CXCL1], cg04988978 [MPO], cg17901584 [DHCR24-DT], cg21161138 [AHRR], and cg12655112 [EHD4]), qPCR and digital PCR, whole blood, algorithm reported as detected or not detected for CHD
→ *CPT Changes: An Insider's View* 2025

● **0441U** Infectious disease (bacterial, fungal, or viral infection), semiquantitative biomechanical assessment (via deformability cytometry), whole blood, with algorithmic analysis and result reported as an index
➔ *CPT Changes: An Insider's View* 2025

● **0442U** Infectious disease (respiratory infection), Myxovirus resistance protein A (MxA) and C-reactive protein (CRP), fingerstick whole blood specimen, each biomarker reported as present or absent
➔ *CPT Changes: An Insider's View* 2025

● **0443U** Neurofilament light chain (NfL), ultra-sensitive immunoassay, serum or cerebrospinal fluid
➔ *CPT Changes: An Insider's View* 2025

● **0444U** Oncology (solid organ neoplasia), targeted genomic sequence analysis panel of 361 genes, interrogation for gene fusions, translocations, or other rearrangements, using DNA from formalin-fixed paraffin-embedded (FFPE) tumor tissue, report of clinically significant variant(s)
➔ *CPT Changes: An Insider's View* 2025

● **0445U** β-amyloid (Abeta42) and phospho tau (181P) (pTau181), electrochemiluminescent immunoassay (ECLIA), cerebral spinal fluid, ratio reported as positive or negative for amyloid pathology
➔ *CPT Changes: An Insider's View* 2025

● **0446U** Autoimmune diseases (systemic lupus erythematosus [SLE]), analysis of 10 cytokine soluble mediator biomarkers by immunoassay, plasma, individual components reported with an algorithmic risk score for current disease activity
➔ *CPT Changes: An Insider's View* 2025

● **0447U** Autoimmune diseases (systemic lupus erythematosus [SLE]), analysis of 11 cytokine soluble mediator biomarkers by immunoassay, plasma, individual components reported with an algorithmic prognostic risk score for developing a clinical flare
➔ *CPT Changes: An Insider's View* 2025

● **0448U** Oncology (lung and colon cancer), DNA, qualitative, next-generation sequencing detection of single-nucleotide variants and deletions in *EGFR* and *KRAS* genes, formalin-fixed paraffin-embedded (FFPE) solid tumor samples, reported as presence or absence of targeted mutation(s), with recommended therapeutic options
➔ *CPT Changes: An Insider's View* 2025

● **0449U** Carrier screening for severe inherited conditions (eg, cystic fibrosis, spinal muscular atrophy, beta hemoglobinopathies [including sickle cell disease], alpha thalassemia), regardless of race or self-identified ancestry, genomic sequence analysis panel, must include analysis of 5 genes *(CFTR, SMN1, HBB, HBA1, HBA2)*
➔ *CPT Changes: An Insider's View* 2025

● **0450U** Oncology (multiple myeloma), liquid chromatography with tandem mass spectrometry (LC-MS/MS), monoclonal paraprotein sequencing analysis, serum, results reported as baseline presence or absence of detectable clonotypic peptides
➔ *CPT Changes: An Insider's View* 2025

● **0451U** Oncology (multiple myeloma), LC-MS/MS, peptide ion quantification, serum, results compared with baseline to determine monoclonal paraprotein abundance
➔ *CPT Changes: An Insider's View* 2025

● **0452U** Oncology (bladder), methylated *PENK* DNA detection by linear target enrichment-quantitative methylation-specific real-time PCR (LTE-qMSP), urine, reported as likelihood of bladder cancer
➔ *CPT Changes: An Insider's View* 2025

● **0453U** Oncology (colorectal cancer), cell-free DNA (cfDNA), methylation-based quantitative PCR assay *(SEPTIN9, IKZF1, BCAT1, Septin9-2, VAV3, BCAN)*, plasma, reported as presence or absence of circulating tumor DNA (ctDNA)
➔ *CPT Changes: An Insider's View* 2025

✷● **0454U** Rare diseases (constitutional/heritable disorders), identification of copy number variations, inversions, insertions, translocations, and other structural variants by optical genome mapping
➔ *CPT Changes: An Insider's View* 2025

▶(For additional PLA codes with identical clinical descriptor, see 0260U, 0264U. See Appendix O or the most current listing on the AMA CPT website to determine appropriate code assignment)◀

● **0455U** Infectious agents (sexually transmitted infection), Chlamydia trachomatis, Neisseria gonorrhoeae, and Trichomonas vaginalis, multiplex amplified probe technique, vaginal, endocervical, gynecological specimens, oropharyngeal swabs, rectal swabs, female or male urine, each pathogen reported as detected or not detected
➔ *CPT Changes: An Insider's View* 2025

● **0456U** Autoimmune (rheumatoid arthritis), next-generation sequencing (NGS), gene expression testing of 19 genes, whole blood, with analysis of anti-cyclic citrullinated peptides (CCP) levels, combined with sex, patient global assessment, and body mass index (BMI), algorithm reported as a score that predicts nonresponse to tumor necrosis factor inhibitor (TNFi) therapy
➔ *CPT Changes: An Insider's View* 2025

● **0457U** Perfluoroalkyl substances (PFAS) (eg, perfluorooctanoic acid, perfluorooctane sulfonic acid), 9 PFAS compounds by LC-MS/MS, plasma or serum, quantitative
➔ *CPT Changes: An Insider's View* 2025

Pathology and Laboratory 80047-89398, 0001U-0520U

● **0458U**   Oncology (breast cancer), S100A8 and S100A9, by enzyme-linked immunosorbent assay (ELISA), tear fluid with age, algorithm reported as a risk score
➔ *CPT Changes: An Insider's View* 2025

● **0459U**   β-amyloid (Abeta42) and total tau (tTau), electrochemiluminescent immunoassay (ECLIA), cerebral spinal fluid, ratio reported as positive or negative for amyloid pathology
➔ *CPT Changes: An Insider's View* 2025

● **0460U**   Oncology, whole blood or buccal, DNA single-nucleotide polymorphism (SNP) genotyping by real-time PCR of 24 genes, with variant analysis and reported phenotypes
➔ *CPT Changes: An Insider's View* 2025

● **0461U**   Oncology, pharmacogenomic analysis of single-nucleotide polymorphism (SNP) genotyping by real-time PCR of 24 genes, whole blood or buccal swab, with variant analysis, including impacted gene-drug interactions and reported phenotypes
➔ *CPT Changes: An Insider's View* 2025

● **0462U**   Melatonin levels test, sleep study, 7 or 9 sample melatonin profile (cortisol optional), enzyme-linked immunosorbent assay (ELISA), saliva, screening/preliminary
➔ *CPT Changes: An Insider's View* 2025

● **0463U**   Oncology (cervix), mRNA gene expression profiling of 14 biomarkers (E6 and E7 of the highest-risk human papillomavirus [HPV] types 16, 18, 31, 33, 45, 52, 58), by real-time nucleic acid sequence-based amplification (NASBA), exo- or endocervical epithelial cells, algorithm reported as positive or negative for increased risk of cervical dysplasia or cancer for each biomarker
➔ *CPT Changes: An Insider's View* 2025

● **0464U**   Oncology (colorectal) screening, quantitative real-time target and signal amplification, methylated DNA markers, including LASS4, LRRC4 and PPP2R5C, a reference marker ZDHHC1, and a protein marker (fecal hemoglobin), utilizing stool, algorithm reported as a positive or negative result
➔ *CPT Changes: An Insider's View* 2025

● **0465U**   Oncology (urothelial carcinoma), DNA, quantitative methylation-specific PCR of 2 genes *(ONECUT2, VIM)*, algorithmic analysis reported as positive or negative
➔ *CPT Changes: An Insider's View* 2025

● **0466U**   Cardiology (coronary artery disease [CAD]), DNA, genome-wide association studies (564856 single-nucleotide polymorphisms [SNPs], targeted variant genotyping), patient lifestyle and clinical data, buccal swab, algorithm reported as polygenic risk to acquired heart disease
➔ *CPT Changes: An Insider's View* 2025

● **0467U**   Oncology (bladder), DNA, next-generation sequencing (NGS) of 60 genes and whole genome aneuploidy, urine, algorithms reported as minimal residual disease (MRD) status positive or negative and quantitative disease burden
➔ *CPT Changes: An Insider's View* 2025

● **0468U**   Hepatology (nonalcoholic steatohepatitis [NASH]), miR-34a-5p, alpha 2-macroglobulin, YKL40, HbA1c, serum and whole blood, algorithm reported as a single score for NASH activity and fibrosis
➔ *CPT Changes: An Insider's View* 2025

● **0469U**   Rare diseases (constitutional/heritable disorders), whole genome sequence analysis for chromosomal abnormalities, copy number variants, duplications/deletions, inversions, unbalanced translocations, regions of homozygosity (ROH), inheritance pattern that indicate uniparental disomy (UPD), and aneuploidy, fetal sample (amniotic fluid, chorionic villus sample, or products of conception), identification and categorization of genetic variants, diagnostic report of fetal results based on phenotype with maternal sample and paternal sample, if performed, as comparators and/or maternal cell contamination
➔ *CPT Changes: An Insider's View* 2025

● **0470U**   Oncology (oropharyngeal), detection of minimal residual disease by next-generation sequencing (NGS) based quantitative evaluation of 8 DNA targets, cell-free HPV 16 and 18 DNA from plasma
➔ *CPT Changes: An Insider's View* 2025

● **0471U**   Oncology (colorectal cancer), qualitative real-time PCR of 35 variants of *KRAS* and *NRAS* genes (exons 2, 3, 4), formalin-fixed paraffin-embedded (FFPE), predictive, identification of detected mutations
➔ *CPT Changes: An Insider's View* 2025

● **0472U**   Carbonic anhydrase VI (CA VI), parotid specific/secretory protein (PSP) and salivary protein (SP1) IgG, IgM, and IgA antibodies, enzyme-linked immunosorbent assay (ELISA), semiqualitative, blood, reported as predictive evidence of early Sjögren's syndrome
➔ *CPT Changes: An Insider's View* 2025

● **0473U**   Oncology (solid tumor), next-generation sequencing (NGS) of DNA from formalin-fixed paraffin-embedded (FFPE) tissue with comparative sequence analysis from a matched normal specimen (blood or saliva), 648 genes, interrogation for sequence variants, insertion and deletion alterations, copy number variants, rearrangements, microsatellite instability, and tumor-mutation burden
➔ *CPT Changes: An Insider's View* 2025

● **0474U**   Hereditary pan-cancer (eg, hereditary sarcomas, hereditary endocrine tumors, hereditary neuroendocrine tumors, hereditary cutaneous melanoma), genomic sequence analysis panel of 88 genes with 20 duplications/deletions using next-generation sequencing (NGS), Sanger sequencing, blood or saliva, reported as positive or negative for germline variants, each gene
➔ *CPT Changes: An Insider's View* 2025

● **0475U** Hereditary prostate cancer-related disorders, genomic sequence analysis panel using next-generation sequencing (NGS), Sanger sequencing, multiplex ligation-dependent probe amplification (MLPA), and array comparative genomic hybridization (CGH), evaluation of 23 genes and duplications/deletions when indicated, pathologic mutations reported with a genetic risk score for prostate cancer
➔ *CPT Changes: An Insider's View* 2025

● **0476U** Drug metabolism, psychiatry (eg, major depressive disorder, general anxiety disorder, attention deficit hyperactivity disorder [ADHD], schizophrenia), whole blood, buccal swab, and pharmacogenomic genotyping of 14 genes and *CYP2D6* copy number variant analysis and reported phenotypes
➔ *CPT Changes: An Insider's View* 2025

● **0477U** Drug metabolism, psychiatry (eg, major depressive disorder, general anxiety disorder, attention deficit hyperactivity disorder [ADHD], schizophrenia), whole blood, buccal swab, and pharmacogenomic genotyping of 14 genes and *CYP2D6* copy number variant analysis, including impacted gene-drug interactions and reported phenotypes
➔ *CPT Changes: An Insider's View* 2025

● **0478U** Oncology (non-small cell lung cancer), DNA and RNA, digital PCR analysis of 9 genes *(EGFR, KRAS, BRAF, ALK, ROS1, RET, NTRK 1/2/3, ERBB2,* and *MET)* in formalin-fixed paraffin-embedded (FFPE) tissue, interrogation for single-nucleotide variants, insertions/deletions, gene rearrangements, and reported as actionable detected variants for therapy selection
➔ *CPT Changes: An Insider's View* 2025

● **0479U** Tau, phosphorylated, pTau217
➔ *CPT Changes: An Insider's View* 2025

● **0480U** Infectious disease (bacteria, viruses, fungi, and parasites), cerebrospinal fluid (CSF), metagenomic next-generation sequencing (DNA and RNA), bioinformatic analysis, with positive pathogen identification
➔ *CPT Changes: An Insider's View* 2025

● **0481U** *IDH1 (isocitrate dehydrogenase 1 [NADP+]), IDH2 (isocitrate dehydrogenase 2 [NADP+]),* and *TERT (telomerase reverse transcriptase)* promoter (eg, central nervous system [CNS] tumors), next-generation sequencing (single-nucleotide variants [SNV], deletions, and insertions)
➔ *CPT Changes: An Insider's View* 2025

● **0482U** Obstetrics (preeclampsia), biochemical assay of soluble fms-like tyrosine kinase 1 (sFlt-1) and placental growth factor (PlGF), serum, ratio reported for sFlt-1/PlGF, with risk of progression for preeclampsia with severe features within 2 weeks
➔ *CPT Changes: An Insider's View* 2025

● **0483U** Infectious disease (Neisseria gonorrhoeae), sensitivity, ciprofloxacin resistance (gyrA S91F point mutation), oral, rectal, or vaginal swab, algorithm reported as probability of fluoroquinolone resistance
➔ *CPT Changes: An Insider's View* 2025

● **0484U** Infectious disease (Mycoplasma genitalium), macrolide sensitivity (23S rRNA point mutation), oral, rectal, or vaginal swab, algorithm reported as probability of macrolide resistance
➔ *CPT Changes: An Insider's View* 2025

● **0485U** Oncology (solid tumor), cell-free DNA and RNA by next-generation sequencing, interpretative report for germline mutations, clonal hematopoiesis of indeterminate potential, and tumor-derived single-nucleotide variants, small insertions/deletions, copy number alterations, fusions, microsatellite instability, and tumor mutational burden
➔ *CPT Changes: An Insider's View* 2025

● **0486U** Oncology (pan-solid tumor), next-generation sequencing analysis of tumor methylation markers present in cell-free circulating tumor DNA, algorithm reported as quantitative measurement of methylation as a correlate of tumor fraction
➔ *CPT Changes: An Insider's View* 2025

● **0487U** Oncology (solid tumor), cell-free circulating DNA, targeted genomic sequence analysis panel of 84 genes, interrogation for sequence variants, aneuploidy-corrected gene copy number amplifications and losses, gene rearrangements, and microsatellite instability
➔ *CPT Changes: An Insider's View* 2025

● **0488U** Obstetrics (fetal antigen noninvasive prenatal test), cell-free DNA sequence analysis for detection of fetal presence or absence of 1 or more of the Rh, C, c, D, E, Duffy (Fya), or Kell (K) antigen in alloimmunized pregnancies, reported as selected antigen(s) detected or not detected
➔ *CPT Changes: An Insider's View* 2025

● **0489U** Obstetrics (single-gene noninvasive prenatal test), cell-free DNA sequence analysis of 1 or more targets (eg, *CFTR, SMN1, HBB, HBA1, HBA2)* to identify paternally inherited pathogenic variants, and relative mutation-dosage analysis based on molecular counts to determine fetal inheritance of maternal mutation, algorithm reported as a fetal risk score for the condition (eg, cystic fibrosis, spinal muscular atrophy, beta hemoglobinopathies [including sickle cell disease], alpha thalassemia)
➔ *CPT Changes: An Insider's View* 2025

● **0490U** Oncology (cutaneous or uveal melanoma), circulating tumor cell selection, morphological characterization and enumeration based on differential CD146, high molecular–weight melanoma-associated antigen, CD34 and CD45 protein biomarkers, peripheral blood
➔ *CPT Changes: An Insider's View* 2025

Pathology and Laboratory 80047-89398, 0001U-0520U

● **0491U**   Oncology (solid tumor), circulating tumor cell selection, morphological characterization and enumeration based on differential epithelial cell adhesion molecule (EpCAM), cytokeratins 8, 18, and 19, CD45 protein biomarkers, and quantification of estrogen receptor (ER) protein biomarker–expressing cells, peripheral blood
➔ *CPT Changes: An Insider's View* 2025

● **0492U**   Oncology (solid tumor), circulating tumor cell selection, morphological characterization and enumeration based on differential epithelial cell adhesion molecule (EpCAM), cytokeratins 8, 18, and 19, CD45 protein biomarkers, and quantification of PD-L1 protein biomarker–expressing cells, peripheral blood
➔ *CPT Changes: An Insider's View* 2025

● **0493U**   Transplantation medicine, quantification of donor-derived cell-free DNA (cfDNA) using next-generation sequencing, plasma, reported as percentage of donor-derived cell-free DNA
➔ *CPT Changes: An Insider's View* 2025

● **0494U**   Red blood cell antigen (fetal RhD gene analysis), next-generation sequencing of circulating cell-free DNA (cfDNA) of blood in pregnant individuals known to be RhD negative, reported as positive or negative
➔ *CPT Changes: An Insider's View* 2025

● **0495U**   Oncology (prostate), analysis of circulating plasma proteins (tPSA, fPSA, KLK2, PSP94, and GDF15), germline polygenic risk score (60 variants), clinical information (age, family history of prostate cancer, prior negative prostate biopsy), algorithm reported as risk of likelihood of detecting clinically significant prostate cancer
➔ *CPT Changes: An Insider's View* 2025

● **0496U**   Oncology (colorectal), cell-free DNA, 8 genes for mutations, 7 genes for methylation by real-time RT-PCR, and 4 proteins by enzyme-linked immunosorbent assay, blood, reported positive or negative for colorectal cancer or advanced adenoma risk
➔ *CPT Changes: An Insider's View* 2025

● **0497U**   Oncology (prostate), mRNA gene-expression profiling by real-time RT-PCR of 6 genes *(FOXM1, MCM3, MTUS1, TTC21B, ALAS1,* and *PPP2CA),* utilizing formalin-fixed paraffin-embedded (FFPE) tissue, algorithm reported as a risk score for prostate cancer
➔ *CPT Changes: An Insider's View* 2025

● **0498U**   Oncology (colorectal), next-generation sequencing for mutation detection in 43 genes and methylation pattern in 45 genes, blood, and formalin-fixed paraffin-embedded (FFPE) tissue, report of variants and methylation pattern with interpretation
➔ *CPT Changes: An Insider's View* 2025

● **0499U**   Oncology (colorectal and lung), DNA from formalin-fixed paraffin-embedded (FFPE) tissue, next-generation sequencing of 8 genes *(NRAS, EGFR, CTNNB1, PIK3CA, APC, BRAF, KRAS,* and *TP53),* mutation detection
➔ *CPT Changes: An Insider's View* 2025

● **0500U**   Autoinflammatory disease (VEXAS syndrome), DNA, *UBA1* gene mutations, targeted variant analysis (M41T, M41V, M41L, c.118-2A>C, c.118-1G>C, c.118-9_118-2del, S56F, S621C)
➔ *CPT Changes: An Insider's View* 2025

● **0501U**   Oncology (colorectal), blood, quantitative measurement of cell-free DNA (cfDNA)
➔ *CPT Changes: An Insider's View* 2025

● **0502U**   Human papillomavirus (HPV), E6/E7 markers for high-risk types (16, 18, 31, 33, 35, 39, 45, 51, 52, 56, 58, 59, 66, and 68), cervical cells, branched-chain capture hybridization, reported as negative or positive for high risk for HPV
➔ *CPT Changes: An Insider's View* 2025

● **0503U**   Neurology (Alzheimer disease), beta amyloid (Aβ40, Aβ42, Aβ42/40 ratio) and tau-protein (ptau217, np-tau217, ptau217/np-tau217 ratio), blood, immunoprecipitation with quantitation by liquid chromatography with tandem mass spectrometry (LC-MS/MS), algorithm score reported as likelihood of positive or negative for amyloid plaques
➔ *CPT Changes: An Insider's View* 2025

● **0504U**   Infectious disease (urinary tract infection), identification of 17 pathologic organisms, urine, real-time PCR, reported as positive or negative for each organism
➔ *CPT Changes: An Insider's View* 2025

● **0505U**   Infectious disease (vaginal infection), identification of 32 pathogenic organisms, swab, real-time PCR, reported as positive or negative for each organism
➔ *CPT Changes: An Insider's View* 2025

● **0506U**   Gastroenterology (Barrett's esophagus), esophageal cells, DNA methylation analysis by next-generation sequencing of at least 89 differentially methylated genomic regions, algorithm reported as likelihood for Barrett's esophagus
➔ *CPT Changes: An Insider's View* 2025

● **0507U**   Oncology (ovarian), DNA, whole-genome sequencing with 5-hydroxymethylcytosine (5hmC) enrichment, using whole blood or plasma, algorithm reported as cancer detected or not detected
➔ *CPT Changes: An Insider's View* 2025

● **0508U**   Transplantation medicine, quantification of donor-derived cell-free DNA using 40 single-nucleotide polymorphisms (SNPs), plasma, and urine, initial evaluation reported as percentage of donor-derived cell-free DNA with risk for active rejection
➔ *CPT Changes: An Insider's View* 2025

● **0509U**   Transplantation medicine, quantification of donor-derived cell-free DNA using up to 12 single-nucleotide polymorphisms (SNPs) previously identified, plasma, reported as percentage of donor-derived cell-free DNA with risk for active rejection
   ➔ *CPT Changes: An Insider's View* 2025

● **0510U**   Oncology (pancreatic cancer), augmentative algorithmic analysis of 16 genes from previously sequenced RNA whole-transcriptome data, reported as probability of predicted molecular subtype
   ➔ *CPT Changes: An Insider's View* 2025

● **0511U**   Oncology (solid tumor), tumor cell culture in 3D microenvironment, 36 or more drug panel, reported as tumor-response prediction for each drug
   ➔ *CPT Changes: An Insider's View* 2025

● **0512U**   Oncology (prostate), augmentative algorithmic analysis of digitized whole-slide imaging of histologic features for microsatellite instability (MSI) status, formalin-fixed paraffin-embedded (FFPE) tissue, reported as increased or decreased probability of MSI-high (MSI-H)
   ➔ *CPT Changes: An Insider's View* 2025

● **0513U**   Oncology (prostate), augmentative algorithmic analysis of digitized whole-slide imaging of histologic features for microsatellite instability (MSI) and homologous recombination deficiency (HRD) status, formalin-fixed paraffin-embedded (FFPE) tissue, reported as increased or decreased probability of each biomarker
   ➔ *CPT Changes: An Insider's View* 2025

● **0514U**   Gastroenterology (irritable bowel disease [IBD]), immunoassay for quantitative determination of adalimumab (ADL) levels in venous serum in patients undergoing adalimumab therapy, results reported as a numerical value as micrograms per milliliter (µg/mL)
   ➔ *CPT Changes: An Insider's View* 2025

● **0515U**   Gastroenterology (irritable bowel disease [IBD]), immunoassay for quantitative determination of infliximab (IFX) levels in venous serum in patients undergoing infliximab therapy, results reported as a numerical value as micrograms per milliliter (µg/mL)
   ➔ *CPT Changes: An Insider's View* 2025

● **0516U**   Drug metabolism, whole blood, pharmacogenomic genotyping of 40 genes and *CYP2D6* copy number variant analysis, reported as metabolizer status
   ➔ *CPT Changes: An Insider's View* 2025

● **0517U**   Therapeutic drug monitoring, 80 or more psychoactive drugs or substances, LC-MS/MS, plasma, qualitative and quantitative therapeutic minimally and maximally effective dose of prescribed and non-prescribed medications
   ➔ *CPT Changes: An Insider's View* 2025

● **0518U**   Therapeutic drug monitoring, 90 or more pain and mental health drugs or substances, LC-MS/MS, plasma, qualitative and quantitative therapeutic minimally effective range of prescribed and non-prescribed medications
   ➔ *CPT Changes: An Insider's View* 2025

● **0519U**   Therapeutic drug monitoring, medications specific to pain, depression, and anxiety, LC-MS/MS, plasma, 110 or more drugs or substances, qualitative and quantitative therapeutic minimally effective range of prescribed, non-prescribed, and illicit medications in circulation
   ➔ *CPT Changes: An Insider's View* 2025

● **0520U**   Therapeutic drug monitoring, 200 or more drugs or substances, LC-MS/MS, plasma, qualitative and quantitative therapeutic minimally effective range of prescribed and non-prescribed medications
   ➔ *CPT Changes: An Insider's View* 2025

Pathology and Laboratory 80047-89398, 0001U-0520U

Notes

Medicine Guidelines

Medicine

The following is a listing of headings and subheadings that appear within the Medicine section of the CPT codebook. The subheadings or subsections denoted with asterisks (*) below have special instructions unique to that subsection. Where these are indicated, special notes or guidelines will be presented preceding those procedural terminology listings, referring to that subsection specifically. Note that all code ranges in each subsection are listed as they appear in the subsection, even if the code numbers are out of numerical sequence and/or repeated in the next subsection.

Medicine 90281-99607

Medicine Guidelines

In addition to the definitions and commonly used terms presented in the **Introduction**, several other items unique to this section on **Medicine** are defined or identified here.

Add-on Codes

Some of the listed procedures are commonly carried out in addition to the primary procedure performed. All add-on codes found in the CPT codebook are exempt from the multiple procedure concept. They are exempt from the use of modifier 51, as these procedures are not reported as stand-alone codes. These additional or supplemental procedures are designated as "add-on" codes. Add-on codes in the CPT codebook can be readily identified by specific descriptor nomenclature which includes phrases such as "each additional" or "(List separately in addition to primary procedure)."

Separate Procedures

Some of the procedures or services listed in the CPT codebook that are commonly carried out as an integral component of a total service or procedure have been identified by the inclusion of the term "separate procedure." The codes designated as "separate procedure" should not be reported in addition to the code for the total procedure or service of which it is considered an integral component.

However, when a procedure or service that is designated as a "separate procedure" is carried out independently or considered to be unrelated or distinct from other procedures/services provided at that time, it may be reported by itself, or in addition to other procedures/services by appending modifier 59 to the specific "separate procedure" code to indicate that the procedure is not considered to be a component of another procedure, but is a distinct, independent procedure. This may represent a different session or patient encounter, different procedure or surgery, different site or organ system, separate incision/excision, separate lesion, or separate injury (or area of injury in extensive injuries).

Unlisted Service or Procedure

A service or procedure may be provided that is not listed in this edition of the CPT codebook. When reporting such a service, the appropriate "Unlisted Procedure" code may be used to indicate the service, identifying it by "Special Report" as discussed on the following page. The "Unlisted Procedures" and accompanying codes for **Medicine** are as follows:

90399	Unlisted immune globulin
90749	Unlisted vaccine/toxoid
90899	Unlisted psychiatric service or procedure
90999	Unlisted dialysis procedure, inpatient or outpatient
91299	Unlisted diagnostic gastroenterology procedure
92499	Unlisted ophthalmological service or procedure
92700	Unlisted otorhinolaryngological service or procedure
93799	Unlisted cardiovascular service or procedure
93998	Unlisted noninvasive vascular diagnostic study
94799	Unlisted pulmonary service or procedure
95199	Unlisted allergy/clinical immunologic service or procedure
95999	Unlisted neurological or neuromuscular diagnostic procedure
96379	Unlisted therapeutic, prophylactic, or diagnostic intravenous or intra-arterial injection or infusion
96549	Unlisted chemotherapy procedure
96999	Unlisted special dermatological service or procedure
97039	Unlisted modality (specify type and time if constant attendance)
97139	Unlisted therapeutic procedure (specify)
97799	Unlisted physical medicine/rehabilitation service or procedure
99199	Unlisted special service, procedure or report
99600	Unlisted home visit service or procedure

Special Report

A service that is rarely provided, unusual, variable, or new may require a special report. Pertinent information should include an adequate definition or description of the nature, extent, and need for the procedure; and the time, effort, and equipment necessary to provide the service.

Imaging Guidance

When imaging guidance or imaging supervision and interpretation is included in a procedure, guidelines for image documentation and report, included in the guidelines for Radiology (including Nuclear Medicine and Diagnostic Ultrasound) will apply. Imaging guidance should not be reported for use of a non-imaging guided tracking or localizing system (eg, radar signals, electromagnetic signals). Imaging guidance should only be reported when an imaging modality (eg, radiography, fluoroscopy, ultrasonography, magnetic resonance imaging, computed tomography, or nuclear medicine) is used and is appropriately documented.

Supplied Materials

Supplies and materials (eg, trays, drug supplies, and materials) over and above those usually included with the procedure(s) rendered are reported separately using code 99070 or a specific supply code.

Foreign Body/Implant Definition

An object intentionally placed by a physician or other qualified health care professional for any purpose (eg, diagnostic or therapeutic) is considered an implant. An object that is unintentionally placed (eg, trauma or ingestion) is considered a foreign body. If an implant (or part thereof) has moved from its original position or is structurally broken and no longer serves its intended purpose or presents a hazard to the patient, it qualifies as a foreign body for coding purposes, unless CPT coding instructions direct otherwise or a specific CPT code exists to describe the removal of that broken/moved implant.

Medicine

Immune Globulins, Serum or Recombinant Products

Codes 90281-90399 identify the serum globulins, extracted from human blood; or recombinant immune globulin products created in a laboratory through genetic modification of human and/or animal proteins. Both are reported in addition to the administration codes 96365, 96366, 96367, 96368, 96369, 96370, 96371, 96372, 96374, 96375, as appropriate. Modifier 51 should not be reported with this section of products codes when performed with another procedure. The serum or recombinant globulin products listed here include broad-spectrum anti-infective immune globulins, antitoxins, various isoantibodies, and monoclonal antibodies. See the Introduction section of the CPT code set for a complete list of the dates of release and implementation.

To assist users in reporting the most recent new or revised immune globulin product codes, the American Medical Association (AMA) currently uses the CPT website (ama-assn.org/cpt-cat-i-immunization-codes) to feature updates from the CPT Editorial Panel actions regarding these products. See the Introduction section of the CPT code set for a complete list of the dates of release and implementation.

In recognition of public health interest in immune globulin products, the CPT Editorial Panel has chosen to publish new immune globulin product codes prior to approval by the US Food and Drug Administration (FDA). These codes are indicated with the ⚯ symbol and will be tracked by the AMA to monitor FDA approval status. Once the FDA status changes to approved, the ⚯ symbol will be removed. CPT code users should refer to the AMA CPT website (ama-assn.org/cpt-cat-i-immunization-codes) for the most up-to-date information on codes with the ⚯ symbol.

90281   Immune globulin (Ig), human, for intramuscular use
➡ *CPT Changes: An Insider's View* 2008
➡ *CPT Assistant* Nov 98:30, Jan 99:3, Sep 99:10

90283   Immune globulin (IgIV), human, for intravenous use
➡ *CPT Changes: An Insider's View* 2008
➡ *CPT Assistant* Nov 98:30, Jan 99:3

90284   Immune globulin (SCIg), human, for use in subcutaneous infusions, 100 mg, each
➡ *CPT Changes: An Insider's View* 2008

90287   Botulinum antitoxin, equine, any route
➡ *CPT Changes: An Insider's View* 2008
➡ *CPT Assistant* Nov 98:30, Jan 99:3

90288   Botulism immune globulin, human, for intravenous use
➡ *CPT Changes: An Insider's View* 2008
➡ *CPT Assistant* Nov 98:30, Jan 99:3

90291   Cytomegalovirus immune globulin (CMV-IgIV), human, for intravenous use
➡ *CPT Changes: An Insider's View* 2008
➡ *CPT Assistant* Nov 98:30, Jan 99:3

90296   Diphtheria antitoxin, equine, any route
➡ *CPT Changes: An Insider's View* 2008
➡ *CPT Assistant* Nov 98:30, Jan 99:3

90371   Hepatitis B immune globulin (HBIg), human, for intramuscular use
➡ *CPT Changes: An Insider's View* 2008
➡ *CPT Assistant* Nov 98:30, Jan 99:3

90375   Rabies immune globulin (RIg), human, for intramuscular and/or subcutaneous use
➡ *CPT Changes: An Insider's View* 2008
➡ *CPT Assistant* Nov 98:30, Jan 99:3

90376   Rabies immune globulin, heat-treated (RIg-HT), human, for intramuscular and/or subcutaneous use
➡ *CPT Changes: An Insider's View* 2008
➡ *CPT Assistant* Nov 98:30, Jan 99:3

90377   Rabies immune globulin, heat- and solvent/detergent-treated (RIg-HT S/D), human, for intramuscular and/or subcutaneous use
➡ *CPT Changes: An Insider's View* 2021

90378   Respiratory syncytial virus, monoclonal antibody, recombinant, for intramuscular use, 50 mg, each
➡ *CPT Changes: An Insider's View* 2000, 2001, 2008, 2010
➡ *CPT Assistant* Jan 99:3, Nov 99:47, Jun 00:10

90380   Respiratory syncytial virus, monoclonal antibody, seasonal dose; 0.5 mL dosage, for intramuscular use
➡ *CPT Changes: An Insider's View* 2024
➡ *CPT Assistant* Nov 23:15, Feb 24:1

90381   1 mL dosage, for intramuscular use
➡ *CPT Changes: An Insider's View* 2024
➡ *CPT Assistant* Nov 23:15, Feb 24:1

▶(Do not report 90380, 90381 in conjunction with 96372)◀

▶(For administration of respiratory syncytial virus, monoclonal antibody, seasonal dose, see 96380, 96381)◀

90384   Rho(D) immune globulin (RhIg), human, full-dose, for intramuscular use
➡ *CPT Changes: An Insider's View* 2008
➡ *CPT Assistant* Nov 98:30, Jan 99:3

90385   Rho(D) immune globulin (RhIg), human, mini-dose, for intramuscular use
➔ *CPT Changes: An Insider's View* 2008
➔ *CPT Assistant* Nov 98:30, Jan 99:3

90386   Rho(D) immune globulin (RhIgIV), human, for intravenous use
➔ *CPT Changes: An Insider's View* 2008
➔ *CPT Assistant* Nov 98:30, Jan 99:3

90389   Tetanus immune globulin (TIg), human, for intramuscular use
➔ *CPT Changes: An Insider's View* 2008
➔ *CPT Assistant* Nov 98:30, Jan 99:3

90393   Vaccinia immune globulin, human, for intramuscular use
➔ *CPT Changes: An Insider's View* 2008
➔ *CPT Assistant* Nov 98:30, Jan 99:3

90396   Varicella-zoster immune globulin, human, for intramuscular use
➔ *CPT Changes: An Insider's View* 2008
➔ *CPT Assistant* Nov 98:30, Jan 99:3

90399   Unlisted immune globulin
➔ *CPT Changes: An Insider's View* 2008
➔ *CPT Assistant* Nov 98:30, Jan 99:3, Feb 99:11, Sep 99:10

Immunization Administration for Vaccines/Toxoids

▶Report vaccine immunization administration codes (90460, 90461, 90471-90474, 90480) in addition to the vaccine and toxoid code(s) (90476-90759, 91304, 91318, 91319, 91320, 91321, 91322).◀

Report codes 90460 and 90461 only when the physician or other qualified health care professional provides face-to-face counseling of the patient/family during the administration of a vaccine other than when performed for severe acute respiratory syndrome coronavirus 2 (SARS-CoV-2) (coronavirus disease [COVID-19]) vaccines. For immunization administration of any vaccine, other than SARS-CoV-2 (coronavirus disease [COVID-19]) vaccines, that is not accompanied by face-to-face physician or other qualified health care professional counseling to the patient/family/guardian or for administration of vaccines to patients over 18 years of age, report codes 90471-90474. (See also **Instructions for Use of the CPT Codebook** for definition of reporting qualifications.)

▶Report 90480 for immunization administration of SARS-CoV-2 (coronavirus disease [COVID-19]) vaccines only. This code is used for administration and counseling that involves the use of COVID-19 vaccines for immunization against contracting disease. This includes administration of COVID-19 vaccine for all age populations.◀

If a significant separately identifiable evaluation and management service (eg, new or established patient office or other outpatient services [99202-99215], office or other outpatient consultations [99242, 99243, 99244, 99245], emergency department services [99281-99285], preventive medicine services [99381-99429]) is performed, the appropriate E/M service code should be reported in addition to the vaccine and toxoid administration codes.

A component refers to all antigens in a vaccine that prevent disease(s) caused by one organism (90460 and 90461). Multi-valent antigens or multiple serotypes of antigens against a single organism are considered a single component of vaccines. Combination vaccines are those vaccines that contain multiple vaccine components. Conjugates or adjuvants contained in vaccines are not considered to be component parts of the vaccine as defined above.

▶For immune globulins and monoclonal antibodies immunizations, see 90281-90399. For administration of immune globulins and monoclonal antibodies immunizations, see 96365, 96366, 96367, 96368, 96369, 96370, 96371, 96372, 96374, 96375, 96380, 96381.◀

(For allergy testing, see 95004 et seq)

(For skin testing of bacterial, viral, fungal extracts, see 86485-86580)

(For therapeutic or diagnostic injections, see 96372-96379)

90460   Immunization administration through 18 years of age via any route of administration, with counseling by physician or other qualified health care professional; first or only component of each vaccine or toxoid administered
➔ *CPT Changes: An Insider's View* 2011, 2012
➔ *CPT Assistant* Mar 11:3, Jun 11:14, Jan 12:43, Jul 12:7, Aug 13:10, Mar 14:10, Apr 15:9, 11, May 15:6, Oct 16:7, Nov 18:7, Jan 20:11, Jun 21:10, Dec 21:20, Jan 23:1, May 23:22, Jul 23:1

+ 90461   each additional vaccine or toxoid component administered (List separately in addition to code for primary procedure)
➔ *CPT Changes: An Insider's View* 2011, 2012
➔ *CPT Assistant* Mar 11:3, Jun 11:14, Jan 12:43, Jul 12:7, Aug 13:10, Mar 14:10, Apr 15:4, May 15:6, Oct 16:7, Nov 18:7, Jan 23:1, Feb 23:1, May 23:22, Feb 24:1

(Use 90460 for each vaccine administered. For vaccines with multiple components [combination vaccines], report 90460 in conjunction with 90461 for each additional component in a given vaccine)

▶(Do not report 90460, 90461 in conjunction with 91304, 91318, 91319, 91320, 91321, 91322, unless both a severe acute respiratory syndrome coronavirus 2 [SARS-CoV-2] [coronavirus disease {COVID-19}] vaccine/toxoid product and at least one vaccine/toxoid product from 90476-90759 are administered at the same encounter)◀

90471   Immunization administration (includes percutaneous, intradermal, subcutaneous, or intramuscular injections); 1 vaccine (single or combination vaccine/toxoid)

➔ *CPT Changes: An Insider's View* 2002, 2005

➔ *CPT Assistant* Nov 98:31, Jan 99:2, Apr 99:10, Oct 99:9, Nov 99:47-48, Nov 00:10, Feb 01:5, Jul 01:2, Nov 02:11, Mar 04:11, Apr 04:14, Apr 05:1, 3, 5, Nov 05:1, Jan 09:8, Jul 09:7, Aug 09:9, Sep 09:7, Oct 09:3, Mar 11:3, Jun 11:14, Jul 12:7, Aug 13:10, Mar 14:10, Apr 15:9, 11, May 15:6, Oct 16:7, Nov 18:7, Jun 19:11, Jan 20:11, Dec 21:20, Jan 23:1, Feb 23:1, May 23:22, Feb 24:1

(Do not report 90471 in conjunction with 90473)

+ 90472   each additional vaccine (single or combination vaccine/toxoid) (List separately in addition to code for primary procedure)

➔ *CPT Changes: An Insider's View* 2000

➔ *CPT Assistant* Nov 98:31, Jan 99:2, Apr 99:10, Oct 99:9, Nov 99:47-48, Nov 00:10, Feb 01:5, Jul 01:2, Nov 02:11, Mar 04:11, Apr 04:14, Apr 05:1, 3, Nov 05:1, Jan 09:3, 8, Jul 09:7, Aug 09:9, Sep 09:7, Oct 09:3, Mar 11:3, Jun 11:14, Jul 12:7, Aug 13:10, Mar 14:10, Apr 15:9, 11, May 15:6, Oct 16:7, Nov 18:7, Jan 20:11, Dec 21:20, Feb 23:1, May 23:22, Feb 24:1

(Use 90472 in conjunction with 90460, 90471, 90473)

▶(Do not report 90471, 90472 in conjunction with 91304, 91318, 91319, 91320, 91321, 91322, unless both a severe acute respiratory syndrome coronavirus 2 [SARS-CoV-2] [coronavirus disease {COVID-19}] vaccine/toxoid product and at least one vaccine/toxoid product from 90476-90759 are administered at the same encounter)◀

(For intravesical administration of BCG vaccine, see 51720, 90586)

90473   Immunization administration by intranasal or oral route; 1 vaccine (single or combination vaccine/toxoid)

➔ *CPT Changes: An Insider's View* 2002

➔ *CPT Assistant* Feb 01:5, Nov 02:11, Apr 04:14, Apr 05:1, 3, Jan 09:3, 8, Jul 09:7, Aug 09:9, Oct 09:3, Mar 11:3, Jun 11:14, Jul 12:7, Aug 13:10, Mar 14:10, Apr 15:9, May 15:6, Nov 18:7, Dec 21:20

(Do not report 90473 in conjunction with 90471)

+ 90474   each additional vaccine (single or combination vaccine/toxoid) (List separately in addition to code for primary procedure)

➔ *CPT Changes: An Insider's View* 2002

➔ *CPT Assistant* Feb 01:5, Nov 02:11, Apr 04:14, Apr 05:1, 3, Jan 09:3, 8, Jul 09:7, Aug 09:9, Oct 09:3, Mar 11:3, Jun 11:14, Jul 12:7, Aug 13:10, Mar 14:10, Apr 15:9, May 15:6, Nov 18:7, Jan 23:1

(Use 90474 in conjunction with 90460, 90471, 90473)

▶(Do not report 90473, 90474 in conjunction with 91304, 91318, 91319, 91320, 91321, 91322, unless both a severe acute respiratory syndrome coronavirus 2 [SARS-CoV-2] [coronavirus disease {COVID-19}] vaccine/toxoid product and at least one vaccine/toxoid product from 90476-90759 are administered at the same encounter)◀

▶(0001A, 0002A, 0003A, 0004A have been deleted. To report administration of COVID-19 vaccine, use 90480)◀

▶(0051A, 0052A, 0053A, 0054A have been deleted. To report administration of COVID-19 vaccine, use 90480)◀

▶(0121A, 0124A have been deleted. To report administration of COVID-19 vaccine, use 90480)◀

▶(0071A, 0072A, 0073A, 0074A have been deleted. To report administration of COVID-19 vaccine, use 90480)◀

▶(0151A, 0154A have been deleted. To report administration of COVID-19 vaccine, use 90480)◀

▶(0081A, 0082A, 0083A have been deleted. To report administration of COVID-19 vaccine, use 90480)◀

▶(0171A, 0172A, 0173A, 0174A have been deleted. To report administration of COVID-19 vaccine, use 90480)◀

▶(0011A, 0012A, 0013A have been deleted. To report administration of COVID-19 vaccine, use 90480)◀

▶(0064A has been deleted. To report administration of COVID-19 vaccine, use 90480)◀

▶(0134A has been deleted. To report administration of COVID-19 vaccine, use 90480)◀

▶(0141A, 0142A, 0144A have been deleted. To report administration of COVID-19 vaccine, use 90480)◀

▶(0091A, 0092A, 0093A, 0094A have been deleted. To report administration of COVID-19 vaccine, use 90480)◀

▶(0021A, 0022A have been deleted. To report administration of COVID-19 vaccine, use 90480)◀

▶(0031A, 0034A have been deleted. To report administration of COVID-19 vaccine, use 90480)◀

▶(0041A, 0042A, 0044A have been deleted. To report administration of COVID-19 vaccine, use 90480)◀

▶(0104A has been deleted. To report administration of COVID-19 vaccine, use 90480)◀

▶(0111A, 0112A, 0113A have been deleted. To report administration of COVID-19 vaccine, use 90480)◀

▶(0164A has been deleted. To report administration of COVID-19 vaccine, use 90480)◀

Medicine / Immunization Administration for Vaccines/Toxoids 90460–90480

Copying, photographing, or sharing this CPT® book violates AMA's copyright

#● **90480** Immunization administration by intramuscular injection of severe acute respiratory syndrome coronavirus 2 (SARS-CoV-2) (coronavirus disease [COVID-19]) vaccine, single dose

➜ *CPT Changes: An Insider's View* 2025
➜ *CPT Assistant* Jan 24:15, Mar 24:29

▶(Report 90480 for the administration of vaccine 91304, 91318, 91319, 91320, 91321, 91322)◀

▶(Do not report 90480 in conjunction with 90476-90759)◀

Vaccines, Toxoids

To assist users to report the most recent new or revised vaccine product codes, the American Medical Association (AMA) currently uses the CPT website (ama-assn.org/cpt-cat-i-immunization-codes), which features updates of CPT Editorial Panel actions regarding these products. See the Introduction section of the CPT code set for a complete list of the dates of release and implementation.

The CPT Editorial Panel, in recognition of the public health interest in vaccine products, has chosen to publish new vaccine product codes prior to approval by the US Food and Drug Administration (FDA). These codes are indicated with the ⚡ symbol and will be tracked by the AMA to monitor FDA approval status. Once the FDA status changes to approval, the ⚡ symbol will be removed. CPT users should refer to the AMA CPT website (ama-assn.org/cpt-cat-i-immunization-codes) for the most up-to-date information on codes with the ⚡ symbol.

▶Codes 90476-90759, 91304, 91318, 91319, 91320, 91321, 91322 identify the vaccine product **only**. To report the administration of a vaccine/toxoid other than SARS-CoV-2 (coronavirus disease [COVID-19]), the vaccine/toxoid product codes (90476-90759) must be used in addition to an immunization administration code(s) (90460, 90461, 90471, 90472, 90473, 90474). To report the administration of a SARS-CoV-2 (coronavirus disease [COVID-19]) vaccine, the vaccine/toxoid product codes 91304, 91318, 91319, 91320, 91321, 91322 should be reported with the corresponding immunization administration code (90480).

Do not report 90476-90759 in conjunction with the SARS-CoV-2 (coronavirus disease [COVID-19]) immunization administration code 90480, unless both a SARS-CoV-2 (coronavirus disease [COVID-19]) vaccine/toxoid product and at least one vaccine/toxoid product from 90476-90759 are administered at the same encounter.

Modifier 51 should not be reported with vaccine/toxoid codes 90476-90759, 91304, 91318, 91319, 91320, 91321, 91322, when reported in conjunction with administration codes 90460, 90461, 90471, 90472, 90473, 90474, 90480.◀

If a significantly separately identifiable Evaluation and Management (E/M) service (eg, office or other outpatient services, preventive medicine services) is performed, the appropriate E/M service code should be reported in addition to the vaccine and toxoid administration codes.

To meet the reporting requirements of immunization registries, vaccine distribution programs, and reporting systems (eg, Vaccine Adverse Event Reporting System) the exact vaccine product administered needs to be reported. Multiple codes for a particular vaccine are provided in the CPT codebook when the schedule (number of doses or timing) differs for two or more products of the same vaccine type (eg, hepatitis A, Hib) or the vaccine product is available in more than one chemical formulation, dosage, or route of administration.

The "when administered to" age descriptions included in CPT vaccine codes are not intended to identify a product's licensed age indication. The term "preservative free" includes use for vaccines that contain no preservative and vaccines that contain trace amounts of preservative agents that are not present in a sufficient concentration for the purpose of preserving the final vaccine formulation. The absence of a designation regarding a preservative does not necessarily indicate the presence or absence of preservative in the vaccine. Refer to the product's prescribing information (PI) for the licensed age indication before administering vaccine to a patient.

Separate codes are available for combination vaccines (eg, Hib-HepB, DTap-IPV/Hib). It is inappropriate to code each component of a combination vaccine separately. If a specific vaccine code is not available, the unlisted procedure code should be reported, until a new code becomes available.

▶The immunization/vaccine/toxoid abbreviations listed in codes 90380, 90381, 90476-90759, 91304, 91318, 91319, 91320, 91321, 91322 reflect the most recent US vaccine abbreviation references used in the Advisory Committee on Immunization Practices (ACIP) recommendations at the time of CPT code set publication. Interim updates to vaccine code descriptors will be made following abbreviation approval by the ACIP on a timely basis via the AMA CPT website (ama-assn.org/cpt-cat-i-immunization-codes). The accuracy of the ACIP vaccine abbreviation designations in the CPT code set does not affect the validity of the vaccine code and its reporting function.◀

▶(For immune globulins and monoclonal antibodies immunizations, see 90281-90399)◀

▶(For administration of immune globulins and monoclonal antibodies immunizations, with the exception of respiratory syncytial virus, monoclonal antibody, seasonal product, see 96365-96375)◀

▶(For administration of respiratory syncytial virus, monoclonal antibody, seasonal product, see 96380, 96381)◀

▶(91300 has been deleted. To report severe acute respiratory syndrome coronavirus 2 [SARS-CoV-2] [coronavirus disease {COVID-19}] vaccine product immunization, see 91318, 91319, 91320, 91321, 91322)◀

▶(91305 has been deleted. To report severe acute respiratory syndrome coronavirus 2 [SARS-CoV-2] [coronavirus disease {COVID-19}] vaccine product immunization, see 91318, 91319, 91320, 91321, 91322)◀

▶(91312 has been deleted. To report severe acute respiratory syndrome coronavirus 2 [SARS-CoV-2] [coronavirus disease {COVID-19}] vaccine product immunization, see 91318, 91319, 91320, 91321, 91322)◀

▶(91307 has been deleted. To report severe acute respiratory syndrome coronavirus 2 [SARS-CoV-2] [coronavirus disease {COVID-19}] vaccine product immunization, see 91318, 91319, 91320, 91321, 91322)◀

▶(91315 has been deleted. To report severe acute respiratory syndrome coronavirus 2 [SARS-CoV-2] [coronavirus disease {COVID-19}] vaccine product immunization, see 91318, 91319, 91320, 91321, 91322)◀

▶(91308 has been deleted. To report severe acute respiratory syndrome coronavirus 2 [SARS-CoV-2] [coronavirus disease {COVID-19}] vaccine product immunization, see 91318, 91319, 91320, 91321, 91322)◀

▶(91317 has been deleted. To report severe acute respiratory syndrome coronavirus 2 [SARS-CoV-2] [coronavirus disease {COVID-19}] vaccine product immunization, see 91318, 91319, 91320, 91321, 91322)◀

▶(91301 has been deleted. To report severe acute respiratory syndrome coronavirus 2 [SARS-CoV-2] [coronavirus disease {COVID-19}] vaccine product immunization, see 91318, 91319, 91320, 91321, 91322)◀

▶(91306 has been deleted. To report severe acute respiratory syndrome coronavirus 2 [SARS-CoV-2] [coronavirus disease {COVID-19}] vaccine product immunization, see 91318, 91319, 91320, 91321, 91322)◀

▶(91313 has been deleted. To report severe acute respiratory syndrome coronavirus 2 [SARS-CoV-2] [coronavirus disease {COVID-19}] vaccine product immunization, see 91318, 91319, 91320, 91321, 91322)◀

▶(91314 has been deleted. To report severe acute respiratory syndrome coronavirus 2 [SARS-CoV-2] [coronavirus disease {COVID-19}] vaccine product immunization, see 91318, 91319, 91320, 91321, 91322)◀

▶(91311 has been deleted. To report severe acute respiratory syndrome coronavirus 2 [SARS-CoV-2] [coronavirus disease {COVID-19}] vaccine product immunization, see 91318, 91319, 91320, 91321, 91322)◀

▶(91316 has been deleted. To report severe acute respiratory syndrome coronavirus 2 [SARS-CoV-2] [coronavirus disease {COVID-19}] vaccine product immunization, see 91318, 91319, 91320, 91321, 91322)◀

▶(91309 has been deleted. To report severe acute respiratory syndrome coronavirus 2 [SARS-CoV-2] [coronavirus disease {COVID-19}] vaccine product immunization, see 91318, 91319, 91320, 91321, 91322)◀

▶(91302 has been deleted. To report severe acute respiratory syndrome coronavirus 2 [SARS-CoV-2] [coronavirus disease {COVID-19}] vaccine product immunization, see 91318, 91319, 91320, 91321, 91322)◀

▶(91303 has been deleted. To report severe acute respiratory syndrome coronavirus 2 [SARS-CoV-2] [coronavirus disease {COVID-19}] vaccine product immunization, see 91318, 91319, 91320, 91321, 91322)◀

#▲ **91304**   Severe acute respiratory syndrome coronavirus 2 (SARS-CoV-2) (coronavirus disease [COVID-19]) vaccine, recombinant spike protein nanoparticle, saponin-based adjuvant, 5 mcg/0.5 mL dosage, for intramuscular use

➔ *CPT Changes: An Insider's View* 2022, 2025
➔ *CPT Assistant* May 21:4, Jun 21:4, 11, Jan 24:1

▶(Report 91304 with administration code 90480)◀

▶(91310 has been deleted. To report severe acute respiratory syndrome coronavirus 2 [SARS-CoV-2] [coronavirus disease {COVID-19}] vaccine product immunization, see 91318, 91319, 91320, 91321, 91322)◀

#● **91318**   Severe acute respiratory syndrome coronavirus 2 (SARS-CoV-2) (coronavirus disease [COVID-19]) vaccine, mRNA-LNP, spike protein, 3 mcg/0.3 mL dosage, tris-sucrose formulation, for intramuscular use

➔ *CPT Changes: An Insider's View* 2025
➔ *CPT Assistant* Oct 23:17

▶(Report 91318 with administration code 90480)◀

#● **91319**   Severe acute respiratory syndrome coronavirus 2 (SARS-CoV-2) (coronavirus disease [COVID-19]) vaccine, mRNA-LNP, spike protein, 10 mcg/0.3 mL dosage, tris-sucrose formulation, for intramuscular use

➔ *CPT Changes: An Insider's View* 2025
➔ *CPT Assistant* Oct 23:17

▶(Report 91319 with administration code 90480)◀

#● **91320**   Severe acute respiratory syndrome coronavirus 2 (SARS-CoV-2) (coronavirus disease [COVID-19]) vaccine, mRNA-LNP, spike protein, 30 mcg/0.3 mL dosage, tris-sucrose formulation, for intramuscular use

➔ *CPT Changes: An Insider's View* 2025
➔ *CPT Assistant* Jan 24:15

▶(Report 91320 with administration code 90480)◀

Medicine / Vaccines, Toxoids 91304-90749

Copying, photographing, or sharing this CPT® book violates AMA's copyright.

#● 91321 Severe acute respiratory syndrome coronavirus 2 (SARS-CoV-2) (coronavirus disease [COVID-19]) vaccine, mRNA-LNP, 25 mcg/0.25 mL dosage, for intramuscular use

➔ *CPT Changes: An Insider's View* 2025

▶(Report 91321 with administration code 90480)◀

#● 91322 Severe acute respiratory syndrome coronavirus 2 (SARS-CoV-2) (coronavirus disease [COVID-19]) vaccine, mRNA-LNP, 50 mcg/0.5 mL dosage, for intramuscular use

➔ *CPT Changes: An Insider's View* 2025

▶(Report 91322 with administration code 90480)◀

90476 Adenovirus vaccine, type 4, live, for oral use

➔ *CPT Changes: An Insider's View* 2008

➔ *CPT Assistant* Nov 98:31, 33, Jan 99:2, Sep 99:10, Oct 99:9, Nov 99:48, Mar 11:4, Aug 13:10, May 15:6, Oct 16:6, Jun 21:10

90477 Adenovirus vaccine, type 7, live, for oral use

➔ *CPT Changes: An Insider's View* 2008

➔ *CPT Assistant* Nov 98:31, 33, Jan 99:2, Oct 99:9, Mar 11:4, Aug 13:10

90480 Code is out of numerical sequence. See 90473-90477

90581 Anthrax vaccine, for subcutaneous or intramuscular use

➔ *CPT Changes: An Insider's View* 2008, 2012

➔ *CPT Assistant* Nov 98:31, 33, Jan 99:2, Oct 99:9, Mar 11:4, Aug 13:10

90584 Code is out of numerical sequence. See 90585-90632

90585 Bacillus Calmette-Guerin vaccine (BCG) for tuberculosis, live, for percutaneous use

➔ *CPT Changes: An Insider's View* 2008

➔ *CPT Assistant* Nov 98:31, 33, Jan 99:2, Oct 99:9, Mar 11:4, Aug 13:10

90586 Bacillus Calmette-Guerin vaccine (BCG) for bladder cancer, live, for intravesical use

➔ *CPT Changes: An Insider's View* 2008

➔ *CPT Assistant* Nov 98:31, 33, Jan 99:2, Oct 99:9, Nov 02:11, Mar 11:4, Aug 13:10

 # 90589 Chikungunya virus vaccine, live attenuated, for intramuscular use

➔ *CPT Changes: An Insider's View* 2024

➔ *CPT Assistant* Feb 24:1

#✒ 90584 Dengue vaccine, quadrivalent, live, 2 dose schedule, for subcutaneous use

➔ *CPT Changes: An Insider's View* 2023

➔ *CPT Assistant* Feb 23:1

90587 Dengue vaccine, quadrivalent, live, 3 dose schedule, for subcutaneous use

➔ *CPT Changes: An Insider's View* 2018

➔ *CPT Assistant* Nov 18:7

90589 Code is out of numerical sequence. See 90585-90632

90611 Code is out of numerical sequence. See 90710-90715

90619 Code is out of numerical sequence. See 90717-90739

90620 Code is out of numerical sequence. See 90717-90739

90621 Code is out of numerical sequence. See 90717-90739

90622 Code is out of numerical sequence. See 90714-90717

90623 Code is out of numerical sequence. See 90717-90739

90624 Code is out of numerical sequence. See 90717-90739

90625 Code is out of numerical sequence. See 90717-90739

90626 Code is out of numerical sequence. See 90714-90717

90627 Code is out of numerical sequence. See 90714-90717

90632 Hepatitis A vaccine (HepA), adult dosage, for intramuscular use

➔ *CPT Changes: An Insider's View* 2008, 2016

➔ *CPT Assistant* Nov 98:31, 33, Jan 99:2, Oct 99:9, Mar 11:4, Aug 13:10

90633 Hepatitis A vaccine (HepA), pediatric/adolescent dosage-2 dose schedule, for intramuscular use

➔ *CPT Changes: An Insider's View* 2008, 2016

➔ *CPT Assistant* Nov 98:31, 33, Jan 99:2, Oct 99:9, Mar 11:4, Aug 13:10

90634 Hepatitis A vaccine (HepA), pediatric/adolescent dosage-3 dose schedule, for intramuscular use

➔ *CPT Changes: An Insider's View* 2008, 2016

➔ *CPT Assistant* Nov 98:31, 33, Jan 99:2, Oct 99:9, Mar 11:4, Aug 13:10

90636 Hepatitis A and hepatitis B vaccine (HepA-HepB), adult dosage, for intramuscular use

➔ *CPT Changes: An Insider's View* 2008

➔ *CPT Assistant* Nov 98:31, 33, Jan 99:2, Oct 99:9, Mar 11:4, Aug 13:10

90637 Code is out of numerical sequence. See 90689-90691

90638 Code is out of numerical sequence. See 90689-90691

90644 Code is out of numerical sequence. See 90717-90739

90647 Haemophilus influenzae type b vaccine (Hib), PRP-OMP conjugate, 3 dose schedule, for intramuscular use

➔ *CPT Changes: An Insider's View* 2008, 2016

➔ *CPT Assistant* Nov 98:31, 33, Jan 99:2, Oct 99:9, Mar 11:4, Aug 13:10

90648 Haemophilus influenzae type b vaccine (Hib), PRP-T conjugate, 4 dose schedule, for intramuscular use

➔ *CPT Changes: An Insider's View* 2008, 2016

➔ *CPT Assistant* Nov 98:31, 33, Jan 99:2, Oct 99:9, Sep 09:7, Mar 11:4, Aug 13:10

90649 Human Papillomavirus vaccine, types 6, 11, 16, 18, quadrivalent (4vHPV), 3 dose schedule, for intramuscular use

➔ *CPT Changes: An Insider's View* 2006, 2008, 2016

➔ *CPT Assistant* Dec 05:9, Jun 06:8, Sep 06:14, Jul 07:13, Mar 11:4, Aug 13:10

90650   Human Papillomavirus vaccine, types 16, 18, bivalent (2vHPV), 3 dose schedule, for intramuscular use
➲ *CPT Changes: An Insider's View* 2009, 2011, 2016
➲ *CPT Assistant* Mar 11:4, Aug 13:10

90651   Human Papillomavirus vaccine types 6, 11, 16, 18, 31, 33, 45, 52, 58, nonavalent (9vHPV), 2 or 3 dose schedule, for intramuscular use
➲ *CPT Changes: An Insider's View* 2015, 2016, 2018
➲ *CPT Assistant* May 15:6, Nov 18:7, Jul 23:1

90653   Influenza vaccine, inactivated (IIV), subunit, adjuvanted, for intramuscular use
➲ *CPT Changes: An Insider's View* 2013, 2016
➲ *CPT Assistant* Aug 13:10, Oct 16:6, Jun 19:11

▶(90654 has been deleted. To report influenza vaccine, see 90653, 90655, 90656, 90657, 90658, 90660, 90661, 90662, 90664, 90666, 90667, 90668, 90672, 90673, 90674, 90682, 90685, 90686, 90687, 90688, 90689, 90694, 90756)◀

▶(90630 has been deleted. To report influenza vaccine, see 90653, 90655, 90656, 90657, 90658, 90660, 90661, 90662, 90664, 90666, 90667, 90668, 90672, 90673, 90674, 90682, 90685, 90686, 90687, 90688, 90689, 90694, 90756)◀

90655   Influenza virus vaccine, trivalent (IIV3), split virus, preservative free, 0.25 mL dosage, for intramuscular use
➲ *CPT Changes: An Insider's View* 2004, 2007, 2008, 2013, 2016, 2017
➲ *CPT Assistant* Oct 99:9, Feb 04:2, Apr 07:12, Apr 08:8, Oct 09:3, Mar 11:4, Aug 13:10, May 16:9, Oct 16:6

90656   Influenza virus vaccine, trivalent (IIV3), split virus, preservative free, 0.5 mL dosage, for intramuscular use
➲ *CPT Changes: An Insider's View* 2005, 2007, 2008, 2013, 2016, 2017
➲ *CPT Assistant* Apr 08:8, Oct 09:3, Mar 11:4, Aug 13:10, May 16:9, Oct 16:6

90657   Influenza virus vaccine, trivalent (IIV3), split virus, 0.25 mL dosage, for intramuscular use
➲ *CPT Changes: An Insider's View* 2004, 2007, 2008, 2013, 2016, 2017
➲ *CPT Assistant* Nov 98:31, 33, Jan 99:2, Oct 99:9, Feb 02:10, Feb 04:2, Apr 05:5, Apr 08:8, Oct 09:3, Mar 11:4, Aug 13:10, May 16:9, Oct 16:6

90658   Influenza virus vaccine, trivalent (IIV3), split virus, 0.5 mL dosage, for intramuscular use
➲ *CPT Changes: An Insider's View* 2004, 2007, 2008, 2013, 2016, 2017
➲ *CPT Assistant* Nov 98:31, 33, Jan 99:2, Oct 99:9, Feb 04:2, Apr 07:12, Apr 08:8, Oct 09:3, Mar 11:4, Aug 13:10, May 16:9, Oct 16:6

90660   Influenza virus vaccine, trivalent, live (LAIV3), for intranasal use
➲ *CPT Changes: An Insider's View* 2008, 2013, 2016
➲ *CPT Assistant* Nov 98:31, 33, Jan 99:2, Oct 99:9, Mar 04:11, Apr 04:14, Oct 09:3, Mar 11:4, Aug 13:10

 # 90672   Influenza virus vaccine, quadrivalent, live (LAIV4), for intranasal use
➲ *CPT Changes: An Insider's View* 2013, 2016
➲ *CPT Assistant* Aug 13:10

▲ **90661**   Influenza virus vaccine, trivalent (ccIIV3), derived from cell cultures, subunit, antibiotic free, 0.5 mL dosage, for intramuscular use
➲ *CPT Changes: An Insider's View* 2008, 2016, 2017, 2025
➲ *CPT Assistant* Apr 08:8, Oct 09:3, Mar 11:4, Aug 13:10, Oct 16:6

 # 90674   Influenza virus vaccine, quadrivalent (ccIIV4), derived from cell cultures, subunit, preservative and antibiotic free, 0.5 mL dosage, for intramuscular use
➲ *CPT Changes: An Insider's View* 2017
➲ *CPT Assistant* Oct 16:6

 # 90756   Influenza virus vaccine, quadrivalent (ccIIV4), derived from cell cultures, subunit, antibiotic free, 0.5 mL dosage, for intramuscular use
➲ *CPT Changes: An Insider's View* 2018
➲ *CPT Assistant* Nov 18:7, Jun 21:10

 # 90673   Influenza virus vaccine, trivalent (RIV3), derived from recombinant DNA, hemagglutinin (HA) protein only, preservative and antibiotic free, for intramuscular use
➲ *CPT Changes: An Insider's View* 2014, 2016
➲ *CPT Assistant* Mar 14:10

90662   Influenza virus vaccine (IIV), split virus, preservative free, enhanced immunogenicity via increased antigen content, for intramuscular use
➲ *CPT Changes: An Insider's View* 2008, 2011, 2016
➲ *CPT Assistant* Apr 08:8, Oct 09:3, 6, Mar 11:4, Aug 13:10

90664   Influenza virus vaccine, live (LAIV), pandemic formulation, for intranasal use
➲ *CPT Changes: An Insider's View* 2011, 2016
➲ *CPT Assistant* Mar 11:4, Aug 13:10

✗ **90666**   Influenza virus vaccine (IIV), pandemic formulation, split virus, preservative free, for intramuscular use
➲ *CPT Changes: An Insider's View* 2011, 2016
➲ *CPT Assistant* May 11:4, Aug 13:10

✗ **90667**   Influenza virus vaccine (IIV), pandemic formulation, split virus, adjuvanted, for intramuscular use
➲ *CPT Changes: An Insider's View* 2011, 2016
➲ *CPT Assistant* Mar 11:4, Aug 13:10

✗ **90668**   Influenza virus vaccine (IIV), pandemic formulation, split virus, for intramuscular use
➲ *CPT Changes: An Insider's View* 2011, 2016
➲ *CPT Assistant* Mar 11:4, Aug 13:10

#✗● **90695**   Influenza virus vaccine, H5N8, derived from cell cultures, adjuvanted, for intramuscular use
➲ *CPT Changes: An Insider's View* 2025

90670 Pneumococcal conjugate vaccine, 13 valent (PCV13), for intramuscular use
➡ *CPT Changes: An Insider's View* 2010, 2011, 2016
➡ *CPT Assistant* Mar 11:4, Aug 13:10

✗ **90671** Pneumococcal conjugate vaccine, 15 valent (PCV15), for intramuscular use
➡ *CPT Changes: An Insider's View* 2022

90677 Pneumococcal conjugate vaccine, 20 valent (PCV20), for intramuscular use
➡ *CPT Changes: An Insider's View* 2022

#● **90684** Pneumococcal conjugate vaccine, 21 valent (PCV21), for intramuscular use
➡ *CPT Changes: An Insider's View* 2025

90672 Code is out of numerical sequence. See 90658-90664

90673 Code is out of numerical sequence. See 90658-90664

90674 Code is out of numerical sequence. See 90658-90664

90675 Rabies vaccine, for intramuscular use
➡ *CPT Changes: An Insider's View* 2008
➡ *CPT Assistant* Nov 98:31, 33, Jan 99:2, Oct 99:9, Mar 11:4, Aug 13:10

90676 Rabies vaccine, for intradermal use
➡ *CPT Changes: An Insider's View* 2008
➡ *CPT Assistant* Nov 98:31, 33, Jan 99:2, Oct 99:9, Mar 11:4, Jul 12:7, Aug 13:10

90677 Code is out of numerical sequence. See 90670-90676

90678 Respiratory syncytial virus vaccine, preF, subunit, bivalent, for intramuscular use
➡ *CPT Changes: An Insider's View* 2023
➡ *CPT Assistant* Feb 23:1, Feb 24:1

90679 Respiratory syncytial virus vaccine, preF, recombinant, subunit, adjuvanted, for intramuscular use
➡ *CPT Changes: An Insider's View* 2024
➡ *CPT Assistant* Feb 24:1

90683 Respiratory syncytial virus vaccine, mRNA lipid nanoparticles, for intramuscular use
➡ *CPT Changes: An Insider's View* 2024
➡ *CPT Assistant* Feb 24:1

▶(For seasonal respiratory syncytial virus [RSV] monoclonal antibodies immunization codes, see 90380, 90381. For administration of seasonal RSV monoclonal antibodies immunizations, see 96380, 96381)◀

90680 Rotavirus vaccine, pentavalent (RV5), 3 dose schedule, live, for oral use
➡ *CPT Changes: An Insider's View* 2006, 2008, 2016
➡ *CPT Assistant* Nov 98:31, 33, Jan 99:2, Oct 99:9, Jun 05:6, Dec 05:9, Jun 06:8, Mar 11:4, Aug 13:10

90681 Rotavirus vaccine, human, attenuated (RV1), 2 dose schedule, live, for oral use
➡ *CPT Changes: An Insider's View* 2009, 2016
➡ *CPT Assistant* Mar 11:4, Jul 12:7, Aug 13:10

90682 Influenza virus vaccine, quadrivalent (RIV4), derived from recombinant DNA, hemagglutinin (HA) protein only, preservative and antibiotic free, for intramuscular use
➡ *CPT Changes: An Insider's View* 2018
➡ *CPT Assistant* Nov 18:7

90683 Code is out of numerical sequence. See 90678-90681

90684 Code is out of numerical sequence. See 90670-90676

90685 Influenza virus vaccine, quadrivalent (IIV4), split virus, preservative free, 0.25 mL dosage, for intramuscular use
➡ *CPT Changes: An Insider's View* 2014, 2016, 2017
➡ *CPT Assistant* Mar 14:10, May 16:9, Oct 16:6

90686 Influenza virus vaccine, quadrivalent (IIV4), split virus, preservative free, 0.5 mL dosage, for intramuscular use
➡ *CPT Changes: An Insider's View* 2014, 2016, 2017
➡ *CPT Assistant* Mar 14:10, May 16:9, Oct 16:6, Dec 21:20

90687 Influenza virus vaccine, quadrivalent (IIV4), split virus, 0.25 mL dosage, for intramuscular use
➡ *CPT Changes: An Insider's View* 2014, 2016, 2017
➡ *CPT Assistant* Mar 14:10, May 16:9, Oct 16:6

90688 Influenza virus vaccine, quadrivalent (IIV4), split virus, 0.5 mL dosage, for intramuscular use
➡ *CPT Changes: An Insider's View* 2014, 2016, 2017
➡ *CPT Assistant* Mar 14:10, May 16:9, Oct 16:6

90689 Influenza virus vaccine, quadrivalent (IIV4), inactivated, adjuvanted, preservative free, 0.25 mL dosage, for intramuscular use
➡ *CPT Changes: An Insider's View* 2019
➡ *CPT Assistant* Nov 18:7, Jul 19:11

90694 Influenza virus vaccine, quadrivalent (aIIV4), inactivated, adjuvanted, preservative free, 0.5 mL dosage, for intramuscular use
➡ *CPT Changes: An Insider's View* 2020
➡ *CPT Assistant* Jul 20:11

#✗● **90637** Influenza virus vaccine, quadrivalent (qIRV), mRNA; 30 mcg/0.5 mL dosage, for intramuscular use
➡ *CPT Changes: An Insider's View* 2025

#✗● **90638** 60 mcg/0.5 mL dosage, for intramuscular use
➡ *CPT Changes: An Insider's View* 2025

90690 Typhoid vaccine, live, oral
➡ *CPT Changes: An Insider's View* 2008
➡ *CPT Assistant* Nov 98:31, 33, Jan 99:2, Oct 99:9, Mar 11:4, Aug 13:10, Jul 20:11

90691 Typhoid vaccine, Vi capsular polysaccharide (ViCPs), for intramuscular use
➡ *CPT Changes: An Insider's View* 2008
➡ *CPT Assistant* Nov 98:31, 33, Jan 99:2, Oct 99:9, Mar 11:4, Aug 13:10, Jul 20:11

90694   Code is out of numerical sequence. See 90688-90691

90695   Code is out of numerical sequence. See 90667-90671

90696   Diphtheria, tetanus toxoids, acellular pertussis vaccine and inactivated poliovirus vaccine (DTaP-IPV), when administered to children 4 through 6 years of age, for intramuscular use
➔ *CPT Changes: An Insider's View* 2009, 2016
➔ *CPT Assistant* Mar 11:4, Aug 13:10

90697   Diphtheria, tetanus toxoids, acellular pertussis vaccine, inactivated poliovirus vaccine, Haemophilus influenzae type b PRP-OMP conjugate vaccine, and hepatitis B vaccine (DTaP-IPV-Hib-HepB), for intramuscular use
➔ *CPT Changes: An Insider's View* 2016

90698   Diphtheria, tetanus toxoids, acellular pertussis vaccine, Haemophilus influenzae type b, and inactivated poliovirus vaccine, (DTaP-IPV/Hib), for intramuscular use
➔ *CPT Changes: An Insider's View* 2008, 2009, 2016
➔ *CPT Assistant* Oct 99:9, Dec 05:9, Jun 06:8, Mar 11:4, Aug 13:10

90700   Diphtheria, tetanus toxoids, and acellular pertussis vaccine (DTaP), when administered to individuals younger than 7 years, for intramuscular use
➔ *CPT Changes: An Insider's View* 2005, 2007, 2008
➔ *CPT Assistant* Jan 96:5, Apr 97:10, Nov 98:31, 33, Jan 99:2, Oct 99:9, Nov 03:13, Mar 11:4, Jul 12:7, Aug 13:10

90702   Diphtheria and tetanus toxoids adsorbed (DT) when administered to individuals younger than 7 years, for intramuscular use
➔ *CPT Changes: An Insider's View* 2001, 2007, 2008, 2016
➔ *CPT Assistant* Jan 96:6, Aug 96:10, Apr 97:10, Nov 98:31, 33, Jan 99:2, Sep 99:10, Oct 99:9, Jun 00:10, Feb 07:11, Mar 11:4, Aug 13:10

90707   Measles, mumps and rubella virus vaccine (MMR), live, for subcutaneous use
➔ *CPT Changes: An Insider's View* 2004, 2008
➔ *CPT Assistant* Jan 96:6, May 96:10, Apr 97:10, Nov 98:31, 33, Jan 99:2, Oct 99:9, Apr 05:1, 5, Mar 11:4, Jul 12:7, Aug 13:10

90710   Measles, mumps, rubella, and varicella vaccine (MMRV), live, for subcutaneous use
➔ *CPT Changes: An Insider's View* 2008
➔ *CPT Assistant* May 96:10, Apr 97:10, Nov 98:31, 33, Jan 99:2, Oct 99:9, Dec 05:9, Jun 06:8, Mar 11:4, Aug 13:10

90713   Poliovirus vaccine, inactivated (IPV), for subcutaneous or intramuscular use
➔ *CPT Changes: An Insider's View* 2006, 2008
➔ *CPT Assistant* Apr 97:10, Nov 98:31, 33, Jan 99:2, Oct 99:9, Jun 05:6, Mar 11:4, Aug 13:10

 # 90611   Smallpox and monkeypox vaccine, attenuated vaccinia virus, live, non-replicating, preservative free, 0.5 mL dosage, suspension, for subcutaneous use
➔ *CPT Changes: An Insider's View* 2024

90714   Tetanus and diphtheria toxoids adsorbed (Td), preservative free, when administered to individuals 7 years or older, for intramuscular use
➔ *CPT Changes: An Insider's View* 2006, 2007, 2008, 2016
➔ *CPT Assistant* Jun 05:6, Mar 11:4, Aug 13:10

90715   Tetanus, diphtheria toxoids and acellular pertussis vaccine (Tdap), when administered to individuals 7 years or older, for intramuscular use
➔ *CPT Changes: An Insider's View* 2006, 2007, 2008
➔ *CPT Assistant* Oct 99:9, Jun 05:6, Dec 05:9, Jun 06:8, Mar 11:4, Aug 13:10

 # 90626   Tick-borne encephalitis virus vaccine, inactivated; 0.25 mL dosage, for intramuscular use
➔ *CPT Changes: An Insider's View* 2022

 # 90627   0.5 mL dosage, for intramuscular use
➔ *CPT Changes: An Insider's View* 2022

 # 90622   Vaccinia (smallpox) virus vaccine, live, lyophilized, 0.3 mL dosage, for percutaneous use
➔ *CPT Changes: An Insider's View* 2024

90716   Varicella virus vaccine (VAR), live, for subcutaneous use
➔ *CPT Changes: An Insider's View* 2008, 2016
➔ *CPT Assistant* Jan 96:6, May 96:10, Apr 97:10, Nov 98:31, 33, Jan 99:2, Oct 99:9, Mar 11:4, Aug 13:10

90717   Yellow fever vaccine, live, for subcutaneous use
➔ *CPT Changes: An Insider's View* 2008
➔ *CPT Assistant* Apr 97:10, Nov 98:31, 33, Jan 99:2, Oct 99:9, Mar 11:4, Aug 13:10

90723   Diphtheria, tetanus toxoids, acellular pertussis vaccine, hepatitis B, and inactivated poliovirus vaccine (DTaP-HepB-IPV), for intramuscular use
➔ *CPT Changes: An Insider's View* 2001, 2008, 2015
➔ *CPT Assistant* Apr 97:10, Oct 99:9, Mar 11:4, Aug 13:10, May 15:6

 # 90625   Cholera vaccine, live, adult dosage, 1 dose schedule, for oral use
➔ *CPT Changes: An Insider's View* 2016
➔ *CPT Assistant* Oct 16:6

90732   Pneumococcal polysaccharide vaccine, 23-valent (PPSV23), adult or immunosuppressed patient dosage, when administered to individuals 2 years or older, for subcutaneous or intramuscular use
➔ *CPT Changes: An Insider's View* 2002, 2007, 2008, 2016
➔ *CPT Assistant* Apr 97:10, Nov 98:31, 33, Jan 99:2, Oct 99:9, Mar 11:4, Aug 13:10

 # 90644   Meningococcal conjugate vaccine, serogroups C & Y and Haemophilus influenzae type b vaccine (Hib-MenCY), 4 dose schedule, when administered to children 6 weeks-18 months of age, for intramuscular use
➔ *CPT Changes: An Insider's View* 2011, 2012, 2016, 2017
➔ *CPT Assistant* Mar 11:4, Aug 13:10

90733   Meningococcal polysaccharide vaccine, serogroups A, C, Y, W-135, quadrivalent (MPSV4), for subcutaneous use

➜ *CPT Changes: An Insider's View* 2001, 2004, 2008, 2016

➜ *CPT Assistant* Apr 97:10, Nov 98:31, 33, Jan 99:2, Oct 99:9, Dec 99:7, Mar 11:4, Aug 13:10

90734   Meningococcal conjugate vaccine, serogroups A, C, W, Y, quadrivalent, diphtheria toxoid carrier (MenACWY-D) or CRM197 carrier (MenACWY-CRM), for intramuscular use

➜ *CPT Changes: An Insider's View* 2008, 2015, 2016, 2017, 2020

➜ *CPT Assistant* Oct 99:9, Mar 11:4, Aug 13:10, May 15:6, Oct 16:6, Jan 20:11

\# **90619**   Meningococcal conjugate vaccine, serogroups A, C, W, Y, quadrivalent, tetanus toxoid carrier (MenACWY-TT), for intramuscular use

➜ *CPT Changes: An Insider's View* 2020

➜ *CPT Assistant* Jan 20:11

\# **90623**   Meningococcal pentavalent vaccine, conjugated Men A, C, W, Y- tetanus toxoid carrier, and Men B-FHbp, for intramuscular use

➜ *CPT Changes: An Insider's View* 2024

➜ *CPT Assistant* Feb 24:1

\#✔● **90624**   Meningococcal pentavalent vaccine, Men B-4C recombinant proteins and outer membrane vesicle and conjugated Men A, C, W, Y-diphtheria toxoid carrier, for intramuscular use

➜ *CPT Changes: An Insider's View* 2025

\# **90620**   Meningococcal recombinant protein and outer membrane vesicle vaccine, serogroup B (MenB-4C), 2 dose schedule, for intramuscular use

➜ *CPT Changes: An Insider's View* 2016, 2018

➜ *CPT Assistant* Nov 18:7

\# **90621**   Meningococcal recombinant lipoprotein vaccine, serogroup B (MenB-FHbp), 2 or 3 dose schedule, for intramuscular use

➜ *CPT Changes: An Insider's View* 2016, 2018

➜ *CPT Assistant* Nov 18:7

90736   Zoster (shingles) vaccine (HZV), live, for subcutaneous injection

➜ *CPT Changes: An Insider's View* 2006, 2008, 2016

➜ *CPT Assistant* Dec 05:9, Jun 06:8, Jul 07:13, Mar 11:4, Aug 13:10, Nov 18:7

\# **90750**   Zoster (shingles) vaccine (HZV), recombinant, subunit, adjuvanted, for intramuscular use

➜ *CPT Changes: An Insider's View* 2018

➜ *CPT Assistant* Nov 18:7

90738   Japanese encephalitis virus vaccine, inactivated, for intramuscular use

➜ *CPT Changes: An Insider's View* 2009, 2010

➜ *CPT Assistant* Mar 11:4, Aug 13:10

90739   Hepatitis B vaccine (HepB), CpG-adjuvanted, adult dosage, 2 dose or 4 dose schedule, for intramuscular use

➜ *CPT Changes: An Insider's View* 2013, 2016, 2023

➜ *CPT Assistant* Aug 13:10, Nov 18:7, Feb 23:1

90740   Hepatitis B vaccine (HepB), dialysis or immunosuppressed patient dosage, 3 dose schedule, for intramuscular use

➜ *CPT Changes: An Insider's View* 2001, 2008, 2016

➜ *CPT Assistant* Apr 97:10, Oct 99:9, Apr 01:10, Mar 11:4, Aug 13:10

90743   Hepatitis B vaccine (HepB), adolescent, 2 dose schedule, for intramuscular use

➜ *CPT Changes: An Insider's View* 2001, 2008, 2016

➜ *CPT Assistant* Apr 97:10, Oct 99:9, Mar 11:4, Aug 13:10

90744   Hepatitis B vaccine (HepB), pediatric/adolescent dosage, 3 dose schedule, for intramuscular use

➜ *CPT Changes: An Insider's View* 2000, 2001, 2008, 2016

➜ *CPT Assistant* Jan 96:5, Apr 97:10, Jun 97:10, Nov 98:31, 33, Jan 99:2, Oct 99:9, Nov 99:48-49, Jun 00:10, Mar 11:4, Aug 13:10

90746   Hepatitis B vaccine (HepB), adult dosage, 3 dose schedule, for intramuscular use

➜ *CPT Changes: An Insider's View* 2008, 2013, 2016

➜ *CPT Assistant* Jan 96:5, Apr 97:10, Nov 98:31, 33, Jan 99:2, Oct 99:9, Mar 11:4, Aug 13:10

\# **90759**   Hepatitis B vaccine (HepB), 3-antigen (S, Pre-S1, Pre-S2), 10 mcg dosage, 3 dose schedule, for intramuscular use

➜ *CPT Changes: An Insider's View* 2022

90747   Hepatitis B vaccine (HepB), dialysis or immunosuppressed patient dosage, 4 dose schedule, for intramuscular use

➜ *CPT Changes: An Insider's View* 2001, 2008, 2016

➜ *CPT Assistant* Jan 96:5, Apr 97:10, Jun 97:10, Nov 98:31, 33, Jan 99:2, Oct 99:9, Jun 00:10, Apr 01:10, Mar 11:4, Aug 13:10

90748   Hepatitis B and Haemophilus influenzae type b vaccine (Hib-HepB), for intramuscular use

➜ *CPT Changes: An Insider's View* 2008, 2016

➜ *CPT Assistant* Apr 97:10, Nov 97:37, Nov 98:31, 33, Jan 99:2, Sep 99:10, Oct 99:9, Mar 11:4, Jul 12:7, Aug 13:10, Oct 16:6

\# **90758**   Zaire ebolavirus vaccine, live, for intramuscular use

➜ *CPT Changes: An Insider's View* 2022

90749   Unlisted vaccine/toxoid

➜ *CPT Changes: An Insider's View* 2008

➜ *CPT Assistant* Jan 96:6, Apr 97:10, Jun 97:10, Nov 98:31, 33, Jan 99:2, Oct 99:9, Nov 02:11, Mar 11:4, May 15:6

90750   Code is out of numerical sequence. See 90717-90739

90756   Code is out of numerical sequence. See 90658-90664

90758   Code is out of numerical sequence. See 90747-90749

90759   Code is out of numerical sequence. See 90744-90748

Psychiatry

Psychiatry services include diagnostic services, psychotherapy, and other services to an individual, family, or group. Patient condition, characteristics, or situational factors may require services described as being with interactive complexity. Services may be provided to a patient in crisis. Services are provided in all settings of care and psychiatry services codes are reported without regard to setting. Services may be provided by a physician or other qualified health care professional. Some psychiatry services may be reported with **evaluation and management services** (99202-99255, 99281-99285, 99304-99316, 99341-99350) or other services when performed. **Evaluation and management services** (99202-99285, 99304-99316, 99341-99350) may be reported for treatment of psychiatric conditions, rather than using **psychiatry services** codes, when appropriate.

Hospital inpatient or observation care in treating a psychiatric inpatient or partial hospitalization may be initial or subsequent in nature (see 99221-99233).

Some patients receive hospital evaluation and management services only and others receive hospital evaluation and management services and other procedures. If other procedures such as electroconvulsive therapy or psychotherapy are rendered in addition to hospital evaluation and management services, these may be listed separately (eg, hospital inpatient or observation care services [99221-99223, 99231-99233] plus electroconvulsive therapy [90870]), or when psychotherapy is done, with appropriate code(s) defining psychotherapy services.

Consultation for psychiatric evaluation of a patient includes examination of a patient and exchange of information with the primary physician and other informants such as nurses or family members, and preparation of a report. These services may be reported using consultation codes (see **Consultations**).

> (Do not report 90785-90899 in conjunction with 90839, 90840, 97151, 97152, 97153, 97154, 97155, 97156, 97157, 97158, 0362T, 0373T)

Interactive Complexity

Code 90785 is an add-on code for interactive complexity to be reported in conjunction with codes for diagnostic psychiatric evaluation (90791, 90792), psychotherapy (90832, 90833, 90834, 90836, 90837, 90838), and group psychotherapy (90853).

Interactive complexity refers to specific communication factors that complicate the delivery of a psychiatric procedure. Common factors include more difficult communication with discordant or emotional family members and engagement of young and verbally undeveloped or impaired patients. Typical patients are those who have third parties, such as parents, guardians, other family members, agencies, court officers, or schools involved in their psychiatric care.

Psychiatric procedures may be reported "with interactive complexity" when at least one of the following is present:

1. The need to manage maladaptive communication (related to, eg, high anxiety, high reactivity, repeated questions, or disagreement) among participants that complicates delivery of care.

2. Caregiver emotions or behavior that interferes with the caregiver's understanding and ability to assist in the implementation of the treatment plan.

3. Evidence or disclosure of a sentinel event and mandated report to third party (eg, abuse or neglect with report to state agency) with initiation of discussion of the sentinel event and/or report with patient and other visit participants.

4. Use of play equipment or other physical devices to communicate with the patient to overcome barriers to therapeutic or diagnostic interaction between the physician or other qualified health care professional and a patient who has not developed, or has lost, either the expressive language communication skills to explain his/her symptoms and response to treatment, or the receptive communication skills to understand the physician or other qualified health care professional if he/she were to use typical language for communication.

Interactive complexity must be reported in conjunction with an appropriate psychiatric diagnostic evaluation or psychotherapy service, for the purpose of reporting increased complexity of the service due to specific communication factors which can result in barriers to diagnostic or therapeutic interaction with the patient.

When provided in conjunction with the psychotherapy services (90832-90838), the amount of time spent by a physician or other qualified health care professional providing interactive complexity services should be reflected in the timed service code for psychotherapy (90832, 90834, 90837) or the psychotherapy add-on code (90833, 90836, 90838) performed with an evaluation and management service and must relate to the psychotherapy service only. Interactive complexity is not a service associated with evaluation and management services when provided without psychotherapy.

★+◄ **90785**   Interactive complexity (List separately in addition to the code for primary procedure)

➔ *CPT Changes: An Insider's View* 2013

➔ *CPT Assistant* May 13:12, Jun 13:3, Apr 14:6, Nov 18:3, Aug 20:3, Jan 22:8

(Use 90785 in conjunction with codes for diagnostic psychiatric evaluation [90791, 90792], psychotherapy [90832, 90833, 90834, 90836, 90837, 90838], and group psychotherapy [90853])

(Use 90785 in conjunction with 90853 for the specified patient when group psychotherapy includes interactive complexity)

(Do not report 90785 in conjunction with psychological and neuropsychological testing [96130, 96131, 96132, 96133, 96136, 96137, 96138, 96139, 96146], or E/M services when no psychotherapy service is also reported)

(Do not report 90785 in conjunction with 90839, 90840, 97151, 97152, 97153, 97154, 97155, 97156, 97157, 97158, 0362T, 0373T)

Psychiatric Diagnostic Procedures

Psychiatric diagnostic evaluation is an integrated biopsychosocial assessment, including history, mental status, and recommendations. The evaluation may include communication with family or other sources and review and ordering of diagnostic studies.

Psychiatric diagnostic evaluation with medical services is an integrated biopsychosocial and medical assessment, including history, mental status, other physical examination elements as indicated, and recommendations. The evaluation may include communication with family or other sources, prescription of medications, and review and ordering of laboratory or other diagnostic studies.

In certain circumstances one or more other informants (family members, guardians, or significant others) may be seen in lieu of the patient. Codes 90791, 90792 may be reported more than once for the patient when separate diagnostic evaluations are conducted with the patient and other informants. Report services as being provided to the patient and not the informant or other party in such circumstances. Codes 90791, 90792 may be reported once per day and not on the same day as an evaluation and management service performed by the same individual for the same patient.

The psychiatric diagnostic evaluation may include interactive complexity services when factors exist that complicate the delivery of the psychiatric procedure. These services should be reported with add-on code 90785 used in conjunction with the diagnostic psychiatric evaluation codes 90791, 90792.

Codes 90791, 90792 are used for the diagnostic assessment(s) or reassessment(s), if required, and do not include psychotherapeutic services. Psychotherapy services, including for crisis, may not be reported on the same day.

(Do not report 90791-90899 in conjunction with 90839, 90840, 97151, 97152, 97153, 97154, 97155, 97156, 97157, 97158, 0362T, 0373T)

★◄ **90791**   Psychiatric diagnostic evaluation

➔ *CPT Changes: An Insider's View* 2013, 2017

➔ *CPT Assistant* May 13:12, Jun 13:3, Dec 13:18, Jun 14:3, Nov 17:3, Nov 18:3, Aug 20:3, Oct 20:15, Aug 22:13

★◄ **90792**   Psychiatric diagnostic evaluation with medical services

➔ *CPT Changes: An Insider's View* 2013, 2017

➔ *CPT Assistant* Jun 13:3, Dec 13:18, Jun 14:3, Nov 17:3, Nov 18:3, Dec 19:15, Aug 20:3, Oct 20:15

▶(Do not report 90791 or 90792 in conjunction with 99202-99316, 99341-99350, 99366-99368, 99401, 99402, 99403, 99404, 99406, 99407, 99408, 99409, 99411, 99412, 97151, 97152, 97153, 97154, 97155, 97156, 97157, 97158, 0362T, 0373T)◀

(Use 90785 in conjunction with 90791, 90792 when the diagnostic evaluation includes interactive complexity services)

Psychotherapy

Psychotherapy is the treatment of mental illness and behavioral disturbances in which the physician or other qualified health care professional, through definitive therapeutic communication, attempts to alleviate the emotional disturbances, reverse or change maladaptive patterns of behavior, and encourage personality growth and development.

The psychotherapy service codes 90832-90838 include ongoing assessment and adjustment of psychotherapeutic interventions, and may include involvement of informants in the treatment process.

Codes 90832, 90833, 90834, 90836, 90837, 90838 describe psychotherapy for the individual patient, although times are for face-to-face services with patient and may include informant(s). The patient must be present for all or a majority of the service.

See codes 90846, 90847 when utilizing family psychotherapy techniques, such as focusing on family dynamics. Do not report 90846, 90847 for family psychotherapy services less than 26 minutes. Codes 90832, 90833, 90834, 90836, 90837, 90838 may be reported on the same day as codes 90846, 90847, when the services are separate and distinct.

In reporting, choose the code closest to the actual time (ie, 16-37 minutes for 90832 and 90833, 38-52 minutes for 90834 and 90836, and 53 or more minutes for 90837 and 90838). Do not report psychotherapy of less than 16 minutes duration. (See instructions for the usage of time in the Introduction of the CPT code set.)

Psychotherapy provided to a patient in a crisis state is reported with codes 90839 and 90840 and cannot be reported in addition to the psychotherapy codes 90832-90838. For psychotherapy for crisis, see "Other Psychotherapy."

Code 90785 is an add-on code to report interactive complexity services when provided in conjunction with the psychotherapy codes 90832-90838. For family psychotherapy, see 90846, 90847. The amount of time spent by a physician or other qualified health care professional providing interactive complexity services should be reflected in the timed service code for psychotherapy (90832, 90834, 90837) or the psychotherapy add-on code performed with an evaluation and management service (90833, 90836, 90838).

Some psychiatric patients receive a medical evaluation and management (E/M) service on the same day as a psychotherapy service by the same physician or other qualified health care professional. To report both E/M and psychotherapy, the two services must be significant and separately identifiable. These services are reported by using codes specific for psychotherapy when performed with evaluation and management services (90833, 90836, 90838) as add-on codes to the evaluation and management service.

Medical symptoms and disorders inform treatment choices of psychotherapeutic interventions, and data from therapeutic communication are used to evaluate the presence, type, and severity of medical symptoms and disorders. For the purposes of reporting, the medical and psychotherapeutic components of the service may be separately identified as follows:

1. The type and level of E/M service is selected based on medical decision making.

2. Time spent on the activities of the E/M service is not included in the time used for reporting the psychotherapy service. Time may not be used as the basis of E/M code selection and prolonged services may not be reported when psychotherapy with E/M (90833, 90836, 90838) are reported.

3. A separate diagnosis is not required for the reporting of E/M and psychotherapy on the same date of service.

★◀ **90832**   Psychotherapy, 30 minutes with patient
> *CPT Changes: An Insider's View* 2013, 2017
> *CPT Assistant* Jan 13:3, May 13:12, Jun 13:3, Aug 13:14, Feb 14:3, Aug 14:5, Oct 15:9, Dec 16:11, Sep 17:12, Nov 18:3, Aug 20:3, Dec 20:14, Apr 22:10

★+◀ **90833**   Psychotherapy, 30 minutes with patient when performed with an evaluation and management service (List separately in addition to the code for primary procedure)
> *CPT Changes: An Insider's View* 2013, 2017
> *CPT Assistant* Jan 13:3, May 13:12, Jun 13:3, Aug 13:14, Aug 14:5, Oct 15:9, Dec 16:11, Nov 18:3, Aug 20:3, Dec 20:14, Apr 22:10, Aug 22:19, Dec 23:49

(Use 90833 in conjunction with 99202-99255, 99304-99316, 99341-99350)

★◀ **90834**   Psychotherapy, 45 minutes with patient
> *CPT Changes: An Insider's View* 2013, 2017
> *CPT Assistant* Jan 13:3, May 13:12, Jun 13:3, Aug 13:14, Jun 14:3, Oct 15:9, Dec 16:11, Nov 18:3, Aug 20:3, Dec 20:14, Apr 22:10

★+◀ **90836**   Psychotherapy, 45 minutes with patient when performed with an evaluation and management service (List separately in addition to the code for primary procedure)
> *CPT Changes: An Insider's View* 2013, 2017
> *CPT Assistant* Jan 13:3, May 13:12, Jun 13:3, Aug 13:14, Oct 15:9, Dec 16:11, Nov 18:3, Aug 20:3, Dec 20:14, Apr 22:10, Aug 22:19

(Use 90836 in conjunction with 99202-99255, 99304-99316, 99341-99350)

★◀ **90837**   Psychotherapy, 60 minutes with patient
> *CPT Changes: An Insider's View* 2013, 2017
> *CPT Assistant* Jan 13:3, May 13:12, Jun 13:3, Aug 13:14, Apr 14:6, Oct 15:3, 9, Dec 16:11, Nov 18:3, Aug 20:3, Dec 20:14, Apr 22:10, Jan 23:33

★+◀ **90838**   Psychotherapy, 60 minutes with patient when performed with an evaluation and management service (List separately in addition to the code for primary procedure)
> *CPT Changes: An Insider's View* 2013, 2017
> *CPT Assistant* Jan 13:3, May 13:12, Jun 13:3, Aug 13:14, Feb 14:3, Apr 14:6, Oct 15:9, Dec 16:11, Nov 18:3, Aug 20:3, Dec 20:14, Apr 22:10, Aug 22:19

(Use 90838 in conjunction with 99202-99255, 99304-99316, 99341-99350)

(Use 90785 in conjunction with 90832, 90833, 90834, 90836, 90837, 90838 when psychotherapy includes interactive complexity services)

Psychotherapy for Crisis

Psychotherapy for crisis is an urgent assessment and history of a crisis state, a mental status exam, and a disposition. The treatment includes psychotherapy, mobilization of resources to defuse the crisis and restore safety, and implementation of psychotherapeutic interventions to minimize the potential for psychological trauma. The presenting problem is typically life threatening or complex and requires immediate attention to a patient in high distress.

Codes 90839, 90840 are used to report the total duration of time face-to-face with the patient and/or family spent by the physician or other qualified health care professional providing psychotherapy for crisis, even if the time spent on that date is not continuous. For any given period of time spent providing psychotherapy for crisis state, the physician or other qualified health care professional must devote his or her full attention to the patient and, therefore, cannot provide services to any other patient during the same time period. The patient must be present for all or some of the service. Do not report with 90791 or 90792.

Code 90839 is used to report the first 30-74 minutes of psychotherapy for crisis on a given date. It should be used only once per date even if the time spent by the physician or other health care professional is not continuous on that date. Psychotherapy for crisis of less than 30 minutes total duration on a given date should be reported with 90832 or 90833 (when provided with evaluation and management services).

Code 90840 is used to report additional block(s) of time, of up to 30 minutes each beyond the first 74 minutes.

★◀ **90839**   Psychotherapy for crisis; first 60 minutes
> *CPT Changes: An Insider's View* 2013
> *CPT Assistant* Jun 13:3, Aug 14:5, Oct 15:9, Nov 18:3, Aug 20:3

★+◀ **90840**   each additional 30 minutes (List separately in addition to code for primary service)
> *CPT Changes: An Insider's View* 2013
> *CPT Assistant* Jun 13:3, Aug 14:5, Oct 15:9, Nov 18:3, Aug 20:3

(Use 90840 in conjunction with 90839)

(Do not report 90839, 90840 in conjunction with 90791, 90792, psychotherapy codes 90832-90838 or other psychiatric services, or 90785-90899)

Other Psychotherapy

★◀ **90845**   Psychoanalysis
> *CPT Changes: An Insider's View* 2017
> *CPT Assistant* Summer 92:15, Nov 97:40-41, Mar 01:8, Mar 02:4, May 05:1, Feb 06:15, Mar 10:6, Oct 15:9, Nov 18:3, Aug 20:3

★◀ **90846**   Family psychotherapy (without the patient present), 50 minutes
> *CPT Changes: An Insider's View* 2017
> *CPT Assistant* Summer 92:15, Nov 97:40-41, Mar 01:8, Mar 02:4, May 05:1, Sep 09:11, Mar 10:6, Jun 13:3, Dec 13:18, Oct 15:9, Dec 16:11, Mar 17:11, Nov 18:3, Aug 20:3

★◀ **90847**   Family psychotherapy (conjoint psychotherapy) (with patient present), 50 minutes
> *CPT Changes: An Insider's View* 2017
> *CPT Assistant* Summer 92:15, Nov 97:40-41, Mar 01:5, Mar 02:4, May 05:1, Mar 10:6, Jun 13:3, Dec 13:18, Oct 15:9, Dec 16:11, Nov 18:3, Aug 20:3

(Do not report 90846, 90847 for family psychotherapy services less than 26 minutes)

(Do not report 90846, 90847 in conjunction with 97151, 97152, 97153, 97154, 97155, 97156, 97157, 97158, 0362T, 0373T)

90849   Multiple-family group psychotherapy
> *CPT Assistant* Summer 92:15, Nov 97:40-41, Mar 01:5, Mar 02:4, May 05:1, Mar 10:6, Aug 14:15, Oct 15:9, Nov 18:3, Aug 20:3

90853   Group psychotherapy (other than of a multiple-family group)
> *CPT Assistant* Summer 92:15, Nov 97:40-41, Mar 01:8, Mar 02:4, May 05:1, Mar 10:6, Jun 13:3, Jun 14:3, Aug 14:15, Oct 15:9, Mar 17:11, Nov 18:3, Aug 20:3, Apr 22:10, Oct 22:7

(Use 90853 in conjunction with 90785 for the specified patient when group psychotherapy includes interactive complexity)

(Do not report 90853 in conjunction with 97151, 97152, 97153, 97154, 97155, 97156, 97157, 97158, 0362T, 0373T)

Other Psychiatric Services or Procedures

(For electronic analysis with programming, when performed, of vagal nerve neurostimulators, see 95970, 95976, 95977)

★+ **90863**   Pharmacologic management, including prescription and review of medication, when performed with psychotherapy services (List separately in addition to the code for primary procedure)
> *CPT Changes: An Insider's View* 2013, 2017
> *CPT Assistant* Jun 13:3, Nov 18:3, Aug 20:3

(Use 90863 in conjunction with 90832, 90834, 90837)

(For pharmacologic management with psychotherapy services performed by a physician or other qualified health care professional who may report evaluation and management codes, use the appropriate evaluation and management codes 99202-99255, 99281-99285, 99304, 99305, 99306, 99307, 99308, 99309, 99310, 99341-99350 and the appropriate psychotherapy with evaluation and management service 90833, 90836, 90838)

(Do not count time spent on providing pharmacologic management services in the time used for selection of the psychotherapy service)

90865   Narcosynthesis for psychiatric diagnostic and therapeutic purposes (eg, sodium amobarbital (Amytal) interview)
> *CPT Assistant* Nov 97:41, Mar 01:5, Mar 02:4, May 05:1, Nov 18:3, Aug 20:3

90867   Therapeutic repetitive transcranial magnetic stimulation (TMS) treatment; initial, including cortical mapping, motor threshold determination, delivery and management
> *CPT Changes: An Insider's View* 2011, 2012
> *CPT Assistant* Nov 18:3, Aug 20:3

(Report only once per course of treatment)

▶(Do not report 90867 in conjunction with 90868, 90869, 95860, 95870, 95928, 95929, 95939, 0889T, 0890T, 0891T, 0892T)◀

(For peripheral nerve transcutaneous magnetic stimulation, see 0766T, 0767T)

90868   subsequent delivery and management, per session

➔ *CPT Changes: An Insider's View* 2011, 2012

➔ *CPT Assistant* Nov 18:3, Aug 20:3

▶(Do not report 90868 in conjunction with 0889T, 0890T, 0891T, 0892T)◀

90869   subsequent motor threshold re-determination with delivery and management

➔ *CPT Changes: An Insider's View* 2012

➔ *CPT Assistant* Nov 18:3, Aug 20:3

▶(Do not report 90869 in conjunction with 90867, 90868, 95860-95870, 95928, 95929, 95939, 0889T, 0890T, 0891T, 0892T)◀

(If a significant, separately identifiable evaluation and management, medication management, or psychotherapy service is performed, the appropriate E/M or psychotherapy code may be reported in addition to 90867-90869. Evaluation and management activities directly related to cortical mapping, motor threshold determination, delivery and management of TMS are not separately reported)

90870   Electroconvulsive therapy (includes necessary monitoring)

➔ *CPT Changes: An Insider's View* 2006

➔ *CPT Assistant* Summer 92:16, Mar 01:5, Mar 02:4, May 05:1, Mar 10:6, Feb 13:3, Nov 18:3, Aug 20:3

90875   Individual psychophysiological therapy incorporating biofeedback training by any modality (face-to-face with the patient), with psychotherapy (eg, insight oriented, behavior modifying or supportive psychotherapy); 30 minutes

➔ *CPT Changes: An Insider's View* 2013

➔ *CPT Assistant* Nov 96:15, Sep 97:11, Nov 97:41, Apr 98:14, Jun 99:5, Mar 01:5, Mar 02:4, Mar 05:16, May 05:1, Nov 18:3, Aug 20:3

90876   45 minutes

➔ *CPT Changes: An Insider's View* 2013

➔ *CPT Assistant* Nov 96:15, Sep 97:11, Nov 97:41, Jun 99:5, Mar 01:5, Mar 05:16, May 05:1, Nov 18:3, Aug 20:3

90880   Hypnotherapy

➔ *CPT Assistant* Summer 92:16, Nov 97:41, Mar 01:5, Mar 02:4, May 05:1, Nov 18:3, Aug 20:3

90882   Environmental intervention for medical management purposes on a psychiatric patient's behalf with agencies, employers, or institutions

➔ *CPT Assistant* Summer 92:16, Mar 01:5, Mar 02:4, May 05:1, Nov 18:3, Aug 20:3

90885   Psychiatric evaluation of hospital records, other psychiatric reports, psychometric and/or projective tests, and other accumulated data for medical diagnostic purposes

➔ *CPT Assistant* Nov 97:41, Mar 01:5, Mar 02:4, Oct 04:10, May 05:1, Nov 18:3, Aug 20:3, Dec 20:14

90887   Interpretation or explanation of results of psychiatric, other medical examinations and procedures, or other accumulated data to family or other responsible persons, or advising them how to assist patient

➔ *CPT Assistant* Summer 92:17, Mar 01:5, Mar 02:4, Oct 02:11, May 05:1, Nov 18:3, Aug 20:3

(Do not report 90887 in conjunction with 97151, 97152, 97153, 97154, 97155, 97156, 97157, 97158, 0362T, 0373T)

90889   Preparation of report of patient's psychiatric status, history, treatment, or progress (other than for legal or consultative purposes) for other individuals, agencies, or insurance carriers

➔ *CPT Changes: An Insider's View* 2013

➔ *CPT Assistant* Summer 92:17, Mar 01:5, Mar 02:4, May 05:1, Nov 18:3, Aug 20:3, Dec 22:18

90899   Unlisted psychiatric service or procedure

➔ *CPT Assistant* Mar 01:5, Mar 02:4, May 05:1, Jan 10:11, Apr 14:6, Nov 18:3, Aug 20:3, Jan 22:8

Biofeedback

(For psychophysiological therapy incorporating biofeedback training, see 90875, 90876)

90901   Biofeedback training by any modality

➔ *CPT Assistant* Sep 97:11, Apr 98:14, Jun 98:10, Jun 99:5, May 02:18, Sep 04:13, Mar 05:16, Jun 20:13

90912   Biofeedback training, perineal muscles, anorectal or urethral sphincter, including EMG and/or manometry, when performed; initial 15 minutes of one-on-one physician or other qualified health care professional contact with the patient

➔ *CPT Changes: An Insider's View* 2020

➔ *CPT Assistant* Jun 20:13

+ **90913**   each additional 15 minutes of one-on-one physician or other qualified health care professional contact with the patient (List separately in addition to code for primary procedure)

➔ *CPT Changes: An Insider's View* 2020

➔ *CPT Assistant* Jun 20:13

(Use 90913 in conjunction with 90912)

(For testing of rectal sensation, tone and compliance, use 91120)

(For incontinence treatment by pulsed magnetic neuromodulation, use 53899)

Dialysis

(For therapeutic apheresis for white blood cells, red blood cells, platelets and plasma pheresis, see 36511, 36512, 36513, 36514)

(For therapeutic apheresis extracorporeal adsorption procedures, use 36516)

(For therapeutic ultrafiltration, use 0692T)

Hemodialysis

Codes 90935, 90937 are reported to describe the hemodialysis procedure with all evaluation and management services related to the patient's renal disease on the day of the hemodialysis procedure. These codes are used for inpatient end-stage renal disease (ESRD) and non-ESRD procedures or for outpatient non-ESRD dialysis services. Code 90935 is reported if only one evaluation of the patient is required related to that hemodialysis procedure. Code 90937 is reported when patient re-evaluation(s) is required during a hemodialysis procedure. Use modifier 25 with evaluation and management codes, including new or established patient office or other outpatient services (99202-99215), office or other outpatient consultations (99242, 99243, 99244, 99245), hospital inpatient or observation care including admission and discharge (99234, 99235, 99236), initial and subsequent hospital inpatient or observation care (99221, 99222, 99223, 99231, 99232, 99233), hospital inpatient or observation discharge services (99238, 99239), new or established patient emergency department services (99281-99285), critical care services (99291, 99292), inpatient neonatal intensive care services and pediatric and neonatal critical care services (99466-99480), nursing facility services (99304, 99305, 99306, 99307, 99308, 99309, 99310, 99315, 99316), and home or residence services (99341-99350), for separately identifiable services unrelated to the dialysis procedure or renal failure that cannot be rendered during the dialysis session.

▶(For home visit hemodialysis services performed by a nonphysician qualified health care professional, use 99512)◀

(For cannula declotting, see 36831, 36833, 36860, 36861)

(For declotting of implanted vascular access device or catheter by thrombolytic agent, use 36593)

(For collection of blood specimen from a partially or completely implantable venous access device, use 36591)

(For prolonged attendance by a physician or other qualified health care professional, use 99360)

90935   Hemodialysis procedure with single evaluation by a physician or other qualified health care professional
➔ *CPT Changes: An Insider's View* 2013
➔ *CPT Assistant* Fall 93:2, May 02:17, Jan 03:22

90937   Hemodialysis procedure requiring repeated evaluation(s) with or without substantial revision of dialysis prescription
➔ *CPT Assistant* Fall 93:2, May 02:17, Jan 03:22

90940   Hemodialysis access flow study to determine blood flow in grafts and arteriovenous fistulae by an indicator method
➔ *CPT Changes: An Insider's View* 2001, 2006
➔ *CPT Assistant* Jan 03:22, May 06:18
➔ *Clinical Examples in Radiology* Summer 06:7, 12

(For duplex scan of hemodialysis access, use 93990)

Miscellaneous Dialysis Procedures

Codes 90945, 90947 describe dialysis procedures other than hemodialysis (eg, peritoneal dialysis, hemofiltration or continuous renal replacement therapies), and all evaluation and management services related to the patient's renal disease on the day of the procedure. Code 90945 is reported if only one evaluation of the patient is required related to that procedure. Code 90947 is reported when patient re-evaluation(s) is required during a procedure. Use modifier 25 with evaluation and management codes, including office or other outpatient services (99202-99215), office or other outpatient consultations (99242, 99243, 99244, 99245), hospital inpatient or observation care including admission and discharge (99234, 99235, 99236), initial and subsequent hospital inpatient or observation care (99221, 99222, 99223, 99231, 99232, 99233), hospital inpatient or observation discharge services (99238, 99239), new or established patient emergency department services (99281-99285), critical care services (99291, 99292), inpatient neonatal intensive care services and pediatric and neonatal critical care services (99466-99480), nursing facility services (99304, 99305, 99306, 99307, 99308, 99309, 99310, 99315, 99316), and home or residence services (99341-99350) for separately identifiable services unrelated to the procedure or the renal failure that cannot be rendered during the dialysis session.

(For percutaneous insertion of intraperitoneal tunneled catheter, use 49418. For open insertion of tunneled intraperitoneal catheter, use 49421)

(For prolonged attendance by a physician or other qualified health care professional, use 99360)

90945   Dialysis procedure other than hemodialysis (eg, peritoneal dialysis, hemofiltration, or other continuous renal replacement therapies), with single evaluation by a physician or other qualified health care professional

➔ *CPT Changes: An Insider's View* 2001, 2013

➔ *CPT Assistant* Fall 93:2, Nov 97:41, Jul 98:10, Oct 01:11, Jan 03:22

(For home infusion of peritoneal dialysis, use 99601, 99602)

90947   Dialysis procedure other than hemodialysis (eg, peritoneal dialysis, hemofiltration, or other continuous renal replacement therapies) requiring repeated evaluations by a physician or other qualified health care professional, with or without substantial revision of dialysis prescription

➔ *CPT Changes: An Insider's View* 2001, 2013

➔ *CPT Assistant* Fall 93:2, Nov 97:41, Jul 98:10, Oct 01:11, Jan 03:22

End-Stage Renal Disease Services

Codes 90951-90962 are reported **once** per month to distinguish age-specific services related to the patient's ESRD performed in an outpatient setting with three levels of service based on the number of face-to-face visits. ESRD-related services by a physician or other qualified health care professional include establishment of a dialyzing cycle, outpatient evaluation and management of the dialysis visits, telephone calls, and patient management during the dialysis provided during a full month. In the circumstances in which the patient has had a complete assessment visit during the month and services are provided over a period of less than a month, 90951-90962 may be used according to the number of visits performed.

Codes 90963-90966 are reported once per month for a full month of service to distinguish age-specific services for end-stage renal disease (ESRD) services for home dialysis patients.

For ESRD and non-ESRD dialysis services performed in an inpatient setting, and for non-ESRD dialysis services performed in an outpatient setting, see 90935-90937 and 90945-90947.

Evaluation and management services unrelated to ESRD services that cannot be performed during the dialysis session may be reported separately.

Codes 90967-90970 are reported to distinguish age-specific services for end-stage renal disease (ESRD) services for less than a full month of service, per day, for services provided under the following circumstances: transient patients, partial month where there was one or more face-to-face visits without the complete assessment, the patient was hospitalized before a complete assessment was furnished, dialysis was stopped due to recovery or death, or the patient received a kidney transplant. For reporting purposes, each month is considered 30 days.

Examples:

ESRD-related services:

ESRD-related services are initiated on July 1 for a 57-year-old male. On July 11, he is admitted to the hospital as an inpatient and is discharged on July 27. He has had a complete assessment and the physician or other qualified health care professional has performed two face-to-face visits prior to admission. Another face-to-face visit occurs after discharge during the month.

In this example, 90961 is reported for the three face-to-face outpatient visits. Report inpatient E/M services as appropriate. Dialysis procedures rendered during the hospitalization (July 11-27) should be reported as appropriate (90935-90937, 90945-90947).

If the patient did not have a complete assessment during the month or was a transient or dialysis was stopped due to recovery or death, 90970 would be used to report each day outside the inpatient hospitalization as described in the home dialysis example below.

ESRD-related services for the home dialysis patient:

Home ESRD-related services are initiated on July 1 for a 57-year-old male. On July 11, he is admitted to the hospital as an inpatient and is discharged on July 27.

Report inpatient E/M services as appropriate. Dialysis procedures rendered during the hospitalization (July 11-27) should be reported as appropriate (90935-90937, 90945-90947).

(Do not report 90951-90970 during the same month in conjunction with 99424, 99425, 99426, 99427, 99437, 99439, 99487, 99489, 99490, 99491)

★ **90951**   End-stage renal disease (ESRD) related services monthly, for patients younger than 2 years of age to include monitoring for the adequacy of nutrition, assessment of growth and development, and counseling of parents; with 4 or more face-to-face visits by a physician or other qualified health care professional per month

➔ *CPT Changes: An Insider's View* 2009, 2013, 2017

➔ *CPT Assistant* Apr 13:3, Nov 13:3, Oct 14:3, Feb 18:12, Jan 24:38

★ **90952**   with 2-3 face-to-face visits by a physician or other qualified health care professional per month

➔ *CPT Changes: An Insider's View* 2009, 2013, 2017

➔ *CPT Assistant* Apr 13:3, Feb 18:12

90953   with 1 face-to-face visit by a physician or other qualified health care professional per month

➔ *CPT Changes: An Insider's View* 2009, 2013

➔ *CPT Assistant* Apr 13:3, Feb 18:12

★ **90954**   End-stage renal disease (ESRD) related services monthly, for patients 2-11 years of age to include monitoring for the adequacy of nutrition, assessment of growth and development, and counseling of parents; with 4 or more face-to-face visits by a physician or other qualified health care professional per month

➔ *CPT Changes: An Insider's View* 2009, 2013, 2017
➔ *CPT Assistant* Apr 13:3, Feb 18:12

★ **90955**   with 2-3 face-to-face visits by a physician or other qualified health care professional per month

➔ *CPT Changes: An Insider's View* 2009, 2013, 2017
➔ *CPT Assistant* Apr 13:3, Feb 18:12

90956   with 1 face-to-face visit by a physician or other qualified health care professional per month

➔ *CPT Changes: An Insider's View* 2009, 2013
➔ *CPT Assistant* Apr 13:3, Feb 18:12

★ **90957**   End-stage renal disease (ESRD) related services monthly, for patients 12-19 years of age to include monitoring for the adequacy of nutrition, assessment of growth and development, and counseling of parents; with 4 or more face-to-face visits by a physician or other qualified health care professional per month

➔ *CPT Changes: An Insider's View* 2009, 2013, 2017
➔ *CPT Assistant* Apr 13:3, Feb 18:12

★ **90958**   with 2-3 face-to-face visits by a physician or other qualified health care professional per month

➔ *CPT Changes: An Insider's View* 2009, 2013, 2017
➔ *CPT Assistant* Apr 13:3, Feb 18:12

90959   with 1 face-to-face visit by a physician or other qualified health care professional per month

➔ *CPT Changes: An Insider's View* 2009, 2013
➔ *CPT Assistant* Apr 13:3, Feb 18:12

★ **90960**   End-stage renal disease (ESRD) related services monthly, for patients 20 years of age and older; with 4 or more face-to-face visits by a physician or other qualified health care professional per month

➔ *CPT Changes: An Insider's View* 2009, 2013, 2017
➔ *CPT Assistant* Apr 13:3, Feb 18:12, Jan 24:38

★ **90961**   with 2-3 face-to-face visits by a physician or other qualified health care professional per month

➔ *CPT Changes: An Insider's View* 2009, 2013, 2017
➔ *CPT Assistant* Apr 13:3, Feb 18:12, Jan 24:38

90962   with 1 face-to-face visit by a physician or other qualified health care professional per month

➔ *CPT Changes: An Insider's View* 2009, 2013
➔ *CPT Assistant* Apr 13:3, Feb 18:12, Jan 24:38

★ **90963**   End-stage renal disease (ESRD) related services for home dialysis per full month, for patients younger than 2 years of age to include monitoring for the adequacy of nutrition, assessment of growth and development, and counseling of parents

➔ *CPT Changes: An Insider's View* 2009
➔ *CPT Assistant* Apr 13:3, Feb 18:12

★ **90964**   End-stage renal disease (ESRD) related services for home dialysis per full month, for patients 2-11 years of age to include monitoring for the adequacy of nutrition, assessment of growth and development, and counseling of parents

➔ *CPT Changes: An Insider's View* 2009
➔ *CPT Assistant* Apr 13:3, Feb 18:12

★ **90965**   End-stage renal disease (ESRD) related services for home dialysis per full month, for patients 12-19 years of age to include monitoring for the adequacy of nutrition, assessment of growth and development, and counseling of parents

➔ *CPT Changes: An Insider's View* 2009
➔ *CPT Assistant* Apr 13:3, Feb 18:12

★ **90966**   End-stage renal disease (ESRD) related services for home dialysis per full month, for patients 20 years of age and older

➔ *CPT Changes: An Insider's View* 2009
➔ *CPT Assistant* Apr 13:3, Feb 18:12

★ **90967**   End-stage renal disease (ESRD) related services for dialysis less than a full month of service, per day; for patients younger than 2 years of age

➔ *CPT Changes: An Insider's View* 2009
➔ *CPT Assistant* Apr 13:3, Feb 18:12

★ **90968**   for patients 2-11 years of age

➔ *CPT Changes: An Insider's View* 2009
➔ *CPT Assistant* Apr 13:3, Feb 18:12

★ **90969**   for patients 12-19 years of age

➔ *CPT Changes: An Insider's View* 2009
➔ *CPT Assistant* Apr 13:3, Feb 18:12

★ **90970**   for patients 20 years of age and older

➔ *CPT Changes: An Insider's View* 2009
➔ *CPT Assistant* Apr 13:3, Nov 13:3, Oct 14:3, Feb 18:12

Other Dialysis Procedures

90989   Dialysis training, patient, including helper where applicable, any mode, completed course

➔ *CPT Assistant* Fall 93:5, Jun 01:10

90993   Dialysis training, patient, including helper where applicable, any mode, course not completed, per training session

➔ *CPT Assistant* Winter 90:11, Fall 93:5, Jun 01:10

90997   Hemoperfusion (eg, with activated charcoal or resin)

90999   Unlisted dialysis procedure, inpatient or outpatient

Gastroenterology

91010   Esophageal motility (manometric study of the esophagus and/or gastroesophageal junction) study with interpretation and report;
➤ *CPT Changes: An Insider's View* 2011, 2012
➤ *CPT Assistant* Nov 97:42

+ 91013   with stimulation or perfusion (eg, stimulant, acid or alkali perfusion) (List separately in addition to code for primary procedure)
➤ *CPT Changes: An Insider's View* 2011, 2012

(Use 91013 in conjunction with 91010)

(Do not report 91013 more than once per session)

(To report esophageal motility studies with high resolution esophageal pressure topography, use 91299)

91020   Gastric motility (manometric) studies
➤ *CPT Assistant* Nov 97:42, Sep 13:13

91022   Duodenal motility (manometric) study
➤ *CPT Changes: An Insider's View* 2006
➤ *CPT Assistant* Sep 13:13

(If gastrointestinal endoscopy is performed, use 43235)

(If fluoroscopy is performed, use 76000)

(If gastric motility study is performed, use 91020)

(Do not report 91020, 91022 in conjunction with 91112)

91030   Esophagus, acid perfusion (Bernstein) test for esophagitis

91034   Esophagus, gastroesophageal reflux test; with nasal catheter pH electrode(s) placement, recording, analysis and interpretation
➤ *CPT Changes: An Insider's View* 2005
➤ *CPT Assistant* May 05:3, Feb 14:11

91035   with mucosal attached telemetry pH electrode placement, recording, analysis and interpretation
➤ *CPT Changes: An Insider's View* 2005
➤ *CPT Assistant* May 05:3, Feb 14:11

91037   Esophageal function test, gastroesophageal reflux test with nasal catheter intraluminal impedance electrode(s) placement, recording, analysis and interpretation;
➤ *CPT Changes: An Insider's View* 2005
➤ *CPT Assistant* May 05:3

91038   prolonged (greater than 1 hour, up to 24 hours)
➤ *CPT Changes: An Insider's View* 2005
➤ *CPT Assistant* May 05:3, Feb 14:11

91040   Esophageal balloon distension study, diagnostic, with provocation when performed
➤ *CPT Changes: An Insider's View* 2005, 2016
➤ *CPT Assistant* May 05:3, Jan 17:7

(Do not report 91040 more than once per session)

Esophageal Acid Reflux Test
91034

A catheter with a pH electrode is placed into the esophagus, either through the nares or swallowed, to measure intraesophageal pH (an indicator of gastric reflux).

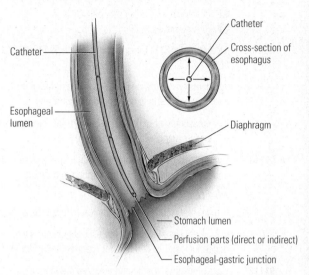

Labels: Catheter · Catheter · Cross-section of esophagus · Esophageal lumen · Diaphragm · Stomach lumen · Perfusion parts (direct or indirect) · Esophageal-gastric junction

91065   Breath hydrogen or methane test (eg, for detection of lactase deficiency, fructose intolerance, bacterial overgrowth, or oro-cecal gastrointestinal transit)
➤ *CPT Changes: An Insider's View* 2005, 2014
➤ *CPT Assistant* May 05:3

(Report 91065 once for each administered challenge)

(For H. pylori breath test analysis, use 83013 for non-radioactive (C-13) isotope or 78268 for radioactive (C-14) isotope)

(To report placement of an esophageal tamponade tube for management of variceal bleeding, use 43460. To report placement of a long intestinal Miller-Abbott tube, use 44500)

(For abdominal paracentesis, see 49082, 49083, 49084; with instillation of medication, see 96440, 96446)

(For peritoneoscopy, use 49320; with biopsy, use 49321)

(For splenoportography, see 38200, 75810)

91110   Gastrointestinal tract imaging, intraluminal (eg, capsule endoscopy), esophagus through ileum, with interpretation and report
➤ *CPT Changes: An Insider's View* 2004, 2013
➤ *CPT Assistant* Oct 04:15, Aug 05:14, May 09:8, Sep 13:13

(Do not report 91110 in conjunction with 91111, 91113, 0651T)

(Incidental visualization of the colon is not reported separately)

(Append modifier 52 if the ileum is not visualized)

91111 Gastrointestinal tract imaging, intraluminal (eg, capsule endoscopy), esophagus with interpretation and report

➔ *CPT Changes: An Insider's View* 2007, 2013

➔ *CPT Assistant* Sep 13:13

(Do not report 91111 in conjunction with 91110, 91113, 0651T)

(Incidental visualization of the stomach, duodenum, ileum, and/or colon is not reported separately)

(For measurement of gastrointestinal tract transit times or pressure using wireless capsule, use 91112)

 # 91113 Gastrointestinal tract imaging, intraluminal (eg, capsule endoscopy), colon, with interpretation and report

➔ *CPT Changes: An Insider's View* 2022

(Do not report 91113 in conjunction with 91110, 91111)

(Incidental visualization of the esophagus, stomach, duodenum, and/or ileum is not reported separately)

91112 Gastrointestinal transit and pressure measurement, stomach through colon, wireless capsule, with interpretation and report

➔ *CPT Changes: An Insider's View* 2013

➔ *CPT Assistant* Sep 13:13

(Do not report 91112 in conjunction with 83986, 91020, 91022, 91117)

91113 Code is out of numerical sequence. See 91110-91117

91117 Colon motility (manometric) study, minimum 6 hours continuous recording (including provocation tests, eg, meal, intracolonic balloon distension, pharmacologic agents, if performed), with interpretation and report

➔ *CPT Changes: An Insider's View* 2011

➔ *CPT Assistant* Sep 13:13

(For wireless capsule pressure measurements, use 91112)

(Do not report 91117 in conjunction with 91120, 91122)

91120 Rectal sensation, tone, and compliance test (ie, response to graded balloon distention)

➔ *CPT Changes: An Insider's View* 2005

➔ *CPT Assistant* May 05:3, Jun 20:13

(For biofeedback training, see 90912, 90913)

(For anorectal manometry, use 91122)

91122 Anorectal manometry

(Do not report 91120, 91122 in conjunction with 91117)

Gastric Physiology

91132 Electrogastrography, diagnostic, transcutaneous;

➔ *CPT Changes: An Insider's View* 2001

91133 with provocative testing

➔ *CPT Changes: An Insider's View* 2001

▶(Do not report 91132, 91133 in conjunction with 0779T, 0868T)◀

Other Procedures

91200 Liver elastography, mechanically induced shear wave (eg, vibration), without imaging, with interpretation and report

➔ *CPT Changes: An Insider's View* 2015

➔ *CPT Assistant* Oct 17:9, Aug 19:3

➔ *Clinical Examples in Radiology* Spring 15:4, Fall 18:3

(Do not report 91200 in conjunction with 76981, 76982, 76983)

91299 Unlisted diagnostic gastroenterology procedure

➔ *CPT Assistant* Aug 05:14

91304 Code is out of numerical sequence. See 90473-90477

91318 Code is out of numerical sequence. See 90473-90477

91319 Code is out of numerical sequence. See 90473-90477

91320 Code is out of numerical sequence. See 90473-90477

91321 Code is out of numerical sequence. See 90473-90477

91322 Code is out of numerical sequence. See 90473-90477

Ophthalmology

(For surgical procedures, see **Surgery**, Eye and Ocular Adnexa, 65091 et seq)

Definitions

Intermediate ophthalmological services describes an evaluation of a new or existing condition complicated with a new diagnostic or management problem not necessarily relating to the primary diagnosis, including history, general medical observation, external ocular and adnexal examination and other diagnostic procedures as indicated; may include the use of mydriasis for ophthalmoscopy.

For example:

a. Review of history, external examination, ophthalmoscopy, biomicroscopy for an acute complicated condition (eg, iritis) not requiring comprehensive ophthalmological services.

b. Review of interval history, external examination, ophthalmoscopy, biomicroscopy and tonometry in established patient with known cataract not requiring comprehensive ophthalmological services.

Comprehensive ophthalmological services describes a general evaluation of the complete visual system. The comprehensive services constitute a single service entity but need not be performed at one session. The service includes history, general medical observation, external and ophthalmoscopic examinations, gross visual fields and basic sensorimotor examination. It often includes, as indicated: biomicroscopy, examination with cycloplegia or mydriasis and tonometry. It always includes initiation of diagnostic and treatment programs.

Intermediate and comprehensive ophthalmological services constitute integrated services in which medical decision making cannot be separated from the examining techniques used. Itemization of service components, such as slit lamp examination, keratometry, routine ophthalmoscopy, retinoscopy, tonometry, or motor evaluation is not applicable.

For example:

The comprehensive services required for diagnosis and treatment of a patient with symptoms indicating possible disease of the visual system, such as glaucoma, cataract or retinal disease, or to rule out disease of the visual system, new or established patient.

Initiation of diagnostic and treatment program includes the prescription of medication, and arranging for special ophthalmological diagnostic or treatment services, consultations, laboratory procedures and radiological services.

Special ophthalmological services describes services in which a special evaluation of part of the visual system is made, which goes beyond the services included under general ophthalmological services, or in which special treatment is given. Special ophthalmological services may be reported in addition to the general ophthalmological services or evaluation and management services.

For example:

Fluorescein angioscopy, quantitative visual field examination, refraction or extended color vision examination (such as Nagel's anomaloscope) should be separately reported.

Prescription of lenses, when required, is included in 92015. It includes specification of lens type (monofocal, bifocal, other), lens power, axis, prism, absorptive factor, impact resistance, and other factors.

Interpretation and report by the physician or other qualified health care professional is an integral part of special ophthalmological services where indicated. Technical procedures (which may or may not be performed personally) are often part of the service, but should not be mistaken to constitute the service itself.

General Ophthalmological Services

New Patient

(For distinguishing between new and established patients, see **Evaluation and Management** guidelines)

92002 Ophthalmological services: medical examination and evaluation with initiation of diagnostic and treatment program; intermediate, new patient

➔ *CPT Assistant* Feb 97:6, Aug 98:3, Jun 05:11, Dec 05:10, Jan 07:30, Jan 08:1, Sep 08:7, Feb 11:10, Aug 12:9, Oct 12:9, Sep 17:15, Feb 18:3, Jan 21:10

(Do not report 92002 in conjunction with 99173, 99174, 99177, 0469T)

92004 comprehensive, new patient, 1 or more visits

➔ *CPT Assistant* Feb 97:6, Aug 98:3, Jun 05:11, Dec 05:10, Jan 07:30, Jan 08:1, Sep 08:7, Nov 10:8, Jan 11:9, Feb 11:10, Aug 12:9, Nov 16:9, Sep 17:15, Feb 18:3, Jan 21:10

(Do not report 92004 in conjunction with 99173, 99174, 99177, 0469T)

Established Patient

(For distinguishing between new and established patients, see **Evaluation and Management** guidelines)

92012 Ophthalmological services: medical examination and evaluation, with initiation or continuation of diagnostic and treatment program; intermediate, established patient

➔ *CPT Assistant* Feb 97:6, Aug 98:3, Jun 05:11, Dec 05:10, Jan 07:30, Jan 08:1, Sep 08:7, Feb 11:10, Aug 12:9, Sep 17:15, Feb 18:3, Jan 21:10

(Do not report 92012 in conjunction with 99173, 99174, 99177, 0469T)

92014 comprehensive, established patient, 1 or more visits

➔ *CPT Assistant* Feb 97:6, Aug 98:3, Dec 99:10, Jun 05:11, Dec 05:10, Jan 07:30, Jan 08:1, Sep 08:7, Nov 10:8, Jan 11:9, Feb 11:10, Aug 12:9, Oct 12:9, Nov 16:9, Sep 17:15, Feb 18:3

(Do not report 92014 in conjunction with 99173, 99174, 99177, 0469T)

(For surgical procedures, see **Surgery**, Eye and Ocular Adnexa, 65091 et seq)

Special Ophthalmological Services

92015 Determination of refractive state
→ *CPT Assistant* Mar 96:11, Feb 97:6, Aug 98:3, Aug 06:11, Mar 13:6, Mar 16:11

(Do not report 92015 in conjunction with 99173, 99174, 99177)

(For instrument-based ocular screening, use 99174, 99177)

92018 Ophthalmological examination and evaluation, under general anesthesia, with or without manipulation of globe for passive range of motion or other manipulation to facilitate diagnostic examination; complete
→ *CPT Assistant* Feb 97:6, Aug 98:3

92019 limited
→ *CPT Assistant* Feb 97:6, Aug 98:3

92020 Gonioscopy (separate procedure)
→ *CPT Assistant* Feb 97:6, Aug 98:3, Sep 21:10

(Do not report 92020 in conjunction with 0621T, 0622T)

(For gonioscopy under general anesthesia, use 92018)

92025 Computerized corneal topography, unilateral or bilateral, with interpretation and report
→ *CPT Changes: An Insider's View* 2007
→ *CPT Assistant* Oct 10:10, Oct 12:9

(Do not report 92025 in conjunction with 65710-65771)

(92025 is not used for manual keratoscopy, which is part of a single system Evaluation and Management or ophthalmological service)

92060 Sensorimotor examination with multiple measurements of ocular deviation (eg, restrictive or paretic muscle with diplopia) with interpretation and report (separate procedure)
→ *CPT Assistant* Feb 97:6, Aug 98:3

92065 Orthoptic training; performed by a physician or other qualified health care professional
→ *CPT Changes: An Insider's View* 2022, 2023
→ *CPT Assistant* Feb 97:6, Jun 98:10, Aug 98:3, Feb 22:11

(Do not report 92065 in conjunction with 92066, 0687T, 0688T, when performed on the same day)

92066 under supervision of a physician or other qualified health care professional
→ *CPT Changes: An Insider's View* 2023
→ *CPT Assistant* Feb 23:14

(Do not report 92066 in conjunction with 92065, 0687T, 0688T, when performed on the same day)

92071 Fitting of contact lens for treatment of ocular surface disease
→ *CPT Changes: An Insider's View* 2012
→ *CPT Assistant* Aug 12:9

(Do not report 92071 in conjunction with 92072)

(Report supply of lens separately with 99070 or appropriate supply code)

92072 Fitting of contact lens for management of keratoconus, initial fitting
→ *CPT Changes: An Insider's View* 2012
→ *CPT Assistant* Aug 12:9, Sep 17:15

(For subsequent fittings, report using evaluation and management services or general ophthalmological services)

(Do not report 92072 in conjunction with 92071)

(Report supply of lens separately with 99070 or appropriate supply code)

92081 Visual field examination, unilateral or bilateral, with interpretation and report; limited examination (eg, tangent screen, Autoplot, arc perimeter, or single stimulus level automated test, such as Octopus 3 or 7 equivalent)
→ *CPT Assistant* Feb 97:6, Aug 98:3, Sep 10:10, Oct 12:9

92082 intermediate examination (eg, at least 2 isopters on Goldmann perimeter, or semiquantitative, automated suprathreshold screening program, Humphrey suprathreshold automatic diagnostic test, Octopus program 33)
→ *CPT Assistant* Feb 97:6, Aug 98:3, Oct 12:9

92083 extended examination (eg, Goldmann visual fields with at least 3 isopters plotted and static determination within the central 30°, or quantitative, automated threshold perimetry, Octopus program G-1, 32 or 42, Humphrey visual field analyzer full threshold programs 30-2, 24-2, or 30/60-2)
→ *CPT Assistant* Feb 97:6, Aug 98:3, Oct 12:9

(Gross visual field testing (eg, confrontation testing) is a part of general ophthalmological services and is not reported separately)

(For visual field assessment by patient activated data transmission to a remote surveillance center, see 0378T, 0379T)

92100 Serial tonometry (separate procedure) with multiple measurements of intraocular pressure over an extended time period with interpretation and report, same day (eg, diurnal curve or medical treatment of acute elevation of intraocular pressure)
→ *CPT Assistant* Feb 97:6, Jun 98:10, Aug 98:3, Aug 12:9, 15, Oct 12:9, May 14:5

(For monitoring of intraocular pressure for 24 hours or longer, use 0329T)

(Ocular blood flow measurements are reported with 0198T. Single-episode tonometry is a component of general ophthalmological service or E/M service)

▲ **92132** Computerized ophthalmic diagnostic imaging (eg, optical coherence tomography [OCT]), anterior segment, with interpretation and report, unilateral or bilateral

⮕ *CPT Changes: An Insider's View* 2011, 2025

⮕ *CPT Assistant* Feb 11:6, Oct 12:9, Mar 13:6, Apr 13:7, May 14:5, Sep 23:42

(Do not report 92132 in conjunction with 0730T)

▶(For computerized ophthalmic diagnostic imaging of the optic nerve and retina, see 92133, 92134, 92137)◀

(For specular microscopy and endothelial cell analysis, use 92286)

(For tear film imaging, use 0330T)

▲ **92133** Computerized ophthalmic diagnostic imaging (eg, optical coherence tomography [OCT]), posterior segment, with interpretation and report, unilateral or bilateral; optic nerve

⮕ *CPT Changes: An Insider's View* 2011, 2025

⮕ *CPT Assistant* Feb 11:6, Oct 12:9, Nov 14:10, Jan 21:10

▲ **92134**   retina

⮕ *CPT Changes: An Insider's View* 2011, 2025

⮕ *CPT Assistant* Feb 11:6, Oct 12:9, Nov 14:10, Jan 21:10, Nov 21:12

#● **92137**   retina, including OCT angiography

⮕ *CPT Changes: An Insider's View* 2025

▶(Do not report 92133, 92134, 92137 at the same patient encounter)◀

▶(Report 92137 separately when performed at same encounter as 92235, 92240, 92242)◀

92136 Ophthalmic biometry by partial coherence interferometry with intraocular lens power calculation

⮕ *CPT Changes: An Insider's View* 2002

⮕ *CPT Assistant* Aug 98:3, Apr 02:18, Sep 09:5, May 14:5

(For tear film imaging, use 0330T)

92137 Code is out of numerical sequence. See 92133-92145

92145 Corneal hysteresis determination, by air impulse stimulation, unilateral or bilateral, with interpretation and report

⮕ *CPT Changes: An Insider's View* 2015

Ophthalmoscopy

Routine ophthalmoscopy is part of general and special ophthalmologic services whenever indicated. It is a non-itemized service and is not reported separately.

92201 Ophthalmoscopy, extended; with retinal drawing and scleral depression of peripheral retinal disease (eg, for retinal tear, retinal detachment, retinal tumor) with interpretation and report, unilateral or bilateral

⮕ *CPT Changes: An Insider's View* 2020

⮕ *CPT Assistant* Dec 19:3

Extended Ophthalmoscopy
92201, 92202

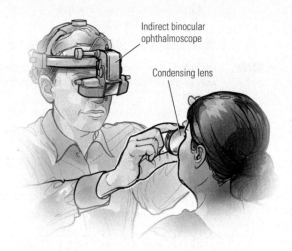

Indirect binocular ophthalmoscope

Condensing lens

Example of clinical drawing of peripheral retinal disease

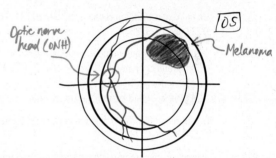

Optic nerve head (ONH)

OS

Melanoma

Example of clinical drawing of optic nerve or macular (posterior pole) pathology

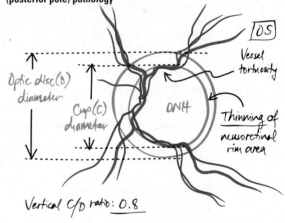

OS

Optic disc (D) diameter

Cup (C) diameter

ONH

Vessel tortuosity

Thinning of neuroretinal rim area

Vertical C/D ratio: 0.8

92202 with drawing of optic nerve or macula (eg, for glaucoma, macular pathology, tumor) with interpretation and report, unilateral or bilateral

➔ *CPT Changes: An Insider's View* 2020

➔ *CPT Assistant* Dec 19:3

(Do not report 92201, 92202 in conjunction with 92250)

★ 92227 Imaging of retina for detection or monitoring of disease; with remote clinical staff review and report, unilateral or bilateral

➔ *CPT Changes: An Insider's View* 2011, 2017, 2020, 2021

➔ *CPT Assistant* Feb 11:7, May 11:9, Oct 12:9, Jul 16:9, Aug 19:11, Jan 21:10, Jun 21:8

(Do not report 92227 in conjunction with 92133, 92134, 92228, 92229, 92250)

★ 92228 with remote physician or other qualified health care professional interpretation and report, unilateral or bilateral

➔ *CPT Changes: An Insider's View* 2011, 2017, 2021

➔ *CPT Assistant* Feb 11:7, May 11:9, Oct 12:9, Jan 21:10, Jun 21:8

(Do not report 92228 in conjunction with 92133, 92134, 92227, 92229, 92250)

92229 point-of-care autonomous analysis and report, unilateral or bilateral

➔ *CPT Changes: An Insider's View* 2021, 2023

➔ *CPT Assistant* Jan 21:10, Jun 21:8, Sep 21:5

(Do not report 92229 in conjunction with 92133, 92134, 92227, 92228, 92250)

92230 Fluorescein angioscopy with interpretation and report

➔ *CPT Assistant* Feb 97:6, Feb 11:6

92235 Fluorescein angiography (includes multiframe imaging) with interpretation and report, unilateral or bilateral

➔ *CPT Changes: An Insider's View* 2017

➔ *CPT Assistant* Feb 97:6, Feb 11:6, Jun 17:8

▶(For optical coherence tomography [OCT] retinal angiography, use 92137)◀

(When fluorescein and indocyanine-green angiography are performed at the same patient encounter, use 92242)

92240 Indocyanine-green angiography (includes multiframe imaging) with interpretation and report, unilateral or bilateral

➔ *CPT Changes: An Insider's View* 2017

➔ *CPT Assistant* Feb 11:6, Oct 12:9, Jun 17:8

▶(For optical coherence tomography [OCT] retinal angiography, use 92137)◀

(When indocyanine-green and fluorescein angiography are performed at the same patient encounter, use 92242)

Fluorescein Angiography
92235

Fluorescein dye is injected in a peripheral vein to enhance imaging. Serial multiframe angiography is performed to evaluate choroidal and retinal circulation. In this illustration, arteries display an even fluorescence, while veins appear striped from the laminar dye flow.

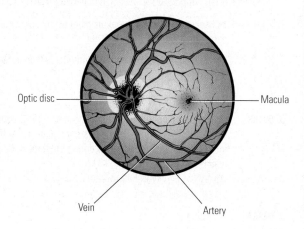

92242 Fluorescein angiography and indocyanine-green angiography (includes multiframe imaging) performed at the same patient encounter with interpretation and report, unilateral or bilateral

➔ *CPT Changes: An Insider's View* 2017

➔ *CPT Assistant* Jun 17:8

▶(For optical coherence tomography [OCT] retinal angiography, use 92137)◀

(To report fluorescein angiography and indocyanine-green angiography not performed at the same patient encounter, see 92235, 92240)

92250 Fundus photography with interpretation and report

➔ *CPT Assistant* Feb 97:6, Apr 99:10, Feb 11:6, Oct 12:9, Nov 14:10, Dec 14:17, May 15:9, Jul 16:9, Jan 21:10, Nov 21:12

92260 Ophthalmodynamometry

➔ *CPT Assistant* Feb 97:6, Feb 11:6

(For ophthalmoscopy under general anesthesia, use 92018)

Other Specialized Services

For prescription, fitting, and/or medical supervision of ocular prosthetic (artificial eye) adaptation by a physician, see evaluation and management services, including office or other outpatient services (99202-99215), office or other outpatient consultations (99242, 99243, 99244, 99245), or general ophthalmological service codes (92002-92014).

Electroretinography (ERG) is used to evaluate function of the retina and optic nerve of the eye, including photoreceptors and ganglion cells. A number of techniques are used which target different areas of the eye, including full field (flash and flicker) (92273) for a global response of photoreceptors of the retina, multifocal (92274) for photoreceptors in multiple separate locations in the retina including the macula, and pattern (0509T) for retinal ganglion cells. Multiple additional terms and techniques are used to describe various types of ERG. If the technique used is not specifically named in the code descriptors for 92273, 92274, or 0509T, use the unlisted procedure code 92499.

92265   Needle oculoelectromyography, 1 or more extraocular muscles, 1 or both eyes, with interpretation and report
➲ *CPT Assistant* Feb 97:6, Oct 12:9

92270   Electro-oculography with interpretation and report
➲ *CPT Assistant* Feb 97:6, Aug 08:12, May 09:9, Oct 12:9, Sep 15:7, Apr 20:7, Feb 21:5

(For vestibular function tests with recording, see 92537, 92538, 92540, 92541, 92542, 92544, 92545, 92546, 92547, 92548)

(Do not report 92270 in conjunction with 92537, 92538, 92540, 92541, 92542, 92544, 92545, 92546, 92547, 92548, 92549)

(To report saccadic eye movement testing with recording, use 92700)

92273   Electroretinography (ERG), with interpretation and report; full field (ie, ffERG, flash ERG, Ganzfeld ERG)
➲ *CPT Changes: An Insider's View* 2019
➲ *CPT Assistant* Jan 19:12

92274   multifocal (mfERG)
➲ *CPT Changes: An Insider's View* 2019
➲ *CPT Assistant* Jan 19:12

(For pattern ERG, use 0509T)

(For electronystagmography for vestibular function studies, see 92541 et seq)

(For ophthalmic echography (diagnostic ultrasound), see 76511-76529)

92283   Color vision examination, extended, eg, anomaloscope or equivalent
➲ *CPT Assistant* Feb 97:6, Oct 12:9

(Color vision testing with pseudoisochromatic plates [such as HRR or Ishihara] is not reported separately. It is included in the appropriate general or ophthalmological service, or 99172)

92284   Diagnostic dark adaptation examination with interpretation and report
➲ *CPT Changes: An Insider's View* 2023
➲ *CPT Assistant* Feb 97:6, Oct 12:9

92285   External ocular photography with interpretation and report for documentation of medical progress (eg, close-up photography, slit lamp photography, goniophotography, stereo-photography)
➲ *CPT Assistant* Feb 97:6, Sep 97:10, Oct 12:9, May 14:5

(For tear film imaging, use 0330T)

(For meibomian gland imaging, use 0507T)

92286   Anterior segment imaging with interpretation and report; with specular microscopy and endothelial cell analysis
➲ *CPT Changes: An Insider's View* 2013
➲ *CPT Assistant* Feb 97:6, Oct 12:9, Mar 13:6

92287   with fluorescein angiography
➲ *CPT Changes: An Insider's View* 2013
➲ *CPT Assistant* Feb 97:6, Mar 13:6

Contact Lens Services

The prescription of contact lens includes specification of optical and physical characteristics (such as power, size, curvature, flexibility, gas-permeability). It is **not** a part of the general ophthalmological services.

The fitting of contact lens includes instruction and training of the wearer and incidental revision of the lens during the training period.

Follow-up of successfully fitted extended wear lenses is reported as part of a general ophthalmological service (92012 et seq).

The supply of contact lenses may be reported as part of the service of fitting. It may also be reported separately by using the appropriate supply codes.

(For therapeutic or surgical use of contact lens, see 68340, 92071, 92072)

92310   Prescription of optical and physical characteristics of and fitting of contact lens, with medical supervision of adaptation; corneal lens, both eyes, except for aphakia
➲ *CPT Assistant* Feb 97:6, Oct 12:9

(For prescription and fitting of 1 eye, add modifier 52)

92311   corneal lens for aphakia, 1 eye
➲ *CPT Assistant* Feb 97:6, Oct 12:9

92312   corneal lens for aphakia, both eyes
➲ *CPT Assistant* Feb 97:6, Oct 12:9

92313   corneoscleral lens
➲ *CPT Assistant* Feb 97:7, Mar 03:1

Medicine / Ophthalmology 92002-92499

92314 Prescription of optical and physical characteristics of contact lens, with medical supervision of adaptation and direction of fitting by independent technician; corneal lens, both eyes except for aphakia

➔ *CPT Assistant* Feb 97:7, Oct 12:9

(For prescription and fitting of 1 eye, add modifier 52)

92315 corneal lens for aphakia, 1 eye

➔ *CPT Assistant* Feb 97:7, Oct 12:9

92316 corneal lens for aphakia, both eyes

➔ *CPT Assistant* Feb 97:7, Oct 12:9

92317 corneoscleral lens

➔ *CPT Assistant* Feb 97:7

92325 Modification of contact lens (separate procedure), with medical supervision of adaptation

➔ *CPT Assistant* Feb 97:7, Oct 12:9

92326 Replacement of contact lens

➔ *CPT Assistant* Feb 97:7

Spectacle Services (Including Prosthesis for Aphakia)

Prescription of lenses, when required, is included in 92015, *Determination of refractive state*. It includes specification of lens type (monofocal, bifocal, other), lens power, axis, prism, absorptive factor, impact resistance, and other factors.

When provided, fitting of spectacles is a separate service and is reported as indicated by 92340-92371.

Fitting includes measurement of anatomical facial characteristics, the writing of laboratory specifications, and the final adjustment of the spectacles to the visual axes and anatomical topography. Presence of the physician or other qualified health care professional is not required.

Supply of materials is a separate service component; it is not part of the service of fitting spectacles.

92340 Fitting of spectacles, except for aphakia; monofocal

➔ *CPT Assistant* Feb 97:7, Aug 98:4, Mar 13:6

92341 bifocal

➔ *CPT Assistant* Feb 97:7, Aug 98:4, Mar 13:6

92342 multifocal, other than bifocal

➔ *CPT Assistant* Feb 97:7, Aug 98:4, Mar 13:6

92352 Fitting of spectacle prosthesis for aphakia; monofocal

➔ *CPT Assistant* Feb 97:7, Aug 98:4, Mar 13:6

92353 multifocal

➔ *CPT Assistant* Feb 97:7, Aug 98:4, Mar 13:6

92354 Fitting of spectacle mounted low vision aid; single element system

➔ *CPT Assistant* Feb 97:7, Aug 98:4, Mar 13:6

92355 telescopic or other compound lens system

➔ *CPT Assistant* Feb 97:7, Aug 98:4, Mar 13:6

92358 Prosthesis service for aphakia, temporary (disposable or loan, including materials)

➔ *CPT Assistant* Feb 97:7, Aug 98:4, Mar 13:6

92370 Repair and refitting spectacles; except for aphakia

➔ *CPT Assistant* Feb 97:7, Mar 13:6

92371 spectacle prosthesis for aphakia

➔ *CPT Assistant* Feb 97:7, Aug 98:4, Mar 13:6

Other Procedures

92499 Unlisted ophthalmological service or procedure

➔ *CPT Assistant* Feb 97:7, Jan 19:12, Aug 20:15, Feb 23:16, Aug 23:14

Special Otorhinolaryngologic Services

Diagnostic or treatment procedures that are reported as evaluation and management services (eg, otoscopy, anterior rhinoscopy, tuning fork test, removal of non-impacted cerumen) are not reported separately.

Special otorhinolaryngologic services are those diagnostic and treatment services not included in an evaluation and management service, including office or other outpatient services (99202-99215) or office or other outpatient consultations (99242, 99243, 99244, 99245).

Codes 92507, 92508, 92520, 92521, 92522, 92523, 92524, and 92526 are used to report evaluation and treatment of speech sound production, receptive language, and expressive language abilities, voice and resonance production, speech fluency, and swallowing. Evaluations may include examination of speech sound production, articulatory movements of oral musculature, oral-pharyngeal swallowing function, qualitative analysis of voice and resonance, and measures of frequency, type, and duration of stuttering. Evaluations may also include the patient's ability to understand the meaning and intent of written and verbal expressions, as well as the appropriate formulation and utterance of expressive thought.

(For laryngoscopy with stroboscopy, use 31579)

92502 Otolaryngologic examination under general anesthesia

➔ *CPT Assistant* Sep 16:6, Dec 21:20

92504 Binocular microscopy (separate diagnostic procedure)

➔ *CPT Assistant* Jul 05:14, Oct 11:10, Oct 13:14, Sep 16:6

★=Telemedicine ◀=Audio-only ✚=Add-on code ✔=FDA approval pending #=Resequenced code ⦸=Modifier 51 exempt ➔➔➔=See p xxi for details

★◀ **92507**   Treatment of speech, language, voice, communication, and/or auditory processing disorder; individual

➔ *CPT Changes: An Insider's View* 2006

➔ *CPT Assistant* Dec 04:14, Jan 06:7, Oct 13:7, Sep 16:6, Nov 18:3, Dec 18:7

(Do not report 92507 in conjunction with 97153, 97155)

★◀ **92508**   group, 2 or more individuals

➔ *CPT Assistant* Dec 04:14, Oct 13:7, Sep 16:6, Nov 18:3

(Do not report 92508 in conjunction with 97154, 97158)

(For auditory rehabilitation, prelingual hearing loss, use 92630)

(For auditory rehabilitation, postlingual hearing loss, use 92633)

(For cochlear implant programming, see 92601-92604)

92511   Nasopharyngoscopy with endoscope (separate procedure)

➔ *CPT Assistant* Sep 16:6, Apr 21:12, Dec 23:23

(Do not report 92511 in conjunction with 31575, 42975, 43197, 43198)

(For nasopharyngoscopy, surgical, with dilation of eustachian tube, see 69705, 69706)

92512   Nasal function studies (eg, rhinomanometry)

➔ *CPT Assistant* Sep 16:6,

92516   Facial nerve function studies (eg, electroneuronography)

➔ *CPT Assistant* Sep 16:6

92517   Code is out of numerical sequence. See 92548-92551

92518   Code is out of numerical sequence. See 92548-92551

92519   Code is out of numerical sequence. See 92548-92551

92520   Laryngeal function studies (ie, aerodynamic testing and acoustic testing)

➔ *CPT Changes: An Insider's View* 2006

➔ *CPT Assistant* Dec 04:17, Jan 06:7, Sep 16:6

(For performance of a single test, use modifier 52)

(To report flexible fiberoptic laryngeal evaluation of swallowing and laryngeal sensory testing, see 92611-92617)

(To report other testing of laryngeal function (eg, electroglottography), use 92700)

★◀ **92521**   Evaluation of speech fluency (eg, stuttering, cluttering)

➔ *CPT Changes: An Insider's View* 2014

➔ *CPT Assistant* Jun 14:3, Sep 16:6, Apr 24:24

★◀ **92522**   Evaluation of speech sound production (eg, articulation, phonological process, apraxia, dysarthria);

➔ *CPT Changes: An Insider's View* 2014

➔ *CPT Assistant* Jun 14:3, Apr 24:24

★◀ **92523**   with evaluation of language comprehension and expression (eg, receptive and expressive language)

➔ *CPT Changes: An Insider's View* 2014

➔ *CPT Assistant* Jun 14:3, Sep 16:6, Apr 24:24

★◀ **92524**   Behavioral and qualitative analysis of voice and resonance

➔ *CPT Changes: An Insider's View* 2014

➔ *CPT Assistant* Jun 14:3, Sep 16:6, Apr 24:24

★ **92526**   Treatment of swallowing dysfunction and/or oral function for feeding

➔ *CPT Assistant* Sep 16:6

Vestibular Function Tests, Without Electrical Recording

92531   Spontaneous nystagmus, including gaze

➔ *CPT Assistant* Aug 20:15

92532   Positional nystagmus test

➔ *CPT Changes: An Insider's View* 2002

➔ *CPT Assistant* Aug 20:15

(Do not report 92531, 92532 with evaluation and management services, including office or other outpatient services [99202-99215], hospital inpatient or observation care services including admission and discharge [99234-99236], hospital inpatient or observation care services [99221-99223, 99231-99233], office or other outpatient consultations [99242, 99243, 99244, 99245], nursing facility services [99304-99316])

92533   Caloric vestibular test, each irrigation (binaural, bithermal stimulation constitutes 4 tests)

➔ *CPT Assistant* May 96:5, Aug 20:15

92534   Optokinetic nystagmus test

➔ *CPT Changes: An Insider's View* 2002

➔ *CPT Assistant* Aug 20:15

Vestibular Function Tests, With Recording (eg, ENG)

92537   Caloric vestibular test with recording, bilateral; bithermal (ie, one warm and one cool irrigation in each ear for a total of four irrigations)

➔ *CPT Changes: An Insider's View* 2016

➔ *CPT Assistant* Aug 20:15

(Do not report 92537 in conjunction with 92270, 92538)

(For three irrigations, use modifier 52)

(For monothermal caloric vestibular testing, use 92538)

92538   monothermal (ie, one irrigation in each ear for a total of two irrigations)

➔ *CPT Changes: An Insider's View* 2016

➔ *CPT Assistant* Aug 20:15

(Do not report 92538 in conjunction with 92270, 92537)

(For one irrigation, use modifier 52)

(For bilateral, bithermal caloric vestibular testing, use 92537)

92540 Basic vestibular evaluation, includes spontaneous nystagmus test with eccentric gaze fixation nystagmus, with recording, positional nystagmus test, minimum of 4 positions, with recording, optokinetic nystagmus test, bidirectional foveal and peripheral stimulation, with recording, and oscillating tracking test, with recording
➔ *CPT Changes: An Insider's View* 2010
➔ *CPT Assistant* Sep 15:7, Aug 20:15

(Do not report 92540 in conjunction with 92270, 92541, 92542, 92544, 92545)

92541 Spontaneous nystagmus test, including gaze and fixation nystagmus, with recording
➔ *CPT Assistant* Feb 05:13, Aug 08:12, May 11:10, Sep 15:7, Aug 20:15

(Do not report 92541 in conjunction with 92270, 92540 or the set of 92542, 92544, and 92545)

92542 Positional nystagmus test, minimum of 4 positions, with recording
➔ *CPT Assistant* Feb 05:13, Aug 08:12, Sep 10:9, Sep 15:7, Aug 20:15

(Do not report 92542 in conjunction with 92270, 92540 or the set of 92541, 92544, and 92545)

92544 Optokinetic nystagmus test, bidirectional, foveal or peripheral stimulation, with recording
➔ *CPT Assistant* Feb 05:13, Aug 08:12, Sep 15:7, Aug 20:15

(Do not report 92544 in conjunction with 92270, 92540 or the set of 92541, 92542, and 92545)

92545 Oscillating tracking test, with recording
➔ *CPT Assistant* Feb 05:13, Aug 08:12, May 11:10, Sep 15:7, Aug 20:15

(Do not report 92545 in conjunction with 92270, 92540 or the set of 92541, 92542, and 92544)

92546 Sinusoidal vertical axis rotational testing
➔ *CPT Assistant* Sep 04:13, Feb 05:13, Aug 08:12, May 11:10, Jun 13:14, Sep 15:7, Aug 20:15

(Do not report 92546 in conjunction with 92270)

+ 92547 Use of vertical electrodes (List separately in addition to code for primary procedure)
➔ *CPT Assistant* May 04:14, Feb 05:13, Aug 08:12, Sep 15:7, Aug 20:15

(Use 92547 in conjunction with 92540-92546)

(For unlisted vestibular tests, use 92700)

(Do not report 92547 in conjunction with 92270)

92548 Computerized dynamic posturography sensory organization test (CDP-SOT), 6 conditions (ie, eyes open, eyes closed, visual sway, platform sway, eyes closed platform sway, platform and visual sway), including interpretation and report;
➔ *CPT Changes: An Insider's View* 2020
➔ *CPT Assistant* May 11:10, Sep 15:7, Apr 20:7, Aug 20:15

92549 with motor control test (MCT) and adaptation test (ADT)
➔ *CPT Changes: An Insider's View* 2020
➔ *CPT Assistant* Apr 20:7, Aug 20:15

(Do not report 92548, 92549 in conjunction with 92270)

 # 92517 Vestibular evoked myogenic potential (VEMP) testing, with interpretation and report; cervical (cVEMP)
➔ *CPT Changes: An Insider's View* 2021
➔ *CPT Assistant* Feb 21:5

(Do not report 92517 in conjunction with 92270, 92518, 92519)

 # 92518 ocular (oVEMP)
➔ *CPT Changes: An Insider's View* 2021
➔ *CPT Assistant* Feb 21:5

(Do not report 92518 in conjunction with 92270, 92517, 92519)

 # 92519 cervical (cVEMP) and ocular (oVEMP)
➔ *CPT Changes: An Insider's View* 2021
➔ *CPT Assistant* Feb 21:5

(Do not report 92519 in conjunction with 92270, 92517, 92518)

Audiologic Function Tests

The audiometric tests listed below require the use of calibrated electronic equipment, recording of results, and a report with interpretation. Hearing tests (such as whispered voice, tuning fork) that are otorhinolaryngologic evaluation and management services are not reported separately. All services include testing of both ears. Use modifier 52 if a test is applied to one ear instead of two ears.

(For evaluation of speech, language, and/or hearing problems through observation and assessment of performance, see 92521, 92522, 92523, 92524)

92550 Tympanometry and reflex threshold measurements
➔ *CPT Changes: An Insider's View* 2010
➔ *CPT Assistant* Aug 14:3

(Do not report 92550 in conjunction with 92567, 92568)

92551 Screening test, pure tone, air only
➔ *CPT Assistant* Aug 14:3

92552 Pure tone audiometry (threshold); air only
➔ *CPT Assistant* Aug 14:3

92553 air and bone
➔ *CPT Assistant* Mar 11:8, Aug 14:3, Apr 22:14

92555 Speech audiometry threshold;
➔ *CPT Assistant* Aug 14:3

★ =Telemedicine ◀ =Audio-only + =Add-on code ✔ =FDA approval pending # =Resequenced code ⊘ =Modifier 51 exempt ➔➔➔ =See p xxi for details

92556   with speech recognition
> *CPT Assistant* Mar 11:8, Aug 14:3, Apr 22:14

92557   Comprehensive audiometry threshold evaluation and speech recognition (92553 and 92556 combined)
> *CPT Assistant* Sep 07:11, Mar 11:8, Aug 14:3, Apr 22:14

(For hearing aid evaluation and selection, see 92590-92595)

(For automated audiometry, see 0208T-0212T)

92558   Code is out of numerical sequence. See 92583-92588

92562   Loudness balance test, alternate binaural or monaural
> *CPT Assistant* Mar 05:7, 9, Aug 14:3

92563   Tone decay test
> *CPT Assistant* Aug 14:3

92565   Stenger test, pure tone
> *CPT Assistant* Aug 14:3

92567   Tympanometry (impedance testing)
> *CPT Assistant* Winter 90:11, Aug 14:3

92568   Acoustic reflex testing, threshold
> *CPT Changes: An Insider's View* 2006, 2010
> *CPT Assistant* Jan 06:7, Sep 07:11, Jun 09:10, Aug 14:3

92570   Acoustic immittance testing, includes tympanometry (impedance testing), acoustic reflex threshold testing, and acoustic reflex decay testing
> *CPT Changes: An Insider's View* 2010
> *CPT Assistant* Aug 14:3

(Do not report 92570 in conjunction with 92567, 92568)

92571   Filtered speech test
> *CPT Assistant* Mar 05:7, Aug 14:3

92572   Staggered spondaic word test
> *CPT Assistant* Mar 05:7, Aug 14:3

92575   Sensorineural acuity level test
> *CPT Assistant* Aug 14:3

92576   Synthetic sentence identification test
> *CPT Assistant* Mar 05:7, Aug 14:3

92577   Stenger test, speech
> *CPT Assistant* Aug 14:3

92579   Visual reinforcement audiometry (VRA)
> *CPT Assistant* Aug 14:3

92582   Conditioning play audiometry
> *CPT Assistant* Aug 14:3

92583   Select picture audiometry

92584   Electrocochleography
> *CPT Assistant* Jul 11:17, Aug 14:3, Oct 21:9

 # 92650   Auditory evoked potentials; screening of auditory potential with broadband stimuli, automated analysis
> *CPT Changes: An Insider's View* 2021
> *CPT Assistant* Oct 20:9

 # 92651   for hearing status determination, broadband stimuli, with interpretation and report
> *CPT Changes: An Insider's View* 2021
> *CPT Assistant* Oct 20:9, Oct 21:9

(Do not report 92651 in conjunction with 92652, 92653)

 # 92652   for threshold estimation at multiple frequencies, with interpretation and report
> *CPT Changes: An Insider's View* 2021
> *CPT Assistant* Oct 21:9

(Do not report 92652 in conjunction with 92651, 92653)

 # 92653   neurodiagnostic, with interpretation and report
> *CPT Changes: An Insider's View* 2021
> *CPT Assistant* Oct 21:9

(Do not report 92653 in conjunction with 92651, 92652)

 # 92558   Evoked otoacoustic emissions, screening (qualitative measurement of distortion product or transient evoked otoacoustic emissions), automated analysis
> *CPT Changes: An Insider's View* 2012
> *CPT Assistant* Aug 14:3

92587   Distortion product evoked otoacoustic emissions; limited evaluation (to confirm the presence or absence of hearing disorder, 3-6 frequencies) or transient evoked otoacoustic emissions, with interpretation and report
> *CPT Changes: An Insider's View* 2012
> *CPT Assistant* Sep 07:11

92588   comprehensive diagnostic evaluation (quantitative analysis of outer hair cell function by cochlear mapping, minimum of 12 frequencies), with interpretation and report
> *CPT Changes: An Insider's View* 2012
> *CPT Assistant* Aug 14:3

(For central auditory function evaluation, see 92620, 92621)

92590   Hearing aid examination and selection; monaural
> *CPT Assistant* Jul 14:4, Aug 14:3, Jul 20:3

92591   binaural
> *CPT Assistant* Jul 20:3

92592   Hearing aid check; monaural
> *CPT Assistant* Jul 20:3

92593   binaural
> *CPT Assistant* Jul 20:3

92594   Electroacoustic evaluation for hearing aid; monaural
> *CPT Assistant* Jul 20:3

92595   binaural
> *CPT Assistant* Aug 14:3, Jul 20:3

92596   Ear protector attenuation measurements

> ➔ *CPT Assistant* Aug 14:3

92597   Code is out of numerical sequence. See 92603-92607

Evaluative and Therapeutic Services

Codes 92601 and 92603 describe post-operative analysis and fitting of previously placed external devices, connection to the cochlear implant, and programming of the stimulator. Codes 92602 and 92604 describe subsequent sessions for measurements and adjustment of the external transmitter and re-programming of the internal stimulator.

> (For placement of cochlear implant, use 69930)

Codes 92622, 92623 describe the analysis, programming, and verification of an auditory osseointegrated sound processor, any type. These services include evaluating the attachment of the processor, device feedback calibration, device programming, and verification of the processor performance. These codes should be used for subsequent reprogramming, when performed.

★ **92601**   Diagnostic analysis of cochlear implant, patient younger than 7 years of age; with programming

> ➔ *CPT Changes: An Insider's View* 2003
> ➔ *CPT Assistant* Mar 03:1, Jan 06:7, Jul 11:17, Oct 13:7, Jul 14:4, Mar 20:15, Jul 20:3, Oct 21:9

★ **92602**   subsequent reprogramming

> ➔ *CPT Changes: An Insider's View* 2003
> ➔ *CPT Assistant* Mar 03:1, 21, Jan 06:7, Oct 13:7, Mar 20:15, Jul 20:3, Oct 21:9

> (Do not report 92602 in addition to 92601)

★ **92603**   Diagnostic analysis of cochlear implant, age 7 years or older; with programming

> ➔ *CPT Changes: An Insider's View* 2003
> ➔ *CPT Assistant* Mar 03:2, 4, Jan 06:7, Jul 11:17, Oct 13:7, Mar 20:15, Jul 20:3, Oct 21:9

★ **92604**   subsequent reprogramming

> ➔ *CPT Changes: An Insider's View* 2003
> ➔ *CPT Assistant* Mar 03:2, 21, Jan 06:7, Jul 11:17, Oct 13:7, Jul 14:4, Mar 20:15, Jul 20:3, Oct 21:9

> (Do not report 92604 in addition to 92603)

> (For diagnostic analysis, programming, and verification of an auditory osseointegrated sound processor, use 92622)

> (For evaluation of auditory function for surgically implanted device[s] candidacy or postoperative status of a surgically implanted device[s], use 92626)

> (For aural rehabilitation services following auditory osseointegrated implant, see 92630, 92633)

> (For initial and subsequent diagnostic analysis and programming of vestibular implant, see 0728T, 0729T)

A View of the Outer Cochlear Implant
92601-92604

An example of the elements that are addressed in the diagnostic analysis and reprogramming of the cochlear implant

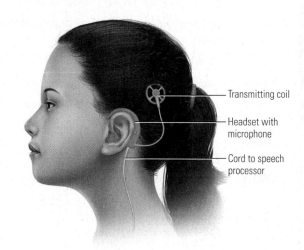

- Transmitting coil
- Headset with microphone
- Cord to speech processor

 # 92597   Evaluation for use and/or fitting of voice prosthetic device to supplement oral speech

> (To report augmentative and alternative communication device services, see 92605, 92607, 92608, 92618)

92605   Evaluation for prescription of non-speech-generating augmentative and alternative communication device, face-to-face with the patient; first hour

> ➔ *CPT Changes: An Insider's View* 2003, 2012
> ➔ *CPT Assistant* Mar 03:2, 4, Oct 13:7

> (To report evaluation for use and/or fitting of voice prosthetic device, use 92597)

#+ 92618   each additional 30 minutes (List separately in addition to code for primary procedure)

> ➔ *CPT Changes: An Insider's View* 2012

> (Use 92618 in conjunction with 92605)

92606   Therapeutic service(s) for the use of non-speech-generating device, including programming and modification

> ➔ *CPT Changes: An Insider's View* 2003
> ➔ *CPT Assistant* Mar 03:2, 4

92607   Evaluation for prescription for speech-generating augmentative and alternative communication device, face-to-face with the patient; first hour

→ *CPT Changes: An Insider's View* 2003

→ *CPT Assistant* Mar 03:2, 4, Dec 04:16, Oct 13:7

(To report evaluation for use and/or fitting of voice prosthetic device, use 92597)

(For evaluation for prescription of a non-speech-generating device, use 92605)

+ 92608   each additional 30 minutes (List separately in addition to code for primary procedure)

→ *CPT Changes: An Insider's View* 2003

→ *CPT Assistant* Mar 03:2, 5, Dec 04:16, Oct 13:7

(Use 92608 in conjunction with 92607)

92609   Therapeutic services for the use of speech-generating device, including programming and modification

→ *CPT Changes: An Insider's View* 2003

→ *CPT Assistant* Mar 03:2, 4, Dec 04:16

(For therapeutic service(s) for the use of a non-speech-generating device, use 92606)

92610   Evaluation of oral and pharyngeal swallowing function

→ *CPT Changes: An Insider's View* 2003

→ *CPT Assistant* Mar 03:2, 5, Dec 04:17

→ *Clinical Examples in Radiology* Spring 18:15

(For motion fluoroscopic evaluation of swallowing function, use 92611)

(For flexible endoscopic examination, use 92612-92617)

92611   Motion fluoroscopic evaluation of swallowing function by cine or video recording

→ *CPT Changes: An Insider's View* 2003

→ *CPT Assistant* Mar 03:2, 5, Dec 04:17, Jan 06:7, Jul 14:5, Apr 17:8, Aug 20:9

→ *Clinical Examples in Radiology* Summer 06:4-5, Spring 18:14

(For radiological supervision and interpretation, use 74230)

(For evaluation of oral and pharyngeal swallowing function, use 92610)

(For flexible diagnostic laryngoscopy, use 31575)

92612   Flexible endoscopic evaluation of swallowing by cine or video recording;

→ *CPT Changes: An Insider's View* 2003, 2017

→ *CPT Assistant* Mar 03:6, Jan 06:7, Apr 17:8

(If flexible endoscopic evaluation of swallowing is performed without cine or video recording, use 92700)

(Do not report 92612 in conjunction with 31575)

92613   interpretation and report only

→ *CPT Changes: An Insider's View* 2003, 2013, 2017

→ *CPT Assistant* Jan 06:7, Apr 17:8

(To report an evaluation of oral and pharyngeal swallowing function, use 92610)

(To report motion fluoroscopic evaluation of swallowing function, use 92611)

92614   Flexible endoscopic evaluation, laryngeal sensory testing by cine or video recording;

→ *CPT Changes: An Insider's View* 2003, 2017

→ *CPT Assistant* Mar 03:6, Jan 06:7, Apr 17:8

(If flexible endoscopic evaluation of swallowing is performed without cine or video recording, use 92700)

(Do not report 92614 in conjunction with 31575)

92615   interpretation and report only

→ *CPT Changes: An Insider's View* 2003, 2013, 2017

→ *CPT Assistant* Mar 03:6, Jan 06:7, Apr 17:8

92616   Flexible endoscopic evaluation of swallowing and laryngeal sensory testing by cine or video recording;

→ *CPT Changes: An Insider's View* 2003, 2017

→ *CPT Assistant* Mar 03:6, Jan 06:7, Apr 17:8

(If flexible endoscopic evaluation of swallowing is performed without cine or video recording, use 92700)

(Do not report 92616 in conjunction with 31575)

92617   interpretation and report only

→ *CPT Changes: An Insider's View* 2003, 2013, 2017

→ *CPT Assistant* Mar 03:6, Jan 06:7, Apr 17:8

92618   Code is out of numerical sequence. See 92603-92607

92620   Evaluation of central auditory function, with report; initial 60 minutes

→ *CPT Changes: An Insider's View* 2005

→ *CPT Assistant* Mar 05:7-8, Aug 14:3

+ 92621   each additional 15 minutes (List separately in addition to code for primary procedure)

→ *CPT Changes: An Insider's View* 2005, 2012

→ *CPT Assistant* Mar 05:7, Aug 14:3

(Use 92621 in conjunction with 92620)

(Do not report 92620, 92621 in conjunction with 92521, 92522, 92523, 92524)

92622   Diagnostic analysis, programming, and verification of an auditory osseointegrated sound processor, any type; first 60 minutes

→ *CPT Changes: An Insider's View* 2024

→ *CPT Assistant* Nov 23:11

+ 92623   each additional 15 minutes (List separately in addition to code for primary procedure)

→ *CPT Changes: An Insider's View* 2024

→ *CPT Assistant* Nov 23:11

(Use 92623 in conjunction with 92622)

(Do not report 92622, 92623 in conjunction with 92626, 92627)

(For diagnostic analysis of cochlear implant, with programming or subsequent reprogramming, see 92601, 92602, 92603, 92604)

(For evaluation of auditory function for surgically implanted device[s] candidacy or postoperative status of a surgically implanted device[s], use 92626)

(For aural rehabilitation services following auditory osseointegrated implant, see 92630, 92633)

92625 Assessment of tinnitus (includes pitch, loudness matching, and masking)

➔ CPT Changes: An Insider's View 2005

➔ CPT Assistant Mar 05:8-9, Aug 14:3

(Do not report 92625 in conjunction with 92562)

(For unilateral assessment, use modifier 52)

92626 Evaluation of auditory function for surgically implanted device(s) candidacy or postoperative status of a surgically implanted device(s); first hour

➔ CPT Changes: An Insider's View 2006, 2020

➔ CPT Assistant Jan 06:7, May 14:10, Jul 14:4, Sep 16:7, Mar 20:15, Jul 20:3, Apr 22:14

+ 92627 each additional 15 minutes (List separately in addition to code for primary procedure)

➔ CPT Changes: An Insider's View 2006, 2020

➔ CPT Assistant Jan 06:7, Jul 14:4, Sep 16:7, Mar 20:15, Jul 20:3, Apr 22:14

(Use 92627 in conjunction with 92626)

(When reporting 92626, 92627, use the face-to-face time with the patient or family)

(Do not report 92626, 92627 in conjunction with 92590, 92591, 92592, 92593, 92594, 92595 for hearing aid evaluation, fitting, follow-up, or selection)

(Do not report 92626, 92627 in conjunction with 92622, 92623)

(For diagnostic analysis of cochlear implant, with programming or subsequent reprogramming, see 92601, 92602, 92603, 92604)

(For diagnostic analysis, programming, and verification of an auditory osseointegrated sound processor, use 92622)

92630 Auditory rehabilitation; prelingual hearing loss

➔ CPT Changes: An Insider's View 2006

➔ CPT Assistant Jan 06:7, Oct 13:7

92633 postlingual hearing loss

➔ CPT Changes: An Insider's View 2006

➔ CPT Assistant Jan 06:7, Oct 13:7

Special Diagnostic Procedures

92640 Diagnostic analysis with programming of auditory brainstem implant, per hour

➔ CPT Changes: An Insider's View 2007

(Report nonprogramming services separately [eg, cardiac monitoring])

92650 Code is out of numerical sequence. See 92583-92588

92651 Code is out of numerical sequence. See 92583-92588

92652 Code is out of numerical sequence. See 92583-92588

92653 Code is out of numerical sequence. See 92583-92588

Other Procedures

92700 Unlisted otorhinolaryngological service or procedure

➔ CPT Changes: An Insider's View 2003

➔ CPT Assistant Sep 04:14, Oct 04:10, Jan 06:7, Sep 06:13, Sep 07:11, Mar 11:10, Jul 11:17, May 14:10, Sep 15:15, Apr 17:8, Feb 21:5, Oct 21:9

Cardiovascular

Therapeutic Services and Procedures

92920 Code is out of numerical sequence. See 92997-93005

92921 Code is out of numerical sequence. See 92997-93005

92924 Code is out of numerical sequence. See 92997-93005

92925 Code is out of numerical sequence. See 92997-93005

92928 Code is out of numerical sequence. See 92997-93005

92929 Code is out of numerical sequence. See 92997-93005

92933 Code is out of numerical sequence. See 92997-93005

92934 Code is out of numerical sequence. See 92997-93005

92937 Code is out of numerical sequence. See 92997-93005

92938 Code is out of numerical sequence. See 92997-93005

92941 Code is out of numerical sequence. See 92997-93005

92943 Code is out of numerical sequence. See 92997-93005

92944 Code is out of numerical sequence. See 92997-93005

Other Therapeutic Services and Procedures

92950 Cardiopulmonary resuscitation (eg, in cardiac arrest)

➔ CPT Assistant Jan 96:7, Oct 04:14, Nov 07:5, Jul 12:13, Sep 12:17

(See also critical care services, 99291, 99292)

92953 Temporary transcutaneous pacing

➔ CPT Changes: An Insider's View 2017

➔ CPT Assistant Nov 99:49, Feb 07:10, Jul 07:1, May 14:4, Aug 19:8, Jan 22:3, Jun 22:19, Dec 22:10

(For direction of ambulance or rescue personnel outside the hospital by a physician or other qualified health care professional, use 99288)

92960 Cardioversion, elective, electrical conversion of arrhythmia; external
➔ *CPT Changes: An Insider's View* 2000, 2017
➔ *CPT Assistant* Summer 93:13, Nov 99:49, Jun 00:5, Nov 00:9, Jul 01:11, Jan 12:13

92961 internal (separate procedure)
➔ *CPT Changes: An Insider's View* 2000, 2017
➔ *CPT Assistant* Summer 93:13, Nov 99:49, Jun 00:5, Jul 00:5, Nov 00:9, Feb 15:3

(Do not report 92961 in conjunction with 93282-93284, 93287, 93289, 93295, 93296, 93618-93624, 93631, 93640-93642, 93650, 93653-93657, 93662)

92970 Cardioassist-method of circulatory assist; internal

92971 external

(For balloon atrial septostomy, use 33741)

(For placement of catheters for use in circulatory assist devices such as intra-aortic balloon pump, use 33970)

92972 Code is out of numerical sequence. See 92997-93005

92973 Code is out of numerical sequence. See 92997-93005

92974 Code is out of numerical sequence. See 92997-93005

92975 Code is out of numerical sequence. See 92997-93005

92977 Code is out of numerical sequence. See 92997-93005

92978 Code is out of numerical sequence. See 92997-93005

92979 Code is out of numerical sequence. See 92997-93005

92986 Percutaneous balloon valvuloplasty; aortic valve
➔ *CPT Changes: An Insider's View* 2017
➔ *CPT Assistant* Jan 13:6, Feb 15:3

92987 mitral valve
➔ *CPT Changes: An Insider's View* 2017
➔ *CPT Assistant* Feb 15:3

92990 pulmonary valve
➔ *CPT Assistant* Winter 91:3, Feb 15:3, Jul 15:11

(For atrial septectomy or septostomy, transvenous method, balloon or blade, use 33741)

92997 Percutaneous transluminal pulmonary artery balloon angioplasty; single vessel
➔ *CPT Assistant* Nov 97:44, Feb 15:3, Mar 16:5

+ 92998 each additional vessel (List separately in addition to code for primary procedure)
➔ *CPT Assistant* Nov 97:44, Feb 15:3, Mar 16:5

(Use 92998 in conjunction with 92997)

Coronary Therapeutic Services and Procedures

Codes 92920-92944 describe percutaneous revascularization services performed for occlusive disease of the coronary vessels (major coronary arteries, coronary artery branches, or coronary artery bypass grafts). These percutaneous coronary intervention (PCI) codes are built on progressive hierarchies with more intensive services inclusive of lesser intensive services. These PCI codes all include the work of accessing and selectively catheterizing the vessel, traversing the lesion, radiological supervision and interpretation directly related to the intervention(s) performed, closure of the arteriotomy when performed through the access sheath, and imaging performed to document completion of the intervention in addition to the intervention(s) performed. These codes include angioplasty (eg, balloon, cutting balloon, wired balloons, cryoplasty), atherectomy (eg, directional, rotational, laser), and stenting (eg, balloon expandable, self-expanding, bare metal, drug eluting, covered). Each code in this family includes balloon angioplasty, when performed. Diagnostic coronary angiography may be reported separately under specific circumstances. Percutaneous transluminal coronary lithotripsy may be reported using 92972 in conjunction with 92920, 92924, 92928, 92933, 92937, 92941, 92943, 92975, as appropriate.

Diagnostic coronary angiography codes (93454-93461) and injection procedure codes (93563-93564) should not be used with percutaneous coronary revascularization services (92920-92944) to report:

1. Contrast injections, angiography, roadmapping, and/or fluoroscopic guidance for the coronary intervention,

2. Vessel measurement for the coronary intervention, **or**

3. Post-coronary angioplasty/stent/atherectomy angiography, as this work is captured in the percutaneous coronary revascularization services codes (92920-92944).

Diagnostic angiography performed at the time of a coronary interventional procedure may be separately reportable if:

1. No prior catheter-based coronary angiography study is available, and a full diagnostic study is performed, and a decision to intervene is based on the diagnostic angiography, **or**

2. A prior study is available, but as documented in the medical record:

a. The patient's condition with respect to the clinical indication has changed since the prior study, **or**

b. There is inadequate visualization of the anatomy and/or pathology, **or**

c. There is a clinical change during the procedure that requires new evaluation outside the target area of intervention.

Diagnostic coronary angiography performed at a separate session from an interventional procedure is separately reportable.

Major coronary arteries: The major coronary arteries are the left main, left anterior descending, left circumflex, right, and ramus intermedius arteries. All PCI procedures performed in all segments (proximal, mid, distal) of a single major coronary artery through the native coronary circulation are reported with one code. When one segment of a major coronary artery is treated through the native circulation and treatment of another segment of the same artery requires access through a coronary artery bypass graft, the intervention through the bypass graft is reported separately.

Coronary artery branches: Up to two coronary artery branches of the left anterior descending (diagonals), left circumflex (marginals), and right (posterior descending, posterolaterals) coronary arteries are recognized. The left main and ramus intermedius coronary arteries do not have recognized branches for reporting purposes. All PCI(s) performed in any segment (proximal, mid, distal) of a coronary artery branch is reported with one code. PCI is reported for up to two branches of a major coronary artery. Additional PCI in a third branch of the same major coronary artery is not separately reportable.

Coronary artery bypass grafts: Each coronary artery bypass graft represents a coronary vessel. A sequential bypass graft with more than one distal anastomosis represents only one graft. A branching bypass graft (eg, Y graft) represents a coronary vessel for the main graft, and each branch off the main graft constitutes an additional coronary vessel. PCI performed on major coronary arteries or coronary artery branches by access through a bypass graft is reported using the bypass graft PCI codes. All bypass graft PCI codes include the use of coronary artery embolic protection devices when performed.

Only one base code from this family may be reported for revascularization of a major coronary artery and its recognized branches. Only one base code should be reported for revascularization of a coronary artery bypass graft, its subtended coronary artery, and recognized branches of the subtended coronary artery. If one segment of a major coronary artery and its recognized branches is treated through the native circulation, and treatment of another segment of the same vessel requires access through a coronary artery bypass graft, an additional base code is reported to describe the intervention performed through the bypass graft. The PCI base codes are 92920, 92924, 92928, 92933, 92937,

92941, and 92943. The PCI base code that includes the most intensive service provided for the target vessel should be reported. The hierarchy of these services is built on an intensity of service ranked from highest to lowest as 92943 = 92941 = 92933 > 92924 > 92937 = 92928 > 92920.

PCI performed during the same session in additional recognized branches of the target vessel should be reported using the applicable add-on code(s). The add-on codes are 92921, 92925, 92929, 92934, 92938, and 92944 and follow the same principle in regard to reporting the most intensive service provided. The intensity of service is ranked from highest to lowest as 92944 = 92938 > 92934 > 92925 > 92929 > 92921.

PCI performed during the same session in additional major coronary or in additional coronary artery bypass grafts should be reported using the applicable additional base code(s). PCI performed during the same session in additional coronary artery branches should be reported using the applicable additional add-on code(s).

If a single lesion extends from one target vessel (major coronary artery, coronary artery bypass graft, or coronary artery branch) into another target vessel, but can be revascularized with a single intervention bridging the two vessels, this PCI should be reported with a single code despite treating more than one vessel. For example, if a left main coronary lesion extends into the proximal left circumflex coronary artery and a single stent is placed to treat the entire lesion, this PCI should be reported as a single vessel stent (92928). In this example, a code for additional vessel treatment (92929) would not be additionally reported.

When bifurcation lesions are treated, PCI is reported for both vessels treated. For example, when a bifurcation lesion involving the left anterior descending artery and the first diagonal artery is treated by stenting both vessels, 92928 and 92929 are both reported.

Target vessel PCI for acute myocardial infarction is inclusive of all balloon angioplasty, atherectomy, stenting, manual aspiration thrombectomy, distal protection, and intracoronary rheolytic agent administration performed. Mechanical thrombectomy is reported separately.

Chronic total occlusion of a coronary vessel is present when there is no antegrade flow through the true lumen, accompanied by suggestive angiographic and clinical criteria (eg, antegrade "bridging" collaterals present, calcification at the occlusion site, no current presentation with ST elevation or Q wave acute myocardial infarction attributable to the occluded target lesion). Current presentation with ST elevation or Q wave acute myocardial infarction attributable to the occluded target lesion, subtotal occlusion, and occlusion with dye staining at the site consistent with fresh thrombus are not considered chronic total occlusion.

Codes 92973 (percutaneous transluminal coronary thrombectomy, mechanical), 92974 (coronary brachytherapy), 92978 and 92979 (intravascular ultrasound/optical coherence tomography), 93571 and 93572 (intravascular Doppler velocity and/or pressure [fractional flow reserve {FFR} or coronary flow reserve {CFR}]), and 92972 (percutaneous transluminal coronary lithotripsy), are add-on codes for reporting procedures performed in addition to coronary and bypass graft diagnostic and interventional services, unless included in the base code. Non-mechanical, aspiration thrombectomy is not reported with 92973, and is included in the PCI code for acute myocardial infarction (92941), when performed.

(To report transcatheter placement of radiation delivery device for coronary intravascular brachytherapy, use 92974)

(For intravascular radioelement application, see 77770, 77771, 77772)

(For nonsurgical septal reduction therapy [eg, alcohol ablation], use 93799)

▶(For percutaneous transcatheter therapeutic drug delivery by intracoronary drug-delivery balloon, see 0913T, 0914T)◀

 # 92920 Percutaneous transluminal coronary angioplasty; single major coronary artery or branch

➡ *CPT Changes: An Insider's View* 2013, 2017

➡ *CPT Assistant* Jan 13:3, Dec 14:6

▶(Do not report 92920 in conjunction with 0913T)◀

#+ 92921 each additional branch of a major coronary artery (List separately in addition to code for primary procedure)

➡ *CPT Changes: An Insider's View* 2013, 2017

➡ *CPT Assistant* Jan 13:3, Sep 14:14, Dec 14:6

(Use 92921 in conjunction with 92920, 92924, 92928, 92933, 92937, 92941, 92943)

▶(For percutaneous transcatheter therapeutic drug delivery by intracoronary drug-delivery balloon, see 0913T, 0914T)◀

 # 92924 Percutaneous transluminal coronary atherectomy, with coronary angioplasty when performed; single major coronary artery or branch

➡ *CPT Changes: An Insider's View* 2013, 2017

➡ *CPT Assistant* Jan 13:3, Dec 14:6

▶(Do not report 92924 in conjunction with 0913T)◀

#+ 92925 each additional branch of a major coronary artery (List separately in addition to code for primary procedure)

➡ *CPT Changes: An Insider's View* 2013, 2017

➡ *CPT Assistant* Jan 13:3, Sep 14:14, Dec 14:6

(Use 92925 in conjunction with 92924, 92928, 92933, 92937, 92941, 92943)

▶(For percutaneous transcatheter therapeutic drug delivery by intracoronary drug-delivery balloon, see 0913T, 0914T)◀

 # 92928 Percutaneous transcatheter placement of intracoronary stent(s), with coronary angioplasty when performed; single major coronary artery or branch

➡ *CPT Changes: An Insider's View* 2013, 2017

➡ *CPT Assistant* Jan 13:3, Jan 14:3, Mar 14:14, Sep 14:14, Dec 14:6, Jan 17:7, Feb 17:15

▶(Do not report 92928 in conjunction with 0913T)◀

#+ 92929 each additional branch of a major coronary artery (List separately in addition to code for primary procedure)

➡ *CPT Changes: An Insider's View* 2013, 2017

➡ *CPT Assistant* Jan 13:3, Sep 14:14, Dec 14:6, Jan 17:7

(Use 92929 in conjunction with 92928, 92933, 92937, 92941, 92943)

▶(For percutaneous transcatheter therapeutic drug delivery by intracoronary drug-delivery balloon, see 0913T, 0914T)◀

 # 92933 Percutaneous transluminal coronary atherectomy, with intracoronary stent, with coronary angioplasty when performed; single major coronary artery or branch

➡ *CPT Changes: An Insider's View* 2013, 2017

➡ *CPT Assistant* Jan 13:3, Dec 14:6, Nov 23:28

▶(Do not report 92933 in conjunction with 0913T)◀

#+ 92934 each additional branch of a major coronary artery (List separately in addition to code for primary procedure)

➡ *CPT Changes: An Insider's View* 2013, 2017 ·

➡ *CPT Assistant* Jan 13:3, Sep 14:14, Dec 14:6, Nov 23:28

(Use 92934 in conjunction with 92933, 92937, 92941, 92943)

▶(For percutaneous transcatheter therapeutic drug delivery by intracoronary drug-delivery balloon, see 0913T, 0914T)◀

 # 92937 Percutaneous transluminal revascularization of or through coronary artery bypass graft (internal mammary, free arterial, venous), any combination of intracoronary stent, atherectomy and angioplasty, including distal protection when performed; single vessel

➡ *CPT Changes: An Insider's View* 2013, 2017

➡ *CPT Assistant* Jan 13:3, Mar 14:14, Dec 14:6, Feb 17:15

▶(Do not report 92937 in conjunction with 0913T)◀

#+ 92938 each additional branch subtended by the bypass graft (List separately in addition to code for primary procedure)

➡ *CPT Changes: An Insider's View* 2013, 2017

➡ *CPT Assistant* Jan 13:3, Mar 14:14, Sep 14:14, Dec 14:6

(Use 92938 in conjunction with 92937)

▶(For percutaneous transcatheter therapeutic drug delivery by intracoronary drug-delivery balloon, see 0913T, 0914T)◀

 # 92941 Percutaneous transluminal revascularization of acute total/subtotal occlusion during acute myocardial infarction, coronary artery or coronary artery bypass graft, any combination of intracoronary stent, atherectomy and angioplasty, including aspiration thrombectomy when performed, single vessel

➔ CPT Changes: An Insider's View 2013, 2017

➔ CPT Assistant Jan 13:3, Jan 14:3, Mar 14:14, Dec 14:6, Feb 17:14, Jul 20:14

▶(Do not report 92941 in conjunction with 0913T for intervention in the same major coronary artery or in the same bypass graft)◀

▶(For additional vessels treated, see 92920-92938, 92943, 92944, 0913T, 0914T)◀

(For transcatheter intra-arterial hyperoxemic reperfusion/supersaturated oxygen therapy [SSO$_2$], use 0659T)

 # 92943 Percutaneous transluminal revascularization of chronic total occlusion, coronary artery, coronary artery branch, or coronary artery bypass graft, any combination of intracoronary stent, atherectomy and angioplasty; single vessel

➔ CPT Changes: An Insider's View 2013, 2017

➔ CPT Assistant Jan 13:3, Dec 14:6

▶(Do not report 92943 in conjunction with 0913T)◀

#+ 92944 each additional coronary artery, coronary artery branch, or bypass graft (List separately in addition to code for primary procedure)

➔ CPT Changes: An Insider's View 2013, 2017

➔ CPT Assistant Jan 13:3, Sep 14:14, Dec 14:6

(Use 92944 in conjunction with 92924, 92928, 92933, 92937, 92941, 92943)

(For intravascular radioelement application, see 77770, 77771, 77772)

(To report transcatheter placement of radiation delivery device for coronary intravascular brachytherapy, use 92974)

▶(For percutaneous transcatheter therapeutic drug delivery by intracoronary drug-delivery balloon, see 0913T, 0914T)◀

#+ 92972 Percutaneous transluminal coronary lithotripsy (List separately in addition to code for primary procedure)

➔ CPT Changes: An Insider's View 2024

(Use 92972 in conjunction with 92920, 92924, 92928, 92933, 92937, 92941, 92943, 92975)

#+ 92973 Percutaneous transluminal coronary thrombectomy mechanical (List separately in addition to code for primary procedure)

➔ CPT Changes: An Insider's View 2002, 2013, 2017

➔ CPT Assistant Mar 02:2, 10, Mar 04:10, Dec 14:6, Feb 17:14, Jul 20:14

(Use 92973 in conjunction with 92920, 92924, 92928, 92933, 92937, 92941, 92943, 92975, 93454-93461, 93563, 93564)

▶(Do not report 92973 in conjunction with 0913T for intervention in the same major coronary artery or in the same bypass graft)◀

(Do not report 92973 for aspiration thrombectomy)

#+ 92974 Transcatheter placement of radiation delivery device for subsequent coronary intravascular brachytherapy (List separately in addition to code for primary procedure)

➔ CPT Changes: An Insider's View 2002, 2017

➔ CPT Assistant Mar 02:2, Dec 14:6, Feb 17:15

(Use 92974 in conjunction with 92920, 92924, 92928, 92933, 92937, 92941, 92943, 93454-93461)

(For intravascular radioelement application, see 77770, 77771, 77772)

 # 92975 Thrombolysis, coronary; by intracoronary infusion, including selective coronary angiography

➔ CPT Changes: An Insider's View 2017

 # 92977 by intravenous infusion

(For thrombolysis of vessels other than coronary, see 37211-37214)

(For cerebral thrombolysis, use 37195)

#+ 92978 Endoluminal imaging of coronary vessel or graft using intravascular ultrasound (IVUS) or optical coherence tomography (OCT) during diagnostic evaluation and/or therapeutic intervention including imaging supervision, interpretation and report; initial vessel (List separately in addition to code for primary procedure)

➔ CPT Changes: An Insider's View 2000, 2017

➔ CPT Assistant Nov 97:43-44, Nov 99:49, Dec 13:18, Dec 14:6

(Use 92978 in conjunction with 92975, 92920, 92924, 92928, 92933, 92937, 92941, 92943, 93454-93461, 93563, 93564)

(Report 92978 once per session)

▶(Do not report 92978 in conjunction with 0913T, 0914T for intervention in the same major coronary artery or in the same bypass graft)◀

#+ 92979 each additional vessel (List separately in addition to code for primary procedure)

➔ CPT Changes: An Insider's View 2000, 2017

➔ CPT Assistant Nov 97:43-44, Nov 99:49, Dec 13:18, Dec 14:6

Intravascular Ultrasound (Coronary Vessel or Graft)
92978

A catheter with a transducer at its tip is inserted and threaded through a selected coronary artery(s) or coronary bypass graft(s).

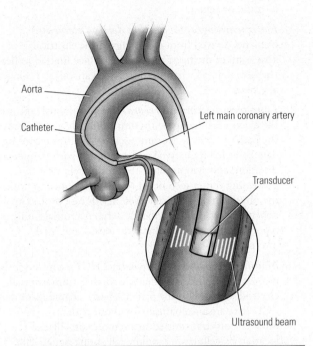

Aorta
Catheter
Left main coronary artery
Transducer
Ultrasound beam

(Report 92979 once per additional vessel)

(Use 92979 in conjunction with 92978)

(Intravascular ultrasound and optical coherence tomography services include all transducer manipulations and repositioning within the specific vessel being examined, both before and after therapeutic intervention [eg, stent placement])

Cardiography

Codes 93040-93042 are appropriate when an order for the test is triggered by an event, the rhythm strip is used to help diagnose the presence or absence of an arrhythmia, and a report is generated. There must be a specific order for an electrocardiogram or rhythm strip followed by a separate, signed, written, and retrievable report. It is not appropriate to use these codes for reviewing the telemetry monitor strips taken from a monitoring system. The need for an electrocardiogram or rhythm strip should be supported by documentation in the patient medical record.

(For echocardiography, see 93303-93350)

(For acoustic cardiography services, use 93799)

93000   Electrocardiogram, routine ECG with at least 12 leads; with interpretation and report
    ➲ *CPT Assistant* Aug 97:9, Feb 05:9, Mar 05:1, 11, Jul 08:3, Dec 20:3

93005   tracing only, without interpretation and report
    ➲ *CPT Assistant* Aug 97:9, Mar 05:1, Apr 16:8, Dec 20:3

93010   interpretation and report only
    ➲ *CPT Assistant* Aug 97:9, Mar 05:1, Apr 07:1, Apr 16:8, Dec 20:3, May 21:9

(For ECG monitoring, use 99418)

(Do not report 93000, 93005, 93010 in conjunction with, 0525T, 0526T, 0527T, 0528T, 0529T, 0530T, 0531T, 0532T)

93015   Cardiovascular stress test using maximal or submaximal treadmill or bicycle exercise, continuous electrocardiographic monitoring, and/or pharmacological stress; with supervision, interpretation and report
    ➲ *CPT Changes: An Insider's View* 2013
    ➲ *CPT Assistant* Apr 96:11, Jun 96:10, Aug 02:10, Jul 08:3, Jan 10:8, May 10:6, Dec 20:3
    ➲ *Clinical Examples in Radiology* Winter 10:12, Winter 24:34

93016   supervision only, without interpretation and report
    ➲ *CPT Changes: An Insider's View* 2013
    ➲ *CPT Assistant* Apr 96:11, Aug 02:10, Jul 08:3, Jan 10:8, May 10:6, Dec 20:3
    ➲ *Clinical Examples in Radiology* Winter 10:12

93017   tracing only, without interpretation and report
    ➲ *CPT Assistant* Aug 02:10, Jul 08:3, Jan 10:8, May 10:6, Dec 20:3
    ➲ *Clinical Examples in Radiology* Winter 10:12

93018   interpretation and report only
    ➲ *CPT Assistant* Apr 96:11, Jun 96:10, Jul 08:3, Jan 10:8, May 10:6, Dec 20:3
    ➲ *Clinical Examples in Radiology* Winter 10:12

93024   Ergonovine provocation test

93025   Microvolt T-wave alternans for assessment of ventricular arrhythmias
    ➲ *CPT Changes: An Insider's View* 2002
    ➲ *CPT Assistant* Mar 02:3

—— *Coding Tip* ——

Instructions for Reporting Electrocardiographic Recording

Codes 93040-93042 are appropriate when an order for the test is triggered by an event, the rhythm strip is used to help diagnose the presence or absence of an arrhythmia, and a report is generated. There must be a specific order for an electrocardiogram or rhythm strip followed by a separate, signed, written, and retrievable report. It is not appropriate to use these codes for reviewing the telemetry monitor strips taken from a monitoring system. The need for an electrocardiogram or rhythm strip should be supported by documentation in the patient medical record.

CPT Coding Guidelines, Cardiovascular, Cardiography

93040 Rhythm ECG, 1-3 leads; with interpretation and report

➔ *CPT Assistant* Apr 04:8, Oct 10:10, Nov 12:6, Sep 20:7, Dec 20:3

93041 tracing only without interpretation and report

➔ *CPT Assistant* Apr 04:8, Oct 10:10, Dec 20:3

93042 interpretation and report only

➔ *CPT Assistant* Apr 04:8, Oct 10:10, Oct 11:7, Dec 20:3

—— *Coding Tip* ——

Instructions for Reporting Electrocardiographic Recording

Do not report 93268-93272 when performing 93260, 93261, 93279-93289, 93291-93296, or 93298. *Do not report 93040, 93041, 93042 when performing 93260, 93261, 93279-93289, 93291-93296, or 93298.*

CPT Coding Guidelines, Cardiovascular, Implantable, Insertable, and Wearable Cardiac Device Evaluations

93050 Arterial pressure waveform analysis for assessment of central arterial pressures, includes obtaining waveform(s), digitization and application of nonlinear mathematical transformations to determine central arterial pressures and augmentation index, with interpretation and report, upper extremity artery, non-invasive

➔ *CPT Changes: An Insider's View* 2016

(Do not report 93050 in conjunction with diagnostic or interventional intra-arterial procedures)

93150 Code is out of numerical sequence. See 93297-93304

93151 Code is out of numerical sequence. See 93297-93304

93152 Code is out of numerical sequence. See 93297-93304

93153 Code is out of numerical sequence. See 93297-93304

Cardiovascular Monitoring Services

Cardiovascular monitoring services are diagnostic medical procedures using in-person and remote technology to assess cardiovascular rhythm (ECG) data. Holter monitors (93224-93227) include up to 48 hours of continuous recording. Mobile cardiac telemetry monitors (93228, 93229) have the capability of transmitting a tracing at any time, always have internal ECG analysis algorithms designed to detect major arrhythmias, and transmit to an attended surveillance center. Event monitors (93268-93272) record segments of ECGs with recording initiation triggered either by patient activation or by an internal automatic, pre-programmed detection algorithm (or both) and transmit the recorded electrocardiographic data when requested (but cannot transmit immediately based upon the patient or algorithmic activation rhythm) and require attended surveillance. Long-term continuous recorders (93241, 93242, 93243, 93244, 93245, 93246, 93247, 93248) continuously record and store for greater than 48 hours and up to 7 days or for greater than 7 days up to 15 days.

Attended surveillance: is the immediate availability of a remote technician to respond to rhythm or device alert transmissions from a patient, either from an implanted or wearable monitoring or therapy device, as they are generated and transmitted to the remote surveillance location or center.

Electrocardiographic rhythm derived elements: elements derived from recordings of the electrical activation of the heart including, but not limited to heart rhythm, rate, ST analysis, heart rate variability, T-wave alternans.

Long-term continuous recorders: Continuously record the electrocardiographic rhythm from a device applied to the patient. The electrocardiographic rhythm recording data collected is analyzed and annotated with frequency, duration, and symptomatic rhythm correlations. The processing center technician reviews the data and notifies the physician or other qualified health care professional depending on the prescribed criteria. An initial findings report is generated for physician review and final interpretation.

Mobile cardiovascular telemetry (MCT): continuously records the electrocardiographic rhythm from external electrodes placed on the patient's body. Segments of the ECG data are automatically (without patient intervention) transmitted to a remote surveillance location by cellular or landline telephone signal. The segments of the rhythm, selected for transmission, are triggered automatically (MCT device algorithm) by rapid and slow heart rates or by the patient during a symptomatic episode. There is continuous real time data analysis by preprogrammed algorithms in the device and attended surveillance of the transmitted rhythm segments by a surveillance center technician to evaluate any arrhythmias and to determine signal quality. The surveillance center technician reviews the data and notifies the physician or other qualified health care professional depending on the prescribed criteria.

ECG rhythm derived elements are distinct from physiologic data, even when the same device is capable of producing both. Implantable cardiovascular physiologic monitor device services are always separately reported from implantable cardioverter-defibrillator (ICD) service.

93224 External electrocardiographic recording up to 48 hours by continuous rhythm recording and storage; includes recording, scanning analysis with report, review and interpretation by a physician or other qualified health care professional

➔ *CPT Changes: An Insider's View* 2009, 2011, 2013

➔ *CPT Assistant* Oct 05:14, Apr 07:3, Mar 08:4, Mar 09:5, Oct 11:5, Nov 11:11

93225   recording (includes connection, recording, and
disconnection)

➜ *CPT Changes: An Insider's View* 2009, 2011

➜ *CPT Assistant* Oct 05:14, Apr 07:3, Mar 09:5, Oct 11:5

93226   scanning analysis with report

➜ *CPT Changes: An Insider's View* 2009, 2011

➜ *CPT Assistant* Oct 05:14, Apr 07:3, Mar 09:5, Oct 11:5

93227   review and interpretation by a physician or other
qualified health care professional

➜ *CPT Changes: An Insider's View* 2009, 2011, 2013

➜ *CPT Assistant* Apr 07:3, Mar 09:5, Apr 09:7, Oct 11:5,
Mar 18:5

(For less than 12 hours of continuous recording, use
modifier 52)

▶(For greater than 48 hours of monitoring, see 93241,
93242, 93243, 93244, 93245, 93246, 93247, 93248,
0937T, 0938T, 0939T, 0940T)◀

93241   External electrocardiographic recording for more than 48
hours up to 7 days by continuous rhythm recording and
storage; includes recording, scanning analysis with
report, review and interpretation

➜ *CPT Changes: An Insider's View* 2021

➜ *CPT Assistant* Nov 20:10

93242   recording (includes connection and initial recording)

➜ *CPT Changes: An Insider's View* 2021

➜ *CPT Assistant* Nov 20:10

93243   scanning analysis with report

➜ *CPT Changes: An Insider's View* 2021

➜ *CPT Assistant* Nov 20:10

93244   review and interpretation

➜ *CPT Changes: An Insider's View* 2021

➜ *CPT Assistant* Nov 20:10

▶(Do not report 93241, 93242, 93243, 93244 in
conjunction with 93224, 93225, 93226, 93227, 93228,
93229, 93245, 93246, 93247, 93248, 93268, 93270,
93271, 93272, 99091, 99453, 99454, 0937T, 0938T, 0939T,
0940T, for the same monitoring period)◀

93245   External electrocardiographic recording for more than 7
days up to 15 days by continuous rhythm recording and
storage; includes recording, scanning analysis with
report, review and interpretation

➜ *CPT Changes: An Insider's View* 2021

➜ *CPT Assistant* Nov 20:10

93246   recording (includes connection and initial recording)

➜ *CPT Changes: An Insider's View* 2021

➜ *CPT Assistant* Nov 20:10

93247   scanning analysis with report

➜ *CPT Changes: An Insider's View* 2021

➜ *CPT Assistant* Nov 20:10

93248   review and interpretation

➜ *CPT Changes: An Insider's View* 2021

➜ *CPT Assistant* Nov 20:10

▶(Do not report 93245, 93246, 93247, 93248 in
conjunction with 93224, 93225, 93226, 93227, 93228,
93229, 93241, 93242, 93243, 93244, 93268, 93270,
93271, 93272, 99091, 99453, 99454, 0937T, 0938T, 0939T,
0940T, for the same monitoring period)◀

★ **93228**   External mobile cardiovascular telemetry with
electrocardiographic recording, concurrent computerized
real time data analysis and greater than 24 hours of
accessible ECG data storage (retrievable with query) with
ECG triggered and patient selected events transmitted to
a remote attended surveillance center for up to 30 days;
review and interpretation with report by a physician or
other qualified health care professional

➜ *CPT Changes: An Insider's View* 2009, 2011, 2013, 2017

➜ *CPT Assistant* Oct 11:5

(Report 93228 only once per 30 days)

(Do not report 93228 in conjunction with 93224, 93227)

★ **93229**   technical support for connection and patient
instructions for use, attended surveillance, analysis
and transmission of daily and emergent data reports
as prescribed by a physician or other qualified health
care professional

➜ *CPT Changes: An Insider's View* 2009, 2011, 2013, 2017

➜ *CPT Assistant* Oct 11:5

(Report 93229 only once per 30 days)

(Do not report 93229 in conjunction with 93224, 93226)

(For external cardiovascular monitors that do not perform
automatic ECG triggered transmissions to an attended
surveillance center, see 93224-93227, 93268-93272)

93241   Code is out of numerical sequence. See 93226-93229

93242   Code is out of numerical sequence. See 93226-93229

93243   Code is out of numerical sequence. See 93226-93229

93244   Code is out of numerical sequence. See 93226-93229

93245   Code is out of numerical sequence. See 93226-93229

93246   Code is out of numerical sequence. See 93226-93229

93247   Code is out of numerical sequence. See 93226-93229

93248   Code is out of numerical sequence. See 93226-93229

93260   Code is out of numerical sequence. See 93283-93291

93261   Code is out of numerical sequence. See 93283-93291

93264   Code is out of numerical sequence. See 93272-93280

★ **93268**   External patient and, when performed, auto activated electrocardiographic rhythm derived event recording with symptom-related memory loop with remote download capability up to 30 days, 24-hour attended monitoring; includes transmission, review and interpretation by a physician or other qualified health care professional

➡ *CPT Changes: An Insider's View* 2003, 2009, 2011, 2013, 2017

➡ *CPT Assistant* Jun 96:2, Nov 99:49-50, Oct 05:14, Apr 07:3, Mar 08:4, Mar 09:5, Oct 11:5

★ **93270**   recording (includes connection, recording, and disconnection)

➡ *CPT Changes: An Insider's View* 2009, 2011, 2017

➡ *CPT Assistant* Jun 96:2, Oct 05:14, Apr 07:3, Mar 09:5, Aug 10:13, Oct 11:5

★ **93271**   transmission and analysis

➡ *CPT Changes: An Insider's View* 2009, 2011, 2017

➡ *CPT Assistant* Jun 96:2, Oct 05:14, Apr 07:3, Mar 09:5, Oct 11:5

★ **93272**   review and interpretation by a physician or other qualified health care professional

➡ *CPT Changes: An Insider's View* 2009, 2011, 2013, 2017

➡ *CPT Assistant* Jun 96:2, Apr 98:14, Nov 99:49-50, Oct 05:14, Apr 07:3, Mar 09:5, Apr 09:7, Oct 11:5, Mar 18:5

(For subcutaneous cardiac rhythm monitoring, see 33285, 93285, 93291, 93298)

93278   Signal-averaged electrocardiography (SAECG), with or without ECG

➡ *CPT Assistant* Oct 11:5

(For interpretation and report only, use 93278 with modifier 26)

(For unlisted cardiographic procedure, use 93799)

Implantable, Insertable, and Wearable Cardiac Device Evaluations

Cardiac device evaluation services are diagnostic medical procedures using in-person and remote technology to assess device therapy and cardiovascular physiologic data. Codes 93260, 93261, 93279-93298 describe this technology and technical/professional and service center practice. Codes 93260, 93261, 93279-93292 are reported per procedure. Codes 93293, 93294, 93295, 93296 are reported no more than **once** every 90 days. Do not report 93293, 93294, 93295, 93296, if the monitoring period is less than 30 days. Codes 93297, 93298 are reported no more than **once** up to every 30 days, per patient. Do not report 93297, 93298, if the monitoring period is less than 10 days. Do not report 93264 if the monitoring period is less than 30 days. Code 93264 is reported no more than once up to every 30 days, per patient.

For body surface–activation mapping to optimize electrical synchrony of a biventricular pacing or biventricular pacing-defibrillator system at the time of follow-up device interrogation or programming

evaluation, also report 0696T in conjunction with the appropriate code (ie, 93279, 93281, 93284, 93286, 93287, 93288, 93289).

A service center may report 93296 during a period in which a physician or other qualified health care professional performs an in-person interrogation device evaluation. The same individual may not report an in-person and remote interrogation of the same device during the same period. Report only remote services when an in-person interrogation device evaluation is performed during a period of remote interrogation device evaluation. A period is established by the initiation of the remote monitoring or the 91st day of a pacemaker or implantable defibrillator monitoring or the 31st day of monitoring a subcutaneous cardiac rhythm monitor or implantable cardiovascular physiologic monitor, and extends for the subsequent 90 or 30 days respectively, for which remote monitoring is occurring. Programming device evaluations and in-person interrogation device evaluations may not be reported on the same date by the same individual. Programming device evaluations and remote interrogation device evaluations may both be reported during the remote interrogation device evaluation period.

For monitoring by wearable devices, see 93224-93272.

ECG rhythm derived elements are distinct from physiologic data, even when the same device is capable of producing both. Implantable cardiovascular physiologic monitor services are always separately reported from implantable defibrillator services. When cardiac rhythm data are derived from an implantable defibrillator or pacemaker, do not report subcutaneous cardiac rhythm monitor services with pacemaker or implantable defibrillator services.

Do not report 93268-93272 when performing 93260, 93261, 93279-93289, 93291-93296, or 93298. Do not report 93040, 93041, 93042 when performing 93260, 93261, 93279-93289, 93291-93296, or 93298.

The pacemaker and implantable defibrillator interrogation device evaluations, peri-procedural device evaluations and programming, and programming device evaluations may not be reported in conjunction with pacemaker or implantable defibrillator device and/or lead insertion or revision services by the same individual.

The following definitions and instructions apply to codes 93260, 93261, 93279-93298.

Attended surveillance: the immediate availability of a remote technician to respond to rhythm or device alert transmissions from a patient, either from an implanted, inserted, or wearable monitoring or therapy device, as they are generated and transmitted to the remote surveillance location or center.

Device, leadless: a leadless cardiac pacemaker system that includes a pulse generator with built-in battery and electrode for implantation into the cardiac chamber via a transcatheter approach.

Device, single lead: a pacemaker or implantable defibrillator with pacing and sensing function in only one chamber of the heart or a subcutaneous electrode.

Device, dual lead: a pacemaker or implantable defibrillator with pacing and sensing function in only two chambers of the heart.

Device, multiple lead: a pacemaker or implantable defibrillator with pacing and sensing function in three or more chambers of the heart.

Electrocardiographic rhythm derived elements: elements derived from recordings of the electrical activation of the heart including, but not limited to heart rhythm, rate, ST analysis, heart rate variability, T-wave alternans.

Implantable cardiovascular physiologic monitor: an implantable cardiovascular device used to assist the physician or other qualified health care professional in the management of non-rhythm related cardiac conditions such as heart failure. The device collects longitudinal physiologic cardiovascular data elements from one or more internal sensors (such as right ventricular pressure, pulmonary artery pressure, left atrial pressure, or an index of lung water) and/or external sensors (such as blood pressure or body weight) for patient assessment and management. The data are stored and transmitted by either local telemetry or remotely to an Internet-based file server or surveillance technician. The function of the implantable cardiovascular physiologic monitor may be an additional function of an implantable cardiac device (eg, implantable defibrillator) or a function of a stand-alone device. When implantable cardiovascular physiologic monitor functionality is included in an implantable defibrillator device or pacemaker, the implantable cardiovascular physiologic monitor data and the implantable defibrillator or pacemaker, heart rhythm data such as sensing, pacing, and tachycardia detection therapy are distinct and, therefore, the monitoring processes are distinct.

Implantable defibrillator: two general categories of implantable defibrillators exist: transvenous implantable pacing cardioverter-defibrillator (ICD) and subcutaneous implantable defibrillator (SICD). An implantable pacing cardioverter-defibrillator device provides high-energy and low-energy stimulation to one or more chambers of the heart to terminate rapid heart rhythms called tachycardia or fibrillation. Implantable pacing cardioverter-

defibrillators also have pacemaker functions to treat slow heart rhythms called bradycardia. In addition to the tachycardia and bradycardia functions, the implantable pacing cardioverter-defibrillator may or may not include the functionality of an implantable cardiovascular physiologic monitor or a subcutaneous cardiac rhythm monitor. The subcutaneous implantable defibrillator uses a single subcutaneous electrode to treat ventricular tachyarrhythmias. Subcutaneous implantable defibrillators differ from transvenous implantable pacing cardioverter-defibrillators in that subcutaneous implantable defibrillators do not provide antitachycardia pacing or chronic pacing. For subcutaneous implantable defibrillator device evaluation, see 93260, 93261.

Interrogation device evaluation: an evaluation of an implantable device such as a cardiac pacemaker, implantable defibrillator, implantable cardiovascular physiologic monitor, or subcutaneous cardiac rhythm monitor. Using an office, hospital, or emergency room instrument or via a remote interrogation system, stored and measured information about the lead(s) when present, sensor(s) when present, battery and the implanted device function, as well as data collected about the patient's heart rhythm and heart rate is retrieved. The retrieved information is evaluated to determine the current programming of the device and to evaluate certain aspects of the device function such as battery voltage, lead impedance, tachycardia detection settings, and rhythm treatment settings.

The components that must be evaluated for the various types of implantable or insertable cardiac devices are listed below. (The required components for both remote and in-person interrogations are the same.)

Pacemaker: programmed parameters, with or without lead(s), battery, capture and sensing function and heart rhythm.

Implantable defibrillator: programmed parameters, lead(s), battery, capture and sensing function, presence or absence of therapy for ventricular tachyarrhythmias and underlying heart rhythm.

Implantable cardiovascular physiologic monitor: programmed parameters and analysis of at least one recorded physiologic cardiovascular data element from either internal or external sensors.

Subcutaneous cardiac rhythm monitor: programmed parameters and the heart rate and rhythm during recorded episodes from both patient initiated and device algorithm detected events, when present.

Interrogation device evaluation (remote): a procedure performed for patients with pacemakers, implantable defibrillators, or subcutaneous cardiac rhythm monitors using data obtained remotely. All device functions, including the programmed parameters, lead(s), battery, capture and sensing function, presence or absence of therapy for ventricular tachyarrhythmias (for implantable defibrillators) and underlying heart rhythm are evaluated.

The components that must be evaluated for the various types of implantable or insertable cardiac devices are listed below. (The required components for both remote and in person interrogations are the same.)

Pacemaker: programmed parameters, with or without lead(s), battery, capture and sensing function, and heart rhythm.

Implantable defibrillator: programmed parameters, lead(s), battery, capture and sensing function, presence or absence of therapy for ventricular tachyarrhythmias, and underlying heart rhythm.

Implantable cardiovascular physiologic monitor: programmed parameters and analysis of at least one recorded physiologic cardiovascular data element from either internal or external sensors.

Subcutaneous cardiac rhythm monitor: programmed parameters and the heart rate and rhythm during recorded episodes from both patient-initiated and device algorithm detected events, when present.

Pacemaker: an implantable device that provides low energy localized stimulation to one or more chambers of the heart to initiate contraction in that chamber. Two general categories of pacemakers exist: (1) pacemakers with a subcutaneous generator plus transvenous/epicardial lead(s); and (2) leadless pacemakers. A leadless pacemaker does not require a subcutaneous pocket for the generator. It combines a miniaturized generator with an integrated electrode for implantation in a heart chamber via a transcatheter approach.

Peri-procedural device evaluation and programming: an evaluation of an implantable device system (either a pacemaker or implantable defibrillator) to adjust the device to settings appropriate for the patient prior to a surgery, procedure, or test. The device system data are interrogated to evaluate the lead(s) when present, sensor(s), and battery in addition to review of stored information, including patient and system measurements. The device is programmed to settings appropriate for the surgery, procedure, or test, as required. A second evaluation and programming are performed after the surgery, procedure, or test to provide settings appropriate to the post procedural situation, as required. If one performs both the pre- and post-evaluation and programming service, the appropriate code, either 93286 or 93287, would be reported two times. If one performs the pre-surgical service and a separate individual performs the post-surgical service, each reports either 93286 or 93287 only one time.

Physiologic cardiovascular data elements: data elements from one or more internal sensors (such as right ventricular pressure, left atrial pressure or an index of lung water) and/or external sensors (such as blood pressure or body weight) for patient assessment and management. It does not include ECG rhythm derived data elements.

Programming device evaluation (in person): a procedure performed for patients with a pacemaker, implantable defibrillator, or subcutaneous cardiac rhythm monitor. All device functions, including the battery, programmable settings and lead(s), when present, are evaluated. To assess capture thresholds, iterative adjustments (eg, progressive changes in pacing output of a pacing lead) of the programmable parameters are conducted. The iterative adjustments provide information that permits the operator to assess and select the most appropriate final program parameters to provide for consistent delivery of the appropriate therapy and to verify the function of the device. The final program parameters may or may not change after evaluation.

The programming device evaluation includes all of the components of the interrogation device evaluation (remote) or the interrogation device evaluation (in person), and it includes the selection of patient specific programmed parameters depending on the type of device.

The components that must be evaluated for the various types of programming device evaluations are listed below. (See also required interrogation device evaluation [remote and in person] components above.)

Pacemaker: programmed parameters, lead(s) when present, battery, capture and sensing function, and heart rhythm. Often, but not always, the sensor rate response, lower and upper heart rates, AV intervals, pacing voltage and pulse duration, sensing value, and diagnostics will be adjusted during a programming evaluation.

Implantable defibrillator: programmed parameters, lead(s), battery, capture and sensing function, presence or absence of therapy for ventricular tachyarrhythmias and underlying heart rhythm. Often, but not always, the sensor rate response, lower and upper heart rates, AV intervals, pacing voltage and pulse duration, sensing value, and diagnostics will be adjusted during a programming evaluation. In addition, ventricular tachycardia detection and therapies are sometimes altered depending on the interrogated data, patient's rhythm, symptoms, and condition.

Subcutaneous cardiac rhythm monitor: programmed parameters and the heart rhythm during recorded episodes from both patient initiated and device algorithm detected events. Often, but not always, the tachycardia and bradycardia detection criteria will be adjusted during a programming evaluation.

Subcutaneous cardiac rhythm monitor: an implantable or insertable device that continuously records the electrocardiographic rhythm triggered automatically by rapid, irregular, and/or slow heart rates or by the patient during a symptomatic episode. The cardiac rhythm monitor function may be the only function of the device or it may be part of a pacemaker or implantable defibrillator device. The data are stored and transmitted by either local telemetry or remotely to an Internet-based file server or surveillance technician. Extraction of data and compilation or report for physician or qualified health care professional interpretation is usually performed in the office setting.

Transtelephonic rhythm strip pacemaker evaluation: service of transmission of an electrocardiographic rhythm strip over the telephone by the patient using a transmitter and recorded by a receiving location using a receiver/recorder (also commonly known as transtelephonic pacemaker monitoring). The electrocardiographic rhythm strip is recorded both with and without a magnet applied over the pacemaker. The rhythm strip is evaluated for heart rate and rhythm, atrial and ventricular capture (if observed) and atrial and ventricular sensing (if observed). In addition, the battery status of the pacemaker is determined by measurement of the paced rate on the electrocardiographic rhythm strip recorded with the magnet applied. For remote monitoring of an implantable wireless pulmonary artery pressure sensor, use 93264.

Implantable wireless pulmonary artery sensor: an implantable cardiovascular device used to assist the physician or other qualified health care professional in monitoring heart failure. The device collects longitudinal physiologic cardiovascular data elements from an internal sensor located in the pulmonary artery. The data are transmitted and stored remotely to an Internet-based file server.

 # 93264 Remote monitoring of a wireless pulmonary artery pressure sensor for up to 30 days, including at least weekly downloads of pulmonary artery pressure recordings, interpretation(s), trend analysis, and report(s) by a physician or other qualified health care professional

➔ *CPT Changes: An Insider's View* 2019
➔ *CPT Assistant* Jun 19:3, Feb 20:7

(Report 93264 only once per 30 days)

(Do not report 93264 if download[s], interpretation[s], trend analysis, and report[s] do not occur at least weekly during the 30-day time period)

(Do not report 93264 if review does not occur at least weekly during the 30-day time period)

(Do not report 93264 if monitoring period is less than 30 days)

▶(For remote monitoring of an implantable wireless left atrial pressure sensor, use 0934T)◀

93279 Programming device evaluation (in person) with iterative adjustment of the implantable device to test the function of the device and select optimal permanent programmed values with analysis, review and report by a physician or other qualified health care professional; single lead pacemaker system or leadless pacemaker system in one cardiac chamber

➔ *CPT Changes: An Insider's View* 2009, 2010, 2013, 2019
➔ *CPT Assistant* Jun 12:4, Jun 13:6, Jul 13:7, Apr 14:3, Jul 14:3, Nov 14:5, Aug 16:5, Mar 19:6, Sep 22:1

(Do not report 93279 in conjunction with 93286, 93288)

93280 dual lead pacemaker system
➔ *CPT Changes: An Insider's View* 2009, 2010, 2013
➔ *CPT Assistant* Jun 12:4, Jun 13:6, Jul 13:7, Apr 14:3, Aug 16:5, Mar 22:13, Sep 22:1

(Do not report 93280 in conjunction with 93286, 93288)

93281 multiple lead pacemaker system
➔ *CPT Changes: An Insider's View* 2009, 2010, 2013
➔ *CPT Assistant* Jun 12:4, Jun 13:6, Jul 13:7, Apr 14:3, Aug 16:5, Sep 22:1

(Use 93281 in conjunction with 0696T when body surface–activation mapping to optimize electrical synchrony is also performed)

(Do not report 93281 in conjunction with 93286, 93288)

93282 single lead transvenous implantable defibrillator system
➔ *CPT Changes: An Insider's View* 2009, 2010, 2013, 2015
➔ *CPT Assistant* Jun 13:6, Jul 13:7, Apr 14:3, Aug 16:5, Sep 22:1

(Do not report 93282 in conjunction with 93260, 93287, 93289, 93745)

93283 dual lead transvenous implantable defibrillator system
➔ *CPT Changes: An Insider's View* 2009, 2010, 2013, 2015
➔ *CPT Assistant* Jun 13:6, Jul 13:7, Apr 14:3, Aug 16:5

(Do not report 93283 in conjunction with 93287, 93289)

93284 multiple lead transvenous implantable defibrillator system
➔ *CPT Changes: An Insider's View* 2009, 2010, 2013, 2015
➔ *CPT Assistant* Jun 13:6, Jul 13:7, Apr 14:3, Aug 16:5

(Use 93284 in conjunction with 0696T when body surface–activation mapping to optimize electrical synchrony is also performed)

(Do not report 93284 in conjunction with 93287, 93289)

93260 implantable subcutaneous lead defibrillator system
➔ *CPT Changes: An Insider's View* 2015
➔ *CPT Assistant* Nov 14:5, Aug 16:5, Sep 22:1

(Do not report 93260 in conjunction with 93261, 93282, 93287)

(Do not report 93260 in conjunction with pulse generator and lead insertion or repositioning codes 33240, 33241, 33262, 33270, 33271, 33272, 33273)

93285 subcutaneous cardiac rhythm monitor system
➔ *CPT Changes: An Insider's View* 2009, 2010, 2013, 2019
➔ *CPT Assistant* Aug 16:5, Sep 22:1

(Do not report 93285 in conjunction with 33285, 93279-93284, 93291, 0650T)

(For programming device evaluation [remote] of subcutaneous cardiac rhythm monitor system, use 0650T)

93286 Peri-procedural device evaluation (in person) and programming of device system parameters before or after a surgery, procedure, or test with analysis, review and report by a physician or other qualified health care professional; single, dual, or multiple lead pacemaker system, or leadless pacemaker system
➔ *CPT Changes: An Insider's View* 2009, 2010, 2013, 2019
➔ *CPT Assistant* Jun 13:6, Jul 13:7, Apr 14:3, Aug 16:5, Mar 19:6, Jul 23:1, Sep 23:48

(Report 93286 once before and once after surgery, procedure, or test, when device evaluation and programming is performed before and after surgery, procedure, or test)

▶(Do not report 93286 in conjunction with 93279, 93280, 93281, 93288, 0408T, 0409T, 0410T, 0411T, 0414T, 0415T, 0915T-0925T)◀

93287 single, dual, or multiple lead implantable defibrillator system
➔ *CPT Changes: An Insider's View* 2009, 2010, 2013, 2015
➔ *CPT Assistant* Jun 13:6, Jul 13:7, Apr 14:3, Jul 14:3, Aug 16:5, Sep 23:48

(Use 93286, 93287 in conjunction with 0696T when body surface–activation mapping to optimize electrical synchrony is also performed)

(Report 93287 once before and once after surgery, procedure, or test, when device evaluation and programming is performed before and after surgery, procedure, or test)

▶(Do not report 93287 in conjunction with 93260, 93261, 93282, 93283, 93284, 93289, 0408T, 0409T, 0410T, 0411T, 0414T, 0415T, 0915T-0925T)◀

93288 Interrogation device evaluation (in person) with analysis, review and report by a physician or other qualified health care professional, includes connection, recording and disconnection per patient encounter; single, dual, or multiple lead pacemaker system, or leadless pacemaker system
➔ *CPT Changes: An Insider's View* 2009, 2013, 2019
➔ *CPT Assistant* Jun 12:4, Jun 13:6, Jul 13:7, Apr 14:3, Aug 16:5, Mar 19:6

(Do not report 93288 in conjunction with 93279-93281, 93286, 93294, 93296)

93289 single, dual, or multiple lead transvenous implantable defibrillator system, including analysis of heart rhythm derived data elements
➔ *CPT Changes: An Insider's View* 2009, 2013, 2015
➔ *CPT Assistant* Jun 13:6, Jul 13:7, Apr 14:3, Aug 16:5

(Use 93288, 93289 in conjunction with 0696T when body surface–activation mapping to optimize electrical synchrony is also performed)

(For monitoring physiologic cardiovascular data elements derived from an implantable defibrillator, use 93290)

(Do not report 93289 in conjunction with 93261, 93282, 93283, 93284, 93287, 93295, 93296)

93261 implantable subcutaneous lead defibrillator system
➔ *CPT Changes: An Insider's View* 2015
➔ *CPT Assistant* Nov 14:5, Aug 16:5

(Do not report 93261 in conjunction with 93260, 93287, 93289)

(Do not report 93261 in conjunction with pulse generator and lead insertion or repositioning codes 33240, 33241, 33262, 33270, 33271, 33272, 33273)

93290 implantable cardiovascular physiologic monitor system, including analysis of 1 or more recorded physiologic cardiovascular data elements from all internal and external sensors
➔ *CPT Changes: An Insider's View* 2009, 2013, 2019
➔ *CPT Assistant* Feb 10:13, Apr 13:11, Aug 16:5, Feb 20:7

(For heart rhythm derived data elements, use 93289)

(Do not report 93290 in conjunction with 93297)

93291 subcutaneous cardiac rhythm monitor system, including heart rhythm derived data analysis
➔ *CPT Changes: An Insider's View* 2009, 2013, 2019
➔ *CPT Assistant* Aug 16:5, Sep 22:1

(Do not report 93291 in conjunction with 33285, 93288-93290, 93298, 0650T)

93292 wearable defibrillator system
➔ *CPT Changes: An Insider's View* 2009, 2013
➔ *CPT Assistant* Aug 16:5

(Do not report 93292 in conjunction with 93745)

—— *Coding Tip* ——

Instructions for Reporting Pacemaker and Interrogation Device Evaluations

Codes 93293-93296 are reported no more than once every 90 days. Do not report 93293-93296 if the monitoring period is less than 30 days.

CPT Coding Guidelines, Cardiovascular, Cardiography Implantable and Wearable Cardiac Device Evaluations

---

93293   Transtelephonic rhythm strip pacemaker evaluation(s) single, dual, or multiple lead pacemaker system, includes recording with and without magnet application with analysis, review and report(s) by a physician or other qualified health care professional, up to 90 days

➔ *CPT Changes: An Insider's View* 2009, 2013

➔ *CPT Assistant* Aug 16:5

(Do not report 93293 in conjunction with 93294)

(For in person evaluation, see 93040, 93041, 93042)

(Report 93293 only once per 90 days)

93294   Interrogation device evaluation(s) (remote), up to 90 days; single, dual, or multiple lead pacemaker system, or leadless pacemaker system with interim analysis, review(s) and report(s) by a physician or other qualified health care professional

➔ *CPT Changes: An Insider's View* 2009, 2013, 2019

➔ *CPT Assistant* Jun 12:4, Aug 16:5, Mar 19:6, Sep 22:1

(Do not report 93294 in conjunction with 93288, 93293)

(Report 93294 only once per 90 days)

93295   single, dual, or multiple lead implantable defibrillator system with interim analysis, review(s) and report(s) by a physician or other qualified health care professional

➔ *CPT Changes: An Insider's View* 2009, 2013, 2015

➔ *CPT Assistant* Aug 16:5, Sep 22:1

(For remote monitoring of physiologic cardiovascular data elements derived from an ICD, use 93297)

(Do not report 93295 in conjunction with 93289)

(Report 93295 only once per 90 days)

(For remote interrogation device evaluation[s] of implantable cardioverter-defibrillator with substernal lead, see 0578T, 0579T)

93296   single, dual, or multiple lead pacemaker system, leadless pacemaker system, or implantable defibrillator system, remote data acquisition(s), receipt of transmissions and technician review, technical support and distribution of results

➔ *CPT Changes: An Insider's View* 2009, 2015, 2019

➔ *CPT Assistant* Aug 16:5, Mar 19:6, Sep 22:1

(Do not report 93296 in conjunction with 93288, 93289)

(Report 93296 only once per 90 days)

(For remote interrogation device evaluation[s] of implantable cardioverter-defibrillator with substernal lead, see 0578T, 0579T)

93297   Interrogation device evaluation(s), (remote) up to 30 days; implantable cardiovascular physiologic monitor system, including analysis of 1 or more recorded physiologic cardiovascular data elements from all internal and external sensors, analysis, review(s) and report(s) by a physician or other qualified health care professional

➔ *CPT Changes: An Insider's View* 2009, 2013, 2019

➔ *CPT Assistant* Feb 09:9, 12, Apr 13:11, Aug 16:5, Oct 19:3, Feb 20:12, Sep 22:1

(For heart rhythm derived data elements, use 93295)

(Do not report 93297 in conjunction with 93264, 93290, 93298, 99091, 99454)

(Report 93297 only once per 30 days)

93298   subcutaneous cardiac rhythm monitor system, including analysis of recorded heart rhythm data, analysis, review(s) and report(s) by a physician or other qualified health care professional

➔ *CPT Changes: An Insider's View* 2009, 2013, 2017, 2019

➔ *CPT Assistant* Feb 09:9, 12, Aug 16:5, Oct 19:3, Feb 20:12, Sep 22:1

(Do not report 93298 in conjunction with 33285, 93291, 93297, 99091, 99454)

(Report 93298 only once per 30 days)

(For remote monitoring of an implantable wireless pulmonary artery pressure sensor, use 93264)

Phrenic Nerve Stimulation System

Phrenic nerve stimulation system–therapy activation (93150) is performed once (after 30 days from implantation to allow for lead stabilization). Activation includes device evaluation and programming services: rate, pulse amplitude; pulse duration; configuration of waveform; battery status; electrode selection output modulation; cycling; impedance; and patient compliance measurements (eg, hours of therapy, sleeping position, and activity [sleep activity, awake activity, time in a sleep position]). Subsequent interrogation only (93153) or interrogation and programming (93151, 93152) may be performed to evaluate device function and to optimize performance incrementally. For patients that require programming during a polysomnogram, report 93152 once, regardless of how many programming changes are made over the course of the polysomnogram.

 # 93150 Therapy activation of implanted phrenic nerve stimulator system, including all interrogation and programming

➲ *CPT Changes: An Insider's View* 2024

➲ *CPT Assistant* Apr 24:9

(Do not report 93150 in conjunction with 33276, 33277, 33278, 33279, 33280, 33281, 93151, 93152, 93153)

 # 93151 Interrogation and programming (minimum one parameter) of implanted phrenic nerve stimulator system

➲ *CPT Changes: An Insider's View* 2024

➲ *CPT Assistant* Apr 24:9

(Do not report 93151 in conjunction with 93150, 93152, 93153)

(For interrogation without programming of implanted phrenic nerve stimulator system, use 93153)

 # 93152 Interrogation and programming of implanted phrenic nerve stimulator system during polysomnography

➲ *CPT Changes: An Insider's View* 2024

➲ *CPT Assistant* Apr 24:9

(Do not report 93152 in conjunction with 33276, 93150, 93151, 93153)

(For polysomnography, see 95808, 95810, 95811, 95782, 95783)

 # 93153 Interrogation without programming of implanted phrenic nerve stimulator system

➲ *CPT Changes: An Insider's View* 2024

➲ *CPT Assistant* Apr 24:9

(Do not report 93153 in conjunction with 33276, 93150, 93151, 93152)

Echocardiography

Echocardiography includes obtaining ultrasonic signals from the heart and great vessels, with real time image and/or Doppler ultrasonic signal documentation, with interpretation and report. When interpretation is performed separately, use modifier 26.

A complete transthoracic echocardiogram without spectral or color flow Doppler (93307) is a comprehensive procedure that includes 2-dimensional and, when performed, selected M-mode examination of the left and right atria, left and right ventricles, the aortic, mitral, and tricuspid valves, the pericardium, and adjacent portions of the aorta. Multiple views are required to obtain a complete functional and anatomic evaluation, and appropriate measurements are obtained and recorded. Despite significant effort, identification and measurement of some structures may not always be possible. In such instances, the reason that an element could not be visualized must be documented. Additional structures that may be visualized (eg, pulmonary veins, pulmonary artery, pulmonic valve, inferior vena cava) would be included as part of the service.

A complete transthoracic echocardiogram with spectral and color flow Doppler (93306) is a comprehensive procedure that includes spectral Doppler and color flow Doppler in addition to the 2-dimensional and selected M-mode examinations, when performed. Spectral Doppler (93320, 93321) and color flow Doppler (93325) provide information regarding intracardiac blood flow and hemodynamics.

A follow-up or limited echocardiographic study (93308) is an examination that does not evaluate or document the attempt to evaluate all the structures that comprise the complete echocardiographic exam. This is typically limited to, or performed in follow-up of a focused clinical concern.

In stress echocardiography, echocardiographic images are recorded from multiple cardiac windows before, after, and in some protocols, during stress. The stress is achieved by (1) walking on a treadmill; (2) using a bicycle (supine or upright); or (3) the administration of pharmacological agents that either simulate exercise (by increasing heart rate, blood pressure, or myocardial contractility) or alter coronary flow (vasodilation). The patient's ECG, heart rate, and blood pressure are monitored at baseline, throughout the procedure and during recovery. Reports are prepared to evaluate (1) the duration of stress, the reason for stopping, and the hemodynamic response to stress; (2) the electrocardiographic response to stress; and (3) the echocardiographic response to stress.

When a stress echocardiogram is performed with a complete cardiovascular stress test (continuous electrocardiographic monitoring, supervision, interpretation and report by a physician or other qualified health care professional), use 93351. When only the professional components of a complete stress test and a stress echocardiogram are provided (eg, in a facility setting) by the same physician, use 93351 with modifier 26. When all professional services of a stress test are not performed by the same physician performing the stress echocardiogram, use 93350 in conjunction with the appropriate codes (93016-93018) for the components of the cardiovascular stress test that are provided.

When left ventricular endocardial borders cannot be adequately identified by standard echocardiographic imaging, echocardiographic contrast may be infused intravenously both at rest and with stress to achieve that purpose. Code 93352 is used to report the administration of echocardiographic contrast agent in conjunction with the stress echocardiography codes (93350 or 93351). Supply of contrast agent and/or drugs used for pharmacological stress is reported separately in addition to the procedure code.

Code 93355 is used to report transesophageal echocardiography (TEE) services during transcatheter intracardiac therapies. Code 93355 is reported once per intervention and only by an individual who is not performing the interventional procedure. Code 93355 includes the work of passing the endoscopic ultrasound transducer through the mouth into the esophagus, when performed by the individual performing the TEE, diagnostic transesophageal echocardiography and ongoing manipulation of the transducer to guide sizing and/or placement of implants, determination of adequacy of the intervention, and assessment for potential complications. Real-time image acquisition, measurements, and interpretation of image(s), documentation of completion of the intervention, and final written report are included in this code.

A range of intracardiac therapies may be performed with TEE guidance. Code 93355 describes TEE during advanced transcatheter structural heart procedures (eg, transcatheter aortic valve replacement [TAVR], left atrial appendage closure [LAA], or percutaneous mitral valve repair).

See 93313 for separate reporting of the probe insertion by a physician other than the physician performing the TEE.

Report of an echocardiographic study, whether complete or limited, includes an interpretation of all obtained information, documentation of all clinically relevant findings including quantitative measurements obtained, plus a description of any recognized abnormalities. Pertinent images, videotape, and/or digital data are archived for permanent storage and are available for subsequent review. Use of echocardiography not meeting these criteria is not separately reportable.

Use of ultrasound, without thorough evaluation of organ(s) or anatomic region, image documentation and final, written report, is not separately reportable.

(For fetal echocardiography, see 76825-76828)

93303   Transthoracic echocardiography for congenital cardiac anomalies; complete
➔ *CPT Assistant* Nov 97:44, Dec 97:5, Sep 05:10-11, Mar 08:4, Oct 10:17, Dec 10:17, Aug 13:3, Dec 13:15, May 15:10, Apr 20:11, Jul 20:12, Jul 21:10, Apr 22:14
➔ *Clinical Examples in Radiology* Fall 06:9-10, Spring 22:15

93304   follow-up or limited study
➔ *CPT Assistant* Nov 97:44, Dec 97:5, Jan 10:8, Oct 10:17, Dec 10:17, Aug 13:3, Dec 13:15, May 15:10, Jul 20:12, Jul 21:10, Apr 22:14
➔ *Clinical Examples in Radiology* Fall 06:9-10, Spring 22:15

93306   Echocardiography, transthoracic, real-time with image documentation (2D), includes M-mode recording, when performed, complete, with spectral Doppler echocardiography, and with color flow Doppler echocardiography
➔ *CPT Changes: An Insider's View* 2009
➔ *CPT Assistant* Oct 10:17, Dec 10:17, Aug 13:3, May 15:10, Apr 16:9, Dec 18:11, May 20:12, Jul 20:12, Jul 21:10

(For transthoracic echocardiography without spectral and color Doppler, use 93307)

93307   Echocardiography, transthoracic, real-time with image documentation (2D), includes M-mode recording, when performed, complete, without spectral or color Doppler echocardiography
➔ *CPT Changes: An Insider's View* 2009
➔ *CPT Assistant* Dec 97:5, Sep 05:11, Oct 10:17, Dec 10:17, Aug 13:3, May 15:10, Apr 16:9, May 20:12, Jul 20:12, Jul 21:10
➔ *Clinical Examples in Radiology* Fall 06:9-10

(Do not report 93307 in conjunction with 93320, 93321, 93325)

93308   Echocardiography, transthoracic, real-time with image documentation (2D), includes M-mode recording, when performed, follow-up or limited study
➔ *CPT Changes: An Insider's View* 2009
➔ *CPT Assistant* Dec 97:5, Sep 05:11, Jan 10:8, Oct 10:17, Dec 10:17, Mar 12:10, Aug 13:3, May 15:10, Apr 16:9, Dec 18:11, Jul 20:12, Jul 21:10
➔ *Clinical Examples in Radiology* Fall 06:9-10, Spring 22:15

93312   Echocardiography, transesophageal, real-time with image documentation (2D) (with or without M-mode recording); including probe placement, image acquisition, interpretation and report
➔ *CPT Changes: An Insider's View* 2017
➔ *CPT Assistant* Dec 97:5, Jan 00:10, Jan 10:8, Oct 12:15, Aug 13:3, Jul 14:9
➔ *Clinical Examples in Radiology* Spring 22:15

(Do not report 93312 in conjunction with 93355)

93313   placement of transesophageal probe only
➔ *CPT Changes: An Insider's View* 2017
➔ *CPT Assistant* Dec 97:5, Mar 08:4, Jan 10:8, Aug 13:3

(The same individual may not report 93313 in conjunction with 93355)

93314   image acquisition, interpretation and report only
➔ *CPT Changes: An Insider's View* 2017
➔ *CPT Assistant* Dec 97:5, Jan 00:10, Jan 10:8, Aug 13:3
➔ *Clinical Examples in Radiology* Spring 22:15

(Do not report 93314 in conjunction with 93355)

93315   Transesophageal echocardiography for congenital cardiac anomalies; including probe placement, image acquisition, interpretation and report
➔ *CPT Changes: An Insider's View* 2017
➔ *CPT Assistant* Nov 97:44, Dec 97:5, Jan 10:8, Aug 13:3, Dec 13:15, Jul 14:9, Apr 22:14
➔ *Clinical Examples in Radiology* Spring 22:15

(Do not report 93315 in conjunction with 93355)

93316   placement of transesophageal probe only

➔ *CPT Changes: An Insider's View* 2017

➔ *CPT Assistant* Nov 97:44, Dec 97:5, Jan 10:8, Aug 13:3, Apr 22:14

(Do not report 93316 in conjunction with 93355)

Transesophageal Echocardiography (TEE)
93312-93318

An endoscopic ultrasound transducer is passed through the mouth into the esophagus and 2-dimensional images are obtained from the posterior aspect of the heart.

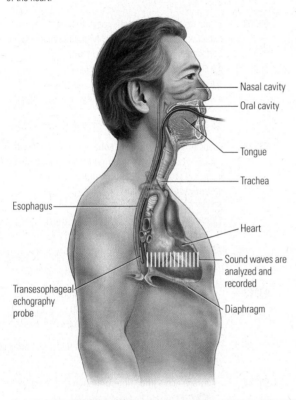

Nasal cavity
Oral cavity
Tongue
Trachea
Esophagus
Heart
Sound waves are analyzed and recorded
Transesophageal echography probe
Diaphragm

93317   image acquisition, interpretation and report only

➔ *CPT Changes: An Insider's View* 2017

➔ *CPT Assistant* Nov 97:44, Dec 97:5, Jan 10:8, Aug 13:3, Dec 13:15, Apr 22:14

➔ *Clinical Examples in Radiology* Spring 22:15

(Do not report 93317 in conjunction with 93355)

#+ 93319   3D echocardiographic imaging and postprocessing during transesophageal echocardiography, or during transthoracic echocardiography for congenital cardiac anomalies, for the assessment of cardiac structure(s) (eg, cardiac chambers and valves, left atrial appendage, interatrial septum, interventricular septum) and function, when performed (List separately in addition to code for echocardiographic imaging)

➔ *CPT Changes: An Insider's View* 2022

(Use 93319 in conjunction with 93303, 93304, 93312, 93314, 93315, 93317)

(Do not report 93319 in conjunction with 76376, 76377, 93325, 93355)

93318   Echocardiography, transesophageal (TEE) for monitoring purposes, including probe placement, real time 2-dimensional image acquisition and interpretation leading to ongoing (continuous) assessment of (dynamically changing) cardiac pumping function and to therapeutic measures on an immediate time basis

➔ *CPT Changes: An Insider's View* 2001, 2017

➔ *CPT Assistant* Jan 10:8, Apr 10:6, Aug 13:3

(Do not report 93318 in conjunction with 93355)

93319   Code is out of numerical sequence. See 93316-93321

+ 93320   Doppler echocardiography, pulsed wave and/or continuous wave with spectral display (List separately in addition to codes for echocardiographic imaging); complete

➔ *CPT Assistant* Nov 97:44, Dec 97:5, Aug 13:3, May 20:12

➔ *Clinical Examples in Radiology* Fall 06:9-10

(Use 93320 in conjunction with 93303, 93304, 93312, 93314, 93315, 93317, 93350, 93351)

(Do not report 93320 in conjunction with 93355)

+ 93321   follow-up or limited study (List separately in addition to codes for echocardiographic imaging)

➔ *CPT Assistant* Nov 97:44, Dec 97:5, Jan 10:8, Aug 13:3

➔ *Clinical Examples in Radiology* Fall 06:9-10

(Use 93321 in conjunction with 93303, 93304, 93308, 93312, 93314, 93315, 93317, 93350, 93351)

(Do not report 93321 in conjunction with 93355)

+ 93325   Doppler echocardiography color flow velocity mapping (List separately in addition to codes for echocardiography)

➔ *CPT Assistant* Nov 97:44, Dec 97:5, Aug 13:3, Jul 16:9, May 20:12, Jun 22:22

➔ *Clinical Examples in Radiology* Fall 06:9-10, Fall 21:16, Spring 22:15

(Use 93325 in conjunction with 76825, 76826, 76827, 76828, 93303, 93304, 93308, 93312, 93314, 93315, 93317, 93350, 93351)

(Do not report 93325 in conjunction with 93355)

93350   Echocardiography, transthoracic, real-time with image documentation (2D), includes M-mode recording, when performed, during rest and cardiovascular stress test using treadmill, bicycle exercise and/or pharmacologically induced stress, with interpretation and report;

➔ *CPT Changes: An Insider's View* 2009

➔ *CPT Assistant* Aug 02:11, Jan 10:8, Oct 10:17, Dec 10:17, Aug 13:3, Jul 14:9, Apr 16:9, Jul 20:12

➔ *Clinical Examples in Radiology* Spring 22:15

(Stress testing codes 93016-93018 should be reported, when appropriate, in conjunction with 93350 to capture the cardiovascular stress portion of the study)

(Do not report 93350 in conjunction with 93015)

93351   including performance of continuous electrocardiographic monitoring, with supervision by a physician or other qualified health care professional

➔ *CPT Changes: An Insider's View* 2009, 2013

➔ *CPT Assistant* Jan 10:8, Oct 10:17, Dec 10:17, Aug 13:3, Jul 14:9, Apr 16:9, Jul 20:12

(Do not report 93351 in conjunction with 93015-93018, 93350. Do not report 93351-26 in conjunction with 93016, 93018, 93350-26)

#+ 93356   Myocardial strain imaging using speckle tracking-derived assessment of myocardial mechanics (List separately in addition to codes for echocardiography imaging)

➔ *CPT Changes: An Insider's View* 2020

➔ *CPT Assistant* Apr 20:11, Jul 20:12

(Use 93356 in conjunction with 93303, 93304, 93306, 93307, 93308, 93350, 93351)

(Report 93356 once per session)

+ 93352   Use of echocardiographic contrast agent during stress echocardiography (List separately in addition to code for primary procedure)

➔ *CPT Changes: An Insider's View* 2009

➔ *CPT Assistant* Jan 10:8, Oct 10:17, Dec 10:17, Aug 13:3

(Do not report 93352 more than once per stress echocardiogram)

(Use 93352 in conjunction with 93350, 93351)

93355   Echocardiography, transesophageal (TEE) for guidance of a transcatheter intracardiac or great vessel(s) structural intervention(s) (eg, TAVR, transcatheter pulmonary valve replacement, mitral valve repair, paravalvular regurgitation repair, left atrial appendage occlusion/closure, ventricular septal defect closure) (peri-and intra-procedural), real-time image acquisition and documentation, guidance with quantitative measurements, probe manipulation, interpretation, and report, including diagnostic transesophageal echocardiography and, when performed, administration of ultrasound contrast, Doppler, color flow, and 3D

➔ *CPT Changes: An Insider's View* 2015

(To report placement of transesophageal probe by separate physician, use 93313)

(Do not report 93355 in conjunction with 76376, 76377, 93312, 93313, 93314, 93315, 93316, 93317, 93318, 93320, 93321, 93325)

93356   Code is out of numerical sequence. See 93350-93355

Cardiac Catheterization

Cardiac catheterization is a diagnostic medical procedure which includes introduction, positioning and repositioning, when necessary, of catheter(s), within the vascular system, recording of intracardiac and/or

intravascular pressure(s), and final evaluation and report of procedure. There are two code families for cardiac catheterization: one for congenital heart disease and one for all other conditions. For cardiac catheterization for congenital heart defects (93593, 93594, 93595, 93596, 93597, 93598), see the **Medicine/Cardiovascular/Cardiac Catheterization for Congenital Heart Defects** subsection. The following guidelines apply to cardiac catheterization performed for indications other than the evaluation of congenital heart defects.

Right heart catheterization for indications other than the evaluation of congenital heart defects (93453, 93456, 93457, 93460, 93461): includes catheter placement in one or more right-sided cardiac chamber(s) or structures (ie, the right atrium, right ventricle, pulmonary artery, pulmonary wedge), obtaining blood samples for measurement of blood gases, and cardiac output measurements (Fick or other method), when performed. For placement of a flow directed catheter (eg, Swan-Ganz) performed for hemodynamic monitoring purposes not in conjunction with other catheterization services, use 93503. Do not report 93503 in conjunction with other diagnostic cardiac catheterization codes. Right heart catheterization does not include right ventricular or right atrial angiography (93566).

For right heart catheterization as part of catheterization to evaluate congenital heart defects, see 93593, 93594, 93596, 93597, 93598. For reporting purposes, when the morphologic left ventricle is in a subpulmonic position (eg, certain cases of transposition of the great arteries) due to congenital heart disease, catheter placement with hemodynamic assessment in this structure during right heart catheterization is considered part of that procedure, and does not constitute left heart catheterization. When the subpulmonic ventricle also connects to the aorta (eg, double outlet right ventricle), catheter placement with hemodynamic assessment of this ventricle during right heart catheterization is considered part of that procedure, while catheter placement with hemodynamic assessment of that same ventricle from the arterial approach is considered left heart catheterization. Report the appropriate code for right and left heart catheterization if catheter placement with hemodynamic assessment of the double outlet right ventricle is performed both during the right heart catheterization and separately from the arterial approach. Right heart catheterization for congenital heart defects does not typically involve thermodilution cardiac output assessments. When thermodilution cardiac output is performed in this setting it may be separately reported using 93598.

Left heart catheterization for indications other than congenital heart defects (93452, 93453, 93458, 93459, 93460, 93461): involves catheter placement in a left-sided (systemic) cardiac chamber(s) (left ventricle or left atrium) and includes left ventricular/left atrial angiography, imaging supervision, and interpretation, when performed. For reporting purposes, when the morphologic right ventricle is in a systemic (subaortic) position due to congenital heart disease (eg, certain cases of transposition of the great arteries), catheter placement with hemodynamic assessment of the subaortic ventricle performed during left heart catheterization is considered part of the procedure and does not constitute right heart catheterization. If additional catheterization of right heart structures (eg, atrium, pulmonary artery) is performed at the same setting, report the appropriate code for right and left heart catheterization. When left heart catheterization is performed using either transapical puncture of the left ventricle or transseptal puncture of an intact septum, report 93462 in conjunction with 93452, 93453, 93458, 93459, 93460, 93461, 93596, 93597. For left heart catheterization services for the evaluation of congenital heart defects, see 93565, 93595, 93596, 93597.

Catheter placement and injection procedures: for a listing of the injection procedures included in specific cardiac catheterization procedures, please refer to the table on pages 810-812.

Cardiac catheterization (93451-93461), other than for the evaluation of congenital heart defects, includes: (a) all roadmapping angiography in order to place the catheters; (b) any injections for angiography of the left ventricle, left atrium, native coronary arteries or bypass grafts listed as inherent to the procedure in the cardiac catheterization table located on pages 810-812; and (c) imaging supervision, interpretation, and report. Do not report 93563, 93564, 93565 in conjunction with 93452, 93453, 93454, 93455, 93456, 93457, 93458, 93459, 93460, 93461. The cardiac catheterization codes do not include contrast injection(s) and imaging supervision, interpretation, and report for imaging that is separately identified by other specific procedure code(s).

Catheter placement(s) in coronary artery(ies) involves selective engagement of the origins of the native coronary artery(ies) for the purpose of coronary angiography. Catheter placement(s) in bypass graft(s) (venous, internal mammary, free arterial graft[s]) involves selective engagement of the origins of the graft(s) for the purpose of bypass angiography. Bypass graft angiography is typically performed only in conjunction with coronary angiography of native vessels.

Codes for catheter placement(s) in native coronary arteries (93454-93461), and bypass graft(s) (93455, 93457, 93459, 93461) include intraprocedural injection(s) for coronary/bypass graft angiography, imaging supervision, and interpretation, except when

these catheter placements are performed during cardiac catheterization for the evaluation of congenital heart defects. Do not report 93563-93565 in conjunction with 93452-93461.

For right ventricular or right atrial angiography performed in conjunction with right heart catheterization for noncongenital heart disease (93451, 93453, 93456, 93457, 93460, 93461) or for the evaluation of congenital heart defects (93593, 93594, 93596, 93597), use 93566. For reporting purposes, angiography of the morphologic right ventricle or morphologic right atrium is reported with 93566, whether these structures are in the standard prepulmonic position or in a systemic (subaortic) position. Left heart catheterization performed for noncongenital heart disease (93452, 93453, 93458, 93459, 93460, 93461) includes left ventriculography, when performed. For reporting purposes, angiography of the morphologic left ventricle or morphologic left atrium is reported with 93565, whether these structures are in the standard systemic (subaortic) position or in a prepulmonic position. Do not report 93565 in conjunction with 93452, 93453, 93454, 93455, 93456, 93457, 93458, 93459, 93460, 93461. For cardiac catheterization performed for the evaluation of congenital heart defects, left ventriculography is separately reported with 93565. For cardiac catheterization for both congenital and noncongenital heart defects, supravalvular aortography is reported with 93567. For cardiac catheterization for both congenital and noncongenital heart defects, pulmonary arterial angiography or selective pulmonary venous angiography is reported with the appropriate pulmonary angiography code(s) (93568, 93569, 93573, 93574, 93575) plus the appropriate cardiac catheterization code.

When contrast injection(s) are performed in conjunction with cardiac catheterization for congenital heart disease (93593, 93594, 93595, 93596, 93597), see 93563, 93564, 93565, 93566, 93567, 93568, 93569, 93573, 93574, 93575. Injection procedures 93563, 93564, 93565, 93566, 93567, 93568, 93569, 93573, 93574, 93575 represent separate identifiable services and may be reported in conjunction with one another when appropriate. Codes 93563, 93564, 93565, 93566, 93567, 93568, 93569, 93573, 93574, 93575 include imaging supervision, interpretation, and report.

For angiography of noncoronary and nonpulmonary arteries and veins, performed as a distinct service, use appropriate codes from the Radiology section and the Vascular Injection Procedures subsection in the Surgery/Cardiovascular System section.

For nonselective pulmonary arterial angiography, use 93568. For selective unilateral or bilateral pulmonary arterial angiography, see 93569, 93573. For selective pulmonary venous angiography, use 93574 for each distinct vessel. For selective pulmonary arterial angiography of major aortopulmonary collateral arteries (MAPCAs) arising off the aorta or its systemic branches, use 93575 for each distinct vessel.

Injection procedures 93574, 93575 represent selective venous and arterial angiography, respectively, for each distinct vessel. Codes 93574, 93575 require evaluation of a distinct, named vessel (eg, right upper pulmonary vein, left lower pulmonary vein, left pulmonary artery via Blalock-Taussig [BT] shunt access, major aortopulmonary collateral artery [MAPCA] vessel #1 from underside of aortic arch) and may be reported for each distinct, named vessel evaluated.

Selective pulmonary angiography codes for cardiac catheterization (93569, 93573, 93574, 93575) include selective angiographic catheter positioning, injection, and radiologic supervision and interpretation).

Adjunctive hemodynamic assessments: when cardiac catheterization is combined with pharmacologic agent administration with the specific purpose of repeating hemodynamic measurements to evaluate hemodynamic response, use 93463 in conjunction with 93451-93453 and 93456-93461, 93593, 93594, 93595, 93596, 93597. Do not report 93463 for intracoronary administration of pharmacologic agents during percutaneous coronary interventional procedures, during intracoronary assessment of coronary pressure, flow or resistance, or during intracoronary imaging procedures. Do not report 93463 in conjunction with 92920-92944, 92975, 92977.

When cardiac catheterization is combined with exercise (eg, walking or arm or leg ergometry protocol) with the specific purpose of repeating hemodynamic measurements to evaluate hemodynamic response, report 93464 in conjunction with 93451-93453, 93456-93461, 93593, 93594, 93595, 93596, 93597.

Contrast injection to image the access site(s) for the specific purpose of placing a closure device is inherent to the catheterization procedure and not separately reportable. Closure device placement at the vascular access site is inherent to the catheterization procedure and not separately reportable.

93451 Right heart catheterization including measurement(s) of oxygen saturation and cardiac output, when performed
➜ *CPT Changes: An Insider's View* 2011, 2017, 2020
➜ *CPT Assistant* Aug 11:5, Mar 12:10, May 13:12, Jul 14:3, Sep 15:3, Mar 16:5, Dec 17:16, Dec 18:11, Mar 19:6, Jun 19:3, May 23:1, Mar 24:1

(Do not report 93451 in conjunction with 33289, 93453, 93456, 93457, 93460, 93461, 0613T, 0632T)

(Do not report 93451 in conjunction with 33418, 0345T, 0483T, 0484T, 0544T, 0545T, 0643T, for diagnostic right heart catheterization procedures intrinsic to the valve repair, annulus reconstruction procedure, or left ventricular restoration device implantation)

Right Heart Catheterization
93451

The physician introduces a cardiac catheter into the venous system. The catheter is directed into the right atrium, right ventricle, and pulmonary artery.

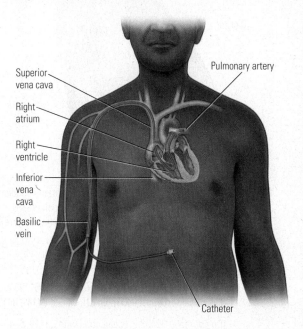

93452 Left heart catheterization including intraprocedural injection(s) for left ventriculography, imaging supervision and interpretation, when performed
➜ *CPT Changes: An Insider's View* 2011, 2017
➜ *CPT Assistant* Aug 11:3, Mar 12:10, Jan 13:6, May 13:12, Sep 15:3, May 23:1

(Do not report 93452 in conjunction with 93453, 93458-93461, 0408T, 0409T, 0410T, 0411T, 0414T, 0415T)

(Do not report 93452 in conjunction with 33418, 0345T, 0483T, 0484T, 0544T, 0545T, 0643T, for diagnostic left heart catheterization procedures intrinsic to the valve repair, annulus reconstruction procedure, or left ventricular restoration device implantation)

Left Heart Catheterization
93452

A catheter is inserted into the arterial system and then into the left ventricle.

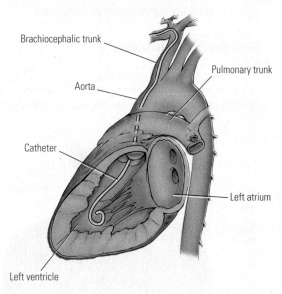

Brachiocephalic trunk
Pulmonary trunk
Aorta
Catheter
Left atrium
Left ventricle

Coronary Angiography Without Concomitant Left Heart Catheterization
93454

Cardiac catheterization procedure performed wherein the catheter does not cross the aortic valve into the left ventricle (left heart catheterization).

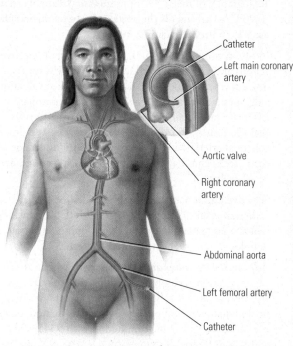

Catheter
Left main coronary artery
Aortic valve
Right coronary artery
Abdominal aorta
Left femoral artery
Catheter

93453 Combined right and left heart catheterization including intraprocedural injection(s) for left ventriculography, imaging supervision and interpretation, when performed

➔ *CPT Changes: An Insider's View* 2011, 2017

➔ *CPT Assistant* Aug 11:3, Mar 12:10, Jan 13:6, May 13:12, Sep 15:3, Mar 16:5, Mar 19:6, Jun 19:3, May 23:1, Mar 24:1

(Do not report 93453 in conjunction with 93451, 93452, 93456-93461, 0408T, 0409T, 0410T, 0411T, 0414T, 0415T)

(Do not report 93453 in conjunction with 33418, 0345T, 0483T, 0484T, 0544T, 0545T, 0643T, for diagnostic left and right heart catheterization procedures intrinsic to the valve repair, annulus reconstruction procedure, or left ventricular restoration device implantation)

93454 Catheter placement in coronary artery(s) for coronary angiography, including intraprocedural injection(s) for coronary angiography, imaging supervision and interpretation;

➔ *CPT Changes: An Insider's View* 2011, 2017

➔ *CPT Assistant* Aug 11:3, Mar 12:10, May 13:12, Dec 14:6, Mar 16:5, Feb 17:15, May 23:1

(Do not report 93454 in conjunction with 33418, 0345T, 0483T, 0484T, 0544T, 0545T, 0643T, for coronary angiography intrinsic to the valve repair, annulus reconstruction procedure, or left ventricular restoration device implantation)

93455 with catheter placement(s) in bypass graft(s) (internal mammary, free arterial, venous grafts) including intraprocedural injection(s) for bypass graft angiography

➔ *CPT Changes: An Insider's View* 2011, 2017

➔ *CPT Assistant* Aug 11:3, Dec 11:9, Mar 12:10, May 13:12, Mar 16:5, May 23:1

(Do not report 93455 in conjunction with 33418, 0345T, 0483T, 0484T, 0544T, 0545T, 0643T, for coronary angiography intrinsic to the valve repair, annulus reconstruction procedure, or left ventricular restoration device implantation)

93456 with right heart catheterization

➔ *CPT Changes: An Insider's View* 2011, 2017, 2020

➔ *CPT Assistant* Aug 11:3, Mar 12:10, May 13:12, Sep 15:3, Mar 16:5, Mar 19:6, Jun 19:3, May 23:1

(Do not report 93456 in conjunction with 33418, 0345T, 0483T, 0484T, 0544T, 0545T, 0643T, for diagnostic coronary angiography or right heart catheterization procedures intrinsic to the valve repair, annulus reconstruction procedure, or left ventricular restoration device implantation)

93457 with catheter placement(s) in bypass graft(s) (internal mammary, free arterial, venous grafts) including intraprocedural injection(s) for bypass graft angiography and right heart catheterization

➔ *CPT Changes: An Insider's View* 2011, 2017

➔ *CPT Assistant* Aug 11:3, Dec 11:9, Mar 12:10, May 13:12, Sep 15:3, Mar 16:5, Mar 19:6, Jun 19:3, May 23:1

(Do not report 93457 in conjunction with 33418, 0345T, 0483T, 0484T, 0544T, 0545T, 0643T, for diagnostic coronary angiography or right heart catheterization procedures intrinsic to the valve repair, annulus reconstruction procedure, or left ventricular restoration device implantation)

93458   with left heart catheterization including intraprocedural injection(s) for left ventriculography, when performed

➔ *CPT Changes: An Insider's View* 2011, 2017

➔ *CPT Assistant* Aug 11:3, Mar 12:10, Jan 13:6, May 13:12, Sep 15:3, Mar 16:5, May 23:1

(Do not report 93458 in conjunction with 33418, 0345T, 0483T, 0484T, 0544T, 0545T, 0643T, for diagnostic coronary angiography or left heart catheterization procedures intrinsic to the valve repair, annulus reconstruction procedure, or left ventricular restoration device implantation)

(Do not report 93458 in conjunction with 0408T, 0409T, 0410T, 0411T, 0414T, 0415T)

93459   with left heart catheterization including intraprocedural injection(s) for left ventriculography, when performed, catheter placement(s) in bypass graft(s) (internal mammary, free arterial, venous grafts) with bypass graft angiography

➔ *CPT Changes: An Insider's View* 2011, 2017

➔ *CPT Assistant* Aug 11:3, Dec 11:11, Mar 12:10, Jan 13:6, May 13:12, Sep 15:3, Mar 16:5, May 23:1

(Do not report 93459 in conjunction with 33418, 0345T, 0483T, 0484T, 0544T, 0545T, 0643T, for diagnostic coronary angiography or left heart catheterization procedures intrinsic to the valve repair, annulus reconstruction procedure, or left ventricular restoration device implantation)

(Do not report 93459 in conjunction with 0408T, 0409T, 0410T, 0411T, 0414T, 0415T)

93460   with right and left heart catheterization including intraprocedural injection(s) for left ventriculography, when performed

➔ *CPT Changes: An Insider's View* 2011, 2017

➔ *CPT Assistant* Aug 11:3, Mar 12:10, Jan 13:6, May 13:12, Sep 15:3, Mar 16:5, Mar 19:6, Jun 19:3, May 23:1

(Do not report 93460 in conjunction with 33418, 0345T, 0483T, 0484T, 0544T, 0545T, 0643T, for diagnostic coronary angiography or left and right heart catheterization procedures intrinsic to the valve repair, annulus reconstruction procedure, or left ventricular restoration device implantation)

(Do not report 93460 in conjunction with 0408T, 0409T, 0410T, 0411T, 0414T, 0415T)

93461   with right and left heart catheterization including intraprocedural injection(s) for left ventriculography, when performed, catheter placement(s) in bypass graft(s) (internal mammary, free arterial, venous grafts) with bypass graft angiography

➔ *CPT Changes: An Insider's View* 2011, 2017

➔ *CPT Assistant* Aug 11:3, Dec 11:9, Mar 12:10, Jan 13:6, May 13:12, Jul 14:3, Dec 14:6, Sep 15:3, Mar 16:5, Mar 19:6, Jun 19:3, May 23:1

(Do not report 93461 in conjunction with 33418, 0345T, 0483T, 0484T, 0544T, 0545T, 0643T, for diagnostic coronary angiography or left and right heart catheterization procedures intrinsic to the valve repair, annulus reconstruction procedure, or left ventricular restoration device implantation)

(Do not report 93461 in conjunction with 0408T, 0409T, 0410T, 0411T, 0414T, 0415T)

+ 93462   Left heart catheterization by transseptal puncture through intact septum or by transapical puncture (List separately in addition to code for primary procedure)

➔ *CPT Changes: An Insider's View* 2011, 2017

➔ *CPT Assistant* Aug 11:3, Mar 12:10, May 13:12, Jun 13:6, Jul 14:3, Sep 15:3, Jul 17:3, Sep 17:3, Nov 20:7

(Use 93462 in conjunction with 33477, 33741, 33745, 93452, 93453, 93458, 93459, 93460, 93461, 93582, 93595, 93596, 93597, 93653, 93654)

(Use 93462 in conjunction with 93590, 93591 for transapical puncture performed for left heart catheterization and percutaneous transcatheter closure of paravalvular leak)

(Use 93462 in conjunction with 93581 for transseptal or transapical puncture performed for percutaneous transcatheter closure of ventricular septal defect)

(Do not report 93462 in conjunction with 93590 for transeptal puncture through intact septum performed for left heart catheterization and percutaneous transcatheter closure of paravalvular leak)

(Do not report 93462 in conjunction with 93656)

(Do not report 93462 in conjunction with 33418, 0345T, 0544T, unless transapical puncture is performed)

+ 93463   Pharmacologic agent administration (eg, inhaled nitric oxide, intravenous infusion of nitroprusside, dobutamine, milrinone, or other agent) including assessing hemodynamic measurements before, during, after and repeat pharmacologic agent administration, when performed (List separately in addition to code for primary procedure)

➔ *CPT Changes: An Insider's View* 2011, 2017

➔ *CPT Assistant* Aug 11:3, Mar 12:10, Dec 14:6

(Use 93463 in conjunction with 33477, 93451-93453, 93456-93461, 93580, 93581, 93582, 93593, 93594, 93595, 93596, 93597)

(Report 93463 only once per catheterization procedure)

(Do not report 93463 for pharmacologic agent administration in conjunction with coronary interventional procedure 92920-92944, 92975, 92977)

+ **93464**   Physiologic exercise study (eg, bicycle or arm ergometry) including assessing hemodynamic measurements before and after (List separately in addition to code for primary procedure)

➜ *CPT Changes: An Insider's View* 2011, 2017
➜ *CPT Assistant* Aug 11:3, Mar 12:10, Jul 14:3

(Use 93464 in conjunction with 33477, 93451-93453, 93456-93461, 93593, 93594, 93595, 93596, 93597)

(Report 93464 only once per catheterization procedure)

(For pharmacologic agent administration, use 93463)

93503   Insertion and placement of flow directed catheter (eg, Swan-Ganz) for monitoring purposes

➜ *CPT Assistant* Winter 91:3, Fall 95:8, Feb 97:5, Apr 98:2, Mar 08:4, Aug 11:3, Dec 11:18, May 23:1

(Do not report 93503 in conjunction with 0632T)

(For subsequent monitoring, use 99418)

93505   Endomyocardial biopsy

➜ *CPT Changes: An Insider's View* 2008, 2017
➜ *CPT Assistant* Apr 98:2, Apr 00:10, Aug 11:3, Dec 17:16

(For radioisotope method of cardiac output, see 78472, 78473, or 78481)

+ **93563**   Injection procedure during cardiac catheterization including imaging supervision, interpretation, and report; for selective coronary angiography during congenital heart catheterization (List separately in addition to code for primary procedure)

➜ *CPT Changes: An Insider's View* 2011, 2017
➜ *CPT Assistant* Aug 11:3, Dec 11:11, Jan 13:6, Dec 14:6, Mar 16:5, Dec 23:47

(Use 93563 in conjunction with 33741, 33745, 93582, 93593, 93594, 93595, 93596, 93597)

+ **93564**   for selective opacification of aortocoronary venous or arterial bypass graft(s) (eg, aortocoronary saphenous vein, free radial artery, or free mammary artery graft) to one or more coronary arteries and in situ arterial conduits (eg, internal mammary), whether native or used for bypass to one or more coronary arteries during congenital heart catheterization, when performed (List separately in addition to code for primary procedure)

➜ *CPT Changes: An Insider's View* 2011, 2017
➜ *CPT Assistant* Aug 11:3, Dec 11:11, Jan 13:6, Dec 14:6, Mar 16:5

(Use 93564 in conjunction with 93582, 93593, 93594, 93595, 93596, 93597)

(Do not report 93563, 93564 in conjunction with 33418, 0345T, 0483T, 0484T, 0544T, 0545T for coronary angiography intrinsic to the valve repair or annulus reconstruction procedure)

+ **93565**   for selective left ventricular or left atrial angiography (List separately in addition to code for primary procedure)

➜ *CPT Changes: An Insider's View* 2011, 2017
➜ *CPT Assistant* Aug 11:3, Dec 11:9, Jan 13:6, Dec 23:47

(Use 93565 in conjunction with 33741, 33745, 93582, 93593, 93594, 93595, 93596, 93597)

(Do not report 93563-93565 in conjunction with 93452-93461)

+ **93566**   for selective right ventricular or right atrial angiography (List separately in addition to code for primary procedure)

➜ *CPT Changes: An Insider's View* 2011, 2017
➜ *CPT Assistant* Aug 11:3, Dec 11:9, Jan 13:6, May 15:3, Mar 16:5, May 16:5, Mar 19:6, Dec 23:47

(Use 93566 in conjunction with 33741, 33745, 93451, 93453, 93456, 93457, 93460, 93461, 93582, 93593, 93594, 93595, 93596, 93597)

(Do not report 93566 in conjunction with 33274, 0795T, 0796T, 0797T, 0801T, 0802T, 0803T, 0823T, 0824T, 0825T, for right ventriculography performed during leadless pacemaker insertion)

(Do not report 93566 in conjunction with 0545T for right ventricular or right atrial angiography procedures intrinsic to the annulus reconstruction procedure)

+ **93567**   for supravalvular aortography (List separately in addition to code for primary procedure)

➜ *CPT Changes: An Insider's View* 2011, 2017
➜ *CPT Assistant* Aug 11:3, Dec 11:9, Jan 13:6, Mar 16:5, Dec 23:47

(Use 93567 in conjunction with 33741, 33745, 93451-93461, 93593, 93594, 93595, 93596, 93597)

(For non-supravalvular thoracic aortography or abdominal aortography performed at the time of cardiac catheterization, use the appropriate radiological supervision and interpretation codes [36221, 75600-75630])

+ **93568**   for nonselective pulmonary arterial angiography (List separately in addition to code for primary procedure)

➜ *CPT Changes: An Insider's View* 2011, 2017, 2023
➜ *CPT Assistant* Aug 11:3, Dec 11:9, Jan 13:6, Mar 16:5, Jun 19:3, May 23:1, Dec 23:47, Feb 24:31

(Use 93568 in conjunction with 33361, 33362, 33363, 33364, 33365, 33366, 33418, 33419, 33477, 33741, 33745, 33894, 33895, 33900, 33901, 33902, 33903, 33904, 37187, 37188, 37236, 37237, 37238, 37246, 37248, 92997, 92998, 93451, 93453, 93456, 93457, 93460, 93461, 93580, 93581, 93582, 93583, 93593, 93594, 93595, 93596, 93597)

(Do not report 93568 in conjunction with 0632T)

(For selective unilateral or bilateral pulmonary arterial angiography, use 93569, 93573, which include catheter placement, injection, and radiologic supervision and interpretation)

+ 93569   for selective pulmonary arterial angiography, unilateral (List separately in addition to code for primary procedure)
> CPT Changes: An Insider's View 2023
> CPT Assistant May 23:1, Dec 23:47, Feb 24:31

#+ 93573   for selective pulmonary arterial angiography, bilateral (List separately in addition to code for primary procedure)
> CPT Changes: An Insider's View 2023
> CPT Assistant May 23:1, Dec 23:47, Feb 24:31

(Use 93569, 93573 in conjunction with 33361, 33362, 33363, 33364, 33365, 33366, 33418, 33419, 33477, 33741, 33745, 37236, 37237, 37238, 37246, 37248, 33894, 33895, 33900, 33901, 33902, 33903, 33904, 37187, 37188, 92997, 92998, 93451, 93453, 93456, 93457, 93460, 93461, 93505, 93580, 93581, 93582, 93583, 93593, 93594, 93595, 93596, 93597)

#+ 93574   for selective pulmonary venous angiography of each distinct pulmonary vein during cardiac catheterization (List separately in addition to code for primary procedure)
> CPT Changes: An Insider's View 2023
> CPT Assistant May 23:1, Dec 23:47, Feb 24:31

(Use 93574 in conjunction with 33361, 33362, 33363, 33364, 33365, 33366, 33418, 33419, 33477, 33741, 33745, 37236, 37237, 37238, 37246, 37248, 33894, 33895, 33900, 33901, 33902, 33903, 33904, 37187, 37188, 92997, 92998, 93451, 93453, 93456, 93457, 93460, 93461, 93505, 93580, 93581, 93582, 93583, 93593, 93594, 93595, 93596, 93597)

#+ 93575   for selective pulmonary angiography of major aortopulmonary collateral arteries (MAPCAs) arising off the aorta or its systemic branches, during cardiac catheterization for congenital heart defects, each distinct vessel (List separately in addition to code for primary procedure)
> CPT Changes: An Insider's View 2023
> CPT Assistant May 23:1, Dec 23:47, Feb 24:31

(Use 93575 in conjunction with 33361, 33362, 33363, 33364, 33365, 33366, 33418, 33419, 33477, 33741, 33745, 37236, 37237, 37238, 37246, 37248, 33894, 33895, 33900, 33901, 33902, 33903, 33904, 37187, 37188, 92997, 92998, 93451, 93453, 93456, 93457, 93460, 93461, 93505, 93580, 93581, 93582, 93583, 93593, 93594, 93595, 93596, 93597)

(93569, 93573, 93574, 93575 include the selective introduction and positioning of the angiographic catheter, injection, and radiologic supervision and interpretation)

+ 93571   Intravascular Doppler velocity and/or pressure derived coronary flow reserve measurement (coronary vessel or graft) during coronary angiography including pharmacologically induced stress; initial vessel (List separately in addition to code for primary procedure)
> CPT Changes: An Insider's View 2017
> CPT Assistant Nov 98:33, Apr 00:2, Mar 08:4, Aug 11:3, Dec 14:6, May 15:10, Dec 15:17, Mar 24:29

▶(Use 93571 in conjunction with 92920, 92924, 92928, 92933, 92937, 92941, 92943, 92975, 93454-93461, 93563, 93564, 93593, 93594, 93595, 93596, 93597, 0913T)◀

(Do not report 93571 in conjunction with 0523T)

Intravascular Distal Blood Flow Velocity
93571

A Doppler guidewire is positioned in a proximal coronary artery with the transducer beam parallel to blood flow to measure blood flow velocity.

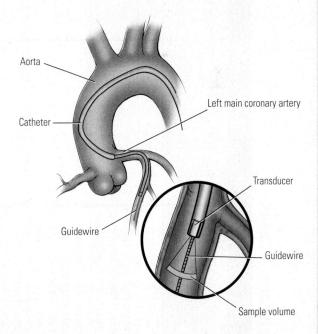

Cardiac Catheterization Codes

CPT Code	Code Descriptor	Catheter Placement Type				Add-on Procedures (Can Be Reported Separately)					
		RHC	LHC	Coronary Artery Placement	Bypass Graft(s)	With Transseptal or Transapical Puncture 93462	With Pharmacological Study 93463	With Exercise Study 93464	Injection Procedure for Selective Right Ventricular or Right Atrial Angiography 93566	Injection Procedure for Supravalvular Aortography 93567	Injection Procedure for Pulmonary Angiography 93568
93451	Right heart catheterization including measurement(s) of oxygen saturation and cardiac output, when performed	X					X	X	X		X
93452	Left heart catheterization including intraprocedural injection(s) for left ventriculography, imaging supervision and interpretation, when performed		X			X	X	X		X	
93453	Combined right and left heart catheterization including intraprocedural injection(s) for left ventriculography, imaging supervision and interpretation, when performed	X	X			X	X	X	X	X	X
93454	Catheter placement in coronary artery(s) for coronary angiography, including intraprocedural injection(s) for coronary angiography, imaging supervision and interpretation;			X						X	
93455	Catheter placement in coronary artery(s) for coronary angiography, including intraprocedural injection(s) for coronary angiography, imaging supervision and interpretation; with catheter placement(s) in bypass graft(s), (internal mammary, free arterial, venous grafts) including intraprocedural injection(s) for bypass graft angiography			X	X					X	

★=Telemedicine ◀=Audio-only ✛=Add-on code ✗=FDA approval pending #=Resequenced code ⊘=Modifier 51 exempt ➲➲➲=See p xxi for details

Cardiac Catheterization Codes, *continued*

CPT Code	Code Descriptor	Catheter Placement Type				Add-on Procedures (Can Be Reported Separately)					
		RHC	LHC	Coronary Artery Placement	Bypass Graft(s)	With Transseptal or Transapical Puncture 93462	With Pharmacological Study 93463	With Exercise Study 93464	Injection Procedure for Selective Right Ventricular or Right Atrial Angiography 93566	Injection Procedure for Supravalvular Aortography 93567	Injection Procedure for Pulmonary Angiography 93568
93456	Catheter placement in coronary artery(s) for coronary angiography, including intraprocedural injection(s) for coronary angiography, imaging supervision and interpretation; with right heart catheterization	X		X			X	X	X	X	X
93457	Catheter placement in coronary artery(s) for coronary angiography, including intraprocedural injection(s) for coronary angiography, imaging supervision and interpretation; with catheter placement(s) in bypass graft(s) (internal mammary, free arterial, venous grafts) including intraprocedural injection(s) for bypass graft angiography and right heart catheterization	X		X	X		X	X	X	X	X
93458	Catheter placement in coronary artery(s) for coronary angiography, including intraprocedural injection(s) for coronary angiography, imaging supervision and interpretation; with left heart catheterization including intraprocedural injection(s) for left ventriculography, when performed		X	X		X	X	X		X	

▲ = Revised code ● = New code ►◄ = Contains new or revised text ✂ = Duplicate PLA test ↕ = Category I PLA   American Medical Association **811**

Medicine / Cardiovascular 92950-93399

Copying, photographing, or sharing this CPT® book violates AMA's copyright.

Medicine / Cardiovascular   92950-93799

Cardiac Catheterization Codes, *continued*

CPT Code	Code Descriptor	Catheter Placement Type				Add-on Procedures (Can Be Reported Separately)					
		RHC	LHC	Coronary Artery Placement	Bypass Graft(s)	With Transseptal or Transapical Puncture 93462	With Pharmacological Study 93463	With Exercise Study 93464	Injection Procedure for Selective Right Ventricular or Right Atrial Angiography 93566	Injection Procedure for Supravalvular Aortography 93567	Injection Procedure for Pulmonary Angiography 93568
93459	Catheter placement in coronary artery(s) for coronary angiography, including intraprocedural injection(s) for coronary angiography, imaging supervision and interpretation; with left heart catheterization including intraprocedural injection(s) for left ventriculography, when performed, catheter placement(s) in bypass graft(s) (internal mammary, free arterial, venous grafts) with bypass graft angiography		X	X	X	X	X	X		X	
93460	Catheter placement in coronary artery(s) for coronary angiography, including intraprocedural injection(s) for coronary angiography, imaging supervision and interpretation; with right and left heart catheterization including intraprocedural injection(s) for left ventriculography, when performed	X	X	X		X	X	X	X	X	X
93461	Catheter placement in coronary artery(s) for coronary angiography, including intraprocedural injection(s) for coronary angiography, imaging supervision and interpretation; with right and left heart catheterization including intraprocedural injection(s) for left ventriculography, when performed, catheter placement(s) in bypass graft(s) (internal mammary, free arterial, venous grafts) with bypass graft angiography	X	X	X	X	X	X	X	X	X	X

★=Telemedicine   ◀=Audio-only   +=Add-on code   ⚡=FDA approval pending   #=Resequenced code   ⊘=Modifier 51 exempt   ➔➔➔=See p xxi for details

+ 93572   each additional vessel (List separately in addition to code for primary procedure)

⮕ *CPT Changes: An Insider's View* 2017

⮕ *CPT Assistant* Nov 98:34, Apr 00:2, Aug 11:5, Dec 14:6, May 15:10, Dec 15:17

(Use 93572 in conjunction with 93571)

(Do not report 93572 in conjunction with 0523T)

(Intravascular distal coronary blood flow velocity measurements include all Doppler transducer manipulations and repositioning within the specific vessel being examined, during coronary angiography or therapeutic intervention [eg, angioplasty])

(For unlisted cardiac catheterization procedure, use 93799)

93573   Code is out of numerical sequence. See 93567-93572

93574   Code is out of numerical sequence. See 93567-93572

93575   Code is out of numerical sequence. See 93567-93572

Repair of Structural Heart Defect

93580   Percutaneous transcatheter closure of congenital interatrial communication (ie, Fontan fenestration, atrial septal defect) with implant

⮕ *CPT Changes: An Insider's View* 2003

⮕ *CPT Assistant* Mar 03:23

(Percutaneous transcatheter closure of atrial septal defect includes a right heart catheterization procedure. Code 93580 includes injection of contrast for atrial and ventricular angiograms. Codes 93451-93453, 93456, 93457, 93458, 93459, 93460, 93461, 93565, 93566, 93593, 93594, 93595, 93596, 93597, 93598 should not be reported separately in addition to 93580)

(For other cardiac angiographic procedures performed at the time of transcatheter atrial septal defect closure, see 93563, 93564, 93567, 93568, as appropriate)

93581   Percutaneous transcatheter closure of a congenital ventricular septal defect with implant

⮕ *CPT Changes: An Insider's View* 2003

⮕ *CPT Assistant* Mar 03:23, Mar 08:4, May 23:1

(Percutaneous transcatheter closure of ventricular septal defect includes a right heart catheterization procedure. Code 93581 includes injection of contrast for atrial and ventricular angiograms. Codes 93451-93453, 93456, 93457, 93458, 93459, 93460, 93461, 93565, 93566, 93593, 93594, 93595, 93596, 93597, 93598 should not be reported separately in addition to 93581)

(For other cardiac angiographic procedures performed at the time of transcatheter closure of ventricular septal defect, see 93563, 93564, 93567, 93568, as appropriate)

(For echocardiographic services performed in addition to 93580, 93581, see 93303-93317, 93662 as appropriate)

93582   Percutaneous transcatheter closure of patent ductus arteriosus

⮕ *CPT Changes: An Insider's View* 2014, 2017

⮕ *CPT Assistant* Jul 14:3

(93582 includes congenital right and left heart catheterization, catheter placement in the aorta, and aortic arch angiography, when performed)

(Do not report 93582 in conjunction with 36013, 36014, 36200, 75600, 75605, 93451, 93453, 93456, 93457, 93458, 93459, 93460, 93461, 93567, 93593, 93594, 93595, 93596, 93597, 93598)

(For other cardiac angiographic procedures performed at the time of transcatheter PDA closure, see 93563, 93564, 93565, 93566, 93568, 93569, 93573, 93574, 93575 as appropriate)

(For repair of patent ductus arteriosus by ligation, see 33820, 33822, 33824)

(For intracardiac echocardiographic services performed at the time of transcatheter PDA closure, use 93662. Other echocardiographic services provided by a separate individual are reported using the appropriate echocardiography service codes, 93315, 93316, 93317)

93583   Percutaneous transcatheter septal reduction therapy (eg, alcohol septal ablation) including temporary pacemaker insertion when performed

⮕ *CPT Changes: An Insider's View* 2014, 2017

(93583 includes insertion of temporary pacemaker, when performed, and left heart catheterization)

(Do not report 93583 in conjunction with 33210, 93452, 93453, 93458, 93459, 93460, 93461, 93565, 93595, 93596, 93597)

(93583 includes left anterior descending coronary angiography for the purpose of roadmapping to guide the intervention. Do not report 93454, 93455, 93456, 93457, 93458, 93459, 93460, 93461, 93563 for coronary angiography performed during alcohol septal ablation for the purpose of roadmapping, guidance of the intervention, vessel measurement, and completion angiography)

(Diagnostic cardiac catheterization procedures may be separately reportable when no prior catheter-based diagnostic study of the treatment zone is available, the prior diagnostic study is inadequate, or the patient's condition with respect to the clinical indication has changed since the prior study or during the intervention. Use the appropriate codes from 93451, 93454, 93455, 93456, 93457, 93563, 93564, 93566, 93567, 93568, 93593, 93594, 93598, 93569, 93573, 93574, 93575)

Medicine / Cardiovascular   92950-93799

Copying, photographing, or sharing this CPT® book violates AMA's copyright.

(Do not report 93583 in conjunction with 33210, 33211)

(Do not report 93463 for the injection of alcohol for this procedure)

(For intracardiac echocardiographic services performed at the time of alcohol septal ablation, use 93662)

(Other echocardiographic services provided by a separate physician are reported using the appropriate echocardiography services codes, 93312, 93313, 93314, 93315, 93316, 93317)

(For surgical ventriculomyotomy [-myectomy] for idiopathic hypertrophic subaortic stenosis, use 33416)

93584 Code is out of numerical sequence. See 93596-93598

93585 Code is out of numerical sequence. See 93596-93598

93586 Code is out of numerical sequence. See 93596-93598

93587 Code is out of numerical sequence. See 93596-93598

93588 Code is out of numerical sequence. See 93596-93598

Transcatheter Closure of Paravalvular Leak

Codes 93590, 93591, 93592 are used to report transcatheter closure of paravalvular leak (PVL). Codes 93590 and 93591 include, when performed, percutaneous access, placing the access sheath(s), advancing the delivery system to the paravalvular leak, positioning the closure device, repositioning the closure device as needed, and deploying the device.

Codes 93590 and 93591 include, when performed, fluoroscopy (76000), angiography, radiological supervision and interpretation services performed to guide the PVL closure (eg, guiding the device placement and documenting completion of the intervention).

Code 93590 includes transseptal puncture and left heart catheterization/left ventriculography (93452, 93453, 93458, 93459, 93460, 93461, 93565, 93595, 93596, 93597), when performed. Transapical left heart catheterization (93462) may be reported separately, when performed.

Code 93591 includes, when performed, supravalvular aortography (93567), left heart catheterization/left ventriculography (93452, 93453, 93458, 93459, 93460, 93461, 93565, 93595, 93596, 93597). Transapical left heart catheterization (93462) may be reported separately, when performed.

Diagnostic right heart catheterization codes (93451, 93456, 93457, 93593, 93594, 93598) and diagnostic coronary angiography codes (93454, 93455, 93456, 93457, 93563, 93564) may be reported with 93590, 93591, representing separate and distinct services from PVL closure, if:

1. No prior study is available and a full diagnostic study is performed, or

2. A prior study is available, but as documented in the medical record:

   a. There is inadequate visualization of the anatomy and/or pathology, or

   b. The patient's condition with respect to the clinical indication has changed since the prior study, or

   c. There is a clinical change during the procedure that requires new evaluation.

Other cardiac catheterization services may be reported separately, when performed for diagnostic purposes not intrinsic to PVL closure.

For same session/same day diagnostic cardiac catheterization services, report the appropriate diagnostic cardiac catheterization code(s) appended with modifier 59 indicating separate and distinct procedural service from PVL closure.

93590 Percutaneous transcatheter closure of paravalvular leak; initial occlusion device, mitral valve

➲ *CPT Changes: An Insider's View* 2017

➲ *CPT Assistant* Sep 17:3

(Do not report 93590 in conjunction with 93462 for transseptal puncture)

(For transapical puncture performed in conjunction with 93590, use 93462)

93591 initial occlusion device, aortic valve

➲ *CPT Changes: An Insider's View* 2017

➲ *CPT Assistant* Sep 17:3

(For transseptal or transapical puncture performed in conjunction with 93591, use 93462)

+ 93592 each additional occlusion device (List separately in addition to code for primary procedure)

➲ *CPT Changes: An Insider's View* 2017

➲ *CPT Assistant* Sep 17:3

(Use 93592 in conjunction with 93590, 93591)

Cardiac Catheterization for Congenital Heart Defects

Cardiac catheterization for the evaluation of congenital heart defect(s) is reported with 93593, 93594, 93595, 93596, 93597, 93598. Cardiac catheterization services for anomalous coronary arteries arising from the aorta or off of other coronary arteries, patent foramen ovale, mitral valve prolapse, and bicuspid aortic valve, in the absence of other congenital heart defects, are reported with 93451-93464, 93566, 93567, 93568. However, when these conditions exist in conjunction with other congenital heart defects, 93593, 93594, 93595, 93596, 93597 may be reported. Evaluation of anomalous coronary arteries arising from the pulmonary arterial system is reported with the cardiac catheterization for congenital heart defects codes.

For additional guidance on reporting cardiac catheterization services for congenital heart defects versus non-congenital indications, see Cardiac Catheterization guidelines.

Right heart catheterization for congenital heart defects (93593, 93594, 93596, 93597): includes catheter placement in one or more right-sided cardiac chamber(s) or structures (ie, the right atrium, right ventricle, pulmonary artery, pulmonary wedge), obtaining blood samples for measurement of blood gases, and Fick cardiac output measurements, when performed. While the morphologic right atrium and morphologic right ventricle are typically the right heart structures supplying blood flow to the pulmonary artery, in congenital heart disease the subpulmonic ventricle may be a morphologic left ventricle and the subpulmonic atrium may be a morphologic left atrium. For reporting purposes, when the morphologic left ventricle or left atrium is in a subpulmonic position due to congenital heart disease, catheter placement in either of these structures is considered part of right heart catheterization and does not constitute left heart catheterization. Right heart catheterization for congenital cardiac anomalies does not typically involve thermodilution cardiac output assessments. When thermodilution cardiac output is performed in this setting, it may be separately reported using add-on code 93598. Right heart catheterization does not include right ventricular or right atrial angiography. When right ventricular or right atrial angiography is performed, use 93566. For reporting purposes, angiography of the morphologic right ventricle or morphologic right atrium is reported with 93566, whether these structures are in the standard pre-pulmonic position or in a systemic (subaortic) position. For placement of a flow directed catheter (eg, Swan-Ganz) performed for hemodynamic monitoring purposes not in conjunction with other catheterization services, use 93503. Do not report 93503 in conjunction with 93453, 93456, 93457, 93460, 93461, 93593, 93594, 93595, 93596, 93597.

Right heart catheterization for congenital heart defects may be performed in patients with normal or abnormal connections. The terms *normal* and *abnormal* native connections are used to define the variations in the anatomic connections from the great veins to the atria, atria to the ventricles, and ventricles to the great arteries. This designation as normal or abnormal is used to determine the appropriate code to report right heart catheterization services in congenital heart disease.

Normal native connections exist when the pathway of blood flow follows the expected course through the right and left heart chambers and great vessels (ie, superior vena cava [SVC]/inferior vena cava [IVC] to right atrium, then right ventricle, then pulmonary arteries for the right heart; left atrium to left ventricle, then aorta for the left heart). Examples of congenital heart defects with normal connections would include acyanotic defects such as isolated atrial septal defect, ventricular septal defect, or patent ductus arteriosus. Services including right heart catheterization for congenital cardiac anomalies with normal connections are reported with 93593, 93596.

Abnormal native connections exist when there are alternative connections for the pathway of blood flow through the heart and great vessels. Abnormal connections are typically present in patients with cyanotic congenital heart defects, any variation of single ventricle anatomy (eg, hypoplastic right or left heart, double outlet right ventricle), unbalanced atrioventricular canal (endocardial cushion) defect, transposition of the great arteries, valvular atresia, tetralogy of Fallot with or without major aortopulmonary collateral arteries (MAPCAs), total anomalous pulmonary veins, truncus arteriosus, and any lesions with heterotaxia and/or dextrocardia. Examples of right heart catheterization through abnormal connections include accessing the pulmonary arteries via surgical shunts, accessing the pulmonary circulation from the aorta via MAPCAs, or accessing isolated pulmonary arteries through a patent ductus arteriosus. Other examples would include right heart catheterization through cavopulmonary anastomoses, Fontan conduits, atrial switch conduits (Mustard/Senning), or any variations of single ventricle anatomy/physiology. Services including right heart catheterization for congenital heart defects with abnormal connections are reported with 93594, 93597.

Left heart catheterization for congenital heart defects (93595, 93596, 93597): involves catheter placement in a left-sided (systemic) cardiac chamber(s) (ventricle or atrium). The systemic chambers channel oxygenated blood to the aorta. In normal physiology, the systemic chambers include the morphologic left atrium and left ventricle. In congenital heart disease, the systemic chambers may include a morphologic right atrium or morphologic right ventricle which is connected to the aorta due to transposition or other congenital anomaly. These may be termed *subaortic* chambers. For the purposes of reporting, the term left ventricle or left atrium is meant to describe the systemic (subaortic) ventricle or atrium. When left heart catheterization is performed using either transapical puncture of the left ventricle or transseptal puncture of an intact septum, report 93462 in conjunction with 93595, 93596, 93597. Left heart catheterization for congenital heart defects does not include left ventricular/left atrial angiography when performed. Left ventriculography or left atrial angiography performed during cardiac catheterization for congenital heart defects is separately reported with 93565. For reporting purposes, angiography of the morphologic left ventricle or morphologic left atrium is reported with 93565, whether these structures are in the standard systemic (subaortic) position or in a pre-pulmonic position. For left heart catheterization only, in patients with congenital heart defects, with either normal or abnormal connections, use 93595. When combined left and right heart catheterization is performed to evaluate congenital heart defects, use 93596 for normal native connections, or 93597 for abnormal native connections.

Catheter placement and injection procedures: The work of imaging guidance, including fluoroscopy and ultrasound guidance for vascular access and to guide catheter placement for hemodynamic evaluation, is included in the cardiac catheterization for congenital heart defects codes, when performed by the same operator.

For cardiac catheterization for congenital heart defects, injection procedures are separately reportable due to the marked variability in the cardiovascular anatomy encountered.

When contrast injection(s) is performed in conjunction with cardiac catheterization for congenital heart defects, see injection procedure codes 93563, 93564, 93565, 93566, 93567, 93568, 93569, 93573, 93574, 93575, 93584, 93585, 93586, 93587, 93588, or use appropriate codes from the Radiology section and the Vascular Injection Procedures subsection in the Surgery/Cardiovascular System section. For venography of the IVC, report 75825. For venography of the SVC, report 75827. Venography of an anomalous or persistent SVC (93584), the azygous/hemiazygous venous system (93585), the coronary sinus (93586), or venovenous collaterals (93587, 93588) requires catheter placement(s) distinct from that required for congenital right and left heart catheterization. Therefore, 93584, 93585, 93586, 93587, 93588 include catheter placement in addition to

venography. Codes 93563, 93564, 93565, 93566, 93567, 93568, 93569, 93573, 93574, 93575, 93584, 93585, 93586, 93587, 93588 include imaging supervision, interpretation, and report.

Injection procedures 93563, 93564, 93565, 93566, 93567, 93568, 93569, 93573, 93574, 93575, 93584, 93585, 93586, 93587, 93588 represent separate, identifiable services and may be reported in conjunction with one another, when appropriate. For angiography of other noncoronary and nonpulmonary arteries and veins, performed as a distinct service, use appropriate codes from the Radiology section and the Vascular Injection Procedures subsection in the Surgery/Cardiovascular System section.

Venography: Catheter placement in a normal SVC and a normal IVC is considered as part of a standard congenital cardiac catheterization. When venography of the normal IVC is performed, report 75825. When venography of the normal SVC is performed, report 75827. For coding purposes, the term "anomalous/persistent left or right SVC" refers to a second SVC on the opposite side of the chest from the first SVC. For example, in a typical cardiac anatomy, the SVC is on the right side and a persistent left SVC would be on the left side. In situs inversus, the SVC would typically be located on the left side of the chest and a persistent right SVC would be on the right side. In heterotaxy, bilateral SVCs are common. In these scenarios, venography of the first SVC would be reported with 75827, and catheter placement and venography of the persistent/anomalous SVC would be reported with 93584.

Selective catheter placement in anomalous congenital venous structures is not included in a standard congenital cardiac catheterization. Therefore, add-on codes 93584, 93585, 93586, 93587, 93588 include selective catheter placement in the specific venous structure(s) being imaged as well as venography and radiologic supervision, interpretation, and report.

Angiography of the native coronary arteries or bypass grafts during cardiac catheterization for congenital heart defects is reported with 93563, 93564. Catheter placement(s) in coronary artery(ies) or bypass grafts involves selective engagement of the origins of the native coronary artery(ies) or bypass grafts for the purpose of coronary angiography.

> (Selective pulmonary angiography codes for cardiac catheterization [93569, 93573, 93574, 93575] include selective catheter positioning of the angiographic catheter, injection, and radiologic supervision and interpretation)

93593   Right heart catheterization for congenital heart defect(s) including imaging guidance by the proceduralist to advance the catheter to the target zone; normal native connections
➔ *CPT Changes: An Insider's View* 2022
➔ *CPT Assistant* Apr 22:14, Apr 24:1

93594   abnormal native connections
➔ *CPT Changes: An Insider's View* 2022
➔ *CPT Assistant* Apr 22:14, Apr 24:1

93595   Left heart catheterization for congenital heart defect(s) including imaging guidance by the proceduralist to advance the catheter to the target zone, normal or abnormal native connections
➔ *CPT Changes: An Insider's View* 2022

93596   Right and left heart catheterization for congenital heart defect(s) including imaging guidance by the proceduralist to advance the catheter to the target zone(s); normal native connections
➔ *CPT Changes: An Insider's View* 2022
➔ *CPT Assistant* Apr 22:14, Apr 24:1

93597   abnormal native connections
➔ *CPT Changes: An Insider's View* 2022
➔ *CPT Assistant* Apr 22:14, Apr 24:1

#+ 93584   Venography for congenital heart defect(s), including catheter placement, and radiological supervision and interpretation; anomalous or persistent superior vena cava when it exists as a second contralateral superior vena cava, with native drainage to heart (List separately in addition to code for primary procedure)
➔ *CPT Changes: An Insider's View* 2024
➔ *CPT Assistant* Apr 24:1

(Use 93584 in conjunction with 93593, 93594, 93596, 93597)

(Report 93584 once per session)

#+ 93585   azygos/hemiazygos venous system (List separately in addition to code for primary procedure)
➔ *CPT Changes: An Insider's View* 2024
➔ *CPT Assistant* Apr 24:1

(Use 93585 in conjunction with 93593, 93594, 93596, 93597)

(Report 93585 once per session)

#+ 93586   coronary sinus (List separately in addition to code for primary procedure)
➔ *CPT Changes: An Insider's View* 2024
➔ *CPT Assistant* Apr 24:1

(Use 93586 in conjunction with 93593, 93594, 93596, 93597)

(Report 93586 once per session)

#+ 93587   venovenous collaterals originating at or above the heart (eg, from innominate vein) (List separately in addition to code for primary procedure)
➔ *CPT Changes: An Insider's View* 2024
➔ *CPT Assistant* Apr 24:1

(Use 93587 in conjunction with 93593, 93594, 93596, 93597)

(Report 93587 once per session)

#+ 93588   venovenous collaterals originating below the heart (eg, from the inferior vena cava) (List separately in addition to code for primary procedure)
➔ *CPT Changes: An Insider's View* 2024
➔ *CPT Assistant* Apr 24:1

(Use 93588 in conjunction with 93593, 93594, 93596, 93597)

(Report 93588 once per session)

+ 93598   Cardiac output measurement(s), thermodilution or other indicator dilution method, performed during cardiac catheterization for the evaluation of congenital heart defects (List separately in addition to code for primary procedure)
➔ *CPT Changes: An Insider's View* 2022
➔ *CPT Assistant* Jan 22:3, Apr 22:14, Jun 22:19, Dec 22:10, May 23:1

(Use 93598 in conjunction with 93593, 93594, 93595, 93596, 93597)

(Do not report 93598 in conjunction with 93451-93461)

(For pharmacologic agent administration during cardiac catheterization for congenital heart defect[s], use 93463)

(For physiological exercise study with cardiac catheterization for congenital heart defect[s], use 93464)

(For indicator dilution studies such as thermodilution for cardiac output measurement during cardiac catheterization for congenital heart defect[s], use 93598)

(For contrast injections during cardiac catheterization for congenital heart defect[s], see 75825, 75827, 93563, 93564, 93565, 93566, 93567, 93568, 93569, 93573, 93574, 93575, 93584, 93585, 93586, 93587, 93588)

(For angiography or venography not described in the 90000 series code section, see appropriate codes from the Radiology section and the Vascular Injection Procedures subsection in the Surgery/Cardiovascular System section)

(For transseptal or transapical access of the left atrium during cardiac catheterization for congenital heart defect[s], use 93462 in conjunction with 93595, 93596, 93597, as appropriate)

Intracardiac Electrophysiological Procedures/Studies

Intracardiac electrophysiologic studies (EPS) are invasive diagnostic medical procedures which include the insertion and repositioning of electrode catheters, recording of electrograms before and during pacing, programmed stimulation of multiple locations in the heart, analysis of recorded information, and report of the procedure. In many circumstances, patients with arrhythmias are evaluated and treated at the same encounter. In this situation, a diagnostic *electrophysiologic study* is performed, induced tachycardia(s) are *mapped*, and on the basis of the diagnostic and mapping information, the tissue is *ablated*.

Definitions

Arrhythmia Induction: In most electrophysiologic studies, an attempt is made to induce arrhythmia(s) from single or multiple sites within the heart. Arrhythmia induction may be achieved by multiple techniques, eg, by performing pacing at different rates or programmed stimulation (introduction of critically timed electrical impulses). Because arrhythmia induction occurs via the same catheter(s) inserted for the electrophysiologic study(ies), catheter insertion and temporary pacemaker codes are not additionally reported. Codes 93600-93603, 93610, 93612, and 93618 are used to describe unusual situations where there may be recording, pacing, or an attempt at arrhythmia induction from only one site in the heart. Code 93619 describes only evaluation of the sinus node, atrioventricular node, and His-Purkinje conduction system, without arrhythmia induction. Codes 93620-93624, 93640-93642, 93653, 93654, and 93656 all include recording, pacing, and attempted arrhythmia induction from one or more site(s) in the heart.

Mapping: When a tachycardia is induced, the site of tachycardia origination or its electrical path through the heart is often defined by mapping. Mapping creates a multidimensional depiction of a tachycardia by recording multiple electrograms obtained sequentially or simultaneously from multiple catheter sites in the heart. Depending upon the technique, certain types of mapping catheters may be repositioned from point-to-point within the heart, allowing sequential recording from the various sites to construct maps. Other types of mapping catheters allow mapping without a point-to-point technique by allowing simultaneous recording from many electrodes on the same catheter and computer-assisted three-dimensional reconstruction of the tachycardia activation sequence.

Mapping is a distinct procedure performed in addition to a diagnostic electrophysiologic study or ablation procedure and may be separately reported using 93609 or 93613. Do not report standard mapping (93609) in addition to 3-dimensional mapping (93613).

▶*Ablation:* Once the part of the heart involved in the tachycardia is localized, the tachycardia may be treated by ablation to the area to selectively destroy cardiac tissue. Ablation procedures (93653-93657) are performed at the same session as electrophysiology studies and therefore represent a combined code descriptor. When reporting ablation therapy codes (93653-93657), the single site electrophysiology studies (93600-93603, 93610, 93612, 93618) and the comprehensive electrophysiology studies (93619, 93620) may not be reported separately. Code 93622 may be reported separately with 93653 and 93656. Code 93623 may be reported separately with 93653, 93654, and 93656. However, 93621 for left atrial pacing and recording from coronary sinus or left atrium should not be reported in conjunction with 93656, as this procedure is a component of 93656. Codes 93653 and 93654 include right ventricular pacing and recording and His bundle recording when clinically indicated. When performance of one or more components is not possible or indicated, document the reason for not performing. Code 93656 includes each of left atrial pacing/recording, right ventricular pacing/recording, and His bundle recording when clinically indicated. When performance of one or more components is not possible or indicated, document the reason for not performing.◄

The differences in the techniques involved for ablation of supraventricular arrhythmias, ventricular arrhythmias, and atrial fibrillation are reflected within the descriptions for 93653-93657. Code 93653 is a primary code for catheter ablation for treatment of supraventricular tachycardia caused by dual atrioventricular nodal pathways, accessory atrioventricular connections, or other atrial foci. Code 93654 describes catheter ablation for treatment of ventricular tachycardia or focus of ventricular ectopy. Code 93656 is a primary code for reporting treatment of atrial fibrillation by ablation to achieve complete pulmonary vein electrical isolation. Codes 93653, 93654, and 93656 are distinct primary procedure codes and may not be reported together.

Codes 93655 and 93657 are add-on codes listed in addition to the primary ablation code to report ablation of sites distinct from the primary ablation site. After ablation of the primary target site, post-ablation electrophysiologic evaluation is performed as part of those ablation services (93653, 93654, 93656) and additional mechanisms of tachycardia may be identified. For example, if the primary tachycardia ablated was atrioventricular nodal reentrant tachycardia and during post-ablation testing an atrial tachycardia, atrial flutter, or accessory pathway with orthodromic reentry tachycardia was identified, this would be considered a separate mechanism of tachycardia. Pacing maneuvers are performed to define the mechanism(s) of the new tachycardia(s). Catheter ablation of this distinct mechanism of tachycardia is then performed at the newly discovered atrial or ventricular origin. Appropriate post-ablation attempts at re-induction and observation are again performed. Code 93655 is listed in conjunction with 93653 when repeat ablation is for treatment of an additional supraventricular tachycardia mechanism and with 93654 when the repeat ablation is for treatment of an additional ventricular tachycardia mechanism. Code 93655 may be reported with 93656 when an additional non-atrial fibrillation tachycardia is separately diagnosed after pulmonary vein isolation. Code 93657 is reported in conjunction with 93656 when successful pulmonary vein isolation is achieved, attempts at re-induction of atrial fibrillation identify an additional left or right atrial focus for atrial fibrillation, and further ablation of this new focus is performed.

In certain circumstances, depending on the chamber of origin, a catheter or catheters may be maneuvered into the left ventricle to facilitate arrhythmia diagnosis. This may be accomplished via a retrograde aortic approach by means of the arterial access or through a transseptal puncture. For ablation treatment of supraventricular tachycardia (93653) and ventricular tachycardia (93654), the left heart catheterization by transseptal puncture through intact septum (93462) may be reported separately as an add-on code. However, for ablation treatment of atrial fibrillation (93656), the transseptal puncture (93462) is a standard component of the procedure and may not be reported separately. Do not report 93462 in conjunction with 93656.

Modifier 51 should not be appended to 93600-93603, 93610, 93612, 93615-93618.

⊘ **93600** Bundle of His recording
> *CPT Assistant* Summer 94:12, Aug 97:9, Apr 04:9, Jul 04:13, Aug 05:13, Dec 07:16, Mar 08:4, Jun 13:6, Jul 13:7, Apr 14:3

(Do not report 93600 in conjunction with 93619, 93620, 93653, 93654, 93656)

⊘ **93602** Intra-atrial recording
> *CPT Assistant* Summer 94:12, Aug 97:9, Apr 04:9, Jul 04:13, Aug 05:13, Jun 13:6, Jul 13:7, Apr 14:3

(Do not report 93602 in conjunction with 93619, 93620, 93653, 93654, 93656)

⊘ **93603** Right ventricular recording
> *CPT Assistant* Summer 94:12, Aug 97:9, Apr 04:9, Jul 04:13, Aug 05:13, Jun 13:6, Jul 13:7, Apr 14:3

(Do not report 93603 in conjunction with 93619, 93620, 93653, 93654, 93656)

+ **93609** Intraventricular and/or intra-atrial mapping of tachycardia site(s) with catheter manipulation to record from multiple sites to identify origin of tachycardia (List separately in addition to code for primary procedure)
> *CPT Changes: An Insider's View* 2002, 2017
> *CPT Assistant* Summer 94:12, Aug 97:9, Apr 04:9, Aug 05:13, Jun 13:6, Jul 13:7, Apr 14:3, May 23:18, Oct 23:23

(Use 93609 in conjunction with 93620, 93653, 93656)

(Do not report 93609 in conjunction with 93613, 93654)

⊘ **93610** Intra-atrial pacing
> *CPT Assistant* Summer 94:12, Aug 97:9, Apr 04:9, Jul 04:13, Jun 13:6, Jul 13:7, Apr 14:3

(Do not report 93610 in conjunction with 93619, 93620, 93653, 93654, 93656)

⊘ **93612** Intraventricular pacing
> *CPT Assistant* Summer 94:12, Aug 97:9, Apr 04:9, Jul 04:13, Jun 13:6, Jul 13:7, Apr 14:3

(Do not report 93612 in conjunction with 93619, 93620, 93621, 93622, 93653, 93654, 93656)

+ **93613** Intracardiac electrophysiologic 3-dimensional mapping (List separately in addition to code for primary procedure)
> *CPT Changes: An Insider's View* 2002, 2017
> *CPT Assistant* Apr 04:8, Aug 05:13, Jun 13:6, Jul 13:7, Apr 14:3, Dec 21:12, Oct 23:23

(Use 93613 in conjunction with 93620)

(Do not report 93613 in conjunction with 93609, 93654)

(For noninvasive arrhythmia localization and mapping, use 0745T)

⊘ **93615** Esophageal recording of atrial electrogram with or without ventricular electrogram(s);
> *CPT Changes: An Insider's View* 2017
> *CPT Assistant* Summer 94:12, Aug 97:9, Apr 04:9, Aug 05:13, Apr 14:3

⊘ **93616**   with pacing
> *CPT Changes: An Insider's View* 2017
> *CPT Assistant* Summer 94:12, Aug 97:9, Apr 04:9, Aug 05:13, Apr 14:3

⊘ **93618** Induction of arrhythmia by electrical pacing
> *CPT Changes: An Insider's View* 2017
> *CPT Assistant* Summer 94:12, Aug 97:9, Oct 97:10, Apr 99:10, Jun 00:5, Nov 00:9, Apr 04:9, Jul 04:13, Aug 05:13, Dec 07:16, Jun 13:6, Jul 13:7, Apr 14:3

(Do not report 93618 in conjunction with 93619, 93620, 93621, 93622, 93653, 93654, 93656)

(For intracardiac phonocardiogram, use 93799)

93619 Comprehensive electrophysiologic evaluation with right atrial pacing and recording, right ventricular pacing and recording, His bundle recording, including insertion and repositioning of multiple electrode catheters, without induction or attempted induction of arrhythmia

➔ *CPT Changes: An Insider's View* 2002, 2008, 2017

➔ *CPT Assistant* Aug 97:9, Oct 97:10, Nov 00:9, Apr 04:9, Jul 04:13, Aug 05:13, Dec 07:16, Nov 12:6, Jun 13:6, Jul 13:7, Apr 14:3, May 23:18

(Do not report 93619 in conjunction with 93600, 93602, 93603, 93610, 93612, 93618, 93620, 93621, 93622, 93653, 93654, 93655, 93656, 93657)

93620 Comprehensive electrophysiologic evaluation including insertion and repositioning of multiple electrode catheters with induction or attempted induction of arrhythmia; with right atrial pacing and recording, right ventricular pacing and recording, His bundle recording

➔ *CPT Changes: An Insider's View* 2002, 2003, 2008, 2017

➔ *CPT Assistant* Summer 94:12, Aug 97:9, Oct 97:10, Jul 98:10, Aug 98:7, Nov 00:9, Apr 04:9, Jul 04:13, Aug 05:13, Dec 07:16, Oct 08:10, Nov 12:6, Jun 13:6, Jul 13:7, Apr 14:3, May 23:18, Oct 23:23

(Do not report 93620 in conjunction with 93600, 93602, 93603, 93610, 93612, 93618, 93619, 93653, 93654, 93655, 93656, 93657)

+ 93621 with left atrial pacing and recording from coronary sinus or left atrium (List separately in addition to code for primary procedure)

➔ *CPT Changes: An Insider's View* 2002, 2017

➔ *CPT Assistant* Summer 94:12, Aug 97:9, Oct 97:10, Jul 98:10, Aug 98:7, Nov 98:34, Nov 00:9, Apr 04:9, Jul 04:13, Aug 05:13, Dec 07:16, Oct 08:10, Nov 12:6, Jun 13:6, Jul 13:7, Apr 14:3, Dec 21:12, May 23:18

(Use 93621 in conjunction with 93620)

(Do not report 93621 in conjunction with 93656)

+ 93622 with left ventricular pacing and recording (List separately in addition to code for primary procedure)

➔ *CPT Changes: An Insider's View* 2002, 2017

➔ *CPT Assistant* Summer 94:14, Aug 97:9, Oct 97:10, Jul 98:10, Aug 98:7, Nov 98:34, Nov 00:9, Apr 04:9, Jul 04:13, Aug 05:13, Dec 07:16, Mar 08:4, Nov 12:6, Jun 13:6, Jul 13:7, Apr 14:3, May 23:18

(Use 93622 in conjunction with 93620, 93653, 93656)

(Do not report 93622 in conjunction with 93654)

(For noninvasive arrhythmia localization and mapping, use 0745T)

+ 93623 Programmed stimulation and pacing after intravenous drug infusion (List separately in addition to code for primary procedure)

➔ *CPT Assistant* Summer 94:14, Aug 97:9, Nov 00:9, Aug 05:13, Dec 07:16, Oct 08:10, Apr 14:3

(Use 93623 in conjunction with 93610, 93612, 93619, 93620, 93653, 93654, 93656)

(Do not report 93623 more than once per day)

93624 Electrophysiologic follow-up study with pacing and recording to test effectiveness of therapy, including induction or attempted induction of arrhythmia

➔ *CPT Changes: An Insider's View* 2008, 2017

➔ *CPT Assistant* Summer 94:14, Aug 97:9, Nov 00:9, Aug 05:13, Dec 07:16

93631 Intra-operative epicardial and endocardial pacing and mapping to localize the site of tachycardia or zone of slow conduction for surgical correction

➔ *CPT Assistant* Summer 94:14, Aug 97:9, Nov 00:9, Aug 05:13, Dec 07:16

(For operative ablation of an arrhythmogenic focus or pathway by a separate individual, see 33250-33261)

93640 Electrophysiologic evaluation of single or dual chamber pacing cardioverter-defibrillator leads including defibrillation threshold evaluation (induction of arrhythmia, evaluation of sensing and pacing for arrhythmia termination) at time of initial implantation or replacement;

➔ *CPT Changes: An Insider's View* 2000, 2008, 2017

➔ *CPT Assistant* Summer 94:14, Aug 97:9, Apr 99:10, Nov 99:50, Nov 00:9, Aug 05:13, Jun 12:3

93641 with testing of single or dual chamber pacing cardioverter-defibrillator pulse generator

➔ *CPT Changes: An Insider's View* 2000, 2008, 2017

➔ *CPT Assistant* Summer 94:14, Aug 97:9, Apr 99:10, Nov 99:50, Jun 00:5, Jul 00:5, Nov 00:9, Aug 05:13, Jun 12:3, Apr 14:3

(For subsequent or periodic electronic analysis and/or reprogramming of single or dual chamber pacing cardioverter-defibrillators, see 93282, 93283, 93289, 93292, 93295, 93642)

93642 Electrophysiologic evaluation of single or dual chamber transvenous pacing cardioverter-defibrillator (includes defibrillation threshold evaluation, induction of arrhythmia, evaluation of sensing and pacing for arrhythmia termination, and programming or reprogramming of sensing or therapeutic parameters)

➔ *CPT Changes: An Insider's View* 2000, 2008, 2015, 2017

➔ *CPT Assistant* Summer 94:14, Aug 97:9, Nov 99:50, Jun 00:5, Nov 00:9, Aug 05:13, Jun 13:6, Jul 13:7, Apr 14:3, Dec 21:12

93644 Electrophysiologic evaluation of subcutaneous implantable defibrillator (includes defibrillation threshold evaluation, induction of arrhythmia, evaluation of sensing for arrhythmia termination, and programming or reprogramming of sensing or therapeutic parameters)

➔ *CPT Changes: An Insider's View* 2015, 2017

(Do not report 93644 in conjunction with 33270 at the time of subcutaneous implantable defibrillator device insertion)

(For subsequent or periodic electrophysiologic evaluation of a subcutaneous implantable defibrillator device, see 93260, 93261)

(For electrophysiological evaluation of subcutaneous implantable defibrillator system, with substernal electrode, use 0577T)

93650   Intracardiac catheter ablation of atrioventricular node function, atrioventricular conduction for creation of complete heart block, with or without temporary pacemaker placement

➡ *CPT Changes: An Insider's View* 2008, 2017

➡ *CPT Assistant* Summer 94:15, Aug 97:9, Nov 00:9, Aug 05:13, Apr 12:18, May 12:15

93653   Comprehensive electrophysiologic evaluation with insertion and repositioning of multiple electrode catheters, induction or attempted induction of an arrhythmia with right atrial pacing and recording and catheter ablation of arrhythmogenic focus, including intracardiac electrophysiologic 3-dimensional mapping, right ventricular pacing and recording, left atrial pacing and recording from coronary sinus or left atrium, and His bundle recording, when performed; with treatment of supraventricular tachycardia by ablation of fast or slow atrioventricular pathway, accessory atrioventricular connection, cavo-tricuspid isthmus or other single atrial focus or source of atrial re-entry

➡ *CPT Changes: An Insider's View* 2013, 2014, 2017, 2022

➡ *CPT Assistant* Jun 13:6, Jul 13:7, Apr 14:3, Dec 21:12, Oct 23:23

(Do not report 93653 in conjunction with 93600, 93602, 93603, 93610, 93612, 93613, 93618, 93619,93620, 93621, 93654, 93656)

93654   with treatment of ventricular tachycardia or focus of ventricular ectopy including left ventricular pacing and recording, when performed

➡ *CPT Changes: An Insider's View* 2013, 2014, 2017, 2022

➡ *CPT Assistant* Jun 13:6, Jul 13:7, Apr 14:3, Dec 21:12

(Do not report 93654 in conjunction with 93279, 93280, 93281, 93282, 93283, 93284, 93286, 93287, 93288, 93289, 93600, 93602, 93603, 93609, 93610, 93612, 93613, 93618, 93619, 93620, 93621, 93622, 93653, 93656)

+ 93655   Intracardiac catheter ablation of a discrete mechanism of arrhythmia which is distinct from the primary ablated mechanism, including repeat diagnostic maneuvers, to treat a spontaneous or induced arrhythmia (List separately in addition to code for primary procedure)

➡ *CPT Changes: An Insider's View* 2013, 2017

➡ *CPT Assistant* Jun 13:6, Jul 13:7

(Use 93655 in conjunction with 93653, 93654, 93656)

▲ **93656**   Comprehensive electrophysiologic evaluation with transseptal catheterizations, insertion and repositioning of multiple electrode catheters, induction or attempted induction of an arrhythmia including left or right atrial pacing/recording, and intracardiac catheter ablation of atrial fibrillation by pulmonary vein isolation, including intracardiac electrophysiologic 3-dimensional mapping, intracardiac echocardiography with imaging supervision and interpretation, right ventricular pacing/recording, and His bundle recording, when performed

➡ *CPT Changes: An Insider's View* 2013, 2014, 2017, 2022, 2025

➡ *CPT Assistant* Jun 13:6, Jul 13:7, Apr 14:3, Sep 19:10, Nov 20:13, Dec 21:12, Sep 22:20, Oct 23:23

(Do not report 93656 in conjunction with 93279, 93280, 93281, 93282, 93283, 93284, 93286, 93287, 93288, 93289, 93462, 93600, 93602, 93603, 93610, 93612, 93613, 93618, 93619, 93620, 93621, 93653, 93654, 93662)

+ 93657   Additional linear or focal intracardiac catheter ablation of the left or right atrium for treatment of atrial fibrillation remaining after completion of pulmonary vein isolation (List separately in addition to code for primary procedure)

➡ *CPT Changes: An Insider's View* 2013, 2017

➡ *CPT Assistant* Jun 13:6, Jul 13:7, Apr 14:3, Sep 19:10, Nov 20:13, Dec 21:19

(Use 93657 in conjunction with 93656)

93660   Evaluation of cardiovascular function with tilt table evaluation, with continuous ECG monitoring and intermittent blood pressure monitoring, with or without pharmacological intervention

➡ *CPT Changes: An Insider's View* 2008

➡ *CPT Assistant* Nov 12:6

(For testing of autonomic nervous system function, see 95921, 95924)

+ 93662   Intracardiac echocardiography during therapeutic/diagnostic intervention, including imaging supervision and interpretation (List separately in addition to code for primary procedure)

➡ *CPT Changes: An Insider's View* 2001

➡ *CPT Assistant* Mar 03:23, Dec 21:12, Sep 22:20

(Use 93662 in conjunction with 33274, 33275, 33340, 33361, 33362, 33363, 33364, 33365, 33366, 33418, 33477, 33741, 33745, 92986, 92987, 92990, 92997, 93451, 93452, 93453, 93454, 93455, 93456, 93457, 93458, 93459, 93460, 93461, 93505, 93580, 93581, 93582, 93583, 93590, 93591, 93593, 93594, 93595, 93596, 93597, 93620, 93653, 93654, 0345T, 0483T, 0484T, 0543T, 0544T, 0545T, 0795T, 0796T, 0797T, 0798T, 0799T, 0800T, 0801T, 0802T, 0803T, 0823T, 0824T, 0825T, as appropriate)

(Do not report 93662 in conjunction with 92961, 0569T, 0570T, 0613T)

Peripheral Arterial Disease Rehabilitation

Peripheral arterial disease (PAD) rehabilitative physical exercise consists of a series of sessions, lasting 45-60 minutes per session, involving use of either a motorized treadmill or a track to permit each patient to achieve symptom-limited claudication. Each session is supervised by an exercise physiologist or nurse. The supervising provider monitors the individual patient's claudication threshold and other cardiovascular limitations for adjustment of workload. During this supervised rehabilitation program, the development of new arrhythmias, symptoms that might suggest angina or the continued inability of the patient to progress to an adequate level of exercise may require review and examination of the patient by a physician or other qualified health care professional. These services would be separately reported with an appropriate level E/M service code, including office or other outpatient services (99202-99215), initial hospital inpatient or observation care (99221-99223), subsequent hospital inpatient or observation care (99231-99233), critical care services (99291-99292).

93668 Peripheral arterial disease (PAD) rehabilitation, per session
> ➔ *CPT Changes: An Insider's View* 2001

Noninvasive Physiologic Studies and Procedures

(For arterial cannulization and recording of direct arterial pressure, use 36620)

(For radiographic injection procedures, see 36000-36299)

(For vascular cannulization for hemodialysis, see 36800-36821)

(For chemotherapy for malignant disease, see 96409-96549)

(For penile plethysmography, use 54240)

93701 Bioimpedance-derived physiologic cardiovascular analysis
> ➔ *CPT Changes: An Insider's View* 2002, 2010
> ➔ *CPT Assistant* Mar 02:3, Mar 08:4

(For bioelectrical impedance analysis whole body composition, use 0358T. For left ventricular filling pressure indirect measurement by computerized calibration of the arterial waveform response to Valsalva, use 93799)

93702 Bioimpedance spectroscopy (BIS), extracellular fluid analysis for lymphedema assessment(s)
> ➔ *CPT Changes: An Insider's View* 2015

(For bioelectrical impedance analysis whole body composition, use 0358T)

(For bioimpedance-derived physiological cardiovascular analysis, use 93701)

93724 Electronic analysis of antitachycardia pacemaker system (includes electrocardiographic recording, programming of device, induction and termination of tachycardia via implanted pacemaker, and interpretation of recordings)
> ➔ *CPT Assistant* Summer 94:23

93740 Temperature gradient studies

93745 Initial set-up and programming by a physician or other qualified health care professional of wearable cardioverter-defibrillator includes initial programming of system, establishing baseline electronic ECG, transmission of data to data repository, patient instruction in wearing system and patient reporting of problems or events
> ➔ *CPT Changes: An Insider's View* 2005, 2013

(Do not report 93745 in conjunction with 93282, 93292)

93750 Interrogation of ventricular assist device (VAD), in person, with physician or other qualified health care professional analysis of device parameters (eg, drivelines, alarms, power surges), review of device function (eg, flow and volume status, septum status, recovery), with programming, if performed, and report
> ➔ *CPT Changes: An Insider's View* 2010, 2013
> ➔ *CPT Assistant* Apr 10:6, Dec 18:11

(Do not report 93750 in conjunction with 33975, 33976, 33979, 33981-33983)

93770 Determination of venous pressure

(For central venous cannulization see 36555-36556, 36500)

93784 Ambulatory blood pressure monitoring, utilizing report-generating software, automated, worn continuously for 24 hours or longer; including recording, scanning analysis, interpretation and report
> ➔ *CPT Changes: An Insider's View* 2020
> ➔ *CPT Assistant* Apr 20:5

93786 recording only
> ➔ *CPT Changes: An Insider's View* 2020
> ➔ *CPT Assistant* Apr 20:5

93788 scanning analysis with report
> ➔ *CPT Changes: An Insider's View* 2020
> ➔ *CPT Assistant* Apr 20:5

93790 review with interpretation and report
> ➔ *CPT Changes: An Insider's View* 2013, 2020
> ➔ *CPT Assistant* Apr 20:5

(For self-measured blood pressure monitoring, see 99473, 99474)

★ =Telemedicine ◀ =Audio-only ✛=Add-on code ✗=FDA approval pending #=Resequenced code ⊘=Modifier 51 exempt ➔➔➔=See p xxi for details

Elements of Cardiac Ablation Codes

Procedure/Services Included with Ablations	SVT Ablation (93653)			VT Ablation (93654)			AF Ablation (93656)		
	Inherent	Bundled	Not bundled; sometimes performed	Inherent	Bundled	Not bundled; sometimes performed	Inherent	Bundled	Not bundled; sometimes performed
Insert/reposition multiple catheters	X			X			X		
Transseptal catheterization(s) (93462)			X			X	X		
Induction or attempted induction of arrhythmia with right atrial pacing and recording	X			X				X	
Intracardiac ablation of arrhythmia	X			X			X		
SVT ablation	X								
VT ablation				X					
AF ablation							X		
Intracardiac 3D mapping (93613)		X			X			X	
Right ventricular pacing and recording		X			X			X	
Left atrial pacing and recording from coronary sinus or left atrium (93621)		X			X			X	
His bundle recording		X			X			X	
Left ventricular pacing and recording					X				
Intracardiac echocardiography (93662)			X			X		X	

Home and Outpatient International Normalized Ratio (INR) Monitoring Services

Home and outpatient international normalized ratio (INR) monitoring services describe the management of warfarin therapy, including ordering, review, and interpretation of new INR test result(s), patient instructions, and dosage adjustments as needed.

If a significantly, separately identifiable evaluation and management (E/M) service is performed on the same day as 93792, the appropriate E/M service may be reported using modifier 25.

Do not report 93793 on the same day as an E/M service.

▶Do not report 93792, 93793 in conjunction with 98012, 98013, 98014, 98015, 98016, 98966, 98967, 98968, 98970, 98971, 98972, 99421, 99422, 99423, when telephone or online digital evaluation and management services address home and outpatient INR monitoring.◀

Do not count time spent in 93792, 93793 in the time of 99439, 99487, 99489, 99490, 99491, when reported in the same calendar month.

93792 Patient/caregiver training for initiation of home international normalized ratio (INR) monitoring under the direction of a physician or other qualified health care professional, face-to-face, including use and care of the INR monitor, obtaining blood sample, instructions for reporting home INR test results, and documentation of patient's/caregiver's ability to perform testing and report results

➔ CPT Changes: An Insider's View 2018

➔ CPT Assistant Mar 18:7

(For provision of test materials and equipment for home INR monitoring, see 99070 or the appropriate supply code)

93793 Anticoagulant management for a patient taking warfarin, must include review and interpretation of a new home, office, or lab international normalized ratio (INR) test result, patient instructions, dosage adjustment (as needed), and scheduling of additional test(s), when performed

➔ CPT Changes: An Insider's View 2018

➔ CPT Assistant Nov 17:11, Mar 18:7, Feb 20:7

(Do not report 93793 in conjunction with 99202, 99203, 99204, 99205, 99211, 99212, 99213, 99214, 99215, 99242, 99243, 99244, 99245)

(Report 93793 no more than once per day, regardless of the number of tests reviewed)

Other Procedures

93797 Physician or other qualified health care professional services for outpatient cardiac rehabilitation; without continuous ECG monitoring (per session)

➔ CPT Changes: An Insider's View 2013

93798 with continuous ECG monitoring (per session)

➔ CPT Changes: An Insider's View 2013

93799 Unlisted cardiovascular service or procedure

➔ CPT Assistant Mar 98:11, Mar 02:10, Nov 05:15, Apr 09:9, Jul 10:10, Oct 11:7, Nov 11:11, Dec 13:18, Aug 18:11, Sep 18:10, Dec 18:11, Nov 20:7, Mar 22:13, Oct 22:19, Mar 24:29

Noninvasive Vascular Diagnostic Studies

Vascular studies include patient care required to perform the studies, supervision of the studies and interpretation of study results with copies for patient records of hard copy output with analysis of all data, including bidirectional vascular flow or imaging when provided.

The use of a simple hand-held or other Doppler device that does not produce hard copy output, or that produces a record that does not permit analysis of bidirectional vascular flow, is considered to be part of the physical examination of the vascular system and is not separately reported. The Ankle-Brachial Index (or ABI) is reportable with 93922 or 93923 as long as simultaneous Doppler recording and analysis of bidirectional blood flow, volume plethysmography, or transcutaneous oxygen tension measurements are also performed.

Duplex scan (eg, 93880, 93882) describes an ultrasonic scanning procedure for characterizing the pattern and direction of blood flow in arteries or veins with the production of real-time images integrating B-mode two-dimensional vascular structure, Doppler spectral analysis, and color flow Doppler imaging.

Physiologic studies Noninvasive physiologic studies are performed using equipment separate and distinct from the duplex ultrasound imager. Codes 93922, 93923, 93924 describe the evaluation of non-imaging physiologic recordings of pressures with Doppler analysis of bi-directional blood flow, plethysmography, and/or oxygen tension measurements appropriate for the anatomic area studied.

Limited studies for lower extremity require either:

(1) ankle/brachial indices at distal posterior tibial and anterior tibial/dorsalis pedis arteries plus bidirectional Doppler waveform recording and analysis at 1-2 levels; or (2) ankle/brachial indices at distal posterior tibial and anterior tibial/dorsalis pedis arteries plus volume plethysmography at 1-2 levels; or (3) ankle/brachial indices at distal posterior tibial and anterior tibial/dorsalis pedis arteries with transcutaneous oxygen tension measurements at 1-2 levels. Potential levels include high thigh, low thigh, calf, ankle, metatarsal and toes.

Limited studies for upper extremity require either:

(1) Doppler-determined systolic pressures and bidirectional Doppler waveform recording and analysis at 1-2 levels; or (2) Doppler-determined systolic pressures and volume plethysmography at 1-2 levels; or (3) Doppler-determined systolic pressures and transcutaneous oxygen tension measurements at 1-2 levels. Potential levels include arm, forearm, wrist, and digits.

Complete studies for lower extremity require either:

(1) ankle/brachial indices at distal posterior tibial and anterior tibial/dorsalis pedis arteries plus bidirectional Doppler waveform recording and analysis at 3 or more levels; or (2) ankle/brachial indices at distal posterior tibial and anterior tibial/dorsalis pedis arteries plus volume plethysmography at 3 or more levels; or (3) ankle/brachial indices at distal posterior tibial and anterior tibial/dorsalis pedis arteries with transcutaneous oxygen tension measurements at 3 or more levels. Alternatively, a complete study may be reported with measurements at a single level if provocative functional maneuvers (eg, measurements with postural provocative tests, or measurements with reactive hyperemia) are performed.

Complete studies for upper extremity require either:

(1) Doppler-determined systolic pressures and bidirectional Doppler waveform recording and analysis at 3 or more levels; or (2) Doppler-determined systolic pressures and volume plethysmography at 3 or more levels; or (3) Doppler-determined systolic pressures and transcutaneous oxygen tension measurements at 3 or more levels. Potential levels include arm, forearm, wrist, and digits. Alternatively, a complete study may be reported with measurements at a single level if provocative functional maneuvers (eg, measurements with postural provocative tests, or measurements with cold stress) are performed.

Cerebrovascular Arterial Studies

A complete transcranial Doppler (TCD) study (93886) includes ultrasound evaluation of the right and left anterior circulation territories and the posterior circulation territory (to include vertebral arteries and basilar artery). In a limited TCD study (93888) there is ultrasound evaluation of two or fewer of these territories. For TCD, ultrasound evaluation is a reasonable and concerted attempt to identify arterial signals through an acoustic window.

▶Use TCD study codes (93886, 93888, 93892, 93893) when a single study is performed. Use 93896, 93897, 93898, when a vasoreactivity study, emboli detection without intravenous microbubble injection, or venous-arterial shunt detection with intravenous microbubble injection is performed in conjunction with a complete TCD on the same day.◀

Code 93895 includes the acquisition and storage of images of the common carotid arteries, carotid bulbs, and internal carotid arteries bilaterally with quantification of intima media thickness (common carotid artery mean and maximal values) and determination of presence of atherosclerotic plaque.

93880   Duplex scan of extracranial arteries; complete bilateral study
- ➡ *CPT Assistant* Jun 96:9, Dec 05:3
- ➡ *Clinical Examples in Radiology* Fall 07:6, Winter 09:2, Winter 13:8, Winter 18:15, Spring 20:12, Summer 20:11, Winter 21:9, Winter 22:3, Summer 22:20, Spring 23:20

(Do not report 93880 in conjunction with 93895)

93882   unilateral or limited study
- ➡ *CPT Assistant* Jun 96:9, Dec 05:3, Dec 22:17
- ➡ *Clinical Examples in Radiology* Fall 07:6, Winter 09:2, Winter 13:8, Winter 18:15, Winter 22:3, Summer 22:20, Spring 23:20

(Do not report 93882 in conjunction with 93895)

93886   Transcranial Doppler study of the intracranial arteries; complete study
- ➡ *CPT Assistant* Jun 96:9, Dec 05:3
- ➡ *Clinical Examples in Radiology* Winter 18:15, Fall 22:19, Spring 23:20

93888   limited study
- ➡ *CPT Assistant* Jun 96:9, Dec 05:3
- ➡ *Clinical Examples in Radiology* Winter 18:15, Fall 22:19, Spring 23:20

▶(Do not report 93888 in conjunction with 93886, 93892, 93893, 93896, 93897, 93898)◀

▶(93890 has been deleted. To report vasoreactivity study, use 93896)◀

93892   emboli detection without intravenous microbubble injection
- ➡ *CPT Changes: An Insider's View* 2005
- ➡ *CPT Assistant* Dec 05:3
- ➡ *Clinical Examples in Radiology* Winter 18:15, Spring 23:20

▲ **93893**   venous-arterial shunt detection with intravenous microbubble injection
- ➡ *CPT Changes: An Insider's View* 2005, 2025
- ➡ *CPT Assistant* Dec 05:3
- ➡ *Clinical Examples in Radiology* Winter 18:15, Spring 23:20

▶(Do not report 93892, 93893 in conjunction with 93886, 93888)◀

\#+● **93896**   Vasoreactivity study performed with transcranial Doppler study of intracranial arteries, complete (List separately in addition to code for primary procedure)
- ➡ *CPT Changes: An Insider's View* 2025

▶(Use 93896 in conjunction with 93886)◀

▶(Do not report 93896 in conjunction with 93888)◀

\#+● **93897**   Emboli detection without intravenous microbubble injection performed with transcranial Doppler study of intracranial arteries, complete (List separately in addition to code for primary procedure)
- ➡ *CPT Changes: An Insider's View* 2025

▶(Use 93897 in conjunction with 93886)◀

▶(Do not report 93897 in conjunction with 93888)◀

\#+● **93898**   Venous-arterial shunt detection with intravenous microbubble injection performed with transcranial Doppler study of intracranial arteries, complete (List separately in addition to code for primary procedure)
- ➡ *CPT Changes: An Insider's View* 2025

▶(Use 93898 in conjunction with 93886)◀

▶(Do not report 93898 in conjunction with 93888)◀

93895   Quantitative carotid intima media thickness and carotid atheroma evaluation, bilateral
- ➡ *CPT Changes: An Insider's View* 2015
- ➡ *Clinical Examples in Radiology* Winter 18:15, Spring 23:20

(Do not report 93895 in conjunction with 93880, 93882)

93896 Code is out of numerical sequence. See 93892-93922

93897 Code is out of numerical sequence. See 93892-93922

93898 Code is out of numerical sequence. See 93892-93922

Extremity Arterial Studies (Including Digits)

93922 Limited bilateral noninvasive physiologic studies of upper or lower extremity arteries, (eg, for lower extremity: ankle/brachial indices at distal posterior tibial and anterior tibial/dorsalis pedis arteries plus bidirectional, Doppler waveform recording and analysis at 1-2 levels, or ankle/brachial indices at distal posterior tibial and anterior tibial/dorsalis pedis arteries plus volume plethysmography at 1-2 levels, or ankle/brachial indices at distal posterior tibial and anterior tibial/dorsalis pedis arteries with, transcutaneous oxygen tension measurement at 1-2 levels)

➲ *CPT Changes: An Insider's View* 2011

➲ *CPT Assistant* Jun 96:9, Dec 05:3, Aug 09:3, Jun 12:16, Jun 13:14, Jan 14:10

➲ *Clinical Examples in Radiology* Spring 11:5-6, Summer 11:11, Winter 18:15, Spring 23:20

(When only 1 arm or leg is available for study, report 93922 with modifier 52 for a unilateral study when recording 1-2 levels. Report 93922 when recording 3 or more levels or performing provocative functional maneuvers)

(Report 93922 only once in the upper extremity(s) and/or once in the lower extremity(s). When both the upper and lower extremities are evaluated in the same setting, 93922 may be reported twice by adding modifier 59 to the second procedure)

(For transcutaneous visible light hyperspectral imaging measurement of oxyhemoglobin, deoxyhemoglobin, and tissue oxygenation, use 0631T)

93923 Complete bilateral noninvasive physiologic studies of upper or lower extremity arteries, 3 or more levels (eg, for lower extremity: ankle/brachial indices at distal posterior tibial and anterior tibial/dorsalis pedis arteries plus segmental blood pressure measurements with bidirectional Doppler waveform recording and analysis, at 3 or more levels, or ankle/brachial indices at distal posterior tibial and anterior tibial/dorsalis pedis arteries plus segmental volume plethysmography at 3 or more levels, or ankle/brachial indices at distal posterior tibial and anterior tibial/dorsalis pedis arteries plus segmental transcutaneous oxygen tension measurements at 3 or more levels), or single level study with provocative functional maneuvers (eg, measurements with postural provocative tests, or measurements with reactive hyperemia)

➲ *CPT Changes: An Insider's View* 2011

➲ *CPT Assistant* Jun 96:9, Jun 01:10, Dec 05:3, Aug 09:3, Jun 12:16, Jan 14:10, Sep 20:15

➲ *Clinical Examples in Radiology* Spring 11:5-6, Summer 11:11, Winter 18:15, Spring 23:20

(When only 1 arm or leg is available for study, report 93922 for a unilateral study when recording 3 or more levels or when performing provocative functional maneuvers)

(Report 93923 only once in the upper extremity(s) and/or once in the lower extremity(s). When both the upper and lower extremities are evaluated in the same setting, 93923 may be reported twice by adding modifier 59 to the second procedure)

(For transcutaneous visible light hyperspectral imaging measurement of oxyhemoglobin, deoxyhemoglobin, and tissue oxygenation, use 0631T)

93924 Noninvasive physiologic studies of lower extremity arteries, at rest and following treadmill stress testing, (ie, bidirectional Doppler waveform or volume plethysmography recording and analysis at rest with ankle/brachial indices immediately after and at timed intervals following performance of a standardized protocol on a motorized treadmill plus recording of time of onset of claudication or other symptoms, maximal walking time, and time to recovery) complete bilateral study

➲ *CPT Changes: An Insider's View* 2011

➲ *CPT Assistant* Jun 96:9, Dec 05:3, Aug 09:3, Jun 12:16, Jan 14:10

➲ *Clinical Examples in Radiology* Spring 11:5-6, Winter 18:15, Spring 23:20

(Do not report 93924 in conjunction with 93922, 93923)

93925 Duplex scan of lower extremity arteries or arterial bypass grafts; complete bilateral study

➲ *CPT Assistant* Jun 96:9, Dec 05:3, Sep 16:9

➲ *Clinical Examples in Radiology* Winter 18:15, Spring 23:20

(Do not report 93925 in conjunction with 93985 for the same extremities)

93926 unilateral or limited study

➲ *CPT Assistant* Jun 96:9, Oct 01:2, Dec 05:3, Sep 16:9

➲ *Clinical Examples in Radiology* Fall 09:4-5, Winter 18:15, Spring 23:20

(Do not report 93926 in conjunction with 93986 for the same extremity)

93930 Duplex scan of upper extremity arteries or arterial bypass grafts; complete bilateral study

➲ *CPT Assistant* Jun 96:9, Dec 05:3, Sep 16:9

➲ *Clinical Examples in Radiology* Winter 18:15, Winter 21:9, Spring 23:20

(Do not report 93930 in conjunction with 93985, 93986 for the same extremity[ies])

93931   unilateral or limited study
> *CPT Assistant* Jun 96:9, Oct 01:2, Dec 05:3, Sep 16:9
> *Clinical Examples in Radiology* Winter 18:15, Winter 21:9, Spring 23:20

(Do not report 93931 in conjunction with 93985, 93986 for the same extremity)

Extremity Venous Studies (Including Digits)

93970   Duplex scan of extremity veins including responses to compression and other maneuvers; complete bilateral study
> *CPT Assistant* Jun 96:9, Dec 05:3, Jan 12:13, Feb 12:11, Oct 14:6, Sep 16:9
> *Clinical Examples in Radiology* Spring 12:8, Spring 17:11, Winter 18:15, Winter 21:9, Spring 23:20

(Do not report 93970 in conjunction with 93985, 93986 for the same extremity[ies])

93971   unilateral or limited study
> *CPT Assistant* Jun 96:9, Oct 01:2, Mar 03:21, Dec 05:3, Jul 10:6, Apr 11:13, Jan 12:13, Feb 12:11, Oct 14:6, Aug 15:8, Sep 16:9
> *Clinical Examples in Radiology* Winter 08:11, Fall 09:4-5, Spring 17:11, Winter 18:15, Winter 21:9, Spring 23:20

(Do not report 93970, 93971 in conjunction with 36475, 36476, 36478, 36479)

(Do not report 93971 in conjunction with 93985, 93986 for the same extremity)

Visceral and Penile Vascular Studies

93975   Duplex scan of arterial inflow and venous outflow of abdominal, pelvic, scrotal contents and/or retroperitoneal organs; complete study
> *CPT Assistant* Apr 96:11, Jun 96:9, Dec 05:3, Jun 14:15, Mar 15:10, Aug 16:10
> *Clinical Examples in Radiology* Winter 08:10, Spring 08:9, Summer 09:12, Summer 12:7, Winter 15:11, Summer 15:10, Winter 18:15, Spring 20:10, Summer 21:5, Fall 22:9-12, Spring 23:20, Fall 23:19

93976   limited study
> *CPT Assistant* Apr 96:11, Jun 96:9, Dec 05:3, Mar 15:10, Aug 16:10
> *Clinical Examples in Radiology* Spring 08:10, Summer 09:12, Summer 12:7, Summer 15:10, Winter 18:15, Spring 20:10, Summer 21:5, Fall 22:9-12, Spring 23:20, Fall 23:19

93978   Duplex scan of aorta, inferior vena cava, iliac vasculature, or bypass grafts; complete study
> *CPT Assistant* Jun 96:9, Dec 05:3
> *Clinical Examples in Radiology* Spring 07:5-6, Spring 17:5, Winter 18:15, Spring 23:18, 20

93979   unilateral or limited study
> *CPT Assistant* Jun 96:9, Dec 05:3, Jun 14:15
> *Clinical Examples in Radiology* Winter 15:11, Spring 17:5, Winter 18:15, Spring 23:18, 20

(For ultrasound screening study for abdominal aortic aneurysm [AAA], real time with image documentation, use 76706)

93980   Duplex scan of arterial inflow and venous outflow of penile vessels; complete study
> *CPT Assistant* Jun 96:9, Dec 05:3
> *Clinical Examples in Radiology* Winter 18:15, Spring 23:20

93981   follow-up or limited study
> *CPT Assistant* Jun 96:9, Dec 05:3
> *Clinical Examples in Radiology* Winter 18:15, Spring 23:20

Extremity Arterial-Venous Studies

A complete extremity duplex scan (93985, 93986) includes evaluation of both arterial inflow and venous outflow for preoperative vessel assessment prior to creation of hemodialysis access. If only an arterial extremity duplex scan is performed, see 93925, 93926, 93930, 93931. If only a venous extremity duplex scan is performed, see 93970, 93971. If a physiologic arterial evaluation of extremities is performed, see 93922, 93923, 93924.

93985   Duplex scan of arterial inflow and venous outflow for preoperative vessel assessment prior to creation of hemodialysis access; complete bilateral study
> *CPT Changes: An Insider's View* 2020
> *CPT Assistant* Oct 19:8
> *Clinical Examples in Radiology* Winter 20:3, Spring 23:20

(Do not report 93985 in conjunction with 93925, 93930, 93970 for the same extremity[ies])

(Do not report 93985 in conjunction with 93990 for the same extremity)

93986   complete unilateral study
> *CPT Changes: An Insider's View* 2020
> *CPT Assistant* Oct 19:8
> *Clinical Examples in Radiology* Winter 20:3, Spring 23:20

(Do not report 93986 in conjunction with 93926, 93931, 93971, 93990 for the same extremity)

93990   Duplex scan of hemodialysis access (including arterial inflow, body of access and venous outflow)
> *CPT Assistant* Jun 96:9, Dec 05:3
> *Clinical Examples in Radiology* Spring 07:5-6, Winter 18:15, Summer 20:11, Winter 21:9, Spring 23:20

(For measurement of hemodialysis access flow using indicator dilution methods, use 90940)

▶(For limited study of body of hemodialysis fistula using computer-aided ultrasound system, use 0876T)◀

Other Noninvasive Vascular Diagnostic Studies

93998   Unlisted noninvasive vascular diagnostic study

     → *CPT Changes: An Insider's View* 2012

     → *CPT Assistant* Sep 12:9, Jan 14:10, Dec 22:17

     → *Clinical Examples in Radiology* Winter 22:3, Summer 22:20

Pulmonary

Ventilator Management

94002   Ventilation assist and management, initiation of pressure or volume preset ventilators for assisted or controlled breathing; hospital inpatient/observation, initial day

     → *CPT Changes: An Insider's View* 2007

     → *CPT Assistant* Feb 07:10, Mar 07:10, Apr 07:3, Jul 07:1, Nov 08:5, May 14:4, Oct 14:9, Aug 19:8, Jan 22:3, Jun 22:19, Dec 22:10

94003   hospital inpatient/observation, each subsequent day

     → *CPT Changes: An Insider's View* 2007

     → *CPT Assistant* Feb 07:10, Apr 07:3, Jul 07:1, Nov 08:5, May 14:4, Aug 19:8, Jan 22:3, Jun 22:19, Dec 22:10

94004   nursing facility, per day

     → *CPT Changes: An Insider's View* 2007

     → *CPT Assistant* Feb 07:10, Apr 07:3, Jul 07:1, Nov 08:5, Aug 19:8, Jan 22:3, Jun 22:19, Dec 22:10

     ►(Do not report 94002-94004 in conjunction with evaluation and management services 98000-98016, 99202-99499)◄

94005   Home ventilator management care plan oversight of a patient (patient not present) in home, domiciliary or rest home (eg, assisted living) requiring review of status, review of laboratories and other studies and revision of orders and respiratory care plan (as appropriate), within a calendar month, 30 minutes or more

     → *CPT Changes: An Insider's View* 2007

     → *CPT Assistant* Mar 07:11, Apr 07:3, Nov 08:5, Oct 14:9

     (Do not report 94005 in conjunction with 99374-99378, 99424, 99425, 99437, 99491)

     (Ventilator management care plan oversight is reported separately from home or domiciliary, rest home [eg, assisted living] services. A physician or other qualified health care professional may report 94005, when performed, including when a different individual reports 99374-99378, 99424, 99425, 99437, 99491, for the same 30 days)

Pulmonary Diagnostic Testing, Rehabilitation, and Therapies

Codes 94010-94799 include laboratory procedure(s) and interpretation of test results. If a separate identifiable evaluation and management service is performed, the appropriate E/M service code, including new or established patient office or other outpatient services (99202-99215), office or other outpatient consultations (99242, 99243, 99244, 99245), emergency department services (99281-99285), nursing facility services (99304-99316), and home or residence services (99341-99350), may be reported in addition to 94010-94799.

Spirometry (94010) measures expiratory airflow and volumes and forms the basis of most pulmonary function testing. When spirometry is performed before and after administration of a bronchodilator, report 94060. Measurement of vital capacity (94150) is a component of spirometry and is only reported when performed alone. The flow-volume loop (94375) is used to identify patterns of inspiratory and/or expiratory obstruction in central or peripheral airways. Spirometry (94010, 94060) includes maximal breathing capacity (94200) and flow-volume loop (94375), when performed.

Measurement of lung volumes may be performed using plethysmography, helium dilution or nitrogen washout. Plethysmography (94726) is utilized to determine total lung capacity, residual volume, functional residual capacity, and airway resistance. Nitrogen washout or helium dilution (94727) may be used to measure lung volumes, distribution of ventilation and closing volume. Oscillometry (94728) assesses airway resistance and may be reported in addition to gas dilution techniques. Spirometry (94010, 94060) and bronchial provocation (94070) are not included in 94726 and 94727 and may be reported separately.

Diffusing capacity (94729) is most commonly performed in conjunction with lung volumes or spirometry and is an add-on code to 94726-94728, 94010, 94060, 94070, and 94375.

Pulmonary function tests (94011-94013) are reported for measurements in infants and young children through 2 years of age.

Pulmonary function testing measurements are reported as actual values and as a percent of predicted values by age, gender, height, and race.

Chest wall manipulation for the mobilization of secretions and improvement in lung function can be performed using manual (94667, 94668) or mechanical (94669) methods. Manual techniques include cupping, percussing, and use of a hand-held vibration device. A mechanical technique is the application of an external vest or wrap that delivers mechanical oscillation.

94010 Spirometry, including graphic record, total and timed vital capacity, expiratory flow rate measurement(s), with or without maximal voluntary ventilation

➲ *CPT Assistant* Summer 91:16, Summer 95:4, Feb 96:9, Mar 96:10, Nov 97:45, Nov 98:35, Jan 99:8, Feb 99:9, Aug 03:15, Jul 05:11, Nov 08:5, Oct 10:15, Dec 10:15, Aug 12:6-7, Nov 12:14, Dec 13:12, Mar 14:11, Sep 15:9, Mar 19:11, Apr 19:11, May 19:10, Dec 20:3

(Do not report 94010 in conjunction with 94150, 94200, 94375, 94728)

94011 Measurement of spirometric forced expiratory flows in an infant or child through 2 years of age

➲ *CPT Changes: An Insider's View* 2010, 2017

➲ *CPT Assistant* May 10:7, Aug 12:6, Dec 13:12

94012 Measurement of spirometric forced expiratory flows, before and after bronchodilator, in an infant or child through 2 years of age

➲ *CPT Changes: An Insider's View* 2010, 2017

➲ *CPT Assistant* May 10:7, Aug 12:6

94013 Measurement of lung volumes (ie, functional residual capacity [FRC], forced vital capacity [FVC], and expiratory reserve volume [ERV]) in an infant or child through 2 years of age

➲ *CPT Changes: An Insider's View* 2010, 2017

➲ *CPT Assistant* May 10:7, Aug 12:6, Dec 13:12

94014 Patient-initiated spirometric recording per 30-day period of time; includes reinforced education, transmission of spirometric tracing, data capture, analysis of transmitted data, periodic recalibration and review and interpretation by a physician or other qualified health care professional

➲ *CPT Changes: An Insider's View* 2000, 2013

➲ *CPT Assistant* Summer 95:4, Nov 98:34, Jan 99:8, Jul 05:11, Nov 08:5, Feb 23:15

94015 recording (includes hook-up, reinforced education, data transmission, data capture, trend analysis, and periodic recalibration)

➲ *CPT Assistant* Summer 95:4, Nov 98:34, Jan 99:8, Jul 05:11, Nov 08:5

94016 review and interpretation only by a physician or other qualified health care professional

➲ *CPT Changes: An Insider's View* 2013

➲ *CPT Assistant* Summer 95:4, Nov 98:34, Jan 99:8, Jul 05:11, Nov 08:5

94060 Bronchodilation responsiveness, spirometry as in 94010, pre- and post-bronchodilator administration

➲ *CPT Changes: An Insider's View* 2005

➲ *CPT Assistant* Summer 95:4, Feb 96:9, Feb 97:10, Nov 98:34, Jan 99:8, Feb 99:9, Jul 05:11, Nov 08:5, Dec 10:15, Aug 12:6-7, Mar 14:11, Sep 15:9, Apr 19:11

(Do not report 94060 in conjunction with 94150, 94200, 94375, 94640, 94728)

(Report bronchodilator supply separately with 99070 or appropriate supply code)

(For exercise test for bronchospasm with pre- and post-spirometry, see 94617, 94619)

94070 Bronchospasm provocation evaluation, multiple spirometric determinations as in 94010, with administered agents (eg, antigen[s], cold air, methacholine)

➲ *CPT Changes: An Insider's View* 2005

➲ *CPT Assistant* Summer 91:16, Summer 95:4, Feb 96:9, Nov 97:45, Jan 99:8, Jul 05:11, Nov 08:5, Aug 12:6, Nov 12:11, Sep 15:9

(Do not report 94070 in conjunction with 94640)

(Report antigen[s] administration separately with 99070 or appropriate supply code)

94150 Vital capacity, total (separate procedure)

➲ *CPT Assistant* Summer 95:4, Feb 96:9, Jul 05:11, Nov 08:5, Dec 10:15, Aug 12:6, Mar 14:11, Sep 18:14

(Do not report 94150 in conjunction with 94010, 94060, 94728. To report thoracic gas volumes, see 94726, 94727)

94200 Maximum breathing capacity, maximal voluntary ventilation

➲ *CPT Assistant* Summer 95:4, Feb 96:9, Aug 03:15, Jul 05:11, Nov 08:5, Dec 10:15, Aug 12:6-7, Mar 14:11

(Do not report 94200 in conjunction with 94010, 94060)

94375 Respiratory flow volume loop

➲ *CPT Assistant* Summer 95:4, Feb 96:9, Oct 03:2, Jul 05:11, Jul 06:4, Jul 07:1, Nov 08:5, Aug 12:6-7, Mar 14:11

(Do not report 94375 in conjunction with 94010, 94060, 94728)

94450 Breathing response to hypoxia (hypoxia response curve)

➲ *CPT Assistant* Summer 95:4, Feb 96:9, Jul 05:11, Nov 08:5

(For high altitude simulation test [HAST], see 94452, 94453)

94452 High altitude simulation test (HAST), with interpretation and report by a physician or other qualified health care professional;

➲ *CPT Changes: An Insider's View* 2005, 2013

➲ *CPT Assistant* Jul 05:11, Nov 08:5

(For obtaining arterial blood gases, use 36600)

(Do not report 94452 in conjunction with 94453, 94760, 94761)

94453 with supplemental oxygen titration

➲ *CPT Changes: An Insider's View* 2005, 2013

➲ *CPT Assistant* Jul 05:11, Nov 08:5

(For obtaining arterial blood gases, use 36600)

(Do not report 94453 in conjunction with 94452, 94760, 94761)

⊘ **94610**   Intrapulmonary surfactant administration by a physician or other qualified health care professional through endotracheal tube
⟶ *CPT Changes: An Insider's View* 2007, 2013
⟶ *CPT Assistant* Apr 07:3, Jul 08:7, Nov 08:5, Dec 10:15

(Do not report 94610 in conjunction with 99468-99472)

(For endotracheal intubation, use 31500)

(Report 94610 once per dosing episode)

94617   Exercise test for bronchospasm, including pre- and post-spirometry and pulse oximetry; with electrocardiographic recording(s)
⟶ *CPT Changes: An Insider's View* 2018, 2021
⟶ *CPT Assistant* Oct 17:3, Mar 19:11, May 19:10, Dec 20:3

94619   without electrocardiographic recording(s)
⟶ *CPT Changes: An Insider's View* 2021
⟶ *CPT Assistant* Dec 20:3

94618   Pulmonary stress testing (eg, 6-minute walk test), including measurement of heart rate, oximetry, and oxygen titration, when performed
⟶ *CPT Changes: An Insider's View* 2018
⟶ *CPT Assistant* Oct 17:3, Mar 19:11, May 19:10

94619   Code is out of numerical sequence. See 94610-94621

94621   Cardiopulmonary exercise testing, including measurements of minute ventilation, CO_2 production, O_2 uptake, and electrocardiographic recordings
⟶ *CPT Changes: An Insider's View* 2018
⟶ *CPT Assistant* Summer 95:4, Nov 98:35, Jan 99:8, Aug 02:10, Jul 05:11, Nov 08:5, Nov 12:14, Oct 17:3, May 19:10

(Do not report 94617, 94619, 94621 in conjunction with 93000, 93005, 93010, 93040, 93041, 93042 for ECG monitoring performed during the same session)

(Do not report 94617, 94619, 94621 in conjunction with 93015, 93016, 93017, 93018)

(Do not report 94621 in conjunction with 94680, 94681, 94690)

(Do not report 94617, 94618, 94619, 94621 in conjunction with 94760, 94761)

94625   Physician or other qualified health care professional services for outpatient pulmonary rehabilitation; without continuous oximetry monitoring (per session)
⟶ *CPT Changes: An Insider's View* 2022
⟶ *CPT Assistant* Jan 22:15

94626   with continuous oximetry monitoring (per session)
⟶ *CPT Changes: An Insider's View* 2022
⟶ *CPT Assistant* Jan 22:15

(Do not report 94625, 94626 in conjunction with 94760, 94761)

94640   Pressurized or nonpressurized inhalation treatment for acute airway obstruction for therapeutic purposes and/or for diagnostic purposes such as sputum induction with an aerosol generator, nebulizer, metered dose inhaler or intermittent positive pressure breathing (IPPB) device
⟶ *CPT Changes: An Insider's View* 2003, 2016
⟶ *CPT Assistant* Summer 95:4, Feb 96:9, May 98:10, Apr 00:11, Jul 05:11, Apr 07:3, Nov 08:5, Sep 10:3, Dec 13:12, Mar 14:11, Sep 15:9

(Do not report 94640 in conjunction with 94060, 94070)

(For more than 1 inhalation treatment performed on the same date, append modifier 76)

(For continuous inhalation treatment of 1 hour or more, see 94644, 94645)

94642   Aerosol inhalation of pentamidine for pneumocystis carinii pneumonia treatment or prophylaxis
⟶ *CPT Assistant* Summer 95:4, Feb 96:9, Jul 05:11, Nov 08:5

94644   Continuous inhalation treatment with aerosol medication for acute airway obstruction; first hour
⟶ *CPT Changes: An Insider's View* 2007
⟶ *CPT Assistant* Apr 07:3, Nov 08:5, Mar 14:11, Sep 15:9, Apr 23:27

(For services of less than 1 hour, use 94640)

+ **94645**   each additional hour (List separately in addition to code for primary procedure)
⟶ *CPT Changes: An Insider's View* 2007
⟶ *CPT Assistant* Apr 07:3, Nov 08:5, Mar 14:11, Sep 15:9, Apr 23:27

(Use 94645 in conjunction with 94644)

94660   Continuous positive airway pressure ventilation (CPAP), initiation and management
⟶ *CPT Assistant* Fall 92:30, Spring 95:4, Summer 95:4, Feb 96:9, Jan 99:10, Aug 00:2, Oct 03:2, Jul 05:11, Jul 06:4, Feb 07:10, Jul 07:1, Nov 08:5, May 14:4, Oct 14:9, Aug 19:8, Jan 22:3, Jun 22:19, Dec 22:10, Jan 24:39

94662   Continuous negative pressure ventilation (CNP), initiation and management
⟶ *CPT Assistant* Fall 92:30, Spring 94:4, Summer 95:4, Feb 96:9, Aug 00:2, Jul 05:11, Feb 07:10, Jul 07:1, Nov 08:5, May 14:4, Aug 19:8, Jan 22:3, Jun 22:19, Dec 22:10

94664   Demonstration and/or evaluation of patient utilization of an aerosol generator, nebulizer, metered dose inhaler or IPPB device
⟶ *CPT Changes: An Insider's View* 2003
⟶ *CPT Assistant* Summer 95:4, Feb 96:9, May 98:10, Apr 00:11, Jul 05:11, Nov 08:5, Sep 10:3, Dec 13:12

(94664 can be reported 1 time only per day of service)

★ = Telemedicine   ◀ = Audio-only   + = Add-on code   ✎ = FDA approval pending   # = Resequenced code   ⊘ = Modifier 51 exempt   ⟶⟶⟶ = See p xxi for details

Medicine / Pulmonary   94002-94799

94667   Manipulation chest wall, such as cupping, percussing, and vibration to facilitate lung function; initial demonstration and/or evaluation
⟳ *CPT Assistant* Summer 95:4, Feb 96:9, Jul 05:11, Nov 08:5, Sep 10:3, Dec 13:12, Mar 14:11, Sep 15:9

94668   subsequent
⟳ *CPT Assistant* Summer 95:4, Feb 96:9, Jul 05:11, Sep 10:3, Dec 13:12, Mar 14:11, Sep 15:9

94669   Mechanical chest wall oscillation to facilitate lung function, per session
⟳ *CPT Changes: An Insider's View* 2014

94680   Oxygen uptake, expired gas analysis; rest and exercise, direct, simple
⟳ *CPT Assistant* Summer 95:4, Feb 96:9, Jul 05:11

94681   including CO_2 output, percentage oxygen extracted
⟳ *CPT Assistant* Summer 95:4, Feb 96:9, Jul 05:11

94690   rest, indirect (separate procedure)
⟳ *CPT Assistant* Summer 95:4, Feb 96:9, Jul 05:11

(For single arterial puncture, use 36600)

(Do not report 94680, 94681, 94690 in conjunction with 94621)

94726   Plethysmography for determination of lung volumes and, when performed, airway resistance
⟳ *CPT Changes: An Insider's View* 2012
⟳ *CPT Assistant* Jan 12:3, Aug 12:6, May 13:11

(Do not report 94726 in conjunction with 94727, 94728)

94727   Gas dilution or washout for determination of lung volumes and, when performed, distribution of ventilation and closing volumes
⟳ *CPT Changes: An Insider's View* 2012
⟳ *CPT Assistant* Jan 12:3, Aug 12:6, May 13:11

(Do not report 94727 in conjunction with 94726)

94728   Airway resistance by oscillometry
⟳ *CPT Changes: An Insider's View* 2012, 2020
⟳ *CPT Assistant* Jan 12:3, Aug 12:6, May 13:11, Mar 14:11

(Do not report 94728 in conjunction with 94010, 94060, 94070, 94375, 94726)

+ 94729   Diffusing capacity (eg, carbon monoxide, membrane) (List separately in addition to code for primary procedure)
⟳ *CPT Changes: An Insider's View* 2012
⟳ *CPT Assistant* Jan 12:3, Aug 12:6, Dec 13:12

(Report 94729 in conjunction with 94010, 94060, 94070, 94375, 94726-94728)

94760   Noninvasive ear or pulse oximetry for oxygen saturation; single determination
⟳ *CPT Assistant* Summer 95:4, Feb 96:9, Feb 97:10, Jul 98:2, Oct 03:2, Jul 05:11, Feb 06:9, Jul 06:4, Feb 07:10, Apr 07:1, Jul 07:1, Dec 10:15, May 14:4, Aug 19:8, Dec 20:3, Jan 22:3, Jun 22:19, Dec 22:10

(For blood gases, see 82803-82810)

94761   multiple determinations (eg, during exercise)
⟳ *CPT Assistant* Summer 95:4, Feb 96:9, Jul 98:2, Jun 99:10, Jul 05:11, Feb 06:9, Jul 06:4, Feb 07:10, Apr 07:1, Jun 07:11, Jul 07:1, Dec 08:5, May 14:4, Aug 19:8, Dec 20:3, Jan 22:3, Jun 22:19, Dec 22:10

(Do not report 94760, 94761 in conjunction with 94617, 94618, 94619, 94621)

94762   by continuous overnight monitoring (separate procedure)
⟳ *CPT Assistant* Summer 95:4, Feb 96:9, Jul 98:2, Oct 03:2, Jul 05:11, Feb 06:9, Jul 06:4, Feb 07:10, Apr 07:1, Jul 07:1, Dec 08:5, May 14:4, Aug 19:8, Jan 22:3, Jun 22:19, Dec 22:10

(For other in vivo laboratory procedures, see 88720-88741)

94772   Circadian respiratory pattern recording (pediatric pneumogram), 12-24 hour continuous recording, infant
⟳ *CPT Assistant* Summer 95:4, Feb 96:9, Jul 05:11

(Separate procedure codes for electromyograms, EEG, ECG, and recordings of respiration are excluded when 94772 is reported)

94774   Pediatric home apnea monitoring event recording including respiratory rate, pattern and heart rate per 30-day period of time; includes monitor attachment, download of data, review, interpretation, and preparation of a report by a physician or other qualified health care professional
⟳ *CPT Changes: An Insider's View* 2007, 2013
⟳ *CPT Assistant* Apr 07:3, Mar 08:4

(Do not report 94774 in conjunction with 94775-94777 during the same reporting period)

94775   monitor attachment only (includes hook-up, initiation of recording and disconnection)
⟳ *CPT Changes: An Insider's View* 2007
⟳ *CPT Assistant* Apr 07:3, Mar 08:4

94776   monitoring, download of information, receipt of transmission(s) and analyses by computer only
⟳ *CPT Changes: An Insider's View* 2007
⟳ *CPT Assistant* Apr 07:3, Mar 08:4

94777   review, interpretation and preparation of report only by a physician or other qualified health care professional
⟳ *CPT Changes: An Insider's View* 2007, 2013
⟳ *CPT Assistant* Apr 07:3, Mar 08:4

(When oxygen saturation monitoring is used in addition to heart rate and respiratory monitoring, it is not reported separately)

(Do not report 94774-94777 in conjunction with 93224-93272)

(Do not report apnea recording device separately)

(For sleep study, see 95805-95811)

94780 Car seat/bed testing for airway integrity, for infants through 12 months of age, with continual clinical staff observation and continuous recording of pulse oximetry, heart rate and respiratory rate, with interpretation and report; 60 minutes

➔ *CPT Changes: An Insider's View* 2012, 2019

➔ *CPT Assistant* Aug 12:6, May 15:11

(Do not report 94780 for less than 60 minutes)

(Do not report 94780 in conjunction with 93040-93042, 94760, 94761, 99468-99472, 99477-99480)

+ 94781 each additional full 30 minutes (List separately in addition to code for primary procedure)

➔ *CPT Changes: An Insider's View* 2012, 2019

➔ *CPT Assistant* Aug 12:6, May 15:11

(Use 94781 in conjunction with 94780)

94799 Unlisted pulmonary service or procedure

➔ *CPT Assistant* Summer 95:4, Feb 96:9, Mar 96:10, Jul 05:11, Dec 10:15, Nov 12:14, Dec 13:12, May 15:11, Dec 15:17, Sep 18:14, Mar 19:11, Dec 20:3, Apr 23:27

Allergy and Clinical Immunology

Definitions

Immunotherapy (desensitization, hyposensitization): is the parenteral administration of allergenic extracts as antigens at periodic intervals, usually on an increasing dosage scale to a dosage which is maintained as maintenance therapy. Indications for immunotherapy are determined by appropriate diagnostic procedures coordinated with clinical judgment and knowledge of the natural history of allergic diseases.

Other therapy: for medical conferences on the use of mechanical and electronic devices (precipitators, air conditioners, air filters, humidifiers, dehumidifiers), climatotherapy, physical therapy, occupational and recreational therapy, see Evaluation and Management services.

Do not report evaluation and management (E/M) services for test interpretation and report. If a significant separately identifiable E/M service is performed, the appropriate E/M service code, which may include new or established patient office or other outpatient services (99202-99215), hospital inpatient or observation care (99221-99223, 99231-99233), consultations (99242, 99243, 99244, 99245, 99252, 99253, 99254, 99255), emergency department services (99281-99285), nursing facility services (99304-99316), home or residence services (99341-99350), or preventive medicine services (99381-99429), should be reported using modifier 25.

Allergy Testing

(For allergy laboratory tests, see 86000-86999)

(For administration of medications [eg, epinephrine, steroidal agents, antihistamines] for therapy for severe or intractable allergic reaction, use 96372)

95004 Percutaneous tests (scratch, puncture, prick) with allergenic extracts, immediate type reaction, including test interpretation and report, specify number of tests

➔ *CPT Changes: An Insider's View* 2007, 2008, 2013

➔ *CPT Assistant* Summer 91:15, May 10:3, Jan 13:9

95012 Nitric oxide expired gas determination

➔ *CPT Changes: An Insider's View* 2007

➔ *CPT Assistant* Mar 07:11, Apr 07:6, Jan 13:9, Mar 14:11

95017 Allergy testing, any combination of percutaneous (scratch, puncture, prick) and intracutaneous (intradermal), sequential and incremental, with venoms, immediate type reaction, including test interpretation and report, specify number of tests

➔ *CPT Changes: An Insider's View* 2013

➔ *CPT Assistant* Jan 13:9, Jul 15:9

95018 Allergy testing, any combination of percutaneous (scratch, puncture, prick) and intracutaneous (intradermal), sequential and incremental, with drugs or biologicals, immediate type reaction, including test interpretation and report, specify number of tests

➔ *CPT Changes: An Insider's View* 2013

➔ *CPT Assistant* Jan 13:9, Jul 15:9

95024 Intracutaneous (intradermal) tests with allergenic extracts, immediate type reaction, including test interpretation and report, specify number of tests

➔ *CPT Changes: An Insider's View* 2003, 2008, 2013

➔ *CPT Assistant* Summer 91:15, May 10:3, Jan 13:9

95027 Intracutaneous (intradermal) tests, sequential and incremental, with allergenic extracts for airborne allergens, immediate type reaction, including test interpretation and report, specify number of tests

➔ *CPT Changes: An Insider's View* 2003, 2008, 2013

➔ *CPT Assistant* Summer 91:15, Jun 97:10, Dec 07:9, May 10:3, Jan 13:9

95028 Intracutaneous (intradermal) tests with allergenic extracts, delayed type reaction, including reading, specify number of tests

➔ *CPT Changes: An Insider's View* 2003

➔ *CPT Assistant* Summer 91:14, May 10:3, Jan 13:9

95044 Patch or application test(s) (specify number of tests)

➔ *CPT Assistant* Summer 91:15, Spring 94:31, Jan 13:9

★=Telemedicine ◀=Audio-only +=Add-on code ⊮=FDA approval pending #=Resequenced code ⊘=Modifier 51 exempt ➔➔➔=See p xxi for details

95052   Photo patch test(s) (specify number of tests)
> *CPT Assistant* Spring 94:31, Jan 13:9

95056   Photo tests
> *CPT Assistant* Summer 91:16, Jan 13:9

95060   Ophthalmic mucous membrane tests
> *CPT Assistant* Summer 91:16, Jan 13:9

95065   Direct nasal mucous membrane test
> *CPT Assistant* Summer 91:15, Jan 13:9

95070   Inhalation bronchial challenge testing (not including necessary pulmonary function tests), with histamine, methacholine, or similar compounds
> *CPT Changes: An Insider's View* 2021
> *CPT Assistant* Summer 91:16, Nov 12:11, Jan 13:9

(For pulmonary function tests, see 94060, 94070)

Ingestion Challenge Testing

Codes 95076 and 95079 are used to report ingestion challenge testing. Report 95076 for initial 120 minutes of testing time (ie, not physician face-to-face time). Report 95079 for each additional 60 minutes of testing time (ie, not physician face-to-face time). For total testing time less than 61 minutes (eg, positive challenge resulting in cessation of testing), report an evaluation and management service, if appropriate. Patient assessment/ monitoring activities for allergic reaction (eg, blood pressure testing, peak flow meter testing) are not separately reported. Intervention therapy (eg, injection of steroid or epinephrine) may be reported separately as appropriate.

For purposes of reporting testing times, if an evaluation and management service is required, then testing time ends.

95076   Ingestion challenge test (sequential and incremental ingestion of test items, eg, food, drug or other substance); initial 120 minutes of testing
> *CPT Changes: An Insider's View* 2013
> *CPT Assistant* Jan 13:9

+ 95079   each additional 60 minutes of testing (List separately in addition to code for primary procedure)
> *CPT Changes: An Insider's View* 2013
> *CPT Assistant* Jan 13:9

(Use 95079 in conjunction with 95076)

Allergen Immunotherapy

Codes 95115-95199 include the professional services necessary for allergen immunotherapy. Office visit codes may be used in addition to allergen immunotherapy if other identifiable services are provided at that time.

95115   Professional services for allergen immunotherapy not including provision of allergenic extracts; single injection
> *CPT Assistant* Fall 91:19, Spring 94:30, Summer 95:4, May 96:1, Nov 98:35, Apr 00:4, Feb 05:10, 12, Nov 05:1, Nov 06:23, Dec 07:9, Jan 13:9, Jun 19:15, Sep 20:15

95117   2 or more injections
> *CPT Assistant* Fall 91:19, Spring 94:30, Summer 95:4, May 96:1, Aug 96:10, Nov 98:35, Apr 00:4, Feb 05:10, 12, Nov 05:1, Nov 06:23, Dec 07:9, Jan 13:9, Jun 19:15, Sep 20:15

95120   Professional services for allergen immunotherapy in the office or institution of the prescribing physician or other qualified health care professional, including provision of allergenic extract; single injection
> *CPT Changes: An Insider's View* 2013
> *CPT Assistant* Fall 91:19, Spring 94:30, Summer 95:4, May 96:2, Nov 98:35, Feb 05:10, 12, Jan 13:9

95125   2 or more injections
> *CPT Changes: An Insider's View* 2013
> *CPT Assistant* Fall 91:19, Spring 94:30, Summer 95:4, May 96:2, Aug 96:10, Nov 98:35, Feb 05:10, 12, Jan 13:9

95130   single stinging insect venom
> *CPT Changes: An Insider's View* 2013
> *CPT Assistant* Fall 91:19, Summer 95:4, May 96:2, Jun 96:10, Nov 98:35, Sep 99:10, Feb 05:10, 12, Jan 13:9

95131   2 stinging insect venoms
> *CPT Changes: An Insider's View* 2013
> *CPT Assistant* Fall 91:19, Summer 95:4, May 96:2, Jun 96:10, Nov 98:35, Sep 99:10, Feb 05:10, 12, Jan 13:9

95132   3 stinging insect venoms
> *CPT Changes: An Insider's View* 2013
> *CPT Assistant* Fall 91:19, Summer 95:4, May 96:2, Nov 98:35, Sep 99:11, Feb 05:10, 12, Jan 13:9

95133   4 stinging insect venoms
> *CPT Changes: An Insider's View* 2013
> *CPT Assistant* Fall 91:19, Summer 95:4, May 96:2, Nov 98:35, Sep 99:11, Feb 05:10, 12, Jan 13:9

95134   5 stinging insect venoms
> *CPT Changes: An Insider's View* 2013
> *CPT Assistant* Fall 91:19, Summer 95:4, May 96:2, Nov 98:35, Sep 99:11, Feb 05:10, 12, Jan 13:9

95144   Professional services for the supervision of preparation and provision of antigens for allergen immunotherapy, single dose vial(s) (specify number of vials)
> *CPT Changes: An Insider's View* 2002
> *CPT Assistant* Fall 91:19, Spring 94:30, Summer 95:4, May 96:11, Nov 98:35, Feb 05:10-11, Jan 13:9

(A single dose vial contains a single dose of antigen administered in 1 injection)

95145   Professional services for the supervision of preparation and provision of antigens for allergen immunotherapy (specify number of doses); single stinging insect venom
> *CPT Changes: An Insider's View* 2002
> *CPT Assistant* Fall 91:19, Summer 95:4, May 96:11, Nov 98:35, Feb 05:10, 12, Jan 13:9

95146   2 single stinging insect venoms
> *CPT Assistant* Fall 91:19, Summer 95:4, May 96:11, Nov 98:35, Feb 05:10, 12, Jan 13:9

95147   3 single stinging insect venoms
> *CPT Assistant* Fall 91:19, Summer 95:4, May 96:11, Nov 98:35, Feb 05:10, 12, Jan 13:9

95148   4 single stinging insect venoms
> *CPT Assistant* Fall 91:19, Summer 95:4, May 96:11, Nov 98:35, Feb 05:10, 12, Jan 13:9

95149   5 single stinging insect venoms
> *CPT Assistant* Fall 91:19, Summer 95:4, May 96:11, Nov 98:35, Feb 05:10, 12, Jan 13:9

95165   Professional services for the supervision of preparation and provision of antigens for allergen immunotherapy; single or multiple antigens (specify number of doses)
> *CPT Changes: An Insider's View* 2002
> *CPT Assistant* Fall 91:19, Spring 94:30, Summer 95:4, May 96:11, Nov 98:35, Apr 00:4, Apr 01:11, Feb 05:10, 12, Jun 05:9, Jan 13:9

95170   whole body extract of biting insect or other arthropod (specify number of doses)
> *CPT Assistant* Fall 91:19, Spring 94:30, Summer 95:4, May 96:12, Apr 01:11, Feb 05:10, 12, Jun 05:9, Jan 13:9

(For allergy immunotherapy reporting, a dose is the amount of antigen[s] administered in a single injection from a multiple dose vial)

95180   Rapid desensitization procedure, each hour (eg, insulin, penicillin, equine serum)
> *CPT Changes: An Insider's View* 2002
> *CPT Assistant* Summer 95:4, Jan 13:9, Jun 19:15

95199   Unlisted allergy/clinical immunologic service or procedure
> *CPT Assistant* Summer 95:4, Nov 98:35, Jan 13:9

(For skin testing of bacterial, viral, fungal extracts, see 86485-86580, 95028)

(For special reports on allergy patients, use 99080)

(For testing procedures such as radioallergosorbent testing [RAST], rat mast cell technique [RMCT], mast cell degranulation test [MCDT], lymphocytic transformation test [LTT], leukocyte histamine release [LHR], migration inhibitory factor test [MIF], transfer factor test [TFT], nitroblue tetrazolium dye test [NTD], see Immunology section in **Pathology** or use 95199)

Endocrinology

Codes 95249 and 95250 are used to report the service for subcutaneous interstitial sensor placement, hook-up of the sensor to the transmitter, calibration of continuous glucose monitoring (CGM) device, patient training on CGM device functions and management, removal of the interstitial sensor, and the print-out of captured data recordings. For the CGM device owned by the physician's or other qualified health care professional's office, use 95250 for the data capture occurring over a **minimum** period of 72 hours.

Code 95249 may be reported only once during the time that a patient owns a given data receiver, including the initial episode of data collection.

Code 95249 may not be reported for subsequent episodes of data collection, unless the patient obtains a new and/or different model of data receiver. Obtaining a new sensor and/or transmitter without a change in receiver may not be reported with 95249.

Code 95249 may not be reported unless the patient brings the data receiver to the physician's or other qualified health care professional's office with the entire initial data collection procedure conducted in the physician's or other qualified health care professional's office.

95249   Code is out of numerical sequence. See 95199-95803

95250   Ambulatory continuous glucose monitoring of interstitial tissue fluid via a subcutaneous sensor for a minimum of 72 hours; physician or other qualified health care professional (office) provided equipment, sensor placement, hook-up, calibration of monitor, patient training, removal of sensor, and printout of recording
> *CPT Changes: An Insider's View* 2002, 2006, 2009, 2016, 2018
> *CPT Assistant* Mar 18:5, Jun 18:6, Feb 22:8, Oct 22:14

(Do not report 95250 more than once per month)

(Do not report 95250 in conjunction with 99091, 0446T)

 # 95249   patient-provided equipment, sensor placement, hook-up, calibration of monitor, patient training, and printout of recording
> *CPT Changes: An Insider's View* 2018
> *CPT Assistant* Jun 18:6

(Do not report 95249 more than once for the duration that the patient owns the data receiver)

(Do not report 95249 in conjunction with 99091, 0446T)

95251   analysis, interpretation and report
> *CPT Changes: An Insider's View* 2006, 2009, 2016, 2018
> *CPT Assistant* Mar 18:5, Jun 18:6

(Do not report 95251 more than once per month)

(Do not report 95251 in conjunction with 99091)

Neurology and Neuromuscular Procedures

Neurologic services are typically consultative, and any of the levels of consultation (99242, 99243, 99244, 99245, 99252, 99253, 99254, 99255) may be appropriate.

In addition, services and skills outlined under **Evaluation and Management** levels of service appropriate to neurologic illnesses should be reported similarly.

The electroencephalogram (EEG), video electroencephalogram (VEEG), autonomic function, evoked potential, reflex tests, electromyography (EMG), nerve conduction velocity (NCV), and magnetoencephalography (MEG) services (95700-95726, 95812-95829, and 95860-95967) include recording, interpretation, and report by a physician or other qualified health care professional. For interpretation only, use modifier 26 with 95812-95829, 95860-95967. For interpretation only for long-term EEG services, report 95717, 95718, 95719, 95720, 95721, 95722, 95723, 95724, 95725, 95726.

Codes 95700-95726 and 95812-95822 use EEG/VEEG recording time as a basis for code use. Recording time is when the recording is underway and diagnostic EEG data is being collected. Recording time excludes set up and take down time. If diagnostic EEG recording is disrupted, recording time stops until diagnostic EEG recording is resumed. Codes 95961-95962 use physician or other qualified health care professional attendance time as a basis for code use.

> (Do not report codes 95860-95875 in addition to 96000-96004)

Sleep Medicine Testing

Sleep medicine services include procedures that evaluate adult and pediatric patients for a variety of sleep disorders. Sleep medicine testing services are diagnostic procedures using in-laboratory and portable technology to assess physiologic data and therapy.

All sleep services (95800-95811) include recording, interpretation, and report. (Report with modifier 52 if less than 6 hours of recording for 95800, 95801 and 95806, 95807, 95810, 95811; if less than 7 hours of recording for 95782, 95783, or if less than four nap opportunities are recorded for 95805).

Definitions

For purposes of CPT reporting of sleep medicine testing services, the following definitions apply:

Actigraphy: the use of a portable, non-invasive, device that continuously records gross motor movement over an extended period of time. The periods of activity and rest are indirect parameters for estimates of the periods of wakefulness and sleep of an individual.

Attended: a technologist or qualified health care professional is physically present (ie, sufficient proximity such that the qualified health care professional can physically respond to emergencies, to other appropriate patient needs or to technical problems at the bedside) throughout the recording session.

Electrooculogram (EOG): a recording of electrical activity indicative of eye movement.

Maintenance of wakefulness test (MWT): a standardized objective test used to determine a person's ability to stay awake. MWT requires sleep staging of the trials that are performed at defined intervals and is attended by a qualified health care professional.

Multiple sleep latency test (MSLT): a standardized objective test of the tendency to fall asleep. MSLT requires sleep staging of the nap opportunities that are performed at defined intervals and is attended by a technologist or qualified health care professional.

Peripheral arterial tonometry (PAT): a plethysmography technique that continuously measures pulsatile volume changes in a digit. This reflects the relative change of blood volume as an indirect measure of sympathetic nervous system activity which is used in respiratory analysis.

Physiological measurements of sleep as used in 95805: the parameters measured are a frontal, central and occipital lead of EEG (3 leads), submental EMG lead and a left and right EOG. These parameters are used together for staging sleep.

Polysomnography: a sleep test involving the continuous, simultaneous, recording of physiological parameters for a period of at least 6 hours that is performed in a sleep laboratory and attended by a technologist or qualified health care professional. The parameters measured are a frontal, central and occipital lead of EEG (3 leads), submental EMG lead and a left and right EOG, (from which sleep is staged), plus four or more additional parameters. The additional parameters typically required in polysomnography are listed below:

a. Electrocardiogram (ECG)

b. Nasal and/or oral airflow

c. Respiratory effort

d. Oxyhemoglobin saturation, SpO_2

e. Bilateral anterior tibialis EMG

Positive airway pressure (PAP): a device used to treat sleep-related breathing disorders with the use of non-invasive delivery of positive pressure to the airway. Examples include but are not limited to: CPAP (continuous positive airway pressure), bilevel PAP, AutoPAP (autotitrating or adjusting PAP), ASV (adaptive-servo ventilation).

Remote: the site of service is distant from the monitoring center. Neither a technologist nor a qualified health care professional is physically present at the testing site.

Respiratory airflow (ventilation): the movement of air during inhaled and exhaled breaths. This is typically assessed using thermistor and nasal pressure sensors.

Respiratory analysis: generation of derived parameters that describe components of respiration obtained by using direct or indirect parameters, eg, by airflow or peripheral arterial tone.

Respiratory effort: contraction of the diaphragmatic and/or intercostal muscles to cause (or attempt to cause) respiratory airflow. This is typically measured using transducers that estimate motion of the thorax and abdomen such as respiratory inductive plethysmography, transducers that estimate pressures generated by breathing muscles such as esophageal manometry, or by contraction of breathing muscles, such as diaphragmatic/intercostal EMG.

Respiratory (thoracoabdominal) movement: movement of the chest and abdomen during respiratory effort.

Sleep latency: the length of time it takes to transition from wakefulness to sleep. In the sleep laboratory it is the time from "lights out" to the first epoch scored as any stage of sleep.

Sleep staging: the delineation of the distinct sleep levels through the simultaneous evaluation of physiologic measures including a frontal, central and occipital lead of EEG (3 leads), submental EMG lead and a left and right EOG.

Sleep testing (or sleep study): the continuous, simultaneous monitoring of physiological parameters during sleep (eg, polysomnography, EEG).

Total sleep time: a derived parameter obtained by sleep staging or may be estimated indirectly using actigraphy or other methods.

Unattended: a technologist or qualified health care professional is not physically present with the patient during the recording session.

(Report with modifier 52 if less than 6 hours of recording or in other cases of reduced services as appropriate)

(For unattended sleep study, use 95806)

95700 Code is out of numerical sequence. See 95966-95971

95705 Code is out of numerical sequence. See 95966-95971

95706 Code is out of numerical sequence. See 95966-95971

95707 Code is out of numerical sequence. See 95966-95971

95708 Code is out of numerical sequence. See 95966-95971

95709 Code is out of numerical sequence. See 95966-95971

95710 Code is out of numerical sequence. See 95966-95971

95711 Code is out of numerical sequence. See 95966-95971

95712 Code is out of numerical sequence. See 95966-95971

95713 Code is out of numerical sequence. See 95966-95971

95714 Code is out of numerical sequence. See 95966-95971

95715 Code is out of numerical sequence. See 95966-95971

95716 Code is out of numerical sequence. See 95966-95971

95717 Code is out of numerical sequence. See 95966-95971

95718 Code is out of numerical sequence. See 95966-95971

95719 Code is out of numerical sequence. See 95966-95971

95720 Code is out of numerical sequence. See 95966-95971

95721 Code is out of numerical sequence. See 95966-95971

95722 Code is out of numerical sequence. See 95966-95971

95723 Code is out of numerical sequence. See 95966-95971

95724 Code is out of numerical sequence. See 95966-95971

95725 Code is out of numerical sequence. See 95966-95971

95726 Code is out of numerical sequence. See 95966-95971

95782 Code is out of numerical sequence. See 95805-95813

95783 Code is out of numerical sequence. See 95805-95813

95800 Code is out of numerical sequence. See 95805-95813

95801 Code is out of numerical sequence. See 95805-95813

95803 Actigraphy testing, recording, analysis, interpretation, and report (minimum of 72 hours to 14 consecutive days of recording)
➔ *CPT Changes: An Insider's View* 2009
➔ *CPT Assistant* Nov 11:3

(Do not report 95803 more than once in any 14 day period)

(Do not report 95803 in conjunction with 95806-95811)

95805 Multiple sleep latency or maintenance of wakefulness testing, recording, analysis and interpretation of physiological measurements of sleep during multiple trials to assess sleepiness
➔ *CPT Assistant* Nov 97:45-46, Nov 98:35, Dec 01:3, Sep 02:2-3, Mar 08:4, Nov 11:3

95806 Sleep study, unattended, simultaneous recording of, heart rate, oxygen saturation, respiratory airflow, and respiratory effort (eg, thoracoabdominal movement)
➔ *CPT Changes: An Insider's View* 2010
➔ *CPT Assistant* Nov 97:45-46, Aug 98:10, Nov 98:35, Jan 11:7, Nov 11:3, Feb 13:14, Jul 13:11

(Do not report 95806 in conjunction with 93041-93227, 93228, 93229, 93268-93272, 95800, 95801)

(For unattended sleep study that measures heart rate, oxygen saturation, respiratory analysis, and sleep time, use 95800)

(For unattended sleep study that measures a minimum heart rate, oxygen saturation, and respiratory analysis, use 95801)

95800   Sleep study, unattended, simultaneous recording; heart rate, oxygen saturation, respiratory analysis (eg, by airflow or peripheral arterial tone), and sleep time

➡ *CPT Changes: An Insider's View* 2011

➡ *CPT Assistant* Jan 11:6, Nov 11:3, Feb 13:14

(Do not report 95800 in conjunction with 93041-93227, 93228, 93229, 93268-93272, 95801, 95803, 95806)

(For unattended sleep study that measures a minimum of heart rate, oxygen saturation, and respiratory analysis, use 95801)

95801   minimum of heart rate, oxygen saturation, and respiratory analysis (eg, by airflow or peripheral arterial tone)

➡ *CPT Changes: An Insider's View* 2011

➡ *CPT Assistant* Jan 11:7, Nov 11:3, Feb 13:14

(Do not report 95801 in conjunction with 93041-93227, 93228, 93229, 93268-93272, 95800, 95806)

(For unattended sleep study that measures heart rate, oxygen saturation, respiratory analysis and sleep time, use 95800)

95807   Sleep study, simultaneous recording of ventilation, respiratory effort, ECG or heart rate, and oxygen saturation, attended by a technologist

➡ *CPT Assistant* Nov 97:46, Nov 98:35, Mar 08:4, Nov 11:3, Feb 13:14

95808   Polysomnography; any age, sleep staging with 1-3 additional parameters of sleep, attended by a technologist

➡ *CPT Changes: An Insider's View* 2013

➡ *CPT Assistant* Sep 96:11, Nov 97:46, Feb 98:6, Nov 98:35, Sep 02:2-3, Mar 08:4, Nov 11:3, Feb 13:14, Apr 24:9

95810   age 6 years or older, sleep staging with 4 or more additional parameters of sleep, attended by a technologist

➡ *CPT Changes: An Insider's View* 2013

➡ *CPT Assistant* Feb 98:6, Nov 98:35, Sep 02:2-3, Nov 11:3, Feb 13:14, Apr 24:9

95811   age 6 years or older, sleep staging with 4 or more additional parameters of sleep, with initiation of continuous positive airway pressure therapy or bilevel ventilation, attended by a technologist

➡ *CPT Changes: An Insider's View* 2013

➡ *CPT Assistant* Nov 97:46, Feb 98:6, Nov 98:35, Sep 02:2-3, Mar 08:4, Nov 11:3, Feb 13:14, Oct 14:9, Apr 24:9

95782   younger than 6 years, sleep staging with 4 or more additional parameters of sleep, attended by a technologist

➡ *CPT Changes: An Insider's View* 2013

➡ *CPT Assistant* Feb 13:14, Apr 24:9

95783   younger than 6 years, sleep staging with 4 or more additional parameters of sleep, with initiation of continuous positive airway pressure therapy or bi-level ventilation, attended by a technologist

➡ *CPT Changes: An Insider's View* 2013

➡ *CPT Assistant* Feb 13:14, Oct 14:9, Apr 24:9

(For interrogation and programming of a phrenic nerve stimulator system during a polysomnogram, use 93152)

Routine Electroencephalography (EEG)

EEG codes 95812-95822 include hyperventilation and/ or photic stimulation when appropriate. Routine EEG codes 95816-95822 include 20 to 40 minutes of recording. Extended EEG codes 95812-95813 include reporting times longer than 40 minutes.

95812   Electroencephalogram (EEG) extended monitoring; 41-60 minutes

➡ *CPT Changes: An Insider's View* 2003

➡ *CPT Assistant* Winter 94:18, Nov 98:35, May 11:3, 10, Dec 18:3, Sep 23:49

(Do not report 95812 in conjunction with 95700-95726)

95813   61-119 minutes

➡ *CPT Changes: An Insider's View* 2020

➡ *CPT Assistant* Winter 94:18, Nov 98:35, May 11:3, 10, Dec 18:3, Sep 23:49

(Do not report 95813 in conjunction with 95700-95726)

(For long-term EEG services [2 hours or more], see 95700-95726)

95816   Electroencephalogram (EEG); including recording awake and drowsy

➡ *CPT Changes: An Insider's View* 2000, 2003

➡ *CPT Assistant* Sep 96:11, Nov 98:35, Nov 99:51, Jul 00:1, May 11:3, Dec 15:17, Dec 18:3, Sep 23:49

(Do not report 95816 in conjunction with 95700-95726)

95819   including recording awake and asleep

➡ *CPT Changes: An Insider's View* 2000, 2003

➡ *CPT Assistant* Nov 98:35, Nov 99:51, Jul 00:1, May 11:3, Dec 15:17, Dec 18:3, Sep 23:49

(Do not report 95819 in conjunction with 95700-95726)

95822   recording in coma or sleep only

➡ *CPT Changes: An Insider's View* 2003

➡ *CPT Assistant* Nov 98:35, May 11:3, May 13:8, Dec 14:19, Dec 18:3, Sep 23:49

(Do not report 95822 in conjunction with 95700-95726)

95824   cerebral death evaluation only
➔ *CPT Assistant* Nov 98:35

(For long-term EEG monitoring, see 95700-95726)

(For EEG during nonintracranial surgery, use 95955)

(For Wada test, use 95958)

95829   Code is out of numerical sequence. See 95824-95852

95830   Insertion by physician or other qualified health care professional of sphenoidal electrodes for electroencephalographic (EEG) recording
➔ *CPT Changes: An Insider's View* 2013

Electrocorticography

Electrocorticography (ECoG) is the recording of EEG from electrodes directly on or in the brain.

Code 95829 describes intraoperative recordings of ECoG from electrode arrays implanted in or placed directly on the brain exposed during surgery. Code 95829 includes review and interpretation during surgery.

Code 95836 describes recording of ECoG from electrodes chronically implanted on or in the brain. Chronically implanted electrodes allow for intracranial recordings to continue after the patient has been discharged from the hospital. Code 95836 includes unattended ECoG recording with storage for later review and interpretation during a single 30-day period. Code 95836 may be reported only once for each 30-day period. The dates encompassed by the 30-day period must be documented in the report.

For report of programming for a brain neurostimulator pulse generator/transmitter during the ECoG (95836) 30-day period, see 95983, 95984.

\# **95829**   Electrocorticogram at surgery (separate procedure)
➔ *CPT Assistant* Nov 98:35, Dec 18:3

\# **95836**   Electrocorticogram from an implanted brain neurostimulator pulse generator/transmitter, including recording, with interpretation and written report, up to 30 days
➔ *CPT Changes: An Insider's View* 2019
➔ *CPT Assistant* Dec 18:3

(Report 95836 only once per 30 days)

(Do not report 95836 in conjunction with 95957)

(For programming a brain neurostimulator pulse generator/transmitter when performed in conjunction with ECoG [95836], see 95983, 95984)

Range of Motion Testing

95836   Code is out of numerical sequence. See 95824-95852

95851   Range of motion measurements and report (separate procedure); each extremity (excluding hand) or each trunk section (spine)
➔ *CPT Assistant* Sep 99:10, Nov 01:5, Apr 03:28, Dec 03:7, Feb 04:5, Dec 07:16, May 08:9, Aug 13:7, Dec 16:16

95852   hand, with or without comparison with normal side
➔ *CPT Assistant* Nov 01:5, Apr 03:28, Dec 03:7, May 08:9, Aug 13:7

95857   Cholinesterase inhibitor challenge test for myasthenia gravis
➔ *CPT Changes: An Insider's View* 2011
➔ *CPT Assistant* Feb 11:3

Intraoperative Electrocorticography (ECoG)
95829

Intraoperative ECoG device and surgical exposure.

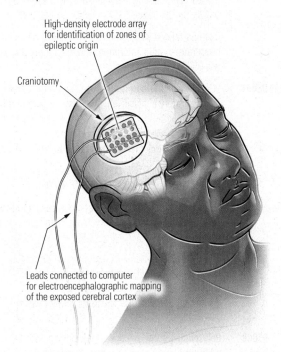

High-density electrode array for identification of zones of epileptic origin

Craniotomy

Leads connected to computer for electroencephalographic mapping of the exposed cerebral cortex

Electromyography

Needle electromyographic (EMG) procedures include the interpretation of electrical waveforms measured by equipment that produces both visible and audible components of electrical signals recorded from the muscle(s) studied by the needle electrode.

Use 95870 or 95885 when four or fewer muscles are tested in an extremity. Use 95860-95864 or 95886 when five or more muscles are tested in an extremity.

Use EMG codes (95860-95864 and 95867-95870) when no nerve conduction studies (95907-95913) are performed on that day. Use 95885, 95886, and 95887 for

EMG services when nerve conduction studies (95907-95913) are performed in conjunction with EMG on the same day.

Extraoperative ECoG
95836

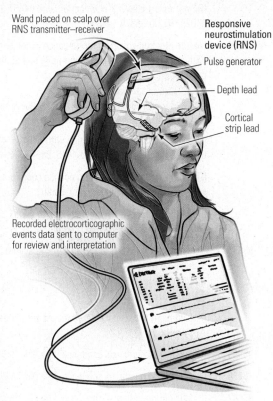

Extraoperative ECoG device with wand placed above head and laptop.

Wand placed on scalp over RNS transmitter–receiver

Responsive neurostimulation device (RNS)

Pulse generator

Depth lead

Cortical strip lead

Recorded electrocorticographic events data sent to computer for review and interpretation

Report either 95885 or 95886 once per extremity. Codes 95885 and 95886 can be reported together up to a combined total of four units of service per patient when all four extremities are tested.

Report 95887 once per anatomic site (ie, cervical paraspinal muscle[s], thoracic paraspinal muscle[s], lumbar paraspinal muscle[s], chest wall muscle[s], and abdominal wall muscle[s]). Use 95887 for a unilateral study of the cranial nerve innervated muscles (excluding extra-ocular and larynx); when performed bilaterally, 95887 may be reported twice.

Use 95887 when a study of the cervical paraspinal muscle(s), or the lumbar paraspinal muscle(s) is performed with no corresponding limb study (95885 or 95886) on the same day.

(For needle electromyography of anal or urethral sphincter, use 51785)

(For non-needle electromyography of anal or urethral sphincter, use 51784)

(For needle electromyography of larynx, use 95865)

(For needle electromyography of hemidiaphragm, use 95866)

(For needle electromyography of extra-ocular muscles, use 92265)

95860 Needle electromyography; 1 extremity with or without related paraspinal areas

➔ *CPT Changes: An Insider's View* 2003

➔ *CPT Assistant* Nov 97:46, Jul 00:2, Apr 02:2, May 03:20, Jun 03:3, Feb 04:4, Jul 04:6, Oct 04:15, Jun 06:8, Sep 06:5, Aug 08:12, Jan 09:8, Oct 10:15, Dec 10:15, Feb 12:8, Mar 13:3, May 13:8, Mar 15:6

95861 2 extremities with or without related paraspinal areas

➔ *CPT Changes: An Insider's View* 2003

➔ *CPT Assistant* Nov 97:46, Jul 00:2, Apr 02:2, May 03:20, Jun 03:3, Feb 04:4, Jul 04:6, Oct 04:15, Jun 05:9, Jun 06:8, Sep 06:5, Aug 08:12, Jan 09:8, Oct 10:15, Dec 10:15, Feb 12:8, Mar 13:3, May 13:8

►(For dynamic electromyography performed during motion analysis studies, use 96002)◄

95863 3 extremities with or without related paraspinal areas

➔ *CPT Changes: An Insider's View* 2003

➔ *CPT Assistant* Nov 97:46, Jul 00:2, Apr 02:2, May 03:20, Jun 03:3, Feb 04:4, Jul 04:6, Oct 04:15, Jun 06:8, Sep 06:5, Oct 10:15, Dec 10:15, Feb 12:8, Mar 13:3, May 13:8

95864 4 extremities with or without related paraspinal areas

➔ *CPT Changes: An Insider's View* 2003

➔ *CPT Assistant* Nov 97:46, Jul 00:2, Jan 02:11, Apr 02:2, May 03:20, Jun 03:3, Feb 04:4, Jul 04:6, Oct 04:15, Jun 06:8, Sep 06:5, Aug 08:12, Jan 09:8, Oct 10:15, Dec 10:15, Feb 12:8, Mar 13:3, May 13:8

95865 larynx

➔ *CPT Changes: An Insider's View* 2006

➔ *CPT Assistant* Sep 06:5, Dec 07:16, Jan 09:8, May 13:8, Jan 14:6

(Do not report modifier 50 in conjunction with 95865)

(For unilateral procedure, report modifier 52 in conjunction with 95865)

95866 hemidiaphragm

➔ *CPT Changes: An Insider's View* 2006

➔ *CPT Assistant* May 13:8

95867 cranial nerve supplied muscle(s), unilateral

➔ *CPT Changes: An Insider's View* 2003

➔ *CPT Assistant* Apr 02:2, May 03:20, Jun 03:3, Jun 06:8, Sep 06:5, Dec 07:16, Aug 08:12, Jan 09:8, Feb 12:8, Mar 13:3, May 13:8

95868 cranial nerve supplied muscles, bilateral

➔ *CPT Changes: An Insider's View* 2003

➔ *CPT Assistant* Apr 02:2, May 03:20, Jun 03:3, Jun 06:8, Sep 06:5, Dec 07:16, Jan 09:8, Feb 12:8, Mar 13:3, May 13:8

95869 thoracic paraspinal muscles (excluding T1 or T12)

➔ *CPT Changes: An Insider's View* 2003

➔ *CPT Assistant* Nov 97:46, Apr 02:2, May 03:20, Jun 03:3, Feb 04:4, Jun 06:8, Sep 06:5, Jan 09:8, May 10:9, Feb 12:8, Mar 13:3, May 13:8

95870 limited study of muscles in 1 extremity or non-limb (axial) muscles (unilateral or bilateral), other than thoracic paraspinal, cranial nerve supplied muscles, or sphincters

➔ *CPT Changes: An Insider's View* 2000

➔ *CPT Assistant* Nov 97:46, Nov 99:51, Jul 00:2, Apr 02:2, May 03:20, Jun 03:3, Feb 04:4, Jul 04:6, Jun 05:9, Jun 06:8, Sep 06:5, Jan 09:8, Feb 12:8, Mar 13:3, May 13:8, Mar 21:12

(To report a complete study of the extremities, see 95860-95864)

(For anal or urethral sphincter, detrusor, urethra, perineum musculature, see 51785-51792)

(For eye muscles, use 92265)

95872 Needle electromyography using single fiber electrode, with quantitative measurement of jitter, blocking and/or fiber density, any/all sites of each muscle studied

➔ *CPT Assistant* Apr 02:2, May 03:20, Jun 03:3, Sep 06:5, Jan 09:8

#+ 95885 Needle electromyography, each extremity, with related paraspinal areas, when performed, done with nerve conduction, amplitude and latency/velocity study; limited (List separately in addition to code for primary procedure)

➔ *CPT Changes: An Insider's View* 2012

➔ *CPT Assistant* Feb 12:8, Mar 13:3, May 13:8, Sep 13:18, Mar 15:6, Jul 17:10, Nov 20:13

#+ 95886 complete, five or more muscles studied, innervated by three or more nerves or four or more spinal levels (List separately in addition to code for primary procedure)

➔ *CPT Changes: An Insider's View* 2012

➔ *CPT Assistant* Feb 12:8, Mar 13:3, May 13:8, Sep 13:18, Mar 15:6, Jul 17:10, Nov 20:13

(Use 95885, 95886 in conjunction with 95907-95913)

(Do not report 95885, 95886 in conjunction with 95860-95864, 95870, 95905)

(Do not report 95885, 95886 for noninvasive nerve conduction guidance used in conjunction with 0766T)

#+ 95887 Needle electromyography, non-extremity (cranial nerve supplied or axial) muscle(s) done with nerve conduction, amplitude and latency/velocity study (List separately in addition to code for primary procedure)

➔ *CPT Changes: An Insider's View* 2012

➔ *CPT Assistant* Feb 12:8, Jul 12:12, Mar 13:3, Jan 14:8, Mar 15:6, Jul 17:11

(Use 95887 in conjunction with 95907-95913)

(Do not report 95887 in conjunction with 95867-95870, 95905)

(Do not report 95887 for noninvasive nerve conduction guidance used in conjunction with 0766T)

Ischemic Muscle Testing and Guidance for Chemodenervation

+ 95873 Electrical stimulation for guidance in conjunction with chemodenervation (List separately in addition to code for primary procedure)

➔ *CPT Changes: An Insider's View* 2006

➔ *CPT Assistant* Apr 13:5, Jan 14:6, Aug 22:18

(Do not report 95873 in conjunction with 64451, 64617, 64625, 95860-95870, 95874)

+ 95874 Needle electromyography for guidance in conjunction with chemodenervation (List separately in addition to code for primary procedure)

➔ *CPT Changes: An Insider's View* 2006

➔ *CPT Assistant* Apr 13:5, Jan 14:6, Oct 14:15, Dec 20:14, Aug 22:18

(Use 95873, 95874 in conjunction with 64612, 64615, 64616, 64642, 64643, 64644, 64645, 64646, 64647)

(Do not report more than one guidance code for each corresponding chemodenervation code)

(Do not report 95874 in conjunction with 64451, 64617, 64625, 95860-95870, 95873)

95875 Ischemic limb exercise test with serial specimen(s) acquisition for muscle(s) metabolite(s)

➔ *CPT Changes: An Insider's View* 2002, 2003

➔ *CPT Assistant* Jun 03:3

(For listing of nerves considered for separate study, see **Appendix J**)

95885 Code is out of numerical sequence. See 95870-95874

95886 Code is out of numerical sequence. See 95870-95874

95887 Code is out of numerical sequence. See 95870-95874

Nerve Conduction Tests

The following applies to nerve conduction tests (95907-95913): Codes 95907-95913 describe nerve conduction tests when performed with individually placed stimulating, recording, and ground electrodes. The stimulating, recording, and ground electrode placement and the test design must be individualized to the patient's unique anatomy. Nerves tested must be limited to the specific nerves and conduction studies needed for the particular clinical question being investigated. The stimulating electrode must be placed directly over the nerve to be tested, and stimulation parameters properly adjusted to avoid stimulating other nerves or nerve branches. In most motor nerve conduction studies, and in some sensory and mixed nerve conduction studies,

★ = Telemedicine ◀ = Audio-only + = Add-on code ✕ = FDA approval pending # = Resequenced code ⊘ = Modifier 51 exempt ➔➔➔ = See p xxi for details

both proximal and distal stimulation will be used. Motor nerve conduction study recordings must be made from electrodes placed directly over the motor point of the specific muscle to be tested. Sensory nerve conduction study recordings must be made from electrodes placed directly over the specific nerve to be tested. Waveforms must be reviewed on site in real time, and the technique (stimulus site, recording site, ground site, filter settings) must be adjusted, as appropriate, as the test proceeds in order to minimize artifact, and to minimize the chances of unintended stimulation of adjacent nerves and the unintended recording from adjacent muscles or nerves. Reports must be prepared on site by the examiner, and consist of the work product of the interpretation of numerous test results, using well-established techniques to assess the amplitude, latency, and configuration of waveforms elicited by stimulation at each site of each nerve tested. This includes the calculation of nerve conduction velocities, sometimes including specialized F-wave indices, along with comparison to normal values, summarization of clinical and electrodiagnostic data, and physician or other qualified health care professional interpretation. Codes 95907-95913 describe one or more nerve conduction studies. For the purposes of coding, a single conduction study is defined as a sensory conduction test, a motor conduction test with or without an F wave test, or an H-reflex test. Each type of study (sensory, motor with or without F wave, H-reflex) for each nerve includes all orthodromic and antidromic impulses associated with that nerve and constitutes a distinct study when determining the number of studies in each grouping (eg, 1-2 or 3-4 nerve conduction studies). Each type of nerve conduction study is counted only once when multiple sites on the same nerve are stimulated or recorded. The numbers of these separate tests should be added to determine which code to use. For a list of nerves, see Appendix J. Use 95885-95887 in conjunction with 95907-95913 when performing electromyography with nerve conduction studies.

Code 95905 describes nerve conduction tests when performed with preconfigured electrodes customized to a specific anatomic site.

⊘ **95905**   Motor and/or sensory nerve conduction, using preconfigured electrode array(s), amplitude and latency/velocity study, each limb, includes F-wave study when performed, with interpretation and report

➔ *CPT Changes: An Insider's View* 2010

➔ *CPT Assistant* Mar 13:3

(Report 95905 only once per limb studied)

(Do not report 95905 in conjunction with 95885, 95886, 95907-95913)

95907   Nerve conduction studies; 1-2 studies

➔ *CPT Changes: An Insider's View* 2013

➔ *CPT Assistant* Mar 13:3, May 13:8, Sep 13:18, Dec 17:15, Aug 18:11, Sep 22:21

95908   3-4 studies

➔ *CPT Changes: An Insider's View* 2013

➔ *CPT Assistant* Mar 13:3, May 13:8, Sep 13:18, Mar 15:6, Aug 18:11, Sep 22:21

95909   5-6 studies

➔ *CPT Changes: An Insider's View* 2013

➔ *CPT Assistant* Mar 13:3, May 13:8, Sep 13:18, Aug 18:11, Sep 22:21

95910   7-8 studies

➔ *CPT Changes: An Insider's View* 2013

➔ *CPT Assistant* Mar 13:3, May 13:8, Sep 13:18, Aug 18:11, Sep 22:21

95911   9-10 studies

➔ *CPT Changes: An Insider's View* 2013

➔ *CPT Assistant* Mar 13:3, May 13:8, Sep 13:18, Aug 18:11, Sep 22:21

95912   11-12 studies

➔ *CPT Changes: An Insider's View* 2013

➔ *CPT Assistant* Mar 13:3, May 13:8, Sep 13:18, Aug 18:11, Sep 22:21

95913   13 or more studies

➔ *CPT Changes: An Insider's View* 2013

➔ *CPT Assistant* Mar 13:3, May 13:8, Sep 13:18, Aug 18:11, Sep 22:21

(Do not report 95905, 95907, 95908, 95909, 95910, 95911, 95912, 95913 for noninvasive nerve conduction guidance used in conjunction with 0766T)

Intraoperative Neurophysiology

Codes 95940, 95941 describe ongoing neurophysiologic monitoring, testing, and data interpretation distinct from performance of specific type(s) of baseline neurophysiologic study(s) performed during surgical procedures. When the service is performed by the surgeon or anesthesiologist, the professional services are included in the surgeon's or anesthesiologist's primary service code(s) for the procedure and are not reported separately. Do not report these codes for automated monitoring devices that do not require continuous attendance by a professional qualified to interpret the testing and monitoring.

Recording and testing are performed either personally or by a technologist who is physically present with the patient during the service. Supervision is performed either in the operating room or by real time connection outside the operating room. The monitoring professional must be solely dedicated to performing the intraoperative neurophysiologic monitoring and must be available to intervene at all times during the service as necessary, for the reported time period(s). For any given period of time spent providing these services, the service takes full attention and, therefore, other clinical activities beyond providing and interpreting of monitoring cannot be provided during the same period of time.

Throughout the monitoring, there must be provisions for continuous and immediate communication directly with the operating room team in the surgical suite. One or more simultaneous cases may be reported (95941). When monitoring more than one procedure, there must be the immediate ability to transfer patient monitoring to another monitoring professional during the surgical procedure should that individual's exclusive attention be required for another procedure. Report 95941 for all remote or non-one-on-one monitoring time connected to each case regardless of overlap with other cases.

Codes 95940, 95941 include only the ongoing neurophysiologic monitoring time distinct from performance of specific type(s) of baseline neurophysiologic study(s), or other services such as intraoperative functional cortical or subcortical mapping. Codes 95940 and 95941 are reported based upon the time spent monitoring only, and not the number of baseline tests performed or parameters monitored. The time spent performing or interpreting the baseline neurophysiologic study(ies) should not be counted as intraoperative monitoring, but represents separately reportable procedures. When reporting 95940 and 95941, the same neurophysiologic study(ies) performed at baseline should be reported not more than once per operative session. Baseline study reporting is based upon the total unique studies performed. For example, if during the course of baseline testing and one-on-one monitoring, two separate nerves have motor testing performed in conjunction with limited single extremity EMG, then 95885 and 95907 would be reported in addition to 95940. Time spent monitoring (95940, 95941) excludes time to set up, record, and interpret the baseline studies, and to remove electrodes at the end of the procedure. To report time spent waiting on standby for a case to start, use 99360. For procedures that last beyond midnight, report services using the day on which the monitoring began and using the total time monitored.

Code 95940 is reported per 15 minutes of service. Code 95940 requires reporting only the portion of time the monitoring professional was physically present in the operating room providing one-on-one patient monitoring, and no other cases may be monitored at the same time. Time spent in the operating room is cumulative. To determine units of service of 95940, use the total minutes monitoring in the operating room one-on-one. Monitoring may begin prior to incision (eg, when positioning on the table is a time of risk). Report

continuous intraoperative neurophysiologic monitoring in the operating room (95940) in addition to the services related to monitoring from outside the operating room (95941).

Code 95941 should be used once per hour even if multiple methods of neurophysiologic monitoring are used during the time. Code 95941 requires the monitoring of neurophysiological data that is collected from the operating room continuously on-line in real time via a secure data link. When reporting 95941, real-time ability must be available through sufficient data bandwidth transfer rates to view and interrogate the neurophysiologic data contemporaneously.

Report 95941 for all cases in which there was no physical presence by the monitoring professional in the operating room during the monitoring time or when monitoring more than one case in an operating room. It is also used to report the time of monitoring physically performed outside of the operating room in those cases where monitoring occurred both within and outside the operating room. Do not report 95941 if the monitoring lasts 30 minutes or less.

Intraoperative neurophysiology monitoring codes 95940 and 95941 are each used to report the total duration of respective time spent providing each service, even if that time is not in a single continuous block.

#+ 95940   Continuous intraoperative neurophysiology monitoring in the operating room, one on one monitoring requiring personal attendance, each 15 minutes (List separately in addition to code for primary procedure)

➔ *CPT Changes: An Insider's View* 2013

➔ *CPT Assistant* May 13:8-10, Apr 14:5, 11, Aug 17:8, Oct 20:14

(Use 95940 in conjunction with the study performed, 92653, 95822, 95860-95870, 95907-95913, 95925, 95926, 95927, 95928, 95929, 95930-95937, 95938, 95939)

#+ 95941   Continuous intraoperative neurophysiology monitoring, from outside the operating room (remote or nearby) or for monitoring of more than one case while in the operating room, per hour (List separately in addition to code for primary procedure)

➔ *CPT Changes: An Insider's View* 2013

➔ *CPT Assistant* Feb 13:16, May 13:8, Apr 14:5, 11, Dec 14:19, Aug 17:8, Oct 20:14

(Use 95941 in conjunction with the study performed, 92653, 95822, 95860-95870, 95907-95913, 95925, 95926, 95927, 95928, 95929, 95930-95937, 95938, 95939)

(For time spent waiting on standby before monitoring, use 99360)

(For electrocorticography, use 95829)

(For intraoperative EEG during nonintracranial surgery, use 95955)

(For intraoperative functional cortical or subcortical mapping, see 95961-95962)

(For intraoperative neurostimulator programming, see 95971, 95972, 95976, 95977, 95983, 95984)

Autonomic Function Tests

The purpose of autonomic nervous system function testing is to determine the presence of autonomic dysfunction, the site of autonomic dysfunction, and the various autonomic subsystems that may be disordered.

Code 95921 should be reported only when electrocardiographic monitoring of heart rate derived from the time elapsing between two consecutive R waves in the electrocardiogram, or the R-R interval, is displayed on a monitor and stored for subsequent analysis of waveforms. Testing is typically performed in the prone position. A tilt table may be used, but is not required equipment for testing of the parasympathetic function. At least two of the following components need to be included in testing:

1. Heart rate response to deep breathing derived from a visual quantitative analysis of recordings with subject breathing at a rate of 5-6 breaths per minute.

2. Valsalva ratio determined by dividing the maximum heart rate by the lowest heart rate. The initial heart rate responses to sustained oral pressure (blowing into a tube with an open glottis) consist of tachycardia followed by a bradycardia at 15-45 seconds after the Valsalva pressure has been released. A minimum of two Valsalva maneuvers are to be performed. The initial cardioacceleration is an exercise reflex while the subsequent tachycardia and bradycardia are baroreflex-mediated.

3. A 30:15 ratio (R-R interval at beat 30)/(R-R interval at beat 15) used as an index of cardiovascular function.

Code 95922 should be reported only when all of the following components are included in testing:

1. Continuous recording of beat-to-beat BP and heart rate. The heart rate needs to be derived from an electrocardiogram (ECG) unit such that an accurate quantitative graphical measurement of the R-R interval is obtained.

2. A period of supine rest of at least 20 minutes prior to testing.

3. The performance and recording of beat-to-beat blood pressure and heart rate during a minimum of two (2) Valsalva maneuvers.

4. The performance of passive head-up tilt with continuous recording of beat-to-beat blood pressure and heart rate for a minimum of five minutes,

followed by passive tilt-back to the supine position. This must be performed using a tilt table.

Code 95924 should be reported only when both the parasympathetic function and the adrenergic function are tested together with the use of a tilt table.

95919   Quantitative pupillometry with physician or other qualified health care professional interpretation and report, unilateral or bilateral
➡ *CPT Changes: An Insider's View* 2023
➡ *CPT Assistant* Aug 23:14

95921   Testing of autonomic nervous system function; cardiovagal innervation (parasympathetic function), including 2 or more of the following: heart rate response to deep breathing with recorded R-R interval, Valsalva ratio, and 30:15 ratio
➡ *CPT Assistant* Nov 98:35-36, Apr 02:2, Oct 03:11, Feb 06:15, Nov 12:6, Sep 20:7

95922   vasomotor adrenergic innervation (sympathetic adrenergic function), including beat-to-beat blood pressure and R-R interval changes during Valsalva maneuver and at least 5 minutes of passive tilt
➡ *CPT Assistant* Nov 98:35-36, Apr 02:2, Jun 03:11, Feb 06:15, Nov 06:23, Dec 08:4, Nov 12:6, Sep 20:7

(Do not report 95922 in conjunction with 95921)

95923   sudomotor, including 1 or more of the following: quantitative sudomotor axon reflex test (QSART), silastic sweat imprint, thermoregulatory sweat test, and changes in sympathetic skin potential
➡ *CPT Assistant* Nov 98:35-36, Apr 02:2, Feb 06:15, Nov 12:6, Sep 20:7

95924   combined parasympathetic and sympathetic adrenergic function testing with at least 5 minutes of passive tilt
➡ *CPT Changes: An Insider's View* 2013
➡ *CPT Assistant* Nov 12:6, Sep 20:7

(Do not report 95924 in conjunction with 95921 or 95922)

Evoked Potentials and Reflex Tests

95925   Short-latency somatosensory evoked potential study, stimulation of any/all peripheral nerves or skin sites, recording from the central nervous system; in upper limbs
➡ *CPT Assistant* Nov 98:35-36, Apr 02:2, Apr 12:17, May 13:8

(Do not report 95925 in conjunction with 95926)

95926   in lower limbs
➡ *CPT Assistant* May 01:11, Apr 02:2, Apr 12:17, May 13:8

(Do not report 95926 in conjunction with 95925)

95938   in upper and lower limbs
➤ *CPT Changes: An Insider's View* 2012
➤ *CPT Assistant* Apr 12:17-18, Feb 13:17, May 13:8

(Do not report 95938 in conjunction with 95925, 95926)

95927   in the trunk or head
➤ *CPT Assistant* Apr 02:2, May 13:8, Oct 20:9

(To report a unilateral study, use modifier 52)

(For auditory evoked potentials, use 92653)

95928   Central motor evoked potential study (transcranial motor stimulation); upper limbs
➤ *CPT Changes: An Insider's View* 2005
➤ *CPT Assistant* May 13:8, Jan 23:31

(Do not report 95928 in conjunction with 95929)

95929   lower limbs
➤ *CPT Changes: An Insider's View* 2005
➤ *CPT Assistant* May 13:8, Jan 23:31

(Do not report 95929 in conjunction with 95928)

95939   in upper and lower limbs
➤ *CPT Changes: An Insider's View* 2012
➤ *CPT Assistant* Apr 12:17-18, May 13:8, Jan 23:31

(Do not report 95939 in conjunction with 95928, 95929)

95930   Visual evoked potential (VEP) checkerboard or flash testing, central nervous system except glaucoma, with interpretation and report
➤ *CPT Changes: An Insider's View* 2018
➤ *CPT Assistant* May 13:8, Aug 14:8, Feb 18:3

(For visual evoked potential testing for glaucoma, use 0464T)

(For screening of visual acuity using automated visual evoked potential devices, use 0333T)

95933   Orbicularis oculi (blink) reflex, by electrodiagnostic testing
➤ *CPT Assistant* Nov 98:35-36, May 13:8, Jul 17:10

95937   Neuromuscular junction testing (repetitive stimulation, paired stimuli), each nerve, any 1 method
➤ *CPT Assistant* Nov 98:35-36, Apr 02:2, Jun 06:8, Mar 13:3, May 13:8, Feb 16:14, Aug 20:15

95938   Code is out of numerical sequence. See 95912-95933

95939   Code is out of numerical sequence. See 95912-95933

95940   Code is out of numerical sequence. See 95912-95933

95941   Code is out of numerical sequence. See 95912-95933

Special EEG Tests

Codes 95961 and 95962 use physician or other qualified health care professional time as a basis for unit of service. Report 95961 for the first hour of attendance. Use modifier 52 with 95961 for 30 minutes or less. Report 95962 for each additional hour of attendance. Codes 95961, 95962 may be reported with 95700-95726 when functional cortical or subcortical mapping is performed with long-term EEG monitoring.

Codes 95700-95726 describe long-term continuous recording services for electroencephalography (EEG), which are performed to differentiate seizures from other abnormalities, determine type or location of seizures, monitor treatment of seizures and status epilepticus, establish if the patient is a candidate for epilepsy surgery, and/or screen for adverse change in critically ill patients.

The set of codes that describe long-term continuous recording EEG services (95700-95726) is divided into two major groups: (1) technical services, and (2) professional services. Codes 95700-95726 may be reported for any site of service. The technical component of the services is reported with 95700-95716. The professional component of the services is reported with 95717, 95718, 95719, 95720, 95721, 95722, 95723, 95724, 95725, 95726. Diagnostic EEG recording time of less than 2 hours (ie, 1 minute, up to 1 hour and 59 minutes) is not reported separately as a long-term EEG service.

Long-term continuous recording EEG services (95700-95726) are different than routine EEGs (95812, 95813, 95816, 95819, 95822). Routine EEGs capture brain-wave activity within a short duration of testing, defined as less than 2 hours. Long-term continuous recording EEGs capture brain-wave activity for durations of time equal to or greater than 2 hours. The length of recording is based on a number of factors, including the clinical indication for the test and the frequency of seizures.

Use of automated spike and seizure detection and trending software is included in 95700-95726, when performed. Do not report 95957 for use of automated software.

Definitions

EEG technologist: An individual who is qualified by education, training, licensure/certification/regulation (when applicable) in seizure recognition. An EEG technologist(s) performs EEG setup, takedown when performed, patient education, technical description, maintenance, and seizure recognition when within his or her scope of practice and as allowed by law, regulation, and facility policy (when applicable).

Unmonitored: Services that have no real-time monitoring by an EEG technologist(s) during the continuous recording. If the criteria for intermittent or continuous monitoring are not met, then the study is an unmonitored study.

Intermittent monitoring (remote or on-site): Requires an EEG technologist(s) to perform and document real-time review of data at least every 2 hours during the entire recording period to assure the integrity and quality of the recording (ie, EEG, VEEG), identify the need for maintenance, and, when necessary, notify the physician or other qualified health care professional of clinical issues. For intermittent monitoring, a single EEG technologist may monitor a maximum of 12 patients concurrently. If the number of intermittently monitored patients exceeds 12, then all of the studies are reported as unmonitored.

Continuous real-time monitoring (may be provided remotely): Requires all elements of intermittent monitoring. In addition, the EEG technologist(s) performs and documents real-time concurrent monitoring of the EEG data and video (when performed) during the entire recording period. The EEG technologist(s) identifies when events occur and notifies, as instructed, the physician or other qualified health care professional. For continuous monitoring, a single EEG technologist may monitor a maximum of four patients concurrently. If the number of concurrently monitored patients exceeds four, then all of the studies are reported as either unmonitored or intermittent studies. If there is a break in the real-time monitoring of the EEG recording, the study is an intermittent study.

Technical description: The EEG technologist(s)'s written documentation of the reviewed EEG/VEEG data, including technical interventions. The technical description is based on the EEG technologist(s)'s review of data and includes the following required elements: uploading and/or transferring EEG/VEEG data from EEG equipment to a server or storage device; reviewing raw EEG/VEEG data and events and automated detection, as well as patient activations; and annotating, editing, and archiving EEG/VEEG data for review by the physician or other qualified health care professional. For unmonitored services, the EEG technologist(s) annotates the recording for review by the physician or other qualified health care professional and creates a single summary.

Maintenance of long-term EEG equipment: Performed by the EEG technologist(s) and involves ensuring the integrity and quality of the recording(s) (eg, camera position, electrode placement, and impedances).

Setup: Performed in person by the EEG technologist(s) and includes preparing supplies and equipment and securing electrodes using the 10/20 system. Code 95700 is reported only once per recording period on the date the setup was performed. "In person" means that the EEG technologist(s) must be physically present with the patient.

Technical Component Services

Code 95700 describes any long-term continuous EEG/VEEG recording setup, takedown when performed, and patient/caregiver education by the EEG technologist(s). To report 95700, the setup must include a minimum of eight channels of EEG. Services with fewer than eight channels may be reported using 95999. Eight to 15 channels are typically used for neonates and when electrodes cannot be placed on certain regions of the scalp that are sterile. Twenty or more channels are typically used for children and adults. If setup is performed by someone who does not meet the definition of an EEG technologist(s), report 95999.

Codes 95705-95716 describe monitoring, maintenance, review of data, and creating a summary technical description. These codes are divided into four groups based on duration and whether video is utilized. Key elements in determining the appropriate technical code (95705-95716) for long-term EEG continuous recording are: (1) whether diagnostic video recording is captured in conjunction and simultaneously with the EEG service, which is referred to as video-EEG (VEEG), and (2) technologist monitoring for the study (ie, unmonitored, intermittently monitored, or continuously monitored). Codes 95711, 95712, 95713, 95714, 95715, 95716 are reported if diagnostic video of the patient is recorded a minimum of 80% of the time of the entire long-term VEEG service, concurrent with diagnostic EEG recording (ie, the entire study is reported as an EEG without video if concurrent diagnostic video occurs less than 80% of the entire study). Diagnostic EEG recording is an essential component of all long-term EEG services. If diagnostic EEG recording stops, timing stops until the diagnostic EEG is resumed.

Codes 95705, 95706, 95707, 95711, 95712, 95713 are reported when total diagnostic recording time is between 2 and 12 hours, or to capture the final increment of a multiple-day service when the final increment extends 2 to 12 hours beyond the time reported by the appropriate greater-than-12-hour-up-to-26-hour code(s) (95708, 95709, 95710, 95714, 95715, 95716). A maximum of one 2-12 hour code may be reported for an entire long-term EEG service. For example, if the testing lasts 48 hours, but diagnostic recording occurs only in the initial 11 hours and the final 11 hours of the testing period, a single greater-than-12-hour-up-to-26-hour technical code is reported, rather than two 2-12 hour code for the 48-hour service (see the Long-Term EEG Monitoring Table).

Professional Component Services

Codes 95717, 95718, 95719, 95720, 95721, 95722, 95723, 95724, 95725, 95726 describe the professional services performed by a physician or other qualified health care professional for reviewing, analyzing, interpreting, and reporting the results of the continuous recording EEG/VEEG with recommendations based on the findings of the studies. These codes do not include E/M services, which may be reported separately.

Codes 95719, 95720 are used for greater than 12 hours (ie, 12 hours and 1 minute) up to 26 hours of recording. Code selection for professional interpretation for long-term EEG is based on: (1) length of the recording being interpreted, and (2) when the physician or other qualified health care professional reports are generated (ie, whether diagnostic interpretations and reports are made daily during the study, or whether the entire professional interpretation is performed after the entire study is completed). Codes 95717, 95718, 95719, 95720 are reported when: (1) daily professional reports are generated during the long-term recording, even if the entire study extends over multiple days or (2) the time of recording for the entire study is between 2 hours and 36 hours. Codes 95717, 95718 are reported once for each 2-12 hour recording and reported a maximum of once for an entire long-term EEG service. Codes 95719, 95720 are reported once for each greater-than-12-hours-up-to-26-hours recording period. Studies lasting 26 to 36 hours or longer are reported using building blocks and reported using one or more of the greater-than-12-hours-up-to-26-hour code with one 2-12 hour code. The recorded data are reviewed, interpreted, and reported daily by the physician or other qualified health care professional, and summary reports are made for the entire multiple-day study. The summary reports are included in each code (95717, 95718, 95719, 95720, 95721, 95722, 95723, 95724, 95725, 95726) and not reported separately (see the Long-Term EEG Monitoring Table).

For 95721, 95722, 95723, 95724, 95725, 95726, the entire professional interpretation (including retrospective daily reports and a summary report) is made after the entire study is recorded and downloaded at the completion of the study. When the entire professional interpretation is provided for a multiple-day study that is greater than 36 hours, 95721, 95722, 95723, 95724, 95725, 95726 are used to report the entire professional service with the appropriate code determined by the span of diagnostic recording time, as defined by the codes. A single code (95721, 95722, 95723, 95724, 95725, 95726) is reported for the multiple-day study. For example, a long-term EEG recording that spans three

days with a total of 50 hours of VEEG recording would be reported with 95722. Sixty hours and one minute of diagnostic VEEG recording is reported with 95724 (see the Long-Term EEG Monitoring Table).

95954 Pharmacological or physical activation requiring physician or other qualified health care professional attendance during EEG recording of activation phase (eg, thiopental activation test)

➲ *CPT Changes: An Insider's View* 2013

➲ *CPT Assistant* Winter 94:18, Nov 98:35

95955 Electroencephalogram (EEG) during nonintracranial surgery (eg, carotid surgery)

➲ *CPT Assistant* Nov 98:35, Dec 14:19

95957 Digital analysis of electroencephalogram (EEG) (eg, for epileptic spike analysis)

➲ *CPT Assistant* Winter 94:18, Nov 98:35, Nov 10:6, Dec 18:3, Mar 20:8, Nov 22:22

(Do not report 95957 for use of automated software. For use of automated spike and seizure detection and trending software when performed with long-term EEG, see 95700-95726)

95958 Wada activation test for hemispheric function, including electroencephalographic (EEG) monitoring

➲ *CPT Assistant* Nov 98:35

95961 Functional cortical and subcortical mapping by stimulation and/or recording of electrodes on brain surface, or of depth electrodes, to provoke seizures or identify vital brain structures; initial hour of attendance by a physician or other qualified health care professional

➲ *CPT Changes: An Insider's View* 2000, 2013

➲ *CPT Assistant* Winter 94:18, Nov 98:35, Nov 99:52-53, Apr 10:10, Aug 10:13, Feb 11:3, Dec 18:3, Oct 23:24

+ 95962   each additional hour of attendance by a physician or other qualified health care professional (List separately in addition to code for primary procedure)

➲ *CPT Changes: An Insider's View* 2013

➲ *CPT Assistant* Winter 94:18, Nov 98:35, Nov 99:52-53, Apr 10:10, Aug 10:13, Feb 11:3, Oct 23:24

(Use 95962 in conjunction with 95961)

95965 Magnetoencephalography (MEG), recording and analysis; for spontaneous brain magnetic activity (eg, epileptic cerebral cortex localization)

➲ *CPT Changes: An Insider's View* 2002

95966   for evoked magnetic fields, single modality (eg, sensory, motor, language, or visual cortex localization)

➲ *CPT Changes: An Insider's View* 2002

+ 95967 for evoked magnetic fields, each additional modality (eg, sensory, motor, language, or visual cortex localization) (List separately in addition to code for primary procedure)

➜ *CPT Changes: An Insider's View* 2002

➜ *CPT Assistant* Oct 20:9

(Use 95967 in conjunction with 95966)

(For electroencephalography performed in addition to magnetoencephalography, see 95812-95824)

(For somatosensory evoked potentials, auditory evoked potentials, and visual evoked potentials performed in addition to magnetic evoked field responses, see 92653, 95925, 95926, and/or 95930)

(For computerized tomography performed in addition to magnetoencephalography, see 70450-70470, 70496)

(For magnetic resonance imaging performed in addition to magnetoencephalography, see 70551-70553)

Long-term EEG Setup

 # 95700 Electroencephalogram (EEG) continuous recording, with video when performed, setup, patient education, and takedown when performed, administered in person by EEG technologist, minimum of 8 channels

➜ *CPT Changes: An Insider's View* 2020

➜ *CPT Assistant* Mar 20:8

(95700 should be reported once per recording period)

(For EEG using patient-placed electrode sets, use 95999)

(For setup performed by non-EEG technologist or remotely supervised by an EEG technologist, use 95999)

Monitoring

 # 95705 Electroencephalogram (EEG), without video, review of data, technical description by EEG technologist, 2-12 hours; unmonitored

➜ *CPT Changes: An Insider's View* 2020

➜ *CPT Assistant* Mar 20:8

 # 95706 with intermittent monitoring and maintenance

➜ *CPT Changes: An Insider's View* 2020

➜ *CPT Assistant* Mar 20:8

 # 95707 with continuous, real-time monitoring and maintenance

➜ *CPT Changes: An Insider's View* 2020

➜ *CPT Assistant* Mar 20:8

 # 95708 Electroencephalogram (EEG), without video, review of data, technical description by EEG technologist, each increment of 12-26 hours; unmonitored

➜ *CPT Changes: An Insider's View* 2020

➜ *CPT Assistant* Mar 20:8

 # 95709 with intermittent monitoring and maintenance

➜ *CPT Changes: An Insider's View* 2020

➜ *CPT Assistant* Mar 20:8

 # 95710 with continuous, real-time monitoring and maintenance

➜ *CPT Changes: An Insider's View* 2020

➜ *CPT Assistant* Mar 20:8

 # 95711 Electroencephalogram with video (VEEG), review of data, technical description by EEG technologist, 2-12 hours; unmonitored

➜ *CPT Changes: An Insider's View* 2020

➜ *CPT Assistant* Mar 20:8

 # 95712 with intermittent monitoring and maintenance

➜ *CPT Changes: An Insider's View* 2020

➜ *CPT Assistant* Mar 20:8

 # 95713 with continuous, real-time monitoring and maintenance

➜ *CPT Changes: An Insider's View* 2020

➜ *CPT Assistant* Mar 20:8

 # 95714 Electroencephalogram with video (VEEG), review of data, technical description by EEG technologist, each increment of 12-26 hours; unmonitored

➜ *CPT Changes: An Insider's View* 2020

➜ *CPT Assistant* Mar 20:8

 # 95715 with intermittent monitoring and maintenance

➜ *CPT Changes: An Insider's View* 2020

➜ *CPT Assistant* Mar 20:8

 # 95716 with continuous, real-time monitoring and maintenance

➜ *CPT Changes: An Insider's View* 2020

➜ *CPT Assistant* Mar 20:8

(95705, 95706, 95707, 95711, 95712, 95713 may be reported a maximum of once for an entire longer-term EEG service to capture either the entire time of service or the final 2-12 hour increment of a service extending beyond 26 hours)

 # 95717 Electroencephalogram (EEG), continuous recording, physician or other qualified health care professional review of recorded events, analysis of spike and seizure detection, interpretation and report, 2-12 hours of EEG recording; without video

➜ *CPT Changes: An Insider's View* 2020

 # 95718 with video (VEEG)

➜ *CPT Changes: An Insider's View* 2020

(For recording greater than 12 hours, see 95719, 95720, 95721, 95722, 95723, 95724, 95725, 95726)

(95717, 95718 may be reported a maximum of once for an entire long-term EEG service to capture either the entire time of service or the final 2-12 hour increment of a service extending beyond 24 hours)

Long-Term EEG Monitoring Table					
	Professional Services		Technical Services		
Duration of Long-Term EEG/VEEG Recording	With Report Each 24 Hours	With Report at Conclusion of Entire Recording Period	Unmonitored	Intermittent	Continuous
Less than 120 minutes (w/video or w/out video)	Not reported separately	See 95812/95813	Not reported separately	Not reported separately	Not reported separately
2 to 12 hours (w/out video)	95717 x 1		95705 x 1	95706 x 1	95707 x 1
2 to 12 hours (w/video)	95718 x 1		95711 x 1	95712 x 1	95713 x 1
12 hours and 1 minute to 26 hours (w/out video)	95719 x 1		95708 x 1	95709 x 1	95710 x 1
12 hours and 1 minute to 26 hours (w/video)	95720 x 1		95714 x 1	95715 x 1	95716 x 1
26 hours and 1 minute to 36 hours (w/out video)	95719 x 1 and 95717 x 1		95708 x 1 and 95705 x 1	95709 x 1 and 95706 x 1	95710 x 1 and 95707 x 1
26 hours and 1 minute to 36 hours (w/video)	95720 x 1 and 95718 x 1		95714 x 1 and 95711 x 1	95715 x 1 and 95712 x 1	95716 x 1 and 95713 x 1
36 hours and 1 minute to 50 hours (w/out video)	95719 x 2	95721 x 1	95708 x 2	95709 x 2	95710 x 2
36 hours and 1 minute to 50 hours (w/video)	95720 x 2	95722 x 1	95714 x 2	95715 x 2	95716 x 2
50 hours and 1 minute to 60 hours (w/out video)	95719 x 2 and 95717 x 1	95721 x 1	95708 x 2 and 95705 x 1	95709 x 2 and 95706 x 1	95710 x 2 and 95707 x 1
50 hours and 1 minute to 60 hours (w/video)	95720 x 2 and 95718 x 1	95722 x 1	95714 x 2 and 95711 x 1	95715 x 2 and 95712 x 1	95716 x 2 and 95713 x 1
60 hours and 1 minute to 74 hours (w/out video)	95719 x 3	95723 x 1	95708 x 3	95709 x 3	95710 x 3
60 hours and 1 minute to 74 hours (w/video)	95720 x 3	95724 x 1	95714 x 3	95715 x 3	95716 x 3
74 hours and 1 minute to 84 hours (w/out video)	95719 x 3 and 95717 x 1	95723 x 1	95708 x 3 and 95705 x 1	95709 x 3 and 95706 x 1	95710 x 3 and 95707 x 1
74 hours and 1 minute to 84 hours (w/video)	95720 x 3 and 95718 x 1	95724 x 1	95714 x 3 and 95711 x 1	95715 x 3 and 95712 x 1	95716 x 3 and 95713 x 1
84 hours and 1 minute to 98 hours (w/out video)	95719 x 4	95725 x 1	95708 x 4	95709 x 4	95710 x 4
84 hours and 1 minute to 98 hours (w/video)	95720 x 4	95726 x 1	95714 x 4	95715 x 4	95716 x 4

★ = Telemedicine   ◀ = Audio-only   ✚ = Add-on code   ✗ = FDA approval pending   # = Resequenced code   ⊘ = Modifier 51 exempt   ➔➔➔ = See p xxi for details

95719   Electroencephalogram (EEG), continuous recording, physician or other qualified health care professional review of recorded events, analysis of spike and seizure detection, each increment of greater than 12 hours, up to 26 hours of EEG recording, interpretation and report after each 24-hour period; without video

➔ *CPT Changes: An Insider's View* 2020

95720   with video (VEEG)

➔ *CPT Changes: An Insider's View* 2020

(95719, 95720 may be reported only once for a recording period greater than 12 hours up to 26 hours. For multiple-day studies, 95719, 95720 may be reported after each 24-hour period during the extended recording period. 95719, 95720 describe reporting for a 26-hour recording period, whether done as a single report or as multiple reports during the same time)

(95717, 95718 may be reported in conjunction with 95719, 95720 for studies lasting greater than 26 hours)

(Do not report 95717, 95718, 95719, 95720 for professional interpretation of long-term EEG studies when the recording is greater than 36 hours and the entire professional report is retroactively generated, even if separate daily reports are rendered after the completion of recording)

(When the entire study includes recording greater than 36 hours, and the professional interpretation is performed after the entire recording is completed, see 95721, 95722, 95723, 95724, 95725, 95726)

95721   Electroencephalogram (EEG), continuous recording, physician or other qualified health care professional review of recorded events, analysis of spike and seizure detection, interpretation, and summary report, complete study; greater than 36 hours, up to 60 hours of EEG recording, without video

➔ *CPT Changes: An Insider's View* 2020

95722   greater than 36 hours, up to 60 hours of EEG recording, with video (VEEG)

➔ *CPT Changes: An Insider's View* 2020

95723   greater than 60 hours, up to 84 hours of EEG recording, without video

➔ *CPT Changes: An Insider's View* 2020

95724   greater than 60 hours, up to 84 hours of EEG recording, with video (VEEG)

➔ *CPT Changes: An Insider's View* 2020

95725   greater than 84 hours of EEG recording, without video

➔ *CPT Changes: An Insider's View* 2020

95726   greater than 84 hours of EEG recording, with video (VEEG)

➔ *CPT Changes: An Insider's View* 2020

(When the entire study includes recording greater than 36 hours, and the professional interpretation is performed after the entire recording is completed, see 95721, 95722, 95723, 95724, 95725, 95726)

(Do not report 95721, 95722, 95723, 95724, 95725, 95726 in conjunction with 95717, 95718, 95719, 95720)

Neurostimulators, Analysis-Programming

Electronic analysis of an implanted neurostimulator pulse generator/transmitter involves documenting settings and electrode impedances of the system parameters prior to programming. Programming involves adjusting the system parameter(s) to address clinical signs and patient symptoms. Parameters available for programming can vary between systems and may need to be adjusted multiple times during a single programming session. The iterative adjustments to parameters provide information that is required for the physician or other qualified health care professional to assess and select the most appropriate final program parameters to provide for consistent delivery of appropriate therapy. The values of the final program parameters may differ from the starting values after the programming session.

Examples of parameters include: contact group(s), interleaving, amplitude, pulse width, frequency (Hz), on/off cycling, burst, magnet mode, dose lockout, patient-selectable parameters, responsive neurostimulation, detection algorithms, closed-loop parameters, and passive parameters. Not all parameters are available for programming in every neurostimulator pulse generator/transmitter.

For coding purposes, a neurostimulator system is considered implanted when the electrode array(s) is inserted into the target area for either permanent or trial placement.

There are several types of implantable neurostimulator pulse generator/transmitters and they are differentiated by the nervous system region that is stimulated. A brain neurostimulator may stimulate either brain surface regions (cortical stimulation) or deep brain structures (deep brain stimulation). A brain neurostimulation system consists of array(s) that targets one or more of these regions.

A cranial nerve neurostimulator targets the fibers of the cranial nerves or their branches and divisions. There are 12 pairs of cranial nerves (see nerve anatomy figure on page 851 [of the codebook]). Each cranial nerve has its origin in the brain and passes through one or more foramina in the skull to innervate extracranial structures.

A cranial nerve neurostimulator stimulates the nerve fibers of either the extracranial or intracranial portion(s) of one or more cranial nerve(s) (eg, vagus nerve, trigeminal nerve).

A spinal cord or peripheral nerve neurostimulator targets nerve(s) that originate in the spinal cord and exit the spine through neural foramina and gives rise to peripheral nerves. The peripheral nervous system consists of the nerves and ganglia outside of the brain and spinal cord. Peripheral nerves may give rise to independent branches or branches that combine with other peripheral nerves in neural plexuses (ie, brachial plexus, lumbosacral plexus). Under the lumbosacral plexus, the sacral nerves (specifically S2, S3, S4) are located in the lower back just above the tailbone. Neurostimulation of the sacral nerves affect pelvic floor muscles and urinary organs (eg, bladder, urinary sphincter).

Cranial nerve, spinal cord, peripheral nerve, and sacral nerve neurostimulator analysis with programming (95971, 95972, 95976, 95977) are reported based on the number of parameters adjusted during a programming session. Brain neurostimulator analysis with programming (95983, 95984) is reported based on physician or other qualified health care professional face-to-face time.

Code 95970 describes electronic analysis of the implanted brain, cranial nerve, spinal cord, peripheral nerve, or sacral nerve neurostimulator pulse generator/transmitter without programming. Electronic analysis is inherent to implantation codes 43647, 43648, 43881, 43882, 61850, 61860, 61863, 61864, 61867, 61868, 61880, 61885, 61886, 61888, 63650, 63655, 63661, 63662, 63663, 63664, 63685, 63688, 64553, 64555, 64561, 64566, 64568, 64569, 64570, 64575, 64580, 64581, 64585, 64590, 64595, and is not separately reportable at the same operative session.

Codes 95971, 95972, 95976, 95977 describe electronic analysis with simple or complex programming of the implanted neurostimulator pulse generator/transmitter. *Simple* programming of a neurostimulator pulse generator/transmitter includes adjustment of one to three parameter(s). *Complex* programming includes adjustment of more than three parameters. For purposes of counting the number of parameters being programmed, a single parameter that is adjusted two or more times during a programming session counts as one parameter.

Code 95971 describes electronic analysis with simple programming of an implanted spinal cord or peripheral nerve (eg, sacral nerve) neurostimulator pulse generator/transmitter.

Code 95972 describes electronic analysis with complex programming of an implanted spinal cord or peripheral nerve (eg, sacral nerve) neurostimulator pulse generator/transmitter.

Code 95976 describes electronic analysis with simple programming of an implanted cranial nerve neurostimulator pulse generator/transmitter.

Code 95977 describes electronic analysis with complex programming of an implanted cranial nerve neurostimulator pulse generator/transmitter.

Codes 95983, 95984 describe electronic analysis with programming of an implanted brain neurostimulator pulse generator/transmitter. Code 95983 is reported for the first 15 minutes of physician or other qualified health care professional face-to-face time for analysis and programming. Code 95984 is reported for each additional 15 minutes. A unit of service is attained when the mid-point is passed. Physician or other qualified health care professional face-to-face time of less than eight minutes is not separately reportable.

Code 95980 describes intraoperative electronic analysis of an implanted gastric neurostimulator pulse generator system, with programming; code 95981 describes subsequent analysis of the device; code 95982 describes subsequent analysis and reprogramming. For electronic analysis and reprogramming of gastric neurostimulator, lesser curvature, see 95980-95982.

Codes 95971, 95972, 95976, 95977, 95983, 95984 are reported when programming a neurostimulator is performed by a physician or other qualified health care professional. Programming may be performed in the operating room, postoperative care unit, inpatient, and/or outpatient setting. Programming a neurostimulator in the operating room is not inherent in the service represented by the implantation code and may be reported by either the implanting surgeon or other qualified health care professional, when performed.

Test stimulations are typically performed during an implantation procedure (43647, 43648, 43881, 43882, 61850, 61860, 61863, 61864, 61867, 61868, 61880, 61885, 61886, 61888, 63650, 63655, 63661, 63662, 63663, 63664, 63685, 63688, 64553, 64555, 64561, 64566, 64568, 64569, 64570, 64575, 64580, 64581, 64582, 64583, 64584, 64585, 64590, 64595) to confirm correct target site placement of the electrode array(s) and/or to confirm the functional status of the system. Test stimulation is not considered electronic analysis or programming of the neurostimulator system (test stimulation is included in the service described by the implantation code) and should not be reported with 95970, 95971, 95972, 95980, 95981, 95982, 95983, 95984. Electronic analysis of a device (95970) is not reported separately at the time of implantation.

★=Telemedicine ◀=Audio-only ✛=Add-on code ✗=FDA approval pending #=Resequenced code ⊘=Modifier 51 exempt ⮞⮞⮞=See p xxi for details

Cranial Nerves

Illustration of the 12 cranial nerves and their areas of innervation.

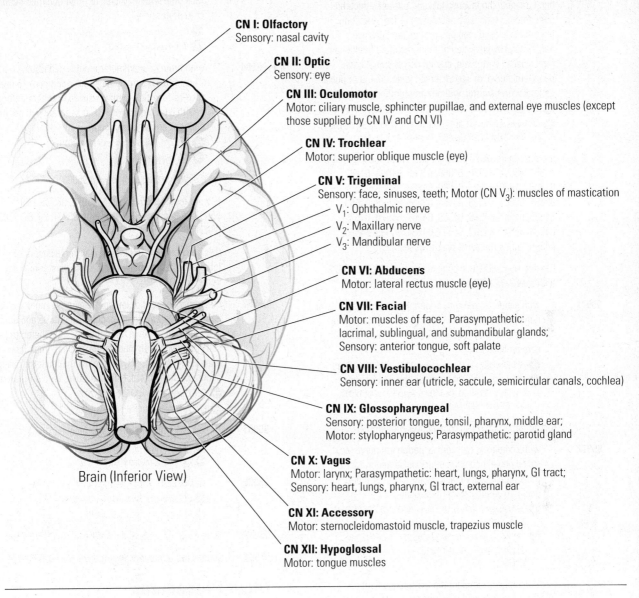

Brain (Inferior View)

CN I: Olfactory
Sensory: nasal cavity

CN II: Optic
Sensory: eye

CN III: Oculomotor
Motor: ciliary muscle, sphincter pupillae, and external eye muscles (except those supplied by CN IV and CN VI)

CN IV: Trochlear
Motor: superior oblique muscle (eye)

CN V: Trigeminal
Sensory: face, sinuses, teeth; Motor (CN V_3): muscles of mastication
V_1: Ophthalmic nerve
V_2: Maxillary nerve
V_3: Mandibular nerve

CN VI: Abducens
Motor: lateral rectus muscle (eye)

CN VII: Facial
Motor: muscles of face; Parasympathetic: lacrimal, sublingual, and submandibular glands; Sensory: anterior tongue, soft palate

CN VIII: Vestibulocochlear
Sensory: inner ear (utricle, saccule, semicircular canals, cochlea)

CN IX: Glossopharyngeal
Sensory: posterior tongue, tonsil, pharynx, middle ear; Motor: stylopharyngeus; Parasympathetic: parotid gland

CN X: Vagus
Motor: larynx; Parasympathetic: heart, lungs, pharynx, GI tract; Sensory: heart, lungs, pharynx, GI tract, external ear

CN XI: Accessory
Motor: sternocleidomastoid muscle, trapezius muscle

CN XII: Hypoglossal
Motor: tongue muscles

(For insertion of neurostimulator pulse generator, see 61885, 61886, 63685, 64568, 64582, 64590)

(For revision or removal of neurostimulator pulse generator or receiver, see 61888, 63688, 64569, 64570, 64583, 64584, 64595)

(For implantation of neurostimulator electrodes, see 43647, 43881, 61850-61868, 63650, 63655, 64553-64581. For revision or removal of neurostimulator electrodes, see 43648, 43882, 61880, 63661, 63662, 63663, 63664, 64569, 64570, 64583, 64584, 64585)

(For analysis and programming of implanted integrated neurostimulation system, posterior tibial nerve, see 0589T, 0590T)

95970 Electronic analysis of implanted neurostimulator pulse generator/transmitter (eg, contact group[s], interleaving, amplitude, pulse width, frequency [Hz], on/off cycling, burst, magnet mode, dose lockout, patient selectable parameters, responsive neurostimulation, detection algorithms, closed loop parameters, and passive parameters) by physician or other qualified health care professional; with brain, cranial nerve, spinal cord, peripheral nerve, or sacral nerve, neurostimulator pulse generator/transmitter, without programming

➜ CPT Changes: An Insider's View 2000, 2012, 2019

➜ CPT Assistant Nov 98:36-37, Sep 99:1, Nov 99:53-54, Aug 05:7, Sep 05:10, Oct 12:15, Jul 16:7, Oct 18:8, Mar 24:11

(Do not report 95970 in conjunction with 43647, 43648, 43881, 43882, 61850, 61860, 61863, 61864, 61867, 61868, 61880, 61885, 61886, 61888, 63650, 63655, 63661, 63662, 63663, 63664, 63685, 63688, 64553, 64555, 64561, 64566, 64568, 64569, 64570, 64575, 64580, 64581, 64582, 64583, 64584, 64585, 64590, 64595, during the same operative session)

(Do not report 95970 in conjunction with 95971, 95972, 95976, 95977, 95983, 95984)

95971 with simple spinal cord or peripheral nerve (eg, sacral nerve) neurostimulator pulse generator/transmitter programming by physician or other qualified health care professional

➜ CPT Changes: An Insider's View 2000, 2005, 2012, 2019

➜ CPT Assistant Nov 98:36-37, Sep 99:1, Nov 99:53-54, Aug 05:7, Oct 10:14, Dec 10:14, Apr 11:11, Oct 12:15, Jul 16:7, Oct 18:8, Mar 24:11

(Do not report 95971 in conjunction with 95972)

95972 with complex spinal cord or peripheral nerve (eg, sacral nerve) neurostimulator pulse generator/transmitter programming by physician or other qualified health care professional

➜ CPT Changes: An Insider's View 2000, 2005, 2012, 2015, 2016, 2019

➜ CPT Assistant Nov 98:36-37, Sep 99:1, Nov 99:53-54, Aug 05:7, Apr 11:10, Oct 12:15, Aug 14:5, Jul 16:7, Oct 18:8, Mar 24:11

(For percutaneous implantation or replacement of integrated neurostimulation system, posterior tibial nerve, use 0587T)

95976 with simple cranial nerve neurostimulator pulse generator/transmitter programming by physician or other qualified health care professional

➜ CPT Changes: An Insider's View 2019

(Do not report 95976 in conjunction with 95977)

95977 with complex cranial nerve neurostimulator pulse generator/transmitter programming by physician or other qualified health care professional

➜ CPT Changes: An Insider's View 2019

 # 95983 with brain neurostimulator pulse generator/transmitter programming, first 15 minutes face-to-face time with physician or other qualified health care professional

➜ CPT Changes: An Insider's View 2019

➜ CPT Assistant Dec 18:3

#+ 95984 with brain neurostimulator pulse generator/transmitter programming, each additional 15 minutes face-to-face time with physician or other qualified health care professional (List separately in addition to code for primary procedure)

➜ CPT Changes: An Insider's View 2019

➜ CPT Assistant Dec 18:3

(Use 95984 in conjunction with 95983)

(Do not report 95970, 95971, 95972, 95976, 95977, 95983, 95984 in conjunction with 0587T, 0588T, 0589T, 0590T)

(For percutaneous implantation or replacement of integrated neurostimulation system, posterior tibial nerve, use 0587T)

95980 Electronic analysis of implanted neurostimulator pulse generator system (eg, rate, pulse amplitude and duration, configuration of wave form, battery status, electrode selectability, output modulation, cycling, impedance and patient measurements) gastric neurostimulator pulse generator/transmitter; intraoperative, with programming

➜ CPT Changes: An Insider's View 2008

➜ CPT Assistant Jan 08:8, Nov 10:8, Jul 16:7

95981 subsequent, without reprogramming

➜ CPT Changes: An Insider's View 2008

➜ CPT Assistant Jan 08:8, Jul 16:7

95982 subsequent, with reprogramming

➜ CPT Changes: An Insider's View 2008

➜ CPT Assistant Jan 08:8, Jul 16:7

95983 Code is out of numerical sequence. See 95976-95981

95984 Code is out of numerical sequence. See 95976-95981

Other Procedures

95990 Refilling and maintenance of implantable pump or reservoir for drug delivery, spinal (intrathecal, epidural) or brain (intraventricular), includes electronic analysis of pump, when performed;

➜ CPT Changes: An Insider's View 2003, 2012

➜ CPT Assistant Nov 02:4, Nov 05:1, Jul 06:1, Jul 12:6, Aug 12:10-12, 15, May 22:18

★ = Telemedicine   ◀ = Audio-only   ✚ = Add-on code   ✗ = FDA approval pending   # = Resequenced code   ⊘ = Modifier 51 exempt   ➜➜➜ = See p xxi for details

Physician or Other Qualified Health Care Professional Face-to-Face Time for Brain Neurostimulator Analysis With Programming	Code(s)
Less than 8 minutes	Not reported
8-22 minutes	95983 X 1
23-37 minutes	95983 X 1 + 95984 X 1
38-52 minutes	95983 X 1 + 95984 X 2
53-67 minutes	95983 X 1 + 95984 X 3
68 minutes or longer	add units of 95984

95991   requiring skill of a physician or other qualified health care professional

> *CPT Changes: An Insider's View* 2004, 2012, 2013

> *CPT Assistant* Nov 05:1, Jul 06:1, Jul 12:6, Aug 12:10-12, 15, May 22:18

(Do not report 95990, 95991 in conjunction with 62367-62370. For analysis and/or reprogramming of implantable infusion pump, see 62367-62370)

(For refill and maintenance of implanted infusion pump or reservoir for systemic drug therapy [eg, chemotherapy], use 96522)

—— *Coding Tip* ——

Instructions for Use of the CPT Codebook

When advanced practice nurses and physician assistants are working with physicians, they are considered as working in the exact same specialty and subspecialty as the physician. A "physician or other qualified health care professional" is an individual who is qualified by education, training, licensure/regulation (when applicable), and facility privileging (when applicable) who performs a professional service within his or her scope of practice and independently reports that professional service. These professionals are distinct from "clinical staff." A clinical staff member is a person who works under the supervision of a physician or other qualified health care professional, and who is allowed by law, regulation, and facility policy to perform or assist in the performance of a specific professional service, but does not individually report that professional service. Other policies may also affect who may report specific services.

CPT Coding Guidelines, Introduction, Instructions for Use of the CPT Codebook

95992   Canalith repositioning procedure(s) (eg, Epley maneuver, Semont maneuver), per day

> *CPT Changes: An Insider's View* 2009, 2020

(Do not report 95992 in conjunction with 92531, 92532)

95999   Unlisted neurological or neuromuscular diagnostic procedure

> *CPT Assistant* Feb 99:11, Jan 02:11, Mar 07:4, Apr 07:7, Dec 08:10, Aug 15:8, Aug 18:11, Mar 20:8

Motion Analysis

▶Codes 96000-96004 describe services performed as part of a major therapeutic or diagnostic decision making process. Motion analysis is performed in a dedicated motion analysis laboratory (ie, a facility capable of performing videotaping from the front, back and both sides, computerized 3D kinematics, 3D kinetics, and dynamic electromyography). Code 96000 may include 3D kinetics and stride characteristics. Code 96002 describes dynamic electromyography.◀

Code 96004 should only be reported once regardless of the number of study(ies) reviewed/interpreted.

(For performance of needle electromyography procedures, see 95860-95870, 95872, 95885-95887)

(For gait training, use 97116)

96000   Comprehensive computer-based motion analysis by video-taping and 3D kinematics;

> *CPT Changes: An Insider's View* 2002

> *CPT Assistant* Aug 02:5, Jun 03:2, Mar 22:14, Oct 23:13

96001   with dynamic plantar pressure measurements during walking

> *CPT Changes: An Insider's View* 2002

> *CPT Assistant* Aug 02:5, Jun 03:2

96002   Dynamic surface electromyography, during walking or other functional activities, 1-12 muscles

> *CPT Changes: An Insider's View* 2002

> *CPT Assistant* Aug 02:5, Jun 03:3, Aug 15:8

▶(Do not report 96002 in conjunction with 95860-95866, 95869-95872, 95885-95887)◀

▶(96003 has been deleted)◀

96004 Review and interpretation by physician or other qualified health care professional of comprehensive computer-based motion analysis, dynamic plantar pressure measurements, dynamic surface electromyography during walking or other functional activities, and dynamic fine wire electromyography, with written report

➜ *CPT Changes: An Insider's View* 2002, 2013

➜ *CPT Assistant* Aug 02:5, Jun 03:3, Aug 15:8, Oct 23:13

Functional Brain Mapping

Code 96020 includes selection and administration of testing of language, memory, cognition, movement, sensation, and other neurological functions when conducted in association with functional neuroimaging, monitoring of performance of this testing, and determination of validity of neurofunctional testing relative to separately interpreted functional magnetic resonance images.

96020 Neurofunctional testing selection and administration during noninvasive imaging functional brain mapping, with test administered entirely by a physician or other qualified health care professional (ie, psychologist), with review of test results and report

➜ *CPT Changes: An Insider's View* 2007, 2013

➜ *CPT Assistant* Feb 07:6

➜ *Clinical Examples in Radiology* Fall 23:13

(For functional magnetic resonance imaging [fMRI], brain, use 70555)

(Do not report 96020 in conjunction with 96112, 96113, 96116, 96121, 96130, 96131, 96132, 96133)

(Do not report 96020 in conjunction with 70554)

(Evaluation and Management services codes should not be reported on the same day as 96020)

Medical Genetics and Genetic Counseling Services

▶These services are provided by trained genetic counselors and may include obtaining a structured family genetic history, pedigree construction, analysis for genetic risk assessment, and counseling of the patient and family.◀

▶Total Time of Medical Genetics and Genetic Counseling Services on the Date of the Encounter	Code(s)
Less than 16 minutes	Not reported separately
16-45 minutes	96041 X 1
46-75 minutes	96041 X 2
76-105 minutes	96041 X 3
106-135 minutes	96041 X 4◀

▶(96040 has been deleted. To report medical genetics and genetic counseling services, use 96041)◀

★◀● **96041** Medical genetics and genetic counseling services, each 30 minutes of total time provided by the genetic counselor on the date of the encounter

➜ *CPT Changes: An Insider's View* 2025

▶(Do not report 96041 for less than 16 minutes of genetic counselor time)◀

▶(For education regarding genetic risks by a nonphysician to a group, see 98961, 98962)◀

▶(For genetic counseling and education to a group by a physician or other qualified health care professional, use 99078)◀

▶(For genetic counseling and/or risk factor reduction intervention provided to patient[s] without symptoms or established disease, by a physician or other qualified health care professional who may report evaluation and management services, see 99401-99412)◀

▶(For genetic counseling and education provided to an individual by a physician or other qualified health care professional who may report evaluation and management services, see the appropriate evaluation and management codes)◀

Adaptive Behavior Services

Adaptive behavior services address deficient adaptive behaviors (eg, impaired social, communication, or self-care skills), maladaptive behaviors (eg, repetitive and stereotypic behaviors, behaviors that risk physical harm to the patient, others, and/or property), or other impaired functioning secondary to deficient adaptive or maladaptive behaviors, including, but not limited to, instruction-following, verbal and nonverbal communication, imitation, play and leisure, social interactions, self-care, daily living, and personal safety.

Definitions

Functional behavior assessment: comprises descriptive assessment procedures designed to identify environmental events that occur just before and just after occurrences of potential target behaviors and that may influence those behaviors. That information may be gathered by interviewing the patient's caregivers; having caregivers complete checklists, rating scales, or questionnaires; and/or observing and recording occurrences of target behaviors and environmental events in everyday situations.

Functional analysis: an assessment procedure for evaluating the separate effects of each of several environmental events on a potential target behavior by systematically presenting and withdrawing each event to a patient multiple times and observing and measuring occurrences of the behavior in response to those events. Graphed data are analyzed visually to determine which events produced relatively high and low occurrences of the behavior.

Standardized instruments and procedures: include, but not limited to, behavior checklists, rating scales, and adaptive skill assessment instruments that comprise a fixed set of items and are administered and scored in a uniform way with all patients (eg, Pervasive Developmental Disabilities Behavior Inventory, Brigance Inventory of Early Development, Vineland Adaptive Behavior Scales).

Nonstandardized instruments and procedures: include, but not limited to, curriculum-referenced assessments, stimulus preference assessment procedures, and other procedures for assessing behaviors and associated environmental events that are specific to the individual patient and behaviors.

Adaptive Behavior Assessments

Behavior identification assessment (97151) is conducted by the physician or other qualified health care professional and may include analysis of pertinent past data (including medical diagnosis), a detailed behavioral history, patient observation, administration of standardized and/or non-standardized instruments and procedures, functional behavior assessment, functional analysis, and/or guardian/caregiver interview to identify and describe deficient adaptive behaviors, maladaptive behaviors, and other impaired functioning secondary to deficient adaptive or maladaptive behaviors. Code 97151 includes the physician's or other qualified health care professional's scoring of assessments, interpretation of results, discussion of findings and recommendations with the primary guardian(s)/caregiver(s), preparation of report, and development of plan of care, which may include behavior identification supporting assessment (97152) or behavior identification–supporting assessment with four required components (0362T).

Behavior identification supporting assessment (97152) is administered by a technician under the direction of a physician or other qualified health care professional. The physician or other qualified health care professional may or may not be on site during the face-to-face assessment process. Code 97152 includes the physician's or other qualified health care professional's interpretation of results and may include functional behavior assessment, functional analysis, and other structured observations and/or standardized and/or nonstandardized instruments and procedures to determine levels of adaptive and maladaptive behavior.

Codes 97152, 0362T may be reported separately with 97151 based on the time that the patient is face-to-face with one or more technician(s). Only count the time of one technician when two or more are present.

For behavior identification–supporting assessment with four required components, use 0362T.

—— *Coding Tip* ——

If the physician or other qualified health care professional personally performs the technician activities, his or her time engaged in these activities should be included as part of the required technician time to meet the components of the code.

97151 **Behavior identification assessment,** administered by a physician or other qualified health care professional, each 15 minutes of the physician's or other qualified health care professional's time face-to-face with patient and/or guardian(s)/caregiver(s) administering assessments and discussing findings and recommendations, and non-face-to-face analyzing past data, scoring/interpreting the assessment, and preparing the report/treatment plan

➔ *CPT Changes: An Insider's View* 2019

➔ *CPT Assistant* Nov 18:3

97152 **Behavior identification-supporting assessment,** administered by one technician under the direction of a physician or other qualified health care professional, face-to-face with the patient, each 15 minutes

➔ *CPT Changes: An Insider's View* 2019

➔ *CPT Assistant* Nov 18:3

(97151, 97152, 0362T may be repeated on the same or different days until the behavior identification assessment [97151] and, if necessary, supporting assessment[s] [97152, 0362T], is complete)

(For psychiatric diagnostic evaluation, see 90791, 90792)

(For speech evaluations, see 92521, 92522, 92523, 92524)

(For occupational therapy evaluation, see 97165, 97166, 97167, 97168)

(For medical team conference, see 99366, 99367, 99368)

(For health and behavior assessment/intervention, see 96156, 96158, 96159, 96164, 96165, 96167, 96168, 96170, 96171)

(For neurobehavioral status exam, see 96116, 96121)

(For neuropsychological testing, see 96132, 96133, 96136, 96137, 96138, 96139, 96146)

Guide to Selection of Codes 97152 and 0362T

	97152	0362T
Physician or other qualified health care professional required to be on site		✓
Physician or other qualified health care professional not required to be on site	✓	
Number of technicians	1	2 or more
Deficient adaptive behavior(s), maladaptive behavior(s), or other impaired functioning secondary to deficient adaptive or maladaptive behaviors	✓	
Destructive behavior(s)		✓
May include functional behavior assessment	✓	✓
May include functional analysis	✓	✓
Environment customized to patient and behavior		✓

Adaptive Behavior Treatment

Adaptive behavior treatment codes 97153, 97154, 97155, 97156, 97157, 97158, 0373T describe services that address specific treatment targets and goals based on results of previous assessments (see 97151, 97152, 0362T), and include ongoing assessment and adjustment of treatment protocols, targets, and goals.

Adaptive behavior treatment by protocol (97153) and **group adaptive behavior treatment by protocol** (97154) are administered by a technician under the direction of a physician or other qualified health care professional, utilizing a treatment protocol designed in advance by the physician or other qualified health care professional, who may or may not provide direction during the treatment. Code 97153 describes face-to-face services with one patient and code 97154 describes face-to-face services with two or more patients. Do not report 97154 if the group is larger than eight patients.

Adaptive behavior treatment with protocol modification (97155) is administered by a physician or other qualified health care professional face-to-face with a single patient. The physician or other qualified health care professional resolves one or more problems with the protocol and may simultaneously direct a technician in administering the modified protocol while the patient is present. Physician or other qualified health care professional direction to the technician without the patient present is not reported separately.

Family adaptive behavior treatment guidance and **multiple-family group adaptive behavior treatment guidance** (97156, 97157) are administered by a physician or other qualified health care professional face-to-face with guardian(s)/caregiver(s) and involve identifying potential treatment targets and training guardian(s)/caregiver(s) of one patient (97156) or multiple patients (97157) to implement treatment protocols designed to address deficient adaptive or maladaptive behaviors. Services described by 97156 may be performed with or without the patient present. Services described by 97157 are performed without the patient present. Do not report 97157 if the group has more than eight patients' guardian(s)/caretaker(s).

Group adaptive behavior treatment with protocol modification (97158) is administered by a physician or other qualified health care professional face-to-face with multiple patients. The physician or other qualified health care professional monitors the needs of individual patients and adjusts the treatment techniques during the group sessions, as needed. In contrast to group adaptive behavior treatment by protocol (97154), protocol adjustments are made in real time rather than for a subsequent service. Do not report 97158 if the group has more than eight patients.

For adaptive behavior treatment with protocol modification with four required components, use 0373T.

—— *Coding Tip* ——

If the physician or other qualified health care professional personally performs the technician activities, his or her time engaged in these activities should be reported as technician time.

 # 97153 **Adaptive behavior treatment by protocol,** administered by technician under the direction of a physician or other qualified health care professional, face-to-face with one patient, each 15 minutes

➔ *CPT Changes: An Insider's View* 2019
➔ *CPT Assistant* Nov 18:3, Jul 20:10

(Do not report 97153 in conjunction with 90785-90899, 92507, 96105-96171, 97129)

 # 97154 **Group adaptive behavior treatment by protocol,** administered by technician under the direction of a physician or other qualified health care professional, face-to-face with two or more patients, each 15 minutes

➔ *CPT Changes: An Insider's View* 2019
➔ *CPT Assistant* Nov 18:3

(Do not report 97154 if the group has more than 8 patients)

(Do not report 97154 in conjunction with 90785-90899, 92508, 96105-96171, 97150)

97155   **Adaptive behavior treatment with protocol modification,** administered by physician or other qualified health care professional, which may include simultaneous direction of technician, face-to-face with one patient, each 15 minutes

➔ *CPT Changes: An Insider's View* 2019

➔ *CPT Assistant* Nov 18:3, Jul 20:10, Jun 23:28

(Do not report 97155 in conjunction with 90785-90899, 92507, 96105-96171, 97129)

97156   **Family adaptive behavior treatment guidance,** administered by physician or other qualified health care professional (with or without the patient present), face-to-face with guardian(s)/caregiver(s), each 15 minutes

➔ *CPT Changes: An Insider's View* 2019

➔ *CPT Assistant* Nov 18:3

(Do not report 97156 in conjunction with 90785-90899, 96105-96171)

97157   **Multiple-family group adaptive behavior treatment guidance,** administered by physician or other qualified health care professional (without the patient present), face-to-face with multiple sets of guardians/caregivers, each 15 minutes

➔ *CPT Changes: An Insider's View* 2019

➔ *CPT Assistant* Nov 18:3

(Do not report 97157 if the group has more than 8 families)

(Do not report 97156, 97157 in conjunction with 90785-90899, 96105-96171)

97158   **Group adaptive behavior treatment with protocol modification,** administered by physician or other qualified health care professional, face-to-face with multiple patients, each 15 minutes

➔ *CPT Changes: An Insider's View* 2019

(Do not report 97158 if the group has more than 8 patients)

(Do not report 97158 in conjunction with 90785-90899, 96105-96171, 92508, 97150)

Central Nervous System Assessments/Tests (eg, Neuro-Cognitive, Mental Status, Speech Testing)

The following codes are used to report the services provided during testing of the central nervous system functions. The central nervous system assessments include, but are not limited to, memory, language, visual motor responses, and abstract reasoning/problem-solving abilities. It is accomplished by the combination of several types of testing procedures. Testing procedures include assessment of aphasia and cognitive performance testing, developmental screening and behavioral assessments and testing, and psychological/neuropsychological testing. The administration of these tests will generate material that will be formulated into a report or an automated result.

(For development of cognitive skills, see 97129, 97533)

(For dementia screens, [eg, Folstein Mini-Mental State Examination, by a physician or other qualified health care professional], see **Evaluation and Management** services codes)

(Do not report assessment of aphasia and cognitive performance testing services [96105, 96125], developmental/behavioral screening and testing services [96110, 96112, 96113, 96127], and psychological/neuropsychological testing services [96116, 96121, 96130, 96131, 96132, 96133, 96136, 96137, 96138, 96139, 96146] in conjunction with 97151, 97152, 97153, 97154, 97155, 97156, 97157, 97158, 0362T, 0373T)

Guide to Selection of Codes 97153, 97155, and 0373T

	97153	97155	0373T
By protocol	✓		
With protocol modification		✓	✓
Physician or other qualified health care professional face-to-face with patient		✓	
Physician or other qualified health care professional required to be on site			✓
Physician or other qualified health care professional not required to be on site	✓		
Number of technicians	1	0-1	2 or more
Deficient adaptive behavior(s), maladaptive behavior(s), or other impaired functioning secondary to deficient adaptive or maladaptive behaviors	✓	✓	
Destructive behavior(s)		✓	✓
Environment customized to patient and behavior			✓

Definitions

Codes in this family (96105-96146) describe a number of services that are defined below:

Cognitive performance testing: assesses the patient's ability to complete specific functional tasks applicable to the patient's environment in order to identify or quantify specific cognitive deficits. The results are used to determine impairments and develop therapeutic goals and objectives.

Interactive feedback: used to convey the implications of psychological or neuropsychological test findings and diagnostic formulation. Based on patient-specific cognitive and emotional strengths and weaknesses, interactive feedback may include promoting adherence to medical and/or psychological treatment plans; educating and engaging the patient about his or her condition to maximize patient collaboration in their care; addressing safety issues; facilitating psychological coping; coordinating care; and engaging the patient in planning given the expected course of illness or condition, when performed.

Interpretation and report: performed by a physician or other qualified health care professional. In some circumstances, a result is generated through the use of a "computer," tablet(s), or other device(s).

Neurobehavioral status examination: a clinical assessment of cognitive functions and behavior, and may include an interview with the patient, other informant(s), and/or staff, as well as integration of prior history and other sources of clinical data with clinical decision making, further assessment and/or treatment planning and report. Evaluation domains may include acquired knowledge, attention, language, memory, planning and problem solving, and visual spatial abilities.

Neuropsychological testing evaluation services: typically include integration of patient data with other sources of clinical data, interpretation, clinical decision making, and treatment planning and report. It may include interactive feedback to the patient, family member(s) or caregiver(s), when performed. Evaluation domains for neuropsychological evaluation may include intellectual function, attention, executive function, language and communication, memory, visual-spatial function, sensorimotor function, emotional and personality features, and adaptive behavior.

Psychological testing evaluation services: typically include integration of patient data with other sources of clinical data, interpretation, clinical decision making, and treatment planning and report. It may include interactive feedback to the patient, family member(s) or caregiver(s) when performed. Evaluation domains for psychological evaluation may include emotional and interpersonal functioning, intellectual function, thought processes, personality, and psychopathology.

Standardized instruments: used in the performance of these services. Standardized instruments are validated tests that are administered and scored in a consistent or "standard" manner consistent with their validation.

Testing: administered by a physician, other qualified health care professional, and technician, or completed by the patient. The mode of completion can be manual (eg, paper and pencil) or via automated means.

Assessment of aphasia and cognitive performance testing, which includes interpretation and report, are described by 96105, 96125.

Developmental screening services are described by 96110. Developmental/behavioral testing services, which include interpretation and report, are described by 96112, 96113.

Neurobehavioral status examination, which includes interpretation and report, is described by 96116, 96121.

Psychological and neuropsychological test evaluation services, which include integration of patient data, interpretation of test results and clinical data, treatment planning and report, and interactive feedback, are described by 96130, 96131, 96132, 96133.

Testing and administration services (96136, 96137) are performed by a physician or other qualified health care professional. For 96136, 96137, do not include time for evaluation services (eg, integration of patient data or interpretation of test results). This time is included with psychological and neuropsychological test evaluation services (96130, 96131, 96132, 96133). Testing and administration services (96138, 96139) are performed by a technician. The tests selected, test administration and method of testing and scoring are the same, regardless whether the testing is performed by a physician, other qualified health care professional, or a technician, for 96136, 96137, 96138, 96139. Automated testing and result code 96146 describes testing performed by a single automated instrument with an automated result.

Some of these services are typically performed together. For example, psychological/neuropsychological testing evaluation services (96130, 96131, 96132, 96133) may be reported with psychological/neuropsychological test administration and scoring services (96136, 96137, 96138, 96139).

A requirement of testing services (96105, 96125, 96112, 96113, 96130, 96131, 96132, 96133, 96146) is that there is an interpretation and report when performed by a qualified health care professional, or a result when generated by automation. These services follow standard CPT time definitions (ie, a minimum of 16 minutes for

30 minutes codes and 31 minutes for 1-hour codes must be provided to report any per hour code). The time reported in 96116, 96121, 96130, 96131, 96132, 96133, 96125 is the face-to-face time with the patient and the time spent integrating and interpreting data.

Report the total time at the completion of the entire episode of evaluation.

> (To report psychological testing evaluation and administration and scoring services, see 96130, 96131, 96136, 96137, 96138, 96139, 96146)

> (To report psychological test administration using a single automated instrument, use 96146)

Assessment of Aphasia and Cognitive Performance Testing

★ **96105** Assessment of aphasia (includes assessment of expressive and receptive speech and language function, language comprehension, speech production ability, reading, spelling, writing, eg, by Boston Diagnostic Aphasia Examination) with interpretation and report, per hour

    ⊙ *CPT Assistant* Jul 96:8, May 05:1, Nov 09:10, Oct 18:5, Nov 18:3

#★ **96125** Standardized cognitive performance testing (eg, Ross Information Processing Assessment) per hour of a qualified health care professional's time, both face-to-face time administering tests to the patient and time interpreting these test results and preparing the report

    ⊙ *CPT Changes: An Insider's View* 2008

    ⊙ *CPT Assistant* Oct 11:4, Oct 18:5, Nov 18:3, Apr 24:24

> (To report neuropsychological testing evaluation and administration and scoring services, see 96132, 96133, 96136, 96137, 96138, 96139, 96146)

Developmental/Behavioral Screening and Testing

◄ **96110** Developmental screening (eg, developmental milestone survey, speech and language delay screen), with scoring and documentation, per standardized instrument

    ⊙ *CPT Changes: An Insider's View* 2012, 2015

    ⊙ *CPT Assistant* Jul 96:9, May 05:1, Nov 09:10, Jun 14:3, Aug 15:5, Feb 17:15, Nov 18:3

> (For an emotional/behavioral assessment, use 96127)

> (To report developmental testing, see 96112, 96113)

96112 Developmental test administration (including assessment of fine and/or gross motor, language, cognitive level, social, memory and/or executive functions by standardized developmental instruments when performed), by physician or other qualified health care professional, with interpretation and report; first hour

    ⊙ *CPT Changes: An Insider's View* 2019

    ⊙ *CPT Assistant* Nov 18:3

+ **96113** each additional 30 minutes (List separately in addition to code for primary procedure)

    ⊙ *CPT Changes: An Insider's View* 2019

    ⊙ *CPT Assistant* Nov 18:3

96127 Brief emotional/behavioral assessment (eg, depression inventory, attention-deficit/hyperactivity disorder [ADHD] scale), with scoring and documentation, per standardized instrument

    ⊙ *CPT Changes: An Insider's View* 2015

    ⊙ *CPT Assistant* Aug 15:5, Feb 17:15, Nov 18:3

> (For developmental screening, use 96110)

Psychological/Neuropsychological Testing

Neurobehavioral Status Examination

★◄ **96116** Neurobehavioral status exam (clinical assessment of thinking, reasoning and judgment, [eg, acquired knowledge, attention, language, memory, planning and problem solving, and visual spatial abilities]), by physician or other qualified health care professional, both face-to-face time with the patient and time interpreting test results and preparing the report; first hour

    ⊙ *CPT Changes: An Insider's View* 2006, 2017, 2019

    ⊙ *CPT Assistant* Oct 11:4, Jun 14:3, Oct 18:5, Nov 18:3

> (To report neuropsychological testing evaluation and administration and scoring services, see 96132, 96133, 96136, 96137, 96138, 96139, 96146)

> (To report psychological test administration using a single automated instrument, use 96146)

★+◄ **96121** each additional hour (List separately in addition to code for primary procedure)

    ⊙ *CPT Changes: An Insider's View* 2019

    ⊙ *CPT Assistant* Nov 18:3

> (Use 96121 in conjunction with 96116)

96125 Code is out of numerical sequence. See 96020-96121

96127 Code is out of numerical sequence. See 96020-96121

Central Nervous System Assessments/Tests (eg, Neuro-Cognitive, Mental Status, Speech Testing) Tables

Assessment of Aphasia and Cognitive Performance Testing

Code	Unit	Cognitive Services		Test Administration/Scoring		Interpretation and Report or Automated Result	
		Evaluation	Interactive Feedback	Physician or Qualified Health Care Professional	Technician	Physician or Qualified Health Care Professional	Automated Result
96105	Per hour	X		X		X	
96125	Per hour	X		X		X	

Developmental/Behavioral Screening and Testing

Code	Unit	Cognitive Services		Test Administration/Scoring		Interpretation and Report or Automated Result	
		Evaluation	Interactive Feedback	Physician or Qualified Health Care Professional	Clinical Staff	Physician or Qualified Health Care Professional	Automated Result
96110	Per instrument				X		
96112	Per hour	X		X		X	
+96113	Per 30 min (add-on)	X		X		X	
96127	Per instrument				X		

Psychological/Neuropsychological Testing

Code	Unit	Cognitive Services		Test Administration/ Scoring		Interpretation and Report or Automated Result	
		Evaluation	Interactive Feedback	Physician or Qualified Health Care Professional	Technician	Physician or Qualified Health Care Professional	Automated Result

Neurobehavioral Status Examination

Code	Unit	Evaluation	Interactive Feedback	Physician or Qualified Health Care Professional	Technician	Physician or Qualified Health Care Professional	Automated Result
96116	Per hour	X		X		X	
+96121	Per hour (add-on)	X		X		X	

Testing Evaluation Services

Code	Unit	Evaluation	Interactive Feedback	Physician or Qualified Health Care Professional	Technician	Physician or Qualified Health Care Professional	Automated Result
96130	Per hour	X	X	Not included in Code	Not included in Code	X	
+96131	Per hour (add-on)	X	X	Not included in Code	Not included in Code	X	
96132	Per hour	X	X	Not included in Code	Not included in Code	X	
+96133	Per hour (add-on)	X	X	Not included in Code	Not included in Code	X	

Test Administration & Scoring

Code	Unit	Evaluation	Interactive Feedback	Physician or Qualified Health Care Professional	Technician	Physician or Qualified Health Care Professional	Automated Result
96136	Per 30 min	Not included in Code	Not included in Code	X		Not included in Code	Not included in Code
+96137	Per 30 min (add-on)	Not included in Code	Not included in Code	X		Not included in Code	Not included in Code
96138	Per 30 min	Not included in Code	Not included in Code		X	Not included in Code	Not included in Code
+96139	Per 30 min (add-on)	Not included in Code	Not included in Code		X	Not included in Code	Not included in Code

Automated Testing and Result

Code	Unit	Evaluation	Interactive Feedback	Physician or Qualified Health Care Professional	Technician	Physician or Qualified Health Care Professional	Automated Result
96146	Automated report(s)	Not included in Code	Not included in Code				X

Testing Evaluation Services

96130 Psychological testing evaluation services by physician or other qualified health care professional, including integration of patient data, interpretation of standardized test results and clinical data, clinical decision making, treatment planning and report, and interactive feedback to the patient, family member(s) or caregiver(s), when performed; first hour

➡ *CPT Changes: An Insider's View* 2019

➡ *CPT Assistant* Nov 18:3, Sep 19:12, Dec 19:15

+ 96131   each additional hour (List separately in addition to code for primary procedure)

➡ *CPT Changes: An Insider's View* 2019

➡ *CPT Assistant* Nov 18:3, Sep 19:12, Dec 19:15

96132 Neuropsychological testing evaluation services by physician or other qualified health care professional, including integration of patient data, interpretation of standardized test results and clinical data, clinical decision making, treatment planning and report, and interactive feedback to the patient, family member(s) or caregiver(s), when performed; first hour

➡ *CPT Changes: An Insider's View* 2019

➡ *CPT Assistant* Nov 18:3, Sep 19:12, Dec 19:15, Jun 23:29

+ 96133   each additional hour (List separately in addition to code for primary procedure)

➡ *CPT Changes: An Insider's View* 2019

➡ *CPT Assistant* Nov 18:3, Sep 19:12, Dec 19:15

Test Administration and Scoring

96136 Psychological or neuropsychological test administration and scoring by physician or other qualified health care professional, two or more tests, any method; first 30 minutes

➡ *CPT Changes: An Insider's View* 2019

➡ *CPT Assistant* Nov 18:3, Sep 19:12, Dec 19:15, Aug 20:3, Jun 23:29

+ 96137   each additional 30 minutes (List separately in addition to code for primary procedure)

➡ *CPT Changes: An Insider's View* 2019

➡ *CPT Assistant* Nov 18:3, Sep 19:12, Dec 19:15, Aug 20:3

(96136, 96137 may be reported in conjunction with 96130, 96131, 96132, 96133 on the same or different days)

96138 Psychological or neuropsychological test administration and scoring by technician, two or more tests, any method; first 30 minutes

➡ *CPT Changes: An Insider's View* 2019

➡ *CPT Assistant* Nov 18:3

+ 96139   each additional 30 minutes (List separately in addition to code for primary procedure)

➡ *CPT Changes: An Insider's View* 2019

➡ *CPT Assistant* Nov 18:3

(96138, 96139 may be reported in conjunction with 96130, 96131, 96132, 96133 on the same or different days)

(For 96136, 96137, 96138, 96139, do not include time for evaluation services [eg, integration of patient data or interpretation of test results]. This time is included in 96130, 96131, 96132, 96133)

Automated Testing and Result

96146 Psychological or neuropsychological test administration, with single automated, standardized instrument via electronic platform, with automated result only

➡ *CPT Changes: An Insider's View* 2019

➡ *CPT Assistant* Nov 18:3, Jun 23:29

(If test is administered by physician, other qualified health care professional, or technician, do not report 96146. To report, see 96127, 96136, 96137, 96138, 96139)

Health Behavior Assessment and Intervention

Health behavior assessment and intervention services are used to identify and address the psychological, behavioral, emotional, cognitive, and interpersonal factors important to the assessment, treatment, or management of physical health problems.

The patient's primary diagnosis is physical in nature and the focus of the assessment and intervention is on factors complicating medical conditions and treatments. These codes describe assessments and interventions to improve the patient's health and well-being utilizing psychological and/or psychosocial interventions designed to ameliorate specific disease-related problems.

Health behavior assessment: includes evaluation of the patient's responses to disease, illness or injury, outlook, coping strategies, motivation, and adherence to medical treatment. Assessment is conducted through health-focused clinical interviews, observation, and clinical decision making.

Health behavior intervention: includes promotion of functional improvement, minimizing psychological and/or psychosocial barriers to recovery, and management of and improved coping with medical conditions. These services emphasize active patient/family engagement and involvement. These interventions may be provided individually, to a group (two or more patients), and/or to the family, with or without the patient present.

Codes 96156, 96158, 96159, 96164, 96165, 96167, 96168, 96170, 96171 describe services offered to patients who present with primary physical illnesses, diagnoses, or symptoms and may benefit from assessments and interventions that focus on the psychological and/or psychosocial factors related to the patient's health status. These services do not represent preventive medicine counseling and risk factor reduction interventions.

For patients that require psychiatric services (90785-90899), adaptive behavior services (97151, 97152, 97153, 97154, 97155, 97156, 97157, 97158, 0362T, 0373T) as well as health behavior assessment and intervention (96156, 96158, 96159, 96164, 96165, 96167, 96168, 96170, 96171), report the predominant service performed. Do not report 96156, 96158, 96159, 96164, 96165, 96167, 96168, 96170, 96171 in conjunction with 90785-90899 on the same date.

Evaluation and management services codes (including counseling risk factor reduction and behavior change intervention [99401-99412]) should not be reported on the same day as health behavior assessment and intervention codes 96156, 96158, 96159, 96164, 96165, 96167, 96168, 96170, 96171 by the same provider.

Health behavior assessment and intervention services (96156, 96158, 96159, 96164, 96165, 96167, 96168, 96170, 96171) can occur and be reported on the same date of service as evaluation and management services (including counseling risk factor reduction and behavior change intervention [99401, 99402, 99403, 99404, 99406, 99407, 99408, 99409, 99411, 99412]), as long as the health behavior assessment and intervention service is reported by a physician or other qualified health care professional and the evaluation and management service is performed by a physician or other qualified health care professional who may report evaluation and management services.

Do not report 96158, 96164, 96167, 96170 for less than 16 minutes of service.

(For health behavior assessment and intervention services [96156, 96158, 96159, 96164, 96165, 96167, 96168, 96170, 96171] performed by a physician or other qualified health care professional who may report evaluation and management services, see **Evaluation and Management** or **Preventive Medicine Services** codes)

(Do not report 96156, 96158, 96159, 96164, 96165, 96167, 96168, 96170, 96171 in conjunction with 97151, 97152, 97153, 97154, 97155, 97156, 97157, 97158, 0362T, 0373T)

★◀ **96156** Health behavior assessment, or re-assessment (ie, health-focused clinical interview, behavioral observations, clinical decision making)
➡ CPT Changes: An Insider's View 2020
➡ CPT Assistant Jul 20:7

★◀ **96158** Health behavior intervention, individual, face-to-face; initial 30 minutes
➡ CPT Changes: An Insider's View 2020
➡ CPT Assistant Jul 20:7, Apr 22:10, Sep 22:22

★+◀ **96159** each additional 15 minutes (List separately in addition to code for primary service)
➡ CPT Changes: An Insider's View 2020
➡ CPT Assistant Jul 20:7, Apr 22:10

(Use 96159 in conjunction with 96158)

(Do not report 96158, 96159 for service time reported in conjunction with 98975, 98978)

#★◀ **96164** Health behavior intervention, group (2 or more patients), face-to-face; initial 30 minutes
➡ CPT Changes: An Insider's View 2020
➡ CPT Assistant Jul 20:7, Oct 22:7

#★+◀ **96165** each additional 15 minutes (List separately in addition to code for primary service)
➡ CPT Changes: An Insider's View 2020
➡ CPT Assistant Jul 20:7, Oct 22:7

(Use 96165 in conjunction with 96164)

#★◀ **96167** Health behavior intervention, family (with the patient present), face-to-face; initial 30 minutes
➡ CPT Changes: An Insider's View 2020

#★+◀ **96168** each additional 15 minutes (List separately in addition to code for primary service)
➡ CPT Changes: An Insider's View 2020

(Use 96168 in conjunction with 96167)

#★◀ **96170** Health behavior intervention, family (without the patient present), face-to-face; initial 30 minutes
➡ CPT Changes: An Insider's View 2020

#★+◀ **96171** each additional 15 minutes (List separately in addition to code for primary service)
➡ CPT Changes: An Insider's View 2020

(Use 96171 in conjunction with 96170)

★◀ **96160** Administration of patient-focused health risk assessment instrument (eg, health hazard appraisal) with scoring and documentation, per standardized instrument
➡ CPT Changes: An Insider's View 2017
➡ CPT Assistant Nov 16:5, Feb 17:15

★◀ **96161** Administration of caregiver-focused health risk assessment instrument (eg, depression inventory) for the benefit of the patient, with scoring and documentation, per standardized instrument
➡ CPT Changes: An Insider's View 2017
➡ CPT Assistant Nov 16:5, Feb 17:15

96164	Code is out of numerical sequence. See 96158-96161
96165	Code is out of numerical sequence. See 96158-96161
96167	Code is out of numerical sequence. See 96158-96161
96168	Code is out of numerical sequence. See 96158-96161
96170	Code is out of numerical sequence. See 96158-96161
96171	Code is out of numerical sequence. See 96158-96161

Behavior Management Services

Behavior modification is defined as the process of altering human-behavior patterns over a long-term period using various motivational techniques, namely, consequences and rewards. More simply, behavior modification is the method of changing the way a person reacts either physically or mentally to a given stimulus.

Behavior modification treatment is based on the principles of operant conditioning. The intended clinical outcome for this treatment approach is to replace unwanted or problematic behaviors with more positive, desirable behaviors through the use of evidence-based techniques and methods.

The purpose of the group-based behavioral management/modification training services is to teach the parent(s)/guardian(s)/caregiver(s) interventions that they can independently use to effectively manage the identified patient's illness(es) or disease(s). Codes 96202, 96203 are used to report the total duration of face-to-face time spent by the physician or other qualified health care professional providing group-based parent(s)/guardian(s)/caregiver(s) behavioral management/modification training services. This service involves behavioral treatment training provided to a multiple-family group of parent(s)/guardian(s)/caregiver(s), without the patient present. These services emphasize active engagement and involvement of the parent(s)/guardian(s)/caregiver(s) in the treatment of a patient with a mental or physical health diagnosis. These services do not represent preventive medicine counseling and risk factor reduction interventions.

During these sessions, the parent(s)/guardian(s)/caregiver(s) are trained, using verbal instruction, video and live demonstrations, and feedback from physician or other qualified health care professional or other parent(s)/guardian(s)/caregiver(s) in group sessions, to use skills and strategies to address behaviors impacting the patient's mental or physical health diagnosis. These skills and strategies help to support compliance with the identified patient's treatment and the clinical plan of care.

For counseling and education provided by a physician or other qualified health care professional to a patient and/or family, see the appropriate evaluation and management codes, including office or other outpatient services (99202, 99203, 99204, 99205, 99211, 99212, 99213, 99214, 99215), hospital inpatient and observation care services (99221, 99222, 99223, 99231, 99232, 99233, 99234, 99235, 99236), new or established patient office or other outpatient consultations (99242, 99243, 99244, 99245), inpatient or observation consultations (99252, 99253, 99254, 99255), emergency department services (99281, 99282, 99283, 99284, 99285), nursing facility services (99304, 99305, 99306, 99307, 99308, 99309, 99310, 99315, 99316), home or residence services (99341, 99342, 99344, 99345, 99347, 99348, 99349, 99350), and counseling risk factor reduction and behavior change intervention (99401-99429). See also **Instructions for Use of the CPT Codebook** for definition of reporting qualifications.

Counseling risk factor reduction and behavior change intervention codes (99401, 99402, 99403, 99404, 99406, 99407, 99408, 99409, 99411, 99412) are included and may not be separately reported on the same day as parent(s)/guardian(s)/caregiver(s) training services codes 96202, 96203 by the same provider.

Medical nutrition therapy (97802, 97803, 97804) provided to the identified patient may be reported on the same date of service as parent(s)/guardian(s)/caregiver(s) training service.

(For health behavior assessment and intervention that is not part of a standardized curriculum, see 96156, 96158, 96159, 96164, 96165, 96167, 96168, 96170, 96171)

(For educational services that use a standardized curriculum provided to patients with an established illness/disease, see 98960, 98961, 98962)

▶(For education provided as genetic counseling services, use 96041. For education to a group regarding genetic risks, see 98961, 98962)◀

96202 Multiple-family group behavior management/modification training for parent(s)/guardian(s)/caregiver(s) of patients with a mental or physical health diagnosis, administered by physician or other qualified health care professional (without the patient present), face-to-face with multiple sets of parent(s)/guardian(s)/caregiver(s); initial 60 minutes

➔ *CPT Changes: An Insider's View* 2023
➔ *CPT Assistant* Oct 22:7

(Do not report 96202 for behavior management services to the patient and the parent[s]/guardian[s]/caregiver[s] during the same session)

(Do not report 96202 for less than 31 minutes of service)

+ 96203 each additional 15 minutes (List separately in addition to code for primary service)

➔ *CPT Changes: An Insider's View* 2023

➔ *CPT Assistant* Oct 22:7

(Use 96203 in conjunction with 96202)

(Do not report 96202, 96203 in conjunction with 97151, 97152, 97153, 97154, 97155, 97156, 97157, 97158, 0362T, 0373T)

(For educational services [eg, prenatal, obesity, or diabetic instructions] rendered to patients in a group setting, use 99078)

(For counseling and/or risk factor reduction intervention provided by a physician or other qualified health care professional to patient[s] without symptoms or established disease, see 99401, 99402, 99403, 99404, 99406, 99407, 99408, 99409, 99411, 99412)

Hydration, Therapeutic, Prophylactic, Diagnostic Injections and Infusions, and Chemotherapy and Other Highly Complex Drug or Highly Complex Biologic Agent Administration

Physician or other qualified health care professional work related to hydration, injection, and infusion services predominantly involves affirmation of treatment plan and direct supervision of staff.

Codes 96360-96379, 96401, 96402, 96409-96425, 96521-96523 are not intended to be reported by the physician in the facility setting. If a significant, separately identifiable office or other outpatient evaluation and management (E/M) service is performed, the appropriate E/M service (99202-99215, 99242, 99243, 99244, 99245) should be reported using modifier 25, in addition to 96360-96549. For same day E/M service, a different diagnosis is not required.

If performed to facilitate the infusion or injection, the following services are included and are not reported separately:

a. Use of local anesthesia

b. IV start

c. Access to indwelling IV, subcutaneous catheter or port

d. Flush at conclusion of infusion

e. Standard tubing, syringes, and supplies

(For declotting a catheter or port, use 36593)

When multiple drugs are administered, report the service(s) and the specific materials or drugs for each.

When administering multiple infusions, injections or combinations, only one "initial" service code should be reported for a given date, unless protocol requires that two separate IV sites must be used. Do not report a second initial service on the same date due to an intravenous line requiring a re-start, an IV rate not being able to be reached without two lines, or for accessing a port of a multi-lumen catheter. If an injection or infusion is of a subsequent or concurrent nature, even if it is the first such service within that group of services, then a subsequent or concurrent code from the appropriate section should be reported (eg, the first IV push given subsequent to an initial one-hour infusion is reported using a subsequent IV push code).

Initial infusion: For physician or other qualified health care professional reporting, an initial infusion is the *key or primary reason for the encounter* reported irrespective of the temporal order in which the infusion(s) or injection(s) are administered. For facility reporting, an initial infusion is based using the hierarchy. For both physician or other qualified health care professional and facility reporting, only one *initial* service code (eg, 96365) should be reported unless the protocol or patient condition requires that two separate IV sites must be utilized. The difference in time and effort in providing this second IV site access is also reported using the *initial* service code with modifier 59 appended (eg, 96365, 96365-59).

Sequential infusion: A sequential infusion is an infusion or IV push of a new substance or drug following a primary or initial service. All sequential services require that there be a new substance or drug, except that facilities may report a sequential intravenous push of the same drug using 96376.

Concurrent infusion: A concurrent infusion is an infusion of a new substance or drug infused at the same time as another substance or drug. A concurrent infusion service is not time based and is only reported once per day regardless of whether an additional new drug or substance is administered concurrently. Hydration may not be reported concurrently with any other service. A separate subsequent concurrent administration of another new drug or substance (the third substance or drug) is not reported.

In order to determine which service should be reported as the initial service when there is more than one type of service, hierarchies have been created. These vary by whether the physician or other qualified health care professional or a facility is reporting. The order of selection for reporting is based upon the physician's or other qualified health care professional's knowledge of the clinical condition(s) and treatment(s). The hierarchy that facilities are to use is based upon a structural algorithm. When these codes are reported by the physician or other qualified health care professional, the "initial" code that best describes the key or primary reason for the encounter should always be reported irrespective of the order in which the infusions or injections occur.

When these codes are reported *by the facility*, the following instructions apply. The initial code should be selected using a hierarchy whereby chemotherapy services are primary to therapeutic, prophylactic, and diagnostic services which are primary to hydration services. Infusions are primary to pushes, which are primary to injections. This hierarchy is to be followed by facilities and supersedes parenthetical instructions for add-on codes that suggest an add-on of a higher hierarchical position may be reported in conjunction with a base code of a lower position. (For example, the hierarchy would not permit reporting 96376 with 96360, as 96376 is a higher order code. IV push is primary to hydration.)

When reporting multiple infusions of the same drug/ substance on the same date of service, the initial code should be selected. The second and subsequent infusion(s) should be reported based on the individual time(s) of each additional infusion(s) of the same drug/ substance using the appropriate add-on code.

Example: In the outpatient observation setting, a patient receives one-hour intravenous infusions of the same antibiotic every 8 hours on the same date of service through the same IV access. The hierarchy for facility reporting permits the reporting of code 96365 for the first one-hour dose administered. Add-on 96366 would be reported twice (once for the second and third one-hour infusions of the same drug).

When reporting codes for which infusion time is a factor, use the actual time over which the infusion is administered. Intravenous or intra-arterial push is defined as: (a) an injection in which the individual who administers the drug/substance is continuously present to administer the injection and observe the patient, or (b) an infusion of 15 minutes or less. If intravenous hydration (96360, 96361) is given from 11 PM to 2 AM, 96360 would be reported once and 96361 twice. For continuous services that last beyond midnight, use the date in which the service began and report the total units of time provided continuously. However, if instead of a continuous infusion, a medication was given by intravenous push at 10 PM and 2 AM, as the service was not continuous, the two administrations would be reported as an initial service (96374) and sequential (96376) as: (1) no other infusion services were performed; and (2) the push of the same drug was performed more than 30 minutes beyond the initial administration. A "keep open" infusion of any type is not separately reported.

Hydration

Codes 96360-96361 are intended to report a hydration IV infusion to consist of a pre-packaged fluid and electrolytes (eg, normal saline, D5-1/2 normal saline+30mEq KCl/liter), but are not used to report infusion of drugs or other substances. Hydration IV infusions typically require direct supervision for purposes of consent, safety oversight, or intraservice supervision of staff. Typically such infusions require little special handling to prepare or dispose of, and staff that administer these do not typically require advanced practice training. After initial set-up, infusion typically entails little patient risk and thus little monitoring. These codes are not intended to be reported by the physician or other qualified health care professional in the facility setting.

Some chemotherapeutic agents and other therapeutic agents require pre- and/or post-hydration to be given in order to avoid specific toxicities. A minimum time duration of 31 minutes of hydration infusion is required to report the service. However, the hydration codes 96360 or 96361 are not used when the purpose of the intravenous fluid is to "keep open" an IV line prior or subsequent to a therapeutic infusion, or as a free-flowing IV during chemotherapy or other therapeutic infusion.

96360   Intravenous infusion, hydration; initial, 31 minutes to 1 hour

➡ *CPT Changes: An Insider's View* 2009

➡ *CPT Assistant* May 10:8, May 11:7, Oct 11:3, Dec 11:3, Oct 13:3, May 14:11, Jun 19:5, Mar 21:3, Jul 21:10

(Do not report 96360 if performed as a concurrent infusion service)

(Do not report intravenous infusion for hydration of 30 minutes or less)

+ 96361   each additional hour (List separately in addition to code for primary procedure)

➡ *CPT Changes: An Insider's View* 2009

➡ *CPT Assistant* May 10:8, May 11:7, Oct 11:3, Dec 11:3, Oct 13:3, May 14:11, Jun 19:5, Jul 21:10

(Use 96361 in conjunction with 96360)

(Report 96361 for hydration infusion intervals of greater than 30 minutes beyond 1 hour increments)

(Report 96361 to identify hydration if provided as a secondary or subsequent service after a different initial service [96360, 96365, 96374, 96409, 96413] is administered through the same IV access)

Therapeutic, Prophylactic, and Diagnostic Injections and Infusions (Excludes Chemotherapy and Other Highly Complex Drug or Highly Complex Biologic Agent Administration)

A therapeutic, prophylactic, or diagnostic IV infusion or injection (other than hydration) is for the administration of substances/drugs. When fluids are used to administer the drug(s), the administration of the fluid is considered incidental hydration and is not separately reportable. These services typically require direct supervision for any or all purposes of patient assessment, provision of consent, safety oversight, and intra-service supervision of staff. Typically, such infusions require special consideration to prepare, dose or dispose of, require practice training and competency for staff who administer the infusions, and require periodic patient assessment with vital sign monitoring during the infusion. These codes are not intended to be reported by the physician or other qualified health care professional in the facility setting.

▶Passive immunizations, such as an immune globulin or monoclonal antibody, provide long-term passive immunization to the patient.◀

See codes 96401-96549 for the administration of chemotherapy or other highly complex drug or highly complex biologic agent services. These highly complex services require advanced practice training and competency for staff who provide these services; special considerations for preparation, dosage or disposal; and commonly, these services entail significant patient risk and frequent monitoring. Examples are frequent changes in the infusion rate, prolonged presence of nurse administering the solution for patient monitoring and infusion adjustments, and frequent conferring with the physician or other qualified health care professional about these issues.

(Do not report 96365-96379 with codes for which IV push or infusion is an inherent part of the procedure [eg, administration of contrast material for a diagnostic imaging study])

(For mechanical scalp cooling, see 0662T, 0663T)

—— *Coding Tip* ——

Instructions for Reporting Medication Administration With Chemotherapy and Other Highly Complex Drug or Highly Complex Biologic Agent Administration

The administration of medications (eg, antibiotics, steroidal agents, antiemetics, narcotics, analgesics) administered independently or sequentially as supportive management of chemotherapy administration, should be separately reported using 96360, 96361, 96365, 96379 as appropriate.

CPT Coding Guidelines, Chemotherapy and Other Highly Complex Drug or Highly Complex Biologic Agent Administration

96365 Intravenous infusion, for therapy, prophylaxis, or diagnosis (specify substance or drug); initial, up to 1 hour
➔ *CPT Changes: An Insider's View* 2009
➔ *CPT Assistant* May 10:8, May 11:7, Oct 11:4, Dec 11:3, May 18:10, Sep 18:15, Dec 18:9, Dec 22:22
➔ *Clinical Examples in Radiology* Spring 10:10

+ 96366   each additional hour (List separately in addition to code for primary procedure)
➔ *CPT Changes: An Insider's View* 2009
➔ *CPT Assistant* May 11:7, Dec 11:3, Sep 18:15, Dec 22:22

(Report 96366 in conjunction with 96365, 96367)

(Report 96366 for additional hour[s] of sequential infusion)

(Report 96366 for infusion intervals of greater than 30 minutes beyond 1 hour increments)

(Report 96366 in conjunction with 96365 to identify each second and subsequent infusions of the same drug/substance)

+ 96367   additional sequential infusion of a new drug/substance, up to 1 hour (List separately in addition to code for primary procedure)
➔ *CPT Changes: An Insider's View* 2009, 2012
➔ *CPT Assistant* May 11:7, Dec 11:3

(Report 96367 in conjunction with 96365, 96374, 96409, 96413 to identify the infusion of a new drug/substance provided as a secondary or subsequent service after a different initial service is administered through the same IV access. Report 96367 only once per sequential infusion of same infusate mix)

+ 96368   concurrent infusion (List separately in addition to code for primary procedure)
➔ *CPT Changes: An Insider's View* 2009
➔ *CPT Assistant* May 10:8, May 11:7, Dec 11:3, Dec 22:22

(Report 96368 only once per date of service)

(Report 96368 in conjunction with 96365, 96366, 96413, 96415, 96416)

96369   Subcutaneous infusion for therapy or prophylaxis (specify substance or drug); initial, up to 1 hour, including pump set-up and establishment of subcutaneous infusion site(s)

➔ *CPT Changes: An Insider's View* 2009

➔ *CPT Assistant* May 11:7

(For infusions of 15 minutes or less, use 96372)

+ 96370   each additional hour (List separately in addition to code for primary procedure)

➔ *CPT Changes: An Insider's View* 2009

➔ *CPT Assistant* May 11:7

(Use 96370 in conjunction with 96369)

(Use 96370 for infusion intervals of greater than 30 minutes beyond 1 hour increments)

+ 96371   additional pump set-up with establishment of new subcutaneous infusion site(s) (List separately in addition to code for primary procedure)

➔ *CPT Changes: An Insider's View* 2009

➔ *CPT Assistant* May 11:7

(Use 96371 in conjunction with 96369)

(Use 96369, 96371 only once per encounter)

96372   Therapeutic, prophylactic, or diagnostic injection (specify substance or drug); subcutaneous or intramuscular

➔ *CPT Changes: An Insider's View* 2009

➔ *CPT Assistant* May 10:9, May 11:7, Jan 13:9, Jan 14:10, Oct 16:9, Dec 18:11, May 22:18

▶(For administration of vaccines/toxoids, see 90460, 90461, 90471, 90472, 90473, 90474, 90480)◀

(Report 96372 for non-antineoplastic hormonal therapy injections)

(Report 96401 for anti-neoplastic nonhormonal injection therapy)

(Report 96402 for anti-neoplastic hormonal injection therapy)

(For intradermal cancer immunotherapy injection, see 0708T, 0709T)

(Do not report 96372 for injections given without direct physician or other qualified health care professional supervision. To report, use 99211. Hospitals may report 96372 when the physician or other qualified health care professional is not present)

(96372 does not include injections for allergen immunotherapy. For allergen immunotherapy injections, see 95115-95117)

96373   intra-arterial

➔ *CPT Changes: An Insider's View* 2009

➔ *CPT Assistant* May 11:7

96374   intravenous push, single or initial substance/drug

➔ *CPT Changes: An Insider's View* 2009

➔ *CPT Assistant* May 10:8, May 11:7, Oct 11:3, Dec 11:4, Feb 13:3, Jun 13:9, Jun 19:9, Sep 22:22

➔ *Clinical Examples in Radiology* Spring 10:10, Summer 16:10, Fall 18:13, Summer 21:11,12

+ 96375   each additional sequential intravenous push of a new substance/drug (List separately in addition to code for primary procedure)

➔ *CPT Changes: An Insider's View* 2009

➔ *CPT Assistant* May 10:8, May 11:7, Feb 13:3

➔ *Clinical Examples in Radiology* Summer 16:10, Fall 18:13

(Use 96375 in conjunction with 96365, 96374, 96409, 96413)

(Report 96375 to identify intravenous push of a new substance/drug if provided as a secondary or subsequent service after a different initial service is administered through the same IV access)

+ 96376   each additional sequential intravenous push of the same substance/drug provided in a facility (List separately in addition to code for primary procedure)

➔ *CPT Changes: An Insider's View* 2009

➔ *CPT Assistant* May 10:6, May 11:7, Dec 11:3, Nov 14:15, Dec 18:9, Sep 22:22

➔ *Clinical Examples in Radiology* Summer 16:10, Fall 18:13

(Do not report 96376 for a push performed within 30 minutes of a reported push of the same substance or drug)

(96376 may be reported by facilities only)

(Report 96376 in conjunction with 96365, 96374, 96409, 96413)

96377   Application of on-body injector (includes cannula insertion) for timed subcutaneous injection

➔ *CPT Changes: An Insider's View* 2017

➔ *CPT Assistant* Oct 16:9

#● 96380   Administration of respiratory syncytial virus, monoclonal antibody, seasonal dose by intramuscular injection, with counseling by physician or other qualified health care professional

➔ *CPT Changes: An Insider's View* 2025

➔ *CPT Assistant* Nov 23:15, Feb 24:1

▶(Report 96380 for administration of respiratory syncytial virus, monoclonal antibody, seasonal dose [90380, 90381])◀

#● 96381   Administration of respiratory syncytial virus, monoclonal antibody, seasonal dose by intramuscular injection

➔ *CPT Changes: An Insider's View* 2025

➔ *CPT Assistant* Nov 23:15, Feb 24:1

▶(Report 96381 for administration of respiratory syncytial virus, monoclonal antibody, seasonal dose [90380, 90381])◀

96379   Unlisted therapeutic, prophylactic, or diagnostic intravenous or intra-arterial injection or infusion

➔ *CPT Changes: An Insider's View* 2009

➔ *CPT Assistant* May 11:7, Dec 11:19, Mar 21:3

(For allergy immunology, see 95004 et seq)

96380   Code is out of numerical sequence. See 96376-96401

96381   Code is out of numerical sequence. See 96376-96401

Chemotherapy and Other Highly Complex Drug or Highly Complex Biologic Agent Administration

Chemotherapy administration codes 96401-96549 apply to parenteral administration of non-radionuclide anti-neoplastic drugs; and also to anti-neoplastic agents provided for treatment of noncancer diagnoses (eg, cyclophosphamide for auto-immune conditions) or to substances such as certain monoclonal antibody agents, and other biologic response modifiers. The highly complex infusion of chemotherapy or other drug or biologic agents requires physician or other qualified health care professional work and/or clinical staff monitoring well beyond that of therapeutic drug agents (96360-96379) because the incidence of severe adverse patient reactions are typically greater. These services can be provided by any physician or other qualified health care professional. Chemotherapy services are typically highly complex and require direct supervision for any or all purposes of patient assessment, provision of consent, safety oversight, and intraservice supervision of staff. Typically, such chemotherapy services require advanced practice training and competency for staff who provide these services; special considerations for preparation, dosage, or disposal; and commonly, these services entail significant patient risk and frequent monitoring. Examples are frequent changes in the infusion rate, prolonged presence of the nurse administering the solution for patient monitoring and infusion adjustments, and frequent conferring with the physician or other qualified health care professional about these issues. When performed to facilitate the infusion of injection, preparation of chemotherapy agent(s), highly complex agent(s), or other highly complex drugs is included and is not reported separately. To report infusions that do not require this level of complexity, see 96360-96379. Codes 96401-96402, 96409-96425, 96521-96523 are not intended to be reported by the individual physician or other qualified health care professional in the facility setting.

The term "chemotherapy" in 96401-96549 includes other highly complex drugs or highly complex biologic agents.

Report separate codes for each parenteral method of administration employed when chemotherapy is administered by different techniques. The administration of medications (eg, antibiotics, steroidal agents, antiemetics, narcotics, analgesics) administered independently or sequentially as supportive management of chemotherapy administration, should be separately reported using 96360, 96361, 96365, 96379 as appropriate.

Report both the specific service as well as code(s) for the specific substance(s) or drug(s) provided. The fluid used to administer the drug(s) is considered incidental hydration and is not separately reportable.

Regional (isolation) chemotherapy perfusion should be reported using the codes for arterial infusion (96420-96425). Placement of the intra-arterial catheter should be reported using the appropriate code from the **Cardiovascular Surgery** section. Placement of arterial and venous cannula(s) for extracorporeal circulation via a membrane oxygenator perfusion pump should be reported using 36823. Code 36823 includes dose calculation and administration of the chemotherapy agent by injection into the perfusate. Do not report 96409-96425 in conjunction with 36823.

(For home infusion services, see 99601-99602)

Injection and Intravenous Infusion Chemotherapy and Other Highly Complex Drug or Highly Complex Biologic Agent Administration

Intravenous or intra-arterial push is defined as: (a) an injection in which the healthcare professional who administers the substance/drug is continuously present to administer the injection and observe the patient, or (b) an infusion of 15 minutes or less.

96401   Chemotherapy administration, subcutaneous or intramuscular; non-hormonal anti-neoplastic

➔ *CPT Changes: An Insider's View* 2006

➔ *CPT Assistant* Nov 05:1, Jan 06:47, Jan 07:30, May 07:3, Jun 07:4, Feb 09:17, Aug 11:9, Dec 11:3, May 22:18, Jan 24:40

➔ *Clinical Examples in Radiology* Winter 18:12, Summer 18:9

(For intradermal cancer immunotherapy injection, see 0708T, 0709T)

96402   hormonal anti-neoplastic

➔ *CPT Changes: An Insider's View* 2006

➔ *CPT Assistant* Nov 05:1, Jan 07:30, May 07:3, Feb 09:17, Dec 11:3, May 22:18, Jan 24:40

➔ *Clinical Examples in Radiology* Winter 18:12, Summer 18:9

★=Telemedicine   ◀=Audio-only   +=Add-on code   ✗=FDA approval pending   #=Resequenced code   ⊘=Modifier 51 exempt   ➔➔➔=See p xxi for details

96405   Chemotherapy administration; intralesional, up to and
including 7 lesions

➔ *CPT Changes: An Insider's View* 2006

➔ *CPT Assistant* Sep 96:5, Aug 97:19, Feb 01:10, Jul 01:2,
Nov 05:1, Jan 07:30, May 07:3, Feb 09:17, May 22:18

➔ *Clinical Examples in Radiology* Summer 18:9

96406   intralesional, more than 7 lesions

➔ *CPT Changes: An Insider's View* 2006

➔ *CPT Assistant* Sep 96:5, Aug 97:19, Feb 01:10, Jul 01:2,
Nov 05:1, Jan 07:30, May 07:3, Feb 09:17, May 22:18

➔ *Clinical Examples in Radiology* Summer 18:9

96409   intravenous, push technique, single or initial
substance/drug

➔ *CPT Changes: An Insider's View* 2006

➔ *CPT Assistant* Nov 05:1, Jan 07:30, May 07:3, Feb 09:17,
May 10:8, May 11:17, Dec 11:3, May 22:18, Oct 22:19

➔ *Clinical Examples in Radiology* Winter 18:12, Summer 18:9

+ 96411   intravenous, push technique, each additional
substance/drug (List separately in addition to code for
primary procedure)

➔ *CPT Changes: An Insider's View* 2006

➔ *CPT Assistant* Nov 05:1, Jan 07:30, May 07:3, Feb 09:17,
Dec 11:3, May 22:18, Oct 22:19

➔ *Clinical Examples in Radiology* Winter 18:12, Summer 18:9

(Use 96411 in conjunction with 96409, 96413)

96413   Chemotherapy administration, intravenous infusion
technique; up to 1 hour, single or initial substance/drug

➔ *CPT Changes: An Insider's View* 2006

➔ *CPT Assistant* Nov 05:1, Jan 07:30, May 07:3, Sep 07:3,
Dec 07:15, Feb 09:17, May 10:8, May 11:7, Dec 11:4, May 22:18,
Oct 22:19

➔ *Clinical Examples in Radiology* Winter 18:12, Summer 18:9

(Report 96361 to identify hydration if administered as a
secondary or subsequent service in association with
96413 through the same IV access)

(Report 96366, 96367, 96375 to identify therapeutic,
prophylactic, or diagnostic drug infusion or injection, if
administered as a secondary or subsequent service in
association with 96413 through the same IV access)

+ 96415   each additional hour (List separately in addition to
code for primary procedure)

➔ *CPT Changes: An Insider's View* 2006, 2007

➔ *CPT Assistant* Nov 05:1, Jan 07:30, May 07:3, Sep 07:3,
Dec 07:15, Feb 09:17, Dec 11:3, May 22:18, Oct 22:19

➔ *Clinical Examples in Radiology* Winter 18:12, Summer 18:9

(Use 96415 in conjunction with 96413)

(Report 96415 for infusion intervals of greater than 30
minutes beyond 1-hour increments)

96416   initiation of prolonged chemotherapy infusion (more
than 8 hours), requiring use of a portable or
implantable pump

➔ *CPT Changes: An Insider's View* 2006

➔ *CPT Assistant* Nov 05:1, Jan 07:30, May 07:3, Sep 07:3,
Dec 07:15, Feb 09:17, Dec 11:3, May 22:18, Oct 22:19

➔ *Clinical Examples in Radiology* Winter 18:12, Summer 18:9

(For refilling and maintenance of a portable pump or an
implantable infusion pump or reservoir for drug delivery,
see 96521-96523)

+ 96417   each additional sequential infusion (different
substance/drug), up to 1 hour (List separately in
addition to code for primary procedure)

➔ *CPT Changes: An Insider's View* 2006

➔ *CPT Assistant* Nov 05:1, Jan 07:30, May 07:3, Jun 07:4,
Feb 09:17, Aug 11:9, Dec 11:3, May 22:18, Oct 22:19

➔ *Clinical Examples in Radiology* Winter 18:12, Summer 18:9

(Use 96417 in conjunction with 96413)

(Report only once per sequential infusion. Report 96415
for additional hour(s) of sequential infusion)

Intra-Arterial Chemotherapy and Other Highly Complex Drug or Highly Complex Biologic Agent Administration

96420   Chemotherapy administration, intra-arterial; push
technique

➔ *CPT Assistant* Aug 97:19, Nov 98:37, Nov 99:54, Feb 01:10,
Jul 01:2, Nov 05:1, Jan 07:30, May 07:3, Jun 07:4, Feb 09:17,
Aug 11:9, Dec 11:3, Nov 13:6

➔ *Clinical Examples in Radiology* Summer 08:1-2, 4, Winter 18:11,
Summer 18:9

96422   infusion technique, up to 1 hour

➔ *CPT Assistant* Dec 96:10, Aug 97:19, Nov 98:37, Feb 01:10,
Jul 01:2, Nov 05:1, Jan 07:30, May 07:3, Dec 07:15,
Feb 09:17, Aug 11:9, Dec 11:3

➔ *Clinical Examples in Radiology* Winter 18:12, Summer 18:9

+ 96423   infusion technique, each additional hour (List
separately in addition to code for primary procedure)

➔ *CPT Changes: An Insider's View* 2006, 2007

➔ *CPT Assistant* Dec 96:10, Nov 98:37, Feb 01:10, Jul 01:2,
Nov 05:1, Jan 07:30, May 07:3, Dec 07:15, Feb 09:17,
Dec 11:3

➔ *Clinical Examples in Radiology* Winter 18:12, Summer 18:9

(Use 96423 in conjunction with 96422)

(Report 96423 for infusion intervals of greater than 30
minutes beyond 1-hour increments)

(For regional chemotherapy perfusion via membrane
oxygenator perfusion pump to an extremity, use 36823)

96425   infusion technique, initiation of prolonged infusion
(more than 8 hours), requiring the use of a portable or
implantable pump

➔ *CPT Assistant* Nov 99:54, Feb 01:10, Jul 01:2, Nov 05:1,
Jan 07:30, May 07:3, Jun 07:4, Feb 09:17, Aug 11:9,
Dec 11:3

➔ *Clinical Examples in Radiology* Winter 18:12, Summer 18:9

(For refilling and maintenance of a portable pump or an implantable infusion pump or reservoir for drug delivery, see 96521-96523)

Other Injection and Infusion Services

Code 96523 does not require direct supervision. Codes 96521-96523 may be reported when these devices are used for therapeutic drugs other than chemotherapy.

(For collection of blood specimen from a completely implantable venous access device, use 36591)

96440   Chemotherapy administration into pleural cavity, requiring and including thoracentesis

➔ *CPT Assistant* Feb 01:10, Jul 01:2, Nov 05:1, Jan 07:30, May 07:3, Jun 07:4, Feb 09:17

➔ *Clinical Examples in Radiology* Summer 18:9

96446   Chemotherapy administration into the peritoneal cavity via implanted port or catheter

➔ *CPT Changes: An Insider's View* 2011, 2024

➔ *CPT Assistant* Oct 10:16, Dec 10:16, Dec 23:27

➔ *Clinical Examples in Radiology* Summer 18:9

(For intraoperative hyperthermic intraperitoneal chemotherapy [HIPEC], see 96547, 96548)

96450   Chemotherapy administration, into CNS (eg, intrathecal), requiring and including spinal puncture

➔ *CPT Changes: An Insider's View* 2002

➔ *CPT Assistant* Feb 01:10, Jul 01:2, Nov 05:1, Jan 07:30, May 07:3, Feb 09:17, Mar 21:3

➔ *Clinical Examples in Radiology* Spring 11:10, Winter 14:10, Summer 18:9, Fall 19:9

(For intravesical (bladder) chemotherapy administration, use 51720)

(For insertion of subarachnoid catheter and reservoir for infusion of drug, see 62350, 62351, 62360-62362; for insertion of intraventricular catheter and reservoir, see 61210, 61215)

(If fluoroscopic guidance is performed, use 77003)

96521   Refilling and maintenance of portable pump

➔ *CPT Changes: An Insider's View* 2006

➔ *CPT Assistant* Nov 05:1, Jan 07:30, May 07:3, Feb 09:17, Dec 11:3

➔ *Clinical Examples in Radiology* Winter 18:12, Summer 18:9

96522   Refilling and maintenance of implantable pump or reservoir for drug delivery, systemic (eg, intravenous, intra-arterial)

➔ *CPT Changes: An Insider's View* 2006

➔ *CPT Assistant* Jul 06:1, Jan 07:30, May 07:3, Feb 09:17, Dec 11:3

➔ *Clinical Examples in Radiology* Winter 18:12, Summer 18:9

(For refilling and maintenance of an implantable infusion pump for spinal or brain drug infusion, use 95990-95991)

96523   Irrigation of implanted venous access device for drug delivery systems

➔ *CPT Changes: An Insider's View* 2006

➔ *CPT Assistant* Jan 07:30, May 07:3, Feb 09:17, Jul 11:16, Dec 11:3

➔ *Clinical Examples in Radiology* Winter 18:12, Summer 18:9

(Do not report 96523 in conjunction with other services. To report collection of blood specimen, use 36591)

96542   Chemotherapy injection, subarachnoid or intraventricular via subcutaneous reservoir, single or multiple agents

➔ *CPT Assistant* Aug 97:19, Jul 01:2, Nov 05:1, Jan 07:30, May 07:3, Feb 09:17

➔ *Clinical Examples in Radiology* Summer 18:9

(For radioactive isotope therapy, use 79005)

Codes 96547, 96548 describe the hyperthermic intraperitoneal chemotherapy (HIPEC) procedure that includes intraoperative perfusion of a heated chemotherapy agent into the abdominal cavity through catheters. The HIPEC procedure is distinct from the primary procedure and may include chemotherapy agent selection, confirmation of perfusion equipment settings for chemotherapy agent delivery, additional incision(s) for catheter and temperature probe placement, perfusion supervision and manual agitation of the heated chemotherapy agent in the abdominal cavity during chemotherapy agent dwell time, irrigation of the chemotherapy agent, closure of wounds related to HIPEC, and documentation of the chemotherapy agent and HIPEC procedure in the medical record. Codes 96547, 96548 are add-on codes and do not include the typical preoperative, intraoperative, and postoperative work related to the primary procedure. Code 96547 is reported for the first 60 minutes of the HIPEC procedure and 96548 is reported for each additional 30 minutes.

+ 96547   Intraoperative hyperthermic intraperitoneal chemotherapy (HIPEC) procedure, including separate incision(s) and closure, when performed; first 60 minutes (List separately in addition to code for primary procedure)

➔ *CPT Changes: An Insider's View* 2024

➔ *CPT Assistant* Dec 23:27, Jan 24:40

+ 96548   each additional 30 minutes (List separately in addition to code for primary procedure)

➔ *CPT Changes: An Insider's View* 2024

➔ *CPT Assistant* Dec 23:27, Jan 24:40

▶(Use 96547, 96548 in conjunction with 38100, 38101, 38102, 38120, 43611, 43620, 43621, 43622, 43631, 43632, 43633, 43634, 44010, 44015, 44110, 44111, 44120, 44121, 44125, 44130, 44139, 44140, 44141, 44143, 44144, 44145, 44146, 44147, 44150, 44151, 44155, 44156, 44157, 44158, 44160, 44202, 44203, 44204, 44207, 44213, 44227, 47001, 47100, 48140, 48145, 48152, 48155, 49000, 49010, 49320, 58200, 58210, 58575, 58940, 58943, 58950, 58951, 58952, 58953, 58954, 58956, 58958, 58960)◀

96549   Unlisted chemotherapy procedure
> CPT Assistant Aug 97:19, Jul 01:2, Nov 05:1, Jan 07:30, May 07:3, Jun 07:4, Oct 10:16, Dec 10:16
> Clinical Examples in Radiology Summer 18:9

Photodynamic Therapy

Codes 96573, 96574 should be used to report nonsurgical treatment of cutaneous lesions using photodynamic therapy by external application of light to destroy premalignant lesion(s) of the skin and adjacent mucosa (eg, face, scalp) by activation of photosensitizing drug(s).

A treatment session is defined as an application of photosensitizer to all lesions within an anatomic area (eg, face, scalp), with or without debridement of all premalignant hyperkeratotic lesions in that area, followed by illumination/activation with an appropriate light source to the same area.

Do not report codes for debridement (11000, 11001, 11004, 11005), lesion shaving (11300-11313), biopsy (11102, 11103, 11104, 11105, 11106, 11107), or lesion excision (11400-11471) within the treatment area(s) on the same day as photodynamic therapy (96573, 96574).

(To report ocular photodynamic therapy, use 67221)

96567   Photodynamic therapy by external application of light to destroy premalignant lesions of the skin and adjacent mucosa with application and illumination/activation of photosensitive drug(s), per day
> CPT Changes: An Insider's View 2018
> CPT Assistant Feb 18:10, Jul 18:15

(Use 96567 for reporting photodynamic therapy when physician or other qualified health care professional is not directly involved in the delivery of the photodynamic therapy service)

+ 96570   Photodynamic therapy by endoscopic application of light to ablate abnormal tissue via activation of photosensitive drug(s); first 30 minutes (List separately in addition to code for endoscopy or bronchoscopy procedures of lung and gastrointestinal tract)
> CPT Changes: An Insider's View 2000, 2010
> CPT Assistant Nov 99:54, Sep 00:5, Oct 11:11, Apr 13:8

(Report 96570 with modifier 52 for service of less than 23 minutes with report)

+ 96571   each additional 15 minutes (List separately in addition to code for endoscopy or bronchoscopy procedures of lung and gastrointestinal tract)
> CPT Changes: An Insider's View 2000, 2010
> CPT Assistant Nov 99:54, Sep 00:5, Oct 11:11, Apr 13:8

(For 23-37 minutes of service, use 96570. For 38-52 minutes of service, use 96570 in conjunction with 96571)

(96570, 96571 are to be used in addition to bronchoscopy, endoscopy codes)

(Use 96570, 96571 in conjunction with 31641, 43229 as appropriate)

96573   Photodynamic therapy by external application of light to destroy premalignant lesions of the skin and adjacent mucosa with application and illumination/activation of photosensitizing drug(s) provided by a physician or other qualified health care professional, per day
> CPT Changes: An Insider's View 2018
> CPT Assistant Feb 18:10, Jul 18:15

(Do not report 96573 in conjunction with 96567, 96574 for the same anatomic area)

96574   Debridement of premalignant hyperkeratotic lesion(s) (ie, targeted curettage, abrasion) followed with photodynamic therapy by external application of light to destroy premalignant lesions of the skin and adjacent mucosa with application and illumination/activation of photosensitizing drug(s) provided by a physician or other qualified health care professional, per day
> CPT Changes: An Insider's View 2018
> CPT Assistant Feb 18:10

(Do not report 96574 in conjunction with 96567, 96573 for the same anatomic area)

Special Dermatological Procedures

See the **Evaluation and Management coding guidelines** for further instructions on reporting that is appropriate for management of dermatologic illnesses.

(For intralesional injections, see 11900, 11901)

(For Tzanck smear, see 88160-88161)

96900   Actinotherapy (ultraviolet light)
> CPT Assistant Jul 12:9, Sep 16:3, Nov 16:9, Mar 22:14

(For rhinophototherapy, intranasal application of ultraviolet and visible light, use 30999)

96902 Microscopic examination of hairs plucked or clipped by the examiner (excluding hair collected by the patient) to determine telogen and anagen counts, or structural hair shaft abnormality

➲ CPT Assistant Nov 97:46-47

96904 Whole body integumentary photography, for monitoring of high risk patients with dysplastic nevus syndrome or a history of dysplastic nevi, or patients with a personal or familial history of melanoma

➲ CPT Changes: An Insider's View 2007

96910 Photochemotherapy; tar and ultraviolet B (Goeckerman treatment) or petrolatum and ultraviolet B

➲ CPT Assistant Jul 12:9, Sep 16:3, Mar 22:14

96912 psoralens and ultraviolet A (PUVA)

➲ CPT Assistant Jul 12:9, Sep 16:3, Mar 22:14

96913 Photochemotherapy (Goeckerman and/or PUVA) for severe photoresponsive dermatoses requiring at least 4-8 hours of care under direct supervision of the physician (includes application of medication and dressings)

➲ CPT Assistant Sep 16:3, Mar 22:14

96920 Excimer laser treatment for psoriasis; total area less than 250 sq cm

➲ CPT Changes: An Insider's View 2003, 2024

➲ CPT Assistant Oct 10:9, Jul 12:9, May 13:12, Sep 16:3, Jul 20:14, Mar 22:14

96921 250 sq cm to 500 sq cm

➲ CPT Changes: An Insider's View 2003, 2024

➲ CPT Assistant Oct 10:9, Jul 12:9, May 13:12, Sep 16:3, Jul 20:14, Mar 22:14

96922 over 500 sq cm

➲ CPT Changes: An Insider's View 2003, 2024

➲ CPT Assistant Oct 10:9, Jul 12:9, May 13:12, Sep 16:3, Jul 20:14, Mar 22:14

(For laser destruction of premalignant lesions, see 17000-17004)

(For laser destruction of cutaneous vascular proliferative lesions, see 17106-17108)

(For laser destruction of benign lesions, see 17110-17111)

(For laser destruction of malignant lesions, see 17260-17286)

Codes 96931, 96932, 96933, 96934, 96935, 96936 describe the acquisition and/or diagnostic interpretation of the device generated stitched image mosaics related to a single lesion. Do not report 96931, 96932, 96933, 96934, 96935, 96936 for a reflectance confocal microscopy examination that does not produce mosaic images. For services rendered using reflectance confocal microscopy not generating mosaic images, use 96999.

96931 Reflectance confocal microscopy (RCM) for cellular and sub-cellular imaging of skin; image acquisition and interpretation and report, first lesion

➲ CPT Changes: An Insider's View 2016

➲ CPT Assistant Sep 17:9

96932 image acquisition only, first lesion

➲ CPT Changes: An Insider's View 2016

➲ CPT Assistant Sep 17:9

96933 interpretation and report only, first lesion

➲ CPT Changes: An Insider's View 2016

➲ CPT Assistant Sep 17:9

+ 96934 image acquisition and interpretation and report, each additional lesion (List separately in addition to code for primary procedure)

➲ CPT Changes: An Insider's View 2016

➲ CPT Assistant Sep 17:9

(Use 96934 in conjunction with 96931)

+ 96935 image acquisition only, each additional lesion (List separately in addition to code for primary procedure)

➲ CPT Changes: An Insider's View 2016

➲ CPT Assistant Sep 17:9

(Use 96935 in conjunction with 96932)

+ 96936 interpretation and report only, each additional lesion (List separately in addition to code for primary procedure)

➲ CPT Changes: An Insider's View 2016

➲ CPT Assistant Sep 17:9

(Use 96936 in conjunction with 96933)

96999 Unlisted special dermatological service or procedure

➲ CPT Assistant Jul 12:9, May 13:12, Sep 17:9, Jul 20:14, Mar 22:14

Physical Medicine and Rehabilitation

Codes 97010-97763 should be used to report each distinct procedure performed. Do not append modifier 51 to 97010-97763.

The work of the physician or other qualified health care professional consists of face-to-face time with the patient (and caregiver, if applicable) delivering skilled services. For the purpose of determining the total time of a service, incremental intervals of treatment at the same visit may be accumulated.

(For range of joint motion, see 95851, 95852)

(For biofeedback training by EMG, use 90901)

(For transcutaneous nerve stimulation [TENS], use 97014 for electrical stimulation requiring supervision only, or use 97032 for electrical stimulation requiring constant attendance)

Physical Therapy Evaluations

Physical therapy evaluations include a patient history and an examination with development of a plan of care, conducted by the physician or other qualified health care professional, which is based on the composite of the patient's presentation.

Coordination, consultation, and collaboration of care with physicians, other qualified health care professionals, or agencies is provided consistent with the nature of the problem(s) and the needs of the patient, family, and/or other caregivers.

At a minimum, each of the following components noted in the code descriptors must be documented, in order to report the selected level of physical therapy evaluation.

Physical therapy evaluations include the following components:

- History
- Examination
- Clinical decision making
- Development of plan of care

Report 97164 for performance of patient re-evaluation that is based on an established and ongoing plan of care.

Definitions

The level of the physical therapy evaluation performed is dependent on clinical decision making and on the nature of the patient's condition (severity). For the purpose of reporting physical therapy evaluations, the body regions and body systems are defined as follows:

Body regions: head, neck, back, lower extremities, upper extremities, and trunk.

Body systems: musculoskeletal, neuromuscular, cardiovascular pulmonary, and integumentary.

A review of body systems include the following:

- For the musculoskeletal system: the assessment of gross symmetry, gross range of motion, gross strength, height, and weight
- For the neuromuscular system: a general assessment of gross coordinated movement (eg, balance, gait, locomotion, transfers, and transitions) and motor function (motor control and motor learning)
- For the cardiovascular pulmonary system: the assessment of heart rate, respiratory rate, blood pressure, and edema
- For the integumentary system: the assessment of pliability (texture), presence of scar formation, skin color, and skin integrity

A review of any of the body systems also includes the assessment of the ability to make needs known, consciousness, orientation (person, place, and time), expected emotional/behavioral responses, and learning preferences (eg, learning barriers, education needs).

Body structures: The structural or anatomical parts of the body, such as organs, limbs, and their components, classified according to body systems.

Personal factors: Factors that include sex, age, coping styles, social background, education, profession, past and current experience, overall behavior pattern, character, and other factors that influence how disability is experienced by the individual. Personal factors that exist but do not impact the physical therapy plan of care are not to be considered, when selecting a level of service.

#★ **97161** Physical therapy evaluation: low complexity, requiring these components:

- A history with no personal factors and/or comorbidities that impact the plan of care;
- An examination of body system(s) using standardized tests and measures addressing 1-2 elements from any of the following: body structures and functions, activity limitations, and/or participation restrictions;
- A clinical presentation with stable and/or uncomplicated characteristics; and
- Clinical decision making of low complexity using standardized patient assessment instrument and/or measurable assessment of functional outcome.

Typically, 20 minutes are spent face-to-face with the patient and/or family.

➔ *CPT Changes: An Insider's View* 2017
➔ *CPT Assistant* Aug 17:3, May 18:5

#★ **97162** Physical therapy evaluation: moderate complexity, requiring these components:

- A history of present problem with 1-2 personal factors and/or comorbidities that impact the plan of care;
- An examination of body systems using standardized tests and measures in addressing a total of 3 or more elements from any of the following: body structures and functions, activity limitations, and/or participation restrictions;
- An evolving clinical presentation with changing characteristics; and
- Clinical decision making of moderate complexity using standardized patient assessment instrument and/or measurable assessment of functional outcome.

Typically, 30 minutes are spent face-to-face with the patient and/or family.

➔ *CPT Changes: An Insider's View* 2017
➔ *CPT Assistant* Aug 17:3, May 18:5

97163 Physical therapy evaluation: high complexity, requiring these components:

- A history of present problem with 3 or more personal factors and/or comorbidities that impact the plan of care;

- An examination of body systems using standardized tests and measures addressing a total of 4 or more elements from any of the following: body structures and functions, activity limitations, and/or participation restrictions;

- A clinical presentation with unstable and unpredictable characteristics; and

- Clinical decision making of high complexity using standardized patient assessment instrument and/or measurable assessment of functional outcome.

Typically, 45 minutes are spent face-to-face with the patient and/or family.

➔ *CPT Changes: An Insider's View* 2017

➔ *CPT Assistant* Aug 17:3, May 18:5

97164 Re-evaluation of physical therapy established plan of care, requiring these components:

- An examination including a review of history and use of standardized tests and measures is required; and

- Revised plan of care using a standardized patient assessment instrument and/or measurable assessment of functional outcome.

Typically, 20 minutes are spent face-to-face with the patient and/or family.

➔ *CPT Changes: An Insider's View* 2017

➔ *CPT Assistant* Aug 17:3, May 18:5

Occupational Therapy Evaluations

Occupational therapy evaluations include an occupational profile, medical and therapy history, relevant assessments, and development of a plan of care, which reflects the therapist's clinical reasoning and interpretation of the data.

Coordination, consultation, and collaboration of care with physicians, other qualified health care professionals, or agencies is provided consistent with the nature of the problem(s) and the needs of the patient, family and/or other caregivers.

At a minimum, each of the following components noted in the code descriptors must be documented, in order to report the selected level of occupational therapy evaluation.

Occupational therapy evaluations include the following components:

- Occupational profile and client history (medical and therapy)
- Assessments of occupational performance
- Clinical decision making
- Development of plan of care

Report 97168 for performance of a re-evaluation that is based on an established and ongoing plan of care.

Definitions

The level of the occupational therapy evaluation performed is determined by patient condition, complexity of clinical decision making, and the scope and nature of the patient's performance deficits relating to physical, cognitive, or psychosocial skills to be assessed. The patient's plan of treatment should reflect assessment of each of the identified performance deficits.

Performance deficits: performance deficits refer to the inability to complete activities due to the lack of skills in one or more of the categories below (ie, relating to physical, cognitive, or psychosocial skills):

- *Physical skills:* Physical skills refer to impairments of body structure or body function (eg, balance, mobility, strength, endurance, fine or gross motor coordination, sensation, dexterity).

- *Cognitive skills:* Cognitive skills refer to the ability to attend, perceive, think, understand, problem solve, mentally sequence, learn, and remember resulting in the ability to organize occupational performance in a timely and safe manner. These skills are observed when: (1) a person attends to and selects, interacts with, and uses task tools and materials; (2) carries out individual actions and steps; and (3) modifies performance when problems are encountered.

- *Psychosocial skills:* Psychosocial skills refer to interpersonal interactions, habits, routines and behaviors, active use of coping strategies, and/or environmental adaptations to develop skills necessary to successfully and appropriately participate in everyday tasks and social situations.

#★ 97165   Occupational therapy evaluation, low complexity, requiring these components:

- An occupational profile and medical and therapy history, which includes a brief history including review of medical and/or therapy records relating to the presenting problem;

- An assessment(s) that identifies 1-3 performance deficits (ie, relating to physical, cognitive, or psychosocial skills) that result in activity limitations and/or participation restrictions; and

- Clinical decision making of low complexity, which includes an analysis of the occupational profile, analysis of data from problem-focused assessment(s), and consideration of a limited number of treatment options. Patient presents with no comorbidities that affect occupational performance. Modification of tasks or assistance (eg, physical or verbal) with assessment(s) is not necessary to enable completion of evaluation component.

Typically, 30 minutes are spent face-to-face with the patient and/or family.
➲ *CPT Changes: An Insider's View* 2017
➲ *CPT Assistant* Feb 17:3, May 18:5

#★ 97166   Occupational therapy evaluation, moderate complexity, requiring these components:

- An occupational profile and medical and therapy history, which includes an expanded review of medical and/or therapy records and additional review of physical, cognitive, or psychosocial history related to current functional performance;

- An assessment(s) that identifies 3-5 performance deficits (ie, relating to physical, cognitive, or psychosocial skills) that result in activity limitations and/or participation restrictions; and

- Clinical decision making of moderate analytic complexity, which includes an analysis of the occupational profile, analysis of data from detailed assessment(s), and consideration of several treatment options. Patient may present with comorbidities that affect occupational performance. Minimal to moderate modification of tasks or assistance (eg, physical or verbal) with assessment(s) is necessary to enable patient to complete evaluation component.

Typically, 45 minutes are spent face-to-face with the patient and/or family.
➲ *CPT Changes: An Insider's View* 2017
➲ *CPT Assistant* Feb 17:3, May 18:5

 # 97167   Occupational therapy evaluation, high complexity, requiring these components:

- An occupational profile and medical and therapy history, which includes review of medical and/or therapy records and extensive additional review of physical, cognitive, or psychosocial history related to current functional performance;

- An assessment(s) that identifies 5 or more performance deficits (ie, relating to physical, cognitive, or psychosocial skills) that result in activity limitations and/or participation restrictions; and

- Clinical decision making of high analytic complexity, which includes an analysis of the patient profile, analysis of data from comprehensive assessment(s), and consideration of multiple treatment options. Patient presents with comorbidities that affect occupational performance. Significant modification of tasks or assistance (eg, physical or verbal) with assessment(s) is necessary to enable patient to complete evaluation component.

Typically, 60 minutes are spent face-to-face with the patient and/or family.
➲ *CPT Changes: An Insider's View* 2017
➲ *CPT Assistant* Feb 17:3, May 18:5

 # 97168   Re-evaluation of occupational therapy established plan of care, requiring these components:

- An assessment of changes in patient functional or medical status with revised plan of care;

- An update to the initial occupational profile to reflect changes in condition or environment that affect future interventions and/or goals; and

- A revised plan of care. A formal reevaluation is performed when there is a documented change in functional status or a significant change to the plan of care is required.

Typically, 30 minutes are spent face-to-face with the patient and/or family.
➲ *CPT Changes: An Insider's View* 2017
➲ *CPT Assistant* Feb 17:3, May 18:5

Athletic Training Evaluations

Athletic training evaluations include a patient history and an examination with development of a plan of care, conducted by the physician or other qualified health care professional.

Coordination, consultation, and collaboration of care with physicians, other qualified health care professionals, or agencies is provided consistent with the nature of the problem(s) and the needs of the patient, family, and/or other caregivers.

At a minimum, each of the following components noted in the code descriptors must be documented, in order to report the selected level of athletic training evaluation.

Athletic training evaluations include the following components:

- History and physical activity profile
- Examination
- Clinical decision making
- Development of plan of care

Report 97172 for performance of patient re-evaluation that is based on an established and ongoing plan of care.

Definitions

For the purpose of reporting athletic training evaluations, the body areas and body systems are defined as follows:

Body areas: head, neck, back, lower extremities, upper extremities, and trunk.

Body systems: musculoskeletal, neuromuscular, cardiovascular pulmonary, and integumentary.

The body systems review includes the following:

- For the musculoskeletal system: the assessment of gross symmetry, gross range of motion, gross strength, height, and weight
- For the neuromuscular system: a general assessment of gross coordinated movement (eg, balance, gait, locomotion, transfers, and transitions) and motor function (motor control and motor learning)
- For the cardiovascular pulmonary system: the assessment of heart rate, respiratory rate, blood pressure, and edema
- For the integumentary system: the assessment of pliability (texture), presence of scar formation, skin color, and skin integrity

 # 97169   Athletic training evaluation, low complexity, requiring these components:

- A history and physical activity profile with no comorbidities that affect physical activity;
- An examination of affected body area and other symptomatic or related systems addressing 1-2 elements from any of the following: body structures, physical activity, and/or participation deficiencies; and
- Clinical decision making of low complexity using standardized patient assessment instrument and/or measurable assessment of functional outcome.

Typically, 15 minutes are spent face-to-face with the patient and/or family.

➔ *CPT Changes: An Insider's View* 2017
➔ *CPT Assistant* Jun 17:6, May 18:5

 # 97170   Athletic training evaluation, moderate complexity, requiring these components:

- A medical history and physical activity profile with 1-2 comorbidities that affect physical activity;
- An examination of affected body area and other symptomatic or related systems addressing a total of 3 or more elements from any of the following: body structures, physical activity, and/or participation deficiencies; and
- Clinical decision making of moderate complexity using standardized patient assessment instrument and/or measurable assessment of functional outcome.

Typically, 30 minutes are spent face-to-face with the patient and/or family.

➔ *CPT Changes: An Insider's View* 2017
➔ *CPT Assistant* Jun 17:6, May 18:5

 # 97171   Athletic training evaluation, high complexity, requiring these components:

- A medical history and physical activity profile, with 3 or more comorbidities that affect physical activity;
- A comprehensive examination of body systems using standardized tests and measures addressing a total of 4 or more elements from any of the following: body structures, physical activity, and/or participation deficiencies;
- Clinical presentation with unstable and unpredictable characteristics; and
- Clinical decision making of high complexity using standardized patient assessment instrument and/or measurable assessment of functional outcome.

Typically, 45 minutes are spent face-to-face with the patient and/or family.

➔ *CPT Changes: An Insider's View* 2017
➔ *CPT Assistant* Jun 17:6, May 18:5

 # 97172   Re-evaluation of athletic training established plan of care requiring these components:

- An assessment of patient's current functional status when there is a documented change; and
- A revised plan of care using a standardized patient assessment instrument and/or measurable assessment of functional outcome with an update in management options, goals, and interventions.

Typically, 20 minutes are spent face-to-face with the patient and/or family.

➔ *CPT Changes: An Insider's View* 2017
➔ *CPT Assistant* Jun 17:6, May 18:5

Modalities

Any physical agent applied to produce therapeutic changes to biologic tissue; includes but not limited to thermal, acoustic, light, mechanical, or electric energy.

Supervised

The application of a modality that does not require direct (one-on-one) patient contact.

97010   Application of a modality to 1 or more areas; hot or cold packs

➔ *CPT Assistant* Summer 95:5, Apr 96:11, Nov 97:47, Dec 98:1, Nov 01:5, Aug 02:11, Aug 06:11, Nov 09:10, Jun 10:8, Aug 10:13, Nov 10:8, Jun 16:9, May 18:5

97012   traction, mechanical

➔ *CPT Assistant* Summer 95:5, Apr 96:11, Nov 97:47, Dec 98:1, May 99:11, Nov 01:5, Aug 02:11, Dec 03:4, Oct 04:9, Jun 10:8, Aug 10:13, Nov 10:8, Jun 16:9, May 18:5, Jul 20:14, Apr 24:37

97014   electrical stimulation (unattended)

➔ *CPT Assistant* Summer 95:5, Apr 96:11, Nov 97:47, May 98:10, Nov 01:5, Jan 02:11, Apr 02:18, Aug 02:11, Dec 03:4, Nov 09:10, Jun 10:8, Aug 10:13, Nov 10:8, Aug 11:6, May 18:5, Oct 18:8, Jul 19:11

(For acupuncture with electrical stimulation, see 97813, 97814)

(For peripheral nerve transcutaneous magnetic stimulation, see 0766T, 0767T)

97016   vasopneumatic devices

➔ *CPT Assistant* Summer 95:6, Apr 96:11, Dec 98:1, Nov 01:5, Aug 02:11, May 05:14, Jun 10:8, Aug 10:13, Nov 10:8, May 18:5

97018   paraffin bath

➔ *CPT Assistant* Summer 95:6, Apr 96:11, Dec 98:1, Nov 01:5, Aug 02:11, Nov 09:10, Jun 10:8, Aug 10:13, Nov 10:8, May 18:5

97022   whirlpool

➔ *CPT Assistant* Summer 95:6, Apr 96:11, May 98:10, Dec 98:1, Nov 01:5, Aug 02:11, Nov 09:10, Jun 10:8, Aug 10:13, Nov 10:8, May 18:5

97024   diathermy (eg, microwave)

➔ *CPT Changes: An Insider's View* 2006
➔ *CPT Assistant* Summer 95:6, Apr 96:11, Dec 98:1, Nov 01:5, Aug 02:11, Nov 09:10, Jun 10:8, Aug 10:13, Nov 10:8, May 18:5

97026   infrared

➔ *CPT Assistant* Summer 95:6, Apr 96:11, Dec 98:1, Nov 01:5, Aug 02:11, Nov 09:10, Feb 10:12, Jun 10:8, Aug 10:13, Nov 10:8, May 18:5

97028   ultraviolet

➔ *CPT Assistant* Summer 95:6, Apr 96:11, Dec 98:1, Nov 01:5, Aug 02:11, Nov 09:10, Jun 10:8, Aug 10:13, Nov 10:8, May 18:5

Constant Attendance

The application of a modality that requires direct (one-on-one) patient contact.

97032   Application of a modality to 1 or more areas; electrical stimulation (manual), each 15 minutes

➔ *CPT Assistant* Summer 95:6, Dec 98:1, Nov 01:5, Apr 02:18, Jul 04:14, Nov 09:10, Jun 10:8, Aug 10:13, Nov 10:8, May 18:5, Oct 18:8, Jul 19:11

(For transcutaneous electrical modulation pain reprocessing [TEMPR/scrambler therapy], use 0278T)

(For peripheral nerve transcutaneous magnetic stimulation, see 0766T, 0767T)

 # 97037   low-level laser therapy (ie, nonthermal and non-ablative) for post-operative pain reduction

➔ *CPT Changes: An Insider's View* 2024

(Do not report 97037 in conjunction with 0552T)

(For dynamic thermokinetic energies therapy, infrared, use 97026)

97033   iontophoresis, each 15 minutes

➔ *CPT Assistant* Summer 95:7, Dec 98:1, Nov 01:5, Nov 09:10, Jun 10:8, Aug 10:13, Nov 10:8, May 18:5

97034   contrast baths, each 15 minutes

➔ *CPT Assistant* Summer 95:7, Dec 98:1, Nov 01:5, Jun 10:8, Aug 10:13, Nov 10:8, May 18:5

97035   ultrasound, each 15 minutes

➔ *CPT Assistant* Summer 95:7, Sep 96:10, Dec 98:1, Nov 01:5, Nov 09:10, Jun 10:8, Aug 10:13, Nov 10:8, May 18:5

97036   Hubbard tank, each 15 minutes

➔ *CPT Assistant* Summer 95:7, Dec 98:1, Nov 01:5, Nov 09:10, Jun 10:8, Aug 10:13, Nov 10:8, May 18:5

97037   Code is out of numerical sequence. See 97028-97034

97039   Unlisted modality (specify type and time if constant attendance)

➔ *CPT Assistant* Summer 95:7, May 98:10, Dec 98:1, Jan 00:10, Nov 01:5, May 05:14, Nov 09:10, Feb 10:12, Jun 10:8, Aug 10:13, Nov 10:8, Jun 16:9, Nov 16:10, May 18:5, Jul 20:14

Therapeutic Procedures

A manner of effecting change through the application of clinical skills and/or services that attempt to improve function.

Physician or other qualified health care professional (eg, therapist) is required to have direct, one-on-one patient contact, except for group therapeutic procedure (97150)

and work hardening/conditioning (97545, 97546) that require direct patient contact, but not one-on-one contact.

★ **97110** Therapeutic procedure, 1 or more areas, each 15 minutes; therapeutic exercises to develop strength and endurance, range of motion and flexibility

➔ *CPT Assistant* Summer 95:7, Feb 97:10, Nov 98:37, Dec 99:11, Mar 05:11, Apr 05:14, Aug 05:11, Dec 05:8, Mar 06:15, Aug 06:11, May 08:13, Dec 09:15, May 10:9, Mar 12:9, Mar 14:15, Aug 14:6, Jun 16:9, Dec 17:15, May 18:5, Dec 18:7, Jun 19:15

★ **97112** neuromuscular reeducation of movement, balance, coordination, kinesthetic sense, posture, and/or proprioception for sitting and/or standing activities

➔ *CPT Changes: An Insider's View* 2002

➔ *CPT Assistant* Summer 95:7, Feb 97:10, Apr 05:14, Aug 05:11, Mar 06:15, Aug 06:11, May 08:13, Oct 09:10, May 10:9, Mar 12:9, Mar 14:15, May 18:5

97113 aquatic therapy with therapeutic exercises

➔ *CPT Assistant* Summer 95:7, Feb 97:10, Apr 05:14, Mar 06:15, Aug 06:11, Oct 09:10, May 10:9, Mar 14:15, May 18:5

★ **97116** gait training (includes stair climbing)

➔ *CPT Assistant* Summer 95:8, Sep 96:7, Feb 97:10, Jun 03:3, Apr 05:14, Mar 06:15, Aug 06:11, Oct 09:10, May 10:9, Mar 14:15, May 18:5

►(Use 96000, 96001, 96002 to report comprehensive gait and motion analysis procedures)◄

(For motor-cognitive, semi-immersive virtual reality–facilitated gait training, use 97116 in conjunction with 0791T)

97124 massage, including effleurage, petrissage and/or tapotement (stroking, compression, percussion)

➔ *CPT Assistant* Summer 95:8, May 96:10, Feb 97:10, Dec 99:7, Apr 05:14, May 05:14, Mar 06:15, Aug 06:11, Oct 09:10, May 10:9, Mar 14:15, Jun 16:9, May 18:5, Jun 19:15, Jul 20:10

(For myofascial release, use 97140)

97129 Therapeutic interventions that focus on cognitive function (eg, attention, memory, reasoning, executive function, problem solving, and/or pragmatic functioning) and compensatory strategies to manage the performance of an activity (eg, managing time or schedules, initiating, organizing, and sequencing tasks), direct (one-on-one) patient contact; initial 15 minutes

➔ *CPT Changes: An Insider's View* 2020

➔ *CPT Assistant* Jul 20:10

(Report 97129 only once per day)

+ **97130** each additional 15 minutes (List separately in addition to code for primary procedure)

➔ *CPT Changes: An Insider's View* 2020

➔ *CPT Assistant* Mar 20:15, Jul 20:10

(Use 97130 in conjunction with 97129)

(Do not report 97129, 97130 in conjunction with 97153, 97155)

97139 Unlisted therapeutic procedure (specify)

➔ *CPT Assistant* Summer 95:8, Feb 97:10, Apr 05:14, Aug 06:11, Mar 14:15, May 18:5

➔ *Clinical Examples in Radiology* Summer 18:9

97140 Manual therapy techniques (eg, mobilization/manipulation, manual lymphatic drainage, manual traction), 1 or more regions, each 15 minutes

➔ *CPT Assistant* Nov 98:37, Feb 99:10, Mar 99:1, Jul 99:11, Aug 01:10, Dec 03:5, May 09:9, Oct 09:10, Mar 14:15, Mar 15:10, Aug 16:11, Sep 16:11, Nov 16:9, May 18:5, Jun 19:15, Feb 20:9

(For needle insertion[s] without injection[s] [eg, dry needling, trigger-point acupuncture], see 20560, 20561)

97150 Therapeutic procedure(s), group (2 or more individuals)

➔ *CPT Assistant* Summer 95:8, Dec 96:10, Feb 97:10, Oct 99:10, Nov 99:54-55, Dec 99:11, Apr 05:14, Aug 06:11, Mar 14:15, Nov 16:9, May 18:5, Nov 18:3, Jul 20:7

(Report 97150 for each member of group)

(Group therapy procedures involve constant attendance of the physician or other qualified health care professional [eg, therapist], but by definition do not require one-on-one patient contact by the same physician or other qualified health care professional)

(For manipulation under general anesthesia, see appropriate anatomic section in **Musculoskeletal System**)

(For osteopathic manipulative treatment [OMT], see 98925-98929)

(Do not report 97150 in conjunction with 97154, 97158)

97151 Code is out of numerical sequence. See 96020-96112

97152 Code is out of numerical sequence. See 96020-96112

97153 Code is out of numerical sequence. See 96020-96112

97154 Code is out of numerical sequence. See 96020-96112

97155 Code is out of numerical sequence. See 96020-96112

97156 Code is out of numerical sequence. See 96020-96112

97157 Code is out of numerical sequence. See 96020-96112

97158 Code is out of numerical sequence. See 96020-96112

97161 Code is out of numerical sequence. See Physical Therapy Evaluations subsection

97162 Code is out of numerical sequence. See Physical Therapy Evaluations subsection

97163 Code is out of numerical sequence. See Physical Therapy Evaluations subsection

97164 Code is out of numerical sequence. See Physical Therapy Evaluations subsection

97165   Code is out of numerical sequence. See Occupational Therapy Evaluations subsection

97166   Code is out of numerical sequence. See Occupational Therapy Evaluations subsection

97167   Code is out of numerical sequence. See Occupational Therapy Evaluations subsection

97168   Code is out of numerical sequence. See Occupational Therapy Evaluations subsection

97169   Code is out of numerical sequence. See Athletic Training Evaluations subsection

97170   Code is out of numerical sequence. See Athletic Training Evaluations subsection

97171   Code is out of numerical sequence. See Athletic Training Evaluations subsection

97172   Code is out of numerical sequence. See Athletic Training Evaluations subsection

★ **97530**   Therapeutic activities, direct (one-on-one) patient contact (use of dynamic activities to improve functional performance), each 15 minutes
➔ *CPT Changes: An Insider's View* 2013
➔ *CPT Assistant* Summer 95:9, Dec 01:6, Apr 03:26, Jul 03:15, Aug 05:11, May 08:13, Mar 14:15, May 18:5, Dec 18:7

97533   Sensory integrative techniques to enhance sensory processing and promote adaptive responses to environmental demands, direct (one-on-one) patient contact, each 15 minutes
➔ *CPT Changes: An Insider's View* 2001, 2013
➔ *CPT Assistant* Dec 01:1, Mar 14:15, May 18:5

★ **97535**   Self-care/home management training (eg, activities of daily living (ADL) and compensatory training, meal preparation, safety procedures, and instructions in use of assistive technology devices/adaptive equipment) direct one-on-one contact, each 15 minutes
➔ *CPT Changes: An Insider's View* 2002, 2013
➔ *CPT Assistant* Sep 96:7, Apr 00:11, Dec 03:6, Mar 14:15, Mar 15:10, Jun 15:11, Aug 16:3, May 18:5, Mar 21:4

97537   Community/work reintegration training (eg, shopping, transportation, money management, avocational activities and/or work environment/modification analysis, work task analysis, use of assistive technology device/adaptive equipment), direct one-on-one contact, each 15 minutes
➔ *CPT Changes: An Insider's View* 2004, 2013
➔ *CPT Assistant* Sep 96:7, Dec 03:6, Mar 14:15, May 18:5, Mar 21:4

(For wheelchair management/propulsion training, use 97542)

97542   Wheelchair management (eg, assessment, fitting, training), each 15 minutes
➔ *CPT Changes: An Insider's View* 2006
➔ *CPT Assistant* Sep 96:8, Mar 14:15, Jun 15:11, May 18:5, Mar 21:4

97545   Work hardening/conditioning; initial 2 hours
➔ *CPT Assistant* Apr 03:26, Jul 03:15, May 08:13, Mar 14:15, May 18:5

+ **97546**   each additional hour (List separately in addition to code for primary procedure)
➔ *CPT Assistant* Mar 14:15, May 18:5

(Use 97546 in conjunction with 97545)

Caregiver Training Without the Patient Present

Caregiver training is direct, skilled intervention for the caregiver(s) to provide strategies and techniques to equip caregiver(s) with knowledge and skills to assist patients living with functional deficits. Codes 97550, 97551 are used to report the total duration of face-to-face time spent by the qualified health care professional providing training to the caregiver(s) of an individual patient without the patient present. Code 97552 is used to report group caregiver training provided to multiple sets of caregivers for multiple patients with similar conditions or therapeutic needs without the patient present.

During a skilled intervention, the caregiver(s) is trained using verbal instructions, video and live demonstrations, and feedback from the qualified health care professional on the use of strategies and techniques to facilitate functional performance and safety in the home or community without the patient present. Skilled training supports a caregiver's understanding of the patient's treatment plan, ability to engage in activities with the patient in between treatment sessions, and knowledge of external resources to assist in areas such as activities of daily living (ADLs), transfers, mobility, safety practices, problem solving, and communication.

These services do not represent therapeutic interventions requiring direct one-to-one patient contact.

97550   Caregiver training in strategies and techniques to facilitate the patient's functional performance in the home or community (eg, activities of daily living [ADLs], instrumental ADLs [iADLs], transfers, mobility, communication, swallowing, feeding, problem solving, safety practices) (without the patient present), face to face; initial 30 minutes
➔ *CPT Changes: An Insider's View* 2024
➔ *CPT Assistant* Nov 23:1

+ **97551**   each additional 15 minutes (List separately in addition to code for primary service)
➔ *CPT Changes: An Insider's View* 2024
➔ *CPT Assistant* Nov 23:1

(Use 97551 in conjunction with 97550)

97552 Group caregiver training in strategies and techniques to facilitate the patient's functional performance in the home or community (eg, activities of daily living [ADLs], instrumental ADLs [iADLs], transfers, mobility, communication, swallowing, feeding, problem solving, safety practices) (without the patient present), face to face with multiple sets of caregivers

➜ *CPT Changes: An Insider's View* 2024

➜ *CPT Assistant* Nov 23:1

Active Wound Care Management

Active wound care procedures are performed to remove devitalized and/or necrotic tissue and promote healing. Chemical cauterization (17250) to achieve wound hemostasis is included in active wound care procedures (97597, 97598, 97602) and should not be separately reported for the same lesion. Services require direct (one-on-one) contact with the patient.

(Do not report 97597-97602 in conjunction with 11042-11047 for the same wound)

(For debridement of burn wounds, see 16020-16030)

97597 Debridement (eg, high pressure waterjet with/without suction, sharp selective debridement with scissors, scalpel and forceps), open wound, (eg, fibrin, devitalized epidermis and/or dermis, exudate, debris, biofilm), including topical application(s), wound assessment, use of a whirlpool, when performed and instruction(s) for ongoing care, per session, total wound(s) surface area; first 20 sq cm or less

➜ *CPT Changes: An Insider's View* 2005, 2011

➜ *CPT Assistant* Jun 05:1, 10, Nov 09:10, Jun 10:8, Nov 10:9, May 11:3, Sep 11:11, Jan 12:8, Mar 12:11, Oct 12:3, Jun 14:11, Aug 16:9, Oct 16:3, May 18:5, Jul 21:3, Aug 22:16

+ 97598 each additional 20 sq cm, or part thereof (List separately in addition to code for primary procedure)

➜ *CPT Changes: An Insider's View* 2005, 2011

➜ *CPT Assistant* Jun 05:1, 10, May 11:3, Sep 11:11, Jan 12:8, Mar 12:11, Jun 14:11, Aug 16:9, Oct 16:3, May 18:5, Aug 22:16

(Use 97598 in conjunction with 97597)

97602 Removal of devitalized tissue from wound(s), non-selective debridement, without anesthesia (eg, wet-to-moist dressings, enzymatic, abrasion, larval therapy), including topical application(s), wound assessment, and instruction(s) for ongoing care, per session

➜ *CPT Changes: An Insider's View* 2001, 2017

➜ *CPT Assistant* May 02:5, Jun 05:1, 10, Sep 08:11, May 11:4, Aug 11:7, Jan 12:9, Mar 12:11, Dec 12:15, Jun 14:11, Oct 16:3, May 18:5

97605 Negative pressure wound therapy (eg, vacuum assisted drainage collection), utilizing durable medical equipment (DME), including topical application(s), wound assessment, and instruction(s) for ongoing care, per session; total wound(s) surface area less than or equal to 50 square centimeters

➜ *CPT Changes: An Insider's View* 2005, 2015

➜ *CPT Assistant* Apr 05:13, Jun 05:1, 10, May 11:4, Nov 14:8, Feb 16:14, May 18:5, Oct 21:14

97606 total wound(s) surface area greater than 50 square centimeters

➜ *CPT Changes: An Insider's View* 2005, 2015

➜ *CPT Assistant* Apr 05:13, Jun 05:1, 10, May 11:4, Nov 14:8, Feb 16:14, May 18:5, Oct 21:14

97607 Negative pressure wound therapy, (eg, vacuum assisted drainage collection), utilizing disposable, non-durable medical equipment including provision of exudate management collection system, topical application(s), wound assessment, and instructions for ongoing care, per session; total wound(s) surface area less than or equal to 50 square centimeters

➜ *CPT Changes: An Insider's View* 2015

➜ *CPT Assistant* Nov 14:8, May 18:5, Oct 21:14

97608 total wound(s) surface area greater than 50 square centimeters

➜ *CPT Changes: An Insider's View* 2015

➜ *CPT Assistant* Nov 14:8, May 18:5, Oct 21:14

(Do not report 97607, 97608 in conjunction with 97605, 97606)

97610 Low frequency, non-contact, non-thermal ultrasound, including topical application(s), when performed, wound assessment, and instruction(s) for ongoing care, per day

➜ *CPT Changes: An Insider's View* 2014

➜ *CPT Assistant* Jun 14:11, May 18:5

Tests and Measurements

Requires direct one-on-one patient contact.

(For joint range of motion, see 95851, 95852; for electromyography, see 95860-95872, 95885, 95886, 95887; for nerve velocity determination, see 95905, 95907, 95908, 95909, 95910, 95911, 95912, 95913)

★ 97750 Physical performance test or measurement (eg, musculoskeletal, functional capacity), with written report, each 15 minutes

➜ *CPT Assistant* Summer 95:5, Feb 97:10, Aug 98:11, Mar 00:11, Nov 01:5, May 02:18, Apr 03:28, Dec 03:7, Feb 04:5, Feb 07:12, May 08:9, Aug 13:7, May 18:5

★ **97755** Assistive technology assessment (eg, to restore, augment or compensate for existing function, optimize functional tasks and/or maximize environmental accessibility), direct one-on-one contact, with written report, each 15 minutes

➤ *CPT Changes: An Insider's View* 2004, 2013

➤ *CPT Assistant* May 18:5, Mar 21:4

(To report augmentative and alternative communication devices, see 92605, 92607)

Orthotic Management and Training and Prosthetic Training

★ **97760** Orthotic(s) management and training (including assessment and fitting when not otherwise reported), upper extremity(ies), lower extremity(ies) and/or trunk, initial orthotic(s) encounter, each 15 minutes

➤ *CPT Changes: An Insider's View* 2006, 2018

➤ *CPT Assistant* Dec 05:8, 11, Feb 07:8, May 18:5

(Code 97760 should not be reported with 97116 for the same extremity[ies])

★ **97761** Prosthetic(s) training, upper and/or lower extremity(ies), initial prosthetic(s) encounter, each 15 minutes

➤ *CPT Changes: An Insider's View* 2006, 2018

➤ *CPT Assistant* Dec 05:8, 11, Feb 07:8, May 18:5

97763 Orthotic(s)/prosthetic(s) management and/or training, upper extremity(ies), lower extremity(ies), and/or trunk, subsequent orthotic(s)/prosthetic(s) encounter, each 15 minutes

➤ *CPT Changes: An Insider's View* 2018

➤ *CPT Assistant* May 18:5

(Do not report 97763 in conjunction with 97760, 97761)

Other Procedures

(For extracorporeal shock wave musculoskeletal therapy, see 0101T, 0102T)

97799 Unlisted physical medicine/rehabilitation service or procedure

➤ *CPT Assistant* Summer 95:5, Oct 99:10, Nov 16:10, May 18:5

Medical Nutrition Therapy

★◀ **97802** Medical nutrition therapy; initial assessment and intervention, individual, face-to-face with the patient, each 15 minutes

➤ *CPT Changes: An Insider's View* 2001, 2017

➤ *CPT Assistant* Apr 03:10, Nov 03:1, Feb 09:13, Jul 20:7

★◀ **97803** re-assessment and intervention, individual, face-to-face with the patient, each 15 minutes

➤ *CPT Changes: An Insider's View* 2001, 2017

➤ *CPT Assistant* Apr 03:10, Nov 03:1, Feb 09:13, Jul 20:7

★◀ **97804** group (2 or more individual(s)), each 30 minutes

➤ *CPT Changes: An Insider's View* 2001, 2017

➤ *CPT Assistant* Apr 03:10, Nov 03:1, Feb 09:13, Jul 20:7

(Physicians and other qualified health care professionals who may report evaluation and management services should use the appropriate evaluation and management codes)

Acupuncture

Acupuncture is reported based on 15-minute increments of personal (face-to-face) contact with the patient, not the duration of acupuncture needle(s) placement.

If no electrical stimulation is used during a 15-minute increment, use 97810, 97811. If electrical stimulation of any needle is used during a 15-minute increment, use 97813, 97814.

Only one code may be reported for each 15-minute increment. Use either 97810 or 97813 for the initial 15-minute increment. Only one initial code is reported per day.

Evaluation and management services may be reported in addition to acupuncture procedures, when performed by physicians or other health care professionals who may report evaluation and management (E/M) services, including new or established patient office or other outpatient services (99202-99215), hospital inpatient or observation care (99221-99223, 99231-99233), office or other outpatient consultations (99242, 99243, 99244, 99245), inpatient or observation consultations (99252, 99253, 99254, 99255), critical care services (99291, 99292), inpatient neonatal intensive care services and pediatric and neonatal critical care services (99466-99480), emergency department services (99281-99285), nursing facility services (99304-99316), and home or residence services (99341-99350), separately using modifier 25 if the patient's condition requires a significant, separately identifiable E/M service above and beyond the usual preservice and postservice work associated with the acupuncture services. The time of the E/M service is not included in the time of the acupuncture service.

For needle insertion(s) without injection(s) (eg, dry needling, trigger point acupuncture), see 20560, 20561.

97810 Acupuncture, 1 or more needles; without electrical stimulation, initial 15 minutes of personal one-on-one contact with the patient

➤ *CPT Changes: An Insider's View* 2005

➤ *CPT Assistant* Jan 05:16-17, Jun 05:5, Jun 06:20, Aug 06:4, Feb 20:9, Feb 24:35

(Do not report 97810 in conjunction with 97813)

+▲ 97811 without electrical stimulation, each additional 15 minutes of personal one-on-one contact with the patient, with insertion of needle(s) (List separately in addition to code for primary procedure)

➜ *CPT Changes: An Insider's View* 2005, 2006, 2025

➜ *CPT Assistant* Jan 05:16, Jun 05:5, Aug 06:4, Feb 20:9, Feb 24:35

(Use 97811 in conjunction with 97810, 97813)

97813 with electrical stimulation, initial 15 minutes of personal one-on-one contact with the patient

➜ *CPT Changes: An Insider's View* 2005, 2006

➜ *CPT Assistant* Jan 05:16, 18, Jun 05:5, Jun 06:20, Aug 06:4, Feb 20:9, Feb 24:35

(Do not report 97813 in conjunction with 97810)

+▲ 97814 with electrical stimulation, each additional 15 minutes of personal one-on-one contact with the patient, with insertion of needle(s) (List separately in addition to code for primary procedure)

➜ *CPT Changes: An Insider's View* 2005, 2006, 2025

➜ *CPT Assistant* Jan 05:16, Jun 05:5, Aug 06:4, Feb 20:9, Feb 24:35

(Use 97814 in conjunction with 97810, 97813)

(Do not report 97810, 97811, 97813, 97814 in conjunction with 20560, 20561. When both time-based acupuncture services and needle insertion[s] without injection[s] are performed, report only the time-based acupuncture codes)

Acupuncture, Needle
97810-97811

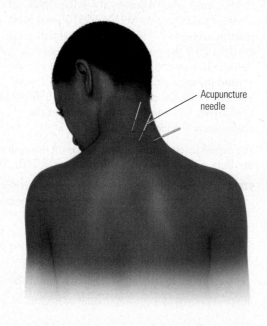

Acupuncture needle

98000 Code is out of numerical sequence. See E/M codes 99214-99222

98001 Code is out of numerical sequence. See E/M codes 99214-99222

98002 Code is out of numerical sequence. See E/M codes 99214-99222

98003 Code is out of numerical sequence. See E/M codes 99214-99222

98004 Code is out of numerical sequence. See E/M codes 99214-99222

98005 Code is out of numerical sequence. See E/M codes 99214-99222

98006 Code is out of numerical sequence. See E/M codes 99214-99222

98007 Code is out of numerical sequence. See E/M codes 99214-99222

98008 Code is out of numerical sequence. See E/M codes 99214-99222

98009 Code is out of numerical sequence. See E/M codes 99214-99222

98010 Code is out of numerical sequence. See E/M codes 99214-99222

98011 Code is out of numerical sequence. See E/M codes 99214-99222

98012 Code is out of numerical sequence. See E/M codes 99214-99222

98013 Code is out of numerical sequence. See E/M codes 99214-99222

98014 Code is out of numerical sequence. See E/M codes 99214-99222

98015 Code is out of numerical sequence. See E/M codes 99214-99222

98016 Code is out of numerical sequence. See E/M codes 99214-99222

Osteopathic Manipulative Treatment

Osteopathic manipulative treatment (OMT) is a form of manual treatment applied by a physician or other qualified health care professional to eliminate or alleviate somatic dysfunction and related disorders. This treatment may be accomplished by a variety of techniques.

Evaluation and management (E/M) services, including new or established patient office or other outpatient services (99202-99215), initial and subsequent hospital inpatient or observation care (99221-99223, 99231-99233), critical care services (99291, 99292), hospital inpatient or observation care services (including admission and discharge services 99234-99236), office or other outpatient consultations (99242, 99243, 99244, 99245), emergency department services (99281-99285), nursing facility services (99304-99316), and home or residence services (99341-99350), may be reported separately using modifier 25 if the patient's condition requires a significant, separately identifiable E/M service above and beyond the usual preservice and postservice work associated with the procedure. The E/M service may be caused or prompted by the same symptoms or condition for which the OMT service was provided. As such, different diagnoses are not required for the reporting of the OMT and E/M service on the same date.

Body regions referred to are: head region; cervical region; thoracic region; lumbar region; sacral region; pelvic region; lower extremities; upper extremities; rib cage region; abdomen and viscera region.

98925   Osteopathic manipulative treatment (OMT); 1-2 body regions involved

> *CPT Assistant* May 96:10, Jan 97:8, 10, Jul 98:10, Aug 00:11, Dec 00:15, Oct 09:10, Dec 17:15, Aug 18:9

98926   3-4 body regions involved

> *CPT Assistant* May 96:10, Jan 97:8, Aug 00:11, Dec 00:15, Oct 09:10, Aug 18:9

98927   5-6 body regions involved

> *CPT Assistant* May 96:10, Jan 97:8, Aug 00:11, Dec 00:15, Oct 09:10, Aug 18:9

98928   7-8 body regions involved

> *CPT Assistant* May 96:10, Jan 97:8, Aug 00:11, Dec 00:15, Oct 09:10, Mar 12:14, May 12:14, Aug 18:9

98929   9-10 body regions involved

> *CPT Assistant* May 96:10, Jan 97:8, 10, Aug 00:11, Oct 09:10, Aug 18:9

Chiropractic Manipulative Treatment

Chiropractic manipulative treatment (CMT) is a form of manual treatment to influence joint and neurophysiological function. This treatment may be accomplished using a variety of techniques.

The chiropractic manipulative treatment codes include a pre-manipulation patient assessment. Additional evaluation and management (E/M) services, including office or other outpatient services (99202-99215), subsequent hospital inpatient or observation care (99231-99233), office or other outpatient consultations (99242, 99243, 99244, 99245), subsequent nursing facility services (99307-99310), and home or residence services

(99341-99350), may be reported separately using modifier 25 if the patient's condition requires a significant, separately identifiable E/M service above and beyond the usual preservice and postservice work associated with the procedure. The E/M service may be caused or prompted by the same symptoms or condition for which the CMT service was provided. As such, different diagnoses are not required for the reporting of the CMT and E/M service on the same date.

For purposes of CMT, the five spinal regions referred to are: cervical region (includes atlanto-occipital joint); thoracic region (includes costovertebral and costotransverse joints); lumbar region; sacral region; and pelvic (sacro-iliac joint) region. The five extraspinal regions referred to are: head (including temporomandibular joint, excluding atlanto-occipital) region; lower extremities; upper extremities; rib cage (excluding costotransverse and costovertebral joints) and abdomen.

98940   Chiropractic manipulative treatment (CMT); spinal, 1-2 regions

> *CPT Assistant* Jan 97:7, 11, Feb 99:10, Dec 00:15, Mar 06:15, Dec 07:16-17, Oct 09:10, May 10:9, Dec 13:15, Nov 18:12

98941   spinal, 3-4 regions

> *CPT Assistant* Jan 97:7, 11, Mar 97:10, Feb 99:10, Dec 00:15, Mar 06:15, Dec 07:16-17, Oct 09:10, May 10:9, Nov 18:12

98942   spinal, 5 regions

> *CPT Assistant* Jan 97:7, 11, Feb 99:10, Dec 00:15, Mar 06:15, Dec 07:16-17, Oct 09:10, May 10:9, Nov 18:12

98943   extraspinal, 1 or more regions

> *CPT Assistant* Jan 97:7, 11, Mar 97:10, Feb 99:10, Dec 00:15, Mar 06:15, Dec 07:16-17, Oct 09:10, May 10:9, Dec 13:15, Nov 18:12

Education and Training for Patient Self-Management

▶The following codes are used to report educational and training services prescribed by a physician or other qualified health care professional and provided by a nonphysician qualified health care professional using a standardized curriculum to an individual or a group of patients for the treatment of established illness(s)/disease(s) or to delay comorbidity(s). Education and training for patient self-management may be reported with these codes only when using a standardized curriculum as described below. This curriculum may be modified as necessary for the clinical needs, cultural norms, and health literacy of the individual patient(s).◄

The purpose of the educational and training services is to teach the patient (may include caregiver[s]) how to effectively self-manage the patient's illness(s)/disease(s) or delay disease comorbidity(s) in conjunction with the patient's professional healthcare team. Education and training related to subsequent reinforcement or due to changes in the patient's condition or treatment plan are reported in the same manner as the original education and training. The type of education and training provided for the patient's clinical condition will be identified by the appropriate diagnosis code(s) reported.

►The qualifications of the nonphysician qualified health care professionals and the content of the educational and training program must be consistent with guidelines or standards established or recognized by a physician society, nonphysician health care professional society/association, or other appropriate source.◄

(For counseling and education provided by a physician to an individual, see the appropriate evaluation and management codes, including office or other outpatient services [99202-99215], initial and subsequent hospital inpatient or observation care [99221-99223, 99231-99233, 99234, 99235, 99236], new or established patient office or other outpatient consultations [99242, 99243, 99244, 99245], inpatient or observation consultations [99252, 99253, 99254, 99255], emergency department services [99281-99285], nursing facility services [99304-99316], home or residence services [99341-99350], and counseling risk factor reduction and behavior change intervention [99401-99429]. See also **Instructions for Use of the CPT Codebook** for definition of reporting qualifications)

(For counseling and education provided by a physician to a group, use 99078)

(For counseling and/or risk factor reduction intervention provided by a physician to patient[s] without symptoms or established disease, see 99401-99412)

(For medical nutrition therapy, see 97802-97804)

(For health behavior assessment and intervention that is not part of a standardized curriculum, see 96156, 96158, 96159, 96164, 96165, 96167, 96168, 96170, 96171)

►(For education provided as genetic counseling services, use 96041. For education to a group regarding genetic risks, see 98961, 98962)◄

★▲ **98960**   Education and training for patient self-management by a nonphysician qualified health care professional using a standardized curriculum, face-to-face with the patient (could include caregiver/family) each 30 minutes; individual patient
➜ *CPT Changes: An Insider's View* 2006, 2017, 2025
➜ *CPT Assistant* Apr 13:3, Nov 13:3, Oct 14:3, Jul 20:7

★▲ **98961**   2-4 patients
➜ *CPT Changes: An Insider's View* 2006, 2017, 2025
➜ *CPT Assistant* Aug 07:9, Aug 08:3, Feb 09:13, Apr 13:3, Jul 20:7

★▲ **98962**   5-8 patients
➜ *CPT Changes: An Insider's View* 2006, 2017, 2025
➜ *CPT Assistant* Aug 07:9, Aug 08:3, Feb 09:13, Apr 13:3, Nov 13:3, Oct 14:3, Jul 20:7

►Non-Face-to-Face Nonphysician Qualified Health Care Professional Services◄

Telephone Services

►Telephone services are non-face-to-face assessment and management services provided by a nonphysician qualified health care professional to a patient using the telephone. These codes are used to report episodes of care by the qualified health care professional initiated by an established patient or guardian of an established patient. If the telephone service ends with a decision to see the patient within 24 hours or the next available urgent visit appointment, the code is not reported; rather the encounter is considered part of the preservice work of the subsequent assessment and management service, procedure, and visit. Likewise, if the telephone call refers to a service performed and reported by the qualified health care professional within the previous seven days (either qualified health care professional requested or unsolicited patient follow-up) or within the postoperative period of the previously completed procedure, then the service(s) are considered part of that previous service or procedure. (Do not report 98966-98968 if reporting 98966-98968 performed in the previous seven days.)◄

►(For telephone services provided by a physician, see 98012, 98013, 98014, 98015, 98016)◄

▲ **98966**   Telephone assessment and management service provided by a nonphysician qualified health care professional to an established patient, parent, or guardian not originating from a related assessment and management service provided within the previous 7 days nor leading to an assessment and management service or procedure within the next 24 hours or soonest available appointment; 5-10 minutes of medical discussion
➜ *CPT Changes: An Insider's View* 2008, 2025
➜ *CPT Assistant* Apr 13:3, Oct 13:11, Nov 13:3, Oct 14:3, Mar 18:7

▲ **98967**   11-20 minutes of medical discussion
➔ *CPT Changes: An Insider's View* 2008, 2025
➔ *CPT Assistant* Apr 13:3, Oct 13:11, Mar 18:7

▲ **98968**   21-30 minutes of medical discussion
➔ *CPT Changes: An Insider's View* 2008, 2025
➔ *CPT Assistant* Apr 13:3, Oct 13:11, Nov 13:3, Oct 14:3, Mar 18:7

(Do not report 98966-98968 during the same month with 99426, 99427, 99439, 99487, 99489, 99490, 99491)

(Do not report 98966, 98967, 98968 in conjunction with 93792, 93793)

▶Nonphysician Qualified Health Care Professional Online Digital Assessment and Management Service◀

▶Nonphysician qualified health care professional online digital assessment and management services are patient-initiated digital services that require patient evaluation and decision making to generate an assessment and subsequent management of the patient. These services are not for the nonevaluative electronic communication of test results, scheduling of appointments, or other communication that does not include assessment and management. While the patient's problem may be new, the patient is an established patient. Patients initiate these services through Health Insurance Portability and Accountability Act (HIPAA)-compliant, secure platforms, such as through the electronic health record (EHR) portal, email, or other digital applications, which allow digital communication.

Nonphysician qualified health care professional online digital assessments are reported once for the nonphysician qualified health care professional's cumulative time devoted to the service during a seven-day period. The seven-day period begins with the personal review of the patient-generated inquiry. The cumulative service time includes review of the initial inquiry, review of patient records or data pertinent to assessment of the patient's problem, personal interaction with clinical staff focused on the patient's problem, development of management plans, including the generation of prescriptions or ordering of tests, and subsequent communication with the patient through online, telephone, email, or other digitally supported communication. All nonphysician qualified health care professionals in the same group practice who are involved in an online digital assessment contribute to the cumulative service time devoted to the patient's online digital assessment. The online digital assessments require visit documentation and permanent storage (electronic or hard copy) of the encounter.

If the patient generates the initial online digital inquiry within seven days of a previous treatment or assessment and management service and both services relate to the same problem, or the online digital inquiry occurs within

the postoperative period of a previously completed procedure, then the online digital assessment may not be reported separately. If the patient generates an initial online digital inquiry for a new problem within seven days of a previous service that addressed a different problem, then the online digital assessment is reported separately. If a separately reported evaluation service occurs within seven days of the initial review of the online digital assessment, codes 98970, 98971, 98972 may not be reported. If the patient presents a new, unrelated problem during the seven-day period of an online digital assessment, then the time spent assessing the additional problem is added to the cumulative service time of the online digital assessment for that seven-day period.◀

▶(Do not report an assessment and management service within 7 days of reporting an online digital assessment and management treatment and/or service)◀

(For an online digital E/M service provided by a physician or other qualified health care professional, see 99421, 99422, 99423)

▲ **98970**   Nonphysician qualified health care professional online digital assessment and management, for an established patient, for up to 7 days, cumulative time during the 7 days; 5-10 minutes
➔ *CPT Changes: An Insider's View* 2020, 2025
➔ *CPT Assistant* Jan 20:3, Mar 20:6, Sep 21:3

▲ **98971**   11-20 minutes
➔ *CPT Changes: An Insider's View* 2020, 2025
➔ *CPT Assistant* Jan 20:3, Mar 20:6, Sep 21:3

▲ **98972**   21 or more minutes
➔ *CPT Changes: An Insider's View* 2020, 2025
➔ *CPT Assistant* Jan 20:3, Mar 20:6, Sep 21:3

(Report 98970, 98971, 98972 once per 7-day period)

▶(Do not report online digital assessment and management services for cumulative visit time less than 5 minutes)◀

(Do not count 98970, 98971, 98972 time otherwise reported with other services)

(Do not report 98970, 98971, 98972 for home and outpatient INR monitoring when reporting 93792, 93793)

(Do not report 98970, 98971, 98972 when using 99091, 99374, 99375, 99377, 99378, 99379, 99380, 99426, 99427, 99437, 99439, 99487, 99489, 99490, 99491, for the same communication[s])

Remote Therapeutic Monitoring Services

Remote therapeutic monitoring services (eg, musculoskeletal system status, respiratory system status, cognitive behavioral therapy, therapy adherence, therapy response) represent the review and monitoring of data related to signs, symptoms, and functions of a therapeutic response. These data may represent objective device-generated integrated data or subjective inputs reported by a patient. These data are reflective of therapeutic responses that provide a functionally integrative representation of patient status.

▶Codes 98976, 98977, 98978 are used to report remote therapeutic monitoring services during a 30-day period. To report 98975, 98976, 98977, 98978, the service(s) must be ordered by a physician or other qualified health care professional. Code 98975 may be used to report the set-up and patient education on the use of any device(s) utilized for therapeutic data collection generated through digital monitoring or digital therapy. Codes 98976, 98977, 98978 may be used to report supply of the device for data access or data transmissions to support monitoring. To report 98975, 98976, 98977, 98978, the device used must be a medical device as defined by the FDA. In addition to its monitoring functionality, the device may also provide a therapeutic intervention. Codes 98975, 98976, 98977, 98978 are not reported if cumulative monitoring is less than 16 days. Do not report 98975, 98976, 98977, 98978 with other physiologic monitoring services (eg, 95250 for continuous glucose monitoring requiring a minimum of 72 hours of monitoring or 99453, 99454 for remote monitoring of physiologic parameter[s]).◀

Code 98975 is reported for each episode of care. For reporting remote therapeutic monitoring parameters, an episode of care is defined as beginning when the remote therapeutic monitoring service is initiated and ends with attainment of targeted treatment goals.

▲ **98975** Remote therapeutic monitoring (eg, therapy adherence, therapy response, digital therapeutic intervention); initial set-up and patient education on use of equipment

➔ *CPT Changes: An Insider's View* 2022, 2023, 2025

➔ *CPT Assistant* Jan 22:12, Feb 22:7-8, Oct 22:14, Feb 23:3, Oct 23:13

(Do not report 98975 more than once per episode of care)

▶(Do not report 98975 for less than 16 days of cumulative monitoring during the 30-day period)◀

▲ **98976** device(s) supply for data access or data transmissions to support monitoring of respiratory system, each 30 days

➔ *CPT Changes: An Insider's View* 2022, 2023, 2025

➔ *CPT Assistant* Jan 22:12, Feb 22:7-8, Oct 22:14, Feb 23:3

▲ **98977** device(s) supply for data access or data transmissions to support monitoring of musculoskeletal system, each 30 days

➔ *CPT Changes: An Insider's View* 2022, 2023, 2025

➔ *CPT Assistant* Jan 22:12, Feb 22:7-8, Oct 22:14, Feb 23:3, Oct 23:13

▲ **98978** device(s) supply for data access or data transmissions to support monitoring of cognitive behavioral therapy, each 30 days

➔ *CPT Changes: An Insider's View* 2023, 2025

➔ *CPT Assistant* Feb 23:3

(Do not report 98975, 98976, 98977, 98978 in conjunction with codes for more specific physiologic parameters [93296, 94760, 99453, 99454])

▶(Do not report 98976, 98977, 98978 for cumulative monitoring of less than 16 days)◀

(For therapeutic monitoring treatment management services, use 98980)

(For remote physiologic monitoring, see 99453, 99454)

(For physiologic monitoring treatment management services, use 99457)

(For self-measured blood pressure monitoring, see 99473, 99474)

Remote Therapeutic Monitoring Treatment Management Services

▶Remote therapeutic monitoring treatment management services are provided when a physician or other qualified health care professional uses the results of remote therapeutic monitoring to manage a patient under a specific treatment plan. To report remote therapeutic monitoring, the service must be ordered by a physician or other qualified health care professional. To report 98980, 98981, any device used must be a medical device as defined by the FDA. Do not use 98980, 98981 for time that can be reported using codes for more specific monitoring services. Codes 98980, 98981 may be reported during the same service period as chronic care management services (99439, 99487, 99489, 99490, 99491), transitional care management services (99495, 99496), principal care management services (99424, 99425, 99426, 99427), behavioral health integration services (99484), psychotherapy services (90832-90853), health behavior assessment and intervention services (96156, 96158, 96159, 96160, 96161, 96164, 96165, 96167, 96168, 96170, 96171), and psychiatric collaborative care services (99492, 99493, 99494). However, time spent performing these services should remain separate and no time should be counted toward the required time for both services in a single month. Codes 98980, 98981 require at least one interactive communication with the patient or caregiver. The interactive communication contributes to the total time, but it does not need to represent the entire cumulative reported time of the treatment management service. For the first completed 20 minutes of physician or other qualified health care professional time in a calendar month, report 98980, and report 98981 for each additional completed 20 minutes. Do not report 98980, 98981 for services of less than 20 minutes. Report 98980 once, regardless of the number of therapeutic monitoring modalities performed in a given calendar month.◀

Do not count any time on a day when the physician or other qualified health care professional reports an E/M service (office or other outpatient services [99202, 99203, 99204, 99205, 99211, 99212, 99213, 99214, 99215], home or residence services [99341, 99342, 99344, 99345, 99347, 99348, 99349, 99350], inpatient or observation care services [99221, 99222, 99223, 99231, 99232, 99233, 99234, 99235, 99236], inpatient consultations [99252, 99253, 99254, 99255]).

▶Do not count any time directly related to other reported services (eg, psychotherapy services [90832, 90833, 90834, 90836, 90837, 90838], interrogation device evaluation services [93290], anticoagulant management services [93793], respiratory monitoring services [94774, 94775, 94776, 94777], health behavior assessment and intervention services [96156, 96158, 96159, 96160, 96161, 96164, 96165, 96167, 96168, 96170, 96171], therapeutic interventions that focus on cognitive function services [97129, 97130], adaptive behavior treatment services [97153, 97154, 97155, 97156, 97157, 97158], therapeutic procedures [97110, 97112, 97116, 97530, 97535], tests and measurements [97750, 97755], .physical therapy evaluation services [97161, 97162, 97163, 97164], occupational therapy evaluations [97165, 97166, 97167, 97168], orthotic management and training and prosthetic training services [97760, 97761, 97763], medical nutrition therapy services [97802, 97803, 97804], medication therapy management services [99605, 99606, 99607], critical care services [99291, 99292], principal care management services [99424, 99425, 99426, 99427]) in the cumulative time of the remote therapeutic monitoring treatment management service during the calendar month of reporting.◀

98980   Remote therapeutic monitoring treatment management services, physician or other qualified health care professional time in a calendar month requiring at least one interactive communication with the patient or caregiver during the calendar month; first 20 minutes

➔ *CPT Changes: An Insider's View* 2022

➔ *CPT Assistant* Jan 22:4, 14, Feb 22:7-9, Oct 22:14, Feb 23:15, Oct 23:13

(Report 98980 once each 30 days, regardless of the number of therapeutic parameters monitored)

(Do not report 98980 for services of less than 20 minutes)

(Do not report 98980 in conjunction with 93264, 99091, 99457, 99458)

(Do not report 98980 in the same calendar month as 99473, 99474)

+ 98981   each additional 20 minutes (List separately in addition to code for primary procedure)

➔ *CPT Changes: An Insider's View* 2022

➔ *CPT Assistant* Jan 22:4, 14, Feb 22:7-9, Oct 22:14, Feb 23:15, Oct 23:13

(Use 98981 in conjunction with 98980)

(Do not report 98981 for services of less than an additional increment of 20 minutes)

Special Services, Procedures and Reports

The procedures with code numbers 99000 through 99082 provide the reporting physician or other qualified health care professional with the means of identifying the completion of special reports and services that are an adjunct to the basic services rendered. The specific number assigned indicates the special circumstances under which a basic procedure is performed.

Codes 99050-99060 are reported in addition to an associated basic service. Do not append modifier 51 to 99050-99060. Typically only a single adjunct code from among 99050-99060 would be reported per patient encounter. However, there may be circumstances in which reporting multiple adjunct codes per patient encounter may be appropriate.

Miscellaneous Services

99000   Handling and/or conveyance of specimen for transfer from the office to a laboratory

➔ *CPT Changes: An Insider's View* 2013

➔ *CPT Assistant* Winter 94:26, Feb 99:10, Oct 99:11, May 02:19, Aug 06:6, Sep 06:15, Jan 07:30

99001   Handling and/or conveyance of specimen for transfer from the patient in other than an office to a laboratory (distance may be indicated)

➔ *CPT Changes: An Insider's View* 2013

➔ *CPT Assistant* Winter 94:26, May 02:19, Aug 06:6, Sep 06:15, Jan 07:30

99002   Handling, conveyance, and/or any other service in connection with the implementation of an order involving devices (eg, designing, fitting, packaging, handling, delivery or mailing) when devices such as orthotics, protectives, prosthetics are fabricated by an outside laboratory or shop but which items have been designed, and are to be fitted and adjusted by the attending physician or other qualified health care professional

➡ *CPT Changes: An Insider's View* 2013

➡ *CPT Assistant* Winter 94:26, May 02:19, Aug 06:6, Sep 06:15, Jan 07:30

(For routine collection of venous blood, use 36415)

99024   Postoperative follow-up visit, normally included in the surgical package, to indicate that an evaluation and management service was performed during a postoperative period for a reason(s) related to the original procedure

➡ *CPT Changes: An Insider's View* 2004

➡ *CPT Assistant* Winter 94:26, Sep 97:10, Aug 98:5, May 02:19, Nov 03:13, Aug 06:6, Sep 06:15, Jan 07:30, Mar 15:3, Jan 17:3, Jul 17:9

(As a component of a surgical "package," see **Surgery Guidelines**)

99026   Hospital mandated on call service; in-hospital, each hour

➡ *CPT Changes: An Insider's View* 2003

➡ *CPT Assistant* Jun 03:10, Aug 06:6, Sep 06:15, Jan 07:30

99027   out-of-hospital, each hour

➡ *CPT Changes: An Insider's View* 2003

➡ *CPT Assistant* Jun 03:10, Aug 06:6, Sep 06:15, Jan 07:30

(For standby services requiring prolonged attendance, use 99360, as appropriate. Time spent performing separately reportable procedure(s) or service(s) should not be included in the time reported as mandated on-call service)

99050   Services provided in the office at times other than regularly scheduled office hours, or days when the office is normally closed (eg, holidays, Saturday or Sunday), in addition to basic service

➡ *CPT Changes: An Insider's View* 2004, 2006

➡ *CPT Assistant* Winter 94:27, May 02:19, Jun 03:10, May 06:18, Aug 06:6, Sep 06:15, Jan 07:30, Aug 10:9

99051   Service(s) provided in the office during regularly scheduled evening, weekend, or holiday office hours, in addition to basic service

➡ *CPT Changes: An Insider's View* 2006

➡ *CPT Assistant* May 06:18, Aug 06:6, Sep 06:15, Jan 07:30, Aug 10:9

99053   Service(s) provided between 10:00 PM and 8:00 AM at 24-hour facility, in addition to basic service

➡ *CPT Changes: An Insider's View* 2006

➡ *CPT Assistant* May 06:18, Aug 06:6, Sep 06:15, Jan 07:30

99056   Service(s) typically provided in the office, provided out of the office at request of patient, in addition to basic service

➡ *CPT Changes: An Insider's View* 2006

➡ *CPT Assistant* Winter 94:27, May 02:19, May 06:18, Aug 06:6, Sep 06:15, Jan 07:30

99058   Service(s) provided on an emergency basis in the office, which disrupts other scheduled office services, in addition to basic service

➡ *CPT Changes: An Insider's View* 2006

➡ *CPT Assistant* Winter 94:27, May 02:19, May 06:18, Aug 06:6, Sep 06:15, Jan 07:30, Aug 10:9

99060   Service(s) provided on an emergency basis, out of the office, which disrupts other scheduled office services, in addition to basic service

➡ *CPT Changes: An Insider's View* 2006

➡ *CPT Assistant* May 06:18, Aug 06:6, Sep 06:15, Jan 07:30

99070   Supplies and materials (except spectacles), provided by the physician or other qualified health care professional over and above those usually included with the office visit or other services rendered (list drugs, trays, supplies, or materials provided)

➡ *CPT Changes: An Insider's View* 2013

➡ *CPT Assistant* Winter 94:28, May 98:10, Jun 99:10, Jun 00:11, Jul 01:2, May 02:19, Aug 02:11, Jun 05:1, Jul 06:1, Aug 06:6, Sep 06:15, Jan 07:30-31, Feb 07:8, Sep 08:11, May 09:8, Sep 09:5, May 10:10, Jun 10:8, Sep 10:11, Apr 12:10, Nov 12:11, Mar 13:6, Dec 13:12, Mar 14:11, Jan 17:6, Sep 17:15, Jan 18:3, Mar 18:7, Jun 18:11, Apr 19:11, Jan 21:7

(For supply of spectacles, use the appropriate supply codes)

(For additional supplies, materials, and clinical staff time required during a Public Health Emergency, as defined by law, due to respiratory-transmitted infectious disease, use 99072)

99071   Educational supplies, such as books, tapes, and pamphlets, for the patient's education at cost to physician or other qualified health care professional

➡ *CPT Changes: An Insider's View* 2013

➡ *CPT Assistant* Winter 94:28, May 02:19, Aug 06:6, Sep 06:15, Jan 07:30, Apr 13:3, Nov 13:3, Oct 14:3

Code 99072 is used to report the additional supplies, materials, and clinical staff time over and above the practice expense(s) included in an office visit or other non-facility service(s) when the office visit or other non-facility service(s) is rendered during a Public Health Emergency (PHE), as defined by law, due to respiratory-transmitted infectious disease. These required additional supplies, materials, and clinical staff time are intended to mitigate the transmission of the respiratory disease for which the PHE was declared. These include, but are not limited to, additional supplies, such as face masks and cleaning supplies, as well as clinical staff time for activities such as pre-visit instructions and office arrival symptom checks that support the safe provision of evaluation, treatment, or procedural service(s) during the respiratory infection–focused PHE. When reporting 99072, report only once per in-person patient encounter per day regardless of the number of services rendered at that encounter. Code 99072 may be reported during a PHE when the additional clinical staff duties as described are performed by the physician or other qualified health care professional in lieu of clinical staff.

99072 Additional supplies, materials, and clinical staff time over and above those usually included in an office visit or other non-facility service(s), when performed during a Public Health Emergency, as defined by law, due to respiratory-transmitted infectious disease
➜ *CPT Changes: An Insider's View* 2022
➜ *CPT Assistant* May 21:7, Jan 22:12, Jun 23:28

99075 Medical testimony
➜ *CPT Assistant* Winter 94:28, May 02:19, Aug 06:6, Sep 06:15, Jan 07:30

99078 Physician or other qualified health care professional qualified by education, training, licensure/regulation (when applicable) educational services rendered to patients in a group setting (eg, prenatal, obesity, or diabetic instructions)
➜ *CPT Changes: An Insider's View* 2013
➜ *CPT Assistant* Winter 94:28, Jan 98:12, May 02:19, Aug 06:6, Sep 06:15, Jan 07:30, Aug 07:9, Apr 13:3, Nov 13:3, Oct 14:3

99080 Special reports such as insurance forms, more than the information conveyed in the usual medical communications or standard reporting form
➜ *CPT Assistant* Winter 94:28, May 02:19, Aug 06:6, Sep 06:15, Jan 07:30, Apr 13:3, Nov 13:3, Oct 14:3

(Do not report 99080 in conjunction with 99455, 99456 for the completion of Workmen's Compensation forms)

99082 Unusual travel (eg, transportation and escort of patient)
➜ *CPT Assistant* May 02:19, Jan 03:24, Nov 03:14, Aug 06:6, Sep 06:15, Jan 07:30

99091 Code is out of numerical sequence. See 99448-99455

Qualifying Circumstances for Anesthesia

(For explanation of these services, see **Anesthesia Guidelines**)

+ 99100 Anesthesia for patient of extreme age, younger than 1 year and older than 70 (List separately in addition to code for primary anesthesia procedure)
➜ *CPT Assistant* Apr 08:3, Dec 17:8, Oct 19:10

(For procedure performed on infants younger than 1 year of age at time of surgery, see 00326, 00561, 00834, 00836)

+ 99116 Anesthesia complicated by utilization of total body hypothermia (List separately in addition to code for primary anesthesia procedure)
➜ *CPT Assistant* Apr 08:3, Dec 17:8, Oct 19:10

+ 99135 Anesthesia complicated by utilization of controlled hypotension (List separately in addition to code for primary anesthesia procedure)
➜ *CPT Assistant* Apr 08:3, Dec 17:8, Oct 19:10

+ 99140 Anesthesia complicated by emergency conditions (specify) (List separately in addition to code for primary anesthesia procedure)
➜ *CPT Assistant* Mar 01:10, Apr 08:3, Dec 17:8, Oct 19:10

(An emergency is defined as existing when delay in treatment of the patient would lead to a significant increase in the threat to life or body part)

Moderate (Conscious) Sedation

Moderate (also known as conscious) sedation is a drug-induced depression of consciousness during which patients respond purposefully to verbal commands, either alone or accompanied by light tactile stimulation. No interventions are required to maintain cardiovascular function or a patent airway, and spontaneous ventilation is adequate.

Moderate sedation codes 99151, 99152, 99153, 99155, 99156, 99157 are not used to report administration of medications for pain control, minimal sedation (anxiolysis), deep sedation, or monitored anesthesia care (00100-01999).

For purposes of reporting, intraservice time of moderate sedation is used to select the appropriate code(s). The following definitions are used to determine intraservice time (compared to pre- and postservice time).

An independent trained observer is an individual who is qualified to monitor the patient during the procedure, who has no other duties (eg, assisting at surgery) during the procedure.

Preservice Work

The preservice activities required for moderate sedation are included in the work described by each of these codes (99151, 99152, 99153, 99155, 99156, 99157) and are not reported separately. The following preservice work components are not included when determining intraservice time for reporting:

- Assessment of the patient's past medical and surgical history with particular emphasis on cardiovascular, pulmonary, airway, or neurological conditions;

- Review of the patient's previous experiences with anesthesia and/or sedation;

- Family history of sedation complications;

- Summary of the patient's present medication list;

- Drug allergy and intolerance history;

- Focused physical examination of the patient with emphasis on:

  - Mouth, jaw, oropharynx, neck and airway for Mallampati score assessment;

  - Chest and lungs;

  - Heart and circulation;

- Vital signs, including heart rate, respiratory rate, blood pressure, and oxygenation with end tidal CO_2 when indicated;

- Review of any pre-sedation diagnostic tests;

- Completion of a pre-sedation assessment form (with an American Society of Anesthesiologists [ASA] Physical Status classification);

- Patient informed consent;

- Immediate pre-sedation assessment prior to first sedating doses; and

- Initiation of IV access and fluids to maintain patency.

Intraservice Work

Intraservice time is used to determine the appropriate CPT code to report moderate sedation services:

- Begins with the administration of the sedating agent(s);

- Ends when the procedure is completed, the patient is stable for recovery status, and the physician or other qualified health care professional providing the sedation ends personal continuous face-to-face time with the patient;

- Includes ordering and/or administering the initial and subsequent doses of sedating agents;

- Requires continuous face-to-face attendance of the physician or other qualified health care professional;

- Requires monitoring patient response to the sedating agents, including:

  - Periodic assessment of the patient;

  - urther administration of agent(s) as needed to maintain sedation; and

  - Monitoring of oxygen saturation, heart rate, and blood pressure.

If the physician or other qualified health care professional who provides the sedation services also performs the procedure supported by sedation (99151, 99152, 99153), the physician or other qualified health care professional

will supervise and direct an independent trained observer who will assist in monitoring the patient's level of consciousness and physiological status throughout the procedure.

Postservice Work

The postservice activities required for moderate sedation are included in the work described by each of these codes (99151, 99152, 99153, 99155, 99156, 99157) and are not reported separately. Once continuous face-to-face time with the patient has ended, additional face-to-face time with the patient is not added to the intraservice time, however, it is considered as part of the postservice work. The following postservice work components are not included, when determining intraservice time for reporting:

- Assessment of the patient's vital signs, level of consciousness, neurological, cardiovascular, and pulmonary stability in the post-sedation recovery period;

- Assessment of the patient's readiness for discharge following the procedure;

- Preparation of documentation regarding sedation service; and

- Communication with family/caregiver regarding sedation service.

Postservice work/times are not used to select the appropriate code.

Do not report 99151, 99152, 99153, 99155, 99156, 99157 in conjunction with 94760, 94761, 94762.

Codes 99151, 99152, 99155, 99156 are reported for the first 15 minutes of intraservice time providing moderate sedation. Codes 99153, 99157 are reported for each additional 15 minutes, in addition to the code for the primary service.

⊘ **99151** Moderate sedation services provided by the same physician or other qualified health care professional performing the diagnostic or therapeutic service that the sedation supports, requiring the presence of an independent trained observer to assist in the monitoring of the patient's level of consciousness and physiological status; initial 15 minutes of intraservice time, patient younger than 5 years of age

➜ *CPT Changes: An Insider's View* 2017

➜ *CPT Assistant* Jan 17:3, May 17:3, Jun 17:3, Sep 17:11, Nov 20:13, Nov 21:14

➜ *Clinical Examples in Radiology* Winter 17:5, Winter 18:11, Spring 18:8, Spring 20:6, Fall 20:4, Fall 21:8, Spring 22:10, Summer 23:27, Fall 23:33

Total Intraservice Time for Moderate Sedation	Patient Age	Moderate Sedation (MS) provided by physician or other qualified health care professional (same physician or qualified health care professional also performing the procedure MS is supporting) Code(s)	MS provided by different physician or other qualified health care professional (not the physician or qualified health care professional who Is performing the procedure MS is supporting) Code(s)
Less than 10 minutes	Any age	Not reported separately	Not reported separately
10-22 minutes	< 5 years	99151	99155
10-22 minutes	5 years or older	99152	99156
23-37 minutes	< 5 years	99151 + 99153 X 1	99155 + 99157 X 1
23-37 minutes	5 years or older	99152 + 99153 X 1	99156 + 99157 X 1
38-52 minutes	< 5 years	99151 + 99153 X 2	99155 + 99157 X 2
38-52 minutes	5 years or older	99152 + 99153 X 2	99156 + 99157 X 2
53-67 minutes (53 min. - 1 hr. 7 min.)	< 5 years	99151 + 99153 X 3	99155 + 99157 X 3
53-67 minutes (53 min. - 1 hr. 7) min.)	5 years or older	99152 + 99153 X 3	99156 + 99157 X 3
68-82 minutes (1 hr. 8 min. - 1 hr. 22 min.)	< 5 years	99151 + 99153 X 4	99155 + 99157 X 4
68-82 minutes (1 hr. 8 min. - 1 hr. 22 min.)	5 years or older	99152 + 99153 X 4	99156 + 99157 X 4
83 minutes or longer (1 hr. 23 min. - etc.)	< 5 years	99153	Add 99157
83 minutes or longer (1 hr. 23 min. - etc.)	5 years or older	Add 99153	Add 99157

⊘ **99152**   initial 15 minutes of intraservice time, patient age 5 years or older

➔ *CPT Changes: An Insider's View* 2017

➔ *CPT Assistant* Jan 17:3, May 17:3, Jun 17:3, Sep 17:11, May 19:10, Nov 20:13, Nov 21:14

➔ *Clinical Examples in Radiology* Winter 17:5, Spring 17:2, Fall 17:2, Winter 18:3, Spring 18:4, Summer 18:2, Spring 19:2, Summer 19:4, Spring 20:6, Fall 20:3-5, Fall 21:8, Winter 22:18, Spring 22:10, Fall 22:21, Winter 23:10, Summer 23:27, Fall 23:33

+ 99153   each additional 15 minutes intraservice time (List separately in addition to code for primary service)

➔ *CPT Changes: An Insider's View* 2017

➔ *CPT Assistant* Jan 17:3, May 17:3, Jun 17:3, Sep 17:11, May 19:10, Nov 20:13, Nov 21:14

➔ *Clinical Examples in Radiology* Winter 17:5, Spring 17:2, Fall 17:2, Winter 18:3, Spring 18:4, Summer 18:2, Spring 19:2, Summer 19:4, Spring 20:6, Fall 20:3-5, Fall 21:8, Winter 22:18, Spring 22:10, Fall 22:21, Winter 23:10, Summer 23:27, Fall 23:33

(Use 99153 in conjunction with 99151, 99152)

(Do not report 99153 in conjunction with 99155, 99156)

99155   Moderate sedation services provided by a physician or other qualified health care professional other than the physician or other qualified health care professional performing the diagnostic or therapeutic service that the sedation supports; initial 15 minutes of intraservice time, patient younger than 5 years of age

➔ *CPT Changes: An Insider's View* 2017

➔ *CPT Assistant* Jan 17:3, May 17:3, Jun 17:3, Sep 17:11, Nov 20:13, Nov 21:14

➔ *Clinical Examples in Radiology* Winter 17:5, Spring 18:10, Spring 20:6, Fall 20:5, Fall 21:8, Summer 23:27, Fall 23:33

99156 initial 15 minutes of intraservice time, patient age 5 years or older

➔ *CPT Changes: An Insider's View* 2017

➔ *CPT Assistant* Jan 17:3, May 17:3, Jun 17:3, Sep 17:11, Nov 20:13, Nov 21:14

➔ *Clinical Examples in Radiology* Winter 17:5, Spring 18:10, Spring 20:6, Fall 20:5, Fall 21:8, Summer 23:27, Fall 23:33

+ 99157 each additional 15 minutes intraservice time (List separately in addition to code for primary service)

➔ *CPT Changes: An Insider's View* 2017

➔ *CPT Assistant* Jan 17:3, May 17:3, Jun 17:3, Sep 17:11, Nov 20:13, Nov 21:14

➔ *Clinical Examples in Radiology* Winter 17:5, Spring 18:10, Spring 20:6, Fall 20:5, Fall 21:8, Summer 23:27, Fall 23:33

(Use 99157 in conjunction with 99155, 99156)

(Do not report 99157 in conjunction with 99151, 99152)

Other Services and Procedures

99170 Anogenital examination, magnified, in childhood for suspected trauma, including image recording when performed

➔ *CPT Changes: An Insider's View* 2014

➔ *CPT Assistant* Nov 99:55, Apr 06:1, Sep 14:7

(For moderate sedation, see 99151, 99152, 99153, 99155, 99156, 99157)

99172 Visual function screening, automated or semi-automated bilateral quantitative determination of visual acuity, ocular alignment, color vision by pseudoisochromatic plates, and field of vision (may include all or some screening of the determination[s] for contrast sensitivity, vision under glare)

➔ *CPT Changes: An Insider's View* 2001

➔ *CPT Assistant* Feb 01:7, Mar 05:1, 3

(This service must employ graduated visual acuity stimuli that allow a quantitative determination of visual acuity [eg, Snellen chart]. This service may not be used in addition to a general ophthalmological service or an E/M service)

(Do not report 99172 in conjunction with 99173, 99174, 99177, 0469T)

99173 Screening test of visual acuity, quantitative, bilateral

➔ *CPT Changes: An Insider's View* 2000

➔ *CPT Assistant* Nov 99:55, May 02:2, Mar 05:1, 3

(The screening test used must employ graduated visual acuity stimuli that allow a quantitative estimate of visual acuity [eg, Snellen chart]. Other identifiable services unrelated to this screening test provided at the same time may be reported separately [eg, preventive medicine services]. When acuity is measured as part of a general ophthalmological service or of an E/M service of the eye, it is a diagnostic examination and not a screening test.)

(Do not report 99173 in conjunction with 99172, 99174, 99177)

99174 Instrument-based ocular screening (eg, photoscreening, automated-refraction), bilateral; with remote analysis and report

➔ *CPT Changes: An Insider's View* 2008, 2013, 2016

➔ *CPT Assistant* Mar 13:6, Mar 16:11, Feb 18:3

(Do not report 99174 in conjunction with 92002-92014, 99172, 99173, 99177)

 # 99177 with on-site analysis

➔ *CPT Changes: An Insider's View* 2016

➔ *CPT Assistant* Mar 16:11, Feb 18:3

(Do not report 99177 in conjunction with 92002-92014, 99172, 99173, 99174)

(For retinal polarization scan, use 0469T)

99175 Ipecac or similar administration for individual emesis and continued observation until stomach adequately emptied of poison

(For diagnostic intubation, see 43754, 43755)

(For gastric lavage for diagnostic purposes, see 43754, 43755)

99177 Code is out of numerical sequence. See 99173-99183

99183 Physician or other qualified health care professional attendance and supervision of hyperbaric oxygen therapy, per session

➔ *CPT Changes: An Insider's View* 2013

➔ *CPT Assistant* Jan 03:23

(Evaluation and Management services and/or procedures [eg, wound debridement] provided in a hyperbaric oxygen treatment facility in conjunction with a hyperbaric oxygen therapy session should be reported separately)

99184 Initiation of selective head or total body hypothermia in the critically ill neonate, includes appropriate patient selection by review of clinical, imaging and laboratory data, confirmation of esophageal temperature probe location, evaluation of amplitude EEG, supervision of controlled hypothermia, and assessment of patient tolerance of cooling

➔ *CPT Changes: An Insider's View* 2015

➔ *CPT Assistant* Oct 15:8

(Do not report 99184 more than once per hospital stay)

99188 Application of topical fluoride varnish by a physician or other qualified health care professional

➔ *CPT Changes: An Insider's View* 2015

99190 Assembly and operation of pump with oxygenator or heat exchanger (with or without ECG and/or pressure monitoring); each hour

99191 45 minutes

99192   30 minutes

99195   Phlebotomy, therapeutic (separate procedure)
> *CPT Assistant* Apr 96:3, Jun 96:10

99199   Unlisted special service, procedure or report
> *CPT Changes: An Insider's View* 2000
> *CPT Assistant* Nov 99:55, Jun 12:16, Sep 12:9

Home Health Procedures/ Services

▶These codes are used by nonphysician qualified health care professionals. Physicians should utilize the home or residence services codes 99341-99350 and utilize CPT codes other than 99500-99600 for any additional procedure/service provided to a patient living in a home or residence.◀

The following codes are used to report services provided in a patient's home or residence (including assisted living facility, group home, custodial care facility, nontraditional private homes, or schools).

Health care professionals who are authorized to use Evaluation and Management (E/M) Home Visit codes (99341-99350) may report 99500-99600 in addition to 99341-99350 if both services are performed. E/M services may be reported separately, using modifier 25, if the patient's condition requires a significant separately identifiable E/M service, above and beyond the home health service(s)/procedure(s) codes 99500-99600.

99500   Home visit for prenatal monitoring and assessment to include fetal heart rate, non-stress test, uterine monitoring, and gestational diabetes monitoring
> *CPT Changes: An Insider's View* 2002
> *CPT Assistant* Oct 03:7, Jan 07:30

99501   Home visit for postnatal assessment and follow-up care
> *CPT Changes: An Insider's View* 2002
> *CPT Assistant* Oct 03:7, Jan 07:30

99502   Home visit for newborn care and assessment
> *CPT Changes: An Insider's View* 2002
> *CPT Assistant* Oct 03:7, Jan 07:30

99503   Home visit for respiratory therapy care (eg, bronchodilator, oxygen therapy, respiratory assessment, apnea evaluation)
> *CPT Changes: An Insider's View* 2002
> *CPT Assistant* Oct 03:7, Jan 07:30

99504   Home visit for mechanical ventilation care
> *CPT Changes: An Insider's View* 2002, 2003
> *CPT Assistant* Oct 03:7, Jan 07:30

99505   Home visit for stoma care and maintenance including colostomy and cystostomy
> *CPT Changes: An Insider's View* 2002
> *CPT Assistant* Oct 03:7, Jan 07:30

99506   Home visit for intramuscular injections
> *CPT Changes: An Insider's View* 2002
> *CPT Assistant* Oct 03:7, Jan 07:30

99507   Home visit for care and maintenance of catheter(s) (eg, urinary, drainage, and enteral)
> *CPT Changes: An Insider's View* 2002
> *CPT Assistant* Oct 03:7, Jan 07:30

99509   Home visit for assistance with activities of daily living and personal care
> *CPT Changes: An Insider's View* 2002
> *CPT Assistant* Oct 03:7, Jan 07:30

(To report self-care/home management training, see 97535)

(To report home medical nutrition assessment and intervention services, see 97802-97804)

(To report home speech therapy services, see 92507-92508)

99510   Home visit for individual, family, or marriage counseling
> *CPT Changes: An Insider's View* 2002
> *CPT Assistant* Oct 03:7, Jan 07:30

99511   Home visit for fecal impaction management and enema administration
> *CPT Changes: An Insider's View* 2002
> *CPT Assistant* Oct 03:7, Jan 07:30

99512   Home visit for hemodialysis
> *CPT Changes: An Insider's View* 2002, 2004
> *CPT Assistant* Oct 03:7, Jan 07:30

(For home infusion of peritoneal dialysis, use 99601, 99602)

99600   Unlisted home visit service or procedure
> *CPT Changes: An Insider's View* 2003
> *CPT Assistant* Oct 03:7, Jan 07:30

Home Infusion Procedures/Services

99601   Home infusion/specialty drug administration, per visit (up to 2 hours);
> *CPT Changes: An Insider's View* 2004
> *CPT Assistant* Nov 05:1

+ 99602   each additional hour (List separately in addition to code for primary procedure)
> *CPT Changes: An Insider's View* 2004
> *CPT Assistant* Nov 05:1

(Use 99602 in conjunction with 99601)

Medication Therapy Management Services

Medication therapy management service(s) (MTMS) describe face-to-face patient assessment and intervention as appropriate, by a pharmacist, upon request. MTMS is provided to optimize the response to medications or to manage treatment-related medication interactions or complications.

MTMS includes the following documented elements: review of the pertinent patient history, medication profile (prescription and nonprescription), and recommendations for improving health outcomes and treatment compliance. These codes are not to be used to describe the provision of product-specific information at the point of dispensing or any other routine dispensing-related activities.

99605　Medication therapy management service(s) provided by a pharmacist, individual, face-to-face with patient, with assessment and intervention if provided; initial 15 minutes, new patient
➲ *CPT Changes: An Insider's View* 2008
➲ *CPT Assistant* Apr 13:3, Nov 13:3, Oct 14:3

99606　　　initial 15 minutes, established patient
➲ *CPT Changes: An Insider's View* 2008
➲ *CPT Assistant* Apr 13:3

+ 99607　　　each additional 15 minutes (List separately in addition to code for primary service)
➲ *CPT Changes: An Insider's View* 2008
➲ *CPT Assistant* Apr 13:3, Nov 13:3, Oct 14:3

(Use 99607 in conjunction with 99605, 99606)

Category II Codes

The following section of *Current Procedural Terminology* (CPT) contains a set of supplemental tracking codes that can be used for performance measurement. It is anticipated that the use of Category II codes for performance measurement will decrease the need for record abstraction and chart review, and thereby minimize administrative burden on physicians, other health care professionals, hospitals, and entities seeking to measure the quality of patient care. These codes are intended to facilitate data collection about the quality of care rendered by coding certain services and test results that support nationally established performance measures and that have an evidence base as contributing to quality patient care.

The use of these codes is optional. The codes are not required for correct coding and may not be used as a substitute for Category I codes.

These codes describe clinical components that may be typically included in evaluation and management services or clinical services and, therefore, do not have a relative value associated with them. Category II codes may also describe results from clinical laboratory or radiology tests and other procedures, identified processes intended to address patient safety practices, or services reflecting compliance with state or federal law.

Category II codes described in this section make use of alphabetical characters as the 5th character in the string (ie, 4 digits followed by the letter **F**). These digits are not intended to reflect the placement of the code in the regular (Category I) part of the CPT code set. To promote understanding of these codes and their associated measures, users are referred to the Alphabetical Clinical Topics Listing, which contains information about performance measurement exclusion modifiers, measures, and the measure's source.

Cross-references to the measures associated with each Category II code and their source are included for reference in the Alphabetical Clinical Topics Listing. In addition, acronyms for the related diseases or clinical condition(s) have been added at the end of each code descriptor to identify the topic or clinical category in which that code is included. A complete listing of the diseases/clinical conditions, and their acronyms are provided in alphabetical order in the Alphabetical Clinical Topics Listing. The Alphabetical Clinical Topics Listing can be accessed on the website at https://www.ama-assn.org/practice-management/cpt/category-ii-codes. Users should review the complete measure(s) associated with each code prior to implementation.

Requests for Category II CPT codes will be reviewed by the CPT/HCPAC Advisory Committee just as requests for Category I CPT codes are reviewed. In developing

new and revised performance measurement codes, requests for codes are considered from:

- measurements that were developed and tested by a national organization;
- evidenced-based measurements with established ties to health outcomes;
- measurements that address clinical conditions of high prevalence, high risk, or high cost; and
- well-established measurements that are currently being used by large segments of the health care industry across the country.

In addition, all of the following are required:

- Definition or purpose of the measure is consistent with its intended use (quality improvement and accountability, or solely quality improvement)
- Aspect of care measured is substantially influenced by the physician (or other qualified health care professional or entity for which the code may be relevant)
- Reduces data collection burden on physicians (or other qualified health care professional or entities)
- Significant
  - Affects a large segment of health care community
  - Tied to health outcomes
  - Addresses clinical conditions of high prevalence, high costs, high risks
- Evidence-based
  - Agreed upon
  - Definable
  - Measurable
- Risk-adjustment specifications and instructions for all outcome measures submitted or compelling evidence as to why risk adjustment is not relevant
- Sufficiently detailed to make it useful for multiple purposes
- Facilitates reporting of performance measure(s)
- Inclusion of select patient history, testing (eg, glycohemoglobin), other process measures, cognitive or procedure services within CPT, or physiologic measures (eg, blood pressure) to support performance measurements

- Performance measure-development process that includes
  - Nationally recognized expert panel
  - Multidisciplinary
  - Vetting process

See the Introduction section of the CPT code set for a complete list of the dates of release and implementation.

The superscripted numbers included at the end of each code descriptor direct users to the measure developers that are associated with these footnotes, whose names and Web addresses are listed below.

1. For more information on measures developed by the Physician Consortium for Performance Improvement (PCPI), see the appropriate payer website.

2. National Committee on Quality Assurance (NCQA), Health Employer Data Information Set (HEDIS®), www.ncqa.org.

3. The Joint Commission (TJC), https://www.jointcommission.org.

4. For more information on measures developed by the National Diabetes Quality Improvement Alliance (NDQIA), see the appropriate payer website.

5. For more information on measures developed as joint measures from Physician Consortium for Performance Improvement (PCPI) and the National Committee on Quality Assurance (NCQA), visit the NCQA website at www.ncqa.org.

6. The Society of Thoracic Surgeons at www.sts.org and National Quality Forum, www.qualityforum.org.

7. Optum, www.optum.com.

8. American Academy of Neurology, https://www.aan.com/practice/quality-measurements or quality@aan.com.

9. College of American Pathologists (CAP), https://www.cap.org/advocacy/quality-payment-program-for-pathologists/mips-for-pathologists/2023-pathology-quality-measures.

10. American Gastroenterological Association (AGA), www.gastro.org/quality.

11. American Society of Anesthesiologists (ASA), www.asahq.org.

12. American College of Gastroenterology (ACG), www.gi.org; American Gastroenterological Association (AGA), www.gastro.org; and American Society for Gastrointestinal Endoscopy (ASGE), www.asge.org.

Modifiers

The following performance measurement modifiers may be used for Category II codes to indicate that a service specified in the associated measure(s) was considered but, due to either medical, patient, or system circumstance(s)

documented in the medical record, the service was not provided. These modifiers serve as denominator exclusions from the performance measure. The user should note that not all listed measures provide for exclusions (see Alphabetical Clinical Topics Listing for more discussion regarding exclusion criteria).

Category II modifiers should only be reported with Category II codes—they should not be reported with Category I or Category III codes. In addition, the modifiers in the Category II section should only be used where specified in the guidelines, reporting instructions, parenthetic notes, or code descriptor language listed in the Category II section (code listing and the Alphabetical Clinical Topics Listing).

1P Performance Measure Exclusion Modifier due to Medical Reasons

Reasons include:

- Not indicated (absence of organ/limb, already received/performed, other)
- Contraindicated (patient allergic history, potential adverse drug interaction, other)
- Other medical reasons

2P Performance Measure Exclusion Modifier due to Patient Reasons

Reasons include:

- Patient declined
- Economic, social, or religious reasons
- Other patient reasons

3P Performance Measure Exclusion Modifier due to System Reasons

Reasons include:

- Resources to perform the services not available
- Insurance coverage/payor-related limitations
- Other reasons attributable to health care delivery system

Modifier 8P is intended to be used as a "reporting modifier" to allow the reporting of circumstances when an action described in a measure's numerator is not performed and the reason is not otherwise specified.

8P Performance measure reporting modifier–action not performed, reason not otherwise specified

Composite Codes

Composite codes combine several measures grouped within a single code descriptor to facilitate reporting for a clinical condition when all components are met. If only some of the components are met or if services are provided in addition to those included in the composite code, they may be reported individually using the corresponding CPT Category II codes for those services.

0001F   Heart failure assessed (includes assessment of all the following components) (CAD)[1]:

Blood pressure measured (2000F)[1]

Level of activity assessed (1003F)[1]

Clinical symptoms of volume overload (excess) assessed (1004F)[1]

Weight, recorded (2001F)[1]

Clinical signs of volume overload (excess) assessed (2002F)[1]

→ *CPT Changes: An Insider's View* 2006, 2007

→ *CPT Assistant* Oct 05:4, 7

(To report blood pressure measured, use 2000F)

0005F   Osteoarthritis assessed (OA)[1]

Includes assessment of all the following components:

Osteoarthritis symptoms and functional status assessed (1006F)[1]

Use of anti-inflammatory or over-the-counter (OTC) analgesic medications assessed (1007F)[1]

Initial examination of the involved joint(s) (includes visual inspection, palpation, range of motion) (2004F)[1]

→ *CPT Changes: An Insider's View* 2006, 2007, 2009

→ *CPT Assistant* Oct 05:4, 11

(To report tobacco use cessation intervention, use 4001F)

0012F   Community-acquired bacterial pneumonia assessment (includes all of the following components) (CAP)[1]:

Co-morbid conditions assessed (1026F)[1]

Vital signs recorded (2010F)[1]

Mental status assessed (2014F)[1]

Hydration status assessed (2018F)[1]

→ *CPT Changes: An Insider's View* 2007

0014F   Comprehensive preoperative assessment performed for cataract surgery with intraocular lens (IOL) placement (includes assessment of all of the following components) (EC)[5]:

Dilated fundus evaluation performed within 12 months prior to cataract surgery (2020F)[5]

Pre-surgical (cataract) axial length, corneal power measurement and method of intraocular lens power calculation documented (must be performed within 12 months prior to surgery) (3073F)[5]

Preoperative assessment of functional or medical indication(s) for surgery prior to the cataract surgery with intraocular lens placement (must be performed within 12 months prior to cataract surgery) (3325F)[5]

→ *CPT Changes: An Insider's View* 2009

0015F   Melanoma follow up completed (includes assessment of all of the following components) (ML)[5]:

History obtained regarding new or changing moles (1050F)[5]

Complete physical skin exam performed (2029F)[5]

Patient counseled to perform a monthly self skin examination (5005F)[5]

→ *CPT Changes: An Insider's View* 2009

Patient Management

Patient management codes describe utilization measures or measures of patient care provided for specific clinical purposes (eg, prenatal care, pre- and post-surgical care).

0500F   Initial prenatal care visit (report at first prenatal encounter with health care professional providing obstetrical care. Report also date of visit and, in a separate field, the date of the last menstrual period [LMP]) (Prenatal)[2]

→ *CPT Changes: An Insider's View* 2005

→ *CPT Assistant* Oct 05:4, 13, Aug 07:1

0501F   Prenatal flow sheet documented in medical record by first prenatal visit (documentation includes at minimum blood pressure, weight, urine protein, uterine size, fetal heart tones, and estimated date of delivery). Report also: date of visit and, in a separate field, the date of the last menstrual period [LMP] (Note: If reporting 0501F Prenatal flow sheet, it is not necessary to report 0500F Initial prenatal care visit) (Prenatal)[1]

→ *CPT Changes: An Insider's View* 2005

→ *CPT Assistant* Oct 05:13

0502F   Subsequent prenatal care visit (Prenatal)[2]

[Excludes: patients who are seen for a condition unrelated to pregnancy or prenatal care (eg, an upper respiratory infection; patients seen for consultation only, not for continuing care)]

→ *CPT Changes: An Insider's View* 2005, 2007

→ *CPT Assistant* Oct 05:13

0503F   Postpartum care visit (Prenatal)[2]

→ *CPT Changes: An Insider's View* 2005

→ *CPT Assistant* Oct 05:13

0505F   Hemodialysis plan of care documented (ESRD, P-ESRD)[1]
> CPT Changes: An Insider's View 2008

0507F   Peritoneal dialysis plan of care documented (ESRD)[1]
> CPT Changes: An Insider's View 2008

0509F   Urinary incontinence plan of care documented (GER)[5]
> CPT Changes: An Insider's View 2008

0513F   Elevated blood pressure plan of care documented (CKD)[1]
> CPT Changes: An Insider's View 2009

0514F   Plan of care for elevated hemoglobin level documented for patient receiving Erythropoiesis-Stimulating Agent therapy (ESA) (CKD)[1]
> CPT Changes: An Insider's View 2009

0516F   Anemia plan of care documented (ESRD)[1]
> CPT Changes: An Insider's View 2009

0517F   Glaucoma plan of care documented (EC)[5]
> CPT Changes: An Insider's View 2009

0518F   Falls plan of care documented (GER)[5]
> CPT Changes: An Insider's View 2009

0519F   Planned chemotherapy regimen, including at a minimum: drug(s) prescribed, dose, and duration, documented prior to initiation of a new treatment regimen (ONC)[1]
> CPT Changes: An Insider's View 2009, 2010

0520F   Radiation dose limits to normal tissues established prior to the initiation of a course of 3D conformal radiation for a minimum of 2 tissue/organ (ONC)[1]
> CPT Changes: An Insider's View 2009, 2010

0521F   Plan of care to address pain documented (COA)[2] (ONC)[1]
> CPT Changes: An Insider's View 2009, 2010

0525F   Initial visit for episode (BkP)[2]
> CPT Changes: An Insider's View 2009

0526F   Subsequent visit for episode (BkP)[2]
> CPT Changes: An Insider's View 2009

0528F   Recommended follow-up interval for repeat colonoscopy of at least 10 years documented in colonoscopy report (End/Polyp)[5]
> CPT Changes: An Insider's View 2010

0529F   Interval of 3 or more years since patient's last colonoscopy, documented (End/Polyp)[5]
> CPT Changes: An Insider's View 2010

0535F   Dyspnea management plan of care, documented (Pall Cr)[5]
> CPT Changes: An Insider's View 2010

0540F   Glucocorticoid Management Plan Documented (RA)[5]
> CPT Changes: An Insider's View 2010

0545F   Plan for follow-up care for major depressive disorder, documented (MDD ADOL)[1]
> CPT Changes: An Insider's View 2011

0550F   Cytopathology report on routine nongynecologic specimen finalized within two working days of accession date (PATH)[9]
> CPT Changes: An Insider's View 2012

0551F   Cytopathology report on nongynecologic specimen with documentation that the specimen was non-routine (PATH)[9]
> CPT Changes: An Insider's View 2012

0555F   Symptom management plan of care documented (HF)[1]
> CPT Changes: An Insider's View 2012

0556F   Plan of care to achieve lipid control documented (CAD)[1]
> CPT Changes: An Insider's View 2012

0557F   Plan of care to manage anginal symptoms documented (CAD)[1]
> CPT Changes: An Insider's View 2012

0575F   HIV RNA control plan of care, documented (HIV)[5]
> CPT Changes: An Insider's View 2010

0580F   Multidisciplinary care plan developed or updated (ALS)[8]
> CPT Changes: An Insider's View 2014

0581F   Patient transferred directly from anesthetizing location to critical care unit (Peri2)[11]
> CPT Changes: An Insider's View 2014

0582F   Patient not transferred directly from anesthetizing location to critical care unit (Peri2)[11]
> CPT Changes: An Insider's View 2014

0583F   Transfer of care checklist used (Peri2)[11]
> CPT Changes: An Insider's View 2014

0584F   Transfer of care checklist not used (Peri2)[11]
> CPT Changes: An Insider's View 2014

Patient History

Patient history codes describe measures for select aspects of patient history or review of systems.

1000F   Tobacco use assessed (CAD, CAP, COPD, PV)[1] (DM)[4]
> CPT Changes: An Insider's View 2005, 2007
> CPT Assistant Oct 05:4, 9

1002F   Anginal symptoms and level of activity assessed (NMA–No Measure Associated)
> CPT Changes: An Insider's View 2005
> CPT Assistant Oct 05:9

1003F   Level of activity assessed (NMA–No Measure Associated)
> CPT Changes: An Insider's View 2006
> CPT Assistant Oct 05:7

1004F   Clinical symptoms of volume overload (excess) assessed (NMA–No Measure Associated)
> CPT Changes: An Insider's View 2006
> CPT Assistant Oct 05:7

1005F Asthma symptoms evaluated (includes documentation of numeric frequency of symptoms or patient completion of an asthma assessment tool/survey/questionnaire) (NMA–No Measure Associated)

➔ *CPT Changes: An Insider's View* 2006, 2013

➔ *CPT Assistant* Oct 05:6

1006F Osteoarthritis symptoms and functional status assessed (may include the use of a standardized scale or the completion of an assessment questionnaire, such as the SF-36, AAOS Hip & Knee Questionnaire) (OA)[1]

[Instructions: Report when osteoarthritis is addressed during the patient encounter]

➔ *CPT Changes: An Insider's View* 2006

➔ *CPT Assistant* Oct 05:11

1007F Use of anti-inflammatory or analgesic over-the-counter (OTC) medications for symptom relief assessed (OA)[1]

➔ *CPT Changes: An Insider's View* 2006

➔ *CPT Assistant* Oct 05:11

1008F Gastrointestinal and renal risk factors assessed for patients on prescribed or OTC non-steroidal anti-inflammatory drug (NSAID) (OA)[1]

➔ *CPT Changes: An Insider's View* 2006

➔ *CPT Assistant* Oct 05:11

1010F Severity of angina assessed by level of activity (CAD)[1]

➔ *CPT Changes: An Insider's View* 2012

1011F Angina present (CAD)[1]

➔ *CPT Changes: An Insider's View* 2012

1012F Angina absent (CAD)[1]

➔ *CPT Changes: An Insider's View* 2012

1015F Chronic obstructive pulmonary disease (COPD) symptoms assessed (Includes assessment of at least 1 of the following: dyspnea, cough/sputum, wheezing), or respiratory symptom assessment tool completed (COPD)[1]

➔ *CPT Changes: An Insider's View* 2007

1018F Dyspnea assessed, not present (COPD)[1]

➔ *CPT Changes: An Insider's View* 2007

1019F Dyspnea assessed, present (COPD)[1]

➔ *CPT Changes: An Insider's View* 2007

1022F Pneumococcus immunization status assessed (CAP, COPD)[1]

➔ *CPT Changes: An Insider's View* 2007

1026F Co-morbid conditions assessed (eg, includes assessment for presence or absence of: malignancy, liver disease, congestive heart failure, cerebrovascular disease, renal disease, chronic obstructive pulmonary disease, asthma, diabetes, other co-morbid conditions) (CAP)[1]

➔ *CPT Changes: An Insider's View* 2007

1030F Influenza immunization status assessed (CAP)[1]

➔ *CPT Changes: An Insider's View* 2007

1031F Smoking status and exposure to second hand smoke in the home assessed (Asthma)[1]

➔ *CPT Changes: An Insider's View* 2012

1032F Current tobacco smoker **or** currently exposed to secondhand smoke (Asthma)[1]

➔ *CPT Changes: An Insider's View* 2012

1033F Current tobacco non-smoker **and** not currently exposed to secondhand smoke (Asthma)[1]

➔ *CPT Changes: An Insider's View* 2012

1034F Current tobacco smoker (CAD, CAP, COPD, PV)[1] (DM)[4]

➔ *CPT Changes: An Insider's View* 2007

1035F Current smokeless tobacco user (eg, chew, snuff) (PV)[1]

➔ *CPT Changes: An Insider's View* 2007

1036F Current tobacco non-user (CAD, CAP, COPD, PV)[1] (DM)[4] (IBD)[10]

➔ *CPT Changes: An Insider's View* 2007

1038F Persistent asthma (mild, moderate or severe) (Asthma)[1]

➔ *CPT Changes: An Insider's View* 2007

➔ *CPT Assistant* Jul 10:3

1039F Intermittent asthma (Asthma)[1]

➔ *CPT Changes: An Insider's View* 2007

➔ *CPT Assistant* Jul 10:3

1040F DSM-5 criteria for major depressive disorder documented at the initial evaluation (MDD, MDD ADOL)[1]

➔ *CPT Changes: An Insider's View* 2008, 2009, 2014, 2015

1050F History obtained regarding new or changing moles (ML)[5]

➔ *CPT Changes: An Insider's View* 2008

1052F Type, anatomic location, and activity all assessed (IBD)[10]

➔ *CPT Changes: An Insider's View* 2013

1055F Visual functional status assessed (EC)[5]

➔ *CPT Changes: An Insider's View* 2008

1060F Documentation of permanent **or** persistent **or** paroxysmal atrial fibrillation (STR)[5]

➔ *CPT Changes: An Insider's View* 2008

1061F Documentation of absence of permanent **and** persistent **and** paroxysmal atrial fibrillation (STR)[5]

➔ *CPT Changes: An Insider's View* 2008

1065F Ischemic stroke symptom onset of less than 3 hours prior to arrival (STR)[5]

➔ *CPT Changes: An Insider's View* 2008

1066F Ischemic stroke symptom onset greater than or equal to 3 hours prior to arrival (STR)[5]

➔ *CPT Changes: An Insider's View* 2008

1070F Alarm symptoms (involuntary weight loss, dysphagia, or gastrointestinal bleeding) assessed; none present (GERD)[5]

➔ *CPT Changes: An Insider's View* 2008

1071F   1 or more present (GERD)[5]
➜ *CPT Changes: An Insider's View* 2008

1090F   Presence or absence of urinary incontinence assessed (GER)[5]
➜ *CPT Changes: An Insider's View* 2008

1091F   Urinary incontinence characterized (eg, frequency, volume, timing, type of symptoms, how bothersome) (GER)[5]
➜ *CPT Changes: An Insider's View* 2008

1100F   Patient screened for future fall risk; documentation of 2 or more falls in the past year or any fall with injury in the past year (GER)[5]
➜ *CPT Changes: An Insider's View* 2008

1101F   documentation of no falls in the past year or only 1 fall without injury in the past year (GER)[5]
➜ *CPT Changes: An Insider's View* 2008

1110F   Patient discharged from an inpatient facility (eg, hospital, skilled nursing facility, or rehabilitation facility) within the last 60 days (GER)[5]
➜ *CPT Changes: An Insider's View* 2008

1111F   Discharge medications reconciled with the current medication list in outpatient medical record (COA)[2] (GER)[5]
➜ *CPT Changes: An Insider's View* 2008

1116F   Auricular or periauricular pain assessed (AOE)[1]
➜ *CPT Changes: An Insider's View* 2009

1118F   GERD symptoms assessed after 12 months of therapy (GERD)[5]
➜ *CPT Changes: An Insider's View* 2009

1119F   Initial evaluation for condition (HEP C)[1] (EPI, DSP)[8]
➜ *CPT Changes: An Insider's View* 2009

1121F   Subsequent evaluation for condition (HEP C)[1] (EPI)[8]
➜ *CPT Changes: An Insider's View* 2009

1123F   Advance Care Planning discussed and documented advance care plan or surrogate decision maker documented in the medical record (DEM)[1] (GER, Pall Cr)[5]
➜ *CPT Changes: An Insider's View* 2009

1124F   Advance Care Planning discussed and documented in the medical record, patient did not wish or was not able to name a surrogate decision maker or provide an advance care plan (DEM)[1] (GER, Pall Cr)[5]
➜ *CPT Changes: An Insider's View* 2009

1125F   Pain severity quantified; pain present (COA)[2] (ONC)[1]
➜ *CPT Changes: An Insider's View* 2009

1126F   no pain present (COA)[2] (ONC)[1]
➜ *CPT Changes: An Insider's View* 2009, 2010

1127F   New episode for condition (NMA–No Measure Associated)
➜ *CPT Changes: An Insider's View* 2009, 2012

1128F   Subsequent episode for condition (NMA–No Measure Associated)
➜ *CPT Changes: An Insider's View* 2009, 2012

1130F   Back pain and function assessed, including all of the following: Pain assessment **and** functional status **and** patient history, including notation of presence or absence of "red flags" (warning signs) **and** assessment of prior treatment and response, **and** employment status (BkP)[2]
➜ *CPT Changes: An Insider's View* 2009

1134F   Episode of back pain lasting 6 weeks or less (BkP)[2]
➜ *CPT Changes: An Insider's View* 2009

1135F   Episode of back pain lasting longer than 6 weeks (BkP)[2]
➜ *CPT Changes: An Insider's View* 2009

1136F   Episode of back pain lasting 12 weeks or less (BkP)[2]
➜ *CPT Changes: An Insider's View* 2009

1137F   Episode of back pain lasting longer than 12 weeks (BkP)[2]
➜ *CPT Changes: An Insider's View* 2009

1150F   Documentation that a patient has a substantial risk of death within 1 year (Pall Cr)[5]
➜ *CPT Changes: An Insider's View* 2010

1151F   Documentation that a patient does not have a substantial risk of death within one year (Pall Cr)[5]
➜ *CPT Changes: An Insider's View* 2010

1152F   Documentation of advanced disease diagnosis, goals of care prioritize comfort (Pall Cr)[5]
➜ *CPT Changes: An Insider's View* 2010

1153F   Documentation of advanced disease diagnosis, goals of care do not prioritize comfort (Pall Cr)[5]
➜ *CPT Changes: An Insider's View* 2010

1157F   Advance care plan or similar legal document present in the medical record (COA)[2]
➜ *CPT Changes: An Insider's View* 2010

1158F   Advance care planning discussion documented in the medical record (COA)[2]
➜ *CPT Changes: An Insider's View* 2010

1159F   Medication list documented in medical record (COA)[2]
➜ *CPT Changes: An Insider's View* 2010

1160F   Review of all medications by a prescribing practitioner or clinical pharmacist (such as, prescriptions, OTCs, herbal therapies and supplements) documented in the medical record (COA)[2]
➜ *CPT Changes: An Insider's View* 2010

1170F   Functional status assessed (COA)[2] (RA)[5]
➜ *CPT Changes: An Insider's View* 2010

1175F   Functional status for dementia assessed and results reviewed (DEM)[1]
➜ *CPT Changes: An Insider's View* 2012

1180F All specified thromboembolic risk factors assessed (AFIB)[1]

   ➔ *CPT Changes: An Insider's View* 2010

1181F Neuropsychiatric symptoms assessed and results reviewed (DEM)[1]

   ➔ *CPT Changes: An Insider's View* 2012

1182F Neuropsychiatric symptoms, one or more present (DEM)[1]

   ➔ *CPT Changes: An Insider's View* 2012

1183F Neuropsychiatric symptoms, absent (DEM)[1]

   ➔ *CPT Changes: An Insider's View* 2012

1200F Seizure type(s) and current seizure frequency(ies) documented (EPI)[8]

   ➔ *CPT Changes: An Insider's View* 2011

1205F Etiology of epilepsy or epilepsy syndrome(s) reviewed and documented (EPI)[8]

   ➔ *CPT Changes: An Insider's View* 2011

1220F Patient screened for depression (SUD)[5]

   ➔ *CPT Changes: An Insider's View* 2010

1400F Parkinson's disease diagnosis reviewed (Prkns)[8]

   ➔ *CPT Changes: An Insider's View* 2011

1450F Symptoms improved or remained consistent with treatment goals since last assessment (HF)[1]

   ➔ *CPT Changes: An Insider's View* 2012

1451F Symptoms demonstrated clinically important deterioration since last assessment (HF)[1]

   ➔ *CPT Changes: An Insider's View* 2012

1460F Qualifying cardiac event/diagnosis in previous 12 months (CAD)[1]

   ➔ *CPT Changes: An Insider's View* 2012

1461F No qualifying cardiac event/diagnosis in previous 12 months (CAD)[1]

   ➔ *CPT Changes: An Insider's View* 2012

1490F Dementia severity classified, mild (DEM)[1]

   ➔ *CPT Changes: An Insider's View* 2012

1491F Dementia severity classified, moderate (DEM)[1]

   ➔ *CPT Changes: An Insider's View* 2012

1493F Dementia severity classified, severe (DEM)[1]

   ➔ *CPT Changes: An Insider's View* 2012

1494F Cognition assessed and reviewed (DEM)[1]

   ➔ *CPT Changes: An Insider's View* 2012

1500F Symptoms and signs of distal symmetric polyneuropathy reviewed and documented (DSP)[8]

   ➔ *CPT Changes: An Insider's View* 2014

1501F Not initial evaluation for condition (DSP)[8]

   ➔ *CPT Changes: An Insider's View* 2014

1502F Patient queried about pain and pain interference with function using a valid and reliable instrument (DSP)[8]

   ➔ *CPT Changes: An Insider's View* 2014

1503F Patient queried about symptoms of respiratory insufficiency (ALS)[8]

   ➔ *CPT Changes: An Insider's View* 2014

1504F Patient has respiratory insufficiency (ALS)[8]

   ➔ *CPT Changes: An Insider's View* 2014

1505F Patient does not have respiratory insufficiency (ALS)[8]

   ➔ *CPT Changes: An Insider's View* 2014

Physical Examination

Physical examination codes describe aspects of physical examination or clinical assessment.

2000F Blood pressure measured (CKD)[1](DM)[2,4]

   ➔ *CPT Changes: An Insider's View* 2005, 2009

   ➔ *CPT Assistant* Oct 05:4, 5, 7, 9, 10, Aug 07:1

2001F Weight recorded (PAG)[1]

   ➔ *CPT Changes: An Insider's View* 2006

   ➔ *CPT Assistant* Oct 05:7

2002F Clinical signs of volume overload (excess) assessed (NMA–No Measure Associated)

   ➔ *CPT Changes: An Insider's View* 2006

   ➔ *CPT Assistant* Oct 05:7, 8

2004F Initial examination of the involved joint(s) (includes visual inspection, palpation, range of motion) (OA)[1]

[Instructions: Report only for initial osteoarthritis visit or for visits for new joint involvement]

   ➔ *CPT Changes: An Insider's View* 2006

   ➔ *CPT Assistant* Oct 05:11

2010F Vital signs (temperature, pulse, respiratory rate, and blood pressure) documented and reviewed (CAP)[1] (EM)[5]

   ➔ *CPT Changes: An Insider's View* 2007, 2008

2014F Mental status assessed (CAP)[1] (EM)[5]

   ➔ *CPT Changes: An Insider's View* 2007, 2008

2015F Asthma impairment assessed (Asthma)[1]

   ➔ *CPT Changes: An Insider's View* 2012

2016F Asthma risk assessed (Asthma)[1]

   ➔ *CPT Changes: An Insider's View* 2012

2018F Hydration status assessed (normal/mildly dehydrated/ severely dehydrated) (CAP)[1]

   ➔ *CPT Changes: An Insider's View* 2007

2019F Dilated macular exam performed, including documentation of the presence or absence of macular thickening or hemorrhage **and** the level of macular degeneration severity (EC)[5]

   ➔ *CPT Changes: An Insider's View* 2008

2020F Dilated fundus evaluation performed within 12 months prior to cataract surgery (EC)[5]

   ➔ *CPT Changes: An Insider's View* 2008, 2009

▲ = Revised code   ● = New code   ▶ ◀ = Contains new or revised text   ✕ = Duplicate PLA test   ↕ = Category I PLA   American Medical Association   **901**

2021F Dilated macular or fundus exam performed, including documentation of the presence or absence of macular edema **and** level of severity of retinopathy (EC)[5]

➔ *CPT Changes: An Insider's View* 2008

2022F Dilated retinal eye exam with interpretation by an ophthalmologist or optometrist documented and reviewed; with evidence of retinopathy (DM)[2]

➔ *CPT Changes: An Insider's View* 2007, 2009, 2020

2023F without evidence of retinopathy (DM)[2]

➔ *CPT Changes: An Insider's View* 2020

2024F 7 standard field stereoscopic retinal photos with interpretation by an ophthalmologist or optometrist documented and reviewed; with evidence of retinopathy (DM)[2]

➔ *CPT Changes: An Insider's View* 2007, 2009, 2020

2025F without evidence of retinopathy (DM)[2]

➔ *CPT Changes: An Insider's View* 2020

2026F Eye imaging validated to match diagnosis from 7 standard field stereoscopic retinal photos results documented and reviewed; with evidence of retinopathy (DM)[2]

➔ *CPT Changes: An Insider's View* 2007, 2009, 2020

 # 2033F without evidence of retinopathy (DM)[2]

➔ *CPT Changes: An Insider's View* 2020

2027F Optic nerve head evaluation performed (EC)[5]

➔ *CPT Changes: An Insider's View* 2008

2028F Foot examination performed (includes examination through visual inspection, sensory exam with monofilament, and pulse exam – report when any of the 3 components are completed) (DM)[4]

➔ *CPT Changes: An Insider's View* 2007

2029F Complete physical skin exam performed (ML)[5]

➔ *CPT Changes: An Insider's View* 2008

2030F Hydration status documented, normally hydrated (PAG)[1]

➔ *CPT Changes: An Insider's View* 2008

2031F Hydration status documented, dehydrated (PAG)[1]

➔ *CPT Changes: An Insider's View* 2008

2033F Code is out of numerical sequence. See 2025F-2028F

2035F Tympanic membrane mobility assessed with pneumatic otoscopy or tympanometry (OME)[1]

➔ *CPT Changes: An Insider's View* 2009

2040F Physical examination on the date of the initial visit for low back pain performed, in accordance with specifications (BkP)[2]

➔ *CPT Changes: An Insider's View* 2009

2044F Documentation of mental health assessment prior to intervention (back surgery or epidural steroid injection) or for back pain episode lasting longer than 6 weeks (BkP)[2]

➔ *CPT Changes: An Insider's View* 2009

2050F Wound characteristics including size **and** nature of wound base tissue **and** amount of drainage prior to debridement documented (CWC)[5]

➔ *CPT Changes: An Insider's View* 2010

2060F Patient interviewed directly on or before date of diagnosis of major depressive disorder (MDD ADOL)[1]

➔ *CPT Changes: An Insider's View* 2011, 2013

Diagnostic/Screening Processes or Results

Diagnostic/screening processes or results codes describe results of tests ordered (clinical laboratory tests, radiological or other procedural examinations, and conclusions of medical decision-making).

3006F Chest X-ray results documented and reviewed (CAP)[1]

➔ *CPT Changes: An Insider's View* 2007

➔ *CPT Assistant* Aug 07:1

3008F Body Mass Index (BMI), documented (PV)[1]

➔ *CPT Changes: An Insider's View* 2011

3011F Lipid panel results documented and reviewed (must include total cholesterol, HDL-C, triglycerides and calculated LDL-C) (CAD)[1]

➔ *CPT Changes: An Insider's View* 2007

3014F Screening mammography results documented and reviewed (PV)[1,2]

➔ *CPT Changes: An Insider's View* 2007, 2009

3015F Cervical cancer screening results documented and reviewed (PV)[1]

➔ *CPT Changes: An Insider's View* 2011

3016F Patient screened for unhealthy alcohol use using a systematic screening method (PV)[1] (DSP)[8]

➔ *CPT Changes: An Insider's View* 2010

3017F Colorectal cancer screening results documented and reviewed (PV)

➔ *CPT Changes: An Insider's View* 2009

3018F Pre-procedure risk assessment **and** depth of insertion **and** quality of the bowel prep **and** complete description of polyp(s) found, including location of each polyp, size, number and gross morphology **and** recommendations for follow-up in final colonoscopy report documented (End/Polyp)[5]

➔ *CPT Changes: An Insider's View* 2010

3019F Left ventricular ejection fraction (LVEF) assessment planned post discharge (HF)[1]

➔ *CPT Changes: An Insider's View* 2012

3020F Left ventricular function (LVF) assessment (eg, echocardiography, nuclear test, or ventriculography) documented in the medical record (Includes quantitative or qualitative assessment results) (NMA–No Measure Associated)

➔ *CPT Changes: An Insider's View* 2007

3021F Left ventricular ejection fraction (LVEF) less than 40% or documentation of moderately or severely depressed left ventricular systolic function (CAD, HF)[1]

➔ *CPT Changes: An Insider's View* 2007

3022F Left ventricular ejection fraction (LVEF) greater than or equal to 40% or documentation as normal or mildly depressed left ventricular systolic function (CAD, HF)[1]

➔ *CPT Changes: An Insider's View* 2007

3023F Spirometry results documented and reviewed (COPD)[1]

➔ *CPT Changes: An Insider's View* 2007

3025F Spirometry test results demonstrate FEV_1/FVC less than 70% with COPD symptoms (eg, dyspnea, cough/sputum, wheezing) (CAP, COPD)[1]

➔ *CPT Changes: An Insider's View* 2007

3027F Spirometry test results demonstrate FEV_1/FVC greater than or equal to 70% or patient does not have COPD symptoms (COPD)[1]

➔ *CPT Changes: An Insider's View* 2007

3028F Oxygen saturation results documented and reviewed (includes assessment through pulse oximetry or arterial blood gas measurement) (CAP, COPD)[1] (EM)[5]

➔ *CPT Changes: An Insider's View* 2007

3035F Oxygen saturation less than or equal to 88% or a PaO_2 less than or equal to 55 mm Hg (COPD)[1]

➔ *CPT Changes: An Insider's View* 2007

3037F Oxygen saturation greater than 88% or PaO_2 greater than 55 mm Hg (COPD)[1]

➔ *CPT Changes: An Insider's View* 2007

3038F Pulmonary function test performed within 12 months prior to surgery (Lung/Esop Cx)[6]

➔ *CPT Changes: An Insider's View* 2011

3040F Functional expiratory volume (FEV_1) less than 40% of predicted value (COPD)[1]

➔ *CPT Changes: An Insider's View* 2007

3042F Functional expiratory volume (FEV_1) greater than or equal to 40% of predicted value (COPD)[1]

➔ *CPT Changes: An Insider's View* 2007

3044F Most recent hemoglobin A1c (HbA1c) level less than 7.0% (DM)[2,4]

➔ *CPT Changes: An Insider's View* 2008

3051F Most recent hemoglobin A1c (HbA1c) level greater than or equal to 7.0% and less than 8.0% (DM)[2]

➔ *CPT Changes: An Insider's View* 2020

3052F Most recent hemoglobin A1c (HbA1c) level greater than or equal to 8.0% and less than or equal to 9.0% (DM)[2]

➔ *CPT Changes: An Insider's View* 2020

3046F Most recent hemoglobin A1c level greater than 9.0% (DM)[4]

➔ *CPT Changes: An Insider's View* 2007

(To report most recent hemoglobin A1c level less than or equal to 9.0%, see 3044F, 3051F, 3052F)

3048F Most recent LDL-C less than 100 mg/dL (CAD)[1] (DM)[4]

➔ *CPT Changes: An Insider's View* 2007

3049F Most recent LDL-C 100-129 mg/dL (CAD)[1] (DM)[4]

➔ *CPT Changes: An Insider's View* 2007

3050F Most recent LDL-C greater than or equal to 130 mg/dL (CAD)[1] (DM)[4]

➔ *CPT Changes: An Insider's View* 2007

3051F Code is out of numerical sequence. See 3042F-3048F

3052F Code is out of numerical sequence. See 3042F-3048F

3055F Left ventricular ejection fraction (LVEF) less than or equal to 35% (HF)[1]

➔ *CPT Changes: An Insider's View* 2012

3056F Left ventricular ejection fraction (LVEF) greater than 35% or no LVEF result available (HF)[1]

➔ *CPT Changes: An Insider's View* 2012

3060F Positive microalbuminuria test result documented and reviewed (DM)[2,4]

➔ *CPT Changes: An Insider's View* 2007

3061F Negative microalbuminuria test result documented and reviewed (DM)[2,4]

➔ *CPT Changes: An Insider's View* 2007

3062F Positive macroalbuminuria test result documented and reviewed (DM)[2,4]

➔ *CPT Changes: An Insider's View* 2007

3066F Documentation of treatment for nephropathy (eg, patient receiving dialysis, patient being treated for ESRD, CRF, ARF, or renal insufficiency, any visit to a nephrologist) (DM)[2,4]

➔ *CPT Changes: An Insider's View* 2007

3072F Low risk for retinopathy (no evidence of retinopathy in the prior year) (DM)[2]

➔ *CPT Changes: An Insider's View* 2007, 2020

3073F Pre-surgical (cataract) axial length, corneal power measurement and method of intraocular lens power calculation documented within 12 months prior to surgery (EC)[5]

➔ *CPT Changes: An Insider's View* 2008, 2009

3074F Most recent systolic blood pressure less than 130 mm Hg (DM)[2,4] (HTN, CKD, CAD)[1]

➔ *CPT Changes: An Insider's View* 2008

▲=Revised code　●=New code　▶◀=Contains new or revised text　✕=Duplicate PLA test　↕=Category I PLA　　　American Medical Association　**903**

3075F   Most recent systolic blood pressure 130-139 mm Hg (DM)[2,4] (HTN, CKD, CAD)[1]
➔ *CPT Changes: An Insider's View* 2008

3077F   Most recent systolic blood pressure greater than or equal to 140 mm Hg (HTN, CKD, CAD)[1] (DM)[2,4]
➔ *CPT Changes: An Insider's View* 2007

3078F   Most recent diastolic blood pressure less than 80 mm Hg (HTN, CKD, CAD)[1] (DM)[2,4]
➔ *CPT Changes: An Insider's View* 2007

3079F   Most recent diastolic blood pressure 80-89 mm Hg (HTN, CKD, CAD)[1] (DM)[2,4]
➔ *CPT Changes: An Insider's View* 2007

3080F   Most recent diastolic blood pressure greater than or equal to 90 mm Hg (HTN, CKD, CAD)[1] (DM)[2,4]
➔ *CPT Changes: An Insider's View* 2007, 2012

3082F   Kt/V less than 1.2 (Clearance of urea [Kt]/volume [V]) (ESRD, P-ESRD)[1]
➔ *CPT Changes: An Insider's View* 2008

3083F   Kt/V equal to or greater than 1.2 and less than 1.7 (Clearance of urea [Kt]/volume [V]) (ESRD, P-ESRD)[1]
➔ *CPT Changes: An Insider's View* 2008

3084F   Kt/V greater than or equal to 1.7 (Clearance of urea [Kt]/volume [V]) (ESRD, P-ESRD)[1]
➔ *CPT Changes: An Insider's View* 2008

3085F   Suicide risk assessed (MDD, MDD ADOL)[1]
➔ *CPT Changes: An Insider's View* 2008

3088F   Major depressive disorder, mild (MDD)[1]
➔ *CPT Changes: An Insider's View* 2008

3089F   Major depressive disorder, moderate (MDD)[1]
➔ *CPT Changes: An Insider's View* 2008

3090F   Major depressive disorder, severe without psychotic features (MDD)[1]
➔ *CPT Changes: An Insider's View* 2008

3091F   Major depressive disorder, severe with psychotic features (MDD)[1]
➔ *CPT Changes: An Insider's View* 2008

3092F   Major depressive disorder, in remission (MDD)[1]
➔ *CPT Changes: An Insider's View* 2008

3093F   Documentation of new diagnosis of initial or recurrent episode of major depressive disorder (MDD)[1]
➔ *CPT Changes: An Insider's View* 2008

3095F   Central dual-energy X-ray absorptiometry (DXA) results documented (OP)[5] (IBD)[10]
➔ *CPT Changes: An Insider's View* 2008

3096F   Central dual-energy X-ray absorptiometry (DXA) ordered (OP)[5] (IBD)[10]
➔ *CPT Changes: An Insider's View* 2008

3100F   Carotid imaging study report (includes direct or indirect reference to measurements of distal internal carotid diameter as the denominator for stenosis measurement) (STR, RAD)[5]
➔ *CPT Changes: An Insider's View* 2008

3110F   Documentation in final CT or MRI report of presence or absence of hemorrhage and mass lesion and acute infarction (STR)[5]
➔ *CPT Changes: An Insider's View* 2008, 2011
➔ *Clinical Examples in Radiology* Winter 08:6

3111F   CT or MRI of the brain performed in the hospital within 24 hours of arrival **or** performed in an outpatient imaging center, to confirm initial diagnosis of stroke, TIA or intracranial hemorrhage (STR)[5]
➔ *CPT Changes: An Insider's View* 2008, 2011, 2012

3112F   CT or MRI of the brain performed greater than 24 hours after arrival to the hospital **or** performed in an outpatient imaging center for purpose other than confirmation of initial diagnosis of stroke, TIA, or intracranial hemorrhage (STR)[5]
➔ *CPT Changes: An Insider's View* 2008, 2011, 2012
➔ *Clinical Examples in Radiology* Winter 08:6

3115F   Quantitative results of an evaluation of current level of activity and clinical symptoms (HF)[1]
➔ *CPT Changes: An Insider's View* 2012

3117F   Heart failure disease specific structured assessment tool completed (HF)[1]
➔ *CPT Changes: An Insider's View* 2012

3118F   New York Heart Association (NYHA) Class documented (HF)[1]
➔ *CPT Changes: An Insider's View* 2012

3119F   No evaluation of level of activity or clinical symptoms (HF)[1]
➔ *CPT Changes: An Insider's View* 2012

3120F   12-Lead ECG Performed (EM)[5]
➔ *CPT Changes: An Insider's View* 2008

3126F   Esophageal biopsy report with a statement about dysplasia (present, absent, or indefinite, and if present, contains appropriate grading) (PATH)[9]
➔ *CPT Changes: An Insider's View* 2015

3130F   Upper gastrointestinal endoscopy performed (GERD)[5]
➔ *CPT Changes: An Insider's View* 2008

3132F   Documentation of referral for upper gastrointestinal endoscopy (GERD)[5]
➔ *CPT Changes: An Insider's View* 2008

3140F   Upper gastrointestinal endoscopy report indicates suspicion of Barrett's esophagus (GERD)[5]
➔ *CPT Changes: An Insider's View* 2008

3141F   Upper gastrointestinal endoscopy report indicates no suspicion of Barrett's esophagus (GERD)[5]
➔ *CPT Changes: An Insider's View* 2008

3142F   Barium swallow test ordered (GERD)[1]

➔ *CPT Changes: An Insider's View* 2008

(To report documentation of barium swallow study, use 3142F)

3150F   Forceps esophageal biopsy performed (GERD)[5]

➔ *CPT Changes: An Insider's View* 2008

3155F   Cytogenetic testing performed on bone marrow at time of diagnosis or prior to initiating treatment (HEM)[1]

➔ *CPT Changes: An Insider's View* 2008

3160F   Documentation of iron stores prior to initiating erythropoietin therapy (HEM)[1]

➔ *CPT Changes: An Insider's View* 2008

3170F   Baseline flow cytometry studies performed at time of diagnosis or prior to initiating treatment (HEM)[1]

➔ *CPT Changes: An Insider's View* 2008, 2021

3200F   Barium swallow test not ordered (GERD)[5]

➔ *CPT Changes: An Insider's View* 2008

3210F   Group A Strep Test Performed (PHAR)[2]

➔ *CPT Changes: An Insider's View* 2008

3215F   Patient has documented immunity to Hepatitis A (HEP-C)[1]

➔ *CPT Changes: An Insider's View* 2009

3216F   Patient has documented immunity to Hepatitis B (HEP-C)[1] (IBD)[10]

➔ *CPT Changes: An Insider's View* 2009

3218F   RNA testing for Hepatitis C documented as performed within 6 months prior to initiation of antiviral treatment for Hepatitis C (HEP-C)[1]

➔ *CPT Changes: An Insider's View* 2009

3220F   Hepatitis C quantitative RNA testing documented as performed at 12 weeks from initiation of antiviral treatment (HEP-C)[1]

➔ *CPT Changes: An Insider's View* 2009

3230F   Documentation that hearing test was performed within 6 months prior to tympanostomy tube insertion (OME)[1]

➔ *CPT Changes: An Insider's View* 2009

3250F   Specimen site other than anatomic location of primary tumor (PATH)[1]

➔ *CPT Changes: An Insider's View* 2010

3260F   pT category (primary tumor), pN category (regional lymph nodes), and histologic grade documented in pathology report (PATH)[1]

➔ *CPT Changes: An Insider's View* 2009

3265F   Ribonucleic acid (RNA) testing for Hepatitis C viremia ordered or results documented (HEP C)[1]

➔ *CPT Changes: An Insider's View* 2009

3266F   Hepatitis C genotype testing documented as performed prior to initiation of antiviral treatment for Hepatitis C (HEP C)[1]

➔ *CPT Changes: An Insider's View* 2009

3267F   Pathology report includes pT category, pN category, Gleason score, and statement about margin status (PATH)[9]

➔ *CPT Changes: An Insider's View* 2012

3268F   Prostate-specific antigen (PSA), **and** primary tumor (T) stage, **and** Gleason score documented prior to initiation of treatment (PRCA)[1]

➔ *CPT Changes: An Insider's View* 2009

3269F   Bone scan performed prior to initiation of treatment or at any time since diagnosis of prostate cancer (PRCA)[1]

➔ *CPT Changes: An Insider's View* 2009

3270F   Bone scan not performed prior to initiation of treatment nor at any time since diagnosis of prostate cancer (PRCA)[1]

➔ *CPT Changes: An Insider's View* 2009

3271F   Low risk of recurrence, prostate cancer (PRCA)[1]

➔ *CPT Changes: An Insider's View* 2009

3272F   Intermediate risk of recurrence, prostate cancer (PRCA)[1]

➔ *CPT Changes: An Insider's View* 2009

3273F   High risk of recurrence, prostate cancer (PRCA)[1]

➔ *CPT Changes: An Insider's View* 2009

3274F   Prostate cancer risk of recurrence not determined or neither low, intermediate nor high (PRCA)[1]

➔ *CPT Changes: An Insider's View* 2009

3278F   Serum levels of calcium, phosphorus, intact Parathyroid Hormone (PTH) and lipid profile ordered (CKD)[1]

➔ *CPT Changes: An Insider's View* 2009

3279F   Hemoglobin level greater than or equal to 13 g/dL (CKD, ESRD)[1]

➔ *CPT Changes: An Insider's View* 2009

3280F   Hemoglobin level 11 g/dL to 12.9 g/dL (CKD, ESRD)[1]

➔ *CPT Changes: An Insider's View* 2009

3281F   Hemoglobin level less than 11 g/dL (CKD, ESRD)[1]

➔ *CPT Changes: An Insider's View* 2009

3284F   Intraocular pressure (IOP) reduced by a value of greater than or equal to 15% from the pre-intervention level (EC)[5]

➔ *CPT Changes: An Insider's View* 2009

3285F   Intraocular pressure (IOP) reduced by a value less than 15% from the pre-intervention level (EC)[5]

➔ *CPT Changes: An Insider's View* 2009

3288F   Falls risk assessment documented (GER)[5]

➔ *CPT Changes: An Insider's View* 2009

3290F   Patient is D (Rh) negative and unsensitized (Pre-Cr)[1]

➔ *CPT Changes: An Insider's View* 2009

3291F Patient is D (Rh) positive or sensitized (Pre-Cr)[1]
➜ *CPT Changes: An Insider's View* 2009

3292F HIV testing ordered or documented and reviewed during the first or second prenatal visit (Pre-Cr)[1]
➜ *CPT Changes: An Insider's View* 2009

3293F ABO and Rh blood typing documented as performed (Pre-Cr)[7]
➜ *CPT Changes: An Insider's View* 2011

3294F Group B Streptococcus (GBS) screening documented as performed during week 35-37 gestation (Pre-Cr)[7]
➜ *CPT Changes: An Insider's View* 2011

3300F American Joint Committee on Cancer (AJCC) stage documented and reviewed (ONC)[1]
➜ *CPT Changes: An Insider's View* 2009

3301F Cancer stage documented in medical record as metastatic and reviewed (ONC)[1]
➜ *CPT Changes: An Insider's View* 2009

(To report measures for cancer staging, see 3321F-3390F)

3315F Estrogen receptor (ER) or progesterone receptor (PR) positive breast cancer (ONC)[1]
➜ *CPT Changes: An Insider's View* 2009

3316F Estrogen receptor (ER) and progesterone receptor (PR) negative breast cancer (ONC)[1]
➜ *CPT Changes: An Insider's View* 2009

3317F Pathology report confirming malignancy documented in the medical record and reviewed prior to the initiation of chemotherapy (ONC)[1]
➜ *CPT Changes: An Insider's View* 2009

3318F Pathology report confirming malignancy documented in the medical record and reviewed prior to the initiation of radiation therapy (ONC)[1]
➜ *CPT Changes: An Insider's View* 2009

3319F 1 of the following diagnostic imaging studies ordered: chest x-ray, CT, Ultrasound, MRI, PET, or nuclear medicine scans (ML)[5]
➜ *CPT Changes: An Insider's View* 2009, 2010

3320F None of the following diagnostic imaging studies ordered: chest X-ray, CT, Ultrasound, MRI, PET, or nuclear medicine scans (ML)[5]
➜ *CPT Changes: An Insider's View* 2009

3321F AJCC Cancer Stage 0 or IA Melanoma, documented (ML)[5]
➜ *CPT Changes: An Insider's View* 2010

3322F Melanoma greater than AJCC Stage 0 or IA (ML)[5]
➜ *CPT Changes: An Insider's View* 2010

3323F Clinical tumor, node and metastases (TNM) staging documented and reviewed prior to surgery (Lung/Esop Cx)[6]
➜ *CPT Changes: An Insider's View* 2011

3324F MRI or CT scan ordered, reviewed or requested (EPI)[8]
➜ *CPT Changes: An Insider's View* 2011

3325F Preoperative assessment of functional or medical indication(s) for surgery prior to the cataract surgery with intraocular lens placement (must be performed within 12 months prior to cataract surgery) (EC)[5]
➜ *CPT Changes: An Insider's View* 2009

3328F Performance status documented and reviewed within 2 weeks prior to surgery (Lung/Esop Cx)[6]
➜ *CPT Changes: An Insider's View* 2011

3330F Imaging study ordered (BkP)[2]
➜ *CPT Changes: An Insider's View* 2009

3331F Imaging study not ordered (BkP)[2]
➜ *CPT Changes: An Insider's View* 2009

3340F Mammogram assessment category of "incomplete: need additional imaging evaluation" documented (RAD)[5]
➜ *CPT Changes: An Insider's View* 2009

3341F Mammogram assessment category of "negative," documented (RAD)[5]
➜ *CPT Changes: An Insider's View* 2009

3342F Mammogram assessment category of "benign," documented (RAD)[5]
➜ *CPT Changes: An Insider's View* 2009

3343F Mammogram assessment category of "probably benign," documented (RAD)[5]
➜ *CPT Changes: An Insider's View* 2009

3344F Mammogram assessment category of "suspicious," documented (RAD)[5]
➜ *CPT Changes: An Insider's View* 2009

3345F Mammogram assessment category of "highly suggestive of malignancy," documented (RAD)[5]
➜ *CPT Changes: An Insider's View* 2009

3350F Mammogram assessment category of "known biopsy proven malignancy," documented (RAD)[5]
➜ *CPT Changes: An Insider's View* 2009

3351F Negative screen for depressive symptoms as categorized by using a standardized depression screening/assessment tool (MDD)[2]
➜ *CPT Changes: An Insider's View* 2009

3352F No significant depressive symptoms as categorized by using a standardized depression assessment tool (MDD)[2]
➜ *CPT Changes: An Insider's View* 2009

3353F Mild to moderate depressive symptoms as categorized by using a standardized depression screening/assessment tool (MDD)[2]
➜ *CPT Changes: An Insider's View* 2009

3354F Clinically significant depressive symptoms as categorized by using a standardized depression screening/assessment tool (MDD)[2]

➲ *CPT Changes: An Insider's View* 2009

3370F AJCC Breast Cancer Stage 0 documented (ONC)[1]

➲ *CPT Changes: An Insider's View* 2010

3372F AJCC Breast Cancer Stage I: T1mic, T1a or T1b (tumor size ≤ 1 cm) documented (ONC)[1]

➲ *CPT Changes: An Insider's View* 2010

3374F AJCC Breast Cancer Stage I: T1c (tumor size > 1 cm to 2 cm) documented (ONC)[1]

➲ *CPT Changes: An Insider's View* 2010

3376F AJCC Breast Cancer Stage II documented (ONC)[1]

➲ *CPT Changes: An Insider's View* 2010

3378F AJCC Breast Cancer Stage III documented (ONC)[1]

➲ *CPT Changes: An Insider's View* 2010

3380F AJCC Breast Cancer Stage IV documented (ONC)[1]

➲ *CPT Changes: An Insider's View* 2010

3382F AJCC colon cancer, Stage 0 documented (ONC)[1]

➲ *CPT Changes: An Insider's View* 2010

3384F AJCC colon cancer, Stage I documented (ONC)[1]

➲ *CPT Changes: An Insider's View* 2010

3386F AJCC colon cancer, Stage II documented (ONC)[1]

➲ *CPT Changes: An Insider's View* 2010

3388F AJCC colon cancer, Stage III documented (ONC)[1]

➲ *CPT Changes: An Insider's View* 2010

3390F AJCC colon cancer, Stage IV documented (ONC)[1]

➲ *CPT Changes: An Insider's View* 2010

3394F Quantitative HER2 immunohistochemistry (IHC) evaluation of breast cancer consistent with the scoring system defined in the ASCO/CAP guidelines (PATH)[9]

➲ *CPT Changes: An Insider's View* 2012

3395F Quantitative non-HER2 immunohistochemistry (IHC) evaluation of breast cancer (eg, testing for estrogen or progesterone receptors [ER/PR]) performed (PATH)[9]

➲ *CPT Changes: An Insider's View* 2012

3450F Dyspnea screened, no dyspnea or mild dyspnea (Pall Cr)[5]

➲ *CPT Changes: An Insider's View* 2010

3451F Dyspnea screened, moderate or severe dyspnea (Pall Cr)[5]

➲ *CPT Changes: An Insider's View* 2010

3452F Dyspnea not screened (Pall Cr)[5]

➲ *CPT Changes: An Insider's View* 2010

3455F TB screening performed and results interpreted within six months prior to initiation of first-time biologic disease modifying anti-rheumatic drug therapy for RA (RA)[5]

➲ *CPT Changes: An Insider's View* 2010

3470F Rheumatoid arthritis (RA) disease activity, low (RA)[5]

➲ *CPT Changes: An Insider's View* 2010

3471F Rheumatoid arthritis (RA) disease activity, moderate (RA)[5]

➲ *CPT Changes: An Insider's View* 2010

3472F Rheumatoid arthritis (RA) disease activity, high (RA)[5]

➲ *CPT Changes: An Insider's View* 2010

3475F Disease prognosis for rheumatoid arthritis assessed, poor prognosis documented (RA)[5]

➲ *CPT Changes: An Insider's View* 2010

3476F Disease prognosis for rheumatoid arthritis assessed, good prognosis documented (RA)[5]

➲ *CPT Changes: An Insider's View* 2010

3490F History of AIDS-defining condition (HIV)[5]

➲ *CPT Changes: An Insider's View* 2010

3491F HIV indeterminate (infants of undetermined HIV status born of HIV-infected mothers) (HIV)[5]

➲ *CPT Changes: An Insider's View* 2010

3492F History of nadir CD4+ cell count <350 cells/mm^3 (HIV)[5]

➲ *CPT Changes: An Insider's View* 2010

3493F No history of nadir CD4+ cell count <350 cells/mm^3 **and** no history of AIDS-defining condition (HIV)[5]

➲ *CPT Changes: An Insider's View* 2010

3494F CD4+ cell count <200 cells/mm^3 (HIV)[5]

➲ *CPT Changes: An Insider's View* 2010

3495F CD4+ cell count 200 – 499 cells/mm^3 (HIV)[5]

➲ *CPT Changes: An Insider's View* 2010

3496F CD4+ cell count ≥500 cells/mm^3 (HIV)[5]

➲ *CPT Changes: An Insider's View* 2010

3497F CD4+ cell percentage <15% (HIV)[5]

➲ *CPT Changes: An Insider's View* 2010

3498F CD4+ cell percentage ≥15% (HIV)[5]

➲ *CPT Changes: An Insider's View* 2010

3500F CD4+ cell count or CD4+ cell percentage documented as performed (HIV)[5]

➲ *CPT Changes: An Insider's View* 2010

3502F HIV RNA viral load below limits of quantification (HIV)[5]

➲ *CPT Changes: An Insider's View* 2010

3503F HIV RNA viral load not below limits of quantification (HIV)[5]

➲ *CPT Changes: An Insider's View* 2010

3510F Documentation that tuberculosis (TB) screening test performed and results interpreted (HIV)[5] (IBD)[10]

➲ *CPT Changes: An Insider's View* 2010

3511F Chlamydia and gonorrhea screenings documented as performed (HIV)[5]

➲ *CPT Changes: An Insider's View* 2010

3512F Syphilis screening documented as performed (HIV)[5]

➲ *CPT Changes: An Insider's View* 2010

3513F   Hepatitis B screening documented as performed (HIV)[5]
➜ *CPT Changes: An Insider's View* 2010

3514F   Hepatitis C screening documented as performed (HIV)[5]
➜ *CPT Changes: An Insider's View* 2010

3515F   Patient has documented immunity to Hepatitis C (HIV)[5]
➜ *CPT Changes: An Insider's View* 2010

3517F   Hepatitis B Virus (HBV) status assessed and results interpreted within one year prior to receiving a first course of anti-TNF (tumor necrosis factor) therapy (IBD)[10]
➜ *CPT Changes: An Insider's View* 2013

3520F   Clostridium difficile testing performed (IBD)[10]
➜ *CPT Changes: An Insider's View* 2013

3550F   Low risk for thromboembolism (AFIB)[1]
➜ *CPT Changes: An Insider's View* 2010

3551F   Intermediate risk for thromboembolism (AFIB)[1]
➜ *CPT Changes: An Insider's View* 2010

3552F   High risk for thromboembolism (AFIB)[1]
➜ *CPT Changes: An Insider's View* 2010

3555F   Patient had International Normalized Ratio (INR) measurement performed (AFIB)[1]
➜ *CPT Changes: An Insider's View* 2010

3570F   Final report for bone scintigraphy study includes correlation with existing relevant imaging studies (eg, X ray, MRI, CT) corresponding to the same anatomical region in question (NUC_MED)[1]
➜ *CPT Changes: An Insider's View* 2010

3572F   Patient considered to be potentially at risk for fracture in a weight-bearing site (NUC_MED)[1]
➜ *CPT Changes: An Insider's View* 2010

3573F   Patient not considered to be potentially at risk for fracture in a weight-bearing site (NUC_MED)[1]
➜ *CPT Changes: An Insider's View* 2010

3650F   Electroencephalogram (EEG) ordered, reviewed or requested (EPI)[8]
➜ *CPT Changes: An Insider's View* 2011

3700F   Psychiatric disorders or disturbances assessed (Prkns)[8]
➜ *CPT Changes: An Insider's View* 2011

3720F   Cognitive impairment or dysfunction assessed (Prkns)[8]
➜ *CPT Changes: An Insider's View* 2011

3725F   Screening for depression performed (DEM)[1]
➜ *CPT Changes: An Insider's View* 2012

3750F   Patient not receiving dose of corticosteroids greater than or equal to 10 mg/day for 60 or greater consecutive days (IBD)[10]
➜ *CPT Changes: An Insider's View* 2013

3751F   Electrodiagnostic studies for distal symmetric polyneuropathy conducted (or requested), documented, and reviewed within 6 months of initial evaluation for condition (DSP)[8]
➜ *CPT Changes: An Insider's View* 2014

3752F   Electrodiagnostic studies for distal symmetric polyneuropathy **not** conducted (or requested), documented, or reviewed within 6 months of initial evaluation for condition (DSP)[8]
➜ *CPT Changes: An Insider's View* 2014

3753F   Patient has clear clinical symptoms and signs that are highly suggestive of neuropathy AND cannot be attributed to another condition, AND has an obvious cause for the neuropathy (DSP)[8]
➜ *CPT Changes: An Insider's View* 2014

3754F   Screening tests for diabetes mellitus reviewed, requested, or ordered (DSP)[8]
➜ *CPT Changes: An Insider's View* 2014

3755F   Cognitive and behavioral impairment screening performed (ALS)[8]
➜ *CPT Changes: An Insider's View* 2014

3756F   Patient has pseudobulbar affect, sialorrhea, or ALS-related symptoms (ALS)[8]
➜ *CPT Changes: An Insider's View* 2014

3757F   Patient does not have pseudobulbar affect, sialorrhea, or ALS-related symptoms (ALS)[8]
➜ *CPT Changes: An Insider's View* 2014

3758F   Patient referred for pulmonary function testing or peak cough expiratory flow (ALS)[8]
➜ *CPT Changes: An Insider's View* 2014

3759F   Patient screened for dysphagia, weight loss, and impaired nutrition, and results documented (ALS)[8]
➜ *CPT Changes: An Insider's View* 2014

3760F   Patient exhibits dysphagia, weight loss, or impaired nutrition (ALS)[8]
➜ *CPT Changes: An Insider's View* 2014

3761F   Patient does not exhibit dysphagia, weight loss, or impaired nutrition (ALS)[8]
➜ *CPT Changes: An Insider's View* 2014

3762F   Patient is dysarthric (ALS)[8]
➜ *CPT Changes: An Insider's View* 2014

3763F   Patient is not dysarthric (ALS)[8]
➜ *CPT Changes: An Insider's View* 2014

3775F   Adenoma(s) or other neoplasm detected during screening colonoscopy (SCADR)[12]
➜ *CPT Changes: An Insider's View* 2015

3776F   Adenoma(s) or other neoplasm not detected during screening colonoscopy (SCADR)[12]
➜ *CPT Changes: An Insider's View* 2015

Therapeutic, Preventive, or Other Interventions

Therapeutic, preventive, or other interventions codes describe pharmacologic, procedural, or behavioral therapies, including preventive services such as patient education and counseling.

4000F Tobacco use cessation intervention, counseling (COPD, CAP, CAD, Asthma)[1] (DM)[4] (PV)[2]
> ➔ *CPT Changes: An Insider's View* 2005
> ➔ *CPT Assistant* Oct 05:4, 9

4001F Tobacco use cessation intervention, pharmacologic therapy (COPD, CAD, CAP, PV, Asthma)[1] (DM)[4] (PV)[2]
> ➔ *CPT Changes: An Insider's View* 2005
> ➔ *CPT Assistant* Oct 05:9

4003F Patient education, written/oral, appropriate for patients with heart failure, performed (NMA–No Measure Associated)[1]
> ➔ *CPT Changes: An Insider's View* 2006
> ➔ *CPT Assistant* Oct 05:8

4004F Patient screened for tobacco use **and** received tobacco cessation intervention (counseling, pharmacotherapy, or both), if identified as a tobacco user (PV, CAD)[1]
> ➔ *CPT Changes: An Insider's View* 2011, 2012

4005F Pharmacologic therapy (other than minerals/vitamins) for osteoporosis prescribed (OP)[5] (IBD)[10]
> ➔ *CPT Changes: An Insider's View* 2008

4008F Beta-blocker therapy prescribed or currently being taken (CAD,HF)[1]
> ➔ *CPT Changes: An Insider's View* 2012

4010F Angiotensin Converting Enzyme (ACE) Inhibitor or Angiotensin Receptor Blocker (ARB) therapy prescribed or currently being taken (CAD, CKD, HF)[1] (DM)[2]
> ➔ *CPT Changes: An Insider's View* 2012

4011F Oral antiplatelet therapy prescribed (CAD)[1]
> ➔ *CPT Changes: An Insider's View* 2005, 2010
> ➔ *CPT Assistant* Oct 05:10

4012F Warfarin therapy prescribed (NMA–No Measure Associated)
> ➔ *CPT Changes: An Insider's View* 2006
> ➔ *CPT Assistant* Oct 05:9

4013F Statin therapy prescribed or currently being taken (CAD)[1]
> ➔ *CPT Changes: An Insider's View* 2012

4014F Written discharge instructions provided to heart failure patients discharged home (Instructions include all of the following components: activity level, diet, discharge medications, follow-up appointment, weight monitoring, what to do if symptoms worsen) (NMA–No Measure Associated)
> ➔ *CPT Changes: An Insider's View* 2006, 2007, 2009
> ➔ *CPT Assistant* Oct 05:9

4015F Persistent asthma, preferred long term control medication or an acceptable alternative treatment, prescribed (NMA–No Measure Associated)
> ➔ *CPT Changes: An Insider's View* 2006, 2007, 2009
> ➔ *CPT Assistant* Oct 05:6

(Note: There are no medical exclusion criteria)

(Do not report modifier 1P with 4015F)

(To report patient reasons for not prescribing, use modifier 2P)

4016F Anti-inflammatory/analgesic agent prescribed (OA)[1]

(Use for prescribed or continued medication[s], including over-the-counter medication[s])
> ➔ *CPT Changes: An Insider's View* 2006
> ➔ *CPT Assistant* Oct 05:12

4017F Gastrointestinal prophylaxis for NSAID use prescribed (OA)[1]
> ➔ *CPT Changes: An Insider's View* 2006
> ➔ *CPT Assistant* Oct 05:12

4018F Therapeutic exercise for the involved joint(s) instructed or physical or occupational therapy prescribed (OA)[1]
> ➔ *CPT Changes: An Insider's View* 2006
> ➔ *CPT Assistant* Oct 05:12

4019F Documentation of receipt of counseling on exercise **and** either both calcium and vitamin D use or counseling regarding both calcium and vitamin D use (OP)[5]
> ➔ *CPT Changes: An Insider's View* 2008

4025F Inhaled bronchodilator prescribed (COPD)[1]
> ➔ *CPT Changes: An Insider's View* 2007

4030F Long-term oxygen therapy prescribed (more than 15 hours per day) (COPD)[1]
> ➔ *CPT Changes: An Insider's View* 2007

4033F Pulmonary rehabilitation exercise training recommended (COPD)[1]
> ➔ *CPT Changes: An Insider's View* 2007

(Report 4033F with 1019F)

4035F Influenza immunization recommended (COPD)[1] (IBD)[10]
> ➔ *CPT Changes: An Insider's View* 2007

4037F Influenza immunization ordered or administered (COPD, PV, CKD, ESRD)(IBD)[10]
> ➔ *CPT Changes: An Insider's View* 2007

4040F Pneumococcal vaccine administered or previously received (COPD)[1] (PV)[1,2] (IBD)[10]
> ➔ *CPT Changes: An Insider's View* 2007, 2009

4041F Documentation of order for cefazolin OR cefuroxime for antimicrobial prophylaxis (PERI 2)[5]
> ➔ *CPT Changes: An Insider's View* 2008

4042F Documentation that prophylactic antibiotics were neither given within 4 hours prior to surgical incision nor given intraoperatively (PERI 2)[5]

➔ CPT Changes: An Insider's View 2008

4043F Documentation that an order was given to discontinue prophylactic antibiotics within 48 hours of surgical end time, cardiac procedures (PERI 2)[5]

➔ CPT Changes: An Insider's View 2008

4044F Documentation that an order was given for venous thromboembolism (VTE) prophylaxis to be given within 24 hours prior to incision time or 24 hours after surgery end time (PERI 2)[5]

➔ CPT Changes: An Insider's View 2008

4045F Appropriate empiric antibiotic prescribed (CAP)[1], (EM)[5]

➔ CPT Changes: An Insider's View 2007, 2008

4046F Documentation that prophylactic antibiotics were given within 4 hours prior to surgical incision or given intraoperatively (PERI 2)[5]

➔ CPT Changes: An Insider's View 2008

4047F Documentation of order for prophylactic parenteral antibiotics to be given within 1 hour (if fluoroquinolone or vancomycin, 2 hours) prior to surgical incision (or start of procedure when no incision is required) (PERI 2)[5]

➔ CPT Changes: An Insider's View 2008, 2011

4048F Documentation that administration of prophylactic parenteral antibiotic was initiated within 1 hour (if fluoroquinolone or vancomycin, 2 hours) prior to surgical incision (or start of procedure when no incision is required) as ordered (PERI 2)[5]

➔ CPT Changes: An Insider's View 2008, 2011

4049F Documentation that order was given to discontinue prophylactic antibiotics within 24 hours of surgical end time, non-cardiac procedure (PERI 2)[5]

➔ CPT Changes: An Insider's View 2008

4050F Hypertension plan of care documented as appropriate (NMA–No Measure Associated)[1]

➔ CPT Changes: An Insider's View 2007

4051F Referred for an arteriovenous (AV) fistula (ESRD, CKD)[1]

➔ CPT Changes: An Insider's View 2008

4052F Hemodialysis via functioning arteriovenous (AV) fistula (ESRD)[1]

➔ CPT Changes: An Insider's View 2008

4053F Hemodialysis via functioning arteriovenous (AV) graft (ESRD)[1]

➔ CPT Changes: An Insider's View 2008

4054F Hemodialysis via catheter (ESRD)[1]

➔ CPT Changes: An Insider's View 2008

4055F Patient receiving peritoneal dialysis (ESRD)[1]

➔ CPT Changes: An Insider's View 2008

4056F Appropriate oral rehydration solution recommended (PAG)[1]

➔ CPT Changes: An Insider's View 2008

4058F Pediatric gastroenteritis education provided to caregiver (PAG)[1]

➔ CPT Changes: An Insider's View 2008

4060F Psychotherapy services provided (MDD, MDD ADOL)[1]

➔ CPT Changes: An Insider's View 2008, 2011

4062F Patient referral for psychotherapy documented (MDD, MDD ADOL)[1]

➔ CPT Changes: An Insider's View 2008

4063F Antidepressant pharmacotherapy considered and not prescribed (MDD ADOL)[1]

➔ CPT Changes: An Insider's View 2011

4064F Antidepressant pharmacotherapy prescribed (MDD, MDD ADOL)[1]

➔ CPT Changes: An Insider's View 2008

4065F Antipsychotic pharmacotherapy prescribed (MDD)[1]

➔ CPT Changes: An Insider's View 2008

4066F Electroconvulsive therapy (ECT) provided (MDD)[1]

➔ CPT Changes: An Insider's View 2008

4067F Patient referral for electroconvulsive therapy (ECT) documented (MDD)[1]

➔ CPT Changes: An Insider's View 2008

4069F Venous thromboembolism (VTE) prophylaxis received (IBD)[10]

➔ CPT Changes: An Insider's View 2013

4070F Deep vein thrombosis (DVT) prophylaxis received by end of hospital day 2 (STR)[5]

➔ CPT Changes: An Insider's View 2008

4073F Oral antiplatelet therapy prescribed at discharge (STR)[5]

➔ CPT Changes: An Insider's View 2008

4075F Anticoagulant therapy prescribed at discharge (STR)[5]

➔ CPT Changes: An Insider's View 2008

4077F Documentation that tissue plasminogen activator (t-PA) administration was considered (STR)[5]

➔ CPT Changes: An Insider's View 2008

4079F Documentation that rehabilitation services were considered (STR)[5]

➔ CPT Changes: An Insider's View 2008

4084F Aspirin received within 24 hours before emergency department arrival or during emergency department stay (EM)[5]

➔ CPT Changes: An Insider's View 2008

4086F Aspirin or clopidogrel prescribed or currently being taken (CAD)[1]

➔ CPT Changes: An Insider's View 2012

4090F　Patient receiving erythropoietin therapy (HEM)[1]
　　　➔ *CPT Changes: An Insider's View* 2008

4095F　Patient not receiving erythropoietin therapy (HEM)[1]
　　　➔ *CPT Changes: An Insider's View* 2008

4100F　Bisphosphonate therapy, intravenous, ordered or received (HEM)[1]
　　　➔ *CPT Changes: An Insider's View* 2008

4110F　Internal mammary artery graft performed for primary, isolated coronary artery bypass graft procedure (CABG)[6]
　　　➔ *CPT Changes: An Insider's View* 2008

4115F　Beta blocker administered within 24 hours prior to surgical incision (CABG)[6]
　　　➔ *CPT Changes: An Insider's View* 2008

4120F　Antibiotic prescribed or dispensed (URI, PHAR)[2], (A-BRONCH)[2]
　　　➔ *CPT Changes: An Insider's View* 2008

4124F　Antibiotic neither prescribed nor dispensed (URI, PHAR)[2], (A-BRONCH)[2]
　　　➔ *CPT Changes: An Insider's View* 2008

4130F　Topical preparations (including OTC) prescribed for acute otitis externa (AOE)[1]
　　　➔ *CPT Changes: An Insider's View* 2009

4131F　Systemic antimicrobial therapy prescribed (AOE)[1]
　　　➔ *CPT Changes: An Insider's View* 2009

4132F　Systemic antimicrobial therapy not prescribed (AOE)[1]
　　　➔ *CPT Changes: An Insider's View* 2009

4133F　Antihistamines or decongestants prescribed or recommended (OME)[1]
　　　➔ *CPT Changes: An Insider's View* 2009

4134F　Antihistamines or decongestants neither prescribed nor recommended (OME)[1]
　　　➔ *CPT Changes: An Insider's View* 2009

4135F　Systemic corticosteroids prescribed (OME)[1]
　　　➔ *CPT Changes: An Insider's View* 2009

4136F　Systemic corticosteroids not prescribed (OME)[1]
　　　➔ *CPT Changes: An Insider's View* 2009

4140F　Inhaled corticosteroids prescribed (Asthma)[1]
　　　➔ *CPT Changes: An Insider's View* 2012

4142F　Corticosteroid sparing therapy prescribed (IBD)[10]
　　　➔ *CPT Changes: An Insider's View* 2013

4144F　Alternative long-term control medication prescribed (Asthma)[1]
　　　➔ *CPT Changes: An Insider's View* 2012

4145F　Two or more anti-hypertensive agents prescribed or currently being taken (CAD, HTN)[1]
　　　➔ *CPT Changes: An Insider's View* 2012

4148F　Hepatitis A vaccine injection administered or previously received (HEP-C)[1]
　　　➔ *CPT Changes: An Insider's View* 2010

4149F　Hepatitis B vaccine injection administered or previously received (HEP-C, HIV)[1] (IBD)[10]
　　　➔ *CPT Changes: An Insider's View* 2010, 2012

4150F　Patient receiving antiviral treatment for Hepatitis C (HEP-C)[1]
　　　➔ *CPT Changes: An Insider's View* 2009

4151F　Patient did not start or is not receiving antiviral treatment for Hepatitis C during the measurement period (HEP-C)[1]
　　　➔ *CPT Changes: An Insider's View* 2009, 2017

4153F　Combination peginterferon and ribavirin therapy prescribed (HEP-C)[1]
　　　➔ *CPT Changes: An Insider's View* 2009

4155F　Hepatitis A vaccine series previously received (HEP-C)[1]
　　　➔ *CPT Changes: An Insider's View* 2009

4157F　Hepatitis B vaccine series previously received (HEP-C)[1]
　　　➔ *CPT Changes: An Insider's View* 2009

4158F　Patient counseled about risks of alcohol use (HEP-C)[1]
　　　➔ *CPT Changes: An Insider's View* 2009, 2010

4159F　Counseling regarding contraception received prior to initiation of antiviral treatment (HEP-C)[1]
　　　➔ *CPT Changes: An Insider's View* 2009

4163F　Patient counseling at a minimum on all of the following treatment options for clinically localized prostate cancer: active surveillance, **and** interstitial prostate brachytherapy, **and** external beam radiotherapy, **and** radical prostatectomy, provided prior to initiation of treatment (PRCA)[1]
　　　➔ *CPT Changes: An Insider's View* 2009

4164F　Adjuvant (ie, in combination with external beam radiotherapy to the prostate for prostate cancer) hormonal therapy (gonadotropin-releasing hormone [GnRH] agonist or antagonist) prescribed/administered (PRCA)[1]
　　　➔ *CPT Changes: An Insider's View* 2009

4165F　3-dimensional conformal radiotherapy (3D-CRT) or intensity modulated radiation therapy (IMRT) received (PRCA)[1]
　　　➔ *CPT Changes: An Insider's View* 2009

4167F　Head of bed elevation (30-45 degrees) on first ventilator day ordered (CRIT)[1]
　　　➔ *CPT Changes: An Insider's View* 2009

4168F　Patient receiving care in the intensive care unit (ICU) and receiving mechanical ventilation, 24 hours or less (CRIT)[1]
　　　➔ *CPT Changes: An Insider's View* 2009

4169F   Patient either not receiving care in the intensive care unit (ICU) OR not receiving mechanical ventilation OR receiving mechanical ventilation greater than 24 hours (CRIT)[1]

→ *CPT Changes: An Insider's View* 2009

4171F   Patient receiving erythropoiesis-stimulating agents (ESA) therapy (CKD)[1]

→ *CPT Changes: An Insider's View* 2009

4172F   Patient not receiving erythropoiesis-stimulating agents (ESA) therapy (CKD)[1]

→ *CPT Changes: An Insider's View* 2009

4174F   Counseling about the potential impact of glaucoma on visual functioning and quality of life, and importance of treatment adherence provided to patient and/or caregiver(s) (EC)[5]

→ *CPT Changes: An Insider's View* 2009

4175F   Best-corrected visual acuity of 20/40 or better (distance or near) achieved within the 90 days following cataract surgery (EC)[5]

→ *CPT Changes: An Insider's View* 2009

4176F   Counseling about value of protection from UV light and lack of proven efficacy of nutritional supplements in prevention or progression of cataract development provided to patient and/or caregiver(s) (NMA–No Measure Associated)

→ *CPT Changes: An Insider's View* 2009

4177F   Counseling about the benefits and/or risks of the Age-Related Eye Disease Study (AREDS) formulation for preventing progression of age-related macular degeneration (AMD) provided to patient and/or caregiver(s) (EC)[5]

→ *CPT Changes: An Insider's View* 2009

4178F   Anti-D immune globulin received between 26 and 30 weeks gestation (Pre-Cr)[1]

→ *CPT Changes: An Insider's View* 2009

4179F   Tamoxifen or aromatase inhibitor (AI) prescribed (ONC)[1]

→ *CPT Changes: An Insider's View* 2009

4180F   Adjuvant chemotherapy referred, prescribed, or previously received for Stage III colon cancer (ONC)[1]

→ *CPT Changes: An Insider's View* 2009, 2010

4181F   Conformal radiation therapy received (NMA–No Measure Associated)

→ *CPT Changes: An Insider's View* 2009

4182F   Conformal radiation therapy not received (NMA–No Measure Associated)

→ *CPT Changes: An Insider's View* 2009

4185F   Continuous (12-months) therapy with proton pump inhibitor (PPI) or histamine H2 receptor antagonist (H2RA) received (GERD)[5]

→ *CPT Changes: An Insider's View* 2009

4186F   No continuous (12-months) therapy with either proton pump inhibitor (PPI) or histamine H2 receptor antagonist (H2RA) received (GERD)[5]

→ *CPT Changes: An Insider's View* 2009

4187F   Disease modifying anti-rheumatic drug therapy prescribed or dispensed (RA)[2]

→ *CPT Changes: An Insider's View* 2009

4188F   Appropriate angiotensin converting enzyme (ACE)/ angiotensin receptor blockers (ARB) therapeutic monitoring test ordered or performed (AM)[2]

→ *CPT Changes: An Insider's View* 2009

4189F   Appropriate digoxin therapeutic monitoring test ordered or performed (AM)[2]

→ *CPT Changes: An Insider's View* 2009

4190F   Appropriate diuretic therapeutic monitoring test ordered or performed (AM)[2]

→ *CPT Changes: An Insider's View* 2009

4191F   Appropriate anticonvulsant therapeutic monitoring test ordered or performed (AM)[2]

→ *CPT Changes: An Insider's View* 2009

4192F   Patient not receiving glucocorticoid therapy (RA)[5]

→ *CPT Changes: An Insider's View* 2010

4193F   Patient receiving <10 mg daily prednisone (or equivalent), or RA activity is worsening, or glucocorticoid use is for less than 6 months (RA)[5]

→ *CPT Changes: An Insider's View* 2010

4194F   Patient receiving ≥10 mg daily prednisone (or equivalent) for longer than 6 months, and improvement or no change in disease activity (RA)[5]

→ *CPT Changes: An Insider's View* 2010

4195F   Patient receiving first-time biologic disease modifying anti-rheumatic drug therapy for rheumatoid arthritis (RA)[5]

→ *CPT Changes: An Insider's View* 2010

4196F   Patient not receiving first-time biologic disease modifying anti-rheumatic drug therapy for rheumatoid arthritis (RA)[5]

→ *CPT Changes: An Insider's View* 2010

4200F   External beam radiotherapy as primary therapy to prostate with or without nodal irradiation (PRCA)[1]

→ *CPT Changes: An Insider's View* 2009, 2010

4201F   External beam radiotherapy with or without nodal irradiation as adjuvant or salvage therapy for prostate cancer patient (PRCA)[1]

→ *CPT Changes: An Insider's View* 2009, 2010

4210F   Angiotensin converting enzyme (ACE) or angiotensin receptor blockers (ARB) medication therapy for 6 months or more (MM)[2]

→ *CPT Changes: An Insider's View* 2009

4220F   Digoxin medication therapy for 6 months or more (MM)[2]

→ *CPT Changes: An Insider's View* 2009

4221F   Diuretic medication therapy for 6 months or more (MM)[2]

➔ *CPT Changes: An Insider's View* 2009

4230F   Anticonvulsant medication therapy for 6 months or more (MM)[2]

➔ *CPT Changes: An Insider's View* 2009

4240F   Instruction in therapeutic exercise with follow-up provided to patients during episode of back pain lasting longer than 12 weeks (BkP)[2]

➔ *CPT Changes: An Insider's View* 2009, 2013

4242F   Counseling for supervised exercise program provided to patients during episode of back pain lasting longer than 12 weeks (BkP)[2]

➔ *CPT Changes: An Insider's View* 2009

4245F   Patient counseled during the initial visit to maintain or resume normal activities (BkP)[2]

➔ *CPT Changes: An Insider's View* 2009

4248F   Patient counseled during the initial visit for an episode of back pain against bed rest lasting 4 days or longer (BkP)[2]

➔ *CPT Changes: An Insider's View* 2009

4250F   Active warming used intraoperatively for the purpose of maintaining normothermia, **or** at least 1 body temperature equal to or greater than 36 degrees Centigrade (or 96.8 degrees Fahrenheit) recorded within the 30 minutes immediately before or the 15 minutes immediately after anesthesia end time (CRIT)[1]

➔ *CPT Changes: An Insider's View* 2009, 2010

4255F   Duration of general or neuraxial anesthesia 60 minutes or longer, as documented in the anesthesia record (CRIT)[5] (Peri2)[11]

➔ *CPT Changes: An Insider's View* 2011

4256F   Duration of general or neuraxial anesthesia less than 60 minutes, as documented in the anesthesia record (CRIT)[5] (Peri2)[11]

➔ *CPT Changes: An Insider's View* 2011

4260F   Wound surface culture technique used (CWC)[5]

➔ *CPT Changes: An Insider's View* 2010

4261F   Technique other than surface culture of the wound exudate used (eg, Levine/deep swab technique, semi-quantitative or quantitative swab technique) **or** wound surface culture technique not used (CWC)[5]

➔ *CPT Changes: An Insider's View* 2010

4265F   Use of wet to dry dressings prescribed or recommended (CWC)[5]

➔ *CPT Changes: An Insider's View* 2010

4266F   Use of wet to dry dressings neither prescribed nor recommended (CWC)[5]

➔ *CPT Changes: An Insider's View* 2010

4267F   Compression therapy prescribed (CWC)[5]

➔ *CPT Changes: An Insider's View* 2010

4268F   Patient education regarding the need for long term compression therapy including interval replacement of compression stockings received (CWC)[5]

➔ *CPT Changes: An Insider's View* 2010

4269F   Appropriate method of offloading (pressure relief) prescribed (CWC)[5]

➔ *CPT Changes: An Insider's View* 2010

4270F   Patient receiving potent antiretroviral therapy for 6 months or longer (HIV)[5]

➔ *CPT Changes: An Insider's View* 2010

4271F   Patient receiving potent antiretroviral therapy for less than 6 months or not receiving potent antiretroviral therapy (HIV)[5]

➔ *CPT Changes: An Insider's View* 2010

4274F   Influenza immunization administered or previously received (HIV)[5] (P-ESRD)[1]

➔ *CPT Changes: An Insider's View* 2010

4276F   Potent antiretroviral therapy prescribed (HIV)[5]

➔ *CPT Changes: An Insider's View* 2010

4279F   Pneumocystis jiroveci pneumonia prophylaxis prescribed (HIV)[5]

➔ *CPT Changes: An Insider's View* 2010

4280F   Pneumocystis jiroveci pneumonia prophylaxis prescribed within 3 months of low CD4+ cell count or percentage (HIV)[5]

➔ *CPT Changes: An Insider's View* 2010

4290F   Patient screened for injection drug use (HIV)[5]

➔ *CPT Changes: An Insider's View* 2010

4293F   Patient screened for high-risk sexual behavior (HIV)[5]

➔ *CPT Changes: An Insider's View* 2010

4300F   Patient receiving warfarin therapy for nonvalvular atrial fibrillation or atrial flutter (AFIB)[1]

➔ *CPT Changes: An Insider's View* 2010

4301F   Patient not receiving warfarin therapy for nonvalvular atrial fibrillation or atrial flutter (AFIB)[1]

➔ *CPT Changes: An Insider's View* 2010

4305F   Patient education regarding appropriate foot care **and** daily inspection of the feet received (CWC)[5]

➔ *CPT Changes: An Insider's View* 2010

4306F   Patient counseled regarding psychosocial **and** pharmacologic treatment options for opioid addiction (SUD)[1]

➔ *CPT Changes: An Insider's View* 2010

4320F   Patient counseled regarding psychosocial **and** pharmacologic treatment options for alcohol dependence (SUD)[5]

➔ *CPT Changes: An Insider's View* 2010

4322F   Caregiver provided with education and referred to additional resources for support (DEM)[1]

➔ *CPT Changes: An Insider's View* 2012

4324F Patient (or caregiver) queried about Parkinson's disease medication related motor complications (Prkns)[8]
➔ *CPT Changes: An Insider's View* 2011

4325F Medical and surgical treatment options reviewed with patient (or caregiver) (Prkns)[8]
➔ *CPT Changes: An Insider's View* 2011

4326F Patient (or caregiver) queried about symptoms of autonomic dysfunction (Prkns)[8]
➔ *CPT Changes: An Insider's View* 2011

4328F Patient (or caregiver) queried about sleep disturbances (Prkns)[8]
➔ *CPT Changes: An Insider's View* 2011

4330F Counseling about epilepsy specific safety issues provided to patient (or caregiver(s)) (EPI)[8]
➔ *CPT Changes: An Insider's View* 2011

4340F Counseling for women of childbearing potential with epilepsy (EPI)[8]
➔ *CPT Changes: An Insider's View* 2011

4350F Counseling provided on symptom management, end of life decisions, and palliation (DEM)[1]
➔ *CPT Changes: An Insider's View* 2012

4400F Rehabilitative therapy options discussed with patient (or caregiver) (Prkns)[8]
➔ *CPT Changes: An Insider's View* 2011

4450F Self-care education provided to patient (HF)[1]
➔ *CPT Changes: An Insider's View* 2012

4470F Implantable cardioverter-defibrillator (ICD) counseling provided (HF)[1]
➔ *CPT Changes: An Insider's View* 2012

4480F Patient receiving ACE inhibitor/ARB therapy and beta-blocker therapy for 3 months or longer (HF)[1]
➔ *CPT Changes: An Insider's View* 2012

4481F Patient receiving ACE inhibitor/ARB therapy and beta-blocker therapy for less than 3 months or patient not receiving ACE inhibitor/ARB therapy and beta-blocker therapy (HF)[1]
➔ *CPT Changes: An Insider's View* 2012

4500F Referred to an outpatient cardiac rehabilitation program (CAD)[1]
➔ *CPT Changes: An Insider's View* 2012

4510F Previous cardiac rehabilitation for qualifying cardiac event completed (CAD)[1]
➔ *CPT Changes: An Insider's View* 2012

4525F Neuropsychiatric intervention ordered (DEM)[1]
➔ *CPT Changes: An Insider's View* 2012

4526F Neuropsychiatric intervention received (DEM)[1]
➔ *CPT Changes: An Insider's View* 2012

4540F Disease modifying pharmacotherapy discussed (ALS)[8]
➔ *CPT Changes: An Insider's View* 2014

4541F Patient offered treatment for pseudobulbar affect, sialorrhea, or ALS-related symptoms (ALS)[8]
➔ *CPT Changes: An Insider's View* 2014

4550F Options for noninvasive respiratory support discussed with patient (ALS)[8]
➔ *CPT Changes: An Insider's View* 2014

4551F Nutritional support offered (ALS)[8]
➔ *CPT Changes: An Insider's View* 2014

4552F Patient offered referral to a speech language pathologist (ALS)[8]
➔ *CPT Changes: An Insider's View* 2014

4553F Patient offered assistance in planning for end of life issues (ALS)[8]
➔ *CPT Changes: An Insider's View* 2014

4554F Patient received inhalational anesthetic agent (Peri2)[11]
➔ *CPT Changes: An Insider's View* 2014

4555F Patient did not receive inhalational anesthetic agent (Peri2)[11]
➔ *CPT Changes: An Insider's View* 2014

4556F Patient exhibits 3 or more risk factors for post-operative nausea and vomiting (Peri2)[11]
➔ *CPT Changes: An Insider's View* 2014

4557F Patient does not exhibit 3 or more risk factors for post-operative nausea and vomiting (Peri2)[11]
➔ *CPT Changes: An Insider's View* 2014

4558F Patient received at least 2 prophylactic pharmacologic anti-emetic agents of different classes preoperatively and intraoperatively (Peri2)[11]
➔ *CPT Changes: An Insider's View* 2014

4559F At least 1 body temperature measurement equal to or greater than 35.5 degrees Celsius (or 95.9 degrees Fahrenheit) recorded within the 30 minutes immediately before or the 15 minutes immediately after anesthesia end time (Peri2)[11]
➔ *CPT Changes: An Insider's View* 2014

4560F Anesthesia technique did not involve general or neuraxial anesthesia (Peri2)[11]
➔ *CPT Changes: An Insider's View* 2014

4561F Patient has a coronary artery stent (Peri2)[11]
➔ *CPT Changes: An Insider's View* 2014

4562F Patient does not have a coronary artery stent (Peri2)[11]
➔ *CPT Changes: An Insider's View* 2014

4563F Patient received aspirin within 24 hours prior to anesthesia start time (Peri2)[11]
➔ *CPT Changes: An Insider's View* 2014

★ = Telemedicine ◀ = Audio-only ✛ = Add-on code ✗ = FDA approval pending # = Resequenced code ⊘ = Modifier 51 exempt ➔➔➔ = See p xxi for details

Follow-up or Other Outcomes

Follow-up or other outcomes codes describe review and communication of test results to patients, patient satisfaction or experience with care, patient functional status, and patient morbidity and mortality.

5005F   Patient counseled on self-examination for new or changing moles (ML)[5]

  → *CPT Changes: An Insider's View* 2008

5010F   Findings of dilated macular or fundus exam communicated to the physician or other qualified health care professional managing the diabetes care (EC)[5]

  → *CPT Changes: An Insider's View* 2008, 2013

5015F   Documentation of communication that a fracture occurred and that the patient was or should be tested or treated for osteoporosis (OP)[5]

  → *CPT Changes: An Insider's View* 2008

5020F   Treatment summary report communicated to physician(s) or other qualified health care professional(s) managing continuing care and to the patient within 1 month of completing treatment (ONC)[1]

  → *CPT Changes: An Insider's View* 2009, 2010, 2013

5050F   Treatment plan communicated to provider(s) managing continuing care within 1 month of diagnosis (ML)[5]

  → *CPT Changes: An Insider's View* 2009

5060F   Findings from diagnostic mammogram communicated to practice managing patient's on-going care within 3 business days of exam interpretation (RAD)[5]

  → *CPT Changes: An Insider's View* 2009

5062F   Findings from diagnostic mammogram communicated to the patient within 5 days of exam interpretation (RAD)[5]

  → *CPT Changes: An Insider's View* 2009

5100F   Potential risk for fracture communicated to the referring physician or other qualified health care professional within 24 hours of completion of the imaging study (NUC_MED)[1]

  → *CPT Changes: An Insider's View* 2010, 2013

5200F   Consideration of referral for a neurological evaluation of appropriateness for surgical therapy for intractable epilepsy within the past 3 years (EPI)[8]

  → *CPT Changes: An Insider's View* 2011

5250F   Asthma discharge plan provided to patient (Asthma)[1]

  → *CPT Changes: An Insider's View* 2012

Patient Safety

Patient safety codes that describe patient safety practices.

6005F   Rationale (eg, severity of illness and safety) for level of care (eg, home, hospital) documented (CAP)[1]

  → *CPT Changes: An Insider's View* 2007
  → *CPT Assistant* Aug 07:1

6010F   Dysphagia screening conducted prior to order for or receipt of any foods, fluids, or medication by mouth (STR)[5]

  → *CPT Changes: An Insider's View* 2008

6015F   Patient receiving or eligible to receive foods, fluids, or medication by mouth (STR)[5]

  → *CPT Changes: An Insider's View* 2008

6020F   NPO (nothing by mouth) ordered (STR)[5]

  → *CPT Changes: An Insider's View* 2008

6030F   All elements of maximal sterile barrier technique, hand hygiene, skin preparation and, if ultrasound is used, sterile ultrasound techniques followed (CRIT)[1]

  → *CPT Changes: An Insider's View* 2009, 2010, 2016

6040F   Use of appropriate radiation dose reduction devices OR manual techniques for appropriate moderation of exposure, documented (RAD)[5]

  → *CPT Changes: An Insider's View* 2009

6045F   Radiation exposure or exposure time in final report for procedure using fluoroscopy, documented (RAD)[5]

  → *CPT Changes: An Insider's View* 2009
  → *Clinical Examples in Radiology* Summer 10:1, Winter 11:2, Spring 11:2, 9-10, Summer 11:2, Fall 11:2-3, Spring 13:2-3, 6, Summer 13:2-3, 5-6, Spring 14:7, Fall 14:6

6070F   Patient queried and counseled about anti-epileptic drug (AED) side effects (EPI)[8]

  → *CPT Changes: An Insider's View* 2011

6080F   Patient (or caregiver) queried about falls (Prkns, DSP)[8]

  → *CPT Changes: An Insider's View* 2011

6090F   Patient (or caregiver) counseled about safety issues appropriate to patient's stage of disease (Prkns)[8]

  → *CPT Changes: An Insider's View* 2011

6100F   Timeout to verify correct patient, correct site, and correct procedure, documented (PATH)[9]

  → *CPT Changes: An Insider's View* 2012

6101F   Safety counseling for dementia provided (DEM)[1]

  → *CPT Changes: An Insider's View* 2012

6102F   Safety counseling for dementia ordered (DEM)[1]

  → *CPT Changes: An Insider's View* 2012

6110F   Counseling provided regarding risks of driving and the alternatives to driving (DEM)[1]

  → *CPT Changes: An Insider's View* 2012

6150F   Patient not receiving a first course of anti-TNF (tumor necrosis factor) therapy (IBD)[10]

  → *CPT Changes: An Insider's View* 2013

Structural Measures

Structural measures codes are used to identify measures that address the setting or system of the delivered care. These codes also address aspects of the capabilities of the organization or health care professional providing the care.

7010F   Patient information entered into a recall system that includes: target date for the next exam specified **and** a process to follow up with patients regarding missed or unscheduled appointments (ML)[5]

➔ *CPT Changes: An Insider's View* 2009, 2011

7020F   Mammogram assessment category (eg, Mammography Quality Standards Act [MQSA], Breast Imaging Reporting and Data System [BI-RADS®], or FDA approved equivalent categories) entered into an internal database to allow for analysis of abnormal interpretation (recall) rate (RAD)[5]

➔ *CPT Changes: An Insider's View* 2009

7025F   Patient information entered into a reminder system with a target due date for the next mammogram (RAD)[5]

➔ *CPT Changes: An Insider's View* 2009

Nonmeasure Code Listing

The following codes are included for reporting of certain aspects of care. These factors are not represented by measures developed by existing measures organizations or recognized measures-development processes at the time they are placed in the CPT code set, but may ultimately be associated with measures approved by an appropriate quality improvement organization.

9001F   Aortic aneurysm less than 5.0 cm maximum diameter on centerline formatted CT or minor diameter on axial formatted CT (NMA–No Measure Associated)

➔ *CPT Changes: An Insider's View* 2014

9002F   Aortic aneurysm 5.0 - 5.4 cm maximum diameter on centerline formatted CT or minor diameter on axial formatted CT (NMA–No Measure Associated)

➔ *CPT Changes: An Insider's View* 2014

9003F   Aortic aneurysm 5.5 - 5.9 cm maximum diameter on centerline formatted CT or minor diameter on axial formatted CT (NMA–No Measure Associated)

➔ *CPT Changes: An Insider's View* 2014

9004F   Aortic aneurysm 6.0 cm or greater maximum diameter on centerline formatted CT or minor diameter on axial formatted CT (NMA–No Measure Associated)

➔ *CPT Changes: An Insider's View* 2014

9005F   Asymptomatic carotid stenosis: No history of any transient ischemic attack or stroke in any carotid or vertebrobasilar territory (NMA–No Measure Associated)

➔ *CPT Changes: An Insider's View* 2014

9006F   Symptomatic carotid stenosis: Ipsilateral carotid territory TIA or stroke less than 120 days prior to procedure (NMA–No Measure Associated)

➔ *CPT Changes: An Insider's View* 2014

9007F   Other carotid stenosis: Ipsilateral TIA or stroke 120 days or greater prior to procedure or any prior contralateral carotid territory or vertebrobasilar TIA or stroke (NMA–No Measure Associated)

➔ *CPT Changes: An Insider's View* 2014

Category III Codes

The following section contains a set of temporary codes for emerging technology, services, procedures, and service paradigms. Category III codes allow data collection for these services/procedures. Use of unlisted codes does not offer the opportunity for the collection of specific data. If a Category III code is available, this code must be reported instead of a Category I unlisted code. This is an activity that is critically important in the evaluation of health care delivery and the formation of public and private policy. The use of the codes in this section allows physicians and other qualified health care professionals, insurers, health services researchers, and health policy experts to identify emerging technology, services, procedures, and service paradigms for clinical efficacy, utilization and outcomes.

The inclusion of a service or procedure in this section does not constitute a finding of support, or lack thereof, with regard to clinical efficacy, safety, applicability to clinical practice, or payer coverage. The codes in this section may not conform to the usual requirements for CPT Category I codes established by the Editorial Panel. For Category I codes, the Panel requires that the service/procedure be performed by many health care professionals in clinical practice in multiple locations and that FDA approval, as appropriate, has already been received. The nature of emerging technology, services, procedures, and service paradigms is such that these requirements may not be met. For these reasons, temporary codes for emerging technology, services, procedures, and service paradigms have been placed in a separate section of the CPT code set and the codes are differentiated from Category I CPT codes by the use of alphanumeric characters.

Services and procedures described in this section make use of alphanumeric characters. These codes have an alpha character as the 5th character in the string (ie, four digits followed by the letter T). The digits are not intended to reflect the placement of the code in the Category I section of CPT nomenclature. Codes in this section may or may not eventually receive a Category I CPT code. In either case, in general, a given Category III code will be archived five years from the date of initial publication or extension unless a modification of the archival date is specifically noted at the time of a revision or change to a code (eg, addition of parenthetical instructions, reinstatement). Services and procedures described by Category III codes which have been archived after five years, without conversion, must be reported using the Category I unlisted code unless another specific cross-reference is established at the time of archiving. New codes or revised codes in this section are released semi-annually via the AMA CPT website to expedite dissemination for reporting. Codes approved for deletion are published annually with the full set of temporary

codes for emerging technology, services, procedures, and service paradigms in the CPT code set. See the Introduction section of the CPT code set for a complete list of the dates of release and implementation.

(For destruction of localized lesion of choroid by transpupillary thermotherapy, use 67299)

(For destruction of macular drusen, photocoagulation, use 67299)

(For application of extracorporeal shock wave involving musculoskeletal system not otherwise specified, use 0101T)

(For application of extracorporeal shock wave involving lateral humeral epicondyle, use 0102T)

(For non-surgical septal reduction therapy, use 93799)

(For lipoprotein, direct measurement, intermediate density lipoproteins [IDL] [remnant lipoprotein], use 84999)

(For endoscopic lysis of epidural adhesions with direct visualization using mechanical means or solution injection [eg, normal saline], use 64999)

(For dual energy x-ray absorptiometry [DXA] body composition study, use 76499)

(For pulsed magnetic neuromodulation incontinence treatment, use 53899)

(To report antiprothrombin [phospholipid cofactor] antibody, use 86849)

(0031T, 0032T have been deleted)

(For speculoscopy, including sampling, use 58999)

(For urinalysis infectious agent detection, semi-quantitative analysis of volatile compounds, use 81099)

0042T   Cerebral perfusion analysis using computed tomography with contrast administration, including post-processing of parametric maps with determination of cerebral blood flow, cerebral blood volume, and mean transit time
Sunset January 2029
➜ *CPT Changes: An Insider's View* 2003
➜ *CPT Assistant* Sep 21:5

(For carbon monoxide, expired gas analysis [eg, ETCO$_c$/hemolysis breath test], use 84999)

(0046T, 0047T have been deleted)

(For mammary duct[s] catheter lavage, use 19499)

+ 0054T Computer-assisted musculoskeletal surgical navigational orthopedic procedure, with image-guidance based on fluoroscopic images (List separately in addition to code for primary procedure)

Sunset January 2029

➔ *CPT Changes: An Insider's View* 2004

➔ *CPT Assistant* May 04:14, Jun 04:8

+ 0055T Computer-assisted musculoskeletal surgical navigational orthopedic procedure, with image-guidance based on CT/MRI images (List separately in addition to code for primary procedure)

Sunset January 2029

➔ *CPT Changes: An Insider's View* 2004, 2005

➔ *CPT Assistant* May 04:14, Jun 04:8

(When CT and MRI are both performed, report 0055T only once)

(For cryopreservation, reproductive tissue, ovarian, use 89398)

(For cryopreservation of mature oocyte(s), use 89337)

(For cryopreservation of immature oocyte[s], use 89398)

(For cryopreservation of embryo(s), sperm and testicular reproductive tissue, see 89258, 89259, 89335)

(For electrical impedance breast scan, use 76499)

(For destruction/reduction of malignant breast tumor, microwave phased array thermotherapy, use 19499)

(0062T, 0063T have been deleted)

(For percutaneous intradiscal annuloplasty, any method other than electrothermal, use 22899)

(For intradiscal electrothermal annuloplasty, see 22526, 22527)

(To report CT colon, screening, use 74263)

(To report CT colon, diagnostic, see 74261-74262)

(0068T-0070T have been deleted)

(For acoustic heart sound recording and computer analysis, use 93799)

0071T Focused ultrasound ablation of uterine leiomyomata, including MR guidance; total leiomyomata volume less than 200 cc of tissue

Sunset January 2030

➔ *CPT Changes: An Insider's View* 2005

➔ *CPT Assistant* Mar 05:1, 5, Dec 05:3

0072T total leiomyomata volume greater or equal to 200 cc of tissue

Sunset January 2030

➔ *CPT Changes: An Insider's View* 2005

➔ *CPT Assistant* Mar 05:1, 5, Dec 05:3

(Do not report 0071T, 0072T in conjunction with 51702 or 77022)

0075T Transcatheter placement of extracranial vertebral artery stent(s), including radiologic supervision and interpretation, open or percutaneous; initial vessel

Sunset January 2030

➔ *CPT Changes: An Insider's View* 2005, 2015

➔ *CPT Assistant* May 05:7, Mar 14:8

+ 0076T each additional vessel (List separately in addition to code for primary procedure)

Sunset January 2030

➔ *CPT Changes: An Insider's View* 2005, 2015

➔ *CPT Assistant* May 05:7, Mar 14:8

(Use 0076T in conjunction with 0075T)

(When the ipsilateral extracranial vertebral arteriogram (including imaging and selective catheterization) confirms the need for stenting, then 0075T and 0076T include all ipsilateral extracranial vertebral catheterization, all diagnostic imaging for ipsilateral extracranial vertebral artery stenting, and all related radiologic supervision and interpretation. If stenting is not indicated, then the appropriate codes for selective catheterization and imaging should be reported in lieu of 0075T or 0076T)

(For breath test for heart transplant rejection, use 84999)

(To report total disc lumbar arthroplasty, use 22857)

+ 0095T Removal of total disc arthroplasty (artificial disc), anterior approach, each additional interspace, cervical (List separately in addition to code for primary procedure)

Sunset January 2029

➔ *CPT Changes: An Insider's View* 2006, 2009

➔ *CPT Assistant* Jun 05:6, Feb 06:1

(Use 0095T in conjunction with 22864)

(To report revision of total disc lumbar arthroplasty, use 22862)

+ 0098T Revision including replacement of total disc arthroplasty (artificial disc), anterior approach, each additional interspace, cervical (List separately in addition to code for primary procedure)

Sunset January 2029

➔ *CPT Changes: An Insider's View* 2006, 2009

➔ *CPT Assistant* Jun 05:6, Feb 06:1

(Use 0098T in conjunction with 22861)

(Do not report 0098T in conjunction with 0095T)

(Do not report 0098T in conjunction with 22853, 22854, 22859 when performed at the same level)

(For decompression, see 63001-63048)

★=Telemedicine ◀=Audio-only ✛=Add-on code ✔=FDA approval pending #=Resequenced code ⊘=Modifier 51 exempt ➔➔➔=See p xxi for details

0100T Placement of a subconjunctival retinal prosthesis receiver and pulse generator, and implantation of intraocular retinal electrode array, with vitrectomy

Sunset January 2026

➔ *CPT Changes: An Insider's View* 2006

➔ *CPT Assistant* Jun 05:6, Feb 06:1, Jun 11:13, Feb 18:3

(For initial programming of implantable intraocular retinal electrode array device, use 0472T)

0101T Extracorporeal shock wave involving musculoskeletal system, not otherwise specified

Sunset January 2026

➔ *CPT Changes: An Insider's View* 2006, 2022

➔ *CPT Assistant* Jun 05:6, Mar 06:1, Jun 11:13, Dec 18:5

(For extracorporeal shock wave therapy involving integumentary system not otherwise specified, see 0512T, 0513T)

(Do not report 0101T in conjunction 0512T, 0513T, when treating same area)

0102T Extracorporeal shock wave performed by a physician, requiring anesthesia other than local, and involving the lateral humeral epicondyle

Sunset January 2026

➔ *CPT Changes: An Insider's View* 2006, 2022

➔ *CPT Assistant* Jun 05:6, Mar 06:1, Jun 11:13, Dec 18:5, Jun 19:11

 # 0512T Extracorporeal shock wave for integumentary wound healing, including topical application and dressing care; initial wound

Sunset January 2029

➔ *CPT Changes: An Insider's View* 2019, 2022

➔ *CPT Assistant* Dec 18:5

#+ 0513T each additional wound (List separately in addition to code for primary procedure)

Sunset January 2029

➔ *CPT Changes: An Insider's View* 2019

➔ *CPT Assistant* Dec 18:5

(Use 0513T in conjunction with 0512T)

(For holotranscobalamin, quantitative, use 84999)

(For inert gas rebreathing for cardiac output measurement during rest, use 93799)

(For inert gas rebreathing for cardiac output measurement during exercise, use 93799)

0106T Quantitative sensory testing (QST), testing and interpretation per extremity; using touch pressure stimuli to assess large diameter sensation

Sunset January 2026

➔ *CPT Changes: An Insider's View* 2006

➔ *CPT Assistant* Jun 05:6, Mar 06:1, May 11:10, Jun 11:13

0107T using vibration stimuli to assess large diameter fiber sensation

Sunset January 2026

➔ *CPT Changes: An Insider's View* 2006

➔ *CPT Assistant* Jun 05:6, Mar 06:1, May 11:10, Jun 11:13

0108T using cooling stimuli to assess small nerve fiber sensation and hyperalgesia

Sunset January 2026

➔ *CPT Changes: An Insider's View* 2006

➔ *CPT Assistant* Jun 05:6, Mar 06:1, May 11:10, Jun 11:13

0109T using heat-pain stimuli to assess small nerve fiber sensation and hyperalgesia

Sunset January 2026

➔ *CPT Changes: An Insider's View* 2006

➔ *CPT Assistant* Jun 05:6, Mar 06:1, May 11:10, Jun 11:13

0110T using other stimuli to assess sensation

Sunset January 2026

➔ *CPT Changes: An Insider's View* 2006

➔ *CPT Assistant* Jun 05:6, Mar 06:1, May 11:10, Jun 11:13

(For very long chain fatty acids, use 82726)

(For long-chain [C20-22] omega-3 fatty acids in red blood cell [RBC] membranes, use 84999)

(For fistulization of sclera for glaucoma, through ciliary body, use 66999)

(For conjunctival incision with posterior extrascleral placement of pharmacological agent, use 68399)

(For common carotid intima-media thickness [IMT] study for evaluation of atherosclerotic burden or coronary heart disease risk factor assessment, use 93998)

(For bilateral quantitative carotid intima media thickness and carotid atheroma evaluation that includes all required elements, use 93895)

(For validated, statistically reliable, randomized, controlled, single-patient clinical investigation of FDA approved chronic care drugs, provided by a pharmacist, interpretation and report to the prescribing health care professional, use 99199)

(0144T-0151T have been deleted. To report, see 75571-75574)

(For laparoscopic implantation, replacement, revision, or removal of gastric stimulation electrodes, lesser curvature, use 43659)

(For open implantation, replacement, revision, or removal of gastric stimulation electrodes, lesser curvature, use 43999)

(0163T has been deleted)

(To report total disc arthroplasty [artificial disc], anterior approach, lumbar, see 22857, 22860)

+ 0164T   Removal of total disc arthroplasty, (artificial disc), anterior approach, each additional interspace, lumbar (List separately in addition to code for primary procedure)
Sunset January 2029

➔ *CPT Changes: An Insider's View* 2007, 2009
➔ *CPT Assistant* Jun 07:1

(Use 0164T in conjunction with 22865)

+ 0165T   Revision including replacement of total disc arthroplasty (artificial disc), anterior approach, each additional interspace, lumbar (List separately in addition to code for primary procedure)
Sunset January 2029

➔ *CPT Changes: An Insider's View* 2007, 2009
➔ *CPT Assistant* Jun 07:1

(Use 0165T in conjunction with 22862)

(Do not report 0164T, 0165T in conjunction with 22853, 22854, 22859, 49010, when performed at the same level)

(For decompression, see 63001-63048)

(For transmyocardial transcatheter closure of ventricular septal defect, with implant, including cardiopulmonary bypass if performed, use 33999)

(For rhinophototherapy, intranasal application of ultraviolet and visible light, use 30999)

(For stereotactic placement of infusion catheter[s] in the brain for delivery of therapeutic agent[s], use 64999)

(To report insertion of interlaminar/interspinous process stabilization/distraction device, without fusion, including image guidance when performed, with open decompression, lumbar, single level, use 22867. To report insertion of interlaminar/interspinous process stabilization/distraction device, without open decompression or fusion, including image guidance when performed, lumbar, single level, use 22869)

(To report insertion of interlaminar/interspinous process stabilization/distraction device, without fusion, including image guidance when performed, with open decompression, lumbar, second level, use 22868. To report insertion of interlaminar/interspinous process stabilization/distraction device, without open decompression or fusion, including image guidance when performed, lumbar, second level use, 22870)

+ 0174T   Computer-aided detection (CAD) (computer algorithm analysis of digital image data for lesion detection) with further physician review for interpretation and report, with or without digitization of film radiographic images, chest radiograph(s), performed concurrent with primary interpretation (List separately in addition to code for primary procedure)
Sunset January 2027

➔ *CPT Changes: An Insider's View* 2008
➔ *CPT Assistant* Apr 18:7, Sep 21:5

(Use 0174T in conjunction with 71045, 71046, 71047, 71048)

0175T   Computer-aided detection (CAD) (computer algorithm analysis of digital image data for lesion detection) with further physician review for interpretation and report, with or without digitization of film radiographic images, chest radiograph(s), performed remote from primary interpretation
Sunset January 2027

➔ *CPT Changes: An Insider's View* 2008
➔ *CPT Assistant* Apr 18:7, Sep 21:5

(Do not report 0175T in conjunction with 71045, 71046, 71047, 71048)

(For electrocardiogram, 64 leads or greater, with graphic presentation and analysis, use 93799)

(For electrocardiogram routine, with at least 12 leads separately performed, see 93000-93010)

0184T   Excision of rectal tumor, transanal endoscopic microsurgical approach (ie, TEMS), including muscularis propria (ie, full thickness)
Sunset January 2029

➔ *CPT Changes: An Insider's View* 2009, 2011
➔ *CPT Assistant* Jun 10:3, Feb 18:11

(For non-endoscopic excision of rectal tumor, see 45160, 45171, 45172)

(Do not report 0184T in conjunction with 45300, 45308, 45309, 45315, 45317, 45320, 69990)

(For multivariate analysis of patient-specific findings with quantifiable computer probability assessment, including report, use 99199)

(For suprachoroidal delivery of pharmacologic agent, use 67299)

(For remote real-time interactive video-conferenced critical care, evaluation and management of the critically ill or critically injured patient, use 99499)

(For placement of intraocular radiation source applicator, use 67299)

(For application of the source by radiation oncologist, see Clinical Brachytherapy section)

(For anterior segment drainage device implantation without concomitant cataract removal, use 0671T)

(For insertion of anterior segment aqueous drainage device without extraocular reservoir, internal approach, see 66989, 66991, 0671T)

 # 0671T Insertion of anterior segment aqueous drainage device into the trabecular meshwork, without external reservoir, and without concomitant cataract removal, one or more
Sunset January 2027
➔ *CPT Changes: An Insider's View* 2022
➔ *CPT Assistant* May 22:17, Jul 22:1, Aug 22:1

(Do not report 0671T in conjunction with 66989, 66991)

(For complex extracapsular cataract removal with intraocular lens implant without concomitant aqueous drainage device, use 66982)

(For extracapsular cataract removal with intraocular lens implant without concomitant aqueous drainage device, use 66984)

(For insertion of anterior segment drainage device into the subconjunctival space, use 0449T)

 # 0253T Insertion of anterior segment aqueous drainage device, without extraocular reservoir, internal approach, into the suprachoroidal space
Sunset January 2029
➔ *CPT Changes: An Insider's View* 2011, 2015
➔ *CPT Assistant* Jul 18:3

(To report insertion of drainage device by external approach, use 66183)

(For arthrodesis, pre-sacral interbody technique, disc space preparation, discectomy, without instrumentation, with image guidance, includes bone graft when performed, L4-L5 interspace, L5-S1 interspace, use 22899)

0198T Measurement of ocular blood flow by repetitive intraocular pressure sampling, with interpretation and report
Sunset January 2030
➔ *CPT Changes: An Insider's View* 2010
➔ *CPT Assistant* Mar 11:10, Aug 12:9

(For tremor measurement with accelerometer(s) and/or gyroscope(s), use 95999)

0200T Percutaneous sacral augmentation (sacroplasty), unilateral injection(s), including the use of a balloon or mechanical device, when used, 1 or more needles, includes imaging guidance and bone biopsy, when performed
Sunset January 2030
➔ *CPT Changes: An Insider's View* 2010, 2015, 2017
➔ *CPT Assistant* Apr 15:8, Dec 15:17
➔ *Clinical Examples in Radiology* Fall 14:3, Fall 22:21

0201T Percutaneous sacral augmentation (sacroplasty), bilateral injections, including the use of a balloon or mechanical device, when used, 2 or more needles, includes imaging guidance and bone biopsy, when performed
Sunset January 2030
➔ *CPT Changes: An Insider's View* 2010, 2015, 2017
➔ *CPT Assistant* Apr 15:8, Dec 15:19
➔ *Clinical Examples in Radiology* Fall 22:21

(Do not report 0200T, 0201T in conjunction with 20225 when performed at the same level)

Minimally Invasive Glaucoma Surgery (Internal Approach)
0253T, 0449T, 0450T, 0474T, 0671T

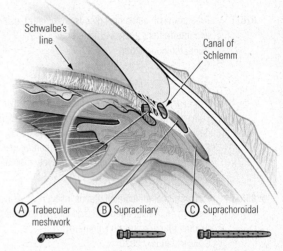

Internal approach

Schwalbe's line — Canal of Schlemm

Ⓐ Trabecular meshwork   Ⓑ Supraciliary   Ⓒ Suprachoroidal

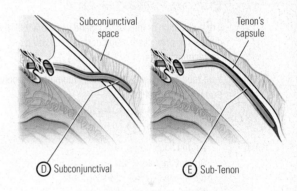

Subconjunctival space   Tenon's capsule

Ⓓ Subconjunctival   Ⓔ Sub-Tenon

0202T Posterior vertebral joint(s) arthroplasty (eg, facet joint[s] replacement), including facetectomy, laminectomy, foraminotomy, and vertebral column fixation, injection of bone cement, when performed, including fluoroscopy, single level, lumbar spine
Sunset January 2030
➔ *CPT Changes: An Insider's View* 2015

(Do not report 0202T in conjunction with 22511, 22514, 22840, 22853, 22854, 22857, 22859, 63005, 63012, 63017, 63030, 63042, 63047, 63056 at the same level)

(For intravascular catheter-based coronary vessel or graft spectroscopy [eg, infrared] during diagnostic evaluation and/or therapeutic intervention including imaging supervision, interpretation, and report, each vessel, use 93799)

(For computerized database analysis of multiple cycles of digitized cardiac electrical data from 2 or more ECG leads, including transmission to a remote center, application of multiple nonlinear mathematical transformations, with coronary artery obstruction severity assessment, use 93799)

0207T Evacuation of meibomian glands, automated, using heat and intermittent pressure, unilateral

Sunset January 2030

➜ *CPT Changes: An Insider's View* 2010

➜ *CPT Assistant* May 14:5

(For evacuation of meibomian glands using heat-delivered through wearable, open-eye eyelid treatment devices and manual gland expression, use 0563T. For evacuation of meibomian gland using manual gland expression only, use the appropriate evaluation and management code)

 # 0563T Evacuation of meibomian glands, using heat delivered through wearable, open-eye eyelid treatment devices and manual gland expression, bilateral

Sunset January 2030

➜ *CPT Changes: An Insider's View* 2020

(For evacuation of meibomian gland using manual gland expression only, use the appropriate evaluation and management code)

0208T Pure tone audiometry (threshold), automated; air only

Sunset January 2026

➜ *CPT Changes: An Insider's View* 2011

➜ *CPT Assistant* Aug 14:3

0209T air and bone

Sunset January 2026

➜ *CPT Changes: An Insider's View* 2011

➜ *CPT Assistant* Mar 11:8, Aug 14:3

0210T Speech audiometry threshold, automated;

Sunset January 2026

➜ *CPT Changes: An Insider's View* 2011

0211T with speech recognition

Sunset January 2026

➜ *CPT Changes: An Insider's View* 2011

➜ *CPT Assistant* Mar 11:8

0212T Comprehensive audiometry threshold evaluation and speech recognition (0209T, 0211T combined), automated

Sunset January 2026

➜ *CPT Changes: An Insider's View* 2011

➜ *CPT Assistant* Mar 11:8, Aug 14:3

(For audiometric testing using audiometers performed manually by a qualified health care professional, see 92551-92557)

0213T Injection(s), diagnostic or therapeutic agent, paravertebral facet (zygapophyseal) joint (or nerves innervating that joint) with ultrasound guidance, cervical or thoracic; single level

Sunset January 2026

➜ *CPT Changes: An Insider's View* 2011

➜ *CPT Assistant* Feb 11:5, Jul 11:14

➜ *Clinical Examples in Radiology* Winter 10:15, Fall 23:33

(To report bilateral procedure, use 0213T with modifier 50)

+ 0214T second level (List separately in addition to code for primary procedure)

Sunset January 2026

➜ *CPT Changes: An Insider's View* 2011

➜ *CPT Assistant* Jul 11:14

➜ *Clinical Examples in Radiology* Winter 10:15, Fall 23:33

(Use 0214T in conjunction with 0213T)

(For bilateral procedure, report 0214T twice. Do not report modifier 50 in conjunction with 0214T)

+ 0215T third and any additional level(s) (List separately in addition to code for primary procedure)

Sunset January 2026

➜ *CPT Changes: An Insider's View* 2011

➜ *CPT Assistant* Jul 11:14

➜ *Clinical Examples in Radiology* Winter 10:14, Fall 23:33

(Do not report 0215T more than once per day)

(Use 0215T in conjunction with 0213T, 0214T)

(For bilateral procedure, report 0215T twice. Do not report modifier 50 in conjunction with 0215T)

0216T Injection(s), diagnostic or therapeutic agent, paravertebral facet (zygapophyseal) joint (or nerves innervating that joint) with ultrasound guidance, lumbar or sacral; single level

Sunset January 2026

➜ *CPT Changes: An Insider's View* 2011

➜ *CPT Assistant* Jul 11:14

➜ *Clinical Examples in Radiology* Winter 10:14, Fall 23:33

(To report bilateral procedure, use 0216T with modifier 50)

+ 0217T second level (List separately in addition to code for primary procedure)

Sunset January 2026

➜ *CPT Changes: An Insider's View* 2011

➜ *CPT Assistant* Jul 11:14

➜ *Clinical Examples in Radiology* Winter 10:14, Fall 23:33

(Use 0217T in conjunction with 0216T)

(For bilateral procedure, report 0217T twice. Do not report modifier 50 in conjunction with 0217T)

+ 0218T   third and any additional level(s) (List separately in addition to code for primary procedure)
Sunset January 2026
➔ *CPT Changes: An Insider's View* 2011
➔ *CPT Assistant* Feb 11:5, Jul 11:14
➔ *Clinical Examples in Radiology* Winter 10:14, Fall 23:33

(Do not report 0218T more than once per day)

(Use 0218T in conjunction with 0216T, 0217T)

(If injection(s) are performed using fluoroscopy or CT, see 64490-64495)

(For bilateral procedure, report 0218T twice. Do not report modifier 50 in conjunction with 0218T)

0219T   Placement of a posterior intrafacet implant(s), unilateral or bilateral, including imaging and placement of bone graft(s) or synthetic device(s), single level; cervical
Sunset January 2026
➔ *CPT Changes: An Insider's View* 2011
➔ *CPT Assistant* Nov 10:8, Jul 11:18

0220T   thoracic
Sunset January 2026
➔ *CPT Changes: An Insider's View* 2011
➔ *CPT Assistant* Nov 10:8, Jul 11:18

0221T   lumbar
Sunset January 2026
➔ *CPT Changes: An Insider's View* 2011
➔ *CPT Assistant* Nov 10:8, Jul 11:18

(Do not report 0219T-0221T in conjunction with any radiological service)

(Do not report 0219T, 0220T, 0221T in conjunction with 20930, 20931, 22600-22614, 22840, 22853, 22854, 22859 at the same level)

+ 0222T   each additional vertebral segment (List separately in addition to code for primary procedure)
Sunset January 2026
➔ *CPT Changes: An Insider's View* 2011
➔ *CPT Assistant* Nov 10:6, Jul 11:18

(Use 0222T in conjunction with 0219T-0221T)

(For posterior or posterolateral arthrodesis technique, see 22600-22614)

(For injection[s], anesthetic agent and/or steroid, transforaminal epidural, with ultrasound guidance, cervical or thoracic, single level, use 64999)

(For transforaminal epidural injections performed under fluoroscopy or CT, see 64479–64484)

0232T   Injection(s), platelet rich plasma, any site, including image guidance, harvesting and preparation when performed
Sunset January 2027
➔ *CPT Changes: An Insider's View* 2011
➔ *CPT Assistant* Oct 10:8, Dec 10:8, May 12:11, Oct 12:14, May 18:3, Apr 19:10, Dec 22:1
➔ *Clinical Examples in Radiology* Spring 18:6

(Do not report 0232T in conjunction with 15769, 15771, 15772, 15773, 15774, 20550, 20551, 20600, 20604, 20605, 20606, 20610, 20611, 36415, 36592, 76942, 77002, 77012, 77021, 86965, 0481T)

(Do not report 38220-38230 for bone marrow aspiration for platelet rich stem cell injection. For bone marrow aspiration for platelet rich stem cell injection, use 0232T)

#● 0901T   Placement of bone marrow sampling port, including imaging guidance when performed
Sunset January 2030
➔ *CPT Changes: An Insider's View* 2025

▶(Do not report 0901T in conjunction with 77002, 77012)◀

Atherectomy (Open or Percutaneous) for Supra-Inguinal Arteries

Codes 0234T-0238T describe atherectomy performed by any method (eg, directional, rotational, laser) in arteries above the inguinal ligaments. These codes are structured differently than the codes describing atherectomy performed below the inguinal ligaments (37225, 37227, 37229, 37231, 37233, 37235).

These supra-inguinal atherectomy codes all include the surgical work of performing the atherectomy plus the radiological supervision and interpretation of the atherectomy. Unlike the atherectomy codes for infra-inguinal arteries, this set of Category III codes does not include accessing and selectively catheterizing the vessel, traversing the lesion, embolic protection if used, other intervention used to treat the same or other vessels, or closure of the arteriotomy by any method. These codes describe endovascular procedures performed percutaneously and/or through an open surgical exposure.

0234T   Transluminal peripheral atherectomy, open or percutaneous, including radiological supervision and interpretation; renal artery
Sunset January 2026
➔ *CPT Changes: An Insider's View* 2011
➔ *CPT Assistant* Jul 11:3
➔ *Clinical Examples in Radiology* Spring 11:3

0235T   visceral artery (except renal), each vessel
Sunset January 2026
➔ *CPT Changes: An Insider's View* 2011
➔ *CPT Assistant* Jul 11:3
➔ *Clinical Examples in Radiology* Spring 11:3

0236T   abdominal aorta
Sunset January 2026
➔ *CPT Changes: An Insider's View* 2011
➔ *CPT Assistant* Jul 11:3
➔ *Clinical Examples in Radiology* Spring 11:3

0237T   brachiocephalic trunk and branches, each vessel
Sunset January 2026
➔ *CPT Changes: An Insider's View* 2011
➔ *CPT Assistant* Jul 11:3
➔ *Clinical Examples in Radiology* Spring 11:3

0238T   iliac artery, each vessel
Sunset January 2026
➔ *CPT Changes: An Insider's View* 2011
➔ *CPT Assistant* Jul 11:3
➔ *Clinical Examples in Radiology* Spring 11:3

(To report esophageal motility studies without high resolution esophageal pressure topography, use 91010 and with stimulant or perfusion, use 91013)

0253T   Code is out of numerical sequence. See 0184T-0200T

0263T   Intramuscular autologous bone marrow cell therapy, with preparation of harvested cells, multiple injections, one leg, including ultrasound guidance, if performed; complete procedure including unilateral or bilateral bone marrow harvest
Sunset January 2027
➔ *CPT Changes: An Insider's View* 2012

(Do not report 0263T in conjunction with 38204-38242, 76942, 93925, 93926)

0264T   complete procedure excluding bone marrow harvest
Sunset January 2027
➔ *CPT Changes: An Insider's View* 2012

(Do not report 0264T in conjunction with 38204-38242, 76942, 93925, 93926, 0265T)

0265T   unilateral or bilateral bone marrow harvest only for intramuscular autologous bone marrow cell therapy
Sunset January 2027
➔ *CPT Changes: An Insider's View* 2012

(Do not report 0265T in conjunction with 38204-38242, 0264T. For complete procedure, use 0263T)

0266T   Implantation or replacement of carotid sinus baroreflex activation device; total system (includes generator placement, unilateral or bilateral lead placement, intra-operative interrogation, programming, and repositioning, when performed)
Sunset January 2027
➔ *CPT Changes: An Insider's View* 2012

0267T   lead only, unilateral (includes intra-operative interrogation, programming, and repositioning, when performed)
Sunset January 2027
➔ *CPT Changes: An Insider's View* 2012

(For bilateral lead implantation or replacement, use 0267T with modifier 50)

0268T   pulse generator only (includes intra-operative interrogation, programming, and repositioning, when performed)
Sunset January 2027
➔ *CPT Changes: An Insider's View* 2012

(Do not report 0267T, 0268T in conjunction with 0266T, 0269T-0273T)

0269T   Revision or removal of carotid sinus baroreflex activation device; total system (includes generator placement, unilateral or bilateral lead placement, intra-operative interrogation, programming, and repositioning, when performed)
Sunset January 2027
➔ *CPT Changes: An Insider's View* 2012

(Do not report 0269T in conjunction with 0266T-0268T, 0270T-0273T)

0270T   lead only, unilateral (includes intra-operative interrogation, programming, and repositioning, when performed)
Sunset January 2027
➔ *CPT Changes: An Insider's View* 2012

(Do not report 0270T in conjunction with 0266T-0269T, 0271T-0273T)

(For bilateral lead removal, use 0270T with modifier 50)

(For removal of total carotid sinus baroreflex activation device, use 0269T)

0271T   pulse generator only (includes intra-operative interrogation, programming, and repositioning, when performed)
Sunset January 2027
➔ *CPT Changes: An Insider's View* 2012

(Do not report 0271T in conjunction with 0266T-0270T, 0272T, 0273T)

(For removal and replacement, see 0266T, 0267T, 0268T)

0272T   Interrogation device evaluation (in person), carotid sinus baroreflex activation system, including telemetric iterative communication with the implantable device to monitor device diagnostics and programmed therapy values, with interpretation and report (eg, battery status, lead impedance, pulse amplitude, pulse width, therapy frequency, pathway mode, burst mode, therapy start/stop times each day);
Sunset January 2027
➔ *CPT Changes: An Insider's View* 2012

(Do not report 0272T in conjunction with 0266T-0271T, 0273T)

0273T   with programming
Sunset January 2027
➔ *CPT Changes: An Insider's View* 2012

(Do not report 0273T in conjunction with 0266T-0272T)

0274T   Percutaneous laminotomy/laminectomy (interlaminar approach) for decompression of neural elements, (with or without ligamentous resection, discectomy, facetectomy and/or foraminotomy), any method, under indirect image guidance (eg, fluoroscopic, CT), single or multiple levels, unilateral or bilateral; cervical or thoracic
Sunset January 2027
➔ *CPT Changes: An Insider's View* 2012, 2017
➔ *CPT Assistant* Jan 12:14, Jul 12:3-4, Feb 17:12

0275T   lumbar
Sunset January 2027
➔ *CPT Changes: An Insider's View* 2012, 2017
➔ *CPT Assistant* Jan 12:14, Jul 12:3-4, Feb 17:12

(For percutaneous decompression of the nucleus pulposus of intervertebral disc utilizing needle based technique, use 62287)

0278T   Transcutaneous electrical modulation pain reprocessing (eg, scrambler therapy), each treatment session (includes placement of electrodes)
Sunset January 2027
➔ *CPT Changes: An Insider's View* 2012

(For peripheral nerve transcutaneous magnetic stimulation, see 0766T, 0767T)

(For implantation of trial or permanent electrode arrays or pulse generators for peripheral subcutaneous field stimulation, use 64999)

(For delivery of thermal energy to the muscle of the anal canal, use 46999)

(For corneal incisions in the recipient cornea created using a laser in preparation for penetrating or lamellar keratoplasty, use 66999)

▶(For greater than 48 hours of monitoring of external electrocardiographic recording, see 93241, 93242, 93243, 93244, 93245, 93246, 93247, 93248, 0937T, 0938T, 0939T, 0940T)◀

(For focused microwave thermotherapy of the breast, use 19499)

0308T   Insertion of ocular telescope prosthesis including removal of crystalline lens or intraocular lens prosthesis
Sunset January 2026
➔ *CPT Changes: An Insider's View* 2013, 2016, 2017
➔ *CPT Assistant* Mar 13:6

(Do not report 0308T in conjunction with 65800-65815, 66020, 66030, 66600-66635, 66761, 66825, 66982-66986, 69990)

(For arthrodesis, pre-sacral interbody technique, including disc space preparation, discectomy, with posterior instrumentation, with image guidance, including bone graft, when performed, lumbar, L4-L5 interspace, use 22899)

(For motor function mapping using non-invasive navigated transcranial magnetic stimulation [nTMS] for therapeutic treatment planning, upper and lower extremity, use 64999)

(0312T, 0313T, 0314T, 0315T, 0316T, 0317T have been deleted)

(For laparoscopic implantation, revision, replacement, or removal of vagus nerve blocking neurostimulator electrode array and/or pulse generator at the esophagogastric junction, use 64999)

0329T   Monitoring of intraocular pressure for 24 hours or longer, unilateral or bilateral, with interpretation and report
Sunset January 2029
➔ *CPT Changes: An Insider's View* 2014
➔ *CPT Assistant* May 14:5

0330T   Tear film imaging, unilateral or bilateral, with interpretation and report
Sunset January 2029
➔ *CPT Changes: An Insider's View* 2014
➔ *CPT Assistant* May 14:5

0331T   Myocardial sympathetic innervation imaging, planar qualitative and quantitative assessment;
Sunset January 2029
➔ *CPT Changes: An Insider's View* 2014
➔ *CPT Assistant* Jun 14:15
➔ *Clinical Examples in Radiology* Summer 13:11

0332T   with tomographic SPECT
Sunset January 2029
➔ *CPT Changes: An Insider's View* 2014
➔ *CPT Assistant* Jun 14:15
➔ *Clinical Examples in Radiology* Summer 13:11

(For myocardial infarct avid imaging, see 78466, 78468, 78469)

0333T   Visual evoked potential, screening of visual acuity, automated, with report
Sunset January 2029
➔ *CPT Changes: An Insider's View* 2014, 2018
➔ *CPT Assistant* Aug 14:8, Feb 18:3

(For visual evoked potential testing for glaucoma, use 0464T)

 # 0464T   Visual evoked potential, testing for glaucoma, with interpretation and report
Sunset January 2028
➔ *CPT Changes: An Insider's View* 2018
➔ *CPT Assistant* Feb 18:3

(For visual evoked potential screening of visual acuity, use 0333T)

(To report percutaneous/minimally invasive [indirect visualization] arthrodesis of the sacroiliac joint with image guidance, use 27279)

0335T   Insertion of sinus tarsi implant
Sunset January 2029

➔ *CPT Changes: An Insider's View* 2019

(Do not report 0335T in conjunction with 28585, 28725, 29907)

 # 0510T   Removal of sinus tarsi implant
Sunset January 2029

➔ *CPT Changes: An Insider's View* 2019

 # 0511T   Removal and reinsertion of sinus tarsi implant
Sunset January 2029

➔ *CPT Changes: An Insider's View* 2019

(For unilateral or bilateral endothelial function assessments, using peripheral vascular response to reactive hyperemia, noninvasive [eg, brachial artery ultrasound, peripheral artery tonometry], use 93998)

0338T   Transcatheter renal sympathetic denervation, percutaneous approach including arterial puncture, selective catheter placement(s) renal artery(ies), fluoroscopy, contrast injection(s), intraprocedural roadmapping and radiological supervision and interpretation, including pressure gradient measurements, flush aortogram and diagnostic renal angiography when performed; unilateral
Sunset January 2029

➔ *CPT Changes: An Insider's View* 2014

0339T   bilateral
Sunset January 2029

➔ *CPT Changes: An Insider's View* 2014

(Do not report 0338T, 0339T in conjunction with 36251, 36252, 36253, 36254)

(For quantitative pupillometry with interpretation and report, unilateral or bilateral, use 95919)

0342T   Therapeutic apheresis with selective HDL delipidation and plasma reinfusion
Sunset January 2029

➔ *CPT Changes: An Insider's View* 2020

Fluoroscopy (76000) and radiologic supervision and interpretation are inherent to the transcatheter mitral valve repair (TMVR) procedure and are not separately reportable. Diagnostic cardiac catheterization (93451, 93452, 93453, 93454, 93455, 93456, 93457, 93458, 93459, 93460, 93461, 93593, 93594, 93595, 93596, 93597, 93598) should **not** be reported with transcatheter mitral valve repair (0345T) for:

- Contrast injections, angiography, roadmapping, and/or fluoroscopic guidance for the transcatheter mitral valve repair (TMVR),
- Left ventricular angiography to assess mitral regurgitation for guidance of TMVR, or

- Right and left heart catheterization for hemodynamic measurements before, during, and after TMVR for guidance of TMVR.

Diagnostic right and left heart catheterization (93451, 93452, 93453, 93456, 93457, 93458, 93459, 93460, 93461, 93593, 93594, 93595, 93596, 93597, 93598) and diagnostic coronary angiography (93454, 93455, 93456, 93457, 93458, 93459, 93460, 93461, 93563, 93564) not inherent to the TMVR may be reported with 0345T, appended with modifier 59, if:

1. No prior study is available and a full diagnostic study is performed, or

2. A prior study is available, but as documented in the medical record:

   a. There is inadequate visualization of the anatomy and/or pathology, or

   b. The patient's condition with respect to the clinical indication has changed since the prior study, or

   c. There is a clinical change during the procedure that requires new evaluation.

Percutaneous coronary interventional procedures may be reported separately, when performed.

Other cardiac catheterization services may be reported separately, when performed for diagnostic purposes not intrinsic to the TMVR.

When transcatheter ventricular support is required, the appropriate code may be reported with the appropriate ventricular assist device (VAD) procedure (33990, 33991, 33992, 33993, 33995, 33997) or balloon pump insertion (33967, 33970, 33973).

0345T   Transcatheter mitral valve repair percutaneous approach via the coronary sinus
Sunset January 2030

➔ *CPT Changes: An Insider's View* 2015
➔ *CPT Assistant* Sep 15:3

(For transcatheter mitral valve repair percutaneous approach including transseptal puncture when performed, see 33418, 33419)

(Do not report 0345T in conjunction with 93451, 93452, 93453, 93456, 93457, 93458, 93459, 93460, 93461 for diagnostic left and right heart catheterization procedures intrinsic to the valve repair procedure)

(Do not report 0345T in conjunction with 93453, 93454, 93563, 93564 for coronary angiography intrinsic to the valve repair procedure)

(For transcatheter mitral valve implantation/replacement [TMVI], see 0483T, 0484T)

(For transcatheter mitral valve annulus reconstruction, use 0544T)

0347T Placement of interstitial device(s) in bone for radiostereometric analysis (RSA)
Sunset January 2030
➔ *CPT Changes: An Insider's View* 2015
➔ *CPT Assistant* Jun 15:8

0348T Radiologic examination, radiostereometric analysis (RSA); spine, (includes cervical, thoracic and lumbosacral, when performed)
Sunset January 2030
➔ *CPT Changes: An Insider's View* 2015
➔ *CPT Assistant* Jun 15:8

0349T upper extremity(ies), (includes shoulder, elbow, and wrist, when performed)
Sunset January 2030
➔ *CPT Changes: An Insider's View* 2015
➔ *CPT Assistant* Jun 15:8

0350T lower extremity(ies), (includes hip, proximal femur, knee, and ankle, when performed)
Sunset January 2030
➔ *CPT Changes: An Insider's View* 2015
➔ *CPT Assistant* Jun 15:8

0351T Optical coherence tomography of breast or axillary lymph node, excised tissue, each specimen; real-time intraoperative
Sunset January 2030
➔ *CPT Changes: An Insider's View* 2015
➔ *CPT Assistant* Apr 15:6

0352T interpretation and report, real-time or referred
Sunset January 2030
➔ *CPT Changes: An Insider's View* 2015
➔ *CPT Assistant* Apr 15:6

(Do not report 0352T in conjunction with 0351T, when performed by the same physician)

0353T Optical coherence tomography of breast, surgical cavity; real-time intraoperative
Sunset January 2030
➔ *CPT Changes: An Insider's View* 2015
➔ *CPT Assistant* Apr 15:6

(Report 0353T once per session)

0354T interpretation and report, real-time or referred
Sunset January 2030
➔ *CPT Changes: An Insider's View* 2015
➔ *CPT Assistant* Apr 15:6

(Do not report 0354T in conjunction with 0353T, when performed by the same physician)

(For gastrointestinal tract imaging, intraluminal [eg, capsule endoscopy] of the colon, use 91113)

(For insertion of drug-eluting implant including punctal dilation, when performed, into the lacrimal canaliculus, use 68841)

(For placement of drug-eluting insert under the eyelid[s], see 0444T, 0445T)

0358T Bioelectrical impedance analysis whole body composition assessment, with interpretation and report
Sunset January 2030
➔ *CPT Changes: An Insider's View* 2020

(For bioimpedance-derived physiological cardiovascular analysis, use 93701)

(For bioimpedance spectroscopy (BIS), use 93702)

Adaptive Behavior Assessments and Treatment

Behavior identification supporting assessment (0362T) and **adaptive behavior treatment with protocol modification** (0373T) include the following required components:

■ administration by the physician or other qualified health care professional who is on-site but not necessarily face-to-face with the patient;

■ with the assistance of two or more technicians;

■ for a patient with destructive behavior that requires the presence of a team;

■ completion in an environment that is customized to the patient's behavior.

"On-site" is defined as immediately available and interruptible to provide assistance and direction throughout the performance of the procedure, however, the physician or other qualified health care professional does not need to be present in the room when the procedure is performed.

Typical patients for 0362T and 0373T present with one or more specific destructive behavior(s) (ie, maladaptive behaviors associated with high risk of medical consequences or property damage [eg, elopement, pica, or self-injury requiring medical attention, aggression with injury to other{s}, or breaking furniture, walls, or windows]). Code 0362T may include functional behavior assessment, functional analysis, other structured observations, and standardized and/or nonstandardized instruments and procedures to determine levels of adaptive and maladaptive behavior as well as other impairments in functioning.

Only count the time of one technician when two or more are present. For assistance with code selection of 97152, 0362T, see the Guide to Selection of Codes 97152 and 0362T on page 856. For assistance with code selection of 97153, 97155, 0373T, see Guide to Selection of Codes 97153, 97155, and 0373T on page 857.

0362T **Behavior identification supporting assessment,** each 15 minutes of technicians' time face-to-face with a patient, requiring the following components:

- administration by the physician or other qualified health care professional who is on site;
- with the assistance of two or more technicians;
- for a patient who exhibits destructive behavior;
- completion in an environment that is customized to the patient's behavior.

Sunset January 2029

➡ *CPT Changes: An Insider's View* 2015, 2019

➡ *CPT Assistant* Jun 14:4, Nov 18:3

(0362T is reported based on a single technician's face-to-face time with the patient and not the combined time of multiple technicians [eg, one hour with three technicians equals one hour of service])

(0362T may be repeated on different days until the behavior identification assessment [97151] and, if necessary, supporting assessment[s] [97152, 0362T], is complete)

(For psychiatric diagnostic evaluation, see 90791, 90792)

(For speech evaluations, see 92521, 92522, 92523, 92524)

(For occupational therapy evaluation, see 97165, 97166, 97167, 97168)

(For medical team conference, see 99366, 99367, 99368)

(For health behavior assessment and intervention, see 96156, 96158, 96159, 96164, 96165, 96167, 96168, 96170, 96171)

(For neurobehavioral status examination, see 96116, 96121)

(For neuropsychological testing, see 96132, 96133, 96136, 96137, 96138, 96139, 96146)

0373T **Adaptive behavior treatment with protocol modification,** each 15 minutes of technicians' time face-to-face with a patient, requiring the following components:

- administration by the physician or other qualified health care professional who is on site;
- with the assistance of two or more technicians;
- for a patient who exhibits destructive behavior;
- completion in an environment that is customized to the patient's behavior.

Sunset January 2029

➡ *CPT Changes: An Insider's View* 2015, 2019

➡ *CPT Assistant* Jun 14:4, 6, 9, Nov 18:3

(0373T is reported based on a single technician's face-to-face time with the patient and not the combined time of multiple technicians)

(Do not report 0373T in conjunction with 90785-90899, 96105, 96110, 96116, 96121, 96156, 96158, 96159, 96164, 96165, 96167, 96168, 96170, 96171)

(For total disc arthroplasty [artificial disc], anterior approach, including discectomy with end-plate preparation [includes osteophytectomy for nerve root or spinal cord decompression and microdissection], cervical, 3 or more levels, use 22899)

(For anoscopy with directed submucosal injection of bulking agent for fecal incontinence, use 46999)

0378T Visual field assessment, with concurrent real time data analysis and accessible data storage with patient initiated data transmitted to a remote surveillance center for up to 30 days; review and interpretation with report by a physician or other qualified health care professional

Sunset January 2030

➡ *CPT Changes: An Insider's View* 2015

0379T   technical support and patient instructions, surveillance, analysis, and transmission of daily and emergent data reports as prescribed by a physician or other qualified health care professional

Sunset January 2030

➡ *CPT Changes: An Insider's View* 2015

(For computer-aided animation and analysis of time series retinal images for the monitoring of disease progression, unilateral or bilateral, with interpretation and report, use 92499)

(For external heart rate and 3-axis accelerometer data recording up to 14 days to assess changes in heart rate and to monitor motion analysis for the purposes of diagnosing nocturnal epilepsy seizure events, including report, scanning analysis with report, review and interpretation by a physician or other qualified health care professional, use 95999)

Pacemaker-Leadless and Pocketless System

(Electronic brachytherapy is a form of radiation therapy in which an electrically generated X-ray source of ionizing radiation is placed inside or in close proximity to the tumor or target tissue to deliver therapeutic radiation dosage)

0394T High dose rate electronic brachytherapy, skin surface application, per fraction, includes basic dosimetry, when performed

Sunset January 2026

➡ *CPT Changes: An Insider's View* 2016

(Do not report 0394T in conjunction with 77261, 77262, 77263, 77300, 77306, 77307, 77316, 77317, 77318, 77332, 77333, 77334, 77336, 77427, 77431, 77432, 77435, 77469, 77470, 77499, 77761, 77762, 77763, 77767, 77768, 77770, 77771, 77772, 77778, 77789)

(For high dose rate radionuclide surface brachytherapy, see 77767, 77768)

(For non-brachytherapy superficial [eg, ≤200 kV] radiation treatment delivery, use 77401)

0395T High dose rate electronic brachytherapy, interstitial or intracavitary treatment, per fraction, includes basic dosimetry, when performed
Sunset January 2026

➡ *CPT Changes: An Insider's View* 2016

(Do not report 0395T in conjunction with 77261, 77262, 77263, 77300, 77306, 77307, 77316, 77317, 77318, 77332, 77333, 77334, 77336, 77427, 77431, 77432, 77435, 77469, 77470, 77499, 77761, 77762, 77763, 77767, 77768, 77770, 77771, 77772, 77778, 77789)

(For skin surface application of high dose rate electronic brachytherapy, use 0394T)

(For intraoperative use of kinetic balance sensor for implant stability during knee replacement arthroplasty, use 27599)

+ 0397T Endoscopic retrograde cholangiopancreatography (ERCP), with optical endomicroscopy (List separately in addition to code for primary procedure)
Sunset January 2026

➡ *CPT Changes: An Insider's View* 2016, 2017

(Use 0397T in conjunction with 43260, 43261, 43262, 43263, 43264, 43265, 43274, 43275, 43276, 43277, 43278)

(Do not report 0397T in conjunction with 88375)

(Do not report optical endomicroscopy more than once per session)

▶(0398T has been deleted)◀

▶(For magnetic resonance image guided high intensity focused ultrasound [MRgFUS], stereotactic ablation lesion, intracranial, use 61715)◀

(For multispectral digital skin lesion analysis of clinically atypical cutaneous pigmented lesions for detection of melanomas and high risk melanocytic atypia, use 96999)

0402T Collagen cross-linking of cornea, including removal of the corneal epithelium, when performed, and intraoperative pachymetry, when performed
Sunset January 2030

➡ *CPT Changes: An Insider's View* 2016, 2020, 2023

➡ *CPT Assistant* Feb 16:12, Jun 18:11

(Report medication separately)

(Do not report 0402T in conjunction with 65435, 69990, 76514)

A diabetes prevention program consists of intensive behavioral counseling that is provided in person, online, or via electronic technology, or a combination of both modalities.

Intensive behavioral counseling consists of care management, lifestyle coaching, facilitation of a peer-support group, and provision of clinically validated educational lessons based on a standardized curriculum that is focused on nutrition, exercise, stress, and weight management. Lifestyle coaches must complete a nationally recognized training program. The lifestyle coach is available to interact with the participants.

Codes 0403T and 0488T describe diabetes prevention programs that use a standardized diabetes prevention curriculum. For educational services that use a standardized curriculum provided to patients with an established illness/disease, see 98960, 98961, 98962. Use 0403T for diabetes prevention programs that are provided only in-person. Use 0488T for programs that are provided online or via electronic technology. Code 0488T includes in person components, if provided.

0403T Preventive behavior change, intensive program of prevention of diabetes using a standardized diabetes prevention program curriculum, provided to individuals in a group setting, minimum 60 minutes, per day
Sunset January 2026

➡ *CPT Changes: An Insider's View* 2016

➡ *CPT Assistant* Aug 18:6, Jul 20:7

(Do not report 0403T in conjunction with 98960, 98961, 98962, 0488T)

 # 0488T Preventive behavior change, online/electronic structured intensive program for prevention of diabetes using a standardized diabetes prevention program curriculum, provided to an individual, per 30 days
Sunset January 2028

➡ *CPT Changes: An Insider's View* 2018

➡ *CPT Assistant* Aug 18:6, Jul 20:7

(Do not report 0488T in conjunction with 98960, 98961, 98962, 0403T)

(0404T has been deleted)

(For transcervical radiofrequency ablation of uterine fibroid[s], including intraoperative ultrasound guidance and monitoring, use 58580)

(For oversight of the care of an extracorporeal liver-assist system patient requiring review of status, review of laboratory and other studies, and revision of orders and liver-assist care plan [as appropriate], within a calendar month, 30 minutes or more of non-face-to-face time, use 99499)

(To report endoscopic placement of a drug-eluting implant in the ethmoid sinus without any other nasal/sinus endoscopic surgical service, use 31299. To report endoscopic placement of a drug-eluting implant in the ethmoid sinus in conjunction with biopsy, polypectomy, or debridement, use 31237)

Codes 0408T-0418T describe procedures related to cardiac contractility modulation systems (CCM). These systems consist of a pulse generator plus one atrial and two ventricular pacemaker electrodes (leads). In contrast to a pacemaker or a defibrillator, which modulate the heart's rhythm, the CCM system's impulses are designed to modulate the strength of contraction of the heart muscle. Unlike pacemakers, these systems stimulate for specific time intervals in order to improve myocardial function.

All catheterization and imaging guidance required to complete a CCM procedure are included in the work of each code. Left heart catheterization with a high fidelity transducer is intrinsic to the CCM procedure. Left heart catheterization codes (93452, 93453, 93458, 93459, 93460, 93461) at the time of CCM placement, replacement, or revision may not be reported separately. Removal of only the CCM pulse generator is reported with 0412T. If only the pulse generator is removed and replaced at the same session without any right atrial and/or right ventricular lead(s) inserted or replaced, report 0414T. For removal and replacement of the pulse generator and leads, individual codes for removal of the generator (0412T) and removal of the leads (0413T for each lead removed) are used in conjunction with the insertion/replacement system code (0408T). When individual transvenous electrodes are inserted or replaced, report using 0410T and 0411T, as appropriate. When the entire system is inserted or replaced, report with 0408T.

Revision of the CCM generator skin pocket is included in 0408T, 0412T, 0414T. Relocation of a skin pocket for a CCM may be necessary for various clinical situations such as infection or erosion. Relocation is reported with 0416T, and follows conventions for pacemaker skin pocket relocation.

Repositioning of a CCM electrode is reported using 0415T.

CCM device evaluation codes 0417T, 0418T may not be reported in conjunction with pulse generator and lead insertion or revision codes.

0408T   Insertion or replacement of permanent cardiac contractility modulation system, including contractility evaluation when performed, and programming of sensing and therapeutic parameters; pulse generator with transvenous electrodes
Sunset January 2027
➲ *CPT Changes: An Insider's View* 2017

0409T   pulse generator only
Sunset January 2027
➲ *CPT Changes: An Insider's View* 2017

0410T   atrial electrode only
Sunset January 2027
➲ *CPT Changes: An Insider's View* 2017

0411T   ventricular electrode only
Sunset January 2027
➲ *CPT Changes: An Insider's View* 2017

(Report 0410T, 0411T once for each transvenous electrode inserted or replaced)

(If the entire system is inserted or replaced, report 0408T)

0412T   Removal of permanent cardiac contractility modulation system; pulse generator only
Sunset January 2027
➲ *CPT Changes: An Insider's View* 2017

0413T   transvenous electrode (atrial or ventricular)
Sunset January 2027
➲ *CPT Changes: An Insider's View* 2017

(Report 0413T once for each transvenous electrode removed)

(For removal of the pulse generator and all 3 leads, use 0412T plus 0413T once for each electrode removed)

(If transvenous electrodes are removed and replaced, report 0413T once for each electrode removed in conjunction with 0410T, 0411T, as appropriate)

0414T   Removal and replacement of permanent cardiac contractility modulation system pulse generator only
Sunset January 2027
➲ *CPT Changes: An Insider's View* 2017

(For removal and replacement of the pulse generator plus all three electrodes, report 0408T in conjunction with 0412T, 0413T once for each transvenous electrode removed)

0415T   Repositioning of previously implanted cardiac contractility modulation transvenous electrode (atrial or ventricular lead)
Sunset January 2027
➲ *CPT Changes: An Insider's View* 2017

(Do not report 0408T, 0409T, 0410T, 0411T, 0414T, 0415T in conjunction with 93286, 93287, 93452, 93453, 93458, 93459, 93460, 93461)

(Do not report 0415T in conjunction with 0408T, 0410T, 0411T)

0416T   Relocation of skin pocket for implanted cardiac contractility modulation pulse generator
Sunset January 2027
➲ *CPT Changes: An Insider's View* 2017

Category III   0042T-0947T

0417T Programming device evaluation (in person) with iterative adjustment of the implantable device to test the function of the device and select optimal permanent programmed values with analysis, including review and report, implantable cardiac contractility modulation system

Sunset January 2027

➔ *CPT Changes: An Insider's View* 2017

(Do not report 0417T in conjunction with 0408T, 0409T, 0410T, 0411T, 0412T, 0413T, 0414T, 0415T, 0418T)

0418T Interrogation device evaluation (in person) with analysis, review and report, includes connection, recording and disconnection per patient encounter, implantable cardiac contractility modulation system

Sunset January 2027

➔ *CPT Changes: An Insider's View* 2017

(Do not report 0418T in conjunction with 0408T, 0409T, 0410T, 0411T, 0412T, 0413T, 0414T, 0415T, 0417T)

0419T Destruction of neurofibroma, extensive (cutaneous, dermal extending into subcutaneous); face, head and neck, greater than 50 neurofibromas

Sunset January 2027

➔ *CPT Changes: An Insider's View* 2017

➔ *CPT Assistant* Apr 16:3

(For excision of neurofibroma, use 64792)

(Report 0419T once per session regardless of the number of lesions treated)

0420T trunk and extremities, extensive, greater than 100 neurofibromas

Sunset January 2027

➔ *CPT Changes: An Insider's View* 2017

➔ *CPT Assistant* Apr 16:3

(For excision of neurofibroma, use 64792)

(Report 0420T once per session regardless of the number of lesions treated)

#▲ **0714T** Transperineal laser ablation of benign prostatic hyperplasia, including imaging guidance; prostate volume less than 50 mL

Sunset January 2028

➔ *CPT Changes: An Insider's View* 2023, 2025

#● **0867T** prostate volume greater or equal to 50 mL

Sunset January 2030

➔ *CPT Changes: An Insider's View* 2025

▶(Do not report 0714T, 0867T in conjunction with 76940, 76942, 77002, 77012, 77021)◀

0421T Transurethral waterjet ablation of prostate, including control of post-operative bleeding, including ultrasound guidance, complete (vasectomy, meatotomy, cystourethroscopy, urethral calibration and/or dilation, and internal urethrotomy are included when performed)

Sunset January 2027

➔ *CPT Changes: An Insider's View* 2017

(Do not report 0421T in conjunction with 52500, 52630, 76872)

0422T Tactile breast imaging by computer-aided tactile sensors, unilateral or bilateral

Sunset January 2027

➔ *CPT Changes: An Insider's View* 2017

(For secretory type II phospholipase A2 [sPLA2-IIA], use 84999)

Phrenic Nerve Stimulation System

(0424T, 0425T, 0426T, 0427T have been deleted)

(For insertion of a phrenic nerve stimulator transvenous sensing lead, use 33277)

(For removal and replacement of phrenic nerve stimulator pulse generator, use 33287)

(For removal and replacement of phrenic nerve stimulator transvenous stimulation or sensing lead[s], use 33288)

(0428T, 0429T, 0430T have been deleted)

(For removal of phrenic nerve stimulator sensing or stimulation lead[s], use 33279)

(For removal of phrenic nerve stimulator pulse generator, use 33280)

(0431T has been deleted)

(For removal and replacement of phrenic nerve stimulator pulse generator, use 33287)

(0432T, 0433T have been deleted)

(For repositioning of phrenic nerve stimulator transvenous lead[s], use 33281)

(0434T has been deleted)

(For interrogation device evaluation of implanted phrenic nerve stimulator system, use 93153)

(0435T, 0436T have been deleted)

(For interrogation and programming of implanted phrenic nerve stimulator system, use 93151)

(For interrogation and programming of implanted phrenic nerve stimulator system during a polysomnography, use 93152)

+ **0437T** Implantation of non-biologic or synthetic implant (eg, polypropylene) for fascial reinforcement of the abdominal wall (List separately in addition to code for primary procedure)

Sunset January 2027

➔ *CPT Changes: An Insider's View* 2017

(For implantation of absorbable mesh or other prosthesis for delayed closure of defect[s] [ie, external genitalia, perineum, abdominal wall] due to soft tissue infection or trauma, use 15778)

Copying, photographing, or sharing this CPT® book violates AMA's copyright.

(For implantation of mesh or other prosthesis for anterior abdominal hernia[s] repair or parastomal hernia repair, see 49591-49622)

+ 0439T Myocardial contrast perfusion echocardiography, at rest or with stress, for assessment of myocardial ischemia or viability (List separately in addition to code for primary procedure)
Sunset January 2027
➔ *CPT Changes: An Insider's View* 2017
➔ *CPT Assistant* Apr 16:9

(Use 0439T in conjunction with 93306, 93307, 93308, 93350, 93351)

0440T Ablation, percutaneous, cryoablation, includes imaging guidance; upper extremity distal/peripheral nerve
Sunset January 2027
➔ *CPT Changes: An Insider's View* 2017
➔ *CPT Assistant* May 17:3, Apr 19:9
➔ *Clinical Examples in Radiology* Winter 17:3, Spring 17:13

0441T lower extremity distal/peripheral nerve
Sunset January 2027
➔ *CPT Changes: An Insider's View* 2017
➔ *CPT Assistant* May 17:3, Apr 19:9
➔ *Clinical Examples in Radiology* Winter 17:2, Spring 17:13

0442T nerve plexus or other truncal nerve (eg, brachial plexus, pudendal nerve)
Sunset January 2027
➔ *CPT Changes: An Insider's View* 2017
➔ *CPT Assistant* May 17:3, Apr 19:9
➔ *Clinical Examples in Radiology* Winter 17:3, Spring 17:13

+ 0443T Real-time spectral analysis of prostate tissue by fluorescence spectroscopy, including imaging guidance (List separately in addition to code for primary procedure)
Sunset January 2027
➔ *CPT Changes: An Insider's View* 2017

(Use 0443T in conjunction with 55700)

(Report 0443T only once per session)

0444T Initial placement of a drug-eluting ocular insert under one or more eyelids, including fitting, training, and insertion, unilateral or bilateral
Sunset January 2027
➔ *CPT Changes: An Insider's View* 2017
➔ *CPT Assistant* Aug 17:7

0445T Subsequent placement of a drug-eluting ocular insert under one or more eyelids, including re-training, and removal of existing insert, unilateral or bilateral
Sunset January 2027
➔ *CPT Changes: An Insider's View* 2017
➔ *CPT Assistant* Aug 17:7

(For insertion and removal of drug-eluting implant into lacrimal canaliculus, use 68841)

0446T Creation of subcutaneous pocket with insertion of implantable interstitial glucose sensor, including system activation and patient training
Sunset January 2027
➔ *CPT Changes: An Insider's View* 2017

(Do not report 0446T in conjunction with 95251, 0447T, 0448T)

0447T Removal of implantable interstitial glucose sensor from subcutaneous pocket via incision
Sunset January 2027
➔ *CPT Changes: An Insider's View* 2017

0448T Removal of implantable interstitial glucose sensor with creation of subcutaneous pocket at different anatomic site and insertion of new implantable sensor, including system activation
Sunset January 2027
➔ *CPT Changes: An Insider's View* 2017

(Do not report 0448T in conjunction with 0446T, 0447T)

(For placement of non-implantable interstitial glucose sensor without pocket, use 95250)

0449T Insertion of aqueous drainage device, without extraocular reservoir, internal approach, into the subconjunctival space; initial device
Sunset January 2027
➔ *CPT Changes: An Insider's View* 2017
➔ *CPT Assistant* Jul 18:3, Sep 18:3

+ 0450T each additional device (List separately in addition to code for primary procedure)
Sunset January 2027
➔ *CPT Changes: An Insider's View* 2017
➔ *CPT Assistant* Jul 18:3

(Use 0450T in conjunction with 0449T)

(For removal of aqueous drainage device without extraocular reservoir, placed into the subconjunctival space via internal approach, use 92499)

(For insertion of intraocular anterior segment drainage device into the trabecular meshwork without concomitant cataract removal with intraocular lens implant, use 0671T)

(For insertion or replacement of a permanently implantable aortic counterpulsation ventricular assist system, endovascular approach, and programming of sensing and therapeutic parameters, use 33999)

(For removal of permanently implantable aortic counterpulsation ventricular assist system, use 33999)

(For relocation of skin pocket with replacement of implanted aortic counterpulsation ventricular assist device, mechano-electrical skin interface and electrodes, use 33999)

(For repositioning of previously implanted aortic counterpulsation ventricular assist device, use 33999)

(For programming device evaluation [in person] with iterative adjustment of the implantable mechano-electrical skin interface and/or external driver, use 33999)

(For interrogation device evaluation [in person] with analysis, review, and report, use 33999)

0464T   Code is out of numerical sequence. See 0332T-0339T

(0465T has been deleted)

(For suprachoroidal injection of a pharmacologic agent, use 67516)

(For insertion, revision or replacement, or removal of chest wall respiratory sensor electrode or electrode array, see 64582, 64583, 64584)

0469T   Retinal polarization scan, ocular screening with on-site automated results, bilateral
Sunset January 2028
➔ *CPT Changes: An Insider's View* 2018
➔ *CPT Assistant* Feb 18:3

(Do not report 0469T in conjunction with 92002, 92004, 92012, 92014)

(For ocular photoscreening, see 99174, 99177)

(0470T, 0471T have been deleted)

(For optical coherence tomography [OCT] for microstructural and morphological imaging of skin, use 96999)

0472T   Device evaluation, interrogation, and initial programming of intraocular retinal electrode array (eg, retinal prosthesis), in person, with iterative adjustment of the implantable device to test functionality, select optimal permanent programmed values with analysis, including visual training, with review and report by a qualified health care professional
Sunset January 2028
➔ *CPT Changes: An Insider's View* 2018
➔ *CPT Assistant* Feb 18:3

0473T   Device evaluation and interrogation of intraocular retinal electrode array (eg, retinal prosthesis), in person, including reprogramming and visual training, when performed, with review and report by a qualified health care professional
Sunset January 2028
➔ *CPT Changes: An Insider's View* 2018
➔ *CPT Assistant* Feb 18:3

(For implantation of intraocular electrode array, use 0100T)

(For reprogramming of implantable intraocular retinal electrode array device, use 0473T)

0474T   Insertion of anterior segment aqueous drainage device, with creation of intraocular reservoir, internal approach, into the supraciliary space
Sunset January 2028
➔ *CPT Changes: An Insider's View* 2018
➔ *CPT Assistant* Feb 18:3, Jul 18:3, Dec 18:9

(0475T, 0476T, 0477T, 0478T have been deleted)

(For recording of fetal magnetic cardiac signal, data scanning, transfer data, signal extraction, review, and interpretation and report, use 93799)

0479T   Fractional ablative laser fenestration of burn and traumatic scars for functional improvement; first 100 cm^2 or part thereof, or 1% of body surface area of infants and children
Sunset January 2028
➔ *CPT Changes: An Insider's View* 2018
➔ *CPT Assistant* Dec 17:13

+ 0480T   each additional 100 cm^2, or each additional 1% of body surface area of infants and children, or part thereof (List separately in addition to code for primary procedure)
Sunset January 2028
➔ *CPT Changes: An Insider's View* 2018
➔ *CPT Assistant* Dec 17:13

(Use 0480T in conjunction with 0479T)

(Report 0479T, 0480T only once per day)

(For excision of cicatricial lesion[s] [eg, full thickness excision, through the dermis], see 11400-11446)

0481T   Injection(s), autologous white blood cell concentrate (autologous protein solution), any site, including image guidance, harvesting and preparation, when performed
Sunset January 2028
➔ *CPT Changes: An Insider's View* 2018
➔ *CPT Assistant* Dec 22:1

(Do not report 0481T in conjunction with 15769, 15771, 15772, 15773, 15774, 20550, 20551, 20600, 20604, 20605, 20606, 20610, 20611, 36415, 36592, 76942, 77002, 77012, 77021, 86965, 0232T)

(Do not report 38220, 38221, 38222, 38230 for bone marrow aspiration for autologous white blood cell concentrate [autologous protein solution] injection. For bone marrow aspiration for autologous white blood cell concentrate [autologous protein solution] injection, use 0481T)

(For absolute quantitation of myocardial blood flow [AQMBF] for cardiac PET, use 78434)

Codes 0483T, 0484T include vascular access, catheterization, balloon valvuloplasty, deploying the valve, repositioning the valve as needed, temporary pacemaker insertion for rapid pacing, and access site closure, when performed.

Angiography, radiological supervision and interpretation, intraprocedural roadmapping (eg, contrast injections, fluoroscopy) to guide the TMVI, left ventriculography (eg, to assess mitral regurgitation for guidance of TMVI), and completion angiography are included in codes 0483T, 0484T.

Diagnostic right and left heart catheterization codes (93451, 93452, 93453, 93456, 93457, 93458, 93459, 93460, 93461, 93593, 93594, 93595, 93596, 93597, 93598) should **not** be used with 0483T, 0484T to report:

1. Contrast injections, angiography, roadmapping, and/or fluoroscopic guidance for the transcatheter mitral valve implantation (TMVI),

2. Left ventricular angiography to assess or confirm valve positioning and function,

3. Right and left heart catheterization for hemodynamic measurements before, during, and after TMVI for guidance of TMVI.

Diagnostic right and left heart catheterization codes (93451, 93452, 93453, 93456, 93457, 93458, 93459, 93460, 93461, 93593, 93594, 93595, 93596, 93597, 93598) and diagnostic coronary angiography codes (93454, 93455, 93456, 93457, 93458, 93459, 93460, 93461, 93563, 93564) performed at the time of TMVI may be separately reportable, if:

1. No prior study is available and a full diagnostic study is performed, or

2. A prior study is available, but as documented in the medical record:

   a. There is inadequate visualization of the anatomy and/or pathology, or

   b. The patient's condition with respect to the clinical indication has changed since the prior study, or

   c. There is a clinical change during the procedure that requires new evaluation.

For same session/same day diagnostic cardiac catheterization services, report the appropriate diagnostic cardiac catheterization code(s) appended with modifier 59, indicating separate and distinct procedural service from TMVI.

When cardiopulmonary bypass is performed in conjunction with TMVI, 0483T, 0484T may be reported with the appropriate add-on code for percutaneous peripheral bypass (33367), open peripheral bypass (33368), or central bypass (33369).

For percutaneous transcatheter tricuspid valve annulus reconstruction, with implantation of adjustable annulus reconstruction device, use 0545T.

0483T   Transcatheter mitral valve implantation/replacement (TMVI) with prosthetic valve; percutaneous approach, including transseptal puncture, when performed
Sunset January 2028
➜ CPT Changes: An Insider's View 2018
➜ CPT Assistant Dec 22:23, Mar 23:37

(For transcatheter mitral valve annulus reconstruction, use 0544T)

(For transcatheter mitral valve repair percutaneous approach including transseptal puncture when performed, see 33418, 33419)

(For transcatheter mitral valve repair percutaneous approach via the coronary sinus, use 0345T)

0484T   transthoracic exposure (eg, thoracotomy, transapical)
Sunset January 2028
➜ CPT Changes: An Insider's View 2018

0485T   Optical coherence tomography (OCT) of middle ear, with interpretation and report; unilateral
Sunset January 2028
➜ CPT Changes: An Insider's View 2018

0486T   bilateral
Sunset January 2028
➜ CPT Changes: An Insider's View 2018

(0487T has been deleted)

(For transvaginal biomechanical mapping, use 58999)

0488T   Code is out of numerical sequence. See 0402T-0408T

0489T   Autologous adipose-derived regenerative cell therapy for scleroderma in the hands; adipose tissue harvesting, isolation and preparation of harvested cells including incubation with cell dissociation enzymes, removal of non-viable cells and debris, determination of concentration and dilution of regenerative cells
Sunset January 2028
➜ CPT Changes: An Insider's View 2018
➜ CPT Assistant Sep 18:12, Dec 22:1

(Do not report 0489T in conjunction with 15769, 15771, 15772, 15773, 15774, 15876, 15877, 15878, 15879, 20600, 20604)

0490T   multiple injections in one or both hands
Sunset January 2028
➜ CPT Changes: An Insider's View 2018
➜ CPT Assistant Sep 18:12

(Do not report 0490T in conjunction with 15769, 15771, 15772, 15773, 15774, 15876, 15877, 15878, 15879, 20600, 20604)

(Do not report 0490T for a single injection)

(For complete procedure, use 0490T in conjunction with 0489T)

(0491T, 0492T have been deleted)

(For non-contact full-field and fractional ablative laser treatment of an open wound, use 17999)

(0493T has been deleted)

(For transcutaneous oxyhemoglobin measurement in a lower extremity wound by near-infrared spectroscopy, use 93998)

Noncontact near-infrared spectroscopy is used to measure cutaneous vascular perfusion. Codes 0640T, 0859T describe noncontact near-infrared spectroscopy for measurement of cutaneous vascular perfusion (other than for screening for peripheral arterial disease) that does not require direct contact of the spectrometer sensors with the patient's skin. Codes 0640T, 0859T may only be reported once, when performing noncontact near-infrared spectroscopy of multiple wounds in one anatomic site (eg, multiple diabetic ulcers involving the plantar surface of the foot). For noncontact near-infrared spectroscopy studies for screening for peripheral arterial disease, use 0860T.

0640T Noncontact near-infrared spectroscopy (eg, for measurement of deoxyhemoglobin, oxyhemoglobin, and ratio of tissue oxygenation), other than for screening for peripheral arterial disease, image acquisition, interpretation, and report; first anatomic site
Sunset January 2027

➡ *CPT Changes: An Insider's View* 2022, 2024

➡ *CPT Assistant* Jun 22:16

(Do not report 0640T in conjunction with 0860T)

#+ **0859T** each additional anatomic site (List separately in addition to code for primary procedure)
Sunset January 2029

➡ *CPT Changes: An Insider's View* 2024

(Use 0859T in conjunction with 0640T)

(Report 0640T, 0859T only once, when performing noncontact near-infrared spectroscopy of multiple wounds in one anatomic site)

(For noncontact near-infrared spectroscopy studies for screening for peripheral arterial disease, use 0860T)

(0641T, 0642T have been deleted)

(For noncontact near-infrared spectroscopy studies other than for screening for peripheral arterial disease, see 0640T, 0859T)

0860T Noncontact near-infrared spectroscopy (eg, for measurement of deoxyhemoglobin, oxyhemoglobin, and ratio of tissue oxygenation), for screening for peripheral arterial disease, including provocative maneuvers, image acquisition, interpretation, and report, one or both lower extremities
Sunset January 2029

➡ *CPT Changes: An Insider's View* 2024

(Do not report 0860T in conjunction with 0640T)

(For noncontact near-infrared spectroscopy studies other than for screening for peripheral arterial disease, see 0640T, 0859T)

0494T Surgical preparation and cannulation of marginal (extended) cadaver donor lung(s) to ex vivo organ perfusion system, including decannulation, separation from the perfusion system, and cold preservation of the allograft prior to implantation, when performed
Sunset January 2028

➡ *CPT Changes: An Insider's View* 2018

0495T Initiation and monitoring marginal (extended) cadaver donor lung(s) organ perfusion system by physician or qualified health care professional, including physiological and laboratory assessment (eg, pulmonary artery flow, pulmonary artery pressure, left atrial pressure, pulmonary vascular resistance, mean/peak and plateau airway pressure, dynamic compliance and perfusate gas analysis), including bronchoscopy and X ray when performed; first two hours in sterile field
Sunset January 2028

➡ *CPT Changes: An Insider's View* 2018

+ **0496T** each additional hour (List separately in addition to code for primary procedure)
Sunset January 2028

➡ *CPT Changes: An Insider's View* 2018

(Report 0496T in conjunction with 0495T)

(0497T, 0498T have been deleted)

(For in-office connection or review and interpretation of an external patient-activated electrocardiographic rhythm–derived event recorder without 24-hour attended monitoring, use 93799)

(0499T has been deleted)

(For cystourethroscopy with mechanical urethral dilation and urethral therapeutic drug delivery by drug-coated balloon catheter for urethral stricture or stenosis, including fluoroscopy, use 52284)

▶(0500T has been deleted)◀

▶(For singular pooled result of high-risk human papillomavirus [HPV] types [eg, 16, 18, 31, 33, 35, 39, 45, 51, 52, 58, 59, 68], use 87624)◀

▶(For separately reported high-risk human papillomavirus [HPV] types 16 and 18 only, including type 45, if performed, use 87625)◀

▶(For high-risk human papillomavirus [HPV] types [eg, 16, 18, 31, 45, 51, 52] individually and high-risk pooled result[s] in a single test, use 87626)◀

(0501T, 0502T, 0503T, 0504T have been deleted)

(For noninvasive estimate of coronary fractional flow reserve [FFR] derived from augmentative software analysis of the data set from a coronary computed tomography angiography, with interpretation and report by a physician or other qualified health care professional, use 75580)

Automated quantification and characterization of coronary atherosclerotic plaque is a service in which coronary computed tomographic angiography (CTA) data are analyzed using computerized algorithms to assess the extent and severity of coronary artery disease. The computer-generated findings are provided in an interactive format to the physician or other qualified health care professional who performs the final review and report. The coronary CTA is performed and interpreted as a separate service and is not included in the service of automated analysis of coronary CTA.

 # 0623T Automated quantification and characterization of coronary atherosclerotic plaque to assess severity of coronary disease, using data from coronary computed tomographic angiography; data preparation and transmission, computerized analysis of data, with review of computerized analysis output to reconcile discordant data, interpretation and report
Sunset January 2026
➔ *CPT Changes: An Insider's View* 2021
➔ *CPT Assistant* Oct 21:3
➔ *Clinical Examples in Radiology* Winter 22:10-12

 # 0624T data preparation and transmission
Sunset January 2026
➔ *CPT Changes: An Insider's View* 2021
➔ *CPT Assistant* Oct 21:3
➔ *Clinical Examples in Radiology* Winter 22:10-12

 # 0625T computerized analysis of data from coronary computed tomographic angiography
Sunset January 2026
➔ *CPT Changes: An Insider's View* 2021
➔ *CPT Assistant* Oct 21:3
➔ *Clinical Examples in Radiology* Winter 22:10-12

 # 0626T review of computerized analysis output to reconcile discordant data, interpretation and report
Sunset January 2026
➔ *CPT Changes: An Insider's View* 2021
➔ *CPT Assistant* Oct 21:3
➔ *Clinical Examples in Radiology* Winter 22:10-12

(Use 0623T, 0624T, 0625T, 0626T one time per coronary computed tomographic angiogram)

(Do not report 0623T in conjunction with 0624T, 0625T, 0626T)

(Do not report 0623T, 0624T, 0625T, 0626T in conjunction with 76376, 76377)

(For noninvasive estimate of coronary fractional flow reserve [FFR] derived from augmentative software analysis of the data set from a coronary computed tomography angiography, with interpretation and report by a physician or other qualified health care professional, use 75580)

#+ 0523T Intraprocedural coronary fractional flow reserve (FFR) with 3D functional mapping of color-coded FFR values for the coronary tree, derived from coronary angiogram data, for real-time review and interpretation of possible atherosclerotic stenosis(es) intervention (List separately in addition to code for primary procedure)
Sunset January 2029
➔ *CPT Changes: An Insider's View* 2019

(Use 0523T in conjunction with 93454, 93455, 93456, 93457, 93458, 93459, 93460, 93461)

(Do not report 0523T more than once per session)

(Do not report 0523T in conjunction with 75580, 76376, 76377, 93571, 93572)

0505T Endovenous femoral-popliteal arterial revascularization, with transcatheter placement of intravascular stent graft(s) and closure by any method, including percutaneous or open vascular access, ultrasound guidance for vascular access when performed, all catheterization(s) and intraprocedural roadmapping and imaging guidance necessary to complete the intervention, all associated radiological supervision and interpretation, when performed, with crossing of the occlusive lesion in an extraluminal fashion
Sunset January 2029
➔ *CPT Changes: An Insider's View* 2019

(0505T includes all ipsilateral selective arterial and venous catheterization, all diagnostic imaging for ipsilateral, lower extremity arteriography, and all related radiological supervision and interpretation)

(Do not report 0505T in conjunction with 37224, 37225, 37226, 37227, 37238, 37239, 37248, 37249, within the femoral-popliteal segment)

(Do not report 0505T in conjunction with 76937, for ultrasound guidance for vascular access)

 # 0620T Endovascular venous arterialization, tibial or peroneal vein, with transcatheter placement of intravascular stent graft(s) and closure by any method, including percutaneous or open vascular access, ultrasound guidance for vascular access when performed, all catheterization(s) and intraprocedural roadmapping and imaging guidance necessary to complete the intervention, all associated radiological supervision and interpretation, when performed
Sunset January 2026
➔ *CPT Changes: An Insider's View* 2021

(0620T includes all ipsilateral selective arterial and venous catheterization, all diagnostic imaging for ipsilateral, lower extremity arteriography, and all related radiological supervision and interpretation)

(Do not report 0620T in conjunction with 37228, 37229, 37230, 37231, 37238, 37239, 37248, 37249 within the tibial-peroneal segment)

0506T Macular pigment optical density measurement by heterochromatic flicker photometry, unilateral or bilateral, with interpretation and report

Sunset January 2029

➔ *CPT Changes: An Insider's View* 2019

➔ *CPT Assistant* Dec 18:6

0507T Near infrared dual imaging (ie, simultaneous reflective and transilluminated light) of meibomian glands, unilateral or bilateral, with interpretation and report

Sunset January 2029

➔ *CPT Changes: An Insider's View* 2019

(For external ocular photography, use 92285)

(For tear film imaging, use 0330T)

(0508T has been deleted)

(For pulse-echo ultrasound bone density measurement resulting in indicator of axial bone mineral density, tibia, use 76999)

Electroretinography (ERG) is used to evaluate function of the retina and optic nerve of the eye, including photoreceptors and ganglion cells. A number of techniques that target different areas of the eye, including full field (flash and flicker) (92273) for a global response of photoreceptors of the retina, multifocal (92274) for photoreceptors in multiple separate locations in the retina, including the macula, and pattern (0509T) for retinal ganglion cells, are used. Multiple additional terms and techniques are used to describe various types of ERG. If the technique used is not specifically named in the code descriptors for 92273, 92274, 0509T, use the unlisted procedure code 92499.

0509T Electroretinography (ERG) with interpretation and report, pattern (PERG)

Sunset January 2029

➔ *CPT Changes: An Insider's View* 2019

➔ *CPT Assistant* Jan 19:12

(For full-field ERG, use 92273)

(For multifocal ERG, use 92274)

0510T Code is out of numerical sequence. See 0332T-0339T

0511T Code is out of numerical sequence. See 0332T-0339T

0512T Code is out of numerical sequence. See 0101T-0107T

0513T Code is out of numerical sequence. See 0101T-0107T

(0514T has been deleted)

Wireless Cardiac Stimulation System for Left Ventricular Pacing

A wireless cardiac stimulator system for left ventricular pacing functions by sensing right ventricular pacing output from a previously implanted conventional device (pacemaker or defibrillator, with univentricular or biventricular leads), and then transmitting an ultrasound pulse to a wireless electrode implanted on the endocardium of the left ventricle, which then emits a left ventricular pacing pulse. In combination, the left ventricular and right ventricular pacemakers provide biventricular cardiac pacing.

The complete wireless left ventricular pacing system consists of a wireless endocardial left ventricle electrode and a pulse generator. The pulse generator has two components: a transmitter and a battery. The electrode is typically implanted transarterially into the left ventricular wall and powered wirelessly using ultrasound delivered by a subcutaneously implanted transmitter. Two subcutaneous pockets are created on the chest wall, one for the battery and one for the transmitter, and these two components are connected by a subcutaneously tunneled cable.

Patients with a wireless cardiac stimulator who also have a conventional pacing device require programming/ interrogation of their existing conventional device, as well as the wireless device. The wireless cardiac stimulator is programmed and interrogated with its own separate programmer and settings.

Code 0515T describes insertion of a complete wireless cardiac stimulator system (electrode and pulse generator, which includes transmitter and battery) for left ventricular pacing, including interrogation, programming, pocket creation, relocation, and all echocardiography, left ventriculography, and fluoroscopic imaging to guide the procedure, when performed. For insertion of only the electrode of a wireless cardiac stimulator for left ventricular pacing, use 0516T. For insertion of both components of a new pulse generator (battery and transmitter), use 0517T.

A wireless cardiac stimulator for left ventricular pacing may need to be removed, relocated, or replaced. The electrode component of the stimulator typically is not removed once implanted. For removal of both components of the pulse generator (battery and transmitter) without replacement, use 0861T. For removal of only the battery component of the pulse generator without replacement, use 0518T. For relocation of the pulse generator, use 0862T for relocation of the battery component or 0863T for relocation of the transmitter component. For removal and replacement of both components of the pulse generator, use 0519T. For removal and replacement of only the battery component, use 0520T.

All catheterization, angiography, and imaging guidance (including transthoracic or transesophageal echocardiography) required to complete a wireless cardiac stimulator procedure is included in 0515T, 0516T, 0517T, 0518T, 0519T, 0520T, 0861T, 0862T, 0863T.

Do not report 76000, 76998, 93303-93355, 93452, 93453, 93458, 93459, 93460, 93461, 93565, 93586, 93595, 93596, 93597 in conjunction with 0515T, 0516T, 0517T, 0518T, 0519T, 0520T, 0795T, 0796T, 0797T, 0798T, 0799T, 0800T, 0801T, 0802T, 0803T, 0823T, 0824T, 0825T, 0861T, 0862T, 0863T.

Do not report left heart catheterization codes (93452, 93453, 93458, 93459, 93460, 93461, 93595, 93596, 93597) for delivery of a wireless cardiac stimulator electrode into the left ventricle.

0515T Insertion of wireless cardiac stimulator for left ventricular pacing, including device interrogation and programming, and imaging supervision and interpretation, when performed; complete system (includes electrode and generator [transmitter and battery])
Sunset January 2029
➡ *CPT Changes: An Insider's View* 2019

0516T electrode only
Sunset January 2029
➡ *CPT Changes: An Insider's View* 2019

0517T both components of pulse generator (battery and transmitter) only
Sunset January 2029
➡ *CPT Changes: An Insider's View* 2019, 2024

(Do not report 0515T, 0516T, 0517T in conjunction with 0518T, 0519T, 0520T, 0521T, 0522T, 0861T, 0862T, 0863T)

 # 0861T Removal of pulse generator for wireless cardiac stimulator for left ventricular pacing; both components (battery and transmitter)
Sunset January 2029
➡ *CPT Changes: An Insider's View* 2024

(Do not report 0861T in conjunction with 0515T, 0516T, 0517T, 0518T, 0519T, 0520T, 0521T, 0522T, 0862T, 0863T)

0518T battery component only
Sunset January 2029
➡ *CPT Changes: An Insider's View* 2019, 2024

(Do not report 0518T in conjunction with 0515T, 0516T, 0517T, 0519T, 0520T, 0521T, 0522T, 0861T, 0862T, 0863T)

 # 0862T Relocation of pulse generator for wireless cardiac stimulator for left ventricular pacing, including device interrogation and programming; battery component only
Sunset January 2029
➡ *CPT Changes: An Insider's View* 2024

(Do not report 0862T in conjunction with 0515T, 0517T, 0518T, 0519T, 0520T, 0521T, 0522T, 0861T)

 # 0863T transmitter component only
Sunset January 2029
➡ *CPT Changes: An Insider's View* 2024

(Do not report 0863T in conjunction with 0515T, 0517T, 0518T, 0519T, 0520T, 0521T, 0522T, 0861T)

0519T Removal and replacement of pulse generator for wireless cardiac stimulator for left ventricular pacing, including device interrogation and programming; both components (battery and transmitter)
Sunset January 2029
➡ *CPT Changes: An Insider's View* 2019, 2024

0520T battery component only
Sunset January 2029
➡ *CPT Changes: An Insider's View* 2019, 2024

(Do not report 0519T, 0520T in conjunction with 0515T, 0516T, 0517T, 0518T, 0521T, 0522T, 0861T, 0862T, 0863T)

0521T Interrogation device evaluation (in person) with analysis, review and report, includes connection, recording, and disconnection per patient encounter, wireless cardiac stimulator for left ventricular pacing
Sunset January 2029
➡ *CPT Changes: An Insider's View* 2019

(Do not report 0521T in conjunction with 0515T, 0516T, 0517T, 0518T, 0519T, 0520T, 0522T, 0861T, 0862T, 0863T)

0522T Programming device evaluation (in person) with iterative adjustment of the implantable device to test the function of the device and select optimal permanent programmed values with analysis, including review and report, wireless cardiac stimulator for left ventricular pacing
Sunset January 2029
➡ *CPT Changes: An Insider's View* 2019

(Do not report 0522T in conjunction with 0515T, 0516T, 0517T, 0518T, 0519T, 0520T, 0521T, 0861T, 0862T, 0863T)

0523T Code is out of numerical sequence. See 0496T-0507T

0524T Endovenous catheter directed chemical ablation with balloon isolation of incompetent extremity vein, open or percutaneous, including all vascular access, catheter manipulation, diagnostic imaging, imaging guidance and monitoring
Sunset January 2029
➡ *CPT Changes: An Insider's View* 2019

0525T Insertion or replacement of intracardiac ischemia monitoring system, including testing of the lead and monitor, initial system programming, and imaging supervision and interpretation; complete system (electrode and implantable monitor)
Sunset January 2029
➔ *CPT Changes: An Insider's View* 2019

0526T   electrode only
Sunset January 2029
➔ *CPT Changes: An Insider's View* 2019

0527T   implantable monitor only
Sunset January 2029
➔ *CPT Changes: An Insider's View* 2019

(Do not report 0525T, 0526T, 0527T in conjunction with 93000, 93005, 93010, 0528T, 0529T)

(For removal and replacement of intracardiac ischemia monitoring system or its components, see 0525T, 0526T, 0527T in conjunction with 0530T, 0531T, 0532T, as appropriate)

0528T Programming device evaluation (in person) of intracardiac ischemia monitoring system with iterative adjustment of programmed values, with analysis, review, and report
Sunset January 2029
➔ *CPT Changes: An Insider's View* 2019

(Do not report 0528T in conjunction with 93000, 93005, 93010, 0525T, 0526T, 0527T, 0529T, 0530T, 0531T, 0532T)

0529T Interrogation device evaluation (in person) of intracardiac ischemia monitoring system with analysis, review, and report
Sunset January 2029
➔ *CPT Changes: An Insider's View* 2019

(Do not report 0529T in conjunction with 93000, 93005, 93010, 0525T, 0526T, 0527T, 0528T, 0530T, 0531T, 0532T)

0530T Removal of intracardiac ischemia monitoring system, including all imaging supervision and interpretation; complete system (electrode and implantable monitor)
Sunset January 2029
➔ *CPT Changes: An Insider's View* 2019

0531T   electrode only
Sunset January 2029
➔ *CPT Changes: An Insider's View* 2019

0532T   implantable monitor only
Sunset January 2029
➔ *CPT Changes: An Insider's View* 2019

(Do not report 0530T, 0531T, 0532T in conjunction with 0528T, 0529T)

(0533T, 0534T, 0535T, 0536T have been deleted)

(For continuous recording of movement disorder symptoms including bradykinesia, dyskinesia, and tremor for 6 days up to 10 days, use 95999)

Cellular and Gene Therapy

▶(0537T, 0538T, 0539T, 0540T have been deleted)◀

▶(For chimeric antigen receptor T-cell [CAR-T] therapy, see 38225, 38226, 38227, 38228)◀

0541T Myocardial imaging by magnetocardiography (MCG) for detection of cardiac ischemia, by signal acquisition using minimum 36 channel grid, generation of magnetic-field time-series images, quantitative analysis of magnetic dipoles, machine learning–derived clinical scoring, and automated report generation, single study;
Sunset January 2029
➔ *CPT Changes: An Insider's View* 2019

0542T   interpretation and report
Sunset January 2029
➔ *CPT Changes: An Insider's View* 2019

0543T Transapical mitral valve repair, including transthoracic echocardiography, when performed, with placement of artificial chordae tendineae
Sunset January 2030
➔ *CPT Changes: An Insider's View* 2020

(For transesophageal echocardiography image guidance, use 93355)

Codes 0544T and 0545T include vascular access, catheterization, deploying and adjusting the reconstruction device(s), temporary pacemaker insertion for rapid pacing if required, and access site closure, when performed.

Angiography, radiological supervision and interpretation, intraprocedural roadmapping (eg, contrast injections, fluoroscopy) to guide the device implantation, ventriculography (eg, to assess target valve regurgitation for guidance of device implantation and adjustment), and completion angiography are included in 0544T and 0545T.

Diagnostic right and left heart catheterization codes (93451, 93452, 93453, 93454, 93455, 93456, 93457, 93458, 93459, 93460, 93461, 93565, 93566, 93593, 93594, 93595, 93596, 93597, 93598) may not be used in conjunction with 0544T, 0545T to report:

1. Contrast injections, angiography, roadmapping, and/or fluoroscopic guidance for the implantation and adjustment of the transcatheter mitral or tricuspid valve annulus reconstruction device, or

2. Right or left ventricular angiography to assess or confirm transcatheter mitral or tricuspid valve annulus reconstruction device positioning and function, or

3. Right and left heart catheterization for hemodynamic measurements before, during, and after transcatheter mitral or tricuspid valve annulus reconstruction for guidance.

Diagnostic right and left heart catheterization codes (93451, 93452, 93453, 93456, 93457, 93458, 93459, 93460, 93461, 93593, 93594, 93595, 93596, 93597, 93598) and diagnostic coronary angiography codes (93454, 93455, 93456, 93457, 93458, 93459, 93460, 93461, 93563, 93564) performed at the time of transcatheter mitral or tricuspid valve annulus reconstruction may be separately reportable, if:

1. No prior study is available and a full diagnostic study is performed, or

2. A prior study is available, but as documented in the medical record:

    a. There is inadequate visualization of the anatomy and/or pathology, or

    b. The patient's condition with respect to the clinical indication has changed since the prior study, or

    c. There is a clinical change during the procedure that requires new evaluation.

Other cardiac catheterization services may be reported separately, when performed for diagnostic purposes not intrinsic to the transcatheter mitral valve annulus reconstruction.

For same session/same day diagnostic cardiac catheterization services, report the appropriate diagnostic cardiac catheterization code(s) appended with modifier 59 indicating separate and distinct procedural service from transcatheter mitral or tricuspid valve annulus reconstruction.

Percutaneous coronary interventional procedures may be reported separately, when performed.

When cardiopulmonary bypass is performed in conjunction with transcatheter mitral valve or tricuspid valve annulus reconstruction, 0544T, 0545T should be reported with the appropriate add-on code for percutaneous peripheral bypass (33367), open peripheral bypass (33368), or central bypass (33369).

When transcatheter ventricular support is required, the appropriate code may be reported with the appropriate ventricular assist device (VAD) procedure (33990, 33991, 33992, 33993) or balloon pump insertion (33967, 33970, 33973).

For percutaneous transcatheter mitral valve repair, use 0345T. For percutaneous transcatheter mitral valve implantation/replacement (TMVI) with prosthetic valve, use 0483T.

0544T   Transcatheter mitral valve annulus reconstruction, with implantation of adjustable annulus reconstruction device, percutaneous approach including transseptal puncture
Sunset January 2030
➲ *CPT Changes: An Insider's View* 2020

(For transcatheter mitral valve repair percutaneous approach including transseptal puncture when performed, see 33418, 33419)

(For transcatheter mitral valve repair percutaneous approach via the coronary sinus, use 0345T)

(For transcatheter mitral valve implantation/replacement [TMVI] with prosthetic valve percutaneous approach, use 0483T)

0545T   Transcatheter tricuspid valve annulus reconstruction with implantation of adjustable annulus reconstruction device, percutaneous approach
Sunset January 2030
➲ *CPT Changes: An Insider's View* 2020
➲ *CPT Assistant* Jul 22:8

(Do not report 0544T, 0545T in conjunction with 76000)

(Do not report 0544T, 0545T in conjunction with 93451, 93452, 93453, 93456, 93457, 93458, 93459, 93460, 93461, 93565, 93566, 93593, 93594, 93595, 93596, 93597, 93598 for diagnostic left and right heart catheterization procedures intrinsic to the annular repair procedure)

(Do not report 0544T, 0545T in conjunction with 93454, 93455, 93456, 93457, 93458, 93459, 93460, 93461, 93563, 93564 for coronary angiography procedures intrinsic to the annular repair procedure)

(For transcatheter left ventricular restoration device implantation from an arterial approach not necessitating transseptal puncture, use 0643T)

Code 0643T includes the primary arterial vascular access and contralateral arterial access and percutaneous access site closure, when performed. Guide catheter(s) and snare wire(s) may be required to advance the device to the treatment zone and are included in 0643T when performed. Left heart catheterization, intracardiac device customization, deploying, cinching, and adjusting the left ventricular restoration device are inherent to the procedure. Right heart catheterization may be performed for guidance of hemodynamics during device placement and is included in the procedure when performed for this purpose. Related angiography, radiological supervision and interpretation, intraprocedural roadmapping (eg, contrast injections, fluoroscopy) to guide the device implantation, ventriculography (eg, to assess ventricular shape, guidance of device implantation and adjustment), and completion angiography are included in 0643T.

Diagnostic right and left heart catheterization codes (93451, 93452, 93453, 93456, 93457, 93458, 93459, 93460, 93461, 93593, 93594, 93595, 93596, 93597), diagnostic coronary angiography codes (93454, 93455,

93456, 93457, 93458, 93459, 93460, 93461, 93563, 93564), and left ventriculography code (93565) may not be used in conjunction with 0643T to report:

1. Contrast injections, angiography, roadmapping, and/or fluoroscopic guidance for the implantation, intracardiac customization, deploying, cinching, and adjustment of the left ventricular restoration device, or

2. Left ventricular angiography to assess or confirm transcatheter left ventricular restoration device positioning and function, or

3. Right and left heart catheterization for hemodynamic measurements before, during, and after transcatheter left ventricular restoration device implantation for guidance.

Diagnostic right and left heart catheterization codes (93451, 93452, 93453, 93456, 93457, 93458, 93459, 93460, 93461, 93593, 93594, 93595, 93596, 93597) and diagnostic coronary angiography codes (93454, 93455, 93456, 93457, 93458, 93459, 93460, 93461, 93563, 93564) performed at the time of transcatheter left ventricular restoration device implantation may be separately reportable, if:

1. No prior study is available and a full diagnostic study is performed, or

2. A prior study is available, but as documented in the medical record:

   a. There is inadequate visualization of the anatomy and/or pathology, or

   b. The patient's condition with respect to the clinical indication has changed since the prior study, or

   c. There is clinical change during the procedure that requires new evaluation.

Other cardiac catheterization services may be reported separately, when performed for diagnostic purposes not intrinsic to transcatheter left ventricular restoration device implantation.

For same session/same day diagnostic cardiac catheterization services not intrinsic to the transcatheter left ventricular restoration device implantation procedure, report the appropriate diagnostic cardiac catheterization code(s) appended with modifier 59, indicating separate and distinct procedural service from transcatheter left ventricular restoration device implantation.

Percutaneous coronary interventional procedures may be reported separately, when performed.

When cardiopulmonary bypass is performed in conjunction with transcatheter left ventricular restoration device implantation, 0643T should be reported with the appropriate add-on code for percutaneous peripheral bypass (33367), open peripheral bypass (33368), or central bypass (33369).

When transcatheter ventricular support is required, the appropriate code may be reported with the appropriate ventricular assist device (VAD) procedure (33990, 33991,

33992, 33993) or balloon pump insertion (33967, 33970, 33973).

For transcatheter mitral valve annulus reconstruction with implantation of adjustable annulus reconstruction device from a venous approach, necessitating transseptal puncture, use 0544T.

 # 0643T   Transcatheter left ventricular restoration device implantation including right and left heart catheterization and left ventriculography when performed, arterial approach
Sunset January 2027

➲ CPT Changes: An Insider's View 2022

(Do not report 0643T in conjunction with 76000)

(Do not report 0643T in conjunction with 93451, 93452, 93453, 93456, 93457, 93458, 93459, 93460, 93461, 93565, 93593, 93594, 93595, 93596, 93597, for diagnostic right and left heart catheterization procedures or ventriculography intrinsic to the left ventricular restoration device implantation procedure)

(Do not report 0643T in conjunction with 93454, 93455, 93456, 93457, 93458, 93459, 93460, 93461, 93563, 93564, for coronary angiography procedures intrinsic to the left ventricular restoration device implantation procedure)

0546T   Radiofrequency spectroscopy, real time, intraoperative margin assessment, at the time of partial mastectomy, with report
Sunset January 2030

➲ CPT Changes: An Insider's View 2020

(Use 0546T only once for each partial mastectomy site)

(Do not report 0546T for re-excision)

0547T   Bone-material quality testing by microindentation(s) of the tibia(s), with results reported as a score
Sunset January 2030

➲ CPT Changes: An Insider's View 2020

(To report unilateral or bilateral insertion, removal, or fluid adjustment of a periurethral adjustable balloon continence device, see 53451, 53452, 53453, 53454)

0552T   Low-level laser therapy, dynamic photonic and dynamic thermokinetic energies, provided by a physician or other qualified health care professional
Sunset January 2030

➲ CPT Changes: An Insider's View 2020

(Do not report 0552T in conjunction with 97037)

(For low-level laser therapy [ie, nonthermal and non-ablative] for post-operative pain, use 97037)

▶(0553T has been deleted)◀

▶(For percutaneous transcatheter placement of iliac arteriovenous anastomosis implant, use 37799)◀

0554T Bone strength and fracture risk using finite element analysis of functional data and bone-mineral density utilizing data from a computed tomography scan; retrieval and transmission of the scan data, assessment of bone strength and fracture risk and bone-mineral density, interpretation and report
Sunset January 2030

➔ *CPT Changes: An Insider's View* 2020
➔ *CPT Assistant* Sep 20:11

(Do not report 0554T in conjunction with 0555T, 0556T, 0557T)

0555T retrieval and transmission of the scan data
Sunset January 2030

➔ *CPT Changes: An Insider's View* 2020
➔ *CPT Assistant* Sep 20:11

0556T assessment of bone strength and fracture risk and bone-mineral density
Sunset January 2030

➔ *CPT Changes: An Insider's View* 2020
➔ *CPT Assistant* Sep 20:11

0557T interpretation and report
Sunset January 2030

➔ *CPT Changes: An Insider's View* 2020
➔ *CPT Assistant* Sep 20:11

(Do not report 0554T, 0555T, 0556T, 0557T in conjunction with 0691T, 0743T)

0558T Computed tomography scan taken for the purpose of biomechanical computed tomography analysis
Sunset January 2030

➔ *CPT Changes: An Insider's View* 2020
➔ *CPT Assistant* Sep 20:11

(Do not report 0558T in conjunction with 71250, 71260, 71270, 71275, 72125, 72126, 72127, 72128, 72129, 72130, 72131, 72132, 72133, 72191, 72192, 72193, 72194, 74150, 74160, 74170, 74174, 74175, 74176, 74177, 74178, 74261, 74262, 74263, 75571, 75572, 75573, 75574, 75635, 78816, 0691T)

Codes 0559T, 0560T represent production of 3D-printed models of individually prepared and processed components of structures of anatomy. These individual components of structures of anatomy include, but are not limited to, bones, arteries, veins, nerves, ureters, muscles, tendons and ligaments, joints, visceral organs, and brain. Each 3D-printed anatomic model of a structure can be made up of one or more separate components. The 3D anatomic printings can be 3D printed in unique colors and/or materials.

Codes 0561T, 0562T represent the production of 3D-printed cutting or drilling guides using individualized imaging data. 3D-printed guides are cutting or drilling tools used during surgery and are 3D printed so that they precisely fit an individual patient's anatomy to guide the surgery. A cutting guide does not have multiple parts, but instead is a unique single tool. It may be necessary to make a 3D-printed model and a 3D-printed cutting or drilling guide on the same patient to assist with surgery.

0559T Anatomic model 3D-printed from image data set(s); first individually prepared and processed component of an anatomic structure
Sunset January 2030

➔ *CPT Changes: An Insider's View* 2020
➔ *CPT Assistant* Mar 22:14
➔ *Clinical Examples in Radiology* Spring 19:6, Spring 23:28-29

+ 0560T each additional individually prepared and processed component of an anatomic structure (List separately in addition to code for primary procedure)
Sunset January 2030

➔ *CPT Changes: An Insider's View* 2020
➔ *CPT Assistant* Mar 22:14
➔ *Clinical Examples in Radiology* Spring 19:6, Spring 23:28-29

(Use 0560T in conjunction with 0559T)

(Do not report 0559T, 0560T in conjunction with 76376, 76377)

0561T Anatomic guide 3D-printed and designed from image data set(s); first anatomic guide
Sunset January 2030

➔ *CPT Changes: An Insider's View* 2020
➔ *CPT Assistant* Mar 22:14
➔ *Clinical Examples in Radiology* Spring 19:6, Spring 23:28-29

+ 0562T each additional anatomic guide (List separately in addition to code for primary procedure)
Sunset January 2030

➔ *CPT Changes: An Insider's View* 2020
➔ *CPT Assistant* Mar 22:14
➔ *Clinical Examples in Radiology* Spring 19:7, Spring 23:28-29

(Use 0562T in conjunction with 0561T)

(Do not report 0561T, 0562T in conjunction with 76376, 76377)

0563T Code is out of numerical sequence. See 0202T-0209T

▶(0564T has been deleted)◀

▶(For chemotherapeutic drug cytotoxicity assay of cancer stem cells, use 89240)◀

0565T Autologous cellular implant derived from adipose tissue for the treatment of osteoarthritis of the knees; tissue harvesting and cellular implant creation

Sunset January 2030

→ *CPT Changes: An Insider's View* 2020

→ *CPT Assistant* Dec 22:1

(Do not report 0565T in conjunction with 15769, 15771, 15772, 15773, 15774)

0566T   injection of cellular implant into knee joint including ultrasound guidance, unilateral

Sunset January 2030

→ *CPT Changes: An Insider's View* 2020

(Do not report 0566T in conjunction with 20610, 20611, 76942, 77002)

(For bilateral procedure, report 0566T with modifier 50)

▶(0567T has been deleted)◀

▶(For permanent fallopian tube occlusion with degradable biopolymer implant, transcervical approach, including transvaginal ultrasound, use 58999)◀

▶(0568T has been deleted)◀

▶(For introduction of mixture of saline and air for sonosalpingography to confirm occlusion of fallopian tubes, transcervical approach, use 58999)◀

Tricuspid Valve Repair

Codes 0569T, 0570T include the work of percutaneous vascular access, placing the access sheath, cardiac catheterization, advancing the repair device system into position, repositioning the prosthesis as needed, deploying the prosthesis, and vascular closure. Code 0569T may only be reported once per session. Add-on code 0570T is reported in conjunction with 0569T for each additional prosthesis placed.

For open tricuspid valve procedures, see 33460, 33463, 33464, 33465, 33468.

Angiography, radiological supervision and interpretation performed to guide transcatheter tricuspid valve repair (TTVr) (eg, guiding device placement and documenting completion of the intervention) are included in these codes.

Intracardiac echocardiography (93662), when performed, is included in 0569T, 0570T. Transesophageal echocardiography (93355) performed by a separate operator for guidance of the procedure may be separately reported.

Fluoroscopy (76000) and diagnostic right and left heart catheterization codes (93451, 93452, 93453, 93456, 93457, 93458, 93459, 93460, 93461, 93566, 93593, 93594, 93595, 93596, 93597, 93598) may **not** be used with 0569T, 0570T to report the following techniques for guidance of TTVr:

1. Contrast injections, angiography, roadmapping, and/or fluoroscopic guidance for the TTVr,

2. Right ventricular angiography to assess tricuspid regurgitation for guidance of TTVr, or

3. Right and left heart catheterization for hemodynamic measurements before, during, and after TTVr for guidance of TTVr.

Diagnostic right and left heart catheterization codes (93451, 93452, 93453, 93456, 93457, 93458, 93459, 93460, 93461, 93566, 93593, 93594, 93595, 93596, 93597, 93598) and diagnostic coronary angiography codes (93454, 93455, 93456, 93457, 93458, 93459, 93460, 93461, 93563, 93564) may be reported with 0569T, 0570T, representing separate and distinct services from TTVr, if:

1. No prior study is available and a full diagnostic study is performed, or

2. A prior study is available but as documented in the medical record:

   a. There is inadequate evaluation of the anatomy and/or pathology, or

   b. The patient's condition with respect to the clinical indication has changed since the prior study, or

   c. There is a clinical change during the procedure that requires new diagnostic evaluation.

Other cardiac catheterization services may be reported separately when performed for diagnostic purposes not intrinsic to TTVr.

For same session/same day diagnostic cardiac catheterization services, report the appropriate diagnostic cardiac catheterization code(s) with modifier 59 indicating separate and distinct procedural service from TTVr.

Diagnostic coronary angiography performed at a separate session from an interventional procedure may be separately reportable.

Percutaneous coronary interventional procedures may be reported separately, when performed.

When transcatheter ventricular support is required in conjunction with TTVr, the procedure may be reported with the appropriate ventricular assist device (VAD) procedure code (33990, 33991, 33992, 33993) or balloon pump insertion code (33967, 33970, 33973).

When cardiopulmonary bypass is performed in conjunction with TTVr, 0569T, 0570T may be reported with the appropriate add-on code for percutaneous peripheral bypass (33367), open peripheral bypass (33368), or central bypass (33369).

0569T Transcatheter tricuspid valve repair, percutaneous approach; initial prosthesis
Sunset January 2030
➔ *CPT Changes: An Insider's View* 2020
➔ *CPT Assistant* Jul 22:8

+ 0570T each additional prosthesis during same session (List separately in addition to code for primary procedure)
Sunset January 2030
➔ *CPT Changes: An Insider's View* 2020
➔ *CPT Assistant* Jul 22:8

(Use 0570T in conjunction with 0569T)

(Do not report 0569T, 0570T in conjunction with 93451, 93452, 93453, 93456, 93457, 93458, 93459, 93460, 93461, 93566 for diagnostic left and right heart catheterization procedures intrinsic to the valve repair procedure)

(Do not report 0569T, 0570T in conjunction with 93454, 93563, 93564 for coronary angiography intrinsic to the valve repair procedure)

Tricuspid Valve Implantation/Replacement

Code 0646T includes vascular access, catheterization, repositioning the valve delivery device as needed, deploying the valve, temporary pacemaker insertion for rapid pacing (33210), and access site closure by any method, when performed.

Angiography (eg, peripheral), radiological supervision and interpretation, intraprocedural roadmapping (eg, contrast injections, fluoroscopy, intracardiac echocardiography) to guide the transcatheter tricuspid valve implantation (TTVI)/replacement, right atrial and/or right ventricular angiography (eg, to assess tricuspid regurgitation for guidance of TTVI), and completion angiography are included in 0646T.

Transesophageal echocardiography (93355) performed by a separate operator for guidance of the procedure may be separately reported. Intracardiac echocardiography (93662) is not separately reportable when performed.

Diagnostic right heart catheterization codes (93451, 93453, 93456, 93457, 93460, 93461, 93593, 93594, 93596, 93597) and right atrial/right ventricular angiography code (93566) should not be used with 0646T to report:

1. Contrast injections, angiography, roadmapping, and/or fluoroscopic guidance for the TTVI,

2. Right atrial and/or ventricular angiography to assess or confirm valve positioning and function,

3. Right heart catheterization for hemodynamic measurements before, during, and after TTVI for guidance of TTVI.

Diagnostic right heart catheterization codes (93451, 93453, 93456, 93457, 93460, 93461, 93593, 93594, 93596, 93597) and right atrial/right ventricular angiography code (93566) performed at the time of TTVI may be separately reportable, if:

1. No prior study is available and a full diagnostic study is performed, or

2. A prior study is available, but as documented in the medical record:

   a. There is inadequate visualization of the anatomy and/or pathology, or

   b. The patient's condition with respect to the clinical indication has changed since the prior study, or

   c. There is a clinical change during the procedure that requires new evaluation.

For same session/same day diagnostic cardiac catheterization services, report the appropriate diagnostic cardiac catheterization code(s) appended with modifier 59, indicating separate and distinct procedural service from TTVI.

When transcatheter ventricular support is required in conjunction with TTVI, the procedure may be reported with the appropriate ventricular assist device (VAD) procedure code (33990, 33991, 33992, 33993) or balloon pump insertion code (33967, 33970, 33973).

 # 0646T Transcatheter tricuspid valve implantation (TTVI)/ replacement with prosthetic valve, percutaneous approach, including right heart catheterization, temporary pacemaker insertion, and selective right ventricular or right atrial angiography, when performed
Sunset January 2027
➔ *CPT Changes: An Insider's View* 2022
➔ *CPT Assistant* Jul 22:8

(Do not report 0646T in conjunction with 33210, 33211 for temporary pacemaker insertion)

(Do not report 0646T in conjunction with 93451, 93453, 93456, 93457, 93460, 93461, 93503, 93566, 93593, 93594, 93596, 93597, for diagnostic right heart catheterization procedures intrinsic to the valve repair procedure)

(Do not report 0646T in conjunction with 93662 for imaging guidance with intracardiac echocardiography)

(For transcatheter tricuspid valve annulus reconstruction, use 0545T)

(For transcatheter tricuspid valve repair, see 0569T, 0570T)

Implantable Cardioverter-Defibrillator with Substernal Electrode

An implantable cardioverter-defibrillator system with substernal electrode (substernal implantable cardioverter-defibrillator) consists of a pulse generator and at least one substernal electrode. The generator is placed in a subcutaneous pocket over the lateral rib cage. The electrode is tunneled subcutaneously and placed into the substernal anterior mediastinum, without entering the pericardial cavity. The electrode performs defibrillation and antitachycardia pacing, but not chronic pacing. The system requires programming and interrogation of the device.

All imaging guidance (eg, fluoroscopy) required to complete the substernal implantable defibrillator procedure is included in 0571T, 0572T, 0573T, 0574T. The work of implantation, removal, repositioning, interrogation, or programming of substernal implantable cardioverter-defibrillator systems, generators, or leads may not be reported using 33202-33275, 93260-93298, 93640, 93641, 93642, 93644.

0571T   Insertion or replacement of implantable cardioverter-defibrillator system with substernal electrode(s), including all imaging guidance and electrophysiological evaluation (includes defibrillation threshold evaluation, induction of arrhythmia, evaluation of sensing for arrhythmia termination, and programming or reprogramming of sensing or therapeutic parameters), when performed
Sunset January 2030
➡ *CPT Changes: An Insider's View* 2020

(Use 0571T in conjunction with 0573T, 0580T for removal and replacement of an implantable defibrillator pulse generator and substernal electrode)

(Do not report 0571T in conjunction with 93260, 93261, 93644, 0572T, 0575T, 0576T, 0577T)

(For insertion or replacement of permanent subcutaneous implantable defibrillator system with subcutaneous electrode, use 33270)

0572T   Insertion of substernal implantable defibrillator electrode
Sunset January 2030
➡ *CPT Changes: An Insider's View* 2020

(Do not report 0572T in conjunction with 93260, 93261, 93644, 0571T, 0575T, 0576T, 0577T, 0580T)

(For insertion of subcutaneous implantable defibrillator electrode, use 33271)

0573T   Removal of substernal implantable defibrillator electrode
Sunset January 2030
➡ *CPT Changes: An Insider's View* 2020

(Use 0573T in conjunction with 0580T for removal of substernal electrode in conjunction with removal of implantable defibrillator pulse generator without replacement)

(Do not report 0573T in conjunction with 93260, 93261, 93644, 0575T, 0576T, 0577T)

(For removal of subcutaneous implantable defibrillator electrode, use 33272)

0574T   Repositioning of previously implanted substernal implantable defibrillator-pacing electrode
Sunset January 2030
➡ *CPT Changes: An Insider's View* 2020

(Do not report 0574T in conjunction with 93260, 93261, 93644, 0572T, 0575T, 0576T, 0577T)

(For repositioning of previously implanted subcutaneous implantable defibrillator electrode, use 33273)

0575T   Programming device evaluation (in person) of implantable cardioverter-defibrillator system with substernal electrode, with iterative adjustment of the implantable device to test the function of the device and select optimal permanent programmed values with analysis, review and report by a physician or other qualified health care professional
Sunset January 2030
➡ *CPT Changes: An Insider's View* 2020

(Do not report 0575T in conjunction with pulse generator or lead insertion, removal or repositioning codes 0571T, 0572T, 0573T, 0574T, 0580T, 0614T)

(Do not report 0575T in conjunction with 93260, 93282, 93287, 0576T)

0576T   Interrogation device evaluation (in person) of implantable cardioverter-defibrillator system with substernal electrode, with analysis, review and report by a physician or other qualified health care professional, includes connection, recording and disconnection per patient encounter
Sunset January 2030
➡ *CPT Changes: An Insider's View* 2020

(Do not report 0576T in conjunction with pulse generator or lead insertion, removal or repositioning codes 0571T, 0572T, 0573T, 0574T, 0580T, 0614T)

(Do not report 0576T in conjunction with 93261, 93289, 0575T)

0577T Electrophysiologic evaluation of implantable cardioverter-defibrillator system with substernal electrode (includes defibrillation threshold evaluation, induction of arrhythmia, evaluation of sensing for arrhythmia termination, and programming or reprogramming of sensing or therapeutic parameters)
Sunset January 2030

➔ *CPT Changes: An Insider's View* 2020, 2021

(Do not report 0577T in conjunction with 93640, 93641, 93642, 93644, 0571T at the time of insertion or replacement of implantable defibrillator system with substernal lead)

(Do not report 0577T in conjunction with 0580T, 0614T)

(For electrophysiologic evaluation of subcutaneous implantable defibrillator system with subcutaneous electrode, use 93644)

0578T Interrogation device evaluation(s) (remote), up to 90 days, substernal lead implantable cardioverter-defibrillator system with interim analysis, review(s) and report(s) by a physician or other qualified health care professional
Sunset January 2030

➔ *CPT Changes: An Insider's View* 2020

(Do not report 0578T in conjunction with 93294, 93295, 93297, 93298, 0576T)

(Report 0578T only once per 90 days)

0579T Interrogation device evaluation(s) (remote), up to 90 days, substernal lead implantable cardioverter-defibrillator system, remote data acquisition(s), receipt of transmissions and technician review, technical support and distribution of results
Sunset January 2030

➔ *CPT Changes: An Insider's View* 2020

(Do not report 0579T in conjunction with 93296, 0576T)

(Report 0579T only once per 90 days)

0580T Removal of substernal implantable defibrillator pulse generator only
Sunset January 2030

➔ *CPT Changes: An Insider's View* 2020

(Use 0580T in conjunction with 0573T for removal of substernal electrode in conjunction with removal of implantable defibrillator pulse generator without replacement)

(Use 0580T in conjunction with 0571T, 0573T for removal and replacement of an implantable cardioverter-defibrillator and substernal electrode[s])

(Do not report 0580T in conjunction with 0575T, 0576T, 0577T, 0614T)

 # 0614T Removal and replacement of substernal implantable defibrillator pulse generator
Sunset January 2026

➔ *CPT Changes: An Insider's View* 2021

(Do not report 0614T in conjunction with 33262, 0571T, 0572T, 0575T, 0576T, 0577T, 0580T)

0581T Ablation, malignant breast tumor(s), percutaneous, cryotherapy, including imaging guidance when performed, unilateral
Sunset January 2030

➔ *CPT Changes: An Insider's View* 2020

(Report 0581T only once per breast treated)

(Do not report 0581T in conjunction with 76641, 76642, 76940, 76942)

(For cryoablation of breast fibroadenoma[s], use 19105)

0582T Transurethral ablation of malignant prostate tissue by high-energy water vapor thermotherapy, including intraoperative imaging and needle guidance
Sunset January 2030

➔ *CPT Changes: An Insider's View* 2020

(Do not report 0582T in conjunction with 52000, 72195, 72196, 72197, 76376, 76377, 76872, 76940, 76942, 77021, 77022)

(For transurethral destruction of prostate tissue by radiofrequency-generated water vapor thermotherapy for benign prostatic hypertrophy [BPH], use 53854)

0583T Tympanostomy (requiring insertion of ventilating tube), using an automated tube delivery system, iontophoresis local anesthesia
Sunset January 2030

➔ *CPT Changes: An Insider's View* 2020

(Do not report 0583T in conjunction with 69209, 69210, 69420, 69421, 69433, 69436, 69990, 92504, 97033)

(For bilateral procedure, report 0583T with modifier 50)

0584T Islet cell transplant, includes portal vein catheterization and infusion, including all imaging, including guidance, and radiological supervision and interpretation, when performed; percutaneous
Sunset January 2030

➔ *CPT Changes: An Insider's View* 2020

0585T laparoscopic
Sunset January 2030

➔ *CPT Changes: An Insider's View* 2020

0586T open
Sunset January 2030

➔ *CPT Changes: An Insider's View* 2020

0587T Percutaneous implantation or replacement of integrated single device neurostimulation system for bladder dysfunction including electrode array and receiver or pulse generator, including analysis, programming, and imaging guidance when performed, posterior tibial nerve
Sunset January 2030

➔ *CPT Changes: An Insider's View* 2020, 2024

(Do not report 0587T in conjunction with 64555, 64566, 64575, 64590, 64596, 95970, 95971, 95972, 0588T, 0589T, 0590T, 0816T, 0817T)

0588T Revision or removal of percutaneously placed integrated single device neurostimulation system for bladder dysfunction including electrode array and receiver or pulse generator, including analysis, programming, and imaging guidance when performed, posterior tibial nerve

Sunset January 2030

➔ *CPT Changes: An Insider's View 2020, 2024*

(Do not report 0588T in conjunction with 64555, 64566, 64575, 64590, 64598, 95970, 95971, 95972, 0587T, 0589T, 0590T, 0818T, 0819T)

0589T Electronic analysis with simple programming of implanted integrated neurostimulation system for bladder dysfunction (eg, electrode array and receiver), including contact group(s), amplitude, pulse width, frequency (Hz), on/off cycling, burst, dose lockout, patient-selectable parameters, responsive neurostimulation, detection algorithms, closed-loop parameters, and passive parameters, when performed by physician or other qualified health care professional, posterior tibial nerve, 1-3 parameters

Sunset January 2030

➔ *CPT Changes: An Insider's View 2020, 2024*

(Do not report 0589T in conjunction with 43647, 43648, 43881, 43882, 61850-61888, 63650, 63655, 63661, 63662, 63663, 63664, 63685, 63688, 64553-64595, 95970, 95971, 95972, 95976, 95977, 95983, 95984, 0587T, 0588T, 0590T, 0788T)

0590T Electronic analysis with complex programming of implanted integrated neurostimulation system for bladder dysfunction (eg, electrode array and receiver), including contact group(s), amplitude, pulse width, frequency (Hz), on/off cycling, burst, dose lockout, patient-selectable parameters, responsive neurostimulation, detection algorithms, closed-loop parameters, and passive parameters, when performed by physician or other qualified health care professional, posterior tibial nerve, 4 or more parameters

Sunset January 2030

➔ *CPT Changes: An Insider's View 2020, 2024*

(Do not report 0590T in conjunction with 43647, 43648, 43881, 43882, 61850-61888, 63650, 63655, 63661, 63662, 63663, 63664, 63685, 63688, 64553-64595, 95970, 95971, 95972, 95976, 95977, 95983, 95984, 0587T, 0588T, 0589T, 0788T)

Health and Well-Being Coaching

Health and well-being coaching is a patient-centered approach wherein patients determine their goals, use self-discovery or active learning processes together with content education to work toward their goals, and self-monitor behaviors to increase accountability, all within the context of an interpersonal relationship with a coach. The health and well-being coach is qualified to perform health and well-being coaching by education, training, national examination and, when applicable, licensure/regulation, and has completed a training program in health and well-being coaching whose content meets standards established by an applicable national credentialing organization. The training includes behavioral change theory, motivational strategies, communication techniques, health education and promotion theories, which are used to assist patients to develop intrinsic motivation and obtain skills to create sustainable change for improved health and well-being.

0591T Health and well-being coaching face-to-face; individual, initial assessment

Sunset January 2030

➔ *CPT Changes: An Insider's View 2020*

➔ *CPT Assistant Jul 20:7*

0592T individual, follow-up session, at least 30 minutes

Sunset January 2030

➔ *CPT Changes: An Insider's View 2020*

➔ *CPT Assistant Jul 20:7*

(Do not report 0592T in conjunction with 96156, 96158, 96159, 98960, 0488T, 0591T)

(For medical nutrition therapy, see 97802, 97803, 97804)

0593T group (2 or more individuals), at least 30 minutes

Sunset January 2030

➔ *CPT Changes: An Insider's View 2020*

➔ *CPT Assistant Jul 20:7*

(Do not report 0593T in conjunction with 96164, 96165, 97150, 98961, 98962, 0403T)

0594T Osteotomy, humerus, with insertion of an externally controlled intramedullary lengthening device, including intraoperative imaging, initial and subsequent alignment assessments, computations of adjustment schedules, and management of the intramedullary lengthening device

Sunset January 2026

➔ *CPT Changes: An Insider's View 2021*

(Do not report 0594T in conjunction with 20696, 24400, 24410, 24420, 24516)

(For revision of externally controlled intramedullary lengthening device, use 24999)

0596T Temporary female intraurethral valve-pump (ie, voiding prosthesis); initial insertion, including urethral measurement

Sunset January 2026

➔ *CPT Changes: An Insider's View 2021*

➔ *CPT Assistant Jan 21:11*

0597T   replacement
Sunset January 2026

➜ *CPT Changes: An Insider's View* 2021

➜ *CPT Assistant* Jan 21:11

(Do not report 0596T, 0597T in conjunction with 51610, 51700, 51701, 51702, 51703, 51705)

0598T   Noncontact real-time fluorescence wound imaging, for bacterial presence, location, and load, per session; first anatomic site (eg, lower extremity)
Sunset January 2026

➜ *CPT Changes: An Insider's View* 2021

➜ *CPT Assistant* Feb 21:14

+ 0599T   each additional anatomic site (eg, upper extremity) (List separately in addition to code for primary procedure)
Sunset January 2026

➜ *CPT Changes: An Insider's View* 2021

➜ *CPT Assistant* Feb 21:14

(Use 0599T in conjunction with 0598T)

0600T   Ablation, irreversible electroporation; 1 or more tumors per organ, including imaging guidance, when performed, percutaneous
Sunset January 2026

➜ *CPT Changes: An Insider's View* 2021

➜ *CPT Assistant* Mar 21:5

(Do not report 0600T in conjunction with 76940, 77002, 77013, 77022)

0601T   1 or more tumors per organ, including fluoroscopic and ultrasound guidance, when performed, open
Sunset January 2026

➜ *CPT Changes: An Insider's View* 2021

➜ *CPT Assistant* Mar 21:5

(Do not report 0601T in conjunction with 76940, 77002)

0602T   Glomerular filtration rate (GFR) measurement(s), transdermal, including sensor placement and administration of a single dose of fluorescent pyrazine agent
Sunset January 2026

➜ *CPT Changes: An Insider's View* 2021

0603T   Glomerular filtration rate (GFR) monitoring, transdermal, including sensor placement and administration of more than one dose of fluorescent pyrazine agent, each 24 hours
Sunset January 2026

➜ *CPT Changes: An Insider's View* 2021

(Do not report 0603T in conjunction with 0602T)

0604T   Optical coherence tomography (OCT) of retina, remote, patient-initiated image capture and transmission to a remote surveillance center, unilateral or bilateral; initial device provision, set-up and patient education on use of equipment
Sunset January 2026

➜ *CPT Changes: An Insider's View* 2021

0605T   remote surveillance center technical support, data analyses and reports, with a minimum of 8 daily recordings, each 30 days
Sunset January 2026

➜ *CPT Changes: An Insider's View* 2021

0606T   review, interpretation and report by the prescribing physician or other qualified health care professional of remote surveillance center data analyses, each 30 days
Sunset January 2026

➜ *CPT Changes: An Insider's View* 2021

(Do not report 0604T, 0605T, 0606T in conjunction with 99457, 99458)

0607T   Remote monitoring of an external continuous pulmonary fluid monitoring system, including measurement of radiofrequency-derived pulmonary fluid levels, heart rate, respiration rate, activity, posture, and cardiovascular rhythm (eg, ECG data), transmitted to a remote 24-hour attended surveillance center; set-up and patient education on use of equipment
Sunset January 2026

➜ *CPT Changes: An Insider's View* 2021

(Do not report 0607T in conjunction with 93224, 93225, 93226, 93227, 93228, 93229, 93264, 93268, 93270, 93271, 93272, 93297, 99453, for same monitoring period)

0608T   analysis of data received and transmission of reports to the physician or other qualified health care professional
Sunset January 2026

➜ *CPT Changes: An Insider's View* 2021

(Report 0608T only once per 30 days)

(Do not report 0608T in conjunction with 93224, 93225, 93226, 93227, 93228, 93229, 93264, 93268, 93270, 93271, 93272, 93297, 99454, for same monitoring period)

0609T   Magnetic resonance spectroscopy, determination and localization of discogenic pain (cervical, thoracic, or lumbar); acquisition of single voxel data, per disc, on biomarkers (ie, lactic acid, carbohydrate, alanine, laal, propionic acid, proteoglycan, and collagen) in at least 3 discs
Sunset January 2026

➜ *CPT Changes: An Insider's View* 2021

➜ *CPT Assistant* Jul 21:6

➜ *Clinical Examples in Radiology* Winter 21:5

0610T   transmission of biomarker data for software analysis
Sunset January 2026

➜ *CPT Changes: An Insider's View* 2021

➜ *CPT Assistant* Jul 21:6

➜ *Clinical Examples in Radiology* Winter 21:5

0611T   postprocessing for algorithmic analysis of biomarker data for determination of relative chemical differences between discs
Sunset January 2026
➔ *CPT Changes: An Insider's View* 2021
➔ *CPT Assistant* Jul 21:6
➔ *Clinical Examples in Radiology* Winter 21:5

0612T   interpretation and report
Sunset January 2026
➔ *CPT Changes: An Insider's View* 2021
➔ *CPT Assistant* Jul 21:6
➔ *Clinical Examples in Radiology* Winter 21:5

(Do not report 0609T, 0610T, 0611T, 0612T in conjunction with 72141, 72142, 72146, 72147, 72148, 72149, 72156, 72157, 72158, 72159, 76390)

0613T   Percutaneous transcatheter implantation of interatrial septal shunt device, including right and left heart catheterization, intracardiac echocardiography, and imaging guidance by the proceduralist, when performed
Sunset January 2026
➔ *CPT Changes: An Insider's View* 2021

(Do not report 0613T in conjunction with 76937, 93313, 93314, 93318, 93355, 93451, 93452, 93453, 93456, 93457, 93458, 93459, 93460, 93461, 93462, 93593, 93594, 93595, 93596, 93597, 93598, 93662)

(For transcatheter atrial septostomy for congenital cardiac abnormality, use 33741)

(For transcatheter intracardiac shunt creation by stent placement for congenital cardiac abnormality, see 33745, 33746)

(For transvenous atrial balloon septectomy or septostomy, see 33741, 33745, 33746)

0614T   Code is out of numerical sequence. See 0579T-0582T

▲ **0615T**   Automated analysis of binocular eye movements without spatial calibration, including disconjugacy, saccades, and pupillary dynamics for the assessment of concussion, with interpretation and report
Sunset January 2029
➔ *CPT Changes: An Insider's View* 2021, 2025

▶(For recording of saccades with electrooculography, see 92499, 92700)◀

▶(0616T, 0617T, 0618T have been deleted)◀

▶(For implantation of iris prosthesis, including suture fixation and repair or removal of iris, when performed, use 66683)◀

0619T   Cystourethroscopy with transurethral anterior prostate commissurotomy and drug delivery, including transrectal ultrasound and fluoroscopy, when performed
Sunset January 2026
➔ *CPT Changes: An Insider's View* 2021

(Do not report 0619T in conjunction with 52000, 52441, 52442, 52450, 52500, 52601, 52630, 52640, 52647, 52648, 52649, 53850, 53852, 53854, 76872)

0620T   Code is out of numerical sequence. See 0496T-0507T

0621T   Trabeculostomy ab interno by laser;
Sunset January 2026
➔ *CPT Changes: An Insider's View* 2021
➔ *CPT Assistant* Sep 21:10, Nov 21:14, Sep 23:42

0622T   with use of ophthalmic endoscope
Sunset January 2026
➔ *CPT Changes: An Insider's View* 2021
➔ *CPT Assistant* Sep 21:10, Nov 21:14, Sep 23:42

(Do not report 0621T, 0622T in conjunction with 92020, 0730T)

0623T   Code is out of numerical sequence. See 0496T-0507T

0624T   Code is out of numerical sequence. See 0496T-0507T

0625T   Code is out of numerical sequence. See 0496T-0507T

0626T   Code is out of numerical sequence. See 0496T-0507T

0627T   Percutaneous injection of allogeneic cellular and/or tissue-based product, intervertebral disc, unilateral or bilateral injection, with fluoroscopic guidance, lumbar; first level
Sunset January 2026
➔ *CPT Changes: An Insider's View* 2021
➔ *CPT Assistant* Oct 21:10
➔ *Clinical Examples in Radiology* Winter 22:18

+ **0628T**   each additional level (List separately in addition to code for primary procedure)
Sunset January 2026
➔ *CPT Changes: An Insider's View* 2021
➔ *CPT Assistant* Oct 21:10
➔ *Clinical Examples in Radiology* Winter 22:18

(Use 0628T in conjunction with 0627T)

(Do not report 0627T, 0628T in conjunction with 77003)

0629T   Percutaneous injection of allogeneic cellular and/or tissue-based product, intervertebral disc, unilateral or bilateral injection, with CT guidance, lumbar; first level
Sunset January 2026
➔ *CPT Changes: An Insider's View* 2021
➔ *CPT Assistant* Oct 21:10
➔ *Clinical Examples in Radiology* Winter 22:19

+ **0630T**   each additional level (List separately in addition to code for primary procedure)
Sunset January 2026
➔ *CPT Changes: An Insider's View* 2021
➔ *CPT Assistant* Oct 21:10
➔ *Clinical Examples in Radiology* Winter 22:19

(Use 0630T in conjunction with 0629T)

(Do not report 0629T, 0630T in conjunction with 77012)

0631T Transcutaneous visible light hyperspectral imaging measurement of oxyhemoglobin, deoxyhemoglobin, and tissue oxygenation, with interpretation and report, per extremity

Sunset January 2026

➔ *CPT Changes: An Insider's View* 2021

(Do not report 0631T in conjunction with 94760, 94761, 94762, 0061U)

0632T Percutaneous transcatheter ultrasound ablation of nerves innervating the pulmonary arteries, including right heart catheterization, pulmonary artery angiography, and all imaging guidance

Sunset January 2026

➔ *CPT Changes: An Insider's View* 2021

(Do not report 0632T in conjunction with 36013, 36014, 36015, 75741, 75743, 75746, 93451, 93453, 93456, 93460, 93503, 93505, 93568, 93593, 93594, 93596, 93597)

(For percutaneous transcatheter thermal ablation of nerves innervating the pulmonary arteries, including right heart catheterization, pulmonary artery angiography, and all imaging guidance, use 0793T)

0633T Computed tomography, breast, including 3D rendering, when performed, unilateral; without contrast material

Sunset January 2026

➔ *CPT Changes: An Insider's View* 2021

➔ *Clinical Examples in Radiology* Summer 21:3

0634T with contrast material(s)

Sunset January 2026

➔ *CPT Changes: An Insider's View* 2021

➔ *Clinical Examples in Radiology* Summer 21:3

0635T without contrast, followed by contrast material(s)

Sunset January 2026

➔ *CPT Changes: An Insider's View* 2021

➔ *Clinical Examples in Radiology* Summer 21:3

(Do not report 0633T, 0634T, 0635T in conjunction with 76376, 76377, 76380, 76497)

0636T Computed tomography, breast, including 3D rendering, when performed, bilateral; without contrast material(s)

Sunset January 2026

➔ *CPT Changes: An Insider's View* 2021

➔ *Clinical Examples in Radiology* Summer 21:3

0637T with contrast material(s)

Sunset January 2026

➔ *CPT Changes: An Insider's View* 2021

➔ *Clinical Examples in Radiology* Summer 21:3

0638T without contrast, followed by contrast material(s)

Sunset January 2026

➔ *CPT Changes: An Insider's View* 2021

➔ *Clinical Examples in Radiology* Summer 21:3

(Do not report 0636T, 0637T, 0638T in conjunction with 76376, 76377, 76380, 76497)

0639T Wireless skin sensor thermal anisotropy measurement(s) and assessment of flow in cerebrospinal fluid shunt, including ultrasound guidance, when performed

Sunset January 2026

➔ *CPT Changes: An Insider's View* 2021

(Do not report 0639T in conjunction with 76998, 76999)

0640T Code is out of numerical sequence. See 0489T-0495T

Code 0644T is for transcatheter percutaneous removal or debulking of intracardiac vegetations (eg, endocarditis) or mass(es) (eg, thrombus) using a suction device. Code 0644T includes the work of percutaneous access, all associated sheath device introduction, manipulation and positioning of guidewires and selective and non-selective catheterizations (eg, 36140, 36200, 36215, 36216, 36217, 36218, 36245, 36246, 36247, 36248), blood vessel dilation, embolic protection if used, percutaneous venous thrombectomy (eg, 37187, 37188), and closure of the blood vessel by pressure or application of an access vessel arterial closure device.

If an axillary, femoral, or iliac conduit is required to facilitate access of the catheter, 34714, 34716, or 34833 may be reported in addition to 0644T.

Extensive repair or replacement of a blood vessel (eg, 35206, 35226, 35231, 35236, 35256, 35266, 35286, 35302, 35371) may be reported separately.

Fluoroscopic and ultrasound guidance used in conjunction with percutaneous intracardiac mass removal is not separately reported. Transesophageal echocardiography guidance may be reported separately when provided by a separate provider.

The insertion and removal of arterial and/or venous cannula(e) (eg, 33951, 33952, 33953, 33954, 33955, 33956, 33965, 33966, 33969, 33984, 33985, 33986) and initiation (eg, 33946, 33947) of the extracorporeal circuit (veno-arterial or veno-venous) for intraoperative reinfusion of aspirated blood is included in the procedure. If prolonged extracorporeal membrane oxygenation (ECMO) or extracorporeal life support (ECLS) is required at the conclusion of the procedure, then the appropriate ECMO cannula(e) insertion code (eg, 33951, 33952, 33953, 33954, 33955, 33956), removal code (33965, 33966, 33969, 33984, 33985, 33986), and initiation code (eg, 33946, 33947) may be reported in addition to 0644T.

Other interventional procedures performed at the time of percutaneous intracardiac mass removal may be reported separately (eg, removal of infected pacemaker leads, removal of tunneled catheters, placement of dialysis catheters, valve repair, or replacement).

★ = Telemedicine ◀ = Audio-only ✦ = Add-on code ✗ = FDA approval pending # = Resequenced code ⊘ = Modifier 51 exempt ➔➔➔ = See p xxi for details

When transcatheter ventricular support is required in conjunction with percutaneous intracardiac mass removal, 0644T may be reported with the appropriate ventricular assist device (VAD) procedure code (33975, 33976, 33990, 33991, 33992, 33993, 33995, 33997, 33999) or balloon pump insertion code (33967, 33970, 33973).

When cardiopulmonary bypass is performed in conjunction with percutaneous intracardiac mass removal, 0644T may be reported with the appropriate add-on code for percutaneous peripheral bypass (33367), open peripheral bypass (33368), or central bypass (33369).

0643T   Code is out of numerical sequence. See 0544T-0547T

0644T   Transcatheter removal or debulking of intracardiac mass (eg, vegetations, thrombus) via suction (eg, vacuum, aspiration) device, percutaneous approach, with intraoperative reinfusion of aspirated blood, including imaging guidance, when performed
Sunset January 2027
➔ CPT Changes: An Insider's View 2022
➔ CPT Assistant Jun 22:22

(Do not report 0644T in conjunction with 37187, 37188)

Code 0645T describes transcatheter implantation of a coronary sinus reduction device and includes vascular access, ultrasound guidance, vascular closure, right heart catheterization, coronary sinus catheterization, venography, coronary sinus angiography, right atrial or right ventricular angiography, any interventions in the coronary sinus, and any other imaging required for guidance of the coronary sinus reduction device placement.

Intracardiac echocardiography (93662), when performed, is included in 0645T. Transesophageal echocardiography (93355) performed by a separate operator for guidance of the procedure may be separately reported.

Diagnostic right heart catheterization codes (93451, 93453, 93456, 93457, 93460, 93461, 93566, 93593, 93594, 93596, 93597, 93598) should **not** be used in conjunction with 0645T to report contrast injections, angiography, roadmapping, fluoroscopic guidance for the coronary sinus reduction device implantation, right atrial, right ventricular, or coronary sinus angiography to assess or confirm device positioning and function, or right heart catheterization for hemodynamic measurements before, during, and after coronary sinus reduction device implantation for guidance of the procedure.

Diagnostic right and left heart catheterization codes (93451, 93452, 93453, 93456, 93457, 93458, 93459, 93460, 93461, 93566, 93593, 93594, 93595, 93596, 93597, 93598) and diagnostic coronary angiography codes (93454, 93455, 93456, 93457, 93458, 93459, 93460, 93461, 93563, 93564) performed at the time of coronary sinus reduction device implantation may be separately reportable, if:

1. No prior study is available and a full diagnostic study is performed, or

2. A prior study is available, but as documented in the medical record:

   a. There is inadequate visualization of the anatomy and/or pathology, or

   b. The patient's condition with respect to the clinical indication has changed since the prior study, or

   c. There is a clinical change during the procedure that requires new evaluation.

For same session/same day diagnostic cardiac catheterization services, report the appropriate diagnostic cardiac catheterization code(s) appended with modifier 59, indicating separate and distinct procedural service from transcatheter coronary sinus reduction implantation.

0645T   Transcatheter implantation of coronary sinus reduction device including vascular access and closure, right heart catheterization, venous angiography, coronary sinus angiography, imaging guidance, and supervision and interpretation, when performed
Sunset January 2027
➔ CPT Changes: An Insider's View 2022

(Do not report 0645T in conjunction with 36010, 36011, 36012, 36013, 37246, 37247, 37252, 37253, 75827, 75860, 76000, 76499, 76937, 77001, 93451, 93453, 93456, 93457, 93460, 93461, 93566, 93593, 93594, 93596, 93597, 93598, 93662)

0646T   Code is out of numerical sequence. See 0569T-0572T

0647T   Insertion of gastrostomy tube, percutaneous, with magnetic gastropexy, under ultrasound guidance, image documentation and report
Sunset January 2027
➔ CPT Changes: An Insider's View 2022

(Do not report 0647T in conjunction with 76942)

0648T   Quantitative magnetic resonance for analysis of tissue composition (eg, fat, iron, water content), including multiparametric data acquisition, data preparation and transmission, interpretation and report, obtained without diagnostic MRI examination of the same anatomy (eg, organ, gland, tissue, target structure) during the same session; single organ
Sunset January 2027
➔ CPT Changes: An Insider's View 2022
➔ CPT Assistant May 22:9,10
➔ Clinical Examples in Radiology Winter 22:6, Fall 22:17, Fall 23:28, Winter 24:12

(Do not report 0648T in conjunction with 0649T, 0697T, 0698T, when also evaluating same organ, gland, tissue, or target structure)

0697T   multiple organs
                 Sunset January 2027

➔ *CPT Changes: An Insider's View* 2022

➔ *CPT Assistant* May 22:9,10

➔ *Clinical Examples in Radiology* Winter 22:6, Fall 22:17, Fall 23:28, Winter 24:12

►(Do not report 0648T, 0697T in conjunction with 70540, 70542, 70543, 70551, 70552, 70553, 71550, 71551, 71552, 72141, 72142, 72146, 72147, 72148, 72149, 72156, 72157, 72158, 72195, 72196, 72197, 73218, 73219, 73220, 73221, 73222, 73223, 73718, 73719, 73720, 73721, 73722, 73723, 74181, 74182, 74183, 75557, 75559, 75561, 75563, 76390, 76498, 77046, 77047, 77048, 77049, when also evaluating same organ, gland, tissue, or target structure)◄

(Do not report 0697T in conjunction with 0648T, 0649T, 0698T, when also evaluating same organ, gland, tissue, or target structure)

+ 0649T   Quantitative magnetic resonance for analysis of tissue composition (eg, fat, iron, water content), including multiparametric data acquisition, data preparation and transmission, interpretation and report, obtained with diagnostic MRI examination of the same anatomy (eg, organ, gland, tissue, target structure); single organ (List separately in addition to code for primary procedure)
                 Sunset January 2027

➔ *CPT Changes: An Insider's View* 2022

➔ *CPT Assistant* May 22:9,10

➔ *Clinical Examples in Radiology* Winter 22:6, Fall 22:17, Fall 23:27, Winter 24:12

(Do not report 0649T in conjunction with 0648T, 0697T, 0698T, when also evaluating same organ, gland, tissue, or target structure)

#+ 0698T   multiple organs (List separately in addition to code for primary procedure)
                 Sunset January 2027

➔ *CPT Changes: An Insider's View* 2022

➔ *CPT Assistant* May 22:9,10

➔ *Clinical Examples in Radiology* Winter 22:7, Fall 22:17, Fall 23:27, Winter 24:12

►(Use 0649T, 0698T in conjunction with 70540, 70542, 70543, 70551, 70552, 70553, 71550, 71551, 71552, 72141, 72142, 72146, 72147, 72148, 72149, 72156, 72157, 72158, 72195, 72196, 72197, 73218, 73219, 73220, 73221, 73222, 73223, 73718, 73719, 73720, 73721, 73722, 73723, 74181, 74182, 74183, 75557, 75559, 75561, 75563, 76390, 76498, 77046, 77047, 77048, 77049, when also evaluating same organ, gland, tissue, or target structure)◄

(Do not report 0698T in conjunction with 0648T, 0649T, 0697T, when also evaluating same organ, gland, tissue, or target structure)

Subcutaneous Cardiac Rhythm Monitor System Programming Device Evaluation (Remote)

The programming evaluation of a subcutaneous cardiac rhythm monitor system may be performed in-person or remotely. Codes 93285, 0650T are reported per procedure. Remote programming device evaluation (0650T) includes in-person device programming (93285), when performed, on the same day. Programming device evaluation includes all components of the interrogation device evaluation. Therefore, 93291 (in-person interrogation) should not be reported in conjunction with 93285, 0650T. Programming device evaluations (93285, 0650T) and remote interrogation device evaluations (93298) may both be reported during the 30-day remote interrogation device evaluation period.

0650T   Programming device evaluation (remote) of subcutaneous cardiac rhythm monitor system, with iterative adjustment of the implantable device to test the function of the device and select optimal permanently programmed values with analysis, review and report by a physician or other qualified health care professional
               Sunset January 2027

➔ *CPT Changes: An Insider's View* 2022

➔ *CPT Assistant* Sep 22:1

(Do not report 0650T in conjunction with 33285, 93260, 93279, 93280, 93281, 93282, 93284, 93285, 93291)

0651T   Magnetically controlled capsule endoscopy, esophagus through stomach, including intraprocedural positioning of capsule, with interpretation and report
               Sunset January 2027

➔ *CPT Changes: An Insider's View* 2022

(Do not report 0651T in conjunction with 91110, 91111)

0652T   Esophagogastroduodenoscopy, flexible, transnasal; diagnostic, including collection of specimen(s) by brushing or washing, when performed (separate procedure)
               Sunset January 2027

➔ *CPT Changes: An Insider's View* 2022

➔ *CPT Assistant* Sep 22:13

0653T   with biopsy, single or multiple
               Sunset January 2027

➔ *CPT Changes: An Insider's View* 2022

➔ *CPT Assistant* Sep 22:13

0654T   with insertion of intraluminal tube or catheter
               Sunset January 2027

➔ *CPT Changes: An Insider's View* 2022

➔ *CPT Assistant* Sep 22:13

(For rigid transoral esophagoscopy services, see 43191, 43192, 43193, 43194, 43195)

(For diagnostic transnasal esophagoscopy, use 43197)

(For transnasal esophagoscopy with biopsy[ies], use 43198)

(For transoral esophagoscopy, esophagogastro-duodenoscopy, see 43200-43232, 43235-43259, 43266, 43270)

(For other transnasal esophagogastroduodenoscopy services, see 43499, 43999, 44799)

0655T   Transperineal focal laser ablation of malignant prostate tissue, including transrectal imaging guidance, with MR-fused images or other enhanced ultrasound imaging
Sunset January 2027
➲ *CPT Changes: An Insider's View* 2022

(Do not report 0655T in conjunction with 52000, 76376, 76377, 76872, 76940, 76942, 76998)

0656T   Anterior lumbar or thoracolumbar vertebral body tethering; up to 7 vertebral segments
Sunset January 2029
➲ *CPT Changes: An Insider's View* 2022, 2024
➲ *CPT Assistant* Jan 24:26

0657T   8 or more vertebral segments
Sunset January 2029
➲ *CPT Changes: An Insider's View* 2022, 2024
➲ *CPT Assistant* Jan 24:26

(Do not report 0656T, 0657T in conjunction with 22800, 22802, 22804, 22808, 22810, 22812, 22818, 22819, 22845, 22846, 22847)

(For vertebral body tethering of the thoracic spine, see 22836, 22837)

 # 0790T   Revision (eg, augmentation, division of tether), replacement, or removal of thoracolumbar or lumbar vertebral body tethering, including thoracoscopy, when performed
Sunset January 2029
➲ *CPT Changes: An Insider's View* 2024
➲ *CPT Assistant* Jan 24:26

(For revision, replacement, or removal of thoracic vertebral body tethering, use 22838)

0658T   Electrical impedance spectroscopy of 1 or more skin lesions for automated melanoma risk score
Sunset January 2027
➲ *CPT Changes: An Insider's View* 2022

0659T   Transcatheter intracoronary infusion of supersaturated oxygen in conjunction with percutaneous coronary revascularization during acute myocardial infarction, including catheter placement, imaging guidance (eg, fluoroscopy), angiography, and radiologic supervision and interpretation
Sunset January 2027
➲ *CPT Changes: An Insider's View* 2022

(Use 0659T in conjunction with 92941)

(Do not report 0659T in conjunction with 92920, 92924, 92928, 92933, 92937, 92943)

0660T   Implantation of anterior segment intraocular nonbiodegradable drug-eluting system, internal approach
Sunset January 2027
➲ *CPT Changes: An Insider's View* 2022

(Report medication separately)

0661T   Removal and reimplantation of anterior segment intraocular nonbiodegradable drug-eluting implant
Sunset January 2027
➲ *CPT Changes: An Insider's View* 2022

(Report medication separately)

0662T   Scalp cooling, mechanical; initial measurement and calibration of cap
Sunset January 2027
➲ *CPT Changes: An Insider's View* 2022
➲ *CPT Assistant* Oct 22:19

(Report 0662T once per chemotherapy treatment period)

+ 0663T   placement of device, monitoring, and removal of device (List separately in addition to code for primary procedure)
Sunset January 2027
➲ *CPT Changes: An Insider's View* 2022
➲ *CPT Assistant* Oct 22:19

(Use 0663T in conjunction with 96409, 96411, 96413, 96415, 96416, 96417)

(Report 0663T once per chemotherapy session)

(For selective head or total body hypothermia in the critically ill neonate, use 99184)

Uterus Transplantation

Uterus allotransplantation involves three distinct components of physician work:

1. *Cadaver donor hysterectomy,* which includes harvesting the uterus allograft from a deceased (eg, brain-dead, cadaver) donor and cold preservation of the uterus allograft (perfusing with cold preservation solution and cold maintenance) (use 0664T). *Living donor hysterectomy,* which includes harvesting the uterus allograft, cold preservation of the uterus allograft (perfusing with cold preservation solution and cold maintenance), and care of the donor (see 0665T, 0666T).

2. ***Backbench work,*** which includes standard preparation of the cadaver or living uterus allograft prior to transplantation, such as dissection and removal of surrounding soft tissues to prepare uterine vein(s) and uterine artery(ies), as necessary (use 0668T). Additional reconstruction of the uterus allograft may include venous and/or arterial anastomosis(es) (see 0669T, 0670T).

3. ***Recipient uterus allotransplantation,*** which includes transplantation of the uterus allograft and care of the recipient (use 0667T).

0664T Donor hysterectomy (including cold preservation); open, from cadaver donor
Sunset January 2027
➡ *CPT Changes: An Insider's View* 2022

0665T open, from living donor
Sunset January 2027
➡ *CPT Changes: An Insider's View* 2022

0666T laparoscopic or robotic, from living donor
Sunset January 2027
➡ *CPT Changes: An Insider's View* 2022

0667T recipient uterus allograft transplantation from cadaver or living donor
Sunset January 2027
➡ *CPT Changes: An Insider's View* 2022

0668T Backbench standard preparation of cadaver or living donor uterine allograft prior to transplantation, including dissection and removal of surrounding soft tissues and preparation of uterine vein(s) and uterine artery(ies), as necessary
Sunset January 2027
➡ *CPT Changes: An Insider's View* 2022

0669T Backbench reconstruction of cadaver or living donor uterus allograft prior to transplantation; venous anastomosis, each
Sunset January 2027
➡ *CPT Changes: An Insider's View* 2022

0670T arterial anastomosis, each
Sunset January 2027
➡ *CPT Changes: An Insider's View* 2022

0671T Code is out of numerical sequence. See 0175T-0200T

0672T Endovaginal cryogen-cooled, monopolar radiofrequency remodeling of the tissues surrounding the female bladder neck and proximal urethra for urinary incontinence
Sunset January 2027
➡ *CPT Changes: An Insider's View* 2022

0673T Ablation, benign thyroid nodule(s), percutaneous, laser, including imaging guidance
Sunset January 2027
➡ *CPT Changes: An Insider's View* 2022

(Do not report 0673T in conjunction with 76940, 76942, 77013, 77022)

Implantable Synchronized Diaphragmatic Stimulation System for Augmentation of Cardiac Function

An implantable synchronized diaphragmatic stimulation system for augmentation of cardiac function consists of a pulse generator and two diaphragmatic leads. The generator is placed in a subcutaneous pocket in the abdomen. The electrodes are affixed to the inferior surface of the diaphragm. The electrodes deliver synchronized diaphragmatic stimulation (SDS) pulses, causing localized contractions of the diaphragm muscle gated to the cardiac cycle, designed to augment intrathoracic pressure and improve cardiac output and left ventricular function.

For laparoscopic insertion or replacement of the complete SDS system (diaphragmatic pulse generator and lead[s]), use 0674T. For laparoscopic insertion of new or replacement of diaphragmatic lead(s), see 0675T, 0676T. For repositioning or relocation of individual components of the SDS system, see 0677T, 0678T for the diaphragmatic lead(s), or use 0681T for the diaphragmatic pulse generator. For laparoscopic removal of diaphragmatic lead(s) without replacement, use 0679T. For insertion or replacement of the diaphragmatic pulse generator only, use 0680T. For removal of the generator only, use 0682T.

Codes 0674T, 0675T, 0676T, 0677T, 0678T, 0680T, 0681T include both interrogation and programming by the implant physician, when performed. Interrogation device evaluation and programming device evaluation include parameters of pulse amplitude, pulse duration, battery status, lead and electrode selectability, impedances, and R-wave sensitivity.

0674T Laparoscopic insertion of new or replacement of permanent implantable synchronized diaphragmatic stimulation system for augmentation of cardiac function, including an implantable pulse generator and diaphragmatic lead(s)
Sunset January 2027
➡ *CPT Changes: An Insider's View* 2022
➡ *CPT Assistant* Apr 22:5,6

(Do not report 0674T in conjunction with 0675T, 0676T, 0677T, 0678T, 0679T, 0680T, 0681T, 0682T, 0683T, 0684T, 0685T)

0675T   Laparoscopic insertion of new or replacement of diaphragmatic lead(s), permanent implantable synchronized diaphragmatic stimulation system for augmentation of cardiac function, including connection to an existing pulse generator; first lead

Sunset January 2027

➔ *CPT Changes: An Insider's View* 2022

➔ *CPT Assistant* Apr 22:5,6

+ 0676T   each additional lead (List separately in addition to code for primary procedure)

Sunset January 2027

➔ *CPT Changes: An Insider's View* 2022

➔ *CPT Assistant* Apr 22:5,6

(Use 0676T in conjunction with 0675T)

(Do not report 0675T, 0676T in conjunction with 0674T, 0677T, 0678T, 0679T, 0680T, 0681T, 0682T, 0683T, 0684T, 0685T)

0677T   Laparoscopic repositioning of diaphragmatic lead(s), permanent implantable synchronized diaphragmatic stimulation system for augmentation of cardiac function, including connection to an existing pulse generator; first repositioned lead

Sunset January 2027

➔ *CPT Changes: An Insider's View* 2022

➔ *CPT Assistant* Apr 22:5,7

+ 0678T   each additional repositioned lead (List separately in addition to code for primary procedure)

Sunset January 2027

➔ *CPT Changes: An Insider's View* 2022

➔ *CPT Assistant* Apr 22:5,7

(Use 0678T in conjunction with 0677T)

(Do not report 0677T, 0678T in conjunction with 0674T, 0675T, 0676T, 0679T, 0680T, 0681T, 0682T, 0683T, 0684T, 0685T)

0679T   Laparoscopic removal of diaphragmatic lead(s), permanent implantable synchronized diaphragmatic stimulation system for augmentation of cardiac function

Sunset January 2027

➔ *CPT Changes: An Insider's View* 2022

➔ *CPT Assistant* Apr 22:5,7

(Use 0679T only once regardless of the number of leads removed)

(Do not report 0679T in conjunction with 0674T, 0677T, 0680T, 0681T, 0682T, 0683T, 0684T, 0685T)

0680T   Insertion or replacement of pulse generator only, permanent implantable synchronized diaphragmatic stimulation system for augmentation of cardiac function, with connection to existing lead(s)

Sunset January 2027

➔ *CPT Changes: An Insider's View* 2022

➔ *CPT Assistant* Apr 22:5,7

(Do not report 0680T in conjunction with 0674T, 0675T, 0676T, 0677T, 0678T, 0679T, 0681T, 0682T, 0683T, 0684T, 0685T)

0681T   Relocation of pulse generator only, permanent implantable synchronized diaphragmatic stimulation system for augmentation of cardiac function, with connection to existing dual leads

Sunset January 2027

➔ *CPT Changes: An Insider's View* 2022

➔ *CPT Assistant* Apr 22:5,7

(Do not report 0681T in conjunction with 0674T, 0675T, 0676T, 0677T, 0678T, 0679T, 0680T, 0682T, 0683T, 0684T, 0685T)

0682T   Removal of pulse generator only, permanent implantable synchronized diaphragmatic stimulation system for augmentation of cardiac function

Sunset January 2027

➔ *CPT Changes: An Insider's View* 2022

➔ *CPT Assistant* Apr 22:5,7

(Do not report 0682T in conjunction with 0674T, 0675T, 0676T, 0677T, 0678T, 0679T, 0680T, 0681T, 0683T, 0684T, 0685T)

0683T   Programming device evaluation (in-person) with iterative adjustment of the implantable device to test the function of the device and select optimal permanent programmed values with analysis, review and report by a physician or other qualified health care professional, permanent implantable synchronized diaphragmatic stimulation system for augmentation of cardiac function

Sunset January 2027

➔ *CPT Changes: An Insider's View* 2022

➔ *CPT Assistant* Apr 22:5,7

(Do not report 0683T in conjunction with 0674T, 0675T, 0676T, 0677T, 0678T, 0679T, 0680T, 0681T, 0682T, 0684T, 0685T, when performed by the same physician or other qualified health care professional)

0684T   Peri-procedural device evaluation (in-person) and programming of device system parameters before or after a surgery, procedure, or test with analysis, review, and report by a physician or other qualified health care professional, permanent implantable synchronized diaphragmatic stimulation system for augmentation of cardiac function

Sunset January 2027

➔ *CPT Changes: An Insider's View* 2022

➔ *CPT Assistant* Apr 22:5,7

(Do not report 0684T in conjunction with 0674T, 0675T, 0677T, 0679T, 0680T, 0681T, 0682T, 0683T, 0685T, when performed by the same physician or other qualified health care professional)

0685T Interrogation device evaluation (in-person) with analysis, review and report by a physician or other qualified health care professional, including connection, recording and disconnection per patient encounter, permanent implantable synchronized diaphragmatic stimulation system for augmentation of cardiac function

Sunset January 2027

➔ *CPT Changes: An Insider's View* 2022

➔ *CPT Assistant* Apr 22:5,7

(Do not report 0685T in conjunction with 0674T, 0675T, 0677T, 0679T, 0680T, 0681T, 0682T, 0683T, 0684T, when performed by the same physician or other qualified health care professional)

0686T Histotripsy (ie, non-thermal ablation via acoustic energy delivery) of malignant hepatocellular tissue, including image guidance

Sunset January 2027

➔ *CPT Changes: An Insider's View* 2022

➔ *CPT Assistant* Jan 24:36

0687T Treatment of amblyopia using an online digital program; device supply, educational set-up, and initial session

Sunset January 2027

➔ *CPT Changes: An Insider's View* 2022

➔ *CPT Assistant* Feb 22:11

0688T assessment of patient performance and program data by physician or other qualified health care professional, with report, per calendar month

Sunset January 2027

➔ *CPT Changes: An Insider's View* 2022

➔ *CPT Assistant* Feb 22:11

(Do not report 0687T, 0688T in conjunction with 92065, when performed on the same day)

0689T Quantitative ultrasound tissue characterization (non-elastographic), including interpretation and report, obtained without diagnostic ultrasound examination of the same anatomy (eg, organ, gland, tissue, target structure)

Sunset January 2027

➔ *CPT Changes: An Insider's View* 2022

➔ *CPT Assistant* Dec 22:17

➔ *Clinical Examples in Radiology* Winter 22:3, Summer 22:19,21

(Do not report 0689T in conjunction with 76536, 76604, 76641, 76642, 76700, 76705, 76770, 76775, 76830, 76856, 76857, 76870, 76872, 76881, 76882, 76981, 76982, 76983, 76999, 93880, 93882, 93998, 0690T)

+ 0690T Quantitative ultrasound tissue characterization (non-elastographic), including interpretation and report, obtained with diagnostic ultrasound examination of the same anatomy (eg, organ, gland, tissue, target structure) (List separately in addition to code for primary procedure)

Sunset January 2027

➔ *CPT Changes: An Insider's View* 2022

➔ *CPT Assistant* Dec 22:17

➔ *Clinical Examples in Radiology* Winter 22:3, Summer 22:19-21

(Use 0690T in conjunction with 76536, 76604, 76641, 76642, 76700, 76705, 76770, 76775, 76830, 76856, 76857, 76870, 76872, 76881, 76882, 76981, 76982, 76999, 93880, 93882, 93998)

(Do not report 0690T in conjunction with 0689T)

0691T Automated analysis of an existing computed tomography study for vertebral fracture(s), including assessment of bone density when performed, data preparation, interpretation, and report

Sunset January 2027

➔ *CPT Changes: An Insider's View* 2022

(Do not report 0691T in conjunction with 71250, 71260, 71270, 71271, 71275, 72125, 72126, 72127, 72128, 72129, 72130, 72131, 72132, 72133, 72191, 72192, 72193, 72194, 74150, 74160, 74170, 74174, 74175, 74176, 74177, 74178, 74261, 74262, 74263, 75571, 75572, 75573, 75574, 75635, 78814, 78815, 78816, 0554T, 0555T, 0556T, 0557T, 0558T, 0743T)

0692T Therapeutic ultrafiltration

Sunset January 2027

➔ *CPT Changes: An Insider's View* 2022

(Use 0692T no more than once per day)

(Do not report 0692T in conjunction with 36511, 36512, 36513, 36514, 36516, 36522, 90935, 90937, 90945, 90947)

(For therapeutic apheresis, see 36511, 36512, 36513, 36514, 36516)

(For extracorporeal photopheresis, use 36522)

(For hemodialysis procedures, see 90935, 90937)

(For dialysis procedures, see 90945, 90947)

0693T Comprehensive full body computer-based markerless 3D kinematic and kinetic motion analysis and report

Sunset January 2027

➔ *CPT Changes: An Insider's View* 2022

0694T 3-dimensional volumetric imaging and reconstruction of breast or axillary lymph node tissue, each excised specimen, 3-dimensional automatic specimen reorientation, interpretation and report, real-time intraoperative

Sunset January 2027

➔ *CPT Changes: An Insider's View* 2022

(Do not report 0694T in conjunction with 76098)

(Report 0694T once per specimen)

0695T Body surface–activation mapping of pacemaker or pacing cardioverter-defibrillator lead(s) to optimize electrical synchrony, cardiac resynchronization therapy device, including connection, recording, disconnection, review, and report; at time of implant or replacement
Sunset January 2027
➔ *CPT Changes: An Insider's View* 2022

(Use 0695T in conjunction with 33224, 33225, 33226)

0696T at time of follow-up interrogation or programming device evaluation
Sunset January 2027
➔ *CPT Changes: An Insider's View* 2022

(Use 0696T in conjunction with 93281, 93284, 93286, 93287, 93288, 93289)

0697T Code is out of numerical sequence. See 0647T-0651T

0698T Code is out of numerical sequence. See 0647T-0651T

The anterior segment of the eye includes the cornea, lens, iris, and aqueous. The aqueous is divided into anterior and posterior chambers. The anterior chamber is by far the larger, including all of the aqueous in front of the lens and iris and behind the cornea. The posterior chamber includes the narrow area behind the iris and in front of the peripheral portion of the lens and lens zonules.

0699T Injection, posterior chamber of eye, medication
Sunset January 2027
➔ *CPT Changes: An Insider's View* 2022

0700T Molecular fluorescent imaging of suspicious nevus; first lesion
Sunset January 2027
➔ *CPT Changes: An Insider's View* 2022
➔ *CPT Assistant* Jul 22:12

+ 0701T each additional lesion (List separately in addition to code for primary procedure)
Sunset January 2027
➔ *CPT Changes: An Insider's View* 2022
➔ *CPT Assistant* Jul 22:12

(Use 0701T in conjunction with 0700T)

(0702T, 0703T have been deleted)

(For remote therapeutic monitoring of a standardized online digital cognitive behavioral therapy program, use 98978)

0704T Remote treatment of amblyopia using an eye tracking device; device supply with initial set-up and patient education on use of equipment
Sunset January 2027
➔ *CPT Changes: An Insider's View* 2022
➔ *CPT Assistant* Feb 22:11

0705T surveillance center technical support including data transmission with analysis, with a minimum of 18 training hours, each 30 days
Sunset January 2027
➔ *CPT Assistant* Feb 22:11

0706T interpretation and report by physician or other qualified health care professional, per calendar month
Sunset January 2027
➔ *CPT Changes: An Insider's View* 2022
➔ *CPT Assistant* Feb 22:11

(Do not report 0704T, 0705T, 0706T in conjunction with 92065, when performed on the same day)

(Do not report 0704T, 0705T, 0706T in conjunction with 0687T, 0688T, when reported during the same period)

0707T Injection(s), bone-substitute material (eg, calcium phosphate) into subchondral bone defect (ie, bone marrow lesion, bone bruise, stress injury, microtrabecular fracture), including imaging guidance and arthroscopic assistance for joint visualization
Sunset January 2027
➔ *CPT Changes: An Insider's View* 2022

(Do not report 0707T in conjunction with 29805, 29860, 29870, 77002)

(For aspiration and injection of bone cysts, use 20615)

0708T Intradermal cancer immunotherapy; preparation and initial injection
Sunset January 2027
➔ *CPT Changes: An Insider's View* 2022

+ 0709T each additional injection (List separately in addition to code for primary procedure)
Sunset January 2027

(Use 0709T in conjunction with 0708T)

(Do not report 0708T, 0709T in conjunction with 96372)

0710T Noninvasive arterial plaque analysis using software processing of data from non-coronary computerized tomography angiography; including data preparation and transmission, quantification of the structure and composition of the vessel wall and assessment for lipid-rich necrotic core plaque to assess atherosclerotic plaque stability, data review, interpretation and report
Sunset January 2027
➔ *CPT Changes: An Insider's View* 2022

(Do not report 0710T in conjunction with 0711T, 0712T, 0713T)

0711T data preparation and transmission
Sunset January 2027

0712T quantification of the structure and composition of the vessel wall and assessment for lipid-rich necrotic core plaque to assess atherosclerotic plaque stability
Sunset January 2027
➔ *CPT Changes: An Insider's View* 2022

0713T   data review, interpretation and report
               Sunset January 2027
               ➔ *CPT Changes: An Insider's View* 2022

(Do not report 0710T, 0711T, 0712T, 0713T in conjunction with 75580, 0623T, 0624T, 0625T, 0626T)

0714T   Code is out of numerical sequence. See 0419T-0422T

(0715T has been deleted)

(For percutaneous transluminal coronary lithotripsy, use 92972)

0716T   Cardiac acoustic waveform recording with automated analysis and generation of coronary artery disease risk score
               Sunset January 2028
               ➔ *CPT Changes: An Insider's View* 2023

0717T   Autologous adipose-derived regenerative cell (ADRC) therapy for partial thickness rotator cuff tear; adipose tissue harvesting, isolation and preparation of harvested cells, including incubation with cell dissociation enzymes, filtration, washing, and concentration of ADRCs
               Sunset January 2028
               ➔ *CPT Changes: An Insider's View* 2023
               ➔ *CPT Assistant* Dec 22:1

(Do not report 0717T in conjunction with 15769, 15771, 15772, 15773, 15774, 15876, 15877, 15878, 15879, 20610, 20611, 76942, 77002, 0232T, 0481T, 0489T, 0565T)

0718T   injection into supraspinatus tendon including ultrasound guidance, unilateral
               Sunset January 2028
               ➔ *CPT Changes: An Insider's View* 2023
               ➔ *CPT Assistant* Dec 22:1

(Do not report 0718T in conjunction with 20610, 20611, 76942, 77002, 0232T, 0481T, 0490T, 0566T)

0719T   Posterior vertebral joint replacement, including bilateral facetectomy, laminectomy, and radical discectomy, including imaging guidance, lumbar spine, single segment
               Sunset January 2028
               ➔ *CPT Changes: An Insider's View* 2023

(Do not report 0719T in conjunction with 22840, 63005, 63012, 63017, 63030, 63042, 63047, 63056, 76000, 76496)

0720T   Percutaneous electrical nerve field stimulation, cranial nerves, without implantation
               Sunset January 2028
               ➔ *CPT Changes: An Insider's View* 2023

0721T   Quantitative computed tomography (CT) tissue characterization, including interpretation and report, obtained without concurrent CT examination of any structure contained in previously acquired diagnostic imaging
               Sunset January 2028
               ➔ *CPT Changes: An Insider's View* 2023
               ➔ *Clinical Examples in Radiology* Spring 22:3

(Do not report 0721T in conjunction with 70450, 70460, 70470, 70480, 70481, 70482, 70486, 70487, 70488, 70490, 70491, 70492, 71250, 71260, 71270, 71271, 72125, 72126, 72127, 72128, 72129, 72130, 72131, 72132, 72133, 72192, 72193, 72194, 73200, 73201, 73202, 73700, 73701, 73702, 74150, 74160, 74170, 74176, 74177, 74178, 74261, 74262, 74263, 75571, 75572, 75573, 76497, 0722T, when performed on the same anatomy)

+ 0722T   Quantitative computed tomography (CT) tissue characterization, including interpretation and report, obtained with concurrent CT examination of any structure contained in the concurrently acquired diagnostic imaging dataset (List separately in addition to code for primary procedure)
               Sunset January 2028
               ➔ *CPT Changes: An Insider's View* 2023
               ➔ *Clinical Examples in Radiology* Spring 22:3

(Use 0722T in conjunction with 70450, 70460, 70470, 70480, 70481, 70482, 70486, 70487, 70488, 70490, 70491, 70492, 71250, 71260, 71270, 71271, 72125, 72126, 72127, 72128, 72129, 72130, 72131, 72132, 72133, 72192, 72193, 72194, 73200, 73201, 73202, 73700, 73701, 73702, 74150, 74160, 74170, 74176, 74177, 74178, 74261, 74262, 74263, 75571, 75572, 75573, 76497, 0721T)

0723T   Quantitative magnetic resonance cholangiopancreatography (QMRCP), including data preparation and transmission, interpretation and report, obtained without diagnostic magnetic resonance imaging (MRI) examination of the same anatomy (eg, organ, gland, tissue, target structure) during the same session
               Sunset January 2028
               ➔ *CPT Changes: An Insider's View* 2023
               ➔ *Clinical Examples in Radiology* Summer 22:2,6,7

(Do not report 0723T in conjunction with 74181, 74182, 74183, 76376, 76377, 0724T, when also evaluating same organ, gland, tissue, or target structure)

+ 0724T   Quantitative magnetic resonance cholangiopancreatography (QMRCP), including data preparation and transmission, interpretation and report, obtained with diagnostic magnetic resonance imaging (MRI) examination of the same anatomy (eg, organ, gland, tissue, target structure) (List separately in addition to code for primary procedure)
               Sunset January 2028
               ➔ *CPT Changes: An Insider's View* 2023
               ➔ *Clinical Examples in Radiology* Summer 22:2,6,7

(Use 0724T in conjunction with 74181, 74182, 74183, when also evaluating same organ, gland, tissue, or target structure)

(Do not report 0724T in conjunction with 76376, 76377, 0723T)

0725T　Vestibular device implantation, unilateral
　　　　Sunset January 2028
　　　　→ *CPT Changes: An Insider's View* 2023
　　　　→ *CPT Assistant* Dec 23:32

(Do not report 0725T in conjunction with 69501, 69502, 69505, 69511, 69601, 69602, 69603, 69604)

0726T　Removal of implanted vestibular device, unilateral
　　　　Sunset January 2028
　　　　→ *CPT Changes: An Insider's View* 2023
　　　　→ *CPT Assistant* Dec 23:32

(Do not report 0726T in conjunction with 69501, 69502, 69505, 69511, 69601, 69602, 69603, 69604)

0727T　Removal and replacement of implanted vestibular device, unilateral
　　　　Sunset January 2028
　　　　→ *CPT Changes: An Insider's View* 2023
　　　　→ *CPT Assistant* Dec 23:32

(Do not report 0727T in conjunction with 69501, 69502, 69505, 69511, 69601, 69602, 69603, 69604)

(For cochlear device implantation, with or without mastoidectomy, use 69930)

0728T　Diagnostic analysis of vestibular implant, unilateral; with initial programming
　　　　Sunset January 2028
　　　　→ *CPT Changes: An Insider's View* 2023
　　　　→ *CPT Assistant* Dec 23:32

0729T　　　with subsequent programming
　　　　Sunset January 2028
　　　　→ *CPT Changes: An Insider's View* 2023
　　　　→ *CPT Assistant* Dec 23:32

(For initial and subsequent diagnostic analysis and programming of cochlear implant, see 92601, 92602, 92603, 92604)

0730T　Trabeculotomy by laser, including optical coherence tomography (OCT) guidance
　　　　Sunset January 2028
　　　　→ *CPT Changes: An Insider's View* 2023
　　　　→ *CPT Assistant* Sep 23:42

(Do not report 0730T in conjunction with 65850, 65855, 92132, 0621T, 0622T)

0731T　Augmentative AI-based facial phenotype analysis with report
　　　　Sunset January 2028
　　　　→ *CPT Changes: An Insider's View* 2023

0732T　Immunotherapy administration with electroporation, intramuscular
　　　　Sunset January 2028
　　　　→ *CPT Changes: An Insider's View* 2023

0733T　Remote real-time, motion capture–based neurorehabilitative therapy ordered by a physician or other qualified health care professional; supply and technical support, per 30 days
　　　　Sunset January 2028
　　　　→ *CPT Changes: An Insider's View* 2023

0734T　　　treatment management services by a physician or other qualified health care professional, per calendar month
　　　　Sunset January 2028
　　　　→ *CPT Changes: An Insider's View* 2023

+ 0735T　Preparation of tumor cavity, with placement of a radiation therapy applicator for intraoperative radiation therapy (IORT) concurrent with primary craniotomy (List separately in addition to code for primary procedure)
　　　　Sunset January 2028
　　　　→ *CPT Changes: An Insider's View* 2023

(Use 0735T in conjunction with 61510, 61512, 61518, 61519, 61521)

0736T　Colonic lavage, 35 or more liters of water, gravity-fed, with induced defecation, including insertion of rectal catheter
　　　　Sunset January 2028
　　　　→ *CPT Changes: An Insider's View* 2023

0737T　Xenograft implantation into the articular surface
　　　　Sunset January 2028
　　　　→ *CPT Changes: An Insider's View* 2023

(Use 0737T once per joint)

(Do not report 0737T in conjunction with 27415, 27416)

0738T　Treatment planning for magnetic field induction ablation of malignant prostate tissue, using data from previously performed magnetic resonance imaging (MRI) examination
　　　　Sunset January 2028
　　　　→ *CPT Changes: An Insider's View* 2023
　　　　→ *CPT Assistant* Apr 23:20

(Do not report 0738T in conjunction with 0739T on the same date of service)

0739T　Ablation of malignant prostate tissue by magnetic field induction, including all intraprocedural, transperineal needle/catheter placement for nanoparticle installation and intraprocedural temperature monitoring, thermal dosimetry, bladder irrigation, and magnetic field nanoparticle activation
　　　　Sunset January 2028
　　　　→ *CPT Changes: An Insider's View* 2023
　　　　→ *CPT Assistant* Apr 23:20

(Do not report 0739T in conjunction with 51700, 51702, 72192, 72193, 72194, 72195, 72196, 72197, 74176, 74177, 74178, 76497, 76498, 76856, 76857, 76872, 76873, 76940, 76942, 76998, 76999, 77011, 77012, 77013, 77021, 77022, 77600, 77605, 77610, 77615, 77620)

0740T   Remote autonomous algorithm-based recommendation system for insulin dose calculation and titration; initial set-up and patient education
Sunset January 2028
➜ *CPT Changes: An Insider's View* 2023

(Do not report 0740T in conjunction with 95249, 95250, 95251, 98975, 99453)

0741T   provision of software, data collection, transmission, and storage, each 30 days
Sunset January 2028
➜ *CPT Changes: An Insider's View* 2023

(Do not report 0741T in conjunction with 95249, 95250, 95251, 99091, 99454)

(Do not report 0741T for data collection less than 16 days)

+ 0742T   Absolute quantitation of myocardial blood flow (AQMBF), single-photon emission computed tomography (SPECT), with exercise or pharmacologic stress, and at rest, when performed (List separately in addition to code for primary procedure)
Sunset January 2028
➜ *CPT Changes: An Insider's View* 2023

(Use 0742T in conjunction with 78451, 78452)

(For absolute quantification of myocardial blood flow [AQMBF] with positron emission tomography [PET], use 78434)

0743T   Bone strength and fracture risk using finite element analysis of functional data and bone mineral density (BMD), with concurrent vertebral fracture assessment, utilizing data from a computed tomography scan, retrieval and transmission of the scan data, measurement of bone strength and BMD and classification of any vertebral fractures, with overall fracture-risk assessment, interpretation and report
Sunset January 2028
➜ *CPT Changes: An Insider's View* 2023

(Do not report 0743T in conjunction with 0554T, 0555T, 0556T, 0557T, 0691T)

 # 0749T   Bone strength and fracture-risk assessment using digital X-ray radiogrammetry-bone mineral density (DXR-BMD) analysis of bone mineral density (BMD) utilizing data from a digital X ray, retrieval and transmission of digital X-ray data, assessment of bone strength and fracture risk and BMD, interpretation and report;
Sunset January 2028
➜ *CPT Changes: An Insider's View* 2023

(When the data from a concurrently performed wrist or hand X ray obtained for another purpose is used for the DXR-BMD analysis, use the appropriate X-ray code in conjunction with 0749T. If a single-view digital X ray of the hand is used as a data source, use 0750T)

 # 0750T   with single-view digital X-ray examination of the hand taken for the purpose of DXR-BMD
Sunset January 2028
➜ *CPT Changes: An Insider's View* 2023

0744T   Insertion of bioprosthetic valve, open, femoral vein, including duplex ultrasound imaging guidance, when performed, including autogenous or nonautogenous patch graft (eg, polyester, ePTFE, bovine pericardium), when performed
Sunset January 2028
➜ *CPT Changes: An Insider's View* 2023

(Do not report 0744T in conjunction with 34501, 34510, 76998, 93971)

0745T   Cardiac focal ablation utilizing radiation therapy for arrhythmia; noninvasive arrhythmia localization and mapping of arrhythmia site (nidus), derived from anatomical image data (eg, CT, MRI, or myocardial perfusion scan) and electrical data (eg, 12-lead ECG data), and identification of areas of avoidance
Sunset January 2028
➜ *CPT Changes: An Insider's View* 2023
➜ *CPT Assistant* May 23:18

(For catheter-based electrophysiologic evaluation, see 93609, 93619, 93620, 93621, 93622)

0746T   conversion of arrhythmia localization and mapping of arrhythmia site (nidus) into a multidimensional radiation treatment plan
Sunset January 2028
➜ *CPT Changes: An Insider's View* 2023
➜ *CPT Assistant* May 23:18

0747T   delivery of radiation therapy, arrhythmia
Sunset January 2028
➜ *CPT Changes: An Insider's View* 2023
➜ *CPT Assistant* May 23:18

0748T   Injections of stem cell product into perianal perifistular soft tissue, including fistula preparation (eg, removal of setons, fistula curettage, closure of internal openings)
Sunset January 2028
➜ *CPT Changes: An Insider's View* 2023

(Report 0748T once per session)

(Report stem cell product separately)

(Do not report 0748T in conjunction with 46030, 46940, 46942)

0749T Code is out of numerical sequence. See 0742T-0745T

0750T Code is out of numerical sequence. See 0742T-0745T

Digital Pathology Digitization Procedures

Digital pathology is a dynamic, image-based environment that enables the acquisition, management, and interpretation of pathology information generated from digitized glass microscope slides.

Glass microscope slides are scanned by clinical staff, and captured whole-slide images (either in real-time or stored in a computer server or cloud-based digital image archival and communication system) are used for digital examination for pathologic diagnosis distinct from direct visualization through a microscope. Static digital photographic and photomicrographic imaging or digital video streaming of any portion of a glass microscope slide on mobile smartphone and tablet devices does not constitute a digital pathology digitization procedure.

Digitization of glass microscope slides enables remote examination by the pathologist and/or in conjunction with the use of artificial intelligence (AI) algorithms. Category III add-on codes 0751T-0763T, 0827T-0856T may be reported in addition to the appropriate Category I service code when the digitization procedure of glass microscope slides is performed and reported in conjunction with the Category I code for the primary service. Each Category III add-on code is reported as a one-to-one unit of service for each primary pathology service code.

Do not report the Category III codes in this subsection solely for archival purposes (eg, after the Category I service has already been performed and reported), solely for educational purposes (eg, when services are not used for individual patient reporting), solely for developing a database for training or validation of AI algorithms, or solely for clinical conference presentations (eg, tumor board interdisciplinary conferences).

+ 0751T Digitization of glass microscope slides for level II, surgical pathology, gross and microscopic examination (List separately in addition to code for primary procedure)
Sunset January 2028
➔ *CPT Changes: An Insider's View* 2023

(Use 0751T in conjunction with 88302)

+ 0752T Digitization of glass microscope slides for level III, surgical pathology, gross and microscopic examination (List separately in addition to code for primary procedure)
Sunset January 2028
➔ *CPT Changes: An Insider's View* 2023

(Use 0752T in conjunction with 88304)

+ 0753T Digitization of glass microscope slides for level IV, surgical pathology, gross and microscopic examination (List separately in addition to code for primary procedure)
Sunset January 2028
➔ *CPT Changes: An Insider's View* 2023
➔ *CPT Assistant* Jun 23:31

(Use 0753T in conjunction with 88305)

+ 0754T Digitization of glass microscope slides for level V, surgical pathology, gross and microscopic examination (List separately in addition to code for primary procedure)
Sunset January 2028
➔ *CPT Changes: An Insider's View* 2023

(Use 0754T in conjunction with 88307)

+ 0755T Digitization of glass microscope slides for level VI, surgical pathology, gross and microscopic examination (List separately in addition to code for primary procedure)
Sunset January 2028
➔ *CPT Changes: An Insider's View* 2023

(Use 0755T in conjunction with 88309)

+ 0756T Digitization of glass microscope slides for special stain, including interpretation and report, group I, for microorganisms (eg, acid fast, methenamine silver) (List separately in addition to code for primary procedure)
Sunset January 2028
➔ *CPT Changes: An Insider's View* 2023

(Use 0756T in conjunction with 88312)

+ 0757T Digitization of glass microscope slides for special stain, including interpretation and report, group II, all other (eg, iron, trichrome), except stain for microorganisms, stains for enzyme constituents, or immunocytochemistry and immunohistochemistry (List separately in addition to code for primary procedure)
Sunset January 2028
➔ *CPT Changes: An Insider's View* 2023

(Use 0757T in conjunction with 88313)

+ 0758T Digitization of glass microscope slides for special stain, including interpretation and report, histochemical stain on frozen tissue block (List separately in addition to code for primary procedure)
Sunset January 2028
➔ *CPT Changes: An Insider's View* 2023

(Use 0758T in conjunction with 88314)

+ 0759T Digitization of glass microscope slides for special stain, including interpretation and report, group III, for enzyme constituents (List separately in addition to code for primary procedure)
Sunset January 2028
➔ *CPT Changes: An Insider's View* 2023

(Use 0759T in conjunction with 88319)

+ 0760T Digitization of glass microscope slides for immunohistochemistry or immunocytochemistry, per specimen, initial single antibody stain procedure (List separately in addition to code for primary procedure)
Sunset January 2028
→ *CPT Changes: An Insider's View* 2023

(Use 0760T in conjunction with 88342)

+ 0761T Digitization of glass microscope slides for immunohistochemistry or immunocytochemistry, per specimen, each additional single antibody stain procedure (List separately in addition to code for primary procedure)
Sunset January 2028
→ *CPT Changes: An Insider's View* 2023

(Use 0761T in conjunction with 88341)

+ 0762T Digitization of glass microscope slides for immunohistochemistry or immunocytochemistry, per specimen, each multiplex antibody stain procedure (List separately in addition to code for primary procedure)
Sunset January 2028
→ *CPT Changes: An Insider's View* 2023

(Use 0762T in conjunction with 88344)

+ 0763T Digitization of glass microscope slides for morphometric analysis, tumor immunohistochemistry (eg, Her-2/neu, estrogen receptor/progesterone receptor), quantitative or semiquantitative, per specimen, each single antibody stain procedure, manual (List separately in addition to code for primary procedure)
Sunset January 2028
→ *CPT Changes: An Insider's View* 2023

(Use 0763T in conjunction with 88360)

#+ 0827T Digitization of glass microscope slides for cytopathology, fluids, washings, or brushings, except cervical or vaginal; smears with interpretation (List separately in addition to code for primary procedure)
Sunset January 2029
→ *CPT Changes: An Insider's View* 2024

(Use 0827T in conjunction with 88104)

#+ 0828T simple filter method with interpretation (List separately in addition to code for primary procedure)
Sunset January 2029
→ *CPT Changes: An Insider's View* 2024

(Use 0828T in conjunction with 88106)

#+ 0829T Digitization of glass microscope slides for cytopathology, concentration technique, smears, and interpretation (eg, Saccomanno technique) (List separately in addition to code for primary procedure)
Sunset January 2029
→ *CPT Changes: An Insider's View* 2024

(Use 0829T in conjunction with 88108)

#+ 0830T Digitization of glass microscope slides for cytopathology, selective-cellular enhancement technique with interpretation (eg, liquid-based slide preparation method), except cervical or vaginal (List separately in addition to code for primary procedure)
Sunset January 2029
→ *CPT Changes: An Insider's View* 2024

(Use 0830T in conjunction with 88112)

#+ 0831T Digitization of glass microscope slides for cytopathology, cervical or vaginal (any reporting system), requiring interpretation by physician (List separately in addition to code for primary procedure)
Sunset January 2029
→ *CPT Changes: An Insider's View* 2024

(Use 0831T in conjunction with 88141)

(Do not report 0831T in conjunction with 88141, when digitization of glass microscope slides is performed using an automated, computer-assisted screening-imaging system)

#+ 0832T Digitization of glass microscope slides for cytopathology, smears, any other source; screening and interpretation (List separately in addition to code for primary procedure)
Sunset January 2029
→ *CPT Changes: An Insider's View* 2024

(Use 0832T in conjunction with 88160)

#+ 0833T preparation, screening and interpretation (List separately in addition to code for primary procedure)
Sunset January 2029
→ *CPT Changes: An Insider's View* 2024

(Use 0833T in conjunction with 88161)

#+ 0834T extended study involving over 5 slides and/or multiple stains (List separately in addition to code for primary procedure)
Sunset January 2029
→ *CPT Changes: An Insider's View* 2024

(Use 0834T in conjunction with 88162)

#+ 0835T Digitization of glass microscope slides for cytopathology, evaluation of fine needle aspirate; immediate cytohistologic study to determine adequacy for diagnosis, first evaluation episode, each site (List separately in addition to code for primary procedure)
Sunset January 2029
→ *CPT Changes: An Insider's View* 2024

(Use 0835T in conjunction with 88172)

(Do not report 0835T in conjunction with 88172, when 0837T is reported in conjunction with 88173)

#+ 0836T   immediate cytohistologic study to determine adequacy for diagnosis, each separate additional evaluation episode, same site (List separately in addition to code for primary procedure)
> Sunset January 2029
> ➔ *CPT Changes: An Insider's View* 2024

(Use 0836T in conjunction with 88177)

(Do not report 0836T in conjunction with 88177, when 0837T is reported in conjunction with 88173)

#+ 0837T   interpretation and report (List separately in addition to code for primary procedure)
> Sunset January 2029
> ➔ *CPT Changes: An Insider's View* 2024

(Use 0837T in conjunction with 88173)

#+ 0838T   Digitization of glass microscope slides for consultation and report on referred slides prepared elsewhere (List separately in addition to code for primary procedure)
> Sunset January 2029
> ➔ *CPT Changes: An Insider's View* 2024

(Use 0838T in conjunction with 88321)

(Do not report 0838T in conjunction with 88321 for referred digitized glass microscope slides prepared elsewhere)

#+ 0839T   Digitization of glass microscope slides for consultation and report on referred material requiring preparation of slides (List separately in addition to code for primary procedure)
> Sunset January 2029
> ➔ *CPT Changes: An Insider's View* 2024

(Use 0839T in conjunction with 88323)

(Do not report 0839T in conjunction with 88323 for referred digitized glass microscope slides prepared elsewhere)

#+ 0840T   Digitization of glass microscope slides for consultation, comprehensive, with review of records and specimens, with report on referred material (List separately in addition to code for primary procedure)
> Sunset January 2029
> ➔ *CPT Changes: An Insider's View* 2024

(Use 0840T in conjunction with 88325)

(Do not report 0840T in conjunction with 88325 for referred digitized glass microscope slides prepared elsewhere)

#+ 0841T   Digitization of glass microscope slides for pathology consultation during surgery; first tissue block, with frozen section(s), single specimen (List separately in addition to code for primary procedure)
> Sunset January 2029
> ➔ *CPT Changes: An Insider's View* 2024

(Use 0841T in conjunction with 88331)

#+ 0842T   each additional tissue block with frozen section(s) (List separately in addition to code for primary procedure)
> Sunset January 2029
> ➔ *CPT Changes: An Insider's View* 2024

(Use 0842T in conjunction with 88332)

#+ 0843T   cytologic examination (eg, touch preparation, squash preparation), initial site (List separately in addition to code for primary procedure)
> Sunset January 2029
> ➔ *CPT Changes: An Insider's View* 2024

(Use 0843T in conjunction with 88333)

#+ 0844T   cytologic examination (eg, touch preparation, squash preparation), each additional site (List separately in addition to code for primary procedure)
> Sunset January 2029
> ➔ *CPT Changes: An Insider's View* 2024

(Use 0844T in conjunction with 88334)

#+ 0845T   Digitization of glass microscope slides for immunofluorescence, per specimen; initial single antibody stain procedure (List separately in addition to code for primary procedure)
> Sunset January 2029
> ➔ *CPT Changes: An Insider's View* 2024

(Use 0845T in conjunction with 88346)

#+ 0846T   each additional single antibody stain procedure (List separately in addition to code for primary procedure)
> Sunset January 2029
> ➔ *CPT Changes: An Insider's View* 2024

(Use 0846T in conjunction with 88350)

#+ 0847T   Digitization of glass microscope slides for examination and selection of retrieved archival (ie, previously diagnosed) tissue(s) for molecular analysis (eg, *KRAS* mutational analysis) (List separately in addition to code for primary procedure)
> Sunset January 2029
> ➔ *CPT Changes: An Insider's View* 2024

(Use 0847T in conjunction with 88363)

(Do not report 0847T in conjunction 88363, when digitization of glass microscope slides has been previously reported)

#+ 0848T   Digitization of glass microscope slides for in situ hybridization (eg, FISH), per specimen; initial single probe stain procedure (List separately in addition to code for primary procedure)
> Sunset January 2029
> ➔ *CPT Changes: An Insider's View* 2024

(Use 0848T in conjunction with 88365)

#+ 0849T   each additional single probe stain procedure (List separately in addition to code for primary procedure)
Sunset January 2029
➡ *CPT Changes: An Insider's View* 2024

(Use 0849T in conjunction with 88364)

#+ 0850T   each multiplex probe stain procedure (List separately in addition to code for primary procedure)
Sunset January 2029
➡ *CPT Changes: An Insider's View* 2024

(Use 0850T in conjunction with 88366)

#+ 0851T   Digitization of glass microscope slides for morphometric analysis, in situ hybridization (quantitative or semiquantitative), manual, per specimen; initial single probe stain procedure (List separately in addition to code for primary procedure)
Sunset January 2029
➡ *CPT Changes: An Insider's View* 2024

(Use 0851T in conjunction with 88368)

#+ 0852T   each additional single probe stain procedure (List separately in addition to code for primary procedure)
Sunset January 2029
➡ *CPT Changes: An Insider's View* 2024

(Use 0852T in conjunction with 88369)

#+ 0853T   each multiplex probe stain procedure (List separately in addition to code for primary procedure)
Sunset January 2029
➡ *CPT Changes: An Insider's View* 2024

(Use 0853T in conjunction with 88377)

#+ 0854T   Digitization of glass microscope slides for blood smear, peripheral, interpretation by physician with written report (List separately in addition to code for primary procedure)
Sunset January 2029
➡ *CPT Changes: An Insider's View* 2024

(Use 0854T in conjunction with 85060)

(Do not report 0854T in conjunction with 85060, when digitization of glass microscope slides is performed using an automated, computer-assisted cell-morphology imaging analyzer)

#+ 0855T   Digitization of glass microscope slides for bone marrow, smear interpretation (List separately in addition to code for primary procedure)
Sunset January 2029
➡ *CPT Changes: An Insider's View* 2024

(Use 0855T in conjunction with 85097)

#+ 0856T   Digitization of glass microscope slides for electron microscopy, diagnostic (List separately in addition to code for primary procedure)
Sunset January 2029
➡ *CPT Changes: An Insider's View* 2024

(Use 0856T in conjunction with 88348)

+ 0764T   Assistive algorithmic electrocardiogram risk-based assessment for cardiac dysfunction (eg, low-ejection fraction, pulmonary hypertension, hypertrophic cardiomyopathy); related to concurrently performed electrocardiogram (List separately in addition to code for primary procedure)
Sunset January 2028
➡ *CPT Changes: An Insider's View* 2023

(Use 0764T in conjunction with 93000, 93010)

(Use 0764T only once for each unique, concurrently performed electrocardiogram tracing)

0765T   related to previously performed electrocardiogram
Sunset January 2028
➡ *CPT Changes: An Insider's View* 2023

(Use 0765T only once for each unique, previously performed electrocardiogram tracing)

Codes 0766T, 0767T describe transcutaneous magnetic stimulation that is performed to treat chronic nerve pain and provided by a physician or other qualified health care professional. The selected nerve is mapped and localized using magnetic stimulation at the time of each treatment and the appropriate amplitude of magnetic stimulation is defined. Noninvasive electroneurography (nerve conduction) may be used as guidance to confirm the precise localization of the selected nerve and, when performed, should not be separately reported as a diagnostic study. A separate diagnostic nerve conduction study performed prior to the decision to treat with transcutaneous magnetic stimulation may be separately reported.

0766T   Transcutaneous magnetic stimulation by focused low-frequency electromagnetic pulse, peripheral nerve, with identification and marking of the treatment location, including noninvasive electroneurographic localization (nerve conduction localization), when performed; first nerve
Sunset January 2028
➡ *CPT Changes: An Insider's View* 2023, 2024

+ 0767T   each additional nerve (List separately in addition to code for primary procedure)
Sunset January 2028
➡ *CPT Changes: An Insider's View* 2023, 2024

(Use 0767T in conjunction with 0766T)

(Do not report 0766T, 0767T in conjunction with 95885, 95886, 95887, 95905, 95907, 95908, 95909, 95910, 95911, 95912, 95913, for nerve conduction used as guidance for transcutaneous magnetic stimulation therapy)

(Do not report 0766T, 0767T in conjunction with 64566, 90867, 90868, 90869, 97014, 97032, 0278T, for the same nerve)

(For posterior tibial neurostimulation, percutaneous needle electrode, use 64566)

(For therapeutic repetitive transcranial magnetic stimulation [TMS] treatment, see 90867, 90868, 90869)

(For application of a modality to one or more areas, electrical stimulation [unattended], use 97014)

(For application of a modality to one or more areas, electrical stimulation [manual], each 15 minutes, use 97032)

(For transcutaneous electrical modulation pain reprocessing [eg, scrambler therapy], each treatment session [includes placement of electrodes], use 0278T)

(0768T, 0769T have been deleted)

(For transcutaneous magnetic stimulation by focused low-frequency electromagnetic pulse, peripheral nerve, see 0766T, 0767T)

Virtual reality (VR) technology may be integrated into multiple types of patient therapy as an adjunct to the base therapy. Code 0770T is an add-on code that represents the practice expense for the software used for the VR technology and may be reported for each session for which the VR technology is used. VR technology is incorporated into the base therapy session and is used to enhance the training or teaching of a skill upon which the therapy is focused. Code 0770T does not incur any additional reported therapist time beyond that already reported with the base therapy code.

+ 0770T   Virtual reality technology to assist therapy (List separately in addition to code for primary procedure)
Sunset January 2028

      ➔ *CPT Changes: An Insider's View* 2023

(Use 0770T only in conjunction with 90832, 90833, 90834, 90836, 90837, 90838, 90847, 90849, 90853, 92507, 92508, 96158, 96159, 96164, 96165, 96167, 96168, 96170, 96171, 97110, 97112, 97129, 97150, 97153, 97154, 97155, 97158, 97530, 97533, 97535, 97537)

(Do not report 0770T more than once per session)

Virtual Reality Patient Procedural Dissociation

Virtual reality (VR) procedural dissociation is a VR-based state of altered consciousness that supports and optimizes the patient's comfort, increases procedural tolerance, and decreases the patient's pain during the associated procedure. VR procedural dissociation establishes a computer-generated audio, visual, and proprioceptive immersive environment in which patients respond purposefully to verbal commands and stimuli, either alone or accompanied by light tactile stimulation. VR procedural dissociation does not involve interventions to maintain cardiovascular function, patent airway, or spontaneous ventilation.

VR procedural dissociation codes 0771T, 0772T, 0773T, 0774T are not used to report administration of medications for pain control, minimal sedation (anxiolysis), moderate sedation (99151, 99152, 99153, 99155, 99156, 99157), deep sedation, or monitored anesthesia care (00100-01999). Time spent administering VR procedural dissociation cannot be used to report moderate sedation or anesthesia services. VR procedural dissociation is not reported for patients younger than 5 years of age.

For 0771T, 0772T, the independent, trained observer is an individual who is qualified to monitor the patient during the procedure and has no other duties (eg, assisting at surgery) during the procedure. This individual has undergone training in immersive technologies and can adjust the technology under the supervision of the physician or other qualified health care professional who is performing the procedure. If the physician or other qualified health care professional who provides the VR also performs the procedure supported by VR (0771T, 0772T), the physician or other qualified health care professional will supervise and direct the independent, trained observer who will assist in monitoring the patient's level of consciousness, procedural disassociation, and physiological status throughout the procedure.

Intraservice time is used to determine the appropriate code to report VR procedural dissociation and is defined as:

- beginning with administration of the immersive VR technology, which at a minimum, includes audio, video, and proprioceptive feedback;

- requiring continuous face-to-face attendance of the physician or other qualified health care professional. Once continuous face-to-face time with the patient has ended, additional face-to-face time with the patient is not added to the intraservice time;

- ending when the procedure and the administration of the VR technology ends and the physician or other qualified health care professional is no longer continuously face-to-face with the patient;

- requiring monitoring patient response to the VR procedural dissociation, including;

  - periodic assessment of the patient;

  - monitoring of procedural tolerance, oxygen saturation, heart rate, pain, neurological status, and global anxiety;

  - altering of and/or adjustment of the VR program to optimize the dissociated state based on patient tolerance of the associated.

- Optimization techniques include:
  - changing the VR baseline software program and/or adjustment of program volume;
  - adjusting the visual virtual environment;
  - altering the visual virtual position of the VR program to enable patient repositioning;
  - changing an embedded video programming in the virtual environment to maintain the dissociated state; and
  - utilizing and adjusting a proprioception, olfactory, or tactile feedback loop that corresponds to the VR program to achieve a proper and/or deeper dissociated state.

Preservice work and time are not reported separately and include the initial ordering and selecting of the VR program, describing VR procedural dissociation to the patient and/or family, and applying the VR device to the patient prior to starting the procedure. Postservice work and time is not reported separately and begins with the end of the procedure, the termination of the VR technology, and when the physician or other qualified health care professional is no longer continuously face-to-face with the patient.

0771T   Virtual reality (VR) procedural dissociation services provided by the same physician or other qualified health care professional performing the diagnostic or therapeutic service that the VR procedural dissociation supports, requiring the presence of an independent, trained observer to assist in the monitoring of the patient's level of dissociation or consciousness and physiological status; initial 15 minutes of intraservice time, patient age 5 years or older
Sunset January 2028
➔ *CPT Changes: An Insider's View* 2023
➔ *CPT Assistant* Oct 23:1
➔ *Clinical Examples in Radiology* Summer 23:5

+ 0772T   each additional 15 minutes intraservice time (List separately in addition to code for primary service)
Sunset January 2028
➔ *CPT Changes: An Insider's View* 2023
➔ *CPT Assistant* Oct 23:1
➔ *Clinical Examples in Radiology* Summer 23:5

(Use 0772T in conjunction with 0771T)

0773T   Virtual reality (VR) procedural dissociation services provided by a physician or other qualified health care professional other than the physician or other qualified health care professional performing the diagnostic or therapeutic service that the VR procedural dissociation supports; initial 15 minutes of intraservice time, patient age 5 years or older
Sunset January 2028
➔ *CPT Changes: An Insider's View* 2023
➔ *CPT Assistant* Oct 23:1
➔ *Clinical Examples in Radiology* Summer 23:5

+ 0774T   each additional 15 minutes intraservice time (List separately in addition to code for primary service)
Sunset January 2028
➔ *CPT Changes: An Insider's View* 2023
➔ *CPT Assistant* Oct 23:1
➔ *Clinical Examples in Radiology* Summer 23:5

(Use 0774T in conjunction with 0773T)

(0775T has been deleted)

(For percutaneous arthrodesis of the sacroiliac joint, see 27278, 27279)

0776T   Therapeutic induction of intra-brain hypothermia, including placement of a mechanical temperature-controlled cooling device to the neck over carotids and head, including monitoring (eg, vital signs and sport concussion assessment tool 5 [SCAT5]), 30 minutes of treatment
Sunset January 2028
➔ *CPT Changes: An Insider's View* 2023

(Do not report 0776T more than once per day)

(For initiation of selective head or total body hypothermia in the critically ill neonate, use 99184)

+ 0777T   Real-time pressure-sensing epidural guidance system (List separately in addition to code for primary procedure)
Sunset January 2028
➔ *CPT Changes: An Insider's View* 2023

(Use 0777T in conjunction with 62320, 62321, 62322, 62323, 62324, 62325, 62326, 62327)

Office-Based Measurement of Mechanomyography and Inertial Measurement Units

Code 0778T represents the measurement and recording of dynamic joint motion and muscle function that includes the incorporation of multiple inertial measurement units (IMUs) with concurrent surface mechanomyography (sMMG) sensors. Code 0778T is not a remote service and measurements are obtained in the office setting while the patient is physically present.

The IMU sensors contain an accelerometer that measures acceleration and velocity of the body during movement, a gyroscope that measures the positioning, rotation, and orientation of the body during movement, and a magnetometer that measures the strength and direction of the magnetic field to orient the body position during movement relative to the earth's magnetic north field. The sMMG sensors measure muscle function by quantifying muscle activation and contraction

		Virtual reality (VR) procedural dissociation by physician or other qualified health care professional (same physician or other qualified health care professional performing the procedure the VR is supporting)	Virtual reality (VR) procedural dissociation by different physician or other qualified health care professional (not the physician or other qualified health care professional who is performing the procedure the VR is supporting)
Total Intraservice Time for VR Procedural Dissociation	**Patient Age**	**Code(s)**	**Code(s)**
Less than 10 minutes	< 5 years	Not reported separately	Not reported separately
	5 years or older	Not reported separately	Not reported separately
10-22 minutes	5 years or older	0771T	0773T
23-37 minutes	5 years or older	0771T + 0772T X 1	0773T + 0774T X 1
38-52 minutes	5 years or older	0771T + 0772T X 2	0773T + 0774T X 2
53-67 minutes	5 years or older	0771T + 0772T X 3	0773T + 0774T X 3

amplitude and duration by recording high-sensitivity volumetric change.

A combination of the sensors is used to dynamically record multi-joint motion and muscle function bilaterally and concurrently during functional movement. Data collected from the wireless-enabled IMUs and sMMGs are then uploaded to a secure, Health Insurance Portability and Accountability Act (HIPAA)-compliant cloud-based processing platform. The cloud-based application immediately processes the data and produces an automated report with digestible chronological data to assist in serial tracking improvement, decline, or plateau of progress during the episode of care. When 0778T is performed on the same day as another therapy, assessment, or evaluation services, those services may be reported separately and in addition to 0778T.

0778T Surface mechanomyography (sMMG) with concurrent application of inertial measurement unit (IMU) sensors for measurement of multi-joint range of motion, posture, gait, and muscle function
Sunset January 2028
➔ CPT Changes: An Insider's View 2023
➔ CPT Assistant Oct 23:13

(Do not report 0778T in conjunction with 96000, 96004, 98975, 98977, 98980, 98981)

0779T Gastrointestinal myoelectrical activity study, stomach through colon, with interpretation and report
Sunset January 2028
➔ CPT Changes: An Insider's View 2023

►(Do not report 0779T in conjunction with 91020, 91022, 91112, 91117, 91122, 91132, 91133, 0868T)◄

0780T Instillation of fecal microbiota suspension via rectal enema into lower gastrointestinal tract
Sunset January 2028
➔ CPT Changes: An Insider's View 2023

(Do not report 0780T in conjunction with 44705, 44799, 45999, 74283)

0781T Bronchoscopy, rigid or flexible, with insertion of esophageal protection device and circumferential radiofrequency destruction of the pulmonary nerves, including fluoroscopic guidance when performed; bilateral mainstem bronchi
Sunset January 2028
➔ CPT Changes: An Insider's View 2023
➔ CPT Assistant Jun 23:21

0782T   unilateral mainstem bronchus
Sunset January 2028
➔ CPT Changes: An Insider's View 2023
➔ CPT Assistant Jun 23:21

(Use 0781T, 0782T only once, regardless of the number of treatments per bronchus)

(Do not report 0781T, 0782T in conjunction with 31622-31638, 31640, 31641, 31643, 31645, 31646, 31647, 31648, 31649, 31651, 31652, 31653, 31654, 31660, 31661)

(For bronchial thermoplasty, see 31660, 31661)

0783T   Transcutaneous auricular neurostimulation, set-up, calibration, and patient education on use of equipment
Sunset January 2028
➔ *CPT Changes: An Insider's View* 2023

0784T   Insertion or replacement of percutaneous electrode array, spinal, with integrated neurostimulator, including imaging guidance, when performed
Sunset January 2029
➔ *CPT Changes: An Insider's View* 2024
➔ *CPT Assistant* Dec 23:1

0785T   Revision or removal of neurostimulator electrode array, spinal, with integrated neurostimulator
Sunset January 2029
➔ *CPT Changes: An Insider's View* 2024
➔ *CPT Assistant* Dec 23:1

0786T   Insertion or replacement of percutaneous electrode array, sacral, with integrated neurostimulator, including imaging guidance, when performed
Sunset January 2029
➔ *CPT Changes: An Insider's View* 2024
➔ *CPT Assistant* Dec 23:1

0787T   Revision or removal of neurostimulator electrode array, sacral, with integrated neurostimulator
Sunset January 2029
➔ *CPT Changes: An Insider's View* 2024
➔ *CPT Assistant* Dec 23:1

0788T   Electronic analysis with simple programming of implanted integrated neurostimulation system (eg, electrode array and receiver), including contact group(s), amplitude, pulse width, frequency (Hz), on/off cycling, burst, dose lockout, patient-selectable parameters, responsive neurostimulation, detection algorithms, closed-loop parameters, and passive parameters, when performed by physician or other qualified health care professional, spinal cord or sacral nerve, 1-3 parameters
Sunset January 2029
➔ *CPT Changes: An Insider's View* 2024
➔ *CPT Assistant* Dec 23:1

(Do not report 0788T in conjunction with 43647, 43648, 43881, 43882, 61850-61888, 63650, 63655, 63661, 63662, 63663, 63664, 63685, 63688, 64553-64595, 64596, 64598, 95970, 95971, 95972, 95976, 95977, 95983, 95984, 0587T, 0588T, 0589T, 0590T, 0784T, 0785T, 0786T, 0787T, 0789T)

0789T   Electronic analysis with complex programming of implanted integrated neurostimulation system (eg, electrode array and receiver), including contact group(s), amplitude, pulse width, frequency (Hz), on/off cycling, burst, dose lockout, patient-selectable parameters, responsive neurostimulation, detection algorithms, closed-loop parameters, and passive parameters, when performed by physician or other qualified health care professional, spinal cord or sacral nerve, 4 or more parameters
Sunset January 2029
➔ *CPT Changes: An Insider's View* 2024
➔ *CPT Assistant* Dec 23:1

(Do not report 0789T in conjunction with 43647, 43648, 43881, 43882, 61850-61888, 63650, 63655, 63661, 63662, 63663, 63664, 63685, 63688, 64553-64595, 64596, 64598, 95970, 95971, 95972, 95976, 95977, 95983, 95984, 0587T, 0588T, 0589T, 0590T, 0784T, 0785T, 0786T, 0787T, 0788T)

0790T   Code is out of numerical sequence. See 0656T-0659T

+ 0791T   Motor-cognitive, semi-immersive virtual reality–facilitated gait training, each 15 minutes (List separately in addition to code for primary procedure)
Sunset January 2029
➔ *CPT Changes: An Insider's View* 2024

(Use 0791T in conjunction with 97116)

0792T   Application of silver diamine fluoride 38%, by a physician or other qualified health care professional
Sunset January 2029
➔ *CPT Changes: An Insider's View* 2024

0793T   Percutaneous transcatheter thermal ablation of nerves innervating the pulmonary arteries, including right heart catheterization, pulmonary artery angiography, and all imaging guidance
Sunset January 2029
➔ *CPT Changes: An Insider's View* 2024

(Do not report 0793T in conjunction with 75746, 93503, 93568)

(For percutaneous transcatheter ultrasound ablation of nerves innervating the pulmonary arteries, including right heart catheterization, pulmonary artery angiography, and all imaging guidance, use 0632T)

Pharmaco-oncologic Algorithmic Treatment Ranking

Code 0794T (pharmaco-oncologic treatment ranking) represents rules based algorithm–generated match scores that rank available monotherapies and drug combinations according to their ability to target the patient's specific cancer biomarkers. These pharmaco-oncologic treatment ranking options are based only on current Food and Drug Administration (FDA)-approved drugs but may include both on-label and off-label uses for targeted therapies, and additional information may also be provided on potential active clinical trials that include specifically matched, currently available, therapy options. Code 0794T includes time spent by the physician, other qualified health care professional, or clinical staff in submitting the patient's clinical and existing molecular, laboratory, or pathology result data for algorithmic assessment. Only existing result data should be submitted without alteration of original results and interpretations (eg, variant calls or expression markers) from those separately reported by the original performing clinical laboratories and should not include genomic sequencing raw data files for re-evaluation. The algorithmic program generates a report that is used by the physician or other qualified health care professional to inform treatment choices.

0794T   Patient-specific, assistive, rules-based algorithm for ranking pharmaco-oncologic treatment options based on the patient's tumor-specific cancer marker information obtained from prior molecular pathology, immunohistochemical, or other pathology results which have been previously interpreted and reported separately
Sunset January 2029
➜ *CPT Changes: An Insider's View* 2024
➜ *CPT Assistant* Nov 23:19

Dual-Chamber Leadless Pacemaker

A complete dual-chamber leadless pacemaker system includes two pulse generators, each with a built-in battery and electrode. Implantation of this system is performed using a catheter under fluoroscopic guidance via transvenous access. One pacemaker is implanted in the right atrium, and one is implanted in the right ventricle. Rarely, for clinical reasons, a complete dual-chamber leadless pacemaker system may be completed in stages, with one pacemaker implanted into the right ventricle at the initial procedure and the other implanted into the right atrium at a subsequent session. An existing single-chamber right ventricular leadless pacemaker may be upgraded to a complete dual-chamber leadless pacemaker system by implantation of a right atrial leadless pacemaker.

For insertion of a complete dual-chamber leadless pacemaker system, report 0795T. For insertion of a leadless pacemaker into the right atrium when a single-chamber right ventricular leadless pacemaker already exists, in order to complete the dual-chamber leadless pacemaker system, report 0796T. For insertion of only the right ventricular pacemaker component of a dual-chamber leadless pacemaker system, report 0797T. For removal of a complete dual-chamber leadless pacemaker system, report 0798T. For removal of only the right atrial leadless pacemaker component of a complete dual-chamber leadless pacemaker, report 0799T. For removal of only the right ventricular leadless pacemaker component of a complete dual-chamber leadless pacemaker, report 0800T. For removal and replacement of a complete dual-chamber leadless pacemaker system, report 0801T. For removal and replacement of only one pacemaker component of a complete dual-chamber leadless pacemaker system, report 0802T for the right atrial pacemaker component or 0803T for the right ventricular pacemaker component.

Right heart catheterization (93451, 93453, 93456, 93457, 93460, 93461, 93593, 93594, 93596, 93597) may not be reported in conjunction with dual-chamber leadless pacemaker codes 0795T, 0796T, 0797T, 0798T, 0799T, 0800T, 0801T, 0802T, 0803T, unless complete right heart catheterization is performed for an indication distinct from the dual-chamber leadless pacemaker procedure.

For programming device evaluation of a dual-chamber leadless pacemaker system, report 0804T. Device evaluation code 93279 may not be reported in conjunction with dual-chamber leadless pacemaker system codes 0795T, 0796T, 0797T, 0798T, 0799T, 0800T, 0801T, 0802T, 0803T.

Radiological supervision and interpretation, fluoroscopy (76000, 77002), ultrasound guidance for vascular access (76937), right ventriculography (93566), and femoral venography (75820) are included in the leadless pacemaker procedures, when performed.

0795T   Transcatheter insertion of permanent dual-chamber leadless pacemaker, including imaging guidance (eg, fluoroscopy, venous ultrasound, right atrial angiography, right ventriculography, femoral venography) and device evaluation (eg, interrogation or programming), when performed; complete system (ie, right atrial and right ventricular pacemaker components)
Sunset January 2029
➜ *CPT Changes: An Insider's View* 2024

(Do not report 0795T in conjunction with 75820, 76000, 76937, 77002, 93566, 0796T, 0797T)

0796T   right atrial pacemaker component (when an existing right ventricular single leadless pacemaker exists to create a dual-chamber leadless pacemaker system)
Sunset January 2029
➜ *CPT Changes: An Insider's View* 2024
➜ *CPT Assistant* Mar 24:1

0797T   right ventricular pacemaker component (when part of a dual-chamber leadless pacemaker system)
Sunset January 2029
➜ *CPT Changes: An Insider's View* 2024

(Do not report 0795T, 0796T, 0797T in conjunction with 33274, 75820, 76000, 76937, 77002, 93566)

(Do not report 0795T, 0796T, 0797T in conjunction with 93451, 93453, 93456, 93457, 93460, 93461, 93593, 93594, 93596, 93597, 93598, unless complete right heart catheterization is performed for indications distinct from the leadless pacemaker procedure)

0798T   Transcatheter removal of permanent dual-chamber leadless pacemaker, including imaging guidance (eg, fluoroscopy, venous ultrasound, right atrial angiography, right ventriculography, femoral venography), when performed; complete system (ie, right atrial and right ventricular pacemaker components)

Sunset January 2029

➔ *CPT Changes: An Insider's View* 2024

0799T   right atrial pacemaker component

Sunset January 2029

➔ *CPT Changes: An Insider's View* 2024

➔ *CPT Assistant* Mar 24:1

0800T   right ventricular pacemaker component (when part of a dual-chamber leadless pacemaker system)

Sunset January 2029

➔ *CPT Changes: An Insider's View* 2024

(Do not report 0798T, 0799T, 0800T in conjunction with 75820, 76000, 76937, 77002, 93451, 93453, 93456, 93457, 93460, 93461, 93566, 93593, 93594, 93596, 93597)

(Do not report 0799T, 0800T in conjunction with 33275, 0798T)

0801T   Transcatheter removal and replacement of permanent dual-chamber leadless pacemaker, including imaging guidance (eg, fluoroscopy, venous ultrasound, right atrial angiography, right ventriculography, femoral venography) and device evaluation (eg, interrogation or programming), when performed; dual-chamber system (ie, right atrial and right ventricular pacemaker components)

Sunset January 2029

➔ *CPT Changes: An Insider's View* 2024

0802T   right atrial pacemaker component

Sunset January 2029

➔ *CPT Changes: An Insider's View* 2024

➔ *CPT Assistant* Mar 24:1

0803T   right ventricular pacemaker component (when part of a dual-chamber leadless pacemaker system)

Sunset January 2029

➔ *CPT Changes: An Insider's View* 2024

(Do not report 0801T, 0802T, 0803T in conjunction with 33274, 33275, 75820, 76000, 76937, 77002, 93451, 93453, 93456, 93457, 93460, 93461, 93566, 0795T, 0796T, 0797T, 0798T, 0799T, 0800T)

(Do not report 33274, 33275 when right ventricular single-chamber leadless pacemaker is part of a dual-chamber leadless pacemaker system)

0804T   Programming device evaluation (in person) with iterative adjustment of implantable device to test the function of device and to select optimal permanent programmed values, with analysis, review, and report, by a physician or other qualified health care professional, leadless pacemaker system in dual cardiac chambers

Sunset January 2029

➔ *CPT Changes: An Insider's View* 2024

(Do not report 0804T in conjunction with 0795T, 0796T, 0797T, 0798T, 0799T, 0800T, 0801T, 0802T, 0803T)

Codes 0805T, 0806T are used to report transcatheter superior and inferior vena cava prosthetic valve implantation (ie, caval valve implantation [CAVI]).

Codes 0805T, 0806T include the work, when performed, of vascular access, placing the access sheath, transseptal puncture, advancing the caval valve delivery systems into position, repositioning the device(s) as needed, and deploying the device(s).

Angiography and radiological supervision and interpretation performed to guide CAVI (eg, guiding device placement and documenting completion of the intervention) are included in these codes.

Diagnostic right and left heart catheterization codes (93451, 93452, 93453, 93456, 93457, 93458, 93459, 93460, 93461, 93593, 93594, 93595, 93596, 93597, 93598) should **not** be used with 0805T, 0806T to report:

1. Contrast injections, angiography, road-mapping, and/or fluoroscopic guidance for the transcatheter CAVI,

2. Left ventricular angiography to assess tricuspid regurgitation for guidance of the transcatheter CAVI, or

3. Right and left heart catheterization for hemodynamic measurements before, during, and after transcatheter superior and inferior vena cava prosthetic valve implantation for guidance.

Diagnostic right and left heart catheterization codes (93451, 93452, 93453, 93456, 93457, 93458, 93459, 93460, 93461, 93593, 93594, 93595, 93596, 93597, 93598) and diagnostic coronary angiography codes (93454, 93455, 93456, 93457, 93458, 93459, 93460, 93461, 93563, 93564) may be reported with 0805T, 0806T, representing separate and distinct services from CAVI, if:

1. No prior study is available and a full diagnostic study is performed, or

2. A prior study is available, but as documented in the medical record:

   a. There is inadequate visualization of the anatomy and/or pathology, or

   b. The patient's condition with respect to the clinical indication has changed since the prior study, or

   c. There is a clinical change during the procedure that requires new evaluation.

For same session or same day diagnostic cardiac catheterization services, the appropriate diagnostic cardiac catheterization code(s) may be reported by appending modifier 59 indicating separate and distinct procedural service from the transcatheter superior and inferior vena cava prosthetic valve implantation procedures.

Percutaneous coronary interventional therapeutic procedures may be reported separately, when performed.

When transcatheter ventricular support is required in conjunction with CAVI, the appropriate ventricular assist device (VAD) procedure codes (33990, 33991, 33992, 33993, 33995, 33997) or balloon pump insertion codes (33967, 33970, 33973) may be reported.

When cardiopulmonary bypass is performed in conjunction with CAVI, 0805T and 0806T may be reported with the appropriate add-on code for percutaneous peripheral bypass (33367), open peripheral bypass (33368), or central bypass (33369).

0805T   Transcatheter superior and inferior vena cava prosthetic valve implantation (ie, caval valve implantation [CAVI]); percutaneous femoral vein approach
Sunset January 2029
➔ *CPT Changes: An Insider's View* 2024

0806T   open femoral vein approach
Sunset January 2029
➔ *CPT Changes: An Insider's View* 2024

(Do not report 0805T, 0806T in conjunction with 33210, 33211, for temporary pacemaker insertion)

(Do not report 0805T, 0806T in conjunction with 93451, 93453, 93456, 93457, 93460, 93461, 93503, 93566, 93593, 93594, 93596, 93597, for diagnostic right heart catheterization procedures intrinsic to the superior and inferior vena cava valve implantations)

(Do not report 0805T, 0806T in conjunction with 93662, for imaging guidance with intracardiac echocardiography)

0807T   Pulmonary tissue ventilation analysis using software-based processing of data from separately captured cinefluorograph images; in combination with previously acquired computed tomography (CT) images, including data preparation and transmission, quantification of pulmonary tissue ventilation, data review, interpretation and report
Sunset January 2029
➔ *CPT Changes: An Insider's View* 2024
➔ *CPT Assistant* Apr 24:30

(Do not report 0807T in conjunction with 76000, 78579, 78582, 78598)

0808T   in combination with computed tomography (CT) images taken for the purpose of pulmonary tissue ventilation analysis, including data preparation and transmission, quantification of pulmonary tissue ventilation, data review, interpretation and report
Sunset January 2029
➔ *CPT Changes: An Insider's View* 2024
➔ *CPT Assistant* Apr 24:30

(Do not report 0808T in conjunction with 71250, 71260, 71270, 71271, 76000, 78579, 78582, 78598)

(0809T has been deleted)

(For percutaneous arthrodesis of the sacroiliac joint, see 27278, 27279)

0810T   Subretinal injection of a pharmacologic agent, including vitrectomy and 1 or more retinotomies
Sunset January 2029
➔ *CPT Changes: An Insider's View* 2024

(Report medication separately)

(Do not report 0810T in conjunction with 67036, 67039, 67040, 67041, 67042, 67043)

0811T   Remote multi-day complex uroflowmetry (eg, calibrated electronic equipment); set-up and patient education on use of equipment
Sunset January 2029
➔ *CPT Changes: An Insider's View* 2024
➔ *CPT Assistant* Feb 24:28

0812T   device supply with automated report generation, up to 10 days
Sunset January 2029
➔ *CPT Changes: An Insider's View* 2024
➔ *CPT Assistant* Feb 24:28

(Do not report 0811T, 0812T more than once per episode of care)

(Do not report 0811T, 0812T in conjunction with 51736, 51741, 99453, 99454)

0813T   Esophagogastroduodenoscopy, flexible, transoral, with volume adjustment of intragastric bariatric balloon
Sunset January 2029
➔ *CPT Changes: An Insider's View* 2024

(Do not report 0813T in conjunction with 43197, 43198, 43235, 43241, 43247, 43290, 43291)

0814T   Percutaneous injection of calcium-based biodegradable osteoconductive material, proximal femur, including imaging guidance, unilateral
Sunset January 2029
➔ *CPT Changes: An Insider's View* 2024
➔ *CPT Assistant* Dec 23:50

(Do not report 0814T in conjunction with 26992, 77002)

0815T   Ultrasound-based radiofrequency echographic multi-spectrometry (REMS), bone-density study and fracture-risk assessment, 1 or more sites, hips, pelvis, or spine
Sunset January 2029
➔ *CPT Changes: An Insider's View* 2024

Category III   0042T-0947T

0816T   Open insertion or replacement of integrated neurostimulation system for bladder dysfunction including electrode(s) (eg, array or leadless), and pulse generator or receiver, including analysis, programming, and imaging guidance, when performed, posterior tibial nerve; subcutaneous
Sunset January 2029
➔ *CPT Changes: An Insider's View* 2024

0817T   subfascial
Sunset January 2029
➔ *CPT Changes: An Insider's View* 2024

0818T   Revision or removal of integrated neurostimulation system for bladder dysfunction, including analysis, programming, and imaging, when performed, posterior tibial nerve; subcutaneous
Sunset January 2029
➔ *CPT Changes: An Insider's View* 2024

0819T   subfascial
Sunset January 2029
➔ *CPT Changes: An Insider's View* 2024

(Do not report 0816T, 0817T, 0818T, 0819T in conjunction with 64555, 64566, 64575, 64590, 64596, 95970, 95971, 95972, 0588T, 0589T, 0590T)

(For percutaneous implantation or replacement of integrated neurostimulation system including electrode array and receiver for bladder dysfunction, posterior tibial nerve, use 0587T)

(For revision or removal of percutaneous integrated neurostimulation system for bladder dysfunction, posterior tibial nerve, use 0588T)

(For electronic analysis with programming of integrated or leadless neurostimulation system for bladder dysfunction, posterior tibial nerve, performed on a day subsequent to the device insertion, replacement, or revision, see 0589T, 0590T)

Continuous In-Person Monitoring and Intervention During Psychedelic Medication Therapy

Continuous in-person monitoring and intervention (eg, psychotherapy, crisis intervention) is provided during and following supervised patient self-administration of a psychedelic medication in a therapeutic setting. Psychedelic medications induce distinctive alterations in perception that may place the patient at risk for emotional vulnerability and physiologic instability. The medications' pharmacologic risks may persist for multiple hours, and during this time, the patient may require continuous in-person monitoring and intervention by a physician or other qualified health care professional (QHP) to support the patient's physical, emotional, and psychological safety and to optimize treatment outcomes.

Code 0820T is used to report the total duration of in-person time with the patient by the physician or other QHP providing continuous monitoring, and intervention as needed, during psychedelic medication therapy. Codes 0821T, 0822T are used to report the concurrent in-person participation of a second physician or other QHP (0821T), or the concurrent in-person participation of clinical staff (0822T) based on a patient's complex presentation, that requires additional personnel in the therapy room (eg, a physician or other QHP monitoring patient needs assistance from additional clinical staff due to a crisis by the psychedelic experience that surfaces past psychological trauma). If necessary, report 0821T, 0822T, as appropriate. It is unlikely that more than two personnel need to be in the room at the same time with the patient (ie, the initial physician or other QHP and one additional physician or other QHP or clinical staff).

Psychotherapy (90832, 90833, 90834, 90836, 90837, 90838), psychotherapy for crisis (90839, 90840), neurobehavioral status examination (96116, 96121), adaptive behavior assessments (97151, 97152), adaptive behavior treatment (97153, 97154, 97155, 97156, 97157, 97158), or prolonged clinical staff services (99415, 99416) may not be reported on the same date of service.

0820T   Continuous in-person monitoring and intervention (eg, psychotherapy, crisis intervention), as needed, during psychedelic medication therapy; first physician or other qualified health care professional, each hour
Sunset January 2029
➔ *CPT Changes: An Insider's View* 2024
➔ *CPT Assistant* Mar 24:18, Apr 24:33

(Do not report 0820T in conjunction with 90832, 90833, 90834, 90836, 90837, 90838, 90839, 90840, 96116, 96121, 97151, 97152, 97153, 97154, 97155, 97156, 97157, 97158, 99415, 99416, on the same date of service)

+ 0821T   second physician or other qualified health care professional, concurrent with first physician or other qualified health care professional, each hour (List separately in addition to code for primary procedure)
Sunset January 2029
➔ *CPT Changes: An Insider's View* 2024
➔ *CPT Assistant* Mar 24:18

+ 0822T clinical staff under the direction of a physician or other qualified health care professional, concurrent with first physician or other qualified health care professional, each hour (List separately in addition to code for primary procedure)

Sunset January 2029

➔ *CPT Changes: An Insider's View* 2024

➔ *CPT Assistant* Mar 24:18

(Use 0821T, 0822T in conjunction with 0820T)

Right Atrial Leadless Pacemaker

A right atrial single-chamber leadless pacemaker includes a pulse generator with a built-in battery and electrode for implantation into the right atrium. Implantation of the atrial leadless pacemaker is performed using a catheter under fluoroscopic guidance via transvenous access.

Codes 0823T, 0824T, 0825T, 0826T only apply to single-chamber leadless pacemakers implanted in the right atrium intended for atrial pacing only and that are not part of a dual-chamber leadless system. For insertion of a right atrial single-chamber leadless pacemaker, report 0823T. For removal of a right atrial single-chamber leadless pacemaker, report 0824T. For removal and replacement of a right atrial single-chamber leadless pacemaker, report 0825T.

Leadless pacemakers are modular systems, and for clinical reasons, a dual-chamber leadless pacemaker may be implanted in stages with one pacemaker implanted into the right ventricle at the initial procedure and one pacemaker implanted into the right atrium at a subsequent session.

When a right atrial leadless pacemaker component of a dual-chamber system is modified or a right atrial leadless pacemaker is implanted to complete a dual-chamber leadless pacemaker system, see 0796T, 0799T, 0802T. For insertion of a leadless pacemaker into the right atrium when a single-chamber right ventricular leadless pacemaker already exists, in order to complete the dual-chamber system, report 0796T. If the right atrial leadless pacemaker is permanently removed when part of a dual-chamber leadless system, report 0799T. If the right atrial leadless pacemaker is removed and replaced when part of a dual-chamber leadless system, report 0802T.

Right heart catheterization (93451, 93453, 93456, 93460, 93461) may not be reported in conjunction with leadless pacemaker insertion, removal, and removal and replacement codes 33274, 33275, 0795T, 0796T, 0797T, 0798T, 0799T, 0800T, 0801T, 0802T, 0803T, 0823T, 0824T, 0825T, unless complete right heart catheterization is performed for an indication distinct from leadless pacemaker procedure.

For programming device evaluation (in person) of a right atrial single-chamber leadless pacemaker, report 0826T. Device evaluation code 93279 may not be reported in conjunction with right atrial single-chamber leadless pacemaker system codes 0823T, 0824T, 0825T.

Fluoroscopy (76000, 77002), ultrasound guidance for vascular access (76937), right ventriculography (93566), and femoral venography (75820) are included in 0823T, 0824T, 0825T, when performed.

0823T Transcatheter insertion of permanent single-chamber leadless pacemaker, right atrial, including imaging guidance (eg, fluoroscopy, venous ultrasound, right atrial angiography and/or right ventriculography, femoral venography, cavography) and device evaluation (eg, interrogation or programming), when performed

Sunset January 2029

➔ *CPT Changes: An Insider's View* 2024

➔ *CPT Assistant* Mar 24:1

(Do not report 0823T in conjunction with 33274, 0795T, 0796T, 0797T, 0802T)

0824T Transcatheter removal of permanent single-chamber leadless pacemaker, right atrial, including imaging guidance (eg, fluoroscopy, venous ultrasound, right atrial angiography and/or right ventriculography, femoral venography, cavography), when performed

Sunset January 2029

➔ *CPT Changes: An Insider's View* 2024

➔ *CPT Assistant* Mar 24:1

(Do not report 0824T in conjunction with 33275, 0799T)

0825T Transcatheter removal and replacement of permanent single-chamber leadless pacemaker, right atrial, including imaging guidance (eg, fluoroscopy, venous ultrasound, right atrial angiography and/or right ventriculography, femoral venography, cavography) and device evaluation (eg, interrogation or programming), when performed

Sunset January 2029

➔ *CPT Changes: An Insider's View* 2024

➔ *CPT Assistant* Mar 24:1

(Do not report 0825T in conjunction with 33274, 0795T, 0796T, 0797T, 0802T)

0826T Programming device evaluation (in person) with iterative adjustment of the implantable device to test the function of the device and select optimal permanent programmed values with analysis, review and report by a physician or other qualified health care professional, leadless pacemaker system in single-cardiac chamber

Sunset January 2029

➔ *CPT Changes: An Insider's View* 2024

➔ *CPT Assistant* Mar 24:1

(Do not report 0826T in conjunction with 0823T, 0824T, 0825T)

0827T Code is out of numerical sequence. See 0762T-0765T

0828T Code is out of numerical sequence. See 0762T-0765T

0829T Code is out of numerical sequence. See 0762T-0765T

0830T Code is out of numerical sequence. See 0762T-0765T

0831T Code is out of numerical sequence. See 0762T-0765T

0832T Code is out of numerical sequence. See 0762T-0765T

0833T Code is out of numerical sequence. See 0762T-0765T

0834T Code is out of numerical sequence. See 0762T-0765T

0835T Code is out of numerical sequence. See 0762T-0765T

0836T Code is out of numerical sequence. See 0762T-0765T

0837T Code is out of numerical sequence. See 0762T-0765T

0838T Code is out of numerical sequence. See 0762T-0765T

0839T Code is out of numerical sequence. See 0762T-0765T

0840T Code is out of numerical sequence. See 0762T-0765T

0841T Code is out of numerical sequence. See 0762T-0765T

0842T Code is out of numerical sequence. See 0762T-0765T

0843T Code is out of numerical sequence. See 0762T-0765T

0844T Code is out of numerical sequence. See 0762T-0765T

0845T Code is out of numerical sequence. See 0762T-0765T

0846T Code is out of numerical sequence. See 0762T-0765T

0847T Code is out of numerical sequence. See 0762T-0765T

0848T Code is out of numerical sequence. See 0762T-0765T

0849T Code is out of numerical sequence. See 0762T-0765T

0850T Code is out of numerical sequence. See 0762T-0765T

0851T Code is out of numerical sequence. See 0762T-0765T

0852T Code is out of numerical sequence. See 0762T-0765T

0853T Code is out of numerical sequence. See 0762T-0765T

0854T Code is out of numerical sequence. See 0762T-0765T

0855T Code is out of numerical sequence. See 0762T-0765T

0856T Code is out of numerical sequence. See 0762T-0765T

+ 0857T Opto-acoustic imaging, breast, unilateral, including axilla when performed, real-time with image documentation, augmentative analysis and report (List separately in addition to code for primary procedure)
Sunset January 2029
➲ *CPT Changes: An Insider's View* 2024

(Use 0857T in conjunction with 76641, 76642)

Code 0858T represents measurement of evoked cortical potentials associated with transcranial magnetic stimulation of two or more cortical areas using multiple, externally applied scalp electrode channels. Upon stimulation, the device performs automated signal processing indicating brain physiological features of connectivity, excitability, and plasticity, which may be impaired with structural and functional brain deficits.

Because these physiological features may be altered in certain types of brain disease, the device's automated report of analyzed data is intended to provide clinical insight of brain function within the context of certain brain disease states.

0858T Externally applied transcranial magnetic stimulation with concomitant measurement of evoked cortical potentials with automated report
Sunset January 2029
➲ *CPT Changes: An Insider's View* 2024

(Do not report 0858T in conjunction with 95836, 95957, 95961, 95965, 95966)

0859T Code is out of numerical sequence. See 0489T-0495T

0860T Code is out of numerical sequence. See 0489T-0495T

0861T Code is out of numerical sequence. See 0516T-0520T

0862T Code is out of numerical sequence. See 0516T-0520T

0863T Code is out of numerical sequence. See 0516T-0520T

0864T Low-intensity extracorporeal shock wave therapy involving corpus cavernosum, low energy
Sunset January 2029
➲ *CPT Changes: An Insider's View* 2024

(Do not report 0864T in conjunction with 0101T when treating the same area)

0865T Quantitative magnetic resonance image (MRI) analysis of the brain with comparison to prior magnetic resonance (MR) study(ies), including lesion identification, characterization, and quantification, with brain volume(s) quantification and/or severity score, when performed, data preparation and transmission, interpretation and report, obtained without diagnostic MRI examination of the brain during the same session
Sunset January 2029
➲ *CPT Changes: An Insider's View* 2024
➲ *Clinical Examples in Radiology* Winter 24:11

(Do not report 0865T in conjunction with 70551, 70552, 70553)

+ 0866T Quantitative magnetic resonance image (MRI) analysis of the brain with comparison to prior magnetic resonance (MR) study(ies), including lesion detection, characterization, and quantification, with brain volume(s) quantification and/or severity score, when performed, data preparation and transmission, interpretation and report, obtained with diagnostic MRI examination of the brain (List separately in addition to code for primary procedure)
Sunset January 2029
➲ *CPT Changes: An Insider's View* 2024
➲ *Clinical Examples in Radiology* Winter 24:10

Category III 0042T-0947T

(Use 0866T in conjunction with 70551, 70552, 70553)

(For quantitative MR for analysis of tissue composition, see 0648T, 0649T, 0697T, 0698T)

(For quantitative computed tomography tissue characterization, see 0721T, 0722T)

(For quantitative MRI analysis of the brain without comparison to prior MR study, report 0865T, 0866T with modifier 52)

0867T   Code is out of numerical sequence. See 0419T-0422T

● **0868T**   High-resolution gastric electrophysiology mapping with simultaneous patient-symptom profiling, with interpretation and report
Sunset January 2030
➔ *CPT Changes: An Insider's View* 2025

▶(Do not report 0868T in conjunction with 91132, 91133, 0779T)◀

● **0869T**   Injection(s), bone-substitute material for bone and/or soft tissue hardware fixation augmentation, including intraoperative imaging guidance, when performed
Sunset January 2030
➔ *CPT Changes: An Insider's View* 2025

▶(Do not report 0869T in conjunction with 0707T)◀

● **0870T**   Implantation of subcutaneous peritoneal ascites pump system, percutaneous, including pump-pocket creation, insertion of tunneled indwelling bladder and peritoneal catheters with pump connections, including all imaging and initial programming, when performed
Sunset January 2030
➔ *CPT Changes: An Insider's View* 2025

▶(Do not report 0870T in conjunction with 49082, 49083, 49405, 49406, 49418, 51100, 51101, 51102, 76942, 76989, 77002, 0871T, 0872T, 0873T, 0874T, 0875T)◀

● **0871T**   Replacement of a subcutaneous peritoneal ascites pump, including reconnection between pump and indwelling bladder and peritoneal catheters, including initial programming and imaging, when performed
Sunset January 2030
➔ *CPT Changes: An Insider's View* 2025

▶(Do not report 0871T in conjunction with 49082, 49083, 75984, 76998, 77002, 0870T, 0873T, 0874T, 0875T)◀

● **0872T**   Replacement of indwelling bladder and peritoneal catheters, including tunneling of catheter(s) and connection with previously implanted peritoneal ascites pump, including imaging and programming, when performed
Sunset January 2030
➔ *CPT Changes: An Insider's View* 2025

▶(Do not report 0872T in conjunction with 49082, 49083, 49405, 49406, 49418, 51100, 51101, 51102, 75984, 76942, 76989, 76998, 77002, 0870T, 0873T, 0874T, 0875T)◀

▶(For single-catheter replacement, report 0872T with modifier 52)◀

● **0873T**   Revision of a subcutaneously implanted peritoneal ascites pump system, any component (ascites pump, associated peritoneal catheter, associated bladder catheter), including imaging and programming, when performed
Sunset January 2030
➔ *CPT Changes: An Insider's View* 2025

▶(Do not report 0873T in conjunction with 0870T, 0871T, 0872T, 0874T, 0875T)◀

● **0874T**   Removal of a peritoneal ascites pump system, including implanted peritoneal ascites pump and indwelling bladder and peritoneal catheters
Sunset January 2030
➔ *CPT Changes: An Insider's View* 2025

▶(Do not report 0874T in conjunction with 0870T, 0871T, 0872T, 0873T, 0875T)◀

● **0875T**   Programming of subcutaneously implanted peritoneal ascites pump system by physician or other qualified health care professional
Sunset January 2030
➔ *CPT Changes: An Insider's View* 2025

▶(Do not report 0875T in conjunction with 0870T, 0871T, 0872T, 0873T)◀

● **0876T**   Duplex scan of hemodialysis fistula, computer-aided, limited (volume flow, diameter, and depth, including only body of fistula)
Sunset January 2030
➔ *CPT Changes: An Insider's View* 2025

▶(Do not report 0876T in conjunction with 76376, 76377, 90940, 90951-90966, 93990)◀

▶(For duplex scan of hemodialysis access, including arterial inflow and venous outflow, use 93990)◀

● **0877T**   Augmentative analysis of chest computed tomography (CT) imaging data to provide categorical diagnostic subtype classification of interstitial lung disease; obtained without concurrent CT examination of any structure contained in previously acquired diagnostic imaging
Sunset January 2030
➔ *CPT Changes: An Insider's View* 2025

▶(Do not report 0877T in conjunction with 71250, 71260, 71270, 71275)◀

● **0878T**   obtained with concurrent CT examination of the same structure
Sunset January 2030
➔ *CPT Changes: An Insider's View* 2025

▶(Use 0878T in conjunction with 71250, 71260, 71270, 71271, 71275, when evaluating same organ, tissue, or target structure)◀

● **0879T**   radiological data preparation and transmission
Sunset January 2030
↪ *CPT Changes: An Insider's View* 2025

● **0880T**   physician or other qualified health care professional interpretation and report
Sunset January 2030
↪ *CPT Changes: An Insider's View* 2025

● **0881T**   Cryotherapy of the oral cavity using temperature regulated fluid cooling system, including placement of an oral device, monitoring of patient tolerance to treatment, and removal of the oral device
Sunset January 2030
↪ *CPT Changes: An Insider's View* 2025

▶(Use 0881T in conjunction with 96409, 96413, 96416, when chemotherapy is also performed)◀

▶(Do not report 0881T more than once per chemotherapy session)◀

+● **0882T**   Intraoperative therapeutic electrical stimulation of peripheral nerve to promote nerve regeneration, including lead placement and removal, upper extremity, minimum of 10 minutes; initial nerve (List separately in addition to code for primary procedure)
Sunset January 2030
↪ *CPT Changes: An Insider's View* 2025

▶(Use 0882T in conjunction with 64702, 64704, 64708, 64713, 64718, 64719, 64721, 64831, 64834, 64835, 64836, 64856, 64857, 64892, 64893, 64895, 64896, 64897, 64898, 64905, 64910, 64911, 64912)◀

+● **0883T**   each additional nerve (List separately in addition to code for primary procedure)
Sunset January 2030
↪ *CPT Changes: An Insider's View* 2025

▶(Use 0883T in conjunction with 0882T)◀

● **0884T**   Esophagoscopy, flexible, transoral, with initial transendoscopic mechanical dilation (eg, nondrug-coated balloon) followed by therapeutic drug delivery by drug-coated balloon catheter for esophageal stricture, including fluoroscopic guidance, when performed
Sunset January 2030
↪ *CPT Changes: An Insider's View* 2025

▶(Do not report 0884T in conjunction with 43191, 43195, 43196, 43200, 43213, 43214, 43220, 43226, 76000)◀

● **0885T**   Colonoscopy, flexible, with initial transendoscopic mechanical dilation (eg, nondrug-coated balloon) followed by therapeutic drug delivery by drug-coated balloon catheter for colonic stricture, including fluoroscopic guidance, when performed
Sunset January 2030
↪ *CPT Changes: An Insider's View* 2025

▶(Do not report 0885T in conjunction with 45378, 45386, 76000, 0886T)◀

▶(For endoscopic balloon dilation of multiple strictures during the same procedure, use 0885T with modifier 59 for each additional stricture dilated)◀

● **0886T**   Sigmoidoscopy, flexible, with initial transendoscopic mechanical dilation (eg, nondrug-coated balloon) followed by therapeutic drug delivery by drug-coated balloon catheter for colonic stricture, including fluoroscopic guidance, when performed
Sunset January 2030
↪ *CPT Changes: An Insider's View* 2025

▶(Do not report 0886T in conjunction with 45300, 45303, 45330, 45340, 76000, 0885T)◀

▶(For endoscopic balloon dilation of multiple strictures during the same procedure, use 0886T with modifier 59 for each additional stricture dilated)◀

+● **0887T**   End-tidal control of inhaled anesthetic agents and oxygen to assist anesthesia care delivery (List separately in addition to code for primary procedure)
Sunset January 2030
↪ *CPT Changes: An Insider's View* 2025

▶(Use 0887T in conjunction with 00100-01999)◀

● **0888T**   Histotripsy (ie, non-thermal ablation via acoustic energy delivery) of malignant renal tissue, including imaging guidance
Sunset January 2030
↪ *CPT Changes: An Insider's View* 2025

● **0889T**   Personalized target development for accelerated, repetitive high-dose functional connectivity MRI–guided theta-burst stimulation derived from a structural and resting-state functional MRI, including data preparation and transmission, generation of the target, motor threshold–starting location, neuronavigation files and target report, review and interpretation
Sunset January 2030
↪ *CPT Changes: An Insider's View* 2025

▶(Report 0889T once per personalized target development)◀

▶(Do not report 0889T in conjunction with 70551, 70552, 70553, 70554, 70555, for the same session)◀

▶(Do not report 0889T in conjunction with 77022)◀

● **0890T**   Accelerated, repetitive high-dose functional connectivity MRI–guided theta-burst stimulation, including target assessment, initial motor threshold determination, neuronavigation, delivery and management, initial treatment day
Sunset January 2030
↪ *CPT Changes: An Insider's View* 2025

▶(Report 0890T once on the first day of the course of treatment)◀

▶(Do not report 0890T in conjunction with 77022)◀

● **0891T** Accelerated, repetitive high-dose functional connectivity MRI–guided theta-burst stimulation, including neuronavigation, delivery and management, subsequent treatment day
Sunset January 2030
➔ *CPT Changes: An Insider's View* 2025

▶(Do not report 0891T in conjunction with 77022)◀

● **0892T** Accelerated, repetitive high-dose functional connectivity MRI–guided theta-burst stimulation, including neuronavigation, delivery and management, subsequent motor threshold redetermination with delivery and management, per treatment day
Sunset January 2030
➔ *CPT Changes: An Insider's View* 2025

▶(Do not report 0892T in conjunction with 77022)◀

▶(Do not report 0892T in conjunction with 0890T, 0891T on the same day)◀

▶(If a significant, separately identifiable evaluation and management, medication management, or psychotherapy service is performed, the appropriate E/M or psychotherapy code may be reported in addition to 0890T, 0891T, 0892T. E/M activities directly related to cortical mapping, motor-threshold determination, delivery and management of accelerated, repetitive high-dose functional connectivity MRI–guided theta-burst stimulation are not separately reported)◀

● **0893T** Noninvasive assessment of blood oxygenation, gas exchange efficiency, and cardiorespiratory status, with physician or other qualified health care professional interpretation and report
Sunset January 2030
➔ *CPT Changes: An Insider's View* 2025

● **0894T** Cannulation of the liver allograft in preparation for connection to the normothermic perfusion device and decannulation of the liver allograft following normothermic perfusion
Sunset January 2030
➔ *CPT Changes: An Insider's View* 2025

● **0895T** Connection of liver allograft to normothermic machine perfusion device, hemostasis control; initial 4 hours of monitoring time, including hourly physiological and laboratory assessments (eg, perfusate temperature, perfusate pH, hemodynamic parameters, bile production, bile pH, bile glucose, biliary bicarbonate, lactate levels, macroscopic assessment)
Sunset January 2030
➔ *CPT Changes: An Insider's View* 2025

+● **0896T** each additional hour, including physiological and laboratory assessments (eg, perfusate temperature, perfusate pH, hemodynamic parameters, bile production, bile pH, bile glucose, biliary bicarbonate, lactate levels, macroscopic assessment) (List separately in addition to code for primary procedure)
Sunset January 2030
➔ *CPT Changes: An Insider's View* 2025

▶(Use 0896T in conjunction with 0895T)◀

● **0897T** Noninvasive augmentative arrhythmia analysis derived from quantitative computational cardiac arrhythmia simulations, based on selected intervals of interest from 12-lead electrocardiogram and uploaded clinical parameters, including uploading clinical parameters with interpretation and report
Sunset January 2030
➔ *CPT Changes: An Insider's View* 2025

▶(Do not report 0897T in conjunction with 93000, 93005, 93010, when performed on the same day)◀

● **0898T** Noninvasive prostate cancer estimation map, derived from augmentative analysis of image-guided fusion biopsy and pathology, including visualization of margin volume and location, with margin determination and physician interpretation and report
Sunset January 2030
➔ *CPT Changes: An Insider's View* 2025

▶(Do not report 0898T in conjunction with 76376, 76377)◀

+● **0899T** Noninvasive determination of absolute quantitation of myocardial blood flow (AQMBF), derived from augmentative algorithmic analysis of the dataset acquired via contrast cardiac magnetic resonance (CMR), pharmacologic stress, with interpretation and report by a physician or other qualified health care professional (List separately in addition to code for primary procedure)
Sunset January 2030
➔ *CPT Changes: An Insider's View* 2025

▶(Use 0899T in conjunction with 75563)◀

▶(Do not report 0899T in conjunction with 0900T)◀

▶(For AQMBF with PET, use 78434)◀

▶(For AQMBF with SPECT, use 0742T)◀

+● **0900T** Noninvasive estimate of absolute quantitation of myocardial blood flow (AQMBF), derived from assistive algorithmic analysis of the dataset acquired via contrast cardiac magnetic resonance (CMR), pharmacologic stress, with interpretation and report by a physician or other qualified health care professional (List separately in addition to code for primary procedure)
Sunset January 2030
➔ *CPT Changes: An Insider's View* 2025

▶(Use 0900T in conjunction with 75563)◀

▶(Do not report 0900T in conjunction with 0899T)◀

▶(For AQMBF with PET, use 78434)◀

▶(For AQMBF with SPECT, use 0742T)◀

0901T Code is out of numerical sequence. See 0222T-0235T

● **0902T**   QTc interval derived by augmentative algorithmic analysis of input from an external, patient-activated mobile ECG device
Sunset January 2030
➔ *CPT Changes: An Insider's View* 2025

▶(Do not report 0902T in conjunction with 93000, 93005, 93010, 93040, 93041, 93042)◀

● **0903T**   Electrocardiogram, algorithmically generated 12-lead ECG from a reduced-lead ECG; with interpretation and report
Sunset January 2030
➔ *CPT Changes: An Insider's View* 2025

▶(Do not report 0903T in conjunction with 93000, 93005, 93010, 0904T, 0905T)◀

● **0904T**   tracing only
Sunset January 2030
➔ *CPT Changes: An Insider's View* 2025

▶(Do not report 0904T in conjunction with 93000, 93005, 93010, 0903T, 0905T)◀

● **0905T**   interpretation and report only
Sunset January 2030
➔ *CPT Changes: An Insider's View* 2025

▶(Do not report 0905T in conjunction with 93000, 93005, 93010, 0903T, 0904T)◀

▶For purposes of reporting 0906T, 0907T for concurrent optical and magnetic stimulation (COMS) therapy, the treatment area is limited to 50 sq cm of skin-surface area per application.◀

● **0906T**   Concurrent optical and magnetic stimulation (COMS) therapy, wound assessment and dressing care; first application, total wound(s) surface area less than or equal to 50 sq cm
Sunset January 2030
➔ *CPT Changes: An Insider's View* 2025

+● **0907T**   each additional application, total wound(s) surface area less than or equal to 50 sq cm (List separately in addition to code for primary procedure)
Sunset January 2030
➔ *CPT Changes: An Insider's View* 2025

▶(Use 0907T in conjunction with 0906T)◀

● **0908T**   Open implantation of integrated neurostimulation system, vagus nerve, including analysis and programming, when performed
Sunset January 2030
➔ *CPT Changes: An Insider's View* 2025

▶(Do not report 0908T in conjunction with 64553, 64568, 0909T, 0910T, 0911T, 0912T)◀

● **0909T**   Replacement of integrated neurostimulation system, vagus nerve, including analysis and programming, when performed
Sunset January 2030
➔ *CPT Changes: An Insider's View* 2025

▶(Do not report 0909T in conjunction with 64570, 0908T, 0910T, 0911T, 0912T)◀

● **0910T**   Removal of integrated neurostimulation system, vagus nerve
Sunset January 2030
➔ *CPT Changes: An Insider's View* 2025

▶(Do not report 0910T in conjunction with 64570, 0908T, 0909T)◀

● **0911T**   Electronic analysis of implanted integrated neurostimulation system, vagus nerve; without programming by physician or other qualified health care professional
Sunset January 2030
➔ *CPT Changes: An Insider's View* 2025

▶(Do not report 0911T in conjunction with 95970, 95971, 95972, 0908T, 0909T, 0912T)◀

● **0912T**   with simple programming by physician or other qualified health care professional
Sunset January 2030
➔ *CPT Changes: An Insider's View* 2025

▶(Do not report 0912T in conjunction with 95970, 95971, 95972, 0908T, 0909T, 0911T)◀

▶Transcatheter Therapeutic Drug Delivery by Intracoronary Drug-Delivery Balloon◀

▶Codes 0913T, 0914T describe percutaneous coronary revascularization services by intracoronary antiproliferative drug delivery, performed for occlusive disease of the coronary vessels (major coronary arteries, coronary artery branches) using drug-delivery balloon (eg, drug-coated, drug-eluting) for intracoronary antiproliferative drug delivery. Code 0913T includes the work of accessing and selectively catheterizing the vessel, coronary angiography and intracoronary imaging (eg, intracoronary ultrasound, intracoronary optical coherence tomography) to guide the intervention, traversing the lesion, radiological supervision and interpretation directly related to the intervention(s) performed, closure of the arteriotomy when performed through the access sheath, and imaging performed to document completion of the intervention in addition to the intervention(s) performed. Code 0914T is an add-on code and includes only the coronary angiography and intracoronary imaging (eg, intracoronary ultrasound, intracoronary optical coherence tomography) to guide the additional intervention, traversing the additional lesion, and radiological supervision and interpretation directly related to the intervention(s) performed on the additional lesion. Codes 0913T, 0914T include mechanical dilation by nondrug-delivery balloon angioplasty followed by therapeutic drug delivery by drug-delivery balloon. Code 0913T may not be reported with 92920, 92924, 92928, 92933, 92937, 92941, 92943, 92973, 92978 for percutaneous coronary interventions (PCI) on the same target lesion in the same major coronary artery or graft as the drug-delivery balloon intervention. For drug delivery by intracoronary drug-delivery balloon (eg, drug-coated, drug-eluting) performed on a separate target lesion in the same major coronary artery or graft, 0914T may be reported for the separate target lesion in conjunction with 92920, 92924, 92928, 92933, 92937, 92941, 92943 for the first target lesion. For PCI in other major coronary arteries, see the appropriate PCI codes (92920, 92924, 92928, 92933, 92937, 92941, 92943, 0913T).

Diagnostic coronary angiography codes (93454, 93455, 93456, 93457, 93458, 93459, 93460, 93461) and injection procedure codes (93563, 93564) should not be used with percutaneous coronary revascularization services by intracoronary antiproliferative drug-delivery balloon services (0913T, 0914T) to report:

1. Contrast injections, angiography, roadmapping, and/or fluoroscopic guidance for the coronary intervention,

2. Vessel measurement for the coronary intervention, or

3. Postcoronary intervention angiography, as this work is captured in the percutaneous coronary revascularization services by intracoronary antiproliferative drug-delivery balloon codes (0913T, 0914T).

Diagnostic angiography performed at the time of a coronary interventional procedure may be separately reportable, if:

1. No prior catheter-based coronary angiography study is available, and a full-diagnostic study is performed, and a decision to intervene is based on the diagnostic angiography, or

2. A prior study is available, but as documented in the medical record:

   a. The patient's condition with respect to the clinical indication has changed since the prior study, or

   b. The prior study provides inadequate visualization of the anatomy and/or pathology, or

   c. There is a clinical change during the procedure that requires new evaluation outside the target area of intervention.

Diagnostic coronary angiography performed at a separate session from an interventional procedure is separately reportable.◄

● **0913T** Percutaneous transcatheter therapeutic drug delivery by intracoronary drug-delivery balloon (eg, drug-coated, drug-eluting), including mechanical dilation by nondrug-delivery balloon angioplasty, endoluminal imaging using intravascular ultrasound (IVUS) or optical coherence tomography (OCT) when performed, imaging supervision, interpretation, and report, single major coronary artery or branch

Sunset January 2030

➔ *CPT Changes: An Insider's View* 2025

►(Do not report 0913T in conjunction with 92920, 92924, 92928, 92933, 92937, 92941, 92943, 92973, 92978, for interventions on the same target lesion in the same major coronary artery or graft as the target lesion treated with drug-delivery balloon intervention)◄

+● **0914T** Percutaneous transcatheter therapeutic drug delivery by intracoronary drug-delivery balloon (eg, drug-coated, drug-eluting) performed on a separate target lesion from the target lesion treated with balloon angioplasty, coronary stent placement or coronary atherectomy, including mechanical dilation by nondrug-delivery balloon angioplasty, endoluminal imaging using intravascular ultrasound (IVUS) or optical coherence tomography (OCT) when performed, imaging supervision, interpretation, and report, single major coronary artery or branch (List separately in addition to code for percutaneous coronary stent or atherectomy intervention)

Sunset January 2030

➔ *CPT Changes: An Insider's View* 2025

►(Use 0914T in conjunction with 92920, 92924, 92928, 92933, 92937, 92941, 92943)◄

►Cardiac Contractility Modulation-Defibrillation◄

►A cardiac contractility modulation-defibrillation (CCM-D) system combines cardiac contractility modulation (CCM) for symptom relief from chronic heart failure with defibrillation protection against sudden cardiac arrhythmia into a single therapy. A CCM-D system consists of a pulse generator and two transvenous electrodes (leads): one defibrillation lead and one pacemaker lead. An implantable CCM-D system's electrodes (leads) are placed transvenously under fluoroscopic guidance. One right ventricular pacing lead is placed on the high septum and a second defibrillation lead is placed in the mid-septum. The pulse generator is implanted in a subcutaneous pocket in the pectoral region.

A CCM-D differs from a CCM system (0408T-0418T). A CCM system consists of a pulse generator and two ventricular pacemaker electrodes (leads) and does not include a defibrillator component. Do not report CCM-D services in conjunction with 0408T-0418T. All services associated with CCM-D implantation, revision, extraction, and follow-up should be reported utilizing Category III codes 0915T-0931T. Do not report CCM-D services with existing Category I codes for pacemaker and defibrillator services (33206-33275).

All catheterization and imaging guidance required to complete a CCM-D procedure are included in the work of each code. Contractility evaluation and programming of sensing and therapeutic parameters (0926T, 0927T) are performed each time a pulse generator or lead is implanted or replaced and cannot be reported separately.

For the implantation of a CCM-D system (generator plus dual leads), report 0915T. If only a pulse generator is implanted without insertion of transvenous electrodes, report 0916T for the implantation or 0923T for the removal and replacement. When CCM-D leads are placed without insertion of a pulse generator, report 0917T for a single-lead insertion or 0918T when both leads are inserted.

In certain circumstances, relocation of the skin pocket is required and is reported using 0925T. Skin pocket relocation includes all services associated with the initial pocket (eg, opening the pocket, incision and drainage of hematoma or abscess if performed, and any closure performed), in addition to the creation of a new pocket for the new generator to be placed.◄

● **0915T** Insertion of permanent cardiac contractility modulation-defibrillation system component(s), including fluoroscopic guidance, and evaluation and programming of sensing and therapeutic parameters; pulse generator and dual transvenous electrodes/leads (pacing and defibrillation)
Sunset January 2030
➔ *CPT Changes: An Insider's View* 2025

● **0916T** pulse generator only
Sunset January 2030
➔ *CPT Changes: An Insider's View* 2025

● **0917T** single transvenous lead (pacing or defibrillation) only
Sunset January 2030
➔ *CPT Changes: An Insider's View* 2025

● **0918T** dual transvenous leads (pacing and defibrillation) only
Sunset January 2030
➔ *CPT Changes: An Insider's View* 2025

►(Do not report 0915T, 0916T, 0917T, 0918T in conjunction with 33206-33275, 0926T, 0927T, 0931T)◄

►(Do not report 0916T, 0917T, 0918T in conjunction with 0915T)◄

● **0919T** Removal of a permanent cardiac contractility modulation-defibrillation system component(s); pulse generator only
Sunset January 2030
➔ *CPT Changes: An Insider's View* 2025

►(Do not report 0919T in conjunction with 33206-33275, 0915T, 0916T, 0923T, 0925T, 0926T, 0927T, 0931T)◄

● **0920T** single transvenous pacing lead only
Sunset January 2030
➔ *CPT Changes: An Insider's View* 2025

● **0921T** single transvenous defibrillation lead only
Sunset January 2030
➔ *CPT Changes: An Insider's View* 2025

● **0922T** dual (pacing and defibrillation) transvenous leads only
Sunset January 2030
➔ *CPT Changes: An Insider's View* 2025

►(Do not report 0920T, 0921T, 0922T in conjunction with 33206-33275, 0926T, 0927T, 0931T)◄

● **0923T** Removal and replacement of permanent cardiac contractility modulation-defibrillation pulse generator only
Sunset January 2030
➔ *CPT Changes: An Insider's View* 2025

►(Do not report 0923T in conjunction with 33206-33275, 0915T, 0916T, 0919T, 0925T, 0926T, 0927T, 0931T)◄

● **0924T** Repositioning of previously implanted cardiac contractility modulation-defibrillation transvenous electrode(s)/lead(s), including fluoroscopic guidance and programming of sensing and therapeutic parameters
Sunset January 2030
➔ *CPT Changes: An Insider's View* 2025

►(Do not report 0924T in conjunction with 33206-33275, 0915T, 0926T, 0927T, 0931T)◄

● **0925T** Relocation of skin pocket for implanted cardiac contractility modulation-defibrillation pulse generator
Sunset January 2030
➔ *CPT Changes: An Insider's View* 2025

►(Do not report 0925T in conjunction with 10140, 10180, 11042, 11043, 11044, 11045, 11046, 11047, 13100, 13101, 13102, 33206-33275, 0915T, 0916T, 0919T, 0923T, 0931T)◄

● **0926T** Programming device evaluation (in person) with iterative adjustment of the implantable device to test the function of the device and select optimal permanent programmed values with analysis, including review and report, implantable cardiac contractility modulation-defibrillation system

Sunset January 2030

➔ *CPT Changes: An Insider's View* 2025

▶(Do not report 0926T in conjunction with 33206-33275, 0915T, 0916T, 0917T, 0918T, 0919T, 0920T, 0921T, 0922T, 0923T, 0924T, 0927T, 0930T, 0931T)◀

● **0927T** Interrogation device evaluation (in person) with analysis, review, and report, including connection, recording, and disconnection, per patient encounter, implantable cardiac contractility modulation-defibrillation system

Sunset January 2030

➔ *CPT Changes: An Insider's View* 2025

▶(Do not report 0927T in conjunction with 33206-33275, 0915T, 0916T, 0917T, 0918T, 0919T, 0920T, 0921T, 0922T, 0923T, 0924T, 0926T, 0930T, 0931T)◀

● **0928T** Interrogation device evaluation (remote), up to 90 days, cardiac contractility modulation-defibrillation system with interim analysis and report(s) by a physician or other qualified health care professional

Sunset January 2030

➔ *CPT Changes: An Insider's View* 2025

▶(Do not report 0928T in conjunction with 33206-33275)◀

● **0929T** Interrogation device evaluation (remote), up to 90 days, cardiac contractility modulation-defibrillation system, remote data acquisition(s), receipt of transmissions, technician review, technical support, and distribution of results

Sunset January 2030

➔ *CPT Changes: An Insider's View* 2025

▶(Do not report 0929T in conjunction with 33206-33275)◀

● **0930T** Electrophysiologic evaluation of cardiac contractility modulation-defibrillator leads, including defibrillation-threshold evaluation (induction of arrhythmia, evaluation of sensing and therapy for arrhythmia termination), at time of initial implantation or replacement with testing of cardiac contractility modulation-defibrillator pulse generator

Sunset January 2030

➔ *CPT Changes: An Insider's View* 2025

▶(Do not report 0930T in conjunction with 33206-33275, 0931T)◀

● **0931T** Electrophysiologic evaluation of cardiac contractility modulation-defibrillator leads, including defibrillation-threshold evaluation (induction of arrhythmia, evaluation of sensing and therapy for arrhythmia termination), separate from initial implantation or replacement with testing of cardiac contractility modulation-defibrillator pulse generator

Sunset January 2030

➔ *CPT Changes: An Insider's View* 2025

▶(Do not report 0931T in conjunction with 33206-33275, 0915T-0927T, 0930T)◀

● **0932T** Noninvasive detection of heart failure derived from augmentative analysis of an echocardiogram that demonstrated preserved ejection fraction, with interpretation and report by a physician or other qualified health care professional

Sunset January 2030

➔ *CPT Changes: An Insider's View* 2025

▶(Use 0932T in conjunction with a concurrent echocardiography [separately reported] or a previously performed transthoracic echocardiography [ie, 93306, 93307, 93308, 93350, 93351])◀

● **0933T** Transcatheter implantation of wireless left atrial pressure sensor for long-term left atrial pressure monitoring, including sensor calibration and deployment, right heart catheterization, transseptal puncture, imaging guidance, and radiological supervision and interpretation

Sunset January 2030

➔ *CPT Changes: An Insider's View* 2025

▶(Do not report 0933T in conjunction with 33289, 36013, 36014, 36015, 75741, 75743, 75746, 76000, 93451, 93453, 93456, 93457, 93460, 93461, 93568, 93569, 93573, 93593, 93594, 93596, 93597, 93598)◀

▶(For implantation of a wireless pulmonary artery pressure sensor, use 33289)◀

● **0934T** Remote monitoring of a wireless left atrial pressure sensor for up to 30 days, including data from daily uploads of left atrial pressure recordings, interpretation(s) and trend analysis, with adjustments to the diuretics plan, treatment paradigm thresholds, medications or lifestyle modifications, when performed, and report(s) by a physician or other qualified health care professional

Sunset January 2030

➔ *CPT Changes: An Insider's View* 2025

▶(Report 0934T only once per 30 days)◀

▶(Do not report 0934T, if monitoring period is less than 16 days)◀

▶(Do not report 0934T in conjunction with 93264)◀

►(For remote monitoring of an implantable wireless pulmonary artery pressure sensor, use 93264)◄

● **0935T** Cystourethroscopy with renal pelvic sympathetic denervation, radiofrequency ablation, retrograde ureteral approach, including insertion of guide wire, selective placement of ureteral sheath(s) and multiple conformable electrodes, contrast injection(s), and fluoroscopy, bilateral

Sunset January 2030

➔ *CPT Changes: An Insider's View* 2025

►(Do not report 0935T in conjunction with 52000, 52005, 76000, 0338T, 0339T)◄

● **0936T** Photobiomodulation therapy of retina, single session

Sunset January 2030

➔ *CPT Changes: An Insider's View* 2025

►(For bilateral procedure, report 0936T with modifier 50)◄

● **0937T** External electrocardiographic recording for greater than 15 days up to 30 days by continuous rhythm recording and storage; including recording, scanning analysis with report, review and interpretation by a physician or other qualified health care professional

Sunset January 2030

➔ *CPT Changes: An Insider's View* 2025

● **0938T** recording (including connection and initial recording)

Sunset January 2030

➔ *CPT Changes: An Insider's View* 2025

● **0939T** scanning analysis with report

Sunset January 2030

➔ *CPT Changes: An Insider's View* 2025

● **0940T** review and interpretation by a physician or other qualified health care professional

Sunset January 2030

➔ *CPT Changes: An Insider's View* 2025

►(Report 0937T, 0938T, 0939T, 0940T for each 30-day period of service)◄

►(Do not report 0938T, 0939T, 0940T in conjunction with 0937T)◄

►(Do not report 0937T, 0938T, 0939T, 0940T in conjunction with 93224, 93225, 93226, 93227, 93228, 93229, 93241, 93242, 93243, 93244, 93245, 93246, 93247, 93248, 93268, 93270, 93271, 93272, 99091, 99453, 99454, for the same monitoring period)◄

● **0941T** Cystourethroscopy, flexible; with insertion and expansion of prostatic urethral scaffold using integrated cystoscopic visualization

Sunset January 2030

➔ *CPT Changes: An Insider's View* 2025

►(For insertion of permanent urethral stent, use 52282)◄

►(For placement of temporary prostatic urethral stent, use 53855)◄

● **0942T** with removal and replacement of prostatic urethral scaffold

Sunset January 2030

➔ *CPT Changes: An Insider's View* 2025

● **0943T** with removal of prostatic urethral scaffold

Sunset January 2030

➔ *CPT Changes: An Insider's View* 2025

►(Do not report 0943T in conjunction with 0942T)◄

►(Do not report 0941T, 0942T, 0943T in conjunction with 52000, 52282, 52310, 52315, 52441, 52442, 53855)◄

►Code 0944T describes three-dimensional (3D) contour simulation of liver lesion(s) performed by a physician or other qualified health care professional to create model probe pathways and locations, as well as to perform simulated volumetric calculations of the ablation cavity, overlaying of proposed ablation volumes on computed tomography (CT) imaging of the liver, and post-ablation volume comparisons requiring pre- and post-procedure CT imaging and guidance. A 3D contour simulation is separate and distinct from intraoperative imaging guidance and other pre-procedure imaging that are typically performed prior to image-guided liver microwave ablation procedures. Code 0944T is reported once per microwave ablation session, regardless of the number of distinct tumors ablated.◄

● **0944T** 3D contour simulation of target liver lesion(s) and margin(s) for image-guided percutaneous microwave ablation

Sunset January 2030

➔ *CPT Changes: An Insider's View* 2025

►(Report 0944T once per liver microwave ablation procedure)◄

►(Do not report 0944T in conjunction with 76376, 76377)◄

+● **0945T** Intraoperative assessment for abnormal (tumor) tissue, in-vivo, following partial mastectomy (eg, lumpectomy) using computer-aided fluorescence imaging (List separately in addition to code for primary procedure)

Sunset January 2030

➔ *CPT Changes: An Insider's View* 2025

►(Use 0945T in conjunction with 19301)◄

►(Report 0945T once per procedure)◄

►(Do not report 0945T in conjunction with 88172, 0546T)◄

★ = Telemedicine ◄ = Audio-only + = Add-on code ⋏ = FDA approval pending # = Resequenced code ⊘ = Modifier 51 exempt ➔➔➔ = See p xxi for details

● **0946T**   Orthopedic implant movement analysis using paired computed tomography (CT) examination of the target structure, including data acquisition, data preparation and transmission, interpretation and report (including CT scan of the joint or extremity performed with paired views)

Sunset January 2030

➜ *CPT Changes: An Insider's View* 2025

▶(Do not report CT scan of the extremity or joint obtained separately)◀

● **0947T**   Magnetic resonance image guided low intensity focused ultrasound (MRgFUS), stereotactic blood-brain barrier disruption using microbubble resonators to increase the concentration of blood-based biomarkers of target, intracranial, including stereotactic navigation and frame placement, when performed

Sunset January 2030

➜ *CPT Changes: An Insider's View* 2025

Notes

Appendix A

Modifiers

This list includes all of the modifiers applicable to CPT 2025 codes.

A modifier provides the means to report or indicate that a service or procedure that has been performed has been altered by some specific circumstance but not changed in its definition or code. Modifiers also enable health care professionals to effectively respond to payment policy requirements established by other entities.

22 Increased Procedural Services: When the work required to provide a service is substantially greater than typically required, it may be identified by adding modifier 22 to the usual procedure code. Documentation must support the substantial additional work and the reason for the additional work (ie, increased intensity, time, technical difficulty of procedure, severity of patient's condition, physical and mental effort required). **Note:** This modifier should not be appended to an E/M service.

➔ *CPT Changes: An Insider's View* 2008

➔ *CPT Assistant* Jan 09:8, Apr 09:8, Jun 09:8, 10, Aug 13:4, Dec 22:20, Jan 23:32, Feb 23:13, Mar 23:34, Nov 23:25, Dec 23:27, Jan 24:17, Feb 24:33, Apr 24:35

➔ *Clinical Examples in Radiology* Spring 21:12

23 Unusual Anesthesia: Occasionally, a procedure, which usually requires either no anesthesia or local anesthesia, because of unusual circumstances must be done under general anesthesia. This circumstance may be reported by adding modifier 23 to the procedure code of the basic service.

24 Unrelated Evaluation and Management Service by the Same Physician or Other Qualified Health Care Professional During a Postoperative Period: The physician or other qualified health care professional may need to indicate that an evaluation and management service was performed during a postoperative period for a reason(s) unrelated to the original procedure. This circumstance may be reported by adding modifier 24 to the appropriate level of E/M service.

➔ *CPT Changes: An Insider's View* 2013

25 Significant, Separately Identifiable Evaluation and Management Service by the Same Physician or Other Qualified Health Care Professional on the Same Day of the Procedure or Other Service: It may be necessary to indicate that on the day a procedure or service identified by a CPT code was performed, the patient's condition required a significant, separately identifiable E/M service above and beyond the other service provided or beyond the usual preoperative and postoperative care associated with the procedure that was performed. A significant, separately identifiable E/M service is defined or substantiated by documentation that satisfies the relevant criteria for the respective E/M service to be reported (see **Evaluation and Management Services Guidelines** for instructions on determining level of E/M service). The E/M service may be prompted by the symptom or condition for which the procedure and/or service was provided. As such, different diagnoses are not required for reporting of the E/M services on the same date. This circumstance may be reported by adding modifier 25 to the appropriate level of E/M service. **Note:** This modifier is not used to report an E/M service that resulted in a decision to perform surgery. See modifier 57. For significant, separately identifiable non-E/M services, see modifier 59.

➔ *CPT Changes: An Insider's View* 2008, 2013

➔ *CPT Assistant* Feb 09:22, Mar 09:3, Apr 09:4, Jun 09:11, Mar 23:1, Jul 23:1, Jan 24:1

➔ *Clinical Examples in Radiology* Spring 23:26

26 Professional Component: Certain procedures are a combination of a physician or other qualified health care professional component and a technical component. When the physician or other qualified health care professional component is reported separately, the service may be identified by adding modifier 26 to the usual procedure number.

➔ *CPT Changes: An Insider's View* 2013

➔ *CPT Assistant* Jan 09:7, Apr 09:4, May 09:7

➔ *Clinical Examples in Radiology* Summer 22:10, Fall 23:5

32 Mandated Services: Services related to *mandated* consultation and/or related services (eg, third party payer, governmental, legislative or regulatory requirement) may be identified by adding modifier 32 to the basic procedure.

➔ *CPT Assistant* Aug 13:12

33 Preventive Services: When the primary purpose of the service is the delivery of an evidence based service in accordance with a US Preventive Services Task Force A or B rating in effect and other preventive services identified in preventive services mandates (legislative or regulatory), the service may be identified by adding 33 to the procedure. For separately reported services specifically identified as preventive, the modifier should not be used.

➔ *CPT Changes: An Insider's View* 2012

47 Anesthesia by Surgeon: Regional or general anesthesia provided by the surgeon may be reported by adding modifier 47 to the basic service. (This does not include local anesthesia.) **Note:** Modifier 47 would not be used as a modifier for the anesthesia procedures.

50 Bilateral Procedure: Unless otherwise identified in the listings, bilateral procedures that are performed at the same session should be identified by adding modifier 50 to the appropriate 5 digit code. **Note:** This modifier should not be appended to designated "add-on" codes (see Appendix D).
➔ *CPT Changes: An Insider's View* 2011, 2020
➔ *CPT Assistant* Apr 09:9, Jun 13:15, Dec 22:20, Mar 23:32, May 23:28, Jul 23:18, Aug 23:14, Sep 23:1, Oct 23:19, Jan 24:17, Feb 24:34
➔ *Clinical Examples in Radiology* Winter 23:8, Fall 23:32, Winter 24:17

51 Multiple Procedures: When multiple procedures, other than E/M services, Physical Medicine and Rehabilitation services or provision of supplies (eg, vaccines), are performed at the same session by the same individual, the primary procedure or service may be reported as listed. The additional procedure(s) or service(s) may be identified by appending modifier 51 to the additional procedure or service code(s). **Note:** This modifier should not be appended to designated "add-on" codes (see Appendix D).
➔ *CPT Changes: An Insider's View* 2008, 2013
➔ *CPT Assistant* Feb 09:6, Mar 09:10, Apr 09:8, Apr 23:26, Jul 23:1, Oct 23:19, Dec 23:39, Jan 24:17
➔ *Clinical Examples in Radiology* Spring 21:3

52 Reduced Services: Under certain circumstances a service or procedure is partially reduced or eliminated at the discretion of the physician or other qualified health care professional. Under these circumstances the service provided can be identified by its usual procedure number and the addition of modifier 52, signifying that the service is reduced. This provides a means of reporting reduced services without disturbing the identification of the basic service. **Note:** For hospital outpatient reporting of a previously scheduled procedure/service that is partially reduced or cancelled as a result of extenuating circumstances or those that threaten the well-being of the patient prior to or after administration of anesthesia, see modifiers 73 and 74 (see modifiers approved for ASC hospital outpatient use).
➔ *CPT Changes: An Insider's View* 2013
➔ *CPT Assistant* Mar 09:11, Apr 09:5, May 09:8, Jun 09:10, Jun 13:17, Nov 22:22, Dec 22:20, Feb 23:6, May 23:28, Jun 23:25, Dec 23:23, Jan 24:17, Apr 24:24
➔ *Clinical Examples in Radiology* Summer 23:23, Winter 24:30

53 Discontinued Procedure: Under certain circumstances, the physician or other qualified health care professional may elect to terminate a surgical or diagnostic procedure. Due to extenuating circumstances or those that threaten the well being of the patient, it may be necessary to indicate that a surgical or diagnostic procedure was started but discontinued. This circumstance may be reported by adding modifier 53 to the code reported by the individual for the discontinued procedure. **Note:** This modifier is not used to report the elective cancellation of a procedure prior to the patient's anesthesia induction and/or surgical preparation in the operating suite. For outpatient hospital/ambulatory surgery center (ASC) reporting of a previously scheduled procedure/service that is partially reduced or cancelled as a result of extenuating circumstances or those that threaten the well being of the patient prior to or after administration

of anesthesia, see modifiers 73 and 74 (see modifiers approved for ASC hospital outpatient use).
➔ *CPT Changes: An Insider's View* 2013
➔ *CPT Assistant* Feb 14:11, Jan 23:31, Dec 23:27, Jan 24:40

54 Surgical Care Only: When 1 physician or other qualified health care professional performs a surgical procedure and another provides preoperative and/or postoperative management, surgical services may be identified by adding modifier 54 to the usual procedure number.
➔ *CPT Changes: An Insider's View* 2013

55 Postoperative Management Only: When 1 physician or other qualified health care professional performed the postoperative management and another performed the surgical procedure, the postoperative component may be identified by adding modifier 55 to the usual procedure number.
➔ *CPT Changes: An Insider's View* 2013
➔ *CPT Assistant* Jul 23:14

56 Preoperative Management Only: When 1 physician or other qualified health care professional performed the preoperative care and evaluation and another performed the surgical procedure, the preoperative component may be identified by adding modifier 56 to the usual procedure number.
➔ *CPT Changes: An Insider's View* 2013

57 Decision for Surgery: An evaluation and management service that resulted in the initial decision to perform the surgery may be identified by adding modifier 57 to the appropriate level of E/M service.
➔ *CPT Assistant* May 09:9, Mar 23:1, Jul 23:1

58 Staged or Related Procedure or Service by the Same Physician or Other Qualified Health Care Professional During the Postoperative Period: It may be necessary to indicate that the performance of a procedure or service during the postoperative period was: (a) planned or anticipated (staged); (b) more extensive than the original procedure; or (c) for therapy following a surgical procedure. This circumstance may be reported by adding modifier 58 to the staged or related procedure. **Note:** For treatment of a problem that requires a return to the operating/procedure room (eg, unanticipated clinical condition), see modifier 78.
➔ *CPT Changes: An Insider's View* 2008, 2013
➔ *CPT Assistant* Nov 22:22

59 Distinct Procedural Service: Under certain circumstances, it may be necessary to indicate that a procedure or service was distinct or independent from other non-E/M services performed on the same day. Modifier 59 is used to identify procedures/services, other than E/M services, that are not normally reported together, but are appropriate under the circumstances. Documentation must support a different session, different procedure or surgery, different site or organ system, separate incision/excision, separate lesion, or separate injury (or area of injury in extensive injuries) not ordinarily encountered or performed on the same day by the same individual. However, when another already established modifier is appropriate it should be used rather than modifier 59. Only if no more descriptive modifier is available, and the use of modifier 59 best explains the circumstances, should modifier 59 be used. **Note:** Modifier 59 should not be appended to an E/M service. To report a separate and distinct E/M service with a non-E/M service performed on the same date, see modifier 25.

➲ *CPT Changes: An Insider's View* 2008

➲ *CPT Assistant* Feb 09:17, Apr 09:4, 8, May 09:6, Jun 09:8, Mar 23:1, Apr 23:24, 26, May 23:24, Jun 23:16, Jul 23:1, Sep 23:1, Oct 23:21, Dec 23:39, Jan 24:17

➲ *Clinical Examples in Radiology* Winter 23:8, Spring 23:20, Summer 23:16, Fall 23:14

62 **Two Surgeons:** When 2 surgeons work together as primary surgeons performing distinct part(s) of a procedure, each surgeon should report his/her distinct operative work by adding modifier 62 to the procedure code and any associated add-on code(s) for that procedure as long as both surgeons continue to work together as primary surgeons. Each surgeon should report the co-surgery once using the same procedure code. If additional procedure(s) (including add-on procedure[s]) are performed during the same surgical session, separate code(s) may also be reported with modifier 62 added. **Note:** If a co-surgeon acts as an assistant in the performance of additional procedure(s), other than those reported with the modifier 62, during the same surgical session, those services may be reported using separate procedure code(s) with modifier 80 or modifier 82 added, as appropriate.

➲ *CPT Changes: An Insider's View* 2013

➲ *CPT Assistant* May 23:27, Jan 24:17

63 **Procedure Performed on Infants less than 4 kg:** Procedures performed on neonates and infants up to a present body weight of 4 kg may involve significantly increased complexity and physician or other qualified health care professional work commonly associated with these patients. This circumstance may be reported by adding modifier 63 to the procedure number. **Note:** Unless otherwise designated, this modifier may only be appended to procedures/services listed in the 20100-69990 code series and 92920, 92928, 92953, 92960, 92986, 92987, 92990, 92997, 92998, 93312, 93313, 93314, 93315, 93316, 93317, 93318, 93452, 93505, 93563, 93564, 93568, 93569, 93573, 93574, 93575, 93580, 93581, 93582, 93590, 93591, 93592, 93593, 93594, 93595, 93596, 93597, 93598, 93615, 93616 from the Medicine/ Cardiovascular section. Modifier 63 should not be appended to any CPT codes listed in the **Evaluation and Management Services, Anesthesia, Radiology, Pathology and Laboratory,** or **Medicine** sections (other than those identified above from the Medicine/Cardiovascular section).

➲ *CPT Changes: An Insider's View* 2013, 2019, 2020, 2022, 2023

➲ *CPT Assistant* May 23:1, Sep 23:47

66 **Surgical Team:** Under some circumstances, highly complex procedures (requiring the concomitant services of several physicians or other qualified health care professionals, often of different specialties, plus other highly skilled, specially trained personnel, various types of complex equipment) are carried out under the "surgical team" concept. Such circumstances may be identified by each participating individual with the addition of modifier 66 to the basic procedure number used for reporting services.

➲ *CPT Changes: An Insider's View* 2013

76 **Repeat Procedure or Service by Same Physician or Other Qualified Health Care Professional:** It may be necessary to indicate that a procedure or service was repeated by the same physician or other qualified health care professional subsequent to the original procedure or service. This circumstance may be reported by adding modifier 76 to the repeated procedure or service. **Note:** This modifier should not be appended to an E/M service.

➲ *CPT Changes: An Insider's View* 2008, 2011, 2013

➲ *CPT Assistant* Feb 09:6, Jul 23:1

77 **Repeat Procedure by Another Physician or Other Qualified Health Care Professional:** It may be necessary to indicate that a basic procedure or service was repeated by another physician or other qualified health care professional subsequent to the original procedure or service. This circumstance may be reported by adding modifier 77 to the repeated procedure or service. **Note:** This modifier should not be appended to an E/M service.

➲ *CPT Changes: An Insider's View* 2008, 2011, 2013

➲ *Clinical Examples in Radiology* Summer 22:10

78 **Unplanned Return to the Operating/Procedure Room by the Same Physician or Other Qualified Health Care Professional Following Initial Procedure for a Related Procedure During the Postoperative Period:** It may be necessary to indicate that another procedure was performed during the postoperative period of the initial procedure (unplanned procedure following initial procedure). When this procedure is related to the first, and requires the use of an operating/procedure room, it may be reported by adding modifier 78 to the related procedure. (For repeat procedures, see modifier 76.)

➲ *CPT Changes: An Insider's View* 2008, 2011, 2013

79 **Unrelated Procedure or Service by the Same Physician or Other Qualified Health Care Professional During the Postoperative Period:** The individual may need to indicate that the performance of a procedure or service during the postoperative period was unrelated to the original procedure. This circumstance may be reported by using modifier 79. (For repeat procedures on the same day, see modifier 76.)

➲ *CPT Changes: An Insider's View* 2013

80 **Assistant Surgeon:** Surgical assistant services may be identified by adding modifier 80 to the usual procedure number(s).

81 **Minimum Assistant Surgeon:** Minimum surgical assistant services are identified by adding modifier 81 to the usual procedure number.

82 **Assistant Surgeon (when qualified resident surgeon not available):** The unavailability of a qualified resident surgeon is a prerequisite for use of modifier 82 appended to the usual procedure code number(s).

90 **Reference (Outside) Laboratory:** When laboratory procedures are performed by a party other than the treating or reporting physician or other qualified health care professional, the procedure may be identified by adding modifier 90 to the usual procedure number.

➔ *CPT Changes: An Insider's View* 2013

91 **Repeat Clinical Diagnostic Laboratory Test:** In the course of treatment of the patient, it may be necessary to repeat the same laboratory test on the same day to obtain subsequent (multiple) test results. Under these circumstances, the laboratory test performed can be identified by its usual procedure number and the addition of modifier 91. **Note:** This modifier may not be used when tests are rerun to confirm initial results; due to testing problems with specimens or equipment; or for any other reason when a normal, one-time, reportable result is all that is required. This modifier may not be used when other code(s) describe a series of test results (eg, glucose tolerance tests, evocative/suppression testing). This modifier may only be used for laboratory test(s) performed more than once on the same day on the same patient.

➔ *CPT Assistant* May 09:6, Sept 13:7

92 **Alternative Laboratory Platform Testing:** When laboratory testing is being performed using a kit or transportable instrument that wholly or in part consists of a single use, disposable analytical chamber, the service may be identified by adding modifier 92 to the usual laboratory procedure code (HIV testing 86701-86703, and 87389). The test does not require permanent dedicated space, hence by its design may be hand carried or transported to the vicinity of the patient for immediate testing at that site, although location of the testing is not in itself determinative of the use of this modifier.

➔ *CPT Changes: An Insider's View* 2008, 2012

93 **Synchronous Telemedicine Service Rendered Via Telephone or Other Real-Time Interactive Audio-Only Telecommunications System:** Synchronous telemedicine service is defined as a real-time interaction between a physician or other qualified health care professional and a patient who is located away at a distant site from the physician or other qualified health care professional. The totality of the communication of information exchanged between the physician or other qualified health care professional and the patient during the course of the synchronous telemedicine service must be of an amount and nature that is sufficient to meet the key components and/or requirements of the same service when rendered via a face-to-face interaction.

➔ *CPT Changes: An Insider's View* 2023

95 **Synchronous Telemedicine Service Rendered Via a Real-Time Interactive Audio and Video Telecommunications System:** Synchronous telemedicine service is defined as a **real-time** interaction between a physician or other qualified health care professional and a patient who is located at a distant site from the physician or other qualified health care professional. The totality of the communication of information exchanged between the physician or other qualified health care professional and the patient during the course of the synchronous telemedicine service must be of an amount and nature that would be sufficient to meet the key components and/or requirements of the same service when rendered via a face-to-face interaction. Modifier 95 may only be appended to the services listed in Appendix P. Appendix P is the list of CPT codes for services that are typically performed face-to-face, but may be rendered via a real-time (synchronous) interactive audio and video telecommunications system.

➔ *CPT Changes: An Insider's View* 2017
➔ *CPT Assistant* Dec 23:49

96 **Habilitative Services:** When a service or procedure that may be either habilitative or rehabilitative in nature is provided for habilitative purposes, the physician or other qualified health care professional may add modifier 96 to the service or procedure code to indicate that the service or procedure provided was a habilitative service. Habilitative services help an individual learn skills and functioning for daily living that the individual has not yet developed, and then keep and/or improve those learned skills. Habilitative services also help an individual keep, learn, or improve skills and functioning for daily living.

➔ *CPT Changes: An Insider's View* 2018

97 **Rehabilitative Services:** When a service or procedure that may be either habilitative or rehabilitative in nature is provided for rehabilitative purposes, the physician or other qualified health care professional may add modifier 97 to the service or procedure code to indicate that the service or procedure provided was a rehabilitative service. Rehabilitative services help an individual keep, get back, or improve skills and functioning for daily living that have been lost or impaired because the individual was sick, hurt, or disabled.

➔ *CPT Changes: An Insider's View* 2018

99 **Multiple Modifiers:** Under certain circumstances 2 or more modifiers may be necessary to completely delineate a service. In such situations modifier 99 should be added to the basic procedure, and other applicable modifiers may be listed as part of the description of the service.

Appendix A

Anesthesia Physical Status Modifiers

The Physical Status modifiers are consistent with the American Society of Anesthesiologists ranking of patient physical status, and distinguishing various levels of complexity of the anesthesia service provided. All anesthesia services are reported by use of the anesthesia five-digit procedure code (00100-01999) with the appropriate physical status modifier appended.

Example: 00100-P1

Under certain circumstances, when another established modifier(s) is appropriate, it should be used in addition to the physical status modifier.

Example: 00100-P4-53

Physical Status Modifier P1: A normal healthy patient

Physical Status Modifier P2: A patient with mild systemic disease

Physical Status Modifier P3: A patient with severe systemic disease

Physical Status Modifier P4: A patient with severe systemic disease that is a constant threat to life

Physical Status Modifier P5: A moribund patient who is not expected to survive without the operation

Physical Status Modifier P6: A declared brain-dead patient whose organs are being removed for donor purposes

Modifiers Approved for Ambulatory Surgery Center (ASC) Hospital Outpatient Use

CPT Level I Modifiers

25 **Significant, Separately Identifiable Evaluation and Management Service by the Same Physician or Other Qualified Health Care Professional on the Same Day of the Procedure or Other Service:** It may be necessary to indicate that on the day a procedure or service identified by a CPT code was performed, the patient's condition required a significant, separately identifiable E/M service above and beyond the other service provided or beyond the usual preoperative and postoperative care associated with the procedure that was performed. A significant, separately identifiable E/M service is defined or substantiated by documentation that satisfies the relevant criteria for the respective E/M service to be reported (see **Evaluation and Management Services Guidelines** for instructions on determining level of E/M service). The E/M service may be prompted by the symptom or condition for which the procedure and/or service was provided. As such, different diagnoses are not required for reporting of the E/M services on the same date. This circumstance may be reported by adding modifier 25 to the appropriate level of E/M service. **Note:** This modifier is not used to report an E/M service

that resulted in a decision to perform surgery. See modifier 57. For significant, separately identifiable non-E/M services, see modifier 59.

> *CPT Changes: An Insider's View* 2008, 2013
> *CPT Assistant* Feb 09:22, Mar 09:3, Apr 09:4, Jun 09:11, Mar 23:1, Jul 23:1, Jan 24:1
> *Clinical Examples in Radiology* Spring 23:26

27 **Multiple Outpatient Hospital E/M Encounters on the Same Date:** For hospital outpatient reporting purposes, utilization of hospital resources related to separate and distinct E/M encounters performed in multiple outpatient hospital settings on the same date may be reported by adding modifier 27 to each appropriate level outpatient and/or emergency department E/M code(s). This modifier provides a means of reporting circumstances involving evaluation and management services provided by physician(s) in more than one (multiple) outpatient hospital setting(s) (eg, hospital emergency department, clinic). **Note:** This modifier is not to be used for physician reporting of multiple E/M services performed by the same physician on the same date. For physician reporting of all outpatient evaluation and management services provided by the same physician on the same date and performed in multiple outpatient setting(s) (eg, hospital emergency department, clinic), see **Evaluation and Management, Emergency Department,** or **Preventive Medicine Services** codes.

33 **Preventive Services:** When the primary purpose of the service is the delivery of an evidence based service in accordance with a US Preventive Services Task Force A or B rating in effect and other preventive services identified in preventive services mandates (legislative or regulatory), the service may be identified by adding 33 to the procedure. For separately reported services specifically identified as preventive, the modifier should not be used.

> *CPT Changes: An Insider's View* 2012

50 **Bilateral Procedure:** Unless otherwise identified in the listings, bilateral procedures that are performed at the same session should be identified by adding modifier 50 to the appropriate 5 digit code. **Note:** This modifier should not be appended to designated "add-on" codes (see Appendix D).

> *CPT Changes: An Insider's View* 2011, 2020
> *CPT Assistant* Apr 09:9, Jun 13:15, Dec 22:20, Mar 23:32, May 23:28, Jul 23:18, Aug 23:14, Sep 23:1, Oct 23:19, Jan 24:17, Feb 24:34
> *Clinical Examples in Radiology* Winter 23:8, Fall 23:32, Winter 24:17

52 **Reduced Services:** Under certain circumstances a service or procedure is partially reduced or eliminated at the discretion of the physician or other qualified health care professional. Under these circumstances the service provided can be identified by its usual procedure number and the addition of modifier 52, signifying that the service

is reduced. This provides a means of reporting reduced services without disturbing the identification of the basic service. **Note:** For hospital outpatient reporting of a previously scheduled procedure/service that is partially reduced or cancelled as a result of extenuating circumstances or those that threaten the well-being of the patient prior to or after administration of anesthesia, see modifiers 73 and 74 (see modifiers approved for ASC hospital outpatient use).

➲ *CPT Changes: An Insider's View* 2013

➲ *CPT Assistant* Mar 09:11, Apr 09:5, May 09:8, Jun 09:10, Jun 13:17, Nov 22:22, Dec 22:20, Feb 23:6, May 23:28, Jun 23:25, Dec 23:23, Jan 24:17, Apr 24:24

➲ *Clinical Examples in Radiology* Summer 23:23, Winter 24:30

58   Staged or Related Procedure or Service by the Same Physician or Other Qualified Health Care Professional During the Postoperative Period: It may be necessary to indicate that the performance of a procedure or service during the postoperative period was: (a) planned or anticipated (staged); (b) more extensive than the original procedure; or (c) for therapy following a surgical procedure. This circumstance may be reported by adding modifier 58 to the staged or related procedure. **Note:** For treatment of a problem that requires a return to the operating/procedure room (eg, unanticipated clinical condition), see modifier 78.

➲ *CPT Changes: An Insider's View* 2008, 2013

➲ *CPT Assistant* Nov 22:22

59   Distinct Procedural Service: Under certain circumstances, it may be necessary to indicate that a procedure or service was distinct or independent from other non-E/M services performed on the same day. Modifier 59 is used to identify procedures/services, other than E/M services, that are not normally reported together, but are appropriate under the circumstances. Documentation must support a different session, different procedure or surgery, different site or organ system, separate incision/excision, separate lesion, or separate injury (or area of injury in extensive injuries) not ordinarily encountered or performed on the same day by the same individual. However, when another already established modifier is appropriate it should be used rather than modifier 59. Only if no more descriptive modifier is available, and the use of modifier 59 best explains the circumstances, should modifier 59 be used. **Note:** Modifier 59 should not be appended to an E/M service. To report a separate and distinct E/M service with a non-E/M service performed on the same date, see modifier 25.

➲ *CPT Changes: An Insider's View* 2008

➲ *CPT Assistant* Feb 09:17, Apr 09:4, 8, May 09:6, Jun 09:8, Mar 23:1, Apr 23:24, 26, May 23:24, Jun 23:16, Jul 23:1, Sep 23:1, Oct 23:21, Dec 23:39, Jan 24:17

➲ *Clinical Examples in Radiology* Winter 23:8, Spring 23:20, Summer 23:16, Fall 23:14

73   Discontinued Out-Patient Hospital/Ambulatory Surgery Center (ASC) Procedure Prior to the Administration of Anesthesia: Due to extenuating circumstances or those that threaten the well being of the patient, the physician may cancel a surgical or diagnostic procedure subsequent to the patient's surgical preparation (including sedation when provided, and being taken to the room where the procedure

is to be performed), but prior to the administration of anesthesia (local, regional block(s) or general). Under these circumstances, the intended service that is prepared for but cancelled can be reported by its usual procedure number and the addition of modifier 73. **Note:** The elective cancellation of a service prior to the administration of anesthesia and/or surgical preparation of the patient should not be reported. For physician reporting of a discontinued procedure, see modifier 53.

➲ *CPT Assistant* Jan 23:31

74   Discontinued Out-Patient Hospital/Ambulatory Surgery Center (ASC) Procedure After Administration of Anesthesia: Due to extenuating circumstances or those that threaten the well being of the patient, the physician may terminate a surgical or diagnostic procedure after the administration of anesthesia (local, regional block(s), general) or after the procedure was started (incision made, intubation started, scope inserted, etc). Under these circumstances, the procedure started but terminated can be reported by its usual procedure number and the addition of modifier 74. **Note:** The elective cancellation of a service prior to the administration of anesthesia and/or surgical preparation of the patient should not be reported. For physician reporting of a discontinued procedure, see modifier 53.

➲ *CPT Assistant* Jun 13:17, Jan 23:31

76   Repeat Procedure or Service by Same Physician or Other Qualified Health Care Professional: It may be necessary to indicate that a procedure or service was repeated by the same physician or other qualified health care professional subsequent to the original procedure or service. This circumstance may be reported by adding modifier 76 to the repeated procedure or service. **Note:** This modifier should not be appended to an E/M service.

➲ *CPT Changes: An Insider's View* 2008, 2011, 2013

➲ *CPT Assistant* Feb 09:6, Jul 23:1

77   Repeat Procedure by Another Physician or Other Qualified Health Care Professional: It may be necessary to indicate that a basic procedure or service was repeated by another physician or other qualified health care professional subsequent to the original procedure or service. This circumstance may be reported by adding modifier 77 to the repeated procedure or service. **Note:** This modifier should not be appended to an E/M service.

➲ *CPT Changes: An Insider's View* 2008, 2011, 2013

➲ *Clinical Examples in Radiology* Summer 22:10

78 Unplanned Return to the Operating/Procedure Room by the Same Physician or Other Qualified Health Care Professional Following Initial Procedure for a Related Procedure During the Postoperative Period: It may be necessary to indicate that another procedure was performed during the postoperative period of the initial procedure (unplanned procedure following initial procedure). When this procedure is related to the first, and requires the use of an operating/procedure room, it may be reported by adding modifier 78 to the related procedure. (For repeat procedures, see modifier 76.)

➔ *CPT Changes: An Insider's View* 2008, 2011, 2013

79 Unrelated Procedure or Service by the Same Physician or Other Qualified Health Care Professional During the Postoperative Period: The individual may need to indicate that the performance of a procedure or service during the postoperative period was unrelated to the original procedure. This circumstance may be reported by using modifier 79. (For repeat procedures on the same day, see modifier 76.)

➔ *CPT Changes: An Insider's View* 2013

91 Repeat Clinical Diagnostic Laboratory Test: In the course of treatment of the patient, it may be necessary to repeat the same laboratory test on the same day to obtain subsequent (multiple) test results. Under these circumstances, the laboratory test performed can be identified by its usual procedure number and the addition of modifier 91. **Note:** This modifier may not be used when tests are rerun to confirm initial results; due to testing problems with specimens or equipment; or for any other reason when a normal, one-time, reportable result is all that is required. This modifier may not be used when other code(s) describe a series of test results (eg, glucose tolerance tests, evocative/suppression testing). This modifier may only be used for laboratory test(s) performed more than once on the same day on the same patient.

➔ *CPT Assistant* May 09:6, Sept 13:7

Category II Modifiers

The following performance measurement modifiers may be used for Category II codes to indicate that a service specified in the associated measure(s) was considered but, due to either medical, patient, or system circumstance(s) documented in the medical record, the service was not provided. These modifiers serve as denominator exclusions from the performance measure. The user should note that not all listed measures provide for exclusions (see Alphabetical Clinical Topics Listing for more discussion regarding exclusion criteria).

Category II modifiers should only be reported with Category II codes—they should not be reported with Category I or Category III codes. In addition, the modifiers in the Category II section should only be used where specified in the guidelines, reporting instructions, parenthetic notes, or code descriptor language listed in the Category II section (code listing and the Alphabetical Clinical Topics Listing).

1P Performance Measure Exclusion Modifier due to Medical Reasons:

Reasons include:

- Not indicated (absence of organ/limb, already received/performed, other)
- Contraindicated (patient allergic history, potential adverse drug interaction, other)
- Other medical reasons

2P Performance Measure Exclusion Modifier due to Patient Reasons:

Reasons include:

- Patient declined
- Economic, social, or religious reasons
- Other patient reasons

3P Performance Measure Exclusion Modifier due to System Reasons:

Reasons include:

- Resources to perform the services not available
- Insurance coverage/payor-related limitations
- Other reasons attributable to health care delivery system

Modifier 8P is intended to be used as a "reporting modifier" to allow the reporting of circumstances when an action described in a measure's numerator is not performed and the reason is not otherwise specified.

8P Performance measure reporting modifier–action not performed, reason not otherwise specified

Level II (HCPCS/National) Modifiers

E1 Upper left, eyelid

E2 Lower left, eyelid

E3 Upper right, eyelid

E4 Lower right, eyelid

FA Left hand, thumb

F1 Left hand, second digit

F2 Left hand, third digit

F3 Left hand, fourth digit

F4 Left hand, fifth digit

F5 Right hand, thumb

F6 Right hand, second digit

F7 Right hand, third digit

F8 Right hand, fourth digit

F9 Right hand, fifth digit

GG Performance and payment of a screening mammogram and diagnostic mammogram on the same patient, same day

GH Diagnostic mammogram converted from screening mammogram on same day

LC Left circumflex coronary artery

LD Left anterior descending coronary artery

LM Left main coronary artery

LT Left side (used to identify procedures performed on the left side of the body)

QM Ambulance service provided under arrangement by a provider of services

QN Ambulance service furnished directly by a provider of services

RC Right coronary artery

RI Ramus intermedius coronary artery

RT Right side (used to identify procedures performed on the right side of the body)

TA Left foot, great toe

T1 Left foot, second digit

T2 Left foot, third digit

T3 Left foot, fourth digit

T4 Left foot, fifth digit

T5 Right foot, great toe

T6 Right foot, second digit

T7 Right foot, third digit

T8 Right foot, fourth digit

T9 Right foot, fifth digit

XE Separate Encounter*

XP Separate Practitioner*

XS Separate Organ/Structure*

XU Unusual Separate Service*

(*HCPCS modifiers for selective identification of subsets of Distinct Procedural Services [59 modifier]

Appendix B

Summary of Additions, Deletions, and Revisions

Appendix B shows the actual changes that were made to the code descriptors. New codes appear with a bullet (●) and are indicated as "Code added." Revised codes are preceded with a triangle (▲). Within revised codes, the deleted language appears with a ~~strikethrough~~, while new text appears <u>underlined</u>. The symbol ⁄ is used to identify codes for vaccines that are pending FDA approval (see **Appendix K**). The symbol # is used to identify codes that have been resequenced (see **Appendix N**). The symbol ℋ is used to identify codes that are duplicate PLA tests. CPT add-on codes are annotated by the symbol ✚ (see **Appendix D**). The symbol ⊘ is used to identify codes that are exempt from the use of modifier 51 (see **Appendix E**). The symbol ★ is used to identify codes that may be used for reporting audio-video telemedicine services (see **Appendix P**). The ⇅ symbol is used to identify Category I PLA codes. The ◀ symbol is used to identify codes that may be used to report audio-only telemedicine services (see **Appendix T**).

Evaluation and Management

#●	98000	Code added
#●	98001	Code added
#●	98002	Code added
#●	98003	Code added
#●	98004	Code added
#●	98005	Code added
#●	98006	Code added
#●	98007	Code added
#●	98008	Code added
#●	98009	Code added
#●	98010	Code added
#●	98011	Code added
#●	98012	Code added
#●	98013	Code added
#●	98014	Code added
#●	98015	Code added
#●	98016	Code added

99441   ~~Telephone evaluation and management service by a physician or other qualified health care professional who may report evaluation and management services provided to an established patient, parent, or guardian not originating from a related E/M service provided within the previous 7 days nor leading to an E/M service or procedure within the next 24 hours or soonest available appointment; 5-10 minutes of medical discussion~~

99442   ~~11-20 minutes of medical discussion~~

99443   ~~21-30 minutes of medical discussion~~

Surgery

●	15011	Code added
✚●	15012	Code added
●	15013	Code added
✚●	15014	Code added
●	15015	Code added
✚●	15016	Code added
●	15017	Code added

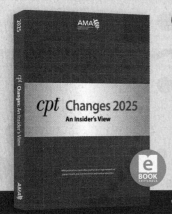

+● **15018**   Code added

15819   ~~Cervicoplasty~~

▲ **21630**   Radical resection of sternum;

21632   ~~with mediastinal lymphadenectomy~~

▲ **25447**   Arthroplasty, ~~interposition,~~ intercarpal or carpometacarpal joints; interposition (eg, tendon)

● **25448**   Code added

33471   ~~Valvotomy, pulmonary valve, closed heart, via pulmonary artery~~

33737   ~~open heart, with inflow occlusion~~

33813   ~~Obliteration of aortopulmonary septal defect; without cardiopulmonary bypass~~

▲ **33814**   Obliteration of aortopulmonary septal defect, with cardiopulmonary bypass; ~~with cardiopulmonary bypass~~

#● **38225**   Code added

#● **38226**   Code added

#● **38227**   Code added

#● **38228**   Code added

47802   ~~U-tube hepaticoenterostomy~~

● **49186**   Code added

● **49187**   Code added

● **49188**   Code added

● **49189**   Code added

● **49190**   Code added

49203   ~~Excision or destruction, open, intra-abdominal tumors, cysts or endometriomas, 1 or more peritoneal, mesenteric, or retroperitoneal primary or secondary tumors; largest tumor 5 cm diameter or less~~

49204   ~~largest tumor 5.1-10.0 cm diameter~~

49205   ~~largest tumor greater than 10.0 cm diameter~~

50135   ~~complicated (eg, secondary operation, congenital kidney abnormality)~~

▲ **51020**   Cystotomy or cystostomy, with fulguration and/or insertion of radioactive material; ~~with fulguration and/or insertion of radioactive material~~

51030   ~~with cryosurgical destruction of intravesical lesion~~

● **51721**   Code added

● **53865**   Code added

● **53866**   Code added

54438   ~~Replantation, penis, complete amputation including urethral repair~~

● **55881**   Code added

● **55882**   Code added

58957   ~~Resection (tumor debulking) of recurrent ovarian, tubal, primary peritoneal, uterine malignancy (intra-abdominal, retroperitoneal tumors), with omentectomy, if performed;~~

▲ **58958**   Resection (tumor debulking) of recurrent ovarian, tubal, primary peritoneal, uterine malignancy (intra-abdominal, retroperitoneal tumors), with omentectomy, if performed, with pelvic lymphadenectomy and limited para-aortic lymphadenectomy; ~~with pelvic lymphadenectomy and limited para-aortic lymphadenectomy~~

● **60660**   Code added

+● **60661**   Code added

● **61715**   Code added

#● **64466**   Code added

#● **64467**   Code added

#● **64468**   Code added

#● **64469**   Code added

#● **64473**   Code added

#● **64474**   Code added

● **66683**   Code added

Radiology

#● **76014**   Code added

#+● **76015**   Code added

#● **76016**   Code added

#⊘● **76017**   Code added

#⊘● **76018**   Code added

#⊘● **76019**   Code added

Pathology and Laboratory

#● **81195**   Code added

▲ **81432**   Hereditary breast cancer-related disorders (eg, hereditary breast cancer, hereditary ovarian cancer, hereditary endometrial cancer, hereditary pancreatic cancer, hereditary prostate cancer), genomic sequence analysis panel, 5 or more genes, interrogation for sequence variants and copy number variants; ~~genomic sequence analysis panel, must include sequencing of at least 10 genes, always including BRCA1, BRCA2, CDH1, MLH1, MSH2, MSH6, PALB2, PTEN, STK11, and TP53~~

81433   ~~Hereditary breast cancer-related disorders (eg, hereditary breast cancer, hereditary ovarian cancer, hereditary endometrial cancer); duplication/deletion analysis panel, must include analyses for BRCA1, BRCA2, MLH1, MSH2, and STK11~~

▲ **81435**   Hereditary colon cancer-related disorders (eg, Lynch syndrome, PTEN hamartoma syndrome, Cowden syndrome, familial adenomatosis polyposis), genomic sequence analysis panel, 5 or more genes, interrogation for sequence variants and copy number variants; genomic sequence analysis panel, must include sequencing of at least 10 genes, including *APC, BMPR1A, CDH1, MLH1, MSH2, MSH6, MUTYH, PTEN, SMAD4,* and *STK11*

   81436   Hereditary colon cancer disorders (eg, Lynch syndrome, PTEN hamartoma syndrome, Cowden syndrome, familial adenomatosis polyposis); duplication/deletion analysis panel, must include analysis of at least 5 genes, including *MLH1, MSH2, EPCAM, SMAD4,* and *STK11*

▲ **81437**   Hereditary neuroendocrine tumor-related disorders (eg, medullary thyroid carcinoma, parathyroid carcinoma, malignant pheochromocytoma or paraganglioma), genomic sequence analysis panel, 5 or more genes, interrogation for sequence variants and copy number variants; genomic sequence analysis panel, must include sequencing of at least 6 genes, including *MAX, SDHB, SDHC, SDHD, TMEM127,* and *VHL*

   81438   Hereditary neuroendocrine tumor disorders (eg, medullary thyroid carcinoma, parathyroid carcinoma, malignant pheochromocytoma or paraganglioma); duplication/deletion analysis panel, must include analyses for *SDHB, SDHC, SDHD,* and *VHL*

● **81515**   Code added

● **81558**   Code added

● **82233**   Code added

● **82234**   Code added

● **83884**   Code added

● **84393**   Code added

● **84394**   Code added

   86327   crossed (2-dimensional assay)

   86490   coccidioidomycosis

● **86581**   Code added

● **87513**   Code added

#▲ **87624**   Human Papillomavirus (HPV), high-risk types (eg, 16, 18, 31, 33, 35, 39, 45, 51, 52, 56, 58, 59, 68), pooled result

#● **87626**   Code added

#● **87564**   Code added

● **87594**   Code added

▲ **88387**   Macroscopic examination, dissection, and preparation of tissue for non-microscopic analytical studies (eg, nucleic acid-based molecular studies), each tissue preparation (eg, a single lymph node); each tissue preparation (eg, a single lymph node)

   88388   Macroscopic examination, dissection, and preparation of tissue for non-microscopic analytical studies (eg, nucleic acid-based molecular studies); in conjunction with a touch imprint, intraoperative consultation, or frozen section, each tissue preparation (eg, a single lymph node) (List separately in addition to code for primary procedure)

   0078U   Pain management (opioid-use disorder) genotyping panel, 16 common variants (ie, *ABCB1, COMT, DAT1, DBH, DOR, DRD1, DRD2, DRD4, GABA, GAL, HTR2A, HTTLPR, MTHFR, MUOR, OPRK1, OPRM1*), buccal swab or other germline tissue sample, algorithm reported as positive or negative risk of opioid-use disorder

   0167U   Gonadotropin, chorionic (hCG), immunoassay with direct optical observation, blood

   0204U   Oncology (thyroid), mRNA, gene expression analysis of 593 genes (including *BRAF, RAS, RET, PAX8,* and *NTRK*) for sequence variants and rearrangements, utilizing fine needle aspirate, reported as detected or not detected

▲ **0248U**   Oncology (brain), spheroid cell culture in a 3D microenvironment, 12-drug panel, tumor brain- or brain metastasis-response prediction for each drug

▲ **0351U**   Infectious disease (bacterial or viral), biochemical assays, tumor necrosis factor-related apoptosis-inducing ligand (TRAIL), interferon gamma-induced protein-10 (IP-10), and C-reactive protein, serum, or venous whole blood, algorithm reported as likelihood of bacterial infection

   0352U   Infectious disease (bacterial vaginosis and vaginitis), multiplex amplified probe technique, for detection of bacterial vaginosis-associated bacteria (BVAB-2, Atopobium vaginae, and Megasphera type 1), algorithm reported as detected or not detected and separate detection of Candida species (C. albicans, C. tropicalis, C. parapsilosis, C. dubliniensis), Candida glabrata/Candida krusei, and trichomonas vaginalis, vaginal-fluid specimen, each result reported as detected or not detected

   0353U   Infectious agent detection by nucleic acid (DNA), Chlamydia trachomatis and Neisseria gonorrhoeae, multiplex amplified probe technique, urine, vaginal, pharyngeal, or rectal, each pathogen reported as detected or not detected

   0354U   Human papilloma virus (HPV), high-risk types (ie, 16, 18, 31, 33, 45, 52 and 58) qualitative mRNA expression of E6/E7 by quantitative polymerase chain reaction (qPCR)

▲ **0356U**   Oncology (oropharyngeal or anal), evaluation of 17 DNA biomarkers using droplet digital PCR (ddPCR), cell-free DNA, algorithm reported as a prognostic risk score for cancer recurrence

0396U ~~Obstetrics (pre-implantation genetic testing), evaluation of 300000 DNA single-nucleotide polymorphisms (SNPs) by microarray, embryonic tissue, algorithm reported as a probability for single-gene germline conditions~~

▲ 0403U Oncology (prostate), mRNA, gene expression profiling of 18 genes, first-catch ~~post-digital rectal examination~~ urine ~~(or processed first-catch urine)~~, algorithm reported as percentage of likelihood of detecting clinically significant prostate cancer

0416U ~~Infectious agent detection by nucleic acid (DNA), genitourinary pathogens, identification of 20 bacterial and fungal organisms, including identification of 20 associated antibiotic-resistance genes, if performed, multiplex amplified probe technique, urine~~

● 0420U Code added
● 0421U Code added
● 0422U Code added
● 0423U Code added
● 0424U Code added
● 0425U Code added
● 0426U Code added
+● 0427U Code added
● 0428U Code added
● 0429U Code added
● 0430U Code added
● 0431U Code added
● 0432U Code added
● 0433U Code added
● 0434U Code added
● 0435U Code added
● 0436U Code added
● 0437U Code added
● 0438U Code added
● 0439U Code added
● 0440U Code added
● 0441U Code added
● 0442U Code added
● 0443U Code added
● 0444U Code added
● 0445U Code added
● 0446U Code added
● 0447U Code added
● 0448U Code added
● 0449U Code added
● 0450U Code added

● 0451U Code added
● 0452U Code added
● 0453U Code added
⌗● 0454U Code added
● 0455U Code added
● 0456U Code added
● 0457U Code added
● 0458U Code added
● 0459U Code added
● 0460U Code added
● 0461U Code added
● 0462U Code added
● 0463U Code added
● 0464U Code added
● 0465U Code added
● 0466U Code added
● 0467U Code added
● 0468U Code added
● 0469U Code added
● 0470U Code added
● 0471U Code added
● 0472U Code added
● 0473U Code added
● 0474U Code added
● 0475U Code added
● 0476U Code added
● 0477U Code added
● 0478U Code added
● 0479U Code added
● 0480U Code added
● 0481U Code added
● 0482U Code added
● 0483U Code added
● 0484U Code added
● 0485U Code added
● 0486U Code added

★=Telemedicine ◀=Audio-only +=Add-on code ✗=FDA approval pending #=Resequenced code ⦸=Modifier 51 exempt ➲➲➲=See p xxi for details

● **0487U**   Code added

● **0488U**   Code added

● **0489U**   Code added

● **0490U**   Code added

● **0491U**   Code added

● **0492U**   Code added

● **0493U**   Code added

● **0494U**   Code added

● **0495U**   Code added

● **0496U**   Code added

● **0497U**   Code added

● **0498U**   Code added

● **0499U**   Code added

● **0500U**   Code added

● **0501U**   Code added

● **0502U**   Code added

● **0503U**   Code added

● **0504U**   Code added

● **0505U**   Code added

● **0506U**   Code added

● **0507U**   Code added

● **0508U**   Code added

● **0509U**   Code added

● **0510U**   Code added

● **0511U**   Code added

● **0512U**   Code added

● **0513U**   Code added

● **0514U**   Code added

● **0515U**   Code added

● **0516U**   Code added

● **0517U**   Code added

● **0518U**   Code added

● **0519U**   Code added

● **0520U**   Code added

Medicine

0001A   Immunization administration by intramuscular injection of severe acute respiratory syndrome coronavirus 2 (SARS-CoV-2) (coronavirus disease [COVID-19]) vaccine, mRNA-LNP, spike protein, preservative free, 30 mcg/0.3 mL dosage, diluent reconstituted; first dose

0002A   second dose

0003A   third dose

0004A   booster dose

0051A   Immunization administration by intramuscular injection of severe acute respiratory syndrome coronavirus 2 (SARS-CoV-2) (coronavirus disease [COVID-19]) vaccine, mRNA-LNP, spike protein, preservative free, 30 mcg/0.3 mL dosage, tris-sucrose formulation; first dose

0052A   second dose

0053A   third dose

0054A   booster dose

0121A   Immunization administration by intramuscular injection of severe acute respiratory syndrome coronavirus 2 (SARS-CoV-2) (coronavirus disease [COVID-19]) vaccine, mRNA-LNP, bivalent spike protein, preservative free, 30 mcg/0.3 mL dosage, tris-sucrose formulation; single dose

0124A   additional dose

0071A   Immunization administration by intramuscular injection of severe acute respiratory syndrome coronavirus 2 (SARS-CoV-2) (coronavirus disease [COVID-19]) vaccine, mRNA-LNP, spike protein, preservative free, 10 mcg/0.2 mL dosage, diluent reconstituted, tris-sucrose formulation; first dose

0072A   second dose

0073A   third dose

0074A   booster dose

0151A   Immunization administration by intramuscular injection of severe acute respiratory syndrome coronavirus 2 (SARS-CoV-2) (coronavirus disease [COVID-19]) vaccine, mRNA-LNP, bivalent spike protein, preservative free, 10 mcg/0.2 mL dosage, diluent reconstituted, tris-sucrose formulation; single dose

0154A   additional dose

0081A   Immunization administration by intramuscular injection of severe acute respiratory syndrome coronavirus 2 (SARS-CoV-2) (coronavirus disease [COVID-19]) vaccine, mRNA-LNP, spike protein, preservative free, 3 mcg/0.2 mL dosage, diluent reconstituted, tris-sucrose formulation; first dose

0082A   second dose

0083A   third dose

0171A   Immunization administration by intramuscular injection of severe acute respiratory syndrome coronavirus 2 (SARS-CoV-2) (coronavirus disease [COVID-19]) vaccine, mRNA-LNP, bivalent spike protein, preservative free, 3 mcg/0.2 mL dosage, diluent reconstituted, tris-sucrose formulation; first dose

0172A   second dose

0173A   third dose

0174A   additional dose

0011A   Immunization administration by intramuscular injection of severe acute respiratory syndrome coronavirus 2 (SARS-CoV-2) (coronavirus disease [COVID-19]) vaccine, mRNA-LNP, spike protein, preservative free, 100 mcg/0.5 mL dosage; first dose

0012A   second dose

0013A   third dose

0064A   Immunization administration by intramuscular injection of severe acute respiratory syndrome coronavirus 2 (SARS-CoV-2) (coronavirus disease [COVID-19]) vaccine, mRNA-LNP, spike protein, preservative free, 50 mcg/0.25 mL dosage, booster dose

0134A   Immunization administration by intramuscular injection of severe acute respiratory syndrome coronavirus 2 (SARS-CoV-2) (coronavirus disease [COVID-19]) vaccine, mRNA-LNP, spike protein, bivalent, preservative free, 50 mcg/0.5 mL dosage, additional dose

0141A   Immunization administration by intramuscular injection of severe acute respiratory syndrome coronavirus 2 (SARS-CoV-2) (coronavirus disease [COVID-19]) vaccine, mRNA-LNP, spike protein, bivalent, preservative free, 25 mcg/0.25 mL dosage; first dose

0142A   second dose

0144A   additional dose

0091A   Immunization administration by intramuscular injection of severe acute respiratory syndrome coronavirus 2 (SARS-CoV-2) (coronavirus disease [COVID-19]) vaccine, mRNA-LNP, spike protein, preservative free, 50 mcg/0.5 mL dosage; first dose, when administered to individuals 6 through 11 years

0092A   second dose, when administered to individuals 6 through 11 years

0093A   third dose, when administered to individuals 6 through 11 years

0094A   booster dose, when administered to individuals 18 years and older

0021A   Immunization administration by intramuscular injection of severe acute respiratory syndrome coronavirus 2 (SARS-CoV-2) (coronavirus disease [COVID-19]) vaccine, DNA, spike protein, chimpanzee adenovirus Oxford 1 (ChAdOx1) vector, preservative free, 5x10¹⁰ viral particles/0.5 mL dosage; first dose

0022A   second dose

0031A   Immunization administration by intramuscular injection of severe acute respiratory syndrome coronavirus 2 (SARS-CoV-2) (coronavirus disease [COVID-19]) vaccine, DNA, spike protein, adenovirus type 26 (Ad26) vector, preservative free, 5x10¹⁰ viral particles/0.5 mL dosage; single dose

0034A   booster dose

0041A   Immunization administration by intramuscular injection of severe acute respiratory syndrome coronavirus 2 (SARS-CoV-2) (coronavirus disease [COVID-19]) vaccine, recombinant spike protein nanoparticle, saponin-based adjuvant, preservative free, 5 mcg/0.5 mL dosage; first dose

0042A   second dose

0044A   booster dose

0104A   Immunization administration by intramuscular injection of severe acute respiratory syndrome coronavirus 2 (SARS-CoV-2) (coronavirus disease [COVID-19]) vaccine, monovalent, preservative free, 5 mcg/0.5 mL dosage, adjuvant AS03 emulsion, booster dose

0111A   Immunization administration by intramuscular injection of severe acute respiratory syndrome coronavirus 2 (SARS-CoV-2) (coronavirus disease [COVID-19]) vaccine, mRNA-LNP, spike protein, preservative free, 25 mcg/0.25 mL dosage; first dose

0112A   second dose

0113A   third dose

0164A   Immunization administration by intramuscular injection of severe acute respiratory syndrome coronavirus 2 (SARS-CoV-2) (coronavirus disease [COVID-19]) vaccine, mRNA-LNP, spike protein, bivalent, preservative free, 10 mcg/0.2 mL dosage, additional dose

#● 90480   Code added

91300   Severe acute respiratory syndrome coronavirus 2 (SARS-CoV-2) (coronavirus disease [COVID-19]) vaccine, mRNA-LNP, spike protein, preservative free, 30 mcg/0.3 mL dosage, diluent reconstituted, for intramuscular use

91305   Severe acute respiratory syndrome coronavirus 2 (SARS-CoV-2) (coronavirus disease [COVID-19]) vaccine, mRNA-LNP, spike protein, preservative free, 30 mcg/0.3 mL dosage, tris-sucrose formulation, for intramuscular use

91312   Severe acute respiratory syndrome coronavirus 2 (SARS-CoV-2) (coronavirus disease [COVID-19]) vaccine, mRNA-LNP, bivalent spike protein, preservative free, 30 mcg/0.3 mL dosage, tris-sucrose formulation, for intramuscular use

91307   Severe acute respiratory syndrome coronavirus 2 (SARS-CoV-2) (coronavirus disease [COVID-19]) vaccine, mRNA-LNP, spike protein, preservative free, 10 mcg/0.2 mL dosage, diluent reconstituted, tris-sucrose formulation, for intramuscular use

91315 ~~Severe acute respiratory syndrome coronavirus 2 (SARS-CoV-2) (coronavirus disease [COVID-19]) vaccine, mRNA-LNP, bivalent spike protein, preservative free, 10 mcg/0.2 mL dosage, diluent reconstituted, tris-sucrose formulation, for intramuscular use~~

91308 ~~Severe acute respiratory syndrome coronavirus 2 (SARS-CoV-2) (coronavirus disease [COVID-19]) vaccine, mRNA-LNP, spike protein, preservative free, 3 mcg/0.2 mL dosage, diluent reconstituted, tris-sucrose formulation, for intramuscular use~~

91317 ~~Severe acute respiratory syndrome coronavirus 2 (SARS-CoV-2) (coronavirus disease [COVID-19]) vaccine, mRNA-LNP, bivalent spike protein, preservative free, 3 mcg/0.2 mL dosage, diluent reconstituted, tris-sucrose formulation, for intramuscular use~~

91301 ~~Severe acute respiratory syndrome coronavirus 2 (SARS-CoV-2) (coronavirus disease [COVID-19]) vaccine, mRNA-LNP, spike protein, preservative free, 100 mcg/0.5 mL dosage, for intramuscular use~~

91306 ~~Severe acute respiratory syndrome coronavirus 2 (SARS-CoV-2) (coronavirus disease [COVID-19]) vaccine, mRNA-LNP, spike protein, preservative free, 50 mcg/0.25 mL dosage, for intramuscular use~~

91313 ~~Severe acute respiratory syndrome coronavirus 2 (SARS-CoV-2) (coronavirus disease [COVID-19]) vaccine, mRNA-LNP, spike protein, bivalent, preservative free, 50 mcg/0.5 mL dosage, for intramuscular use~~

91314 ~~Severe acute respiratory syndrome coronavirus 2 (SARS-CoV-2) (coronavirus disease [COVID-19]) vaccine, mRNA-LNP, spike protein, bivalent, preservative free, 25 mcg/0.25 mL dosage, for intramuscular use~~

91311 ~~Severe acute respiratory syndrome coronavirus 2 (SARS-CoV-2) (coronavirus disease [COVID-19]) vaccine, mRNA-LNP, spike protein, preservative free, 25 mcg/0.25 mL dosage, for intramuscular use~~

91316 ~~Severe acute respiratory syndrome coronavirus 2 (SARS-CoV-2) (coronavirus disease [COVID-19]) vaccine, mRNA-LNP, spike protein, bivalent, preservative free, 10 mcg/0.2 mL dosage, for intramuscular use~~

91309 ~~Severe acute respiratory syndrome coronavirus 2 (SARS-CoV-2) (coronavirus disease [COVID-19]) vaccine, mRNA-LNP, spike protein, preservative free, 50 mcg/0.5 mL dosage, for intramuscular use~~

91302 ~~Severe acute respiratory syndrome coronavirus 2 (SARS-CoV-2) (coronavirus disease [COVID-19]) vaccine, DNA, spike protein, chimpanzee adenovirus Oxford 1 (ChAdOx1) vector, preservative free, 5x10^{10} viral particles/0.5 mL dosage, for intramuscular use~~

91303 ~~Severe acute respiratory syndrome coronavirus 2 (SARS-CoV-2) (coronavirus disease [COVID-19]) vaccine, DNA, spike protein, adenovirus type 26 (Ad26) vector, preservative free, 5x10^{10} viral particles/0.5 mL dosage, for intramuscular use~~

\#▲ **91304** Severe acute respiratory syndrome coronavirus 2 (SARS-CoV-2) (coronavirus disease [COVID-19]) vaccine, recombinant spike protein nanoparticle, saponin-based adjuvant ~~preservative free~~ 5 mcg/0.5 mL dosage, for intramuscular use

91310 ~~Severe acute respiratory syndrome coronavirus 2 (SARS-CoV-2) (coronavirus disease [COVID-19]) vaccine, monovalent, preservative free, 5 mcg/0.5 mL dosage, adjuvant AS03 emulsion, for intramuscular use~~

\#● **91318** Code added

\#● **91319** Code added

\#● **91320** Code added

\#● **91321** Code added

\#● **91322** Code added

90654 ~~Influenza virus vaccine, trivalent (IIV3), split virus, preservative-free, for intradermal use~~

90630 ~~Influenza virus vaccine, quadrivalent (IIV4), split virus, preservative free, for intradermal use~~

▲ **90661** Influenza virus vaccine, trivalent (ccIIV3), derived from cell cultures, subunit, ~~preservative and~~ antibiotic free, 0.5 mL dosage, for intramuscular use

\#✖● **90695** Code added

\#● **90684** Code added

\#✖● **90637** Code added

\#✖● **90638** Code added

\#✖● **90624** Code added

▲ **92132** ~~Scanning c~~Computerized ophthalmic diagnostic imaging (eg, optical coherence tomography [OCT]), anterior segment, with interpretation and report, unilateral or bilateral

▲ **92133** ~~Scanning c~~Computerized ophthalmic diagnostic imaging (eg, optical coherence tomography [OCT]), posterior segment, with interpretation and report, unilateral or bilateral; optic nerve

▲ **92134** retina

\#● **92137** Code added

Appendix B

▲ 93656   Comprehensive electrophysiologic evaluation ~~including~~with transseptal catheterizations, insertion and repositioning of multiple electrode catheters, induction or attempted induction of an arrhythmia including left or right atrial pacing/recording, ~~with~~and intracardiac catheter ablation of atrial fibrillation by pulmonary vein isolation, including intracardiac electrophysiologic 3-dimensional mapping, intracardiac echocardiography ~~including~~with imaging supervision and interpretation,- ~~induction or attempted induction of an arrhythmia including left or right atrial pacing/recording,~~ right ventricular pacing/recording, and His bundle recording, when performed

   93890   ~~vasoreactivity study~~

▲ 93893   ~~emboli~~venous-arterial shunt detection with intravenous microbubble injection

#+● 93896   Code added

#+● 93897   Code added

#+● 93898   Code added

   96003   ~~Dynamic fine wire electromyography, during walking or other functional activities, 1 muscle~~

   96040   ~~Medical genetics and genetic counseling services, each 30 minutes face-to-face with patient/family~~

★◀● 96041   Code added

#● 96380   Code added

#● 96381   Code added

+▲ 97811   without electrical stimulation, each additional 15 minutes of personal one-on-one contact with the patient, with re-insertion of needle(s) (List separately in addition to code for primary procedure)

+▲ 97814   with electrical stimulation, each additional 15 minutes of personal one-on-one contact with the patient, with re-insertion of needle(s) (List separately in addition to code for primary procedure)

★▲ 98960   Education and training for patient self-management by a nonphysician qualified; ~~nonphysician~~health care professional using a standardized curriculum, face-to-face with the patient (could include caregiver/family) each 30 minutes; individual patient

★▲ 98961   2-4 patients

★▲ 98962   5-8 patients

▲ 98966   Telephone assessment and management service provided by a nonphysician qualified ~~nonphysician~~health care professional to an established patient, parent, or guardian not originating from a related assessment and management service provided within the previous 7 days nor leading to an assessment and management service or procedure within the next 24 hours or soonest available appointment; 5-10 minutes of medical discussion

▲ 98967   11-20 minutes of medical discussion

▲ 98968   21-30 minutes of medical discussion

▲ 98970   Nonphysician Θqualified ~~nonphysician~~health care professional online digital assessment and management, for an established patient, for up to 7 days, cumulative time during the 7 days; 5-10 minutes

▲ 98971   11-20 minutes

▲ 98972   21 or more minutes

▲ 98975   Remote therapeutic monitoring (eg, therapy adherence, therapy response, digital therapeutic intervention); initial set-up and patient education on use of equipment

▲ 98976   device(s) supply for data access or data transmissions to support monitoring of~~with scheduled (eg, daily) recording(s) and/or programmed alert(s) transmission to monitor~~ respiratory system, each 30 days

▲ 98977   device(s) supply for data access or data transmissions to support monitoring of~~with scheduled (eg, daily) recording(s) and/or programmed alert(s) transmission to monitor~~ musculoskeletal system, each 30 days

▲ 98978   device(s) supply for data access or data transmissions to support monitoring of~~with scheduled (eg, daily) recording(s) and/or programmed alert(s) transmission to monitor~~ cognitive behavioral therapy, each 30 days

Category III Codes

#● 0901T   Code added

   0398T   ~~Magnetic resonance image guided high intensity focused ultrasound (MRgFUS), stereotactic ablation lesion, intracranial for movement disorder including stereotactic navigation and frame placement when performed~~

#▲ 0714T   Transperineal laser ablation of benign prostatic hyperplasia, including imaging guidance; prostate volume less than 50 mL

#● 0867T   Code added

   0500T   ~~Infectious agent detection by nucleic acid (DNA or RNA), Human Papillomavirus (HPV) for five or more separately reported high-risk HPV types (eg, 16, 18, 31, 33, 35, 39, 45, 51, 52, 56, 58, 59, 68) (ie, genotyping)~~

   0537T   ~~Chimeric antigen receptor T-cell (CAR-T) therapy; harvesting of blood-derived T lymphocytes for development of genetically modified autologous CAR-T cells, per day~~

   0538T   ~~preparation of blood-derived T lymphocytes for transportation (eg, cryopreservation, storage)~~

   0539T   ~~receipt and preparation of CAR-T cells for administration~~

   0540T   ~~CAR-T cell administration, autologous~~

0553T ~~Percutaneous transcatheter placement of iliac arteriovenous anastomosis implant, inclusive of all radiological supervision and interpretation, intraprocedural roadmapping, and imaging guidance necessary to complete the intervention~~

0564T ~~Oncology, chemotherapeutic drug cytotoxicity assay of cancer stem cells (CSCs), from cultured CSCs and primary tumor cells, categorical drug response reported based on percent of cytotoxicity observed, a minimum of 14 drugs or drug combinations~~

0567T ~~Permanent fallopian tube occlusion with degradable biopolymer implant, transcervical approach, including transvaginal ultrasound~~

0568T ~~Introduction of mixture of saline and air for sonosalpingography to confirm occlusion of fallopian tubes, transcervical approach, including transvaginal ultrasound and pelvic ultrasound~~

▲ 0615T Automated~~Eye-movement~~ analysis of binocular eye movements without spatial calibration, including disconjugacy, saccades, and pupillary dynamics for the assessment of concussion, with interpretation and report

0616T ~~Insertion of iris prosthesis, including suture fixation and repair or removal of iris, when performed; without removal of crystalline lens or intraocular lens, without insertion of intraocular lens~~

0617T ~~with removal of crystalline lens and insertion of intraocular lens~~

0618T ~~with secondary intraocular lens placement or intraocular lens exchange~~

● 0868T Code added

● 0869T Code added

● 0870T Code added

● 0871T Code added

● 0872T Code added

● 0873T Code added

● 0874T Code added

● 0875T Code added

● 0876T Code added

● 0877T Code added

● 0878T Code added

● 0879T Code added

● 0880T Code added

● 0881T Code added

+● 0882T Code added

+● 0883T Code added

● 0884T Code added

● 0885T Code added

● 0886T Code added

+● 0887T Code added

● 0888T Code added

● 0889T Code added

● 0890T Code added

● 0891T Code added

● 0892T Code added

● 0893T Code added

● 0894T Code added

● 0895T Code added

+● 0896T Code added

● 0897T Code added

● 0898T Code added

+● 0899T Code added

+● 0900T Code added

● 0902T Code added

● 0903T Code added

● 0904T Code added

● 0905T Code added

● 0906T Code added

+● 0907T Code added

● 0908T Code added

● 0909T Code added

● 0910T Code added

● 0911T Code added

● 0912T Code added

● 0913T Code added

+● 0914T Code added

● 0915T Code added

● 0916T Code added

● 0917T Code added

● 0918T Code added

● 0919T Code added

● 0920T Code added

● 0921T Code added

● 0922T Code added

● 0923T Code added

- 0924T   Code added
- 0925T   Code added
- 0926T   Code added
- 0927T   Code added
- 0928T   Code added
- 0929T   Code added
- 0930T   Code added
- 0931T   Code added
- 0932T   Code added
- 0933T   Code added
- 0934T   Code added
- 0935T   Code added
- 0936T   Code added
- 0937T   Code added
- 0938T   Code added
- 0939T   Code added
- 0940T   Code added
- 0941T   Code added
- 0942T   Code added
- 0943T   Code added
- 0944T   Code added
+● 0945T   Code added
- 0946T   Code added
- 0947T   Code added

Administrative Multianalyte Assays with Algorithmic Analyses (MAAA)

- 0020M   Code added

Appendix C

Clinical Examples

The clinical examples for CPT evaluation and management (E/M) services codes (formerly Appendix C) have been removed from the CPT code set. For information or guidance on reporting E/M services, refer to the E/M Guidelines.

Appendix D

Summary of CPT Add-on Codes

This listing is a summary of CPT add-on codes for CPT 2025. The codes listed below are identified in CPT 2025 with a + symbol.

01953	13153	15274	19288
01968	14302	15276	19294
01969	15003	15278	19297
10004	15005	15772	20700
10006	15012	15774	20701
10008	15014	15777	20702
10010	15016	15787	20703
10012	15018	15847	20704
10036	15101	15853	20705
11001	15111	15854	20930
11008	15116	16036	20931
11045	15121	17003	20932
11046	15131	17312	20933
11047	15136	17314	20934
11103	15151	17315	20936
11105	15152	19001	20937
11107	15156	19082	20938
11201	15157	19084	20939
11732	15201	19086	20985
11922	15221	19126	22103
13102	15241	19282	22116
13122	15261	19284	22208
13133	15272	19286	22216

22226	32506	34808	37252	60512
22328	32507	34812	37253	60661
22512	32667	34813	38102	61316
22515	32668	34820	38746	61517
22527	32674	34833	38747	61611
22534	33141	34834	38900	61641
22552	33225	35306	43273	61642
22585	33257	35390	43283	61651
22614	33258	35400	43338	61781
22632	33259	35500	43635	61782
22634	33268	35572	44015	61783
22840	33277	35681	44121	61797
22841	33367	35682	44128	61799
22842	33368	35683	44139	61800
22843	33369	35685	44203	61864
22844	33370	35686	44213	61868
22845	33419	35697	44701	62148
22846	33508	35700	44955	62160
22847	33517	36218	47001	63035
22848	33518	36227	47542	63043
22853	33519	36228	47543	63044
22854	33521	36248	47544	63048
22858	33522	36474	47550	63052
22859	33523	36476	48400	63053
22860	33530	36479	49326	63057
22868	33572	36483	49327	63066
22870	33746	36907	49412	63076
26125	33768	36908	49435	63078
26861	33866	36909	49623	63082
26863	33884	37185	49905	63086
27358	33904	37186	50606	63088
27692	33924	37222	50705	63091
29826	33929	37223	50706	63103
31627	33987	37232	51797	63295
31632	34709	37233	52442	63308
31633	34711	37234	56606	63621
31637	34713	37235	57267	64421
31649	34714	37237	57465	64462
31651	34715	37239	58110	64480
31654	34716	37247	58611	64484
32501	34717	37249	59525	64491

▲ = Revised code   ● = New code   ▶ ◀ = Contains new or revised text   ✖ = Duplicate PLA test   ↕ = Category I PLA

Appendix C

64492	76812	0075U	92944	93657	96423	0055T	0753T	0848T
64494	76814	0076U	92972	93662	96547	0076T	0754T	0849T
64495	76937	0130U	92973	93896	96548	0095T	0755T	0850T
64597	76979	0131U	92974	93897	96570	0098T	0756T	0851T
64629	76983	0132U	92978	93898	96571	0164T	0757T	0852T
64634	77001	0133U	92979	94645	96934	0165T	0758T	0853T
64636	77002	0134U	92998	94729	96935	0174T	0759T	0854T
64643	77003	0135U	93319	94781	96936	0214T	0760T	0855T
64645	77063	0136U	93320	95079	97130	0215T	0761T	0856T
64727	77293	0137U	93321	95873	97546	0217T	0762T	0857T
64778	78020	0138U	93325	95874	97551	0218T	0763T	0859T
64783	78434	0157U	93352	95885	97598	0222T	0764T	0866T
64787	78496	0158U	93356	95886	97811	0397T	0767T	0882T
64832	78730	0159U	93462	95887	97814	0437T	0770T	0883T
64837	78835	0160U	93463	95940	98981	0439T	0772T	0887T
64859	80506	0161U	93464	95941	99100	0443T	0774T	0896T
64872	81266	0162U	93563	95962	99116	0450T	0777T	0899T
64874	81416	0207U	93564	95967	99135	0480T	0791T	0900T
64876	81426	0427U	93565	95984	99140	0496T	0821T	0907T
64901	81536	90461	93566	96113	99153	0513T	0822T	0914T
64902	82952	90472	93567	96121	99157	0523T	0827T	0945T
64913	86826	90474	93568	96131	99292	0560T	0828T	
65757	87187	90785	93569	96133	99359	0562T	0829T	
66990	87503	90833	93571	96137	99415	0570T	0830T	
67225	87904	90836	93572	96139	99416	0599T	0831T	
67320	88155	90838	93573	96159	99417	0628T	0832T	
67331	88177	90840	93574	96165	99418	0630T	0833T	
67332	88185	90863	93575	96168	99425	0649T	0834T	
67334	88311	90913	93584	96171	99427	0663T	0835T	
67335	88314	91013	93585	96203	99437	0676T	0836T	
67340	88332	92547	93586	96361	99439	0678T	0837T	
69990	88334	92608	93587	96366	99458	0690T	0838T	
74248	88341	92618	93588	96367	99459	0698T	0839T	
74301	88350	92621	93592	96368	99467	0701T	0840T	
74713	88364	92623	93598	96370	99486	0709T	0841T	
75565	88369	92627	93609	96371	99489	0722T	0842T	
75774	88373	92921	93613	96375	99494	0724T	0843T	
76015	0071U	92925	93621	96376	99498	0735T	0844T	
76125	0072U	92929	93622	96411	99602	0742T	0845T	
76802	0073U	92934	93623	96415	99607	0751T	0846T	
76810	0074U	92938	93655	96417	0054T	0752T	0847T	

★ = Telemedicine ◀ = Audio-only + = Add-on code ✗ = FDA approval pending # = Resequenced code ⊘ = Modifier 51 exempt ➲➲➲ = See p xxi for details

Appendix E

Summary of CPT Codes Exempt from Modifier 51

This listing is a summary of CPT codes that are exempt from the use of modifier 51. Procedures on this list are typically performed with another procedure but may be a stand-alone procedure and not always performed with other specified procedures. For add-on codes, see Appendix D. This is not an exhaustive list of procedures that are typically exempt from multiple procedure reductions. The codes listed below are identified in CPT 2025 with a ⊘ symbol.

20697	76018	93616
20974	76019	93618
20975	93600	94610
33509	93602	95905
35600	93603	99151
44500	93610	99152
61107	93612	
76017	93615	

Appendix F

Summary of CPT Codes Exempt from Modifier 63

This listing is a summary of CPT codes that are exempt from the use of modifier 63. The codes listed below are additionally identified in CPT 2025 with the parenthetical instruction "(Do not report modifier 63 in conjunction with…)."

30540	33750	43314	49491
30545	33755	43520	49492
31520	33762	43831	49495
33502	33778	44055	49496
33503	33786	44126	49600
33505	33922	44127	49605
33506	33946	44128	49606
33610	33947	46070	49610
33611	33948	46705	49611
33619	33949	46715	53025
33647	36415	46716	54000
33670	36420	46730	54150
33690	36450	46735	54160
33694	36456	46740	63700
33730	36460	46742	63702
33732	36510	46744	63704
33735	36660	47700	63706
33736	39503	47701	65820
33741	43313	49215	

Appendix G

Summary of CPT Codes That Include Moderate (Conscious) Sedation

The summary of CPT codes that include moderate (conscious) sedation (formerly Appendix G) has been removed from the CPT code set.

The codes that were previously included in the former **Appendix G** have been revised with the removal of the moderate (conscious) sedation symbol. For information/guidance on reporting moderate (conscious) sedation services with codes formerly listed in **Appendix G**, please refer to the guidelines for codes 99151, 99152, 99153, 99155, 99156, 99157.

Appendix H

Alphabetical Clinical Topics Listing (AKA – Alphabetical Listing)

The Alphabetical Clinical Topics Listing (formerly Appendix H) has been removed from the CPT codebook. Since this document is a dynamic and rapidly expanding source of information to link CPT Category II codes, clinical conditions, and measure abstracts, the Alphabetical Listing is now solely accessed on the AMA CPT website at https://www.ama-assn.org/system/files/2020-01/cpt-cat2-codes-alpha-listing-clinical-topics.pdf.

In addition, new codes for the publication cycle (ie, the **Update to the List of Category II Codes**) will continue to be located on the AMA CPT website prior to publication in the next edition of the CPT codebook (subsequent to its listing on the Web).

Appendix I

Genetic Testing Code Modifiers

The **Genetic Testing Code Modifiers** (formerly Appendix I) has been removed from the CPT code set.

The addition of more than 100 molecular pathology codes to the 2012 code set and still more codes to the 2013 CPT code set resulted in the deletion of the stacking codes (83890–83914). The genetic testing code modifiers formerly described in Appendix I applied to those stacking codes, and therefore, the Appendix and modifiers have been removed from the code set.

For the most up-to-date information on future updates for molecular pathology coding in the CPT code set, see the AMA CPT website (https://www.ama-assn.org/practice-management/cpt/molecular-pathology-tier-2-codes).

Appendix J

Electrodiagnostic Medicine Listing of Sensory, Motor, and Mixed Nerves

This summary assigns each sensory, motor, and mixed nerve with its appropriate nerve conduction study code in order to enhance accurate reporting of codes 95907-95913. Each nerve constitutes one unit of service.

Motor Nerves Assigned to Codes 95907-95913

I. Upper extremity, cervical plexus, and brachial plexus motor nerves
  A. Axillary motor nerve to the deltoid
  B. Long thoracic motor nerve to the serratus anterior
  C. Median nerve
    1. Median motor nerve to the abductor pollicis brevis
    2. Median motor nerve, anterior interosseous branch, to the flexor pollicis longus
    3. Median motor nerve, anterior interosseous branch, to the pronator quadratus
    4. Median motor nerve to the first lumbrical
    5. Median motor nerve to the second lumbrical
  D. Musculocutaneous motor nerve to the biceps brachii
  E. Radial nerve
    1. Radial motor nerve to the extensor carpi ulnaris
    2. Radial motor nerve to the extensor digitorum communis
    3. Radial motor nerve to the extensor indicis proprius
    4. Radial motor nerve to the brachioradialis
  F. Suprascapular nerve
    1. Suprascapular motor nerve to the supraspinatus
    2. Suprascapular motor nerve to the infraspinatus
  G. Thoracodorsal motor nerve to the latissimus dorsi
  H. Ulnar nerve
    1. Ulnar motor nerve to the abductor digiti minimi
    2. Ulnar motor nerve to the palmar interosseous
    3. Ulnar motor nerve to the first dorsal interosseous
    4. Ulnar motor nerve to the flexor carpi ulnaris
  I. Other

II. Lower extremity motor nerves
  A. Femoral motor nerve to the quadriceps
    1. Femoral motor nerve to vastus medialis
    2. Femoral motor nerve to vastus lateralis
    3. Femoral motor nerve to vastus intermedialis
    4. Femoral motor nerve to rectus femoris
  B. Ilioinguinal motor nerve
  C. Peroneal (fibular) nerve
    1. Peroneal motor nerve to the extensor digitorum brevis
    2. Peroneal motor nerve to the peroneus brevis
    3. Peroneal motor nerve to the peroneus longus
    4. Peroneal motor nerve to the tibialis anterior
  D. Plantar motor nerve
  E. Sciatic nerve
  F. Tibial nerve
    1. Tibial motor nerve, inferior calcaneal branch, to the abductor digiti minimi
    2. Tibial motor nerve, medial plantar branch, to the abductor hallucis
    3. Tibial motor nerve, lateral plantar branch, to the flexor digiti minimi brevis
  G. Other

III. Cranial nerves and trunk
  A. Cranial nerve VII (facial motor nerve)
    1. Facial nerve to the frontalis
    2. Facial nerve to the nasalis
    3. Facial nerve to the orbicularis oculi
    4. Facial nerve to the orbicularis oris
  B. Cranial nerve XI (spinal accessory motor nerve)
  C. Cranial nerve XII (hypoglossal motor nerve)
  D. Intercostal motor nerve
  E. Phrenic motor nerve to the diaphragm
  F. Recurrent laryngeal nerve
  G. Other

IV. Nerve Roots
  A. Cervical nerve root stimulation
    1. Cervical level 5 (CT)
    2. Cervical level 6 (C6)
    3. Cervical level 7 (C7)
    4. Cervical level 8 (C8)

B. Thoracic nerve root stimulation
   1. Thoracic level 1 (T1)
   2. Thoracic level 2 (T2)
   3. Thoracic level 3 (T3)
   4. Thoracic level 4 (T4)
   5. Thoracic level 5 (T5)
   6. Thoracic level 6 (T6)
   7. Thoracic level 7 (T7)
   8. Thoracic level 8 (T8)
   9. Thoracic level 9 (T9)
   10. Thoracic level 10 (T10)
   11. Thoracic level 11 (T11)
   12. Thoracic level 12 (T12)
C. Lumbar nerve root stimulation
   1. Lumbar level 1 (L1)
   2. Lumbar level 2 (L2)
   3. Lumbar level 3 (L3)
   4. Lumbar level 4 (L4)
   5. Lumbar level 5 (L5)
D. Sacral nerve root stimulation
   1. Sacral level 1 (S1)
   2. Sacral level 2 (S2)
   3. Sacral level 3 (S3)
   4. Sacral level 4 (S4)

Sensory and Mixed Nerves Assigned to Codes 95907-95913

I. Upper extremity sensory and mixed nerves
  A. Lateral antebrachial cutaneous sensory nerve
  B. Medial antebrachial cutaneous sensory nerve
  C. Medial brachial cutaneous sensory nerve
  D. Median nerve
    1. Median sensory nerve to the first digit
    2. Median sensory nerve to the second digit
    3. Median sensory nerve to the third digit
    4. Median sensory nerve to the fourth digit
    5. Median palmar cutaneous sensory nerve
    6. Median palmar mixed nerve
  E. Posterior antebrachial cutaneous sensory nerve
  F. Radial sensory nerve
    1. Radial sensory nerve to the base of the thumb
    2. Radial sensory nerve to digit 1
  G. Ulnar nerve
    1. Ulnar dorsal cutaneous sensory nerve
    2. Ulnar sensory nerve to the fourth digit
    3. Ulnar sensory nerve to the fifth digit
    4. Ulnar palmar mixed nerve
  H. Intercostal sensory nerve
  I. Other

II. Lower extremity sensory and mixed nerves
  A. Lateral femoral cutaneous sensory nerve
  B. Medial calcaneal sensory nerve
  C. Medial femoral cutaneous sensory nerve
  D. Peroneal nerve
    1. Deep peroneal sensory nerve
    2. Superficial peroneal sensory nerve, medial dorsal cutaneous branch
    3. Superficial peroneal sensory nerve, intermediate dorsal cutaneous branch
  E. Posterior femoral cutaneous sensory nerve
  F. Saphenous nerve
    1. Saphenous sensory nerve (distal technique)
    2. Saphenous sensory nerve (proximal technique)
  G. Sural nerve
    1. Sural sensory nerve, lateral dorsal cutaneous branch
    2. Sural sensory nerve
  H. Tibial sensory nerve (digital nerve to toe 1)
  I. Tibial sensory nerve (medial plantar nerve)
  J. Tibial sensory nerve (lateral plantar nerve)
  K. Other

III. Head and trunk sensory nerves
  A. Dorsal nerve of the penis
  B. Greater auricular nerve
  C. Ophthalmic branch of the trigeminal nerve
  D. Pudendal sensory nerve
  E. Suprascapular sensory nerves
  F. Other

★=Telemedicine   ◀=Audio-only   +=Add-on code   ✔=FDA approval pending   #=Resequenced code   ⊘=Modifier 51 exempt   ➔➔➔=See p xxi for details

The following table provides a reasonable maximum number of studies performed per diagnostic category necessary for a physician to arrive at a diagnosis in 90% of patients with that final diagnosis. The numbers in each column represent the number of studies recommended. The appropriate number of studies to be performed is based upon the physician's discretion.

	Type of Study/Maximum Number of Studies		
Indication	**Limbs Studied by Needle EMG (95860-95864, 95867-95870, 95885-95887)**	**Nerve Conduction Studies (Total Nerves Studied, 95907-95913)**	**Neuromuscular Junction Testing (Repetitive Stimulation, 95937)**
Carpal Tunnel (Unilateral)	1	7	—
Carpal Tunnel (Bilateral)	2	10	—
Radiculopathy	2	7	—
Mononeuropathy	1	8	—
Polyneuropathy/Mononeuropathy Multiplex	3	10	—
Myopathy	2	4	2
Motor Neuronopathy (eg, ALS)	4	6	2
Plexopathy	2	12	—
Neuromuscular Junction	2	4	3
Tarsal Tunnel Syndrome (Unilateral)	1	8	—
Tarsal Tunnel Syndrome (Bilateral)	2	11	—
Weakness, Fatigue, Cramps, or Twitching (Focal)	2	7	2
Weakness, Fatigue, Cramps, or Twitching (General)	4	8	2
Pain, Numbness, or Tingling (Unilateral)	1	9	—
Pain, Numbness, or Tingling (Bilateral)	2	12	—

Appendix K

Product Pending FDA Approval

Some vaccine and immune globulin products have been assigned a CPT Category I code in anticipation of future approval from the Food and Drug Administration (FDA). Following is a list of the vaccine and immune globulin product codes pending FDA approval status that are identified in the CPT code set with the ⁄ symbol. Upon revision of the approval status by the FDA, notation of this revision will be provided via the AMA CPT "Category I Vaccine Codes" website listing (ama-assn.org/cpt-cat-i-immunization-codes) and in subsequent publications of the CPT code set.

90584

90624

90637

90638

90666

90667

90668

90671

90695

Appendix L

Vascular Families

Appendix L is a vascular branching model that assumes the aorta, vena cava, pulmonary artery, or portal vein is the starting point of catheterization. Accordingly, branches have been categorized into first, second, third order, and beyond. (Note that this categorization does not apply, for instance, if a femoral or carotid artery were catheterized directly in an antegrade direction.) Common branching patterns of typical anatomy are shown in the charts and illustrations.

No specific coding instructions should be inferred from Appendix L. End-users must determine how best to code any specific procedure based on variant anatomy and different vascular access point relative to vessel(s) selectively catheterized (eg, antegrade femoral artery, radial artery, retrograde femoral to ipsilateral internal iliac artery catheterization, transsplenic splenic vein access to portal venous system, etc).

Arterial Vascular Family

Abbreviations:

R = Right	Asc = Ascending
L = Left	Desc = Descending
Ant = Anterior	Lat = Lateral
Post = Posterior	Int = Internal
Sup = Superior	Ext = External
Inf = Inferior	Transv = Transverse
	Tr = Trunk

Beyond Third Order

- R. vidian
- R. caroticotympanic
- R. meningohypophyseal tr.
- R. inferolateral tr.
- R. inf. hypophyseal
- R. ophthalmic
- R. sup. hypophyseal
- R. ant. choroidal
- R. post. communicating
- R. middle cerebral
- R. ant. cerebral

- R. sup. thyroid
- R. asc. pharyngeal
- R. lingual
- R. facial
- R. occipital
- R. post. auricular
- R. superficial temporal
- R. internal maxillary
  - R. middle meningeal

Third Order

- R. int. carotid
- R. ext. carotid

- R. vertebral → Basilar and branches / Post. cerebral
- R. int. thoracic (int. mammary) → R. sup. epigastric
- R. thyrocervical tr. → R. inf. thyroid / R. asc. cervical / R. transv. cervical / R. suprascapular
- R. costocervical tr. → R. deep cervical / R. supreme intercostal

- R. sup. thoracic
- R. thoracoacromial
- R. lat. thoracic
- R. ant. & post. circumflex humeral
- R. subscapular → R. circumflex scapular / R. thoracodorsal
- R. brachial → R. profunda brachii / R. ulnar → R. common interosseous / R. radial → R. deep palmar arch / R. superficial palmar arch / R. metacarpal(s) / R. digital(s)

- L. vidian
- L. caroticotympanic
- L. meningohypophyseal tr.
- L. inferolateral tr.
- L. inf. hypophyseal
- L. ophthalmic
- L. sup. hypophyseal
- L. ant. choroidal
- L. post. communicating
- L. middle cerebral
- L. ant. cerebral

- L. sup. thyroid
- L. asc. pharyngeal
- L. lingual
- L. facial
- L. occipital
- L. post. auricular
- L. superficial temporal
- L. internal maxillary → L. middle meningeal

Second Order

- R. common carotid → R. int. carotid / R. ext. carotid
- R. subclavian → R. vertebral / R. int. thoracic / R. thyrocervical tr. / R. costocervical tr.
- R. axillary (Considered 1 vessel for coding purposes) → R. sup. thoracic / R. thoracoacromial / R. lat. thoracic / R. ant. & post. circumflex humeral / R. subscapular / R. brachial
- L. int. carotid
- L. ext carotid

First Order

- R. & L. coronary
- Innominate (brachiocephalic)
- L. common carotid

Thoracic aorta

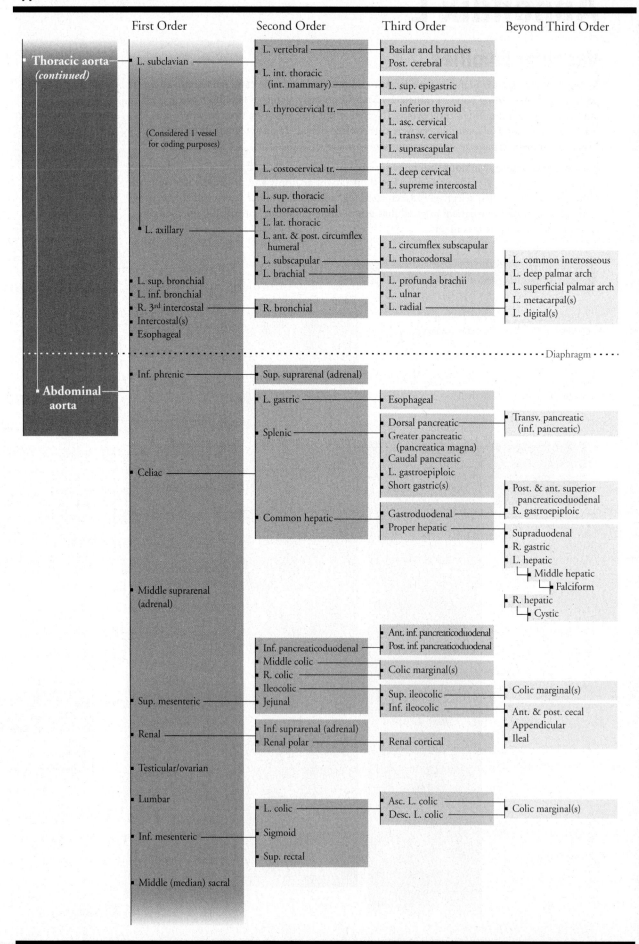

★ = Telemedicine   ◀ = Audio-only   ✛ = Add-on code   ✗ = FDA approval pending   # = Resequenced code   ⊘ = Modifier 51 exempt   ➋➋➋ = See p xxi for details

First Order Second Order Third Order Beyond Third Order

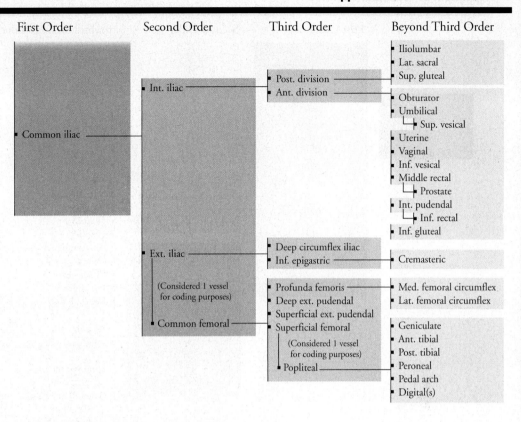

Iliolumbar
Lat. sacral
Sup. gluteal

Int. iliac → Post. division
Ant. division

Obturator
Umbilical
└ Sup. vesical
Uterine
Vaginal
Inf. vesical
Middle rectal
└ Prostate
Int. pudendal
└ Inf. rectal
Inf. gluteal

Common iliac

Ext. iliac → Deep circumflex iliac
Inf. epigastric → Cremasteric

(Considered 1 vessel
for coding purposes)

Profunda femoris → Med. femoral circumflex
Deep ext. pudendal → Lat. femoral circumflex
Superficial ext. pudendal
Common femoral → Superficial femoral

(Considered 1 vessel
for coding purposes)

Geniculate
Ant. tibial
Post. tibial
Popliteal → Peroneal
Pedal arch
Digital(s)

Venous Vascular Family

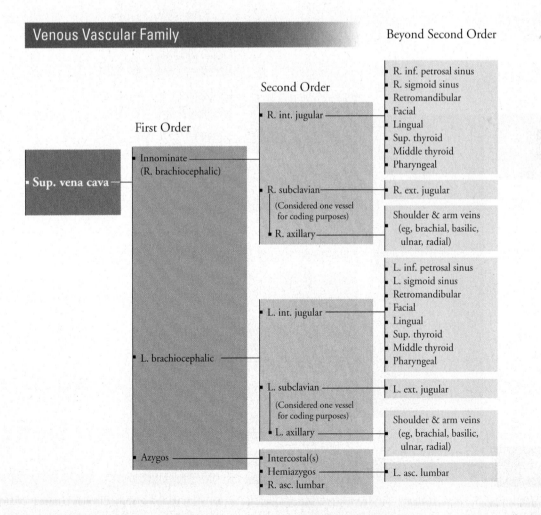

Beyond Second Order

Second Order

R. int. jugular → R. inf. petrosal sinus
R. sigmoid sinus
Retromandibular
Facial
Lingual
Sup. thyroid
Middle thyroid
Pharyngeal

First Order

Innominate
(R. brachiocephalic)

R. subclavian → R. ext. jugular

(Considered one vessel
for coding purposes)

Sup. vena cava

R. axillary → Shoulder & arm veins
(eg, brachial, basilic,
ulnar, radial)

L. int. jugular → L. inf. petrosal sinus
L. sigmoid sinus
Retromandibular
Facial
Lingual
Sup. thyroid
Middle thyroid
Pharyngeal

L. brachiocephalic

L. subclavian → L. ext. jugular

(Considered one vessel
for coding purposes)

L. axillary → Shoulder & arm veins
(eg, brachial, basilic,
ulnar, radial)

Azygos → Intercostal(s)
Hemiazygos → L. asc. lumbar
R. asc. lumbar

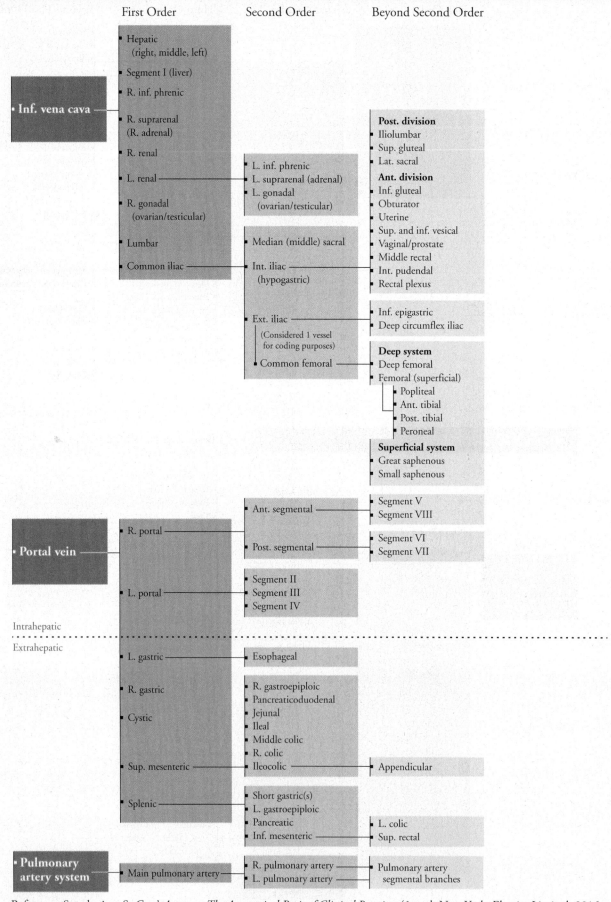

First Order   Second Order   Beyond Second Order

- **Inf. vena cava**
  - Hepatic (right, middle, left)
  - Segment I (liver)
  - R. inf. phrenic
  - R. suprarenal (R. adrenal)
  - R. renal
  - L. renal
    - L. inf. phrenic
    - L. suprarenal (adrenal)
    - L. gonadal (ovarian/testicular)
  - R. gonadal (ovarian/testicular)
  - Lumbar
  - Common iliac
    - Median (middle) sacral
    - Int. iliac (hypogastric)
      - **Post. division**
      - Iliolumbar
      - Sup. gluteal
      - Lat. sacral
      - **Ant. division**
      - Inf. gluteal
      - Obturator
      - Uterine
      - Sup. and inf. vesical
      - Vaginal/prostate
      - Middle rectal
      - Int. pudendal
      - Rectal plexus
    - Ext. iliac
      (Considered 1 vessel for coding purposes)
      - Inf. epigastric
      - Deep circumflex iliac
    - Common femoral
      - **Deep system**
      - Deep femoral
      - Femoral (superficial)
        - Popliteal
        - Ant. tibial
        - Post. tibial
        - Peroneal
      - **Superficial system**
      - Great saphenous
      - Small saphenous

- **Portal vein**
  - R. portal
    - Ant. segmental
      - Segment V
      - Segment VIII
    - Post. segmental
      - Segment VI
      - Segment VII
  - L. portal
    - Segment II
    - Segment III
    - Segment IV

Intrahepatic
·····································
Extrahepatic

  - L. gastric
    - Esophageal
  - R. gastric
  - Cystic
  - Sup. mesenteric
    - R. gastroepiploic
    - Pancreaticoduodenal
    - Jejunal
    - Ileal
    - Middle colic
    - R. colic
    - Ileocolic
      - Appendicular
  - Splenic
    - Short gastric(s)
    - L. gastroepiploic
    - Pancreatic
    - Inf. mesenteric
      - L. colic
      - Sup. rectal

- **Pulmonary artery system**
  - Main pulmonary artery
    - R. pulmonary artery
    - L. pulmonary artery
      - Pulmonary artery segmental branches

Reference: Standstring, S. *Gray's Anatomy: The Anatomical Basis of Clinical Practice.* 41st ed. New York: Elsevier Limited; 2016

Arterial Vascular Family: Thorax and Abdomen

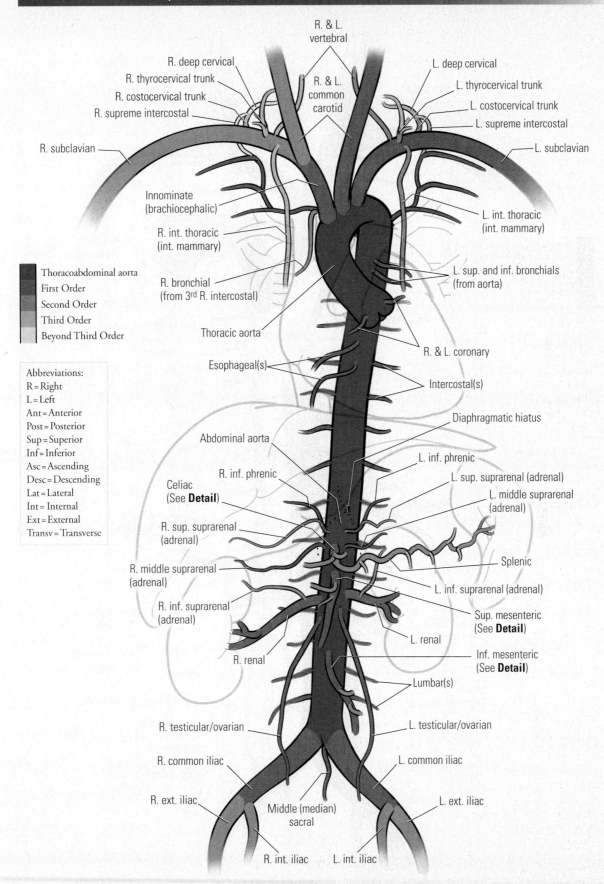

R. & L. vertebral

R. deep cervical
R. thyrocervical trunk
R. costocervical trunk
R. supreme intercostal

R. & L. common carotid

L. deep cervical
L. thyrocervical trunk
L. costocervical trunk
L. supreme intercostal

R. subclavian

L. subclavian

Innominate (brachiocephalic)

L. int. thoracic (int. mammary)

R. int. thoracic (int. mammary)

Thoracoabdominal aorta
First Order
Second Order
Third Order
Beyond Third Order

R. bronchial (from 3rd R. intercostal)

L. sup. and inf. bronchials (from aorta)

Thoracic aorta

R. & L. coronary

Abbreviations:
R = Right
L = Left
Ant = Anterior
Post = Posterior
Sup = Superior
Inf = Inferior
Asc = Ascending
Desc = Descending
Lat = Lateral
Int = Internal
Ext = External
Transv = Transverse

Esophageal(s)

Intercostal(s)

Diaphragmatic hiatus

Abdominal aorta

L. inf. phrenic

R. inf. phrenic

L. sup. suprarenal (adrenal)

Celiac (See **Detail**)

L. middle suprarenal (adrenal)

R. sup. suprarenal (adrenal)

Splenic

R. middle suprarenal (adrenal)

L. inf. suprarenal (adrenal)

R. inf. suprarenal (adrenal)

Sup. mesenteric (See **Detail**)

L. renal

R. renal

Inf. mesenteric (See **Detail**)

Lumbar(s)

R. testicular/ovarian

L. testicular/ovarian

R. common iliac

L. common iliac

R. ext. iliac

L. ext. iliac

Middle (median) sacral

R. int. iliac   L. int. iliac

Venous Vascular Family: Thorax and Abdomen

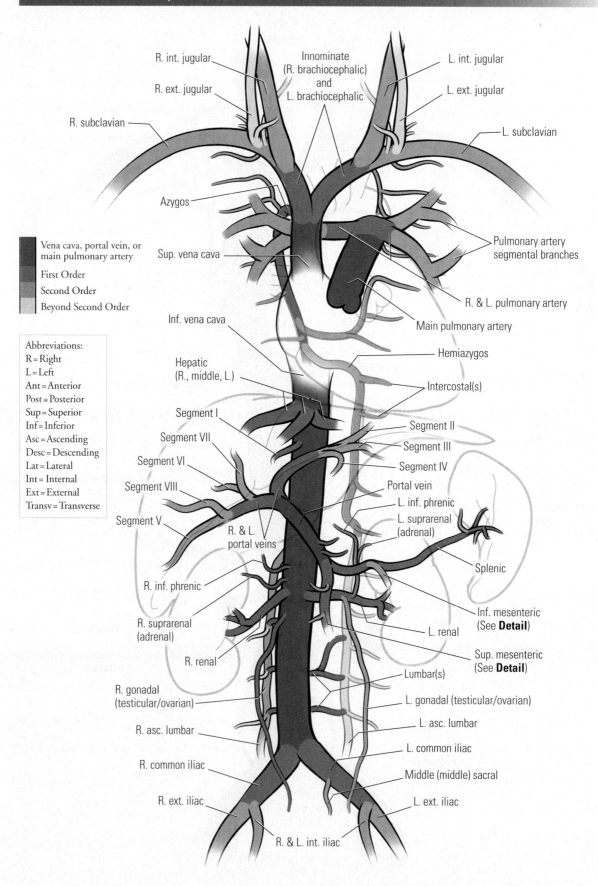

R. int. jugular

Innominate
(R. brachiocephalic)
and
L. brachiocephalic

L. int. jugular

R. ext. jugular

L. ext. jugular

R. subclavian

L. subclavian

Azygos

Pulmonary artery
segmental branches

Sup. vena cava

R. & L. pulmonary artery

Main pulmonary artery

Inf. vena cava

Hemiazygos

Hepatic
(R., middle, L.)

Intercostal(s)

Segment I

Segment II

Segment VII

Segment III

Segment VI

Segment IV

Segment VIII

Portal vein

L. inf. phrenic

Segment V

L. suprarenal
(adrenal)

R. & L.
portal veins

Splenic

R. inf. phrenic

Inf. mesenteric
(See **Detail**)

R. suprarenal
(adrenal)

L. renal

Sup. mesenteric
(See **Detail**)

R. renal

Lumbar(s)

R. gonadal
(testicular/ovarian)

L. gonadal (testicular/ovarian)

R. asc. lumbar

L. asc. lumbar

R. common iliac

L. common iliac

Middle (middle) sacral

R. ext. iliac

L. ext. iliac

R. & L. int. iliac

Vena cava, portal vein, or
main pulmonary artery

First Order

Second Order

Beyond Second Order

Abbreviations:
R = Right
L = Left
Ant = Anterior
Post = Posterior
Sup = Superior
Inf = Inferior
Asc = Ascending
Desc = Descending
Lat = Lateral
Int = Internal
Ext = External
Transv = Transverse

★ = Telemedicine   ◀ = Audio-only   ✦ = Add-on code   ✗ = FDA approval pending   # = Resequenced code   ⊘ = Modifier 51 exempt   ➲➲➲ = See p xxi for details

Arterial Vascular Family: Abdomen, Detail

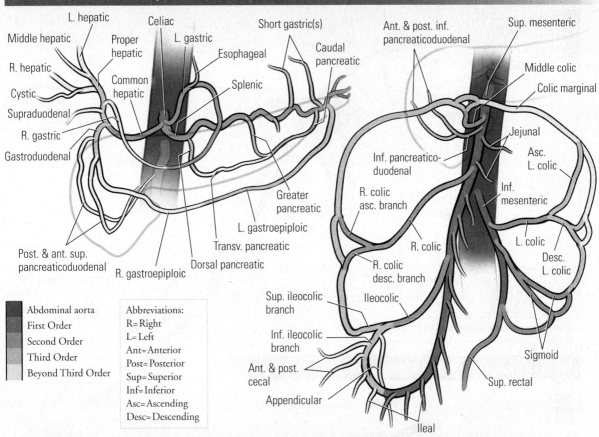

Venous Vascular Family: Abdomen, Detail

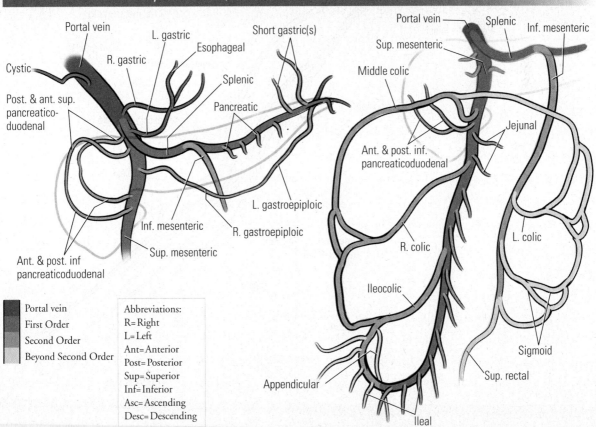

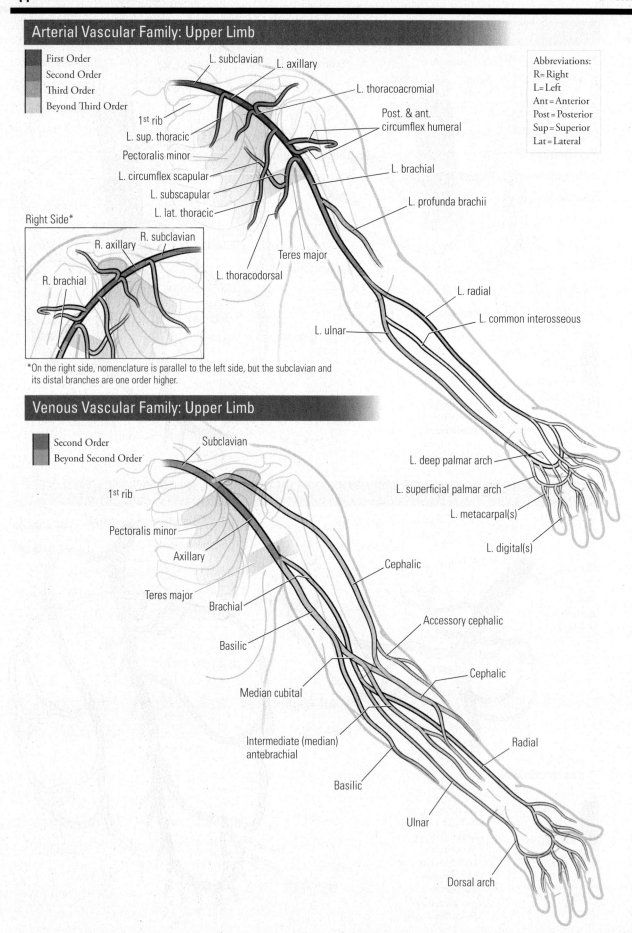

Arterial Vascular Family: Upper Limb

First Order
Second Order
Third Order
Beyond Third Order

Abbreviations:
R = Right
L = Left
Ant = Anterior
Post = Posterior
Sup = Superior
Lat = Lateral

L. subclavian
L. axillary
L. thoracoacromial
Post. & ant. circumflex humeral
1st rib
L. sup. thoracic
Pectoralis minor
L. circumflex scapular
L. subscapular
L. lat. thoracic
L. brachial
L. profunda brachii
Teres major
L. thoracodorsal
L. radial
L. common interosseous
L. ulnar

Right Side*
R. axillary
R. subclavian
R. brachial

*On the right side, nomenclature is parallel to the left side, but the subclavian and its distal branches are one order higher.

Venous Vascular Family: Upper Limb

Second Order
Beyond Second Order

Subclavian
1st rib
Pectoralis minor
Axillary
Teres major
Brachial
Basilic
Median cubital
Intermediate (median) antebrachial
Basilic
Cephalic
Accessory cephalic
Cephalic
L. deep palmar arch
L. superficial palmar arch
L. metacarpal(s)
L. digital(s)
Radial
Ulnar
Dorsal arch

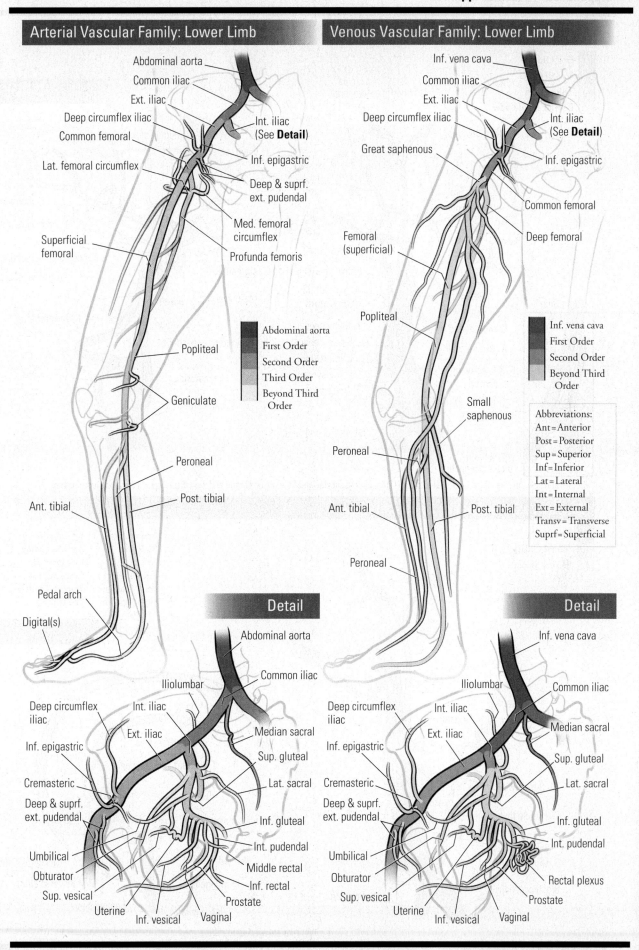

Arterial Vascular Family: Lower Limb

- Abdominal aorta
- Common iliac
- Ext. iliac
- Deep circumflex iliac
- Common femoral
- Int. iliac (See **Detail**)
- Inf. epigastric
- Lat. femoral circumflex
- Deep & suprf. ext. pudendal
- Med. femoral circumflex
- Superficial femoral
- Profunda femoris
- Popliteal
- Geniculate
- Peroneal
- Post. tibial
- Ant. tibial
- Pedal arch
- Digital(s)

Legend:
- Abdominal aorta
- First Order
- Second Order
- Third Order
- Beyond Third Order

Detail
- Abdominal aorta
- Iliolumbar
- Int. iliac
- Common iliac
- Deep circumflex iliac
- Ext. iliac
- Median sacral
- Inf. epigastric
- Sup. gluteal
- Cremasteric
- Lat. sacral
- Deep & suprf. ext. pudendal
- Inf. gluteal
- Umbilical
- Int. pudendal
- Obturator
- Middle rectal
- Sup. vesical
- Inf. rectal
- Uterine
- Prostate
- Inf. vesical
- Vaginal

Venous Vascular Family: Lower Limb

- Inf. vena cava
- Common iliac
- Ext. iliac
- Deep circumflex iliac
- Int. iliac (See **Detail**)
- Great saphenous
- Inf. epigastric
- Common femoral
- Deep femoral
- Femoral (superficial)
- Popliteal
- Small saphenous
- Peroneal
- Ant. tibial
- Post. tibial
- Peroneal

Legend:
- Inf. vena cava
- First Order
- Second Order
- Beyond Third Order

Abbreviations:
Ant = Anterior
Post = Posterior
Sup = Superior
Inf = Inferior
Lat = Lateral
Int = Internal
Ext = External
Transv = Transverse
Suprf = Superficial

Detail
- Inf. vena cava
- Iliolumbar
- Int. iliac
- Common iliac
- Deep circumflex iliac
- Ext. iliac
- Median sacral
- Inf. epigastric
- Sup. gluteal
- Cremasteric
- Lat. sacral
- Deep & suprf. ext. pudendal
- Inf. gluteal
- Umbilical
- Int. pudendal
- Obturator
- Rectal plexus
- Sup. vesical
- Prostate
- Uterine
- Inf. vesical
- Vaginal

Arterial Vascular Family: Head and Neck

First Order
Second Order
Third Order
Beyond Third Order

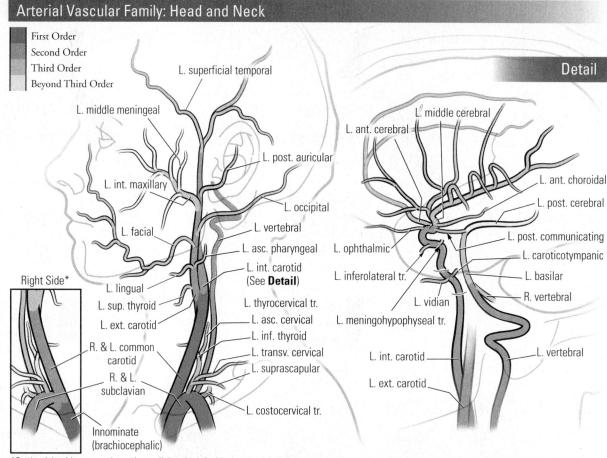

Detail

L. superficial temporal
L. middle meningeal
L. post. auricular
L. int. maxillary
L. occipital
L. facial
L. vertebral
L. asc. pharyngeal
L. int. carotid (See **Detail**)
L. lingual
Right Side*
L. sup. thyroid
L. thyrocervical tr.
L. ext. carotid
L. asc. cervical
R. & L. common carotid
L. inf. thyroid
L. transv. cervical
R. & L. subclavian
L. suprascapular
L. costocervical tr.
Innominate (brachiocephalic)

L. middle cerebral
L. ant. cerebral
L. ant. choroidal
L. post. cerebral
L. post. communicating
L. ophthalmic
L. caroticotympanic
L. inferolateral tr.
L. basilar
R. vertebral
L. vidian
L. meningohypophyseal tr.
L. int. carotid
L. vertebral
L. ext. carotid

*On the right side, nomenclature is parallel to the left side, but the subclavian and common carotid and their distal branches are one order higher.

Venous Vascular Family: Head and Neck

First Order
Second Order
Beyond Second Order

Abbreviations:	
R = Right	Inf = Inferior
L = Left	Asc = Ascending
Ant = Anterior	Int = Internal
Post = Posterior	Ext = External
Sup = Superior	Transv = Transverse
	Tr = Trunk

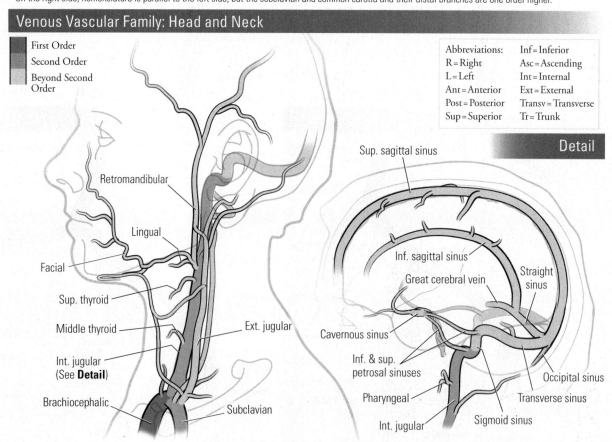

Detail

Sup. sagittal sinus
Retromandibular
Lingual
Inf. sagittal sinus
Facial
Great cerebral vein
Straight sinus
Sup. thyroid
Middle thyroid
Ext. jugular
Cavernous sinus
Int. jugular (See **Detail**)
Inf. & sup. petrosal sinuses
Occipital sinus
Brachiocephalic
Subclavian
Pharyngeal
Transverse sinus
Int. jugular
Sigmoid sinus

Appendix M

Renumbered CPT Codes–Citations Crosswalk

This listing is a summary of crosswalked deleted and renumbered codes and descriptors with the associated *CPT Assistant* references for the deleted codes. This listing includes codes deleted and renumbered from 2007 to 2009. Additional codes will not be added, since the principle of deleting and renumbering is no longer being utilized in the CPT code set.

Current Code(s)	Deleted/Former Code	Year Code Deleted	Citations Referencing Former Code—Applicable to Current Code(s)
89240	0058T	2009	Jun 04:8 CPT Changes: An Insider's View 2004
89240	0059T	2009	CPT Changes: An Insider's View 2004
41530	0088T	2009	May 05:7, Sep 05:9 CPT Changes: An Insider's View 2005
95803	0089T	2009	Jun 05:6, Feb 06:1 CPT Changes: An Insider's View 2006
22856	0090T	2009	Jun 05:6, Feb 06:1 CPT Changes: An Insider's View 2006, 2007
22864	0093T	2009	Jun 05:6, Feb 06:1 CPT Changes: An Insider's View 2006, 2007
22861	0096T	2009	Jun 05:6, Feb 06:1 CPT Changes: An Insider's View 2006, 2007
55706	0137T	2009	CPT Changes: An Insider's View 2006
95980-95982	0162T	2009	CPT Changes: An Insider's View 2007
1123F, 1124F	1080F	2009	CPT Changes: An Insider's View 2008
0054T, 0055T	20986	2009	CPT Changes: An Insider's View 2008
0054T, 0055T	20987	2009	CPT Changes: An Insider's View 2008
4177F	4007F	2009	CPT Changes: An Insider's View 2008
52214	52606	2009	Apr 01:4
52601	52612	2009	Apr 01:4
52601	52614	2009	Apr 01:4
52630	52620	2009	Apr 01:4
61796-61800, 63620, 63621	61793	2009	Nov 97:23, May 03:19, Apr 04:15, Jan 06:46
88720	88400	2009	Aug 05:9
96360	90760	2009	Nov 05:1, Jul 06:4, Sep 06:14, Dec 06:14 CPT Changes: An Insider's View 2006, 2008
96361	90761	2009	Nov 05:1, Jul 06:4, Sep 06:14, Dec 06:14, Mar 07:10 CPT Changes: An Insider's View 2006, 2007
96365	90765	2009	Nov 05:1, Sep 06:14, Nov 06:22, Dec 06:14 CPT Changes: An Insider's View 2006
96366	90766	2009	Nov 05:1, Sep 06:14, Dec 06:14, Mar 07:10 CPT Changes: An Insider's View 2006, 2007
96367	90767	2009	Nov 05:1, Sep 06:14, Nov 06:22, Dec 06:14 CPT Changes: An Insider's View 2006
96368	90768	2009	Nov 05:1, Aug 06:11, Sep 06:14, Nov 06:22, Dec 06:14 CPT Changes: An Insider's View 2006
96369	90769	2009	CPT Changes: An Insider's View 2008
96370	90770	2009	CPT Changes: An Insider's View 2008

Current Code(s)	Deleted/Former Code	Year Code Deleted	Citations Referencing Former Code—Applicable to Current Code(s)
96371	90771	2009	CPT Changes: An Insider's View 2008
96372	90772	2009	Nov 05:1, Sep 06:14, Dec 06:14 CPT Changes: An Insider's View 2006
96373	90773	2009	Nov 05:1, Sep 06:14, Dec 06:14 CPT Changes: An Insider's View 2006
96374	90774	2009	Nov 05:1, Sep 06:14, Dec 06:14 CPT Changes: An Insider's View 2006
96375	90775	2009	Nov 05:1, Sep 06:14, Dec 06:14 CPT Changes: An Insider's View 2006
96376	90776	2009	CPT Changes: An Insider's View 2008
96379	90779	2009	Nov 05:1, Sep 06:14, Dec 06:14 CPT Changes: An Insider's View 2006
90951-90953, 90963, 90967	90918	2009	Fall 93:5, May 96:4, May 02:17, Jan 03:22
90954-90956, 90964, 90968	90919	2009	Fall 93:5, May 96:5, May 02:17, Jan 03:22
90957-90959, 90965, 90969	90920	2009	Fall 93:5, May 96:5, May 02:17, Jan 03:22
90960-90962, 90966, 90970	90921	2009	Fall 93:5, May 96:5, May 02:17, Jan 03:22
90951-90953, 90963, 90967	90922	2009	Fall 93:5, May 96:5, May 02:17, Jan 03:22
90954-90956, 90964, 90968	90923	2009	May 96:5, May 02:17, Jan 03:22
90957-90959, 90965, 90969	90924	2009	May 96:5, May 02:17, Jan 03:22
90960-90962, 90966, 90970	90925	2009	May 96:5, May 02:17, Jan 03:22
93285, 93291, 93298	93727	2009	Nov 99:50, Jul 00:5, CPT Changes: An Insider's View 2000
93280, 93288, 93294	93731	2009	Summer 94:23, Feb 98:11
93280, 93288, 93294	93732	2009	Summer 94:23, Feb 98:11, Mar 00:10
93293	93733	2009	Summer 94:23
93279, 93288, 93294	93734	2009	Summer 94:23, Feb 98:11
93279, 93288, 93294	93735	2009	Summer 94:23, Feb 98:11
93293	93736	2009	Summer 94:23
93282, 93289, 93292, 93295	93741	2009	Nov 99:50-51, Jul 00:5, Nov 00:9, Sep 05:8 CPT Changes: An Insider's View 2000, 2005
93282, 93289, 93292, 93295	93742	2009	Nov 99:50-51, Jul 00:5, Nov 00:9 CPT Changes: An Insider's View 2000, 2005
93283, 93289, 93295	93743	2009	Nov 99:50-51, Jul 00:5, Nov 00:9, Sep 05:8 CPT Changes: An Insider's View 2000
93283, 93289, 93295	93744	2009	Nov 99:50-51, Jul 00:5, Nov 00:9 CPT Changes: An Insider's View 2000
99466	99289	2009	May 05:1, Jul 06:4 CPT Changes: An Insider's View 2002, 2003
99467	99290	2009	CPT Changes: An Insider's View 2002
99468	99295	2009	Summer 93:1, Nov 97:4-5, Mar 98:11, Nov 99:5-6, Dec 00:14, Feb 03:15, Oct 03:1, May 05:1, Nov 05:10, CPT Changes: An Insider's View 2000, 2003, 2004, 2005

Current Code(s)	Deleted/Former Code	Year Code Deleted	Citations Referencing Former Code—Applicable to Current Code(s)
99469	99296	2009	Summer 93:1, Nov 97:4-5, Mar 98:11, Nov 99:5-6, Dec 00:14, Feb 03:15, Oct 03:1, Nov 05:10, CPT Changes: An Insider's View 2000, 2003, 2004, 2005, 2008
99471	99293	2009	Feb 03:15, Oct 03:2, Aug 04:7, 10, May 05:1, Nov 05:10, Jul 06:4, Apr 07:3 CPT Changes: An Insider's View 2003, 2004, 2005
99472	99294	2009	Feb 03:15, Oct 03:2, Aug 04:7, Nov 05:10, Jul 06:4, Apr 07:3 CPT Changes: An Insider's View 2003, 2004, 2005
99478	99298	2009	Nov 98:2-3, Nov 99: 5-6, Aug 00:4, Dec 00:15, Oct 03:2, May 05:1, Nov 05:10; CPT Changes: An Insider's View 2000, 2003
99479	99299	2009	Oct 03:2, Nov 05:10; CPT Changes: An Insider's View 2003
99480	99300	2009	CPT Changes: An Insider's View 2006
99460	99431	2009	Apr 97:10, Nov 97:9, Sep 98:5, Apr 04:14, May 05:1
99461	99432	2009	Sep 98:5, May 99:11, Apr 04:14
99462	99433	2009	Sep 98:5, Apr 03:27
99463	99435	2009	Sep 98:5, Apr 04:14
99464	99436	2009	Nov 97:9-10, Sep 98:5, Nov 99:5-6, Aug 00:3, Aug 04:9, Nov 05:15
99465	99440	2009	Summer 93:3, Mar 96:10, Nov 97:9, Sep 98:5, Nov 99:5-6, Aug 00:3, Oct 03:3, Aug 04:9, Apr 07:3
20985	0054T	2008	May 04:14, Jun 04:8 CPT Changes: An Insider's View 2004
20985	0055T	2008	May 04:14, Jun 04:8 CPT Changes: An Insider's View 2004, 2005
20985	0056T	2008	May 04:14, Jun 04:8 CPT Changes: An Insider's View 2004
99174	0065T	2008	Mar 05:1, 3-4 CPT Changes: An Insider's View 2005
99605-99607	0115T	2008	CPT Changes: An Insider's View 2006
99605-99607	0116T	2008	CPT Changes: An Insider's View 2006
99605-99607	0117T	2008	CPT Changes: An Insider's View 2006
50593	0135T	2008	CPT Changes: An Insider's View 2006, Clinical Examples in Radiology Winter 06:18
24357-24359	24350	2008	
24357-24359	24351	2008	
24357-24359	24352	2008	
24357-24359	24354	2008	
24357-24359	24356	2008	
3044F	3047F	2008	CPT Changes: An Insider's View 2007
3074F-3075F	3076F	2008	CPT Changes: An Insider's View 2007
32560	32005	2008	
32550	32019	2008	CPT Changes: An Insider's View 2005
32551	32020	2008	Fall 92:13, Nov 03:14
36591	36540	2008	Jan 02:11, Nov 02:3, Apr 03:26, Nov 05:1 CPT Changes: An Insider's View 2001, 2003
36593	36550	2008	Nov 99:20, Nov 05:1 CPT Changes: An Insider's View 2000
58958	49200	2008	CPT Changes: An Insider's View 2003
58958	49201	2008	
51100	51000	2008	Nov 99:32-33, Aug 00:3, Oct 03:2

Current Code(s)	Deleted/Former Code	Year Code Deleted	Citations Referencing Former Code—Applicable to Current Code(s)
51101	51005	2008	
51102	51010	2008	
60300	60001	2008	
67041, 67042, 67043	67038	2008	Aug 03:15, Sep 05:12
75557, 75559, 75561, 75563	75552	2008	Fall 95:2
75557, 75559, 75561, 75563	75553	2008	Fall 95:2
75557, 75559, 75561, 75563	75554	2008	Fall 95:2
75557, 75559, 75561, 75563	75555	2008	Fall 95:2
75557, 75559, 75561, 75563	75556	2008	Fall 95:2
78610	78615	2008	CPT Changes: An Insider's View 2002
86356, 86486	86586	2008	Jul 98:11
99366-99368	99361	2008	May 05:1
99366-99368	99362	2008	
96904	0044T	2007	CPT Changes: An Insider's View 2003, 2004
96904	0045T	2007	Jul 04:7 CPT Changes: An Insider's View 2004
77371-77373	0082T	2007	CPT Changes: An Insider's View 2005
77371-77373	0083T	2007	CPT Changes: An Insider's View 2005
22857	0091T	2007	CPT Changes: An Insider's View 2006
22865	0094T	2007	CPT Changes: An Insider's View 2006
22862	0097T	2007	CPT Changes: An Insider's View 2006
19105	0120T	2007	CPT Changes: An Insider's View 2006
15002, 15004	15000	2007	Fall 93:7, Apr 97:4, Aug 97:6, Sep 97:2, Nov 98:5, Jan 99:4, Apr 99:10, May 99:10, Nov 02:7, Aug 03:14 CPT Changes: An Insider's View 2001, 2006
15003, 15005	15001	2007	Nov 98:5-6, Jan 99:4, May 99:10, Aug 03:14
15830, 15847, 17999	15831	2007	May 01:11 CPT Changes: An Insider's View 2007
17311	17304	2007	Winter 94:19, Mar 99:11, Jun 99:10, Nov 02:7, Nov 03:15, Feb 04:11, Jul 04:2 CPT Changes: An Insider's View 2003
17312, 17314	17305	2007	Winter 94:19, Mar 99:11, Jun 99:10, Nov 02:7, Feb 04:11, Jul 04:3
17312, 17314	17306	2007	Winter 94:19, Mar 99:11, Jun 99:10, Nov 02:7, Feb 04:11, Jul 04:4
17312, 17314	17307	2007	Winter 94:19, Mar 99:11, Jun 99:10, Nov 02:7, Nov 03:15, Feb 04:11, Jul 04:4
17315	17310	2007	Winter 94:19, Mar 99:11, Jun 99:10, Nov 02:7, Feb 04:11, May 04:14, Jul 04:4 CPT Changes: An Insider's View 2003
19300	19140	2007	Feb 96:9, Apr 05:13
19301	19160	2007	Apr 05:7 CPT Changes: An Insider's View 2005
19302	19162	2007	Jun 00:11, Apr 05:7
19303	19180	2007	Apr 05:7

Current Code(s)	Deleted/Former Code	Year Code Deleted	Citations Referencing Former Code—Applicable to Current Code(s)
19305	19200	2007	Apr 05:7
19306	19220	2007	Apr 05:7
19307	19240	2007	Apr 05:7
25606	25611	2007	Fall 93:23, Oct 99:5
25607-25609	25620	2007	
26390	26504	2007	
27325	27315	2007	
27326	27320	2007	
28055	28030	2007	
33254-33256	33253	2007	
35302-35306	35381	2007	
35506	35507	2007	
35537, 35538	35541	2007	
35539, 35540	35546	2007	
35637, 35638	35641	2007	Dec 01:7
44799	44152	2007	
44799	44153	2007	
48105	48005	2007	
48548	48180	2007	
49402	49085	2007	
54150	54152	2007	Sep 96:11, Dec 96:10, May 98:11, Apr 03:27 CPT Changes: An Insider's View 2007
54865	54820	2007	Oct 01:8
55875	55859	2007	Apr 04:6
56442	56720	2007	
57558	57820	2007	
67346	67350	2007	
77001	75998	2007	Dec 04:12-13 CPT Changes: An Insider's View 2004 Clinical Examples in Radiology Inaugural 04:1-2, Winter 05:9
77002	76003	2007	Fall 93:14, Jul 01:7 CPT Changes: An Insider's View 2001 Clinical Examples in Radiology Spring 05:5-6
77003	76005	2007	Nov 99:32, 34, 41, Jan 00:2, Feb 00:6, Aug 00:8, Sep 02:11, Sep 04:5 CPT Changes: An Insider's View 2000
77071	76006	2007	Nov 98:21 CPT Changes: An Insider's View 2003
77072	76020	2007	
77073	76040	2007	
77074	76061	2007	
77075	76062	2007	
77076	76065	2007	
77077	76066	2007	CPT Changes: An Insider's View 2002

Current Code(s)	Deleted/Former Code	Year Code Deleted	Citations Referencing Former Code—Applicable to Current Code(s)
77078	76070	2007	Nov 97:24 CPT Changes: An Insider's View 2002, 2003
77080	76075	2007	Nov 97:24, Jun 03:11 CPT Changes: An Insider's View 2005
77081	76076	2007	Nov 97:24
77053	76086	2007	
77054	76088	2007	
77011	76355	2007	CPT Changes: An Insider's View 2002, 2003
77012	76360	2007	Fall 93:12, Fall 94:2, Jan 01:9-10, Mar 05:2 CPT Changes: An Insider's View 2001, 2002, 2003
77013	76362	2007	Oct 02:4 CPT Changes: An Insider's View 2002, 2004
77014	76370	2007	Fall 91:12 CPT Changes: An Insider's View 2002, 2003
77021	76393	2007	Jan 01:10, Mar 05:2 CPT Changes: An Insider's View 2001, 2002
77022	76394	2007	Oct 02:4, Mar 05:5 CPT Changes: An Insider's View 2002, 2004
77084	76400	2007	
76775, 76776	76778	2007	CPT Changes: An Insider's View 2002
76998	76986	2007	CPT Changes: An Insider's View 2001
78707-78709	78704	2007	
78701, 78707, 78708, 78709	78715	2007	
78761	78760	2007	
92700	92573	2007	
94002, 94004	94656	2007	Fall 92:30, Spring 95:4, Summer 95:4, Feb 96:9, Aug 00:2, Oct 03:2
94003, 94004	94657	2007	Fall 92:30, Spring 95:4, Summer 95:4, Feb 96:9, Aug 00:2, Oct 03:2

Appendix N

Summary of Resequenced CPT Codes

This is a table of CPT codes that do not appear in numeric sequence in the listing of CPT codes and the code ranges with their corresponding locations. Rather than deleting and renumbering, resequencing allows existing codes to be relocated to an appropriate location for the code concept, regardless of the numeric sequence. The codes listed below are identified in the CPT 2025 code set with a # symbol for the location of the resequenced number within the family of related concepts. Numerically placed references (eg, **Code is out of numerical sequence. See...**) are used as navigational alerts to direct the user to the location of an out-of-sequence code.

Resequenced Code	Corresponding Locations of Resequenced Code	Resequenced Code	Corresponding Locations of Resequenced Code	Resequenced Code	Corresponding Locations of Resequenced Code	Resequenced Code	Corresponding Locations of Resequenced Code
10004	10021-10035	27337	27326-27331	33269	33259-33266	34834	34712-34716
10005	10021-10035	27339	27326-27331	33270	33244-33251	36465	36470-36474
10006	10021-10035	27632	27616-27625	33271	33244-33251	36466	36470-36474
10007	10021-10035	27634	27616-27625	33272	33244-33251	36482	36478-36500
10008	10021-10035	28039	28035-28047	33273	33244-33251	36483	36478-36500
10009	10021-10035	28041	28035-28047	33274	33244-33251	36572	36568-36571
10010	10021-10035	28295	28292-28298	33275	33244-33251	36573	36568-36571
10011	10021-10035	29914	29862-29867	33276	33244-33251	36836	36832-36838
10012	10021-10035	29915	29862-29867	33277	33244-33251	36837	36832-36838
11045	11012-11047	29916	29862-29867	33278	33244-33251	37246	37234-37237
11046	11012-11047	31242	31235-31239	33279	33244-33251	37247	37234-37237
15769	15760-15772	31243	31235-31239	33280	33244-33251	37248	37234-37237
15853	15851-15860	31253	31254-31267	33281	33244-33251	37249	37234-37237
15854	15851-15860	31257	31254-31267	33287	33244-33251	38225	38129-38205
20560	20552-20600	31259	31254-31267	33288	33244-33251	38226	38129-38205
20561	20552-20600	31551	31579-31587	33440	33406-33412	38227	38129-38205
21552	21550-21558	31552	31579-31587	33962	33958-33968	38228	38129-38205
21554	21550-21558	31553	31579-31587	33963	33958-33968	38243	38240-38300
22836	22846-22849	31554	31579-31587	33964	33958-33968	43210	43254-43261
22837	22846-22849	31572	31577-31580	33965	33958-33968	43211	43216-43227
22838	22846-22849	31573	31577-31580	33966	33958-33968	43212	43216-43227
22858	22853-22861	31574	31577-31580	33969	33958-33968	43213	43216-43227
22859	22853-22861	31651	31646-31649	33984	33958-33968	43214	43216-43227
23071	23066-23078	32994	32997-32999	33985	33958-33968	43233	43248-43251
23073	23066-23078	33221	33212-33215	33986	33958-33968	43266	43254-43261
24071	24066-24079	33227	33226-33244	33987	33958-33968	43270	43254-43261
24073	24066-24079	33228	33226-33244	33988	33958-33968	43274	43264-43279
25071	25066-25078	33229	33226-33244	33989	33958-33968	43275	43264-43279
25073	25066-25078	33230	33226-33244	33995	33982-33991	43276	43264-43279
26111	26110-26118	33231	33226-33244	33997	33991-33993	43277	43264-43279
26113	26110-26118	33262	33226-33244	34717	34707-34711	43278	43264-43279
27043	27041-27052	33263	33226-33244	34718	34707-34711	43290	43246-43249
27045	27041-27052	33264	33226-33244	34812	34712-34716	43291	43246-43249
27059	27041-27052	33267	33259-33266	34820	34712-34716	44381	44380-44385
27329	27358-27365	33268	33259-33266	34833	34712-34716	44401	44391-44402

▲ = Revised code ● = New code ▶ ◀ = Contains new or revised text ✖ = Duplicate PLA test ↑↓ = Category I PLA   American Medical Association   **1027**

Resequenced Code	Corresponding Locations of Resequenced Code	Resequenced Code	Corresponding Locations of Resequenced Code	Resequenced Code	Corresponding Locations of Resequenced Code	Resequenced Code	Corresponding Locations of Resequenced Code
45346	45337-45341	64629	64610-64612	80171	80168-80173	80328	See Definitive Drug Testing subsection
45388	45381-45385	64633	64617-64632	80176	80170-80183		
45390	45391-45397	64634	64617-64632	80179	80192-80197		
45398	45391-45397	64635	64617-64632	80181	80168-80173	80329	See Definitive Drug Testing subsection
45399	45910-45999	64636	64617-64632	80189	80173-80175		
46220	46200-46255	66987	66940-66984	80193	80170-80183	80330	See Definitive Drug Testing subsection
46320	46200-46255	66988	66983-66986	80204	80170-80183		
46945	46200-46255	66989	66940-66984	80210	80192-80195		
46946	46200-46255	66991	66983-66986	80220	80170-80175	80331	See Definitive Drug Testing subsection
46947	46760-46910	67810	67710-67801	80230	80170-80183		
46948	46200-46255	69714	69670-69705	80235	80170-80183		
49613	49595-49605	69716	69670-69705	80280	80201-80299	80332	See Definitive Drug Testing subsection
49614	49595-49605	69717	69670-69705	80285	80201-80299		
49615	49595-49605	69719	69670-69705	80305	See Presumptive Drug Class Screening subsection	80333	See Definitive Drug Testing subsection
49616	49595-49605	69726	69670-69705				
49617	49595-49605	69727	69670-69705			80334	See Definitive Drug Testing subsection
49618	49595-49605	69728	69670-69705				
49621	49595-49605	69729	69670-69705	80306	See Presumptive Drug Class Screening subsection	80335	See Definitive Drug Testing subsection
49622	49595-49605	69730	69670-69705				
49623	49595-49605	76014	75984-76010				
50430	50390-50405	76015	75984-76010			80336	See Definitive Drug Testing subsection
50431	50390-50405	76016	75984-76010	80307	See Presumptive Drug Class Screening subsection		
50432	50390-50405	76017	75984-76010			80337	See Definitive Drug Testing subsection
50433	50390-50405	76018	75984-76010				
50434	50390-50405	76019	75984-76010				
50435	50390-50405	77085	77080-77261			80338	See Definitive Drug Testing subsection
50436	50390-50405	77086	77080-77261	80320	See Definitive Drug Testing subsection		
50437	50390-50405	77295	77293-77301				
51797	51728-51741	77385	77412-77427			80339	See Definitive Drug Testing subsection
52356	52352-52355	77386	77412-77427	80321	See Definitive Drug Testing subsection		
58353	58578-58600	77387	77412-77427				
58356	58578-58600	77424	77412-77427			80340	See Definitive Drug Testing subsection
58674	58520-58542	77425	77412-77427	80322	See Definitive Drug Testing subsection		
62328	62269-62280	78429	78458-78468				
62329	62269-62280	78430	78483-78496	80323	See Definitive Drug Testing subsection	80341	See Definitive Drug Testing subsection
63052	63047-63051	78431	78483-78496				
63053	63047-63051	78432	78483-78496				
64461	64483-64487	78433	78483-78496	80324	See Definitive Drug Testing subsection	80342	See Definitive Drug Testing subsection
64462	64483-64487	78434	78483-78496				
64463	64483-64487	78804	78801-78811				
64466	64483-64487	78830	78801-78811	80325	See Definitive Drug Testing subsection	80343	See Definitive Drug Testing subsection
64467	64483-64487	78831	78801-78811				
64468	64483-64487	78832	78801-78811				
64469	64483-64487	78835	78801-78811	80326	See Definitive Drug Testing subsection	80344	See Definitive Drug Testing subsection
64473	64483-64487	80081	80053-80069				
64474	64483-64487	80161	80156-80159				
64624	64605-64612	80164	80200-80203	80327	See Definitive Drug Testing subsection	80345	See Definitive Drug Testing subsection
64625	64605-64612	80165	80200-80203				
64628	64610-64612	80167	80168-80173				

★=Telemedicine   ◀=Audio-only   ✚=Add-on code   ✗=FDA approval pending   #=Resequenced code   ⊘=Modifier 51 exempt   ➲➲➲=See p xxi for details

Resequenced Code	Corresponding Locations of Resequenced Code	Resequenced Code	Corresponding Locations of Resequenced Code	Resequenced Code	Corresponding Locations of Resequenced Code	Resequenced Code	Corresponding Locations of Resequenced Code
80346	See Definitive Drug Testing subsection	80364	See Definitive Drug Testing subsection	81162	81182-81216	81264	81255-81270
				81163	81182-81216	81265	81223-81226
				81164	81182-81216	81266	81223-81226
80347	See Definitive Drug Testing subsection	80365	See Definitive Drug Testing subsection	81165	81182-81216	81267	81223-81226
				81166	81182-81216	81268	81223-81226
				81167	81215-81220	81269	81253-81256
80348	See Definitive Drug Testing subsection	80366	See Definitive Drug Testing subsection	81168	81215-81220	81271	81255-81270
				81173	81171-81176	81274	81255-81270
80349	See Definitive Drug Testing subsection	80367	See Definitive Drug Testing subsection	81174	81171-81176	81277	81228-81235
				81184	81215-81220	81278	81255-81260
80350	See Definitive Drug Testing subsection	80368	See Definitive Drug Testing subsection	81185	81215-81220	81279	81260-81273
				81186	81215-81220	81283	81255-81270
				81187	81223-81226	81284	81243-81248
80351	See Definitive Drug Testing subsection	80369	See Definitive Drug Testing subsection	81188	81223-81226	81285	81243-81248
				81189	81223-81226	81286	81243-81248
				81190	81223-81226	81287	81276-81297
80352	See Definitive Drug Testing subsection	80370	See Definitive Drug Testing subsection	81191	81310-81314	81288	81276-81297
				81192	81310-81314	81289	81243-81248
				81193	81310-81314	81291	81299-81310
80353	See Definitive Drug Testing subsection	80371	See Definitive Drug Testing subsection	81194	81310-81314	81292	81276-81297
				81195	81228-81235	81293	81276-81297
				81200	81171-81176	81294	81276-81297
80354	See Definitive Drug Testing subsection	80372	See Definitive Drug Testing subsection	81201	81171-81176	81295	81276-81297
				81202	81171-81176	81301	81276-81297
				81203	81171-81176	81302	81276-81297
80355	See Definitive Drug Testing subsection	80373	See Definitive Drug Testing subsection	81204	81171-81176	81303	81276-81297
				81205	81182-81216	81304	81276-81297
80356	See Definitive Drug Testing subsection	80374	See Definitive Drug Testing subsection	81206	81182-81216	81306	81310-81316
				81207	81182-81216	81307	81310-81316
				81208	81182-81216	81308	81310-81316
80357	See Definitive Drug Testing subsection	80375	See Definitive Drug Testing subsection	81209	81182-81216	81309	81310-81316
				81210	81182-81216	81312	81310-81316
				81219	81215-81220	81320	81310-81316
80358	See Definitive Drug Testing subsection	80376	See Definitive Drug Testing subsection	81227	81223-81226	81324	81310-81318
				81230	81225-81229	81325	81310-81318
80359	See Definitive Drug Testing subsection	80377	See Definitive Drug Testing subsection	81231	81225-81229	81326	81310-81318
				81233	81215-81220	81332	81318-81335
				81234	81228-81235	81334	81318-81335
80360	See Definitive Drug Testing subsection	81105	81255-81270	81238	81240-81248	81336	81318-81335
		81106	81255-81270	81239	81228-81235	81337	81318-81335
		81107	81255-81270	81245	81240-81248	81338	81276-81297
80361	See Definitive Drug Testing subsection	81108	81255-81270	81246	81240-81248	81339	81276-81297
		81109	81255-81270	81250	81243-81248	81343	81318-81335
		81110	81255-81270	81257	81253-81256	81344	81318-81335
80362	See Definitive Drug Testing subsection	81111	81255-81270	81258	81253-81256	81345	81318-81335
		81112	81255-81270	81259	81253-81256	81347	81327-81329
80363	See Definitive Drug Testing subsection	81120	81255-81270	81261	81255-81270	81348	81330-81340
		81121	81255-81270	81262	81255-81270	81349	81228-81235
		81161	81228-81235	81263	81255-81270	81351	81330-81340

Resequenced Code	Corresponding Locations of Resequenced Code	Resequenced Code	Corresponding Locations of Resequenced Code	Resequenced Code	Corresponding Locations of Resequenced Code	Resequenced Code	Corresponding Locations of Resequenced Code
81352	81330-81340	86413	86376-86386	90759	90744-90748	93247	93226-93229
81353	81330-81340	87154	87149-87153	91113	91110-91117	93248	93226-93229
81357	81342-81355	87428	87425-87430	91304	90473-90477	93260	93283-93291
81361	81253-81256	87484	87496-87500	91318	90473-90477	93261	93283-93291
81362	81253-81256	87564	87561-87580	91319	90473-90477	93264	93272-93280
81363	81253-81256	87623	87538-87541	91320	90473-90477	93319	93316-93321
81364	81253-81256	87624	87538-87541	91321	90473-90477	93356	93350-93355
81418	81414-81416	87625	87538-87541	91322	90473-90477	93573	93567-93572
81419	81413-81416	87626	87538-87541	92137	92133-92145	93574	93567-93572
81441	81437-81442	87806	87802-87903	92517	92548-92551	93575	93567-93572
81443	81420-81426	87811	87804-87809	92518	92548-92551	93584	93596-93598
81448	81437-81442	87906	87802-87903	92519	92548-92551	93585	93596-93598
81462	81458-81465	87910	87802-87903	92558	92583-92588	93586	93596-93598
81463	81458-81465	87912	87802-87903	92597	92603-92607	93587	93596-93598
81464	81458-81465	87913	87899-87904	92618	92603-92607	93588	93596-93598
81479	81407-81411	88177	88172-88175	92650	92583-92588	93896	93892-93922
81500	81536-81541	88341	88334-88372	92651	92583-92588	93897	93892-93922
81503	81536-81541	88350	88334-88372	92652	92583-92588	93898	93892-93922
81504	81542-81554	88364	88334-88372	92653	92583-92588	94619	94610-94621
81522	81513-81520	88373	88334-88372	92920	92997-93005	95249	95199-95803
81540	81542-81554	88374	88334-88372	92921	92997-93005	95700	95966-95971
81546	81542-81554	88377	88334-88372	92924	92997-93005	95705	95966-95971
81595	81490-81506	90480	90473-90477	92925	92997-93005	95706	95966-95971
81596	81513-81520	90584	90585-90632	92928	92997-93005	95707	95966-95971
82042	82044-82077	90589	90585-90632	92929	92997-93005	95708	95966-95971
82652	82300-82310	90611	90710-90715	92933	92997-93005	95709	95966-95971
82653	82642-82658	90619	90717-90739	92934	92997-93005	95710	95966-95971
82681	82668-82672	90620	90717-90739	92937	92997-93005	95711	95966-95971
83529	83525-83540	90621	90717-90739	92938	92997-93005	95712	95966-95971
83992	See Definitive Drug Testing subsection	90622	90714-90717	92941	92997-93005	95713	95966-95971
		90623	90717-90739	92943	92997-93005	95714	95966-95971
		90624	90717-90739	92944	92997-93005	95715	95966-95971
84433	84425-84432	90625	90717-90739	92972	92997-93005	95716	95966-95971
86015	85810-86001	90626	90714-90717	92973	92997-93005	95717	95966-95971
86041	85810-86001	90627	90714-90717	92974	92997-93005	95718	95966-95971
86042	85810-86001	90637	90689-90691	92975	92997-93005	95719	95966-95971
86043	85810-86001	90638	90689-90691	92977	92997-93005	95720	95966-95971
86051	86060-86078	90644	90717-90739	92978	92997-93005	95721	95966-95971
86052	86060-86078	90672	90658-90664	92979	92997-93005	95722	95966-95971
86053	86060-86078	90673	90658-90664	93150	93297-93304	95723	95966-95971
86152	86146-86155	90674	90658-90664	93151	93297-93304	95724	95966-95971
86153	86146-86155	90677	90670-90676	93152	93297-93304	95725	95966-95971
86328	86317-86325	90683	90678-90681	93153	93297-93304	95726	95966-95971
86362	86355-86360	90684	90670-90676	93241	93226-93229	95782	95805-95813
86363	86355-86360	90694	90688-90691	93242	93226-93229	95783	95805-95813
86364	86355-86360	90695	90667-90671	93243	93226-93229	95800	95805-95813
86366	86355-86360	90750	90717-90739	93244	93226-93229	95801	95805-95813
86408	86376-86386	90756	90658-90664	93245	93226-93229	95829	95824-95852
86409	86376-86386	90758	90747-90749	93246	93226-93229	95836	95824-95852

★ = Telemedicine　◀ = Audio-only　+ = Add-on code　✗ = FDA approval pending　# = Resequenced code　⊘ = Modifier 51 exempt　➡➡➡ = See p xxi for details

Appendix N

Resequenced Code	Corresponding Locations of Resequenced Code	Resequenced Code	Corresponding Locations of Resequenced Code	Resequenced Code	Corresponding Locations of Resequenced Code	Resequenced Code	Corresponding Locations of Resequenced Code
95885	95870-95874	97167	See Occupational Therapy Evaluations subsection	98015	See E/M codes 99214-99222	0625T	0496T-0507T
95886	95870-95874					0626T	0496T-0507T
95887	95870-95874			98016	See E/M codes 99214-99222	0640T	0489T-0495T
95938	95912-95933					0643T	0544T-0547T
95939	95912-95933	97168	See Occupational Therapy Evaluations subsection	99091	99448-99455	0646T	0569T-0572T
95940	95912-95933			99177	99173-99183	0671T	0175T-0200T
95941	95912-95933			99415	99358-99366	0697T	0647T-0651T
95983	95976-95981	97169	See Athletic Training Evaluations subsection	99416	99358-99366	0698T	0647T-0651T
95984	95976-95981			99417	99358-99366	0714T	0419T-0422T
96125	96020-96121			99418	99358-99366	0749T	0742T-0745T
96127	96020-96121			99421	99412-99447	0750T	0742T-0745T
96164	96158-96161	97170	See Athletic Training Evaluations subsection	99422	99412-99447	0790T	0656T-0659T
96165	96158-96161			99423	99412-99447	0827T	0762T-0765T
96167	96158-96161			99424	99487-99493	0828T	0762T-0765T
96168	96158-96161			99425	99487-99493	0829T	0762T-0765T
96170	96158-96161	97171	See Athletic Training Evaluations subsection	99426	99487-99493	0830T	0762T-0765T
96171	96158-96161			99427	99487-99493	0831T	0762T-0765T
96380	96376-96401			99437	99480-99489	0832T	0762T-0765T
96381	96376-96401			99439	99480-99489	0833T	0762T-0765T
97037	97028-97034	97172	See Athletic Training Evaluations subsection	99451	99448-99455	0834T	0762T-0765T
97151	96020-96112			99452	99448-99455	0835T	0762T-0765T
97152	96020-96112			99453	99448-99455	0836T	0762T-0765T
97153	96020-96112			99454	99448-99455	0837T	0762T-0765T
97154	96020-96112	98000	See E/M codes 99214-99222	99457	99448-99455	0838T	0762T-0765T
97155	96020-96112			99458	99448-99455	0839T	0762T-0765T
97156	96020-96112	98001	See E/M codes 99214-99222	99459	99497-99499	0840T	0762T-0765T
97157	96020-96112			99473	99448-99455	0841T	0762T-0765T
97158	96020-96112	98002	See E/M codes 99214-99222	99474	99448-99455	0842T	0762T-0765T
97161	See Physical Therapy Evaluations subsection			99484	99497-99499	0843T	0762T-0765T
		98003	See E/M codes 99214-99222	99485	99466-99469	0844T	0762T-0765T
				99486	99466-99469	0845T	0762T-0765T
97162	See Physical Therapy Evaluations subsection	98004	See E/M codes 99214-99222	99490	99480-99489	0846T	0762T-0765T
				99491	99480-99489	0847T	0762T-0765T
		98005	See E/M codes 99214-99222	2033F	2025F-2028F	0848T	0762T-0765T
97163	See Physical Therapy Evaluations subsection	98006	See E/M codes 99214-99222	3051F	3042F-3048F	0849T	0762T-0765T
				3052F	3042F-3048F	0850T	0762T-0765T
		98007	See E/M codes 99214-99222	0253T	0184T-0200T	0851T	0762T-0765T
97164	See Physical Therapy Evaluations subsection	98008	See E/M codes 99214-99222	0464T	0332T-0339T	0852T	0762T-0765T
				0488T	0402T-0408T	0853T	0762T-0765T
		98009	See E/M codes 99214-99222	0510T	0332T-0339T	0854T	0762T-0765T
		98010	See E/M codes 99214-99222	0511T	0332T-0339T	0855T	0762T-0765T
97165	See Occupational Therapy Evaluations subsection	98011	See E/M codes 99214-99222	0512T	0101T-0107T	0856T	0762T-0765T
				0513T	0101T-0107T	0859T	0489T-0495T
		98012	See E/M codes 99214-99222	0523T	0496T-0507T	0860T	0489T-0495T
				0563T	0202T-0209T	0861T	0516T-0520T
97166	See Occupational Therapy Evaluations subsection	98013	See E/M codes 99214-99222	0614T	0579T-0582T	0862T	0516T-0520T
				0620T	0496T-0507T	0863T	0516T-0520T
		98014	See E/M codes 99214-99222	0623T	0496T-0507T	0867T	0419T-0422T
				0624T	0496T-0507T	0901T	0222T-0235T

▲ = Revised code   ● = New code   ▶ ◀ = Contains new or revised text   ✕ = Duplicate PLA test   ↕ = Category I PLA   American Medical Association

Appendix O

Multianalyte Assays with Algorithmic Analyses and Proprietary Laboratory Analyses

The following list includes three types of CPT codes:

1. Multianalyte assays with algorithmic analyses (MAAA) administrative codes

2. Category I MAAA codes

3. Proprietary laboratory analyses (PLA) codes

1. Multianalyte assays with algorithmic analyses (MAAAs) are procedures that utilize multiple results derived from assays of various types, including molecular pathology assays, fluorescent in situ hybridization assays and non-nucleic acid based assays (eg, proteins, polypeptides, lipids, carbohydrates). Algorithmic analysis using the results of these assays as well as other patient information (if used) is then performed and reported typically as a numeric score(s) or as a probability. MAAAs are typically unique to a single clinical laboratory or manufacturer. The results of individual component procedure(s) that are inputs to the MAAAs may be provided on the associated laboratory report, however these assays are not reported separately using additional codes. MAAAs, by nature, are typically unique to a single clinical laboratory or manufacturer.

The list includes a proprietary name and clinical laboratory or manufacturer in the first column, an alpha-numeric code in the second column and code descriptor in the third column. The format for the code descriptor usually includes (in order):

- Disease type (eg, oncology, autoimmune, tissue rejection),

- Chemical(s) analyzed (eg, DNA, RNA, protein, antibody),

- Number of markers (eg, number of genes, number of proteins),

- Methodology(s) (eg, microarray, real-time [RT]-PCR, in situ hybridization [ISH], enzyme linked immunosorbent assays [ELISA]),

- Number of functional domains (if indicated),

- Specimen type (eg, blood, fresh tissue, formalin-fixed paraffin-embedded),

- Algorithm result type (eg, prognostic, diagnostic),

- Report (eg, probability index, risk score).

MAAA procedures that have been assigned a Category I code are noted in the list below and additionally listed in the Category I MAAA section (81500-81599). The Category I MAAA section introductory language and associated parenthetical instruction(s) should be used to govern the appropriate use for Category I MAAA codes. If a specific MAAA procedure has not been assigned a Category I code, it is indicated as a four-digit number followed by the letter M.

When a specific MAAA procedure is not included in either the list below or in the Category I MAAA section, report the analysis using the Category I MAAA unlisted code (81599). The codes below are specific to the assays identified in Appendix O by proprietary name. In order to report an MAAA code, the analysis performed must fulfill the code descriptor **and**, if proprietary, must be the test represented by the proprietary name listed in Appendix O. When an analysis is performed that may potentially fall within a specific descriptor, however the proprietary name is not included in the list below, the MAAA unlisted code (81599) should be used.

Additions in this section may be released tri-annually (or quarterly for PLA codes) via the AMA CPT website to expedite dissemination for reporting. See the Introduction section of the CPT code set for a complete list of the dates of release and implementation.

These administrative codes encompass all analytical services required for the algorithmic analysis (eg, cell lysis, nucleic acid stabilization, extraction, digestion, amplification, hybridization and detection) in addition to the algorithmic analysis itself, when applicable. Procedures that are required prior to cell lysis (eg, microdissection, codes 88380 and 88381) should be reported separately.

The codes in this list are provided as an administrative coding set to facilitate accurate reporting of MAAA services. The minimum standard for inclusion in this list is that an analysis is generally available for patient care. The AMA has not reviewed procedures in the administrative coding set for clinical utility. The list is not a complete list of all MAAA procedures.

2. Category I MAAA codes are included below along with their proprietary names. These codes are also listed in the Pathology and Laboratory section of the CPT code set (81490-81599).

3. PLA codes created in response to the Protecting Access to Medicare Act (PAMA) of 2014 are listed along with their proprietary names. These codes are also located at the end of the Pathology and Laboratory section of the CPT code set. In some instances, the descriptor language of PLA codes may be identical, which are differentiated only by the listed propriety names.

The accuracy of a PLA code is to be maintained by the original applicant, or the current owner of the test kit or laboratory performing the proprietary test.

A new PLA code is required when:

1. Additional nucleic acid (DNA or RNA) and/or protein analysis(es) are added to the current PLA test, or
2. The name of the PLA test has changed in association with changes in test performance or test characteristics.

The addition or modification of the therapeutic applications of the test require submission of a code change application, but it may not require a new code number.

Proprietary Name and Clinical Laboratory or Manufacturer	Alpha-Numeric Code	Code Descriptor
Administrative Codes for Multianalyte Assays with Algorithmic Analyses (MAAA)		
ASH FibroSURE™, BioPredictive S.A.S	0002M	Liver disease, ten biochemical assays (ALT, A2-macroglobulin, apolipoprotein A-1, total bilirubin, GGT, haptoglobin, AST, glucose, total cholesterol and triglycerides) utilizing serum, prognostic algorithm reported as quantitative scores for fibrosis, steatosis and alcoholic steatohepatitis (ASH)
NASH FibroSURE™, BioPredictive S.A.S	0003M	Liver disease, ten biochemical assays (ALT, A2-macroglobulin, apolipoprotein A-1, total bilirubin, GGT, haptoglobin, AST, glucose, total cholesterol and triglycerides) utilizing serum, prognostic algorithm reported as quantitative scores for fibrosis, steatosis and nonalcoholic steatohepatitis (NASH)
ScoliScore™ Transgenomic	0004M	Scoliosis, DNA analysis of 53 single nucleotide polymorphisms (SNPs), using saliva, prognostic algorithm reported as a risk score
HeproDX™, GoPath Laboratories, LLC	0006M	Oncology (hepatic), mRNA expression levels of 161 genes, utilizing fresh hepatocellular carcinoma tumor tissue, with alpha-fetoprotein level, algorithm reported as a risk classifier
NETest, Wren Laboratories, LLC	0007M	Oncology (gastrointestinal neuroendocrine tumors), real-time PCR expression analysis of 51 genes, utilizing whole peripheral blood, algorithm reported as a nomogram of tumor disease index
NeoLAB™ Prostate Liquid Biopsy, NeoGenomics Laboratories	0011M	Oncology, prostate cancer, mRNA expression assay of 12 genes (10 content and 2 housekeeping), RT-PCR test utilizing blood plasma and urine, algorithms to predict high-grade prostate cancer risk

(Continued on page 1034)

Cxbladder™ Detect, Pacific Edge Diagnostics USA, Ltd	0012M	Oncology (urothelial), mRNA, gene expression profiling by real-time quantitative PCR of five genes (*MDK, HOXA13, CDC2 [CDK1], IGFBP5,* and *CXCR2),* utilizing urine, algorithm reported as a risk score for having urothelial carcinoma
Cxbladder™ Monitor, Pacific Edge Diagnostics USA, Ltd	0013M	Oncology (urothelial), mRNA, gene expression profiling by real-time quantitative PCR of five genes (*MDK, HOXA13, CDC2 [CDK1], IGFBP5,* and *CXCR2),* utilizing urine, algorithm reported as a risk score for having recurrent urothelial carcinoma
—	(0014M has been deleted) (For multianalyte assay with algorithmic analysis [MAAA] for liver disease using analysis of 3 biomarkers, use 81517)	—
Adrenal Mass Panel, 24 Hour, Urine, Mayo Clinic Laboratories (MCL), Mayo Clinic	0015M	Adrenal cortical tumor, biochemical assay of 25 steroid markers, utilizing 24-hour urine specimen and clinical parameters, prognostic algorithm reported as a clinical risk and integrated clinical steroid risk for adrenal cortical carcinoma, adenoma, or other adrenal malignancy
Decipher Bladder, Veracyte Labs SD	0016M	Oncology (bladder), mRNA, microarray gene expression profiling of 219 genes, utilizing formalin-fixed paraffin-embedded tissue, algorithm reported as molecular subtype (luminal, luminal infiltrated, basal, basal claudin-low, neuroendocrine-like)
Lymph2Cx, Mayo Clinic Arizona Molecular Diagnostics Laboratory	0017M	Oncology (diffuse large B-cell lymphoma [DLBCL]), mRNA, gene expression profiling by fluorescent probe hybridization of 20 genes, formalin-fixed paraffin-embedded tissue, algorithm reported as cell of origin (Do not report 0017M in conjunction with 0120U)
Pleximark™, Plexision, Inc	0018M	Transplantation medicine (allograft rejection, renal), measurement of donor and third-party-induced CD154+T-cytotoxic memory cells, utilizing whole peripheral blood, algorithm reported as a rejection risk score (Do not report 0018M in conjunction with 81560, 85032, 86353, 86821, 88184, 88185, 88187, 88230, 88240, 88241)
SOMAmer®, SomaLogic	0019M	Cardiovascular disease, plasma, analysis of protein biomarkers by aptamer-based microarray and algorithm reported as 4-year likelihood of coronary event in high-risk populations

★=Telemedicine ◀=Audio-only +=Add-on code ✗=FDA approval pending #=Resequenced code ⊘=Modifier 51 exempt ⊝⊝⊝=See p xxi for details

▶Epignostix CNS Tumor Methylation Classifier, Heidelberg Epignostix GmbH◀	●0020M	▶Oncology (central nervous system), analysis of 30000 DNA methylation loci by methylation array, utilizing DNA extracted from tumor tissue, diagnostic algorithm reported as probability of matching a reference tumor subclass◀
Category I Codes for Multianalyte Assays with Algorithmic Analyses (MAAA)		
Vectra®, Labcorp	81490	Autoimmune (rheumatoid arthritis), analysis of 12 biomarkers using immunoassays, utilizing serum, prognostic algorithm reported as a disease activity score (Do not report 81490 in conjunction with 86140)
AlloMap®, CareDx, Inc	#81595	Cardiology (heart transplant), mRNA, gene expression profiling by real-time quantitative PCR of 20 genes (11 content and 9 housekeeping), utilizing subfraction of peripheral blood, algorithm reported as a rejection risk score
Corus® CAD, CardioDx, Inc	81493	Coronary artery disease, mRNA, gene expression profiling by real-time RT-PCR of 23 genes, utilizing whole peripheral blood, algorithm reported as a risk score
PreDx Diabetes Risk Score™, Tethys Clinical Laboratory	81506	Endocrinology (type 2 diabetes), biochemical assays of seven analytes (glucose, HbA1c, insulin, hs-CRP, adiponectin, ferritin, interleukin 2-receptor alpha), utilizing serum or plasma, algorithm reporting a risk score (Do not report 81506 in conjunction with constituent components [ie, 82728, 82947, 83036, 83525, 86141], 84999 [for adopectin], and 83520 [for interleukin 2-receptor alpha])
Harmony™ Prenatal Test, Ariosa Diagnostics	81507	Fetal aneuploidy (trisomy 21, 18, and 13) DNA sequence analysis of selected regions using maternal plasma, algorithm reported as a risk score for each trisomy (Do not report 81228, 81229, 88271 when performing genomic sequencing procedures or other molecular multianalyte assays for copy number analysis)

(Continued on page 1036)

No proprietary name and clinical laboratory or manufacturer. Maternal serum screening procedures are well-established procedures and are performed by many laboratories throughout the country. The concept of prenatal screens has existed and evolved for over 10 years and is not exclusive to any one facility.	81508	Fetal congenital abnormalities, biochemical assays of two proteins (PAPP-A, hCG [any form]), utilizing maternal serum, algorithm reported as a risk score (Do not report 81508 in conjunction with 84163, 84702)
	81509	Fetal congenital abnormalities, biochemical assays of three proteins (PAPP-A, hCG [any form], DIA), utilizing maternal serum, algorithm reported as a risk score (Do not report 81509 in conjunction with 84163, 84702, 86336)
	81510	Fetal congenital abnormalities, biochemical assays of three analytes (AFP, uE3, hCG [any form]), utilizing maternal serum, algorithm reported as a risk score (Do not report 81510 in conjunction with 82105, 82677, 84702)
	81511	Fetal congenital abnormalities, biochemical assays of four analytes (AFP, uE3, hCG [any form], DIA) utilizing maternal serum, algorithm reported as a risk score (may include additional results from previous biochemical testing) (Do not report 81511 in conjunction with 82105, 82677, 84702, 86336)
	81512	Fetal congenital abnormalities, biochemical assays of five analytes (AFP, uE3, total hCG, hyperglycosylated hCG, DIA) utilizing maternal serum, algorithm reported as a risk score (Do not report 81512 in conjunction with 82105, 82677, 84702, 86336)
Aptima® BV Assay, Hologic, Inc	81513	Infectious disease, bacterial vaginosis, quantitative real-time amplification of RNA markers for Atopobium vaginae, Gardnerella vaginalis, and Lactobacillus species, utilizing vaginal-fluid specimens, algorithm reported as a positive or negative result for bacterial vaginosis

BD MAX™ Vaginal Panel, Becton Dickinson and Company	81514	Infectious disease, bacterial vaginosis and vaginitis, quantitative real-time amplification of DNA markers for Gardnerella vaginalis, Atopobium vaginae, Megasphaera type 1, Bacterial Vaginosis Associated Bacteria-2 (BVAB-2), and Lactobacillus species (L. crispatus and L. jensenii), utilizing vaginal-fluid specimens, algorithm reported as a positive or negative for high likelihood of bacterial vaginosis, includes separate detection of Trichomonas vaginalis and/or Candida species (C. albicans, C. tropicalis, C. parapsilosis, C. dubliniensis), Candida glabrata, Candida krusei, when reported (Do not report 81514 in conjunction with 87480, 87481, 87482, 87510, 87511, 87512, 87660, 87661)
▶Xpert® Xpress MVP, Cepheid®◀	●81515	▶Infectious disease, bacterial vaginosis and vaginitis, real-time PCR amplification of DNA markers for Atopobium vaginae, Atopobium species, Megasphaera type 1, and Bacterial Vaginosis Associated Bacteria-2 (BVAB-2), utilizing vaginal-fluid specimens, algorithm reported as positive or negative for high likelihood of bacterial vaginosis, includes separate detection of Trichomonas vaginalis and Candida species (C. albicans, C. tropicalis, C. parapsilosis, C. dubliniensis), Candida glabrata/Candida krusei, when reported◀
HCV FibroSURE™, FibroTest™, BioPredictive S.A.S.	#81596	Infectious disease, chronic hepatitis C virus (HCV) infection, six biochemical assays (ALT, A2-macro-globulin, apolipoprotein A-1, total bilirubin, GGT, and haptoglobin) utilizing serum, prognostic algorithm reported as scores for fibrosis and necroinflammatory activity in liver
Enhanced Liver Fibrosis™ (ELF™) Test, Siemens Healthcare Diagnostics Inc/Siemens Healthcare Laboratory LLC	81517	Liver disease, analysis of 3 biomarkers (hyaluronic acid [HA], procollagen III amino terminal peptide [PIIINP], tissue inhibitor of metalloproteinase 1 [TIMP-1]), using immunoassays, utilizing serum, prognostic algorithm reported as a risk score and risk of liver fibrosis and liver-related clinical events within 5 years (Do not report 81517 in conjunction with 83520 for identification of biomarkers included for liver disease analysis)
Breast Cancer Index, Biotheranostics, Inc	81518	Oncology (breast), mRNA, gene expression profiling by real-time RT-PCR of 11 genes (7 content and 4 housekeeping), utilizing formalin-fixed paraffin-embedded tissue, algorithms reported as percentage risk for metastatic recurrence and likelihood of benefit from extended endocrine therapy

(Continued on page 1038)

▲ = Revised code   ● = New code   ▶◀ = Contains new or revised text   ✕ = Duplicate PLA test   ⇅ = Category I PLA   American Medical Association   **1037**

EndoPredict®, Myriad Genetic Laboratories, Inc	#81522	Oncology (breast), mRNA, gene expression profiling by RT-PCR of 12 genes (8 content and 4 housekeeping), utilizing formalin-fixed paraffin-embedded tissue, algorithm reported as recurrence risk score
Oncotype DX®, Genomic Health	81519	Oncology (breast), mRNA, gene expression profiling by real-time RT-PCR of 21 genes, utilizing formalin-fixed paraffin-embedded tissue, algorithm reported as recurrence score
Prosigna® Breast Cancer Assay, NanoString Technologies, Inc	81520	Oncology (breast), mRNA gene expression profiling by hybrid capture of 58 genes (50 content and 8 housekeeping), utilizing formalin-fixed paraffin-embedded tissue, algorithm reported as a recurrence risk score
MammaPrint®, Agendia, Inc	81521	Oncology (breast), mRNA, microarray gene expression profiling of 70 content genes and 465 housekeeping genes, utilizing fresh frozen or formalin-fixed paraffin-embedded tissue, algorithm reported as index related to risk of distant metastasis (Do not report 81521 in conjunction with 81523 for the same specimen)
MammaPrint®, Agendia, Inc	81523	Oncology (breast), mRNA, next-generation sequencing gene expression profiling of 70 content genes and 31 housekeeping genes, utilizing formalin-fixed paraffin-embedded tissue, algorithm reported as index related to risk to distant metastasis (Do not report 81523 in conjunction with 81521 for the same specimen)
Oncotype DX® Colon Cancer Assay, Genomic Health	81525	Oncology (colon), mRNA, gene expression profiling by real-time RT-PCR of 12 genes (7 content and 5 housekeeping), utilizing formalin-fixed paraffin-embedded tissue, algorithm reported as a recurrence score
Cologuard™, Exact Sciences, Inc	81528	Oncology (colorectal) screening, quantitative real-time target and signal amplification of 10 DNA markers (*KRAS* mutations, promoter methylation of *NDRG4* and *BMP3*) and fecal hemoglobin, utilizing stool, algorithm reported as a positive or negative result (Do not report 81528 in conjunction with 81275, 82274)
DecisionDx® Melanoma, Castle Biosciences, Inc	81529	Oncology (cutaneous melanoma), mRNA, gene expression profiling by real-time RT-PCR of 31 genes (28 content and 3 housekeeping), utilizing formalin-fixed paraffin-embedded tissue, algorithm reported as recurrence risk, including likelihood of sentinel lymph node metastasis

ChemoFX®, Helomics, Corp	81535	Oncology (gynecologic), live tumor cell culture and chemotherapeutic response by DAPI stain and morphology, predictive algorithm reported as a drug response score; first single drug or drug combination
	+81536	each additional single drug or drug combination (List separately in addition to code for primary procedure) (Use 81536 in conjunction with 81535)
VeriStrat, Biodesix, Inc	81538	Oncology (lung), mass spectrometric 8-protein signature, including amyloid A, utilizing serum, prognostic and predictive algorithm reported as good versus poor overall survival
Risk of Ovarian Malignancy Algorithm (ROMA)™, Fujirebio Diagnostics	#81500	Oncology (ovarian), biochemical assays of two proteins (CA-125 and HE4), utilizing serum, with menopausal status, algorithm reported as a risk score (Do not report 81500 in conjunction with 86304, 86305)
OVA1™, Vermillion, Inc	#81503	Oncology (ovarian), biochemical assays of five proteins (CA-125, apolipoprotein A1, beta-2 microglobulin, transferrin, and pre-albumin), utilizing serum, algorithm reported as a risk score (Do not report 81503 in conjunction with 82172, 82232, 84134, 84466, 86304)
4Kscore test, OPKO Health, Inc	81539	Oncology (high-grade prostate cancer), biochemical assay of four proteins (Total PSA, Free PSA, Intact PSA, and human kallikrein-2 [hK2]), utilizing plasma or serum, prognostic algorithm reported as a probability score
Prolaris®, Myriad Genetic Laboratories, Inc	81541	Oncology (prostate), mRNA gene expression profiling by real-time RT-PCR of 46 genes (31 content and 15 housekeeping), utilizing formalin-fixed paraffin-embedded tissue, algorithm reported as a disease-specific mortality risk score
Decipher® Prostate, Decipher® Biosciences	81542	Oncology (prostate), mRNA, microarray gene expression profiling of 22 content genes, utilizing formalin-fixed paraffin-embedded tissue, algorithm reported as metastasis risk score
ConfirmMDx® for Prostate Cancer, MDxHealth, Inc	81551	Oncology (prostate), promoter methylation profiling by real-time PCR of 3 genes (*GSTP1, APC, RASSF1*), utilizing formalin-fixed paraffin-embedded tissue, algorithm reported as a likelihood of prostate cancer detection on repeat biopsy
Afirma® Genomic Sequencing Classifier, Veracyte, Inc	#81546	Oncology (thyroid), mRNA, gene expression analysis of 10,196 genes, utilizing fine needle aspirate, algorithm reported as a categorical result (eg, benign or suspicious)

(*Continued on page 1040*)

Appendix O

Tissue of Origin Test Kit-FFPE, Cancer Genetics, Inc	#81504	Oncology (tissue of origin), microarray gene expression profiling of > 2000 genes, utilizing formalin-fixed paraffin-embedded tissue, algorithm reported as tissue similarity scores
CancerTYPE ID, bioTheranostics, Inc	#81540	Oncology (tumor of unknown origin), mRNA, gene expression profiling by real-time RT-PCR of 92 genes (87 content and 5 housekeeping) to classify tumor into main cancer type and subtype, utilizing formalin-fixed paraffin-embedded tissue, algorithm reported as a probability of a predicted main cancer type and subtype
DecisionDx®-UM test, Castle Biosciences, Inc	81552	Oncology (uveal melanoma), mRNA, gene expression profiling by real-time RT-PCR of 15 genes (12 content and 3 housekeeping), utilizing fine needle aspirate or formalin-fixed paraffin-embedded tissue, algorithm reported as risk of metastasis
Envisia® Genomic Classifier, Veracyte, Inc	81554	Pulmonary disease (idiopathic pulmonary fibrosis [IPF]), mRNA, gene expression analysis of 190 genes, utilizing transbronchial biopsies, diagnostic algorithm reported as categorical result (eg, positive or negative for high probability of usual interstitial pneumonia [UIP])
▶TruGraf® Kidney, Eurofins Transplant Genomics, Inc◀	●81558	▶Transplantation medicine (allograft rejection, kidney), mRNA, gene expression profiling by quantitative polymerase chain reaction (qPCR) of 139 genes, utilizing whole blood, algorithm reported as a binary categorization as transplant excellence, which indicates immune quiescence, or not transplant excellence, indicating subclinical rejection◀
Pleximmune™, Plexision, Inc	81560	Transplantation medicine (allograft rejection, pediatric liver and small bowel), measurement of donor and third-party-induced CD154+T-cytotoxic memory cells, utilizing whole peripheral blood, algorithm reported as a rejection risk score (Do not report 81560 in conjunction with 85032, 86353, 86821, 88184, 88185, 88187, 88230, 88240, 88241, 0018M)
—	81599	Unlisted multianalyte assay with algorithmic analysis (Do not use 81599 for multianalyte assays with algorithmic analyses listed in Appendix O)
Proprietary Laboratory Analyses (PLA)		
PreciseType® HEA Test, Immucor, Inc	0001U	Red blood cell antigen typing, DNA, human erythrocyte antigen gene analysis of 35 antigens from 11 blood groups, utilizing whole blood, common RBC alleles reported

PolypDX™, Atlantic Diagnostic Laboratories, LLC, Metabolomic Technologies, Inc	0002U	Oncology (colorectal), quantitative assessment of three urine metabolites (ascorbic acid, succinic acid and carnitine) by liquid chromatography with tandem mass spectrometry (LC-MS/MS) using multiple reaction monitoring acquisition, algorithm reported as likelihood of adenomatous polyps
Overa (OVA1 Next Generation), Asprira Labs, Inc, Vermillion, Inc	0003U	Oncology (ovarian) biochemical assays of five proteins (apolipoprotein A-1, CA 125 II, follicle stimulating hormone, human epididymis protein 4, transferrin), utilizing serum, algorithm reported as a likelihood score
ExosomeDx® Prostate (IntelliScore), Exosome Diagnostics, Inc, Exosome Diagnostics, Inc	0005U	Oncology (prostate) gene expression profile by real-time RT-PCR of 3 genes (*ERG, PCA3,* and *SPDEF*), urine, algorithm reported as risk score
ToxProtect, Genotox Laboratories LTD	0007U	Drug test(s), presumptive, with definitive confirmation of positive results, any number of drug classes, urine, includes specimen verification including DNA authentication in comparison to buccal DNA, per date of service
AmHPR® H. pylori Antibiotic Resistance Panel, American Molecular Laboratories, Inc	0008U	Helicobacter pylori detection and antibiotic resistance, DNA, 16S and 23S rRNA, gyrA, pbp1, rdxA and rpoB, next generation sequencing, formalin-fixed paraffin-embedded or fresh tissue or fecal sample, predictive, reported as positive or negative for resistance to clarithromycin, fluoroquinolones, metronidazole, amoxicillin, tetracycline, and rifabutin
DEPArray™ HER2, PacificDx	0009U	Oncology (breast cancer), *ERBB2* (HER2) copy number by FISH, tumor cells from formalin-fixed paraffin-embedded tissue isolated using image-based dielectrophoresis (DEP) sorting, reported as *ERBB2* gene amplified or non-amplified
Bacterial Typing by Whole Genome Sequencing, Mayo Clinic	0010U	Infectious disease (bacterial), strain typing by whole genome sequencing, phylogenetic-based report of strain relatedness, per submitted isolate
Cordant CORE™, Cordant Health Solutions	0011U	Prescription drug monitoring, evaluation of drugs present by LC-MS/MS, using oral fluid, reported as a comparison to an estimated steady-state range, per date of service including all drug compounds and metabolites
—	(0012U has been deleted)	—
—	(0013U has been deleted)	—
—	(0014U has been deleted)	—
BCR-ABL1 major and minor breakpoint fusion transcripts, University of Iowa, Department of Pathology, Asuragen	0016U	Oncology (hematolymphoid neoplasia), RNA, *BCR/ABL1* major and minor breakpoint fusion transcripts, quantitative PCR amplification, blood or bone marrow, report of fusion not detected or detected with quantitation

(Continued on page 1042)

▲=Revised code   ●=New code   ►◄=Contains new or revised text   ✕=Duplicate PLA test   ⇅=Category I PLA   American Medical Association   **1041**

JAK2 Mutation, University of Iowa, Department of Pathology	0017U	Oncology (hematolymphoid neoplasia), JAK2 mutation, DNA, PCR amplification of exons 12-14 and sequence analysis, blood or bone marrow, report of JAK2 mutation not detected or detected
ThyraMIR™, Interpace Diagnostics	0018U	Oncology (thyroid), microRNA profiling by RT-PCR of 10 microRNA sequences, utilizing fine needle aspirate, algorithm reported as a positive or negative result for moderate to high risk of malignancy
OncoTarget/OncoTreat, Columbia University Department of Pathology and Cell Biology, Darwin Health	0019U	Oncology, RNA, gene expression by whole transcriptome sequencing, formalin-fixed paraffin-embedded tissue or fresh frozen tissue, predictive algorithm reported as potential targets for therapeutic agents
Apifiny®, Armune BioScience, Inc	0021U	Oncology (prostate), detection of 8 autoantibodies (ARF 6, NKX3-1, 5'-UTR-BMI1, CEP 164, 3'-UTR-Ropporin, Desmocollin, AURKAIP-1, CSNK2A2), multiplexed immunoassay and flow cytometry serum, algorithm reported as risk score
Oncomine™ Dx Target Test, Thermo Fisher Scientific, Thermo Fisher Scientific	0022U	Targeted genomic sequence analysis panel, non-small cell lung neoplasia, DNA and RNA analysis, 23 genes, interrogation for sequence variants and rearrangements, reported as presence or absence of variants and associated therapy(ies) to consider
LeukoStrat® CDx FLT3 Mutation Assay, LabPMM LLC, an Invivoscribe Technologies, Inc Company, Invivoscribe Technologies, Inc	0023U	Oncology (acute myelogenous leukemia), DNA, genotyping of internal tandem duplication, p.D835, p.I836, using mononuclear cells, reported as detection or non-detection of FLT3 mutation and indication for or against the use of midostaurin
GlycA, Laboratory Corporation of America, Laboratory Corporation of America	0024U	Glycosylated acute phase proteins (GlycA), nuclear magnetic resonance spectroscopy, quantitative
UrSure Tenofovir Quantification Test, Synergy Medical Laboratories, UrSure Inc	0025U	Tenofovir, by liquid chromatography with tandem mass spectrometry (LC-MS/MS), urine, quantitative
Thyroseq Genomic Classifier, CBLPath, Inc, University of Pittsburgh Medical Center	0026U	Oncology (thyroid), DNA and mRNA of 112 genes, next-generation sequencing, fine needle aspirate of thyroid nodule, algorithmic analysis reported as a categorical result ("Positive, high probability of malignancy" or "Negative, low probability of malignancy")
JAK2 Exons 12 to 15 Sequencing, Mayo Clinic, Mayo Clinic	0027U	JAK2 (Janus kinase 2) (eg, myeloproliferative disorder) gene analysis, targeted sequence analysis exons 12-15
Focused Pharmacogenomics Panel, Mayo Clinic, Mayo Clinic	0029U	Drug metabolism (adverse drug reactions and drug response), targeted sequence analysis (ie, CYP1A2, CYP2C19, CYP2C9, CYP2D6, CYP3A4, CYP3A5, CYP4F2, SLCO1B1, VKORC1 and rs12777823)

Warfarin Response Genotype, Mayo Clinic, Mayo Clinic	0030U	Drug metabolism (warfarin drug response), targeted sequence analysis (ie, *CYP2C9, CYP4F2, VKORC1,* rs12777823)
Cytochrome P450 1A2 Genotype, Mayo Clinic, Mayo Clinic	0031U	*CYP1A2 (cytochrome P450 family 1, subfamily A, member 2)* (eg, drug metabolism) gene analysis, common variants (ie, *1F, *1K, *6, *7)
Catechol-O-Methyltransferase (*COMT*) Genotype, Mayo Clinic, Mayo Clinic	0032U	*COMT (catechol-O-methyltransferase)* (eg, drug metabolism) gene analysis, c.472G>A (rs4680) variant
Serotonin Receptor Genotype (*HTR2A* and *HTR2C*), Mayo Clinic, Mayo Clinic	0033U	*HTR2A (5-hydroxytryptamine receptor 2A), HTR2C (5-hydroxytryptamine receptor 2C)* (eg, citalopram metabolism) gene analysis, common variants (ie, *HTR2A* rs7997012 [c.614-2211T>C], *HTR2C* rs3813929 [c.-759C>T] and rs1414334 [c.551-3008C>G])
Thiopurine Methyltransferase (*TPMT*) and Nudix Hydrolase (*NUDT15*) Genotyping, Mayo Clinic, Mayo Clinic	0034U	*TPMT (thiopurine S-methyltransferase), NUDT15 (nudix hydroxylase 15)* (eg, thiopurine metabolism) gene analysis, common variants (ie, *TPMT* *2, *3A, *3B, *3C, *4, *5, *6, *8, *12; *NUDT15* *3, *4, *5)
Real-time quaking-induced conversion for prion detection (RT-QuIC), National Prion Disease Pathology Surveillance Center	0035U	Neurology (prion disease), cerebrospinal fluid, detection of prion protein by quaking-induced conformational conversion, qualitative
EXaCT-1 Whole Exome Testing, Lab of Oncology-Molecular Detection, Weill Cornell Medicine-Clinical Genomics Laboratory	0036U	Exome (ie, somatic mutations), paired formalin-fixed paraffin-embedded tumor tissue and normal specimen, sequence analyses
FoundationOne CDx™ (F1CDx), Foundation Medicine, Inc, Foundation Medicine, Inc	0037U	Targeted genomic sequence analysis, solid organ neoplasm, DNA analysis of 324 genes, interrogation for sequence variants, gene copy number amplifications, gene rearrangements, microsatellite instability and tumor mutational burden
Sensieva™ Droplet 25OH Vitamin D2/D3 Microvolume LC/MS Assay, InSource Diagnostics, InSource Diagnostics	0038U	Vitamin D, 25 hydroxy D2 and D3, by LC-MS/MS, serum microsample, quantitative
Anti-dsDNA, High Salt/Avidity, University of Washington, Department of Laboratory Medicine, Bio-Rad	0039U	Deoxyribonucleic acid (DNA) antibody, double stranded, high avidity
MRDx BCR-ABL Test, MolecularMD, MolecularMD	0040U	*BCR/ABL1 (t(9;22))* (eg, chronic myelogenous leukemia) translocation analysis, major breakpoint, quantitative
Lyme ImmunoBlot IgM, IGeneX Inc, ID-FISH Technology Inc (ASR) (Lyme ImmunoBlot IgM Strips Only)	0041U	Borrelia burgdorferi, antibody detection of 5 recombinant protein groups, by immunoblot, IgM

(*Continued on page 1044*)

Lyme ImmunoBlot IgG, IGeneX Inc, ID-FISH Technology Inc (ASR) (Lyme ImmunoBlot IgG Strips Only)	0042U	Borrelia burgdorferi, antibody detection of 12 recombinant protein groups, by immunoblot, IgG
Tick-Borne Relapsing Fever (TBRF) Borrelia ImmunoBlots IgM Test, IGeneX Inc, ID-FISH Technology (Provides TBRF ImmunoBlot IgM Strips)	0043U	Tick-borne relapsing fever Borrelia group, antibody detection to 4 recombinant protein groups, by immunoblot, IgM
Tick-Borne Relapsing Fever (TBRF) Borrelia ImmunoBlots IgG Test, IGeneX Inc, ID-FISH Technology Inc (Provides TBRF ImmunoBlot IgG Strips)	0044U	Tick-borne relapsing fever Borrelia group, antibody detection to 4 recombinant protein groups, by immunoblot, IgG
The Oncotype DX® Breast DCIS Score™ Test, Genomic Health, Inc, Genomic Health, Inc	0045U	Oncology (breast ductal carcinoma in situ), mRNA, gene expression profiling by real-time RT-PCR of 12 genes (7 content and 5 housekeeping), utilizing formalin-fixed paraffin-embedded tissue, algorithm reported as recurrence score
FLT3 ITD MRD by NGS, LabPMM LLC, an Invivoscribe Technologies, Inc Company	0046U	*FLT3 (fms-related tyrosine kinase 3)* (eg, acute myeloid leukemia) internal tandem duplication (ITD) variants, quantitative
▶Genomic Prostate Score® (GPS) Test, MDxHealth, Inc, MDxHealth, Inc◀	0047U	Oncology (prostate), mRNA, gene expression profiling by real-time RT-PCR of 17 genes (12 content and 5 housekeeping), utilizing formalin-fixed paraffin-embedded tissue, algorithm reported as a risk score
MSK-IMPACT (Integrated Mutation Profiling of Actionable Cancer Targets), Memorial Sloan Kettering Cancer Center	0048U	Oncology (solid organ neoplasia), DNA, targeted sequencing of protein-coding exons of 468 cancer-associated genes, including interrogation for somatic mutations and microsatellite instability, matched with normal specimens, utilizing formalin-fixed paraffin-embedded tumor tissue, report of clinically significant mutation(s)
NPM1 MRD by NGS, LabPMM LLC, an Invivoscribe Technologies, Inc Company	0049U	*NPM1 (nucleophosmin)* (eg, acute myeloid leukemia) gene analysis, quantitative
MyAML NGS Panel, LabPMM LLC, an Invivoscribe Technologies, Inc Company	0050U	Targeted genomic sequence analysis panel, acute myelogenous leukemia, DNA analysis, 194 genes, interrogation for sequence variants, copy number variants or rearrangements
UCompliDx, Elite Medical Laboratory Solutions, LLC, Elite Medical Laboratory Solutions, LLC (LDT)	0051U	Prescription drug monitoring, evaluation of drugs present by liquid chromatography tandem mass spectrometry (LC-MS/MS), urine or blood, 31 drug panel, reported as quantitative results, detected or not detected, per date of service

VAP Cholesterol Test, VAP Diagnostics Laboratory, Inc, VAP Diagnostics Laboratory, Inc	0052U	Lipoprotein, blood, high resolution fractionation and quantitation of lipoproteins, including all five major lipoprotein classes and subclasses of HDL, LDL, and VLDL by vertical auto profile ultracentrifugation
—	(0053U has been deleted)	—
AssuranceRx Micro Serum, Firstox Laboratories, LLC, Firstox Laboratories, LLC	0054U	Prescription drug monitoring, 14 or more classes of drugs and substances, definitive tandem mass spectrometry with chromatography, capillary blood, quantitative report with therapeutic and toxic ranges, including steady-state range for the prescribed dose when detected, per date of service
myTAIHEART, TAI Diagnostics, Inc, TAI Diagnostics, Inc	0055U	Cardiology (heart transplant), cell-free DNA, PCR assay of 96 DNA target sequences (94 single nucleotide polymorphism targets and two control targets), plasma
—	(0056U has been deleted)	—
Merkel SmT Oncoprotein Antibody Titer, University of Washington, Department of Laboratory Medicine	0058U	Oncology (Merkel cell carcinoma), detection of antibodies to the Merkel cell polyoma virus oncoprotein (small T antigen), serum, quantitative
Merkel Virus VP1 Capsid Antibody, University of Washington, Department of Laboratory Medicine	0059U	Oncology (Merkel cell carcinoma), detection of antibodies to the Merkel cell polyoma virus capsid protein (VP1), serum, reported as positive or negative
Twins Zygosity PLA, Natera, Inc, Natera, Inc	0060U	Twin zygosity, genomic-targeted sequence analysis of chromosome 2, using circulating cell-free fetal DNA in maternal blood
Transcutaneous multispectral measurement of tissue oxygenation and hemoglobin using spatial frequency domain imaging (SFDI), Modulated Imaging, Inc, Modulated Imaging, Inc	0061U	Transcutaneous measurement of five biomarkers (tissue oxygenation [StO$_2$], oxyhemoglobin [ctHbO$_2$], deoxyhemoglobin [ctHbR], papillary and reticular dermal hemoglobin concentrations [ctHb1 and ctHb2]), using spatial frequency domain imaging (SFDI) and multi-spectral analysis
SLE-key® Rule Out, Veracis Inc, Veracis Inc	0062U	Autoimmune (systemic lupus erythematosus), IgG and IgM analysis of 80 biomarkers, utilizing serum, algorithm reported with a risk score
NPDX ASD ADM Panel I, Stemina Biomarker Discovery, Inc, Stemina Biomarker Discovery, Inc d/b/a NeuroPointDX	0063U	Neurology (autism), 32 amines by LC-MS/MS, using plasma, algorithm reported as metabolic signature associated with autism spectrum disorder
BioPlex 2200 Syphilis Total & RPR Assay, Bio-Rad Laboratories, Bio-Rad Laboratories	0064U	Antibody, Treponema pallidum, total and rapid plasma reagin (RPR), immunoassay, qualitative
BioPlex 2200 RPR Assay, Bio-Rad Laboratories, Bio-Rad Laboratories	0065U	Syphilis test, non-treponemal antibody, immunoassay, qualitative (RPR)
—	(0066U has been deleted)	—

(Continued on page 1046)

▲=Revised code   ●=New code   ▶ ◀=Contains new or revised text   ✖=Duplicate PLA test   ↕=Category I PLA   American Medical Association   **1045**

BBDRisk Dx™, Silbiotech, Inc, Silbiotech, Inc	0067U	Oncology (breast), immunohistochemistry, protein expression profiling of 4 biomarkers (matrix metalloproteinase-1 [MMP-1], carcinoembryonic antigen-related cell adhesion molecule 6 [CEACAM6], hyaluronoglucosaminidase [HYAL1], highly expressed in cancer protein [HEC1]), formalin-fixed paraffin-embedded precancerous breast tissue, algorithm reported as carcinoma risk score
MYCODART-PCR™ Dual Amplification Real Time PCR Panel for 6 Candida species, RealTime Laboratories, Inc/MycoDART, Inc, RealTime Laboratories, Inc	0068U	Candida species panel (*C. albicans, C. glabrata, C. parapsilosis, C. kruseii, C. tropicalis,* and *C. auris*), amplified probe technique with qualitative report of the presence or absence of each species
miR-31*now*™, GoPath Laboratories, GoPath Laboratories	0069U	Oncology (colorectal), microRNA, RT-PCR expression profiling of miR-31-3p, formalin-fixed paraffin-embedded tissue, algorithm reported as an expression score
CYP2D6 Common Variants and Copy Number, Mayo Clinic, Laboratory Developed Test	0070U	*CYP2D6 (cytochrome P450, family 2, subfamily D, polypeptide 6)* (eg, drug metabolism) gene analysis, common and select rare variants (ie, *2, *3, *4, *4N, *5, *6, *7, *8, *9, *10, *11, *12, *13, *14A, *14B, *15, *17, *29, *35, *36, *41, *57, *61, *63, *68, *83, *xN)
CYP2D6 Full Gene Sequencing, Mayo Clinic, Laboratory Developed Test	+0071U	*CYP2D6 (cytochrome P450, family 2, subfamily D, polypeptide 6)* (eg, drug metabolism) gene analysis, full gene sequence (List separately in addition to code for primary procedure) (Use 0071U in conjunction with 0070U)
CYP2D6-2D7 Hybrid Gene Targeted Sequence Analysis, Mayo Clinic, Laboratory Developed Test	+0072U	*CYP2D6 (cytochrome P450, family 2, subfamily D, polypeptide 6)* (eg, drug metabolism) gene analysis, targeted sequence analysis (ie, *CYP2D6-2D7* hybrid gene) (List separately in addition to code for primary procedure) (Use 0072U in conjunction with 0070U)
CYP2D7-2D6 Hybrid Gene Targeted Sequence Analysis, Mayo Clinic, Laboratory Developed Test	+0073U	*CYP2D6 (cytochrome P450, family 2, subfamily D, polypeptide 6)* (eg, drug metabolism) gene analysis, targeted sequence analysis (ie, *CYP2D7-2D6* hybrid gene) (List separately in addition to code for primary procedure) (Use 0073U in conjunction with 0070U)
CYP2D6 trans-duplication/ multiplication non-duplicated gene targeted sequence analysis, Mayo Clinic, Laboratory Developed Test	+0074U	*CYP2D6 (cytochrome P450, family 2, subfamily D, polypeptide 6)* (eg, drug metabolism) gene analysis, targeted sequence analysis (ie, non-duplicated gene when duplication/multiplication is trans) (List separately in addition to code for primary procedure) (Use 0074U in conjunction with 0070U)

CYP2D6 5' gene duplication/ multiplication targeted sequence analysis, Mayo Clinic, Laboratory Developed Test	+0075U	CYP2D6 (cytochrome P450, family 2, subfamily D, polypeptide 6) (eg, drug metabolism) gene analysis, targeted sequence analysis (ie, 5' gene duplication/ multiplication) (List separately in addition to code for primary procedure) (Use 0075U in conjunction with 0070U)
CYP2D6 3' gene duplication/ multiplication targeted sequence analysis, Mayo Clinic, Laboratory Developed Test	+0076U	CYP2D6 (cytochrome P450, family 2, subfamily D, polypeptide 6) (eg, drug metabolism) gene analysis, targeted sequence analysis (ie, 3' gene duplication/ multiplication) (List separately in addition to code for primary procedure) (Use 0076U in conjunction with 0070U)
M-Protein Detection and Isotyping by MALDI-TOF Mass Spectrometry, Mayo Clinic, Laboratory Developed Test	0077U	Immunoglobulin paraprotein (M-protein), qualitative, immunoprecipitation and mass spectrometry, blood or urine, including isotype
—	▶(0078U has been deleted)◀	—
ToxLok™, InSource Diagnostics, InSource Diagnostics	0079U	Comparative DNA analysis using multiple selected single-nucleotide polymorphisms (SNPs), urine and buccal DNA, for specimen identity verification
BDX-XL2, Biodesix®, Inc, Biodesix®, Inc	0080U	Oncology (lung), mass spectrometric analysis of galectin-3-binding protein and scavenger receptor cysteine-rich type 1 protein M130, with five clinical risk factors (age, smoking status, nodule diameter, nodule-spiculation status and nodule location), utilizing plasma, algorithm reported as a categorical probability of malignancy
NextGen Precision™ Testing, Precision Diagnostics, Precision Diagnostics LBN Precision Toxicology, LLC	0082U	Drug test(s), definitive, 90 or more drugs or substances, definitive chromatography with mass spectrometry, and presumptive, any number of drug classes, by instrument chemistry analyzer (utilizing immunoassay), urine, report of presence or absence of each drug, drug metabolite or substance with description and severity of significant interactions per date of service
Onco4D™, Animated Dynamics, Inc, Animated Dynamics, Inc	0083U	Oncology, response to chemotherapy drugs using motility contrast tomography, fresh or frozen tissue, reported as likelihood of sensitivity or resistance to drugs or drug combinations
BLOODchip® ID CORE XT™, Grifols Diagnostic Solutions Inc	0084U	Red blood cell antigen typing, DNA, genotyping of 10 blood groups with phenotype prediction of 37 red blood cell antigens

(Continued on page 1048)

Accelerate PhenoTest™ BC kit, Accelerate Diagnostics, Inc	0086U	Infectious disease (bacterial and fungal), organism identification, blood culture, using rRNA FISH, 6 or more organism targets, reported as positive or negative with phenotypic minimum inhibitory concentration (MIC)-based antimicrobial susceptibility
Molecular Microscope® MMDx—Heart, Kashi Clinical Laboratories	0087U	Cardiology (heart transplant), mRNA gene expression profiling by microarray of 1283 genes, transplant biopsy tissue, allograft rejection and injury algorithm reported as a probability score
Molecular Microscope® MMDx—Kidney, Kashi Clinical Laboratories	0088U	Transplantation medicine (kidney allograft rejection), microarray gene expression profiling of 1494 genes, utilizing transplant biopsy tissue, algorithm reported as a probability score for rejection
Pigmented Lesion Assay (PLA), DermTech	0089U	Oncology (melanoma), gene expression profiling by RTqPCR, *PRAME* and *LINC00518*, superficial collection using adhesive patch(es)
myPath® Melanoma, Castle Biosciences, Inc	0090U	Oncology (cutaneous melanoma), mRNA gene expression profiling by RT-PCR of 23 genes (14 content and 9 housekeeping), utilizing formalin-fixed paraffin-embedded (FFPE) tissue, algorithm reported as a categorical result (ie, benign, intermediate, malignant)
FirstSight^CRC, CellMax Life	0091U	Oncology (colorectal) screening, cell enumeration of circulating tumor cells, utilizing whole blood, algorithm, for the presence of adenoma or cancer, reported as a positive or negative result
REVEAL Lung Nodule Characterization, MagArray, Inc	0092U	Oncology (lung), three protein biomarkers, immunoassay using magnetic nanosensor technology, plasma, algorithm reported as risk score for likelihood of malignancy
ComplyRX, Claro Labs	0093U	Prescription drug monitoring, evaluation of 65 common drugs by LC-MS/MS, urine, each drug reported detected or not detected
RCIGM Rapid Whole Genome Sequencing, Rady Children's Institute for Genomic Medicine (RCIGM)	0094U	Genome (eg, unexplained constitutional or heritable disorder or syndrome), rapid sequence analysis
Esophageal String Test™ (EST), Children's Hospital Colorado Department of Pathology and Laboratory Medicine	0095U	Eosinophilic esophagitis (Eotaxin-3 *[CCL26 {C-C motif chemokine ligand 26}]* and major basic protein *[PRG2 {proteoglycan 2, pro eosinophil major basic protein}]*), enzyme-linked immunosorbent assays (ELISA), specimen obtained by esophageal string test device, algorithm reported as probability of active or inactive eosinophilic esophagitis
HPV, High-Risk, Male Urine, Molecular Testing Labs	0096U	Human papillomavirus (HPV), high-risk types (ie, 16, 18, 31, 33, 35, 39, 45, 51, 52, 56, 58, 59, 66, 68), male urine

★=Telemedicine ◀=Audio-only ✚=Add-on code ✔=FDA approval pending #=Resequenced code ⊘=Modifier 51 exempt ➲➲➲=See p xxi for details

—	(0097U has been deleted)	—
ColoNext®, Ambry Genetics®, Ambry Genetics®	0101U	Hereditary colon cancer disorders (eg, Lynch syndrome, *PTEN* hamartoma syndrome, Cowden syndrome, familial adenomatosis polyposis), genomic sequence analysis panel utilizing a combination of NGS, Sanger, MLPA, and array CGH, with mRNA analytics to resolve variants of unknown significance when indicated (15 genes [sequencing and deletion/duplication], *EPCAM* and *GREM1* [deletion/duplication only])
BreastNext®, Ambry Genetics®, Ambry Genetics®	0102U	Hereditary breast cancer-related disorders (eg, hereditary breast cancer, hereditary ovarian cancer, hereditary endometrial cancer), genomic sequence analysis panel utilizing a combination of NGS, Sanger, MLPA, and array CGH, with mRNA analytics to resolve variants of unknown significance when indicated (17 genes [sequencing and deletion/duplication])
OvaNext®, Ambry Genetics®, Ambry Genetics®	0103U	Hereditary ovarian cancer (eg, hereditary ovarian cancer, hereditary endometrial cancer), genomic sequence analysis panel utilizing a combination of NGS, Sanger, MLPA, and array CGH, with mRNA analytics to resolve variants of unknown significance when indicated (24 genes [sequencing and deletion/duplication], *EPCAM* [deletion/duplication only])
KidneyIntelX™, RenalytixAI, RenalytixAI	0105U	Nephrology (chronic kidney disease), multiplex electrochemiluminescent immunoassay (ECLIA) of tumor necrosis factor receptor 1A, receptor superfamily 2 *(TNFR1, TNFR2),* and kidney injury molecule-1 (KIM-1) combined with longitudinal clinical data, including *APOL1* genotype if available, and plasma (isolated fresh or frozen), algorithm reported as probability score for rapid kidney function decline (RKFD)
13C-Spirulina Gastric Emptying Breath Test (GEBT), Cairn Diagnostics d/b/a Advanced Breath Diagnostics, LLC, Cairn Diagnostics d/b/a Advanced Breath Diagnostics, LLC	0106U	Gastric emptying, serial collection of 7 timed breath specimens, non-radioisotope carbon-13 (^{13}C) spirulina substrate, analysis of each specimen by gas isotope ratio mass spectrometry, reported as rate of $^{13}CO_2$ excretion
Singulex Clarity C. diff toxins A/B Assay, Singulex	0107U	Clostridium difficile toxin(s) antigen detection by immunoassay technique, stool, qualitative, multiple-step method

(Continued on page 1050)

TissueCypher® Barrett's Esophagus Assay, Cernostics, Cernostics	0108U	Gastroenterology (Barrett's esophagus), whole slide–digital imaging, including morphometric analysis, computer-assisted quantitative immunolabeling of 9 protein biomarkers (p16, AMACR, p53, CD68, COX-2, CD45RO, HIF1a, HER-2, K20) and morphology, formalin-fixed paraffin-embedded tissue, algorithm reported as risk of progression to high-grade dysplasia or cancer
MYCODART Dual Amplification Real Time PCR Panel for 4 Aspergillus species, RealTime Laboratories, Inc/MycoDART, Inc	0109U	Infectious disease (Aspergillus species), real-time PCR for detection of DNA from 4 species (*A. fumigatus, A. terreus, A. niger,* and *A. flavus),* blood, lavage fluid, or tissue, qualitative reporting of presence or absence of each species
Oral OncolyticAssuranceRX, Firstox Laboratories, LLC, Firstox Laboratories, LLC	0110U	Prescription drug monitoring, one or more oral oncology drug(s) and substances, definitive tandem mass spectrometry with chromatography, serum or plasma from capillary blood or venous blood, quantitative report with steady-state range for the prescribed drug(s) when detected
Praxis™ Extended RAS Panel, Illumina, Illumina	0111U	Oncology (colon cancer), targeted *KRAS* (codons 12, 13, and 61) and *NRAS* (codons 12, 13, and 61) gene analysis, utilizing formalin-fixed paraffin-embedded tissue
MicroGenDX qPCR & NGS For Infection, MicroGenDX, MicroGenDX	0112U	Infectious agent detection and identification, targeted sequence analysis (16S and 18S rRNA genes) with drug-resistance gene
MyProstateScore, Lynx DX, Lynx DX	0113U	Oncology (prostate), measurement of *PCA3* and *TMPRSS2-ERG* in urine and PSA in serum following prostatic massage, by RNA amplification and fluorescence-based detection, algorithm reported as risk score
EsoGuard™, Lucid Diagnostics, Lucid Diagnostics	0114U	Gastroenterology (Barrett's esophagus), *VIM* and *CCNA1* methylation analysis, esophageal cells, algorithm reported as likelihood for Barrett's esophagus
ePlex Respiratory Pathogen (RP) Panel, GenMark Diagnostics, Inc, GenMark Diagnostics, Inc	0115U	Respiratory infectious agent detection by nucleic acid (DNA and RNA), 18 viral types and subtypes and 2 bacterial targets, amplified probe technique, including multiplex reverse transcription for RNA targets, each analyte reported as detected or not detected
Snapshot Oral Fluid Compliance, Ethos Laboratories	0116U	Prescription drug monitoring, enzyme immunoassay of 35 or more drugs confirmed with LC-MS/MS, oral fluid, algorithm results reported as a patient-compliance measurement with risk of drug to drug interactions for prescribed medications

Foundation PI^{SM}, Ethos Laboratories	0117U	Pain management, analysis of 11 endogenous analytes (methylmalonic acid, xanthurenic acid, homocysteine, pyroglutamic acid, vanilmandelate, 5-hydroxyindoleacetic acid, hydroxymethylglutarate, ethylmalonate, 3-hydroxypropyl mercapturic acid (3-HPMA), quinolinic acid, kynurenic acid), LC-MS/MS, urine, algorithm reported as a pain-index score with likelihood of atypical biochemical function associated with pain
▶Eurofins TRAC™ dd-cfDNA, Transplant Genomics Inc, Transplant Genomics Inc◀	0118U	Transplantation medicine, quantification of donor-derived cell-free DNA using whole genome next-generation sequencing, plasma, reported as percentage of donor-derived cell-free DNA in the total cell-free DNA
MI-HEART Ceramides, Plasma, Mayo Clinic, Laboratory Developed Test	0119U	Cardiology, ceramides by liquid chromatography–tandem mass spectrometry, plasma, quantitative report with risk score for major cardiovascular events
Lymph3Cx Lymphoma Molecular Subtyping Assay, Mayo Clinic, Laboratory Developed Test	0120U	Oncology (B-cell lymphoma classification), mRNA, gene expression profiling by fluorescent probe hybridization of 58 genes (45 content and 13 housekeeping genes), formalin-fixed paraffin-embedded tissue, algorithm reported as likelihood for primary mediastinal B-cell lymphoma (PMBCL) and diffuse large B-cell lymphoma (DLBCL) with cell of origin subtyping in the latter (Do not report 0120U in conjunction with 0017M)
Flow Adhesion of Whole Blood on VCAM-1 (FAB-V), Functional Fluidics, Functional Fluidics	0121U	Sickle cell disease, microfluidic flow adhesion (VCAM-1), whole blood
Flow Adhesion of Whole Blood to P-SELECTIN (WB-PSEL), Functional Fluidics, Functional Fluidics	0122U	Sickle cell disease, microfluidic flow adhesion (P-Selectin), whole blood
Mechanical Fragility, RBC by shear stress profiling and spectral analysis, Functional Fluidics, Functional Fluidics	0123U	Mechanical fragility, RBC, shear stress and spectral analysis profiling
BRCAplus, Ambry Genetics	0129U	Hereditary breast cancer–related disorders (eg, hereditary breast cancer, hereditary ovarian cancer, hereditary endometrial cancer), genomic sequence analysis and deletion/duplication analysis panel *(ATM, BRCA1, BRCA2, CDH1, CHEK2, PALB2, PTEN*, and *TP53)*

(Continued on page 1052)

+RNAinsight™ for ColoNext®, Ambry Genetics	+0130U	Hereditary colon cancer disorders (eg, Lynch syndrome, PTEN hamartoma syndrome, Cowden syndrome, familial adenomatosis polyposis), targeted mRNA sequence analysis panel (*APC, CDH1, CHEK2, MLH1, MSH2, MSH6, MUTYH, PMS2, PTEN,* and *TP53*) (List separately in addition to code for primary procedure) (Use 0130U in conjunction with 81435, 0101U)
+RNAinsight™ for BreastNext®, Ambry Genetics	+0131U	Hereditary breast cancer–related disorders (eg, hereditary breast cancer, hereditary ovarian cancer, hereditary endometrial cancer), targeted mRNA sequence analysis panel (13 genes) (List separately in addition to code for primary procedure) (Use 0131U in conjunction with 81162, 81432, 0102U)
+RNAinsight™ for OvaNext®, Ambry Genetics	+0132U	Hereditary ovarian cancer–related disorders (eg, hereditary breast cancer, hereditary ovarian cancer, hereditary endometrial cancer), targeted mRNA sequence analysis panel (17 genes) (List separately in addition to code for primary procedure) (Use 0132U in conjunction with 81162, 81432, 0103U)
+RNAinsight™ for ProstateNext®, Ambry Genetics	+0133U	Hereditary prostate cancer–related disorders, targeted mRNA sequence analysis panel (11 genes) (List separately in addition to code for primary procedure) (Use 0133U in conjunction with 81162)
+RNAinsight™ for CancerNext®, Ambry Genetics	+0134U	Hereditary pan cancer (eg, hereditary breast and ovarian cancer, hereditary endometrial cancer, hereditary colorectal cancer), targeted mRNA sequence analysis panel (18 genes) (List separately in addition to code for primary procedure) (Use 0134U in conjunction with 81162, 81432, 81435)
+RNAinsight™ for GYNPlus®, Ambry Genetics	+0135U	Hereditary gynecological cancer (eg, hereditary breast and ovarian cancer, hereditary endometrial cancer, hereditary colorectal cancer), targeted mRNA sequence analysis panel (12 genes) (List separately in addition to code for primary procedure) (Use 0135U in conjunction with 81162)
+RNAinsight™ for *ATM*, Ambry Genetics	+0136U	*ATM (ataxia telangiectasia mutated)* (eg, ataxia telangiectasia) mRNA sequence analysis (List separately in addition to code for primary procedure) (Use 0136U in conjunction with 81408)

+RNAinsight™ for *PALB2*, Ambry Genetics	**+**0137U	*PALB2 (partner and localizer of BRCA2)* (eg, breast and pancreatic cancer) mRNA sequence analysis (List separately in addition to code for primary procedure) (Use 0137U in conjunction with 81307)
+RNAinsight™ for *BRCA1/2*, Ambry Genetics	**+**0138U	*BRCA1 (BRCA1, DNA repair associated), BRCA2 (BRCA2, DNA repair associated)* (eg, hereditary breast and ovarian cancer) mRNA sequence analysis (List separately in addition to code for primary procedure) (Use 0138U in conjunction with 81162)
ePlex® BCID Fungal Pathogens Panel, GenMark Diagnostics, Inc, GenMark Diagnostics, Inc	0140U	Infectious disease (fungi), fungal pathogen identification, DNA (15 fungal targets), blood culture, amplified probe technique, each target reported as detected or not detected
ePlex® BCID Gram-Positive Panel, GenMark Diagnostics, Inc, GenMark Diagnostics, Inc	0141U	Infectious disease (bacteria and fungi), gram-positive organism identification and drug resistance element detection, DNA (20 gram-positive bacterial targets, 4 resistance genes, 1 pan gram-negative bacterial target, 1 pan Candida target), blood culture, amplified probe technique, each target reported as detected or not detected
ePlex® BCID Gram-Negative Panel, GenMark Diagnostics, Inc, GenMark Diagnostics, Inc	0142U	Infectious disease (bacteria and fungi), gram-negative bacterial identification and drug resistance element detection, DNA (21 gram-negative bacterial targets, 6 resistance genes, 1 pan gram-positive bacterial target, 1 pan Candida target), amplified probe technique, each target reported as detected or not detected
—	(0143U has been deleted)	—
—	(0144U has been deleted)	—
—	(0145U has been deleted)	—
—	(0146U has been deleted)	—
—	(0147U has been deleted)	—
—	(0148U has been deleted)	—
—	(0149U has been deleted)	—
—	(0150U has been deleted)	—
—	(0151U has been deleted)	—
Karius® Test, Karius Inc, Karius Inc	0152U	Infectious disease (bacteria, fungi, parasites, and DNA viruses), microbial cell-free DNA, plasma, untargeted next-generation sequencing, report for significant positive pathogens
Insight TNBCtype™, Insight Molecular Labs	0153U	Oncology (breast), mRNA, gene expression profiling by next-generation sequencing of 101 genes, utilizing formalin-fixed paraffin-embedded tissue, algorithm reported as a triple negative breast cancer clinical subtype(s) with information on immune cell involvement

(*Continued on page 1054*)

therascreen® *FGFR* RGQ RT-PCR Kit, QIAGEN, QIAGEN GmbH	0154U	Oncology (urothelial cancer), RNA, analysis by real-time RT-PCR of the *FGFR3 (fibroblast growth factor receptor 3)* gene analysis (ie, p.R248C [c.742C>T], p. S249C [c.746C>G], p.G370C [c.1108G>T], p. Y373C [c.1118A>G], FGFR3-TACC3v1, and FGFR3-TACC3v3), utilizing formalin-fixed paraffin-embedded urothelial cancer tumor tissue, reported as *FGFR* gene alteration status
therascreen *PIK3CA* RGQ PCR Kit, QIAGEN, QIAGEN GmbH	0155U	Oncology (breast cancer), DNA, *PIK3CA (phosphatidylinositol-4,5-bisphosphate 3-kinase, catalytic subunit alpha)* (eg, breast cancer) gene analysis (ie, p.C420R, p.E542K, p.E545A, p.E545D [g.1635G>T only], p.E545G, p.E545K, p.Q546E, p. Q546R, p.H1047L, p.H1047R, p.H1047Y), utilizing formalin-fixed paraffin-embedded breast tumor tissue, reported as *PIK3CA* gene mutation status
SMASH™, New York Genome Center, Marvel Genomics™	0156U	Copy number (eg, intellectual disability, dysmorphology), sequence analysis
CustomNext + RNA: *APC*, Ambry Genetics®, Ambry Genetics®	+0157U	*APC (APC regulator of WNT signaling pathway)* (eg, familial adenomatosis polyposis [FAP]) mRNA sequence analysis (List separately in addition to code for primary procedure) (Use 0157U in conjunction with 81201)
CustomNext + RNA: *MLH1*, Ambry Genetics®, Ambry Genetics®	+0158U	*MLH1 (mutL homolog 1)* (eg, hereditary non-polyposis colorectal cancer, Lynch syndrome) mRNA sequence analysis (List separately in addition to code for primary procedure) (Use 0158U in conjunction with 81292)
CustomNext + RNA: *MSH2*, Ambry Genetics®, Ambry Genetics®	+0159U	*MSH2 (mutS homolog 2)* (eg, hereditary colon cancer, Lynch syndrome) mRNA sequence analysis (List separately in addition to code for primary procedure) (Use 0159U in conjunction with 81295)
CustomNext + RNA: *MSH6*, Ambry Genetics®, Ambry Genetics®	+0160U	*MSH6 (mutS homolog 6)* (eg, hereditary colon cancer, Lynch syndrome) mRNA sequence analysis (List separately in addition to code for primary procedure) (Use 0160U in conjunction with 81298)
CustomNext + RNA: *PMS2*, Ambry Genetics®, Ambry Genetics®	+0161U	*PMS2 (PMS1 homolog 2, mismatch repair system component)* (eg, hereditary non-polyposis colorectal cancer, Lynch syndrome) mRNA sequence analysis (List separately in addition to code for primary procedure) (Use 0161U in conjunction with 81317)

Appendix O

CustomNext + RNA: Lynch *(MLH1, MSH2, MSH6, PMS2)*, Ambry Genetics®, Ambry Genetics®	+0162U	Hereditary colon cancer (Lynch syndrome), targeted mRNA sequence analysis panel *(MLH1, MSH2, MSH6, PMS2)* (List separately in addition to code for primary procedure) (Use 0162U in conjunction with 81292, 81295, 81298, 81317, 81435)
BeScreened™-CRC, Beacon Biomedical Inc, Beacon Biomedical Inc	0163U	Oncology (colorectal) screening, biochemical enzyme-linked immunosorbent assay (ELISA) of 3 plasma or serum proteins (teratocarcinoma derived growth factor-1 [TDGF-1, Cripto-1], carcinoembryonic antigen [CEA], extracellular matrix protein [ECM]), with demographic data (age, gender, CRC-screening compliance) using a proprietary algorithm and reported as likelihood of CRC or advanced adenomas
ibs-smart™, Gemelli Biotech, Gemelli Biotech	0164U	Gastroenterology (irritable bowel syndrome [IBS]), immunoassay for anti-CdtB and anti-vinculin antibodies, utilizing plasma, algorithm for elevated or not elevated qualitative results
VeriMAP™ Peanut Dx – Bead-based Epitope Assay, AllerGenis™ Clinical Laboratory, AllerGenis™ LLC	0165U	Peanut allergen-specific quantitative assessment of multiple epitopes using enzyme-linked immunosorbent assay (ELISA), blood, individual epitope results and probability of peanut allergy
LiverFASt™, Fibronostics	0166U	Liver disease, 10 biochemical assays (α2-macroglobulin, haptoglobin, apolipoprotein A1, bilirubin, GGT, ALT, AST, triglycerides, cholesterol, fasting glucose) and biometric and demographic data, utilizing serum, algorithm reported as scores for fibrosis, necroinflammatory activity, and steatosis with a summary interpretation
—	▶(0167U has been deleted)◀	—
NT *(NUDT15* and *TPMT)* genotyping panel, RPRD Diagnostics	0169U	*NUDT15 (nudix hydrolase 15)* and *TPMT (thiopurine S-methyltransferase)* (eg, drug metabolism) gene analysis, common variants
Clarifi™, Quadrant Biosciences, Inc, Quadrant Biosciences, Inc	0170U	Neurology (autism spectrum disorder [ASD]), RNA, next-generation sequencing, saliva, algorithmic analysis, and results reported as predictive probability of ASD diagnosis
MyMRD® NGS Panel, Laboratory for Personalized Molecular Medicine, Laboratory for Personalized Molecular Medicine	0171U	Targeted genomic sequence analysis panel, acute myeloid leukemia, myelodysplastic syndrome, and myeloproliferative neoplasms, DNA analysis, 23 genes, interrogation for sequence variants, rearrangements and minimal residual disease, reported as presence/absence

(Continued on page 1056)

---

myChoice® CDx, Myriad Genetics Laboratories, Inc, Myriad Genetics Laboratories, Inc	0172U	Oncology (solid tumor as indicated by the label), somatic mutation analysis of *BRCA1 (BRCA1, DNA repair associated), BRCA2 (BRCA2, DNA repair associated)* and analysis of homologous recombination deficiency pathways, DNA, formalin-fixed paraffin-embedded tissue, algorithm quantifying tumor genomic instability score
Psych HealthPGx Panel, RPRD Diagnostics, RPRD Diagnostics	0173U	Psychiatry (ie, depression, anxiety), genomic analysis panel, includes variant analysis of 14 genes
LC-MS/MS Targeted Proteomic Assay, OncoOmicDx Laboratory, LDT	0174U	Oncology (solid tumor), mass spectrometric 30 protein targets, formalin-fixed paraffin-embedded tissue, prognostic and predictive algorithm reported as likely, unlikely, or uncertain benefit of 39 chemotherapy and targeted therapeutic oncology agents
Genomind® Professional PGx Express™ CORE, Genomind, Inc, Genomind, Inc	0175U	Psychiatry (eg, depression, anxiety), genomic analysis panel, variant analysis of 15 genes
IB*Schek*®, Commonwealth Diagnostics International, Inc, Commonwealth Diagnostics International, Inc	0176U	Cytolethal distending toxin B (CdtB) and vinculin IgG antibodies by immunoassay (ie, ELISA)
therascreen® *PIK3CA* RGQ PCR Kit, QIAGEN, QIAGEN GmbH	0177U	Oncology (breast cancer), DNA, *PIK3CA (phosphatidylinositol-4,5-bisphosphate 3-kinase catalytic subunit alpha)* gene analysis of 11 gene variants utilizing plasma, reported as *PIK3CA* gene mutation status
VeriMAP™ Peanut Reactivity Threshold–Bead Based Epitope Assay, AllerGenis™ Clinical Laboratory, AllerGenis™ LLC	0178U	Peanut allergen-specific quantitative assessment of multiple epitopes using enzyme-linked immunosorbent assay (ELISA), blood, report of minimum eliciting exposure for a clinical reaction
Resolution ctDx Lung™, Resolution Bioscience, Resolution Bioscience, Inc	0179U	Oncology (non-small cell lung cancer), cell-free DNA, targeted sequence analysis of 23 genes (single nucleotide variations, insertions and deletions, fusions without prior knowledge of partner/breakpoint, copy number variations), with report of significant mutation(s)
Navigator ABO Sequencing, Grifols Immunohematology Center, Grifols Immunohematology Center	0180U	Red cell antigen (ABO blood group) genotyping (ABO), gene analysis Sanger/chain termination/conventional sequencing, *ABO (ABO, alpha 1-3-N-acetylgalactosaminyltransferase and alpha 1-3-galactosyltransferase)* gene, including subtyping, 7 exons
Navigator CO Sequencing, Grifols Immunohematology Center, Grifols Immunohematology Center	0181U	Red cell antigen (Colton blood group) genotyping (CO), gene analysis, *AQP1 (aquaporin 1 [Colton blood group])* exon 1

Navigator CROM Sequencing, Grifols Immunohematology Center, Grifols Immunohematology Center	0182U	Red cell antigen (Cromer blood group) genotyping (CROM), gene analysis, *CD55 (CD55 molecule [Cromer blood group])* exons 1-10
Navigator DI Sequencing, Grifols Immunohematology Center, Grifols Immunohematology Center	0183U	Red cell antigen (Diego blood group) genotyping (DI), gene analysis, *SLC4A1 (solute carrier family 4 member 1 [Diego blood group])* exon 19
Navigator DO Sequencing, Grifols Immunohematology Center, Grifols Immunohematology Center	0184U	Red cell antigen (Dombrock blood group) genotyping (DO), gene analysis, *ART4 (ADP-ribosyltransferase 4 [Dombrock blood group])* exon 2
Navigator FUT1 Sequencing, Grifols Immunohematology Center, Grifols Immunohematology Center	0185U	Red cell antigen (H blood group) genotyping (FUT1), gene analysis, *FUT1 (fucosyltransferase 1 [H blood group])* exon 4
Navigator FUT2 Sequencing, Grifols Immunohematology Center, Grifols Immunohematology Center	0186U	Red cell antigen (H blood group) genotyping (FUT2), gene analysis, *FUT2 (fucosyltransferase 2)* exon 2
Navigator FY Sequencing, Grifols Immunohematology Center, Grifols Immunohematology Center	0187U	Red cell antigen (Duffy blood group) genotyping (FY), gene analysis, *ACKR1 (atypical chemokine receptor 1 [Duffy blood group])* exons 1-2
Navigator GE Sequencing, Grifols Immunohematology Center, Grifols Immunohematology Center	0188U	Red cell antigen (Gerbich blood group) genotyping (GE), gene analysis, *GYPC (glycophorin C [Gerbich blood group])* exons 1-4
Navigator GYPA Sequencing, Grifols Immunohematology Center, Grifols Immunohematology Center	0189U	Red cell antigen (MNS blood group) genotyping (GYPA), gene analysis, *GYPA (glycophorin A [MNS blood group])* introns 1, 5, exon 2
Navigator GYPB Sequencing, Grifols Immunohematology Center, Grifols Immunohematology Center	0190U	Red cell antigen (MNS blood group) genotyping (GYPB), gene analysis, *GYPB (glycophorin B [MNS blood group])* introns 1, 5, pseudoexon 3
Navigator IN Sequencing, Grifols Immunohematology Center, Grifols Immunohematology Center	0191U	Red cell antigen (Indian blood group) genotyping (IN), gene analysis, *CD44 (CD44 molecule [Indian blood group])* exons 2, 3, 6
Navigator JK Sequencing, Grifols Immunohematology Center, Grifols Immunohematology Center	0192U	Red cell antigen (Kidd blood group) genotyping (JK), gene analysis, *SLC14A1 (solute carrier family 14 member 1 [Kidd blood group])* gene promoter, exon 9
Navigator JR Sequencing, Grifols Immunohematology Center, Grifols Immunohematology Center	0193U	Red cell antigen (JR blood group) genotyping (JR), gene analysis, *ABCG2 (ATP binding cassette subfamily G member 2 [Junior blood group])* exons 2-26
Navigator KEL Sequencing, Grifols Immunohematology Center, Grifols Immunohematology Center	0194U	Red cell antigen (Kell blood group) genotyping (KEL), gene analysis, *KEL (Kell metallo-endopeptidase [Kell blood group])* exon 8
Navigator *KLF1* Sequencing, Grifols Immunohematology Center, Grifols Immunohematology Center	0195U	*KLF1 (Kruppel-like factor 1)*, targeted sequencing (ie, exon 13)
Navigator LU Sequencing, Grifols Immunohematology Center, Grifols Immunohematology Center	0196U	Red cell antigen (Lutheran blood group) genotyping (LU), gene analysis, *BCAM (basal cell adhesion molecule [Lutheran blood group])* exon 3

(Continued on page 1058)

Navigator LW Sequencing, Grifols Immunohematology Center, Grifols Immunohematology Center	0197U	Red cell antigen (Landsteiner-Wiener blood group) genotyping (LW), gene analysis, *ICAM4 (intercellular adhesion molecule 4 [Landsteiner-Wiener blood group])* exon 1
Navigator RHD/CE Sequencing, Grifols Immunohematology Center, Grifols Immunohematology Center	0198U	Red cell antigen (RH blood group) genotyping (RHD and RHCE), gene analysis Sanger/chain termination/conventional sequencing, *RHD (Rh blood group D antigen) exons 1-10 and RHCE (Rh blood group CcEe antigens)* exon 5
Navigator SC Sequencing, Grifols Immunohematology Center, Grifols Immunohematology Center	0199U	Red cell antigen (Scianna blood group) genotyping (SC), gene analysis, *ERMAP (erythroblast membrane associated protein [Scianna blood group])* exons 4, 12
Navigator XK Sequencing, Grifols Immunohematology Center, Grifols Immunohematology Center	0200U	Red cell antigen (Kx blood group) genotyping (XK), gene analysis, *XK (X-linked Kx blood group)* exons 1-3
Navigator YT Sequencing, Grifols Immunohematology Center, Grifols Immunohematology Center	0201U	Red cell antigen (Yt blood group) genotyping (YT), gene analysis, *ACHE (acetylcholinesterase [Cartwright blood group])* exon 2
BioFire® Respiratory Panel 2.1 (RP2.1), BioFire® Diagnostics, BioFire® Diagnostics, LLC	#0202U	Infectious disease (bacterial or viral respiratory tract infection), pathogen-specific nucleic acid (DNA or RNA), 22 targets including severe acute respiratory syndrome coronavirus 2 (SARS-CoV-2), qualitative RT-PCR, nasopharyngeal swab, each pathogen reported as detected or not detected

(For additional PLA code with identical clinical descriptor, see 0223U. See Appendix O or the most current listing on the AMA CPT website to determine appropriate code assignment) |
PredictSURE IBD™ Test, KSL Diagnostics, PredictImmune Ltd	0203U	Autoimmune (inflammatory bowel disease), mRNA, gene expression profiling by quantitative RT-PCR, 17 genes (15 target and 2 reference genes), whole blood, reported as a continuous risk score and classification of inflammatory bowel disease aggressiveness
—	▶(0204U has been deleted)◀	—
Vita Risk®, Arctic Medical Laboratories, Arctic Medical Laboratories	0205U	Ophthalmology (age-related macular degeneration), analysis of 3 gene variants (2 *CFH* gene, 1 *ARMS2* gene), using PCR and MALDI-TOF, buccal swab, reported as positive or negative for neovascular age-related macular-degeneration risk associated with zinc supplements

DISCERN™, NeuroDiagnostics, NeuroDiagnostics	0206U	Neurology (Alzheimer disease); cell aggregation using morphometric imaging and protein kinase C-epsilon (PKCe) concentration in response to amylospheroid treatment by ELISA, cultured skin fibroblasts, each reported as positive or negative for Alzheimer disease
	+0207U	quantitative imaging of phosphorylated *ERK1* and *ERK2* in response to bradykinin treatment by in situ immunofluorescence, using cultured skin fibroblasts, reported as a probability index for Alzheimer disease (List separately in addition to code for primary procedure)
		(Use 0207U in conjunction with 0206U)
—	(0208U has been deleted)	—
CNGnome™, PerkinElmer Genomics, PerkinElmer Genomics	0209U	Cytogenomic constitutional (genome-wide) analysis, interrogation of genomic regions for copy number, structural changes and areas of homozygosity for chromosomal abnormalities
BioPlex 2200 RPR Assay – Quantitative, Bio-Rad Laboratories, Bio-Rad Laboratories	0210U	Syphilis test, non-treponemal antibody, immunoassay, quantitative (RPR)
MI Cancer Seek™ - NGS Analysis, Caris MPI d/b/a Caris Life Sciences, Caris MPI d/b/a Caris Life Sciences	0211U	Oncology (pan-tumor), DNA and RNA by next-generation sequencing, utilizing formalin-fixed paraffin-embedded tissue, interpretative report for single nucleotide variants, copy number alterations, tumor mutational burden, and microsatellite instability, with therapy association
Genomic Unity® Whole Genome Analysis – Proband, Variantyx Inc, Variantyx Inc	0212U	Rare diseases (constitutional/heritable disorders), whole genome and mitochondrial DNA sequence analysis, including small sequence changes, deletions, duplications, short tandem repeat gene expansions, and variants in non-uniquely mappable regions, blood or saliva, identification and categorization of genetic variants, proband
		(Do not report 0212U in conjunction with 81425)
Genomic Unity® Whole Genome Analysis – Comparator, Variantyx Inc, Variantyx Inc	0213U	Rare diseases (constitutional/heritable disorders), whole genome and mitochondrial DNA sequence analysis, including small sequence changes, deletions, duplications, short tandem repeat gene expansions, and variants in non-uniquely mappable regions, blood or saliva, identification and categorization of genetic variants, each comparator genome (eg, parent, sibling)
		(Do not report 0213U in conjunction with 81426)

(*Continued on page 1060*)

Genomic Unity® Exome Plus Analysis – Proband, Variantyx Inc, Variantyx Inc	0214U	Rare diseases (constitutional/heritable disorders), whole exome and mitochondrial DNA sequence analysis, including small sequence changes, deletions, duplications, short tandem repeat gene expansions, and variants in non-uniquely mappable regions, blood or saliva, identification and categorization of genetic variants, proband (Do not report 0214U in conjunction with 81415)
Genomic Unity® Exome Plus Analysis – Comparator, Variantyx Inc, Variantyx Inc	0215U	Rare diseases (constitutional/heritable disorders), whole exome and mitochondrial DNA sequence analysis, including small sequence changes, deletions, duplications, short tandem repeat gene expansions, and variants in non-uniquely mappable regions, blood or saliva, identification and categorization of genetic variants, each comparator exome (eg, parent, sibling) (Do not report 0215U in conjunction with 81416)
Genomic Unity® Ataxia Repeat Expansion and Sequence Analysis, Variantyx Inc, Variantyx Inc	0216U	Neurology (inherited ataxias), genomic DNA sequence analysis of 12 common genes including small sequence changes, deletions, duplications, short tandem repeat gene expansions, and variants in non-uniquely mappable regions, blood or saliva, identification and categorization of genetic variants
Genomic Unity® Comprehensive Ataxia Repeat Expansion and Sequence Analysis, Variantyx Inc, Variantyx Inc	0217U	Neurology (inherited ataxias), genomic DNA sequence analysis of 51 genes including small sequence changes, deletions, duplications, short tandem repeat gene expansions, and variants in non-uniquely mappable regions, blood or saliva, identification and categorization of genetic variants
Genomic Unity® DMD Analysis, Variantyx Inc, Variantyx Inc	0218U	Neurology (muscular dystrophy), *DMD* gene sequence analysis, including small sequence changes, deletions, duplications, and variants in non-uniquely mappable regions, blood or saliva, identification and characterization of genetic variants
Sentosa® SQ HIV-1 Genotyping Assay, Vela Diagnostics USA, Inc, Vela Operations Singapore Pte Ltd	0219U	Infectious agent (human immunodeficiency virus), targeted viral next-generation sequence analysis (ie, protease [PR], reverse transcriptase [RT], integrase [INT]), algorithm reported as prediction of antiviral drug susceptibility
PreciseDx™ Breast Cancer Test, PreciseDx, PreciseDx	0220U	Oncology (breast cancer), image analysis with artificial intelligence assessment of 12 histologic and immunohistochemical features, reported as a recurrence score
Navigator ABO Blood Group NGS, Grifols Immunohematology Center, Grifols Immunohematology Center	0221U	Red cell antigen (ABO blood group) genotyping (ABO), gene analysis, next-generation sequencing, *ABO (ABO, alpha 1-3-N-acetylgalactosaminyltransferase and alpha 1-3-galactosyltransferase) gene*

Appendix O

Navigator Rh Blood Group NGS, Grifols Immunohematology Center, Grifols Immunohematology Center	0222U	Red cell antigen (RH blood group) genotyping (RHD and RHCE), gene analysis, next-generation sequencing, RH proximal promoter, exons 1-10, portions of introns 2-3
QIAstat-Dx Respiratory SARS CoV-2 Panel, QIAGEN Sciences, QIAGEN GmbH	✕0223U	Infectious disease (bacterial or viral respiratory tract infection), pathogen-specific nucleic acid (DNA or RNA), 22 targets including severe acute respiratory syndrome coronavirus 2 (SARS-CoV-2), qualitative RT-PCR, nasopharyngeal swab, each pathogen reported as detected or not detected (For additional PLA code with identical clinical descriptor, see 0202U. See Appendix O or the most current listing on the AMA CPT website to determine appropriate code assignment)
COVID-19 Antibody Test, Mt Sinai, Mount Sinai Laboratory	0224U	Antibody, severe acute respiratory syndrome coronavirus 2 (SARS-CoV-2) (coronavirus disease [COVID-19]), includes titer(s), when performed (Do not report 0224U in conjunction with 86769)
ePlex® Respiratory Pathogen Panel 2, GenMark Dx, GenMark Diagnostics, Inc	0225U	Infectious disease (bacterial or viral respiratory tract infection) pathogen-specific DNA and RNA, 21 targets, including severe acute respiratory syndrome coronavirus 2 (SARS-CoV-2), amplified probe technique, including multiplex reverse transcription for RNA targets, each analyte reported as detected or not detected
Tru-Immune™, Ethos Laboratories, GenScript® USA Inc	0226U	Surrogate viral neutralization test (sVNT), severe acute respiratory syndrome coronavirus 2 (SARS-CoV-2) (coronavirus disease [COVID-19]), ELISA, plasma, serum
Comprehensive Screen, Aspenti Health	0227U	Drug assay, presumptive, 30 or more drugs or metabolites, urine, liquid chromatography with tandem mass spectrometry (LC-MS/MS) using multiple reaction monitoring (MRM), with drug or metabolite description, includes sample validation
PanGIA Prostate, Genetics Institute of America, Entopsis, LLC	0228U	Oncology (prostate), multianalyte molecular profile by photometric detection of macromolecules adsorbed on nanosponge array slides with machine learning, utilizing first morning voided urine, algorithm reported as likelihood of prostate cancer
Colvera®, Clinical Genomics Pathology Inc	0229U	*BCAT1 (Branched chain amino acid transaminase 1)* and *IKZF1 (IKAROS family zinc finger 1)* (eg, colorectal cancer) promoter methylation analysis

(Continued on page 1062)

Genomic Unity® AR Analysis, Variantyx Inc, Variantyx Inc	0230U	*AR (androgen receptor)* (eg, spinal and bulbar muscular atrophy, Kennedy disease, X chromosome inactivation), full sequence analysis, including small sequence changes in exonic and intronic regions, deletions, duplications, short tandem repeat (STR) expansions, mobile element insertions, and variants in non-uniquely mappable regions
Genomic Unity® CACNA1A Analysis, Variantyx Inc, Variantyx Inc	0231U	*CACNA1A (calcium voltage-gated channel subunit alpha 1A)* (eg, spinocerebellar ataxia), full gene analysis, including small sequence changes in exonic and intronic regions, deletions, duplications, short tandem repeat (STR) gene expansions, mobile element insertions, and variants in non-uniquely mappable regions
Genomic Unity® CSTB Analysis, Variantyx Inc, Variantyx Inc	0232U	*CSTB (cystatin B)* (eg, progressive myoclonic epilepsy type 1A, Unverricht-Lundborg disease), full gene analysis, including small sequence changes in exonic and intronic regions, deletions, duplications, short tandem repeat (STR) expansions, mobile element insertions, and variants in non-uniquely mappable regions
Genomic Unity® FXN Analysis, Variantyx Inc, Variantyx Inc	0233U	*FXN (frataxin)* (eg, Friedreich ataxia), gene analysis, including small sequence changes in exonic and intronic regions, deletions, duplications, short tandem repeat (STR) expansions, mobile element insertions, and variants in non-uniquely mappable regions
Genomic Unity® MECP2 Analysis, Variantyx Inc, Variantyx Inc	0234U	*MECP2 (methyl CpG binding protein 2)* (eg, Rett syndrome), full gene analysis, including small sequence changes in exonic and intronic regions, deletions, duplications, mobile element insertions, and variants in non-uniquely mappable regions
Genomic Unity® PTEN Analysis, Variantyx Inc, Variantyx Inc	0235U	*PTEN (phosphatase and tensin homolog)* (eg, Cowden syndrome, PTEN hamartoma tumor syndrome), full gene analysis, including small sequence changes in exonic and intronic regions, deletions, duplications, mobile element insertions, and variants in non-uniquely mappable regions
Genomic Unity® SMN1/2 Analysis, Variantyx Inc, Variantyx Inc	0236U	*SMN1 (survival of motor neuron 1, telomeric)* and *SMN2 (survival of motor neuron 2, centromeric)* (eg, spinal muscular atrophy) full gene analysis, including small sequence changes in exonic and intronic regions, duplications, deletions, and mobile element insertions

Genomic Unity® Cardiac Ion Channelopathies Analysis, Variantyx Inc, Variantyx Inc	0237U	Cardiac ion channelopathies (eg, Brugada syndrome, long QT syndrome, short QT syndrome, catecholaminergic polymorphic ventricular tachycardia), genomic sequence analysis panel including *ANK2, CASQ2, CAV3, KCNE1, KCNE2, KCNH2, KCNJ2, KCNQ1, RYR2,* and *SCN5A,* including small sequence changes in exonic and intronic regions, deletions, duplications, mobile element insertions, and variants in non-uniquely mappable regions
Genomic Unity® Lynch Syndrome Analysis, Variantyx Inc, Variantyx Inc	0238U	Oncology (Lynch syndrome), genomic DNA sequence analysis of *MLH1, MSH2, MSH6, PMS2,* and *EPCAM,* including small sequence changes in exonic and intronic regions, deletions, duplications, mobile element insertions, and variants in non-uniquely mappable regions
FoundationOne® Liquid CDx, Foundation Medicine, Inc, Foundation Medicine, Inc	0239U	Targeted genomic sequence analysis panel, solid organ neoplasm, cell-free DNA, analysis of 311 or more genes, interrogation for sequence variants, including substitutions, insertions, deletions, select rearrangements, and copy number variations
Xpert® Xpress CoV-2/Flu/RSV plus (SARS-CoV-2 and Flu targets), Cepheid®	0240U	Infectious disease (viral respiratory tract infection), pathogen-specific RNA, 3 targets (severe acute respiratory syndrome coronavirus 2 [SARS-CoV-2], influenza A, influenza B), upper respiratory specimen, each pathogen reported as detected or not detected
Xpert® Xpress CoV-2/Flu/RSV plus (all targets), Cepheid®	0241U	Infectious disease (viral respiratory tract infection), pathogen-specific RNA, 4 targets (severe acute respiratory syndrome coronavirus 2 [SARS-CoV-2], influenza A, influenza B, respiratory syncytial virus [RSV]), upper respiratory specimen, each pathogen reported as detected or not detected
Guardant360® CDx, Guardant Health Inc, Guardant Health Inc	0242U	Targeted genomic sequence analysis panel, solid organ neoplasm, cell-free circulating DNA analysis of 55-74 genes, interrogation for sequence variants, gene copy number amplifications, and gene rearrangements
PlGF Preeclampsia Screen, PerkinElmer Genetics, PerkinElmer Genetics, Inc	0243U	Obstetrics (preeclampsia), biochemical assay of placental-growth factor, time-resolved fluorescence immunoassay, maternal serum, predictive algorithm reported as a risk score for preeclampsia
Oncotype MAP™ Pan-Cancer Tissue Test, Paradigm Diagnostics, Inc, Paradigm Diagnostics, Inc	0244U	Oncology (solid organ), DNA, comprehensive genomic profiling, 257 genes, interrogation for single-nucleotide variants, insertions/deletions, copy number alterations, gene rearrangements, tumor-mutational burden and microsatellite instability, utilizing formalin-fixed paraffin-embedded tumor tissue

(*Continued on page 1064*)

ThyGeNEXT® Thyroid Oncogene Panel, Interpace Diagnostics, Interpace Diagnostics	0245U	Oncology (thyroid), mutation analysis of 10 genes and 37 RNA fusions and expression of 4 mRNA markers using next-generation sequencing, fine needle aspirate, report includes associated risk of malignancy expressed as a percentage
PrecisionBlood™, San Diego Blood Bank, San Diego Blood Bank	0246U	Red blood cell antigen typing, DNA, genotyping of at least 16 blood groups with phenotype prediction of at least 51 red blood cell antigens
PreTRM®, Sera Prognostics, Sera Prognostics, Inc®	0247U	Obstetrics (preterm birth), insulin-like growth factor–binding protein 4 (IBP4), sex hormone–binding globulin (SHBG), quantitative measurement by LC-MS/MS, utilizing maternal serum, combined with clinical data, reported as predictive-risk stratification for spontaneous preterm birth
3D Predict Glioma, KIYATEC®, Inc	▲0248U	▶Oncology, spheroid cell culture in 3D microenvironment, 12-drug panel, brain- or brain metastasis–response prediction for each drug◀
Theralink® Reverse Phase Protein Array (RPPA), Theralink® Technologies, Inc, Theralink® Technologies, Inc	0249U	Oncology (breast), semiquantitative analysis of 32 phosphoproteins and protein analytes, includes laser capture microdissection, with algorithmic analysis and interpretative report
PGDx elio™ tissue complete, Personal Genome Diagnostics, Inc, Personal Genome Diagnostics, Inc	0250U	Oncology (solid organ neoplasm), targeted genomic sequence DNA analysis of 505 genes, interrogation for somatic alterations (SNVs [single nucleotide variant], small insertions and deletions, one amplification, and four translocations), microsatellite instability and tumor-mutation burden
Intrinsic Hepcidin IDx™ Test, IntrinsicDx, Intrinsic LifeSciences™ LLC	0251U	Hepcidin-25, enzyme-linked immunosorbent assay (ELISA), serum or plasma
POC (Products of Conception), Igenomix®, Igenomix® USA	0252U	Fetal aneuploidy short tandem–repeat comparative analysis, fetal DNA from products of conception, reported as normal (euploidy), monosomy, trisomy, or partial deletion/duplication, mosaicism, and segmental aneuploidy
ERA® (Endometrial Receptivity Analysis), Igenomix®, Igenomix® USA	0253U	Reproductive medicine (endometrial receptivity analysis), RNA gene expression profile, 238 genes by next-generation sequencing, endometrial tissue, predictive algorithm reported as endometrial window of implantation (eg, pre-receptive, receptive, post-receptive)

SMART PGT-A (Pre-implantation Genetic Testing - Aneuploidy), Igenomix®, Igenomix® USA	0254U	Reproductive medicine (preimplantation genetic assessment), analysis of 24 chromosomes using embryonic DNA genomic sequence analysis for aneuploidy, and a mitochondrial DNA score in euploid embryos, results reported as normal (euploidy), monosomy, trisomy, or partial deletion/duplication, mosaicism, and segmental aneuploidy, per embryo tested
Cap-Score™ Test, Androvia LifeSciences, Avantor Clinical Services (previously known as Therapak)	0255U	Andrology (infertility), sperm-capacitation assessment of ganglioside GM1 distribution patterns, fluorescence microscopy, fresh or frozen specimen, reported as percentage of capacitated sperm and probability of generating a pregnancy score
Trimethylamine (TMA) and TMA N-Oxide, Children's Hospital Colorado Laboratory	0256U	Trimethylamine/trimethylamine N-oxide (TMA/TMAO) profile, tandem mass spectrometry (MS/MS), urine, with algorithmic analysis and interpretive report
Very-Long Chain Acyl-CoA Dehydrogenase (VLCAD) Enzyme Activity, Children's Hospital Colorado Laboratory	0257U	Very long chain acyl-coenzyme A (CoA) dehydrogenase (VLCAD), leukocyte enzyme activity, whole blood
Mind.Px, Mindera, Mindera Corporation	0258U	Autoimmune (psoriasis), mRNA, next-generation sequencing, gene expression profiling of 50-100 genes, skin-surface collection using adhesive patch, algorithm reported as likelihood of response to psoriasis biologics
GFR by NMR, Labtech™ Diagnostics	0259U	Nephrology (chronic kidney disease), nuclear magnetic resonance spectroscopy measurement of myo-inositol, valine, and creatinine, algorithmically combined with cystatin C (by immunoassay) and demographic data to determine estimated glomerular filtration rate (GFR), serum, quantitative
Augusta Optical Genome Mapping, Georgia Esoteric and Molecular (GEM) Laboratory, LLC, Bionano Genomics Inc	⯒0260U	Rare diseases (constitutional/heritable disorders), identification of copy number variations, inversions, insertions, translocations, and other structural variants by optical genome mapping ▶(For additional PLA codes with identical clinical descriptor, see 0264U, 0454U. See Appendix O or the most current listing on the AMA CPT website to determine appropriate code assignment)◀
Immunoscore®, HalioDx, HalioDx	0261U	Oncology (colorectal cancer), image analysis with artificial intelligence assessment of 4 histologic and immunohistochemical features (CD3 and CD8 within tumor-stroma border and tumor core), tissue, reported as immune response and recurrence-risk score

(*Continued on page 1066*)

OncoSignal 7 Pathway Signal, Protean BioDiagnostics, Philips Electronics Nederland BV	0262U	Oncology (solid tumor), gene expression profiling by real-time RT-PCR of 7 gene pathways *(ER, AR, PI3K, MAPK, HH, TGFB,* Notch), formalin-fixed paraffin-embedded (FFPE), algorithm reported as gene pathway activity score
NPDX ASD and Central Carbon Energy Metabolism, Stemina Biomarker Discovery, Inc, Stemina Biomarker Discovery, Inc	0263U	Neurology (autism spectrum disorder [ASD]), quantitative measurements of 16 central carbon metabolites (ie, α-ketoglutarate, alanine, lactate, phenylalanine, pyruvate, succinate, carnitine, citrate, fumarate, hypoxanthine, inosine, malate, S-sulfocysteine, taurine, urate, and xanthine), liquid chromatography tandem mass spectrometry (LC-MS/MS), plasma, algorithmic analysis with result reported as negative or positive (with metabolic subtypes of ASD)
Praxis Optical Genome Mapping, Praxis Genomics LLC	#0264U	Rare diseases (constitutional/heritable disorders), identification of copy number variations, inversions, insertions, translocations, and other structural variants by optical genome mapping ▶(For additional PLA codes with identical clinical descriptor, see 0260U, 0454U. See Appendix O or the most current listing on the AMA CPT website to determine appropriate code assignment)◀
Praxis Whole Genome Sequencing, Praxis Genomics LLC	0265U	Rare constitutional and other heritable disorders, whole genome and mitochondrial DNA sequence analysis, blood, frozen and formalin-fixed paraffin-embedded (FFPE) tissue, saliva, buccal swabs or cell lines, identification of single nucleotide and copy number variants
Praxis Transcriptome, Praxis Genomics LLC	0266U	Unexplained constitutional or other heritable disorders or syndromes, tissue-specific gene expression by whole-transcriptome and next-generation sequencing, blood, formalin-fixed paraffin-embedded (FFPE) tissue or fresh frozen tissue, reported as presence or absence of splicing or expression changes
Praxis Combined Whole Genome Sequencing and Optical Genome Mapping, Praxis Genomics LLC	0267U	Rare constitutional and other heritable disorders, identification of copy number variations, inversions, insertions, translocations, and other structural variants by optical genome mapping and whole genome sequencing
Versiti™ aHUS Genetic Evaluation, Versiti™ Diagnostic Laboratories, Versiti™	0268U	Hematology (atypical hemolytic uremic syndrome [aHUS]), genomic sequence analysis of 15 genes, blood, buccal swab, or amniotic fluid
Versiti™ Autosomal Dominant Thrombocytopenia Panel, Versiti™ Diagnostic Laboratories, Versiti™	0269U	Hematology (autosomal dominant congenital thrombocytopenia), genomic sequence analysis of 22 genes, blood, buccal swab, or amniotic fluid

Versiti™ Coagulation Disorder Panel, Versiti™ Diagnostic Laboratories, Versiti™	0270U	Hematology (congenital coagulation disorders), genomic sequence analysis of 20 genes, blood, buccal swab, or amniotic fluid
Versiti™ Congenital Neutropenia Panel, Versiti™ Diagnostic Laboratories, Versiti™	0271U	Hematology (congenital neutropenia), genomic sequence analysis of 24 genes, blood, buccal swab, or amniotic fluid
Versiti™ Comprehensive Bleeding Disorder Panel, Versiti™ Diagnostic Laboratories, Versiti™	0272U	Hematology (genetic bleeding disorders), genomic sequence analysis of 60 genes and duplication/deletion of *PLAU*, blood, buccal swab, or amniotic fluid, comprehensive
Versiti™ Fibrinolytic Disorder Panel, Versiti™ Diagnostic Laboratories, Versiti™	0273U	Hematology (genetic hyperfibrinolysis, delayed bleeding), analysis of 9 genes (*F13A1, F13B, FGA, FGB, FGG, SERPINA1, SERPINE1, SERPINF2* by next-generation sequencing, and *PLAU* by array comparative genomic hybridization), blood, buccal swab, or amniotic fluid
Versiti™ Comprehensive Platelet Disorder Panel, Versiti™ Diagnostic Laboratories, Versiti™	0274U	Hematology (genetic platelet disorders), genomic sequence analysis of 62 genes and duplication/deletion of *PLAU*, blood, buccal swab, or amniotic fluid
Versiti™ Heparin-Induced Thrombocytopenia Evaluation – PEA, Versiti™ Diagnostic Laboratories, Versiti™	0275U	Hematology (heparin-induced thrombocytopenia), platelet antibody reactivity by flow cytometry, serum
Versiti™ Inherited Thrombocytopenia Panel, Versiti™ Diagnostic Laboratories, Versiti™	0276U	Hematology (inherited thrombocytopenia), genomic sequence analysis of 42 genes, blood, buccal swab, or amniotic fluid
Versiti™ Platelet Function Disorder Panel, Versiti™ Diagnostic Laboratories, Versiti™	0277U	Hematology (genetic platelet function disorder), genomic sequence analysis of 40 genes and duplication/deletion of *PLAU*, blood, buccal swab, or amniotic fluid
Versiti™ Thrombosis Panel, Versiti™ Diagnostic Laboratories, Versiti™	0278U	Hematology (genetic thrombosis), genomic sequence analysis of 14 genes, blood, buccal swab, or amniotic fluid
Versiti™ VWF Collagen III Binding, Versiti™ Diagnostic Laboratories, Versiti™	0279U	Hematology (von Willebrand disease [VWD]), von Willebrand factor (VWF) and collagen III binding by enzyme-linked immunosorbent assays (ELISA), plasma, report of collagen III binding
Versiti™ VWF Collagen IV Binding, Versiti™ Diagnostic Laboratories, Versiti™	0280U	Hematology (von Willebrand disease [VWD]), von Willebrand factor (VWF) and collagen IV binding by enzyme-linked immunosorbent assays (ELISA), plasma, report of collagen IV binding
Versiti™ VWF Propeptide Antigen, Versiti™ Diagnostic Laboratories, Versiti™	0281U	Hematology (von Willebrand disease [VWD]), von Willebrand propeptide, enzyme-linked immunosorbent assays (ELISA), plasma, diagnostic report of von Willebrand factor (VWF) propeptide antigen level

(Continued on page 1068)

Versiti™ Red Cell Genotyping Panel, Versiti™ Diagnostic Laboratories, Versiti™	0282U	Red blood cell antigen typing, DNA, genotyping of 12 blood group system genes to predict 44 red blood cell antigen phenotypes
Versiti™ VWD Type 2B Evaluation, Versiti™ Diagnostic Laboratories, Versiti™	0283U	von Willebrand factor (VWF), type 2B, platelet-binding evaluation, radioimmunoassay, plasma
Versiti™ VWD Type 2N Binding, Versiti™ Diagnostic Laboratories, Versiti™	0284U	von Willebrand factor (VWF), type 2N, factor VIII and VWF binding evaluation, enzyme-linked immunosorbent assays (ELISA), plasma
RadTox™ cfDNA test, DiaCarta Clinical Lab, DiaCarta Inc	0285U	Oncology, response to radiation, cell-free DNA, quantitative branched chain DNA amplification, plasma, reported as a radiation toxicity score
CNT (*CEP72, TPMT* and *NUDT15*) genotyping panel, RPRD Diagnostics	0286U	*CEP72 (centrosomal protein, 72-KDa), NUDT15 (nudix hydrolase 15)* and *TPMT (thiopurine S-methyltransferase)* (eg, drug metabolism) gene analysis, common variants
ThyroSeq® CRC, CBLPath, Inc, University of Pittsburgh Medical Center	0287U	Oncology (thyroid), DNA and mRNA, next-generation sequencing analysis of 112 genes, fine needle aspirate or formalin-fixed paraffin-embedded (FFPE) tissue, algorithmic prediction of cancer recurrence, reported as a categorical risk result (low, intermediate, high)
DetermaRx™, Oncocyte Corporation	0288U	Oncology (lung), mRNA, quantitative PCR analysis of 11 genes (*BAG1, BRCA1, CDC6, CDK2AP1, ERBB3, FUT3, IL11, LCK, RND3, SH3BGR, WNT3A*) and 3 reference genes (*ESD, TBP, YAP1*), formalin-fixed paraffin-embedded (FFPE) tumor tissue, algorithmic interpretation reported as a recurrence risk score
MindX Blood Test™ - Memory/Alzheimer's, MindX Sciences™ Laboratory, MindX Sciences™ Inc	0289U	Neurology (Alzheimer disease), mRNA, gene expression profiling by RNA sequencing of 24 genes, whole blood, algorithm reported as predictive risk score
MindX Blood Test™ - Pain, MindX Sciences™ Laboratory, MindX Sciences™ Inc	0290U	Pain management, mRNA, gene expression profiling by RNA sequencing of 36 genes, whole blood, algorithm reported as predictive risk score
MindX Blood Test™ - Mood, MindX Sciences™ Laboratory, MindX Sciences™ Inc	0291U	Psychiatry (mood disorders), mRNA, gene expression profiling by RNA sequencing of 144 genes, whole blood, algorithm reported as predictive risk score
MindX Blood Test™ - Stress, MindX Sciences™ Laboratory, MindX Sciences™ Inc	0292U	Psychiatry (stress disorders), mRNA, gene expression profiling by RNA sequencing of 72 genes, whole blood, algorithm reported as predictive risk score
MindX Blood Test™ - Suicidality, MindX Sciences™ Laboratory, MindX Sciences™ Inc	0293U	Psychiatry (suicidal ideation), mRNA, gene expression profiling by RNA sequencing of 54 genes, whole blood, algorithm reported as predictive risk score

MindX Blood Test™ - Longevity, MindX Sciences™ Laboratory, MindX Sciences™ Inc	0294U	Longevity and mortality risk, mRNA, gene expression profiling by RNA sequencing of 18 genes, whole blood, algorithm reported as predictive risk score
DCISionRT®, PreludeDx™, Prelude Corporation	0295U	Oncology (breast ductal carcinoma in situ), protein expression profiling by immunohistochemistry of 7 proteins (COX2, FOXA1, HER2, Ki-67, p16, PR, SIAH2), with 4 clinicopathologic factors (size, age, margin status, palpability), utilizing formalin-fixed paraffin-embedded (FFPE) tissue, algorithm reported as a recurrence risk score
mRNA CancerDetect™, Viome Life Sciences, Inc, Viome Life Sciences, Inc	0296U	Oncology (oral and/or oropharyngeal cancer), gene expression profiling by RNA sequencing of at least 20 molecular features (eg, human and/or microbial mRNA), saliva, algorithm reported as positive or negative for signature associated with malignancy
Praxis Somatic Whole Genome Sequencing, Praxis Genomics LLC	0297U	Oncology (pan tumor), whole genome sequencing of paired malignant and normal DNA specimens, fresh or formalin-fixed paraffin-embedded (FFPE) tissue, blood or bone marrow, comparative sequence analyses and variant identification
Praxis Somatic Transcriptome, Praxis Genomics LLC	0298U	Oncology (pan tumor), whole transcriptome sequencing of paired malignant and normal RNA specimens, fresh or formalin-fixed paraffin-embedded (FFPE) tissue, blood or bone marrow, comparative sequence analyses and expression level and chimeric transcript identification
Praxis Somatic Optical Genome Mapping, Praxis Genomics LLC	0299U	Oncology (pan tumor), whole genome optical genome mapping of paired malignant and normal DNA specimens, fresh frozen tissue, blood, or bone marrow, comparative structural variant identification
Praxis Somatic Combined Whole Genome Sequencing and Optical Genome Mapping, Praxis Genomics LLC	0300U	Oncology (pan tumor), whole genome sequencing and optical genome mapping of paired malignant and normal DNA specimens, fresh tissue, blood, or bone marrow, comparative sequence analyses and variant identification
Bartonella ddPCR, Galaxy Diagnostics, Inc	0301U	Infectious agent detection by nucleic acid (DNA or RNA), Bartonella henselae and Bartonella quintana, droplet digital PCR (ddPCR);
Bartonella Digital ePCR™, Galaxy Diagnostics, Inc	0302U	following liquid enrichment
Hypoxic BioChip Adhesion, BioChip Labs™, BioChip Labs™	0303U	Hematology, red blood cell (RBC) adhesion to endothelial/subendothelial adhesion molecules, functional assessment, whole blood, with algorithmic analysis and result reported as an RBC adhesion index; hypoxic
Normoxic BioChip Adhesion, BioChip Labs™, BioChip Labs™	0304U	normoxic

(*Continued on page 1070*)

Ektacytometry, BioChip Labs™, BioChip Labs™	0305U	Hematology, red blood cell (RBC) functionality and deformity as a function of shear stress, whole blood, reported as a maximum elongation index
Invitae PCM Tissue Profiling and MRD Baseline Assay, Invitae Corporation, Invitae Corporation	0306U	Oncology (minimal residual disease [MRD]), next-generation targeted sequencing analysis, cell-free DNA, initial (baseline) assessment to determine a patient-specific panel for future comparisons to evaluate for MRD (Do not report 0306U in conjunction with 0307U)
Invitae PCM MRD Monitoring, Invitae Corporation, Invitae Corporation	0307U	Oncology (minimal residual disease [MRD]), next-generation targeted sequencing analysis of a patient-specific panel, cell-free DNA, subsequent assessment with comparison to previously analyzed patient specimens to evaluate for MRD (Do not report 0307U in conjunction with 0306U)
HART CADhs®, Atlas Genomics, Prevencio, Inc	0308U	Cardiology (coronary artery disease [CAD]), analysis of 3 proteins (high sensitivity [hs] troponin, adiponectin, and kidney injury molecule-1 [KIM-1]) with 3 clinical parameters (age, sex, history of cardiac intervention), plasma, algorithm reported as a risk score for obstructive CAD
HART CVE®, Atlas Genomics, Prevencio, Inc	0309U	Cardiology (cardiovascular disease), analysis of 4 proteins (NT-proBNP, osteopontin, tissue inhibitor of metalloproteinase-1 [TIMP-1], and kidney injury molecule-1 [KIM-1]), plasma, algorithm reported as a risk score for major adverse cardiac event
HART KD®, Atlas Genomics, Prevencio, Inc	0310U	Pediatrics (vasculitis, Kawasaki disease [KD]), analysis of 3 biomarkers (NT-proBNP, C-reactive protein, and T-uptake), plasma, algorithm reported as a risk score for KD
Accelerate PhenoTest® BC kit, AST configuration, Accelerate Diagnostics, Inc, Accelerate Diagnostics, Inc	0311U	Infectious disease (bacterial), quantitative antimicrobial susceptibility reported as phenotypic minimum inhibitory concentration (MIC)–based antimicrobial susceptibility for each organism identified (Do not report 0311U in conjunction with 87076, 87077, 0086U)
Avise® Lupus, Exagen Inc, Exagen Inc	0312U	Autoimmune diseases (eg, systemic lupus erythematosus [SLE]), analysis of 8 IgG autoantibodies and 2 cell-bound complement activation products using enzyme-linked immunosorbent immunoassay (ELISA), flow cytometry and indirect immunofluorescence, serum, or plasma and whole blood, individual components reported along with an algorithmic SLE-likelihood assessment

PancreaSeq® Genomic Classifier, Molecular and Genomic Pathology Laboratory, University of Pittsburgh Medical Center	0313U	Oncology (pancreas), DNA and mRNA next-generation sequencing analysis of 74 genes and analysis of CEA (CEACAM5) gene expression, pancreatic cyst fluid, algorithm reported as a categorical result (ie, negative, low probability of neoplasia or positive, high probability of neoplasia)
DecisionDx® DiffDx™-Melanoma, Castle Biosciences, Inc, Castle Biosciences, Inc	0314U	Oncology (cutaneous melanoma), mRNA gene expression profiling by RT-PCR of 35 genes (32 content and 3 housekeeping), utilizing formalin-fixed paraffin-embedded (FFPE) tissue, algorithm reported as a categorical result (ie, benign, intermediate, malignant)
DecisionDx®-SCC, Castle Biosciences, Inc, Castle Biosciences, Inc	0315U	Oncology (cutaneous squamous cell carcinoma), mRNA gene expression profiling by RT-PCR of 40 genes (34 content and 6 housekeeping), utilizing formalin-fixed paraffin-embedded (FFPE) tissue, algorithm reported as a categorical risk result (ie, Class 1, Class 2A, Class 2B)
Lyme Borrelia Nanotrap® Urine Antigen Test, Galaxy Diagnostics Inc	0316U	Borrelia burgdorferi (Lyme disease), OspA protein evaluation, urine
LungLB®, LungLife AI®, LungLife AI®	0317U	Oncology (lung cancer), four-probe FISH (3q29, 3p22.1, 10q22.3, 10cen) assay, whole blood, predictive algorithm-generated evaluation reported as decreased or increased risk for lung cancer
EpiSign Complete, Greenwood Genetic Center	0318U	Pediatrics (congenital epigenetic disorders), whole genome methylation analysis by microarray for 50 or more genes, blood
Clarava™, Verici Dx, Verici Dx, Inc	0319U	Nephrology (renal transplant), RNA expression by select transcriptome sequencing, using pretransplant peripheral blood, algorithm reported as a risk score for early acute rejection
Tuteva™, Verici Dx, Verici Dx, Inc	0320U	Nephrology (renal transplant), RNA expression by select transcriptome sequencing, using posttransplant peripheral blood, algorithm reported as a risk score for acute cellular rejection
Bridge Urinary Tract Infection Detection and Resistance Test, Bridge Diagnostics	0321U	Infectious agent detection by nucleic acid (DNA or RNA), genitourinary pathogens, identification of 20 bacterial and fungal organisms and identification of 16 associated antibiotic-resistance genes, multiplex amplified probe technique
NPDX ASD Test Panel III, Stemina Biomarker Discovery d/b/a NeuroPointDX, Stemina Biomarker Discovery d/b/a NeuroPointDX	0322U	Neurology (autism spectrum disorder [ASD]), quantitative measurements of 14 acyl carnitines and microbiome-derived metabolites, liquid chromatography with tandem mass spectrometry (LC-MS/MS), plasma, results reported as negative or positive for risk of metabolic subtypes associated with ASD

(*Continued on page 1072*)

Johns Hopkins Metagenomic Next-Generation Sequencing Assay for Infectious Disease Diagnostics, Johns Hopkins Medical Microbiology Laboratory	0323U	Infectious agent detection by nucleic acid (DNA and RNA), central nervous system pathogen, metagenomic next-generation sequencing, cerebrospinal fluid (CSF), identification of pathogenic bacteria, viruses, parasites, or fungi
—	(0324U has been deleted)	—
—	(0325U has been deleted)	—
Guardant360®, Guardant Health, Inc, Guardant Health, Inc	0326U	Targeted genomic sequence analysis panel, solid organ neoplasm, cell-free circulating DNA analysis of 83 or more genes, interrogation for sequence variants, gene copy number amplifications, gene rearrangements, microsatellite instability and tumor mutational burden
Vasistera™, Natera, Inc, Natera, Inc	0327U	Fetal aneuploidy (trisomy 13, 18, and 21), DNA sequence analysis of selected regions using maternal plasma, algorithm reported as a risk score for each trisomy, includes sex reporting, if performed
CareView360, Newstar Medical Laboratories, LLC, Newstar Medical Laboratories, LLC	0328U	Drug assay, definitive, 120 or more drugs and metabolites, urine, quantitative liquid chromatography with tandem mass spectrometry (LC-MS/MS), includes specimen validity and algorithmic analysis describing drug or metabolite and presence or absence of risks for a significant patient-adverse event, per date of service
Oncomap™ ExTra, Exact Sciences, Inc, Genomic Health Inc	0329U	Oncology (neoplasia), exome and transcriptome sequence analysis for sequence variants, gene copy number amplifications and deletions, gene rearrangements, microsatellite instability and tumor mutational burden utilizing DNA and RNA from tumor with DNA from normal blood or saliva for subtraction, report of clinically significant mutation(s) with therapy associations
Bridge Women's Health Infectious Disease Detection Test, Bridge Diagnostics, Thermo Fisher and Hologic Test Kit on Panther Instrument	0330U	Infectious agent detection by nucleic acid (DNA or RNA), vaginal pathogen panel, identification of 27 organisms, amplified probe technique, vaginal swab
Augusta Hematology Optical Genome Mapping, Georgia Esoteric and Molecular Labs, Augusta University, Bionano	0331U	Oncology (hematolymphoid neoplasia), optical genome mapping for copy number alterations and gene rearrangements utilizing DNA from blood or bone marrow, report of clinically significant alterations
EpiSwitch® CiRT (Checkpoint-inhibitor Response Test), Next Bio-Research Services, LLC, Oxford BioDynamics, PLC	0332U	Oncology (pan-tumor), genetic profiling of 8 DNA-regulatory (epigenetic) markers by quantitative polymerase chain reaction (qPCR), whole blood, reported as a high or low probability of responding to immune checkpoint–inhibitor therapy

★=Telemedicine ◀=Audio-only ✚=Add-on code ✗=FDA approval pending #=Resequenced code ⊘=Modifier 51 exempt ➤➤➤=See p xxi for details

HelioLiver™ Test, Fulgent Genetics, LLC, Helio Health, Inc	0333U	Oncology (liver), surveillance for hepatocellular carcinoma (HCC) in high-risk patients, analysis of methylation patterns on circulating cell-free DNA (cfDNA) plus measurement of serum of AFP/AFP-L3 and oncoprotein des-gamma-carboxy-prothrombin (DCP), algorithm reported as normal or abnormal result
Guardant360 TissueNext™, Guardant Health, Inc, Guardant Health, Inc	0334U	Oncology (solid organ), targeted genomic sequence analysis, formalin-fixed paraffin-embedded (FFPE) tumor tissue, DNA analysis, 84 or more genes, interrogation for sequence variants, gene copy number amplifications, gene rearrangements, microsatellite instability and tumor mutational burden
IriSight™ Prenatal Analysis – Proband, Variantyx, Inc, Variantyx, Inc	0335U	Rare diseases (constitutional/heritable disorders), whole genome sequence analysis, including small sequence changes, copy number variants, deletions, duplications, mobile element insertions, uniparental disomy (UPD), inversions, aneuploidy, mitochondrial genome sequence analysis with heteroplasmy and large deletions, short tandem repeat (STR) gene expansions, fetal sample, identification and categorization of genetic variants (Do not report 0335U in conjunction with 81425, 0212U)
IriSight™ Prenatal Analysis – Comparator, Variantyx, Inc, Variantyx, Inc	0336U	Rare diseases (constitutional/heritable disorders), whole genome sequence analysis, including small sequence changes, copy number variants, deletions, duplications, mobile element insertions, uniparental disomy (UPD), inversions, aneuploidy, mitochondrial genome sequence analysis with heteroplasmy and large deletions, short tandem repeat (STR) gene expansions, blood or saliva, identification and categorization of genetic variants, each comparator genome (eg, parent) (Do not report 0336U in conjunction with 81426, 0213U)
CELLSEARCH® Circulating Multiple Myeloma Cell (CMMC) Test, Menarini Silicon Biosystems, Inc, Menarini Silicon Biosystems, Inc	0337U	Oncology (plasma cell disorders and myeloma), circulating plasma cell immunologic selection, identification, morphological characterization, and enumeration of plasma cells based on differential CD138, CD38, CD19, and CD45 protein biomarker expression, peripheral blood
CELLSEARCH® HER2 Circulating Tumor Cell (CTC-HER2) Test, Menarini Silicon Biosystems, Inc, Menarini Silicon Biosystems, Inc	0338U	Oncology (solid tumor), circulating tumor cell selection, identification, morphological characterization, detection and enumeration based on differential EpCAM, cytokeratins 8, 18, and 19, and CD45 protein biomarkers, and quantification of HER2 protein biomarker–expressing cells, peripheral blood

(Continued on page 1074)

SelectMDx® for Prostate Cancer, MDxHealth®, Inc, MDxHealth®, Inc	0339U	Oncology (prostate), mRNA expression profiling of *HOXC6* and *DLX1*, reverse transcription polymerase chain reaction (RT-PCR), first-void urine following digital rectal examination, algorithm reported as probability of high-grade cancer
Signatera™, Natera, Inc, Natera, Inc	0340U	Oncology (pan-cancer), analysis of minimal residual disease (MRD) from plasma, with assays personalized to each patient based on prior next-generation sequencing of the patient's tumor and germline DNA, reported as absence or presence of MRD, with disease-burden correlation, if appropriate
Single Cell Prenatal Diagnosis (SCPD) Test, Luna Genetics, Inc, Luna Genetics, Inc	0341U	Fetal aneuploidy DNA sequencing comparative analysis, fetal DNA from products of conception, reported as normal (euploidy), monosomy, trisomy, or partial deletion/duplication, mosaicism, and segmental aneuploid
IMMray® PanCan-d, Immunovia, Inc, Immunovia, Inc	0342U	Oncology (pancreatic cancer), multiplex immunoassay of C5, C4, cystatin C, factor B, osteoprotegerin (OPG), gelsolin, IGFBP3, CA125 and multiplex electrochemiluminescent immunoassay (ECLIA) for CA19-9, serum, diagnostic algorithm reported qualitatively as positive, negative, or borderline
miR Sentinel™ Prostate Cancer Test, miR Scientific, LLC, miR Scientific, LLC	0343U	Oncology (prostate), exosome-based analysis of 442 small noncoding RNAs (sncRNAs) by quantitative reverse transcription polymerase chain reaction (RT-qPCR), urine, reported as molecular evidence of no-, low-, intermediate- or high-risk of prostate cancer
OWLiver®, CIMA Sciences, LLC	0344U	Hepatology (nonalcoholic fatty liver disease [NAFLD]), semiquantitative evaluation of 28 lipid markers by liquid chromatography with tandem mass spectrometry (LC-MS/MS), serum, reported as at-risk for nonalcoholic steatohepatitis (NASH) or not NASH
GeneSight® Psychotropic, Assurex Health, Inc, Myriad Genetics, Inc	#0345U	Psychiatry (eg, depression, anxiety, attention deficit hyperactivity disorder [ADHD]), genomic analysis panel, variant analysis of 15 genes, including deletion/duplication analysis of *CYP2D6* (For additional PLA code with identical clinical descriptor, see 0411U. See Appendix O to determine appropriate code assignment)
QUEST AD-Detect™, Beta-Amyloid 42/40 Ratio, Plasma, Quest Diagnostics	0346U	Beta amyloid, Aβ40 and Aβ42 by liquid chromatography with tandem mass spectrometry (LC-MS/MS), ratio, plasma
RightMed® PGx16 Test, OneOme®, OneOme®, LLC	0347U	Drug metabolism or processing (multiple conditions), whole blood or buccal specimen, DNA analysis, 16 gene report, with variant analysis and reported phenotypes

RightMed® Comprehensive Test Exclude F2 and F5, OneOme®, OneOme®, LLC	0348U	Drug metabolism or processing (multiple conditions), whole blood or buccal specimen, DNA analysis, 25 gene report, with variant analysis and reported phenotypes
RightMed® Comprehensive Test, OneOme®, OneOme®, LLC	0349U	Drug metabolism or processing (multiple conditions), whole blood or buccal specimen, DNA analysis, 27 gene report, with variant analysis, including reported phenotypes and impacted gene-drug interactions
RightMed® Gene Report, OneOme®, OneOme®, LLC	0350U	Drug metabolism or processing (multiple conditions), whole blood or buccal specimen, DNA analysis, 27 gene report, with variant analysis and reported phenotypes
MeMed BV®, MeMed Diagnostics, Ltd, MeMed Diagnostics, Ltd	▲0351U	►Infectious disease (bacterial or viral), biochemical assays, tumor necrosis factor-related apoptosis-inducing ligand (TRAIL), interferon gamma-induced protein-10 (IP-10), and C-reactive protein, serum, or venous whole blood, algorithm reported as likelihood of bacterial infection◄
—	►(0352U has been deleted. To report infectious disease, bacterial vaginosis and vaginitis, real-time PCR amplification of DNA markers for algorithm reported as high likelihood of bacterial vaginosis, use 81515)◄	—
—	►(0353U has been deleted)◄	—
—	►(0354U has been deleted)◄	—
Apolipoprotein L1 (APOL1) Renal Risk Variant Genotyping, Quest Diagnostics®, Quest Diagnostics®	0355U	APOL1 (apolipoprotein L1) (eg, chronic kidney disease), risk variants (G1, G2)
NavDx®, Naveris, Inc, Naveris, Inc	▲0356U	►Oncology (oropharyngeal or anal), evaluation of 17 DNA biomarkers using droplet digital PCR (ddPCR), cell-free DNA, algorithm reported as a prognostic risk score for cancer recurrence◄
—	(0357U has been deleted)	—
Lumipulse® G β-Amyloid Ratio (1-42/1-40) Test, Fujirebio Diagnostics, Inc, Fujirebio Diagnostics, Inc	0358U	Neurology (mild cognitive impairment), analysis of β-amyloid 1-42 and 1-40, chemiluminescence enzyme immunoassay, cerebral spinal fluid, reported as positive, likely positive, or negative

(Continued on page 1076)

IsoPSA®, Cleveland Diagnostics, Inc, Cleveland Diagnostics, Inc	0359U	Oncology (prostate cancer), analysis of all prostate-specific antigen (PSA) structural isoforms by phase separation and immunoassay, plasma, algorithm reports risk of cancer
Nodify CDT®, Biodesix, Inc, Biodesix, Inc	0360U	Oncology (lung), enzyme-linked immunosorbent assay (ELISA) of 7 autoantibodies (p53, NY-ESO-1, CAGE, GBU4-5, SOX2, MAGE A4, and HuD), plasma, algorithm reported as a categorical result for risk of malignancy
Neurofilament Light Chain (NfL), Mayo Clinic, Mayo Clinic	0361U	Neurofilament light chain, digital immunoassay, plasma, quantitative
Thyroid GuidePx®, Protean BioDiagnostics, Qualisure Diagnostics	0362U	Oncology (papillary thyroid cancer), gene-expression profiling via targeted hybrid capture–enrichment RNA sequencing of 82 content genes and 10 housekeeping genes, fine needle aspirate or formalin-fixed paraffin-embedded (FFPE) tissue, algorithm reported as one of three molecular subtypes
Cxbladder™ Triage, Pacific Edge Diagnostics USA, Ltd, Pacific Edge Diagnostics USA, Ltd	0363U	Oncology (urothelial), mRNA, gene-expression profiling by real-time quantitative PCR of 5 genes (MDK, HOXA13, CDC2 [CDK1], IGFBP5, and CXCR2), utilizing urine, algorithm incorporates age, sex, smoking history, and macrohematuria frequency, reported as a risk score for having urothelial carcinoma
clonoSEQ® Assay, Adaptive Biotechnologies	0364U	Oncology (hematolymphoid neoplasm), genomic sequence analysis using multiplex (PCR) and next-generation sequencing with algorithm, quantification of dominant clonal sequence(s), reported as presence or absence of minimal residual disease (MRD) with quantitation of disease burden, when appropriate
Oncuria® Detect, DiaCarta Clinical Lab, DiaCarta, Inc	0365U	Oncology (bladder), analysis of 10 protein biomarkers (A1AT, ANG, APOE, CA9, IL8, MMP9, MMP10, PAI1, SDC1, and VEGFA) by immunoassays, urine, algorithm reported as a probability of bladder cancer
Oncuria® Monitor, DiaCarta Clinical Lab, DiaCarta, Inc	0366U	Oncology (bladder), analysis of 10 protein biomarkers (A1AT, ANG, APOE, CA9, IL8, MMP9, MMP10, PAI1, SDC1, and VEGFA) by immunoassays, urine, algorithm reported as a probability of recurrent bladder cancer
Oncuria® Predict, DiaCarta Clinical Lab, DiaCarta, Inc	0367U	Oncology (bladder), analysis of 10 protein biomarkers (A1AT, ANG, APOE, CA9, IL8, MMP9, MMP10, PAI1, SDC1, and VEGFA) by immunoassays, urine, diagnostic algorithm reported as a risk score for probability of rapid recurrence of recurrent or persistent cancer following transurethral resection

ColoScape™ Colorectal Cancer Detection, DiaCarta Clinical Lab, DiaCarta, Inc	0368U	Oncology (colorectal cancer), evaluation for mutations of *APC, BRAF, CTNNB1, KRAS, NRAS, PIK3CA, SMAD4,* and *TP53,* and methylation markers (MYO1G, KCNQ5, C9ORF50, FLI1, CLIP4, ZNF132, and TWIST1), multiplex quantitative polymerase chain reaction (qPCR), circulating cell-free DNA (cfDNA), plasma, report of risk score for advanced adenoma or colorectal cancer
GI assay (Gastrointestinal Pathogen with ABR), Lab Genomics LLC, Thermo Fisher Scientific	0369U	Infectious agent detection by nucleic acid (DNA and RNA), gastrointestinal pathogens, 31 bacterial, viral, and parasitic organisms and identification of 21 associated antibiotic-resistance genes, multiplex amplified probe technique
Lesion Infection (Wound), Lab Genomics LLC, Thermo Fisher Scientific	0370U	Infectious agent detection by nucleic acid (DNA and RNA), surgical wound pathogens, 34 microorganisms and identification of 21 associated antibiotic-resistance genes, multiplex amplified probe technique, wound swab
Qlear UTI, Lifescan Labs of Illinois, Thermo Fisher Scientific	0371U	Infectious agent detection by nucleic acid (DNA or RNA), genitourinary pathogen, semiquantitative identification, DNA from 16 bacterial organisms and 1 fungal organism, multiplex amplified probe technique via quantitative polymerase chain reaction (qPCR), urine
Qlear UTI - Reflex ABR, Lifescan Labs of Illinois, Thermo Fisher Scientific	0372U	Infectious disease (genitourinary pathogens), antibiotic-resistance gene detection, multiplex amplified probe technique, urine, reported as an antimicrobial stewardship risk score
Respiratory Pathogen with ABR (RPX), Lab Genomics LLC, Thermo Fisher Scientific	0373U	Infectious agent detection by nucleic acid (DNA and RNA), respiratory tract infection, 17 bacteria, 8 fungus, 13 virus, and 16 antibiotic-resistance genes, multiplex amplified probe technique, upper or lower respiratory specimen
Urogenital Pathogen with Rx Panel (UPX), Lab Genomics LLC, Thermo Fisher Scientific	0374U	Infectious agent detection by nucleic acid (DNA or RNA), genitourinary pathogens, identification of 21 bacterial and fungal organisms and identification of 21 associated antibiotic-resistance genes, multiplex amplified probe technique, urine
OvaWatch™, Aspira Women's Health™, Aspira Labs, Inc	0375U	Oncology (ovarian), biochemical assays of 7 proteins (follicle stimulating hormone, human epididymis protein 4, apolipoprotein A-1, transferrin, beta-2 macroglobulin, prealbumin [ie, transthyretin], and cancer antigen 125), algorithm reported as ovarian cancer risk score

(Continued on page 1078)

ArteraAI Prostate Test, Artera Inc®, Artera Inc®	0376U	Oncology (prostate cancer), image analysis of at least 128 histologic features and clinical factors, prognostic algorithm determining the risk of distant metastases, and prostate cancer-specific mortality, includes predictive algorithm to androgen deprivation-therapy response, if appropriate
Liposcale®, CIMA Sciences, LLC	0377U	Cardiovascular disease, quantification of advanced serum or plasma lipoprotein profile, by nuclear magnetic resonance (NMR) spectrometry with report of a lipoprotein profile (including 23 variables)
UCGSL *RFC1* Repeat Expansion Test, University of Chicago Genetic Services Laboratories	0378U	*RFC1 (replication factor C subunit 1),* repeat expansion variant analysis by traditional and repeat-primed PCR, blood, saliva, or buccal swab
Solid Tumor Expanded Panel, Quest Diagnostics®, Quest Diagnostics®	0379U	Targeted genomic sequence analysis panel, solid organ neoplasm, DNA (523 genes) and RNA (55 genes) by next-generation sequencing, interrogation for sequence variants, gene copy number amplifications, gene rearrangements, microsatellite instability, and tumor mutational burden
PersonalisedRX, Lab Genomics LLC, Agena Bioscience, Inc	0380U	Drug metabolism (adverse drug reactions and drug response), targeted sequence analysis, 20 gene variants and *CYP2D6* deletion or duplication analysis with reported genotype and phenotype
Branched-Chain Amino Acids, Self-Collect, Blood Spot, Mayo Clinic, Laboratory Developed Test	0381U	Maple syrup urine disease monitoring by patient-collected blood card sample, quantitative measurement of allo-isoleucine, leucine, isoleucine, and valine, liquid chromatography with tandem mass spectrometry (LC-MS/MS)
Phenylalanine and Tyrosine, Self-Collect, Blood Spot, Mayo Clinic, Laboratory Developed Test	0382U	Hyperphenylalaninemia monitoring by patient-collected blood card sample, quantitative measurement of phenylalanine and tyrosine, liquid chromatography with tandem mass spectrometry (LC-MS/MS)
Tyrosinemia Follow-Up Panel, Self-Collect, Blood Spot, Mayo Clinic, Laboratory Developed Test	0383U	Tyrosinemia type I monitoring by patient-collected blood card sample, quantitative measurement of tyrosine, phenylalanine, methionine, succinylacetone, nitisinone, liquid chromatography with tandem mass spectrometry (LC-MS/MS)
NaviDKD™ Predictive Diagnostic Screening for Kidney Health, Journey Biosciences, Inc, Journey Biosciences, Inc	0384U	Nephrology (chronic kidney disease), carboxymethyl-lysine, methylglyoxal hydroimidazolone, and carboxy-ethyl lysine by liquid chromatography with tandem mass spectrometry (LC-MS/MS) and HbA1c and estimated glomerular filtration rate (GFR), with risk score reported for predictive progression to high-stage kidney disease

PromarkerD, Sonic Reference Laboratory, Proteomics International Pty Ltd	0385U	Nephrology (chronic kidney disease), apolipoprotein A4 (ApoA4), CD5 antigen-like (CD5L), and insulin-like growth factor binding protein 3 (IGFBP3) by enzyme-linked immunoassay (ELISA), plasma, algorithm combining results with HDL, estimated glomerular filtration rate (GFR) and clinical data reported as a risk score for developing diabetic kidney disease
—	(0386U has been deleted)	—
AMBLor® melanoma prognostic test, Avero® Diagnostics	0387U	Oncology (melanoma), autophagy and beclin 1 regulator 1 (AMBRA1) and loricrin (AMLo) by immunohistochemistry, formalin-fixed paraffin-embedded (FFPE) tissue, report for risk of progression (Do not report 0387U in conjunction with 88341, 88342)
InVisionFirst®-Lung Liquid Biopsy, Inivata, Inc, Inivata, Inc	0388U	Oncology (non-small cell lung cancer), next-generation sequencing with identification of single nucleotide variants, copy number variants, insertions and deletions, and structural variants in 37 cancer-related genes, plasma, with report for alteration detection
KawasakiDx, OncoOmicsDx Laboratory, mProbe	0389U	Pediatric febrile illness (Kawasaki disease [KD]), interferon alpha-inducible protein 27 (IFI27) and mast cell-expressed membrane protein 1 (MCEMP1), RNA, using quantitative reverse transcription polymerase chain reaction (RT-qPCR), blood, reported as a risk score for KD
PEPredictDx, OncoOmicsDx Laboratory, mProbe	0390U	Obstetrics (preeclampsia), kinase insert domain receptor (KDR), Endoglin (ENG), and retinol-binding protein 4 (RBP4), by immunoassay, serum, algorithm reported as a risk score
Strata Select™, Strata Oncology, Inc, Strata Oncology, Inc	0391U	Oncology (solid tumor), DNA and RNA by next-generation sequencing, utilizing formalin-fixed paraffin-embedded (FFPE) tissue, 437 genes, interpretive report for single nucleotide variants, splice-site variants, insertions/deletions, copy number alterations, gene fusions, tumor mutational burden, and microsatellite instability, with algorithm quantifying immunotherapy response score
Medication Management Neuropsychiatric Panel, RCA Laboratory Services LLC d/b/a GENETWORx, GENETWORx	0392U	Drug metabolism (depression, anxiety, attention deficit hyperactivity disorder [ADHD]), gene-drug interactions, variant analysis of 16 genes, including deletion/duplication analysis of *CYP2D6*, reported as impact of gene-drug interaction for each drug

(Continued on page 1080)

SYNTap® Biomarker Test, Amprion Clinical Laboratory, Amprion Clinical Laboratory	0393U	Neurology (eg, Parkinson disease, dementia with Lewy bodies), cerebrospinal fluid (CSF), detection of misfolded β-synuclein protein by seed amplification assay, qualitative
PFAS Testing & PFASure™, National Medical Services, NMS Labs, Inc	0394U	Perfluoroalkyl substances (PFAS) (eg, perfluorooctanoic acid, perfluorooctane sulfonic acid), 16 PFAS compounds by liquid chromatography with tandem mass spectrometry (LC-MS/MS), plasma or serum, quantitative
OncobiotaLUNG, Micronoma™, Micronoma™	0395U	Oncology (lung), multi-omics (microbial DNA by shotgun next-generation sequencing and carcinoembryonic antigen and osteopontin by immunoassay), plasma, algorithm reported as malignancy risk for lung nodules in early-stage disease
—	▶(0396U has been deleted)◀	—
—	(0397U has been deleted)	—
ESOPREDICT® Barrett's Esophagus Risk Classifier Assay, Capsulomics, Inc d/b/a Previse	0398U	Gastroenterology (Barrett's esophagus), *P16, RUNX3, HPP1,* and *FBN1* DNA methylation analysis using PCR, formalin-fixed paraffin-embedded (FFPE) tissue, algorithm reported as risk score for progression to high-grade dysplasia or cancer
FRAT® (Folate Receptor Antibody Test), Religen Inc, Religen Inc	0399U	Neurology (cerebral folate deficiency), serum, detection of anti-human folate receptor IgG-binding antibody and blocking autoantibodies by enzyme-linked immunoassay (ELISA), qualitative, and blocking autoantibodies, using a functional blocking assay for IgG or IgM, quantitative, reported as positive or not detected
Genesys Carrier Panel, Genesys Diagnostics, Inc	0400U	Obstetrics (expanded carrier screening), 145 genes by next-generation sequencing, fragment analysis and multiplex ligation-dependent probe amplification, DNA, reported as carrier positive or negative
CARDIO inCode-Score (CIC-SCORE), GENinCode U.S. Inc, GENinCode U.S. Inc	0401U	Cardiology (coronary heart disease [CHD]), 9 genes (12 variants), targeted variant genotyping, blood, saliva, or buccal swab, algorithm reported as a genetic risk score for a coronary event
Abbott Alinity™ m STI Assay, Abbott Molecular, Inc	0402U	Infectious agent (sexually transmitted infection), Chlamydia trachomatis, Neisseria gonorrhoeae, Trichomonas vaginalis, Mycoplasma genitalium, multiplex amplified probe technique, vaginal, endocervical, or male urine, each pathogen reported as detected or not detected
MyProstateScore 2.0, LynxDX, LynxDX	▲0403U	▶Oncology (prostate), mRNA, gene expression profiling of 18 genes, first-catch urine, algorithm reported as percentage of likelihood of detecting clinically significant prostate cancer◀

DiviTum®TKa, Biovica Inc, Biovica International AB	0404U	Oncology (breast), semiquantitative measurement of thymidine kinase activity by immunoassay, serum, results reported as risk of disease progression
BTG Early Detection of Pancreatic Cancer, Breakthrough Genomics, Breakthrough Genomics	0405U	Oncology (pancreatic), 59 methylation haplotype block markers, next-generation sequencing, plasma, reported as cancer signal detected or not detected
CyPath® Lung, Precision Pathology Services, bioAffinity Technologies, Inc	0406U	Oncology (lung), flow cytometry, sputum, 5 markers (meso-tetra [4-carboxyphenyl] porphyrin [TCPP], CD206, CD66b, CD3, CD19), algorithm reported as likelihood of lung cancer
▶kidneyintelX.dkd™◀, Renalytix Inc, Renalytix Inc, NYC, NY	0407U	Nephrology (diabetic chronic kidney disease [CKD]), multiplex electrochemiluminescent immunoassay (ECLIA) of soluble tumor necrosis factor receptor 1 (sTNFR1), soluble tumor necrosis receptor 2 (sTNFR2), and kidney injury molecule 1 (KIM-1) combined with clinical data, plasma, algorithm reported as risk for progressive decline in kidney function
Omnia™ SARS-CoV-2 Antigen Test, Qorvo Biotechnologies, Qorvo Biotechnologies	0408U	Infectious agent antigen detection by bulk acoustic wave biosensor immunoassay, severe acute respiratory syndrome coronavirus 2 (SARS-CoV-2) (coronavirus disease [COVID-19])
LiquidHALLMARK®, Lucence Health, Inc	0409U	Oncology (solid tumor), DNA (80 genes) and RNA (36 genes), by next-generation sequencing from plasma, including single nucleotide variants, insertions/deletions, copy number alterations, microsatellite instability, and fusions, report showing identified mutations with clinical actionability
Avantect™ Pancreatic Cancer Test, ClearNote™ Health, ClearNote™ Health	0410U	Oncology (pancreatic), DNA, whole genome sequencing with 5-hydroxymethylcytosine enrichment, whole blood or plasma, algorithm reported as cancer detected or not detected
IDgenetix®, Castle Biosciences, Inc, Castle Biosciences, Inc	⋇0411U	Psychiatry (eg, depression, anxiety, attention deficit hyperactivity disorder [ADHD]), genomic analysis panel, variant analysis of 15 genes, including deletion/duplication analysis of *CYP2D6* (For additional PLA code with identical clinical descriptor, see 0345U. See Appendix O to determine appropriate code assignment)
PrecivityAD® blood test, C2N Diagnostics LLC, C2N Diagnostics LLC	0412U	Beta amyloid, Aβ42/40 ratio, immunoprecipitation with quantitation by liquid chromatography with tandem mass spectrometry (LC-MS/MS) and qualitative ApoE isoform-specific proteotyping, plasma combined with age, algorithm reported as presence or absence of brain amyloid pathology

(Continued on page 1082)

DH Optical Genome Mapping/ Digital Karyotyping Assay, The Clinical Genomics and Advanced Technology (CGAT) Laboratory at Dartmouth Health, Bionano Genomics	0413U	Oncology (hematolymphoid neoplasm), optical genome mapping for copy number alterations, aneuploidy, and balanced/complex structural rearrangements, DNA from blood or bone marrow, report of clinically significant alterations
LungOI, Imagene	0414U	Oncology (lung), augmentative algorithmic analysis of digitized whole slide imaging for 8 genes (*ALK, BRAF, EGFR, ERBB2, MET, NTRK1-3, RET, ROS1*), and *KRAS* G12C and PD-L1, if performed, formalin-fixed paraffin-embedded (FFPE) tissue, reported as positive or negative for each biomarker
SmartHealth Vascular Dx™, Morningstar Laboratories, LLC, SmartHealth DX	0415U	Cardiovascular disease (acute coronary syndrome [ACS]), IL-16, FAS, FASLigand, HGF, CTACK, EOTAXIN, and MCP-3 by immunoassay combined with age, sex, family history, and personal history of diabetes, blood, algorithm reported as a 5-year (deleted risk) score for ACS
—	▶(0416U has been deleted)◀	—
Genomic Unity® Comprehensive Mitochondrial Disorders Analysis, Variantyx Inc, Variantyx Inc	0417U	Rare diseases (constitutional/heritable disorders), whole mitochondrial genome sequence with heteroplasmy detection and deletion analysis, nuclear-encoded mitochondrial gene analysis of 335 nuclear genes, including sequence changes, deletions, insertions, and copy number variants analysis, blood or saliva, identification and categorization of mitochondrial disorder–associated genetic variants
PreciseDx Breast Biopsy Test, PreciseDx, PreciseDx, Inc NYC, NY	0418U	Oncology (breast), augmentative algorithmic analysis of digitized whole slide imaging of 8 histologic and immunohistochemical features, reported as a recurrence score
Tempus nP, Tempus Labs, Inc, Tempus Labs, Inc	0419U	Neuropsychiatry (eg, depression, anxiety), genomic sequence analysis panel, variant analysis of 13 genes, saliva or buccal swab, report of each gene phenotype
▶Cxbladder Detect+, Pacific Edge Diagnostics USA LTD, Pacific Edge Diagnostics USA LTD◀	●0420U	▶Oncology (urothelial), mRNA expression profiling by real-time quantitative PCR of *MDK, HOXA13, CDC2, IGFBP5,* and *CXCR2* in combination with droplet digital PCR (ddPCR) analysis of 6 single-nucleotide polymorphisms (SNPs) of genes *TERT* and *FGFR3,* urine, algorithm reported as a risk score for urothelial carcinoma◀
▶Colosense™, Geneoscopy, Inc, Geneoscopy, Inc◀	●0421U	▶Oncology (colorectal) screening, quantitative real-time target and signal amplification of 8 RNA markers (*GAPDH, SMAD4, ACY1, AREG, CDH1, KRAS, TNFRSF10B, EGLN2*) and fecal hemoglobin, algorithm reported as a positive or negative for colorectal cancer risk◀

▶Guardant360 Response™, Guardant Health, Inc, Guardant Health, Inc◀	●0422U	▶Oncology (pan-solid tumor), analysis of DNA biomarker response to anti-cancer therapy using cell-free circulating DNA, biomarker comparison to a previous baseline pre-treatment cell-free circulating DNA analysis using next-generation sequencing, algorithm reported as a quantitative change from baseline, including specific alterations, if appropriate◀
▶Genomind® Pharmacogenetics Report – Full, Genomind®, Inc, Genomind®, Inc◀	●0423U	▶Psychiatry (eg, depression, anxiety), genomic analysis panel, including variant analysis of 26 genes, buccal swab, report including metabolizer status and risk of drug toxicity by condition◀
▶miR Sentinel™ Prostate Cancer Test, miR Scientific®, LLC, miR Scientific®, LLC◀	●0424U	▶Oncology (prostate), exosome-based analysis of 53 small noncoding RNAs (sncRNAs) by quantitative reverse transcription polymerase chain reaction (RT-qPCR), urine, reported as no molecular evidence, low-, moderate-, or elevated-risk of prostate cancer◀
▶RCIGM Rapid Whole Genome Sequencing, Comparator Genome, Rady Children's Institute for Genomic Medicine, Rady Children's Institute for Genomic Medicine◀	●0425U	▶Genome (eg, unexplained constitutional or heritable disorder or syndrome), rapid sequence analysis, each comparator genome (eg, parents, siblings)◀
▶RCIGM Ultra-Rapid Whole Genome Sequencing, Rady Children's Institute for Genomic Medicine, Rady Children's Institute for Genomic Medicine◀	●0426U	▶Genome (eg, unexplained constitutional or heritable disorder or syndrome), ultra-rapid sequence analysis◀
▶Early Sepsis Indicator, Beckman Coulter, Inc◀	+●0427U	▶Monocyte distribution width, whole blood (List separately in addition to code for primary procedure)◀ ▶(Use 0427U in conjunction with 85004, 85025)◀
▶Epic Sciences ctDNA Metastatic Breast Cancer Panel, Epic Sciences, Inc, Epic Sciences, Inc◀	●0428U	▶Oncology (breast), targeted hybrid-capture genomic sequence analysis panel, circulating tumor DNA (ctDNA) analysis of 56 or more genes, interrogation for sequence variants, gene copy number amplifications, gene rearrangements, microsatellite instability, and tumor mutation burden◀
▶Omnipathology Oropharyngeal HPV PCR Test, OmniPathology Solutions, Medical Corporation, OmniPathology Solutions, Medical Corporation◀	●0429U	▶Human papillomavirus (HPV), oropharyngeal swab, 14 high-risk types (ie, 16, 18, 31, 33, 35, 39, 45, 51, 52, 56, 58, 59, 66, and 68)◀

(Continued on page 1084)

▲=Revised code   ●=New code   ▶◀=Contains new or revised text   ✕=Duplicate PLA test   ↑↓=Category I PLA

▶Malabsorption Evaluation Panel, Mayo Clinic/Mayo Clinic Laboratories, Mayo Clinic/Mayo Clinic Laboratories◀	●0430U	▶Gastroenterology, malabsorption evaluation of alpha-1-antitrypsin, calprotectin, pancreatic elastase and reducing substances, feces, quantitative◀
▶Glycine Receptor Alpha1 IgG, Mayo Clinic/Mayo Clinic Laboratories, Mayo Clinic/Mayo Clinic Laboratories◀	●0431U	▶Glycine receptor alpha1 IgG, serum or cerebrospinal fluid (CSF), live cell-binding assay (LCBA), qualitative◀
▶Kelch-Like Protein 11 Antibody, Mayo Clinic/Mayo Clinic Laboratories, Mayo Clinic/Mayo Clinic Laboratories◀	●0432U	▶Kelch-like protein 11 (KLHL11) antibody, serum or cerebrospinal fluid (CSF), cell-binding assay, qualitative◀
▶EpiSwitch® Prostate Screening Test (PSE), Oxford BioDynamics Inc, Oxford BioDynamics PLC◀	●0433U	▶Oncology (prostate), 5 DNA regulatory markers by quantitative PCR, whole blood, algorithm, including prostate-specific antigen, reported as likelihood of cancer◀
▶RightMed® Gene Test Exclude F2 and F5, OneOme® LLC, OneOme® LLC◀	●0434U	▶Drug metabolism (adverse drug reactions and drug response), genomic analysis panel, variant analysis of 25 genes with reported phenotypes◀
▶ChemoID®, ChemoID® Lab, Cordgenics, LLC◀	●0435U	▶Oncology, chemotherapeutic drug cytotoxicity assay of cancer stem cells (CSCs), from cultured CSCs and primary tumor cells, categorical drug response reported based on cytotoxicity percentage observed, minimum of 14 drugs or drug combinations◀
▶PROphet® NSCLC Test, OncoHost, Inc, OncoHost, Inc◀	●0436U	▶Oncology (lung), plasma analysis of 388 proteins, using aptamer-based proteomics technology, predictive algorithm reported as clinical benefit from immune checkpoint inhibitor therapy◀
▶MindX One™ Blood Test – Anxiety, MindX Sciences, MindX Sciences◀	●0437U	▶Psychiatry (anxiety disorders), mRNA, gene expression profiling by RNA sequencing of 15 biomarkers, whole blood, algorithm reported as predictive risk score◀
▶EffectiveRX™ Comprehensive Panel, RCA Laboratory Services LLC d/b/a GENETWORx, GENETWORx◀	●0438U	▶Drug metabolism (adverse drug reactions and drug response), buccal specimen, gene-drug interactions, variant analysis of 33 genes, including deletion/duplication analysis of *CYP2D6*, including reported phenotypes and impacted gene-drug interactions◀

▶Epi+Gen CHD™, Cardio Diagnostics, Inc, Cardio Diagnostics, Inc◀	●0439U	▶Cardiology (coronary heart disease [CHD]), DNA, analysis of 5 single-nucleotide polymorphisms (SNPs) (rs11716050 [LOC105376934], rs6560711 [WDR37], rs3735222 [SCIN/LOC107986769], rs6820447 [intergenic], and rs9638144 [ESYT2]) and 3 DNA methylation markers (cg00300879 [transcription start site {TSS200} of CNKSR1], cg09552548 [intergenic], and cg14789911 [body of SPATC1L]), qPCR and digital PCR, whole blood, algorithm reported as a 4-tiered risk score for a 3-year risk of symptomatic CHD◀
▶PrecisionCHD™, Cardio Diagnostics, Inc, Cardio Diagnostics, Inc◀	●0440U	▶Cardiology (coronary heart disease [CHD]), DNA, analysis of 10 single-nucleotide polymorphisms (SNPs) (rs710987 [LINC010019], rs1333048 [CDKN2B-AS1], rs12129789 [KCND3], rs942317 [KTN1-AS1], rs1441433 [PPP3CA], rs2869675 [PREX1], rs4639796 [ZBTB41], rs4376434 [LINC00972], rs12714414 [TMEM18], and rs7585056 [TMEM18]) and 6 DNA methylation markers (cg03725309 [SARS1], cg12586707 [CXCL1], cg04988978 [MPO], cg17901584 [DHCR24-DT], cg21161138 [AHRR], and cg12655112 [EHD4]), qPCR and digital PCR, whole blood, algorithm reported as detected or not detected for CHD◀
▶IntelliSep® test, Cytovale®◀	●0441U	▶Infectious disease (bacterial, fungal, or viral infection), semiquantitative biomechanical assessment (via deformability cytometry), whole blood, with algorithmic analysis and result reported as an index◀
▶FebriDx® Bacterial/Non-Bacterial Point-of-Care Assay, Lumos Diagnostics, LLC, Lumos Diagnostics, LLC◀	●0442U	▶Infectious disease (respiratory infection), Myxovirus resistance protein A (MxA) and C-reactive protein (CRP), fingerstick whole blood specimen, each biomarker reported as present or absent◀
▶Neurofilament Light Chain (NfL), Neuromuscular Clinical Laboratory at Washington University in St. Louis School of Medicine, Neuromuscular Clinical Laboratory at Washington University in St. Louis School of Medicine◀	●0443U	▶Neurofilament light chain (NfL), ultra-sensitive immunoassay, serum or cerebrospinal fluid◀
▶Aventa FusionPlus™, Aventa Genomics, LLC◀	●0444U	▶Oncology (solid organ neoplasia), targeted genomic sequence analysis panel of 361 genes, interrogation for gene fusions, translocations, or other rearrangements, using DNA from formalin-fixed paraffin-embedded (FFPE) tumor tissue, report of clinically significant variant(s)◀

(Continued on page 1086)

▶Elecsys® Phospho-Tau (181P) CSF (pTau181) and β-Amyloid (1-42) CSF II (Abeta 42) Ratio, Roche Diagnostics Operations, Inc (US owner/operator)◀	●0445U	▶β-amyloid (Abeta42) and phospho tau (181P) (pTau181), electrochemiluminescent immunoassay (ECLIA), cerebral spinal fluid, ratio reported as positive or negative for amyloid pathology◀
▶aisle® DX Disease Activity Index, Progentec Diagnostics, Inc, Progentec Diagnostics, Inc◀	●0446U	▶Autoimmune diseases (systemic lupus erythematosus [SLE]), analysis of 10 cytokine soluble mediator biomarkers by immunoassay, plasma, individual components reported with an algorithmic risk score for current disease activity◀
▶aisle® DX Flare Risk Index, Progentec Diagnostics, Inc, Progentec Diagnostics, Inc◀	●0447U	▶Autoimmune diseases (systemic lupus erythematosus [SLE]), analysis of 11 cytokine soluble mediator biomarkers by immunoassay, plasma, individual components reported with an algorithmic prognostic risk score for developing a clinical flare◀
▶oncoReveal™ DX Lung and Colon Cancer Assay, Pillar® Biosciences, Pillar® Biosciences◀	●0448U	▶Oncology (lung and colon cancer), DNA, qualitative, next-generation sequencing detection of single-nucleotide variants and deletions in *EGFR* and *KRAS* genes, formalin-fixed paraffin-embedded (FFPE) solid tumor samples, reported as presence or absence of targeted mutation(s), with recommended therapeutic options◀
▶UNITY Carrier Screen™, BillionToOne Laboratory, BillionToOne, Inc◀	●0449U	▶Carrier screening for severe inherited conditions (eg, cystic fibrosis, spinal muscular atrophy, beta hemoglobinopathies [including sickle cell disease], alpha thalassemia), regardless of race or self-identified ancestry, genomic sequence analysis panel, must include analysis of 5 genes *(CFTR, SMN1, HBB, HBA1, HBA2)*◀
▶M-inSight® Patient Definition Assay, Corgenix Clinical Laboratory, Sebia◀	●0450U	▶Oncology (multiple myeloma), liquid chromatography with tandem mass spectrometry (LC-MS/MS), monoclonal paraprotein sequencing analysis, serum, results reported as baseline presence or absence of detectable clonotypic peptides◀
▶M-inSight® Patient Follow-Up Assessment, Corgenix Clinical Laboratory, Sebia◀	●0451U	▶Oncology (multiple myeloma), LC-MS/MS, peptide ion quantification, serum, results compared with baseline to determine monoclonal paraprotein abundance◀
▶EarlyTect® Bladder Cancer Detection (EarlyTect® BCD), Promis Diagnostics, Inc, Promis Diagnostics, Inc◀	●0452U	▶Oncology (bladder), methylated *PENK* DNA detection by linear target enrichment-quantitative methylation-specific real-time PCR (LTE-qMSP), urine, reported as likelihood of bladder cancer◀
▶ColonAiQ®, Breakthrough Genomics, Singlera Genomics, Inc◀	●0453U	▶Oncology (colorectal cancer), cell-free DNA (cfDNA), methylation-based quantitative PCR assay *(SEPTIN9, IKZF1, BCAT1,* Septin9-2, *VAV3, BCAN)*, plasma, reported as presence or absence of circulating tumor DNA (ctDNA)◀

▶Chromosome Genome Mapping, UR Medicine Labs, Bionano Genomics, Inc◀	✣●0454U	▶Rare diseases (constitutional/heritable disorders), identification of copy number variations, inversions, insertions, translocations, and other structural variants by optical genome mapping◀
		▶(For additional PLA codes with identical clinical descriptor, see 0260U, 0264U. See Appendix O or the most current listing on the AMA CPT website to determine appropriate code assignment)◀
▶Abbott Alinity™ m STI Assay, Abbott Molecular, Inc◀	●0455U	▶Infectious agents (sexually transmitted infection), Chlamydia trachomatis, Neisseria gonorrhoeae, and Trichomonas vaginalis, multiplex amplified probe technique, vaginal, endocervical, gynecological specimens, oropharyngeal swabs, rectal swabs, female or male urine, each pathogen reported as detected or not detected◀
▶PrismRA®, Scipher Medicine®, Scipher Medicine®◀	●0456U	▶Autoimmune (rheumatoid arthritis), next-generation sequencing (NGS), gene expression testing of 19 genes, whole blood, with analysis of anti-cyclic citrullinated peptides (CCP) levels, combined with sex, patient global assessment, and body mass index (BMI), algorithm reported as a score that predicts nonresponse to tumor necrosis factor inhibitor (TNFi) therapy◀
▶PFAS (Forever Chemicals) 9 Panel, Quest Diagnostics®, Quest Diagnostics®◀	●0457U	▶Perfluoroalkyl substances (PFAS) (eg, perfluorooctanoic acid, perfluorooctane sulfonic acid), 9 PFAS compounds by LC-MS/MS, plasma or serum, quantitative◀
▶Auria®, Namida Lab, Inc, Namida Lab, Inc◀	●0458U	▶Oncology (breast cancer), S100A8 and S100A9, by enzyme-linked immunosorbent assay (ELISA), tear fluid with age, algorithm reported as a risk score◀
▶Elecsys® Total Tau CSF (tTau) and β-Amyloid (1-42) CSF II (Abeta 42) Ratio, Roche Diagnostics Operations, Inc (US owner/operator)◀	●0459U	▶β-amyloid (Abeta42) and total tau (tTau), electrochemiluminescent immunoassay (ECLIA), cerebral spinal fluid, ratio reported as positive or negative for amyloid pathology◀
▶RightMed® Oncology Gene Report, OneOme® LLC, OneOme® LLC◀	●0460U	▶Oncology, whole blood or buccal, DNA single-nucleotide polymorphism (SNP) genotyping by real-time PCR of 24 genes, with variant analysis and reported phenotypes◀
▶RightMed® Oncology Medication Report, OneOme® LLC, OneOme® LLC◀	●0461U	▶Oncology, pharmacogenomic analysis of single-nucleotide polymorphism (SNP) genotyping by real-time PCR of 24 genes, whole blood or buccal swab, with variant analysis, including impacted gene-drug interactions and reported phenotypes◀

(Continued on page 1088)

►Salimetrics® Salivary Melatonin Profile (Circadian Phase Assessment), Salimetrics® Clinical Laboratory, Salimetrics®, LLC◄	●0462U	►Melatonin levels test, sleep study, 7 or 9 sample melatonin profile (cortisol optional), enzyme-linked immunosorbent assay (ELISA), saliva, screening/preliminary◄
►Proofer '7 HPV mRNA E6 and E7 Biomarker Test, Global Diagnostics Labs, LLC, PreTect AS, a Mel-Mont Medical, Inc, wholly owned subsidiary◄	●0463U	►Oncology (cervix), mRNA gene expression profiling of 14 biomarkers (E6 and E7 of the highest-risk human papillomavirus [HPV] types 16, 18, 31, 33, 45, 52, 58), by real-time nucleic acid sequence-based amplification (NASBA), exo- or endocervical epithelial cells, algorithm reported as positive or negative for increased risk of cervical dysplasia or cancer for each biomarker◄
►Cologuard Plus™, Exact Sciences Laboratories, LLC, Exact Sciences Corporation◄	●0464U	►Oncology (colorectal) screening, quantitative real-time target and signal amplification, methylated DNA markers, including LASS4, LRRC4 and PPP2R5C, a reference marker ZDHHC1, and a protein marker (fecal hemoglobin), utilizing stool, algorithm reported as a positive or negative result◄
►UriFind® Urothelial Carcinoma Assay, DiaCarta, Inc, AnchorDx◄	●0465U	►Oncology (urothelial carcinoma), DNA, quantitative methylation-specific PCR of 2 genes *(ONECUT2, VIM)*, algorithmic analysis reported as positive or negative◄
►CardioRisk+, Gene by Gene, Ltd, OpenDNA, Ltd◄	●0466U	►Cardiology (coronary artery disease [CAD]), DNA, genome-wide association studies (564856 single-nucleotide polymorphisms [SNPs], targeted variant genotyping), patient lifestyle and clinical data, buccal swab, algorithm reported as polygenic risk to acquired heart disease◄
►UroAmp MRD, Convergent Genomics, Inc, Convergent Genomics, Inc◄	●0467U	►Oncology (bladder), DNA, next-generation sequencing (NGS) of 60 genes and whole genome aneuploidy, urine, algorithms reported as minimal residual disease (MRD) status positive or negative and quantitative disease burden◄
►NASHnext™ (NIS4™), Labcorp, Labcorp◄	●0468U	►Hepatology (nonalcoholic steatohepatitis [NASH]), miR-34a-5p, alpha 2-macroglobulin, YKL40, HbA1c, serum and whole blood, algorithm reported as a single score for NASH activity and fibrosis◄

Appendix O

▶IriSight™ CNV Analysis, Variantyx Inc, Variantyx Inc◀	●0469U	▶Rare diseases (constitutional/heritable disorders), whole genome sequence analysis for chromosomal abnormalities, copy number variants, duplications/deletions, inversions, unbalanced translocations, regions of homozygosity (ROH), inheritance pattern that indicate uniparental disomy (UPD), and aneuploidy, fetal sample (amniotic fluid, chorionic villus sample, or products of conception), identification and categorization of genetic variants, diagnostic report of fetal results based on phenotype with maternal sample and paternal sample, if performed, as comparators and/or maternal cell contamination◀
▶HPV-SEQ Test, Sysmex Inostics, Inc, Sysmex Inostics, Inc◀	●0470U	▶Oncology (oropharyngeal), detection of minimal residual disease by next-generation sequencing (NGS) based quantitative evaluation of 8 DNA targets, cell-free HPV 16 and 18 DNA from plasma◀
▶CRCdx® RAS Mutation Detection Kit, EntroGen, Inc, EntroGen, Inc◀	●0471U	▶Oncology (colorectal cancer), qualitative real-time PCR of 35 variants of *KRAS* and *NRAS* genes (exons 2, 3, 4), formalin-fixed paraffin-embedded (FFPE), predictive, identification of detected mutations◀
▶Early Sjögren's Syndrome Profile, Immco Diagnostics, Inc, Immco Diagnostics, Inc◀	●0472U	▶Carbonic anhydrase VI (CA VI), parotid specific/secretory protein (PSP) and salivary protein (SP1) IgG, IgM, and IgA antibodies, enzyme-linked immunosorbent assay (ELISA), semiqualitative, blood, reported as predictive evidence of early Sjögren's syndrome◀
▶xT CDx, Tempus AI, Inc, Tempus AI, Inc◀	●0473U	▶Oncology (solid tumor), next-generation sequencing (NGS) of DNA from formalin-fixed paraffin-embedded (FFPE) tissue with comparative sequence analysis from a matched normal specimen (blood or saliva), 648 genes, interrogation for sequence variants, insertion and deletion alterations, copy number variants, rearrangements, microsatellite instability, and tumor-mutation burden◀
▶GeneticsNow® Comprehensive Germline Panel, GoPath Diagnostics, Inc, GoPath Diagnostics, Inc◀	●0474U	▶Hereditary pan-cancer (eg, hereditary sarcomas, hereditary endocrine tumors, hereditary neuroendocrine tumors, hereditary cutaneous melanoma), genomic sequence analysis panel of 88 genes with 20 duplications/deletions using next-generation sequencing (NGS), Sanger sequencing, blood or saliva, reported as positive or negative for germline variants, each gene◀

(Continued on page 1090)

▶ProstateNow™ Prostate Germline Panel, GoPath Diagnostics, Inc, GoPath Diagnostics, Inc◀	●0475U	▶Hereditary prostate cancer-related disorders, genomic sequence analysis panel using next-generation sequencing (NGS), Sanger sequencing, multiplex ligation-dependent probe amplification (MLPA), and array comparative genomic hybridization (CGH), evaluation of 23 genes and duplications/deletions when indicated, pathologic mutations reported with a genetic risk score for prostate cancer◀
▶RightMed® Mental Health Gene Report, OneOme, LLC, OneOme, LLC◀	●0476U	▶Drug metabolism, psychiatry (eg, major depressive disorder, general anxiety disorder, attention deficit hyperactivity disorder [ADHD], schizophrenia), whole blood, buccal swab, and pharmacogenomic genotyping of 14 genes and *CYP2D6* copy number variant analysis and reported phenotypes◀
▶RightMed® Mental Health Medication Report, OneOme, LLC, OneOme, LLC◀	●0477U	▶Drug metabolism, psychiatry (eg, major depressive disorder, general anxiety disorder, attention deficit hyperactivity disorder [ADHD], schizophrenia), whole blood, buccal swab, and pharmacogenomic genotyping of 14 genes and *CYP2D6* copy number variant analysis, including impacted gene-drug interactions and reported phenotypes◀
▶Lung HDPCR™, Protean BioDiagnostics, Protean BioDiagnostics◀	●0478U	▶Oncology (non-small cell lung cancer), DNA and RNA, digital PCR analysis of 9 genes (*EGFR, KRAS, BRAF, ALK, ROS1, RET, NTRK 1/2/3, ERBB2,* and *MET*) in formalin-fixed paraffin-embedded (FFPE) tissue, interrogation for single-nucleotide variants, insertions/deletions, gene rearrangements, and reported as actionable detected variants for therapy selection◀
▶ALZpath pTau217, Neurocode USA, Inc, Quanterix/ALZpath◀	●0479U	▶Tau, phosphorylated, pTau217◀
▶Bacteria, Viruses, Fungus, and Parasite Metagenomic Sequencing, Spinal Fluid (MSCSF), Mayo Clinic, Laboratory Developed Test◀	●0480U	▶Infectious disease (bacteria, viruses, fungi, and parasites), cerebrospinal fluid (CSF), metagenomic next-generation sequencing (DNA and RNA), bioinformatic analysis, with positive pathogen identification◀
▶IDH1, IDH2, and TERT Mutation Analysis, Next-Generation Sequencing, Tumor (IDTRT), Mayo Clinic, Laboratory Developed Test◀	●0481U	▶*IDH1 (isocitrate dehydrogenase 1 [NADP+]), IDH2 (isocitrate dehydrogenase 2 [NADP+]),* and *TERT (telomerase reverse transcriptase)* promoter (eg, central nervous system [CNS] tumors), next-generation sequencing (single-nucleotide variants [SNV], deletions, and insertions)◀
▶Preeclampsia sFlt-1/PlGF Ratio (PERA), Mayo Clinic, Laboratory Developed Test◀	●0482U	▶Obstetrics (preeclampsia), biochemical assay of soluble fms-like tyrosine kinase 1 (sFlt-1) and placental growth factor (PlGF), serum, ratio reported for sFlt-1/PlGF, with risk of progression for preeclampsia with severe features within 2 weeks◀

▶Ciprofloxacin Susceptibility of Neisseria gonorrhoeae, MedArbor Diagnostics, SpeeDx, Inc◀	●0483U	▶Infectious disease (Neisseria gonorrhoeae), sensitivity, ciprofloxacin resistance (gyrA S91F point mutation), oral, rectal, or vaginal swab, algorithm reported as probability of fluoroquinolone resistance◀
▶Macrolide Resistance of Mycoplasma genitalium, MedArbor Diagnostics, SpeeDx, Inc◀	●0484U	▶Infectious disease (Mycoplasma genitalium), macrolide sensitivity (23S rRNA point mutation), oral, rectal, or vaginal swab, algorithm reported as probability of macrolide resistance◀
▶Caris Assure™, Caris MPI, Inc d/b/a Caris Life Sciences®, Caris MPI, Inc d/b/a Caris Life Sciences®◀	●0485U	▶Oncology (solid tumor), cell-free DNA and RNA by next-generation sequencing, interpretative report for germline mutations, clonal hematopoiesis of indeterminate potential, and tumor-derived single-nucleotide variants, small insertions/deletions, copy number alterations, fusions, microsatellite instability, and tumor mutational burden◀
▶Northstar Response™, BillionToOne Laboratory, BillionToOne, Inc◀	●0486U	▶Oncology (pan-solid tumor), next-generation sequencing analysis of tumor methylation markers present in cell-free circulating tumor DNA, algorithm reported as quantitative measurement of methylation as a correlate of tumor fraction◀
▶Northstar Select™, BillionToOne Laboratory, BillionToOne, Inc◀	●0487U	▶Oncology (solid tumor), cell-free circulating DNA, targeted genomic sequence analysis panel of 84 genes, interrogation for sequence variants, aneuploidy-corrected gene copy number amplifications and losses, gene rearrangements, and microsatellite instability◀
▶UNITY Fetal Antigen™ NIPT, BillionToOne Laboratory, BillionToOne, Inc◀	●0488U	▶Obstetrics (fetal antigen noninvasive prenatal test), cell-free DNA sequence analysis for detection of fetal presence or absence of 1 or more of the Rh, C, c, D, E, Duffy (Fya), or Kell (K) antigen in alloimmunized pregnancies, reported as selected antigen(s) detected or not detected◀
▶UNITY Fetal Risk Screen™, BillionToOne Laboratory, BillionToOne, Inc◀	●0489U	▶Obstetrics (single-gene noninvasive prenatal test), cell-free DNA sequence analysis of 1 or more targets (eg, *CFTR, SMN1, HBB, HBA1, HBA2*) to identify paternally inherited pathogenic variants, and relative mutation-dosage analysis based on molecular counts to determine fetal inheritance of maternal mutation, algorithm reported as a fetal risk score for the condition (eg, cystic fibrosis, spinal muscular atrophy, beta hemoglobinopathies [including sickle cell disease], alpha thalassemia)◀

(Continued on page 1092)

▶CELLSEARCH® Circulating Melanoma Cell (CMC) Test, Menarini Silicon Biosystems Inc, Menarini Silicon Biosystems Inc◀	●0490U	▶Oncology (cutaneous or uveal melanoma), circulating tumor cell selection, morphological characterization and enumeration based on differential CD146, high molecular–weight melanoma-associated antigen, CD34 and CD45 protein biomarkers, peripheral blood◀
▶CELLSEARCH® ER Circulating Tumor Cell (CTC-ER) Test, Menarini Silicon Biosystems Inc, Menarini Silicon Biosystems Inc◀	●0491U	▶Oncology (solid tumor), circulating tumor cell selection, morphological characterization and enumeration based on differential epithelial cell adhesion molecule (EpCAM), cytokeratins 8, 18, and 19, CD45 protein biomarkers, and quantification of estrogen receptor (ER) protein biomarker–expressing cells, peripheral blood◀
▶CELLSEARCH® PD-L1 Circulating Tumor Cell (CTC-PD-L1) Test, Menarini Silicon Biosystems Inc, Menarini Silicon Biosystems Inc◀	●0492U	▶Oncology (solid tumor), circulating tumor cell selection, morphological characterization and enumeration based on differential epithelial cell adhesion molecule (EpCAM), cytokeratins 8, 18, and 19, CD45 protein biomarkers, and quantification of PD-L1 protein biomarker–expressing cells, peripheral blood◀
▶Prospera™, Natera™◀	●0493U	▶Transplantation medicine, quantification of donor-derived cell-free DNA (cfDNA) using next-generation sequencing, plasma, reported as percentage of donor-derived cell-free DNA◀
▶Rh Test, Natera™◀	●0494U	▶Red blood cell antigen (fetal RhD gene analysis), next-generation sequencing of circulating cell-free DNA (cfDNA) of blood in pregnant individuals known to be RhD negative, reported as positive or negative◀
▶Stockholm3, BioAgilytix Diagnostics◀	●0495U	▶Oncology (prostate), analysis of circulating plasma proteins (tPSA, fPSA, KLK2, PSP94, and GDF15), germline polygenic risk score (60 variants), clinical information (age, family history of prostate cancer, prior negative prostate biopsy), algorithm reported as risk of likelihood of detecting clinically significant prostate cancer◀
▶ColoScape™ PLUS, DiaCarta, Inc, DiaCarta, Inc◀	●0496U	▶Oncology (colorectal), cell-free DNA, 8 genes for mutations, 7 genes for methylation by real-time RT-PCR, and 4 proteins by enzyme-linked immunosorbent assay, blood, reported positive or negative for colorectal cancer or advanced adenoma risk◀
▶OncoAssure™ Prostate, DiaCarta, Inc, DiaCarta, Inc◀	●0497U	▶Oncology (prostate), mRNA gene-expression profiling by real-time RT-PCR of 6 genes (*FOXM1, MCM3, MTUS1, TTC21B, ALAS1,* and *PPP2CA*), utilizing formalin-fixed paraffin-embedded (FFPE) tissue, algorithm reported as a risk score for prostate cancer◀

▶OptiSeq™ Colorectal Cancer NGS Panel, DiaCarta, Inc, DiaCarta, Inc◀	●0498U	▶Oncology (colorectal), next-generation sequencing for mutation detection in 43 genes and methylation pattern in 45 genes, blood, and formalin-fixed paraffin-embedded (FFPE) tissue, report of variants and methylation pattern with interpretation◀
▶OptiSeq™ Dual Cancer Panel Kit, DiaCarta, Inc, DiaCarta, Inc◀	●0499U	▶Oncology (colorectal and lung), DNA from formalin-fixed paraffin-embedded (FFPE) tissue, next-generation sequencing of 8 genes (*NRAS, EGFR, CTNNB1, PIK3CA, APC, BRAF, KRAS,* and *TP53*), mutation detection◀
▶QClamp® Plex VEXAS UBA1 Mutation Test, DiaCarta, Inc, DiaCarta, Inc◀	●0500U	▶Autoinflammatory disease (VEXAS syndrome), DNA, *UBA1* gene mutations, targeted variant analysis (M41T, M41V, M41L, c.118-2A>C, c.118-1G>C, c.118-9_118-2del, S56F, S621C)◀
▶QuantiDNA™ Colorectal Cancer Triage Test, DiaCarta, Inc, DiaCarta, Inc◀	●0501U	▶Oncology (colorectal), blood, quantitative measurement of cell-free DNA (cfDNA)◀
▶QuantiVirus™ HPV E6/E7 mRNA Test for Cervical Cancer, DiaCarta, Inc, DiaCarta, Inc◀	●0502U	▶Human papillomavirus (HPV), E6/E7 markers for high-risk types (16, 18, 31, 33, 35, 39, 45, 51, 52, 56, 58, 59, 66, and 68), cervical cells, branched-chain capture hybridization, reported as negative or positive for high risk for HPV◀
▶PrecivityAD2™, C2N Diagnostics, LLC, C2N Diagnostics, LLC◀	●0503U	▶Neurology (Alzheimer disease), beta amyloid (Aβ40, Aβ42, Aβ42/40 ratio) and tau-protein (ptau217, np-tau217, ptau217/np-tau217 ratio), blood, immunoprecipitation with quantitation by liquid chromatography with tandem mass spectrometry (LC-MS/MS), algorithm score reported as likelihood of positive or negative for amyloid plaques◀
▶Urinary Tract Infection Testing, NxGen MDx LLC, NxGen MDx LLC◀	●0504U	▶Infectious disease (urinary tract infection), identification of 17 pathologic organisms, urine, real-time PCR, reported as positive or negative for each organism◀
▶Vaginal Infection Testing, NxGen MDx LLC, NxGen MDx LLC◀	●0505U	▶Infectious disease (vaginal infection), identification of 32 pathogenic organisms, swab, real-time PCR, reported as positive or negative for each organism◀
▶EndoSign® Barrett's Esophagus Test, Cyted Health Inc, Cyted Health Inc◀	●0506U	▶Gastroenterology (Barrett's esophagus), esophageal cells, DNA methylation analysis by next-generation sequencing of at least 89 differentially methylated genomic regions, algorithm reported as likelihood for Barrett's esophagus◀
▶Avantect Ovarian Cancer Test, ClearNote® Health◀	●0507U	▶Oncology (ovarian), DNA, whole-genome sequencing with 5-hydroxymethylcytosine (5hmC) enrichment, using whole blood or plasma, algorithm reported as cancer detected or not detected◀

(*Continued on page 1094*)

▶VitaGraft™ Kidney Baseline + 1st Plasma Test, Oncocyte Corporation, Oncocyte Corporation◀	●0508U	▶Transplantation medicine, quantification of donor-derived cell-free DNA using 40 single-nucleotide polymorphisms (SNPs), plasma, and urine, initial evaluation reported as percentage of donor-derived cell-free DNA with risk for active rejection◀
▶VitaGraft™ Kidney Subsequent, Oncocyte Corporation, Oncocyte Corporation◀	●0509U	▶Transplantation medicine, quantification of donor-derived cell-free DNA using up to 12 single-nucleotide polymorphisms (SNPs) previously identified, plasma, reported as percentage of donor-derived cell-free DNA with risk for active rejection◀
▶PurIST℠, Tempus AI, Inc, Tempus AI, Inc◀	●0510U	▶Oncology (pancreatic cancer), augmentative algorithmic analysis of 16 genes from previously sequenced RNA whole-transcriptome data, reported as probability of predicted molecular subtype◀
▶PARIS, Tempus AI, Inc, Tempus AI, Inc (by its wholly owned subsidiary SEngine Precision Medicine, LLC)◀	●0511U	▶Oncology (solid tumor), tumor cell culture in 3D microenvironment, 36 or more drug panel, reported as tumor-response prediction for each drug◀
▶Tempus p-MSI, Tempus AI, Inc, Tempus AI, Inc◀	●0512U	▶Oncology (prostate), augmentative algorithmic analysis of digitized whole-slide imaging of histologic features for microsatellite instability (MSI) status, formalin-fixed paraffin-embedded (FFPE) tissue, reported as increased or decreased probability of MSI-high (MSI-H)◀
▶Tempus p-Prostate, Tempus AI, Inc, Tempus AI, Inc◀	●0513U	▶Oncology (prostate), augmentative algorithmic analysis of digitized whole-slide imaging of histologic features for microsatellite instability (MSI) and homologous recombination deficiency (HRD) status, formalin-fixed paraffin-embedded (FFPE) tissue, reported as increased or decreased probability of each biomarker◀
▶Procise ADL™, ProciseDx Inc◀	●0514U	▶Gastroenterology (irritable bowel disease [IBD]), immunoassay for quantitative determination of adalimumab (ADL) levels in venous serum in patients undergoing adalimumab therapy, results reported as a numerical value as micrograms per milliliter (μg/mL)◀
▶Procise IFX™, ProciseDx Inc◀	●0515U	▶Gastroenterology (irritable bowel disease [IBD]), immunoassay for quantitative determination of infliximab (IFX) levels in venous serum in patients undergoing infliximab therapy, results reported as a numerical value as micrograms per milliliter (μg/mL)◀
▶MyGenVar Pharmacogenomics Test, Geisinger Medical Laboratories, Geisinger Medical Laboratories◀	●0516U	▶Drug metabolism, whole blood, pharmacogenomic genotyping of 40 genes and *CYP2D6* copy number variant analysis, reported as metabolizer status◀

▶PrecisView® CNS, Phenomics Health™ Inc, Phenomics Health™ Inc◀	●0517U	▶Therapeutic drug monitoring, 80 or more psychoactive drugs or substances, LC-MS/MS, plasma, qualitative and quantitative therapeutic minimally and maximally effective dose of prescribed and non-prescribed medications◀
▶SyncView® Pain, Phenomics Health™ Inc, Phenomics Health™ Inc◀	●0518U	▶Therapeutic drug monitoring, 90 or more pain and mental health drugs or substances, LC-MS/MS, plasma, qualitative and quantitative therapeutic minimally effective range of prescribed and non-prescribed medications◀
▶SyncView® PainPlus, Phenomics Health™ Inc, Phenomics Health™ Inc◀	●0519U	▶Therapeutic drug monitoring, medications specific to pain, depression, and anxiety, LC-MS/MS, plasma, 110 or more drugs or substances, qualitative and quantitative therapeutic minimally effective range of prescribed, non-prescribed, and illicit medications in circulation◀
▶SyncView® Rx, Phenomics Health™ Inc, Phenomics Health™ Inc◀	●0520U	▶Therapeutic drug monitoring, 200 or more drugs or substances, LC-MS/MS, plasma, qualitative and quantitative therapeutic minimally effective range of prescribed and non-prescribed medications◀

Appendix P

CPT Codes That May Be Used for Synchronous Real-Time Interactive Audio-Video Telemedicine Services

This listing is a summary of CPT codes that are typically rendered in person but may be used for reporting synchronous (real-time) interactive audio-video telemedicine services when appended with modifier 95. Procedures on this list involve electronic communication using interactive telecommunications equipment that includes, at a minimum, audio and video. The codes listed below are identified in CPT 2025 with the ★ symbol.

90785	90970	96164	99243
90791	92227	96165	99244
90792	92228	96167	99245
90832	92507	96168	99252
90833	92508	96170	99253
90834	92521	96171	99254
90836	92522	97110	99255
90837	92523	97112	99307
90838	92524	97116	99308
90839	92526	97161	99309
90840	92601	97162	99310
90845	92602	97165	99406
90846	92603	97166	99407
90847	92604	97530	99408
90863	93228	97535	99409
90951	93229	97750	99417
90952	93268	97755	99418
90954	93270	97760	99495
90955	93271	97761	99496
90957	93272	97802	99497
90958	96041	97803	99498
90960	96105	97804	
90961	96116	98960	
90963	96121	98961	
90964	96125	98962	
90965	96156	99211	
90966	96158	99231	
90967	96159	99232	
90968	96160	99233	
90969	96161	99242	

★=Telemedicine   ◀=Audio-only   +=Add-on code   ✗=FDA approval pending   #=Resequenced code   ⊘=Modifier 51 exempt   ➔➔➔=See p xxi for details

Appendix Q

Severe Acute Respiratory Syndrome Coronavirus 2 (SARS-CoV-2) (coronavirus disease [COVID-19]) Vaccines

►The crosswalk of COVID-19 vaccine and administration codes and their associated patient age, vaccine manufacturer, vaccine name(s), NDC Labeler Product ID, and interval between doses instructions (formerly Appendix Q) have been removed from the CPT code set. For information and guidance on reporting for COVID-19 immunization services, refer to the E/M and Medicine section guidelines.◄

Appendix R

Digital Medicine–Services Taxonomy

Appendix R is a listing of digital medicine services described in the CPT code set. The digital medicine–services taxonomy table in this appendix classifies CPT codes that are related to digital medicine services into discrete categories of clinician-to-patient services (eg, visit), clinician-to-clinician services (eg, consultation), patient-monitoring services, and digital diagnostic services. The clinician-to-patient services and clinician-to-clinician services categories are differentiated by the nature of their services, ie, synchronous and asynchronous communication. The patient-monitoring services represent ongoing, extended monitoring that produces data that require physician assessment and interpretation and are further categorized into device/software set-up and education, data transfer, and data-interpretation services. The digital diagnostic services differentiate automated/autonomous, algorithmically enabled diagnostic-support services into patient-directed and image/specimen-directed services. The term "clinician" in the table represents a physician or other qualified health care professional (QHP) who may use the specific code(s).

This taxonomy is intended to support increased awareness and understanding of approaches to patient care through the multifaceted digital medicine services available for reporting in the CPT code set. The taxonomy is not intended to be a complete representation of all applicable digital medicine service codes in the CPT code set and does not supersede specific coding guidance listed in specific sections of the CPT code set. Furthermore, the table does not denote services that are currently payable through coverage policies by either public or commercial payers.

For purposes of this appendix, the following terms should be understood as:

- Digital medicine services represent the use of technologies for measurement and intervention in the service of patient health.
- Synchronous services represent real-time interactions between a distant-site physician or other QHP and a patient and/or family located at a remote originating site.
- Asynchronous services represent store-and-forward transmissions of health information over periods of time using a secure Web server, encrypted email, specially designed store-and-forward software, or electronic health record. Asynchronous services enable a patient to share health information for later review by the physician or other QHP. These services also allow a physician or other QHP to share a patient's medical history, images, physiologic/non-physiologic clinical data and/or pathology and laboratory reports with a specialist physician for diagnostic and treatment expertise.

Digital Medicine—Services Taxonomy*

(*Note that the codes listed in this table are examples and not meant to be an exhaustive list)

	Clinician*-to-Patient Services (Eg, visit)		Clinician-to-Clinician Services (Eg, consultation)		Patient Monitoring and/or Therapeutic Services			Digital Diagnostic Services	
	Synchronous	Asynchronous	Synchronous	Asynchronous	Device/Software Set-Up and Education	Data Transfer	Data Interpretation	Patient Directed	Image/Specimen Directed
Encounter Activity	Real-time audiovisual interaction	Store-and-forward digital communication	Real-time consultative communication between requesting and consulting clinicians	Store-and-forward consultative digital exchange of clinical information between requesting and consulting clinicians	In-person, virtual face-to-face, telephone, or other modalities of communication with patient to support device set-up education/supply	Acquisition of patient data with transfer to managing or interpreting physician/other QHP/clinical staff	Data review, interpretation, and patient management by clinical staff/physician/other QHP with associated patient communication	Automated and autonomous algorithmically enabled diagnostic support	Automated and autonomous algorithmically enabled diagnostic support
CPT Service	▲Synchronous audio-video visit (98000-98007)▼ ▲Synchronous audio-only visit (98008-98015) Brief communication technology-based service (98016)▼	Online digital evaluation & management (99421-99423) (98970-98972)	Interprofessional telephone/Internet/EHR consultation (Typically via telephone) (99446-99449, 99451) If patient is present at originating site→ transition to virtual face-to-face E/M consultation (Use modifier 95)	Interprofessional telephone/Internet/EHR consultation (99446-99449, 99451, 99452)	Remote physiologic monitoring initial set-up/education (99453)	Remote physiologic monitoring device supply (99454)	Physiologic data collection/interpretation by physician/other QHP (99091) Remote physiologic monitoring treatment management by clinical staff/physician/other QHP (99457, 99458)	Autonomous retinopathy screening (92229)	Multianalyte assays with algorithmic analyses (MAAA)

(Continued on page 1100)

▲ = Revised code   ● = New code   ► ◄ = Contains new or revised text   ✕ = Duplicate PLA test   ↑↓ = Category I PLA   American Medical Association   **1099**

Digital Medicine–Services Taxonomy* (cont'd)

(*Note that the codes listed in this table are examples and not meant to be an exhaustive list)

CPT Service	Clinician*-to-Patient Services (Eg. visit)		Clinician-to-Clinician Services (Eg. consultation)		Patient Monitoring and/or Therapeutic Services			Digital Diagnostic Services	
	Synchronous	Asynchronous	Synchronous	Asynchronous	Device/Software Set-Up and Education	Data Transfer	Data Interpretation	Patient Directed	Image/Specimen Directed
					Remote therapeutic monitoring initial set-up/education (98975)	Remote therapeutic monitoring device supply (98976 for respiratory system; 98977 for musculo-skeletal system)	Remote therapeutic monitoring treatment management by physician/other QHP (98980, 98981)		Computer-aided detection (CAD) imaging (77048, 77049, 77065-77067, 0042T, 0174T, 0175T)
					Remote pulmonary artery pressure sensor monitoring treatment management by physician/other QHP (93264)				
					Ambulatory continuous glucose monitoring hook-up, education, recording print-out (95250 for office-equipped; 95249 for patient-equipped)		Ambulatory continuous glucose monitoring analysis (95251)		
					External electrocardiographic recording (Recording, scanning analysis with report, review and interpretation) (93224, 93241, 93245)				
					External electrocardiographic recording (Recording) (93224, 93225, 93241, 93242, 93245, 93246)	External electrocardiographic recording (Scanning analysis with report only) (93226, 93241, 93243, 93247)	External electrocardiographic recording (Review and interpretation) (93224, 93227, 93241, 93244, 93245, 93248)	External electrocardiographic recording (Autonomous algorithms used to analyze/create report) (93241-93243, 93245-93247)	

Digital Medicine–Services Taxonomy* (cont'd)
(*Note that the codes listed in this table are examples and not meant to be an exhaustive list)

CPT Service	Clinician*-to-Patient Services (Eg, visit)		Clinician-to-Clinician Services (Eg, consultation)		Patient Monitoring and/or Therapeutic Services			Digital Diagnostic Services	
	Synchronous	Asynchronous	Synchronous	Asynchronous	Device/Software Set-Up and Education	Data Transfer	Data Interpretation	Patient Directed	Image/Specimen Directed
						External mobile cardiovascular telemetry technical support (93229)	External mobile cardiovascular telemetry review and interpretation (93228)		
						Digital amblyopia services (0704T for initial set-up/education; 0705T for surveillance center technical support, including data transmission)	Digital amblyopia services (Assessment of patient performance, program data) (0706T)		
						Automated analysis of CT study (Data preparation, interpretation and report) (0691T)			

*The term "clinician" in the table represents a physician or other qualified health care professional (QHP) by whom the specific code may be used.

Appendix S

Artificial Intelligence Taxonomy for Medical Services and Procedures

This taxonomy provides guidance for classifying various artificial intelligence (AI) applications (eg, expert systems, machine learning, algorithm-based services) for medical services and procedures into one of these three categories: assistive, augmentative, and autonomous. AI as applied to health care may differ from AI in other public and private sectors (eg, banking, energy, transportation). Note that there is no single product, procedure, or service for which the term "AI" is sufficient or necessary to describe its intended clinical use or utility; therefore, the term "AI" is not defined in the code set. In addition, the term "AI" is not intended to encompass or constrain the full scope of innovations that are characterized as "work done by machines." Classification of AI medical services and procedures as assistive, augmentative, and autonomous is based on the clinical procedure or service provided to the patient and the work performed by the machine on behalf of the physician or other qualified health care professional (QHP).

Assistive: The work performed by the machine for the physician or other QHP is assistive when the machine **detects** clinically relevant data without analysis or generated conclusions. Requires physician or other QHP interpretation and report.

Augmentative: The work performed by the machine for the physician or other QHP is augmentative when the machine **analyzes** and/or **quantifies** data to yield clinically meaningful output. Requires physician or other QHP interpretation and report.

Autonomous: The work performed by the machine for the physician or other QHP is autonomous when the machine automatically **interprets** data and independently generates clinically meaningful conclusions without concurrent physician or other QHP involvement. Autonomous medical services and procedures include interrogating and analyzing data. The work of the algorithm may or may not include acquisition, preparation, and/or transmission of data. The clinically meaningful conclusion may be a characterization of data (eg, likelihood of pathophysiology) to be used to establish a diagnosis or to implement a therapeutic intervention. There are three levels of autonomous AI medical services and procedures with varying physician or other QHP professional involvement:

Level I. The autonomous AI draws conclusions and offers diagnosis and/or management options, which are contestable and require physician or other QHP action to implement.

Level II. The autonomous AI draws conclusions and initiates diagnosis and/or management options with alert/opportunity for override, which may require physician or other QHP action to implement.

Level III. The autonomous AI draws conclusions and initiates management, which requires physician or other QHP initiative to contest.

Service Components	AI Category: Assistive	AI Category: Augmentative	AI Category: Autonomous
Primary objective	Detects clinically relevant data	Analyzes and/or quantifies data to yield clinically meaningful output	Interprets data and independently generates clinically meaningful conclusions
Provides independent diagnosis and/or management decision	No	No	Yes
Analyzes data	No	Yes	Yes
Requires physician or other QHP interpretation and report	Yes	Yes	No
Examples in CPT code set	Algorithmic electrocardiogram risk-based assessment for cardiac dysfunction (0764T, 0765T)	Noninvasive estimate of coronary fractional flow reserve (FFR) (75580)	Retinal imaging (92229)

Appendix T

CPT Codes That May Be Used for Synchronous Real-Time Interactive Audio-Only Telemedicine Services

This listing is a summary of CPT codes that are typically rendered in person but may be used for reporting audio-only services when appended with modifier 93. Procedures on this list involve electronic communication using interactive telecommunications equipment that includes, at a minimum, audio. The codes listed below are identified in CPT 2025 with the ◀ symbol.

90785	92508	96165
90791	92521	96167
90792	92522	96168
90832	92523	96170
90833	92524	96171
90834	96041	97802
90836	96110	97803
90837	96116	97804
90838	96121	99406
90839	96156	99407
90840	96158	99408
90845	96159	99409
90846	96160	99497
90847	96161	99498
92507	96164	

Notes

Index

Instructions for the Use of the CPT Index

The alphabetic index is **not** a substitute for the main text of the CPT codebook. Even if only one code is present, the user must refer to the main text to ensure that the code selected accurately identifies the service(s) performed.

Main Terms

The index is organized by main terms. Each main term can stand alone or can be followed by up to three modifying terms. There are four primary classes of main entries:

1. Procedure or service.
   For example: Endoscopy; Anastomosis; Splint

2. Organ or other anatomical site.
   For example: Tibia; Colon; Salivary Gland

3. Condition.
   For example: Abscess; Entropion; Tetralogy of Fallot

4. Synonyms, Eponyms, and Abbreviations.
   For example: EEG; Brock Operation; Clagett Procedure

The Anesthesia section codes are indexed under the Anesthesia main entry and are not double-entered under the anatomical sites. Only codes within the Surgery, Medicine, Category II, and Category III sections that specifically reference the service of anesthesia are indexed under the anatomical sites.

Modifying Terms

A main term may be followed by up to three indented terms that modify the terms they follow. For example, the main term *Endoscopy* is subdivided by the anatomical sites in which the procedure is used, and within these anatomical sites, the specific purpose of the procedure is identified. In the following example, the code for an endoscopic removal of a foreign body from the bile duct could be located:

Bile Duct
   Removal
      Foreign Body 43275

Note that in this entry, the inclusion of a subentry under "Removal" implies the reading "Removal [of]" the term that follows it. If no subheads followed "Removal," the procedure would relate to the subhead that preceded it, as in this entry for the endoscopic removal of the spleen:

Spleen
   Removal 38120

When modifying terms appear, one should review the list, as these subterms further qualify the selection of the appropriate code for the procedure.

Code Ranges

Whenever more than one code applies to a given index entry, a code range is listed. If several nonsequential codes apply, they will be separated by a comma. In the following example, three nonsequential codes apply:

Esophagus
   Reconstruction 43300, 43310, 43313

If three or more sequential codes apply, they will be separated by a hyphen. If more than one code range applies, the code ranges will be separated by a comma as in the following example:

Anesthesia
   Forearm 01810-01820, 01830-01860

Conventions

As a space-saving convention, certain terms carry meaning inferred from the context. This convention is primarily used when a procedure or service is listed as a subterm. For example:

Knee
   Exploration [of] 27310, 27331

In this example, the bracketed qualifier "[of]" does not appear in the index; "of" is understood in the context of the term "Exploration." As another example:

Pelvis
   Halo [Application of] 20662

In this example, as there is no such entity as "pelvis halo," the bracketed words are inferred.

Pathology and Laboratory

The Pathology and Laboratory listing in the index presents the headings, subheadings, procedures, and analytes in the Pathology and Laboratory section of the CPT codebook. Analytes are either listed alphabetically (for example, the Chemistry analytes) or cross-referenced to the index main heads where they are alphabetically listed (for example, to reference infectious agent analytes, the entry will indicate "*See* Infectious-Agent Detection").

A

Abbe-Estlander Procedure
Lip Reconstruction 40527, 40761

Abdomen
See also Abdominal
Abdominal Wall
  Debridement
    Infected................. 11005, 11006
  Fascial Reinforcement
    with Implant..................... 0437T
  Implantation
    Non-Biologic or Synthetic Implant.... 0437T
  Removal
    Mesh....................... 11008
    Prosthesis.................. 11008
  Repair
    Hernia
      See Hernia Repair
  Tumor
    Excision................. 22900-22903
    Radical Resection.......... 22904, 22905
Abscess
  Incision and Drainage
    Open.................... 49020, 49040
Angiography........ 74174, 74175, 74185, 75635
Aorta
  See Aorta, Abdominal
Aortic Aneurysm
  See Aorta, Abdominal, Aneurysm
Artery
  Ligation 37617
Biopsy............................ 49000
Bypass Graft
  Excision 35907
Catheter
  Removal 49422
Celiotomy
  Exploratory.................... 49000
CT Scan............... 74150, 74160, 74170,
        74174-74178, 75635
Cyst
  Destruction/Excision 49186-49190
Deliveries
  See Cesarean Delivery
Drainage
  Fluid 49082, 49083
Ectopic Pregnancy..................... 59130
Exploration 49000, 49010
  Blood Vessel................... 35840
  Staging........................ 58960
Hysterectomy
  See Hysterectomy, Abdominal
Incision 49000-49084
  Staging........................ 58960
Incision and Drainage
  Pancreatitis 48000
Infraumbilical Panniculectomy 15830
Injection
  Air............................ 49400
  Contrast Material................ 49400
Insertion
  Catheter........ 49324, 49418, 49419, 49421
  Venous Shunt................... 49425
Intraperitoneal
  Catheter Exit Site............... 49436
  Catheter Insertion 49418-49421, 49435
  Catheter Removal 49422

Catheter Revision.................. 49325
Shunt
  Insertion 49425
  Ligation....................... 49428
  Removal 49429
  Revision 49426
Laparoscopy 49320-49327, 49329
Laparotomy
  Exploratory.................... 49000
  Reopening 49002
  Staging........................ 58960
Lymphangiogram
  See Lymphangiography, Abdomen
Magnetic Resonance Imaging (MRI).. 74181-74183
Needle Biopsy (Mass).................. 49180
Paracentesis 49082, 49083
Radiation Therapy
  Placement of Guidance Devices .. 49411, 49412
Radical Resection 51597
Radiographies
  See Abdomen, X ray
Repair
  Blood Vessel................... 35221
    with Other Graft............... 35281
    with Vein Graft................ 35251
  Hernia.......... 49591-49596, 49613-49618
  Suture........................ 49900
Revision
  Venous Shunt.................. 49426
Suture 49900
Tumor
  Destruction/Excision 49186-49190
Ultrasound..................... 76700-76705
Unlisted Services and Procedures 49999
Wall
  Debridement 11005, 11006
  Prosthetic Mesh
    Implantation.................. 15778
    Removal 11008
  Tumor
    Excision.................. 22900-22903
    Radical Resection.......... 22904, 22905
Wound Exploration
  Penetrating.................... 20102
X ray 74018, 74019, 74021, 74022

Abdominal
See also Abdomen
Aorta
  See Aorta, Abdominal
Aortic Aneurysm
  See Aorta, Abdominal, Aneurysm
Deliveries
  See Cesarean Delivery
Hysterectomy
  See Hysterectomy, Abdominal
Lymphangiogram
  See Lymphangiography, Abdomen
Paracentesis
  See Abdomen, Drainage
Radiographies
  See Abdomen, X ray

Abdominohysterectomy
See Hysterectomy, Abdominal

Abdominopelvic Amputation
Interpelviabdominal Amputation 27290

Abdominoplasty
Excision, Skin and Tissue 15830, 15847
Unlisted Procedure 17999

Ablation
Anus
  Polyp......................... 46615
  Tumor 46615
Bone
  Tumor
    with Adjacent Soft Tissue 20982, 20983
Breast
  Malignant Tumor 0581T
Colon
  Lesion............... 44401, 45346, 45388
  Polyp............... 44401, 45346, 45388
  Tumor.............. 44401, 45346, 45388
Cryosurgical
  Breast Tumor 0581T
  Fibroadenoma 19105
  Liver Tumor............... 47381, 47383
  Renal Mass.................... 50250
  Renal Tumor
    Percutaneous 50593
CT Scan Guidance..................... 77013
Electroporation 0600T-0601T
Endometrial............ 58353, 58356, 58563
  with Ultrasound Guidance........... 58356
Heart
  Arrhythmogenic Focus
    See Arrhythmogenic Focus
  Atrioventricular 93650, 93654
  Atrioventricular Pathway......... 93653
High Intensity Focused Ultrasound (HIFU)
  Prostate Tissue.................... 55880
Histotripsy
  Hepatocellular Tissue 0686T
  Renal Tissue..................... 0888T
Intracranial Lesion
  Magnetic Resonance Image-Guided High
  Intensity Focused Ultrasound (MRgFUS) 61715
Larynx
  Lesion........................ 31572
Laser
  Prostate Malignancy 0655T
  Prostatic Hyperplasia......... 0714T, 0867T
Liver Lesion
  3D Contour Simulation for Microwave
  Ablation...................... 0944T
Liver Tumor
  Cryosurgical............... 47381, 47383
  Laparoscopic 47370, 47371
  Radiofrequency 47380-47382
Lung Tumor
  Radiofrequency 32998
Magnetic Field Induction
  Prostate 0738T
Nasal Sinuses................. 31242, 31243
Nerve
  Percutaneous................ 0440T-0442T
  Radiofrequency 64625
  Thermal 0793T
  Ultrasound 0632T
Parenchymal Tissue
  CT Scan Guidance 77013
  Magnetic Resonance Imaging Guidance 77022
  Ultrasound Guidance.............. 76940
Prostate
  Cryosurgical 55873
  High Intensity Focused Ultrasound
  (HIFU)........................ 55880
  Laser, Transperineal.......... 0714T, 0867T
  Magnetic Field Induction....... 0738T, 0739T

Index

Index

Anesthesia, Local

Aneurysm Repair

Angina Assessment

Angiocardiographies

Angiography

Angioma

Angioplasty

Index

Antibody Identification

Antibody Neutralization Test

See Neutralization Test

Antibody Screening

Anticoagulant

See Clotting Inhibitors

Anticoagulant Management

Anti-D Immunoglobulin

See Immune Globulins, Rho(D)

Antidiabetic Hormone

See Glucagon

Antidiuretic Hormone (ADH)

Measurement

Anti-DNA Autoantibody

See Antinuclear Antibodies (ANA)

Antigen

See also Antigen Detection

Antigen, Australia

See Hepatitis B Surface Antigen (HBsAg)

Antigen, CD4

See CD4

Antigen, CD8

See CD8

Antigen, CD142

See Thromboplastin

Antigen, CD143

See Angiotensin Converting Enzyme (ACE)

Antigen Bronchial Provocation Tests

See Bronchial Challenge Test

Antigen Detection

Direct Fluorescence
Immunoassay
Immunoassay with Direct Optical Observation
Immunofluorescence

Index

Index

with Synovectomy
    Glenohumeral Joint 23105
    Sternoclavicular Joint 23106
Tarsometatarsal Joint 28020, 28050
Temporomandibular Joint 21010
Wrist 25040, 25100-25107

Arthrotomy for Removal of Prosthesis of Ankle
See Ankle, Removal, Implant

Arthrotomy for Removal of Prosthesis of Hip
See Hip, Removal, Prosthesis

Arthrotomy for Removal of Prosthesis of Wrist
See Wrist, Removal, Prosthesis

Articular Ligament
See Ligament

Artificial Abortion
See Abortion

Artificial Cardiac Pacemaker
See Pacemaker

Artificial Eye
See Eye, Prosthesis

Artificial Genitourinary Sphincter
See Prosthesis, Urethral Sphincter

Artificial Insemination
Intracervical 58321
Intrauterine 58322
Sperm Washing 58323

Artificial Intelligence (AI) Medical Services
Algorithmic Electrocardiogram Risk
Assessment. 0764T, 0765T
Algorithmically Generated 12-Lead
ECG 0903T-0905T
Augmentative Algorithmic Analyses
    Absolute Quantitation of Myocardial Blood
    Flow (AQMBF) 0899T, 0900T
    Algorithm-Derived QTc Interval from
    Electrocardiogram 0902T
    Cardiac Arrhythmia 0897T
    Heart Failure Detection 0932T
    Prostate Cancer Estimation Map. 0898T
Facial Phenotype Analysis 0731T

Artificial Knee Joints
See Prosthesis, Knee

Artificial Penis
See Penile Prosthesis

Artificial Pneumothorax
See Pneumothorax, Therapeutic

Arytenoid
Excision 31400, 31560
Fixation 31400

Arytenoidectomy
Arytenoid Excision 31400
Endoscopic 31560

Arytenoidopexy
Arytenoid Fixation. 31400

Ascorbic Acid
Blood. 82180

Aspartate Aminotransferase
See Transaminase, Glutamic-Oxaloacetic

Aspergillus
Detection
    Antibody. 86606
    Antigen. 87305

Aspiration
Abdomen 49322
Amniotic Fluid
    Diagnostic 59000
    Therapeutic 59001
Aspirate Evaluation. 88172, 88173, 88177
Bladder 51100-51102
Bone Marrow 38220, 38222
    Spine Surgery. 20939
Brain Lesion 61750, 61751
Breast 19000, 19001
Bronchi 31629, 31633, 31645, 31646, 31725
Bursa . . 20600, 20604, 20605, 20606, 20610, 20611
    with Recording and Reporting 20604,
                               20606, 20611
    with Ultrasound Guidance 20604,
                               20606, 20611
Catheter
    Nasotracheal 31720
    Tracheobronchial 31725
Cyst
    Bone. 20615
    Breast. 19000, 19001
    Ganglion. 20612
    Kidney 50390
    Pelvis 50390
    Spinal Cord. 62268
    Thyroid 60300
Duodenum. 43756, 43757
Fetal Fluid 59074
Fine Needle 67415
    Aspirate Evaluation 88172, 88173, 88177
Fine Needle, Biopsy
    See Fine Needle Aspiration (FNA) Biopsy
Gastric. 43753, 43754
Hydrocele
    Tunica Vaginalis 55000
Joint 20600, 20604-20606, 20610, 20611
    with Recording and Reporting 20604,
                               20606, 20611
    with Ultrasound Guidance 20604,
                               20606, 20611
Laryngoscopy 31515
Lens Material 66840
Liver. 47015
Orbital Contents 67415
Pericardium. 33016
Pleural Cavity 32554, 32555
    with Imaging Guidance 32555
Puncture
    See Puncture Aspiration
Spinal Cord
    Syrinx 62268
Stomach
    Diagnostic 43754, 43755
    Therapeutic 43753
Syrinx
    Spinal Cord. 62268
Thyroid 60300
Trachea 31612, 31629
    Nasotracheal 31720
    Tracheobronchial 31645, 31646, 31725
Tunica Vaginalis
    Hydrocele 55000

Vertebral
    Disc 62267
    Nucleus Pulposus. 62267
    Tissue. 62267
Vitreous. 67015

Aspiration, Chest
Thoracentesis 32554, 32555
    with Imaging Guidance 32555

Aspiration, Nail
See Evacuation, Hematoma, Subungual

Aspiration, Spinal Puncture
Lumbar 62272, 62328

Aspiration Lipectomies
Liposuction 15876-15879

Aspiration of Bone Marrow from Donor for Transplant
See Bone Marrow, Harvesting

Assay, Tobramycin
See Tobramycin

Assay, Very Long Chain Fatty Acids
See Fatty Acid, Very Long Chain

Assisted Circulation
See Circulation Assist

AST
See Transaminase, Glutamic-Oxaloacetic

Astragalectomy
Talectomy 28130

Astragalus
See Talus

Asymmetry, Face
See Hemifacial Microsomia

Ataxia Telangiectasia
Chromosome Analysis 88248
Cytogenetic Study. 88248
Gene Test .0136U, 81408

Ataxy, Telangiectasia
See Ataxia Telangiectasia

Atherectomies, Coronary
See Artery, Coronary, Atherectomy

Atherectomy
See also Revascularization, Artery
Abdominal Aorta. 0236T
Brachiocephalic. 0237T
Coronary 92924, 92925, 92937,
                  92938, 92941, 92943, 92944
Femoral 37225, 37227
Iliac 0238T
Peroneal 37229, 37231, 37233, 37235
Popliteal 37225, 37227
Renal. 0234T
Tibial 37229, 37231, 37233, 37235
Visceral 0235T

Athletic Training
Evaluation 97169-97171
Re-evaluation 97172

ATLV (Adult T Cell Leukemia Virus)
See HTLV-I

ATLV Antibodies
See HTLV-I, Antibody

Atomic Absorption Spectroscopy
Each Analyte. 82190

Index

Index

Index

Index

Index

Index

Index

Index

Index

Index

Index

with Rectal Repair 45563, 45805, 45825
Revision. 44340, 44345, 44346

Colotomy
Biopsy 44025
Exploration 44025
Foreign Body Removal 44025

Colpectomy
See Vaginectomy

Colpoceliocentesis
See Colpocentesis

Colpocentesis 57020

Colpocleisis 57120

Colpocleisis Complete
See Vagina, Closure

Colpohysterectomies
See Hysterectomy, Vaginal

Colpoperineorrhaphy 57210

Colpopexy
Abdominal. 57280
Laparoscopic. 57425
Vaginal 57282, 57283

Colpoplasty
See Repair, Vagina

Colporrhaphy
Anterior. 57240, 57289
   with Insertion of Mesh 57267
   with Insertion of Prosthesis. 57267
Anteroposterior. 57260-57265
   with Enterocele Repair 57265
   with Insertion of Mesh 57267
   with Insertion of Prosthesis. 57267
Nonobstetrical 57200
Posterior 57250
   with Insertion of Mesh 57267
   with Insertion of Prosthesis. 57267

Colposcopy
Biopsy
   Cervix 57421, 57454, 57455
      Loop Electrode Biopsy 57460
      Loop Electrode Conization 57461
   Endometrium 58110
Cervix . . 57420, 57421, 57454-57456, 57460, 57461
   with Computer-aided Mapping 57465
   and Upper/Adjacent Vagina 57452
Endometrium. 58110
Exploration 57452
Vagina 57420, 57421, 57452
Vulva 56820
   Biopsy. 56821

Colpotomy
Exploration 57000
Pelvic Abscess Drainage. 57010

Colpo-Urethrocystopexy
with Hysterectomy 58152, 58267
Marshall-Marchetti-Krantz Type. 58152, 58267
Pereyra Type 58267

Colprosterone
See Progesterone

Column Chromatography/Mass Spectrometry
See also Pathology and Laboratory, Chemistry
Unspecified Non-Drug Analyte. 82542

Columna Vertebralis
See Spine

Combined Heart-Lung Transplantation
See Transplantation, Heart-Lung

Combined Right and Left Heart Cardiac Catheterization
See Cardiac Catheterization, Combined Left and Right Heart

Comedones
Removal 10040

Commissurotomy
Right Ventricle 33476, 33478

Common Sensory Nerve
Repair/Suture 64834

Common Truncus
See Truncus Arteriosus

Communication Device
Non-Speech-Generating. 92605, 92606, 92618
Speech-Generating. 92607-92609

Community/Work Reintegration
Training 97537

Comparative Analysis (Short Tandem Repeat)
Patient and Comparative Specimen . . 81265, 81266

Compatibility Test
Blood. 86920, 86923
Specimen Pretreatment 86970-86972

Complement
Antigen 86160
Fixation Test 86171
Functional Activity 86161
Total Hemolytic. 86162

Complete Blood Count (CBC)
See Blood Cell Count

Complete Colectomy
See Colectomy, Total

Complete Pneumonectomy
See Pneumonectomy, Completion

Complete Transposition of Great Vessels
See Transposition, Great Arteries

Complex, Factor IX
See Christmas Factor

Component Removal, Blood
See Apheresis

Composite Graft . . 15760-15770, 35681-35683

Compound B
See Corticosterone

Compound F
See Cortisol

Compression, Nerve, Median
See Carpal Tunnel Syndrome

Computed Tomographic Angiography (CTA)
Abdomen. 74174, 74175
Abdominal Aorta. 75635
Arm 73206
Chest. 71275
Coronary Artery. 75574
   Automated Data Analysis 0623T-0626T
   Software Analysis for Fractional Flow Reserve
   (FFR) 75580

Head 70496
Heart 75571-75574
Leg. 73706
Neck 70498
Non-Coronary Artery
   Software Analysis
      Arterial Plaque Quantification . . .0710T-0713T
Pelvis. 72191, 74174

Computed Tomographic Scintigraphy
See SPECT

Computed Tomography (CT)
See CT Scan

Computer Analysis
Acoustic Recording
   Heart Sounds 93799
Digital Image Data
   Mammography. 77065-77067
Electrocardiographic Data 93228
Morphometric Analysis. 88121
Motion Analysis 96000-96004
   Full Body. 0693T
Pediatric Home Apnea Monitor 94776

Computer Data Analysis
Electrocardiographic. 93228

Computer-Aided Detection (CAD)
Lesion
   Chest Radiograph. 0174T, 0175T
   Mammography 77065-77067
   Magnetic Resonance Imaging
   (MRI). 77048, 77049

Computer-Assisted Navigation
Bronchoscopy 31627
Cranial Procedure 61781, 61782
Musculoskeletal Procedure . . 0054T, 0055T, 20985
Spinal Procedure. 61783

Computer-Assisted Testing 96146
Cytopathology. 88121
Morphometric Analysis. 88121
Motion Analysis 96000-96004
Neuropsychological 96146
Psychological 96146

Computerized Emission Tomography
See SPECT

Concentration, Hydrogen-Ion
See Blood Gases, pH

Concentration, Minimum Inhibitory
See Minimum Inhibitory Concentration

Concentration of Specimen
Cytopathology. 88108
Electrophoretic Fractionation
and Quantitation. 84166
Immunoelectrophoresis 86325
Immunofixation Electrophoresis. 86335
Infectious Agent 87015
Ova and Parasites. 87177

Concentric Procedure 28296

Concha Bullosa Resection
with Nasal/Sinus Endoscopy 31240

Conchae Nasale
See Nasal Turbinate

Concurrent Optical and Magnetic Stimulation (COMS)
Wound Therapy. 0906T, 0907T

Index

Index

Index

Index

Index

Index

Index

Index

Index

Index

Index

Index

Index

Index

Glutamic Aspartic Transaminase
Glutamic-Oxaloacetic 84450

Glutamic Dehydrogenase
Glutamate Dehydrogenase.............. 82965

Glutamyltransferase, Gamma 82977

Glutathione 82978

Glutathione Reductase 82979

Glycanhydrolase, N-Acetylmuramide
Lysozyme.......................... 85549

Glycated Hemoglobins
Glycosylated Hemoglobin.............. 83036

Glycated Protein................. 82985

Glycerol, Phosphatidyl
Phosphatidylglycerol................. 84081

Glycerol Phosphoglycerides
Phosphatidylglycerol................. 84081

Glycerophosphatase
See Alkaline Phosphatase

Glycinate, Theophylline Sodium
Theophylline 80198

Glycocholic Acid
Cholylglycine....................... 82240

Glycohemoglobin
Glycosylated Hemoglobin.............. 83036

Glycosaminoglycan
Mucopolysaccharides.................. 83864

Goeckerman Treatment
Photochemotherapy 96910, 96912, 96913

Goldwaite Procedure
Knee 27422

Golfer's Elbow
Tenotomy...................... 24357-24359

Gol-Vernet Operation
Pyelotomy, Exploration 50120

Gonadectomy, Female
See Oophorectomy

Gonadectomy, Male
See Orchiectomy

Gonadotropin
Chorionic..................... 84702-84704
    Stimulation Panel.................. 80414
FSH 83001
ICSH 83002
LH 83002
Stimulation Panel 80426

Gonadotropin Panel
Stimulation 80426

Gonioscopy
Ophthalmic 92020

Goniotomy
Congenital Glaucoma 65820

Gonococcus
Neisseria Gonorrhoeae...... 87590-87592, 87850

GOTT
Transaminase, Glutamic-Oxaloacetic....... 84450

GPUT
Galactose-1-Phosphate, Uridyl Transferase.. 82776
Uridyl Transferase................... 82775

Graft
Allograft
    See Allograft
Anal................................. 46753
Aorta
    See Aorta, Graft
Artery
    Bypass Graft
       See Bypass Graft, Arterial; Bypass Graft,
       Arterial-Venous
       Coronary......................... 33503
Bone and Skin....... 20969, 20970, 20972, 20973
Bone Marrow
    Aspiration....................... 20939
    Transplantation 38240-38242
Cartilage
    See Cartilage Graft
Conjunctiva........................... 65782
    Harvesting 68371
Cornea
    with Lesion Excision 65426
Cornea Transplant
    See Cornea, Transplantation
Dura
    Cranial
       Anterior Cranial Fossa 61601
       Middle Cranial Fossa 61606, 61608
       Posterior Cranial Fossa........... 61616
       Suboccipital Craniectomy.......... 61343
    Spinal Cord...................... 63710
Ear
    Dermal Autograft............ 15135, 15136
    Epidermal Autograft.......... 15115, 15116
    Fat Autograft 15773, 15774
    Full-thickness Graft, Free....... 15260, 15261
    Preparation of Recipient Site.... 15004, 15005
    Skin Substitute Graft 15275-15278
    Split-thickness Autograft....... 15120, 15121
    Tissue Cultured Skin Autograft .. 15155-15157
Eye
    Amniotic Membrane 65778-65780
    Conjunctiva 65782
    Stem Cell 65781
for Facial Nerve Paralysis
    Fascia.......................... 15840
    Muscle 15841, 15842, 15845
Fascia
    See Fascial Graft
Fascia Lata
    Harvesting 20920, 20922
Fat.......................... 15771-15774
Gum Mucosa........................... 41870
Intestine 43116, 46748
Muscle
    See Muscle Flaps; Muscle Grafts
Nail Bed
    Reconstruction................... 11762
Nerve
    See Nerve Graft
Oral Mucosa 40818
Organ
    See Transplantation
Pancreas
    See Pancreas, Transplantation
Patency
    Blood Flow Check................. 15860
    Vascular Flow Check 15860
Skin
    See Skin Graft and Flap

Skin Substitute
    See Skin Substitute Graft
Tendon
    Finger 26392, 26416, 26420, 26428, 26434
    Hand............... 26392, 26412, 26416
    Harvesting 20924
Vein
    Bypass Graft
       See Bypass Graft, Venous
    Cross-Over 34520

Grain Alcohol
Drug Assay, Alcohols 80320

Granulation Tissue
Cauterization, Chemical 17250

Gravis, Myasthenia
Cholinesterase Inhibitor Challenge Test..... 95857

Gravities, Specific
Specific Gravity...................... 84315

Great Toe
Arthrodesis
    Interphalangeal Joint.............. 28755
       with Tendon Transfer 28760
    Metatarsophalangeal Joint.......... 28750
Fracture
    Closed Treatment................. 28490
    Open Treatment.................. 28505
    Skeletal Fixation................. 28496
Osteocutaneous Flap 20973
Toe-to-Hand Transfer 20973
    Wrap-around with Bone Graft........ 26551

Great Vessels
Graft Insertion.................. 33330, 33335
Shunts
    Aorta to Pulmonary Artery
       Ascending...................... 33755
       Descending..................... 33762
    Central 33764
    Subclavian to Pulmonary Artery 33750
    Vena Cava to Pulmonary Artery.. 33766, 33767
Suture Repair 33320-33322
Translocation
    Aortic Root................. 33782, 33783
Transposition Repair
    Aortic Pulmonary Artery
       Reconstruction.............. 33778-33781
    Atrial Baffle Procedure 33774-33777
    with Subpulmonary Stenosis.... 33770, 33771
    with Ventricular Septal Defect .. 33770, 33771
Unlisted Services and Procedures 33999

Great Vessels Transposition
See Transposition, Great Arteries

Greater Tuberosity Fracture
Humeral
    Closed Treatment....... 23620, 23625, 23665
    Open Treatment............. 23630, 23670
with Shoulder Dislocation
    Closed Treatment................. 23665
    Open Treatment.................. 23670

Greater Vestibular Gland
See Bartholin's Gland

Grippe, Balkan
Q Fever 86000, 86638

Gritti Operation
Amputation, Thigh, through Femur........ 27590

Index

Index

Index

Incision and Drainage

Index

Incisional Hernia Repair
See Hernia Repair, Incisional

Inclusion Bodies

Indicator Dilution Studies

Induced Abortion
See Abortion, Induced

Induced Hyperthermia
See Thermotherapy

Induratio Penis Plastica
See Peyronie Disease

Indwelling Catheter
Percutaneous, Lung
    See Pleural Cavity, Catheterization

Infant, Newborn, Intensive Care
See Intensive Care, Neonate

Infantile Paralysis
See Polio

Infection

Infection, Actinomyces
See Actinomycosis

Infection, Bone
See Osteomyelitis

Infection, Filarioidea
See Filariasis

Infection, Postoperative Wound

Infection, Wound

Index

Index

Index

Index

Index

Index

Index

Index

Lip, Reconstruction (continued)

Reconstruction 40525-40527
Repair 40650-40654
   Cleft Lip 40700-40761
   Complex 13151-13153
   Fistula 42260
Resection 40530
Shave 40500
Suture
   Tongue to Lip 41510
Unlisted Services and Procedures 40799
Vermilionectomy 40500

Lip, Cleft
See Cleft Lip

Lipase 83690

Lipectomy
Excision 15830-15839, 15847
Suction Assisted 15876-15879

Lipectomy, Aspiration
Liposuction 15876-15879

Lipids
Feces 82705-82710
Panel 80061
Phospholipid
   Antibody 86147, 86148
   Neutralization 85597, 85598

Lipo-Lutin
Progesterone 84144

Lipolysis, Aspiration
Liposuction 15876-15879

Lipophosphodiesterase I
See Tissue, Typing

Lipoprotein
(a) 83695
Apolipoprotein 82172
Blood 83695, 83700-83721
Delipidation
   HDL 0342T
HDL 83718
LDL 83700-83704, 83721, 83722
Phospholipase A2 83698
VLDL 83719

Lipoprotein, Alpha
See Lipoprotein

Lipoprotein, Pre-Beta
See Lipoprotein, Blood

Liposuction
for Autologous Fat Grafting 15876-15879

Listeria monocytogenes
Antibody 86723

Lithium
Assay 80178

Litholapaxy 52317, 52318

Lithotripsy
Bile Duct Calculi (Stone)
   Endoscopy 43265
Bladder 52353
Coronary Lesions 92972
with Cystourethroscopy 52353
with Indwelling Ureteral Stent Insertion 52356
Kidney 50080, 50081, 50590, 52353
Pancreatic Duct Calculi (Stone)
   Endoscopy 43265
Ureter 52353
Urethra 52353

Lithotrity
Litholapaxy 52317, 52318

Liver
See also Hepatic Duct
Ablation
   Malignant Cellular Tissue
      Histotripsy 0686T
   Tumor 47380-47383
      Laparoscopic 47370, 47371
Abscess
   Aspiration 47015
   Incision and Drainage
      Open 47010
      Injection 47015
Aspiration 47015
Biopsy 47700
   Needle 47000, 47001
   Wedge 47100
Cyst
   Aspiration 47015
   Incision and Drainage
      Open 47010
      Injection 47015
Drainage 47400
   Image Guided Fluid Collection 49405
Excision
   Extensive 47122
   Partial 47120, 47125-47130
   Donor 47140-47142
   Total
      Donor 47133
Exploration 47400
Hemorrhage 47350-47362
Injection 47015
Lesion
   See Lesion, Liver
Lobectomy 47125-47130
   Partial 47120
Needle Biopsy 47000, 47001
Nuclear Medicine
   Imaging 78201-78216
   Vascular Flow 78202
Removal
   Calculus 47400
Repair
   Abscess 47300
   Cyst 47300
   Wound 47350-47362
Suture
   Wound 47350-47362
Transplantation
   Allograft Preparation 47143-47147
      Cannulation/Decannulation 0894T
      Lobe Split 47145
      Mechanical Perfusion 0895T, 0896T
      Trisegment Split 47144
   Partial 47135, 47144, 47145
   Whole 47135
Trisegmentectomy 47122
Ultrasound
   Elastography, Shear Wave 91200
Unlisted Services and Procedures . . . 47379, 47399

Living Activities, Daily
See Activities of Daily Living

L-Leucylnaphthylamidase
Leucine Aminopeptidase 83670

Lobectomy
Brain 61323, 61537-61540
   Partial 61539, 61540
   Temporal Lobe 61537, 61538
Contralateral Subtotal
   Thyroid Gland 60212, 60225
Liver 47120-47130
   Donor 47141, 47142
Lung 32480-32482
   Sleeve 32486
   Thoracoscopic 32663, 32670
Parotid Gland 42410-42415
Sleeve 32486
Temporal Lobe 61537, 61538
Thoracoscopic
   Lung 32663, 32670
Thyroid Gland
   Partial 60210-60212
   Total 60220-60225

Local Excision Mastectomies
See Breast, Excision, Lesion

Local Excision of Lesion or Tissue of Femur
See Tumor, Femur

Localization of Nodule
Breast
   Device Placement
      with Magnetic Resonance Guidance . . 19085,
                19086, 19287, 19288
      with Mammographic Guidance 19281, 19282
      with Stereotactic Guidance . . 19081, 19082,
                19283, 19284
      with Ultrasound Guidance . . . 19083, 19084,
                19285, 19286
Soft Tissue
   Device Placement 10035, 10036

Log Hydrogen Ion Concentration
Blood Gases, pH 82800, 82803, 82930

Long-Acting Thyroid Stimulator
Thyrotropin Releasing Hormone
(TRH) 80438, 80439

Longmire Operation
Anastomosis, Hepatic Duct to Intestines 47765

Long-Term Care Facility Visits
See Nursing Facility Services

Loop Recorder System, Implantable
See Subcutaneous Cardiac Rhythm Monitor System

Loose Body
Removal
   Ankle Joint 27620, 29894
   Carpometacarpal Joint 26070
   Elbow Joint 24101, 29834
   Glenohumeral Joint 23107
   Hip Joint 27033
   Interphalangeal Joint 28024
   Intertarsal Joint 28020
   Knee Joint 27331
   Metatarsophalangeal Joint 28022
   Shoulder Joint 29819
   Subtalar Joint 29904
   Tarsometatarsal Joint 28020
   Toe 28022
   Wrist Joint 25101

Lord Procedure
Anal Sphincter Dilation 45905

Index

Index

Lysis of Adhesions 30560
Polyp
   Excision
      Endoscopic 31237
      Extensive 30115
      Simple. 30110
Reconstruction
   Cleft Lip/Cleft Palate 30460-30462
   Complete 30410
   Dermatoplasty 30620
   Primary 30400, 30420
   Secondary 30430-30450
   Septum 30520
Removal
   Foreign Body 30300
      with Anesthesia 30310
      by Lateral Rhinotomy 30320
Repair
   Adhesions 30560
   Choanal Atresia 30540, 30545
   Cleft Lip 40700-40761
   Complex 13151-13153
   Fistula 30580-30600, 42260
   Nasal Valve Collapse 30468, 30469
   Rhinophyma 30120
   Septum 30540-30545, 30630
   Synechia 30560
   Vestibular Stenosis 30465
Skin
   Excision 30120
   Surgical Planing 30120
Submucous Resection Turbinate
   Excision 30140
Turbinate
   Excision 30130-30140
   Fracture 30930
   Injection 30200
Turbinate Mucosa
   Cauterization 30801, 30802
Unlisted Services and Procedures 30999

Nose Bleed
Cauterization 30901-30906
Packs 30901-30906
   Endoscopic 31237

NTD
Nitroblue Tetrazolium Dye Test 86384

Nuclear Antigen
Antibody 86235

Nuclear Imaging
See Nuclear Medicine

Nuclear Magnetic Resonance Imaging
See Magnetic Resonance Imaging (MRI)

Nuclear Magnetic Resonance Spectroscopy
See Magnetic Resonance Spectroscopy

Nuclear Matrix Protein 22 86386

Nuclear Medicine
Diagnostic
   Adrenal Gland Imaging 78075
   Bile Duct
      Imaging 78226, 78227
   Bladder
      Residual Study 78730
   Blood Pool Imaging 78472, 78473,
                        78481, 78483

Bone and Joint
   Bone Density Study 78350, 78351
   Imaging 78300, 78305, 78306, 78315, 78803
   SPECT 78803
   Ultrasound 76977
Bone Marrow
   Imaging 78102-78104
Brain
   Blood Flow 78610
   Cerebrospinal Fluid Imaging . . . 78630-78650
   Imaging 78600-78609
   PET Imaging 78608, 78609
   Vascular Flow 78601, 78606, 78610
Endocrine System
   Parathyroid Gland Imaging 78070-78072
   Unlisted Services and Procedures 78099
Esophagus
   Imaging (Motility) 78258
   Reflux Study 78262
Flow Imaging 78445
   Plasma Volume 78110-78121
   Platelet Survival 78191
   Red Cell Sequestration 78140
   Red Cell Survival 78130
   Red Cell Volume 78120, 78121
   Unlisted Services and Procedures 78199
   Whole Blood Volume 78122
Function Study 78725
   Imaging 78700-78709
   Imaging, SPECT 78803
Gallbladder
   Imaging 78226, 78227
Gastric
   Emptying Imaging Study 78264-78266
   Mucosa Imaging 78261
   Urea Breath Test 78267, 78268
Gastroesophageal Reflux Study 78262
Gastrointestinal
   Blood Loss Imaging 78278
   Intestine Imaging 78290
   Peritoneal-Venous Shunt Patency 78291
   Protein Loss Study 78282
   Unlisted Services and Procedures 78299
Genitourinary System
   Unlisted Services and Procedures 78799
Heart
   Angiography 78445
   Blood Flow 78414
   Blood Pool Imaging 78472, 78473,
                        78481-78483
   Blood Pool SPECT Imaging 78494-78496
   Myocardial Imaging . . . 78459, 78466-78469
   Myocardial Perfusion Imaging . . 78451-78454
   Myocardial PET Imaging 78429-78434,
                  78459, 78491, 78492
   Shunt Detection 78428
   Unlisted Services and Procedures 78499
   Vascular Flow Imaging 78445
   Venography 78445
   Venous Thrombosis Imaging . . 78456-78458
Hepatic Duct
   Imaging 78226, 78227
Inflammatory Process 78800-78804,
                       78830-78832
   Injection Procedure 78808
Intestines
   Imaging 78290
Lacrimal Gland Tear Flow 78660

Liver
   Imaging 78201-78216
   Vascular Flow 78202, 78216
Lung
   Imaging, Perfusion 78580, 78597, 78598
   Imaging, Ventilation . . . 78579, 78582, 78598
   Unlisted Respiratory Procedure 78599
Lymphatics and Lymph Nodes
   Imaging 78195
Positron Emission Tomography
(PET) 78811-78816
   with Computed Tomography . . 78814-78816
Pulmonary Perfusion 78580, 78597, 78598
Pulmonary Ventilation 78579, 78582
Quantification Measurement 78835
Salivary Gland
   Function Study 78232
   Imaging 78230, 78231
Spleen
   Imaging 78185, 78215, 78216
   Unlisted Services and Procedures 78199
Testes
   Imaging 78761
Thyroid
   Imaging for Metastases 78015-78018
   Imaging with Flow 78013
   Metastases Uptake 78020
   Uptake 78012, 78014
Tumor Localization
   by Radiopharmaceuticals 78800-78804,
                 78808, 78830-78832
   by SPECT 78803, 78830-78832
Unlisted Diagnostic Procedures
   Cardiovascular 78499
   Endocrine 78099
   Gastrointestinal 78299
   Genitourinary 78799
   Hematopoietic, Reticuloendothelial, and
      Lymphatic 78199
   Miscellaneous 78999
   Musculoskeletal 78399
   Nervous System 78699
   Respiratory 78599
Urea Breath Test 78267, 78268
Ureter
   Reflux Study 78740
Vascular Flow 78701-78709
Vein
   Thrombosis Imaging 78456-78458
Therapeutic
   Radiopharmaceutical, Administration
      Interstitial Radioactive Colloid 79300
      Intra-Arterial 79445
      Intra-Articular 79440
      Intracavitary 79200
      Intravenous 79101
      Intravenous Infusion 79403
      Oral 79005
      Thyroid 79200-79300
      Unlisted Radiopharmaceutical
      Procedure 79999

Nucleases, DNA
DNAse Antibody 86215

Nucleic Acid Probe
Amplified Probe Detection
   Helicobacter pylori Clarithromycin
   Resistance 87513

Nucleolysis, Intervertebral Disc

Nucleotidase

Nursemaid Elbow

Nursing Facility Discharge Services

Nursing Facility Services

Nuss Procedure

Nutrition Therapy

Nystagmus Tests

O

Obliteration

Oblongata, Medulla

Observation Hospital Services

Observational Behavioral Follow-Up Assessment

Obstetrical Care

Obstruction

Obstruction, Colon

Obstruction Clearance

Obturator Nerve

Obturator Prosthesis

Index

Index

Index

Index

Index

Index

Index

Index

Retina
  Placement
    Pulse Generator 0100T
    Receiver 0100T
Shoulder
  Removal 23334, 23335
Skull Plate
  Removal 62142
  Replacement 62143
Spectacle
  Fitting 92352, 92353
  Repair 92371
Speech Aid
  Insertion 31611
Spine
  Insertion 22853, 22854, 22859
Synthetic 69633, 69637
Temporomandibular Joint
  Arthroplasty 21243
Testis
  Insertion 54520, 54660
Tissue Expander, Other than Breast
  Insertion 11960
Training 97761
Unlisted Maxillofacial Prosthetic Procedure . . 21089
Urethral Sphincter
  Insertion 53444, 53445
  Removal 53446, 53447
  Repair 53449
  Replacement 53448
Urethral Voiding Valve-Pump
  Insertion 0596T
  Replacement 0597T
Vagina
  Insertion 57267
  Removal 57295, 57296, 57426
  Revision 57295, 57296, 57426
Voiding
  Female Intraurethral Valve-Pump
    Insertion 0596T
    Replacement 0597T
Wrist
  Insertion 25443-25446
  Removal 25250, 25251

Prosthetic Valve, Aortic Valve
Replacement 33361-33369, 33405

Protease F
Plasmin 85400

Protein
A, Plasma (PAPP-A) 84163
S
  Free 85306
  Total 85305
C
  Activated (APC) 85307
  Activator 85337
  Activity 85303
  Antigen 85302
  Reactive 86140, 86141
  Resistance Assay 85307
CA-125 . . . . 81500, 81503
Analysis, Tissue
  Western Blot 88371
Apoliproprotein A1 81503
Beta-2 Microglobulin 81503
Cerebrospinal Fluid 83873
DIA 81509

Electrophoresis 84165, 84166
  Other Fluids 84166
  Western Blot 84181, 84182
Glycated 82985
hCG 81508, 81509
HE4 81500
Human Epididymis Protein 4 86305
Myelin Basic 83873
Nuclear Matrix Protein 22 (NMP22) 86386
Osteocalcin 83937
PAPP-A 81508, 81509
Prealbumin 81503, 84134
Serum, Plasma or Whole Blood 84155, 84165
Total 84155-84157
  by Refractometry 84160
Transferrin 81503
  Urine 84156
Urine 84156
  Dipstick 81000
Western Blot 84181, 84182, 88371, 88372

Protein Analysis, Tissue
Western Blot 88371

Protein Blotting
Western Blot 88371

Protein C Activator 85337

Protein C Antigen 85302

Protein C Assay 85303

Protein C Resistance Assay 85307

Protein S
Assay 85306
Total 85305

Prothrombase
Thrombokinase 85260

Prothrombin 85210

Prothrombin Time 85610, 85611

Prothrombinase
See Thromboplastin

Prothrombokinase 85230

Protime
See Prothrombin Time

Proton Treatment Delivery
Complex 77525
Intermediate 77523
Simple 77520-77522

Protoporphyrin 84202, 84203

Protozoa
Antibody 86753

Provitamin A
Vitamin A 84590

Provocation Test
Allergy
  Bronchial Challenge Tests 95070
    Ingestion Challenge Tests 95076, 95079
Bronchospasm, Evaluation 94070
with Electrogastrography 91133
Ergonovine 93024
Esophageal Balloon Distension Study 91040

Prower Factor 85260

PSA (Prostate Specific
Antigen) 84152-84154

Pseudocyst
Esophagus
  Drainage 43240
Pancreas
  Drainage 48510

Pseudophakia
See Keratoplasty

PSG
See Polysomnography

Psoriasis Treatment
Excimer Laser Treatment 96920-96922

Psychiatric Diagnosis
Assessment
  Behavior Identification . . . 0362T, 97151, 97152
  Brief Emotional/Behavioral 96127
Evaluation 90791
  with Medical Services 90792
Evaluation of Records or Reports 90885
Interactive Complexity 90785
Neurobehavioral Status Exam 96116, 96121
Performance Measures
  Dementia
    See Performance Measures, Dementia
  Major Depressive Disorder (MDD)
    See Performance Measures, Major
      Depressive Disorder
Psychological Testing 96130-96133,
                                      96136-96139, 96146
Suicide Risk Assessment 3085F
Unlisted Services and Procedures 90899

Psychiatric Treatment
See also Adaptive Behavior Treatment
Biofeedback Training 90875, 90876
Consultation with Family 90887
Drug Management 90863
Electroconvulsive Therapy 4066F, 90870
  Referral, Documented 4067F
Environmental Intervention 90882
Family 90846-90849, 99510
Group 90853
Hypnotherapy 90880
Narcosynthesis Analysis 90865
Pharmacotherapy
  Antidepressant 4063F, 4064F
  Antipsychotic 4065F
  Drug Management 90863
Psychedelic Medication Therapy
  Monitoring and Intervention 0820T-0822T
Psychoanalysis 90845
Psychotherapy
  See Psychotherapy
Report Preparation 90889
Suicide Risk Assessment 3085F
Theta-Burst Stimulation 0889T-0892T
Transcranial Magnetic Stimulation
(TMS) 90867-90869
Unlisted Services and Procedures 90899

Psychoanalysis 90845

Psychological/Neuropsychological
Testing
Neurobehavioral Status Exam 96116, 96121
Test Administration 96136-96139, 96146
Testing Evaluation 96130-96133

Psychophysiologic Feedback
See Biofeedback Training

Aorta 33320-33322, 33802, 33803
 Coarctation. 33840-33851
 Graft. 33858, 33859, 33877
 Infrarenal Abdominal
 Endovascular 34701-34706, 34845-34848
 Sinus of Valsalva 33702-33720
 Thoracic 75956-75959
 Endovascular 33880-33891
 Visceral
 Endovascular 34841-34848
 Physician Planning 34839
Aortic Arch
 with Cardiopulmonary Bypass 33853
 without Cardiopulmonary Bypass 33852
Aortic Valve. 33390, 33391
 Obstruction
 Outflow Tract 33414
 Septic Hypertrophy 33416
 Stenosis 33415
Arm
 Lower 25260-25263, 25270
 Fasciotomy 24495
 Secondary. 25265, 25272-25274
 Tendon 25290
 Tendon Sheath 25275
 Muscle 24341
 Tendon 24332, 24341, 25280,
 25295, 25310-25316
 Upper
 Muscle Revision 24330, 24331
 Muscle Transfer 24301, 24320
 Tendon Lengthening 24305
 Tendon Revision 24320
 Tendon Transfer 24301
 Tenotomy 24310
Arteriovenous Fistula
 Abdomen
 Acquired or Traumatic 35189
 Congenital 35182
 Extremity
 Acquired or Traumatic 35190
 Congenital 35184
 Head
 Acquired or Traumatic 35188
 Congenital 35180
 Neck
 Acquired or Traumatic 35188
 Congenital 35180
 Thorax
 Acquired or Traumatic 35189
 Congenital 35182
Arteriovenous Malformation
 Intracranial 61680-61692
 Intracranial Artery 61705-61708
 Spinal Artery 62294
 Spinal Cord. 63250-63252
Artery
 Angioplasty
 Aorta 37246-37247
 Axillary 37246-37247
 Brachiocephalic 37246-37247
 Bypass Graft. 35501-35571,
 35601-35683, 35691-35695, 35700
 Bypass In-Situ 35583-35587
 Bypass Venous Graft 33510-33516,
 35510-35525
 Coronary. 33507
 Direct Repair for Aneurysm
 Axillary-Brachial. 35011, 35013

Carotid 35001, 35002
Celiac 35121, 35122
Femoral. 35141, 35142
Hepatic 35121, 35122
Iliac 35131, 35132
Innominate 35021, 35022
Mesenteric 35121, 35122
Popliteal 35151, 35152
Radial 35045
Renal. 35121, 35122
Splenic 35111, 35112
Subclavian . . . 35001, 35002, 35021, 35022
Ulnar 35045
Vertebral. 35005
Femoral 37224
Iliac 37220-37222, 37227
Popliteal 37224
Pulmonary 33690
Renal 37246, 37247
Renal or Visceral 37246, 37247
Subclavian 37246, 37247
Thromboendarterectomy 35301-35321,
 35341-35390
Tibioperoneal 37228-37235
Viscera 37246, 37247
Arytenoid Cartilage. 31400
Atria
 Laparoscopic 33265, 33266
 Open. 33254-33256
Bile Duct 47701
 with Intestines 47760, 47780-47785
 Wound 47900
Bladder
 Exstrophy 51940
 Fistula. 44660, 44661,
 45800-45805, 51880-51925
 Neck. 51845
 Resection 52500
 Wound 51860-51865
Blepharoptosis
 Frontalis Muscle Technique with Fascial
 Sling. 67902
Blood Vessel
 Abdomen 35221
 with Other Graft 35281
 with Vein Graft 35251
 Chest 35211-35216
 with Other Graft 35271-35276
 with Vein Graft 35241-35246
 Finger 35207
 Graft Defect 35870
 Hand. 35207
 Kidney 50100
 Lower Extremity 35226
 with Other Graft 35286
 with Vein Graft 35256
 Neck. 35201
 with Other Graft 35261
 with Vein Graft 35231
 Upper Extremity 35206
 with Other Graft 35266
 with Vein Graft 35236
Body Cast 29720
Brain
 Wound 61571
Breast
 Mastopexy 19316
 Suspension. 19316

Bronchi
 Fistula. 32815
Brow Ptosis 67900
Bunion. 28292, 28295-28299
Bypass Graft 35901-35907
 Fistula. 35870
Calcaneus
 Osteotomy 28300
Cannula. 36860, 36861
Carpal 25440
Carpal Bone. 25431
Cervix
 Cerclage 57700
 Abdominal 59320-59325
 Suture. 57720
Chest Wall 32905
 Closure 32810
 Fistula. 32906
Chin
 Augmentation 21120, 21123
 Osteotomy 21121-21123
Clavicle
 Osteotomy 23480-23485
Cleft Hand. 26580
Cleft Lip. 40525-40527, 40700-40761
 Nasal Deformity. . 40700, 40701, 40720-40761
Cleft Palate 42200, 42205, 42210,
 42215, 42220, 42225
Colon
 Fistula. 44650-44661
 Hernia. 44050
 Malrotation 44055
 Obstruction. 44050
Cornea
 See Cornea, Repair
Coronary Chamber Fistula. 33500, 33501
Cyst
 Bartholin's Gland 56440
 Liver 47300
Diaphragm
 for Eventration 39545
 Hernia. 39503, 39540, 39541
 Laceration 39501
Ductus Arteriosus 33820-33824, 93582
Ear, Middle
 Oval Window Fistula 69666
 Round Window Fistula. 69667
Elbow
 Hemiepiphyseal Arrest 24470
 Ligament 24343-24346
 Muscle 24341
 Muscle Transfer 24301
 Tendon 24340-24342
 Each 24341
 Tendon Lengthening. 24305
 Tendon Transfer 24301
 Tennis Elbow 24357-24359
Encephalocele. 62121
Endovascular
 See Endovascular Repair
Enterocele
 Hysterectomy. 58270, 58294
Epididymis. 54900, 54901
Epiphysis
 Femur 27177-27181, 27475, 27479,
 27485, 27516-27519, 27742
 Fibula 27477, 27479, 27485,
 27732, 27734, 27740, 27742
 Tibia 27477-27485, 27730-27742

Index

Index

Index

Index

Index

Index

Index

Index

Positron Emission Tomography (PET) .. 78811-78816
Pubis 27065-27067
Pulmonary
  Ablation
    Cryoablation 32994
    Radiofrequency 32998
Radiation Therapy
  See Brachytherapy; Interstitial Radiation
  Therapy
Radius 25120-25126, 25170
  with Allograft
    Excision 24126
  with Autograft
    Excision 24125
  Excision 24120
Rectum
  Ablation 45346
  Destruction 45190, 45320
  Excision 45160-45172
Renal
  Ablation 50592, 50593
Retroperitoneal Area
  Destruction/Excision 49186-49190
Sacrum 49215
Scapula
  Excision 23140, 23210
    with Allograft 23146
    with Autograft 23145
Shoulder
  Soft Tissue
    Excision 23071-23076
    Radical Resection 23077, 23078
Skin
  Mohs Micrographic Surgery 17311-17315
Skull
  Excision 61500
Spinal Cord
  Excision 63275-63290
Stomach
  Excision 43610, 43611
Talus
  Excision 28100-28103
  Radical Resection 27647
Tarsal
  Excision 28104-28107
  Radical Resection 28171
Temporal Bone
  Removal 69970
Testis
  Excision 54530-54535
Thigh
  Excision 27327, 27328, 27337, 27339
  Radical Resection 27329, 27364, 27365
Thorax
  Excision 21552-21558
  Radical Resection 21557, 21558
Thyroid
  Excision 60200
Tibia 27365, 27635-27638
  Radical Resection 27645
Toe
  Excision 28039-28045
  Radical Resection 28046, 28047
Torus Mandibularis 21031
Trachea
  Excision
    Cervical 31785
    Thoracic 31786

Ulna 25120-25126, 25170
  with Allograft
    Excision 24126
  with Autograft
    Excision 24125
  Excision 24120
Ureter
  Excision 52355
Urethra
  Excision 52355, 53220
  Fulguration 52234-52240
Uterus
  Ablation 0071T, 0072T
  Excision 58140-58146
  Resection 58951, 58952, 58958
Vagina
  Excision 57135
Vertebra
  Additional Segment
    Excision 22116
  Cervical
    Excision 22100
  Lumbar 22102
  Thoracic
    Excision 22101
Wrist
  Bone
    Curettage 25130, 25135, 25136
    Excision 25130, 25135, 25136
    Radical Resection 25077, 25078
  Subcutaneous
    Excision 25071, 25075
  Subfascial
    Excision 25073, 25076

Tunica Vaginalis
Hydrocele
  Aspiration 55000
  Excision 55040, 55041
  Repair 55060

Turbinate
Excision 30130-30140
Fracture
  Therapeutic 30930
Injection 30200
Submucous Resection
  Nose Excision 30140

Turbinate Mucosa
Cauterization 30801, 30802

Turcica, Sella
CT Scan 70480, 70482
X ray 70240

TURP
Transurethral Prostatectomy 52601, 52630

Tylectomy
Breast Lumpectomy 19301

Tympanic Membrane
Create Stoma 0583T, 69433, 69436
  Myringoplasty 69620
  Myringotomy 69421
  Neurectomy 69676
  Repair 69610
  Tympanolysis 69450
  Tympanoplasty
    See Tympanoplasty
  Tympanostomy 0583T, 69433, 69436
    Removal of Tube 69424

Tympanic Nerve
Excision 69676

Tympanolysis 69450

Tympanomastoidectomy 69641-69646

Tympanometry 92550, 92567, 92570

Tympanoplasty 69631-69633
See also Myringoplasty
with Antrotomy or Mastoidotomy . . . 69635-69637
with Mastoidectomy 69641, 69642
    Intact or Reconstructed Wall 69643, 69644
    Radical or Complete 69645
with Ossicular Chain Reconstruction 69632,
    69633, 69636, 69637, 69642, 69644, 69646
with Synthetic Prosthesis 69633, 69637

Tympanostomy
with Automated Tube Delivery System 0583T
with General Anesthesia 69436
with Iontophoresis Anesthesia 0583T
with Local Anesthesia 0583T, 69433
Removal of Tube 69424

Tympanotomy
Myringotomy 69420, 69421

Typhoid Vaccine
Intramuscular 90691
Oral 90690

Typhus
Endemic 86000
Mite-Borne 86000
Sao Paulo 86000
Tropical 86000

Typing, Blood
See Blood Typing, Serologic

Typing, HLA
Tissue Typing . . 86812, 86813, 86816, 86817, 86821
Typing 81370-81383

Typing, Tissue
See Tissue, Typing

Tyrosine 84510

Tzank Smear 88160, 88161

U

UDP Galactose Pyrophosphorylase
Galactose-1-Phosphate, Uridyl
Transferase 82775, 82776

UFR
See Uroflowmetry

Ulcer
Anal Fissure
  Destruction 46940, 46942
  Excision 46200
Decubitus
  Excision
    Coccygeal 15920, 15922
    Ischial 15940, 15941, 15944-15946
    Sacral 15931, 15933-15937
    Trochanteric . . . 15950-15953, 15956, 15958
    Unlisted Procedure 15999
Pinch Graft 15050
Pressure 15920-15999
Stomach
  Excision 43610

Index

Index

Excision

Decompression 63081-63103
Lesion. 63300-63308
with Skull Base Surgery. 61597

Fracture/Dislocation
Closed Treatment
without Manipulation. 22310

Insertion
Stabilization/Distraction Device . . 22867-22870
Kyphectomy. 22818, 22819

Repair
Injection
Cervicothoracic. 22510, 22512
Lumbosacral 22511, 22512

Tethering
Lumbar/Thoracolumbar . . 0656T, 0657T, 0790T
Thoracic 22836-22838

Vertebral Column
See Spine

Vertebral Disc
See Intervertebral Disc

Vertebral Fracture
See Fracture, Vertebra

Vertebral Joints
Arthroplasty 0202T
Facetectomy 62380, 63020,
63045-63048, 63052, 63053
Injection 64490-64495
Placement, Implant. 0219T-0222T
Replacement. 0719T

Very Low Density Lipoprotein 83695,
83700-83721

Vesication
See Bulla

Vesicle, Seminal
See Seminal Vesicle

Vesico-Psoas Hitch. 50785

Vesicostomy
Cutaneous. 51980

Vesicourethropexy 51840, 51841

Vesicovaginal Fistula
Closure 51900, 57300, 57320

Vesiculectomy. 55650

Vesiculogram, Seminal 55300

Vesiculography 55300

Vesiculotomy 55600-55605
Complicated 55605

Vessel, Blood
See Blood Vessels

Vessels Transposition, Great
See Transposition, Great Arteries

Vestibular Function
Tests
Caloric 92533, 92537, 92538
Computerized Dynamic Posturography (CDP),
Sensory Organization Test
(CDP-SOT). 92548, 92549
Foveal Stimulation. 92540
Nystagmus. 92531, 92532, 92534, 92540,
92541, 92542, 92544, 92547
Peripheral Stimulation. 92540
Sinusoidal Vertical Axis Rotation 92546

Torsion Swing Test. 92546
Tracking Test 92540, 92545
Vestibular Device Implant. 0725T-0729T

Vestibular Nerve
Section
Transcranial Approach. 69950
Translabyrinthine Approach. 69915

Vestibule of Mouth
See Mouth, Vestibule

Vestibuloplasty 40840-40845

Video
Esophagus. 74230
Pharynx 70371, 74230
Speech Evaluation 70371
Swallowing Evaluation. 74230

Video-Assisted Thoracoscopic Surgery (VATS)
See Thoracoscopy, Surgical

Videoradiography
Esophagus. 74230
Pharynx 70371, 74230
Site Unspecified 76120-76125
Speech Evaluation 70371
Swallowing Evaluation. 74230

VII, Coagulation Factor 85230

VII, Cranial Nerve
See Facial Nerve

VIII, Coagulation Factor
See Clotting Factor, Factor VIII

Villus, Chorionic
Biopsy 59015

Villusectomy
See Synovectomy

VIP
Vasoactive Intestinal Peptide 84586

Viral Antibodies 86280

Viral Warts
Flat
Destruction. 17110, 17111

Virtual Appointment
See Telemedicine, Synchronous Care

Virtual Reality (VR) Therapy
Dissociation Services 0771T-0774T
Therapy Assist 0770T

Virus
AIDS
See HIV-1
Burkitt Lymphoma
See Epstein-Barr Virus
Human Immunodeficiency
See HIV
Influenza
See Influenza Virus
Respiratory Syncytial
See Respiratory Syncytial Virus
Salivary Gland
See Cytomegalovirus

Virus Identification
Immunofluorescence. 87254

Virus Isolation 87250-87255

Visceral Larval Migrans 86280

Viscosity, Blood 85810

Visible Light Hyperspectral Imaging (VLHI) 0631T

Visit, Home
See Home Services

Visual Acuity Screen
Automated 99172, 99173
Evoked Potentials 0333T

Visual Field
Assessment. 0378T, 0379T
Exam 92081-92083

Visual Function Screen 1055F, 99172

Visual Reinforcement Audiometry 92579

Visualization
Ileal Conduit 50690

Vital Capacity Measurement 94150

Vitamins
A 84590
B Complex
B1 (Thiamine). 84425
B2 (Riboflavin) 84252
B3 (Niacin) 84591
B5 (Pantothenic Acid). 84591
B6 (Pyroxidine) 84207
B7 (Biotin). 84591
B9 (Folic Acid) 82746, 82747
B12 (Cyanocobalamin) 82607, 82608
B-1. 84425
B-2. 84252
B-6. 84207
B-6 Measurement
Pyridoxal Phosphate. 84207
B-12. . . . . 82607, 82608
Holotranscobalamin. 84999
BC
Folic Acid 82746, 82747
C 82180
D
Blood Serum Level
1, 25 dihydroxy 82652
25 hydroxy 82306
Counseling 4019F
E 84446
K 84597
K-Dependent Bone Protein 83937
K-Dependent Protein S 85305, 85306
Other, Unspecified 84591

Vitelline Duct
Omphalomesenteric Duct. 44800

Vitrectomy
Anterior Approach
Partial. 67005
Subtotal 67010
with Endolaser Panretinal Photocoagulation 67040
with Focal Endolaser Photocoagulation 67039
with Implantation or Replacement
Drug Delivery System 67027
Retinal Electrodes 0100T
with Lens Material Removal. 66852
Pars Plana Approach. 67036-67043
for Retinal Detachment. 67108, 67113
by Sampling 0198T
with Retinal Prosthesis Placement. 0100T

Index

X

Index

Notes

Code Changes Beyond the Annual Code Set Release Cycle

The CPT® code set contains all codes effective for the upcoming year. However, some CPT® code sections undergo more frequent updates.

The following chart serves as the perfect quick reference, especially when coordinating updates to your processes, policies, and/or coding and billing software.

Code Type	Release Dates	Effective Dates
Immune Globulins, Serum or Recombinant Products and Vaccines, Toxoids	Update 1: Apr. 2025 Update 2: Jul. 2025 Update 3: Oct. 2025	Update 1: Jul. 2025 Update 2: Oct. 2025 Update 3: Jan. 2026
ama-assn.org/cpt-cat-i-vaccine-codes		
Proprietary Lab Analyses (PLA)	Update: Jan. 2025 Update: Apr. 2025 Update: Jul. 2025 Update: Oct. 2025	Update: Apr. 2025 Update: Jul. 2025 Update: Oct. 2025 Update: Jan. 2026
ama-assn.org/cpt-pla-codes		
AAdministrative Multianalyte Assays Algorithmic Analyses (MAAA)	Update 1: Apr. 2025 Update 2: Jul. 2025 Update 3: Oct. 2025	Update 1: Jul. 2025 Update 2: Oct. 2025 Update 3: Jan. 2026
ama-assn.org/maaa-codes		
Molecular Pathology Tier 2	Update 1: Apr. 2025 Update 2: Jul. 2025 Update 3: Oct. 2025	Update 1: Jul. 2025 Update 2: Oct. 2025 Update 3: Jan. 2026
ama-assn.org/mo-path-tier-2-codes		
CPT® Category III	Update 1: Jan. 2025 Update 2: Jul. 2025	Update 1: Jul. 2025 Update 2: Jan. 2026
ama-assn.org/cpt-cat-iii-codes		

Subscribe to or update your preferences for "CPT Updates" to get the latest CPT® change notifications and more.

ama-assn.org/life-career/email-newsletter-publications